P9-CRF-438

Pharmacology and Therapeutics for Dentistry

Pharmacology and Therapeutics for Dentistry

Fifth Edition

John A. Yagiela, DDS, PhD
Professor and Chair, Division of Diagnostic and Surgical Sciences,
School of Dentistry;
Professor of Anesthesiology, School of Medicine
University of California, Los Angeles
Los Angeles, California

Frank J. Dowd, DDS, PhD
Professor and Chairman, Department of Pharmacology,
Professor, Department of Oral Biology,
School of Dentistry,
Creighton University School of Medicine
Omaha, Nebraska

Enid A. Neidle, PhD
Professor Emeritus, Pharmacology, New York University
New York, New York;
Former Assistant Executive Director, Scientific Affairs
American Dental Association
Chicago, Illinois

With 700 illustrations

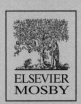

ELSEVIER
MOSBY
An Affiliate of Elsevier

11830 Westline Industrial Drive
St. Louis, Missouri 63146

Pharmacology and Therapeutics for Dentistry:
Fifth Edition

NOTICE
Dentistry is an ever-changing field. Standard safety precautions must be followed, but as new research and clinical experience broaden our knowledge, changes in treatment and drug therapy may become necessary or appropriate. Readers are advised to check the most current product information provided by the manufacturer of each drug to be administered to verify the recommended dose, the method and duration of administration, and contraindications. It is the responsibility of the licensed prescriber, relying on experience and knowledge of the patient, to determine dosages and the best treatment for each individual patient. Neither the publisher nor the author assumes any liability for any injury and/or damage to persons or property arising from this publication.

Previous editions copyrighted 1998, 1989, 1985, 1980

Library of Congress Cataloging in Publication Data

Pharmacology and therapeutics for dentistry / [edited by] John A. Yagiela, Frank J. Dowd,
Enid A. Neidle.—5th ed.
p. cm.
Previous ed. cataloged under: Yagiela, John A.
Includes bibliographical references and index.
ISBN-13: 978-0-323-01618-6 ISBN-10: 0-323-01618-9
1. Dental pharmacology. 2. Dental therapeutics. I. Yagiela, John A. II. Dowd, Frank J., 1939- III. Neidle, Enid Anne.

RK701.N44 2004
615'.1'0246176—dc22

2004052408

ISBN-13: 978-0-323-01618-6
ISBN-10: 0-323-01618-9

Publishing Director: Linda L. Duncan
Executive Editor: Penny Rudolph
Senior Developmental Editor: Jaime Pendill
Publishing Services Manager: Linda McKinley
Project Manager: Jennifer Furey
Design Manager: Mark Bernard
Cover Art: Teri McDermott

Printed in the United States of America

Last digit is the print number: 9 8 7 6 5 4 3

CONTRIBUTORS

Peter W. Abel, PhD
Professor
Department of Pharmacology
School of Medicine
Creighton University
Omaha, Nebraska

Jeffrey D. Bennett, DMD
Professor and Chair
Department of Oral Surgery and Hospital Dentistry
School of Dentistry
Indiana University
Indianapolis, Indiana

Mark Blumenthal, BA
Adjunct Associate Professor, Medicinal Chemistry
College of Pharmacy
University of Texas
Austin, Texas
Founder and Executive Director,
American Botanical Council
Publisher and Editor, *HerbalGram*

Charles S. Bockman, PhD
Assistant Professor
Department of Pharmacology
School of Medicine
Creighton University
Omaha, Nebraska

Gretchen J. Bruce, DDS, MBA
Assistant Professor
Department of Periodontics
Arthur A. Dugoni School of Dentistry
University of the Pacific
San Francisco, California

Richard P. Cohan, AB, DDS, MS, MA, MBA
Associate Professor
Course Director of Orientation to Comprehensive Patient Care
Department of Diagnostic and Emergency Services
Arthur A. Dugoni School of Dentistry
University of the Pacific
San Francisco, California

George A. Cook, PhD
Professor
Department of Pharmacology
University of Tennessee Health Science Center
Memphis, Tennessee

Stephen A. Cooper
Senior Vice President, Global, Clinical, and Medical Affairs
Wyeth Consumer Healthcare
Madison, New Jersey

Paul J. Desjardins, DMD, PhD
Executive Vice President, Clinical Analgesic Research
Scirex Corporation
Austin, Texas;
Clinical Professor
Department of Oral and Maxillofacial Surgery
University of Medicine and Dentistry of New Jersey
Newark, New Jersey

Raymond A. Dionne, DDS, PhD
Chief, Pain and Neurosensory Mechanisms Branch
National Institute of Dental and Craniofacial Research
National Institutes of Health
Bethesda, Maryland

Joel B. Epstein, DMD, MSD
Professor and Head
Department of Oral Medicine and Diagnostic Sciences;
Director, Interdisciplinary Program in Oral Cancer Detection, Biology and Treatment
University of Illinois
Chicago, Illinois

Gail T. Galasko, MSc, PhD
Associate Professor and Section Head of Pharmacology
Department of Applied Dental Medicine
School of Dental Medicine
Southern Illinois University
Alton, Illinois;
Adjunct Faculty
Department of Pharmacological and Physiological Sciences
St. Louis University
St. Louis, Missouri

Gerald F. Gebhart, PhD
Professor and Head
Department of Pharmacology
College of Medicine
University of Iowa
Iowa City, Iowa

Michael J. Gleason, DDS, PhD
Associate Professor
Department of Biomedical Sciences
School of Dentistry
University of Detroit Mercy
Detroit, Michigan

Daniel A. Haas, DDS, PhD, FRCD(c)
Associate Dean, Clinical Sciences
Chapman Chair in Clinical Sciences
Professor and Head of Anaesthesia
Faculty of Dentistry;
Department of Pharmacology
Faculty of Medicine
University of Toronto
Toronto, Canada

Kenneth M. Hargreaves, DDS, PhD
Professor and Chairman
Department of Endodontics;
Professor
Department of Pharmacology
School of Dentistry
University of Texas Health Sciences Center
San Antonio, Texas

Marc W. Heft, DMD, PhD
Professor and Program Director
Department of Oral and Maxillofacial Surgery and Diagnostic Sciences;
Director
Claude D. Pepper Center for Research on Oral Health and Aging;
Professor
Department of Neuroscience
College of Medicine
University of Florida
Gainesville, Florida

David W. Hein, PhD
Peter K. Knoefel Professor and Chairman
Department of Pharmacology and Toxicology
School of Medicine
University of Louisville
Louisville, Kentucky

Elliot V. Hersh, DMD, MS, PhD
Professor and Director
Division of Pharmacology and Therapeutics;
Associate Dean of Clinical Research
Department of Oral Surgery and Pharmacology
School of Dental Medicine
University of Pennsylvania
Philadelphia, Pennsylvania

Harrell E. Hurst, MS, PhD
Professor
Department of Pharmacology and Toxicology
School of Medicine
University of Louisville
Louisville, Kentucky

Douglass L. Jackson, DMD, MS, PhD
Assistant Professor
Department of Oral Medicine
School of Dentistry
University of Washington
Seattle, Washington

Peter L. Jacobsen, PhD, DDS
Professor
Department of Pathology and Medicine;
Director
Oral Medicine Clinic
Authur A. Dugoni School of Dentistry
University of the Pacific
San Francisco, California

William B. Jeffries, PhD
Associate Professor
Department of Pharmacology;
Associate Dean for Medical Education
School of Medicine
Creighton University
Omaha, Nebraska

Barton S. Johnson, DDS, MS
Associate Professor
Department of Restorative/Hospital Dentistry
School of Dentistry
University of Washington
Seattle, Washington

Mo K. Kang, DDS, PhD
Assistant Professor
Section of Endodontics
School of Dentistry
University of California, Los Angeles
Los Angeles, California

Hyungsuk Kim, DDS, PhD
Pain and Neurosensory Mechanisms Branch
National Institute of Dental and Craniofacial Research
National Institutes of Health
Bethesda, Maryland

Bruno Kreiner, DMD, MSc
Department of Oral and Maxillofacial Surgery
School of Dental Medicine
Hadassah Medical Organization
Kyriat Hadassah
Jerusalum, Israel

Karl K. Kwok, PharmD
Clinical Professor
School of Pharmacy
University of Washington;
Clinical Pharmacist-Oncology
Department of Pharmacy
University of Washington Medical Center
Seattle, Washington

Vahn A. Lewis, PharmD, PhD
Associate Professor
Department of Neurobiology and Anatomy
Medical School
University of Texas-Houston Health Science Center
Houston, Texas

Angelo J. Mariotti, DDS, PhD
Professor and Chair
Department of Periodontology
College of Dentistry
Ohio State University
Columbus, Ohio

Michael D. Martin, DMD, MPH, MA, MSD, PhD
Associate Professor
Department of Oral Medicine
University of Washington
Seattle, Washington

Robert L. Merrill, DDS, MS
Adjunct Associate Professor
Division of Oral Biology and Medicine
School of Dentistry
University of California, Los Angeles
Los Angeles, California

Kenneth T. Miyasaki, DDS, PhD
Associate Professor
Department of Oral Biology and Medicine
School of Dentistry
University of California, Los Angeles
Los Angeles, California

John A. Molinari, PhD
Professor and Chairman
Department of Biomedical Sciences
School of Dentistry
University of Detroit Mercy
Detroit, Michigan

Paul A. Moore, DMD, PhD, MPH
Professor
Department of Pharmacology;
Director
Oral Health Science Institute
School of Dental Medicine
University of Pittsburgh
Pittsburgh, Pennsylvania

Ernest Newbrun, DMD, PhD, Dodont(hc), DDSc(hc)
Professor Emeritus
Oral Biology and Periodontology
Department of Stomatology
University of California, San Francisco
San Francisco, California

Thomas J. Pallasch, DDS, MS
Professor Emeritus of Dentistry
University of Southern California
Los Angeles, California

No-Hee Park, DMD, PhD
Dean and Professor
School of Dentistry
University of California, Los Angeles
Los Angeles, California

Douglas E. Peterson, DMD, PhD
Professor and Head
Department of Oral Diagnosis
School of Medicine;
Associate Director
Cancer Center
University of Connecticut Health Center
Farmington, Connecticut

Michael T. Piascik, PhD
Professor
Department of Pharmacology
College of Medicine
University of Kentucky
Lexington, Kentucky

Morton B. Rosenberg, DMD
Professor
Department of Oral and Maxillofacial Surgery;
Head
Division of Anesthesia and Pain Control;
Associate Professor of Anesthesia
Tufts University Schools of Medicine and Dental Medicine
Boston, Massachusetts

Mark T. Roszkowski, DDS
Assistant Professor
Department of Oral and Maxillofacial Surgery
School of Dentistry
University of Texas Health Sciences Center
San Antonio, Texas

Joel D. Schiff, PhD
Associate Professor
Division of Biological Science, Medicine, and Surgery
David B. Kriser College of Dentistry
New York University
New York, New York

Mark M. Schubert, DDS, MSD
Professor
Department of Oral Medicine
School of Dentistry
University of Washington;
Director
Department of Oral Medicine
Seattle Cancer Care Alliance/Fred Hutchinson Cancer Research Center
Seattle, Washington

David H. Shaw, PhD
Professor and Chairman
Department of Oral Biology
College of Dentistry
University of Nebraska Medical Center
Lincoln, Nebraska

Ania U. Sweet, PharmD
Clinical Oncology Pharmacist
Department of Pharmacy
University of Washington Medical Center
Seattle, Washington

Clarence L. Trummel, DDS, PhD
Professor
Department of Periodontology
School of Dental Medicine
University of Connecticut Health Center
Farmington, Connecticut

Eileen L. Watson, RPh, PhD
Professor
Departments of Oral Biology and Pharmacology
University of Washington
Seattle, Washington

Dennis W. Wolff, PhD
President and Chief Executive Officer
Medical Diagnoses Explained, Inc.
Omaha, Nebraska

PREFACE

This fifth edition marks 24 years for *Pharmacology and Therapeutics for Dentistry*. The changes in this edition reflect the continuous and accelerating advances in the discipline of pharmacology and its application to clinical dentistry. Study of the human genome and related investigation of the molecular mechanisms of drug action have continued to drive updates in the text. This influence is apparent throughout the book, with new information on receptor structure and function, signaling pathways, and drugs designed to influence them. Meanwhile, elucidation of the isoenzymes and transporter proteins that support human drug metabolism and excretion has revolutionized our understanding of pharmacokinetic drug interactions.

Many chapters have undergone major revisions. New drugs and revised drug lists have been incorporated in every chapter. This edition has enhanced coverage of such topics as pharmacogenetics and alternative medicine, both of which are of strong contemporary interest. Serotonin and related drugs have also received greater emphasis. The ever-expanding area of immunology is reflected in major changes in the chapters on immunotherapy and cancer chemotherapy. A hot topic is the burgeoning therapeutic application of monoclonal antibodies as therapeutic agents and as delivery vehicles for cytotoxins and radiologicals. Toxicology coverage has been expanded to answer the need for greater appreciation of this increasingly vital field. New figures have been added to most chapters in an effort to assist in the learning of increasingly complex subject matter.

Throughout this revision, we have continued to emphasize dental applications of pharmacology and have expanded the discussion of dental aspects in several relevant areas. There is, for instance, more expansive coverage of pain control for both acute problems and chronic disorders. The reader should find the updated chapter on prescription writing and drug regulations helpful in the practice of dentistry. We have added website references in several chapters. Such references provide valuable access to online information in rapidly changing fields.

Although Dr. Enid Neidle scaled back her duties as editor for this edition, she continued to provide insightful scientific and stylistic critiques of our editorial effort. Life changes have caused some long-term authors to cease their participation. We are most grateful for their previous efforts. In particular, we wish to acknowledge the many fine contributions of Drs. Leslie Felpel, Glenn Housholder, Edward Montgomery, Anthony Picozzi, and William Warner. We are most fortunate to welcome back our returning authors and to add a group of new contributors for this edition.

Despite these changes, this quote from the preface of the first edition still applies:

> *. . . we feel it fair to characterize* Pharmacology and Therapeutics for Dentistry *as a standard, basic, thorough textbook of pharmacology* and *therapeutics, written specifically with the needs of the dentist in mind. With this new edition, the dentist should be able to understand basic pharmacology, to know how and when to use specific drugs and what dosage of these drugs to use, and to know how a patient's pharmacologic status will determine the treatment and medicine prescribed for that patient.*

John A. Yagiela
Frank J. Dowd
Enid A. Neidle

ACKNOWLEDGMENTS

We wish to thank several individuals who made special contributions to this work. Ms. Penny Rudolph, Executive Editor; Ms. Jaime Pendill, Senior Developmental Editor; Ms. Jennifer Furey, Senior Project Manager; and Ms. Courtney Sprehe, Associate Developmental Editor, of Elsevier played crucial roles in the completion of this edition. We acknowledge the fine artistic talents of Ms. Teri McDermott, who rendered the cover art for this book, and Mr. Patrick Masson, who prepared new illustrations for some of the chapters. Finally, we wish to thank Ms. Claudia Hernandez and Dr. Chris Hague for their assistance in checking chapter references and Ms. Betty Schopperth for helping with manuscript preparation.

John A. Yagiela
Frank J. Dowd
Enid A. Neidle

CONTENTS

INTRODUCTION

Pharmacology may be defined as the science of drugs, their preparation, uses, and effects. The term derives from *pharmakon*, the Greek word for drug or medicine, and *logia*, the Latin suffix traditionally used to designate a body of knowledge and its study. As an organized discipline, pharmacology is of recent origin, but the study of medicinal substances is as old as civilization itself.

HISTORY

Sir William Osler once said, "The desire to take medicine is perhaps the greatest feature which distinguishes man from animals." Although this argument has been vitiated by experiments involving self-medication in rats and other laboratory species, it nevertheless serves to illustrate the historic relationship between drugs and humankind. The use of natural products to cure disease and alter mentation dates back to the dawn of time. By the writing of the Ebers papyrus (circa 1550 BC), more than 700 prescriptions for various ailments were known. Many of the ingredients incorporated in these preparations—lizard's blood, virgin's hair, fly excreta—are humorous by modern standards, but also included were many compounds recognized today as pharmacologically active. A summary of folk remedies and other medicinals that have withstood scientific scrutiny would list such substances as opium (morphine), belladonna (atropine), squill and foxglove (digitalis), cinchona bark (quinine and quinidine), coca leaves (cocaine), and ma huang (ephedrine). The empirical study of plant derivatives and animal products must have been quite extensive to have been so fruitful.

A major hindrance to the effective use of these drugs, however, was the large number of materials usually present in apothecary formulations. For example, the most popular drug of the fifteenth century, triaca, contained more than 100 separate components. Aureolus Paracelsus (1493-1541) was the first to recognize that the indiscriminate mixing of numerous substances did little but dilute whatever effective compounds may have been present initially. The focus of Paracelsus on single agents was refined by Felice Fontana (1720-1805), who deduced from his own experiments that each crude drug contains an "active principle" that, when administered, yields a characteristic effect on the body. One of the greatest scientific achievements of the nineteenth century was the isolation and objective evaluation of such active principles.

In 1803, a young German pharmacist, Frederick Sertürner (1780-1841), extracted the alkaloid morphine from opium. This singular achievement not only marked the beginning of pharmaceutical chemistry, but also led to a revolution in experimental biology. The availability of newly purified drugs and the standardization of existing biologic preparations encouraged pioneers like Francois Magendie (1783-1855) and Claude Bernard (1813-1878) to employ pharmacologic agents as probes in the study of physiologic processes. The use of curare by Bernard for the elucidation of the neuromuscular junction is but one example of the successes obtained with this approach. Perhaps because drugs became associated with several biologic sciences and were of course considered under the domain of the various medical specialties, the development of pharmacology as a separate discipline was delayed.

Rudolf Buchheim (1820-1879) and Oswald Schmiedeberg (1838-1921) were the two individuals most responsible for establishing pharmacology as a science in its own right. Buchheim organized the first laboratory exclusively devoted to pharmacology and became the first professor of his discipline. A student of Buchheim's, Schmiedeberg founded the first scientific journal of pharmacology. More importantly, through his tutelage Schmiedeberg helped spread acceptance of pharmacology throughout the world. One protégé of Schmiedeberg was John Abel (1857-1938), generally regarded as the father of American pharmacology.

Once an obscure experimental science, pharmacology has expanded its purview to such an extent that the subject has become an important area of study for all health professionals and holds certain interests for the lay public as well. In dentistry, the impact of pharmacology was formally recognized by the American Dental Association in 1934 with publication of the first edition of *Accepted Dental Remedies.*

SCOPE OF PHARMACOLOGY

Pharmacology is one of the few medical sciences that straddles the division between the basic and the clinical. The scope of pharmacology is so extensive that several subdivisions have come to be recognized. *Pharmacodynamics* is the study of the biologic activity that a drug has on a living system. It includes a study of the mechanisms of action of the drug and the exact processes that are affected by it. The influence of chemical structure on drug action (the structure-activity relationship) is also a concern of this branch of pharmacology. *Pharmacokinetics* deals with the magnitude and time course of drug effect, and it attempts to explain these aspects of drug action through a consideration of dosage and the absorption, distribution, and fate of chemicals in living systems. *Pharmacotherapeutics* is the proper selection of an agent whose biologic effect on a living organism is most appropriate to treat a particular disease state. It requires a consideration of, among many other things, dose, duration of therapy, and side effects of drug treatment. The practice of *pharmacy* involves the preparation and dispensing of medicines. Although pharmacists today are rarely called on to actually prepare drug products, they can serve as a useful source of drug information for both the clinician and the patient. *Toxicology* is that aspect of pharmacology dealing with poisons, their actions, their detection, and the treatment of conditions produced by them. The importance of toxicology to modern life is continually underscored by new discoveries of chemical hazards in the environment. As the various disciplines of science and medicine have continued to evolve, fruitful areas of inquiry have emerged from the union of fields with overlapping interest. For example, study of the interrelationships between drugs and heredity, aging, and the immune system has led to the respective development of *pharmacogenetics, geriatric pharmacology,* and *immunopharmacology.* A final subdivision of pharmacology, *pharmacognosy,* is now a somewhat vestigial science.

Essential at a time when most drugs were derived from plants, it literally means "drug recognition" and deals with the characteristics of plants and how to identify those with pharmacologic activity. Most drugs today are synthesized chemically, but phytochemistry, especially the synthesis of complex chemical structures by plants, remains of interest. On the other hand, herbal medicine as a discipline has gained in importance since 1994. The use of products in this area has spurred interest in the active components of herbal medicines, their clinical efficacy, and their potential liabilities.

After a description of how the study of drugs is classified, it is appropriate to discuss what is meant by the word *drug.* To the pharmacologist, a drug is any chemical agent that has an effect on the processes associated with life. This definition is obviously quite broad and ill-suited for many parties who define the term more restrictively to better serve their particular needs. The therapist, for example, considers as drugs those chemicals that are effective in treating disease states. To the lay public, drugs generally connote those substances that cause mental and psychologic alterations. Finally, governmental agencies are concerned with the revenue derived from the taxes levied against the sale of certain substances or with public health problems associated with their use. Some of these agents, such as tobacco and alcohol, are legally sequestered; that is, by law they are considered "nondrugs." Although pharmacologists have long recognized these agents as potent drugs, they are exempted from the usual governmental restraints and are not subject to normal scrutiny by the Food and Drug Administration. There are other substances that have gained such special status not by historical accident, as did some of those previously mentioned, but by considerations of public health. Examples of these include chlorine and fluoride added to community water supplies and iodides mixed with table salt. Lawsuits over the question of whether these public measures constitute an illegal form of "mass medication" have been resolved by the courts, at least in part, through the categorization of these chemicals as legal nondrugs when they are employed in a specific manner for the public good.

Drugs to be covered in this text include almost exclusively only those substances with a known therapeutic application. Even so, the potential number of agents for consideration is large—several thousand drugs marketed in a multiplicity of dosage forms and, in some instances, in a bewildering variety of combinations. To limit confusion, emphasis is placed on single, prototypical agents that are representative of their respective drug classes. By this approach, an understanding of the properties of related agents can be more readily achieved: at the same time, differences that may exist between them can be highlighted. Finally, it is important to recognize that there are certain generalizations that apply to all drugs. These principles of drug action are the subject of the first four chapters of this text. A mastery of the concepts presented in these chapters is necessary for a thorough understanding of pharmacology, for the rational use of therapeutic agents, and for the objective evaluation of new drugs.

PART I

Principles of Pharmacology

CHAPTER • 1

Pharmacodynamics: Mechanisms of Drug Action

John A. Yagiela

DRUG-RECEPTOR INTERACTIONS

The actions of most therapeutic agents are imbued with a certain degree of specificity. In conventional doses, for example, drugs are generally selective in action; that is, they influence a narrow spectrum of biologic events. The pharmacologic profile of such agents is, in addition, often markedly dependent on chemical structure; thus simple molecular modifications may drastically alter drug activity. These attributes of drug action suggest that the tissue components with which drugs interact to cause observable effects are uniquely individualized. Such tissue elements must have highly ordered physicochemical properties to permit particular compounds to combine with them while prohibiting all others from doing so. Furthermore, they must be intimately involved with discrete processes of life in order for drug interactions to exert specific physiologic influences. These "biologic partners" of drug action are given the term *receptors*.

The existence of receptors for exogenously administered drugs implies that drugs often mimic or inhibit the actions of endogenous ligands for these receptors. Thus drugs rarely produce novel effects; instead, they modify existing physiologic functions.

Receptor Characterization

For many years after their postulation a century ago, receptors remained an enigma to pharmacologists. Little was known about them other than the probability that they were complex macromolecules possessing a ligand-binding site to interact with specific drugs and an effector site to initiate the pharmacologic response. With the development of biochemical methods for the isolation, solubilization, and characterization of proteins, however, enzymes became available as model systems for the study of drug-receptor interactions. Enzymes exhibit many of the properties that are ascribed to receptors. They are, for example, macromolecules having measurable biologic functions and possessing specific reactive sites for selected substrates. The close association between enzymes and receptors was underscored in the early 1940s when it became apparent that some enzymes are, in fact, drug receptors.[1] The list of drugs that alter known enzymatic activities is fairly extensive and includes the angiotensin-converting enzyme inhibitors, allopurinol, anticholinesterases, carbidopa, carbonic anhydrase inhibitors, disulfiram, entacapone, monoamine oxidase inhibitors, protease inhibitors, reverse transcriptase inhibitors, sulfonamides, trimethoprim, and various antimetabolites used in cancer chemotherapy.

Besides enzymes (including coenzymes) and certain other easily solubilized proteins, there are at least two additional classes of receptors that have been identified and are of clinical significance: nucleic acids and membrane constituents. Nucleic acids serve as receptors for a limited number of agents. Certain antibiotics and antineoplastic compounds interfere with replication, transcription, or translation of genetic material by binding, sometimes irreversibly, to the nucleic acids involved. Other drugs, including thyroid hormones, vitamin D analogues, sex steroids, and adrenal corticosteroids, also modify transcription, but here the affected deoxyribonucleic acid (DNA) becomes activated or inhibited as a consequence of drug interaction with a separate receptor in the cytosol or nucleus of the cell. Generally, binding of the drug to its receptor permits the receptor to interact with its own specific response element in the DNA.

By far the most common receptors of drugs are those located on or within the various membranes of the cell. These receptors resisted characterization until the late 1970s. A brief description of some of the difficulties involved in their isolation and study will help explain why tissue-bound receptors proved difficult to investigate. Even when prevalent, membrane receptors are sparsely distributed. It is estimated, for example, that each intestinal smooth muscle cell contains approximately 16,000 receptors for acetylcholine (ACh), the major chemical transmitter of the peripheral nervous system.[25] Assuming that these receptors are scattered over a smooth plasma membrane, only 0.002% of the available surface area is involved with the binding of ACh. Calculations with other drugs, such as histamine and epinephrine, also show them to occupy an equally small fraction of the cell surface when present at effective concentrations.[20] Although a considerable number of enzymes have been solubilized from native tissues and consequently made accessible for further study, few membrane-bound receptors have. Attempts to remove the receptor macromolecule from its natural setting may inactivate it. Even if inactivation does not occur, a problem is always posed by isolation of the receptor per se, because in the isolated state the usual method of measuring its response (e.g., muscle contraction) is no longer possible.

Finally, although receptors bind drugs selectively, drugs often adhere to other tissue constituents rather indiscriminately. Plasma proteins, especially albumin, represent a common binding site for pharmacologically active molecules. In high concentrations, drugs can also be taken up nonselectively by a wide range of tissues. Because binding of this type is not saturable, the total amount of drug sequestered can be large. Fortunately, this nonspecific uptake can be differentiated from specific (e.g., receptor) binding because the latter is capacity limited and operates at low drug concentrations.

Despite these impediments, it has become possible to study membrane receptors directly through the isolation, purification, and synthesis of macromolecules that have many, if not all, of the properties of specific drug receptors. Because these receptors are tightly bound to tissues, it is first necessary to disrupt the cellular elements.[15] The chemical dissection of membranes and the release of receptor moieties are accomplished through the use of chelating agents, salts, phospholipases, and detergents. The mixture of macromolecules so derived must then be purified. An important technique for this process is affinity chromatography, in which a ligand (a compound that is complementary to the receptor and binds to it) is attached covalently to an insoluble polysaccharide matrix. Ligands that have proved useful in this regard include specific and potent drugs, snake toxins, and monoclonal antibodies.[15,34] When passed through a column of this matrix, the receptors become bound to their ligands. After several washings to remove contaminants, the receptors are eluted by one of several methods, including the addition of free ligand. The recovered receptors can then be studied in vitro, but special methods, such as incorporation of the receptors into artificial or natural plasma membranes and use of radioactively labeled drug ligands, are needed to examine drug-receptor interactions.

The development of molecular biology has proved revolutionary to the study of drug receptors. Since the early 1980s, the amino acid sequences of many important receptors have been deduced, and research in this area is progressing rapidly. The basic strategy of receptor characterization[36] begins with the isolation of the receptor in pure form, as already described. Next, small portions of the receptor protein are identified and sequenced, and oligonucleotides that encode for these peptide lengths are synthesized and used as DNA probes to hybridize with, and therefore identify, the gene equivalents in DNA libraries previously developed by recombinant DNA techniques. (Alternatively, specific ligands for the receptor may be used to identify its expression in cells containing its complementary DNA.) Based on the sequence of the genomic clones, the entire amino acid sequence of the receptor protein can be derived. Moreover, plasmids containing DNA encoding the receptor can be introduced into cells, which then synthesize the receptor protein in large quantities. This strategy provides sufficient protein for such analytical techniques as x-ray crystallography. It also facilitates the study of receptor function in defined cell cultures. An unanticipated benefit of molecular biologic approaches to the study of receptors was the finding that the vast majority of membrane-bound receptors could be grouped into several receptor superfamilies of homologous proteins. This conservation of receptor structure has led to the rapid elucidation of receptor subtypes and the identification of novel receptors with unknown functions.

The characterization of drug receptors continues to provide great benefits for pharmacology. For the scientist, the examination of receptors and their distribution provides insight into the mechanisms by which cells communicate and clues to the existence of unknown neurotransmitters and other mediators. For the clinician, receptor investigations lead to a deeper understanding of disease states and to new methods of drug treatment. The isolation of opioid receptors in the central nervous system (CNS) and the subsequent discovery of endogenous morphinelike compounds is but one example of how the study of receptors can yield basic scientific information while concurrently opening new avenues for drug therapy.[10]

Receptor Classification

As mentioned previously, membrane-linked receptors, which constitute the majority of drug receptors, can be grouped by molecular structure and functional characteristics into several superfamilies. These receptors have one or more extracellular ligand-binding domains linked by one or more lipophilic membrane-spanning segments to an effector domain often, but not always, located on the cytoplasmic side of the membrane. This arrangement is ideal for the translation of an extracellular signal into an intracellular response. Usually, the endogenous ligand "signal" is hydrophilic and incapable of passive diffusion through the cell membrane. For lipophilic regulatory ligands, such as for thyroid hormone and various steroids, a separate superfamily of intracellular receptors exists. Commonly, drug binding exposes a DNA-binding site on the receptor protein, allowing the receptor to interact with DNA and alter transcription. These major classes of receptors are illustrated in Figure 1-1 and described below.

Ion channel–linked receptors

There are two general classes of ion channels: voltage gated and ligand gated. Voltage-gated ion channels are activated by alterations in membrane voltage. For example, voltage-gated Na^+ channels open when the membrane is depolarized to a threshold potential and contribute to further membrane depolarization by allowing Na^+ influx into the cell. As described in Chapter 16, local anesthetics such as lidocaine bind to voltage-gated Na^+ channels, leading to blockade of neuronal depolarization. In contrast, ligand-gated ion channels are activated in response to the binding of specific ligands or drugs. Many neurotransmitters and drugs activate membrane-bound ligand-gated ion channels, including several types of glutamate receptors (promoting Na^+, K^+, and/or Ca^{++} movements), as well as certain γ-aminobutyric acid and glycine receptors (both promoting Cl^- influx). Depending on the ionic charge and the direction of flow, ligand-gated ion channels can either depolarize or hyperpolarize the cell membrane.

The nicotinic receptor (Figure 1-2), the first membrane-bound drug receptor to be fully characterized,[12,26] is an important example of a ligand-gated ion channel. An oligomeric structure, the polypeptide constituents of the nicotinic receptor are arranged concentrically to form a channel through which small ions can traverse the plasma membrane when the receptor is activated by ACh.

G protein–linked receptors

G protein–linked receptors, sometimes referred to as *metabotropic receptors*, consist of a large class of membrane-bound receptors that collectively serve as targets for approximately half of all nonantimicrobial prescription drugs.[4,9,31] The protein structure of these receptors includes a common seven-membered transmembrane domain. In general, metabotropic receptors greatly amplify extracellular biologic signals because they activate G proteins that, in turn, activate ion channels or, more commonly, other enzymes (e.g., adenylyl cyclase), leading to the introduction or formation of a host of internal second messengers for each extracellular signal molecule detected.[3,27] This amplification system, which also usually involves an extended duration of activation of G proteins relative to the binding of drug to the receptor, may explain why maximal pharmacologic effects are often observed when only a small proportion of receptors are activated.

G proteins are heterotrimers consisting of α, β, and γ subunits. After receptor activation, guanosine diphosphate attached to the α subunit is replaced by guanosine triphosphate, and the heterotrimer splits into the α monomer and βγ dimer. Many, but not all, of the observed cellular actions are caused by the α subunit (see Figure 5-7). For example, $G_{\alpha s}$, the specific α subunit for the G protein associated with β-adrenergic receptors, activates adenylyl cyclase, which, in turn, catalyzes the synthesis of cyclic adenosine 3′,5′-monophosphate (cAMP).[9] cAMP then activates protein kinase A, which catalyzes the phosphorylation of serine and

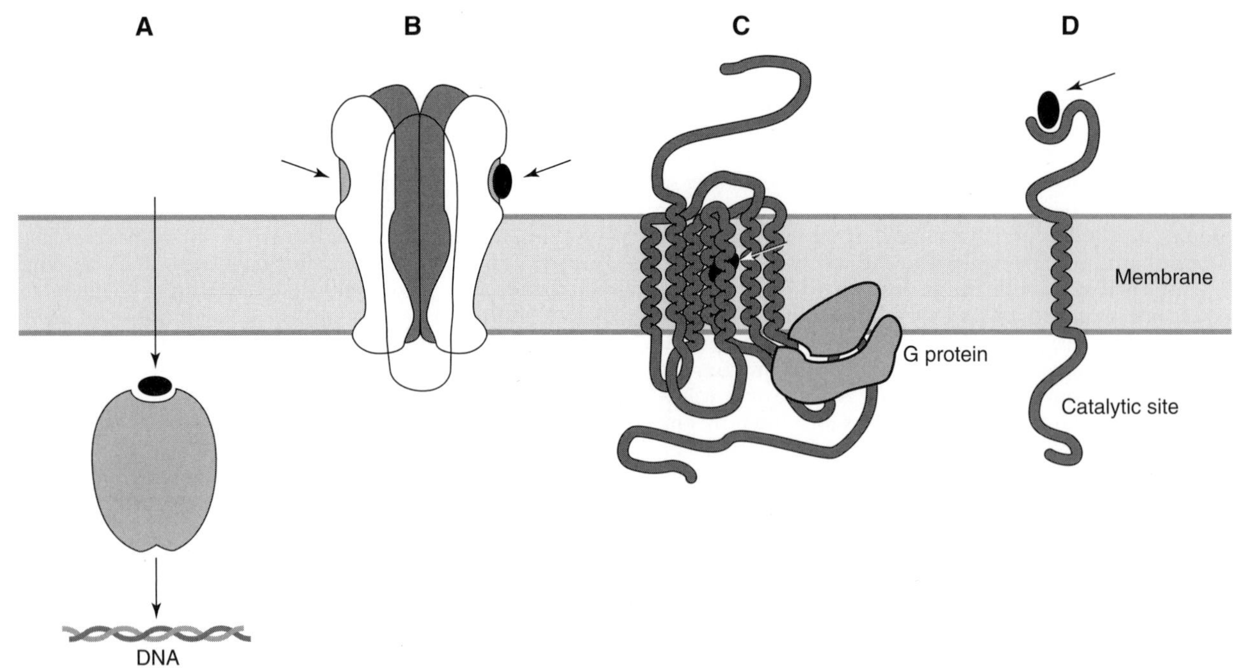

Fig. 1-1 Illustration of the four major classes of receptors and signal transduction mechanisms. *Arrows* denote the receptor ligand-binding sites. **A,** Intracellular receptors. Lipophilic substances such as steroids can cross the plasma membrane and activate intracellular receptors that, after translocation to the nucleus, alter gene transcription and, ultimately, synthesis of new protein. **B,** Ion channel–linked receptors. Drugs such as nicotine can activate ligand-gated ion channels, leading to depolarization (or hyperpolarization) of the plasma membrane. **C,** G protein–linked receptors. Many drugs can activate G protein–linked receptors, causing release of the α and βγ subunits of associated G proteins. **D,** Enzyme-linked receptors. Drugs such as insulin promote dimerization of its receptor and activation of the catalytic site on the intracellular end of the receptor.

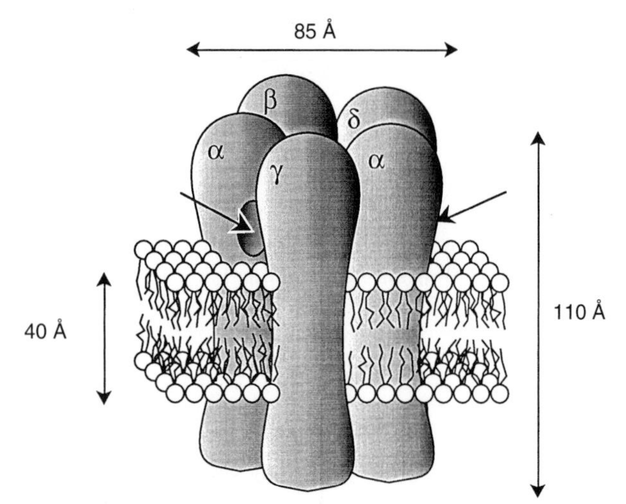

Fig. 1-2 Structural model of the nicotinic ACh receptor from the electric organ of *Torpedo californica.* Five polypeptide units consisting of four different types (α, β, γ [or ε], and δ) form a rosette with a hydrophilic pore spanning the center of the oligomer. A single ACh binding site *(arrow)* is present on the extracellular surface of each α subunit. Each polypeptide subunit is believed to include four α-helical sequences that traverse the plasma membrane. The dimensions shown were determined by electron microscopy and by x-ray and neutron scattering analysis.[12,26]

threonine residues of certain intracellular proteins, leading to altered cellular function.

The G protein system is complex and still incompletely understood. For example, one receptor subtype may activate different G proteins, several receptor subtypes may activate the same G protein, and the ultimate target protein can exist in tissue-specific isoforms with differing susceptibility to secondary effector systems. Moreover, the different G protein pathways can interact with one another. The complexity of G protein signal transduction provides a sophisticated regulatory system by which cellular responses can vary, depending on the combination of receptors activated as well as the cell-specific expression of distinct regulatory and target proteins. Several specific membrane-bound G proteins are discussed in Chapter 5.

Figure 1-3 depicts the structure of the mammalian β_2 receptor and how it is believed to be arranged within the plasma membrane.[16,24] Binding sites for epinephrine (the endogenous receptor ligand) and the G_s protein are also indicated.

Enzyme-linked receptors

Enzyme-linked receptors have only one transmembrane domain per protein subunit, with an enzymatic catalytic site on the cytoplasmic side of the receptor. Dimerization of activated receptors usually provides the conformational change required for expression of enzymatic activity. The catalytic sites are commonly protein kinases that phosphorylate

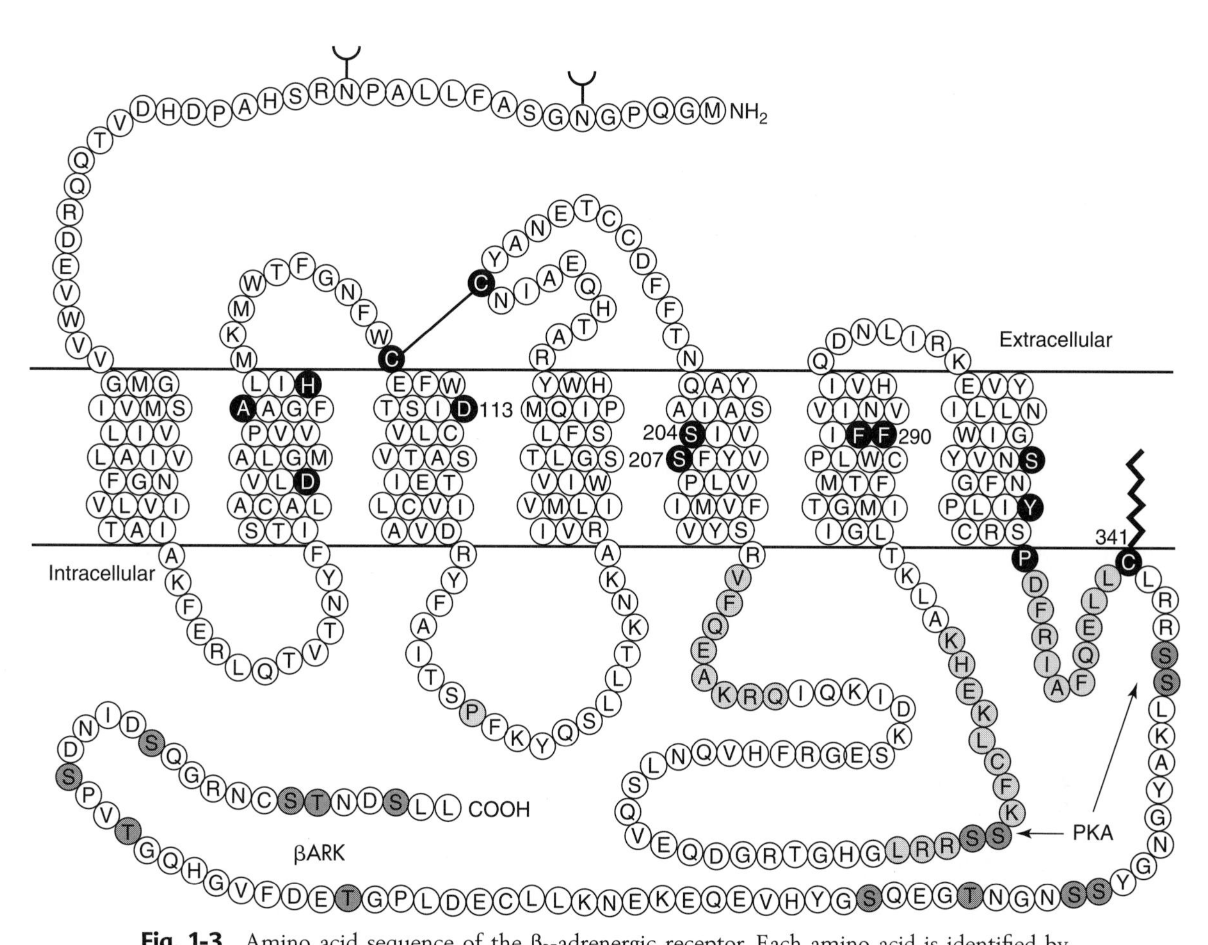

Fig. 1-3 Amino acid sequence of the β_2-adrenergic receptor. Each amino acid is identified by the single letter code. Seven regions of hydrophobic sequences form α helixes within the plasma membrane. Amino acid residues critical for binding the agonist epinephrine are shown in black; residues involved in G protein interactions are shaded. Phosphorylation sites (serine *[S]* and threonine *[T]* residues) for protein kinase A *(PKA)* and β-adrenergic receptor kinase *(βARK)* are darkly shaded. Sites for glycosylation of asparagine residues *(N)* and palmitoylation of the cysteine[341] residue *(C)* are also indicated. (Adapted from Schwinn DA, Caron MG, Lefkowitz RJ: The beta-adrenergic receptor as a model for molecular structure-function relationships in G-protein-coupled receptors. In Fozzard HA, Haber E, Jennings RB, et al, eds: *The heart and cardiovascular system: scientific foundation*, ed 2, New York, 1991, Raven Press.)

tyrosine or, less commonly, serine or threonine residues on target proteins. Autophosphorylation of the receptor also occurs. Some catalytic receptors have guanylyl cyclase or tyrosine phosphatase activity. Insulin, atrial natriuretic peptide, and various growth factors (e.g., epidermal growth factor) activate catalytic receptors. A closely related group of receptors responsible for the action of numerous peptides, including various neurotrophic peptides and cytokines, lacks enzymatic activity. In such cases, the catalytic site is supplied by a separate intracellular protein that interacts with the dimerized receptor.

Many forms of cancer appear to involve mutant forms of enzyme-linked receptors in which the catalytic site is continually activated.[7] In fact, approximately half of all oncogenes discovered to date appear to encode for continually activated protein kinases.

Intracellular receptors

Lipophilic substances capable of crossing the plasma membrane may activate intracellular receptors. Sex steroids, mineralocorticoids, glucocorticoids, thyroid hormones, and vitamin D derivatives all activate specific intracellular receptors that influence DNA transcription.[23,32] The typical receptor is composed of three major subunits. The carboxyl end of the receptor forms the ligand-binding site; the adjacent segment includes the DNA-binding region; and the amino terminus constitutes the transcription-modulating domain. When a drug (or hormone) binds to the receptor, associated proteins are released from the receptor, allowing it to fold into the active configuration. The conformational change results in a dramatic increase in binding to specific DNA sequences. For example, binding of thyroid hormone to its receptor produces more than a tenfold increase in receptor affinity for binding to DNA.[32] DNA binding of the activated receptor often initiates transcription, leading to increased production of specific proteins. Because this type of signal transduction requires protein synthesis, drugs that activate intracellular receptors typically have a delay of several hours before the onset of their pharmacologic effect. (It is for this reason that glucocorticoids cannot be used as primary drugs for the management of anaphylaxis.) In some systems, the binding of the drug-receptor complex inhibits transcription. Regardless of the specific mechanism involved, however, the intensity and duration of drug effect is temporally independent of the plasma concentration.

In addition to these intracellular receptors, other enzymes and proteins involved in gene expression and cellular regulation are receiving increasing scrutiny as potential targets for drug therapy. Nitric oxide, which stimulates guanylyl cyclase directly to form cyclic guanosine 3′,5′-monophosphate (cGMP), and sildenafil, which inhibits the breakdown of cGMP by cGMP-specific phosphodiesterase-5, are two examples of currently available agents acting intracellularly on regulatory enzymes.

Drug-Binding Forces

Implicit in the interaction of a drug with its receptor is the chemical binding of that drug to one or more specific sites on the receptor molecule. There are five basic types of binding that may be involved (Figure 1-4).

Covalent bonds

Covalent bonds arise from the sharing of electrons by a pair of atoms. Although covalent bonds are required for the structural integrity of molecules, they are generally not involved in drug-receptor interactions. Most drugs reversibly associate with their receptors. As described in Chapter 2, the duration of action of these agents is related to how long an effective drug concentration remains in the vicinity of the drug receptors. This time may vary from a few minutes to many days but usually is on the order of several hours. With bond energies of 250 to 500 kJ/mole, the stability of covalent linkages is so great that, once formed, drug-receptor complexes are often irreversible. In these instances, the duration of action is not influenced by the concentration of unbound drug vicinal to the receptors. Instead, it may depend on the synthesis of new receptors or on the turnover of the affected cells, processes that often take days to weeks. When the receptors happen to compose the genetic material of a cell, drug effects may be permanent.

Ionic bonds

Ionic bonds result from the electrostatic attraction between ions of opposite charge. Such associations are relatively weak in an aqueous environment, having bond energies of approximately 20 kJ/mole. Nevertheless, many drugs have a formal charge at physiologic pH, and it is likely that ionic bonds are commonly made with ionized groups located at receptor sites. Because the attraction between ions is inversely proportional to the square of the distance separating them, ionic influences operate over much greater distances than do other interatomic forces. It is reasonable to assume, therefore, that ionic bonds initiate many drug-receptor combinations.

Cation-π interactions

Although benzene and similar aromatic compounds are hydrophobic solvents, their π electron clouds are capable of interacting with positively charged ions.[8] Phenylalanine, tyrosine, and tryptophan—amino acids with aromatic side groups—retain this ability. These amino acids are common constituents at receptor sites for such positively charged drugs as ACh, dopamine, epinephrine, and 5-hydroxytryptamine. Individual bond energies are similar to those of hydrogen bonds; however, interactions between multiple aromatic amino acids and a single cationic moiety commonly strengthen the overall interaction.

Hydrogen bonds

The hydrogen bond represents a special type of interaction between polar molecules. When a hydrogen atom is covalently attached to a strongly electronegative atom such as oxygen or nitrogen, it becomes partially stripped of its electron and takes on some of the characteristics of a bare proton. Strongly electropositive and with an exceedingly small atomic radius, the hydrogen nucleus is able to associate closely with additional electronegative atoms. Hydrogen linkages are generally weaker than ionic bonds (approximately 5 kJ) and are more sensitive to interatomic separation. However, functional groups capable of forming hydrogen bonds are common to both drugs and receptor sites, and, if multiple unions occur, the resultant stabilizing force could far outweigh that of a single ionic bond.

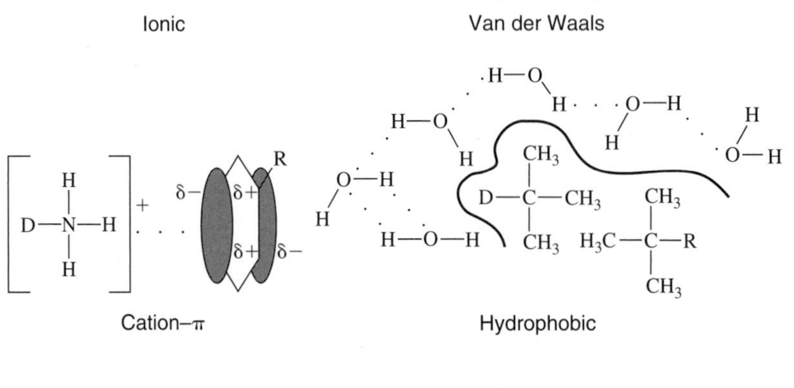

Fig. 1-4 Major chemical bonds associated with drug-receptor interactions, where *D* is drug and *R* is receptor.

Van der Waals forces

Van der Waals forces collectively describe the weak interactions that develop when two atoms are placed in close proximity. The electrostatic attractions that comprise these forces result from reciprocal perturbations in the electron clouds of the atoms involved. These "bonds" are the weakest of the five types described (approximately 0.5 kJ); in addition, they decrease in strength according to the seventh power of the interatomic distance. Paradoxic as it may seem, van der Waals forces are of primary importance in conferring specificity to drug-receptor interactions. Because even electroneutral carbon atoms can participate in such associations, the number of these bonds that connect a drug to its receptor may be large and the total binding force considerable. When minor steric influences prevent an exact fit between a drug and its receptor, the sensitivity of van der Waals forces to interatomic separation forestalls their development, and drug-receptor stability markedly suffers.

Hydrophobic interactions

In addition to the bonding forces already described, hydrophobic interactions between the drug, its receptor, and the aqueous environment can play a major role in stabilizing drug-receptor binding. Water is an unusual liquid with respect to its ability to form hydrogen bonds with itself as well as with various solutes. The association of a drug with its receptor is enhanced if the drug is hydrophobic or if the surface area of a nonpolar region of the receptor is reduced by drug binding. In either case, stability occurs because of the reduced perturbation of the normal water structure.

Cooperation of binding forces

The binding of a drug to its receptor is generally not related to a particular attractive force but results from the conjoint action of ionic, cation-π, hydrogen, van der Waals, and (rarely) covalent linkages, as well as hydrophobic interactions. Each type of association contributes differently to the drug-receptor complex. When random movement causes a drug molecule to approach or collide with the receptor surface, ionic attractions, closely followed by cation-π interactions, are the first to develop. Unable to convey specificity or stability to a drug-receptor union by themselves, these forces nevertheless serve to draw in and partially orient the drug to its receptor. As the intermolecular separation diminishes, hydrophobic influences, hydrogen bonding, and subsequently van der Waals forces become prominent. In concert, these interactions provide for the specificity of drug action; without an exact fit, binding is impaired and the drug cannot adhere well enough to influence receptor function. Covalent linkage confers a high degree of permanency to the drug-receptor complex. It is fortunate, however, that irreversible binding is uncommon in therapeutics. Many agents are used to produce a single, temporary effect; covalent attachment would preclude such use. Furthermore, covalent bonding would, in many instances, make drug regimens more difficult to administer and adverse reactions more troublesome to treat.

Structure-Activity Relationships

Examination of structure-activity relationships (SAR) is a time-honored method of studying drug-receptor interactions. In SAR investigations, specific features of the structure of a drug molecule are identified and then altered systematically to determine their influence on pharmacologic activity. The chemical features that are most often involved in these considerations are the presence and type of ionic charge, the effect of neighboring groups on the degree of ionization, hydrogen-bonding capability, and steric factors such as the size of alkyl side chains, the distance between reactive groups, and the three-dimensional configuration of such groups. SAR studies of closely related agents (congeners) have led to an understanding of the chemical prerequisites for pharmacologic activity and, on a practical level, made possible the molecular modification of drugs to provide enhanced or even novel therapeutic effects while reducing the incidence and severity of toxic reactions. In addition, they serve to illustrate how the combined action of the various binding forces described above are necessary for maximal drug activity and yield certain clues concerning the physicochemical properties of the receptor sites involved that are of value to investigators seeking to unravel the exact structure of these sites.[11]

A typical example of SAR is provided by the study of epinephrine and its binding to the β-adrenergic receptor (Figure 1-5). The epinephrine molecule is composed of a catechol residue (a benzene ring with two hydroxyl groups in the ortho position) connected by a two-carbon intermediate chain to a methylated nitrogen terminus that is positively charged at physiologic pH. The presence of a cationic nitrogen locus is essential for full activity; loss of the ionic charge by replacing the nitrogen with a nonionic carbon atom virtually eliminates drug action. The nitrogen-bound methyl group is also involved in binding; its removal, yielding norepinephrine, results in almost complete loss of β_2-adrenergic activity. Conversely, increasing the size of the alkyl moiety increases β-adrenergic selectivity. Because alkyl moieties do not form hydrogen or ionic bonds, this finding implies that van der Waals forces and/or hydrophobic interactions contribute significantly to the binding of epinephrine and congeners with selective β-adrenergic properties. Hydrogen bonds involving both ring hydroxyl groups greatly increase potency but preclude entry of the drug into the CNS. Replacement of a hydroxyl with a larger group generally eliminates agonist activity at β receptors but may result in antagonistic effects. The distance separating the catechol and nitrogen moieties of the molecule is likewise critical for full activity. Electrostatic interactions involving the benzene ring and aromatic amino acid residues of the receptor protein have also been postulated as contributing to the binding of epinephrine.

An important source of support for the concept of specificity in drug-receptor interactions comes from the differences so often observed in the activity of optical isomers, such as *d*- and *l*-epinephrine. It is common for virtually all the activity in a racemic mixture to reside in one of the two stereoisomers. In the case of epinephrine, the levorotatory isomer is highly active, whereas the other member of the pair is almost devoid of activity. The presence of only a single atom with an opposite configuration is apparently sufficient to bring about dramatic differences in binding efficiency. Such critical sensitivity can occur only if the drug and receptor fit together with some degree of precision. The optical isomers quinine and quinidine are of interest because both are used therapeutically but for different purposes. Quinidine (dextro) and quinine (levo) differ from each other only in the configuration of a single secondary alcohol group that serves as the connector of the two halves of the molecule. Both isomers are approximately equal in antimalarial activity, a property that depends on the drug reacting with the DNA of the plasmodial parasites responsible for the disease. The antiarrhythmic action on cardiac muscle, however, is greater for quinidine than for quinine. The enantiomers of D-mannose are another example of two molecules that differ only in the spatial arrangement of a single hydroxyl group and yet vary in their biologic activity. α-D-Mannose is sweet when applied to chemoreceptors of the tongue, whereas β-D-mannose is bitter.[30]

Consequences of Drug Binding

The combination of a drug with its receptor represents the incipient event in a series of reactions that culminate in a pharmacologic effect. Of prime importance is the second step

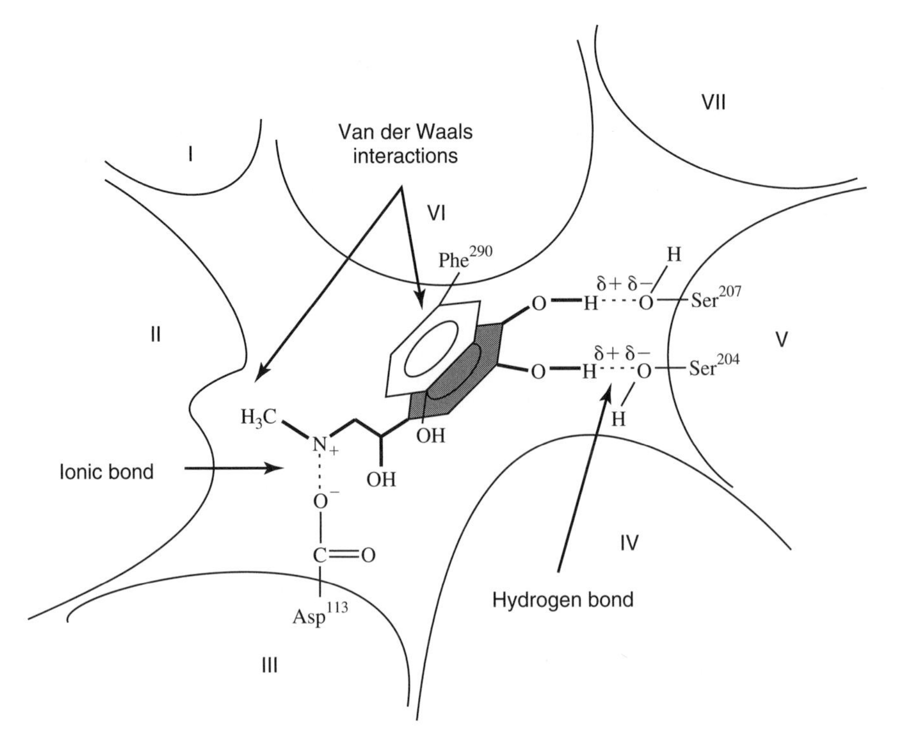

Fig. 1-5 Interaction of epinephrine with the β-adrenergic receptor. The seven transmembrane segments (*I* through *VII*) are shown in cross-section along with specific amino acid residues implicated in drug binding.

in this chain—the receptor response to drug binding. Drugs generally are not highly reactive compounds in the chemical sense; they exert their influences indirectly by altering, through receptor attachment, the activity of an important regulator of a biologic process. The mechanism of action of a drug refers to this initial perturbation of normal function.

Of the various receptor-based mechanisms of drug action, perhaps the most readily observed are those involving enzymes. Certain drugs are analogues of natural enzyme substrates. These antimetabolites compete with the substrate for the same catalytic site on the enzyme molecule, the result of this competition being a decrease in the rate of product formation. As a general rule, however, such inhibitions are likely to be of little biologic consequence unless the magnitude of inhibition approaches 50%. This phenomenon appears to be explained best by the concept that the number of enzyme molecules present usually exceeds what is necessary for adequate catalysis. A 20% inhibition therefore might produce no observable response because the remaining fraction of uninhibited enzyme is still capable of providing enough product. The enzyme carbonic anhydrase represents an extreme example of this situation. To reduce by half the enzymatic hydration of carbon dioxide, 99.7% of the carbonic anhydrase activity must be abolished.[18] Another consideration related to antimetabolites is the often greater affinity of the reactive site for the natural substrate. This difference may be as much as 1000-fold and has some significance for pharmacology. If the substrate to be interfered with is abundant, such as glucose, the dose of inhibitor needed to obtain a body fluid concentration a thousand times that of the metabolite would be formidable indeed. Substrates that are in more limited supply, such as vitamin derivatives or chemical mediators, are more reasonable targets for therapy based on this form of inhibition.

Many drugs that influence enzyme activity are not structurally related to native substrates. These drugs affect catalysis by serving as allosteric regulators; that is, by binding elsewhere on the enzyme, they induce conformational changes at the active center. These disturbances may lead to an increased affinity for the substrate, but it is more likely for the effect to be one of inhibition. Although the basis of drug-induced allosteric changes in enzymes is poorly understood, hydrophobic interactions involving the surrounding hydration layer appear to be involved. As with other macromolecules, enzymes are covered by a surface film of water. When a drug is bound to its receptor, it upsets the microenvironment around the binding site. Alkyl groups common to many drugs are especially proficient at disturbing the hydration layer; as a result, they promote conformational changes in the drug-receptor complex that minimize their impact. It should be noted that the quaternary structure of proteins is greatly influenced by the state of the surrounding water molecules and that enzymes subject to allosteric regulation have quaternary structures of exceptional conformational sensitivity. The requirement described above that a certain percentage of enzyme be affected before an observable effect is achieved also holds for allosteric regulation, but the need for the drug concentration to be in excess of the substrate does not because the two compounds are not in direct competition for binding.

The concept of allostericism may be of particular relevance to the membrane-bound receptors previously described. The allosteric concept suggests that a receptor, whether stimulated by its natural effector or by a drug substitute, becomes morphologically distorted. This disturbance then causes a change in a particular enzyme activity or transport mechanism or an alteration of membrane permeability. An illustration of the consequences of drug binding is provided by epinephrine.[28] Incorporated into local anesthetic solutions to prolong the duration of anesthesia, epinephrine mimics the action of the neurotransmitter norepinephrine. As a result of epinephrine attachment to α_1-adrenergic receptors of vascular smooth muscle cells, the G protein known as G_q is activated, phospholipase C_β activity is stimulated, and the membrane lipid phosphatidylinositol-4,5-bisphosphate is broken down to yield the second messengers diacylglycerol and inositol-1,4,5-trisphosphate (IP_3). Diacylglycerol initiates a cascade of metabolic events that support muscle contraction. IP_3 causes the release of Ca^{++} from intracellular storage sites, which ultimately induces the activation of actomyosin and initiates vasoconstriction.

Drugs can directly alter processes controlled by membrane-bound receptors without resorting to mimicry of natural messengers. As is the case with enzymes, drugs can act either by physically interfering with messenger binding or by adjusting receptor affinity for the messenger through an allosteric mechanism.

DOSE-RESPONSE RELATIONSHIPS

One of the most fundamental aspects of drug action is the relationship between the dose administered and the effect obtained. Common experience dictates that the magnitude of a chemical's effect on a system is positively correlated with the quantity or concentration of that chemical present. To increase the saltiness of a food, for example, more salt must be added. Within certain limits, the addition of salt yields a graded response, but very small increments have no effect on taste, and if the food is quite salty to begin with, further additions, no matter how great, will have no effect either. There is reason to expect, therefore, that the dose-effect relationship of a drug is not a linear function throughout the entire dose range. Below a minimum threshold there can be no incremental effect from a dose, because there is no observable effect to begin with. Above a certain ceiling, even a large dose will exert no demonstrable influence because the maximal effect has already been reached.

Occupation Theory

Clark attempted in the 1920s to quantitate drug effects through application of the law of mass action.[6] Out of his efforts and the contributions of others emerged the occupation theory of drug action.[17] The occupation theory holds that the magnitude of a pharmacologic response elicited by a drug that reversibly combines with its receptor is directly proportional to the number (or fraction) of receptors occupied by the drug. The relationship can be written as follows:

$$D + R \underset{k_2}{\overset{k_1}{\rightleftharpoons}} DR \rightarrow \text{Effect}$$

where D is the drug, R the receptor, and k_1 and k_2 are rate constants. This reaction is analogous to the interaction of an enzyme with a single substrate yielding a single product. Hence, a derivative of the Michaelis-Menton equation can be used to quantify drug effects as follows:

$$\text{Effect} = \frac{\text{Maximal effect} \times [D]}{K_D + [D]}$$

where K_D (the dissociation constant) = k_2/k_1.

This mathematic relationship between the dose (or concentration) of a drug and its response may be demonstrated visually by an experiment in which an isolated muscle is exposed to increasing concentrations of a drug while the force of contraction is measured (Figure 1-6). When a drug is introduced into a tissue, it binds to its receptor in accordance with the K_D. For various reasons, very small quantities will not elicit a measurable response. For example, each muscle cell may require a minimal number of receptors to be occupied before it contracts, or technical difficulties in detecting small contractions may make such determinations inaccurate or impossible to obtain. The lowest concentration to elicit a measurable response is termed the *threshold concentration.* As higher concentrations are used, the number of receptors occupied rises, as does the intensity of response. An increase in the fraction of receptors occupied necessarily reduces the number available for subsequent binding, so that at high concentrations each increment produces progressively smaller additions to the magnitude of contraction. At very high concentrations, the receptor population becomes saturated, and further drug administration will no longer influence contraction. A maximal muscle response for the drug, termed the *ceiling effect,* is achieved.

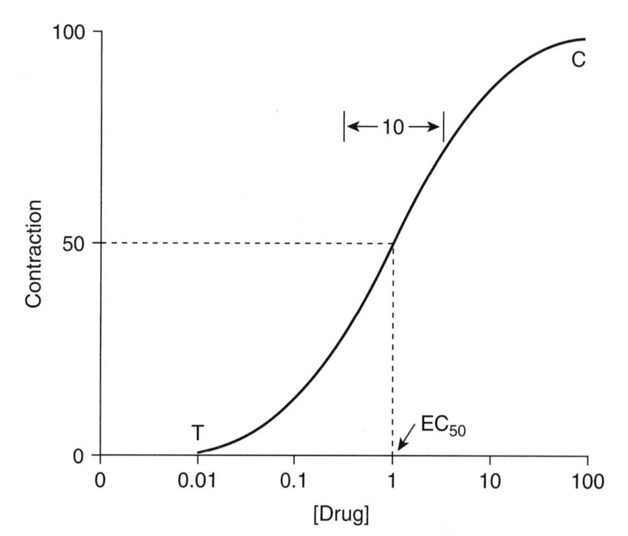

Fig. 1-6 Theoretic dose-response curve (log scale) for a smooth muscle stimulant. The threshold and ceiling effects are represented by *T* and C, respectively. As shown, the linear portion of the sigmoid curve, extending from approximately 25% to 75% of the maximal effect, is encompassed by a 10-fold concentration range. A range of 10,000 times is required, however, to depict the curve in its entirety (from 1% to 99% of the maximal effect). The concentration yielding 50% of the maximal response *(EC_{50})* is also shown.

The most useful concentration range for a drug falls between the threshold and the ceiling. By expressing data as the logarithm of the concentration versus the degree of response, this important, normally hyperbolic segment of the concentration-effect relationship becomes a sigmoid curve with the linear central portion extending over a tenfold concentration range. The advantage of plotting with the log scale instead of the arithmetic scale is that it greatly simplifies drug study. For example, the concentration of a drug that produces a half-maximal response (EC_{50}) is often used in comparisons with like agents. (In classic occupation theory, the EC_{50} equals the K_D). When data from several experiments are expressed on a single graph with the log dose, this value can be accurately determined for each drug from the linear portion of the respective curve. If the concentration data were not logarithmically transformed, statistical analysis would become more complex. Figure 1-7 illustrates the difficulties encountered if two drugs differing only in receptor affinity are examined on an arithmetic scale. The curve for drug A is so compressed that the concentration yielding the EC_{50} cannot be easily ascertained; for drug B, it cannot even be represented on the same page.

Agonists

Drugs that elicit a response from a tissue are known as *agonists.* Agonists that produce ceiling effects—effects that are not exceeded by other drugs—are called *full agonists,* and drugs whose maximal effects are less than those of full agonists are referred to as *partial agonists.* It should be stressed that the distinction between full and partial agonists is unrelated to variances in receptor affinity; the relatively low ceiling effect of a partial agonist cannot be raised by increasing its

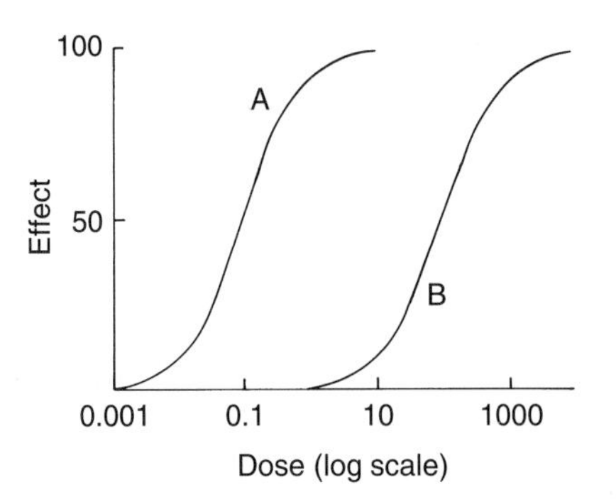

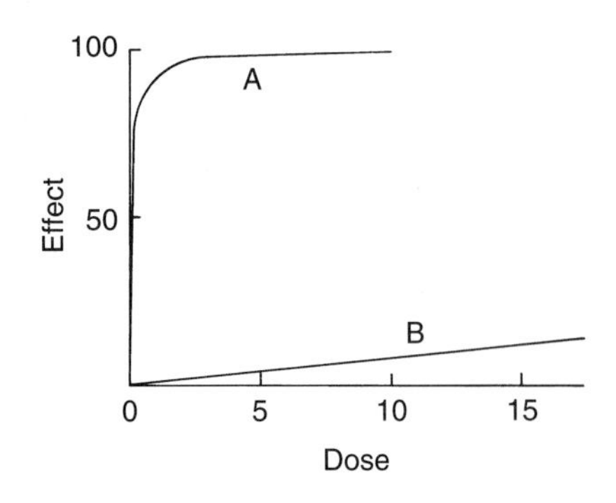

Fig. 1-7 Dose-effect curves for two drugs differing in receptor affinity by a factor of 1000. *Left,* A log scale. Note the identical shapes of the two dose-effect relationships. *Right,* An arithmetic scale. The lack of correspondence between the two curves hinders drug comparison.

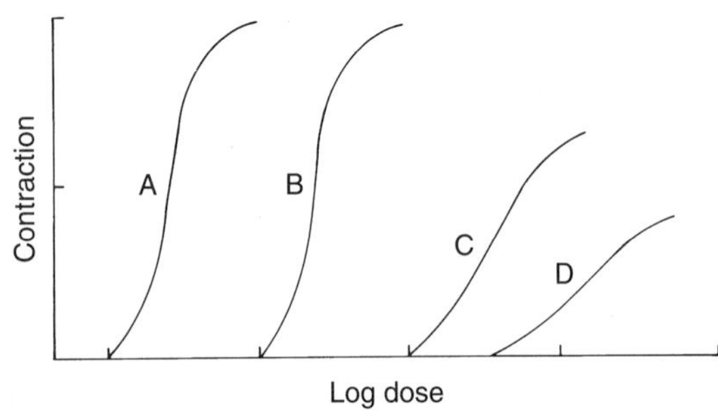

Fig. 1-8 Effects of four catecholamines on muscle contraction in the vas deferens of the rat. Drugs *A* and *B* differ in affinity but not in intrinsic activity. Drugs C and *D* differ from each other and from A and B in both affinity and intrinsic activity. (Adapted from Ariëns EJ, Simonis AM, van Rossum JM: Drug-receptor interactions: interaction of one or more drugs with one receptor system. In Ariëns EJ, ed: *Molecular pharmacology: the mode of action of biologically active compounds,* New York, 1964, Academic Press.)

dose. The difference between these two classes of agonists lies in their unequal intrinsic activities. *Intrinsic activity* is an empirical term used in classic occupation theory to describe the ability of a drug to activate a receptor once the drug-receptor complex has formed. Incorporating intrinsic activity into the concentration-effect equation yields:

$$\text{Effect} = \frac{a \times [D]}{K_D + [D]}$$

where a is the intrinsic activity. Drugs with a low intrinsic activity not only have a relatively low ceiling effect, but each fraction of receptors occupied elicits a response that is smaller than that produced by a similar degree of receptor binding by a full agonist. In other words, the log dose–response curve of a partial agonist has a lower maximum and a smaller slope than does that of a full agonist.

These precepts of occupation theory are demonstrated in Figure 1-8, which presents data from a study of four agonists of muscle contraction.[2] The muscle to be investigated was removed from the animal, placed in a bath containing an oxygenated physiologic salt solution, and attached to a strain gauge to measure isometric contractions. In such experiments, conditions can be manipulated to ensure that each drug tested has equal access to the receptor. (This condition, which greatly simplifies the interpretation of experimental results, cannot be duplicated in whole-animal investigations.) The most potent drug shown is A, with drugs B, C, and D exhibiting progressively decreasing potencies. The potency of a drug is the dose required to elicit an arbitrarily determined level of response (commonly the EC_{50}). Potency is usually a matter of little importance, because a drug that is very potent regarding its desirable effects is often equally potent regarding those that are undesirable. In the intact animal (or patient), potency is influenced by the affinity of a drug for its receptor and its intrinsic activity as well as its ability to reach the receptor (determined by the rate of absorption and the patterns of distribution and elimination). A very active drug will appear to have low potency if it is not well absorbed, becomes bound to nonspecific sites, or cannot reach the target organ.

Drugs A and B are full agonists (assuming no other drug with an affinity for this particular receptor can produce a greater ceiling effect), and drugs C and D are partial agonists. Drug D has the smallest intrinsic activity. Note that the consequences of the low potency of drug B can be completely overcome by increasing its dose. According to classic receptor theory, drug B exhibits a lower potency than drug A solely because it has a weaker affinity for its receptor. Drugs C and D represent a more complex problem. Obviously, these agents are less potent than drugs A and B, which suggests that they possess lesser affinities. Part of their reduced potency, however, is a consequence of their lower intrinsic activities.

Antagonists

Drugs that bind to a receptor at the same site as the agonist but have an intrinsic activity of zero (no receptor activation; $a = 0$) are competitive antagonists. By making receptors less available for agonist binding, a competitive antagonist will depress the response to a given dose or concentration of agonist. The result is a parallel shift to the right of the agonist dose-response curve. The most important aspect of this type of inhibition is that it is completely surmountable by a high enough dose of agonist. As in enzymology, the presence of a competitive antagonist produces an apparent reduction in the affinity of an agonist for its receptor. A functionally similar reduction (described as negative cooperativity) can occur by allosteric distortion of the site to reduce binding efficiency for the agonist. Competitive antagonisms are quite common in pharmacology, and numerous examples are cited in succeeding chapters: histamine versus antihistamines, morphine versus naloxone, ACh versus atropine, epinephrine versus propranolol, diazepam versus flumazenil. By virtue of its small intrinsic activity, a partial agonist can also serve as a competitive antagonist of a full agonist. The aggregate receptor stimulation from the combination will depend on the relative concentrations, receptor affinities, and intrinsic activities of the two agents.

Another type of antagonism commonly encountered is the noncompetitive variety. The noncompetitive blockade is insurmountable in that the ceiling effect of an agonist can never be reattained, regardless of the dose administered. A noncompetitive antagonist may decrease the effective number of receptors, either by irreversibly binding to the receptor site or by binding elsewhere and eliminating receptor sites through allosteric influences. Alternatively, the antagonist may interfere with the ability of the drug-receptor complex to create the measured effect, effectively decreasing intrinsic

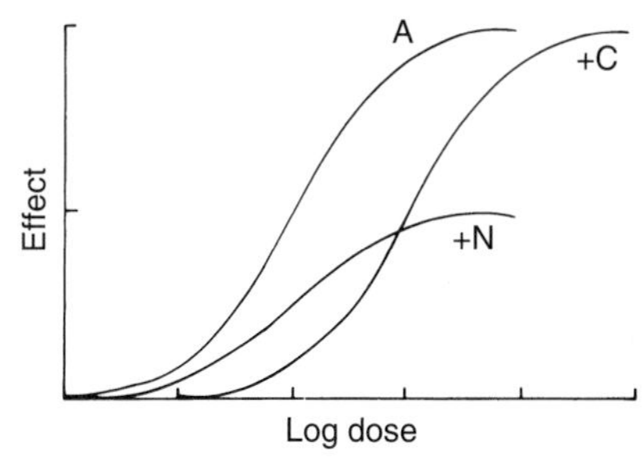

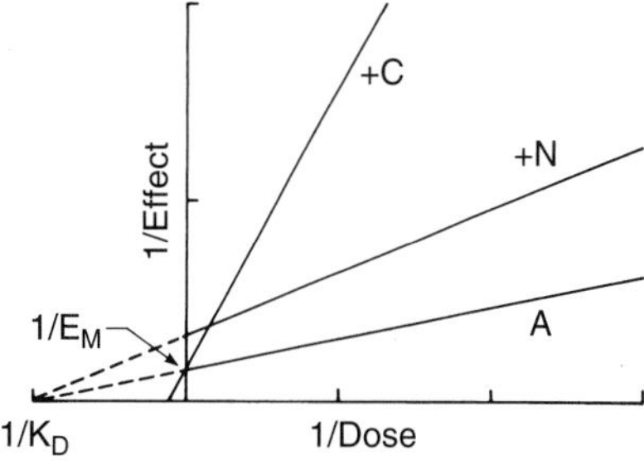

Fig. 1-9 Modification of a pharmacologic effect by drug antagonism. *Left, Curve A* depicts the dose-effect relationship of a full agonist; *Curves* C and *N* represent the influences of a competitive and noncompetitive antagonist, respectively. Note the shift to the right of the agonist dose-response curve by the competitive inhibitor and its downward displacement by the noncompetitive variety. *Right,* A double-reciprocal plot of the same curves; the competitive antagonist increases the apparent dissociation constant *(K_D)* without influencing the maximum effect obtainable by the agonist *(E_M)*. The noncompetitive inhibitor selectively decreases E_M.

activity. In none of these cases can the agonist successfully "compete" against the block, and the result is a downward displacement of the agonist log dose–response curve. Figure 1-9 reviews the dissimilarities between the two major types of drug blockade as represented in occupation theory.

Limitations of occupation theory

The occupation theory provides a good conceptual framework to understand receptor-mediated drug effects. However, it must be recognized that basic to the foregoing discussion are several assumptions about the interactions between a drug and its receptor:

1. One drug molecule reversibly combines with a single receptor.
2. This binding is independent of other drug-receptor interactions.
3. The receptors are identical and equally accessible to the drug.
4. Only a small portion of the total drug is involved in forming complexes with the receptor.
5. The biologic response is proportional to the degree of receptor occupancy and independent of time.

Research findings over the last four decades have made obvious the fact that all these assumptions are usually not valid regarding individual dose-response relationships. It has already been mentioned that equal access of receptors to drugs is unlikely in vivo. Moreover, as illustrated for the nicotinic receptor in Figure 1-2, some receptors require the binding of more than one drug molecule to become active. Systematic exploration of these assumptions has led to a fuller understanding of the complexities involved in dose-response relationships and improved models of drug action.

Stimulus-Response Coupling

One representative failure of classic occupation theory is its inability to account for the inhibition of ACh by atropine. Atropine is typically classified as a competitive antagonist of ACh. It binds to the ACh receptor and causes an inhibition that can be surmounted by increasing the concentration of agonist present. Surprisingly, the association of atropine with its receptor in some tissues is practically irreversible; neither ACh nor extensive washing will remove the drug once it is bound. Thus atropine would be expected to behave as a noncompetitive antagonist of ACh. To explain the paradox presented by atropine, pharmacologists borrowed from the phenomenon of enzyme excess described earlier in this chapter to postulate the existence of *spare receptors.*[29] This amendment to the occupation theory states that for many agonists there are more receptors available than are required to yield a maximal response. Although atropine completely blocks a number of receptors from binding ACh, a sufficient quantity remains to produce a ceiling effect, albeit at a higher agonist concentration. As one might predict, the competitive inhibition obtained with a conventional dose of an antagonist such as atropine gradually takes on the characteristics of a noncompetitive block as larger doses of the antagonist deplete the spare receptor pool.[22]

Another observation that cannot be reconciled with classic occupation theory is the finding that various ligands for the same receptor can behave as full agonists in one tissue but not in another expressing the same receptor. For example, the α-adrenergic agonists norepinephrine and oxymetazoline display essentially identical potencies and ceiling effects in contracting the anococcygeus muscle in the rat. In the vas deferens, however, norepinephrine remains a full agonist, albeit with less potency, whereas oxymetazoline loses in both potency and ceiling effect to become a weak partial agonist.[14]

These two examples give only a taste of the complexities that can arise from the gulf that often separates the binding of a drug by its receptor and the resultant development of a biologic effect. Even if the assumptions basic to the occupation theory hold for the initial action of a drug, they often do not apply to an observed effect that is removed from drug binding by several intermediate events and where the magnitude of drug effect holds a complex relationship to the degree of receptor occupancy. One useful approach to resolving these findings with classic occupation theory is to consider the binding of a drug to its receptor as an initial stimulus, which is then translated by the affected tissue into a response, as illustrated by the following equation[13]:

$$\text{Response} = f\left[\frac{\varepsilon \times R_t \times [D]}{K_D + [D]}\right]$$

Here, the "effect" of classic occupation theory (see the Equation on p. 10) becomes the stimulus (in brackets), with the intrinsic activity replaced by the product of the intrinsic efficacy (ε) and the total number of receptors available for binding the drug (R_t). The function *f* couples the stimulus to the response. Intrinsic efficacy refers to the number of receptors that must be activated to yield a maximal response. A drug with high efficacy needs to stimulate only a small percentage of receptors, whereas a drug with lesser efficacy (but still considered to be a full agonist) must activate a larger proportion. In the case of a partial agonist, insufficient receptors exist even when fully occupied to yield a maximal response.

Because full agonists can differ in efficacy and in receptor affinity, potency differences between drugs such as A and B in Figure 1-8 cannot simply be ascribed to unequal affinities for the receptor. Indeed, curves similar to Figure 1-8 can be generated by drugs that differ from each other solely in intrinsic efficacy, and affinity constants calculated according to classic occupation theory would be grossly in error.

Figure 1-10 depicts the influence of stimulus-response coupling on three drugs that have identical dissociation constants (K_D) for the same receptor but differ significantly in

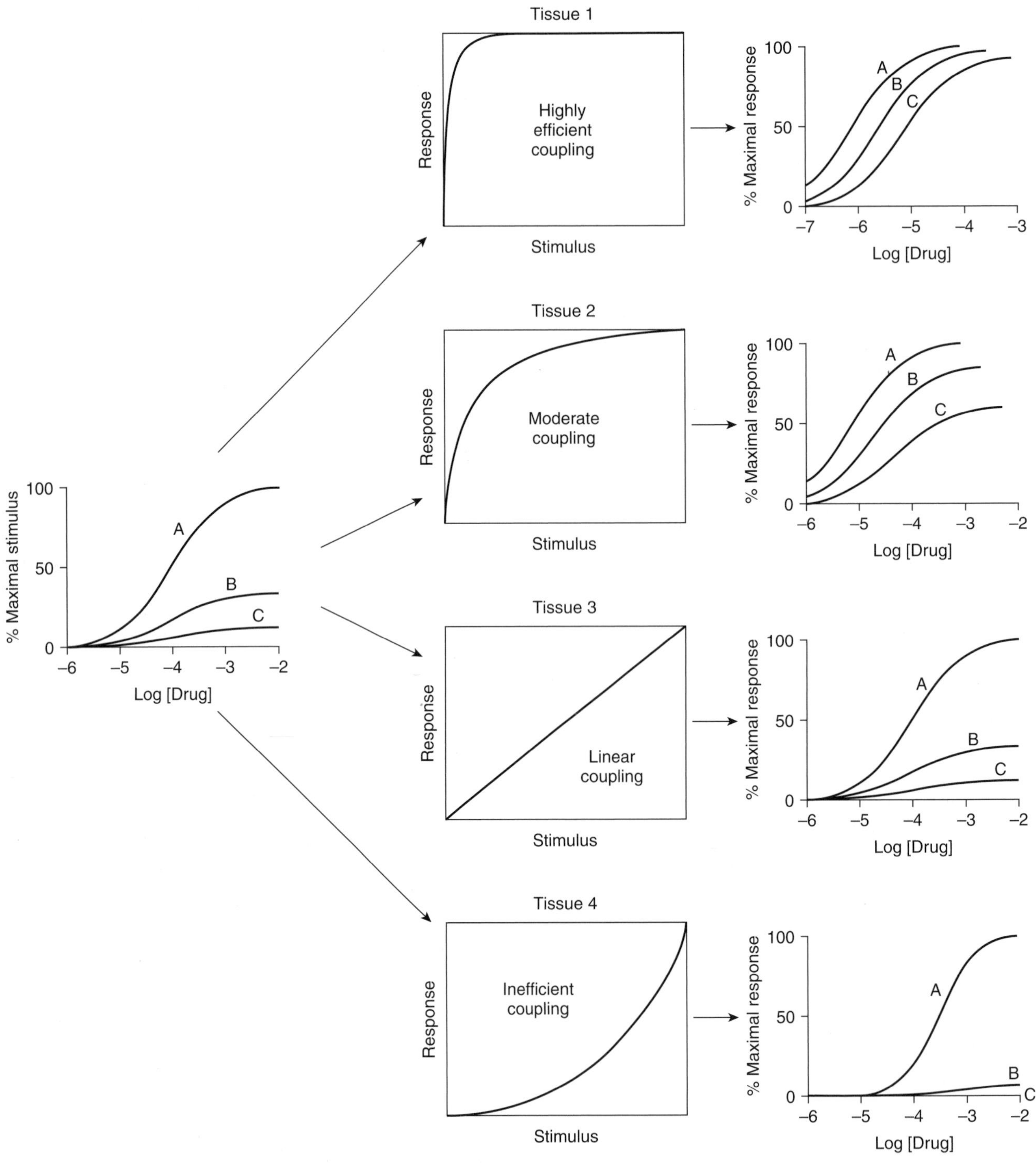

Fig. 1-10 Stimulus-response coupling. *Left,* The dose-stimulus curves (representing the initial effect of receptor binding) for three drugs with identical receptor affinity but differing sequentially in relative efficacy by a factor of 3 ($A > B > C$). *Middle,* The tissue-dependent coupling between the initial stimulus and the evoked response in four different tissues. *Right,* The dose-response curves for the three drugs in each tissue. Note the different abscissa for *Tissue 1*, reflecting the increased potency of drugs in a highly coupled stimulus-response system. (Adapted from Ross EM, Kenakin TP: Pharmacodynamics: mechanisms of drug action and the relationship between drug concentration and effect. In Hardman JG, Limbird LE, Gilman AG, eds: *Goodman & Gilman's The pharmacological basis of therapeutics,* ed 10, 2001, McGraw-Hill.)

intrinsic efficacy. In a highly coupled system (Tissue 1), all three drugs behave essentially as full agonists. However, in systems with less efficient coupling (Tissues 2 and 3), drugs B and C are revealed as partial agonists. Finally, in a system with inefficient coupling (Tissue 4), drug A remains a full agonist, drug B is a weak partial agonist, and drug C exhibits no agonistic effect at all but instead serves as a purely competitive antagonist. The selective estrogen receptor modulator tamoxifen illustrates how differences in tissue response elements can greatly alter drug activity. Tamoxifen behaves as a full estrogen receptor agonist in some tissues (e.g., mouse uterus), a partial agonist in others (e.g., rat uterus), and competitive antagonist in still others (e.g., mouse and rat pituitary gland). Figure 1-10 helps explain these diverse responses to tamoxifen.[19] Clinically, selective estrogen receptor modulators are used both to block estrogen receptors in breast tumors and to stimulate estrogen receptors in managing osteoporosis.

Competitive antagonists always act in stimulus-response systems by decreasing the apparent affinity of an agonist for its receptor without altering the maximal effect that the agonist can generate. However, noncompetitive antagonists can present different patterns of action based on the coupling function. Figure 1-11 displays the influence of increasing concentrations of a noncompetitive antagonist in a highly coupled stimulus-response system. As previously described for atropine, low concentration of the antagonist cause a rightward shift of the agonist's dose-response curve, whereas higher concentrations also depress the maximal effect. For noncompetitive antagonists that essentially remove receptors from the system (i.e., reduce R_t in the Equation on p. 11) by irreversibly associating with the ligand binding site, a complete loss of drug effect can be obtained by giving enough antagonist. However, for noncompetitive antagonists that reduce intrinsic efficacy (i.e., reduce ε in the Equation on p. 11) to some value other than zero through an allosteric mechanism, some agonist activity may be retained in highly coupled systems despite massive doses of the antagonist.

Receptor Diversity

In addition to the fact that pharmacologic responses are usually not linearly related to receptor occupancy, situations exist in which the receptors for a drug are not identical to one another. For example, a repeating theme in the elucidation of the autonomic nervous system has been the division of receptor classes into an increasing array of subtypes with differing drug sensitivities. Part of the explanation for the unusual pharmacology of tamoxifen was made clear by the discovery that there were two subtypes of estrogen receptors in various tissues that responded differently to the agent.[19] Individuals may harbor differences in receptor structure based on single point mutations. An important example is the β_2-adrenergic receptor, for which a number of single nucleotide polymorphisms have been identified that may alter drug responsiveness in diseases such as bronchial asthma.[33] As more refined techniques are developed to study drug-receptor interactions, it is possible that subtle differences in configuration and/or membrane location will be found to negate generally the assumption that all receptors are identical and equally accessible to a drug.

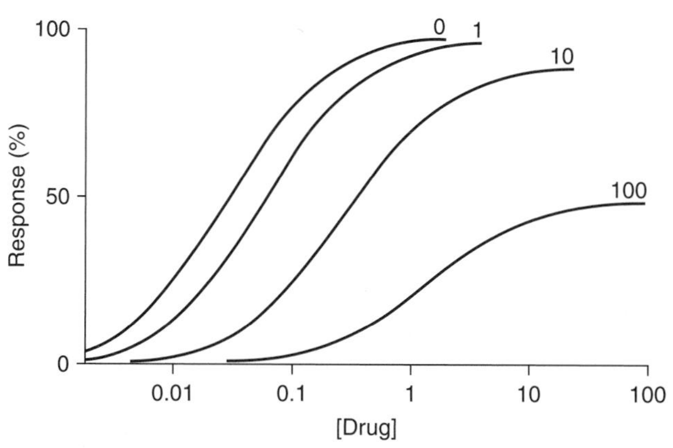

Fig. 1-11 Noncompetitive antagonism in a highly coupled stimulus-response system. The relative concentration of the noncompetitive antagonist for each agonist dose-response curve is shown at *right*. Low concentrations of antagonist (*1* and *10*) cause a rightward shift in the agonist dose-response curve with little or no effect on the agonist-induced maximal response. Higher concentrations (*100*), however, increasingly depress the maximal agonist response.

Receptors with Multiple Ligand-Binding Sites

The aforementioned isolation of the nicotinic receptor for ACh provides an important exception to the assumption of the occupation theory that a single drug molecule binds to a single receptor. To activate the nicotinic receptor, two ACh molecules must be bound at the same time, although at different sites on the molecule.[12,26] Evidence suggests that positive cooperativity occurs (the binding of one ACh molecule improves the binding of the second). The requirement for more than one agonist to bind the receptor before a response can occur is not uncommon; other ligand-gated ion channels commonly share this characteristic, as does the insulin receptor[35] and various receptors that must dimerize to become active (e.g., estrogen receptors[21]).

Pharmacodynamic Tolerance

The preceding discussion of dose-response relationships was predicated on the often erroneous assumption that the intensity of drug effect is not influenced by the passage of time. Pharmacodynamic tolerance is a general term for situations in which drug effects dissipate with time despite the continued presence of the agonist at a fixed concentration. At the receptor level, various processes in addition to the primary drug effect are often invoked that subsequently limit pharmacologic responses. In the case of the β-adrenergic receptor (Figure 1-12), phosphorylation of specific amino acid constituents leads to a loss of drug action, a process termed *desensitization*. The effect is temporary; removal of the agonist for a certain interval reestablishes tissue responsiveness to receptor activation. A longer-lasting loss of drug effect may occur in response to *downregulation*. In this process, membrane-bound receptors are internalized by the cell, where they may be sequestered for later use or destroyed by lysosomal enzymes. Pharmacodynamic tolerance may also occur independently of any change in the drug receptor or stimulus-response system. As an illustration of this point, consider a drug that increases blood pressure by causing vasoconstriction in selected vascular beds. In response to the hypertensive effect of the drug, various cardiovascular reflexes are evoked that tend to lower blood pressure, including activation of the parasympathetic nervous system, which leads to bradycardia. The buildup of lactate and other metabolites in the affected tissues also limits vasoconstriction. Eventually, additional changes, such as decreased salt and water retention, may further reduce drug responses. These and other mechanisms of drug tolerance are described more fully in Chapter 3.

ALLOSTERIC MODEL OF DRUG ACTION

Most early attempts to model drug action assumed the receptor was in a quiescent state until activated by an agonist. However, as has been shown for ion channels and increasingly for other receptor families, receptors in general may exist

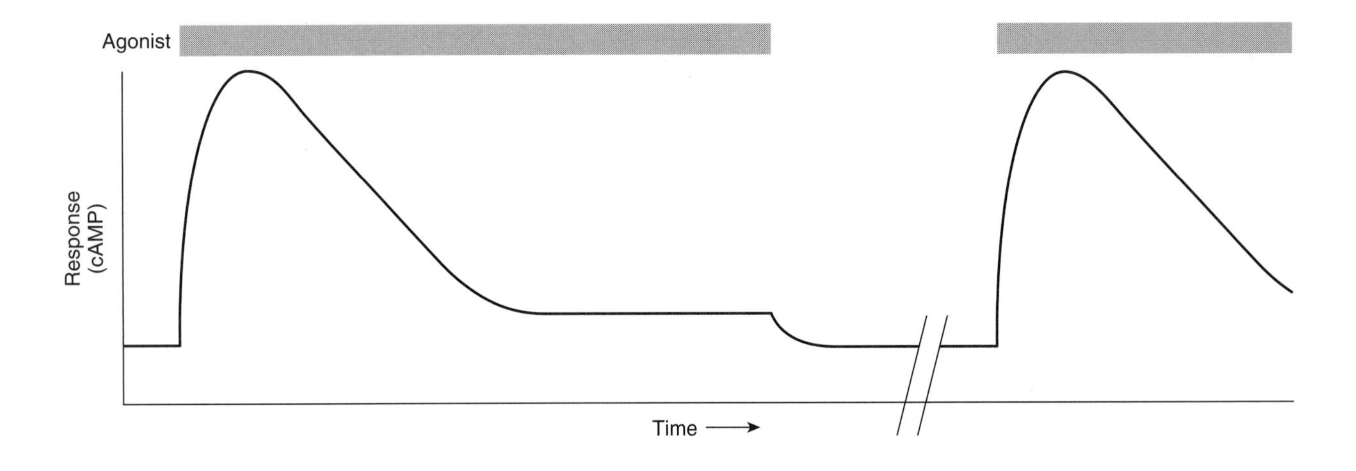

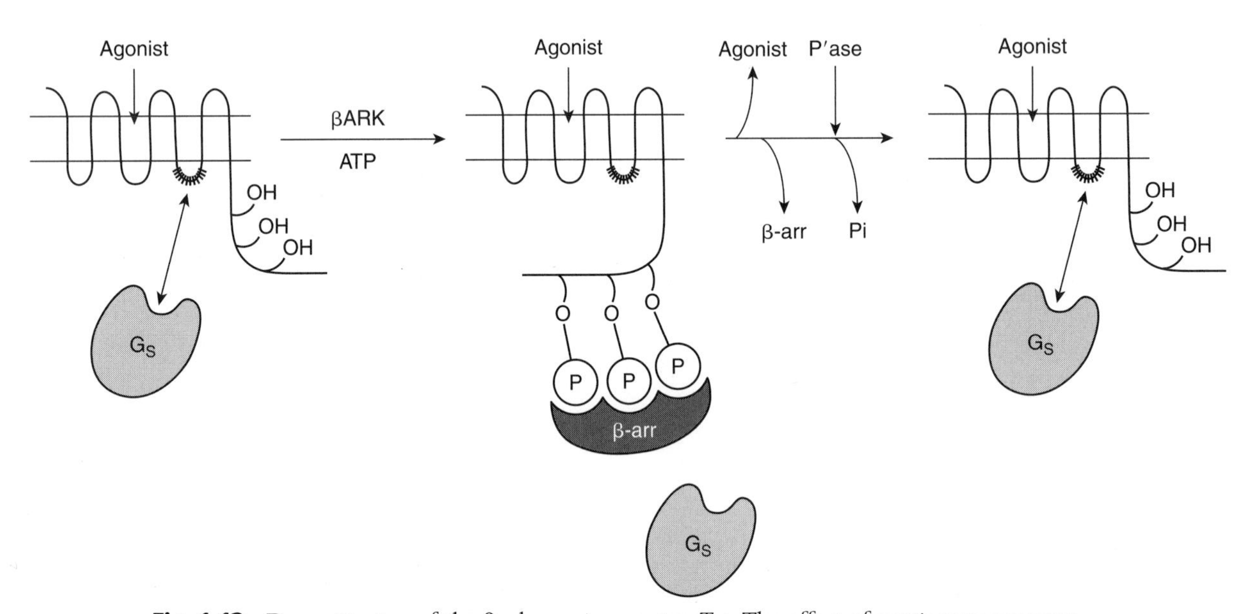

Fig. 1-12 Desensitization of the β-adrenergic receptor. *Top,* The effect of continuous exposure of the receptor to a fixed concentration of agonist *(shaded bar at left)* on the synthesis of cAMP, followed by the removal of agonist *(no bar)* and, after a delay, reintroduction of the agonist *(shaded bar at right)*. Desensitization is reflected in the decreased production of cAMP despite continuous receptor binding. Tissue responsiveness is restored after removal of agonist. *Bottom,* The events involved in desensitization. Initially, agonist binding activates G_s and subsequent cAMP production. However, agonist binding also stimulates phosphorylation *(P)* of the receptor by β-adrenergic receptor kinase *(βARK)*. The subsequent binding of the protein β-arrestin *(β-arr)* prevents receptor interaction with G_s. Removal of the agonist allows dissociation of β-arr, removal of phosphate *(Pi)* by phosphatase activity *(P′ase)*, and restoration of the receptor's normal responsiveness to the agonist. (From Bourne HR, von Zastrow M: Drug receptors & pharmacodynamics. In Katzung BG: *Basic & clinical pharmacology,* ed 8, New York, 2001, McGraw-Hill.)

individually in more than one configuration, with or without the presence of an agonist. According to the allosteric model of drug action, these forms of receptors are in equilibrium, and drugs act by altering their relative distributions.[17] Figure 1-13 illustrates a simple two-state version in which the receptor can exist in an active or inactive configuration. In this model, both full and partial agonists increase the proportion of receptors that exist in the active state. The model does not distinguish between agonists whose binding tends to force a conformational change in the receptor to the active form and agonists that bind preferentially with active receptors, stabilizing their configuration and altering their number through the law of mass action. Drugs with high efficacy would produce the highest ratios of active to inactive species; partial agonist binding would result in the presence of insufficient active form to yield a maximal response (Figure 1-14). Competitive antagonists would associate with receptors irrespective of—and without influencing—their conformational state. Noncompetitive antagonists would limit the ability of agonist binding to elevate the proportion of receptors in the active state (either by decreasing agonist efficacy or by reducing the total number of available receptors).

The major attractions of the allosteric model are that it gives a physical solution for differences in efficacy between

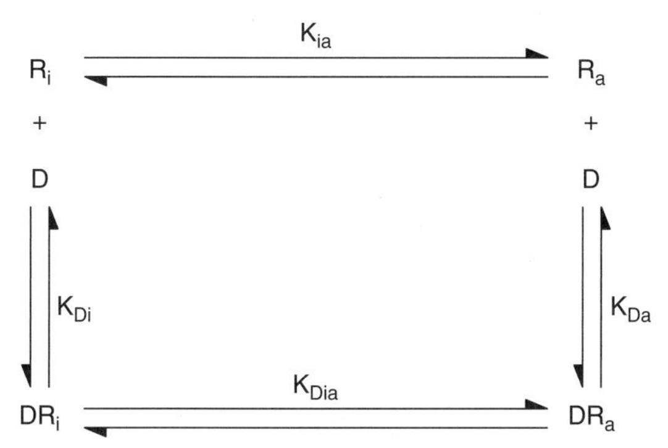

Fig. 1-13 Two-state model of drug-receptor interaction. The receptor can exist in an active *(R_a)* or inactive *(R_i)* state, as governed by the equilibrium constant K_{ia}. Unless the receptor mediates a tonically active process, K_{ia} greatly favors the inactive form. Drugs *(D)* may bind to R_a, R_i, or both. Agonist binding alters the proportion of active ($R_a + DR_a$) to inactive ($R_i + DR_i$) receptors.

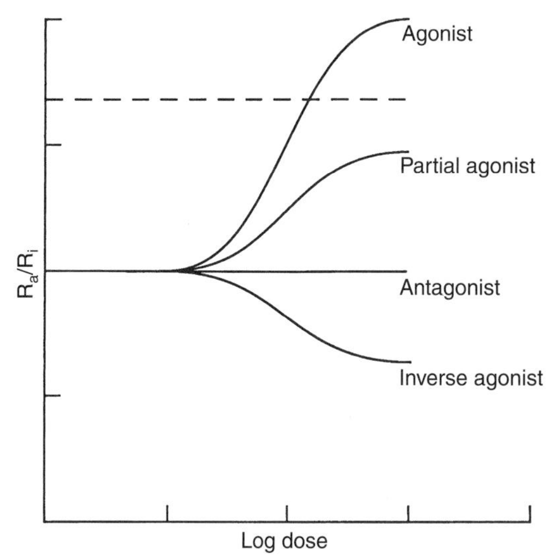

Fig. 1-14 Dose-effect relationships according to the two-state model. In this example, a tonically active process is depicted. Full agonists can increase the ratio of active to inactive receptors *(R_a/R_i)* above that which causes the ceiling effect *(dotted line)*; partial agonists also increase the ratio, but to a lesser maximal degree. Antagonists bind without disturbing the existing R_a/R_i ratio, and inverse agonists exert an opposite effect by lowering the R_a/R_i ratio and inhibiting a normally active pathway. In this example, all the drugs are assumed to have the same receptor affinity.

congeners and that it affords a simple mechanism for the pharmacologic response elicited by drug binding. It also provides an excellent explanation for drugs known as *inverse agonists.* An inverse agonist causes an effect opposite to that of the agonist, in contrast to a competitive antagonist that simply blocks the agonist (or the inverse agonist for that matter) but has no inherent effect of its own. In a tonically active pathway, a drug that preferentially binds to the inactive configuration would behave as an inverse agonist. Such agents (e.g., β-carboline) have been described for the benzodiazepine receptor. In contrast to sedative benzodiazepines such as diazepam, these experimental drugs cause anxiety and CNS arousal. Flumazenil, a competitive antagonist of the benzodiazepine receptor, reverses the effects of both agonists and inverse agonists.[11] A final advantage of the allosteric model is that it can accommodate desensitization and time-dependent actions of drugs such as nicotine. Nicotine exhibits a complex pharmacologic profile. Initially, this natural alkaloid acts like an agonist: it stimulates ACh receptors at autonomic ganglia and in skeletal muscle. The stimulation is temporary, however, and in a matter of minutes the action of nicotine transforms from that of excitation to one of antagonism. This metamorphosis can be adequately explained if one assumes that a third, or "desensitized," configuration of the receptor exists to which active receptors are slowly converted and from which they even more slowly recover. Nicotine, by increasing the proportion of active receptors, causes both an initial stimulation and a subsequent prolonged loss of activity as receptors are progressively trapped in the desensitized state.

RECEPTOR-INDEPENDENT DRUG ACTIONS

No description of drug action would be complete without a consideration of those agents that exert pharmacologic effects through receptor-independent mechanisms. Aside from the fact that these drugs act without the benefit of receptor intermediaries, there are no common traits serving to link this miscellaneous array of compounds. It has also proved impossible to derive a quantitative description of drug responses akin to that presented for receptor-based agents. The very diversity of these drugs precludes any unifying relationship between dose and effect. Nevertheless, concentration-effect curves similar to those previously discussed are often obtained with these drugs, and general concepts such as potency and efficacy still apply. For the sake of discussion, these drugs are grouped arbitrarily into three categories: chemically reactive agents, physically active agents, and counterfeit biochemical constituents.

Chemically Reactive Agents

Chemically reactive drugs include a wide variety of compounds, some of which interact with small molecules or ions, whereas others attack proteins and other macromolecules. Gastric antacids and metallic ion chelators are two kinds of drugs that combine with inorganic substances within the body. Of particular importance to dentistry is dimercaprol, a chelating agent capable of forming coordination complexes with mercury and other heavy metals. Drugs affecting macromolecules include most germicides and the antineoplastic alkylating agents. Sodium hypochlorite solutions provide antisepsis and facilitate canal debridement during endodontic therapy because they release hypochlorous acid, a potent chemical disrupter of biologic matter. In general, these compounds can be readily distinguished from drugs that are receptor mediated. With the exception of certain chelating agents, they lack specificity and may individually react with a variety of substances, organic or otherwise. Minor structural modifications also do not usually influence drug activity. Finally, the reactions of these drugs rely heavily on covalent bonding or on strong ionic attachments; they do not usually depend on hydrophobic or weak electrostatic interactions.

Physically Active Agents

Physically active agents, in contrast, are often useful therapeutically because they are chemically inert and can safely be used for their colligative properties. Thus magnesium sulfate is an effective cathartic because it is not absorbed from the gastrointestinal tract and exerts an osmotic effect, causing retention of large amounts of water within the intestinal lumen. The colon becomes distended and is stimulated to undergo expulsive contraction. Through a similar osmotic mechanism, mannitol helps reverse cerebral edema in the patient with traumatic brain injury. A totally unrelated physical mechanism is evoked by hydrogen peroxide. Although highly reactive, hydrogen peroxide finds use in wound debridement because of its effervescent action. The release of gas bubbles promotes the physical removal of debris from injured tissues.

The physically active agents, in general, exhibit a surprising lack of structural specificity. For many agents, the major requirements for activity appear to be a certain pharmacologic inertness coupled with the ability to be administered in high concentrations (compared with most other drugs) without causing undue toxicity.

Counterfeit Biochemical Constituents

The counterfeit biochemical constituents resemble antimetabolite drugs inasmuch as they are artificial analogues of natural substrates. Hence, they have to meet the same rigid structural requirements as do their receptor-based counterparts. Counterfeit agents, however, do not affect enzymes; they are instead incorporated into specific macromolecules by the cell. The resulting drug effects arise from an altered biologic activity of the affected macromolecules or from their increased susceptibility to destruction. The thymine analogue 5-bromouracil is representative of this group.[5] The effect of 5-bromouracil incorporation into the genetic material of a cell is an elevation in the mutation rate and an increased frequency of chromosomal disturbances. Agents of this type are used therapeutically in the treatment of several neoplasias and microbial infections.

Cited References

1. Albert A: Relations between molecular structure and biological activity: stages in the evolution of current concepts, *Annu Rev Pharmacol Toxicol* 11:13-36, 1971.
2. Ariëns EJ, Simonis AM, van Rossum JM: Drug-receptor interactions: interaction of one or more drugs with one receptor system. In Ariëns EJ, ed: *Molecular pharmacology: mode of action of biologically active compounds,* New York, 1964, Academic Press.
3. Asano T, Pedersen SE, Scott CW, et al: Reconstitution of catecholamine-stimulated binding of guanosine 5′-O-(3-thiotriphosphate) to the stimulatory GTP-binding protein of adenylate cyclase, *Biochemistry* 23:5460-5467, 1984.
4. Berridge MJ: Inositol triphosphate and diacylglycerol: two interacting second messengers, *Annu Rev Biochem* 56:159-193, 1987.
5. Brockman RW, Anderson EP: Pyrimidine analogues. In Hochster RM, Quastel JH, eds: *Metabolic inhibitors, a comprehensive treatise,* vol 1, New York, 1963, Academic Press.
6. Clark AJ: *The mode of action of drugs on cells,* London, 1933, E Arnold & Co.
7. Deuel TF: Polypeptide growth factors: roles in normal and abnormal cell growth, *Annu Rev Cell Biol* 3:443-492, 1987.
8. Dougherty DA: Cation-π interactions in chemistry and biology: a new view of benzene, Phe, Tyr, and Trp, *Science* 271:163-168, 1996.
9. Gilman AG: G proteins: transducers of receptor-generated signals, *Annu Rev Biochem* 56:615-649, 1987.
10. Goldstein A: Opioid peptide endorphins in pituitary and brain, *Science* 193:1081-1086, 1976.
11. Haefely WE: The benzodiazepine receptor and its clinically useful ligands, *Clin Neuropharmacol* 9(suppl 4):398-400, 1986.
12. Karlin A, Cox RN, Dipaola M, et al: Functional domains of the nicotinic acetylcholine receptor, *Ann NY Acad Sci* 463:53-69, 1986.
13. Kenakin T: Efficacy: molecular mechanisms and operational methods of measurement. In Kenakin T, Angus JA, eds: *The pharmacology of functional, biochemical, and recombinant receptor systems. Handbook of experimental pharmacology,* vol 148, Berlin, 2000, Springer-Verlag.
14. Kenakin TP: The relative contribution of affinity and efficacy to agonist activity: organ selectivity of noradrenaline and oxymetazoline with reference to the classification of drug receptors, *Br J Pharmacol* 81:131-143, 1984.
15. Laduron PM, Ilien B: Solubilization of brain muscarinic, dopaminergic and serotonergic receptors: a critical analysis, *Biochem Pharmacol* 31:2145-2151, 1982.
16. Lefkowitz RJ, Caron MG: Molecular and regulatory properties of adrenergic receptors, *Recent Prog Horm Res* 43:469-497, 1987.
17. Mackay D: A critical survey of receptor theories of drug action. In van Rossum JM, ed: *Kinetics of drug action. Handbook of experimental pharmacology,* vol 47, Berlin, 1977, Springer-Verlag.
18. Maren TH: The relation between enzyme inhibition and physiological response in the carbonic anhydrase system, *J Pharmacol Exp Ther* 139:140-153, 1963.
19. McDonnell DP, Wijayaratne A, Chang CY, et al: Elucidation of the molecular mechanism of action of selective estrogen receptor modulators, *Am J Cardiol* 90:35F-43F, 2002.
20. Miller JW, Lewis JE: Drugs affecting smooth muscle, *Annu Rev Pharmacol* 9:147-172, 1969.
21. Mulvihill ER, Palmiter RD: Relationship of nuclear estrogen receptor levels to induction of ovalbumin and conalbumin mRNA in chick oviduct, *J Biol Chem* 252:2060-2068, 1977.
22. Nickerson M: Receptor occupancy and tissue response, *Nature* 178:697-698, 1956.
23. O'Malley BW, Schwartz RJ, Schrader WT: A review of regulation of gene expression by steroid hormone receptors, *J Steroid Biochem* 7:1151-1159, 1976.
24. Ostrowski J, Kjelsberg MA, Caron MG, et al: Mutagenesis of the β_2-adrenergic receptor: how structure elucidates function, *Annu Rev Pharmacol Toxicol* 32:167-183, 1992.
25. Paton WDM, Rang HP: The uptake of atropine and related drugs by intestinal smooth muscle of the guinea pig in relation to acetylcholine receptors, *Proc R Soc Lond* [Biol] 163:1-44, 1965.
26. Popot J-L, Changeux J-P: Nicotinic receptor of acetylcholine: structure of an oligomeric integral membrane protein, *Physiol Rev* 64:1162-1239, 1984.
27. Ross EM: Signal sorting and amplification through G protein-coupled receptors, *Neuron* 3:141-152, 1989.
28. Ruffolo RR, Jr, Nichols AJ, Stadel JM, et al: Structure and function of α-adrenoceptors, *Pharmacol Rev* 43:475-505, 1991.
29. Stephenson RP: A modification of receptor theory, *Br J Pharmacol Chemother* 11:379-393, 1956.
30. Stewart RA, Carrico CK, Webster RL, et al: Physicochemical stereospecificity in taste perception of α-D-mannose and β-D-mannose, *Nature* 234:220, 1971.

31. Stryer L, Bourne HR: G proteins: a family of signal transducers, *Annu Rev Cell Biol* 2:391-419, 1986.

32. Surks MI, Oppenheimer JH: Concentration of L-thyroxine and L-triiodothyronine specifically bound to nuclear receptors in rat liver and kidney. Quantitative evidence favoring a major role of T3 in thyroid hormone action, *J Clin Invest* 60:555-562, 1977.

33. Taylor DR, Kennedy MA: Genetic variation of the β_2-adrenoceptor: its functional and clinical importance in bronchial asthma, *Am J Pharmacogenomics* 1:165-174, 2001.

34. Venter JC, Fraser CM, Soiefer AI, et al: Autoantibodies and monoclonal antibodies to β-adrenergic receptors: their use in receptor purification and characterization, *Adv Cyclic Nucleotide Res* 14:135-143, 1981.

35. Virkamäki A, Ueki K, Kahn CR: Protein-protein interaction in insulin signaling and the molecular mechanisms of insulin resistance, *J Clin Invest* 103:931-943, 1999.

36. Weinberg RA: The molecules of life, *Sci Am* 253:48-57, 1985.

General References

Bourne HR, von Zastrow M: Drug receptors & pharmacodynamics. In Katzung BG: *Basic & clinical pharmacology,* ed 8, New York, 2001, McGraw-Hill.

Derendorf H, Hochhaus G, eds: *Handbook of pharmacokinetic/pharmacodynamic correlation,* Boca Raton, FL, 1995, CRC Press.

Kenakin T, Angus JA, eds: *The pharmacology of functional, biochemical, and recombinant receptor systems. Handbook of experimental pharmacology,* vol 148, Berlin, 2000, Springer-Verlag.

Neubig RR: Membrane organization in G-protein mechanisms, *FASEB J* 8:939-946, 1994.

Pratt WB, Taylor P, eds: *Principles of drug action: the basis of pharmacology,* ed 3, New York, 1990, Churchill Livingstone.

Ross EM, Kenakin TP: Pharmacodynamics: mechanisms of drug action and the relationship between drug concentration and effect. In Hardman JG, Limbird LE, Gilman AG, eds: *Goodman & Gilman's The pharmacological basis of therapeutics,* ed 10, 2001, McGraw-Hill.

CHAPTER • 2

Pharmacokinetics: The Absorption, Distribution, and Fate of Drugs

John A. Yagiela

When the magnitude of a drug's pharmacologic effect is quantified as a function of dose, the tacit assumption is that the drug concentration vicinal to the site of action is linearly related to the amount administered. Although this assumption may strictly apply to an in vitro test, it ignores the temporal factors that modify drug effects in vivo. Drug concentrations are rarely static; they rise and fall as dictated by the processes of absorption, distribution, metabolism, and excretion. The following discussion examines these processes (Figure 2-1) and how they influence the passage of drugs in the body.

PASSAGE OF DRUGS ACROSS MEMBRANES

For a drug to be absorbed, reach its site of action, and eventually be eliminated, it must cross one or more biologic membrane barriers. These may consist of a single plasma membrane or constitute a layer of closely packed cells. Because such barriers to drugs behave similarly, the cell membrane can serve as a prototype for all. The plasma membrane is approximately 100 Å thick. It is composed of a bimolecular sheet of lipids (primarily cholesterol and phospholipids) and a variety of proteins. Although early models depicted the protein as covering essentially the entire membrane surface, subsequent observations suggest a more fluid model with proteins interspersed throughout and extending beyond the lipid phase of the membrane (Figure 2-2).[7,47] The presence of protein molecules spanning the entire thickness of the membrane provides a necessary link between the extracellular environment and the cell interior, which is consistent with the concept that drug activation of a membrane-bound receptor on the external surface of a cell can be directly translated into an intracellular response.

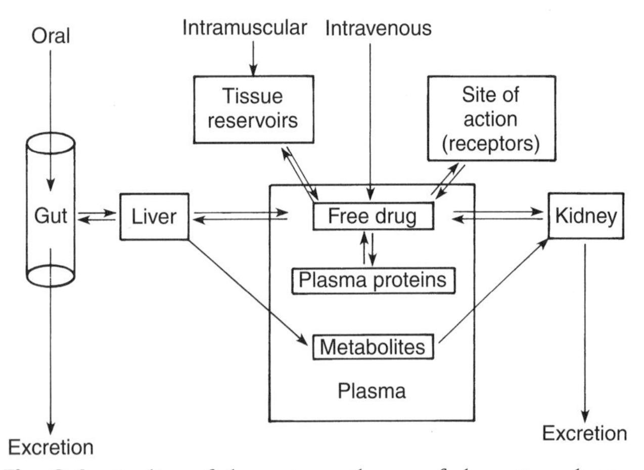

Fig. 2-1 Outline of the major pathways of absorption, distribution, metabolism, and excretion of drugs. Compounds taken orally must pass through the liver before reaching the systemic circulation. Once in the bloodstream, agents are distributed throughout the body and come in contact with their respective sites of action. Drugs are filtered by the kidney, only to be reabsorbed if lipid soluble. Metabolism of many drugs occurs primarily in the liver, after which the metabolites are excreted in bile or urine. Some agents eliminated in the bile are subject to reabsorption and may participate in an enterohepatic cycle.

Passive Diffusion

The passage of drugs across membranes can involve several different mechanisms. Of these, passive diffusion is the most commonly encountered. Studies by Overton and Meyer at the turn of this century demonstrated that the cell membrane acts for the most part as a lipoid barrier. As shown by Collander (Figure 2-3),[8] the rate of transfer of nonelectrolytes across a membrane is directly proportional to the lipid/water partition coefficient. (The partition coefficient is a measure of the relative solubility of an agent in a fat solvent versus its solubility in water.) A drug with a high partition coefficient readily enters the lipid phase of the membrane and passes down its concentration gradient to the aqueous phase on the other side. More molecules are then free to enter the membrane and continue the transfer process. With poorly lipid-soluble compounds, however, few molecules enter the membrane per unit of time, and the rate of passage is depressed.

The absence of an ionic charge is one major factor favoring lipid solubility. Drugs with a fixed charge, such as those containing a quaternary nitrogen atom, permeate membranes slowly if at all. The reason for the relative solubility of nonionized molecules in lipids relates to their exclusion from polar media. Simple ions and charged molecules are stabilized in water by the hydration shells that surround them, a consequence of the tendency of charged species to orient polar molecules. This process excludes nonpolar substances, and the resulting segregation causes them to coalesce in a manner analogous to the formation of oil droplets on the surface of water. The term *hydrophobic bonding,* introduced in Chapter 1, refers to the tendency for water-insoluble molecules to be drawn together; this behavior is responsible for the preferential tendency of lipid-soluble drugs to penetrate cell membranes by way of the lipid components. Ionized compounds, on the other hand, are so stabilized by their interaction with water that movement into a lipid phase is markedly restricted.

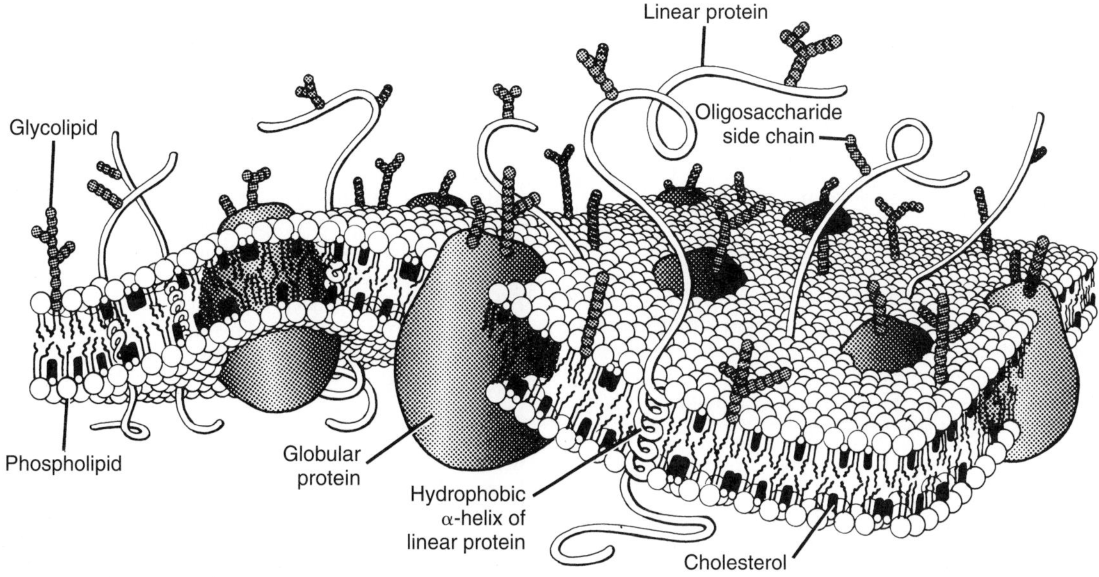

Fig. 2-2 The plasma membrane depicting the lipid bilayer, composed of phospholipids and cholesterol, and the globular and linear proteins, which are anchored within the membrane by α-helical segments and extend beyond the 40-Å thick bilayer on both the extracellular and cytoplasmic surfaces. For clarity, the ratio of lipid to protein is much larger than exists in natural membranes. Glycolipid components of the membrane and saccharide polymers attached to proteins are also shown. (Redrawn from Bretscher MS: The molecules of the cell membrane, *Sci Am* 253:100-108, 1985.)

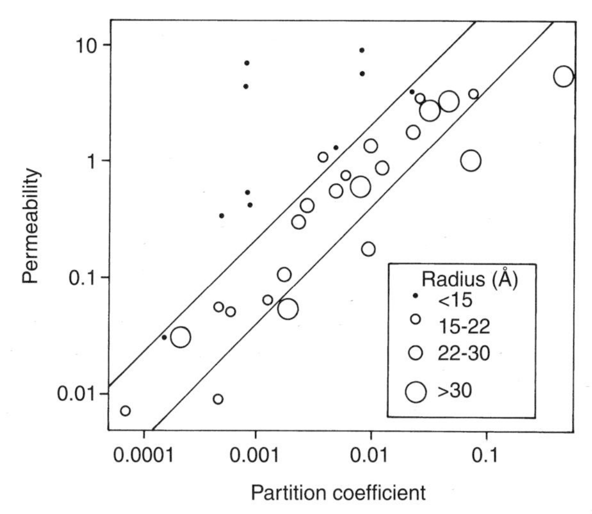

Fig. 2-3 Relationship between membrane permeability and lipid (olive oil)/water partition coefficient in *Chara certatophylla*. Each *circle* represents a single nonelectrolyte with a molecular radius as indicated in the key. Small compounds permeate more readily than their partition coefficient would indicate; the reverse is true for large molecules. (Adapted from Collander R: The permeability of plant protoplasts to small molecules, *Physiol Plantarum* 2:300-311, 1949.)

Many therapeutic agents are weak electrolytes; depending on the pH of their aqueous environment, they can exist in both ionized and neutral forms. Because charged molecules penetrate membranes with considerable difficulty, the rate of movement of these drugs is governed by the partition coefficient of the neutral species as well as the degree of ionization. As illustrated in Figure 2-4, acidic conditions favor the transport of weak acids, and the opposite holds true for basic compounds.

The same concept of water interaction used to explain the aqueous solubility of ions also applies to many nonionic molecules. Although unsubstituted aliphatic and aromatic hydrocarbons have little or no tendency to react with water, affinity for water molecules is not restricted to structures with a formal charge. Organic residues possessing electronegative atoms such as oxygen, nitrogen, and sulfur can interact with water through the formation of hydrogen bonds to provide some degree of aqueous solubility.

Examination of Figure 2-3 reveals that lipid solubility is not the only factor influencing the passive diffusion of uncharged drugs across cell membranes; molecular size is also important. Water, glycerol, and some other small molecules permeate much more readily than would be predicted from their respective partition coefficients. This finding led to the postulation of channels that extend through the plasma membrane and allow these compounds to enter the cell interior without having to cross a lipoid barrier. Aquaporin 1, discovered in 1991, was the first such channel to be identified.[2] Aquaporin 1 is a 28,000-dalton polypeptide that forms a 3-Å channel through which water can enter or leave cells. More than 10 aquaporins have been discovered in mammalian tissues and are especially prominent in cells and organs involved with the transcellular movement of water: kidneys, capillaries, secretory glands, red blood cells, choroid plexus, brain glia, eyes, and lungs.[2,25] Some aquaporins are selective for water only, increasing its membrane permeability by a factor of 10 to 100; others permit the passage of glycerol and several other molecules in addition to water.

Figure 2-3 also shows that some large organic molecules diffuse more slowly than expected. Nonelectrolytes containing a number of hydrophobic groups are often so insoluble in water that their transit across the lipid/water interface may be retarded despite a favorable partition coefficient.[27] This finding suggests that some degree of water solubility is necessary for the passive diffusion of drugs across membranes. No matter how lipid soluble an agent is, it will never cross a

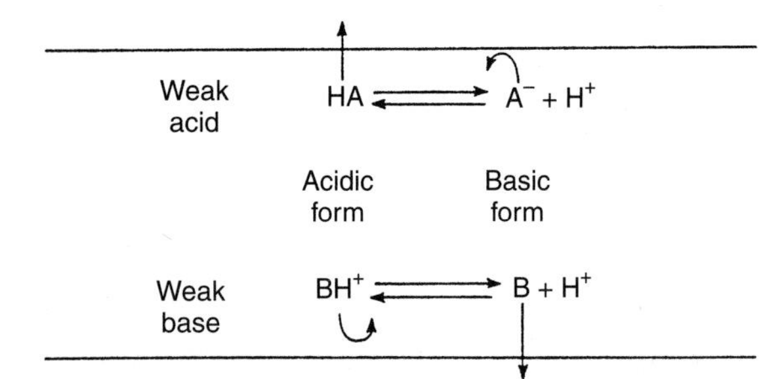

Fig. 2-4 Membrane penetration by weak electrolytes. The nonionic species of drugs *(HA, B)* permeate membranes much more efficiently than do the charged forms *(A^-, BH^+)*. Acidic conditions shift the dissociation curves to the left, favoring the diffusion of weak acids. An increase in pH favors the loss of hydrogen *(H^+)* and the diffusion of weak bases.

membrane if it cannot first dissolve in the extracellular fluid and be carried to the structure. Thus benzocaine, an active local anesthetic when applied directly to nerves, is ineffective after injection because its water insolubility precludes significant diffusion away from the administration site and toward its locus of action within the neuronal membrane. Once inside the membrane, a drug with an extremely high partition coefficient may be so soluble in the lipid phase that it has little tendency, regardless of its water solubility, to diffuse outward down its concentration gradient.[37]

In various tissues, the movement of specific ions (e.g., Na^+ and K^+) across the cell membrane is facilitated by the presence of transmembrane channels, such as the nicotinic receptor described in Figure 1-2 and the Na^+ channel illustrated in Figures 16-3 and 16-4. The opening of these channels is often regulated by the electrical potential across the membrane or by the presence of specific ligands, such as neurotransmitters. When a channel is open, passive diffusion of an ion capable of traversing it depends on the electrical potential across the membrane as well as the ion's own chemical gradient. Boosting the electrochemical gradient by manipulating the voltage across the cell membrane is an effective method of increasing ionic flow. Even in the absence of specific ion channels, the transport of both fixed ions and weak electrolytes across tissue barriers can be facilitated by the appropriate use of electrical current (as in iontophoresis, discussed later in this chapter).

In summary, the passive diffusion of most drugs across lipoid barriers is largely a function of their lipid/water partition coefficients. A modicum of water solubility is required, though, for drugs to reach and cross membranes in concentrations sufficient to permit a reasonable rate of diffusion. Because ions do not generally penetrate membranes well, the passage of weak electrolytes is further governed by their degree of ionization.

Specialized Transport Processes

Several mechanisms besides passive diffusion are responsible for the movement of drugs across membranes. Many compounds too large and too hydrophilic for passive diffusion across membranes nevertheless migrate through without difficulty. These anomalies are especially prevalent in tissues specialized for the transport of chemicals and fluids (e.g., intestinal mucosa, capillary endothelium, choroid plexus, renal tubule). Drugs resembling important endogenous compounds (e.g., metabolites, neurotransmitters) are the most likely to receive special handling.

Carrier-mediated transport

A number of lipid-insoluble substances are shuttled across plasma membranes by forming complexes with specific membrane constituents called *carriers* or *transporters.* Carriers are like receptors in many ways; they are proteins, often quite selective in the agents with which they combine, and subject to competitive inhibition. Because the number of carriers is finite, carrier-mediated transport can be saturated at high drug concentrations. *Facilitated diffusion* is the term given to carrier-based transfer when the driving force is simply the concentration difference of the drug across the membrane. Frequently, however, carriers move substances against their electrochemical gradients. This *active transport,* in addition to exhibiting selectivity and saturability, requires the expenditure of energy and may be blocked by inhibitors of cellular metabolism. Active transport permits the efficient absorption of materials vital for cellular function and the selective elimination of waste products. The Na^+ pump, by maintaining a large Na^+ gradient across the membrane, indirectly serves as the energy source for the active transport of many drugs whose movement is coupled in some way to the influx of Na^+. Other transport systems use adenosine triphosphate directly as the energy source.

The organic anion transporting polypeptide family is responsible for the cellular uptake of acidic drugs into the liver, kidney, intestine, lung, and brain; elements of an analogous transport system for organic bases have also been identified.[24] Active transport of drugs out of cells often involves the P-glycoprotein family of proteins. P-glycoproteins are associated with the excretion of numerous amphipathic hydrophobic substances (e.g., erythromycin, ritonavir, and verapamil) into the bile and urine and with the removal of the agents from the central nervous system (CNS) and intestine. Drug resistance in some cancer cells has been linked to overexpression of P-glycoprotein.

Filtration

The endothelial lining of most capillaries behaves as though it were fenestrated by holes (i.e., gaps between the endothelial cells) up to 80 Å in diameter. Fluids move through these spaces by bulk flow according to the pressure differential across the membrane. Because materials are excluded from passage only on the basis of size, this type of drug transfer (often referred to as *paracellular transport*) is in fact a form of filtration. Filtration is involved in the distribution and elimination of almost all drugs and is often the only mechanism of membrane penetration available to lipid-insoluble compounds.

Endocytosis and exocytosis

The processes of endocytosis and exocytosis are, together, the most complex methods of drug transfer across a biologic membrane. The term *endocytosis* refers to a series of events in which a substance is engulfed and internalized by the cell. Because a small amount of extracellular fluid is also taken up, *pinocytosis* (literally "cell drinking") is an appropriate synonym. (*Phagocytosis,* or "cell eating," is a variant of endocytosis associated more with the removal of particulate matter by macrophages than with drug transport.)

Endocytosis begins with the binding of the compound to be absorbed by its receptor on the membrane surface. Two good examples are the attachment of low-density lipoprotein (LDL) and insulin to their respective receptors. With time, the bound agent-receptor complex is concentrated in an indentation of the membrane called a *coated pit.* (This migration also occurs spontaneously with the LDL receptor.) Clathrin, a cytoplasmic protein that attaches to the internal surface of the plasma membrane, serves to capture the receptors within the pit while excluding other surface proteins.[45] Internal rearrangement of its structure then deepens the pit, forming a coated bud. A second protein, termed *dynamin,* is believed to congregate around the collar of the invaginated bud and initiate separation from the membrane. Once released, the vesicle loses its clathrin coat and fuses with an organelle called the *endosome.* Some of the captured contents, such as LDL receptors, are recycled back to the plasma membrane by transport vesicles; the remainder undergo lysosomal processing and release into the cytoplasm.

The complementary process of *exocytosis* occurs when vesicles, such as those produced by the Golgi apparatus, fuse with the plasma membrane and discharge their contents outside the cell. Exocytosis is the primary method by which cellular products such as regulatory hormones are secreted by the cell. The term *transcytosis* is descriptive of a coupled form of endocytosis and exocytosis leading to the transfer of drug from one epithelial surface of a cell to the other. In this scenario the endosomal vesicle described above avoids lysosomal capture, is transported across the cell, and fuses with the plasma membrane to release its contents extracellularly.

Cells generally are capable of endocytosis; however, exocytosis and transcytosis are most intensive in tissues adapted for the absorption, distribution, and export of important foodstuffs, regulatory hormones, and secretory products. Endocytosis/transcytosis is probably responsible for the absorption of antigenic proteins and certain toxins from the small intestine and for the transfer of certain large molecules between tissue compartments. It plays a minor role in the transport of most drugs.

ABSORPTION

Absorption refers to the transfer of a drug from its site of administration into the bloodstream. Obviously, the particular route of administration selected greatly influences the rate and perhaps even the extent of drug absorption.

Oral Ingestion

Oral ingestion was the first and is still the most commonly used method for the administration of therapeutic agents. The major advantages of the oral route lie in three areas: convenience, economics, and safety. Patient acceptance of oral medication is good because the technique itself is painless and trained personnel are not required for its accomplishment. The convenience and low cost with respect to other modes of therapy are especially prominent for drugs that must be given several times daily on a long-term basis. The oral route is relatively safe because drug absorption is comparatively slow. Sudden high blood concentrations are not nearly as likely to be achieved by the ingestion of drugs as they are by parenteral injection. Allergic reactions are also less likely to occur, especially those of a serious nature. The oral route, however, does have some drawbacks. Because self-administration is the rule, patient compliance is required for optimal therapy. Drug absorption is likely to be delayed (on a clinical average of 30 to 60 minutes) and may be incomplete. Metabolic inactivation or complex formation may also occur before the drug has a chance to reach the systemic circulation. These limitations to the oral route translate into an increased variability in patient response. Finally, the spectrum of adverse reactions caused by oral medication can extend from one end of the gastrointestinal tract to the other.

Drugs taken orally may be absorbed along the entire alimentary canal, but the relative degree of contact with the mucosa determines the amount of uptake in each segment. Variables affecting absorption include the duration of exposure, the concentration of the drug, and the surface area available for absorption. Under normal circumstances, the oral and esophageal mucosa are exposed too briefly to a drug during the process of swallowing for any absorption to take place. The colon normally plays no role in the uptake of orally administered compounds because, with the exception of some sustained-release preparations, little absorbable drug usually reaches it. By exclusion, the bulk of drug absorption must take place in the stomach and small intestine.

Influence of pH

As previously discussed, absorption is favored when the drug ingested is lipid soluble. For weak electrolytes, the pH of the surrounding medium affects the degree of ionization and therefore drug absorption. Because the H^+ concentrations of the stomach and small intestine diverge widely, the two structures appear to be qualitatively dissimilar in their respective patterns of drug absorption. Figure 2-5 illustrates this difference and its effect on the once commonly used analgesic combination of aspirin plus codeine. Aspirin is an organic acid with a pK_a (negative log of the dissociation constant) of 3.49. In gastric juice (pH 1 to 3), aspirin remains nonionized, and its passage across the stomach mucosa and into the bloodstream is favored. The plasma, however, has a pH of 7.4. On entering this environment, the aspirin becomes ionized to such an extent that return of the drug to the gastrointestinal tract is prevented by the low lipid solubility of the anionic species. When equilibrium is established, the concentration of nonionized aspirin molecules on both sides of the membrane is the same, but the total amount of drug (ionized plus neutral forms) is much greater on the plasma side. The relative concentration of drug in each compartment can be calculated with the Henderson-Hasselbalch equation, as follows:

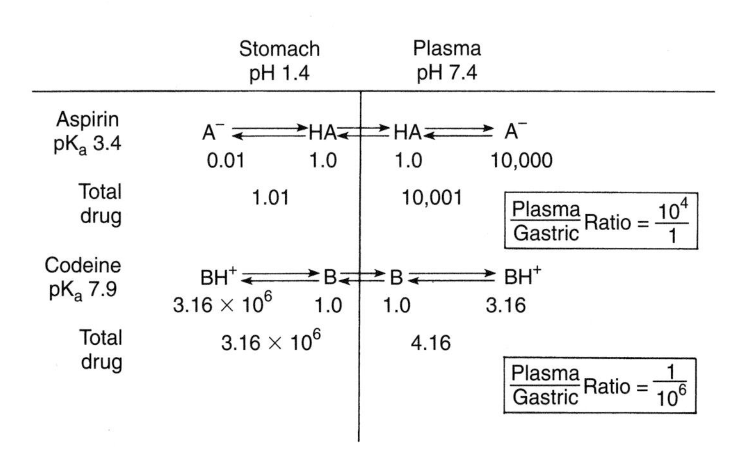

Fig. 2-5 Gastric absorption of aspirin, a weak acid, and codeine, a weak base. The absorption of aspirin is promoted by ion trapping within the plasma; the low pH of stomach fluid favors gastric retention of codeine. (The 3.49 pK_a of aspirin was truncated to 3.4 for purposes of illustration.)

$$\mathrm{Log}\frac{\mathrm{base}\ (A^-)}{\mathrm{acid}\ (HA)} = pH - pk_a$$

This unequal distribution of drug molecules based on the pH gradient across the gastric membrane is an example of ion trapping. The biologic process that sustains this partitioning is the energy-consuming secretion of H^+ by the gastric parietal cells. Because few organic acids have a pK_a low enough to permit significant ionization at stomach pH, almost all acidic drugs should theoretically be effectively absorbed across the gastric mucosa.

For bases such as codeine (pK_a 7.9), the opposite applies. Codeine is almost completely ionized in the acidic environment of the stomach; hence absorption is negligible. At equilibrium, virtually all the drug remains within the stomach. Only very weak bases are nonionized at gastric pH and available for absorption. The ion trapping of basic compounds within the gastric lumen is sometimes useful in forensic medicine. Many drugs subject to abuse are organic bases (e.g., heroin, cocaine, and amphetamine). Even when injected intravenously, they tend to accumulate in the stomach by crossing the gastric mucosa in the reverse direction. Questions of intravenous overdosage can often be answered from the analysis of stomach contents.

When the gastric fluid passes into the small intestine, it is quickly neutralized by pancreatic, biliary, and intestinal secretions. The pH of the proximal one fourth of the intestine varies from 3 to 6, but it reaches neutrality in more distal segments. Under these more alkaline conditions, aspirin converts to the anionic form, whereas a significant fraction of the codeine molecules give up their positive charge. Although basic drugs are favored for absorption over acids in the small intestine, ion trapping is not as extensive because the pH differential across the intestinal mucosa is small. Therefore differences in intestinal absorption based on pH are more concerned with the rate of uptake than with its extent. As one might expect, neutralization of gastric contents by the administration of antacids removes the qualitative disparity in electrolyte absorption normally observed between the stomach and the small intestine.

Mucosal surface area

A second major difference between absorption in the stomach and absorption in the small intestine relates to the intraluminal surface areas involved in drug uptake. Aside from certain mucosal irregularities (rugae), the stomach lining approximates that of a smooth pouch with a thick mucous layer. The mucosa of the small intestine, however, is uniquely adapted for absorption. Contributions by the folds of Kerckring, villi, and microvilli combine to increase the effective surface area 600-fold.[53] Assuming a small intestine 280 cm in length and 4 cm in diameter, approximately 200 m^2 are available for drug absorption. The surface/volume ratio in the small intestine is so great that drugs ionized even to the extent of 99% may still be effectively absorbed. Many studies have shown, in fact, that acidic drugs with a pK_a greater than 3.0 and basic compounds with a pK_a less than 8.0 readily pass from the intestinal fluid into the plasma.[20] Although pH considerations favor the gastric absorption of aspirin, as much as 90% of the drug when given in tablet form is actually absorbed from the small intestine in vivo.[9] Experimentally, nonelectrolytes such as ethanol are also absorbed from the intestine many times faster than from the stomach.[30]

Gastric emptying

Because almost any substance that can penetrate the gastrointestinal epithelium is best absorbed in the small intestine, the rate of gastric emptying can significantly affect drug absorption, particularly for organic bases that are not absorbed at all from the stomach. Gastric emptying is accomplished by contraction of the antrum of the stomach, an event that occurs roughly three times per minute. A mixed meal of solids and liquids requires approximately 4 hours to completely leave the stomach, but liquids alone are removed in about 1.5 hours. As a general rule, approximately 10 ml of liquid are passed into the duodenum per minute.

A major variable in delaying gastric emptying is the presence of fat. Unless drug-induced irritation of the gastric mucosa must be avoided, oral medications should be taken in the absence of food but with a full glass of water. This procedure speeds drug entry into the small intestine and provides maximum access to the gastrointestinal mucosa. Occasionally, the presence of a fatty meal promotes the absorption of a drug that has a high lipid but low water solubility. The antifungal agent griseofulvin and the fat-soluble vitamins are examples of substances that are better absorbed in the presence of lipids. In these instances, the delay in gastric emptying produced by the high fat content of the chyme is compensated for by a more complete absorption.[49]

Additional situations in which food enhances drug uptake have been reviewed.[33] Nevertheless, because gastric emptying is often a limiting factor in the rate of drug absorption, many unrelated drugs exhibit latency periods (the lag phase between oral ingestion and onset of drug effect) of a similar magnitude.

Influence of dosage form

Although the times required for gastric emptying and for diffusion across the mucosal barrier undoubtedly contribute to the delayed onset of action of drugs taken orally, situations exist in which these events are not rate limiting. Most drugs intended for oral use are marketed in the form of capsules or solid tablets. Unlike solutions, these preparations must first dissolve in the gastrointestinal fluid before absorption can occur. If dissolution is very slow, it can become the controlling factor in drug absorption.

The first step in the dissolution process is the disintegration of the tablet (or the capsule and its granules) to yield the primary drug particles. Various excipients are usually included in solid drug preparations to promote disintegration and particle dispersion. Obviously, if disintegration is impaired, drug absorption is depressed accordingly. The dissolution of drug particles occurs by a diffusion-limited mechanism. The diffusion layer of solvent surrounding each particle becomes saturated very quickly with drug molecules escaping from the solid. Because saturation of the diffusion layer occurs far more rapidly than does diffusion from it into the bulk solution, the entire process proceeds no faster than the rate of drug diffusion. Several methods can be used, however, to accelerate the dissolution rate. Because the total surface area of the particles determines the area available for diffusion, reducing the mean particle size through the process of micronization promotes solubilization. A decrease in particle size of 85% with a compensating increase in particle number, for example, doubles the rate of dissolution.[28] Another useful approach is to manufacture drugs in the form of water-soluble salts. The concentration of drug in the dissolution layer is enhanced (often by many times) and the rate of diffusion increased.

The dissolution process may be considered rate limiting whenever a drug solution produces a systemic effect faster than does a solid formulation of the same agent. Sometimes discrepancies in absorption between dosage forms are of such magnitude that clinical differences are noted. With aspirin, the concentration of drug in the plasma 30 minutes after administration can be twice as high for a solution as for a solid tablet.[28] Although it is not clear whether this difference results solely from drug dissolution or from other factors, such as the more rapid gastric emptying typical of liquids, dissolution is probably at least partially responsible.

The influence of dosage form on drug absorption is quite often taken advantage of by drug manufacturers. For instance, some drugs (e.g., erythromycin) are unstable at a low pH and others (e.g., ammonium chloride) are irritating to the gastric mucosa. To avoid release of these drugs within the stomach, they are often prepared in the form of enteric-coated tablets. An enteric coat consists of a film of shellac or some polymeric substitute. The covering is insoluble under acidic conditions but does break down to permit tablet disintegration in the more alkaline environment of the small intestine. Although these preparations are often beneficial, their usefulness nevertheless suffers from an increased variability in patient response. Because drug absorption cannot begin until the tablet passes into the duodenum, the time required for gastric transit becomes an important variable. The passage of a single insoluble tablet from the stomach into the intestine is a random event that can take anywhere from several minutes to more than 6 hours.[16]

Sustained-release preparations represent another method of capitalizing on the influence of formulation on drug absorption. These products are usually designed to release a steady amount of drug within the gastrointestinal tract for a period of 12 to 24 hours. In addition, some preparations also provide an initial loading dose that is readily available for absorption. Sustained release may be accomplished by using a porous matrix, with the drug located both in the interior spaces and on the external surface. An alternative is to make spheres of drug that dissolve at different rates because of various coatings. An intriguing form of sustained-release tablet is the "elementary osmotic pump," in which the drug is enclosed in a semipermeable membrane that lets water in but restricts drug egress. Constant release through a small hole in the membrane is achieved by the osmotic pressure that builds up within the tablet as the drug is slowly dissolved. Advantages claimed for these drug products include greater patient compliance and smaller fluctuations in blood concentration between dosages. Studies with some preparations, however, have documented a greater variability in performance than is normally encountered with conventional dosage forms. Because sustained-release products contain several conventional doses of medication, a danger exists that a too-rapid release of drug from these preparations might cause unexpected toxic concentrations. Conversely, inordinately slow or incomplete release could lead to inadequate drug therapy. Uncertainty over the effects of these formulations is recognized by the Food and Drug Administration (FDA), which regards them as new drugs and requires that both efficacy and safety be demonstrated before they can be marketed. In general, orally administered agents are taken three or four times each day, rarely a hardship for most patients. The additional cost of sustained-release preparations may also influence decisions about their use in place of more conventional forms.

The sensitivity of gastrointestinal absorption to variations in drug formulation is best exemplified by the concern over bioavailability. In a number of instances, chemically identical drugs have proved to be biologically inequivalent. In one study of tetracycline hydrochloride, for example, nine preparations of different manufacture were compared with an aqueous solution of the same drug.[29] Although seven brands produced blood concentrations ranging from 70% to 100% of the reference solution, two products exhibited relative bioavailabilities of only 20% to 30%. Differences in bioavailability are most likely to be clinically important with drugs that are poorly absorbed, have low margins of safety, and are inactivated by capacity-limited processes. Federal law has required since 1977 that bioequivalence testing be performed on all new drugs, and the FDA has mandated such testing of existing products for which a problem of inequivalence is known to exist. Bioavailability considerations related to drug selection are considered further in Chapter 55.

Drug inactivation

One of the shortcomings of oral ingestion is the inactivation of drugs before they reach the systemic circulation. The destruction of some agents (e.g., epinephrine and insulin) is sufficiently great to preclude their administration by this route. With other drugs (e.g., penicillin G), losses may be smaller but still large enough to make oral administration inefficient. Gastric acid is one of the principal causes of drug breakdown within the gastrointestinal tract, but degradation also results from enzymatic activity. For instance, vasopressin, insulin, calcitonin, and other polypeptides are subject to hydrolysis by pancreatic and intestinal peptidases. Intestinal cells also contain intracellular enzymes for metabolizing drugs. Of particular importance is the presence of monoamine oxidase for the inactivation of biogenic amines and of CYP3A4/5 enzymes (described later) for the oxidation of numerous compounds. Enteric bacterial enzymes may also destroy certain ingested agents, such as chlorpromazine. Finally, intestinal contents can alter the effectiveness of many orally administered drugs. Binding to constituents of chyme, chelation with divalent cations, or formation of insoluble salts may decrease the amount of drug available for absorption.

A special fate exists for substances that are successfully absorbed from the gastrointestinal tract. The venous drainage of the stomach, small intestine, and colon is routed by the hepatic portal system to the liver. A first pass of high drug concentration through this enzyme-laden organ can significantly reduce the quantity of agent reaching the systemic circulation. Lidocaine, in fact, is metabolized so rapidly in the liver that virtually all of an oral dose is destroyed during its first pass. Although less pronounced, disparities in opioid analgesic and antibiotic efficacies observed between the oral route and other modes of administration are of clinical importance to the practice of dentistry.

Other enteral routes

The oral and rectal mucosae are occasionally used as sites of drug absorption. Sublingual administration, in which a tablet or troche is allowed to dissolve completely in the oral cavity, takes advantage of the permeability of the oral epithelium and is the preferred route for a few potent, lipophilic drugs, such as nitroglycerin and oxytocin. The oral and intestinal mucosal layers do not differ qualitatively as absorbing surfaces, and comparable absorption has been shown for many agents.[5] One reason for selecting the sublingual route is to avoid drug destruction. Because gastric acid and intestinal and hepatic enzymes are bypassed, sublingual absorption can be more efficient overall for certain drugs than is intestinal uptake. The onset of drug effect may also be quicker than with oral ingestion.

Rectal administration may be used when other enteral routes are precluded, as in the unconscious or nauseated patient. Although a significant fraction of absorbed drug enters the circulation without having to pass through the liver, uptake is often unpredictable. Several drugs irritating to the gastric mucosa (e.g., xanthines) may be given rectally; for others, rectal sensitivity prohibits administration by this route.

Inhalation

The alveolar membrane is an important route of entry for some drugs and many noxious substances. Although the alveolar lining is highly permeable, it is accessible only to agents that are in a gaseous state or are inhaled in sufficiently fine powders or droplets to reach the deepest endings of the respiratory tree. Included in the first category are the therapeutic gases, carbon monoxide, the inhalation anesthetics, and a number of volatile organic solvents. The second category of alveolar membrane penetrants are collectively known as *aerosols*. This term refers to liquid or solid particles small enough (usually 10 μm or less in diameter) to remain suspended in air for prolonged periods. Particles of this sort include bacteria, viruses, smoke, pollens, sprays, and dusts. Any such finely divided material, when inhaled, reaches some portion of the respiratory tree and is affected by the processes of sedimentation and inertial precipitation. Most aerosols contain a mixture of particle sizes. Relatively large particles (greater than 6 μm) impact on the terminal bronchioles and larger branches of the respiratory tree and are removed from the lungs by a cilia-driven blanket of mucus flowing continuously toward the pharynx. Smaller particles, which do reach the alveolar sacs, can be absorbed through the lining cells into the bloodstream, taken up by the process of phagocytosis, or carried by an aqueous film covering the alveolar cells to the terminal bronchioles where they join the mucous blanket. Although two of these three possible fates involve particle uptake, the mechanism for removing solids is remarkably efficient. Only a minute portion of the inhaled dusts of a lifetime fails to be removed by ciliary transport.

Therapeutic use of aerosols is not widespread, but some emergency medications are prepared in this form. Because the onset of effect is extremely rapid after inhalation of an aerosol drug, this route can provide a means of quick self-medication for persons in danger of acute allergic reactions to venoms or drugs. Epinephrine is one such emergency agent that is marketed as an aerosol. Many respiratory drugs are also prepared in aerosol form because they are highly effective by this route while minimizing systemic exposure. However, the rapidity and efficiency of alveolar membrane absorption can, on occasion, pose problems for therapy, as illustrated by the use of pressurized aerosols containing isoproterenol. Although up to 97% of an isoproterenol spray is swallowed under normal conditions and inactivated by various enzymes, overmedication can produce toxic effects. Data gathered over a 7-year period in the United Kingdom suggested that the undisciplined use of these preparations produced an increased mortality rate in asthmatic patients. Restriction of over-the-counter sales and warnings to physicians were accompanied by a fall in mortality rate.[22] Findings such as these reflect the hazards of aerosols when abused and provide a caveat for uncontrolled self-medication with any potentially dangerous drug. Concern over aerosols is also related to questions of toxicology, such as the absorption of heavy metal dusts by industrial workers.

Parenteral Injection

Drugs are frequently given by parenteral injection when oral ingestion is precluded by the patient's condition, when a rapid onset of effect is necessary, or when blood concentrations in excess of those obtainable with the enteral route are required. The method of injection selected varies with the particular drug and therapeutic need of the patient.

Intravenous route

The administration of drugs by infusion or injection directly into the bloodstream is particularly useful when immediate effects or exact blood concentrations are desired. Because absorption is bypassed, intravenous injection circumvents the delays and variations in drug response characteristically associated with other modes of administration. Rapid dilution in the bloodstream and the relative insensitivity of the venous endothelium to drugs often permit the successful administration of compounds or solutions too irritating for other routes (e.g., alkylating anticancer drugs and hypertonic fluids). Also, through the technique of titration, the intravenous route provides an avenue for the controlled administration of drugs that have a very narrow margin of safety between therapeutic and toxic concentrations. The infusion of lidocaine to prevent ventricular arrhythmias and the incremental injection of antianxiety drugs during intravenous sedation are two examples in which titration is used to achieve a desired effect while avoiding adverse reactions. Although many intravenous agents do not require titration and may be given in standardized doses, they should still be injected slowly. If administered too quickly, a dose may move initially through the heart, lungs, and major arteries as a bolus of high drug concentration. Nonspecific but potentially disastrous cardiopulmonary side effects may result, even from the rapid injection of simple salt solutions. Most drugs should be administered over a period of 1 minute, which approximates the circulation time of blood through the body. This procedure avoids high, transient concentrations and permits discontinuance if any untoward effect is observed during the course of injection.

A major disadvantage of the intravenous route is that after the drug is injected, very little can be done to remove it from the bloodstream. When an adverse response is noted with another route, further absorption can usually be delayed or perhaps even prevented. Toxic reactions to drugs given intravenously are often instantaneous and severe. Life-threatening anaphylactic events are also more likely because of the possibility of a massive antigen-antibody reaction. Other complications of intravenous injection include vasculitis and embolism (either from drug irritation, particulate matter in the injected solution, or needle trauma), fever (from injection of pyrogens such as bacterial lipopolysaccharides), infection, and hematoma formation.

Intramuscular route

The intramuscular route is often selected for drugs that cannot be given orally because of slow or erratic absorption, high percentage of drug inactivation, or lack of patient cooperation. The rate of absorption from an intramuscular site is governed by the same factors influencing gastrointestinal uptake, such as lipid/water partition coefficient, degree of ionization, and molecular size. Many drugs, however, are absorbed at approximately the same rate, regardless of these factors. The only barrier separating a drug deposited intramuscularly from the bloodstream is the capillary endothelium, a multicellular membrane with large intercellular gaps. Many lipid-insoluble substances can enter the vascular compartment through these gaps, and even proteins are capable of being absorbed. In these circumstances, blood flow through the tissue is often the primary determinant of the rate of drug absorption. Thus muscles with high blood flows (e.g., deltoid) provide faster absorption rates than muscles with lesser flows (e.g., gluteus maximus). In general, 5 to 30 minutes is required for the onset of drug effect, but this latency period can be controlled to some extent. Exercise markedly speeds absorption by stimulating local circulation. Conversely, uptake may be minimized by the application of ice packs or (in an emergency) tourniquets.

With the exception of a few drugs that are relatively insoluble at tissue pH (e.g., diazepam, phenytoin), absorption from an intramuscular injection is usually rapid and complete. Formulations have therefore been developed to provide for prolonged and steady drug release. These depot preparations consist of drugs manufactured as insoluble salts or dispensed in oil vehicles, or both, such as procaine penicillin suspended in peanut oil. Relatively large volumes of solution may be given by this route, but soreness at the injection site is frequent, and some drugs (e.g., doxycycline) are too irritating to be administered in this manner.

Subcutaneous route

Injection of drugs into the subcutaneous connective tissue is a widely used method of administration for agents that can be given in small volumes (2 ml or less) and are not locally damaging. Subcutaneous absorption is similar to that of resting muscle, and onset times are often comparable. As with the intramuscular route, absorption can be delayed by diminishing blood flow, either through the application of pressure or by surface cooling. Pharmacologic interruption of circulation with vasoconstrictors is also a common strategy, especially in local anesthesia. Because of the ease of subcutaneous implantation, compressed pellets of drugs, sometimes mixed with insoluble matrix material, can be inserted to provide nearly constant drug release for weeks or months. Testosterone and several progestational contraceptive agents (e.g., levonorgestrel) have been successfully administered by this approach. Slow absorption can be achieved, too, through the use of depot forms as described for intramuscular injections.

When subcutaneous administration is chosen for a systemic effect, the hastening of drug absorption is sometimes advantageous. Toward this end, warming the tissue promotes drug uptake by improving local circulation. Massage of the injection site, in addition to stimulating blood flow, helps spread the drug and provides an increased surface area for absorption. This latter effect can also be accomplished through the coadministration of hyaluronidase, an enzyme that breaks down the mucopolysaccharide matrix of connective tissue. The lateral spread of aqueous solutions is so enhanced, in fact, that hyaluronidase is sometimes used to permit the injection of large fluid volumes in situations in which continuous intravenous infusion is difficult or impossible.

Other parenteral injection routes

Intraarterial injections are occasionally performed when a localized effect on a particular organ or area of the body is desired. Injections of radiopaque dyes for diagnostic purposes and antineoplastic agents to control localized tumors are the most commonly encountered examples. Intrathecal administration is used when the direct access of drug to the CNS is necessary. Indications for injection into the subarachnoid space include the production of spinal anesthesia with local anesthetics and the resolution of acute CNS infections with antibiotics. The intraperitoneal infusion of fluids is a useful substitute for hemodialysis in the treatment of drug poisoning. Although intraperitoneal injection is commonly used in animal experimentation, the risk of infection usually precludes such use in human beings. Lastly, intraosseous (anterior tibial) injection of emergency drugs can be used in pediatric patients when intravenous access cannot be obtained quickly.

All these specialized injection techniques are potentially dangerous to the patient. They should be performed only when expressly indicated and then only by qualified personnel.

Topical Application

Drugs are often applied to epithelial surfaces for local effects and less frequently for systemic absorption. Penetration of drugs across the epithelium is strongly influenced by the degree of keratinization.

Skin

The epidermis is a highly modified tissue that isolates the body from the external environment. The outer layer of skin (stratum corneum) is densely packed with the protein keratin. This layer is impervious to water and therefore water-soluble drugs, and its relative thickness and paucity of lipids in contrast to other biologic membranes retards even the diffusion of strongly lipophilic agents. The impermeable nature of skin to water-soluble drugs often requires that agents (e.g., antibiotics, fungicides) intended for dermatologic conditions be administered by a systemic route despite the obvious accessibility of the skin. For lipid-soluble drugs, however, the percutaneous route is often successful for local problems. Moreover, when the keratinized layer is disrupted, drug absorption, especially of hydrophilic compounds, is markedly enhanced. The underlying connective tissue (dermis) is quite permeable to many solutes, although it differs from most tissues in having an abundant supply of arteriovenous shunts, which may cause systemic absorption to be particularly sensitive to changes in temperature.

The general resistance of the intact skin to drugs does not invalidate the need for caution when dealing with potentially toxic chemicals. Sufficient documentation of epidermal absorption of foreign substances has established that certain compounds may readily penetrate the skin to cause systemic effects. These drugs include organic solvents, organophosphate and nicotine-based insecticides, and some nerve gases. Severe poisoning has also resulted from the excessive application of sunburn creams containing local anesthetics. Even lipid-insoluble substances such as inorganic mercury can diffuse across skin if exposure is prolonged.

The obvious benefits of improving and sufficiently controlling percutaneous absorption to make it a reliable route of drug administration have prompted several strategies. For example, a "transdermal therapeutic system" has been developed to provide continuous systemic uptake of nitroglycerin, scopolamine, fentanyl, and nicotine, respectively, for prophylaxis of angina pectoris and motion sickness, management of chronic pain, and assistance with smoking cessation. The system is a complex patch that consists of an outer impermeable backing, a reservoir containing the drug in a suspended form, a semipermeable membrane, and an inner adhesive seal.

In the early 1960s, it was discovered that the industrial solvent dimethyl sulfoxide promotes the percutaneous absorption of water-soluble drugs. The potential of simplified therapy for arthritic and other patients that this drug carrier offered generated much enthusiasm. Subsequent reports of adverse reactions in animals caused interest to wane, however, until the late 1970s when it was promoted as an effective agent for the symptomatic relief of a wide variety of musculoskeletal and collagen disorders. Although widely available as an herbal remedy, dimethyl sulfoxide is currently approved by the FDA only for the treatment of interstitial cystitis.

Another approach to improving drug penetration through the epidermis is the use of occlusive dressings. These dressings retain moisture and break down the horny layer through the process of maceration. A final technique, iontophoresis, is covered below.

Mucous membranes

The topical application of drugs to mucous membranes offers several potential advantages for local therapy. The tissues can often be visualized by the clinician, permitting accurate drug placement. The use of this route generally minimizes systemic effects while providing an optimal concentration of drug in the area being treated. Unlike the case with skin, drugs have little trouble permeating mucous membranes to affect localized conditions. Indeed, systemic absorption of lipophilic drugs from mucous membranes readily occurs. Before this fact was widely appreciated, the topical application of tetracaine to the pharyngeal and tracheal mucosae was a leading cause of local anesthetic overdosage.[1] In dentistry, the use of corticosteroids to ameliorate inflammatory conditions has also given rise to systemic responses, such as the suppression of adrenocortical function by triamcinolone.[26] Although these effects are generally mild and transient, they can create problems for patients with hypertension, diabetes mellitus, or peptic ulcer. Local therapies can also affect systemic health by serving as antigenic stimulants and, in the case of antibiotics, by disturbing the normal microbial ecology and promoting the emergence of resistant microorganisms.

Drugs are sometimes applied mucosally for their systemic effects. In addition to the previously discussed sublingual and rectal routes of administration, the nasal mucosa offer a suitable avenue for the uptake of certain agents. Desmopressin, used in the treatment of diabetes insipidus, and butorphanol, a potent analgesic, are examples of drugs that can be given intranasally.

Iontophoresis

Iontophoresis is the electrical transport of positively or negatively charged drugs across surface tissues. The technique involves passing a direct electrical current of appropriate polarity through the drug solution and patient. Permeation of mucous membranes and even skin and hard tissues is possible with this approach, yet the total dose delivered is small, and systemic toxicity is unlikely. In dental therapeutics, iontophoretic application of drugs has been used in several situations. Loose deciduous teeth have been extracted successfully after the iontophoretic administration of lidocaine with epinephrine for soft tissue anesthesia.[14] For the treatment of herpes orolabialis, galvanic current increases the tissue concentration of idoxuridine up to three times that obtainable with topical application alone.[15] Probably the most common use of iontophoresis in dentistry, however, is the promotion of F^- uptake into exposed hypersensitive dentin. A 1% solution of sodium fluoride administered in this manner produced better results than did a 33% paste.[34]

DISTRIBUTION

Distribution refers to the movement of drugs throughout the body. The rate, sequence, and extent of distribution depend on many factors: the physicochemical properties of the drug, cardiac output and regional blood flow, anatomic characteristics of membranes, transmembrane electrical and pH gradients, binding to plasma proteins and tissue reservoirs, and occasionally active transport, facilitated diffusion, or endocytosis/transcytosis. For all but the very few drugs that act intravascularly, the capillary membrane constitutes the first tissue barrier to be crossed in the journey of a drug from the bloodstream to its site of action.

Capillary Penetration

After a drug gains access to the systemic circulation, it becomes diluted by the plasma volume of the entire vascular compartment. For a compound administered intravenously, this process requires only several minutes for completion; for drugs given by other routes, intravascular distribution takes place concurrently with absorption. The transfer of drugs out of the bloodstream is governed by the same factors that control its entrance. Lipophilic drugs, for example, diffuse across the capillary membrane extremely rapidly. The transfer is so expeditious, in fact, that equilibrium with interstitial fluid is practically instantaneous. Under these conditions, the rate of drug uptake is determined by the blood flow through the tissue under consideration. Thus well-perfused organs are saturated with drug long before many other tissues have had a chance to reach even a fraction of the equilibrium concentration. Water-soluble drugs diffuse through gaps located between adjacent endothelial cells. With these agents, transcapillary movement is slower than for drugs that have high lipid/water partition coefficients and is inversely proportional to molecular weight. As drug size increases, aqueous diffusion becomes less important, and filtration takes over as the primary motive force behind drug transport. Substances with molecular weights greater than 60,000 pass across capillary membranes very slowly. Electron microscopic evidence suggests that transcytosis is involved in their distribution.[40]

Entry of Drugs into Cells

As previously discussed, the cell membrane acts as a semipermeable barrier, admitting some drugs into the cell while excluding others. Nonpolar, lipid-soluble compounds distribute evenly across plasma membranes, but distribution of weak electrolytes at equilibrium is somewhat more complex. The intracellular pH is approximately 7.0, differing slightly from the 7.4 pH of extracellular fluid. Acids with a pK_a less than 8.0 tend to remain outside the cell, whereas basic drugs with a pK_a greater than 6.0 tend to accumulate within. Because the concentration differential across the cell membrane based on a pH gradient of 0.4 can equal 2.5 : 1, the acid-base status of a patient can significantly affect the dose response of weak electrolytes acting intracellularly. (The influence of pH on the distribution of local anesthetics across nerve membranes is described in Chapter 16.) Ions, unless very small in size (molecular weights of 60 or less) or transported by membrane-bound carriers, penetrate cell membranes with difficulty or not at all. Charged drugs that do gain access to the cell by passive diffusion are distributed at equilibrium according to their electrochemical gradient across the membrane.

Distribution into Special Fluid Compartments

In some tissues or organs, anatomic components permit the sequestration of interstitial or transcellular fluids from the general extracellular space. The most important examples for therapeutics involve the CNS, the fetal circulation, and, insofar as dentistry is concerned, saliva.

Central nervous system

Entry of drugs into the CNS is unusually dependent on lipid solubility. Drugs with high lipid/water partition coefficients are taken up very fast, as exemplified by the immediate onset of general anesthesia after the intravenous injection of thiopental. The rapid distribution of lipophilic drugs into the brain and spinal cord arises from the fact that the CNS receives approximately 15% of the cardiac output yet composes only 2% of total body weight. Despite this favorable blood supply, drugs that are sparingly lipid soluble are largely excluded from the extracellular space of the brain. In contrast to the capillaries of most tissues, the endothelial cells of the CNS are joined together by tight junctions that limit the entry of water-soluble drugs to those with an effective molecular radius of 8 Å or less. Thus relatively large molecules (e.g., inulin, with a molecular weight of 5000) that normally pass without difficulty into the interstitial space are completely barred, and most other drugs dependent on aqueous channels for penetration and weighing more than 100 to 200 daltons are slowed considerably. A relative absence of endocytosis/transcytosis is also notable in CNS capillaries.

A second impediment to the transfer of ions and other water-soluble substances is the cellular sheath that surrounds the capillaries of the brain. This investing layer is made up of processes extending from connective tissue astrocytes. Although the area of capillary surface coverage is not complete, it nevertheless is sufficient to retard the diffusion of all but highly lipid-soluble compounds.

A third factor limiting access of drugs to the CNS is an extensive collection of membrane transporters, such as

P-glycoprotein, that efficiently export drugs gaining entry into the endothelial cells. Together, the modified capillary endothelium, astrocytic sheath, and export carrier system constitute the blood-brain barrier.

Drugs may also gain access to the CNS by way of the choroid plexuses. Each choroid plexus is composed of a network of small blood vessels and capillaries projecting into a ventricular space and covered by a layer of epithelial cells specifically adapted for the secretion of cerebrospinal fluid. Diffusion of drugs across the choroid plexus epithelium and into the cerebrospinal fluid is largely restricted to highly lipid-soluble drugs, indicating the functionally analogous existence of a barrier between blood and cerebrospinal fluid. The choroid plexus and cerebrospinal fluid are actually more closely involved with the removal of drugs from the CNS than with their entry. Secreted into the third, fourth, and lateral ventricles, the cerebrospinal fluid moves by bulk flow through the ventriculocisternal system to bathe the surfaces of the brain and spinal cord before exiting through the arachnoid villi. Drugs present in the extracellular fluid of the CNS are free to diffuse into the cerebrospinal fluid. Because the total quantity of cerebrospinal fluid (150 ml) approximates the volume of the interstitial space and because it has a moderately fast turnover rate (10% per hour), the removal of drugs by bulk flow through the arachnoid villi can prevent an agent in the brain from ever reaching equilibrium with the blood. The active transport of organic ions from the cerebrospinal fluid back into the systemic circulation by the lining cells of the choroid plexus also promotes the removal of many drugs from the brain.

The selective distribution of compounds into the CNS has several important therapeutic ramifications. Some alkaloids intended for peripheral nervous system effects, for example, may cause central disturbances on entry into the brain. Conversion of such drugs (e.g., scopolamine) to positively charged quaternary ammonium derivatives (e.g., methscopolamine) prevent CNS influences yet allow essential peripheral nervous system activity. Conversely, drugs used for their central effects may benefit by molecular modifications that enhance their entry into the brain. Lower total doses can then be given and peripheral effects minimized. Sometimes the blood-brain barrier is a hindrance to therapy. Penicillin G, a water-soluble organic acid with a pK_a of 2.6, diffuses slowly into the CNS and is subject to active removal by the choroid plexus. For persons with bacterial encephalitis, this lack of drug penetration can complicate treatment. (Capillary permeability in the brain fortunately often increases during meningeal inflammation.) A clever approach to circumventing the blood-brain barrier is embodied in the treatment of parkinsonism. This condition is associated with a deficiency of dopamine within selected portions of the brain. Replacement therapy with dopamine is ineffective, however, because the drug is excluded by the blood-brain barrier. To avoid this problem, levodopa, the amino acid precursor of dopamine, is used instead. Levodopa readily enters the brain, where it is subsequently decarboxylated to the active drug. A more drastic and potentially dangerous method of breaking through the blood-brain barrier is to disrupt it temporarily by infusing hypertonic solution into the carotid artery. An osmotically induced shrinkage of cerebrovascular endothelial cells causes the tight junctions to pull apart and permits the uptake of water-soluble drugs.[41] Current strategies include attaching the drug to a carrier substance, or vector, that is transported into the brain. Such vectors may consist of naturally transported molecules or involve monoclonal antibodies targeted for these molecules.[46] Other peptide vectors have been identified that promote transcytosis. Coupling of drugs such as penicillin and doxorubicin greatly improves their uptake across the blood-brain barrier.

Placental transfer

Obstetric delivery of conscious infants from anesthetized mothers was once misconstrued as evidence for a unique placental barrier excluding even lipid-soluble drugs from the fetus. It is now understood that such observations largely result from the finite rate of drug transfer from the maternal circulation to fetal tissues. Fetal blood vessels projecting into sinuses filled with maternal blood are covered by a single layer of cells called *trophoblasts*. The movement of drugs across the placenta is limited by the trophoblastic membrane, which is qualitatively similar to plasma membranes elsewhere. Although trophoblasts are known to actively secrete amino acids and other nutrients into the fetal circulation, the entry of most drugs depends on passive diffusion across the lipoid barrier. For highly lipophilic drugs such as thiopental, distribution is retarded only by the rate of maternal blood flow through the placenta and by peculiarities in the fetal circulation that limit tissue perfusion. Even so, it has been calculated that 40 minutes are required for fetal tissues to attain 90% equilibration with a constant maternal arterial concentration.[40] Limited by a sluggish transmembrane diffusion, the transfer of water-soluble compounds is so inefficient that virtually no drug from a single administration may gain access to the fetus. As in the CNS, P-glycoprotein in the placenta also tends to prevent potentially dangerous substances from entering the fetal circulation. Nevertheless, even sparingly lipid-soluble agents will eventually accumulate in the fetus if administered to the mother in multiple doses.

Concern over the placental transfer of drugs arises from the possibility of inducing toxic manifestations in the newborn and developmental defects in the embryo and fetus. These topics are discussed further in Chapter 3.

Salivary secretion

The distribution of drugs into saliva is of pharmacologic interest in two respects. First, drugs gaining access to the oral environment from the systemic circulation can affect microorganisms or tissue surfaces within the mouth. Although these influences are usually undesirable, a drug developed for a local effect, such as caries prevention, could conceivably be administered systemically to achieve a sustained therapeutic concentration in the saliva while obviating the necessity of repeated mouth rinsing. The second pharmacologic interest in saliva stems from the fact that salivary drug determinations can provide a noninvasive measure of the free plasma concentration of drugs. Because the free drug concentration in plasma is normally the primary determinant of patient response, the benefit of salivary drug quantitation to therapeutics is potentially great. However, clinical studies have documented a complex relationship between plasma and salivary drug titers, one that must be fully understood before salivary monitoring can be successfully used.[4,44]

Drugs may enter the oral fluids from several sources: (1) passive diffusion across the alveolar and ductal cells of salivary glands, (2) passive diffusion across the oral epithelium, and (3) bulk flow of fluid from the gingival crevice. Of these avenues, the first is the most important and the third is the least (except for drugs that cannot gain entry by either of the other two routes). As shown in Table 2-1, the salivary concentration of a drug is influenced by many factors.[12] Agents that are relatively lipid soluble (e.g., diazepam) or very small in size (e.g., ethanol) encounter little difficulty in equilibrating with saliva. Because only the unbound portion of a drug is involved in distribution across membranes and the salivary compartment is quite small with respect to the total intravascular space, protein binding does not affect the saliva/plasma ratio of the free drug (e.g., diazepam and acetaminophen). Regarding weak electrolytes, the disparity in pH between the plasma and the more acidic saliva results in the concentration

Table • 2-1

Distribution of Drugs into Saliva

DRUG	L*	PROTEIN BINDING (%)	pK_a	SALIVA/PLASMA RATIO† RESTING	STIMULATION
Quinidine	3000	89	8.8 (b)	3.1	1.3
Sulfamerazine	0.4	88	7.1 (a)	0.69	0.55
Diazepam	820	99	3.3 (b)	1.0	1.0
Ethanol	0.5	0	—	1.0	1.0

Adapted from Feller K, le Petit G: On the distribution of drugs in saliva and blood plasma, *Int J Clin Pharmacol Biopharm* 15:468–469, 1977.
a, Acid; *b*, base.
*Lipid/water partition coefficient (*n*-octanol as the lipid).
†Refers to the unbound drug.

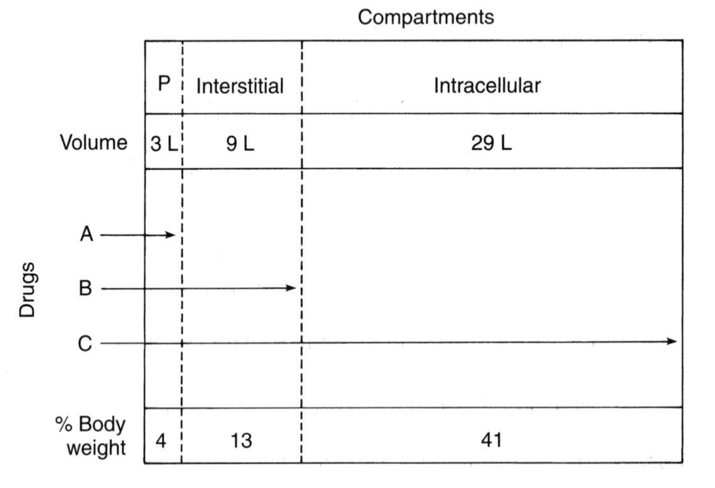

Fig. 2-6 Body water compartments. The membrane barriers that separate plasma from interstitial fluid and interstitial fluid from intracellular water are indicated by *dashed lines*. The upper set of figures are the respective volumes for a 70-kg man; the lower set are percentages of total body weight. Of the drugs shown, *A* is restricted to the plasma, *B* is distributed within the extracellular compartment (plasma + interstitial fluid), and C is disseminated throughout the total body water.

of bases with a pK_a greater than 5.5 in saliva (e.g., quinidine) and an opposite effect on acids with a pK_a less than 8.5 (e.g., sulfamerazine). Finally, the rate of salivary flow can alter intraoral concentrations in at least two ways. Increased salivary production may outpace the diffusion rate of drugs with moderate to low lipid solubility (e.g., acetaminophen), thus lowering the saliva/plasma ratio. Additionally, the pH of stimulated saliva tends to approach 7.4, thus eliminating the unequal distribution of drugs based on pH (e.g., quinidine). With some weak acids, these two influences on drug concentration may tend to cancel each other out (e.g., sulfamerazine).

Volume of Distribution

It should be obvious from the foregoing discussion that drugs are not distributed equally throughout the body. Although lipophilic substances tend to penetrate all tissue compartments (provided they have a modicum of water solubility), hydrophilic compounds are often disseminated more restrictively. The volume of distribution (V_d) is a useful indicator of how drugs are dispersed among the various body compartments. In its simplest form, the V_d is calculated from the equation $V_d = Q/C$, where Q is the quantity of drug administered and C is the plasma concentration of the drug at equilibrium. The V_d is therefore the amount of water by which a particular dose would have to be diluted to produce a given plasma concentration, assuming that no drug has been lost through incomplete absorption or by metabolism or excretion.

Evans blue dye is typical of the few drugs that are distributed only within the vascular space. Several minutes after an intravenous injection, Evans blue becomes thoroughly mixed within the blood, and a V_d of 3 L is obtained. This value represents the total plasma volume of a 70-kg man of average build. Most compounds, however, pass readily from the vascular tree into the interstitial compartment. At equilibrium, these drugs are distributed in an extracellular volume of 12 L, which includes the vascular and interstitial fluids. Ionic drugs (e.g., aminoglycosides) are generally contained in this V_d. Molecules that can freely penetrate all membranes are diluted by the water of the entire body, approximately 41 L. Figure 2-6 depicts the major body fluid volumes, and Table 2-2 provides a list of agents with representative V_d values.

It is apparent from Table 2-2 that the V_d of many compounds does not correspond to any definable anatomic fluid compartment. Accepting that the measurements were made correctly and that problems in drug absorption and elimination were successfully avoided, several explanations remain for these results. The V_d equation actually provides only an apparent distribution, partly because it assumes that drugs are evenly dispersed. To illustrate this point, Na^+ is present in all body fluids (with an actual V_d of 41 L), but the apparent (calculated) V_d for Na^+ is only 18 L. This discrepancy arises because Na^+ is actively but incompletely extruded from intracellular water. Dissimilarities between true and calculated volumes of distribution based on unequal compartment concentrations arise whenever ions are distributed across

Table • 2-2

Volumes of Distribution of Various Agents

AGENT	V_d (L)	CORRESPONDING FLUID COMPARTMENT
Evans blue	3	Plasma water
Iodine 131–albumin	3	
Mannitol	12	Extracellular water
Inulin	11	
Urea	41	Total body water
Enalapril	40	
Amoxicillin	15	
Na^+	18	
Lidocaine	77	
Tetracycline	100	
Atropine	120	
Meperidine	300	
Chlorpromazine	1500	
Propofol	4000	
Chloroquine	13,000	

electrically polarized membranes, weak electrolytes are present in fluids of different pH, or drugs are actively transported into or out of a water space.

The enormous V_d values recorded for drugs such as propofol and chloroquine generally result from tissue binding. The sequestration of compounds within cells or certain tissues necessarily reduces the concentration of drug in the plasma, leading to an abnormally high calculation of V_d. (Obviously, no drug can have a true V_d greater than approximately 41 L.) Plasma protein binding can also affect V_d determinations. Because the total drug in plasma is usually measured, binding artificially inflates the drug concentration and depresses V_d. If free drug is measured, significant binding by plasma proteins has the same effect as binding at extravascular sites.

Drug Binding and Storage

The sojourn of drugs in the body is considerably influenced by binding to proteins and other tissue components. Reducing the concentration of free solute causes a decrease in the rate of passage across membrane barriers and may, as reflected in V_d determinations, alter drug distribution at equilibrium as well. Drug sequestration can also affect the processes of absorption, metabolism, and elimination.

Plasma protein binding

Many drugs become associated with plasma proteins, especially albumin. The predominant protein in plasma, albumin contains roughly 200 ionized functional groups per molecule and has the capacity to bind a number of different substances concurrently. A second plasma protein, α_1-acid glycoprotein (also known as *orosomucoid*), is a major "acceptor" of basic, or cationic, agents. Transcortin (which is specific for corticosteroids and a few other agents), other globulins, and various lipoproteins play more limited roles in drug binding.

The reversible attachment of drugs to plasma proteins is reminiscent of drug-receptor combinations in that the reaction obeys the law of mass action, as follows:

$$\text{Drug} + \text{Protein} \rightleftharpoons \text{Drug–protein complex}$$

This binding is capacity limited because the number of binding sites is finite. At concentrations less than the binding dissociation constant, the fraction bound is a fixed value; at concentrations greater than the dissociation constant, the fraction of drug bound varies inversely with the drug concentration. Clinically, the percentage of bound drug usually does not change over the dosage ranges used clinically, and assigning most drugs a fixed value is permissible (e.g., 99% for diazepam; see Table 2-1). Drugs differ tremendously in their affinity for plasma proteins; the percentage of binding of individual agents ranges from 0% to 100%.

The binding of agents within the vascular compartment reduces the concentration gradient of free drug across the capillary membrane and slows egress from the plasma into the extravascular space. As free molecules leave the circulation, a portion of the bound drug dissociates according to the law of mass action and becomes available for further transport. Hence the rate but not the extent of distribution is generally altered by plasma protein binding. There are, of course, exceptions. The attachment of Evans blue is so tight, for example, that the compound is retained virtually in toto within the bloodstream. For a drug that is 95% bound in plasma, a little more than half of the total dose remains intravascular, assuming that the agent is not sequestered elsewhere. However, drugs that are extensively but reversibly bound to plasma proteins generally bind to tissue elements as well, decreasing the fraction of drug in the plasma to less than one third the total even in the most extreme cases.

The reversibility of binding causes the plasma proteins to act as a kind of drug reservoir. Agents must occasionally be administered in large loading doses to saturate binding sites as a prelude to achieving therapeutic concentrations at the site of action. Once accommodated, though, reservoirs of bound drug can provide certain benefits. For instance, fluctuations in drug concentration resulting from intermittent dosage schedules are kept to a minimum. As the dose is absorbed, a portion becomes bound, only to be released later as metabolism and excretion lower free drug titers. Drug binding additionally often prolongs the duration of action, which may permit administrations to be spaced more conveniently than would otherwise be possible. Both glomerular filtration and passive hepatic uptake are ineffective against the bound fraction; significant binding, therefore, may depress the metabolism and excretion of drugs. When compounds are actively or otherwise rapidly taken up by organs of elimination, however, the instantaneous reversibility of binding can lead to a faster than normal elimination rate. Penicillin G, for example, is secreted into the urine so efficiently that blood flowing through the kidney is almost completely cleared of the antibiotic in a single pass. Because albumin binding presents the kidney with more total drug per unit time, secretion is quicker than would be the case if the drug were more evenly distributed throughout the body.

Two potential clinical concerns related to plasma protein binding involve patient variability in binding efficacy and the possibility for drug interaction. Differences in drug binding affect the concentration of free drug within the bloodstream and may lead to insufficient therapy on the one hand and overdosage on the other. The unusual susceptibility to diazepam exhibited by patients with hypoalbuminemia should be considered when the drug is used for intravenous sedation.[17] Inasmuch as the attachment of drugs to plasma proteins is generally less selective than are drug-receptor associations, competition between drugs for binding sites is relatively common. Such interactions may reach clinical significance, though, only when the drugs are highly bound, are administered in large doses, and have a narrow margin of safety or a small V_d.

Tissue binding

As previously mentioned, drugs capable of associating with plasma proteins are also likely to bind to tissue constituents.

Such binding does not impede the movement of drugs out of the bloodstream, but it does slow the rate of elimination. By virtue of its aggregate size, muscle tissue is a significant reservoir for many drugs. Fat is also quantitatively important, especially for highly lipid-soluble compounds. Although uptake into fat is limited by a parsimonious blood supply, adipose tissue constitutes from 10% to more than 50% of total body weight, and most of an administered dose of a lipophilic drug may accumulate in fat over the course of several hours. Certain tissues display unusual affinities for particular drugs. The antimalarial agents chloroquine and quinacrine are heavily concentrated in the liver. Guanethidine and other quaternary ammonium compounds adhere to negatively charged residues in mucous secretions of the gastrointestinal tract.

The attachment of drugs to drug receptors deserves special comment. Obviously important in the pharmacologic sense, the contribution of drug-receptor interactions to the total amount of binding is usually quite small. When distribution throughout the body and the various types of sequestration are considered, the percentage of drug administered that actually reaches its receptor to evoke a response is quantitatively negligible.

Storage

The association between drugs and tissue elements is sometimes so stable that discussing such binding in terms of storage is appropriate. When drugs are stored, they are not readily available for release and thus do not effectively prolong the duration of action. Some of the most common examples of storage involve mineralized tissues and fat. Bone-seeking ions such as F^- and lead, and Ca^{++} chelators such as the tetracyclines, may be deposited with bone salts during mineralization or become associated with existing hydroxyapatite crystals. Essentially in an insoluble state, these substances are difficult or impossible to remove completely. Bone and tooth mineralization may benefit from appropriate concentrations of F^-, but most drug-induced alterations are detrimental. In the case of radioactive metals (e.g., strontium 90), storage in bone can lead to the development of leukemia, osteogenic sarcoma, and other forms of neoplasia. Several general anesthetics (e.g., halothane) and some lipophilic insecticides (e.g., chlorophenothane, otherwise known as DDT) are commonly sequestered in fat. Although not usually dangerous when stored, the slow release of these substances has been linked to a variety of health problems.[31,40] Plasma proteins are generally not associated with drug storage, yet the now-obsolete radiocontrast medium 3-hydroxy-2,4,6-triiodo-α-ethylhydrocinnamic acid exhibited a binding half-life to albumin of approximately 2.5 years.

Redistribution

Strongly lipophilic drugs, especially when administered intravenously in bolus form, characteristically go through several phases of distribution: an initial transfer into vessel-rich organs (brain, heart, kidneys, liver, and lungs) followed by progressive redistribution to less highly vascularized tissues (muscle, skin, and eventually fat). When the target organ of a drug happens to have a high blood flow per unit mass, redistribution can result in the abrupt termination of drug effect. Thiopental has been extensively studied in this regard (Figure 2-7).[32] The onset of anesthesia with thiopental is almost instantaneous; however, consciousness is lost only temporarily, and the patient normally awakens in approximately 15 minutes. The quick onset and brief duration of thiopental reflect the rapidity by which the agent equilibrates between the blood and the CNS. Soon after a peak brain titer is reached (in 30 to 90 seconds), the concentration begins to fall as thiopental continues to be absorbed by the relatively large mass of muscle. Consciousness returns at about the same time muscle reaches

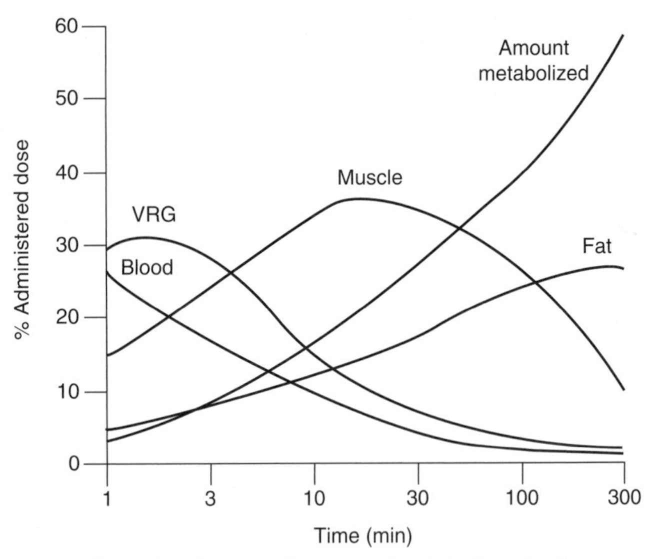

Fig. 2-7 Redistribution of thiopental. *VRG*, Vessel-rich group tissues, including the brain, heart, lungs, kidneys, and liver. (Redrawn from Saidman LJ: Uptake, distribution and elimination of barbiturates. In Eger E II, ed: *Anesthetic uptake and action*, Baltimore, 1974, Williams & Wilkins.)

equilibrium with the blood. Thereafter, both the brain and muscle concentrations parallel the plasma decay curve as the drug slowly passes into adipose tissue. With a metabolic half-life of approximately 10 hours, thiopental would be a relatively long-acting drug if not for redistribution. Indeed, when repetitive injections saturate the fat reservoir, thiopental assumes the characteristics of a long-duration anesthetic.

METABOLISM

Metabolism is a major pathway for the termination of pharmacologic effects of drugs and is often a prerequisite for the excretion of lipid-soluble chemicals. From an evolutionary standpoint, mechanisms for the biotransformation of lipophilic substances to compounds with reduced lipid/water partition coefficients appear necessary for terrestrial vertebrate life. The constraint imposed on land animals to eliminate waste products in limited volumes of water precludes the excretion of drugs with high lipid solubility. In human beings, the kidney represents the major pathway for drug excretion. All drugs that exist free in the plasma are present in the glomerular filtrate. But, whereas polar compounds tend to remain within the renal tubule during the resorptive phase of urine formation, lipophilic chemicals diffuse back into the systemic circulation. Because the urinary concentration of a lipid-soluble nonelectrolyte should theoretically equal the free plasma titer, the rate of renal excretion (given a normal urinary output of 1 to 1.5 L/day) is small for a drug having a reasonably large V_d. Creatures in an aquatic habitat, however, have little difficulty in eliminating lipophilic chemicals. Substances with a high lipid/water partition coefficient readily diffuse across the gill membrane and are lost to the surrounding water. Therefore, the highly developed enzyme systems for metabolizing drugs in terrestrial species are often absent in marine and freshwater organisms.

Historically, the term *detoxification* was used in reference to drug metabolism. Although many compounds are rendered pharmacologically inert by metabolic attack, this is not always the case. Numerous drugs yield metabolites with full or partial activity, and some provide derivatives with novel or highly

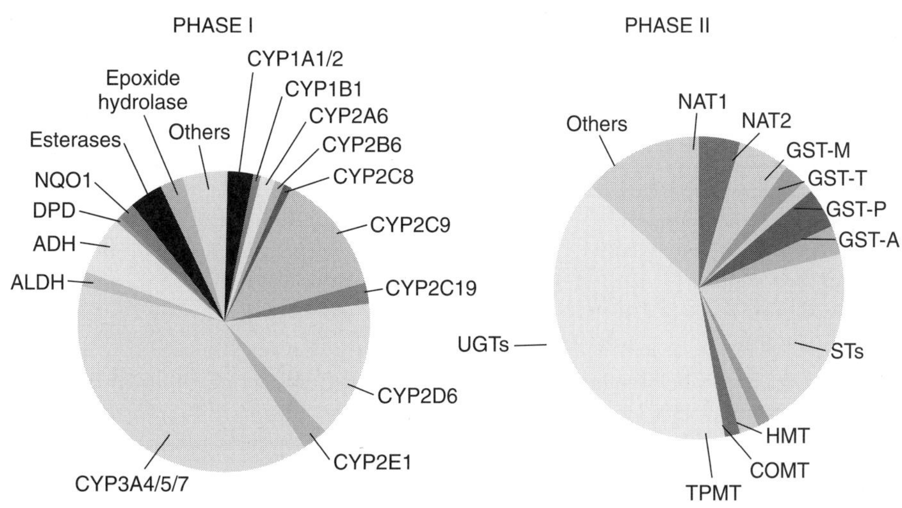

Fig. 2-8 Major enzymes involved in drug metabolism. The percentage of phase I and phase II metabolism of drugs contributed by each enzyme is represented by the relative size of each section of the corresponding chart. *ADH,* Alcohol dehydrogenase; *ALDH,* aldehyde dehydrogenase; *CYP,* cytochrome P450; *DPD,* dihydropyrimidine dehydrogenase; *NQ01,* NADPH:quinone oxidoreductase (or DT diaphorase); *COMT,* catechol O-methyltransferase; *GST,* glutathione-S-transferase; *HMT,* histamine methyltransferase; *NAT,* N-acetyltransferase; *UGTs,* uridine diphosphate glucuronosyltransferases. (Adapted from Evans WE, Relling MV: Pharmacogenomics: translating functional genomics into rational therapeutics, *Science* 286:487-491, 1999.)

toxic drug effects. An increasing number of agents even require chemical activation to be of therapeutic benefit (e.g., cyclophosphamide, mercaptopurine, methyldopa, and sulindac). The best generalization that can be drawn concerning drug metabolism is that agents are eventually converted to polar, relatively lipid-insoluble compounds that are susceptible to renal or biliary excretion or both.

Drug metabolism can be categorized according to the types of reactions involved and where they take place. *Nonsynthetic reactions* include the various transformations of molecular structure: oxidation, reduction, and hydrolysis. These events are also called *phase I reactions* because they often represent the initial stage of biotransformation. *Synthetic,* or *phase II, reactions* consist of the conjugation of drugs or their metabolites with functional groups provided by endogenous cofactors. Drugs may be metabolized by virtually any tissue of the body, but quantitatively the most important enzyme systems for the biotransformation of exogenous substances are located in the liver.

Hepatic Microsomal Metabolism

Each hepatocyte contains an extensive network of smooth endoplasmic reticulum that catalyzes the metabolism of a variety of endogenous chemicals (e.g., bilirubin, thyroxine, and steroids). Studies of fragmented reticular elements isolated along with other membrane structures in the form of microsomes have demonstrated that numerous drugs are also chemically altered by enzymes located within this subcellular organelle. The greatest number of reactions involve oxidation; however, reduction, hydrolysis, and conjugation with glucuronic acid also occur.

Oxidation

The oxidation of drugs results in compounds that are more polar, relatively more hydrophilic, and less likely to penetrate cells and bind to tissue elements. Microsomal oxidations are catalyzed by a set of mixed-function oxidases, so named because one atom of an oxygen dimer is incorporated into the drug while the other is converted to water through the addition of two hydrogen atoms. Of particular significance to microsomal oxidation is the component that actually binds the drug during metabolism, cytochrome P450 (CYP). This hemoprotein, actually a group of closely related isoenzymes, was designated P450 because of its absorption peak at 450 Å when combined in the reduced state with carbon monoxide. Some 18 distinct CYP families, encoded in 57 genes, have been identified in human beings[35]; the major enzymes involved in drug metabolism are represented in Figure 2-8.[11]

In aggregate, the CYP superfamily constitutes up to 20% of the total protein content of liver microsomes. It acts as the terminal acceptor of electrons in a transport chain that also includes the reduced coenzyme nicotinamide adenine dinucleotide phosphate (NADPH) and the flavoprotein NADPH-cytochrome P450 reductase. A unique ability of the CYP enzymes is their collective capacity to react with a diverse array of chemicals. In fact, the only identified requirement for microsomal oxidation is that the drug sufficiently penetrate the cell membranes to reach the hemoprotein. Table 2-3 lists the major CYP enzymes in human beings along with some drugs that are metabolized by them and drugs that can inhibit or induce their activities.

The general pathway for oxidation of drugs by the hepatic microsomal enzyme system is depicted in Figure 2-9. The drug initially attaches to an oxidized (Fe^{+++}) CYP enzyme. This complex then accepts an electron from the flavoprotein-catalyzed oxidation of NADPH. A ternary structure is produced next by the inclusion of molecular oxygen, and the addition of a second electron and two protons causes the complex to break down, yielding the CYP enzyme, a water molecule, and the oxidized drug.

The oxidation of an agent may lead to several different derivatives. Oxygen may be incorporated in the form of an alcohol, aldehyde, epoxide, ketone, or carboxylic acid in such structures as aliphatic residues, aromatic rings, amino groups, and sulfur moieties. Oxygen may also replace a sulfur atom

Table 2-3

Major Cytochrome P450 Enzymes and Representative Substrates, Inhibitors, and Inducers

CYP	SUBSTRATES	INHIBITORS	INDUCERS
1A1/2	Acetaminophen, amitriptyline, caffeine, clozapine, estradiol, haloperidol, imipramine, mexiletine, naproxen, ondansetron, propranolol, ropivacaine, tamoxifen, theophylline, *R*-warfarin, zileuton	Amiodarone, cimetidine, ciprofloxacin, clarithromycin, erythromycin, grapefruit juice, insulin, ticlopidine	Benzo[*a*]pyrene, chargrilled meat, modafinil, nafcillin, omeprazole, rifampin
2A6	Acetaminophen, coumarin, halothane, nicotine, nitrosamines, valproic acid	Azole antifungals, pilocarpine, tranylcypromine	Barbiturates, dexamethasone, rifampin
2B6	Bupropion, cyclophosphamide, ifosfamide, methadone	Amlodipine, methimazole, thiotepa, tretinoin	Barbiturates, dihydropyridines, ifosfamide, lovastatin, rifampin
2C8/9	Amitriptyline, celecoxib, fluoxetine, fluvastatin, losartan, nonsteroidal anti-inflammatories, oral hypoglycemics, phenobarbital, phenytoin, sulfaphenazole, *S*-warfarin, tamoxifen	Amiodarone, azole antifungals, fluvastatin, lovastatin, metronidazole, paroxetine, ritonavir, sertraline, trimethoprim, zafirlukast	Barbiturates, dihydropyridines, ifosfamide, rifampin
2C18/19	Amitriptyline, citalopram, indomethacin, diazepam, naproxen, phenobarbital, phenytoin, primidone, progesterone, propranolol, proton pump inhibitors	Chloramphenicol, cimetidine, fluoxetine, fluvoxamine, ketoconazole, modafinil, omeprazole, paroxetine, ticlopidine, topiramate	Aspirin, barbiturates, carbamazepine, norethindrone, rifampin
2D6	Amphetamine, β-adrenergic blockers, chlorpheniramine, clomipramine, clozapine, codeine, dextromethorphan, encainide, flecainide, fluoxetine, haloperidol, hydrocodone, metoclopramide, mexiletine, ondansetron, oxycodone, paroxetine, propoxyphene, risperidone, selegiline, thioridazine, tramadol, tricyclic antidepressants, venlafaxine	Amiodarone, antipsychotics, celecoxib, cimetidine, cocaine, fluoxetine, methadone, metoclopramide, paroxetine, quinidine, ritonavir, sertraline, terbinafine, ticlopidine, venlafaxine	Dexamethasone, rifampin
2E1	Acetaminophen, ethanol, sildenafil, theophylline, volatile inhalation anesthetics	Disulfiram, propofol, tricyclic antidepressants	Colchicine, ethanol, isoniazid, tretinoin
3A4/5/7	Acetaminophen, alfentanil, alprazolam, amiodarone, atorvastatin, buspirone, chlorpheniramine, cocaine, cortisol, cyclosporine, dapsone, diazepam, dihydroergotamine, dihydropyridines, diltiazem, dronabinol, ethinyl estradiol, fentanyl, indinavir, lidocaine, lovastatin, macrolides, methadone, miconazole, midazolam, mifepristone, modafinil, ondansetron, paclitaxel, progesterone, quinidine, ritonavir, saquinavir, sildenafil, spironolactone, sulfamethoxazole, sufentanil, tacrolimus, tamoxifen, testosterone, trazodone, triazolam, verapamil, zaleplon, zolpidem	Amiodarone, chloramphenicol, cimetidine, ciprofloxacin, clarithromycin, diltiazem, dihydroergotamine, doxycycline, erythromycin, felodipine, fluoxetine, fluvoxamine, glucocorticoids, grapefruit juice, HIV antivirals, itraconazole, ketoconazole, nefazodone, sildenafil, verapamil	Barbiturates, carbamazepine, glucocorticoids, ifosfamide, modafinil, nevirapine, phenytoin, rifampin, St. John's wort (hypericum), troleandomycin

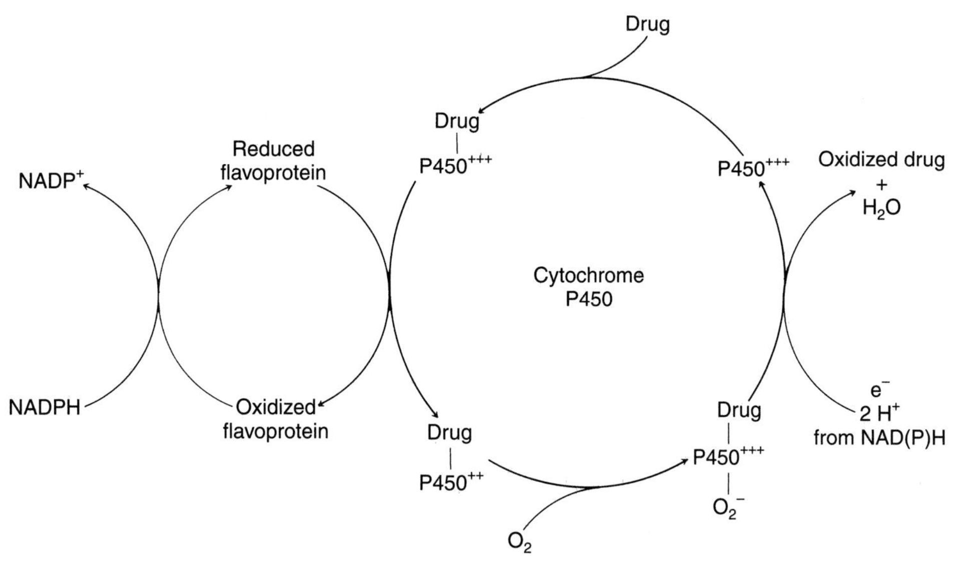

Fig. 2-9 Microsomal enzyme oxidation system. In the electron transport chain, the initial electron is passed from *NADPH* by the flavoprotein NADPH-cytochrome P450 reductase to the complex of drug and cytochrome P450. The second electron may come from the same source or from nicotinamide adenine dinucleotide *(NADH)* by the cytochrome b_5 pathway.

(desulfuration) or an amino group (deamination), or it may not appear in the metabolite at all but become attached to a hydrocarbon unit released during the dealkylation of nitrogen, oxygen, or sulfur. The various types of microsomal oxidations are reviewed along with other phase I reactions in Table 2-4.

Reduction

The microsomal reduction of drugs is limited to molecules with nitro or carbonyl groups or azo linkages. Similar reactions may also be mediated by nonmicrosomal enzymes of the body, but most reductions of this variety appear to result primarily from the action of enteric bacteria. When reduction occurs at one site in a molecule, oxidation usually takes place elsewhere, and the final product is more polar despite the initial addition of hydrogen atoms.

Hydrolysis

The hydrolysis of ester or amide compounds resulting in the production of two smaller entities, each with a polar end, occasionally depends on microsomal enzymes. The hydrolysis of the ester meperidine and the cleavage of amide local anesthetics and their oxidized metabolites are two important examples of microsomal hydrolysis. Epoxide hydrolase, responsible for the biotransformation of highly reactive and toxic intermediates formed during microsomal oxidation reactions, yields inactive dihydrodiol products.

Dehalogenation

Various compounds, such as chlorophenothane and some volatile general anesthetics (e.g., halothane and sevoflurane), are dehalogenated by microsomal enzymes. The reactions are complex, may involve oxidative as well as reductive steps, and may result in the formation of potentially toxic metabolites.[31]

Glucuronide conjugation

The combination of compounds with glucuronic acid is the only phase II reaction catalyzed by microsomal enzymes (in this case, by a group of glucuronosyltransferases). Originally derived from glucose, glucuronic acid is transferred from its donor, uridine diphosphate, to an appropriate reactive center on the drug molecule (Table 2-5). The glucuronide conjugate produced is then excreted, often by active secretion, into the bile or urine. Unlike many phase I reactions, conjugation with glucuronic acid almost invariably results in a total loss of pharmacologic activity. An important exception to this rule is morphine-6-glucuronide, which is 100 times more potent than morphine as an analgesic when injected into the CNS.[39] Some glucuronides excreted in the bile are subject to hydrolysis by bacterial and intestinal β-glucuronidase enzymes. If it has sufficient lipid solubility, the released drug may then be absorbed once again. Glucuronidation is a quantitatively significant metabolic pathway for many drugs and their metabolites; for agents like morphine, it represents the primary mode of metabolism.

Nonmicrosomal Metabolism

The pattern of drug metabolism mediated by nonmicrosomal enzymes is considerably different from that of the microsomal system. Although important, the liver is not always predominant in nonmicrosomal biotransformations. The various major types of nonsynthetic reactions already described take place, but their relative frequencies of occurrence are dissimilar. In general, drugs must resemble natural substrates to be metabolized by most nonmicrosomal enzymes; certainly, the spectacular lack of specificity displayed in microsomal oxidation has no counterpart here. Although cytosolic enzymes are most commonly involved, enzymes associated with the nucleus, mitochondria, and plasma membrane also play limited roles. Plasma esterase is an important example of an extracellular enzyme involved in drug metabolism.

Oxidation

Nonmicrosomal enzymes are responsible for the oxidation of a number of compounds. Selected alcohols and aldehydes are oxidized by dehydrogenases present in the cytosol of the liver. Other oxidation reactions include the oxidative deamination of drugs such as tyramine and phenylephrine by mitochondrial enzymes found in the liver, kidneys, and other organs and the hydroxylation of the purine derivatives theophylline and allopurinol by xanthine oxidase.

Reduction

Nonmicrosomal enzymes promote the hydrogenation of double bonds and, through a reversal of the normal dehydro-

Table • 2-4

Phase I Reactions—Metabolic Transformations

REACTION	EXAMPLE
MICROSOMAL ENZYME SYSTEM	
Oxidation	
$RCH_2R' \rightarrow RCH(OH)R'$ **Aliphatic hydroxylation** $R-C_6H_5 \rightarrow R-C_6H_4-OH$ **Aromatic hydroxylation** $RNHR' \rightarrow RN(OH)R'$ **N-hydroxylation**	$C_6H_5NHCOCH_3$ **Acetanilid** $\xrightarrow{[O]}$ $HO-C_6H_4-NHCOCH_3$ **Acetaminophen**
$RCH=CHR' \rightarrow RCH(-O-)CHR'$ **Epoxidation**	**Naphthalene** $\xrightarrow{[O]}$ naphthalene epoxide (H, O, H)
$RNHR' \rightarrow RNH_2 + R'=O$ **N-dealkylation** $ROR' \rightarrow ROH + R'=O$ **O-dealkylation** $RSCH_3 \rightarrow RSH + CH_2O$ **S-demethylation**	$C_2H_5O-C_6H_4-NHCOCH_3$ **Phenacetin** $\xrightarrow{[O]}$ $HO-C_6H_4-NHCOCH_3 + CH_3CHO$ **Acetaminophen**
$(R)_3N \rightarrow (R)_3N=O$ **N-oxidation** $RSR' \rightarrow RS(=O)R'$ **Sulfoxidation**	**Chlorpromazine** (S, N, Cl; $CH_2CH_2CH_2N(CH_3)_2$) $\xrightarrow{[O]}$ chlorpromazine sulfoxide (S=O, N, Cl; $CH_2CH_2CH_2N(CH_3)_2$)
$R_2CHNH_2 \rightarrow R_2CO + NH_3$ **Deamination** $RSH \rightarrow ROH$ **Desulfuration**	$C_6H_5-CH_2CH(CH_3)NH_2$ **Amphetamine** $\xrightarrow{[O]}$ $C_6H_5-CH_2C(CH_3)=O + NH_3$
Reduction	
$RC(=O)R' \rightarrow RCH(OH)R'$ **Carbonyl reduction** $RNO_2 \rightarrow RNH_2$ **Nitro reduction** $RN=NR' \rightarrow RNH_2 + R'NH_2$ **Azo reduction**	$O_2N-C_6H_4-CH(OH)CH(CH_2OH)NHC(=O)CHCl_2$ **Chloramphenicol** $\xrightarrow{[H]}$ $H_2N-C_6H_4-CH(OH)CH(CH_2OH)NHC(=O)CHCl_2$

Table • 2-4

Phase I Reactions—Metabolic Transformations—cont'd

REACTION	EXAMPLE
Hydrolysis $RCOOR' \rightarrow RCOOH + R'OH$ **Ester hydrolysis** $RNHCOR' \rightarrow RNH_2 + R'COOH$ **Amide hydrolysis**	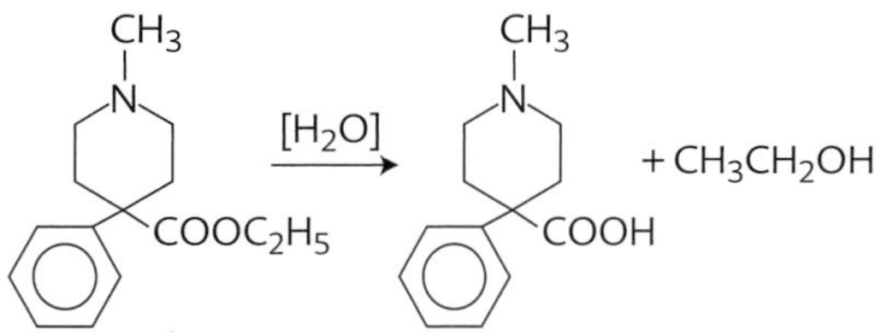 CH_3, N, $COOC_2H_5$ $\xrightarrow{[H_2O]}$ CH_3, N, $COOH$ + CH_3CH_2OH **Meperidine**
Dehalogenation Various reactions	$CF_3CHBrCl \xrightarrow{[O]} CF_3COOH$ **Halothane**
NONMICROSOMAL ENZYMES	
Oxidation $RCH_2OH \rightarrow RCHO$ **Alcohol dehydrogenation** $RCHO \rightarrow RCOOH$ **Aldehyde oxidation**	$CH_3CH_2OH \xrightarrow{[O]} CH_3CHO$ **Ethanol**
$RCH_2R' \rightarrow RCH(OH)R'$ **Aliphatic hydroxylation** 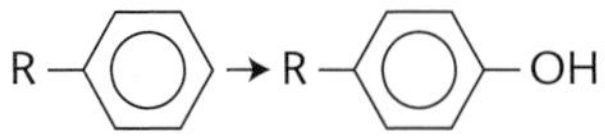 R–(benzene) → R–(benzene)–OH **Aromatic hydroxylation**	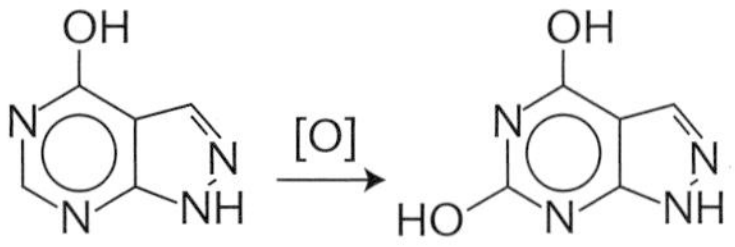 OH, N, N, N, NH $\xrightarrow{[O]}$ OH, N, N, N, NH, HO **Allopurinol**
$RCH_2NH_2 \rightarrow RCHO + NH_3$ **Deamination**	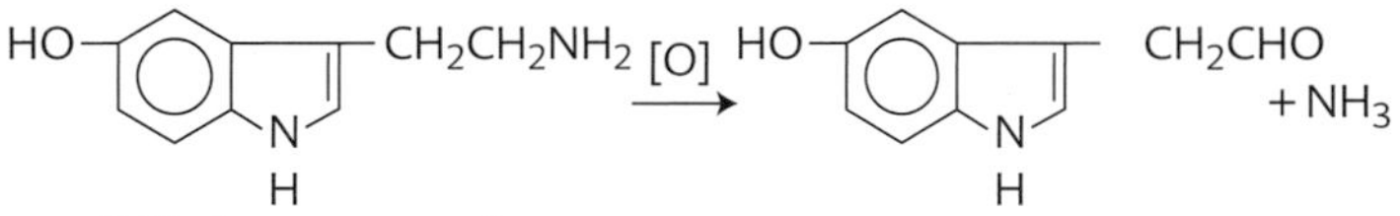 HO–(indole, N, H)–$CH_2CH_2NH_2$ $\xrightarrow{[O]}$ HO–(indole, N, H)–CH_2CHO + NH_3 **5-Hydroxytryptamine**
Reduction $ROH \rightarrow RH$ **Alcohol reduction**	$Cl_3C{-}CH(OH)OH \xrightarrow{[H]} Cl_3C{-}CH_2OH + H_2O$ **Chloral hydrate** **Trichloroethanol**
Various Reactions	$(C_2H_5)_2NC(=S){-}S{-}S{-}C(=S)N(C_2H_5)_2 \xrightarrow{[H]} 2(C_2H_5)_2NC(=S)SH$ **Disulfiram**
Hydrolysis $RCOOR' \rightarrow RCOOH + R'OH$ **Ester hydrolysis** $RNHCOR' \rightarrow RNH_2 + R'COOH$ **Amide hydrolysis**	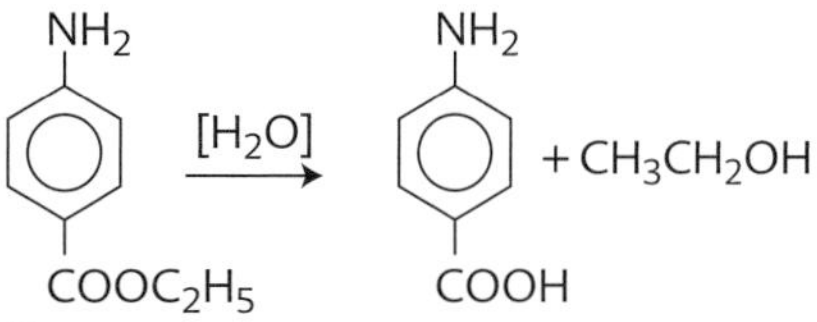 NH_2–(benzene)–$COOC_2H_5$ $\xrightarrow{[H_2O]}$ NH_2–(benzene)–$COOH$ + CH_3CH_2OH **Benzocaine**

Table 2-5

Phase II Reactions—Conjugations

CONJUGATION REACTION (COFACTOR)	SUBSTRATES	EXAMPLE
Glucuronide synthesis (uridine diphosphate)	Amines Carboxylic acids Alcohols Phenols Mercaptans	**Salicylic acid** (UDP-glucuronide)
Acetylation (coenzyme A)	Amines Hydrazines	**Sulfanilamide** (Acetyl-CoA)
Glycine conjugation (coenzyme A)	Carboxylic acids	**Salicylic acid** (CoA + Glycine)
Methylation (S-adenosyl-methionine)	Amines Phenols Mercaptans	**Norepinephrine** (SAM)
Sulfate addition (3′-phosphoadenosine-5′-phosphosulfate)	Aromatic amines Alcohols Phenols	**Acetaminophen** (PAPS)
Other reactions (various)	Purines Pyrimidines Epoxides and other reactive metabolites	**Naphthalene epoxide** (Glutathione)

genase pathway, the removal of oxygen atoms. The reduction of chloral hydrate to trichloroethanol by alcohol dehydrogenase is an often cited example of this latter type of reaction.

Hydrolysis

Most hydrolytic reactions of foreign substances depend on nonmicrosomal esterase and amidase enzymes. Nonspecific esterases are found throughout the body but the two most important sites, by virtue of their hydrolytic capacity and availability to drugs, are the liver and plasma. Ester local anesthetics such as procaine and benzocaine are hydrolyzed by these enzymes. Except for blood and other tissue peptidases responsible for the breakdown of pharmacologically active polypeptides, most amidase activities reside in the liver.

Conjugation reactions

A number of synthetic reactions are catalyzed by nonmicrosomal transferase enzymes. As with the microsomal synthesis of glucuronides, the body usually supplies an acidic moiety (e.g., sulfate, acetate, cysteine, glycine, glutamine, or riboside phosphate) attached to a particular cofactor or carrier molecule. The addition of methyl groups to phenols, mercaptans, and amines may lead to less polar compounds, but even here subsequent oxidation or conjugation reactions decrease lipid solubility. With amines, methylation may even increase polarity, as in the formation of a quaternary ammonium cation. The quantitative contributions of the various phase II reactions are illustrated in Figure 2-8.

Conjugation with glutathione is unusual in that it is directed against highly reactive metabolites, such as epoxides and quinones, and may occur with or without enzymatic support. Although a quantitatively minor pathway, glutathione conjugation may be of major importance in preventing metabolism-induced drug toxicity.

Phase II reactions can be expected whenever a drug carries one or more of the reactive centers listed in Table 2-5. Such conjugations generally result in the termination of drug effect, restriction in the apparent V_d, and acceleration of drug excretion, often through active secretory processes.

Nonhepatic Metabolism

Although focusing on the liver when considering biotransformation in general is appropriate, other tissues also contain drug-metabolizing enzymes, including members of the CYP family, and contribute to the microsomal and nonmicrosomal metabolism of drugs. This ability is occasionally taken advantage of by preparing prodrugs that become metabolically activated in target tissues. The aforementioned use of levodopa to circumvent the blood-brain barrier is an example of this approach; administration of acyclovir, an antiviral prodrug that is converted to the active nucleotide form in diseased cells (see Chapter 40), is another. By virtue of location and blood supply, certain organs play special roles in drug metabolism. As previously discussed in the context of bioavailability, the intestine, working alone or in concert with the liver, can metabolize some drugs so completely that the oral route cannot be used for their administration. CYP3A4 is the principal enzyme involved. The kidney is well suited for drug metabolism because it has a well-developed microsomal enzyme system and receives a bountiful blood supply. Glucuronidation is an especially prominent activity.

In recent years, the role of the lung in drug disposition has been an active area of investigation. By means of the pulmonary circulation, virtually all the blood is exposed to lung tissue with each circulation. Studies have shown that the lung is a primary site for metabolism of endogenous blood-borne compounds such as bradykinin, angiotensin I, prostaglandins, and biogenic amines.[43] Its role in the biotransformation of purely exogenous compounds was discounted because the liver has such a high content of drug-metabolizing enzymes. However, this reasoning fails to account for the important influence of blood flow or drug delivery on the metabolism of some drugs. Thus whereas the activity of arylhydrocarbon hydroxylase in the liver is more than 1000 times that of the lung, the pulmonary metabolism of benzo[*a*]pyrene by this enzyme in vivo may approach or even exceed the hepatic rate.[43]

Factors Affecting Drug Metabolism

The rate of drug biotransformation depends on numerous variables. These include access to the site of metabolism, the concentration and phenotype of the enzyme present, and the effect of certain agents on enzymatic activity. Because most drugs are metabolized in the liver, attention is centered on factors influencing hepatic drug biotransformation.

Entry into the liver

As stated previously, plasma protein binding can significantly reduce the rate of uptake and metabolism of drugs by the liver. Inverse correlations between the rate of biotransformation and the degree of protein binding have been reported for sulfonamides, warfarin, and phenytoin, among others.[16] A similar relationship also holds for drugs bound to extravascular reservoirs. For some compounds, however, plasma protein binding does not hinder metabolism and may even enhance it. Lidocaine and propranolol are so effectively absorbed by hepatic tissues that, even with significant binding, the clearance of these drugs from the body is primarily limited by hepatic blood flow. Because protein binding retains extra drug within the vascular compartment, more is presented to the liver per unit of time for metabolism.

Certain disease states and drug interactions can affect the accessibility of liver enzymes to pharmacologic agents. Uremia, by reducing the binding capacity of albumin, promotes the biotransformation of some highly bound drugs. Because inflammation and stress increase the plasma concentration of α_1-acid glycoprotein, the opposite effect may occur with some basic drugs.[54] Hepatic damage can affect drug delivery to the liver in several ways. For example, it may lead to reduced plasma protein concentrations and altered drug binding. Decreased metabolism of bilirubin and other substrates may also alter distribution of a drug and its availability for hepatic uptake. Entry into the liver may further be slowed by decreased carrier-mediated transport. Finally, cirrhosis, cardiac insufficiency, and other conditions that reduce hepatic blood flow may significantly retard the metabolism of lidocaine and like agents whose biotransformation is normally limited by the rate of drug delivery to the liver.

Enzyme inhibition

Drug-metabolizing enzymes are subject to competitive and noncompetitive antagonism. Because so many drugs are acted on by the CYP system, competitive inhibition of microsomal oxidation is easily demonstrated in the laboratory. Fortunately, drug interactions of this type are usually not clinically important. In many instances, the rate of biotransformation is limited not by the CYP electron transport chain but by the movement of drugs into the smooth endoplasmic reticulum. Some compounds, however, exhibit saturation kinetics and are restricted in metabolism by the rate of binding to specific CYP enzymes. Competition involving these agents (e.g., phenytoin and dicumarol competing for CYP2C9) is of practical significance.

A variety of metabolic poisons—carbon monoxide, cyanide, heavy metals—noncompetitively inhibit microsomal biotransformation. These actions are only of experimental interest, though, because effects on respiration and other vital processes take precedence in vivo. A much more specific inhibition of microsomal oxidation is achieved with proadifen, which avidly binds to the heme iron of CYP. This compound blocks the metabolism of a great number of agents dependent on CYP enzymes; it can also inhibit glucuronidation. The effect on most drugs is a prolongation of action, but compounds requiring microsomal activation may have a loss of potency. The plethora of substances affected by proadifen prohibits its use in human beings; however, similar compounds find application as potentiators of insecticides that are inactivated by microsomal biotransformation. Clinically useful drugs that inhibit the metabolism of numerous other agents by inactivating various CYP enzymes include the macrolide antibiotics (other than azithromycin), chloramphenicol, certain imidazole derivatives (cimetidine and the azole antifungals), and amiodarone (see Table 2-3). These drugs—or their metabolites—react covalently or otherwise strongly with specific sites on the CYP molecule. St. John's wort and grapefruit juice are herbal and dietary constituents, respectively, that powerfully inhibit certain classes of CYP enzymes.

Several drugs are used specifically as inhibitors of selected nonmicrosomal enzymes. When the enzyme affected happens to be responsible for the inactivation of other therapeutic agents, drug interactions are likely to develop. Examples of such enzymes are monoamine oxidase, pseudocholinesterase, and xanthine oxidase. The inhibition of aldehyde dehydrogenase by disulfiram is exceptional because that drug's primary indication is to interrupt the metabolism of another foreign compound, ethanol (see Chapter 43).

Enzyme induction

Microsomal drug-metabolizing enzymes are inducible; under an appropriate chemical stimulus, catalytic activity will increase. Many chemicals, including therapeutic agents, "social" drugs, and environmental toxins, are capable of stimulating their own biotransformation and that of closely related compounds. In addition, some chemicals can augment the breakdown of a whole host of diverse substances. Phenobarbital illustrates this latter type of induction. On reaching the cytosol of the hepatocyte, phenobarbital binds to a transcription factor termed the *constitutive androstane receptor*, which then migrates into the nucleus to activate genes with the appropriate response elements. Several hours thereafter, an elevation in hepatic protein synthesis becomes apparent. Reductions in the metabolic half-lives of affected drugs are paralleled by increases in microsomal weight and in the concentrations of NADPH-cytochrome P450 reductase and several CYP enzymes (most importantly CYP2B6, 2C8/9, 2C18/19, and 3A4/5). The liver eventually hypertrophies, and hepatic blood flow and bile secretion are likewise enhanced. Rifampin, another broad-spectrum inducer, binds to a closely related protein termed the *pregnane X receptor* to initiate a similar response.

By way of contrast, benzo[*a*]pyrene exemplifies agents with a more restrictive form of induction. Although benzo[*a*]pyrene requires new enzyme formation for its stimulation of metabolism (inhibitors of protein synthesis block its action), structural changes in the smooth endoplasmic reticulum are not prominent and may be undetectable. Enzyme induction in this case principally involves the CYP1 gene family (CYP1A1/2 and CYP1B1). The transcription factor for benzo[*a*]pyrene and many other aromatic hydrocarbons and heterocyclics is the *aryl hydrocarbon receptor*.

No matter the pattern of induction, the rate of metabolism of affected compounds may be enhanced experimentally by as much as seven times the baseline. Stimulation is usually less pronounced clinically; nevertheless, enzyme induction has many important therapeutic ramifications. It is, for instance, a major cause of drug interactions. A classic example of this form of drug interaction is the stimulation by phenobarbital of the metabolism of the anticoagulant dicumarol, which causes standard doses of the anticoagulant to be ineffective.[10] Induction of microsomal enzymes leading to a loss of pharmacologic responsiveness is referred to as *pharmacokinetic tolerance*. Finally, enzyme induction may affect the function of endogenous chemicals metabolized microsomally. Acceleration of vitamin D oxidation to yield inactive products is the leading cause of rickets and osteomalacia in epileptic patients receiving medications such as phenytoin and phenobarbital.[19]

It would seem an obvious outcome that enzyme induction should decrease drug toxicity in concert with any reduction in drug potency. Surprisingly, this is not always the case. Of strong concern in the field of toxicology is the potential danger posed by highly reactive intermediary substances produced during microsomal oxidation of drugs such as acetaminophen, halothane, and benzo[*a*]pyrene.[38] These substances are normally synthesized in such limited quantities that succeeding reactions, including hydrolysis and glutathione conjugation, inactivate the compounds before cellular injury can ensue. Selective microsomal enzyme induction, however, may so increase their synthesis that subsequent protective reactions become overwhelmed. In agreement with this thesis is the estimate that cigarette smokers who exhibited high inducibility of arylhydrocarbon hydroxylase activity, which converts benzo[*a*]pyrene and related polycyclic hydrocarbons into epoxide intermediates, were estimated to have a 36-fold increased risk of developing bronchogenic carcinoma than people having low inducibility.[23]

Genetic factors

Individuals vary in their ability to metabolize drugs. Although differences can result from the environmental induction of microsomal enzymes (as seen in chemical factory workers and cigarette smokers), studies comparing identical and fraternal twins have conclusively established the preeminent influence of heredity on the rate of biotransformation.[51] For some drugs, the range in metabolic half-life may exceed an order of magnitude, but usually this figure is restricted to a value of two or three. The ability to metabolize a particular type of compound at an abnormal rate does not usually signify anything concerning the biotransformation of unrelated substances. However, normal individuals exhibiting the lowest microsomal metabolism rates are the most likely to undergo profound enzyme induction after phenobarbital treatment.[51]

Genetic influences on metabolism are most easily characterized when single genes are involved. A good example of this principle is provided by the plasma enzyme pseudocholinesterase. Approximately one individual in 3000 is homozygous for an atypical gene whose enzyme product metabolizes esters very slowly. A conventional dose of the muscle relaxant succinylcholine produces prolonged apnea in these patients. Those with a combination of typical and atypical genes (heterozygotes) still have enough normal enzyme to hydrolyze the drug fast enough to avoid unusual clinical manifestations. Since the discovery of the atypical gene for pseudocholinesterase, other novel genotypes have been described, including one that is "silent" (its product has no enzymatic activity whatsoever)[3] and one that yields an enzyme so effective in catalysis that patients with it exhibit a remarkable innate resistance to the paralyzing effect of succinylcholine.[36] The pharmacogenetics of drug metabolism are explored more fully in Chapter 4.

Age

Neonates, especially premature infants, often lack certain functional drug-metabolizing systems. The relative inability to conjugate bilirubin with glucuronic acid and the resultant development of hyperbilirubinemia is a commonly observed example of this deficiency in biotransformation. The failure to account for marked quantitative differences in neonatal metabolism is tragically highlighted by the "gray syndrome" and infant death associated with chloramphenicol.[52] Unlike newborn infants, children are often more adept at metabolizing drugs on a weight basis than are young adults.[48] Thereafter, biotransformation capacity appears to diminish with age; the elderly may often exhibit retarded rates of drug metabolism.

Pathology

Obviously, significant destruction of the hepatic parenchyma with loss of drug-metabolizing enzymes can directly depress the biotransformation of many agents. The clinical effect, however, may be quite small because of the liver's reserve metabolic capacity and because of enzyme induction in the unaffected tissue. (See Chapter 3 for further discussion of hepatic dysfunction and patient response.)

A more subtle effect of pathology is exemplified by the influence of infection on hepatic metabolism.[42] Viral illnesses have been linked to depression of CYP activity and inhibition of the microsomal oxidation of theophylline and a few other drugs. Interferons produced in response to these diseases or to vaccines prepared from disrupted virions may actually cause the inhibition. Several nonviral infections, such as malaria, leprosy, and various forms of pneumonia, have also been associated with impaired drug biotransformation.

Finally, endocrine derangements may alter drug metabolism. Hypothyroidism may slow biotransformation of certain drugs; hyperthyroidism tends to have the opposite effect. In animals, derangements of the pituitary gland, adrenal cortex, and gonads have been shown to affect drug metabolism; whether similar effects occur in human beings is unknown.

EXCRETION

Foreign substances, including therapeutic medications, are prevented from building up in the body by the combined action of metabolism and excretion. Drugs and their metabolites may be eliminated by a number of routes: urine, bile, sweat, saliva and other gastrointestinal secretions, pulmonary exhalation, tears, and breast milk. Quantitative considerations make the kidney the major organ of drug excretion.

Renal Excretion

Three processes—glomerular filtration, tubular reabsorption, and active transport—control the urinary elimination of drugs. Although all drugs are subject to filtration, the percentage filtered varies inversely according to the degree of plasma protein binding and to the V_d. Once filtered, agents tend to be resorbed in relation to their lipid/water partition coefficients. These considerations favor the renal excretion of highly polar compounds, but the exact rate of elimination also depends on whether active transport into (or, rarely, out of) the tubular fluid also occurs.

Glomerular filtration

Each day the kidneys filter approximately 180 L of plasma. Arterial blood entering Bowman's capsule is routed through a tuft of capillaries collectively described as the *glomerulus.* These capillaries are uniquely modified for filtration, having large numbers of pores with an effective diameter to 80 Å penetrating through the endothelium. Approximately one fifth of the plasma entering the glomerular apparatus is actually filtered, the remainder exiting by way of efferent arterioles to supply other portions of the nephron. In general, molecules smaller than albumin (molecular weight 69,000) appear in the tubular fluid. Because plasma proteins are almost completely retained within the bloodstream, bound drugs are not subject to filtration.

Tubular reabsorption

Because only approximately 1.5 L of urine is actually excreted every 24 hours (less than 1% of the daily filtered load), the kidney must have an efficient reabsorption system. Indeed, were this not the case, a person would lose valuable fluid and nutrients and quickly die. Approximately 80% of the glomerular filtrate is reclaimed by the proximal convoluted tubule. A high-capacity pump actively transports Na^+ back into the bloodstream, with anions (principally Cl^-) and water following passively. This process continues throughout the nephron and is aided by specific transport systems, such as in the ascending loop of Henle, where co-transport of Na^+, K^+, and Cl^- occurs. In addition, the reabsorption of Na^+ is aided by its exchange with H^+ and, in the distal convoluted tubule, K^+. The resultant concentration of the tubular fluid creates a chemical gradient for the diffusion of drugs back into the systemic circulation. Agents with a favorable lipid/water partition coefficient then readily traverse the tubular epithelium and escape from the urine.

A major factor influencing the reabsorption of weak electrolytes from renal tubular fluid is the pH. Depending on the rate of H^+ secretion, the urinary pH may vary from 4.5 to 8.0. Weak acids such as aspirin and phenobarbital are reabsorbed more effectively under acidic conditions; the reverse is true for weak bases such as amphetamine and ephedrine. On occasion, the influence of pH on drug excretion is used to clinical advantage. Thus a common strategy in the face of aspirin toxicity is to promote salicylate elimination through alkalization of the urine by the systemic administration of sodium bicarbonate. For the sulfonamides (also weak acids), alkalization of the urine may reduce the plasma half-life by 50% and prevent the development of crystalluria by increasing aqueous solubility.[16] Of course, attempts to enhance renal excretion are of little value for agents whose inactivation depends largely on biotransformation.

Active secretion

Numerous organic cations and anions are actively secreted by cells of the proximal convoluted tubule. The anionic transport system, responsible for the secretion of amphipathic anions and conjugated metabolites (e.g., glucuronides, sulfates), involves transporters such as P-glycoprotein and multidrug resistance–associated protein type 2. The cationic transport mechanism moves compounds with charged amino groups. Because each transport carrier is rather nonselective, competition for binding sites is sometimes observed. Probenecid, an acidic anion, has been used to block the active secretion of another acid, penicillin G. The inhibition of penicillin excretion was beneficial at a time when the drug was in short supply and still finds use when it is necessary to maintain a high concentration of the antibiotic for prolonged periods.

Specific carrier systems of the kidney, found principally in the distal convoluted tubule, actively reabsorb certain agents. The most important active resorption of organic ions by this mechanism involves uric acid. Because probenecid can compete with urate ions as readily as it can with penicillin, probenecid finds application in gout as a promoter of uric acid excretion.

Active secretion of substances into the urine is not adversely affected by plasma protein binding. The transport is often so effective that drug dissociation takes place instantly, making available more drug for secretion, until all the drug has been cleared from the local blood supply. Binding to extravascular tissues, however, does reduce the rate of renal elimination, regardless of the mechanisms involved.

Clearance

The amount of drug removed by the kidney per unit of time is often evaluated as a function of the plasma water "cleared" of drug. Mathematically, the volume of plasma cleared per minute (CL) can be written as $CL = U \times V/P$, where U is the urinary concentration of drug, V is the volume of urine produced per minute, and P is the plasma concentration. The clearance and V_d are related by the simple formula $CL = k_e \times V_d$, where k_e is the elimination rate constant. Agents that are filtered but not resorbed or secreted, such as inulin, yield a clearance of 130 ml/min (assuming no plasma protein binding) and serve as a measure of the glomerular filtration rate. With a V_d of 12 L, this clearance rate translates into a plasma half-life for inulin of 64 minutes. Compounds actively secreted into the urine and not reabsorbed, such as penicillin G and *p*-aminohippurate, may approach a clearance of 650 ml/min, which is the rate of total plasma flow through the kidneys. Assuming a V_d of 12 L, such a drug would have a plasma half-life of approximately 13 minutes. By way of contrast, drugs that are highly bound and subject to passive reabsorption may exhibit clearance rates approaching 0.

Biliary Excretion

A number of cationic, anionic, and steroidlike molecules are selectively removed from the blood for excretion into the bile and eventually the feces. In general, these substances have molecular weights exceeding 500 daltons. The transport process is an active one in which the dissolved substance is transferred from the plasma to the hepatocytes and then to the bile. As in all situations of this kind, special energy-requiring mechanisms for such transfers exist.[24] The aforementioned organic anion transporting polypeptide family of transporters includes members that facilitate uptake into the liver cytoplasm of such diverse chemicals as bile acids, digoxin, and methotrexate. Other carrier systems exist for cationic molecules but have not been as well characterized. P-glycoprotein and multidrug resistance–associated protein type 2 are important transporters for moving drugs from liver cells to the bile. These proteins are also involved in the transfer of acidic metabolites produced by hepatic CYP3A and phase II reactions into the bile, plasma, or both.

Biliary excretion is responsible for all but a small portion of the fecal elimination of drugs. The remainder results from direct transmucosal passage into the gastrointestinal tract from the bloodstream or represents compounds dissolved in one or more gastrointestinal tract secretions. Of course, the feces may also contain a variable amount of unabsorbed drug as well. Reabsorption of molecules excreted through the bile can occur, such as with the laxative phenolphthalein. Such enterohepatic recycling can prolong the duration of action and may continue ad infinitum until the system is interrupted (e.g., by metabolism, curtailment of bile flow, or ingestion of drug chelator).

Other Routes of Excretion

Pulmonary excretion is a primary route for the elimination of gases and some volatile compounds. Except for the inhalation anesthetics, however, excretion of chemicals into the respiratory tree may be of more esthetic concern than pharmacokinetic interest. For example, halitosis produced by odoriferous agents (e.g., paraldehyde) may impair clinical suitability.

Elimination of drugs by breast milk is important, not because of any quantitative significance, but because it represents a potential danger to the nursing baby. Drugs of particular concern include lithium, various anticancer agents, and isoniazid.[6] The primary variable influencing the passage of drugs into milk is lipid solubility.

Other minor routes of excretion include sweat; tears; saliva; and gastric, pancreatic, and intestinal secretions. In all cases, excretion is limited by the lipid/water partition coefficient. For saliva and related gastrointestinal fluids, drugs are deposited into the gastrointestinal tract after secretion and are available for reabsorption into the systemic circulation.

TIME COURSE OF DRUG ACTION

The close correspondence between the plasma concentration of an agent and its magnitude of effect has already been emphasized. Because drug administration usually encompasses the linear midrange of the log dose–response curve, the relationship between plasma titer and patient reaction is often straightforward. Thus a temporal description of drug concentration on the basis of pharmacokinetic principles is useful in illustrating how absorption, distribution, metabolism, and excretion influence drug effects in concert and in providing guidance for adjusting dosage schedules to achieve therapeutic results with a minimum of drug toxicity.

Kinetics of Absorption and Elimination

Most biologic events involving the fate of drugs can be described in simple kinetic terms: zero order, first order, or capacity limited (a combination of the two).

Zero-order kinetics

Zero-order kinetics define processes that occur at a constant rate per unit of time. Mathematically this can be written as $dC/dt = k_o$, where dC/dt is the rate of change in concentration and k_o is a constant in units of amount per time. A good example of zero-order input of drugs is the continuous intravenous infusion in which the quantity of compound entering the bloodstream each minute is held constant (e.g., 5 mg/min). Another example of zero-order absorption is provided by the intramuscular or subcutaneous injection of a depot form of drug. Poor aqueous solubility of the preparation permits a constant rate of drug release for hours. With oral administration, essentially zero-order absorption is realized whenever the rate-limiting factor is the dissolution of the primary drug particles. Finally, topical therapy often results in zero-order uptake. As long as the agent is in great excess, a relatively fixed quantity of drug permeates the skin per unit of time.

First-order kinetics

First-order kinetics relate to events that occur at a constant fractional rate per unit of time (e.g., 5%/min). Here $dC/dt = k_1C$, with k_1 representing the fractional rate constant in units of $time^{-1}$ and C representing the drug concentration. The absorption, distribution, and elimination of compounds commonly exhibit this type of kinetics because they generally rely on processes that are first-order in character: passive diffusion, filtration, blood flow, or drug transport or metabolism operating well below saturation. Because the fraction of drug affected per unit of time is independent of concentration, referring to the reaction rate by its half-life ($t_{1/2}$), the period required for the process to reach 50% of completion, is often useful. The half-life is related to the fractional rate constant by the formula $t_{1/2} = 0.693/k_1$. Thus the greater the rate constant, the shorter the half-life and the faster the reaction. It is easily shown that first-order processes are essentially complete (94%) after four half-lives. Figure 2-10 provides an example of the first-order elimination of a drug with a $t_{1/2}$ of 2 hours, and Table 2-6 lists the elimination half-lives of some commonly used categories of drugs in dentistry.

Capacity-limited reactions

Capacity-limited reactions involve enzymes responsible for the metabolism of drugs and carrier molecules concerned with drug transport across membranes. This kind of process initially displays zero-order kinetics when the endogenous factor (enzyme or carrier) is saturated with drug; it gradually takes on the features of a first-order reaction as the drug concentration falls. As already stated, doses used clinically are usually below those required for saturation. Some exceptions exist, however, in which saturation kinetics are evident. Alcohol, even in moderately intoxicating doses, is metabolized at a constant rate of approximately 8 g/hr. Only when the concentration falls far below that producing any observable effect does alcohol dehydrogenation assume a first-order rate.

Another important instance of capacity-limited biotransformation involves aspirin. Aspirin is quickly deacetylated to salicylate, the anion responsible for much of the drug's pharmacologic activity. The salicylate is then eliminated through several metabolic pathways and by renal excretion, yielding an overall elimination half-life of approximately 3 hours. Some of the inactivation routes, though, are easily saturated, so that when an overdose is ingested the toxicity problem is compounded by a relative loss in elimination efficiency. Elimination half-lives can be calculated for drugs displaying capac-

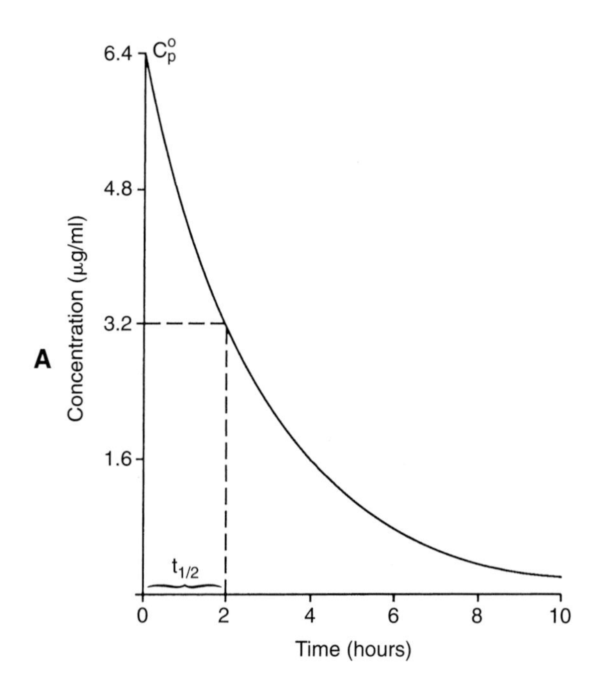

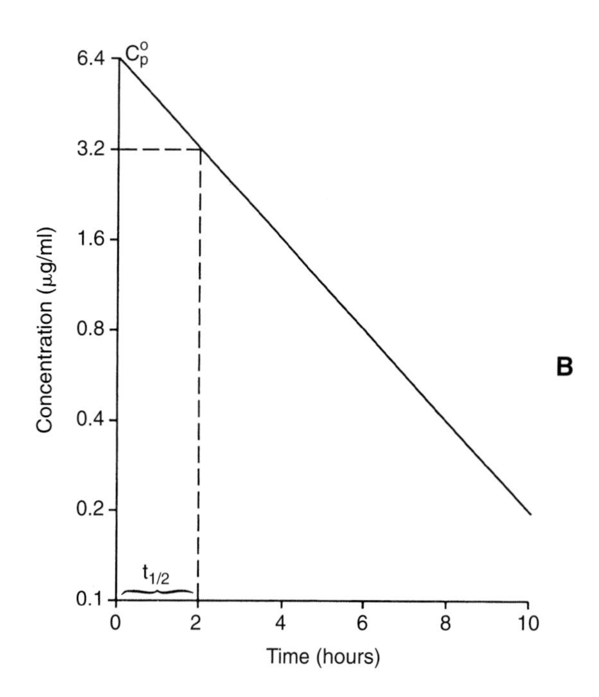

Fig. 2-10 First-order elimination of a drug given as an intravenous bolus. In this example of a plasma concentration-time curve, it is assumed that the body behaves as a single compartment and that the distribution of the drug is essentially instantaneous. In **A,** the plasma concentration is plotted on an arithmetic scale; in **B,** a logarithmic scale is used to yield a straight line. The elimination half-life *($t_{1/2}$)* is determined by the time interval required (2 hours in this case) for the plasma concentration to fall by 50%. C_p^o indicates the interpolated concentration of drug immediately after drug injection.

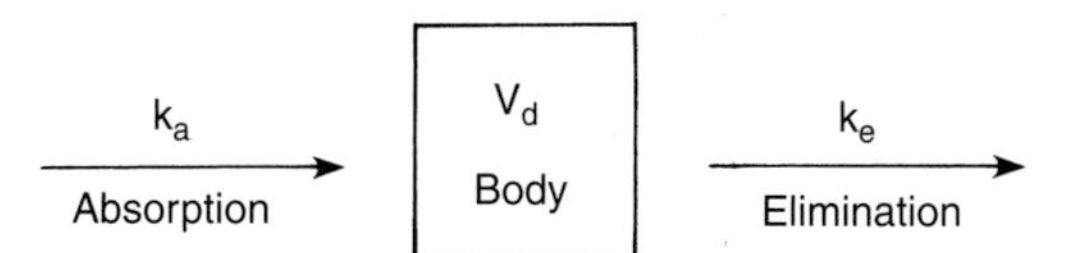

Fig. 2-11 Single-compartment model of drug kinetics. Absorption into and elimination from the body are each assigned a single first-order rate constant. Distribution, assumed to be rapid regarding both absorption and elimination, is not considered.

ity-limited kinetics, but the values obtained vary continuously according to the drug concentration (see Table 2-6). Thus salicylate has a plasma half-life of 20 hours when a very high concentration is present in the bloodstream. As the salicylate titer falls into the therapeutic range, the elimination half-life decreases to a constant of 3 hours.

Single-Compartment Model

In its entirety, the body's disposition of an administered drug involves such a complex temporal interplay of biochemical and physiologic processes, each with its own unique set of kinetic parameters, that a full quantitative description of the time course of drug action may be impossible to achieve. However, for practical purposes, the sojourn of many agents can be described by a simple model system (Figure 2-11) in which the body is depicted as a single compartment whose size corresponds to the V_d and whose elimination is based on first-order kinetics. In this model, which assumes rapid distribution regarding absorption and elimination, the relationships among elimination half-life, total body clearance (CL, or the volume of blood "cleared" of the drug per unit of time by the combined processes of metabolism and excretion), and V_d are straightforward, as follows:

$$t_{1/2} = 0.693 \times V_d/CL$$

The unknowns of this equation are best determined by injecting the drug intravenously (thus eliminating the absorption variable) and then measuring the plasma concentration at regular intervals sufficient to construct a plasma concentration-time curve, as shown in Figure 2-10. Given an initial dose of 500 mg (Q) and an initial plasma concentration of 6.4 µg/ml (C_p^o), determined by extrapolating the plasma concentration curve back to the moment of injection, V_d equals Q/C_p^o or approximately 78 L. With a $t_{1/2}$ of 2 hours, CL approximates 27 L/hr or 450 ml/min.

The elimination half-life is a dependent variable based on two independent attributes: the V_d and drug clearance. If a drug exhibits an increased half-life in a patient, this could mean that tissue binding of the drug is greater than normal just as easily as it could indicate a reduction in the rate of metabolism or excretion of the agent. Similarly, a significant reduction in V_d, which can occur in some diseases, could have the curious result of reducing the half-life of a drug even in the face of impaired clearance.

Plasma concentration—single doses

Therapeutic agents are often administered in dental practice as single doses. Whether the drug is lidocaine injected for regional anesthesia, atropine to control salivation, or midazolam to provide preoperative sedation, the plasma concentration rises to a peak during the absorptive phase and subsequently falls, eventually to zero, as the drug is eliminated from the bloodstream. By using the single-compartment

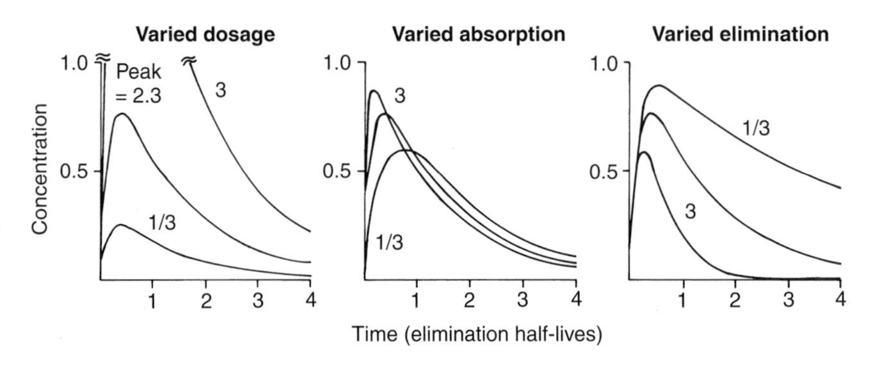

Fig. 2-12 Time course of plasma concentration after single doses of drug. The various curves illustrate the influence of threefold increases (3) or decreases (1/3) of dosage, absorption, and elimination on drug titers. The standard curve reproduced in all three graphs represents an agent whose first-order absorption rate is 10 times faster than elimination. A concentration of 1.0 is the value that would result if the drug were absorbed instantaneously, as with an intravenous injection.

model, it is possible to construct theoretical plasma concentration curves and observe how modifications of dosage, absorption, or elimination can alter drug concentrations and, presumably, drug effects. (Similar curves can also be generated by zero-order absorption.) As shown in Figure 2-12, the plasma concentration is at all times directly proportional to the dose. This relationship, of course, does not hold for agents that are capacity limited in absorption, binding, metabolism, or excretion.

As long as absorption is several times faster than elimination, changes in the rate of drug uptake have little effect other than to alter somewhat the peak concentration. The duration of action is hardly influenced at all. A different pattern emerges, however, in those instances in which the rate of absorption approximates that of elimination (not shown in Figure 2-12), either because a timed-release formulation is used to slow absorption or because the drug is quickly metabolized or excreted. As exemplified by penicillin G ($t_{1/2}$ of 30 minutes), the slow absorption achieved by oral ingestion relative to its swift excretion results in a peak concentration that is much reduced and considerably delayed compared with intravenous injection. On the positive side, oral administration can result in a duration of effect that is significantly prolonged.

Variations in the elimination rate markedly affect the postabsorptive phase of drug action. As shown in Figure 2-12, a threefold decrease in elimination can be more effective than a similar increase in the dose in extending the duration of effect. Because the peak titer is generally not nearly as sensitive to changes in elimination as it is to alterations in dosage, retarding elimination may be the better approach to lengthening the duration of effect of compounds with a low or moderate margin of safety. For penicillin G, retarding of elimination can be accomplished by inhibiting urinary excretion through the coadministration of probenecid. Once again, however, penicillin G is an exception to the rule. This antibiotic has such a low toxicity that the drug's rapid elimination can be offset by simply multiplying the dose several times.

Table • 2-6

Approximate Half-Lives of Some Common Drugs

DRUG	ELIMINATION HALF-LIFE (hr)
Antibiotics	
Amoxicillin	1.7
Clindamycin	3
Erythromycin	1.5
Penicillin G	0.5
Tetracycline	10
Analgesics	
Acetaminophen	3
Aspirin (as salicylate)	3 to 20*
Codeine	3†
Meperidine	3
Morphine	2†
Local Anesthetics	
Articaine	0.4
Bupivacaine	2.4
Lidocaine	1.8†
Procaine	0.01
Sedative Agents	
Alcohol	1.4 to 20*
Diazepam	45†
Pentobarbital	30
Triazolam	3

*Capacity-limited metabolism.
†Converted to active metabolite.

Plasma concentration—repeated doses

Whenever a drug is administered more than once every four elimination half-lives, accumulation of the compound occurs within the body. Figure 2-13 demonstrates the result of continued use of a drug given either by intravenous infusion (a zero-order process) or by repetitive administration (first-order absorption of each dose). Regardless of the administration format, a plateau concentration is reached in approximately four elimination half-lives. The periodic fluctuations obtained with intermittent administration are a function of the absorption rate and the dosage interval. Approaching 50% of the peak concentration when absorption is very rapid and the dosage period equals the elimination half-life, such variations can be minimized by increasing the frequency of administration or retarding the rate of absorption.

The average steady-state concentration relative to the peak value obtainable after an initial dose can be determined by multiplying the number of doses administered per elimination half-life by 1.44. Thus the steady-state concentration of a drug given once every half-life equals 144% of the initial peak concentration. For diazepam ingested three times per day, the average equilibrium concentration approximates (assuming a half-life of 2 days) 1.44×6, or 8.6 times the peak concentration after a single dose. Of course, at least 8 days (four half-lives) are required to reach this final drug titer.

The gradual approach to steady-state concentrations associated with slowly eliminated drugs can either benefit or

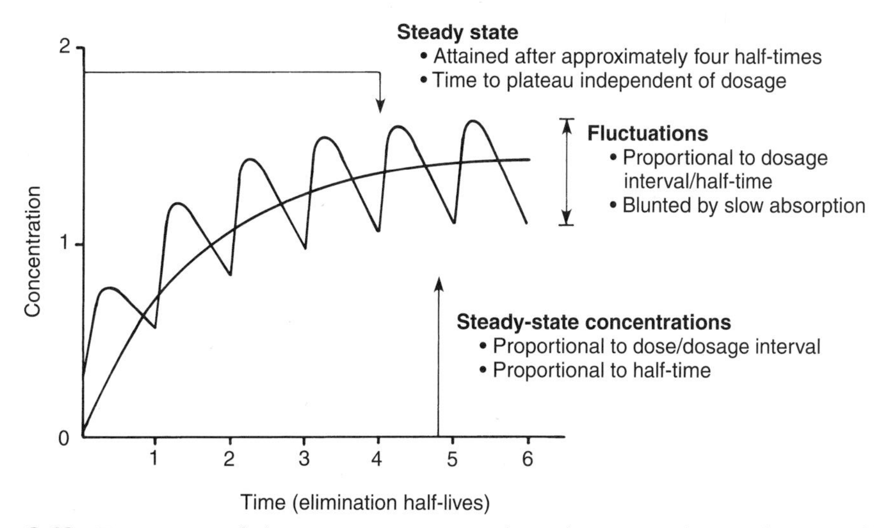

Fig. 2-13 Time course of plasma concentration involving drug accumulation. The *serrated line* reflects the pattern of accumulation observed during the repeated administration of a drug at intervals equal to its elimination half-life, when drug absorption is 10 times as rapid as elimination. As the relative rate of absorption increases, the concentration maximums approach twice the minimums during the steady state. The *smooth line* depicts drug accumulation during the administration of an equivalent dosage by continuous intravenous infusion. (Adapted from Benet LZ, Kroetz DL, Sheiner LB: Pharmacokinetics: the dynamics of drug absorption, distribution, and elimination. In Hardman JG, Limbird LE, Gilman AG, eds: *Goodman & Gilman's The pharmacological basis of therapeutics*, ed 9, New York, 1996, McGraw-Hill.)

hinder therapy. On the positive side, a long half-life permits the clinician to administer the drug at convenient intervals, perhaps once a day, without having to be concerned with wide swings in plasma concentration. If patient monitoring reveals an unusual buildup of drug because of impaired metabolism or excretion or some other cause, time is available to adjust the dose before toxic effects ensue. On the debit side, however, the attainment of a therapeutic effect is delayed by the time required for drug accumulation to proceed. If an immediate pharmacologic effect is needed, a loading dose of the drug must be administered. A loading dose is a large, initial quantity of drug substituted for the normal amount to quickly produce a concentration approximating the steady state. For an agent given once each half-life, the loading dose equals twice the maintenance dose; for drugs given more frequently, the loading dose is relatively larger. Dividing a loading dose into several smaller fractions is often wise. The sacrifice of some speed in attaining a therapeutic concentration is usually more than compensated for by the ability to evaluate patient responses during the early phase of therapy. Indeed, the fact that elimination rates, which help regulate steady-state concentrations, can vary greatly among individuals should dictate caution whenever cumulative drug effects are sought.

Multiple-Compartment Models

For many drugs the simple single-compartment model does not adequately describe the early time course of plasma concentration. Large discrepancies are particularly likely to be observed when a relatively lipophilic drug is given intravenously, as in the use of CNS depressants for conscious sedation. In that situation, the assumption that the body acts as a single compartment does not hold, and one or more additional drug reservoirs must be postulated.

Figure 2-14 depicts a two-compartment model in which the drug is administered into a small central compartment. The agent may leave the central compartment either by distribution to a larger peripheral compartment or by processes of elimination. With time, a quasi–steady state is established between the central and peripheral reservoirs in which net redistribution back into the central compartment occurs as the drug is metabolized or excreted. In the example provided, which is analogous to the scenario in Figure 2-10, the initial high concentration (C_p^o) after a 500-mg dose reflects the smaller volume of distribution of the central compartment (V_c = 9.8 L). The central compartment consists of organs, such as the brain, heart, lungs, and kidneys, that receive a large blood supply. A terminal half-life is determined from the log-linear portion of the curve, but in this case the term reflects both distribution and elimination functions. Other parameters, such as the total V_d, are likewise more complex in derivation and interpretation than are their counterparts in the single-compartment model.[16] This complexity is compounded as the number of compartments in the model is increased. Nevertheless, multicompartment models are quite useful in understanding how the duration of a drug's effect after a single injection may be largely independent of the clearance rate or elimination half-life. In Figure 2-14, if the threshold concentration for a sedative effect of the drug was 10 µg/ml, a patient would recover from the sedation within 30 minutes, even if metabolism and excretion were completely blocked, simply by distribution into less well perfused tissues.

Context-Sensitive Half-Lives

The numerous variables of the multicompartment model make it impossible to predict intuitively the influence of individual pharmacokinetic parameters such as half-lives, V_d values, and clearance rates on the plasma-concentration profile of a highly lipid-soluble drug given repeatedly or continuously for a period of time. This situation poses a problem when intravenous agents are administered by continuous infusion for anesthesia or sedation. A partial solution involves the use of computer modeling to estimate context-sensitive half-

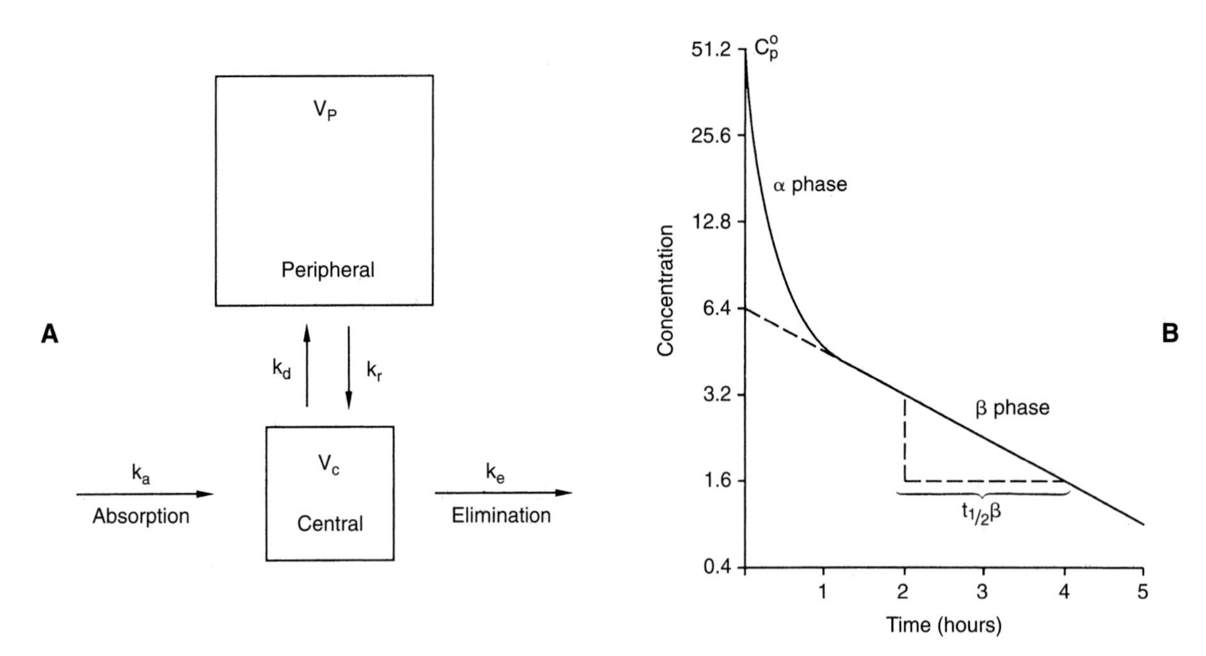

Fig. 2-14 Two-compartment model of drug kinetics. In this model **(A)**, drugs are absorbed into and eliminated from a central compartment that is linked by distribution processes (having rate constants of k_d and k_r) to a second, peripheral compartment. The central compartment includes the blood, from which drug determinations are taken. The plasma concentration-time curve **(B)** consists of two phases: an early distribution or *α phase*, during which the concentration falls largely as a result of distribution out of the central compartment, and a late elimination or *β phase* during which metabolism and excretion predominate. The terminal half-life *($t_{1/2}β$)* is calculated from the log-linear portion of the elimination curve.

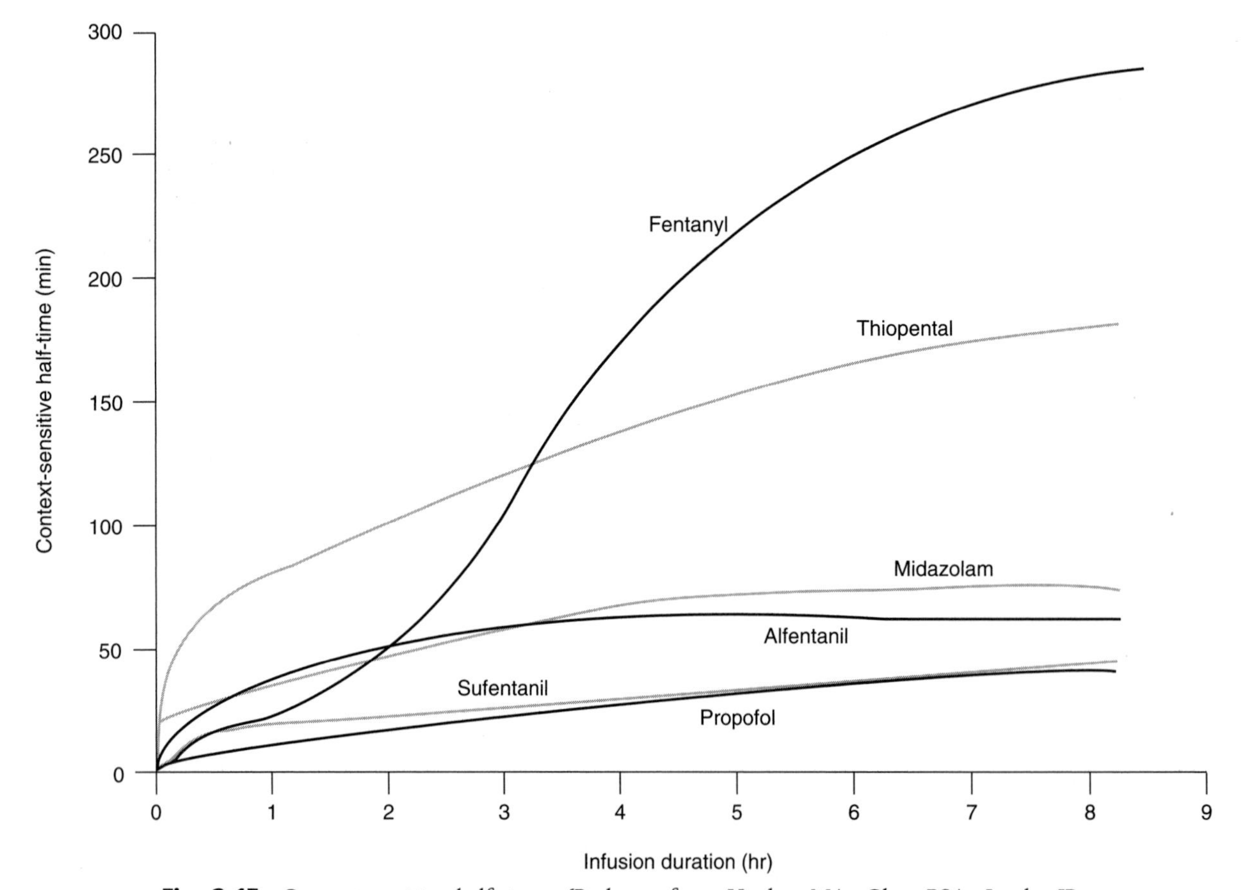

Fig. 2-15 Context-sensitive half-times. (Redrawn from Hughes MA, Glass PSA, Jacobs JR: Context-sensitive half-time in multicompartment pharmacokinetic models for intravenous anesthetic drugs, *Anesthesiology* 76:334-341, 1992.)

lives.[21] The context-sensitive half-life is the time required for the plasma concentration of a drug to fall by 50% when consideration is given to how long the drug has been infused. As illustrated in Figure 2-15, fentanyl demonstrates a significant rise in this parameter as the duration of infusion exceeds 2 hours. This phenomenon is the result of saturation of redistribution sites. Conversely, propofol, with its enormous capacity for redistribution, experiences only a slow rise over time. Such information is useful clinically in selecting the appropriate agent for use and in estimating the changing duration of drug effect. Similar context-sensitive curves can be generated for recovery to different percentages (e.g., 25%) of the plasma concentration, depending on what value best predicts recovery of function. Further advances in computer modeling will undoubtedly help address other limitations of the multicompartment model, such as the oscillations in arterial plasma concentrations that occur with bolus injection of drug and errors associated with the fact that some drugs are metabolized in more than a single compartment.[13]

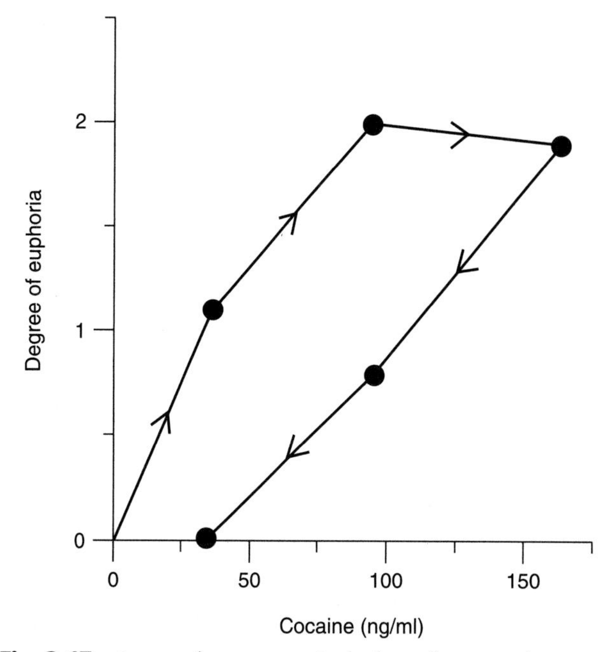

Fig. 2-17 Acute tolerance to a single dose of intranasal cocaine. The clockwise hysteresis loop indicates a loss of subjective drug effect as a function of the plasma concentration over time. (Data from Van Dyke C, Jatlow P, Ungerer J, et al: Oral cocaine: plasma concentrations and central effects, *Science* 200:211-213, 1978.)

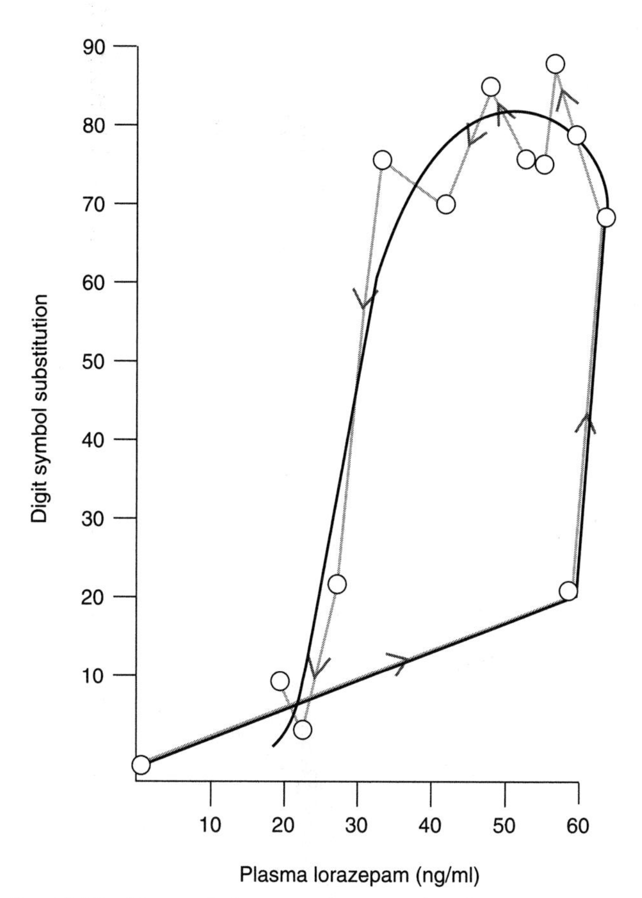

Fig. 2-16 Temporal distortion between the plasma concentration of lorazepam and cognition as measured by the digit symbol substitution test. The counterclockwise hysteresis loop indicates a delay in the distribution of lorazepam to its site of action within the brain. (Adapted from Gupta SK, Ellinwood EH, Nikaido AM, et al: Simultaneous modeling of the pharmacokinetic and pharmacodynamic properties of benzodiazepines. 1. Lorazepam, *J Pharmacokinet Biopharm* 18:89-102, 1990.)

PHARMACOKINETIC-PHARMACODYNAMIC MODELING

Two basic assumptions underlying pharmacokinetic studies are that the plasma concentration of a drug is predictive of the concentration around the site of drug action, and the magnitude of drug effect depends on this concentration. Although these assumptions generally hold, important exceptions to them do exist. As previously stated, drugs that bind covalently to their receptors produce effects that far outlast the drugs' passage in the bloodstream. Drugs that rely on transcription and protein synthesis are delayed in effect because of the time required for these processes to occur. Additional discrepancies between plasma concentration and drug effect arise because of delays in reaching the site of action and temporal changes that occur in receptor responsiveness. Pharmacokinetic-pharmacodynamic modeling seeks to account for these discrepancies.

Lorazepam provides a good example of a drug whose effects are temporally delayed (Figure 2-16). Lorazepam, a benzodiazepine used for relief of anxiety, must gain access to the CNS to stimulate its receptor and produce its characteristic CNS effects. The drug's modest lipid solubility, however, ensures that the peak plasma concentration after oral administration occurs before the drug has had any significant effect in the brain.[18]

Cocaine produces the opposite relationship in that maximal drug effects after oral administration precede the peak plasma concentration (Figure 2-17).[50] In this case, receptors that mediate the pharmacologic effect of cocaine undergo desensitization. Desensitization often involves a change in receptor sensitivity, either by phosphorylation of a regulatory subunit of the receptor or uncoupling of the receptor from its intracellular response system. Longer-lasting losses of drug responsiveness may include downregulation of receptors, in which the number of receptors decreases on continuous exposure to the drug.

CITED REFERENCES

1. Adriani J, Campbell D: Fatalities following topical application of local anesthetics to mucous membranes, *JAMA* 162:1527-1530, 1956.
2. Agre P, King LS, Yasui M, et al: Aquaporin water channels—from atomic structure to clinical medicine, *J Physiol* 542.1:3-16, 2002.
3. Altland K, Goedde HW: Heterogeneity in the silent gene phenotype of pseudocholinesterase of human serum, *Biochem Genet* 4:321-338, 1970.
4. Barchowsky A, Stargel WW, Shand DG, et al: Saliva concentrations of lidocaine and its metabolites in man, *Ther Drug Monit* 4:335-339, 1982.
5. Beckett AH, Hossie RD: Buccal absorption of drugs. In Brodie BB, Gillette JR, eds: *Handbook of experimental pharmacology*, Berlin, 1971, Springer-Verlag.
6. Berlin CM, Jr: Pharmacologic considerations of drug use in the lactating mother, *Obstet Gynecol* 58(suppl):17S-23S, 1981.
7. Bretscher MS: The molecules of the cell membrane, *Sci Am* 253:100-108, 1985.
8. Collander R: The permeability of plant protoplasts to small molecules, *Physiol Plantarum* 2:300-311, 1949.
9. Cooke AR, Hunt JN: Absorption of acetylsalicylic acid from unbuffered and buffered gastric contents, *Am J Dig Dis* 15:95-102, 1970.
10. Cucinell SA, Conney AH, Sansur M, et al: Drug interactions in man. I. Lowering effect of phenobarbital on plasma levels of bishydroxycoumarin (Dicumarol) and diphenylhydantoin (Dilantin), *Clin Pharmacol Ther* 6:420-429, 1965.
11. Evans WE, Relling MV: Pharmacogenomics: translating functional genomics into rational therapeutics, *Science* 286:487-491, 1999.
12. Feller K, le Petit G: On the distribution of drugs in saliva and blood plasma, *Int J Clin Pharmacol Biopharm* 15:468-469, 1977.
13. Fisher DM: (Almost) everything you learned about pharmacokinetics was (somewhat) wrong! *Anesth Analg* 83:901-903, 1996.
14. Gangarosa LP, Sr: Iontophoresis for surface local anesthesia, *J Am Dent Assoc* 88:125-128, 1974.
15. Gangarosa LP, Park NH, Hill JM: Iontophoretic assistance of 5-iodo-2-deoxyuridine penetration into neonatal mouse skin and effects on DNA synthesis, *Proc Soc Exp Biol Med* 154:439-443, 1977.
16. Gibaldi M: *Biopharmaceutics and clinical pharmacokinetics*, ed 3, Philadelphia, 1984, Lea & Febiger.
17. Greenblatt DJ, Koch-Weser J: Clinical toxicity of chlordiazepoxide and diazepam in relation to serum albumin concentration: a report from the Boston Collaborative Drug Surveillance Program, *Eur J Clin Pharmacol* 7:259-262, 1974.
18. Gupta SK, Ellinwood EH, Nikaido AM, et al: Simultaneous modeling of the pharmacokinetic and pharmacodynamic properties of benzodiazepines. 1. Lorazepam, *J Pharmacokinet Biopharm* 18:89-102, 1990.
19. Hahn TJ, Hendin BA, Scharp CR, et al: Serum 25-hydroxycalciferol levels and bone mass in children on chronic anticonvulsant therapy, *N Engl J Med* 292:550-553, 1975.
20. Hogben CAM, Tocco DJ, Brodie BB, et al: On the mechanism of intestinal absorption of drugs, *J Pharmacol Exp Ther* 125:275-282, 1959.
21. Hughes MA, Glass PSA, Jacobs JR: Context-sensitive half-time in multicompartment pharmacokinetic models for intravenous anesthetic drugs, *Anesthesiology* 76:334-341, 1992.
22. Inman WHW, Adelstein AM: Rise and fall of asthma mortality in England and Wales in relation to use of pressurized aerosols, *Lancet* 2:279-285, 1969.
23. Kellermann G, Shaw CR, Luyten-Kellerman M: Aryl hydrocarbon hydroxylase inducibility and bronchogenic carcinoma, *N Engl J Med* 289:934-937, 1973.
24. Kim RB: Transporters and xenobiotic disposition, *Toxicology* 181-182:291-297, 2002.
25. King LS, Yasui M: Aquaporins and disease: lessons from mice to humans, *Trends Endocrinol Metab* 13:355-360, 2002.
26. Lehner T, Lyne C: Adrenal function during topical oral treatment with triamcinolone acetonide, *Br Dent J* 129:164-167, 1970.
27. Levine RR: *Pharmacology: drug actions and reactions*, ed 4, Boston, 1990, Little, Brown.
28. Levy G: Kinetics and implications of dissolution rate. Limited gastrointestinal absorption of drugs. In Ariens EJ, ed: *Physico-chemical aspects of drug action*, Oxford, 1968, Pergamon Press.
29. Lovering EG, McGilveray IJ, McMillan I, et al: The bioavailability and dissolution behavior of nine brands of tetracycline tablets, *Can J Pharm Sci* 10:36-39, 1975.
30. Magnussen MP: The effect of ethanol on the gastrointestinal absorption of drugs in the rat, *Acta Pharmacol Toxicol* (Copenhagen) 26:130-144, 1968.
31. Marier JR: Halogenated hydrocarbon environmental pollution: the special case of halogenated anesthetics, *Environ Res* 28:212-239, 1982.
32. Mark LC: Thiobarbiturates. In Papper EM, Kitz RJ, eds: *Uptake and distribution of anesthetic agents*, New York, 1963, McGraw-Hill.
33. Melander A: Influence of food on the bioavailability of drugs. In Gibaldi M, Prescott L, eds: *Handbook of clinical pharmacokinetics*, New York, 1983, ADIS Health Science Press.
34. Murthy KS, Talim ST, Singh I: A comparative evaluation of topical application and iontophoresis of sodium fluoride for desensitization of hypersensitive dentin, *Oral Surg Oral Med Oral Pathol* 36:448-458, 1973.
35. Nebert DW, Russell DW: Clinical importance of the cytochromes P450, *Lancet* 360:1155-1162, 2002.
36. Neitlich HW: Increased plasma cholinesterase activity and succinylcholine resistance: a genetic variant, *J Clin Invest* 45:380-387, 1966.
37. Ohki S, Gravis C, Pant H: Permeability of axon membranes to local anesthetics, *Biochim Biophys Acta* 643:495-507, 1981.
38. Okey AB, Roberts EA, Harper PA, et al: Induction of drug-metabolizing enzymes: mechanisms and consequences, *Clin Biochem* 19:132-141, 1986.
39. Portenoy RK, Khan E, Layman M, et al: Chronic morphine therapy for cancer pain: plasma and cerebrospinal fluid morphine and morphine-6-glucuronide concentrations, *Neurology* 41:1457-1461, 1991.

40. Pratt WB: The entry, distribution, and elimination of drugs. In Pratt WB, Taylor P, eds: *Principles of drug action: the basis of pharmacology*, ed 3, New York, 1990, Churchill Livingstone.
41. Rapoport SI, Robinson PJ: Tight-junctional modification as the basis of osmotic opening of the blood-brain barrier, *Ann NY Acad Sci* 481:250-267, 1986.
42. Renton KW: Factors affecting drug biotransformation, *Clin Biochem* 19:72-75, 1986.
43. Roth RA: Biochemistry, physiology and drug metabolism—implications regarding the role of the lungs in drug disposition, *Clin Physiol Biochem* 3:66-79, 1985.
44. Rylance GW, Moreland TA: Saliva carbamazepine and phenytoin level monitoring, *Arch Dis Child* 56:637-640, 1981.
45. Schekman R, Orci L: Coat proteins and vesicle budding, *Science* 271:1526-1533, 1996.
46. Scherrmann J-M: Drug delivery to brain via the blood-brain barrier, *Vasc Pharmacol* 38:349-354, 2002.
47. Singer SJ, Nicholson GL: The fluid mosaic model of the structure of cell membranes, *Science* 175:720-731, 1972.
48. Tanaka E: In vivo age-related changes in hepatic drug-oxidizing capacity in humans, *J Clin Pharm Ther* 23:247-255, 1998.
49. Van der Reis L, Lazar HP: *The human digestive system: its functions and disorders*, Basel, Switzerland, 1972, S Karger AG.
50. Van Dyke C, Jatlow P, Ungerer J, et al: Oral cocaine: plasma concentrations and central effects, *Science* 200:211-213, 1978.
51. Vesell ES: Advances in pharmacogenetics, *Prog Med Genet* 9:291-367, 1973.
52. Weiss CF, Glazko AJ, Weston JK: Chloramphenicol in the newborn infant. A physiologic explanation of its toxicity when given in excessive doses, *N Engl J Med* 262:787-794, 1960.
53. Wilson TH: *Intestinal absorption*, Philadelphia, 1962, WB Saunders.
54. Wood M: Plasma drug binding: implications for anesthesiologists, *Anesth Analg* 65:786-804, 1986.

General References

Chernow B, ed: *The pharmacologic approach to the critically ill patient*, ed 3, Baltimore, 1994, Williams & Wilkins.

Correia MA: Drug biotransformation. In Katzung BG, ed: *Basic & clinical pharmacology*, ed 8, New York, 2001, McGraw-Hill.

Derendorf H, Hochhaus G, eds: *Handbook of pharmacokinetic/pharmacodynamic correlation*, Boca Raton, FL, 1995, CRC Press.

Gibaldi M: *Biopharmaceutics and clinical pharmacokinetics*, ed 4, Philadelphia, 1991, Lea & Febiger.

Levine RR: *Pharmacology: drug actions and reactions*, ed 6, New York, 2000, Parthenon.

Pratt WB, Taylor P, eds: *Principles of drug action: the basis of pharmacology*, ed 3, New York, 1990, Churchill Livingstone.

Rendic S: Summary of information on human CYP enzymes: human P450 metabolism data, *Drug Metab Rev* 34:83-448, 2002.

Rowland M, Tozer TN: *Clinical pharmacokinetics: concepts and applications*, ed 3, Baltimore, 1995, Williams & Wilkins.

Wilkinson GR: Pharmacokinetics: the dynamics of drug absorption, distribution, and elimination. In Hardman JG, Limbird LE, Gilman AG, eds: *Goodman & Gilman's The pharmacological basis of therapeutics*, ed 10, New York, 2001, McGraw-Hill.

CHAPTER • 3

Pharmacotherapeutics: The Clinical Use of Drugs

John A. Yagiela and Frank J. Dowd

The primary goal of drug treatment is to achieve a desired pharmacologic effect without causing adverse reactions. Because no therapeutic regimen is without risk, the clinician must weigh the benefits expected from a drug against the dangers inherent in its use. If drugs are to be properly selected and administered, a number of factors should be considered that complicate both the attainment of therapeutic responses and the avoidance of unwanted effects.

As stated in Chapter 1, drugs are often selective in the effects they produce because they activate or inhibit specific drug receptors. However, even the most selective agents generally evoke a spectrum of reactions rather than a single pharmacologic outcome. Atropine in therapeutic concentrations, for example, specifically prevents the stimulation of muscarinic receptors by acetylcholine. Because these receptors are vital to the normal function of the entire parasympathetic nervous system, their blockade can result in a wide range of autonomic responses. Although specific in action, atropine is thus rather nonselective in effect. In addition, specificity of receptor binding is usually a matter of dose; in concentrations greater than therapeutic, atropine will block the nonmuscarinic effects of acetylcholine and may inhibit the actions of other chemicals, such as histamine and 5-hydroxytryptamine. Finally, nonspecific effects unrelated to receptor blockade may be observed. Large concentrations of atropine have local anesthetic activity and may directly affect the central nervous system (CNS) and peripheral vasculature.

In addition to the fact that single agents can produce multiple effects, pharmacotherapeutics is complicated by variations in patient responsiveness. A therapeutic dose of drug for one person may be ineffective for a second person and toxic to a third. Even highly inbred laboratory species display measurable biologic variations in drug sensitivity. Figure 3-1 is a quantal dose-effect graph illustrating the percentage of subjects responding to an agent as a logarithmic function of the dose. The graph is constructed by counting the number of animals or patients exhibiting a specified effect at various doses. With low amounts of drug, very few individuals react; as the dose is increased, however, more are affected until a dose is reached at which the response is universal. Although similar in appearance, this *quantal* dose-effect relation must not be confused with the *graded* dose-response curve described in Chapter 1 (see Figure 1-6). The quantal dose-response curve is sigmoidal because of the log-normal distribution of drug sensitivities found in most populations (see Figure 3-1). The median effective dose (ED_{50}) is the amount of drug required to produce a particular effect in 50% of the persons treated. Although potency is represented in both quantal and graded relationships by the position of the curve on the abscissa, intrinsic activity or efficacy is apparent only in graded responses. On the other hand, biologic variation, which is inversely correlated with the slope of the quantal dose-effect curve, cannot be estimated from a single graded dose-response graph.[32]

Patients who are unusually sensitive to a drug are said to be *hyperreactive.* Terms more or less synonymous with hyperreactivity include *hypersusceptibility* and *drug intolerance.* The term *hypersensitivity* is also used on occasion, but this usage can be misleading because hypersensitivity commonly indicates drug allergy. Persons unexpectedly resistant to conventional doses of drug are referred to as being *hyporeactive.* Tolerance, tachyphylaxis, and several additional types of hyporeactivity are discussed later. Many variables influence the responsiveness of individuals to drugs. Some of these are readily apparent and under the control of the clinician; others are often hidden from view and not amenable to modification. Because it is impossible to predict how a given patient will respond to a particular agent, appropriate monitoring of drug effects is usually necessary to achieve optimal therapy.

FACTORS INFLUENCING DRUG EFFECTS

Differences between patients in reaction to a therapeutic agent may arise from disparities in drug concentration obtained with a standardized dose (pharmacokinetic differences), from variations in individual responsiveness to a given drug concentration (pharmacodynamic differences), or from secondary factors such as the failure of patients to take their medication as prescribed (noncompliance). Figure 3-2 shows the lack of correlation that can develop clinically between the prescribed dose of a drug, in this case the anticonvulsant phenytoin, and the resultant plasma concentration and pharmacologic response. Even with the daily dose corrected for body weight, this study revealed that the steady-state concentration of phenytoin differed 20-fold or more.[36] It is apparent that, given a therapeutic concentration range of 10 to 20 μg/ml (the plasma concentration of phenytoin supposed to provide seizure protection with minimal adverse effects[17]), the majority of patients were prescribed or took on their own either insufficient medication or an overdose. Although pharmacokinetic dissimilarities undoubtedly account for many differences in patient responsiveness, the fact that phenytoin has a "therapeutic range" rather than a single effective concentration indicates that there also exists some variation in pharmacodynamic sensitivity to the anticonvulsant. Indeed, a small percentage of persons have nystagmus, an early indication of drug toxicity, at plasma concentrations barely sufficient to control convulsions in other patients.[28]

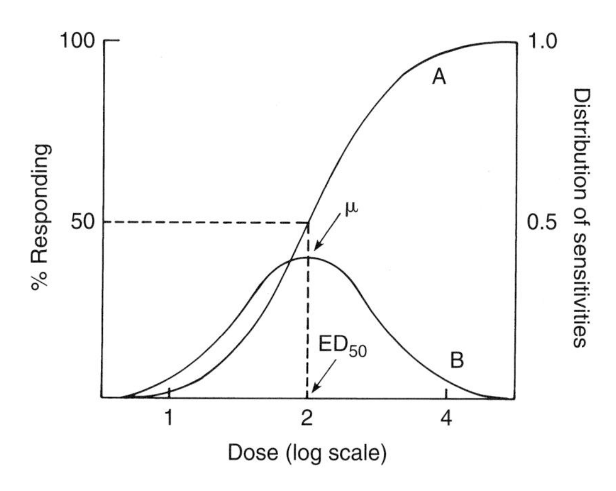

Fig. 3-1 Quantal dose-response curves (log scale). *Curve A* represents the cumulative distribution and *curve B* the frequency distribution of patient responses in a normal population. As shown, the mean (μ) and median (50% responding) sensitivities fall on the same dose (median effective dose, ED_{50}). (Adapted from Goldstein A, Aronow L, Kalman SM: *Principles of drug action: the basis of pharmacology,* ed 2, New York, 1974, John Wiley & Sons.)

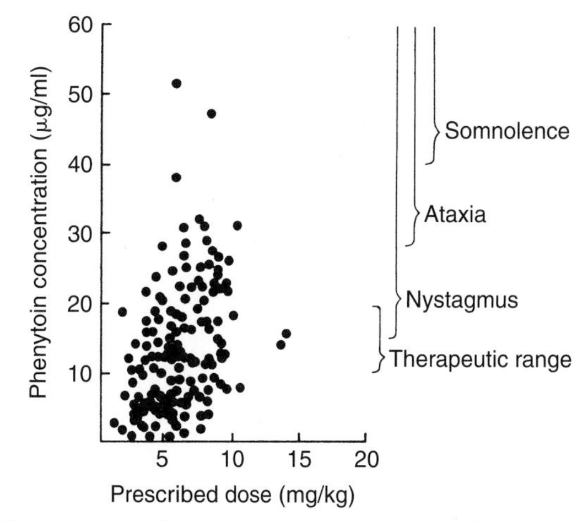

Fig. 3-2 Plasma phenytoin concentration as a function of the prescribed dose. Each *dot* represents a single patient ($n = 294$). *Closed bracket* indicates the accepted therapeutic concentration range for phenytoin in plasma; *open-ended brackets* denote concentrations at which the various toxic manifestations listed may occur. (Data from Lund L: Effects of phenytoin in patients with epilepsy in relation to its concentration in plasma. In Davies DS, Prichard BNC, eds: *Biological effects of drugs in relation to their plasma concentrations,* Baltimore, 1973, University Park Press; and Kutt H, Winters W, Kokenge R, et al: Diphenylhydantoin metabolism, blood levels, and toxicity, *Arch Neurol* 11:642-648, 1964.)

Patient Factors

Many factors that can influence drug effects clinically are highly variable in individual patients. Although attributes such as size, age, and genetic makeup are not amenable to modification, they must be taken into account whenever drug therapy is planned.

Body weight and composition

Adults may differ three times or more in weight. Because the volume of distribution of a drug is a function of body mass, extremes in patient size may result in significant differences in plasma concentration when drugs are administered in the form of a "standard adult dose." Body composition is also an important variable here. Two equally heavy patients, one obese and the other muscular, may react quite differently to certain agents. Because adipose tissue contributes very little to body water, the obese person will be more susceptible to a drug distributed essentially within one or more body fluid compartments. On the other hand, the same person may demonstrate unusual resistance to a highly lipophilic agent such as thiopental, especially when it is given in repeated doses.

Age

Pediatric patients generally cannot be given adult dosages of drugs. The primary reason for this difference is body size, and various formulas (discussed in Chapter 55) have been devised to calculate pediatric fractions of the adult dose. For the following reasons, however, children must not be thought of as merely miniature adults. First, even with the size differential taken into account, neonates display an unusual hyperreactivity to drugs. Immature hepatic and renal systems during the first weeks of life tend to promote drug accumulation, and the relative inefficiency of drug binding by albumin (sometimes because of competition for binding sites by bilirubin[8]) may also lead to abnormal concentrations of drug in the vicinity of receptors. In addition, distribution of compounds into the CNS may be enhanced by an incomplete maturation of the blood-brain barrier. Second, in contrast to neonates, children and infants older than 6 months often require large milligram per kilogram body weight doses of drugs during therapy. This relative hyporeactivity is mostly attributable to an enhancement in the rate of elimination.[15] Dosage adjustment on the basis of surface area (see Figure 55-6) rather than body weight is empirically a useful strategy in correcting for age-related differences in elimination.

Pharmacodynamic differences also exist in the young. Incomplete maturation renders children especially vulnerable to the toxic effects of certain agents. For example, benzocaine is especially likely to cause methemoglobinemia in infants younger than 6 months, tetracyclines pose the risk of tooth discoloration up to the age of 8 years, and sex steroids and other hormones administered before puberty may impair normal growth and development. In part because of the young child's high metabolic rate, atropine intoxication may readily cause hyperthermia, and salicylate overdosage may quickly lead to acid-base and electrolyte disturbances. The association of Reye's syndrome with aspirin and excitement reactions with antihistamines give added proof that children respond differently than do adults to certain drugs.

Obviously, there is no method of pediatric dosage calculation suitable for all drugs and therapeutic situations. In older children, adjustments based on age, weight, or (preferably) surface area may be satisfactory, but no general guide is possible for the very young. Dosages for neonates and infants should be based on clinical trials; unfortunately, studies of this nature are often not done and dosage schedules for small children not provided.

Geriatric patients are frequently hyperreactive to drugs. Although increased sensitivity may result from organic pathologic conditions or from drug interactions, both more likely to occur in the elderly, age-related functional changes in drug disposition and cellular responsiveness are also involved. Because patients older than 65 years are twice as likely to have adverse reactions as are young adults, careful selection of dosage schedules is necessary, especially with drugs of low safety. Geriatric pharmacology is becoming increasingly important to the dentist as the general population ages and as a higher proportion of the elderly retain their teeth (thanks to improved oral hygiene and professional care); the subject is therefore covered in its entirety in Chapter 53.

Sex, pregnancy, and lactation

The sex of a patient is sometimes important with respect to drug effects. Because women tend to be smaller than men and have a higher percentage of body fat, dosage adjustments may be necessary for some agents. Hepatic disposition of drugs is affected by the ratio of female to male sex hormones. Women appear to be more susceptible to drug-induced blood dyscrasias, and those taking systemic contraceptives may be more prone to some drug interactions. For obvious reasons, side effects such as hirsutism are less tolerable in women, and gynecomastia is more disconcerting in men. In 1998, the Food and Drug Administration (FDA) mandated that information pertaining to safety and effectiveness of new drugs include data for demographic subgroups who would benefit from these drugs. This ruling includes women, who were previously often excluded from trials, making it difficult to evaluate the influence of sex on drug safety and clinical efficacy.

Pregnancy is a major concern in pharmacotherapeutics. Alterations in liver and renal function are common and may delay the metabolism and excretion of numerous substances. The hepatic toxicity of tetracycline and certain other compounds is markedly accentuated by pregnancy. When present, toxemia may increase drug effects by reducing the binding capacity of albumin. Of primary importance are the actions of drugs on the unborn child. Spontaneous abortion, teratogenesis, mental retardation, drug dependence, and cancer have resulted from drug administration during pregnancy. Because few, if any, agents have been proved totally safe for the fetus, it is best to avoid all medications when possible. Drug administration should also be conservative in women of child-bearing age, because pregnancy is often undiagnosed during the first trimester (the most critical period of fetal development). Many drugs (e.g., methadone) are excreted in the milk. Because some of these agents may cause unwanted effects in the nursing infant, it is advisable to review carefully drug exposure during lactation as well. Toxicologic concerns related to pregnancy are explored more fully later in this chapter.

Environmental factors

Factors such as ambient temperature, sunlight, and altitude are capable of influencing responses to certain drugs. As prime examples, children given atropine on a warm day are especially susceptible to drug-induced hyperthermia, toxic skin reactions to sulfonamides increase with exposure to sunlight, and nitrous oxide loses efficacy in mountainous regions. Probably the most important environmental factor influencing drug effects is the diet. The timing of meals and the types of food eaten can markedly affect drug absorption. For example, the gastrointestinal absorption of most tetracyclines is impaired when taken with milk or other dairy products.

Numerous chemicals that are ingested, inhaled, or absorbed through the skin can influence the body's disposition of, or response to, various drugs. Patients receiving monoamine oxidase inhibitors, for instance, risk severe hypertension and death if they eat foods containing tyramine (e.g., certain cheeses, beers, and wines). The therapeutic effects of levodopa in parkinsonism may be prevented by pyridoxine (vitamin B_6), present in foods and multivitamin supplements. Grapefruit juice contains substances that downregulate the CYP3A enzymes responsible for metabolizing a host of drugs. Finally, the use of insulin must be carefully matched to the patient's dietary intake to avoid complications associated with hypoglycemia and hyperglycemia.

The indigenous microflora represents a special kind of environmental variable. Several drugs given orally are metabolized by bacterial enzymes to such an extent that absorption may be significantly impaired. The dose of coumarin anticoagulants is partially governed by the amount of vitamin K produced by enteric bacteria. During antibiotic therapy, the type and number of microorganisms surviving play a large role in determining whether superinfection develops in patients.

Physiologic variables

Numerous physiologic factors can modify clinical responses to drugs. Fluctuations in gastric, plasma, and urinary pH, for instance, may alter the pharmacokinetics of weak electrolytes. Salt and water balance, exercise, sleep, body temperature, blood pressure, and many other factors also influence patient reactions. The effects of blocking agents are particularly sensitive to variations in physiologic or biochemical events. Thus isoproterenol, an adrenergic agonist, increases heart rate irrespective of autonomic nervous system tone, but atropine, an acetylcholine antagonist, increases heart rate only in the face of tonic vagal activity.

Many physiologic functions reveal a daily periodicity of intensity. These circadian rhythms often result in daily fluctuations of drug responsiveness. In dentistry, the duration of local anesthesia after nerve blockade varies by a factor of two during the course of a day, with the greatest effect occurring in the afternoon in patients with normal sleep patterns.[51]

Pathologic factors

Diseases may influence pharmacotherapeutics by modifying drug disposition or tissue responsiveness. Pathologic states most commonly associated with altered patient reactivity involve the organs of absorption, distribution, metabolism, and excretion. Diarrhea, malabsorption syndromes, and other disturbances of the gastrointestinal tract may depress the absorption of ingested agents. Although data are few, it is probable that actively absorbed substances are more likely to be affected by gastrointestinal disease than are drugs that reach the systemic circulation by passive diffusion.[41]

The distribution of drugs is sensitive to pathologic changes in the blood and circulatory system and to perturbations in anatomic barriers to diffusion. Disturbances in the concentration of plasma proteins (e.g., hypoalbuminemia) or in their function (as in uremia) may lead to drug toxicity or to a loss of therapeutic benefit. Congestive heart failure and arteriosclerosis may so diminish tissue perfusion that drug elimination is significantly retarded. Meningeal inflammation permits entry into the CNS of many drugs (e.g., penicillins) normally excluded by the blood-brain barrier.

Renal disease is a common modifier of drug effects. The plasma half-lives of agents eliminated in the urine are often greatly prolonged by renal failure. Even for compounds completely destroyed in the liver, inadequate excretion of metabolites may increase the incidence of untoward reactions.[17] A good measure of renal status is provided by the endogenous creatinine clearance. By way of illustration, a 50% drop in creatinine clearance should theoretically indicate a twofold increase in the elimination half-life of a drug that is removed from the blood solely by renal excretion. For a drug partially eliminated in the urine, the increase in plasma half-life should be correspondingly less. The customary approach to avoiding excessive drug accumulation in patients with renal disease is to lengthen the dosage interval in accordance with the degree of impaired elimination. Table 3-1 lists, for several drugs (including some commonly used in dentistry), the approximate dosage intervals indicated for patients with moderate or severe renal disability.[55]

Hepatic dysfunction, whether caused by specific hepatic disease, infection, or other ailments, can markedly reduce the metabolism and biliary excretion of drugs.[27] Unfortunately, standard liver function tests are of little prognostic value regarding drug biotransformation. Some patients with demonstrable cirrhosis or hepatitis may show surprisingly little metabolic deficit, whereas others may exhibit marked hyper-reactivity to standard doses of drugs. Within the same

Table • 3-1

Dosage Adjustments in Renal Failure

DRUG	ROUTE OF ELIMINATION	DOSE INTERVAL IN HOURS (AND PERCENTAGE OF NORMAL DOSE) ACCORDING TO DEGREE OF RENAL FAILURE*		
		NORMAL FUNCTION	MODERATE IMPAIRMENT	SEVERE IMPAIRMENT
Antibiotics				
Cefoxitin	Mainly renal	6	8 to 12	24
Erythromycin	Hepatic	6	6	12
Penicillin G	Mainly renal	4 to 6	4 to 6 (50%)	8 (33% to 50%)
Tetracycline†	Renal/hepatic	12	12 to 24	Avoid use
Analgesics				
Acetaminophen†	Hepatic	4	6	6
Aspirin†	Hepatic/renal	4	4 to 6	Avoid use
Codeine‡	Mainly hepatic	4 to 6	4 to 6 (75% to 100%)	4 to 6 (25% to 50%)
Meperidine‡	Hepatic	3 to 4	3 to 4 (50% to 100%)	Avoid use
Cardiovascular Agents				
Diltiazem	Hepatic	8	8	8
Furosemide	Renal/hepatic	12	12	12
Lisinopril	Fecal/renal	24	24 (50% to 75%)	24 (25% to 50%)
Propranolol	Hepatic	8	8	8 (75% to 100%)
CNS Depressants				
Alprazolam	Hepatic	8	8	8
Lorazepam	Hepatic	12	12	12
Pentobarbital	Hepatic/renal	8	8	8
Phenobarbital	Hepatic/renal	8	8	8 (75% to 100%)
Others				
Diphenhydramine	Hepatic	6 to 8	6 to 8	6 to 8
Insulin	Hepatic/renal	Variable	Variable (75%)	Variable (50%)
Prednisone	Hepatic	12	12	12
Ranitidine	Renal/hepatic	8	12	24

Data from St. Peter WL, Halstenson CE: Pharmacologic approach in patients with renal failure. In Chernow B, ed: *The pharmacologic approach to the critically ill patient,* ed 3, Baltimore, 1994, Williams & Wilkins.
*The degree of renal failure as defined by creatinine clearance: normal function to minimal impairment, >50 ml/min; moderate impairment, 10 to 50 ml/min; severe impairment, <10 ml/min.
†Drugs that may accentuate renal damage.
‡Accumulation of active metabolite limits dosing.

individual, the metabolism of some drugs but not others may be impaired. Because the liver is responsible for the synthesis of plasma proteins such as albumin and pseudocholinesterase, and for the breakdown of compounds such as bilirubin that compete for drug binding sites in plasma and various tissues, hepatitis may significantly alter (up or down) a drug's volume of distribution and elimination half-life independently of its specific effects on hepatic drug metabolism. For drugs with high hepatic clearance, metabolism will be decreased by cirrhosis-induced reductions in total liver blood flow. The uncertainties of drug metabolism introduced by hepatic disease require that substances inactivated in the liver be used cautiously in affected patients and that careful monitoring of drug effects be performed to avoid serious adverse reactions.

An insidious form of interaction between pathologic factors and drug effects occurs with agents potentially toxic to their primary organs of elimination. Acetaminophen accumulation permitted by liver disease may result in hepatic necrosis and further impairment of drug metabolism.[47] A similar vicious cycle involving the kidney has been observed with a variety of drugs.

Exaggeration of the systemic effects of epinephrine and reduction in the analgesic potency of morphine in uncontrolled hyperthyroidism are two examples of drug effects modified by disease states through nonpharmacokinetic means. Although pathologic factors may influence drug-receptor interactions directly, as in myasthenia gravis (in which receptor reactivity to acetylcholine is reduced), most alterations of patient response occur indirectly through the augmentation of overt disease or the unmasking of latent physiologic deficits. Thus agents that promote hyperuricemia may cause an acute exacerbation of gout, and propranolol may induce heart failure in patients with a severely compromised myocardium.

Genetic influences

Without question, genetic variables contribute greatly to the differences in drug responsiveness illustrated in Figure

3-1. Although the importance of heredity is underscored by the evolution of pharmacogenetics into a recognized field of study, the elucidation of multigenetic factors that lead to log-normal distributions in drug reactivity has proved difficult. Previously, the only variations in drug effects that had been unequivocally linked to genetic differences were those that exhibit simple inheritance patterns and yield bimodal or otherwise discontinuous distribution curves and those that can be associated with certain groups of people on the basis of blood type, race, ethnic background, and so on. Now, studies of gene expression and polymorphisms are helping to uncover an increasingly broad array of genetically determined differences in drug responsiveness. Genetic factors are responsible for idiosyncratic reactions and determine, in part, the relative likelihood of a patient having an allergic response to an administered agent. Genetic influences can alter drug effects quantitatively; they may also result in the appearance of novel pharmacologic outcomes (see below). Genetic influences affecting drug metabolism and drug receptors are discussed in Chapter 4.

Drug Factors

In addition to individual variations in patient reactivity, certain drug factors, namely the formulation and dosage regimen of an agent and the development of tolerance, can markedly influence the success of drug therapy.

Variables in drug administration

Of all the factors influencing pharmacologic responses clinically, only those involved with drug selection and administration are totally under the control of the clinician. Some of these variables are discussed in detail in previous chapters: dose, drug formulation, route of administration, and drug accumulation. Two additional factors worthy of comment are the time of administration and the duration of therapy. Many disturbing side effects are minimized if an agent can be given shortly before sleep. These include the autonomic effects of the belladonna alkaloids, the vestibular component of nausea associated with opioid analgesics, and the sedative properties of the antihistamines. Conversely, agents producing mild CNS stimulation are better tolerated in the daytime. The scheduling of doses with or between meals to limit gastrointestinal upset or to enhance absorption is mentioned in Chapter 2.

The duration of therapy has several important ramifications. Treatment must, of course, be sufficiently long to be effective. This is particularly true with antimicrobial agents, in which an inadequate duration of coverage can lead to reinfection. However, because adverse drug reactions are more likely to occur during extended courses of therapy, treatment should never be unduly prolonged. It is generally inappropriate, for example, to continue a patient on medication after the condition requiring therapy has subsided. The duration of administration should be monitored especially carefully when drugs capable of producing physical or psychologic dependence are being used.

Drug tolerance

In pharmacology, tolerance to a drug refers to a state of decreased responsiveness that develops on repeated or continuous exposure to the agent or one of its congeners. Two major categories of tolerance are recognized: pharmacokinetic or drug-disposition tolerance, in which the effective concentration of the drug is diminished, and pharmacodynamic or cellular tolerance, in which the activity of a given concentration of the drug is reduced.

Most documented cases of drug-disposition tolerance involve agents that stimulate their own metabolism through the induction of microsomal enzymes. Other mechanisms are possible, such as an immune tolerance, in which circulating antibodies produced in response to an antigenic substance (e.g., bovine insulin) combine with the agent, thereby decreasing its effective concentration at the receptor site. When pharmacokinetic tolerance is encountered, clinical effectiveness can usually be restored through simple adjustment of the dose or administration interval.

Cellular tolerance is commonly observed with drugs that alter mood, perception, or thought; opioid analgesics, barbiturates, benzodiazepines, alcohol, amphetamines, caffeine, and cocaine are examples. Tolerance is usually acquired gradually, depending on the drug, its dose, and how often it is administered. Generally, cellular tolerance does not develop equally to all effects of a drug. Sometimes this is beneficial, as when undesirable side effects of an agent are lost but therapeutic activity is retained. Unfortunately, differences in tolerance can also promote adverse reactions. Alcoholics, for example, become tolerant to the "therapeutic" effect of ethanol yet remain normally susceptible to the lethal effect. Continual use of ethanol leads to a potentially dangerous reduction in the drug's margin of safety because the user is forced to approach toxic concentrations to achieve the desired level of inebriety. (The ability of alcoholics to walk a straight line while inebriated also involves a "learned tolerance" in which they develop coping skills to mask their inebriation.) A similar phenomenon occurs with other CNS depressants. Clinical management of pharmacodynamic tolerance can often be accomplished by increasing the dose; however, this approach is occasionally ineffective in restoring drug activity and may result in serious toxicity or drug dependence. Normal sensitivity in a tolerant person can be restored eventually through abstention from the drug.

Although the bases for most types of cellular tolerance are not well understood, it appears that adaptive changes to oppose drugs acting on specific receptor systems administered long term are a common phenomenon. Receptor responsiveness is not static; in the case of agonist drugs, receptors may become diminished in both activity and number through the respective processes of desensitization and downregulation, as described in Chapter 1. Response elements downstream from the primary receptor may be similarly affected. Other adaptive changes may include alterations in endogenous mediator synthesis, storage, release, and reuptake.

Specific mechanisms of tolerance have been established for certain drugs that evoke a rapidly developing form of tolerance known as *tachyphylaxis*. The sympathomimetic agent tyramine provides a classic example of tachyphylaxis. Administered intravenously to an animal whose vagal innervation of the heart has been interrupted, tyramine indirectly increases heart rate and blood pressure by causing the release of norepinephrine from adrenergic nerves. A subsequent dose given after the effects of the first have disappeared generates a smaller response, and, after a series of repetitions, the drug may lose essentially all activity. Acute tolerance to tyramine is produced by rapid depletion of the functional norepinephrine stores of the adrenergic nerve terminals. Two additional examples of tachyphylaxis are associated with histamine. Because endogenous stores of histamine can be quickly depleted but take a long time to be replenished, drugs that cause histamine release (e.g., morphine and tubocurarine) will generate tolerance in much the same manner as does tyramine. Tachyphylaxis may also occur to histamine itself. Repetition of increasing doses of intravenous histamine can produce in several hours a hyporeactivity of 100-fold less than normal. Other drugs capable of evoking acute tolerance include the benzodiazepines, nitrites, cholinergics, and anticholinergics. Pharmacodynamic sensitization, in which the individual becomes increasingly responsive to drugs administered on a regular basis, has been documented for several CNS stimulants. For example, cocaine given in single daily doses to rats causes increased motor activity after a week of treatment. This effect, associated with increased release of dopamine in the brain, is a conditioned response, because placebo substitution for cocaine after 1 week elicits a similar response.[23]

Factors Associated with the Therapeutic Regimen

Some factors influencing drug effects are related to the therapeutic context in which the agent is administered or prescribed. Attitudes, for example, toward the drug regimen or practitioner may determine whether an agent proves effective or even if it is taken. Concurrent use of other medicines may alter drug effects directly through pharmacologic mechanisms or indirectly by promoting errors in drug administration.

Placebo effects

A placebo effect is any effect attributable to a medication or procedure that is not related to its pharmacodynamic or specific properties.[65] The term *placebo* is derived from the Latin verb *placere*, meaning "to please." In pharmacotherapeutics, a placebo may be either "pure," in which the preparation is pharmacologically inert (e.g., a lactose tablet), or "impure," in which the drug has pharmacologic activity but is given for a condition or in a manner such that no benefit can be obtained from its specific properties. Two commonly held misconceptions are that placebos provide nothing more than a means of placating patients and that they may help in psychosomatic illness but are worthless when symptoms are organically based. Numerous studies have revealed, however, that placebo medication is effective in treating the subjective responses to a variety of "real" medical conditions (e.g., the pain of cancer, angina pectoris, headache, and surgical wounds).[4] Actually, the distinction between psychogenic and organic illness has become blurred by the realization that psychologic disturbances often produce physiologic or pathologic manifestations and that organic diseases, or at least their signs and symptoms, can be influenced by the CNS through regulation of hormonal secretion and peripheral nervous system activity. Placebo effects are not merely subjective in nature; the administration of pharmacologically inert substances has led to measurable changes in gastric acid secretion, in heart rate and blood pressure, in the number of circulating leukocytes, and in the plasma concentrations of various compounds, including adrenal steroids, catecholamines, electrolytes, and glucose.[4] Even so-called subjective responses to placebos may have a biochemical basis. It has been argued, for example, that placebo analgesia can be blocked by naloxone, a specific opioid antagonist,[31] and that the placebo effect may involve the dopaminergic reward system.[11]

Placebo responses to drugs arise from expectations by the patient concerning their effects and from a wish to obtain benefit or relief. Expectations develop at the conscious and subconscious levels and are influenced by many factors. The patient, of course, must be aware that treatment is being rendered. It is the symbolic association of receiving medication in a therapeutic environment that generates placebo reactions. The patient must also be anxious about the problem and desirous of being cured. Placebo effects are unlikely if there is patient indifference to the condition or to the therapeutic regimen. Past experience is another important variable. Previous drug exposure informs a patient of what to expect from a drug; repeated administrations evoking prompt, noticeable effects may, in fact, produce conditioned reflexes. Because suggestion is involved, placebo effects are subject to modification by the practitioner's attitudes (to the patient, to the patient's illness, and to the drug or placebo) and how these feelings are communicated. In one study, a 45% reduction in placebo response occurred solely as a result of the administrators' negative bias toward the placebo medication.[3]

Several important similarities and differences between placebo and specific effects of drugs must be remembered if clinicians are to avoid being deceived by the preparations they use. Therapeutic responses to placebos and to active agents may resemble each other in magnitude and duration. For example, the pain relief and cough suppression afforded by a placebo may parallel that of codeine. Toxicities can also overlap. Pure placebos are associated with many common side effects—nausea, drowsiness, sweating, xerostomia—and may occasionally call forth such life-threatening emergencies as bronchial asthma, acute hypotension, and cardiac arrhythmia. By way of contrast, placebos have a relative lack of predictability. Although some drugs can be relied on to produce a given effect in essentially all patients, only approximately one third of persons receiving placebos usually react. Attempts to identify placebo responders on the basis of psychologic profile or other characteristics have been unfruitful; it appears that anyone may respond to placebos in the appropriate situation. Finally, there are many classes of drugs, such as the general anesthetics and the antibiotics, whose effects placebos cannot duplicate.

The placebo effect has recently been more carefully scrutinized. Because most studies using placebo controls have not adequately distinguished between the effects they produce and the natural course of a symptom, disease, or healing process, the placebo effect may have been overemphasized.[22] Moreover, the administration of a placebo necessarily involves both the placebo intervention (such as the giving of a lactose tablet) and the remainder of the patient-doctor interaction.[21] Determining the relative contributions of each experience may be especially difficult.

Placebos are valid, often necessary inclusions in clinical trials, especially in studies such as analgesic drug trials, in which the placebo effect is well documented. Studies involving other subjective outcomes also represent a strong argument for placebo use.[22] Placebo effects advantageous to therapy—in addition to beneficial pharmacologic effects—should also be sought whenever a drug is administered clinically. Sometimes the effective communication of confidence and other positive attitudes by the practitioner can make the difference between therapeutic success and failure. The clinical application of placebo drugs, however, should be restricted to those conditions for which no other agent is superior. Even then, the evolution of informed consent into a basic patient right has, at best, complicated the clinical administration of placebo medication. There appears to be no justification for the therapeutic use of placebo medication in routine dental practice.

Medication errors and patient noncompliance

Medication errors commonly result in suboptimal therapy and occasionally life-threatening responses. Poor pharmacotherapeutic decisions by the clinician may stem from a lack of knowledge about the patient, disease, or drug. In addition, drugs are often not used in the manner intended by the prescriber. Occasionally, the clinician may miswrite the prescription, or the pharmacist may supply the wrong drug or incorrectly transcribe the instructions to the patient. In the hospital setting, the nursing or house staff may administer the drug incorrectly, neglect to administer it, or administer it to the wrong patient. The vast preponderance of medication errors, though, arise from the failure of patients to take their preparations as directed. Drug defaulting is a major problem in therapeutics; most studies document a noncompliance rate of 25% to 60%.[57] The reasons for noncompliance are varied: a lack of understanding of the drug, the purpose for which it was prescribed, or how it is to be administered; economic factors; negative feelings toward the drug or prescriber; development of adverse reactions; forgetfulness or carelessness; and resolution of the problem before the drug regimen is complete or, conversely, failure to notice any therapeutic benefit. Although infrequent omissions and minor mistakes in dosage or time of administration are often innocuous, complete failure to take the prescribed drug, premature discontinuance, or ingestion of excessive amounts can be disastrous. The possibility of noncompliance should be considered whenever a drug is seemingly without activity. Unfortunately, patients are notoriously inaccurate in reporting their own compliance, and physicians are not much better in estimating its occurrence.[53] When effective therapy is essential, direct assay of the patient's blood, urine, saliva, or feces for the drug or its metabolites may be necessary to detect noncompliance.

As with the placebo responder, attempts have been made to characterize the potential drug defaulter on the basis of such factors as age, sex, education, race, and socioeconomic status. Although some correlations have been drawn (e.g., elderly patients are more apt to forget their medicine or to confuse one type of pill with another), many investigations have been either inconclusive or contradictory. The most important variables relate not to the patient but to the illness, the drug administered, the overall therapeutic regimen, and the doctor-patient relationship. Administration schedules are followed more faithfully by patients with life-threatening diseases than by those with minor ailments. However, even with serious illnesses such as essential hypertension or chronic infection, compliance is generally poor (approximately 50%) when the benefits of therapy are not superficially apparent.[6] Other things being equal, drugs that produce unwanted side effects are more likely to be discontinued. Deviations in self-administration tend to increase progressively with drugs that are taken long term. Also, the more complex the therapeutic regimen in terms of doses and drugs, the higher the incidence of drug defaulting. The quality of the doctor-patient relationship is important in several respects. Patients who trust and respect their physician are more likely to take prescribed medications. Effective communication further promotes compliance and reduces the possibility of a patient unilaterally terminating the drug if adverse effects occur. Measures that the clinician may use to enhance patient compliance are discussed in Chapter 55.

Drug interactions

The effect of a drug may be increased, decreased, or otherwise altered by the concurrent administration of another compound. Because agents routinely used in dental practice have been implicated in drug interactions, the topic is of considerable interest to the clinician and is considered separately in Chapter 4 (see also Appendix 1).

ADVERSE DRUG REACTIONS

It has been estimated that 5% to 17% of all patients hospitalized in the United States each year are admitted because of adverse reactions to drugs.[7,39,50] In addition, a survey of hospitalized patients between 1966 and 1996 revealed that 7% had a serious adverse drug reaction.[29] Estimates of the annual cost of managing these reactions range from $3 billion to $7 billion.[39,50] The introduction of new, highly efficacious compounds into pharmacotherapy during the past few decades has led to a disturbing increase in the incidence of adverse reactions; indeed, drug toxicity is now considered a major cause of iatrogenic disease. Reductions in mortality rate associated with certain drugs (e.g., aspirin) demonstrate, however, that toxic responses to therapeutic agents can be minimized through concerted efforts by health professionals, the pharmaceutical industry, government, and lay public.

Classification of Adverse Drug Reactions

Drug toxicity may come in many forms: acute versus chronic, mild versus severe, predictable versus unpredictable, and local versus systemic. Therapeutic agents also differ widely in their tendency to elicit adverse reactions. Acetaminophen, for example, used to relieve headache rarely causes undesired responses, but many agents used in cancer chemotherapy invariably produce some degree of toxicity. Agents quite safe for some individuals may be life-threatening to others. Thus penicillin G, which normally enjoys an exceptionally high margin of safety, can, in small doses, initiate fatal anaphylaxis in allergic patients. Although no classification of adverse drug reactions is universally accepted, a taxonomy based on mechanism of toxicity is the most useful in promoting the recognition, management, and prevention of untoward responses to drugs.

Extension effects

Many drugs are used clinically in dosages that provide an intensity of effect that is less than maximal. The reason for this conservatism is simple: increasing drug effects beyond a certain point may be dangerous. The anticoagulant warfarin provides a typical example of a drug whose therapeutic action must be held in check to avoid serious toxicity. For the treatment of peripheral vascular thrombosis, warfarin is administered in doses that sufficiently increase the prothrombin time to yield an international normalized ratio (see Chapter 31) of 2 to 3. Warfarin could be given in larger amounts to further inhibit clotting, but the risk of spontaneous bleeding would be unacceptably high. Even with conventional therapy, hemorrhage, the toxic extension of warfarin's anticoagulant effect, occurs in 2% to 4% of the patients treated. Inadvertent overmedication is, of course, one cause of warfarin toxicity; however, many additional factors influencing drug effects may also be involved: diet; heredity; drug interactions; renal, hepatic, or cardiac insufficiency; gastrointestinal ulceration; and variable patient compliance. It is obvious that the "normal dose" has little meaning regarding warfarin because a therapeutic dose to one patient may represent an overdose to another.

Adverse responses arising from an extension of the therapeutic effect are dose related and predictable. Theoretically, they are the only toxic reactions that can always be avoided without loss of therapeutic benefit by properly adjusting the dosage regimen. Additional examples of drugs that display this form of toxicity are provided in Table 3-2.

Side effects

Predictable, dose-dependent reactions unrelated to the goal of therapy are referred to as *side effects.* As illustrated in Table 3-3, drugs can produce a huge array of deleterious side reactions. Although many such effects are associated with only a single agent or class of drugs, others appear to be almost universal in occurrence. It is questionable, however, whether frequently noted side effects such as nausea and drowsiness are always drug related; similar symptoms are also commonly observed in patients after placebo administration and are even reported by persons receiving no medication whatsoever.[49] Side effects may be produced by the same drug-receptor interaction responsible for the therapeutic effect, differing only in the tissue or organ affected. In these instances, the categorization of drug responses as toxic or therapeutic may depend on the purpose of treatment. Xerostomia induced by atropine is a side reaction during the management of gastrointestinal hypermotility but is a desired effect when the drug is used to control excessive salivation. Side effects unrelated pharmacodynamically to the therapeutic action are also quite common, and they too may occasionally be useful. Table 3-4 lists some drugs whose side effects were found sufficiently noteworthy

Table • 3-2

Examples of Drug Toxicity as an Extension of the Therapeutic Effect

DRUG	MEDICAL INDICATION	THERAPEUTIC EFFECT	TOXIC EXTENSION OF THERAPEUTIC EFFECT
Modafinil	Narcolepsy	Wakefulness	Insomnia
Furosemide	Edema	Diuresis	Hypovolemia
Heparin	Thromboembolic disorders	Inhibition of coagulation	Spontaneous bleeding
Insulin	Diabetes mellitus	Reduction of blood glucose concentration	Hypoglycemia
Zolpidem	Insomnia	Hypnosis	Unconsciousness
Vecuronium	Abdominal surgery	Skeletal muscle relaxation	Prolonged respiratory paralysis

Table • 3-3

Some Side Effects of Drugs

DRUG	EFFECT	DRUG	EFFECT
Oral Cavity		**Neuromuscular System**	
Diphenhydramine	Xerostomia	Atorvastatin	Myalgia
Griseofulvin	Black hairy tongue	Chlorpromazine	Tardive dyskinesia
Phenytoin	Gingival hyperplasia	Dantrolene	Weakness
Tetracycline	Pigmentation, hypoplasia of the teeth	Lidocaine	Convulsions
		Theophylline	Tremors
Skin and Hair		**Central Nervous System**	
Amoxicillin	Dermatitis	Clonidine	Drowsiness and lethargy
Cyclophosphamide	Alopecia	Dexamethasone	Mental depression
Methandrostenolone	Acne	Diazepam	Confusion
Minoxidil	Hypertrichosis	Levodopa	Mania
Bone and Joints		**Cardiovascular System**	
Ciprofloxacin	Arthralgia	Bupivacaine	Bradycardia
Hydralazine	Arthralgia	Phenelzine	Hypertensive crisis
Phenobarbital	Osteomalacia	Propofol	Hypotension
Prednisolone	Osteoporosis	Propranolol	Cardiac failure
Sensory Apparatus		**Respiratory System**	
Baclofen	Blurred vision	Ketamine	Laryngospasm
Digoxin	Yellow vision	Meperidine	Respiratory depression
Gentamicin	Ototoxicity	Methohexital	Hiccough
Thioridazine	Pigmentary retinopathy	Propranolol	Bronchospasm
Blood		**Gastrointestinal Tract**	
Cytarabine	Pancytopenia	Aspirin	Melena
Prilocaine	Methemoglobinemia	Erythromycin	Diarrhea
Valproic acid	Thrombocytopenia	Lithium	Nausea and vomiting
Zidovudine	Granulocytopenia	Morphine	Constipation
Metabolic Effects		**Genitourinary System**	
Aspirin	Metabolic acidosis	Ergonovine	Abortion
Furosemide	Hyperglycemia	Guanethidine	Impotence
Nadolol	Hypoglycemia	Sulfadiazine	Crystalluria
Rifampin	Jaundice	Testosterone	Priapism

Table 3-4

Useful Side Effects of Some Drugs

DRUG	ORIGINAL USE	SUBSEQUENT USE
Amantadine	Antiviral	Parkinsonism
Amphetamine	CNS stimulant	Attention deficit—hyperactivity disorder
Chlorothiazide	Diuretic	Antihypertensive
Diphenhydramine	Antihistaminic	Sedative
Lidocaine	Local anesthetic	Antiarrhythmic
Methadone	Analgesic	Heroin substitute
Metronidazole	Antiparasitic	Antibacterial
Phenytoin	Anticonvulsant	Antiarrhythmic
Probenecid	Inhibition of penicillin excretion	Uricosuric
Quinidine	Antimalarial	Antiarrhythmic

to provide new and unanticipated indications for therapeutic use.

Many side effects, particularly the more dangerous forms, develop only with drug overdose. Careful alteration of the administration regimen will usually resolve these problems while maintaining effective treatment. Many other side effects, however, appear at therapeutic or even subtherapeutic concentrations and cannot be avoided by dosage adjustment without loss of drug benefit. Such reactions can be tolerated, though, if they are mild, brief in duration, reversible, and compatible with therapy. Occasionally, even disturbing side effects will be accepted if the need for medication is great. Drugs used in the treatment of various cancers, for example, produce severe toxic effects that must be tolerated because no therapeutic alternative is available.

When two drugs share a common desired effect but cause different side effects, it is sometimes possible to limit toxic responses by using reduced doses of the agents in combination. Another pharmacologic approach to avoiding side effects is to add a secondary agent that is capable of blocking or otherwise compensating for the unwanted activity of the principal drug. These strategies presuppose that no additional toxicity will be generated by the combination over that produced by a single effective drug. The association of renal papillary necrosis with long-term abuse of analgesic mixtures that formerly contained aspirin, phenacetin, and caffeine is highly instructive regarding the noncritical acceptance of this assumption.[54] Undoubtedly, the most fruitful pharmacologic approach to eliminating undesired side effects is through the development of more selective drugs. Studies of structure-activity relationships have proved invaluable in removing side effects unrelated to therapeutic actions and in reducing side effects that are related.

Idiosyncratic reactions

An idiosyncratic reaction may be defined as a genetically determined abnormal response to a drug. Although dose dependent, such reactions are unpredictable in most instances because exceedingly few patients given an agent respond idiosyncratically and because the genetic trait responsible for an atypical reaction may be completely "silent" in the absence of drug challenge. When confronted with an unexpected response to a drug, it is a common, although erroneous, practice to describe the event as an idiosyncrasy. This habit may explain why the idiosyncratic reaction is jocularly defined as a reaction the "idiots can't explain." Most responses lying outside the normal range of drug reactivity are not truly idiosyncratic in nature but represent allergic manifestations or reflect extension or side effects in patients intolerant to the drug by virtue of age, weight, existing disease, and so on. In dentistry, the majority of idiosyncratic reactions to local anesthetics are actually the result of accidental intravascular injections or anxiety reactions to the process of injection.

An idiosyncratic reaction is often manifested as abnormal drug sensitivity in which the agent produces its characteristic effect at an unconventional dose. Drug effects may be unusually strong or weak in intensity or brief or prolonged in duration. In most such instances (e.g., involving succinylcholine, isoniazid, vitamin D, or phenytoin), altered drug metabolism is responsible for the abnormal responses; however, additional mechanisms have also been identified, such as abnormal distribution (iron, thyroxine) and unusual receptor affinity (coumarin anticoagulants). In addition to perturbing characteristic drug responses, genetic singularities can produce novel drug effects that, regardless of dose, may never occur in normal individuals. One example of a novel drug effect is the hemolytic anemia caused by the antimalarial drug primaquine. Red blood cells of sensitive individuals are deficient in glucose-6-phosphate dehydrogenase, an enzyme involved in the intermediary metabolism of glucose. Lacking the ability to produce normal amounts of reducing equivalents, these erythrocytes are susceptible to oxidative destruction by primaquine and several dozen other compounds. The genetic basis of primaquine hemolysis is clear: the reaction occurs almost exclusively in men of certain racial and ethnic groups (e.g., African Americans, Sardinians, Sephardic Jews, Iranians, Filipinos).[40]

Several idiosyncrasies are known to be associated with drugs. Some examples are listed in Table 3-5. If an adverse response is suspected of having a genetic basis, it becomes important to determine whether the patient has a personal or familial history of atypical reactivity to the drug. Because idiosyncratic reactions are quite reproducible within any individual, a single episode of serious toxicity should preclude future use of the inciting compound. Examination of the patient's family is helpful in establishing the hereditary nature of the reaction and identifying other individuals at risk.

Drug allergy

Adverse responses of immunologic origin account for approximately 10% of all untoward reactions to drugs. Allergy can be distinguished from other forms of drug toxicity in several respects. First, prior exposure to the drug or a closely related compound is necessary to elicit the reaction. Second,

Table • 3-5

Idiosyncratic Reactions to Drugs Used in Dentistry

GENETIC ABNORMALITY	DRUGS AFFECTED	IDIOSYNCRATIC RESPONSE
NADH-methemoglobin reductase deficiency	Benzocaine, prilocaine	Methemoglobinemia
Glucose-6-phosphate dehydrogenase deficiency	Aspirin, primaquine, sulfonamides	Hemolytic anemia
Abnormal heme synthesis	Barbiturates, sulfonamides	Porphyria
Low plasma cholinesterase activity	Procaine and other ester local anesthetics	Local anesthetic toxicity
Altered muscle calcium homeostasis	Volatile inhalation anesthetics, succinylcholine	Malignant hyperthermia
Prolonged QT interval	Cisapride, some antipsychotics and antiarrhythmics	*Torsades de pointes*

NADH, Reduced nicotinamide adenine dinucleotide.

the severity of response is seemingly dose independent. Third, the nature of the unfavorable effect is a function not of the offending drug but of the immune mechanism involved. Finally, the reaction is unpredictable; it usually occurs in a small portion of the population, sometimes in patients who had been previously treated on numerous occasions without mishap.

Drugs differ enormously in antigenic potential. Certain compounds (e.g., caffeine and epinephrine) never cause drug allergy; others (e.g., phenylethylhydantoin) have proved too allergenic for human use. With drugs commonly implicated clinically in allergic reactions (e.g., penicillins, sulfonamides, quinidine), the incidence of such responses is approximately 5%. On occasion, it is not the drug itself that causes the reaction but some other substance in the preparation, such as a preservative or coloring agent.

Aside from agents of high molecular weight (insulin, dextran, polypeptides), drugs are usually not antigenic in the free state but must be covalently linked to endogenous carrier molecules, normally proteins such as albumin, to generate immunologic responses. Because these therapeutic agents are often chemically inert, they generally require activation by metabolism or by sunlight (photoallergy) before serving as haptens in the formation of antigen. Penicillins, which are responsible for most fulminating reactions, are exceptional in that they spontaneously convert to highly reactive derivatives in addition to undergoing in vivo metabolism to a small degree.

Four types of drug allergy have been differentiated on the basis of the immune reactions that cause them and the loci of their actions.[10] Type I reactions, otherwise known as reaginic or anaphylactic responses, include the immediate forms of drug allergy, in which disturbances appear within minutes or hours of taking the drug. The underlying immune reactions are initiated by the attachment of antigen to immunoglobulin (Ig) E antibodies bound to the surface of mast cells and basophils. Subsequent cellular degranulation and release of histamine, leukotrienes, cytokines, and other mediators are responsible for the undesired effects. Major signs and symptoms of type I allergy involve the gastrointestinal tract (cramps and diarrhea), skin and mucous membranes (erythema, urticaria, angioneurotic edema), lungs (bronchoconstriction), and blood vessels (vasodilatation, increased permeability). In its most severe form, anaphylaxis can cause death by airway obstruction or by cardiovascular collapse within a few minutes after drug exposure. Parenteral injection of the drug is more likely to produce life-threatening reactions than is oral or topical use. Nevertheless, patients have died from topical application of less than 1 µg of penicillin. It is believed that patients with allergic diathesis (noted by a history of hay fever or bronchial asthma) are more prone to develop serious type I reactions. The immediate anaphylactic response is the only type of drug allergy that the dentist may be forced to treat without the benefit of medical backup. Epinephrine is the drug of choice to reverse the manifestations of a severe response; antihistamines and adrenal corticosteroids are useful as adjunctive medications (see Chapter 54).

Type II, or cytotoxic, reactions are caused by circulating antibodies (IgG and IgM). When a plasma membrane constituent serves as the hapten carrier, or when a complete antigen is adsorbed on the membrane surface, the binding of immunoglobulin is followed by complement fixation and lysis of the cell. Many forms of drug-induced hemolytic anemia, leukopenia, and thrombocytopenia are the result of this form of immunologic destruction. Type II responses are usually delayed and manifest from several hours to days after drug administration.

Type III, or immune-complex, reactions occur when soluble antigen-antibody complexes form in intravascular or interstitial spaces. Eventual deposition of the complexes on the walls of small blood vessels is followed by activation of complement and migration of neutrophils into the area. These cells degranulate in attempts to remove the complexes, releasing lysosomal enzymes that cause local tissue damage and promote thrombosis of affected vessels. Type III reactions can induce a number of unpleasant sequelae, some of which can be quite serious (neuropathy, glomerulonephritis, serum sickness). Reactions indistinguishable from disease states such as lupus erythematosus and erythema multiforme are also observed. Finally, soluble antigen-antibody complexes can attach to cell membranes and cause cytotoxicity indistinguishable from type II reactions. (Because of the close correspondence between cytotoxic and immune-complex reactions in general, the identification of type II and type III reactions as separate entities may have more historic than biologic significance.[20])

Type IV reactions are synonymous with cell-mediated immunity. Sensitized T lymphocytes exposed to the drug hapten or its conjugate release lymphokines that attract additional cells (lymphocytes, macrophage, cytotoxic T cells) to the antigenic site. Lysozymes and other substances (including toxic lymphokines) elaborated by the recruited cells produce local tissue necrosis. Type IV reactions are usually delayed because of the time required for effector cells to concentrate in the area involved. For dentists, an important cellular immune reaction is the contact dermatitis acquired from repeated exposure of the hands to ester local anesthetics such as procaine. Before the availability of amide anesthetic drugs, allergy to procaine markedly complicated clinical practice. Even today, allergy to ester-based local anesthetics presents a problem for some patients because of the variety of substances that may cross-react to elicit an eczematoid rash: methylparaben, a pharmaceutical preservative in widespread use; *p*-phenylenediamine, a component of hair dyes; and dichlorophene, a germicide in soaps.[1]

Although drug allergies cannot always be prevented, their frequency of occurrence can be minimized by observing the following precautions:

1. *Take an adequate medical history.* If a patient has a presumptive history of drug allergy, it is important to discover the identity of the inciting preparation and to determine whether the reaction is, in fact, consistent with an immunologic cause.
2. *Avoid the offending drug and likely cross-reactors.* A patient truly allergic to a drug should not receive the agent or congener again unless need for the particular medication is great.
3. *Avoid inappropriate drug administration.* In one study, a review of 30 fatalities to penicillin revealed that the antibiotic was not even indicated in more than 50% of the cases examined.[52]
4. *Promote oral use and limit topical exposure.* At least with the penicillins, the oral and topical routes are, respectively, the least and most allergenic avenues of drug administration.
5. *Request allergy testing when appropriate.* Although such methods are generally unreliable and can be dangerous, skin tests for penicillin allergy have proved highly predictive,[46] and success has also been claimed regarding local anesthetics.[2] Allergy testing may be necessary when suitable alternatives to the drug in question are not available.

Adherence to these recommendations will reduce the incidence of allergic reactions to drugs. It is encouraging to note that a more prudent use of penicillin in recent years may have led to a decline in the drug's mortality rate, once estimated to be as high as 500 persons per year.[45]

Pseudoallergic and secondary reactions

Pseudoallergic reactions are adverse drug responses caused by mediators of allergy that are released through antibody-independent processes. In the case of macromolecules, the alternate pathway of complement fixation may lead to various cytotoxic and immune-complex reactions. Much more common, though, are *anaphylactoid* reactions that mimic one or more aspects of anaphylaxis. Some opioid analgesics, neuromuscular blocking drugs, and intravenous anesthetic agents can cause the release of histamine from mast cells. Also, aspirin, ibuprofen, and related inhibitors of prostaglandin synthesis can result in the overproduction of bronchospastic leukotrienes. As with true allergies, these reactions are unpredictable; however, they do not require prior sensitization and may occur on initial exposure to the drug.

Secondary reactions are indirect (and often unpredictable) consequences of a drug's primary pharmacologic action.[13] Antibiotics provide the best examples. One possible outcome of antibiotic administration is the development of superinfection, a secondary microbial disease made possible by the antibiotic-induced suppression of the normal microflora (see Chapters 38 and 39). Alternatively, the rapid lysis of susceptible bacteria may result in the Jarisch-Herxheimer phenomenon, a serum sickness–like syndrome caused by the release of microbial antigens, endotoxins, or both.

Carcinogenesis

One aspect of drug toxicity that has had a strong impact on public awareness is carcinogenesis. Although most attention has been focused on environmental pollutants, including those chemicals that pose an occupational hazard, the association of leukemia with various anticancer agents and uterine neoplasia with diethylstilbestrol underscores the tumorigenic potential of certain therapeutic drugs. Of course, the most pervasive cancer-producing substances in our society are derived from a "social" drug—the cigarette.[12]

Virtually any agent capable of altering the structure of DNA is a potential carcinogen. Agents known to be carcinogenic include radioactive substances, alkylating agents, nitrosamines, and various aromatic amines and polycyclic hydrocarbons. With the exception of radioactive materials, most drugs capable of initiating neoplastic change must become chemically activated. This process occurs spontaneously with some alkylating substances, but it usually depends on metabolic biotransformation. Cytochrome P450 enzymes are commonly involved, yielding highly reactive electrophilic intermediates. These activated molecules can then interact with DNA at specific sites. For example, alkylating drugs can form covalent linkages with the 7-nitrogen atom of guanine. If replication occurs before the damage can be repaired, a transversion may occur in which the alkylated guanine-cytosine pair is replaced by a thymine-adenine. Such transversions are not randomly distributed throughout the genome but are clustered at specific loci.[14] Neoplastic transformation occurs when mutations develop in genes regulating cellular growth.

Compelling evidence has accumulated since 1980 implicating two groups of genes in chemical carcinogenesis: oncogenes and tumor suppressor genes.[56] Oncogenes are derived from normal genes, or protooncogenes, whose function is to promote growth and development. Several mechanisms for neoplastic transformation of protooncogenes have been discovered, including point mutation, which would seem to be the most likely candidate for chemical carcinogenesis. The *ras* group of protooncogenes is frequently transformed in human cancer. Each *ras* gene codes for a protein that helps convey stimulatory signals from membrane-bound tyrosine kinase receptors to the nucleus.[12] Ras proteins are activated by binding guanosine triphosphate (GTP) and inactivated by autohydrolysis of the bound GTP to guanosine diphosphate. *Ras* oncogene products differ from the natural protein by a single amino acid substitution at one of several key points that are apparently involved in nucleotide binding and protein regulation. The net result is a protein that loses its ability to split GTP and remains activated at all times. Other oncogenes that have been identified code for various tyrosine kinases, serine/threonine-specific protein kinases, and gene regulatory proteins.

Tumor suppressor genes code for proteins that normally inhibit cell growth. An important example involved in a majority of human cancers is the *p53* gene. Its protein derivative, p53, is a nuclear regulatory protein that activates transcription of a gene whose protein product prevents the cell from replicating. When the *p53* gene is rendered inactive or mutated, this important inhibitory pathway is lost and the affected cell may begin to multiply. Spontaneous errors in replication may also accumulate as rapid cellular division leaves insufficient time for DNA repair.

Cancer is normally a multistage phenomenon involving multiple genetic mutations. In the case of colorectal cancer, three to seven separate defects must accumulate for the full expression of malignancy.[62] Collectively, these changes are responsible for both the initiation of neoplastic transformation and the subsequent promotion of cellular growth.

Certain compounds cause tumors only after prior treatment with another agent. The first chemical appears to initiate the neoplastic transformation, and the second promotes tumor growth. The latter are called *promoters* or *nongenotoxic carcinogens*. It is hypothesized in these instances that the promoter removes the control of growth that distinguishes normal from cancerous cells. Examples of promoters in experimental models include phorbol esters, saccharin, chlorophenothane, and phenobarbital.[19] Irrespective of initiating or promoting factors, immunosuppressive drugs may foster cancer development generally by interfering with immunologic surveillance mechanisms responsible for the elimination of transformed neoplastic cells.

Carcinogens are often detected by screening for mutagenicity by the Ames test. However, major difficulties are encountered in assessing the carcinogenicity of agents intended for human use. First, the latency period between the initiation and clinical appearance of neoplasia may extend for years to decades. Second, although the incidence of tumor induction is dose dependent, it is not established whether a dose or duration of exposure below which tumors will not be produced can be found for any drug. Third, because an administered agent usually requires metabolism for activation, interspecies differences in biotransformation severely limit the use of animal testing in such instances. Without a foolproof method of screening drugs, continued appraisal of cancer rates regarding drug intake is a necessary, if not ideal, approach to identifying carcinogenic compounds. In view of the prolonged latency of cancer development and the flood of agents introduced into pharmacology in recent decades, it would be surprising not to witness the discovery of new carcinogens among therapeutic agents now in use.

Special Problems

Hazards of medication pertaining to abuse, poisoning, and effects on the unborn child deserve special comment inasmuch as the persons affected are generally not exposed to the agent for therapeutic purposes. In these situations, the prevention and management of adverse reactions can be complicated by matters such as the intent of the person taking the drug, an inability to identify the offending agent, and the unique susceptibility of the embryo to drug toxicity.

Drug abuse

Typified by persistent and excessive self-administration, drug abuse refers to the inappropriate and deviant use of any drug. Drug abuse presents a special problem in toxicology because, in addition to the hazards of taking pharmacologically active agents without proper medical supervision (drug toxicity, infection from inadequate antisepsis), adverse consequences may arise from the acts involved in procuring and using such compounds. Compulsive behavior is especially strong with drugs that act on the CNS, and, except for substances to which little stigma is attached (e.g., coffee and tobacco products), the attendant social, economic, and legal costs of the abuse of these agents can be enormous. Moreover, abstinence from drugs producing physical dependence results in the appearance of withdrawal symptoms characteristic of the substance involved and the intensity of previous use. A thorough discussion of drug abuse involving centrally acting agents is presented in Chapter 51.

Drug poisoning

As revealed by data from the American Association of Poison Control Centers, more than 2 million poisonings were reported in 2001.[34] Of the more than 1000 poisoning deaths in the same report, more than half were believed to be the result of suicide. Drug poisoning accounts for a significant percentage of reported episodes and therefore is a major concern for health professionals and laypersons alike.[5] Drugs most commonly implicated in fatal poisonings are analgesics, antidepressants, alcohol, CNS stimulants, and cardiovascular agents.

Children younger than 5 years account for the majority of poisonings and for approximately 2% of the deaths. Against this backdrop of statistics, however, it is pleasing to note that fatal poisonings of small children have actually decreased by more than 70% since the early 1960s.[63] Aspirin, historically the leading cause of drug toxicity in the very young, provides a noteworthy example of how unintentional poisoning can be controlled. Recognizing the special hazard of flavored baby aspirin, the pharmaceutical industry voluntarily limited the number of aspirin tablets per bottle to a (normally) sublethal total of 36. Safety packaging, which became mandatory after the passage of the Poison-Prevention Packaging Act of 1970,[63] further reduced the incidence of fatal ingestion. Finally, increased public awareness concerning the danger of aspirin overdose, engendered in part by the proliferation of poison control centers throughout the country, led to safer storage of aspirin in the home. In combination, these events reduced aspirin fatalities by 83% between 1959 and 1974.[61] Further decrements in the aspirin mortality rate have occurred (no deaths in 1998), aided in part by the increased reliance on liquid acetaminophen and ibuprofen preparations for analgesia and antipyresis. As one might predict, however, acetaminophen and ibuprofen poisonings, once quite rare, are now relatively common. The principles of toxicology and the prevention and management of drug poisoning are covered in Chapter 52.

Drugs and pregnancy

The hazard to the unborn child of administering drugs during pregnancy has received considerable attention in the lay and professional literature. Over the years, certain compounds have been implicated in the development of congenital abnormalities. These teratogens disturb organogenesis in the developing embryo so that defects in one or more structures are produced. If the defects are incompatible with life, fetal death and either resorption or spontaneous abortion ensues; if they are less severe, the result is a malformed child.

Very little is known about the teratogenic potential of most drugs in human beings, but the thalidomide disaster of 1960 to 1962 proved that an ordinary drug, extremely safe in adults, could induce extensive malformation of the human fetus. Thalidomide is a sedative-hypnotic that was released for clinical use in Europe and elsewhere in the late 1950s. The drug quickly gained wide acceptance and was commonly used by women to relieve the nausea of "morning sickness." Shortly after its introduction, however, there occurred an epidemic of infants born with phocomelia, or "seal limb" malformation of the arms and legs. Retrospective studies determined that phocomelia was caused by thalidomide when the agent was taken 24 to 29 days after conception.[30] Other defects were also produced by thalidomide (e.g., absence of external ears, cranial nerve dysfunction, anorectal stenosis), depending on the time of administration. Surprisingly, thalidomide has made a comeback in therapy. It is currently approved for treating certain forms of leprosy; it is also used clinically to manage various sequelae of HIV infection, and it is potentially useful as an immune modulator in disorders such as Crohn's disease.

Laboratory experiments in animals and investigations of accidental teratogenesis in human beings have found that drug-induced malformation is governed by the sequential pattern of embryonic and fetal development. From fertilization to approximately 20 days, an embryo will either survive or succumb to a chemical insult. No malformations will occur, though, because the cells remain undifferentiated during this period. Beginning at day 21 (when the somites appear) and continuing until the end of the first trimester (when differentiation and organogenesis are well established), malformations are possible when the embryo is exposed to a teratogen. The defects produced will vary with the toxic action of the agent and with the time of administration. Certain malformations, such as cleft palate, may be produced by a variety of

Table • 3-6

Toxic Effects of Selected Drugs during Pregnancy

		MOST SUSCEPTIBLE PERIOD*			
		TRIMESTER			
DRUG	TOXIC EFFECT TO THE FETUS	1ST	2ND	3RD	TERM
Anticancer drugs	Cleft palate, extremity defects, severe stunting, death	✓			
Chloramphenicol	Gray syndrome, death				✓
Cortisone	Cleft palate	✓			
Coumarin anticoagulants	Hemorrhage, death				
Diazepam	Cleft palate, respiratory depression	✓			✓
Local anesthetics	Bradycardia, respiratory depression				✓
Lysergic acid diethylamide	Chromosomal damage, stunted growth	✓			
Opioid analgesics	Respiratory depression, neonatal death				✓
Potassium iodide	Goiter, mental retardation				
Quinine	Deafness, thrombocytopenia			✓	✓
Sex steroids	Masculinization, vaginal carcinoma (delayed)				
Streptomycin	Eighth nerve damage, micromelia, multiple skeletal abnormalities				
Tetracyclines	Inhibition of bone growth, tooth discoloration, micromelia, syndactyly				
Thalidomide	Phocomelia, multiple defects	✓			
Thiazide diuretics	Thrombocytopenia, neonatal death			✓	✓

Adapted from Underwood T, Iturrian EB, Cadwallader DE: Some aspects of chemical teratogenesis, *Am J Hosp Pharm* 27:115-122, 1970.
*Coumarins and other drugs with no indication mark are approximately evenly toxic throughout pregnancy.

substances; some teratogens, such as antifolate drugs, can evoke a wide spectrum of structural defects.[59] Selective toxicity of drugs to the unborn child does not end after 3 months' gestation. Although gross malformation may not occur, normal development may be retarded or otherwise affected throughout pregnancy. Immaturities in physiology and biochemistry may promote adverse reactions in the fetus at doses quite safe to the mother. The administration of drugs at the time of delivery is commonly associated with exaggerated effects in the neonate. Table 3-6 lists several agents known to elicit toxic effects during pregnancy and indicates when their administration is most dangerous to the fetus. In an attempt to classify drugs on the basis of their toxic potential during pregnancy, the FDA instituted a pregnancy category rating, as summarized in Table 3-7. Many older drugs have not yet been rated; of those that have, most fall into categories indicating a lack of definitive information regarding safety in human beings.

Despite uncertainties concerning most drugs and the fetus, pharmacologic agents have been extensively used by pregnant women. In a 1973 survey, 82% of the women questioned received prescription drugs and 65% took over-the-counter medications.[16] The major drug categories included (in decreasing order of usage) iron supplements, analgesics, vitamins, sedative-hypnotics, diuretics, antiemetics, antimicrobials, cold remedies, hormones, "tranquilizers," bronchodilators, and appetite suppressants. More than half of the women smoked, and more than 85% used alcohol. Even though women and health care professionals are now more aware of the risks posed by drugs, the admonition to restrict usage of therapeutic agents, especially during the first trimester, bears reiteration. For dentistry, only emergency treatment should be rendered during the critical period of fetal development. Regular dental care need not be postponed, however, during the second and most of the third trimester, as long as reasonable attention and care are given to avoiding undue physical and emotional stress in the patient and drugs that pose a known risk to the fetus.

DEVELOPMENT OF NEW DRUGS

Advances in pharmacotherapy ultimately depend on the discovery, evaluation, and marketing of new drugs. The past several decades have witnessed an unprecedented proliferation of medicinal agents, and major revisions in how drugs intended for human use are evaluated have contributed to the manufacture of safer as well as more effective compounds. As a prescriber of drugs, however, the practitioner should be aware of the attendant problems and costs of developing therapeutic agents and of the unavoidable limitations in assessing drug safety before widespread use. Only with this knowledge can the clinician arrive at a balanced attitude toward new drugs and claims made for them.

Sources of New Drugs

For many years, considerable effort in pharmacology was devoted to the purification of active constituents from natural plant and animal products previously used for medicinal purposes. With the possible exception of various herbal medicines, these traditional sources of drugs are, for the most part, depleted.

Many new therapeutic agents are discovered by empirical screening. In screening tests, thousands of compounds from natural materials or synthetic chemistry are examined for a particular pharmacologic activity. Microplate, microarray, and other types of high-throughput technology have made screening an important method of finding new drugs capable of producing a defined drug effect. With the exception of penicillin, all the antibiotic groups have been isolated by the screening

Table • 3-7

FDA Pregnancy Risk Categories

CATEGORY	DEFINITION	EXAMPLE DRUGS
A	Adequate and well-controlled studies have failed to demonstrate a risk to the fetus in the first trimester of pregnancy (and there is no evidence of risk in later trimesters).	Levothyroxine, magnesium sulfate (injectable), sodium fluoride*
B	Either (1) adequate and well-controlled studies have failed to demonstrate a risk to the fetus in the first trimester of pregnancy and there is no evidence of risk in later trimesters, but animal reproduction studies have shown an adverse effect on the fetus; or (2) human studies are lacking, but animal studies have failed to demonstrate a risk to the fetus.	Acetaminophen*, amoxicillin and clavulanate, cefaclor, erythromycin, etidocaine, lidocaine, naproxen, penicillin V*
C	No adequate and well-controlled studies have been performed in pregnant women, but animal reproduction studies are lacking or have shown an adverse effect on the fetus. Potential benefit may warrant use of the drug in pregnant women despite potential risk.	Atropine, bupivacaine, butorphanol, codeine, diflunisal, epinephrine, hydrocortisone (topical), mepivacaine, morphine, thiopental
D	Positive evidence exists of human fetal risk based on adverse reaction data from investigational or marketing experience or studies in human beings. Potential benefit may warrant use of the drug in pregnant women despite potential risk.	Aspirin*, hydrocortisone (systemic)*, lorazepam, midazolam, pentobarbital, valproic acid
X	Studies in animals or human beings have demonstrated fetal abnormalities, and/or there is positive evidence of human fetal risk based on adverse reaction data from investigational or marketing experience, and the potential risk of the drug in pregnant women clearly outweighs the potential benefit.	Ergotamine, estradiol, isotretinoin, temazepam, triazolam, warfarin

Adapted from *USP dispensing information—drug information for the health care provider,* ed 23, Rockville, MD, 2003, The United States Pharmacopeial Convention, Inc.
*Estimated ranking based on current information and FDA category definitions.

of soils and other materials for antimicrobial activity. In recent years, advances in synthetic chemistry and molecular biology have led to a proliferation of screening tests in which cells engineered to express receptors of interest and easily measured biologic responses to receptor activation are exposed to large collections of chemicals and examined for activity.

One of the more productive techniques of finding new drugs is to alter the molecular structure of an existing agent. Obviously, structure-activity relationship studies are intimately involved in this approach. When derivatives are produced, they are frequently little more than "me too" drugs—agents that, although similar in activity to the parent compound, offer no therapeutic advantage but are marketed anyway for economic reasons. Less often, a drug is synthesized that differs substantially from its predecessor in pharmacokinetic properties. Penicillin V, which is nearly identical in antimicrobial activity to its precursor, penicillin G, is nevertheless preferred for oral use because its absorption is two to five times better. Pharmacokinetic differences are especially prominent among the benzodiazepine congeners, with elimination half-lives ranging from several hours to several days. The least common but usually most desirable outcome of molecular modification is the synthesis of a derivative that differs qualitatively from the parent drug in pharmacodynamic effect. Such discoveries are generally the result of attempts to enhance one aspect of an agent's spectrum of activity over all others. Thus the observations that sulfonamides used in chemotherapy of bacterial infections could lower blood glucose concentrations and promote urine flow under appropriate conditions eventually led to the manufacture of several new classes of drugs: carbonic anhydrase inhibitors, thiazide diuretics, and sulfonylurea hypoglycemic agents.

Increasingly, discoveries of new drugs are evolving from advances in our understanding of basic physiology and biochemistry. It has occasionally been possible to tailor compounds for a specific purpose. Nowhere is this approach more apparent than in the synthesis of antimetabolites for antiviral and cancer chemotherapy. The extraction of some natural effectors (e.g., insulin, calcitonin, and adrenocorticotropin) and the synthesis of others (e.g., adrenal and sex steroids, epinephrine, vitamin D derivatives, and prostaglandins) have provided a host of new therapeutic agents. Recombinant DNA technology, by which bacteria or even mammalian cells can be altered genetically to synthesize foreign proteins, is fulfilling its promise[38] for the large-scale production of human biologic agents (e.g., interferons, insulin, calcitonin, growth hormone, and hematopoietic growth factors) that were previously obtainable only in small amounts. Undoubtedly, this source of drugs will continue to grow, and it is expected that hitherto unknown protein agents will become available for pharmacotherapy as studies of the human genome progress.

A burgeoning source of new pharmaceutical products comes from the development of novel delivery systems for existing drugs. The use of prodrugs to provide for improved gastrointestinal absorption (e.g., enalapril), regional distribution (e.g., levodopa, when given with carbidopa), or greater safety (e.g., acyclovir) is a well-established strategy. More complex approaches, such as drug-laden liposomes, may provide a safer parenteral delivery of drugs such as amphotericin B, a highly toxic antifungal agent.[48] Monoclonal antibodies, whose production is outlined in Chapter 41, are now being used in cancer patients as vehicles for cytotoxic substances (e.g., diphtheria toxin) and various anticancer drugs and radioactive isotopes.[26,43] The antibody attaches to tumor-associated surface antigens; the active ligand provides the tumoricidal effect. Similar drug-carrying monoclonal antibodies directed against discrete cellular elements of the immune system have found use in preventing transplant rejection and in the treatment of autoimmune diseases.[37] Attaching drugs, often covalently, to polymeric carriers is proving effective in localizing and prolonging drug effects, either because the controlled release of free drug from the immobilized matrix permits only local effects or because the drug is active in the bound state.[60] In either case, the distribution of drug action is determined by the properties of the carrier. There are many potential applications for such systems; in dentistry, the controlled release of antibiotics is useful in treating certain forms of periodontitis.[25]

The last major source of new drugs is serendipity. Probably the greatest single breakthrough in pharmacotherapeutics in the twentieth century was the isolation of penicillin, made possible by the chance, but astute observation of Fleming, that bacteria in a culture dish were lysed by a mold contaminant of the genus *Penicillium*. Other classes of agents that originated by accident include the antiarrhythmic drugs (quinine) and the oral anticoagulants (dicumarol). Table 3-4 lists several drugs for which new therapeutic applications were fortuitously discovered after marketing.

Evaluation of New Drugs

Before a drug can be released for general use, it must pass a rigorous evaluation program established by the FDA (Figure 3-3). This program, although subject to some modification depending on the drug's intended use, invariably includes a series of animal and human investigations to ensure the product's safety and efficacy. (See Chapter 55 for a review of drug regulations pertaining to the FDA and the development of new drugs.)

Preclinical testing

The first step in evaluating a newly discovered compound is to ascertain its pharmacologic activity in animals. Initially, a few rats may be given several different doses of the chemical and observed for any disturbances that may occur in physiology or behavior. If the drug is being developed for a given purpose (e.g., to lower blood pressure), it would be tested for that particular effect as well. Agents that appear to have a useful action are then enrolled in more extensive examinations. Graded dose-response curves are constructed to determine the potency and intrinsic activity of the compound (see Chapter 1). When a specific therapeutic effect is identified, quantal dose-effect relationships are drawn to estimate the compound's relative safety. As shown in Figure 3-4, quantal dose-effect curves can be prepared for both desired and toxic responses.

When one is working with laboratory animals, one of the most convenient toxic effects to monitor is lethality. Death is universal, all drugs are capable of producing it, and it represents a definite end point that can be quickly and unequivocally recognized. The dose causing death in 50% of the test animals in a given period of time is designated as the median lethal dose (LD_{50}). The ratio of this dose to the median effective dose (LD_{50}/ED_{50}) defines the therapeutic index, a crude but useful measure of drug safety. Other things being equal, a drug with a large therapeutic index is safer than an agent with a smaller value. Indeed, when many congeners are being tested concurrently, those with the most favorable therapeutic indexes are given preference in further investigations and are considered the most promising candidates for clinical application. Unfortunately, the LD_{50}/ED_{50} ratio is not fully predictive of relative safety. Drugs produce many toxic effects besides death that can prevent their use in human beings. An agent that has a large therapeutic index regarding one adverse reaction may fare poorly in regard to another type of toxicity.

Table 3-8 compares a group of local anesthetics in their propensity to elicit two separate toxic effects—death and local tissue irritation—as a function of the anesthetic concentration.[35] Each test was performed in a different species: lethality in mice, irritability in rabbits, and anesthesia in guinea pigs. With procaine used as a standard, propoxycaine was 4.6 times safer regarding tissue irritation but essentially equivalent in relation to lethality. From these data, cocaine would appear to be the safest local anesthetic for human administration; however, cocaine has some additional liabilities (CNS stimulation, abuse potential) not shared by the other agents that severely restrict its medical usefulness.

A second limitation of the therapeutic index is that biologic variability is not taken into account. In Figure 3-4, drug B has a larger therapeutic index than drug A but is nevertheless clinically inferior. The goal of pharmacotherapy is to achieve a desired effect in virtually all patients without producing toxicity in any. Because the slopes of the quantal dose-effect curves of drug A are steep (indicating little variation in responsiveness to the drug), a dose effective in 99% of the population (ED_{99}) can be administered with little risk to the recipients. Although drug B exhibits a therapeutic index five times greater than drug A, the biologic variability to it is so great that an ED_{99} would produce toxicity in a significant fraction of the population. Estimates of relative safety that take biologic variation into account include the *certain safety factor*, which is the LD_{01}/ED_{99} ratio (with LD_{01} being the lethal dose in 1% of the population), and the *standard safety margin*, which is the percent increase over the ED_{99} needed to reach the LD_{01}, calculated as follows:

$$\frac{LD_{01} - ED_{99}}{ED_{99}} \times 100$$

The disadvantage of these measures compared with the therapeutic index is the larger number of animals required for their determination.

To thoroughly evaluate drug safety in animals, acute, subacute, and chronic toxicity testing must be carried out in several different species and by several different routes of administration. Special studies are performed to detect carcinogenic and teratogenic activity, and adjuvants (e.g., Freund's) are used to test new products for their propensity to cause contact dermatitis. In addition to toxicity evaluations, pharmacokinetic investigations are run to determine the rate and extent of drug absorption, pattern of distribution, plasma half-life, and routes of elimination. Correlation of pharmacologic effect with plasma titer has some predictive value for the therapeutic concentration in human beings and can indicate if the parent drug or a metabolite is the active moiety. Some of the more protracted and costly investigations may be run concurrently with human studies to save time and expense (if the drug proves unsuitable during initial clinical trials).

Regardless of the number, size, or sophistication of animal tests used, studies in human beings are necessary to establish the clinical worth of any drug. Primarily because of unpredictable differences in biotransformation, pharmacokinetic studies in animals cannot be relied on to determine the correct dose or the duration of action of a drug in human beings. Of even greater importance is the inability of preclinical studies to detect many forms of drug toxicity that occur in human beings. Most revealing in this regard was a retrospective compilation of adverse reactions to six unrelated drugs, each used in human beings, rats, and dogs.[33] Considering only toxic signs that are observable in animals as well as human beings, 43% of the various kinds of human toxicity caused by the drugs were not found in either of the test species. When subjective

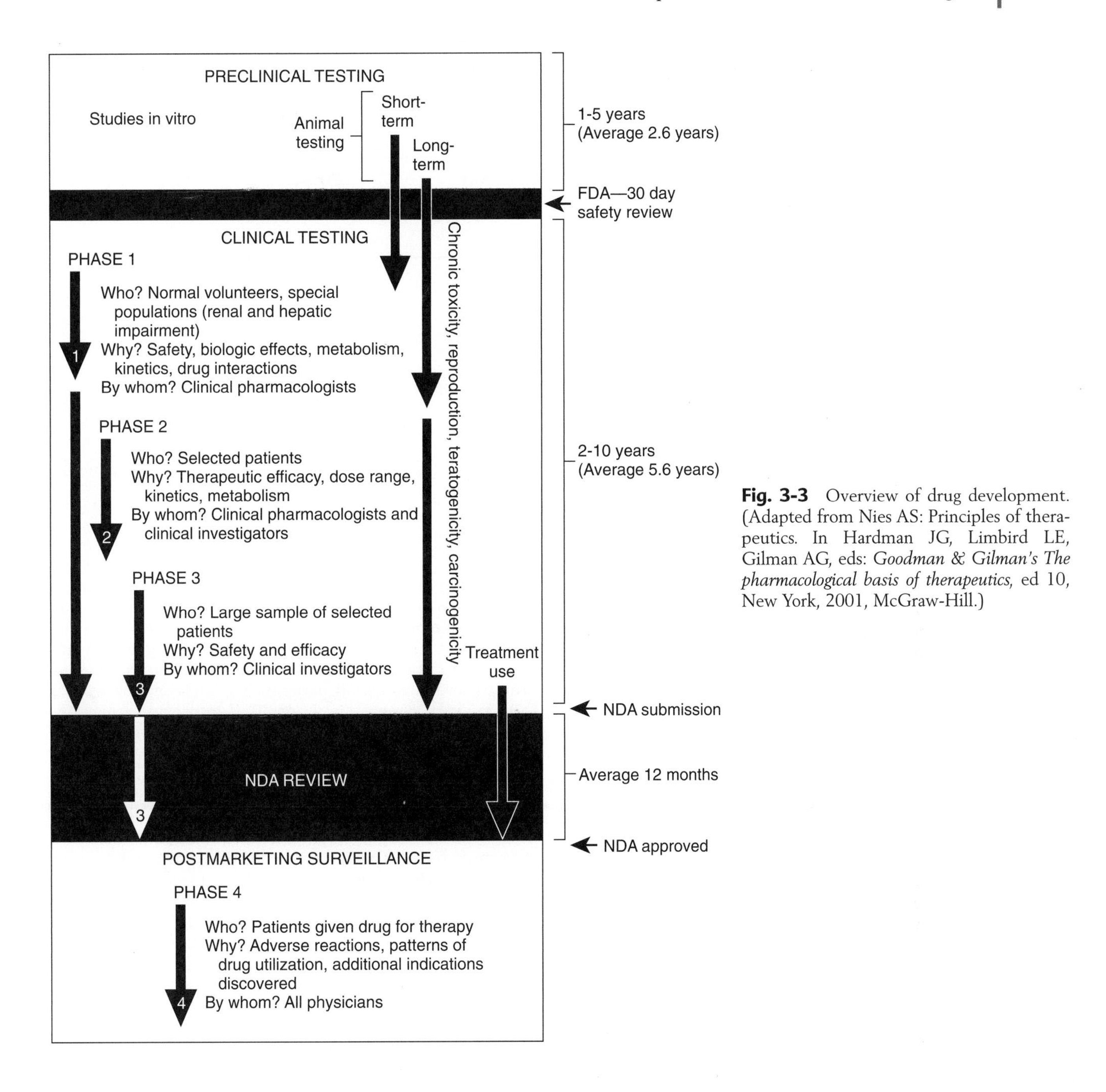

Fig. 3-3 Overview of drug development. (Adapted from Nies AS: Principles of therapeutics. In Hardman JG, Limbird LE, Gilman AG, eds: *Goodman & Gilman's The pharmacological basis of therapeutics*, ed 10, New York, 2001, McGraw-Hill.)

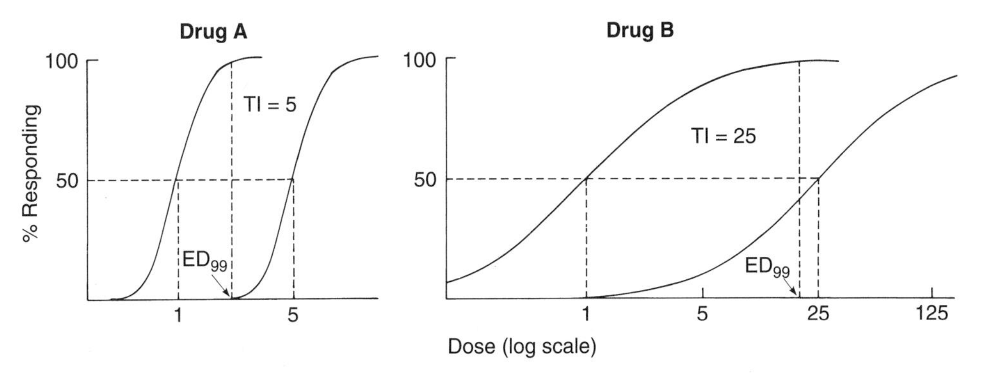

Fig. 3-4 Quantal dose-response relationships (log scale) of two drugs, *A* and *B*. For each drug, the curve on the left reflects therapeutic responses and the curve on the right represents toxic reactions. *TI*, Therapeutic index; ED_{99}, dose effective in 99% of the population.

Table • 3-8

Comparison of Potency, Irritancy, and Lethality of Several Local Anesthetics

		LOCAL IRRITANCY†		LETHALITY‡	
DRUG	ANESTHESIA* TAC (mmol/L)	TIC (mmol/L)	RELATIVE SAFETY	LD_{50} (μmol/L)	RELATIVE SAFETY
Procaine	8.8	176	1.0	220	1.0
Tetracaine	0.69	12	0.9	27	1.6
Propoxycaine	0.81	75	4.6	22	1.1
Lidocaine	2.69	62	1.2	85	1.3
Cocaine	1.16	79	3.4	62	2.1

Data from Luduena FP, Hoppe JO: 2-Alkoxy benzoate and thiolbenzoate derivatives as local anesthetics, *J Pharmacol Exp Ther* 117:89-96, 1956.
*Intracutaneous wheal test in guinea pigs.
†Trypan blue test in rabbits.
‡Intravenous injection in mice.
LD_{50}, Median lethal dose; *TAC*, threshold anesthetic concentration; *TIC*, threshold irritant concentration.

responses (e.g., depression and giddiness) and other effects not detectable in animals (e.g., urticaria, nausea, headache) are taken into account, it becomes apparent that at least half of the untoward responses frequently caused by drugs cannot be ascertained preclinically. Thus the need for human experimentation in drug development is unassailable.

Clinical trials

If an agent appears sufficiently promising on the basis of its preclinical evaluation to warrant testing in human beings, the drug sponsor (generally a large pharmaceutical company) must first submit an application to the FDA in the form of a *Notice of Claimed Investigational Exemption for a New Drug* (IND application) detailing, among other things: (1) the identity of the drug and how it is prepared; (2) all results of preclinical investigations to date; (3) the intended use of the agent, dosage form, and route of administration; and (4) the procedures to be followed in assessing the drug's safety and effectiveness in human beings. On FDA approval of the IND application, the first phase of clinical evaluation can begin.

Phase I trials represent an intensive study of the drug in a few, usually healthy volunteers. The safe or tolerable human dose is arrived at by cautiously administering increasing increments of the drug to subjects until the desired response is obtained or a toxic side effect intervenes. Pharmacokinetic data from single as well as repeated administrations are collected to determine the bioavailability of the compound, its time course of action, and how it is eliminated from the body. Careful attention is given to any adverse effects that may appear. As with subsequent clinical studies, informed consent must be obtained from all subjects involved in phase I trials. Regulations by the FDA involving human experimentation conform to the principles incorporated in the Nuremberg Code and Declaration of Helsinki of the World Medical Association.[18]

The second phase of clinical evaluation involves administration of the drug to a small number of targeted patients. Phase II trials are the first real attempt to establish efficacy, and many drugs are withdrawn from further investigation at this point. The exact studies made during phase II are determined in large measure by the drug. However, the major goals of investigation are constant: to establish efficacy and safety in patients and to arrive at the therapeutic dose. These first two phases are conducted exclusively by professionals trained and experienced in clinical pharmacology.

The decision to proceed to phase III trials commits the drug sponsor to a large-scale, controlled study of the drug. In phase III, the agent must be proved to be relatively safe and effective in a clinical setting. Such proof may require the combined efforts of more than 100 practitioners administering the drug to several thousand patients. It is most important that these trials be designed and organized to provide a scientifically sound appraisal of the drug's therapeutic value. There must, for example, be a clearly defined end point of treatment so that drug effectiveness can be accurately determined. Proper controls (placebos when appropriate, active drugs when available) must be run concurrently to provide the necessary comparisons of drugs, and sufficient numbers of subjects must be used in the study to make such comparisons meaningful. The assignment of subjects to control and test categories must be unbiased. This generally requires either a randomized allotment of patients, in which each volunteer has an equal chance of being in any treatment group, or a crossover design, in which every subject receives each treatment in a balanced order. Bias in reporting drug effects must also be avoided. This can often only be accomplished by performing the trial under "blind" conditions. In a single-blind study, patients are not informed of which drug they receive; in a double-blind investigation, the identity of the medication is concealed from all persons directly engaged in the study. Finally, appropriate statistical methods must be used to verify any conclusions reached about the drug.

Drug approval and continued surveillance

At the conclusion of phase III, a considerable body of information will have been gathered about the drug. These data are submitted to the FDA in the form of a *New Drug Application* (NDA). If accepted as "complete," the drug will be approved for marketing as a prescription drug or as an over-the-counter item, depending on the need for professional supervision to ensure user safety. More often than not, however, the NDA is labeled "incomplete," and the sponsor is advised of additional evaluations that must be performed for it to be accepted. Even with approval of the agent, the sponsor must continue to submit reports to the FDA at regular intervals describing the quantity of drug distributed and detailing any unusual responses to the preparation, such as allergic reactions, idiosyncratic responses, or unanticipated drug interactions. This review constitutes phase IV of the clinical investigation. Continued surveillance of the drug after general release is often the only method available for identifying uncommon or delayed toxic effects. For instance, chloramphenicol was extensively used for 2 years before it was discovered to be capable of inducing severe blood dyscrasias (in approximately 0.002% of treated patients)[42] and for 17 years before it was recognized to be capable of causing visual impairment.[9] It seems an ever-repeating cycle that a new drug is initially hailed as being essentially nontoxic, only to have enthusiasm dampened several years later by the realization that adverse effects are, in fact, an integral part of the agent's pharmacologic profile.

Impact of FDA regulations on the development of new drugs

Regulations by the FDA governing the development and marketing of therapeutic agents exist largely as a result of public concern over the toxic liabilities of drugs. Indeed, had similar regulations been in force in Europe before 1959, the thalidomide disaster affecting some 10,000 children could probably have been averted. There are, however, several disadvantages to the present evaluation system used in the United States. It may take an average of 15 years for a new chemical entity (an agent unrelated to other drugs) to successfully negotiate the obstacle course of preclinical and clinical testing and, including the development costs associated with unfruitful compounds, cost more than $1 billion.

The delay in introducing new drugs into pharmacotherapeutics after 1962 opened up a "drug lag" between the United States and other countries.[64] In response to this problem (and more specifically to pressure from AIDS advocates), the FDA established new regulations that allowed patients to receive investigational drugs targeted against serious or life-threatening disease outside clinical trials when no satisfactory alternative therapy was available.[24] In the most extreme example, several promising drugs against the HIV virus were made available to patients immediately after completion of phase I trials. Other strategies were instituted within the FDA to speed the review process. The FDA Modernization Act of 1997 incorporated these and other changes to streamline drug development.

The uncertainty and expense of bringing new drugs to market in recent years have had a striking influence on the pharmaceutical industry. Only the largest drug manufacturers have the resources to meet FDA guidelines for new drugs. Because pharmaceutical companies are profit-oriented enterprises, the enormous cost of developing a drug will be incurred only if a reasonable return on the investment can be anticipated. Thus, without some additional incentive, the development of drugs for rare diseases has been priced out of consideration. It is also to be expected that agents under patent protection will be highly priced and heavily promoted.

Two laws pertaining to drug development have been enacted in an effort to stimulate therapies for "orphan" diseases and to reduce the cost of pharmaceuticals. The Orphan Drug Act of 1983 provided tax incentives and other considerations to companies for the development of drugs for rare disorders (afflicting fewer than 200,000 people in the United States) and for more common diseases in which there is no reasonable expectation for recovery of development costs. Examples of orphan drugs that have been marketed under this legislation include levocarnitine for primary carnitine deficiency, pentamidine for the treatment of *Pneumocystis carinii* pneumonia, and naltrexone for support of abstinence in former heroin addicts. The Drug Price Competition and Patent Term Restoration Act of 1984 extended the period of patent protection for drugs whose introduction is delayed by the FDA approval process, and it abbreviated the requirements for NDA approval of generic versions of drugs approved after 1962 that are pharmaceutically identical and have equivalent bioavailability.

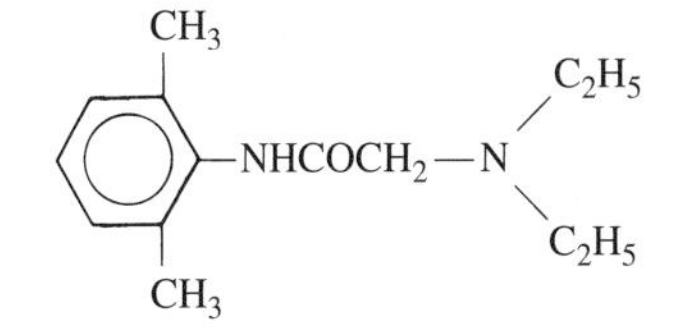

CH_3 / $-NHCOCH_2-N(C_2H_5)_2$ / CH_3

Chemical name:	Diethylaminoaceto-2,6-xylidide
Code name:	LL 30
Nonproprietary name:	Lidocaine
Official name:	Lidocaine
Trade names:	Xylocaine, Dilocaine, Lignospan, Nervocaine, Octocaine

Fig. 3-5 Full nomenclature of a local anesthetic.

Drug Nomenclature

During the course of development and marketing, a drug acquires a variety of names or designations (Figure 3-5). The first identification of a drug is the formal chemical name. Although descriptive of the molecular structure of the compound, the chemical name is usually too unwieldy for practical purposes. Often, therefore, a newly synthesized drug is given a simple code name by the parent pharmaceutical firm to denote the agent during the various stages of drug evaluation. If the drug manufacturer intends to request approval by the FDA for distributing the agent, a nonproprietary name, or United States Adopted Name, will be assigned to the drug by the United States Adopted Name Council, an organization jointly sponsored by the United States Pharmacopeial Convention, the American Medical Association, and the American Pharmaceutical Association. The nonproprietary name is commonly referred to as the "generic" name, but, by definition, the generic designation should be reserved to indicate a family of compounds (e.g., penicillins) rather than a single entity (e.g., ampicillin). If the drug is eventually admitted to the *United States Pharmacopeia* (USP), its nonproprietary name then becomes the official name.

Much confusion over drug nomenclature arises because a single drug may be marketed under many different trade names. A trade, or proprietary, name is given to a drug by the manufacturer when the agent is approved for general release. Unlike the nonproprietary name, which is publicly owned, a trade name receives copyright protection and is the sole property of the drug company. On occasion, a manufacturer may distribute the agent under several different trade names to promote separate uses of the drug. In addition, the manufacturer may arrange with other pharmaceutical firms to sell the drug, each using its own trade name. A profusion of trade names may develop when the drug patent expires and all companies are permitted by law to produce the agent. Assignment of trade names to drug combination products contributes yet another voice to the babel of drug names.

Confusion often arises when the manufacturer of a popular drug uses an extension of the drug's trade name to market additional, sometimes unrelated, products. For example, Chlor-Trimeton is a well-known brand name for the antihistamine chlorpheniramine.[44] The marketing of the adrenergic vasoconstrictor pseudoephedrine in the 1990s as Chlor-Trimeton Non-Drowsy raised the potential for ineffective therapy in the allergic patient and hypertension and angina pectoris in the patient with cardiovascular disease. Today, chlorpheniramine is marketed by the manufacturer with the label Chlor-Trimeton Allergy; the combination of chlorpheniramine and pseudoephedrine is sold as Chlor-Trimeton Allergy-D.

Throughout this book, nonproprietary names are emphasized in discussions of the various drugs. This practice reduces confusion and equips the reader to use other sources of drug information to the best advantage. The benefits and debits of using nonproprietary designations in prescription writing are presented in Chapter 55.

SOURCES OF DRUG INFORMATION

The continued development of new drugs and the acquisition of new information about existing agents make pharmacology a discipline requiring continual study. Various resources are available to aid the clinician in keeping abreast of advances in pharmacotherapeutics.

Official Compendia

The *USP* and The *National Formulary (NF)* were designated as official compendia of drugs in the United States by the Pure Food and Drug Act of 1906. First published in 1820, the *USP* is revised every 5 years, with interim supplementation as needed, by the Committee on Revision of the United States Pharmacopeial Convention, Inc. Members of the Council on Scientific Affairs of the American Dental Association serve in an advisory capacity to the Committee on Revision. Before 1975, only single-entity drugs (preparations with a single active ingredient) of proven therapeutic value were considered for inclusion in the *USP*. The *NF*, first released in 1888, was a publication of the American Pharmaceutical Association. In addition to single-entity agents of therapeutic value, the *NF* admitted combination products when their use provided a therapeutic advantage to the patient. After publication of the fourteenth edition in 1975, the *NF* was consolidated with the *USP* under the management of the *USP* organization. With this consolidation, the *USP* was expanded to include "all drugs having proven efficiency as therapeutic agents," including selected combination products, whereas the *NF* was restricted to describing pharmaceutical ingredients used in the formulation of marketed products.[58] The USP-NF is not a good source of information about the clinical use of drugs. However, it provides an invaluable service to the practitioner by defining criteria for the manufacture of pharmaceutical preparations. It ensures that when a prescription is written for an official drug, the medication supplied to the patient will meet certain standards of strength, purity, and chemical and physical properties.

A number of other nations have their own official compendia. In addition, the *International Pharmacopoeia* is issued by the World Health Organization. Although not official in the sense of the *USP*, the *International Pharmacopoeia* is instrumental in promoting the standardization and unification of the various national compendia.

Unofficial Compendia

The *Physicians' Desk Reference (PDR)* is perhaps the most widely distributed source of prescribing information available to health professionals. The *PDR* is published annually (with interim revisions as necessary) by the Medical Economics Company in cooperation with more than 200 pharmaceutical manufacturing and distributing concerns. More than 4000 preparations are listed by proprietary name in an alphabetical arrangement according to drug distributor. (The cost of including a drug deters many companies from listing all their products.) Although the *PDR* is well indexed, its organization makes the comparison of similar agents difficult. The product information, which is largely derived from phase III trials and must legally conform to FDA regulations, contains concise summaries of the uses, dosage forms and schedules, contraindications, and adverse effects of the drugs listed. Nevertheless, the lack of critical appraisals of, or relative comparisons between, the various preparations included in the *PDR* limits its use as a reliable guide for the rational selection of drugs in therapy. The *PDR for Herbal Medicines*, the *PDR for Nutritional Supplements*, and the *PDR for Nonprescription Drugs and Dietary Supplements* are specialized sources of information.

A suitable alternative to the *PDR* is *Facts and Comparisons*. Published independently of the pharmaceutical industry, *Facts and Comparisons* contains monographs in a format designed to facilitate comparisons between drugs. Constructed as a loose-leaf binder, the compendium readily incorporates page revisions, which are distributed monthly to keep the drug information up to date. A less expensive book version published annually is also available.

Mosby's Drug Consult is a compilation of full prescribing information for 21,000 drug products. Because drug entries in *Mosby's Drug Consult* are not paid for by pharmaceutical companies, the book contains information on unlabeled uses, older drugs no longer under patent, investigational drugs, and international brand names. *Mosby's Drug Consult* has a single keyword index that lists information by nonproprietary and trade names, indications, and pharmacologic and therapeutic class. *Mosby's Drug Consult* provides cost comparison information for brand and generic products. Comparative tables aid in selecting an appropriate drug within a therapeutic class.

In 1975, the *USP* organization decided to directly assist and benefit health care practitioners in the use of drugs. Publication of the *USP Dispensing Information (USPDI)* was a major outcome of that decision. In its current form, the *USPDI* comprises three separate volumes. Volume I, *Drug Information for the Health Care Professional*, contains useful clinical information for numerous drugs. Volume II, *Advice for the Patient*, includes information for the patient regarding the proper use of specific medications, precautions to consider, and adverse effects that may occur. Drug monographs from this volume may be reproduced and distributed without prior authorization by the *USP* organization to patients receiving the medications. Volume III, *Approved Drug Products and Legal Requirements*, contains information on the therapeutic equivalence of drugs and various regulatory issues.

Books on Pharmacology and Therapeutics

Textbooks of general pharmacology usually present basic principles of drug action and pharmacologic profiles of the various classes of therapeutic agents. Descriptions of relationships between pathophysiologic characteristics and drug effects contained in textbooks significantly contribute to the understanding of pharmacotherapeutics. Although textbooks can provide perhaps the best overview of pharmacology, for clarity of presentation and because of limitations of space, detailed coverage of individual agents in each drug category is generally restricted to a limited number of prototypical compounds. Thus epinephrine may be discussed in depth while other sympathomimetic amines commonly used by practitioners (e.g., levonordefrin as a vasoconstrictor in local anesthetic solutions) or patients (e.g., pseudoephedrine as a vasoconstrictor in cold remedies) need not be as extensively discussed. Textbooks are also limited in that they cannot include information on the most recent advances in pharmacotherapeutics, such as the introduction of new drugs.

The *Handbook of Nonprescription Drugs*, published by the American Pharmaceutical Association, is one of the few sources of information concerning over-the-counter drugs. The handbook presents critical evaluations of the various preparations available to the public. Of special interest to dentists are the chapters on headache and muscle and joint pain, herbal remedies, and oral pain and discomfort.

Periodicals

A number of journals and reviews are expressly devoted to pharmacology and therapeutics. *The Journal of Pharmacology and Experimental Therapeutics* and *Molecular Pharmacology* offer in-depth treatment of all areas of pharmacology. These journals are primarily concerned with the experimental aspects of pharmacodynamics. *Clinical Pharmacology and Therapeutics* has articles dealing with drug effects in human beings. Journals that review pharmacologic information of direct clinical relevance include *Drugs* and the *Annual Review of Pharmacology and Toxicology*. Although not restricted in scope to drugs, the *New England Journal of Medicine* is noteworthy for its excellent coverage of pharmacotherapeutics. Specialty journals of significance to dentistry include *Anesthesiology*, *Anesthesia and Analgesia*, and *Pain*.

The *Medical Letter on Drugs and Therapeutics* provides a unique service to practitioners in this country. Published biweekly, *The Medical Letter* offers current, concise, and critical reviews of new drugs and pharmaceutical preparations. Expert opinion is also provided regarding the therapeutic and toxic effects of established drugs. In this respect, the periodic updates on drug interactions and on clinical selection of antimicrobial agents are especially helpful.

Dental Sources of Information

The American Dental Association *Guide to Dental Therapeutics* is published by the Council on Scientific Affairs of the American Dental Association. It is an excellent reference for the therapeutic application of drugs in dentistry. This resource has information on drugs listed by both proprietary and nonproprietary names. Drugs pertaining predominantly to dentistry are also extensively covered.

Mosby's Dental Drug Reference and *Drug Information Handbook for Dentistry* are reference handbooks useful for the quick identification of drugs and their dental implications. Both sources are published annually. The former is more compact and easier to use; the latter is more comprehensive in its coverage and is now available for downloading to handheld electronic devices.

Although there is currently no dental periodical solely concerned with pharmacology, a number of journals feature articles dealing with drugs in dental practice. *Anesthesia Progress* is the official journal of the American Dental Society of Anesthesiology. It publishes papers on drugs useful in pain and anxiety control and prints abstracts from other periodicals of related papers of interest. The *Journal of the American Dental Association* is also a good source of information about dental pharmacotherapeutics. In addition to publishing original contributions and review articles, the *Journal of the American Dental Association* provides evaluations from the Council on Scientific Affairs on issues pertaining to drugs and dentistry. *Critical Reviews in Oral Biology and Medicine* publishes quarterly reviews, some of which relate to drug therapy in dentistry. Specialty journals, such as the *Journal of Oral and Maxillofacial Surgery* and the *Journal of Periodontology* occasionally publish papers on dental pharmacotherapeutics.

Electronic Media

Computerization of sources of drug information is rapidly progressing. Most of the sources of information described above, or the databases from which they are derived, are now available on compact disk. These formats permit the use of Boolean descriptors and hypertext links to facilitate searches within a single source or among several sources at the same time. Digital book systems, incorporating one or more sources of information in a palm-sized reader, facilitate immediate access to drug information in all clinical settings. ePocrates Rx (www.epocrates.com) is a free resource on drugs that includes concise information ranging from pharmacodynamics to cost of drugs. It is available exclusively for Palm handheld electronic devices and is designed for quick reference.

The Internet is increasingly becoming a vital source of drug information. A number of sites on the World Wide Web provide information regarding specific issues pertaining to dental therapeutics. Some of these are free; others charge a monthly or connect fee. Many of the book titles listed previously are also available online. Some other sources are as follows. PubMed (www.ncbi.nlm.nih.gov/PubMed) is the National Library of Medicine's interface to MEDLINE and other information sources. It provides access, for a fee, to a large number of scientific journals. Free access to numerous journal articles may be obtained through PubMed Central (www.pubmedcentral.gov). Micromedex (www.micromedex.com) is a reference that provides useful drug information for the health care professional. Lexi-Comp online (www.lexi.com) has a useful drug identification and vocal pronunciation guide for drugs as well as information on pharmacokinetics, adverse effects, and drug interactions. eMedicine (www.emedicine.com) is an extensive online resource that presents a discussion of disorders and treatment options. RxList (www.rxlist.com) is a handy and valuable online resource concentrating on the clinical aspects of drugs. xPharm (www.xpharm.com) is a comprehensive online resource in pharmacology. xPharm is extensively linked both internally and externally, offering significant search capabilities. Principles of pharmacology as well as drug and receptor characteristics are covered in depth. This resource also has extensive discussions of disorders for which the drugs are used.

Cited References

1. Adams RM: *Occupational contact dermatitis*, Philadelphia, 1969, JB Lippincott.
2. Arora S, Aldrete JA: Investigation of possible allergy to local anesthetic drugs: correlation of intradermal with intramuscular injections, *Anesth Rev* 3:13-16, 1976.
3. Beck FM: Placebos in dentistry: their profound potential effects, *J Am Dent Assoc* 95:1122-1126, 1977.
4. Beecher HK: The powerful placebo, *JAMA* 159:1602-1606, 1955.
5. Blanc PD, Jones MR, Olson KR: Surveillance of poisoning and drug overdose through hospital discharge coding, poison control center reporting, and the Drug Abuse Warning Network, *Am J Emerg Med* 11:14-19, 1993.
6. Bourne HR: The placebo—a poorly understood and neglected therapeutic agent, *Rational Drug Ther* 5:1-6, 1971.
7. Bretherton A, Day L, Lewis G: Polypharmacy and older people, *Nurs Times* 99:54-55, 2003.
8. Chignell CF, Vesell ES, Starkweather DK, et al: The binding of sulfaphenazole to fetal, neonatal, and adult human plasma albumin, *Clin Pharmacol Ther* 12:897-901, 1971.
9. Cocke JG, Jr, Brown RE, Geppert LJ: Optic neuritis with prolonged use of chloramphenicol. Case report and relationship to fundus changes in cystic fibrosis, *J Pediatr* 68:27-31, 1966.
10. Coombs RRA, Gell PGH: Classification of allergic reactions responsible for clinical hypersensitivity and disease. In Gell PGH, Coombs RRA, Lachmann PJ, eds: *Clinical aspects of immunology*, ed 3, Oxford, 1975, Blackwell Scientific.
11. de la Fuente-Fernandez R, Schulzer M, Stoessl AJ: The placebo effect in neurological disorders, *Lancet Neurol* 1:85-91, 2002.
12. Denissenko MF, Pao A, Tang M, et al: Preferential formation of benzo[*a*]pyrene adducts at lung cancer mutational hotspots in *P53*, *Science* 274:430-432, 1996.

13. DeSwarte RD: Drug allergy. In Patterson R, ed: *Allergic diseases: diagnosis and management*, ed 3, Philadelphia, 1985, JB Lippincott.
14. de Vos AM, Tong L, Milburn MV, et al: Three-dimensional structure of an oncogene protein: catalytic domain of human c-H-*ras* p21, *Science* 239:888-893, 1988.
15. Done AK, Cohen SN, Strebel L: Pediatric clinical pharmacology and the "therapeutic orphan," *Annu Rev Pharmacol Toxicol* 17:561-573, 1977.
16. Forfar JO, Nelson MM: Epidemiology of drugs taken by pregnant women: drugs that may affect the fetus adversely, *Clin Pharmacol Ther* 14:632-642, 1973.
17. Gibaldi M: *Biopharmaceutics and clinical pharmacokinetics*, ed 3, Philadelphia, 1984, Lea & Febiger.
18. Grilley B: Investigational drugs. In Malone PM, Wilkinson Mosdell K, et al, eds: *Drug information: a guide for pharmacists*, ed 2, New York, 2001, McGraw-Hill.
19. Hathway DE: *Mechanisms of chemical carcinogenesis*, London, 1986, Butterworth.
20. Henson PM: Antibody and immune-complex-mediated allergic and inflammatory reactions. In Lachmann PJ, Peters DK, eds: *Clinical aspects of immunology*, ed 4, Oxford, 1982, Blackwell Scientific.
21. Hrobjartsson A: What are the main methodological problems in the estimation of placebo effects? *J Clin Epidemiol* 55:430-435, 2002.
22. Hrobjartsson A, Gotzsche PC: Is the placebo powerless? An analysis of clinical trials comparing placebo with no treatment, *N Engl J Med* 344:1594-1602, 2001.
23. Kalivas PW, Duffy P: Effect of acute and daily cocaine treatment on extracellular dopamine in the nucleus acumbens, *Synapse* 5:48-58, 1990.
24. Kessler DA, Hass AE, Feiden KL, et al: Approval of new drugs in the United States. Comparison with the United Kingdom, Germany, and Japan, *JAMA* 276:1826-1831, 1996.
25. Killoy WJ, Polson AM: Controlled local delivery of antimicrobials in the treatment of periodontitis, *Dent Clin North Am* 42:263-283, 1998.
26. Kreitman RJ: Recombinant toxins for the treatment of cancer, *Curr Opin Mol Ther* 5:44-51, 2003.
27. Kubisty CA, Arns PA, Wedlund PJ, et al: Adjustment of medications in liver failure. In Chernow B, ed: *The pharmacologic approach to the critically ill patient*, ed 3, Baltimore, 1994, Williams & Wilkins.
28. Kutt H: Diphenylhydantoin metabolism, blood levels, and toxicity, *Arch Neurol* 11:642-648, 1964.
29. Lazarou J, Pomeranz BH, Corey PN: Incidence of adverse drug reactions in hospitalized patients: a meta-analysis of prospective studies, *JAMA* 279:1200-1205, 1998.
30. Lenz W: Epidemiology of congenital malformations, *Ann NY Acad Sci* 123:228-236, 1965.
31. Levine JD, Gordon NC, Fields HL: The mechanism of placebo analgesia, *Lancet* 2:654-657, 1978.
32. Levine RR: *Pharmacology: drug actions and reactions*, ed 6, Boston, 2000, Little, Brown.
33. Litchfield JT, Jr: Evaluation of the safety of new drugs by means of tests in animals, *Clin Pharmacol Ther* 3:665-672, 1962.
34. Litovitz TL, Klein-Schwartz W, Rogers GC, Jr, et al: 2001 Annual report of the American Association of Poison Control Centers Toxic Exposure Surveillance System, *Am J Emerg Med* 20:391-452, 2002.
35. Luduena FP, Hoppe JO: 2-Alkoxy benzoate and thiolbenzoate derivatives as local anesthetics, *J Pharmacol Exp Ther* 117:89-96, 1956.
36. Lund L: Effects of phenytoin in patients with epilepsy in relation to its concentration in plasma. In Davies DS, Prichard BNC, eds: *Biological effects of drugs in relation to their plasma concentrations*, Baltimore, 1973, University Park Press.
37. Macek C: Monoclonal antibodies: key to a revolution in clinical medicine, *JAMA* 247:2463-2470, 1982.
38. Malik VS: Recombinant DNA technology, *Adv Appl Microbiol* 27:1-84, 1981.
39. Malone PM, Kier KL: Pharmacy and therapeutics committee. In Malone PM, Wilkinson Mosdell K, Kier KL, et al, eds: *Drug information: a guide for pharmacists*, ed 2, New York, 2001, McGraw-Hill.
40. Marks PA, Banks J: Drug-induced hemolytic anemias associated with glucose-6-phosphate dehydrogenase deficiency: a genetically heterogeneous trait, *Ann NY Acad Sci* 123:198-206, 1965.
41. Mattila MJ, Jussila J, Takki S: Drug absorption in patients with intestinal villous atrophy, *Arzneimittelforschung* 23:583-585, 1973.
42. McCurdy PR: Chloramphenicol bone marrow toxicity, *JAMA* 176:588-593, 1961.
43. Moolten FL, Schreiber BM, Zajdel SH: Antibodies conjugated to potent cytotoxins as specific antitumor agents, *Immunol Rev* 62:47-73, 1982.
44. *OTC names: an invitation to err?* USP Quality Review, no. 54, Rockville, MD, 1996, United States Pharmacopeial Convention.
45. Parker CW: Drug allergy, part 1, *N Engl J Med* 292:511-514, 1975.
46. Parker CW: Drug allergy, part 3, *N Engl J Med* 292:957-960, 1975.
47. Prescott LF, Roscoe P, Wright N, et al: Plasma-paracetamol half-life and hepatic necrosis in patients with paracetamol overdosage, *Lancet* 1:519-522, 1971.
48. Raymond CA: Liposomes embark on rescue mission to make highly toxic drugs more useful, *JAMA* 257:1143-1144, 1987.
49. Reidenberg MM, Lowenthal DT: Adverse nondrug reactions, *N Engl J Med* 279:678-679, 1968.
50. Reider MJ: Mechanisms of unpredictable adverse drug reactions, *Drug Saf* 11:196-212, 1994.
51. Reinberg A, Reinberg MA: Circadian changes of the duration of action of local anaesthetic agents, *Naunyn Schmiedebergs Arch Pharmacol* 297:149-152, 1977.
52. Rosenthal A: Follow-up study of fatal penicillin reactions, *JAMA* 167:1118-1121, 1958.
53. Roth HP, Caron HS: Accuracy of doctors' estimates and patients' statements on adherence to a drug regimen, *Clin Pharmacol Ther* 23:361-370, 1978.
54. Shelley JH: Phenacetin, through the looking glass, *Clin Pharmacol Ther* 8:427-471, 1967.
55. St. Peter WL, Halstenson CE: Pharmacologic approach in patients with renal failure. In Chernow B, ed: *The pharmacologic approach to the critically ill patient*, ed 3, Baltimore, 1994, Williams & Wilkins.
56. Stanley LA: Molecular aspects of chemical carcinogenesis: the roles of oncogenes and tumour suppressor genes, *Toxicology* 96:173-194, 1996.

57. Stewart RB, Cluff LE: A review of medication errors and compliance in ambulant patients, *Clin Pharmacol Ther* 13:463-468, 1972.
58. *The United States Pharmacopeia*, rev 26, and *The National Formulary*, ed 21, Rockville, MD, 2002, The United States Pharmacopeial Convention.
59. Underwood T, Iturrian WB, Cadwallader DE: Some aspects of chemical teratogenesis, *Am J Hosp Pharm* 27:115-122, 1970.
60. Venter JC: Immobilized and insolubilized drugs, hormones, and neurotransmitters: properties, mechanisms of action and applications, *Pharmacol Rev* 34:153-187, 1982.
61. *Vital statistics—special reports, national summaries*, Washington, DC, 1959-1974, National Office of Vital Statistics, US Department of Health, Education, and Welfare.
62. Vogelstein B, Kinsler KW: The multistep nature of cancer, *Trends Genet* 9:138-141, 1993.
63. Walton WW: An evaluation of the Poison Prevention Packaging Act, *Pediatrics* 69:363-370, 1982.
64. Wardell WM: Therapeutic implications of the drug lag, *Clin Pharmacol Ther* 15:73-96, 1974.
65. Wolf S: The pharmacology of placebos, *Pharmacol Rev* 11:689-704, 1959.

General References

Chernow B, ed: *The pharmacologic approach to the critically ill patient*, ed 3, Baltimore, 1994, Williams & Wilkins.

Hanston PD, Horn JR: *Hanston and Horn's Drug interactions analysis and management*, Vancouver, WA, 1997, Applied Therapeutics.

Levine RR: *Pharmacology: drug actions and reactions*, ed 6, Boston, 2000, Little, Brown.

Malone PM, Wilkinson Mosdell K, Kier KL, et al, eds: *Drug information: a guide for pharmacists*, ed 2, New York, 2001, McGraw-Hill.

Nielsen JR: *Handbook of federal drug law*, ed 2, Philadelphia, 1992, Lea & Febiger.

Pratt WB, Taylor P, eds: *Principles of drug action: the basis of pharmacology*, ed 3, New York, 1990, Churchill Livingstone.

Rowland M, Tozer TN: *Clinical pharmacokinetics: concepts and applications*, ed 3, Baltimore, 1995, Williams & Wilkins.

CHAPTER • 4

Pharmacogenetics and General Mechanisms of Drug Interactions*

John A. Yagiela and David W. Hein

Individual patient differences in drug responsiveness are well recognized by health care professionals. Understanding the basis for these differences is of major clinical and economic importance because of the high frequency of both therapeutic failure and adverse reactions to drugs. A recent study reported the incidence of severe adverse drug reactions in the United States at 6.7%, or more than 2 million cases annually.[18] Furthermore, the incidence of fatal drug reactions among hospitalized patients in the United States was 0.32%, or more than 100,000 cases annually, making it the fourth leading cause of death after heart disease, cancer, and stroke. Millions more receive inadequate or suboptimal benefit from drug treatment. In this chapter, we describe pharmacogenetics and drug interactions as two important mechanisms for differences in drug responsiveness.

PHARMACOGENETICS/PHARMACOGENOMICS

Pharmacogenetics is the branch of pharmacology that seeks to understand the genetic basis for differences in drug responsiveness among the human population. The ability to select the safest and most effective drug and dose for a patient on the basis of the patient's pharmacogenetic profile should minimize the need to adjust the therapeutic regimen to achieve the desired clinical response. The term *pharmacogenomics* is sometimes used interchangeably with *pharmacogenetics* but more precisely refers to the application of genomic information toward the discovery and development of drugs with new and more specific targets. Both pharmacogenetics and pharmacogenomics are areas of intense interest and development within the biotechnology and pharmaceutical industries. Many pharmaceutical companies are beginning to genotype patients in their clinical trials to exclude individuals predisposed to adverse effects or therapeutic failure. A consortium that includes major pharmaceutical companies is assembling a high-density map of single nucleotide polymorphisms (SNPs) to construct pharmacogenetic profiles that predict drug responsiveness. SNPs occur, on average, about once every 100 to 300 bases in the 3 billion base human genome. A website sponsored by the National Center for Biotechnology Information maintains an updated listing of these SNPs (http://www.ncbi.nlm.nih.gov/SNP).

This chapter presents basic principles and mechanisms that account for pharmacogenetic differences in drug therapy and toxicity. The pharmacogenetic examples included are of historic or clinical interest; they are not intended to be exhaustive because, with the recent sequencing of the human genome, tabular listings of pharmacogenetic traits of clinical interest fall rapidly out of date. For more comprehensive and contemporary information, readers are directed, respectively, to a comprehensive monograph on pharmacogenetics[32] and to the regularly updated Pharmacogenetics and Pharmacogenomics Knowledge Base (http://www.pharmgkb.org).

The genome determines the structure, configuration, and even the concentration of endogenous proteins. In most cases, for a drug to produce a therapeutic or toxic response, it must interact with one or more proteins, which in turn are subject to genetic variation in the human population. For example, genetic differences in plasma proteins may affect the affinity and the extent of drug binding. Genetic differences in the enzymes that metabolize a drug may confer differences in the concentrations of the parent compound, its active metabolites, and toxic derivatives. Genetic differences in cell membrane proteins or drug transporter proteins may influence drug absorption, distribution, and excretion. Finally, patients may have drug receptors mediating therapeutic or adverse effects that are genetically more or less abundant or sensitive than is the norm.

The influence of genetic differences on drug responsiveness has been highlighted in the popular press:

> *Every year, more than 100,000 people die in the U.S. because they carry "misspelled" genes that make medications either ineffective or deadly. Now doctors can test for the genes before prescribing . . . Imagine a lawyer asking: "Doctor, did you know this drug would kill your patient? Did you know there is a test that would have predicted that? And why did you not give your patient the test?"*[3]

Such statements, widely read by the lay public (and their lawyers), underscore the need for dental professionals to understand the role of pharmacogenetic factors in drug responsiveness. Indeed, patient malpractice claims have already alleged negligence in the use of pharmacogenetic information.[29]

Pharmacokinetics/Pharmacodynamics

Proteins affect both drug concentration (pharmacokinetics) and response (pharmacodynamics). Historically, genetic variation most often has been identified in pharmacokinetics, particularly in drug-metabolizing enzymes.[32] Genetic variation in pharmacokinetic profile often necessitates a change in the dosage regimen of a drug but not in its selection. Pharmacogenetic differences in drug responsiveness are less well understood but will potentially have the greater impact on patient outcomes in the years ahead. In these instances, certain drugs will be contraindicated for patients with particular

* The authors wish to recognize Dr. Anthony Picozzi for his past contributions to this chapter. See the Acknowledgments.

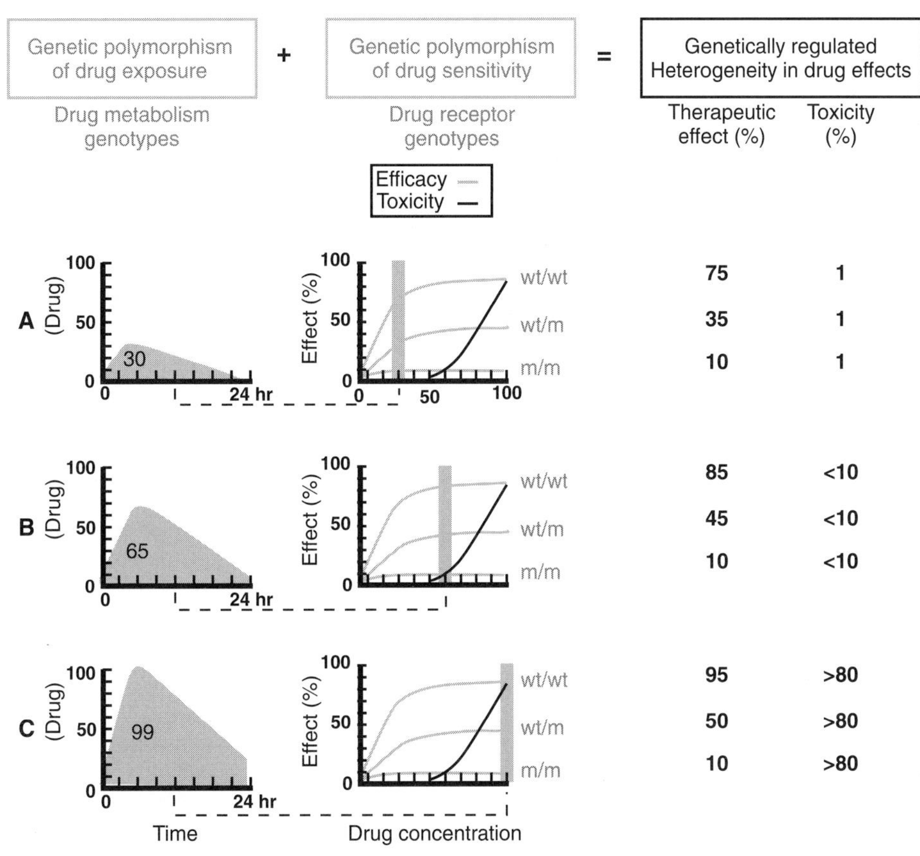

Fig. 4-1 The potential consequences of administering the same dose of drug to individuals with genetic polymorphisms in both pharmacokinetics (drug-metabolizing enzymes) and pharmacodynamics (drug receptors). Active drug concentrations in the systemic circulation are determined by the individual's drug metabolism genotype, with **(A)** homozygous wild type *(wt/wt)* converting 70% of a dose to the inactive metabolite, leaving 30% to exert an effect on the target receptor. **B,** For the patient with heterozygous *(wt/m)* drug metabolism genotype, 35% is inactivated, whereas the patient with homozygous mutant *(m/m)* drug metabolism inactivates only 1% of the drug dose **(C)**, yielding the three drug concentration time curves. The drug response is further influenced by drug receptor genotypes. Patients with a wt/wt receptor genotype exhibit a greater effect at any given drug concentration compared with those with a wt/m receptor genotype, whereas those with m/m receptor genotypes are relatively refractory to drug effects at any plasma drug concentration. The combination of genetic polymorphisms in drug metabolism and receptor yields nine different theoretical patterns of drug effect. The therapeutic ratio (efficacy versus toxicity) ranges from very favorable in a patient with wt/wt genotypes for drug metabolism and drug receptor to very unfavorable in the patient with m/m genotypes. (Redrawn from Evans WE, Relling MV: Pharmacogenomics: translating functional genomics into rational therapeutics, *Science* 286:487-491, 1999.)

genotypes. Just as drug prescribers are currently responsible for avoiding adverse drug-drug interactions as described later in this chapter, they increasingly will be held accountable for avoiding gene-drug interactions in clinical practice. Genetic differences in both pharmacokinetics and pharmacodynamics are anticipated for many if not most drugs, yielding important consequences for drug responsiveness, especially for agents with a narrow therapeutic index. Figure 4-1 illustrates the separate and combined influences of genetic polymorphisms in pharmacokinetics and pharmacodynamics.[8]

Many gene-drug interactions are important to dentistry. For example, codeine—one of the most commonly prescribed opioid analgesics for pain relief—depends on its activation to morphine by CYP2D6, a drug-metabolizing enzyme known to exhibit a common genetic polymorphism in human beings. Thus codeine is an ineffective analgesic in a significant genetic subset (up to 10% depending on ethnic group) of the population.[26] Genetic polymorphisms in opioid receptors or in second messenger systems mediating opioid receptor actions also are expected. If a patient inherits deficiencies in both CYP2D6 and the opioid receptor, codeine is unlikely to be of any therapeutic benefit. Increasing the dose of codeine to compensate for the genetic deficiency in enzymatic activation in a patient who also has the deficient opioid receptor will most likely not result in analgesia but in an adverse reaction mediated by an alternative receptor responsive to codeine.

Phenotype/Genotype

A person's *genotype* is a genetic trait defined by the DNA sequences (i.e., alleles) inherited from the mother and the father. An individual can inherit two copies of the same allele (homozygous genotype) or a different allele from each of the parents (heterozygous genotype). The *phenotype* is a biologic or measurable expression of the genetic trait that depends on the level of penetrance of the gene as well as the accuracy and selectivity of the method used to measure it. Historically, one of the most easily measured phenotypes was plasma drug concentration, which is probably why most pharmacogenetic traits identified to date are pharmacokinetic phenotypes. Determination of drug concentration, however, is relatively invasive, requiring administration of a drug or surrogate chemical and collection of blood samples over time. The drug concentration also depends to varying degrees on patient age, general health, nutritional status, and other factors such as exposure to enzyme inducers and inhibitors. Determination of a patient's genotype is much less invasive because it does not require administration of a test drug or collection of blood samples over time. Instead, the genotype is determined from a small sample of DNA easily obtained from a buccal swab, hair follicle, or other ready source and is not affected by age, general health, nutritional status, or other factors. Many methods to determine the genotype have been developed in the past decade, including restriction fragment length polymorphism analysis, allele-specific amplification, and sequencing. Most methods rely on amplification techniques to yield millions of copies of the specific target gene by the polymerase chain reaction. New high-throughput methods promise to make determination of multiple genotypes readily available to health care professionals.[22] Understanding the relationship between genotype and phenotype is important and has fostered research in functional genomics and proteomics.

Monogenic/Polygenic Phenotypes

A discussion of genetic polymorphisms in enzymes and receptors would be incomplete without consideration of the differences inherent between monogenic and polygenic phenotypes. *Monogenic* phenotypes derive from a single gene. Thus monogenic traits often separate populations into discontinuous (polymorphic) distributions of phenotypes. Different drugs or dosing regimens may be appropriate for specific phenotypes. *Polygenic* traits, in contrast, are phenotypes that derive from multiple genes. Clearly distinct or discontinuous phenotypes are not observed in a studied population. Instead, a single continuous (monomorphic) distribution is noted. A monomorphic distribution of drug response is observed for most drugs metabolized by multiple enzymes and/or transported by multiple proteins and/or acting through multiple receptors and/or second messenger systems. This does not mean an absence of genetic variation in one or all of these proteins, but rather that multiple genes determine the drug-response phenotype. Because each of the genes is potentially subject to genetic variation, the utility of genetic information in predicting therapeutic and toxic responses is more complicated. Until recently, polygenic phenotypes were too complex to consider in optimizing drug therapy.

Ethnic Differences in Pharmacogenetics

The frequency of alleles, genotypes, and phenotypes for drug-metabolizing enzymes varies widely with ethnic origin.[32] A similar variance is expected for drug receptors. Thus clinical trials are best conducted within ethnically diverse study populations to capture differences among ethnic groups. Some genotype methods were originally designed to identify only alleles prevalent in whites. However, because of the documented ethnic heterogeneity within the human population, genotyping should identify all relevant alleles of a particular gene regardless of ethnic frequency.

Pharmacogenetics of Drug Metabolism

As indicated above, most of the pharmacogenetic traits identified to date occur in genes encoding drug-metabolizing enzymes. It is anticipated that genetic polymorphisms may be identified in all drug-metabolizing enzymes. A number of these genetic polymorphisms are already known to be important in therapeutics, and selected examples of historic and clinical interest are highlighted below.

Acetylation polymorphisms

N-acetylation is an important phase II conjugation reaction for many drugs that possess an aromatic amine (e.g., procainamide, dapsone, many sulfonamides) or hydrazine (e.g., isoniazid, hydralazine) moiety. The acetylation polymorphism was originally discovered by studying the development of peripheral neuropathy in patients administered isoniazid.[32] N-acetylation of aromatic amine- and hydrazine-containing drugs is catalyzed by two different N-acetyltransferase isozymes, NAT1 and NAT2.[12,32] Genetic polymorphisms have been identified in both enzymes, but genetic polymorphisms in NAT2 are more common and important for the metabolism of many drugs in common use.[32,33] Human populations can be distinguished as rapid and slow acetylator phenotypes by measuring production of N-acetylated metabolites after administration of drugs such as isoniazid or dapsone.[32,33] SNPs have been identified in the NAT2 gene affecting protein expression and/or stability.[9] Acetylator genotypes derived from more than 25 different NAT2 alleles have been identified in human beings. A listing of these alleles is regularly updated at http://www.louisville.edu/medschool/pharmacology/NAT.html.

As is the case for most drug-metabolizing enzyme polymorphisms, the frequencies of these SNPs, genotypes, and acetylator phenotypes vary markedly with ethnic origin. For example, the frequency of slow acetylator phenotypes is approximately 10% in Asian populations, roughly 50% in many white and African populations, and more than 85% among Egyptians.[32,33] Slow acetylator phenotypes exhibit higher plasma concentrations of parent drug and higher incidences of peripheral neuropathy from isoniazid and systemic lupus erythematosus syndrome from procainamide or hydralazine.[32,33] In contrast, rapid acetylator phenotypes exhibit greater myelosuppression after treatment with amonafide.[27] Genetic polymorphisms in NAT2 are associated with cancer predisposition after environmental and occupational exposure to aromatic and heterocyclic amine carcinogens.[12,32]

Oxidation polymorphisms

The CYP system, as described in Chapter 2, is a family of microsomal enzymes with selective but frequently overlapping substrate specificities. The system is the predominant pathway for phase I metabolism (both activation and deactivation) and is responsible for the oxidation of a very large diversity of therapeutic drugs and environmental carcinogens. Genetic polymorphisms in many of the CYP enzymes have been identified in human populations.[14,32] A continuously updated listing of these polymorphisms and alleles is available at http://www.imm.ki.se/cypalleles. Variant alleles possess gene deletions; gene conversions with related pseudogenes; or SNPs yielding frameshift, missense, nonsense, or alternative splice sites. The phenotypic consequences of variant alleles and genotypes include absent, diminished, qualitatively altered, and enhanced CYP enzymatic activities. Three drug oxidation polymorphisms that have received the most clinical attention involve CYP2D6, CYP2C9, and CYP2C19. The different CYPs are products of separate genes. Thus genetic deficiency in one CYP should not infer genetic deficiencies in the others.

The oxidation polymorphism in CYP2D6 was originally discovered by the toxic responses observed in some patients after administration of debrisoquine and sparteine.[32] However, human populations with this genetic defect differ in their capacity to oxidize not only debrisoquine and sparteine but up to 25% of all drugs.[14] Poor metabolizer CYP2D6 phenotypes result from defective splicing causing inactive enzyme, gene deletion resulting in absence of protein, and missense SNPs yielding enzyme with reduced stability or reduced substrate affinity.[14] An ultrarapid phenotype resulting from gene duplication has also been identified.[14] Poor metabolizer phenotypes have higher concentrations of parent drug after administration and consequently have greater adverse effects.[14,32] When CYP2D6 is required for activation to a more efficacious metabolite (e.g., codeine to morphine), poor metabolizer phenotypes often exhibit therapeutic failure.[26] The opposite effects can occur in the ultrarapid metabolizer phenotype. For example, severe abdominal pain attributable to morphine has been observed in an ultrarapid metabolizer treated with codeine.[6]

CYP2C9 catalyzes the oxidation of S-warfarin (the more potent enantiomer of warfarin) and other drugs, including phenytoin, tolbutamide, and losartan.[14,32] Allelic variants of CYP2C9 possess missense SNPs leading to enzymes with reduced or altered affinities.[14] Individuals homozygous for these variant CYP2C9 alleles exhibit a 90% reduction in S-warfarin clearance, resulting in bleeding complications during warfarin therapy.[1]

CYP2C19 catalyzes the oxidation of drugs such as mephenytoin and omeprazole.[14,32] Individuals with genetic deficiencies may have increased sedation and ataxia with the anticonvulsant mephenytoin[32] and enhanced therapeutic efficacy with omeprazole used for the treatment of peptic ulcer.[10]

Plasma cholinesterase polymorphisms

Plasma cholinesterase is an enzyme that catalyzes the hydrolysis of choline esters. Succinylcholine is an important neuromuscular blocking agent frequently used to produce muscular relaxation for endotracheal intubation and brief operative procedures. As described in Chapter 2, individuals with genetic deficiency in plasma cholinesterase have prolonged apnea when treated with succinylcholine, which is potentially fatal unless appropriate respiratory support is provided. The primary atypical form of plasma cholinesterase possesses a SNP that changes an amino acid (aspartic acid to glycine) in the anionic site of the esterase, reducing affinity for succinylcholine.[17]

Thiopurine-S-methyltransferase polymorphism

Thiopurine-S-methyltransferase is a phase II conjugation enzyme that catalyzes the S-methylation (deactivation) of anticancer and antiinflammatory drugs such as 6-mercaptopurine, 6-thioguanine, and azathioprine. The gene encoding this enzyme exhibits genetic polymorphism in human populations; the frequency of the homozygous deficient phenotype is approximately 0.33% in whites and blacks. More than 10 variant alleles have been identified that encode enzymes with reduced stability or catalytic activity.[17] Treatment of acute lymphoblastic leukemia often requires long-term treatment with 6-mercaptopurine. Individuals with the homozygous deficient phenotype frequently develop severe hematopoietic toxicity when treated with standard doses of 6-mercaptopurine, requiring substantial reductions in dose. Individuals with heterozygous genotypes have milder levels of toxicity.[15]

Dihydropyrimidine dehydrogenase polymorphism

5-Fluorouracil is used extensively in the chemotherapy of solid tumors. Dihydropyrimidine dehydrogenase catalyzes the rate-limiting step in the deactivation of 5-fluorouracil. Patients with genetic deficiency of this enzyme have a 90% lower clearance of 5-fluorouracil and may have severe toxicity from even modest doses of 5-fluorouracil.[7] The toxicity depends on route of administration but involves rapidly dividing tissues such as bone marrow and the mucosal lining of the gastrointestinal tract. Life-threatening neurotoxicity also has been observed.[7]

Pharmacogenetic Polymorphisms in Drug Targets

Because the therapeutic response is more difficult to quantify than is the drug concentration, much less is known regarding genetic polymorphisms in drug targets. However, genetic polymorphisms exist in most proteins, including drug receptors. Several genetic polymorphisms reported in recent years are provided here as examples. Many more clinically relevant genetic polymorphisms in drug receptors are likely to be discovered in the near future.

Malignant hyperthermia

Malignant hyperthermia is perhaps the first pharmacogenetic trait identified resulting from genetic polymorphism in a drug target (receptor).[32] Malignant hyperthermia is triggered in susceptible persons by the administration of inhalation anesthetics such as halothane and the depolarizing muscle relaxant succinylcholine.[20] The syndrome presents with tachycardia, hypercarbia, hypoxia, muscular rigidity, arrhythmias, and, eventually, high fever. The molecular basis of the phenotype, at least in some individuals, is a variant ryanodine receptor acting as a Ca^{++}-release channel that bridges the gap between the sarcoplasmic reticulum and the t-tubular system in skeletal muscle. Administration of a volatile anesthetic to predisposed individuals disturbs Ca^{++} regulation and release in the sarcoplasmic reticulum.[20] If appropriate therapy is not initiated immediately, the patient may die within minutes from ventricular fibrillation, within hours from pulmonary edema or coagulopathy, or within days from neurologic damage or renal failure. Malignant hyperthermia is treated by administration of the muscle relaxant dantrolene.[32]

β-Adrenergic receptor polymorphisms

β-Adrenergic receptors mediate critical sympathetic responses in the cardiovascular, pulmonary, metabolic, and central nervous systems. β_2-Adrenergic agonists such as albuterol are potent bronchodilators widely used to treat asthma. Other β-adrenergic agonists are administered to increase cardiac output in the emergency management of cardiogenic shock and decompensated congestive heart failure. Antagonists of β-adrenergic receptors are used in the long-term treatment of heart failure.

Genetic polymorphisms in both β_1 and β_2 receptors have been identified in human populations.[19] β_2-adrenergic receptor genotype variation has been shown to affect therapeutic response to β_2-selective agonists such as albuterol.[19] Polymorphisms in β receptors potentially influence drug treatment of cardiovascular diseases in two ways. The primary effect is alteration of agonist or antagonist efficacy because of a variant β_1 or β_2 receptor. However, the influence on drug efficacy also may be a secondary effect of the polymorphism on cardiovascular function. For example, a β_2-receptor variant is associated with lower systemic vascular resistance and a greater vasodilatory response. Thus individuals with this β_2-receptor variant might be more sensitive to a vasodilator (such as captopril) acting by another mechanism, secondary to the altered systemic vascular tone.

Dopamine receptor polymorphisms

Genetic polymorphisms in dopamine receptors are associated with drug abuse and the reinforcing effects of alcohol, cocaine, and nicotine.[5] Genetically variant dopamine receptors are also associated with increased therapeutic response and tardive dyskinesia after long-term treatment with dopamine receptor antagonists.[5]

Pharmacogenetics and schizophrenia

Schizophrenia is a complex set of diseases that is not adequately managed in many patients.[5] Clozapine has been found to be effective in some, but not all, patients with schizophrenia. Genetic polymorphisms in clozapine receptor targets (adrenergic, serotonergic, histaminergic receptor subtypes) have been associated with different clinical responses to clozapine.[2] Combinations of these polymorphisms may form the basis for targeting genetic subgroups of patients with schizophrenia for effective treatment with clozapine.[2]

Miscellaneous drug targets

Many additional genetic polymorphisms in drug targets have been reported recently, and many more are expected. For example, a genetic polymorphism in the cholesterol transport protein apolipoprotein E is associated with a loss of efficacy of acetylcholinesterase inhibitors such as tacrine in the treatment of Alzheimer's disease.[25] Genetic polymorphisms in cholesteryl ester transfer proteins have been found to alter the benefits of 3-hydroxy-3-methylglutaryl coenzyme A reductase inhibitors such as pravastatin in the treatment of coronary atherosclerosis.[16]

GENERAL MECHANISMS OF DRUG INTERACTIONS

Numerous studies have documented that drugs are rarely taken in isolation. For example, adults in contemporary society may take an average of four to five drugs daily and hospitalized patients may receive from nine to 13 different agents every 24 hours, depending on the institution, the patient's status, and the intercommunication among attending physicians.[28] As the number of administered drugs increases arithmetically, the risk of an adverse drug reaction increases geometrically (Figure 4-2).[30] Although some of this increase undoubtedly reflects a greater severity of disease and reduced physiologic reserve in patients requiring multidrug therapy, it also underscores the fact that drugs may interact with each other in producing toxicologic effects. Drug interactions, in fact, account for 5% to 10% of all adverse reactions to drugs and may be responsible for extending the hospital stay of approximately 15% of admitted patients. However, not all drug interactions are clinically significant or undesired, and some are actively sought in pharmacotherapeutics to increase drug effectiveness, decrease toxicity, or both. This section reviews the basic principles and general mechanisms of drug interactions and illustrates these interactions with selected examples. Some interactions are not included here, for example, medication interference with laboratory tests and metabolic interactions with environmental chemicals, such as pesticides that alter in vivo enzyme activity. Interactions involving herbal products are described in Chapter 56. Finally, it is generally assumed for the sake of simplicity that only two agents are interacting concurrently.

The sources of drugs that may be involved in drug interactions are varied. They may be prescribed or administered by a single physician or dentist or by several practitioners. Patients may also medicate themselves with over-the-counter preparations, with drugs provided by relatives or friends, or with medication remaining from a previous prescription. Finally, certain substances in foods and in cigarette smoke[31] may interact with administered drugs. Potential interactions between concurrently administered drugs are both dose and duration dependent; nevertheless, the degree or severity of an adverse interaction is seldom predictable.

In the discussion that follows, drug interactions are reviewed according to type and mechanism, and examples of each are included for illustration. More comprehensive references of interactions that involve common drugs used in dental practice (antibiotics, analgesics, local anesthetics, and antianxiety-sedative agents) are provided in Appendix I and in a series of articles published in the *Journal of the American Dental Association*.[11,13,23,24,36]

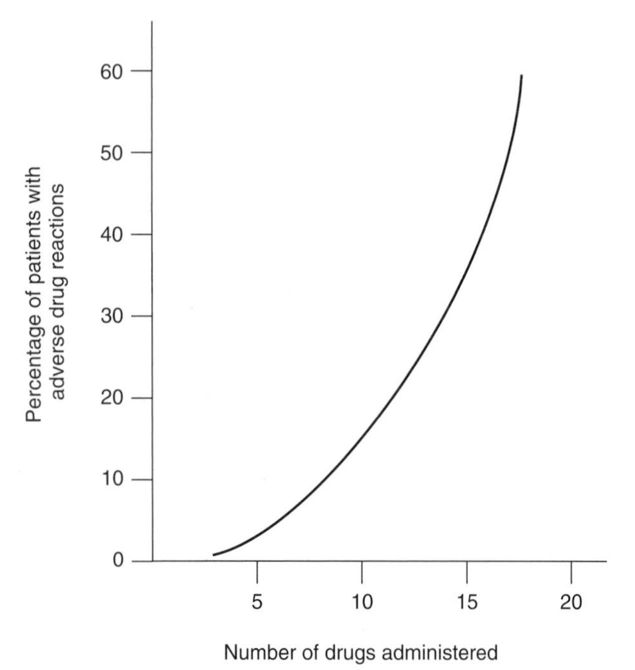

Fig. 4-2 Relationship of rate of adverse reactions to number of drugs administered. The *exponential curve* indicates that drug interactions contribute to episodes of toxicity during multiple drug therapy. (Redrawn from Smith JW, Seidl LG, Cluff LE: Studies on the epidemiology of adverse drug reactions. V. Clinical factors influencing susceptibility, *Ann Intern Med* 65:629-640, 1966.)

Classification of Drug Interactions

Drug interactions are expressed in a bewildering diversity of altered responses. Quantitative changes in reactions to one or more drugs can occur, and complex systems of nomenclature and mathematic description have been developed to characterize the combined effects of drugs. Although such approaches are of theoretic and experimental value, they are less useful in the clinical setting and fail to take into account some qualitative changes in drug effect that can occur.

The simplest clinical classification scheme recognizes three basic types of drug interactions: *antagonism*, *potentiation*, and *unexpected drug effect*. Implicit in this classification is a primary or "object" drug whose effects are modified (i.e., reduced, increased, or transformed) and an interacting or "precipitant" drug responsible for altering the effects of the object drug. Omitted, however, are drugs that produce identical or similar actions, yielding a *summation* of drug effects when the drugs are administered together.[21] Inasmuch as summation is commonly exploited in therapeutics and is often responsible for adverse drug reactions, it is included here. A last category, *synergism*, is used to identify agonist combinations that yield a magnitude of effect beyond that obtainable with a single agonist regardless of dose.

Antagonism

Antagonism indicates that the biologic or clinical response to a drug is reduced by administering a second agent. In some cases, the action of one or both of the drugs might be diminished or completely lost. An example of this type of interaction is occasionally seen in antibiotic therapy, where the combined use of a drug that acts by inhibiting the synthesis of bacterial cell walls, such as penicillin, and one that acts by inhibiting bacterial protein synthesis, such as tetracycline, results in less antimicrobial activity than might have been obtained by adequate doses of either antibiotic used alone.

Antagonism can directly occur when an antagonist produces a physical or chemical change in the agonist, reducing or abolishing its activity. An example of this is the chelation of divalent cations in antacids by tetracycline, reducing the absorption and therefore the therapeutic effectiveness of that antibiotic. A second form of antagonism may develop when one drug modifies the disposition of a second agent. An antagonism of this nature is caused by a compound that stimulates drug metabolism and shortens the biologic half-life of the agonist. Third, competition can develop between drugs for the same receptor site, diminishing or even abolishing the effectiveness of the active drug. Such pharmacologic antagonisms frequently occur with drugs that act on the autonomic nervous system, such as the blockade of sympathomimetic amines by α- and β-adrenergic antagonists. Fourth, antagonism of receptor activation may be of a noncompetitive nature, such as when one drug allosterically modifies the affinity of a receptor for a second agent. Finally, drugs having opposing actions at different receptor sites may partially or completely antagonize the effects of either or both drugs. Examples of this type of antagonism are the opposing effects of simultaneous administration of central nervous system (CNS) stimulants and depressants or the physiologic antagonism of glucocorticoids and insulin.

Potentiation

Potentiation is said to occur when a combination of two drugs that do not share similar pharmacologic activities results in an effect of one of the drugs that is greater than expected. Although not active in producing the effect by itself, the precipitant or potentiating drug sensitizes the person to the active object drug. Quite often, this form of interaction occurs when the precipitant drug elevates the free concentration of the active drug by increasing its absorption, altering its distribution, or inhibiting its elimination. A typical example of potentiation is the increased neuromuscular blocking activity of succinylcholine occurring in patients receiving a pseudocholinesterase inhibitor, such as neostigmine, which inhibits the inactivation of succinylcholine.

Unexpected drug effect

On occasion, the combination of two or more drugs can result in a response typically not observed when any of the drugs is given singly, even in overdose. One possible way in which such a novel drug effect may occur involves perturbation of the metabolism of one drug by another, leading to the formation of a highly active metabolite. For instance, disulfiram inhibits the intermediary metabolism of alcohol, resulting in the accumulation of acetaldehyde if alcohol is ingested by the patient. The symptoms of acetaldehyde intoxication—throbbing headache, blurred vision, pronounced hypotension, chest pain, dysphoria, and mental confusion—constitute a syndrome that does not normally occur with either drug administered alone.

Summation

Summation refers to the combined activities of two or more drugs that elicit identical or related pharmacologic effects. If the drugs act at the same site and produce simple arithmetic summation of effects, they are said to be *additive*. In this case, the drugs are interchangeable when the dose of each drug is expressed as a percentage of that drug's median effective dose. *Infraadditive* and *supraadditive effects* indicate, respectively, interactions that yield less than or more than an expected additive response. In all these situations, however, the maximum effect that can be obtained is no greater than what can be achieved by sufficient doses of a single drug. Examples of drugs that summate by acting at identical and at different sites include the opioid analgesics morphine and meperidine and the general anesthetics midazolam and halothane. Figure 4-3 illustrates the three forms of summation as observed with agents used for intravenous sedation-anesthesia.

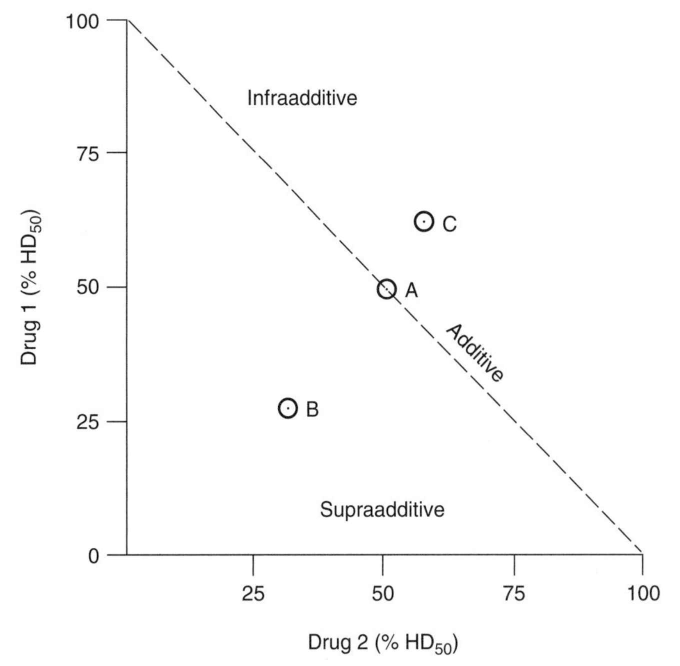

Fig. 4-3 Isobologram of the summation of intravenous anesthetic agents. Drug dosages are indicated as the percentage of the median hypnotic dose *(HD_{50})* for each drug given singly. The *dashed line* indicates a purely additive relationship of two drugs. *A,* Thiopental *(y axis)* and thiamylal *(x axis)*. With identical mechanisms of action, these drugs produce additive effects. *B,* Midazolam and propofol: supraadditive effects. C, Thiopental and ketamine: infraadditive effects. (Data from Vinik HR, Bradley EL, Jr, Kissin I: Triple anesthetic combination: propofol-midazolam-alfentanil, *Anesth Analg* 78:354-358, 1994; Manani G, Valenti S, Vincenti E, et al: Interaction between thiopentone and subhypnotic doses of ketamine, *Eur J Anaesthesiol* 9:43-47, 1992.)

Synergism

Occasionally, the combination of two or more agonists produces an effect that is greater quantitatively than what can be achieved by maximally effective doses of any one drug given alone. Common examples of *synergism* used therapeutically include the combination of chemotherapeutic agents to treat certain infections (e.g., tuberculosis) and neoplastic diseases. In these situations, the emergence of drug resistance is reduced and the cure rate is enhanced. The combination of alcohol and carbon tetrachloride provides an example of synergism leading to acute toxicity. Here, hepatotoxicity is much greater than what is typically associated with either drug given alone.

Mechanisms of Drug Interactions

Drug interactions can occur at any point along the pharmacologic pathway of the agonist, from even before the drug is administered to a patient, to the period when it is in contact with its site of action, to the point at which it is eliminated. The various mechanisms involved in drug interactions can be grouped taxonomically into three broad categories: pharmaceutical, pharmacokinetic, and pharmacodynamic interactions.

Table • 4-1

Examples of Pharmaceutical Drug Interactions

DRUG A	WITH	DRUG B
Gentamicin		Ampicillin
Diazepam		Intravenous fluids
Barbiturates		Opioid analgesics
Bupivacaine		Sodium bicarbonate
Hydroxyzine		Pentobarbital
Metaraminol		Hydrocortisone

Mixing of any of the above pairs of drugs in the same bottle, tubing, syringe, or intravenous drip may result in the precipitation or destruction of one or both constituents.

Pharmaceutical interactions

Pharmaceutical interactions represent drug incompatibilities of a physical or chemical nature (Table 4-1). In general, pharmaceutical interactions can be anticipated between organic acids and bases, resulting in precipitation of one or both drugs. Chemical reactions between drugs may also occur, but these are less common. Most pharmaceutical interactions of importance to dentistry involve drugs that are given parenterally for intravenous sedation. As a general rule, drugs should not be mixed within the same syringe.

Pharmacokinetic interactions

Pharmacokinetic interactions derive from the influence of one drug on the absorption, distribution, biotransformation, or excretion of another drug (Table 4-2).

Absorption Many times an interaction affects the rate or extent of effective absorption of a drug into the systemic circulation, causing a decrease or increase in that drug's effect. Factors influencing absorption include the pH of lumen fluids, enzyme activity, and intestinal motility. Familiar examples of interactions that decrease drug absorption include the previously mentioned chelation by tetracycline of multivalent cations (Ca^{++}, Mg^{++}, Fe^{++}, and Al^{+++}) in dairy products, antacids, or ferrous salts and the hydrolysis of penicillin G by fruit juice acids, resulting in a decrease in the amount of antibiotic available for absorption and therefore a decrease in the therapeutic effect. Dentists are familiar with combining vasoconstrictors with local anesthetics to retard absorption of the anesthetic from the site of administration.

A well-known example of an interaction that facilitates or increases absorption occurs in patients taking monoamine oxidase (MAO) inhibitors. Tyramine in beer, ripened cheese, red wine, and many other fermented foods is normally not absorbed because it is enzymatically inactivated by MAOs in the intestinal mucosa and liver. When MAO inhibitors suppress these enzymes, tyramine, a sympathomimetic amine, is absorbed in excessive amounts, releasing norepinephrine from sympathetic nerve endings. The effect frequently results in drug toxicity, including severe headache and, occasionally, hypertensive crisis and death.

Distribution After a drug is absorbed, an interaction may modify its distribution or the rate of transfer of the drug from one location to another. Drugs may be free in the bloodstream or become reversibly bound to plasma or tissue components. Plasma proteins, primarily albumin and α_1-acid glycoprotein, act as acceptor or storage sites for many drugs. Protein-bound drugs are inactive, being unavailable for active combination with a receptor site, for biotransformation, or for glomerular filtration. Because a bound drug is in equilibrium with the free drug in plasma and tissue fluids, an interacting drug that displaces an agonist from its protein-binding sites raises the plasma concentration of the pharmacologically active, unbound agonist. This potentially increases its pharmacologic activity; it may also increase the amount available for metabolism and excretion, thus shortening its duration of action. Warfarin, which is highly protein bound, is displaced from its plasma protein binding sites by chloral hydrate (specifically, the trichloroethanol metabolite), transiently potentiating the anticoagulant effect and increasing the possibility of spontaneous hemorrhage. Of course, this interaction is more likely to become clinically evident in patients with a variant CYP2C9 phenotype.

Distribution across cellular membranes can be influenced by drugs that compete for or otherwise block active transport mechanisms such as the P-glycoprotein transporter, alter pH gradients, or disrupt membrane diffusion barriers. Inhibition of the active uptake of adrenergic vasoconstrictors into sympathetic nerve terminals by tricyclic antidepressants increases the concentration of the adrenergic drugs in the synaptic cleft. Drugs that cause acute respiratory acidosis tend to shift the distribution of opioid analgesics from intracellular locations to the extracellular space. Because the opioid receptors are located on the external surface of the plasma membrane, increased opioid effects result. The intraarterial administration of osmotic agents to shrink the endothelial cells forming the bulk of the blood-brain barrier increases the entry of anticancer drugs into the CNS.

Metabolism The degree and duration of activity of a drug are often functions of its metabolism; therefore an interacting drug can modify the effect of an agonist by altering its rate of biotransformation. The majority of drugs used therapeutically are metabolized in the liver by the microsomal enzyme system. As discussed in Chapter 2, the CYP family of enzymes is commonly involved in these reactions. Inhibition of CYP isozymes provides a rich source of drug interactions. Erythromycin, for instance, irreversibly inhibits CYP3A4; its nitrosoalkane metabolite forms complexes with the CYP3A4 iron, blocking the metabolism of other drugs dependent on the same CYP.[34] These agents include the opioid agonist alfentanyl, the hypnotic agent triazolam, the immunosuppressant cyclosporine, and a host of other pharmacologically unrelated compounds. Additional agents that are capable of inhibiting the metabolism of multiple drugs include amiodarone, cimetidine, fluvoxamine, disulfiram, and the MAO inhibitors. In the latter two cases, nonmicrosomal enzymes are the targets of inhibition (alcohol dehydrogenase and MAO, respectively).

The anticonvulsants phenobarbital, phenytoin, and carbamazepine are known to induce the production of hepatic microsomal enzymes that are responsible for their own biotransformation. These same microsomal enzymes, however, also metabolize other drugs, such as oral anticoagulants, resulting in an increase in the rate of biotransformation of the anticoagulant and a consequent decrease in the active free form, with a resultant loss of therapeutic effectiveness. Because the effect of the enzyme-inducing agent is not permanent, care must be taken to reassess the anticoagulant dosage when the inducer is withdrawn, because effective doses of the anticoagulant in the presence of enzyme induction may lead to spontaneous hemorrhage after the induction is lost. The antibiotic rifampin also causes enzyme induction, resulting, for instance, in a decreased efficiency of hydrocortisone used in the treatment of acute asthma. See Table 2-3 for a list of common inhibitors and inducers of the various human CYP enzymes involved in drug metabolism.

The hepatic biotransformation of some drugs may be indirectly affected by other agents that influence hepatic

Table • 4-2

Examples of Pharmacokinetic Drug Interactions

MECHANISM OF DRUG INTERACTION	DRUG A GIVEN WITH	DRUG B OR DIETARY CONSTITUENT	PRODUCES	NET EFFECT
Inhibition of drug absorption	Penicillin G	Acidic fruit juices	Decreased gastric pH; hydrolysis of penicillin	Less antibiotic is absorbed, and blood concentrations are reduced
	Ketoconazole	Antacids, H_2 antihistamines	Increased gastric pH	Decreased absorption and blood concentrations of ketoconazole
	Many oral medications	Antimuscarinics, opioid analgesics	Delay in gastric emptying	Retarded absorption of drugs normally absorbed in the small intestine
	Cimetidine	Metoclopramide	Enhanced gastric emptying	Decreased absorption of cimetidine
	Many oral medications	Cathartics	Increased gastrointestinal motility	Decreased absorption and blood concentrations of oral medications
	Tetracyclines	Drugs containing multivalent cations	Chelation by tetracycline	Formation of insoluble tetracycline complexes that are poorly absorbed
	Vitamins A, D, K	Mineral oil	Sequestration of vitamins in the oil; inadequate contact with intestinal epithelium	Decreased absorption of vitamins
	Local anesthetic	Epinephrine, levonordefrin	Vasoconstriction in the area of injection	Decreased absorption of anesthetic with prolongation of anesthesia
Enhancement of drug absorption	Enteric-coated medications	Antacids, H_2 antihistamines	Increased gastric pH	Premature loss of coating and increased rate of drug absorption
	Mexiletine	Metoclopramide	Enhanced gastric emptying	Increased absorption of mexiletine
	Tyramine in dietary constituents (e.g., wine, beer, aged cheese)	MAO inhibitors	Decreased gastrointestinal breakdown of tyramine	Increased tyramine absorption and norepinephrine release from adrenergic nerve terminals
	Triazolam	Erythromycin, clarithromycin	Decreased gastrointestinal breakdown of triazolam	Increased triazolam absorption and sedation
Alteration of binding	Warfarin	Chloral hydrate	Displacement of oral anticoagulant from protein binding sites	Activity of anticoagulant transiently increased; spontaneous bleeding possible
	Digoxin	Quinidine	Displacement of digoxin from tissue binding sites	Increased risk of digoxin intoxication
Alteration of distribution	Guanethidine	Tricyclic antidepressants	Uptake of guanethidine into sympathetic nerve terminals is inhibited	Decreased antihypertensive effect of guanethidine
	Anticancer drugs	Hypertonic solution	Disruption of blood-brain barrier by osmotic shrinkage of endothelial cells	Anticancer drugs gain access to brain tumor
	Anticancer drugs	Verapamil	Inhibition of P-glycoprotein efflux of anticancer drugs from cells	Increased anticancer activity
Induction of drug-metabolizing enzymes	Warfarin	Barbiturates, carbamazepine, phenytoin	Induction of enzymes for inactivation of warfarin	Decreased blood concentrations of warfarin
	Barbiturates	Alcohol	Induction of enzymes for inactivation of barbiturates	Decreased blood concentration of barbiturates

Continued

Table • 4-2

Examples of Pharmacokinetic Drug Interactions—cont'd

MECHANISM OF DRUG INTERACTION	DRUG A GIVEN WITH	DRUG B OR DIETARY CONSTITUENT	PRODUCES	NET EFFECT
Induction of drug-metabolizing enzymes—cont'd	Valproic acid	Phenobarbital	Induction of hepatic microsomal enzymes for valproic acid	Formation of toxic metabolite of valproic acid leading to hepatotoxicity
	Diazepam	Cigarette smoking	Induction of hepatic microsomal enzymes for diazepam	Decreased diazepam concentrations with long-term administration
Inhibition of biotransformation	Levodopa	Carbidopa	Prevention of levodopa destruction before it reaches the brain	Reduction in dosage of levodopa and decreased cardiovascular toxicity
	Tolbutamide	Cyclosporine	Inhibition of microsomal enzymes for metabolism of tolbutamide	Increased blood concentrations of tolbutamide; hypoglycemia
	Alcohol	Disulfiram	Inhibition of acetaldehyde dehydrogenase	Increased blood concentrations of acetaldehyde; unpleasant side effects
	Diazepam	Cimetidine	Inhibition of microsomal enzymes for metabolism of diazepam	Excessive accumulation of diazepam; increased toxicity
	Lidocaine	Propranolol	Decreased hepatic blood flow and uptake of lidocaine	Increased blood concentrations of lidocaine; increased toxicity
Alteration of excretion	Aspirin, phenobarbital	Sodium bicarbonate	Alkalization of urine	Acidic drugs are less readily reabsorbed by kidneys; excretion enhanced
	Penicillins	Probenecid	Competition with penicillins for renal tubular secretory pathway	Half-lives of penicillins are increased; enhanced antibacterial effects
	Ciprofloxacin	Probenecid	Inhibition of renal secretion of ciprofloxacin	Decreased antibiotic effect in urinary tract infections
	Digoxin	Erythromycin, clarithromycin	Inhibition of renal P-glycoprotein activity	Decreased renal excretion of digoxin; increased toxicity

blood flow. Part of the inhibition of lidocaine clearance by the liver in patients receiving propranolol, for example, is believed to result from the fact that propranolol reduces cardiac output, hepatic blood flow, and therefore the transport of lidocaine to the liver, its primary site of elimination.

Excretion Increasing or decreasing the rate of excretion, or renal or biliary clearance, of a drug also alters its elimination rate constant and therefore the amount of drug available in the circulating plasma, thus affecting the duration as well as the degree of activity of the drug. Renal excretion is influenced by urinary pH and tubular reabsorption as well as inhibition of active transport. For example, weak acids such as aspirin are more rapidly excreted in an alkaline urine produced by sodium bicarbonate, whereas weak bases such as amphetamine are more readily excreted in a urine acidified by ammonium chloride. Tubular secretion of an object drug might also be decreased by an interacting agent. A common example is that of probenecid, which, by competing for the same renal transport system as the penicillins, increases the serum concentration and the duration of action of the penicillins.

Pharmacodynamic interactions

Pharmacodynamic interactions represent modifications in the pharmacologic effects of a drug independent of any change in the quantitative disposition of that drug (Table 4-3). Such interactions may increase, diminish, or qualitatively alter the therapeutic effect.

Many interactions take place at or near receptor sites. The mechanisms involved can include competition for the receptor or alterations of either the receptor or its natural ligand. This type of interaction is especially common among autonomic drugs. For instance, phenoxybenzamine and propranolol are specific competitive antagonists for epinephrine at α- and β-adrenergic receptors. A drug such as guanethidine affects the synthesis, storage, release, and reuptake of norepinephrine, resulting in depletion of norepinephrine in the neuronal vesicles. Subsequent administration of an agent that acts by evoking the release of norepinephrine (e.g., ephedrine or amphetamine) is less effective. An example of the opposite effect is that of MAO inhibitors, such as pargyline, which permit the accumulation of norepinephrine by forming complexes with the enzyme that metabolizes the neuromediator within the nerve terminals. In this instance,

Table • 4-3

Examples of Pharmacodynamic Drug Interactions

MECHANISM OF DRUG INTERACTION	DRUG A GIVEN WITH	DRUG B	PRODUCES	NET EFFECT
Competition for same receptor	Pilocarpine	Atropine receptor	Competition for the muscarinic parasympathetic nerve	Responses to muscarinic drugs and stimulation are blocked
	Histamine	Diphenhydramine	Competition for the H_1 receptor	Responses of the H_1 receptor are blocked; many manifestations of allergy are prevented
	Epinephrine	Propranolol	Competition for the β-adrenergic receptor	Some responses to epinephrine are blocked; unopposed α receptor activity causes hypertension
Opposing pharmacologic effects on different systems	Histamine	Epinephrine	Physiologic antagonism of histamine by opposite effects, on different receptors, of epinephrine	Epinephrine is an effective physiologic antidote to histamine overdose
	Barbiturates	Amphetamines	Opposing CNS depression and stimulation but at different sites in the brain	A mixture of CHS depressant and stimulant effects occur; amphetamine administration actually worsens survival from barbiturate overdose
Antagonism involving enzyme inactivation	Atropine	Physostigmine	Reversible inactivation of AChE; excess ACh competes with atropine for muscarinic receptors	Physostigmine antagonizes the effects of atropine at muscarinic receptors and vice versa; each drug is an antidote for the other
	Tubocurarine	Neostigmine	Inhibition of AChE and build-up of ACh at the motor endplate	Neuromuscular blockade produced by tubocurarine is terminated
Summation of effects on the same receptor	Diazepam	Zolpidem	Added stimulation of the benzodiazepine receptor	Increased CNS depression
	Promazine	Amitriptyline	Added blockade of muscarinic receptors	Xerostomia and increased incidence of caries
Summation of pharmacologic effects on different systems	Heparin	Aspirin	Complementary inhibition of hemostatic mechanisms	Increased risk of hemorrhage
	Vecuronium	Sevoflurane	Potentiation of neuromuscular blockade by central depression of motor pathways	Intensification and prolongation of neuromuscular blockade by vecuronium
	Vecuronium	Lidocaine	Stabilization of the prejunctional and postjunctional membranes by lidocaine	Intensification and prolongation of neuromuscular blockade by vecuronium
	Epinephrine	Halothane	Sensitization of the myocardium to epinephrine	Cardiac arrhythmias
	Acetaminophen	Hydrocodone	Summation of analgesic effects	Increased pain relief
Potentiation involving enzyme inactivation	Succinylcholine	Neostigmine	Accumulation of ACh at the motor endplate	Potentiation of neuromuscular blocking effects of succinylcholine
	Amphetamine	Phenelzine	MAO inhibition by phenelzine increases norepinephrine release by amphetamine	Potentiation of stimulant effects of amphetamine; hypertensive emergency

ACh, Acetylcholine; *AChE,* acetylcholinesterase.

ephedrine or amphetamine produces markedly exaggerated effects.

Interacting drugs may also exert their effects at sites of action in different locations. A previously cited example of this phenomenon is the physiologic antagonism of CNS stimulants, such as caffeine or amphetamine, by CNS depressants, such as the benzodiazepines or anticonvulsants. When the agents are administered simultaneously, these drug groups produce opposing actions. Probably the most common interactions involve drugs that evoke similar pharmacologic effects. Combinations of alcohol, barbiturates, benzodiazepines, phenothiazines, antihistamines, bromides, or other drugs capable of producing CNS depression are sometimes unwittingly consumed by people, resulting in somnolence, unconsciousness, or even death.

Factors Influencing Drug Interactions

Several variables can affect the occurrence and intensity of potential drug interactions. Prime among these are variations in the handling of and reaction to administered drugs, including the genetic-based differences previously described in this chapter. Drug interactions and drug effects are both dose dependent and duration dependent; thus an interaction may not be clinically discernible each time interacting drugs are administered. The higher the dosage and the longer the administration, the greater the chance that an interaction may occur. Previous exposure affecting drug transport, metabolism, or responsiveness may alter the potential for interaction. In addition, many drugs have a long biologic half-life, and effective concentrations may be present in the blood or tissue for many days after the cessation of therapy; interactions may occur, therefore, days and occasionally weeks after discontinuation of therapy with one of the interacting drugs.

Drug Interactions Used in Pharmacotherapeutics

Combinations of drugs are used in therapy to provide enhanced effects and to prevent adverse reactions.[4] Purposeful drug interactions are especially common in the treatment of certain diseases, such as essential hypertension, tuberculosis, and cancer, in which the concurrent administration of two or more drugs is routine. Drugs may also be given sequentially so the second agent abruptly terminates the action of the first. Thus edrophonium, a cholinesterase inhibitor, is administered to reverse the neuromuscular blockade of vecuronium, and leucovorin (folinic acid) is administered to "rescue" patients given potentially lethal doses of methotrexate, a folic acid analogue used in cancer chemotherapy. Agents useful as specific antidotes in accidental drug overdosage include protamine for heparin, naloxone for opioid analgesics, and atropine for anticholinesterases.

Particular mention should be made of fixed-dose combination products. Such preparations make up a significant fraction of all drugs sold in the United States, from over-the-counter remedies to prescription items to agents administered by practitioners. The fixed combination of a local anesthetic with epinephrine to provide more effective and more prolonged anesthesia is a notable example. In general, drug mixtures include a principal ingredient for the main therapeutic effect; adjuvants that summate with, potentiate, or otherwise complement the first drug; and correctives that antagonize or minimize undesired side effects.

The major criticisms of fixed-dose combinations are (1) the inability to adjust the dosages of the individual ingredients to the needs of a particular patient; (2) discrepancies in half-lives of individual agents, leading to the accumulation of some, but not other, constituents during repeated administration; (3) the likelihood of taking unnecessary drugs; (4) the possibility of increased toxicity or allergenicity without correspondingly increased therapeutic efficacy; and (5) the possibility of a higher cost from the manufacturer. However, fixed-dose combinations have certain potential advantages. Certain mixtures offer therapeutic gains in effectiveness or safety (e.g., acetaminophen with hydrocodone combinations, local anesthetic-vasoconstrictor solutions, and hydrochlorothiazide with triamterene). In addition, drug combinations may improve patient compliance by reducing the number of medications the patient must take. Finally, the reduced number of individual prescriptions can be less expensive to the patient.

Although certain fixed-dose combinations are useful, such preparations should be avoided as a general rule, and only those mixtures that have been demonstrated to be therapeutically advantageous to the patient should be used.

IMPLICATIONS FOR DENTISTRY

The elucidation of the human genome—coupled with advancements in DNA array technology, high-throughput genotyping, and bioinformatics—will soon enable rapid elucidation of complex genetic factors necessary for optimization of drug therapy. Pharmacogenomics will increasingly result in the development of drugs targeted to specific, genetically identifiable subgroups of the population. Some drugs previously abandoned for clinical use because they proved toxic in some patients will return to clinical use, but with restrictions for specific genetic groups. Health care providers, including dentists, will be accountable for prescribing the drug appropriately to genetic subgroups. Automated genotyping systems and easily accessible genetic information will provide crucial information necessary for optimal drug therapy in the individual patient. The determination and accessibility of human genetic information have potential ethical and legal concerns.[29] One proposed solution is to use "abbreviated pharmacogenetic chips" that assess anonymous genetic information specific to each drug rather than a comprehensive genetic profile determined for each patient.[35] Although the ways in which pharmacogenetic information is accessed remain to be fully developed, a one size fits all mode of drug therapy that fails to consider pharmacogenetic information will be increasingly considered substandard clinical care.

As a prescriber and administrator of drugs, the dentist is already responsible for ensuring that adverse drug interactions do not arise as a consequence of the dentist's therapeutic intervention. The dentist must therefore know what drugs the patient is currently taking and how these drugs may interact with whatever medications the dentist is thinking about using. An accurate medical history easily solves the first part of the problem; the second is less tractable. It is virtually impossible for the dentist to be cognizant of all drug interactions that may be relevant to dental practice. Hundreds of such interactions exist, and new drugs are constantly being marketed and new drug interactions discovered. All the dentist can realistically do is be familiar with the common, important interactions that involve the few drugs the dentist routinely uses or prescribes, maintain access to an appropriately updated information source on drug interactions, and consult that source whenever confronted with a patient taking a medication with which the dentist is unfamiliar.

A number of publications—from books and periodicals to computer database programs and websites—contain information on drug interactions. The best of these provide concise descriptions of each drug interaction, the frequency and seriousness of the interaction, the quality of the documentation for the interaction, a recommended course of action to follow, and a complete cross-reference for related drugs that might produce the same interaction. Services that provide periodic updates in the form of loose-leaf inserts are advantageous in keeping the source reference up to date. For the computerized office, a database program or website service is ideal. The list of drugs the patient is taking can be entered along with the agent being considered by the dentist. The potential interactions are automatically listed by the computer.

Cited References

1. Aithal GP, Day CP, Kesteven PJL, et al: Association of polymorphisms in the cytochrome P450 CYP2C9 with warfarin dose requirement and risk of bleeding complications, *Lancet* 353:717-719, 1999.
2. Arranz MJ, Munro J, Birkett J, et al: Pharmacogenetic prediction of clozapine response, *Lancet* 355:1615-1616, 2000.
3. Begley S: Screening for genes: matching medications to your genetic heritage, *Newsweek* February 8, 1999.
4. Caranasos GJ, Stewart RB, Cluff LE: Clinically desirable drug interactions, *Annu Rev Pharmacol Toxicol* 25:67-95, 1985.
5. Cichon S, Nothen MM, Rietschel M, et al: Pharmacogenetics of schizophrenia, *Am J Med Genet* 97:98-106, 2000.
6. Dalen P, Frengell C, Dahl ML, et al: Quick onset of severe abdominal pain after codeine in an ultrarapid metabolizer of debrisoquine, *Ther Drug Monit* 19:543-544, 1997.
7. Diasio RB, Johnson MR: The role of pharmacogenetics and pharmacogenomics in cancer chemotherapy with 5-fluorouracil, *Pharmacology* 61:199-203, 2000.
8. Evans WE, Relling MV: Pharmacogenomics: translating functional genomics into rational therapeutics, *Science* 286:487-491, 1999.
9. Fretland AJ, Leff MA, Doll MA, et al: Functional characterization of human N-acetyltransferase 2 (NAT2) single nucleotide polymorphisms, *Pharmacogenetics* 11207-11215, 2001.
10. Furuta T, Ohashi K, Kamata T, et al: Effect of genetic differences in omeprazole metabolism on cure rates for *Helicobacter pylori* infection and peptic ulcer, *Ann Intern Med* 129:1027-1030, 1998.
11. Haas DA: Adverse drug interactions in dental practice: interactions associated with analgesics. Part III in a series, *J Am Dent Assoc* 130:397-407, 1999.
12. Hein DW, Doll MA, Fretland AJ, et al: Molecular genetics and epidemiology of the NAT1 and NAT2 acetylation polymorphisms, *Cancer Epidemiol Biomarkers Prev* 9:29-42, 2000.
13. Hersh HV: Adverse drug interactions in dental practice: interactions involving antibiotics. Part II of a series, *J Am Dent Assoc* 130:236-251, 1999.
14. Ingelman-Sundberg M, Oscarson M, McLellan RA: Polymorphic human cytochrome P450 enzymes: an opportunity for individualized drug treatment, *Trends Pharmacol Sci* 20:342-349, 1999.
15. Krynetski EY, Evans WE: Genetic polymorphism of thiopurine S-methyltransferase: molecular mechanisms and clinical importance, *Pharmacology* 61:136-146, 2000.
16. Kuivenhoven JA, Jukema JW, Zwinderman AH, et al: The role of a common variant of the cholesteryl ester transfer protein gene in the progression of coronary atherosclerosis. The Regression Growth Evaluation Statin Study Group, *New Engl J Med* 338:86-93, 1998.
17. La Du BN, Bartels CF, Nogueira CP, et al: Phenotypic and molecular biological analysis of human butyrylcholinesterase variants, *Clin Biochem* 23:423-431, 1990.
18. Lazarou J, Pomeranz BH, Corey PN: Incidence of adverse drug reactions in hospitalized patients: a meta-analysis of prospective studies, *JAMA* 279:1200-1205, 1998.
19. Liggett SB: Pharmacogenetics of beta-1 and beta-2-adrenergic receptors, *Pharmacology* 61:167-173, 2000.
20. MacLennan DH, Phillips MS: Malignant hyperthermia, *Science* 256:789-794, 1992.
21. McInnes GT, Brodie MJ: Drug interactions that matter: a critical reappraisal, *Drugs* 36:83-110, 1988.
22. McLeod HL, Evans WE: Pharmacogenomics: unlocking the human genome for better drug therapy, *Annu Rev Pharmacol Toxicol* 41:101-121, 2001.
23. Moore PA: Adverse drug interactions in dental practice: interactions associated with local anesthetics, sedatives and anxiolytics. Part IV of a series, *J Am Dent Assoc* 130:541-554, 1999.
24. Moore PA, Gage TW, Hersh EV, et al: Adverse drug interactions in dental practice: professional and educational implications. Part I of a series, *J Am Dent Assoc* 130:47-54, 1999.
25. Poirier J, Delisle M-C, Quirion R, et al: Apolipoprotein E4 allele as a predictor of cholinergic deficits and treatment outcome in Alzheimer disease, *Proc Natl Acad Sci USA* 92:12260-12264, 1995.
26. Poulsen L, Brosen K, Arendt-Nielsen L, et al: Codeine and morphine in extensive and poor metabolizers of sparteine: pharmacokinetics, analgesic effect and side effects, *Eur J Clin Pharmacol* 51:289-295, 1996.
27. Ratain MJ, Rosner G, Allen SL, et al: Population pharmacodynamic study of amonafide: a Cancer and Leukemia Group B study, *J Clin Oncol* 13:741-747, 1995.
28. Ross NM: General mechanisms of drug interactions. In Bourgault PC, Ross NM, eds: *Drug interactions,* vol 3, the third symposium of the Pharmacology, Therapeutics, and Toxicology Group, International Association for Dental Research, 1976.
29. Rothstein MA, Epps PG: Ethical and legal implications of pharmacogenomics, *Nat Rev Genet* 2:228-231, 2001.
30. Smith JW, Seidl LG, Cluff LE: Studies on the epidemiology of adverse drug reactions. V. Clinical factors influencing susceptibility, *Ann Intern Med* 65:629-640, 1966.
31. Vestal RE, Wood AJJ: Influence of age and smoking on drug kinetics in man: studies using model compounds, *Clin Pharmacokinet* 5:309-319, 1980.
32. Weber WW: *Pharmacogenetics,* New York, 1997, Oxford University Press.
33. Weber WW, Hein DW: N-acetylation pharmacogenetics, *Pharmacol Rev* 37:25-79, 1985.
34. Westphal JF: Macrolide-induced clinically relevant drug interactions with cytochrome P-450A (CYP) 3A4: an update focused on clarithromycin, azithromycin and dirithromycin, *Br J Clin Pharmacol* 50:285-295, 2000.
35. Wilkins MR, Roses AD, Clifford CP: Pharmacogenetics and the treatment of cardiovascular disease, *Heart* 84:353-354, 2000.
36. Yagiela JA: Adverse drug interactions in dental practice: interactions associated with vasoconstrictors. Part V of a series, *J Am Dent Assoc* 130:701-709, 1999.

General References

Evans WE, McLeod HL: Pharmacogenomics: drug disposition, drug targets, and side effects, *New Engl J Med* 348:538-549, 2003.

Hansten PD, Horn JR, Hansten PD: *Managing clinically important drug interactions,* St Louis, 2002, Facts and Comparisons.

Hardman JG, Limbird LE, Gilman AG, eds: *Goodman & Gilman's The pharmacological basis of therapeutics,* ed 10, New York, 2001, McGraw-Hill.

Stockley IH: *Drug interactions: a source book of adverse interactions, their mechanisms, clinical importance, and management,* ed 5, London, 1999, Pharmaceutical Press.

Vesell ES: Advances in pharmacogenetics and pharmacogenomics, *J Clin Pharmacol* 40:930-938, 2000.

Weber WW: *Pharmacogenetics,* New York, 1997, Oxford University Press.

Wolf CR, Smith G: Pharmacogenetics, *Br Med Bull* 55:366-388, 1999.

Zucchero FJ, Hogan MJ, Sommer CD, et al: *Evaluations of drug interactions,* St Louis, 2003, First DataBank.

PART II

Pharmacology of Specific Drug Groups

CHAPTER • 5

Introduction to Autonomic Nervous System Drugs

Peter W. Abel and Michael T. Piascik

The autonomic nervous system (ANS) and the endocrine system are the major regulatory systems for controlling homeostatic functions. These two systems collectively regulate and coordinate the cardiovascular, respiratory, gastrointestinal, renal, reproductive, metabolic, and immunologic systems. Accordingly, drugs that alter the activity of either the ANS or the endocrine system often exhibit multiple actions and side effects. This chapter introduces the pharmacology of the ANS; the endocrine system and drugs are reviewed in Chapters 34 through 37. An understanding of the pharmacology of agents affecting the ANS rests on two basic foundations: a knowledge of the structural and functional organization of the ANS and an understanding of where certain neurotransmitters are located and how these neurotransmitters affect cellular function.

AUTONOMIC NERVOUS SYSTEM

The ANS, also referred to as the visceral, vegetative, or involuntary nervous system, regulates the function of involuntary structures: smooth muscle, the heart, and secretory glands. These structures possess intrinsic mechanisms that allow them to function in the absence of neuronal input, but the ANS contributes a regulatory and coordinating function. Most of our knowledge of the ANS is restricted to efferent functions; much less is known about the afferent limb other than that sensory fibers carry impulses that are received and organized centrally, often at an unconscious level. Thus a person is not aware of impulses generated at the baroreceptors, although these impulses may trigger a generalized body response, such as a reflex fall in blood pressure, that the person may sense. It has been estimated that approximately 80% of the vagus nerve consists of primary afferent fibers and that the effects of certain drugs (e.g., opioids) may be mediated, in part, by altering autonomic sensory inputs.[16,30] Nevertheless, most currently available ANS drugs influence efferent activity.

Anatomy

The structural organization of the efferent arm of the ANS differs from that of the somatic nervous system in that somatic efferent fibers originate from cell bodies located in the central nervous system (CNS) and innervate skeletal (striated) muscle without intervening synapses (Figure 5-1). In contrast, the ANS consists of a two-neuron system in which preganglionic nerves emanating from cell bodies in the cerebrospinal axis synapse with postganglionic nerves originating in autonomic ganglia outside the CNS. The ANS is divided into two parts on the basis of the anatomic characteristics of each division. The sympathetic division includes nerve pathways that originate in the thoracolumbar regions of the spinal cord, whereas the parasympathetic division includes nerve pathways from the craniosacral regions of the cerebrospinal axis.

Sympathetic nervous system

The organizational anatomy of the two divisions of the ANS is shown in greater detail in Figure 5-2. The sympathetic division originates from neurons with cell bodies located in the intermediolateral columns of the spinal cord, extending from the first thoracic to the third lumbar segments. The myelinated preganglionic fibers emerge with the ventral roots of the spinal nerves and synapse with second neurons in one of three possible types of ganglia: paravertebral (vertebral or lateral), prevertebral, or terminal. The paravertebral ganglia are composed of 22 pairs of ganglia lying on either side of the spinal cord and connected to each other by communicating nerve fibers. The superior cervical ganglia (the topmost pair) innervate structures in the head and neck, including the submandibular glands, whereas the superior, middle, and inferior cervical ganglia all innervate the heart. The prevertebral ganglia are located in the abdomen and pelvis and include the celiac, superior mesenteric, and inferior mesenteric, which innervate the stomach, the small intestine, and the colon. The few terminal ganglia lie near the organs they innervate, principally the urinary bladder and rectum.

One of the striking anatomic aspects of the sympathetic nervous system, and one that has great functional significance, is that a single preganglionic nerve may contact as many as 20 or more postganglionic nerves. This means that impulses arising in one preganglionic neuron of the sympathetic nervous system may ultimately affect many postganglionic neurons, which explains the diffuse and widespread character of sympathetic nervous system responses. Stimulation of the sympathetic nervous system also activates preganglionic nerves that innervate the adrenal medulla and cause it to release a mixture of the catecholamines epinephrine and norepinephrine. This release provides an additional basis for the widespread effects of the sympathetic nervous system.

Parasympathetic nervous system

The parasympathetic nervous system, or craniosacral division, has its origin in neurons with cell bodies located in the brainstem nuclei of four cranial nerves—the oculomotor (III), the facial (VII), the glossopharyngeal (IX), and the vagus (X)—and in the second, third, and fourth segments of the sacral spinal cord. The preganglionic nerves arising from the brainstem form part of the cranial nerves and travel with them to synapse with postganglionic neurons located in ganglia near or actually within the structures innervated. The midbrain outflow from the nucleus of the oculomotor nerve synapses

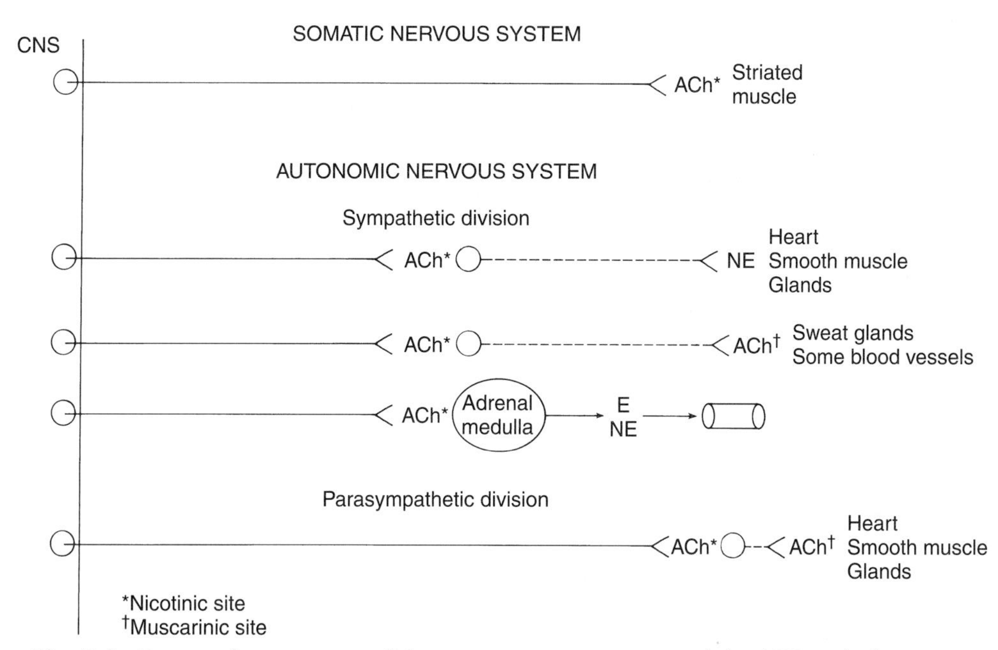

Fig. 5-1 Functional organization of the somatic nervous system and the ANS, with the structures innervated by the different nerves and the chemical mediators responsible for transmission at the various sites. Solid lines indicate somatic motor or preganglionic autonomic nerves; dashed lines indicate postganglionic autonomic nerves. *ACh*, Acetylcholine; *E*, epinephrine; *NE*, norepinephrine.

in the ciliary ganglion located in the orbit. The ganglion gives rise to nerves that supply the ciliary muscle and the sphincter muscle of the eye. Neurons of the facial nerve that synapse in the sublingual and submandibular ganglia form the chorda tympani and provide innervation to the sublingual and submandibular glands, respectively. Other neurons of the facial nerve synapse in the sphenopalatine ganglion; postganglionics then terminate in the lacrimal gland and in mucus-secreting glands of the nose, palate, and pharynx. Nerves originating in the glossopharyngeal nuclei synapse in the otic ganglion; its postganglionic neurons innervate the parotid gland. A major component of the cranial outflow is the vagus nerve, which originates from vagal nuclei in the medulla oblongata. Preganglionic nerves pass to ganglia located within the heart and the viscera of the thorax and abdomen. Postganglionic nerves, very short in length, arise from these ganglia to terminate in the aforementioned structures. Neurons originating from sacral segments form the pelvic nerves, which synapse in terminal ganglia lying near or within the uterus, bladder, rectum, and sex organs.

Unlike the arrangement in the sympathetic nervous system, there is little overlap or divergence in the parasympathetic nervous system. With few exceptions (e.g., in Auerbach's plexus in the gastrointestinal tract, where one preganglionic nerve exists for every 8000 postganglionic nerves), there is a one-to-one relation between preganglionic and postganglionic nerves, which makes possible discrete and limited responses in the parasympathetic nervous system. The parasympathetic nervous system is characterized by relatively long preganglionic and very short postganglionic nerves and, with only a few exceptions, an absence of well-defined, anatomically distinct ganglia.

Functional Characteristics

Many organs are dually innervated by both the sympathetic and parasympathetic nervous systems, such as the salivary glands, heart, lungs (bronchial muscle), and abdominal and pelvic viscera, whereas other organs receive innervation from only one division. The sweat glands, adrenal medulla, piloerector muscles, and most blood vessels receive innervation from only the sympathetic nervous system. On the other hand, the parenchyma of the parotid, lacrimal, and nasopharyngeal glands are supplied only with parasympathetic nerves. Table 5-1 lists the organs to which nerve fibers of the parasympathetic and sympathetic nervous systems are distributed, the effects of stimulation of these nerves, and the autonomic receptors that are activated by neurotransmitters released from autonomic nerves.

To understand or predict the effects of autonomic drugs on a specific organ, it is necessary to know how each division of the ANS affects that organ as well as whether the organ is singly or dually innervated and, if dually, which of the two systems is dominant in the organ. In certain circumstances, one or the other of the two divisions of the ANS may provide the dominant influence, but it should be noted that often neither division is totally dominant in many of the dually innervated organs. The fact that both divisions of the ANS modulate the intrinsic activity of the various tissues cannot be overemphasized.

The anatomic and functional characteristics of the two divisions of the ANS should make it clear that there are striking differences between the sympathetic and parasympathetic nervous systems. Cannon was the first to recognize that the sympathetic nervous system is capable of producing the kind of widespread and massive response that would enable an organism confronted with a stressor (such as pain, asphyxia, or strong emotions) to mount an appropriate response ("fright, fight, or flight").[11] Controlled clinical trials in dental patients indicate that oral surgical procedures constitute physiologically significant stressors for stimulating the sympathetic nervous system, with noticeable increases in circulating norepinephrine concentrations observed in patients during surgery and with the development of postsurgical pain (Figure 5-3). The stress of oral surgery is mediated by the CNS because drugs that reduce anxiety (e.g., diazepam) also reduce the sympathetic response to surgical stress and postoperative

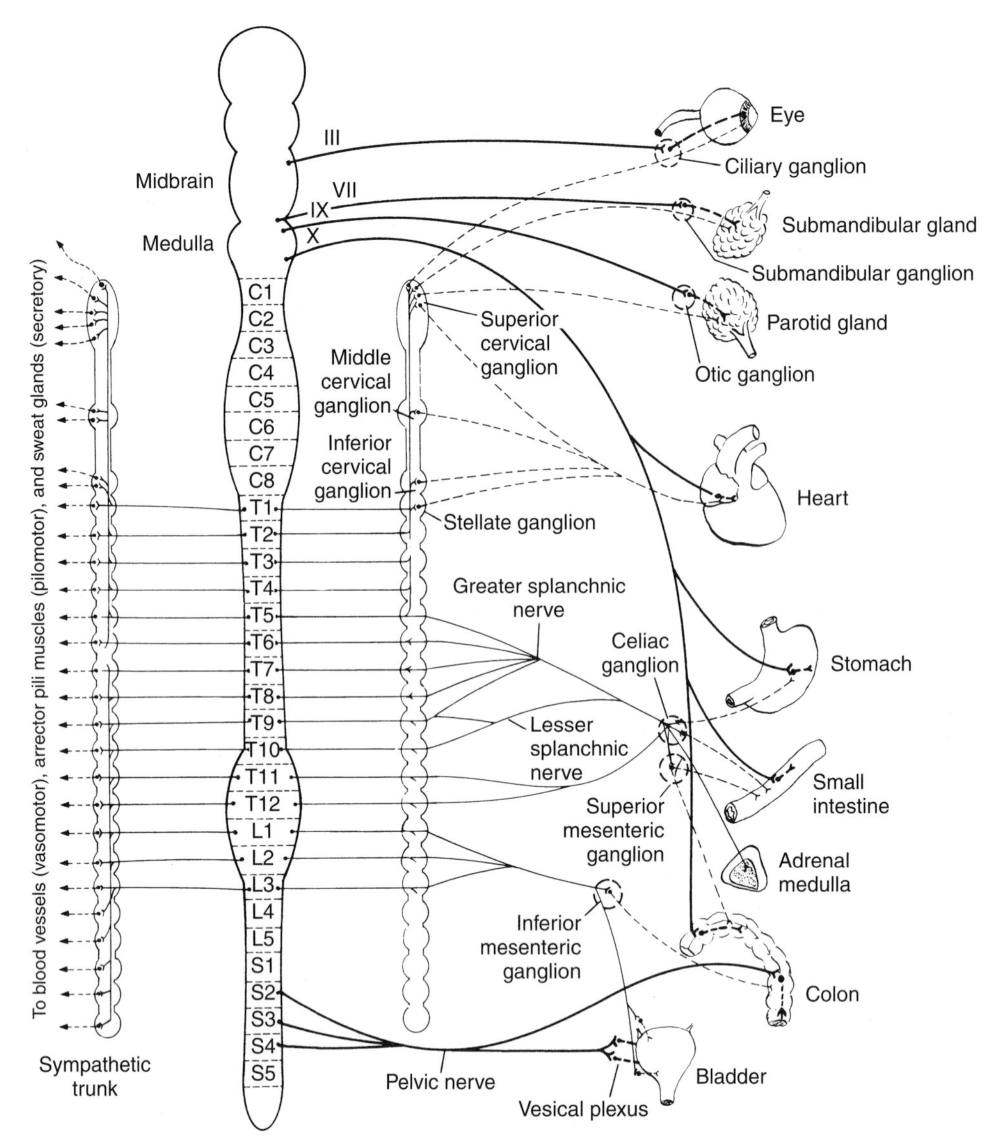

Fig. 5-2 General arrangement of the ANS showing one side of the bilateral outflow. On either side of the spinal cord (*C1* to *S5*) are pictured the two chains of the paravertebral sympathetic ganglia. Preganglionic nerves of the sympathetic nervous system are indicated by *light solid lines*; postganglionic nerves of the sympathetic nervous system are indicated by *light dashed lines*. Preganglionic nerves of the parasympathetic nervous system, originating from the brain and sacral spinal cord, are shown in *bold solid lines*; postganglionic nerves of the parasympathetic nervous system are shown in *bold dashed lines.* (Adapted from Copenhaver WM, ed: *Bailey's Textbook of histology*, ed 15, Baltimore, 1964, Williams & Wilkins.)

pain.[15,19] On the other hand, the parasympathetic division is primarily concerned with the protection, conservation, and restoration of bodily resources. These differences in function are subserved by some of the anatomic characteristics that have already been mentioned, including the involvement of the adrenal medulla and the high ratio of postganglionic to preganglionic nerves in the sympathetic, but not the parasympathetic, nervous system.

NEUROTRANSMITTERS

The concept that chemical mediators were responsible for transmission of information in the ANS emerged at the end of the nineteenth and the beginning of the twentieth century. Acetylcholine was identified as the primary neurotransmitter released from preganglionic nerves and from postganglionic nerves in the parasympathetic nervous system. Norepinephrine was found to be the neurotransmitter released from the majority of postganglionic sympathetic nerves, whereas both norepinephrine and epinephrine are released after sympathetic stimulation of the adrenal medulla. More recently dopamine has also been found to be an important neurotransmitter at some sites in the ANS. Although acetylcholine, norepinephrine, epinephrine, and possibly dopamine have come to be recognized as the principal mediators of ANS activity, evidence exists that other molecules may also serve as chemical transmitters for specific neuronal circuits. Among these are histamine, 5-hydroxytryptamine (5-HT, serotonin),

Table • 5-1

Responses of Various Effectors to Stimulation by Autonomic Nerves

EFFECTOR	SYMPATHETIC RESPONSE	SYMPATHETIC RECEPTOR	PARASYMPATHETIC RESPONSE*
Eye			
Radial muscle of the iris	Contraction (mydriasis)	α_1	—
Sphincter muscle of the iris	—		Contraction (miosis)
Ciliary muscle	Slight relaxation (far vision)	β_2	Contraction (near vision)
Heart†			
Sinoatrial node	Increase in rate	β_1, β_2	Decrease in rate
Atria	Increased contractility and conduction velocity	β_1, β_2	Decreased contractility, usually increased conduction velocity
Atrioventricular node	Increase in automaticity and conduction velocity	β_1, β_2	Decrease in conduction velocity
Ventricles	Increased contractility, conduction velocity, and automaticity	β_1, β_2	—
Blood vessels‡			
Coronary	Functional significance is doubtful	α_1, α_2, β_2	Same as sympathetic
Skin and mucosa	Constriction	α_1, α_2	Dilation, but of questionable significance
Skeletal muscle	Constriction; dilation	α, β_2§	—
Abdominal viscera	Constriction; dilation	α_1, β_2	—
Salivary glands	Constriction	α_1, α_2	Dilation
Erectile tissue	Constriction	α	Dilation
Lungs			
Bronchial smooth muscle	Relaxation	β_2	Contraction
Bronchial glands	Decreased secretion; increased secretion	α_1, β_2	Increased secretion
Gastrointestinal tract			
Smooth muscle	Decreased motility and tone	α_1, α_2, β_1, β_2	Increased motility and tone
Sphincters	Contraction	α_1	Relaxation
Secretion	Inhibition	α_2	Stimulation
Salivary glands	Watery secretion; viscous and amylase secretion‖	α_1, β_1, β_2	Profuse, watery secretion
Spleen capsule	Contraction; mild relaxation	α_1, β_2	—
Urinary bladder			
Detrusor	Relaxation	β_2	Contraction
Trigone and sphincter	Contraction	α_1	Relaxation
Ureter			
Motility and tone	Increased	α_1	Increased (?)
Uterus	Variable, depending on species, endocrine status, etc.	α_1, β_2	Variable
Skin			
Pilomotor muscles	Contraction	α_1	—
Sweat glands	Secretion¶		—
Liver	Glycogenolysis, gluconeogenesis, etc.	α_1, β_2	Glycogen synthesis
Adipose tissue	Lipolysis	α_2, β_1, β_3	—

*All parasympathetic responses are mediated by activation of muscarinic receptors.
†Norepinephrine released from sympathetic nerves to the heart activates only β_1 receptors; epinephrine released from the adrenal medulla stimulates both β_1 and β_2 receptors. The predominant adrenergic receptor in the heart is β_1.
‡In most smooth muscles, including blood vessels, α_1 receptors contract (constrict), whereas β_2 receptors relax (dilate). Prejunctional α_2 receptors on sympathetic nerve terminals inhibit norepinephrine release which will relax blood vessels and cause vasodilation.
§Blood vessels in skeletal muscle are innervated by some sympathetic nerves that release acetylcholine, which acts on muscarinic receptors to cause vasodilation.
‖The human parotid glands do not receive sympathetic innervation.
¶The sweat glands receive sympathetic innervation, but with few exceptions (e.g., the sweat glands of the palms of the hands, which are activated by α_1-receptor stimulation) the transmitter is acetylcholine and the receptors activated are muscarinic.

γ-aminobutyric acid (GABA), prostanoids, aspartate, adenosine triphosphate (ATP), glutamate, glycine, and a variety of peptides, including neuropeptide Y, cholecystokinin, enkephalin and opioids, substance P, calcitonin gene-related peptide, and vasoactive intestinal peptide.

Location of Adrenergic and Cholinergic Junctions

Figure 5-1 shows the sites at which the neurotransmitters acetylcholine and norepinephrine and the hormone epinephrine act as chemical mediators. With the exception of effectors (smooth muscle, the heart, and secretory glands) that are

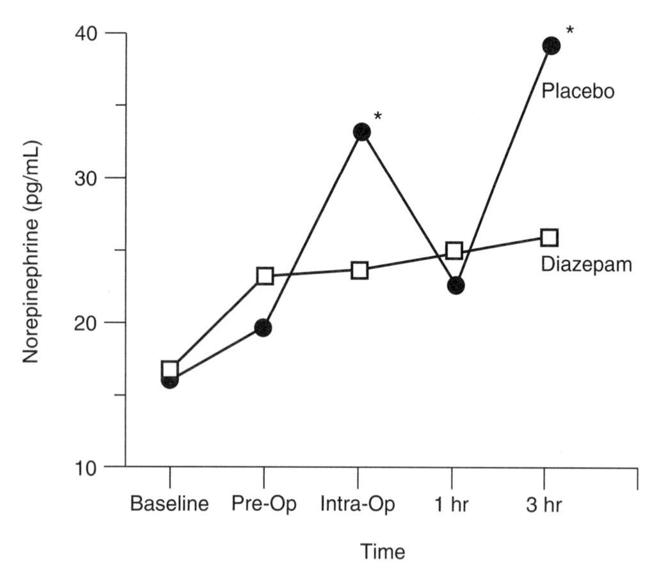

Fig. 5-3 Response of the sympathetic nervous system to the stress of oral surgery, as indicated by the circulating concentration of norepinephrine. Plasma norepinephrine was measured 1 week before surgery (baseline) and on the day of surgery at the indicated time points. Patients were randomly injected intravenously with either placebo or diazepam (0.3 mg/kg), followed by intraoral injections of 2% lidocaine with 1 : 100,000 epinephrine before surgical removal of impacted third molars. Placebo-treated patients demonstrated significant increases *(asterisks)* in norepinephrine at the intraoperative and 3-hour postoperative periods, whereas diazepam-treated patients did not. (Adapted from Hargreaves KM, Dionne RA, Mueller GP, et al: Naloxone, fentanyl, and diazepam modify plasma β-endorphin levels during surgery, *Clin Pharmacol Ther* 40:165-171, 1986.)

innervated by postganglionic sympathetic nerves where the neurotransmitter is norepinephrine, all other sites are innervated by cholinergic nerves, including the ganglia of the ANS, the adrenal medulla, a few effectors of the sympathetic nervous system, and all the effectors of the parasympathetic nervous system. At cholinergic junctions, cholinergic nerves release acetylcholine, which acts on cholinergic receptors to produce an effect. These ubiquitous cholinergic receptors are composed of two structurally unrelated types, called *muscarinic* and *nicotinic,* that are located at specific sites in the ANS. Muscarinic receptors are located on effectors innervated by cholinergic nerves. This includes effectors at postganglionic parasympathetic junctions and a few postganglionic sympathetic junctions (some sweat glands and blood vessels). Nicotinic receptors are found at different anatomic sites, including postganglionic nerve cell bodies at all autonomic ganglia, the adrenal medulla, and skeletal muscle. There are also different types of structurally related[37] adrenergic receptors (α_1, α_2, β_1, β_2, β_3)[10] that are found at postganglionic sympathetic junctions where norepinephrine is released from postganglionic sympathetic nerves. However, these adrenergic receptors do not have a precise anatomic distribution; some effector organs have only a single adrenergic receptor, whereas other organs have two or more adrenergic receptor subtypes. The fact that there are significant differences in autonomic receptor subtypes is supported by the discovery that there are agonists that stimulate one receptor subtype but not others and blocking drugs or antagonists that block one receptor but not others. Research has revealed the existence of additional subtypes for both adrenergic and cholinergic receptors, and it is anticipated that drugs highly selective for these receptor subtypes will be developed for future clinical use.

Mechanism of Neurotransmitter Release

Our current understanding of exocytotic neurotransmitter release has arisen from the work of many different investigators. Although several mechanisms for neurotransmitter release may exist, as summarized in reviews on the subject,[26,36] one main model has been developed for the secretion of classic neurotransmitters, such as acetylcholine (Figure 5-4) and norepinephrine (Figure 5-5). It has been proposed that when an action potential reaches the axon terminal it depolarizes the membrane, leading to the opening of voltage-gated Ca^{++} channels.[31] (This activation of Ca^{++} channels causes high, but transient, increases in intracellular Ca^{++} concentrations near the neurotransmitter storage vesicles. Intracellular Ca^{++} activates calmodulin, a small Ca^{++}-binding protein found in nearly all cells.[14] In turn, calmodulin activates an enzyme called Ca^{++}/calmodulin-dependent protein kinase. This enzyme, found in extremely high concentrations in neurons (approximately 1% of total protein), then catalyzes the phosphorylation of several proteins associated with the storage vesicle, including synapsin I. Synapsin I binds to actin present on the cytoskeleton and is thought to interact with other proteins (e.g., synaptobrevin, synaptophysin, and synaptoporin) to initiate docking and fusion of the storage vesicle with the cell membrane, followed by exocytotic neurotransmitter release. The neurotransmitter crosses the junctional or synaptic cleft and binds to its receptor on the nerve or effector cell membrane, which could be located on a ganglionic neuron, a skeletal muscle fiber, an autonomic effector, or a cell in the CNS.

ADRENERGIC NEUROTRANSMISSION

Catecholamine Synthesis

The catecholamines norepinephrine and epinephrine are the primary neurotransmitters/hormones released after stimulation of the sympathetic nervous system. The synthesis and storage of the catecholamines can be modified by a number of clinically useful drugs. The synthetic process, shown in Figure 5-6, involves a number of enzymes that are synthesized in the nerve cell body and carried by axoplasmic transport to the nerve endings. The enzyme tyrosine hydroxylase, which catalyzes the conversion of tyrosine to dihydroxyphenylalanine, is the rate-limiting enzyme in this process; any drug that inhibits the function of tyrosine hydroxylase will reduce the rate at which norepinephrine is produced in the nerve terminal. It also appears that the concentration of norepinephrine in the cytoplasm is one of the factors that regulates its own formation, principally by feedback inhibition on tyrosine hydroxylase activity.[27] The enzyme phenylethanolamine-N-methyltransferase, which catalyzes the conversion of norepinephrine to epinephrine, occurs almost exclusively in the chromaffin cells of the adrenal medulla and is therefore missing in peripheral nerve terminals.[3] Hence, norepinephrine is the final product in most adrenergic nerves, whereas mainly epinephrine (80%), with some norepinephrine (20%), is produced in adrenal chromaffin cells in human beings.

Catecholamine Release

Evidence suggests that 90% to 95% of intracellular norepinephrine is stored in small granulated vesicles, where it is protected from intracellular enzymatic destruction until it is released by depolarization, whereas 5% to 10% is found in the cytoplasm. Thus most norepinephrine is stored in vesicles complexed with the protein chromogranin, the enzyme dopamine β-hydroxylase, and ATP. There are two different norepinephrine pools inside the neuron: a mobile and a reserve pool. Membrane depolarization causes release of transmitter from the mobile pool. Newly synthesized

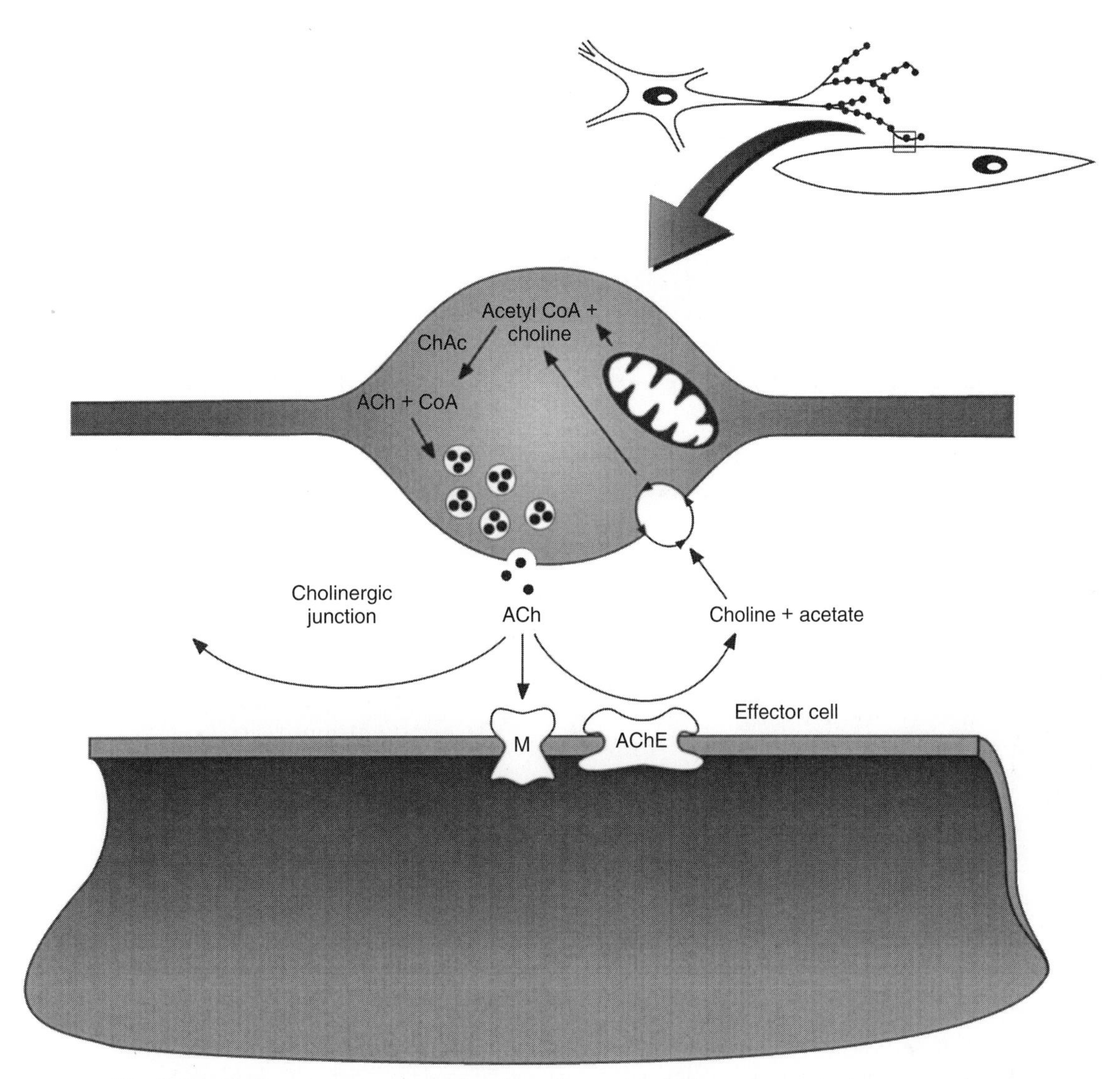

Fig. 5-4 Cholinergic nerve terminal and its effector, in which are shown the intraneuronal synthesis of acetylcholine *(ACh)*, the vesicles containing ACh, the release of ACh into the junctional cleft, its removal by the action of acetylcholinesterase *(AChE)* and diffusion, and the subsequent reuptake of choline back into the nerve terminal. *CoA*, Coenzyme A; *ChAc*, choline acetyltransferase; *M*, muscarinic receptor. (Adapted from Hubbard JI: Mechanism of transmitter release from nerve terminals, *Ann NY Acad Sci* 183:131-146, 1971.)

norepinephrine would appear to constitute the mobile pool because it is preferentially released during depolarization.[40] The function of the small cytoplasmic pool, as well as its relationship to vesicular norepinephrine, is not well understood. A diagrammatic representation of the adrenergic nerve terminal is shown in Figure 5-5.

Autonomic neuroeffector junctions are less structurally organized than the classic neuromuscular junction. The autonomic axon resembles a string of beads as it passes among smooth muscle fibers in blood vessels, intestines, and other sites (see the top right of Figure 5-5). The beaded varicosities release neurotransmitter near relatively few directly innervated effector cells. Most of the effector cells are either directly or indirectly coupled to those cells that are innervated. As the nerve impulse passes down the axon and depolarization successively involves each varicosity, extracellular Ca^{++} enters into the nerve terminals and norepinephrine is released into the junctional cleft by the process of exocytosis, as previously described. The cleft distances in both the sympathetic and parasympathetic nervous systems are quite variable, ranging from 15 nm up to many hundred nanometers, depending on the specific neuroeffector junction.[6] After crossing the junctional cleft by passive diffusion, the transmitter binds to receptor sites on the effector organ and elicits an appropriate response.

Adrenergic Receptors

In 1948, Ahlquist proposed the existence of two kinds of adrenergic receptors. He called these alpha (α) and beta (β).[1] Two subtypes of the β-adrenergic receptor, called β_1 and β_2, were identified, followed by two different α-adrenergic receptors: α_1, the predominant postjunctional membrane receptor, and α_2, located both prejunctionally[33] and postjunctionally.[5] The presence or absence of these different adrenergic receptors provides an explanation for the seemingly contradictory (or opposing) actions of the adrenergic transmitters (e.g., vasodilation in some vascular beds and vasoconstriction in others; see Table 5-1) and is supported by experiments with synthetic drugs (both agonists and antagonists) that have a

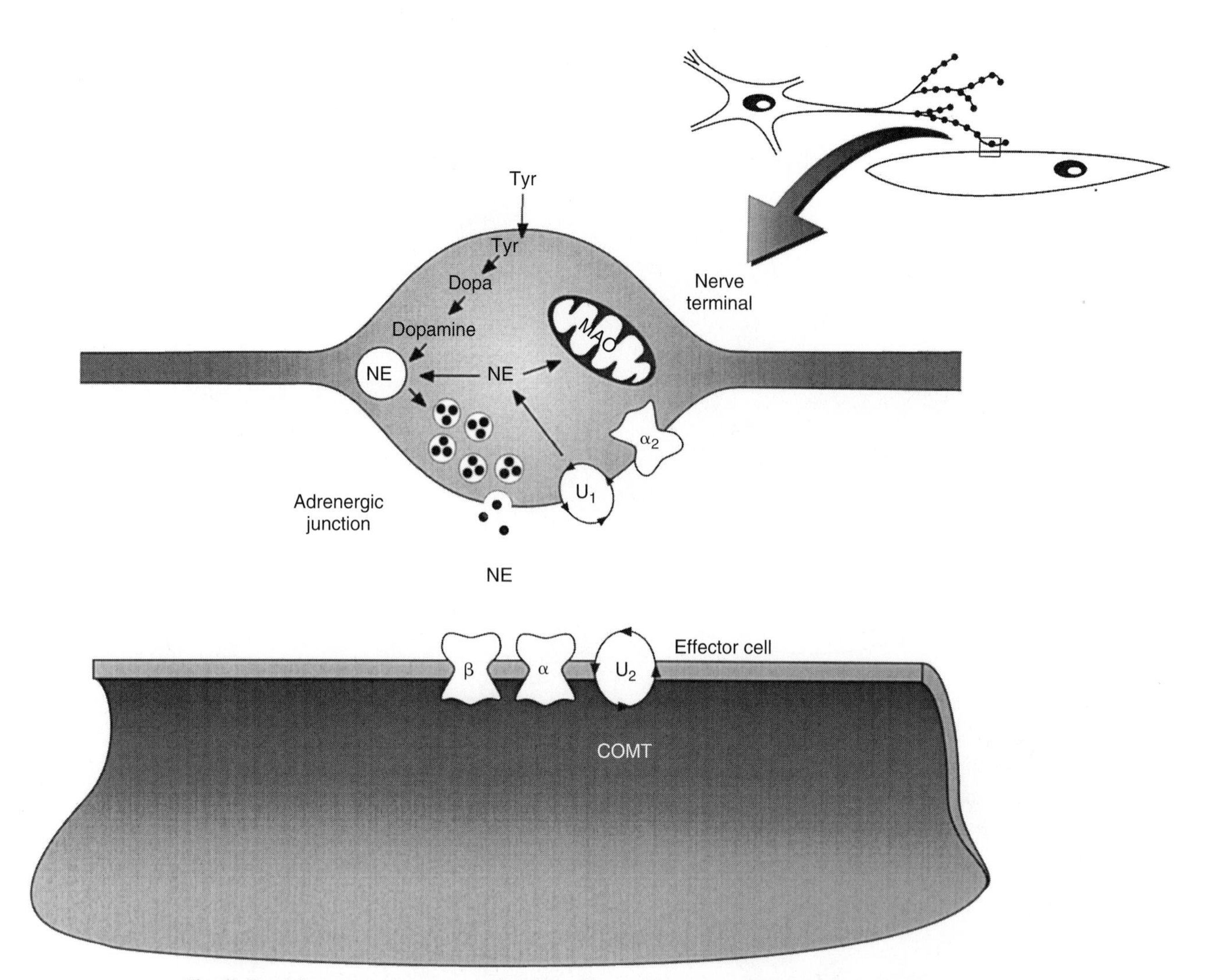

Fig. 5-5 Adrenergic nerve terminal and its effector. Shown are the precursors of norepinephrine *(NE)*, the sites of synthesis and storage of dopamine and NE, and the location of prejunctional and postjunctional adrenergic receptors *(α_2, α, β)*. It also shows the enzymatic (catechol-O-methyltransferase *[COMT]*, monoamine oxidase *[MAO]*) and uptake-1 *(U_1)* and uptake-2 *(U_2)* mechanisms by which the action of NE is terminated. *Tyr,* Tyrosine; *Dopa,* dihydroxyphenylalanine.

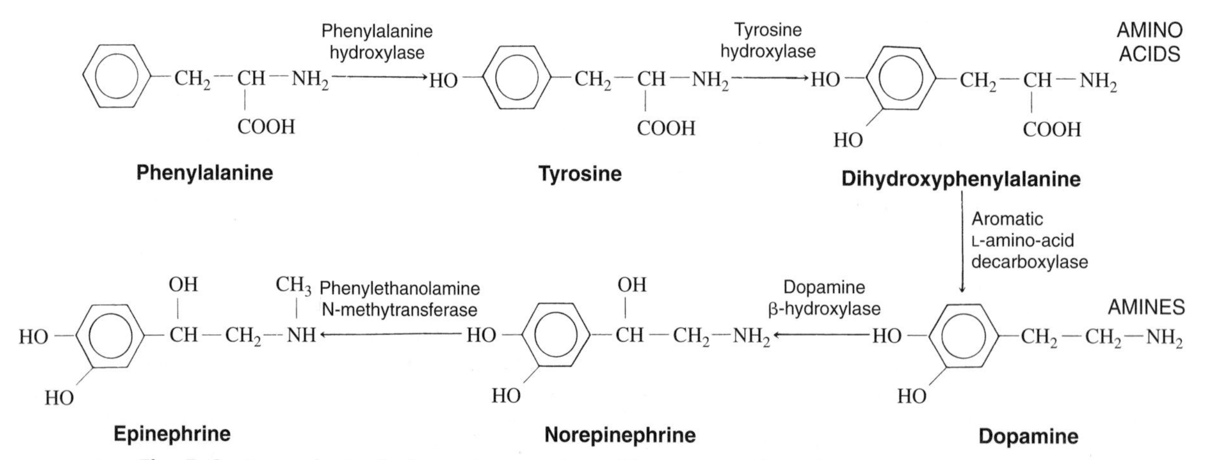

Fig. 5-6 Biosynthesis of adrenergic transmitters. The amino acids in the top row can penetrate the blood-brain barrier, whereas the amines shown in the bottom row cannot. Conversion of dopamine into norepinephrine takes place in the storage vesicles of adrenergic nerves and the adrenal medulla, whereas conversion of norepinephrine to epinephrine occurs only in storage vesicles in the adrenal medulla and in some neurons of the CNS. The enzyme tyrosine hydroxylase is the rate-limiting regulatory enzyme in the synthesis of catecholamines and is a target for the enzyme inhibitor metyrosine.

high degree of selectivity for an individual adrenergic receptor type.

More recent molecular cloning and pharmacologic studies have demonstrated the existence of multiple subtypes of adrenergic receptors. For example, the α_1-adrenergic receptor family consists of three subtypes, classified as α_{1A}, α_{1B}, and α_{1D}.[28,42] Similar studies have demonstrated the existence of multiple subtypes of the α_2 receptor (α_{2A}, α_{2B}, α_{2C}) and the β-adrenergic receptor (β_1, β_2, β_3).[10] It is now possible, by using molecular biologic techniques, to define a protein structure for these receptors.[37] Thus the human β_2 receptor is a protein of 413 amino acids, with seven transmembrane spanning domains (see Figure 1-3). This heptihelical structure is a general characteristic of many cell surface neurotransmitter receptors. Because many of these receptors appear to have substantial differences in tissue distribution and function, considerable research is being directed toward the development of drugs with selectivity at individual receptor subtypes.[4,28] These drugs may possess greater specificity of action compared with currently used adrenergic agonists or antagonists.

As can be seen in Table 5-1, some organs express only one type of adrenergic receptor, whereas others have several types. α_1-Adrenergic receptors mediate smooth muscle contraction and glandular secretion and are often excitatory. The function of α_2 receptors at postjunctional sites includes regulation of several metabolic functions (e.g., glycogenolysis, lipolysis, and water absorption)[4] and vascular smooth muscle contraction. Norepinephrine acts on prejunctional α_2 receptors to inhibit transmitter release. This negative feedback control is supported by the observation that antagonists for these receptors (e.g., phentolamine) cause an increase in the release of transmitter in response to nerve stimulation.[33] Centrally, α_2 receptors are known to be involved in the regulation of blood pressure. Although several important exceptions exist, β_1 receptors are generally associated with excitatory cellular responses and β_2 receptors with relaxation. β_3 Receptors are primarily associated with stimulation of lipolysis in fat cells.

Catecholamine Fate

The fate of the released catecholamines and systems responsible for termination of their action are quite different from mechanisms of neurotransmitter termination at cholinergic junctions. At adrenergic junctions, enzymatic destruction of the transmitter normally plays a relatively minor role. Uptake of the transmitter accounts for the greatest proportion of transmitter loss, with enzymatic breakdown and diffusion away from the junction responsible for only a small percentage of the total. As depicted in Figure 5-5, uptake can be neuronal (uptake-1) or extraneuronal (uptake-2).[21] Uptake-1 is an active process that requires energy and extracellular Na^+ and exhibits stereospecificity. Amphetamines, tyramine, and levonordefrin (α-methylnorepinephrine) are examples of drugs that are taken up by this transporter system. Inhibitors of neuronal uptake include cocaine and imipramine. Uptake-2 has a greater capacity but lower affinity than uptake-1. At high concentrations of norepinephrine, uptake-2 results in the relatively rapid removal of the transmitter. Uptake-2 is sometimes referred to as the cocaine-insensitive uptake.

Within the nerve terminal, uptake of norepinephrine into the storage vesicles also takes place. It is an active process, requiring ATP and Mg^{++}, and it is by this mechanism that norepinephrine and structurally related compounds (such as some vasoconstrictors added to local anesthetic solutions) ultimately enter the storage vesicles. The drug best known for its ability to inhibit this transfer of norepinephrine and related compounds from the neuronal cytoplasm into storage vesicles is reserpine.

In the cytoplasmic pool, the neurotransmitter is susceptible to the enzymatic action of a mitochondrial enzyme, monoamine oxidase (MAO), which is capable of deaminating the molecule. MAO is widely distributed throughout the body, especially in the liver, kidney, and brain, and is associated with the mitochondria of the adrenergic nerve terminals. It is the principal intraneuronal enzyme concerned with the breakdown of norepinephrine. Certain drugs are capable of inhibiting MAO, leading to an accumulation of the transmitter in the nerve terminal, an effect that has both physiologic and therapeutic implications. A second enzyme concerned with the breakdown of norepinephrine is catechol-O-methyltransferase (COMT). It is widely distributed in many tissues and is the principal extraneuronal enzyme involved with the metabolism of norepinephrine.

CHOLINERGIC TRANSMISSION

Synthesis, Release, and Fate of Acetylcholine

The general concept of transmitter synthesis, storage, and removal also applies to acetylcholine at cholinergic junctions of the ANS. As shown in Figure 5-4, the conversion of choline to acetylcholine in the nerve terminal is accomplished by the enzyme choline acetyltransferase. The mitochondrial cofactor acetyl coenzyme A serves as the acetyl group donor for the reaction. The newly synthesized acetylcholine is then stored in vesicles.[20] The vesicles are transported toward the presynaptic membrane and make contact with specialized docking proteins, and the contents of the vesicles are released by exocytosis,[20] as described previously. Acetylcholine crosses the junctional cleft and attaches reversibly to the postjunctional receptor, which exists in close proximity to a highly specific enzyme, acetylcholinesterase (AChE). Acetylcholine becomes bound to the enzyme at two primary sites (see Figure 8-6) and is hydrolyzed to choline and acetate at such a rapid rate that the nerve can respond to another stimulus milliseconds later. The choline produced by the action of AChE is then returned to the nerve terminal by a carrier mechanism and is once more used in the synthesis of acetylcholine.

Even in the total absence of AChE activity, the action of acetylcholine can be terminated very quickly by pseudocholinesterase, a nonspecific plasma enzyme also known as butyrocholinesterase, which is found in many tissues, including blood. Clinically, a subpopulation of patients lacks plasma pseudocholinesterase activity and can have prolonged paralysis with muscle-relaxing agents such as succinylcholine, which is metabolized primarily by this enzyme (see Chapter 10). Acetylcholine is also removed from the junctional cleft by the simple process of diffusion.

Cholinergic Receptors

As with the adrenergic receptors, receptors for acetylcholine can be separated into two major categories: nicotinic and muscarinic. The anatomic distribution and functional significance of these receptors has been described (see Table 5-1 and Figures 5-1 and 5-2). Nicotinic receptors outside the CNS are located on postganglionic nerves in autonomic ganglia, on chromaffin cells in the adrenal medulla, and on skeletal muscle in neuromuscular junctions. Nicotinic receptors on postganglionic neurons and in the adrenal medulla are classified as N_N (nerve) receptors; N_M (muscle) receptors are found on skeletal muscle in neuromuscular junctions. In contrast to adrenergic receptors and muscarinic receptors, nicotinic receptors are ion channel receptors composed of an allosteric protein containing four different subunits—α, β, δ, and γ—gathered together in a transmembrane pentamer.[24] Each of the subunits has an intracellular and extracellular exposure, and together they surround a central channel. Recognition sites for acetylcholine and other agonists, cholinergic antagonists, and certain snake venom toxins are located primarily on the α subunits.

Muscarinic receptors of the ANS are located primarily on effector cells—smooth muscle, the heart, and secretory glands—that are innervated by postganglionic parasympathetic nerves. Molecular cloning studies have deduced the amino acid sequence of five subtypes of muscarinic receptors classified as M_1 to M_5.[12] As with adrenergic receptors, muscarinic receptors all have seven transmembrane-spanning domains and display the same general structure as the β_2-adrenergic receptor shown in Figure 1-3.

SIGNAL TRANSDUCTION AND SECOND MESSENGERS

The binding of an autonomic neurotransmitter to its receptor on the plasma membrane surface of a target cell initials a signaling cascade that alters the physiologic activity of the cell. The exact response elicited depends not on the neurotransmitter per se but on the type of receptor activated. As previously described, there are two general classes of membrane-bound receptors that interact with autonomic drugs: ion channel–linked and G protein–linked receptors.

Ion Channel—Linked Receptors

Ion channel–linked receptors, otherwise known as ionotropic receptors, are ligand-gated ion channels that undergo binding-dependent conformational changes leading to an opening of the ion channel (see Chapter 1). For example, the nicotinic receptor was first isolated and purified from the electric organ of the eel, *Electrophorus torpedo*, and by 1984 it had become the first receptor for which complete structural data had been obtained.[13] The nicotinic receptor is a ligand-gated ion channel that, when activated, leads to rapid membrane depolarization as a result of the passage of Na^+ and Ca^{++} through the channel. Ligand-gated ion channels may increase permeability of the membrane to all ions or selectively increase permeability only to certain ions. In the case of a ligand-gated Na^+ channel in neurons, channel opening produces an excitatory postsynaptic potential, and, in the case of a ligand-gated K^+ or Cl^- channel, an inhibitory postsynaptic potential. An excitatory postsynaptic potential will activate a neuron, whereas an inhibitory postsynaptic potential inhibits neuronal activity.

G Protein—Linked Receptors

Adrenergic and muscarinic receptors belong to a large family of receptors characterized by their functional dependence on G proteins (shorthand for guanine nucleotide-binding proteins) to initiate cellular signaling. G proteins are heterotrimers, so named because they consist of three different proteins: the α subunit, which activates target proteins (enzymes, ion channels) and hydrolyzes guanosine triphosphate (GTP) to guanosine diphosphate (GDP), and the β and γ subunits, which attach the G protein to the cell membrane and have signaling properties distinctly different from the α subunit.[7,38] G proteins are signal transducers in that they convert the external signal of neurotransmitter binding into an alteration of cellular function. Molecular cloning studies suggest that there are many different types of G protein heterotrimers consisting of different varieties of α, β, and γ subunits.

As an immediate result of G protein actions, intracellular signaling molecules are generated that serve as "second messengers" for the neurotransmitters, which are the primary messengers. Figure 5-7 depicts two major second messenger pathways: the cyclic 3′,5′-adenosine monophosphate (cAMP) and the Ca^{++}/inositol phospholipid pathway. These two pathways mediate many of the actions of the G protein–coupled adrenergic and muscarinic receptors.[7,22,41]

G_s protein–dependent events

In the example illustrated in Figure 5-7, activation of the β_1-adrenergic receptor by norepinephrine leads to the receptor's association with a membrane-bound G protein heterotrimer called G_s ("s" implies a stimulatory effect). This binding activates G_s, causing the G_s α subunit to exchange its bound GDP for GTP and to dissociate from the adrenergic receptor and from the $\beta\gamma$ subunit pair. The free $G_{\alpha s}$ complexed with GTP is capable of binding to and activating effector enzymes such as adenylyl cyclase, leading to the production of cAMP. In turn, cAMP activates protein kinase A, which phosphorylates a number of target proteins. This phosphorylation step alters the ongoing activity of the cell, because many of these target proteins are either enzymes or ion channels. For example, protein kinase A can activate the enzyme glycogen phosphorylase, leading to increased glycogen breakdown and release of glucose. Some other responses linked to increased cAMP synthesis include relaxation of vascular smooth muscle, increased contractile force of the myocardium, and secretion of amylase and other proteins by salivary glands.[9,32,34] In addition to β receptors, many receptors activate the cAMP pathway, including dopamine D_1 and D_5 receptors, 5-HT_4 receptors, histamine H_2 receptors, adenosine A_2 receptors, and certain peptide and prostanoid receptors.[38,39] These receptors are discussed in other chapters.

Hydrolysis of the bound GTP by $G_{\alpha s}$ leads to inactivation of the subunit. $G_{\alpha s}$, complexed with GDP, now reassociates with the β and γ subunits. The heterotrimer can then be reactivated by an appropriate stimulus. Cholera toxin blocks the ability of $G_{\alpha s}$ to hydrolyze GTP. Thus $G_{\alpha s}$ is permanently activated, contributing to the signs and symptoms of cholera. Once formed, cAMP is subject to breakdown by a second enzyme, cAMP phosphodiesterase. Inhibition of this enzyme blocks the breakdown of cAMP and accentuates the adrenergic response. Caffeine and related methylxanthines are effective inhibitors of phosphodiesterase, at least in vitro.[2] A particular form of cAMP phosphodiesterase is the site of action for inamrinone and milrinone, agents used to treat congestive heart failure (see Chapter 25).

The G protein system serves to greatly amplify the biologic response to a drug or neurotransmitter. Because of the large degree of signal amplification, stimulation of only a small proportion of the total receptors may be required to elicit a maximal biologic response. It has been estimated, for example, that binding of only 1% of the insulin receptors can produce maximal rates of glycogenolysis in liver cells. Amplification of the biologic response by second messenger systems may contribute to the phenomenon of "spare receptors" described in Chapter 1 in which maximal responses are observed after activation of only a small proportion of the available receptors.

G_i protein–dependent events

Different biologic responses can occur when receptors activate different G_α protein subunits. Stimulation of α_2-adrenergic receptors, for example (see Figure 5-7), leads to the release of $G_{\alpha i}$ ("i" for inhibitory). $G_{\alpha i}$ inhibits adenylyl cyclase and therefore causes decreased cAMP concentrations.[23] Other receptors that act by reducing cAMP include adenosine A_1 receptors; dopamine D_2 receptors; 5-HT_1 receptors; $GABA_B$ receptors; M_2- and M_4-muscarinic receptors; and several glutamate, opioid, and other peptide receptors.[39] In addition, certain toxins, such as pertussis toxin, inactivate $G_{\alpha i}$ so that it cannot inhibit adenylyl cyclase, which promotes an increase in cAMP and contributes to many of the signs and symptoms of whooping cough.

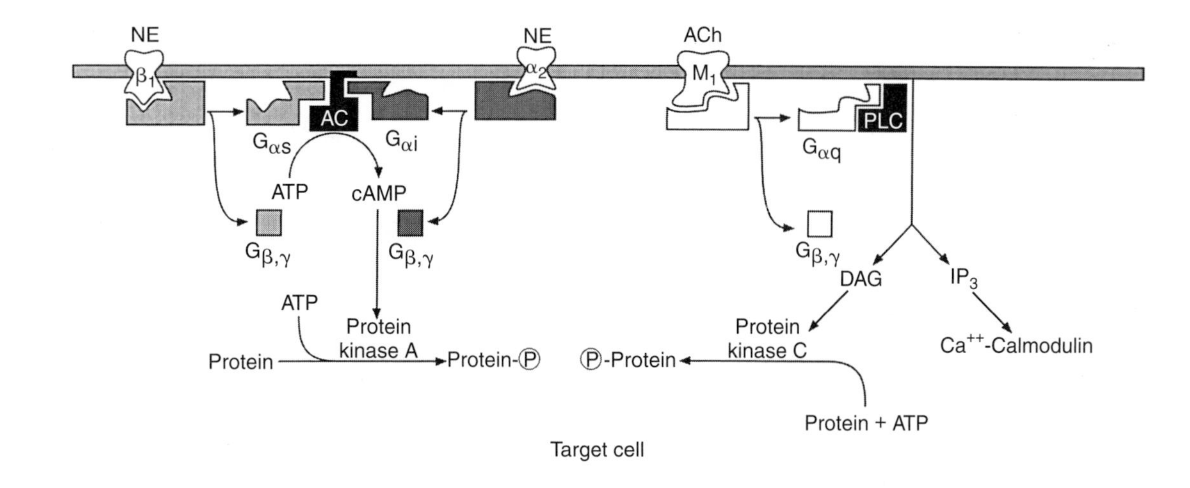

Fig. 5-7 Sites of action of primary messengers, such as norepinephrine *(NE)* and acetylcholine *(ACh)*, and their role in regulating the formation of second messengers in target cells. The binding of the agonist to its receptor (in this example, β_1- or α_2-adrenergic, or M_1-muscarinic) leads to release of the α subunit of the associated G protein ($G_{\alpha s}$, $G_{\alpha i}$, or $G_{\alpha q}$). $G_{\alpha s}$ activates adenylyl cyclase *(AC)*, leading to the production of *cAMP*. Elevated cAMP activates protein kinase A, which in turn catalyzes the phosphorylation of a number of target proteins. $G_{\alpha i}$ inhibits AC, leading to a reduction in cAMP. Receptor activation of $G_{\alpha q}$ leads to stimulation of the enzyme phospholipase C *(PLC)*. PLC catalyzes the hydrolysis of phosphatidylinositol 4,5-bisphosphate *(PIP_2)* in the cell membrane, yielding diacylglycerol *(DAG)* and inositol 1,4,5-trisphosphate *(IP_3)*. DAG activates protein kinase C, which in turn catalyzes the phosphorylation of a number of target proteins. IP_3 increases intracellular Ca^{++} release from intracellular storage sites, resulting in activation of calmodulin and other Ca^{++}-dependent events.

G_q protein–dependent events

$G_{\alpha q}$, a third G_α subunit important in ANS responses, activates the Ca^{++}/inositol phospholipid pathway. In the example illustrated in Figure 5-7, acetylcholine stimulation of the M_1-muscarinic receptor leads to release of $G_{\alpha q}$ from its associated β and γ subunits. $G_{\alpha q}$ activates the enzyme phospholipase C, which hydrolyzes phosphatidylinositol 4,5-bisphosphate (PIP_2), a minor phospholipid found on the cytoplasmic surface of the cell membrane. The hydrolysis of PIP_2 yields two biologically active products, diacylglycerol (DAG) and inositol 1,4,5-trisphosphate (IP_3). DAG stimulates the enzyme protein kinase C, which phosphorylates target proteins generally consisting of other enzymes or ion channels. In addition, DAG can itself be hydrolyzed to yield prostanoids, resulting in activation of additional cellular responses. IP_3 releases Ca^{++} from intracellular binding sites, leading to increased activation of protein kinase C and to other biologic responses, including activation of calmodulin-mediated events.

α_1 Receptors activate the second messenger system linked to $G_{\alpha q}$, namely Ca^{++}, DAG, and IP_3. Additional receptors that activate this second messenger system include histamine H_1 receptors; M_1- and M_3-muscarinic receptors; leukotriene receptors; several 5-HT_2 receptors; and certain receptors for glutamate and various peptides, including angiotensin, bradykinin, cholecystokinin, and substance P.[38,39]

Additional second messenger systems

Other second messenger systems exist besides those mentioned, and the roles of cyclic 3′,5′-guanosine monophosphate, Ca^{++}, calmodulin, nitric oxide, prostanoids, peptides, and other mediators of cellular function are currently under extensive investigation.

DOPAMINERGIC TRANSMISSION

Dopamine receptors exist outside the CNS, in the kidney (where their activation leads to vasodilation), the mesenteric vascular bed, the coronary blood vessels, and other vascular and nonvascular smooth muscle. The discovery of dopamine receptors in the periphery has led to the application of dopamine to a number of clinical situations, such as the treatment of cardiogenic shock and renal failure, where it has the capacity to increase cardiac contractility (by stimulating β_1-adrenergic receptors) and renal blood flow without causing marked systemic vasodepressor effects.[17] The existence of dopaminergic nerves in the peripheral nervous system is less settled; one location where dopamine may be a neurotransmitter is the gastrointestinal tract. The possible role of dopamine in sympathetic ganglionic transmission is outlined in Chapter 10. Most of the evidence to date indicates that dopamine is synthesized, stored, released, and taken up in a manner identical to that of norepinephrine.[17] Molecular cloning studies indicate that there are five subtypes of dopamine receptors (D_1 to D_5), all of which resemble adrenergic receptors in overall structure and use G protein–mediated second messenger systems.[38]

PURINERGIC TRANSMISSION

Evidence has accumulated that there are noncholinergic, nonadrenergic nerves, designated as purinergic, that are found in the gastrointestinal tract of all vertebrates as well as in certain areas of the CNS, the vasculature, and the lungs, trachea, and bladder.[8] ATP is stored in vesicles in purinergic nerve endings and, when released, directly activates purinergic receptors of

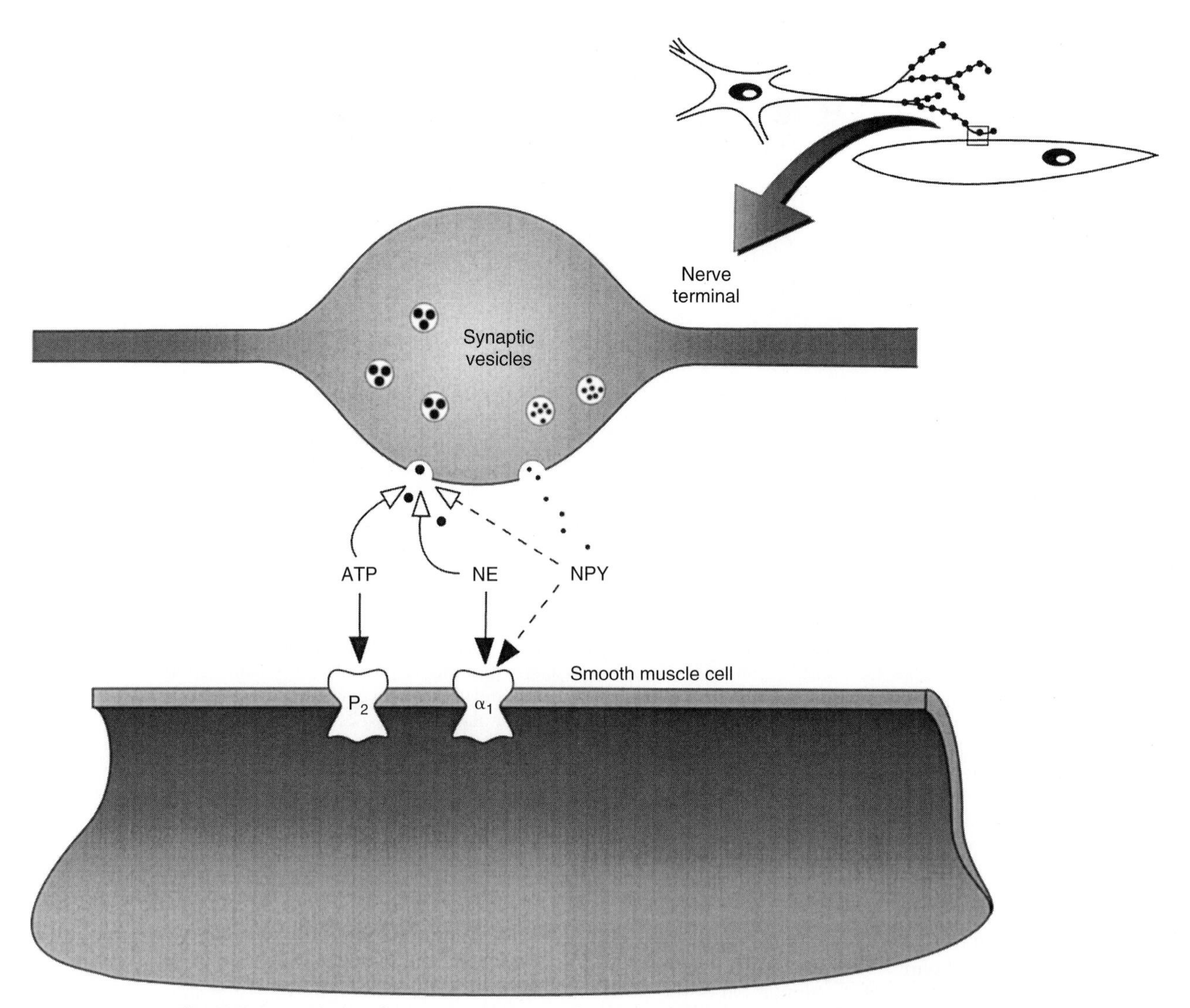

Fig. 5-8 Co-release of neurotransmitters and neuromodulators. Norepinephrine *(NE)* and *ATP*, stored in the same storage vesicles, are released together from the sympathetic nerve varicosity to stimulate *(solid arrows)* their respective α_1 and P_2 receptors on smooth muscle. Neuropeptide Y *(NPY)*, stored in separate vesicles, is also released during sympathetic nerve stimulation. Here, NPY serves as a neuromodulator *(dashed arrows)*, increasing the activity of NE. All three agents inhibit further release *(open arrowheads)* through effects on prejunctional receptors (not shown).

the P2 type, or it is broken down to adenosine, which activates P1 or adenosine receptors. There are four types of adenosine receptors (A_1, A_{2A}, A_{2B}, A_3), which are all linked to either $G_{\alpha s}$ or $G_{\alpha i}$, and two major groups of P2 receptors ($P2X_{1\text{-}7}$ and $P2Y_{1,2,4,6,11}$), which are either ligand-gated ion channels (P2X) or G protein–linked receptors (P2Y).[29] The demonstration that adenosine and its nucleotides inhibit norepinephrine release from adrenergic nerves has led to the hypothesis that purines may act as neuromodulators, regulating the release of norepinephrine through a feedback mechanism.[35] ATP can also act as a neurotransmitter or as a cotransmitter with norepinephrine and acetylcholine (Figure 5-8).

PEPTIDE TRANSMISSION AND CO-RELEASE OF NEUROTRANSMITTERS

Certain neurons release more than one neurotransmitter, such as norepinephrine with ATP. Often, co-release is automatic because both substances are found in the same storage vesicle. Simultaneous release of transmitters may also occur when they are stored separately. In recent years, it has become increasingly clear that various peptides in particular are co-released with classic ANS transmitters through both these mechanisms.

When co-release occurs, it is thought that the two substances may have slightly different functions, with one substance functioning as a neurotransmitter and the other functioning as a neuromodulator, or that they act cooperatively as transmitters to elicit some physiologic response. For example, cholinergic neurons in the cat submandibular gland contain and release vasoactive intestinal peptide, a transmitter that potentiates the salivary secretion induced by acetylcholine, possibly by enhancing the binding of acetylcholine to its receptor.[25] Similarly, neuropeptide Y enhances vasoconstriction by a direct action on the vasculature as well as by potentiating the effects of norepinephrine (see Figure 5-8).[18] The recognition of the existence of multiple peptide neurotransmitters affecting the ANS offers additional new targets for drug development.

Table • 5-2

Mechanism of Action of Representative Drugs Affecting the Autonomic Nervous System

	SITE OF ACTION	
MECHANISM OF ACTION	CHOLINERGIC JUNCTIONS	ADRENERGIC JUNCTIONS
Interfere with synthesis of transmitter	Hemicholinium	Metyrosine
Cause formation of "false" transmitter	—	Methyldopa
Prevent release of transmitter	Botulinum toxin	Guanethidine
Prevent reuptake of transmitter	—	Imipramine, cocaine
Prevent incorporation of transmitter in storage vesicles	Vesamicol	Reserpine
Cause release of transmitter	Carbachol	Tyramine, amphetamine
Activate postjunctional receptor	Muscarinic: choline esters, cholinomimetic alkaloids Nicotinic: nicotine	α_1 Receptor: phenylephrine; α_2 receptor: clonidine; β_1 and β_2 receptors: isoproterenol; β_2 receptor: albuterol
Block access of transmitter to receptor	Muscarinic: atropine Nicotinic: tubocurarine, trimethaphan	α_1 and α_2 Receptors: phentolamine; α_1 receptor: prazosin; α_2 receptor: yohimbine; β_1 and β_2 receptors: propranolol; β_1 receptor: metoprolol
Inhibit enzymatic breakdown of transmitter	Acetylcholinesterase inhibitors (physostigmine, isoflurophate)	MAO inhibitors (tranylcypromine, selegiline); COMT inhibitors (entacapone, tolcapone)

CENTRAL CONTROL OF AUTONOMIC FUNCTION

Virtually all levels of the CNS contribute significantly to the regulation of the ANS. This includes the spinal cord and brainstem, where reflexes regulating blood pressure are integrated, to the higher centers in the hypothalamus, limbic system, and cerebral cortex, which integrate highly complex autonomic responses involved in behavior, reproduction, and emotional states. Indeed, the finding that benzodiazepines reduce sympathetic responses to oral surgery (see Figure 5-3) emphasizes the role of the CNS in initiating and coordinating sympathetic responses to stress. The location of centers in the CNS that directly regulate functions such as blood pressure, respiration, micturition, and sweating are known. The ANS modulates the activity of these centers by the hypothalamus, which plays a very important role in the integration of responses to changes in temperature, emotional states, and patterns of sexual and reproductive activity, all of which involve integration of the endocrine, autonomic, and somatic nervous systems. Furthermore, the limbic system has been shown through stimulation experiments to cause changes in blood pressure, sexual activity, ragelike responses, and a host of other reactions characteristic of ANS stimulation. Thus it is believed that the limbic system plays an important role in patterns of sexual activity and states of rage and fear and that its effects may be superimposed on those exerted by the hypothalamus. The cerebellum and the cerebral cortex also make contributions to patterns of autonomic activity, but their importance is less than that of the hypothalamus (see Chapter 11).

SPECIFIC SITES AND MECHANISMS OF ACTION OF AUTONOMIC DRUGS

The foregoing discussion in this chapter has shown that neurotransmission in the ANS, and therefore normal function of the two divisions of the ANS, depends on a number of integrated steps, including synthesis of transmitter, release of transmitter, combination of the transmitter with the receptor, and destruction by highly specific enzymes or reuptake and reuse of the transmitter in the nerve terminal. The explosion of knowledge about the function of the ANS at the neuronal and molecular levels has been accompanied by the discovery and development of drugs that interfere with one or several steps in the complex processes described in the earlier sections on cholinergic and adrenergic transmission.

Some of these drugs and their specific mechanisms and sites of action are listed in Table 5-2. Their pharmacology is described in the appropriate chapters of the text. But, with a working knowledge of the ANS and the role it plays in the normal function of various organs, it is possible to predict what effects a drug with a known mechanism of action would have. For example, if a drug (e.g., reserpine) prevents norepinephrine from being transferred from the cytoplasm of the neuron into storage vesicles, it is reasonable to expect that the norepinephrine that has been taken up from the neuroeffector junction will remain in the cytoplasm. Here it will be subject to destruction by MAO, and in time (a relatively short time, in fact) the stores of norepinephrine will be reduced, leaving adrenergic nerve terminals throughout the body depleted of norepinephrine. It is now possible to predict that the depletion of norepinephrine throughout the sympathetic nervous system will place the animal under the unopposed control of the parasympathetic nervous system. Thus the pupils are constricted, postural hypotension occurs, and gastrointestinal motility and secretion are increased.

CITED REFERENCES

1. Ahlquist RP: A study of adrenotropic receptors, *Am J Physiol* 153:586-600, 1948.
2. Andersson R: Cyclic AMP as a mediator of the relaxing action of papaverine, nitroglycerine, diazoxide, and hydralazine in intestinal and vascular smooth muscle, *Acta Pharmacol Toxicol* 32:321-336, 1973.
3. Axelrod J: Purification and properties of phenylethanolamine-N-methyl-transferase, *J Biol Chem* 237:1657-1660, 1962.

4. Berlan M, Montastruc JL, Lafontan M: Pharmacological prospects for α2-adrenoreceptor antagonist therapy, *Trends Pharmacol Sci* 13:277-282, 1992.
5. Berthelsen S, Pettinger WA: A functional basis for classification of α-adrenergic receptors, *Life Sci* 21:595-606, 1977.
6. Bevan JA: Some functional consequences of variation in adrenergic synaptic cleft width and on nerve density and distribution, *Fed Proc* 36:2439-2443, 1978.
7. Birnbaumer L: G proteins in signal transduction, *Annu Rev Pharmacol Toxicol* 30:675-705, 1990.
8. Burnstock G: A basis for distinguishing two types of purinergic receptor. In Straub RW, Bolis L, eds: *Cell membrane receptors for drugs and hormones: a multidisciplinary approach*, New York, 1978, Raven Press.
9. Butcher FR: The role of calcium and cyclic nucleotides in α-amylase release from slices of rat parotid: studies with the divalent cation ionophore A-23187, *Metabolism* 24:409-418, 1975.
10. Bylund DB, Eikenberg DC, Hieble JP, et al: International Union of Pharmacology nomenclature of adrenoceptors, *Pharmacol Rev* 46:121-136, 1994.
11. Cannon WB: *Bodily changes in pain, hunger, fear, and rage,* ed 2, New York, 1929, Appleton-Century.
12. Caulfield MP, Birdsall JM: International union of pharmacology. XVII. Classification of muscarinic acetylcholine receptors, *Pharmacol Rev* 50:279-290, 1998.
13. Changeux J-P, Devillers-Thiery A, Cemouilli P: Acetylcholine receptor: an allosteric protein, *Science* 225:1335-1345, 1984.
14. DeLorenzo RJ, Freedman SD, Yohe WB, et al: Stimulation of Ca^2-dependent neurotransmitter release and presynaptic nerve terminal protein phosphorylation by calmodulin and a calmodulin-like protein isolated from synaptic vesicles, *Proc Natl Acad Sci USA* 76:1838-1842, 1979.
15. Dionne RA, Goldstein DS, Wirdzek PJ: Effects of diazepam premedication and epinephrine-containing local anesthetic on cardiovascular and plasma catecholamine responses to oral surgery, *Anesth Analg* 63:640-646, 1984.
16. Fitzgerald M: The course and termination of primary afferent fibres. In Wall P, Melzack R, eds: *Textbook of pain,* New York, 1984, Churchill Livingstone.
17. Goldberg LI, Hsieh Y-Y, Resnekov L: Newer catecholamines for treatment of heart failure and shock: an update on dopamine and a first look at dobutamine, *Prog Cardiovasc Dis* 19:327-340, 1977.
18. Han C, Abel PW: Neuropeptide Y potentiates contraction and inhibits relaxation of rabbit coronary arteries, *J Cardiovasc Pharmacol* 9:675-681, 1987.
19. Hargreaves KM, Dionne RA, Mueller GP, et al: Naloxone, fentanyl, and diazepam modify plasma β-endorphin levels during surgery, *Clin Pharmacol Ther* 40:165-171, 1986.
20. Hubbard JI, Kwanbumbumpen S: Evidence for the vesicle hypothesis, *J Physiol* (London) 194:407-420, 1968.
21. Iversen LL: Catecholamine uptake processes, *Br Med Bull* 29:130-135, 1973.
22. Kobilka B: Adrenergic receptors as models for G protein-coupled receptors, *Annu Rev Neurosci* 15:87-114, 1992.
23. Limbird LE: α_2-Adrenergic systems: models for exploring hormonal inhibition of adenylate cyclase, *Trends Pharmacol Sci* 4:135-138, 1983.
24. Lukas RJ, Changeux J-P, le Novère N, et al: International Union of Pharmacology. XX. Current status of the nomenclature for nicotinic acetylcholine receptors and their subunits, *Pharmacol Rev* 51:379-401, 1999.
25. Lundberg JM, Hedlund B, Bartfai T: Vasoactive intestinal polypeptide enhances muscarinic ligand binding in cat submandibular salivary gland, *Nature* 295:147-149, 1982.
26. Matteoli M, DeCamilli P: Molecular mechanisms in neurotransmitter release, *Curr Opinion Neurobiol* 1:91-97, 1991.
27. Mueller RA, Thoenen H, Axelrod J: Increase in tyrosine hydroxylase activity after reserpine administration, *J Pharmacol Exp Ther* 169:74-79, 1969.
28. Piascik MT, Perez DM: α_1-Adrenergic receptors: new insights and directions, *J Pharmacol Exp Ther* 298:403-410, 2001.
29. Ralevic V, Burnstock G: Receptors for purines and pyrimidines, *Pharmacol Rev* 50:413-492, 1998.
30. Randich A, Maixner W: [D-Ala2]-methionine enkephalinamide reflexively induces antinociception by activating vagal afferents, *Pharmacol Biochem Behav* 21:441-448, 1984.
31. Robitaille R, Adler EM, Charlton MP: Strategic location of calcium channels at transmitter release sites of frog neuromuscular synapses, *Neuron* 5:773-779, 1990.
32. Schramm M, Selinger Z: The functions of cyclic AMP and calcium as alternative second messengers in parotid gland and pancreas, *J Cyclic Nucleotide Res* 1:181-192, 1975.
33. Starke K: Regulation of noradrenaline release by presynaptic receptor systems, *Rev Physiol Biochem Pharmacol* 77:1-24, 1977.
34. Sutherland EW, Robison GA, Butcher RW: Some aspects of the biological role of adenosine 3′,5′-monophosphate (cyclic AMP), *Circulation* 37:279-306, 1968.
35. Todorov LD, Bjur RA, Westfall DP: Inhibitory and facilitatory effects of purines on transmitter release from sympathetic nerves, *J Pharmacol Exp Ther* 268:985-989, 1994.
36. Trimble WS, Linial M, Scheller RH: Cellular and molecular biology of the presynaptic nerve terminal, *Annu Rev Neurosci* 14:93-122, 1991.
37. Venter JC, Fraser CM: The structure of α- and β-adrenergic receptors, *Trends Pharmacol Sci* 4:256-258, 1983.
38. Watson S, Arkinstall S: *The G-protein linked receptor factsbook,* London, 1994, Academic Press.
39. Watson S, Girdlestone D: 1995 receptor and ion channel nomenclature supplement, *Trends Pharmacol Sci* 15(suppl):1-73, 1995.
40. Weiner N, Clotier G, Bjur R, et al: Modification of norepinephrine synthesis in intact tissue by drugs and during short-term adrenergic nerve stimulation, *Pharmacol Rev* 24:203-221, 1972.
41. Yuen PS, Garbers DL: Guanylyl cyclase-linked receptors, *Annu Rev Neurosci* 15:193-225, 1992.
42. Zhong H, Minneman KP: α_1-Adrenoceptor subtypes, *Eur J Pharmacol* 375:261-276, 1999.

General References

Alberts B, Johnson A, Lewis J, et al: *Molecular biology of the cell,* ed 4, New York, 2002, Garland Publishing.

Cooper JR, Bloom FE, Roth R: *The biochemical basis of neuropharmacology,* ed 7, New York, 1996, Oxford University Press.

Hoffman BB, Taylor P: Neurotransmission: the autonomic and somatic motor nervous systems. In Hardman JG, Limbird LE, Gilman AG, eds: *Goodman & Gilman's The pharmacological basis of therapeutics,* ed 10, New York, 2001, McGraw-Hill.

Kalsner S, ed: *Trends in autonomic pharmacology,* vol 2, Baltimore, 1982, Urban & Schwarzenberg.

Kandel ER, Schwartz JH, Jessell TM: *Principles of neural science,* ed 4, New York, 2000, McGraw-Hill.

Nester EJ, Hyman SE, Malenka RC: *Molecular neuropharmacology: a foundation for clinical neuroscience,* New York, 2001, McGraw-Hill.

CHAPTER • 6

Adrenergic Agonists

Peter W. Abel and Michael T. Piascik

The endogenous catecholamines norepinephrine, epinephrine, and dopamine compose an important class of neurotransmitters and hormones. By activating adrenergic receptors, these biochemicals mediate a large number of functions in the periphery and in the central nervous system (CNS). Thus these and other adrenergic agonists represent an important group of drugs with a broad spectrum of actions. These agents are also referred to as *sympathomimetic drugs* because they mimic the effects caused by stimulation of the sympathetic nervous system. There are several therapeutic uses for these compounds: as vasoconstrictors in local anesthetic solutions and for hemostasis; as decongestants in ophthalmic and nasal preparations; as vasopressor agents to maintain blood pressure in some types of shock; and as bronchodilators for asthmatic attacks and for allergic reactions, including anaphylaxis. Centrally acting adrenergic agonists are used to treat essential hypertension, narcolepsy, and attention deficit–hyperactivity disorder.

HISTORY

The first recorded study of an adrenergic agent resulted in the isolation in 1887 of ephedrine from the herb *ma huang*, which had been grown and used in China for centuries. At the same time, investigators were making extracts of all the organs of the body in an attempt to discover new hormones. Studies by Oliver and Schafer in the early 1890s demonstrated a potent vasopressor substance in extracts of the adrenal gland. The active agent, epinephrine, was soon isolated by J. J. Abel, prepared commercially, and marketed in the United States under the trade name of Adrenalin(e). By 1905, it had been synthesized and was being incorporated with local anesthetics. In fact, in that year an account was published of the results of mixing procaine with epinephrine to obtain dental anesthesia.[3] With the explosive increase in the sale of herbal products over the last few years, various plant products containing adrenergic agonists, including *ma huang*, have been used with increased frequency.

CLASSIFICATION OF ADRENERGIC DRUGS AND RECEPTORS

Since the identification of norepinephrine as the neurotransmitter at adrenergic neuroeffector junctions and of epinephrine and norepinephrine as the two adrenergic agents released by the adrenal medulla, a number of agonists with adrenergic activity have been developed. Direct-acting adrenergic agonists are those that directly bind to adrenergic receptors and activate those receptors to produce their effects. Indirect-acting agonists act by increasing the amount of norepinephrine available to stimulate adrenergic receptors. While indirect-acting agonists may act through a number of different mechanisms, their most common action is to cause the release of the neurotransmitter norepinephrine from sympathetic nerve terminals. Mixed-acting adrenergic agonists have both direct and indirect mechanisms of action. One common feature of all these drugs is that their effects are mediated through activation of adrenergic receptors.

Adrenergic receptors have been classified into three major types: α_1-, α_2-, and β-adrenergic receptors. In recent years a number of receptor subtypes (α_{1A}, α_{1B}, α_{1D}; α_{2A}, α_{2B}, α_{2C}; β_1, β_2, β_3) have been discovered by molecular cloning and pharmacologic techniques.[4,19,33,40] Several dopamine receptors have also been identified (D_1, D_2, D_3, D_4, D_5).[14,41] These receptor subtypes are distinguished by differences in their amino acid sequences as determined from gene-cloning experiments[4,41] and by their affinity for subtype-selective drugs. Many adrenergic agonists activate more than one of the major adrenergic receptor types. In contrast, some agonists selectively activate α receptors, others activate β receptors, and some are even selective for an individual adrenergic receptor subtype (e.g., β_1 or β_2). Similarly, as is discussed in Chapter 7, there are antagonists for the various adrenergic receptors, some of which are receptor type or subtype selective and some nonselective. The development of receptor-selective agonists and antagonists remains an active area of research.[30,34,37,40] Whereas most adrenergic agonists have prominent peripheral actions that form the basis for their therapeutic applications, some of these drugs have important actions in the CNS. It is certainly true that adrenergic drugs such as amphetamine and ephedrine are capable of causing stimulation of adrenergic receptors in the CNS. Several drugs have been developed, including the antihypertensive agent clonidine, that have their principal action on CNS α_2 receptors, whose stimulation results in a decrease in sympathetic outflow from the brain.

CHEMISTRY AND STRUCTURE-ACTIVITY RELATIONSHIPS

The chemical structures of the three endogenous adrenergic amines, namely dopamine, norepinephrine, and epinephrine, are illustrated in Figure 6-1. These compounds are synthesized sequentially in adrenergic nerve terminals and adrenal chromaffin cells (see Chapter 5). These three agents, all derived from tyrosine, are also referred to as *catecholamines* because they are catechol derivatives of phenylethylamine.

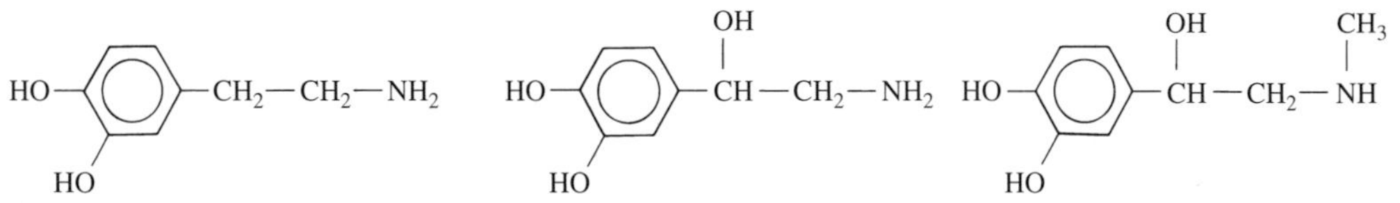

HO, HO — $CH_2—CH_2—NH_2$ HO, HO — $CH(OH)—CH_2—NH_2$ HO, HO — $CH(OH)—CH_2—NH(CH_3)$

Dopamine   **Norepinephrine**   **Epinephrine**

Fig. 6-1 Chemical structures of three naturally occurring adrenergic agonists.

Table • 6-1

Structure-Activity Relationships of Selected Adrenergic Agonists

AGONIST	RECEPTOR PREFERENCE	STRUCTURE (PHENYLETHYLAMINE NUCLEUS)			
		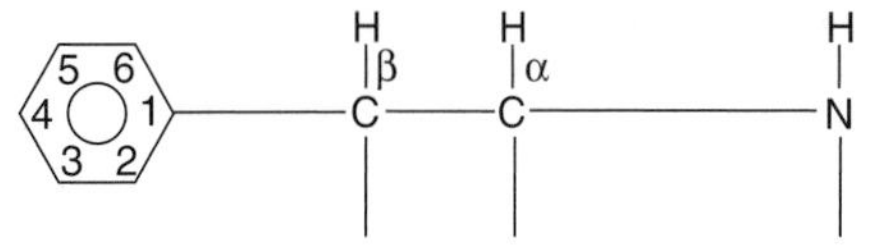 Ring (positions 1–6)	H–Cβ	H–Cα	H–N
Direct Action					
Dopamine	D*, α_1, β_1	3—OH, 4—OH	H	H	H
Dobutamine	β_1†	3—OH, 4—OH	H	H	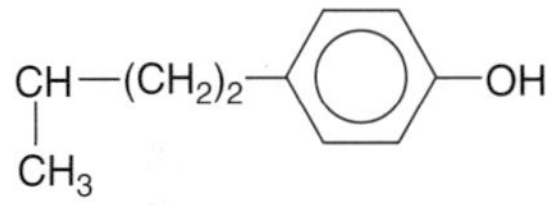 $CH(CH_3)—(CH_2)_2—C_6H_4—OH$
Norepinephrine	α, β_1	3—OH, 4—OH	OH	H	H
Levonordefrin	α_2, β_1	3—OH, 4—OH	OH	CH_3	H
Epinephrine	α, β	3—OH, 4—OH	OH	H	CH_3
Isoproterenol	β	3—OH, 4—OH	OH	H	$CH(CH_3)_2$
Metaproterenol	β_2	3—OH, 5—OH	OH	H	$CH(CH_3)_2$
Terbutaline	β_2	3—OH, 5—OH	OH	H	$C(CH_3)_3$
Albuterol	β_2	3—CH_2OH, 4—OH	OH	H	$C(CH_3)_3$
Ritodrine	β_2	— 4—OH	OH	CH_3	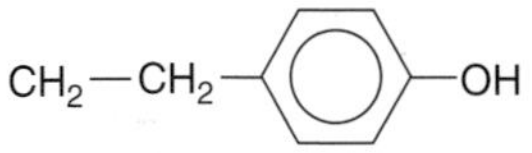 $CH_2—CH_2—C_6H_4—OH$
Isoetharine	β_2	3—OH, 4—OH	OH	CH_2CH_3	$CH(CH_3)_2$
Mainly Direct Action					
Methoxamine	α_1	2—OCH_3, 5—OCH_3	OH	CH_3	H
Phenylephrine	α_1	3—OH —	OH	H	CH_3
Mixed Action					
Ephedrine	α, α (CNS), β	— —	OH	CH_3	CH_3
Metaraminol	α, β	3—OH —	OH	CH_3	H
Mainly Indirect Action					
Tyramine	α, β	4—OH —	H	H	H
Hydroxyamphetamine	α, β	4—OH —	H	CH_3	H
Amphetamine	α, α (CNS), β	— —	H	CH_3	H
Methamphetamine	α, α (CNS), β	— —	H	CH_3	CH_3

*Dopaminergic.
†Different stereoisomers have opposing actions on α_1 receptors and β_2 receptors; thus β_1 selectivity is more apparent than real.

Table 6-1 lists some of the adrenergic agonists currently in use and illustrates certain major alterations in biologic activity that occur with structural modifications. The following conclusions about the relationship between structure and activity can be drawn:

1. Direct-acting agonists (those that bind to adrenergic receptors) generally require a hydroxyl group at positions 3 and 4 of the aromatic ring plus a hydroxyl group on the β-carbon atom of the side chain for maximal stimulation of α and β receptors. The two hydroxyl groups on the ring are believed to form hydrogen bonds with serine residues in the fifth membrane-spanning region of the receptor.[42]
2. Indirect-acting agonists (those that cause release of norepinephrine) have no β-hydroxyl group and either no or one hydroxyl group on the ring. Those agents devoid

of hydroxyl substitutions can better penetrate the blood-brain barrier and exert prominent CNS effects.

3. Mixed-acting agonists (those having both actions already described) generally have a β-hydroxyl group and a single ring hydroxyl group.
4. Dopamine, which lacks the β-carbon hydroxyl moiety present in other endogenous catecholamines, stimulates dopamine receptors in addition to α_1 and β_1 receptors. Low concentrations of systemically administered dopamine selectively stimulate D_1 receptors.
5. Slight modifications in chemical structure can confer significant differences in pharmacodynamics. For example, therapeutic agents can be designed to provide specific responses by selective action on receptor subtypes.[30] Other structural modifications yield differences in pharmacokinetics. For example, methyl substitution on the α carbon yields orally active compounds able to resist enzymatic destruction by monoamine oxidase (MAO) in the stomach and small intestine.
6. As the alkyl substitution on the nitrogen is increased in molecular weight, a shift in drug affinity toward the β_2-adrenergic receptor is observed. The affinity of norepinephrine, with no alkyl substitution, is much greater for α-adrenergic receptors than for β_2-adrenergic receptors; the affinity of epinephrine, with a methyl group, is similar for α- and β_2-adrenergic receptors; and that of isoproterenol, with an isopropyl group, is much greater for β_2 receptors than for α receptors. All three drugs have significant β_1-adrenergic receptor effects. Changes in the position of ring hydroxyl groups (to the 3 and 5 positions, or a single hydroxyl group in the 4 position) lead to compounds (e.g., terbutaline and ritodrine) with selective affinity for the β_2-adrenergic receptor.
7. Besides structural modifications, many of the compounds listed exist as optical isomers. Substitutions on either the α- or β-carbon atom of the phenylethylamine nucleus produce stereoisomeric pairs. Levorotatory substitution on the β carbon enhances adrenergic receptor effects. Dextrorotatory substitution on the α carbon increases CNS stimulant activity (e.g., *d*-amphetamine).

The catecholamine nucleus is extremely sensitive to oxidation. This chemical reaction results in the formation of a quinone, adrenochrome, which accounts for inactivation and color changes that may occur in solutions of catecholamines, such as in dental anesthetic cartridges. A sulfite salt (e.g., sodium metabisulfite) is incorporated in such solutions as an antioxidant to prevent catecholamine degradation.

PHARMACOLOGIC EFFECTS

The pharmacology of the adrenergic agonists is complicated by the diversity of the drugs in this group. They differ in mode of action (direct, indirect, or mixed), receptor selectivity, and relative predominance of their peripheral and CNS effects. Predicting the pharmacologic activity of any adrenergic agonist is possible by knowing whether it is direct acting or indirect acting and what receptors it affects. The density of the receptor population in a particular organ or organ system also influences the effectiveness of adrenergic agonists. Thus a smooth muscle with a high density of α-adrenergic receptors will be strongly contracted by a drug that is efficacious in activating α-adrenergic receptors, but another smooth muscle, expressing few or no α receptors, would be minimally or not at all affected by the same agonist. Table 6-2 summarizes the relative receptor preferences of several adrenergic drugs.

Of the many adrenergic agonists that have been isolated or synthesized and are used clinically, only a few will be considered in detail here. The discussion that follows begins with agents that are endogenous transmitters or hormones, capable of interacting with both α and β receptors, and then focuses successively on other direct-acting agonists that are more selective in receptor preference. This discussion concludes with indirect- and mixed-acting drugs that cause the release of norepinephrine as their primary mode of action. Where appropriate, additional drugs are mentioned in the sections on therapeutic applications and adverse effects.

Endogenous Catecholamines: Norepinephrine and Epinephrine

Vascular effects

The net effect of systemic administration of norepinephrine or epinephrine on the cardiovascular system depends on a variety of factors, including the route and rate of administration, the dose given, and the presence or absence of interacting drugs. When injected locally, both norepinephrine and epinephrine cause contraction of vascular smooth muscle and vasoconstriction in the surrounding tissues by stimulating α-adrenergic receptors. Systemic effects on the vasculature

Table • 6-2

Receptor Selectivity of Adrenergic Receptor Agonists

Epinephrine (1)	Epinephrine	Epinephrine	Epinephrine
Levonordefrin (3)	Levonordefrin	Levonordefrin	
Norepinephrine (10)	Norepinephrine	Norepinephrine	
		Isoproterenol	Isoproterenol (0.05)
α_1-AR	**α_2-AR**	**β_1-AR**	**β_2-AR**
Phenylephrine (20)	Oxymetazoline	Dobutamine	Albuterol
Methoxamine	Tetrahydrozoline		Terbutaline
	Brimonidine		Bitolterol
	Clonidine		Salmeterol
	Guanabenz		Ritodrine

Drugs listed in the same column as an adrenergic receptor *(AR)* activate that receptor. At low doses, the drugs below the receptors selectively activate a single receptor type. However, as the dose of these selective drugs is increased, they can also activate some of the other receptor types. Numbers in *parentheses* indicate the potency ratio of α- to β_2-receptor–mediated effects, with epinephrine having equal potency at α- and β_2-adrenergic receptors. Potency ratios are approximate only and vary with the tissue and species studied.

occurring after absorption of these catecholamines into the circulation depend on the plasma concentrations achieved and on the drugs' actions at α- and β-adrenergic receptors. With plasma concentrations attained by an intravenous infusion of 0.2 μg/kg per minute or more, the response to norepinephrine reflects stimulation of α receptors causing increased systolic and diastolic blood pressures, with a reflex bradycardia caused by activation of the baroreceptor reflex. The bradycardia occurs despite the direct stimulation of cardiac β_1 receptors by norepinephrine, which tends to increase heart rate.

Although the same infusion of epinephrine stimulates both α- and β_2-adrenergic receptors in the vasculature, the more robust α-receptor–mediated vasoconstrictor response masks the vasodilatory effect of β_2-receptor stimulation, and the net result is usually vasoconstriction, similar to that of norepinephrine. However, at low plasma concentrations, as achieved by an intravenous administration of 0.1 μg/kg per minute or less, the effect of epinephrine on α-adrenergic receptors is less, allowing the β_2-receptor vasodilator response to become manifest. Under these conditions, a fall in mean arterial blood pressure may occur, and the direct stimulant effect of epinephrine on the myocardium (tachycardia) is observed. This effect is not shared by norepinephrine because it does not stimulate β_2 receptors.

Figure 6-2 portrays the typical cardiovascular responses to the intravenous bolus injection of these catecholamines. The qualitatively different effects of high versus low doses of epinephrine on blood pressure and heart rate described above are apparent as the initially high concentration of drug declines over the course of several minutes into the low dose range.

Cardiac effects

Norepinephrine and epinephrine both stimulate β_1-adrenergic receptors located in cardiac muscle, pacemaker, and conducting tissues of the heart; β_2 receptors, also located in these tissues but in smaller numbers, contribute to the cardiac effects of epinephrine. Not only is the strength of contraction increased by β-receptor stimulation (positive inotropic effect), but the rate of force development and subsequent relaxation is accentuated, resulting in a shorter systolic interval. The spread of the excitatory action potential through the conductile tissues is also increased (positive dromotropic action). Pacemaker cells increase their firing rate (positive chronotropic effect), and automaticity is enhanced in normally quiescent muscle (latent pacemaker cells are activated).

All the effects described are effectively antagonized by β-receptor blockade. However, simulation of α_1-adrenergic receptors has been shown to enhance myocardial contraction and prolong the refractory period and has been implicated in certain ventricular arrhythmias occurring during general anesthesia.[38]

β-Adrenergic receptor stimulation increases the work of the heart, which elevates cardiac oxygen consumption. Overall, cardiac efficiency (cardiac work done relative to oxygen consumption) is diminished. The delivery of oxygen to the heart by the coronary arteries is variably affected by the relative amounts of α- and β-receptor activation produced by each adrenergic agonist (see Table 6-2) as well as by metabolic regulators of local blood flow.

Effects on nonvascular smooth muscle

The effect of adrenergic agonists on smooth muscle in the organs of the thoracic and abdominal cavities is usually

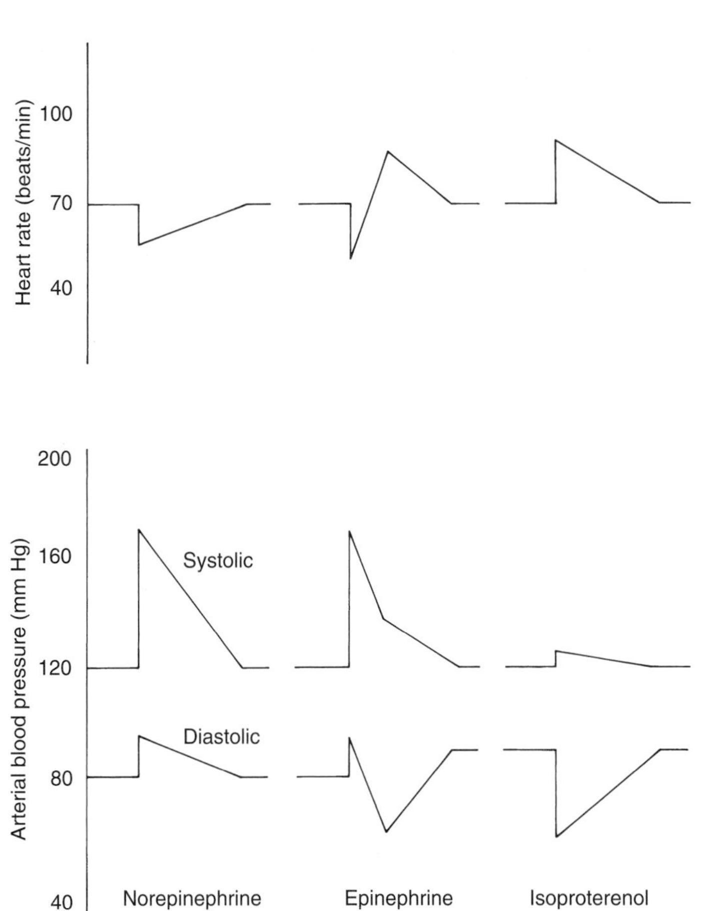

Fig. 6-2 Schematic representation of the effects of three catecholamines on heart rate and arterial blood pressure in the dog. The drugs were administered intravenously by bolus injection at a dose of 1 μg/kg. Note the biphasic effect of epinephrine. Initially the drug resembles norepinephrine by causing an increase in blood pressure and reduction in heart rate. As the concentration of epinephrine falls into the physiologic range, however, β-adrenergic receptor activation predominates. There is a fall in diastolic pressure, and direct cardiac effects are unmasked. The decreased heart rate seen with norepinephrine and at the beginning of the epinephrine response are produced indirectly by the baroreceptor reflex. The drug effects shown here last for approximately 5 minutes.

relaxation. The gastrointestinal tract shows decreased motility from activation of β_2-adrenergic receptors on smooth muscle, causing relaxation, and α_2-adrenergic receptors located on excitatory parasympathetic nerves that inhibit acetylcholine release. The sphincters are constricted through α_1-receptor stimulation. A similar situation exists for the urinary bladder. The sphincter and trigone muscles contract as a result of α_1-receptor stimulation, whereas the detrusor muscle is relaxed by β_2-receptor stimulation, causing urinary retention. The response of the uterus varies with the species, the stage of the estrous cycle, and pregnancy. Generally, α_1-adrenergic receptor activation leads to contraction, whereas β_2-receptor activation leads to relaxation. In either case, these effects require doses of epinephrine or norepinephrine that result in significant cardiovascular stimulation and are too evanescent to be useful therapeutically. However, selective β_2-adrenergic receptor agonists with longer half-lives than epinephrine are used clinically to temporarily relax the uterus.

Bronchodilation is another example of smooth muscle relaxation that is of major therapeutic importance. The β_2-adrenergic receptors of the bronchioles are stimulated by epinephrine. Whereas epinephrine is a drug of choice to counteract bronchospasm associated with hypotension, as in anaphylactic shock, β_2-receptor–selective drugs such as albuterol produce bronchodilation with less concomitant β_1-receptor stimulation of the heart and are preferred in asthmatic patients.

Epinephrine and norepinephrine stimulate α_1 receptors to cause the splenic capsule to contract, although in human beings this does not appear to play an important role in increasing the hematocrit. The pilomotor muscles of the skin contract to cause piloerection, and the radial muscle of the iris contracts to cause mydriasis in response to norepinephrine and epinephrine activation of α_1 receptors.

Effects on salivary glands

Epinephrine and norepinephrine affect secretion by salivary glands through activation of adrenergic receptors on secretory cells and by stimulation of vascular adrenergic receptors that alter blood flow to the glands. Secretory cells of the major salivary glands contain α_1-, β_1-, and some β_2-adrenergic receptors. The principal adrenergic receptor linked to protein secretion is the β_1 receptor, although α_1 receptors also play a secretory role, and some evidence supports a role for β_2 receptors, at least in some species. The primary effect of α_1-receptor stimulation on secretory cells resembles qualitatively that of muscarinic receptor stimulation in that water and electrolyte (i.e., K^+) secretion is stimulated. Salivary glands also contain myoepithelial cells, in which α_1-receptor stimulation causes contraction around secretory acinar units, contributing to secretion. β-Receptor stimulation causes a more protein-rich (e.g., amylase) secretion. Overall, the predominant characteristic of epinephrine and norepinephrine stimulation of the salivary glands is a modest secretion with a high concentration of protein.

Metabolic responses

Metabolic responses to β_2- and α_1-adrenergic receptor stimulation lead to a transitory increase in circulating blood glucose as a result of liver glycogenolysis and increased glucagon secretion.[1] An α_2-receptor–mediated inhibition of insulin secretion contributes to the hyperglycemia caused by epinephrine. Stimulation of β_1 and β_3 receptors is involved in the hydrolysis of triglycerides, causing an increase in triglyceride lipase activity and subsequently in the concentration of circulating free fatty acids. The specific receptors that mediate metabolic effects vary among species.

Central nervous system effects

Although the catecholamines are extensively involved in neurotransmission in the CNS, peripherally administered catecholamines gain little access to the CNS because hydroxyl groups on the aromatic ring deter passage across the blood-brain barrier. Intravenous injection of epinephrine does, however, produce a variety of apparently central effects, including feelings of anxiety, jitteriness, and apprehension. Most, if not all, of these effects are thought to be indirect, resulting from sensory input to the brain from the periphery. Centrally mediated reflex respiratory apnea is induced by drugs that cause an increase in blood pressure.

Dopamine

Although dopamine is primarily a CNS neurotransmitter, it also has effects in the periphery, where dopamine receptors have been identified in a variety of tissues. Molecular cloning studies have revealed at least five subtypes of the dopamine receptor (D_1 to D_5). Although the D_1 receptor subtype is thought to cause peripheral vasodilation, other dopamine receptor subtypes may also contribute to the various peripheral effects of dopamine. Peripheral dopamine-containing neurons have been found in autonomic ganglia in the form of small, intensely fluorescent cells and in kidney glomeruli. Evidence suggests that dopamine neurons help regulate sympathetic nervous system transmission, promote gastrointestinal relaxation, and cause vasodilation in some vascular beds.

Cardiovascular effects

Dopamine interacts with a variety of receptor types to influence vascular function. In low doses, dopamine produces responses caused by activation of D_1 receptors located in renal, mesenteric, and coronary blood vessels. The celiac, hepatic, and mesenteric vasculatures are dilated, resulting in increased blood flow to the abdominal organs. Low doses of dopamine also increase renal blood flow, glomerular filtration, and the excretion of Na^+.[15] Accordingly, dopamine agonists are used therapeutically for maintaining renal function in cases of shock associated with compromised cardiac output. In moderate doses, dopamine acts at myocardial β_1-adrenergic receptors to increase contractile force. In higher doses, dopamine stimulates α_1-adrenergic receptors, which produces vasoconstriction. Despite the fact that dopamine stimulates β_1 receptors, therapeutic doses do not produce a significant increase in heart rate. However, as with all catecholamines, excessive doses of dopamine can cause tachycardia and generate arrhythmias. In addition to stimulating α_1 and β_1 receptors directly, dopamine in moderate to high doses causes the release of norepinephrine from sympathetic nerve terminals.

Fenoldopam, a pharmacologic congener of dopamine, selectively activates D_1 receptors at therapeutic doses. It lowers mean blood pressure, increases renal blood flow, and causes diuresis and natriuresis. It is used intravenously for acute treatment of severe hypertension (see Chapter 28).

Other effects

Dopamine is involved with the sensory division of the autonomic nervous system. The high concentration of dopamine in the glomus cells of the carotid body and the effects of hypoxia on these cells suggest that dopamine is an inhibitory transmitter that modulates the frequency of discharge of the sensory fibers from that structure.[18] It is theorized that, by this mechanism, dopamine may affect cardiovascular and respiratory responses.

Dopamine itself does not penetrate the blood-brain barrier. However, levodopa, which is converted into dopamine, does enter the CNS and is used to treat Parkinson's disease (see Chapter 15). Approximately 95% of an oral dose of levodopa is normally decarboxylated in the periphery to dopamine,[8] leading to significant peripheral side effects attributable to dopamine. Dopamine can also produce nausea and vomiting as a result of excitation of the medullary chemoreceptor trigger zone, which lies outside the blood-brain barrier.

Another physiologic role for dopamine is modulation of the release of several anterior pituitary hormones. Dopamine acts as a prolactin release–inhibiting hormone by binding to D_2 receptors on the lactotrope cells of the anterior pituitary. Although dopamine itself is limited therapeutically by its inability to penetrate the blood-brain barrier, bromocriptine and other dopamine receptor agonists that are sufficiently lipid soluble to enter the CNS have been used successfully in the treatment of female infertility and other health problems resulting from hyperprolactinemia. Bromocriptine has also proved effective in controlling excessive secretion of growth hormone associated with pituitary adenomas. This last therapeutic application is surprising inasmuch as dopamine is a stimulant of growth hormone release in the normal pituitary.

α-Adrenergic Receptor Agonists

The group of drugs classified as α-adrenergic receptor agonists is growing increasingly diverse. These drugs stimulate α-adrenergic receptors but have low affinity for β-adrenergic receptors. Phenylephrine and methoxamine differ from epinephrine and norepinephrine by being selective agonists at α_1-adrenergic receptors. Their primary pharmacologic effect is to cause contraction of vascular smooth muscle, resulting in an increase in systolic and diastolic blood pressures and reflex bradycardia. They have no direct CNS actions. Other agonists with actions similar to phenylephrine and methoxamine include mephentermine and metaraminol, although they are mixed-acting agonists (discussed later) because they release catecholamines in addition to directly stimulating α_1-adrenergic receptors. (Mephentermine also stimulates β_2-adrenergic receptors.) Midorine is a newer synthetic drug that selectively activates α_1-adrenergic receptors. It also causes vasoconstriction and is used to treat postural hypotension caused by impaired autonomic nervous system function.

The α_2-adrenergic receptor agonists clonidine, guanabenz, guanfacine, and methyldopa (Figure 6-3) effectively enter into the CNS and stimulate α_2-adrenergic receptors in the brain. They are, in varying degrees, selective agonists at α_2 receptors. Methyldopa, an α-methyl derivative of dopa (dihydroxyphenylalanine, an important intermediate in the synthesis of norepinephrine), enters into the nerve terminal and is converted into the α_2-receptor–selective agonist α-methylnorepinephrine by the same synthetic process that converts dopa into norepinephrine. Although α-methylnorepinephrine is then present in neuronal storage vesicles in peripheral sympathetic nerves, this metabolite of methyldopa is nearly equipotent to norepinephrine as a vasoconstrictor in human beings. In fact, this agent has been developed as the drug levonordefrin, which is used as a vasoconstrictor in local anesthetic solutions. Because it is not metabolized by MAO, it has a longer duration of action than does norepinephrine. Clonidine was first used as a nasal decongestant, but it was soon found to lower blood pressure. An imidazoline derivative, clonidine is a selective α_2-adrenergic receptor agonist with relatively weak peripheral effects. Guanabenz and guanfacine are guanidine derivatives that, like clonidine, also selectively activate α_2-adrenergic receptors.

These centrally acting agonists are thought to exert their antihypertensive effect by acting on α_2 receptors in the nucleus tractus solitarius of the brainstem, leading to a decrease in sympathetic outflow. This proposed mechanism of action is supported by experiments involving the stereotactic administration of α_2-receptor agonists into the nucleus tractus solitarius followed by inhibition of drug effects by α-receptor antagonists injected into the cerebrospinal fluid. Blocking the conversion of methyldopa to α-methylnorepinephrine prevents the antihypertensive action of this drug.

The administration of these centrally acting drugs in human beings results in moderate decreases in the mean arterial blood pressure. This effect usually occurs without increases in heart rate, because a decrease in CNS sympathetic outflow tends to reduce venous return, heart rate, and cardiac output. Guanfacine, for instance, decreases peripheral vascular resistance without affecting cardiac output.[17] Intravenous administration of these drugs may actually increase blood pressure acutely as a result of stimulation of peripheral vasoconstrictor α_2 receptors. This effect is not usually seen with oral administration.

Serendipity has played a role in the use of clonidine to treat the withdrawal symptoms of opioid addiction.[27] Clonidine, when given to addicts undergoing withdrawal, blocks the nausea, vomiting, sweating, diarrhea, and other symptoms of excessive autonomic discharge (see Chapter 51). Evidence indicates that either systemic or intracerebral injection of opioids inhibits neuronal activity in the locus ceruleus of the dorsolateral pons. When the opioids are withdrawn, certain neurons are thought to be disinhibited and release excessive norepinephrine, which gives rise to the symptoms of withdrawal. Clonidine, by stimulating presynaptic α_2 receptors on these same neurons, causes inhibition of neurotransmitter release. The current clinical practice is to follow abrupt withdrawal of the opioid with oral administration of clonidine for

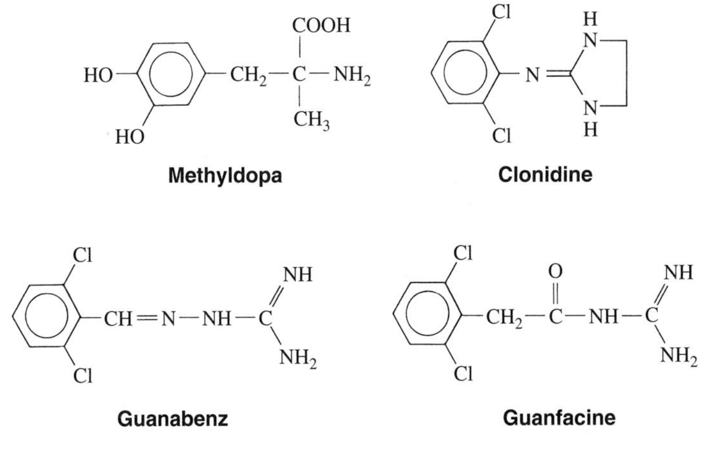

Methyldopa

Clonidine

Guanabenz

Guanfacine

Fig. 6-3 Structural formulas of some centrally acting α_2-adrenergic receptor agonists.

2 weeks or until opioid detoxification is complete. Similarly, patients with alcohol abuse problems, certain neurologic diseases, or some forms of psychotic illness show some improvement in their condition with clonidine. Other studies have found that clonidine has analgesic and sedative effects when given alone or in combination with opioids, and clonidine has been used as an adjunct in general anesthesia and for treating some patients with chronic pain. Dexmedetomidine is the first α_2 agonist specifically developed as a sedative for patients receiving intensive care (see Chapter 18).

Oxymetazoline is also an imidazoline derivative selective for α_{2A} receptors, causing contraction of smooth muscle in certain blood vessels. It is used as a nasal decongestant. Other imidazoline agonists available for the same therapeutic indication include tetrahydrozoline, xylometazoline, and naphazoline. Brimonidine and apraclonidine are newer α_2-receptor agonists that are used to lower intraocular pressure in patients with glaucoma.

β-Adrenergic Receptor Agonists: Isoproterenol

Isoproterenol, a synthetic catecholamine, is a potent nonselective β-receptor agonist. It does not appreciably distinguish among the β_1-, β_2-, and β_3-receptor subtypes but has very low affinity for α-adrenergic receptors and thus has no significant effect resulting from α-receptor stimulation.

Cardiac and vascular effects

The actions of isoproterenol on the cardiovascular system are based solely on the stimulation of β-adrenergic receptors (see Figure 6-2). It causes a marked fall in diastolic blood pressure from β_2-receptor–mediated vasodilation, primarily caused by relaxation of blood vessels in skeletal muscle, with some additional vasodilation in the renal and mesenteric vascular beds. There is also an increase in systolic blood pressure largely resulting from the increase in cardiac output caused by β_1-receptor stimulation of contractility. Because of the effects on systolic (slight increase) and diastolic (decrease) pressures, the mean arterial blood pressure is only modestly affected. Heart rate is increased by the stimulation of β_1 receptors in pacemaker cells. The drug's ability to increase excitability and conduction velocity in the heart may induce palpitation and arrhythmias. The powerful inotropic and chronotropic actions may increase myocardial oxygen demand sufficiently to cause ischemia.

Effects on bronchial smooth muscle

As an agonist of β_2-adrenergic receptors, isoproterenol relaxes bronchial smooth muscle in the lungs to relieve and/or prevent bronchoconstriction. Disadvantages of the use of isoproterenol for relief of bronchospastic disorders that limit its clinical use are its nonselectivity for β-adrenergic receptor subtypes, which can result in β_1-receptor–induced tachycardia, palpitation, and arrhythmias, and the development of tolerance and even refractoriness with frequent use.[36] The introduction of selective β_2-receptor agonists has provided an important alternative class of drugs for bronchodilation. It must be remembered, however, that even though the β_2-receptor–selective drugs will have weaker cardiac effects than isoproterenol, they still have the potential to cause cardiac acceleration and tachyarrhythmias.

Metabolic and other effects

Although the β-receptor agonist activity of isoproterenol stimulates glycogenolysis and gluconeogenesis in the liver, it is not as effective as epinephrine in elevating plasma glucose. Isoproterenol stimulates the secretion of a saliva that is rich in amylase and other proteins. The drug is also capable of causing CNS excitation at doses higher than are conventionally used clinically.

Dobutamine

A synthetic analogue of dopamine, dobutamine acts as an adrenergic receptor agonist with little or no effect on dopamine receptors.[31] The two stereoisomers of the racemic drug preparation have different effects on the various adrenergic receptor types, which together account for β_1- and α_1-receptor stimulation and α_1-receptor inhibition. The primary action of dobutamine is to increase myocardial contractility and cardiac output without significantly raising the heart rate. The inotropic effect results primarily from direct β_1-receptor stimulation in the heart, with lesser contributions from β_2-receptor activation. Peripheral vascular resistance is usually changed very little. However, because blood pressure effects of this drug are a function of the combination of α_1- and β_2-receptor activation and α_1-receptor blockade, some patients may show a greater pressor effect, whereas others may experience a moderate reduction in ventricular filling pressure and peripheral vascular resistance. Dobutamine is used for short-term treatment of acute myocardial insufficiency resulting from congestive heart failure, myocardial infarction, or cardiac surgery.[28]

Selective β_2-Adrenergic Receptor Agonists

Although isoproterenol and epinephrine are capable of relaxing bronchial smooth muscle, both drugs (especially isoproterenol) can also cause dangerous tachycardia and arrhythmias. These side effects limit the therapeutic use of these drugs and stimulated a search for selective agonists capable of stimulating β_2-adrenergic receptors in bronchial and uterine smooth muscle, while having less effect on the β_1 receptors of the heart. However, even with the selective β_2-receptor agonists, especially at higher doses, effects on the heart are substantial. Metaproterenol, terbutaline, albuterol, isoetharine, bitolterol, pirbuterol, and salmeterol are relatively selective β_2-receptor agonists that are effective in decreasing airway resistance without causing as much cardiac acceleration as does isoproterenol. These drugs are usually inhaled; however, oral administration of metaproterenol, albuterol, and terbutaline may be useful under certain limited conditions. Systemic adverse effects are usually greater by the oral route. Bitolterol, an inactive prodrug, is inhaled and is converted in the lung to colterol, which is a selective β_2-receptor agonist. Ritodrine, another selective β_2-receptor agonist, is used as a uterine relaxant in the short-term management of preterm labor. The drug is initially given intravenously, followed in some cases by oral dosing. The use of β_2 agonists in the therapy of bronchospastic disorders is discussed in Chapter 32.

Mixed- and Indirect-Acting Adrenergic Agonists

A number of adrenergic agonist drugs produce some or all of their effects by causing the release of norepinephrine from adrenergic nerve terminals. They do so by being transported into the adrenergic nerve ending or adrenal chromaffin cells, where they are then transported into the storage vesicles. These drugs displace catecholamines from their vesicular storage sites into a cytoplasmic pool in the nerve endings or chromaffin cells, from which norepinephrine or epinephrine is then released. This cytoplasmic pool is distinct from that of the storage vesicles from which release occurs during nerve stimulation. Thus these drugs have a pharmacologic profile similar to that of norepinephrine. Differences that do exist are associated with the relative ability of the various drugs to stimulate α or β receptors directly and with the ease by which these agents gain access to the CNS. In contrast to norepinephrine, these drugs are generally not subject to rapid inactivation and are usually effective by the oral route.

Ephedrine is an example of an orally active, mixed-acting drug. In addition to releasing norepinephrine, ephedrine is a direct α- and β-receptor agonist. Thus it can cause bronchodilation, vasoconstriction, increased heart rate, and modest CNS stimulation. Amphetamine, a more lipophilic drug, is primarily a purely indirect-acting drug that easily enters the brain and stimulates the release of catecholamines in the CNS. Amphetamine is a potent CNS stimulant that causes a number of effects, including increased alertness, relief of fatigue, enhanced athletic performance, and euphoria. Although a person taking amphetamine may work more rapidly, there is a disproportionate increase in mistakes. Furthermore, the need for sleep can only be delayed with amphetamine, not diminished. Drugs related to amphetamine include dextroamphetamine and methamphetamine. Compared with amphetamine, both tend to have more effects on the CNS relative to the periphery. The addition of a single hydroxyl group (4-OH) to yield hydroxyamphetamine produces a drug with less CNS activity.

Acute tolerance (tachyphylaxis) is a common outcome of repeated administration of indirect-acting adrenergic drugs. Multiple doses of either mixed- or indirect-acting adrenergic agonists may lead to a depletion of the neurotransmitter, resulting in a reduction or loss of activity in response to nerve stimulation. These drugs are also susceptible as a class to several drug interactions. Compounds such as the tricyclic antidepressants and some adrenergic neuron–blocking drugs interfere competitively with the uptake of indirect-acting agonists into adrenergic nerve terminals and therefore block their subsequent release of norepinephrine. MAO inhibitors, on the other hand, promote the accumulation of intraneuronal catecholamines, which are released by these agonists. The combination of an MAO inhibitor and an indirect-acting or mixed-acting sympathomimetic drug typically results in excessive release of catecholamines with serious consequences. Some indirect-acting compounds, such as tyramine, occur naturally in several foods and beverages and therefore pose a great risk to patients taking MAO inhibitors.

ABSORPTION, FATE, AND EXCRETION

As noted in the section on chemistry and structure-activity relationships, the route for administering adrenergic agonists is determined by the chemical structure. All catecholamines and certain other drugs, unless specifically modified at the α carbon of the side chain, are subject to enzymatic destruction in the gastrointestinal tract. Catecholamines are usually administered systemically by parenteral injection or intravenous infusion. Topical instillation and inhalation are the preferred routes of administration for ocular and respiratory applications, respectively.

The inactivation and metabolic disposal of catecholamines can involve many processes, as illustrated by the fate of endogenous norepinephrine (Figure 6-4). After neuronal release, a large portion (up to 80% in some cases) of the adrenergic neurotransmitter is returned to the nerve terminal by an active neuronal uptake process. What remains in the junctional cleft is subjected to O-methylation by catechol-O-methyltransferase (COMT) after uptake by postjunctional effector cells. Norepinephrine that diffuses out of the junction may be taken up by other cells and metabolized by COMT. Once the transmitter is O-methylated to normetanephrine, it can no longer be transported into the adrenergic nerve terminal but is instead carried by the blood to the liver, where it is largely deaminated by hepatic MAO.[11] Some portion of the released neurotransmitter also diffuses away from the junctional cleft to enter the circulation intact.

Of the norepinephrine that is actively transported back into the neuron, a large part is actively returned to the storage vesicles from which it can again be released upon neuronal stimulation. A smaller portion is deaminated by MAO located in the outer membrane of the mitochondria to form 3,4-dihydroxyphenylglycoaldehyde. Most of the aldehyde is converted to an acid, the remainder to a glycol. Both metabolites enter the circulation and are eventually O-methylated by COMT. The major metabolic products of norepinephrine resulting from the combined action of MAO and COMT are 3-methoxy-4-hydroxymandelic acid, also referred to as *vanillylmandelic acid,* and 3-methoxy-4-hydroxyphenylethylene glycol. About 90% of the total endogenous norepinephrine load excreted in the urine is in the form of vanillylmandelic acid and 3-methoxy-4-hydroxyphenylethylene glycol, with the remainder consisting of other O-methylated compounds and lesser quantities of other derivatives and unmetabolized norepinephrine.[26] Variable amounts of these products may be

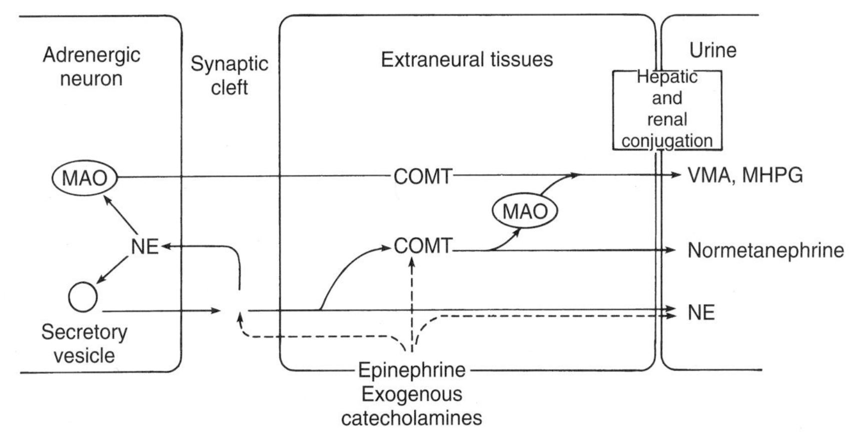

Fig. 6-4 Biotransformation and excretion of catecholamines. After release, up to 80% of norepinephrine *(NE)* is taken up by a reuptake process into the nerve terminal, where most is recycled into storage vesicles and some is metabolized by mitochondrial *MAO*. Extraneuronal effector tissues metabolize catecholamines through MAO and catechol-O-methyl transferase *(COMT)*. Excreted substances include the metabolites 3-methoxy-4-hydroxymandelic acid *(VMA)*, 3-methoxy-4-hydroxyphenylethylene glycol *(MHPG)*, as well as normetanephrine, NE, and related glucuronide and sulfate conjugates. Epinephrine and some other adrenergic agonists are also biotransformed and excreted by some of these same pathways.

conjugated as the glucuronide or sulfate before being excreted by the kidney.

Exogenously administered catecholamines and endogenous dopamine and epinephrine are transported and metabolized in much the same manner as norepinephrine. Nevertheless, there are some differences. The metabolic inactivation of epinephrine and most injected catecholamines (including norepinephrine) largely depends on COMT because COMT is widely distributed throughout the body, and the administration of exogenous catecholamines allows them to be distributed far beyond the adrenergic neuroeffector junctions. The relative shift toward COMT for the initial enzymatic attack ensures the recovery of high concentrations of O-methylated derivatives in the urine. In patients with a pheochromocytoma, a relatively large percentage of catecholamines released by the adrenal medulla is recovered unmetabolized in the urine. As with norepinephrine and epinephrine, dopamine is a substrate for both MAO and COMT. The metabolite formed by the combined action of these enzymes is homovanillic acid. In contrast to the other endogenous catecholamines, dopamine, when given by intravenous infusion, is significantly potentiated by MAO inhibitors.

A small percentage of epinephrine injected as a vasoconstrictor during local anesthesia will ultimately reside in the patient's adrenergic nerve terminals and be released during sympathetic nerve stimulation.[13] Similarly, a small amount of administered dopamine may be converted to norepinephrine by β hydroxylation in the adrenergic nerve terminal.

Noncatecholamines are not subject to metabolism by COMT and typically have durations of action significantly longer than the catecholamines. The centrally acting α_2-receptor agonists are all given orally and are eliminated largely as unchanged drug (e.g., clonidine), are extensively metabolized (e.g., guanabenz), or are partly metabolized and partly excreted as the parent compound (e.g., guanfacine, methyldopa). Several of the selective β_2-receptor agonists are excreted in the urine as conjugates of sulfate or glucuronic acid.

The indirect-acting adrenergic agonists, which act by displacing the neurotransmitter norepinephrine from the cytoplasmic pool, must first enter the neuron to evoke this release. While in the cytoplasm, these compounds may be subjected to deamination by MAO and other enzymes. A small amount of tyramine in the neuron is oxidized at the β carbon to form octopamine. Octopamine, which has only weak adrenergic activity, can, in turn, be transported into the storage vesicles, where it may act as a false transmitter.[25] Other avenues for the metabolism of these noncatecholamines include *p*-hydroxylation, N-demethylation, deamination, conjugation in the liver and kidney, or a combination of all these. Amphetamine and ephedrine, which are resistant to the actions of MAO (also found in abundance in the gastrointestinal tract), can be administered orally.

GENERAL THERAPEUTIC USES

Clinical applications of the adrenergic agonists can be divided into eight major categories: local vasoconstriction, vasoconstriction in the treatment of hypotension and shock, bronchodilation, relaxation of uterine smooth muscle, ophthalmic uses, relief of allergic states (including anaphylaxis), CNS stimulation, and control of hypertension. The choice of a specific drug for each of these uses depends on the relative contribution of α- and/or β-adrenergic receptors or dopamine receptors to the response in these tissues as well as the drug's receptor subtype selectivity. Other factors that determine the choice of a drug include the therapeutic effect versus adverse effects profile as well as pharmacokinetic factors such as the rate and routes of absorption, duration of action, and metabolic fate. Most of the commercially available adrenergic agonists are marketed as water-soluble salts. The following section examines all of these therapeutic uses, indicating in each case one or more preferred drugs.

Local Vasoconstriction

Various drops, sprays, aerosols, and even oral dosage forms of several adrenergic agonists have proved useful in providing temporary symptomatic relief of nasal congestion associated with a variety of causes. These compounds are agonists at α receptors (α_1 or α_2, or both) and have minimal CNS-stimulant effects. Common examples include phenylephrine, pseudoephedrine, and oxymetazoline.

An adverse effect associated with the local administration of nasal decongestants is rebound congestion, a chronic swelling of the nasal mucous membranes after the effect of the drugs wears off. This response is more likely with the longer-acting α_2-receptor–selective nasal decongestants that have the imidazoline structure. Overdose, with systemic effects, is frequently manifested by signs of excessive adrenergic stimulation. Imidazoline derivatives, such as tetrahydrozoline and oxymetazoline, can paradoxically produce drowsiness, comatose sleep with hypotension, and bradycardia. These effects are thought to be caused by the entry of the drugs into the CNS, where they stimulate central α_2-adrenergic receptors. Children and infants are especially prone to these adverse effects.

Decongestants have also been used to constrict dilated conjunctival vessels and to relieve itching in hyperemic (bloodshot) eyes. Such agents include naphazoline and tetrahydrozoline. Sometimes these drugs are mixed with other agents used to treat disorders of the conjunctiva or corneal epithelium.

Adrenergic agonists are often used to produce hemostasis for surgery and to enhance local anesthesia. Whether applied topically or administered by injection with or without a local anesthetic, adrenergic agonists can, in certain situations, significantly improve visibility in the operative field. Because vasoconstriction is temporary, however, the use of these drugs is no substitute for the adequate surgical control of bleeding. Furthermore, adrenergic agonists must often be used with special caution during general anesthesia because certain inhalation anesthetics (e.g., halothane) predispose the heart to the arrhythmogenic action of the adrenergic agonists.[12,22] Finally, the injection of vasoconstrictors into appendages supplied by end arteries is commonly listed as an absolute contraindication. Failure to heed this admonition has been reported to cause tissue necrosis and gangrene of the fingers, toes, ears, and penis. However, a recent study found that epinephrine with lidocaine produced no adverse sequelae when administered for local anesthesia of the digits.[46] Employment of vasoconstrictors for surgical hemostasis and as adjuvants for local anesthetics is discussed later in the section on dental uses.

Treatment of Hypotension and Shock

Shock is a condition caused by inadequate tissue perfusion. It is usually associated with a fall in arterial blood pressure and, if not treated, may quickly lead to multiorgan system failure. Shock has a number of causes, including hemorrhage; fluid losses from diarrhea or third-degree burns; internal fluid derangements from sepsis or anaphylaxis; disruption of autonomic tone as a result of drugs or spinal damage; and inadequate cardiac output because of myocardial infarction, arrhythmia, mechanical defects, or outflow obstruction. In most cases of hypotension, baroreceptor reflex–mediated sympathetic stimulation occurs, causing tachycardia, peripheral vasoconstriction, dyspnea, excessive sweating, and mental disturbances.

Treatment of shock includes specific therapies aimed at reversing the underlying problem and nonspecific measures to sustain an effective circulation. If hypotension is the result of blood or fluid loss (hypovolemic shock), the intravascular volume should be restored with blood and/or other intravenous fluids. Additional specific treatments include antibiotics for sepsis, surgery to correct reparable myocardial defects, and antidotes to reverse the effects of drug overdose. Lastly, adrenergic agonists may prove useful in restoring blood pressure and in correcting the distribution of blood flow, especially to the vital organs, whenever shock develops under normovolemic conditions.

The pharmacologic management of shock has three general goals: (1) constriction of capacitance vessels to reduce venous pooling, (2) dilation of resistance vessels to increase perfusion of vital organs, and (3) improvement of myocardial contractility to increase cardiac output. Adrenergic agonists are used to treat various conditions associated with hypotension. α-Adrenergic receptor agonists (e.g., methoxamine and phenylephrine), which increase blood pressure by causing vasoconstriction, are most useful during episodes of inadequate sympathetic nervous system function that may result from spinal anesthesia or hypotensive drug overdose. However, such drugs are less beneficial in other shock states associated with hypotension because they may impair blood flow to the kidneys and mesenteric organs.

In cardiogenic shock, which is most often caused by acute myocardial infarction, the β_1-adrenergic receptor agonists should be useful, but unfortunately the improvement in tissue perfusion and coronary blood flow is often accompanied by increased myocardial oxygen demand. Thus a drug such as isoproterenol, which typically causes tachycardia, may actually worsen the myocardial ischemia and predispose an already damaged heart to arrhythmias. Dopamine is therefore often used for initial therapy of cardiogenic shock because it causes less generalized vasodilation than typical β-receptor agonists and, through stimulation of dopamine receptors, may improve renal and mesenteric perfusion.[15,35] The ability to increase contractile force without a concomitant increase in heart rate is an additional advantage of dopamine. It also has use in certain other types of shock, such as septic shock. Dobutamine, like dopamine, can increase the force of myocardial contraction without producing changes in heart rate and thus is also used in patients with heart failure.

Bronchodilation

Acute and chronic obstructive pulmonary diseases are marked by increased inspiratory and expiratory resistance, and the adrenergic agonists have historically played an important role in the relief of these conditions. Epinephrine or isoproterenol, given by spray or aerosol, promptly relieves constricted bronchial passageways. However, the β_1-receptor stimulation by these drugs is associated with cardiac palpitation and arrhythmias that severely limit their usefulness. Epinephrine also causes an undesired drying effect because of decreased secretions.

Currently, the adrenergic agents most useful in the treatment of bronchospastic disease are agonists with selectivity for β_2-adrenergic receptors, because they produce marked bronchodilation with less effect on the heart than do nonselective β-receptor agonists. The selective β_2-receptor agonists used for bronchodilation include isoetharine (least selective), metaproterenol, terbutaline, albuterol, bitolterol, pirbuterol, salmeterol, and formoterol. Salmeterol and formoterol have durations of action of up to 24 hours.[39] This extended duration can be of significant benefit in treating those with asthma.[36] For instance, the shorter-acting drugs are used to reverse acute bronchoconstriction, whereas salmeterol and formoterol are used prophylactically to prevent bronchoconstriction. See Chapter 32 for a more complete discussion of the use of these agents in bronchial asthma.

Uterine Relaxation

Selective β_2-adrenergic receptor agonists are administered to arrest premature labor by relaxing uterine smooth muscle. Drugs that control premature labor are often termed *tocolytics*. Ritodrine is used almost exclusively to cause uterine relaxation. Terbutaline and other β_2-receptor–selective agonists have also been used as tocolytic drugs. Unfortunately, these drugs are effective in relaxing the uterus for only a few days. Stimulation of β receptors in the heart can cause palpitation and arrhythmias, which limit the usefulness of these drugs.

Ophthalmic Uses

The two major ocular indications for adrenergic agonists are for the production of mild mydriasis and the reduction of intraocular pressure. The former is mediated by stimulation of α_1-adrenergic receptors in the radial muscle of the eye. Although muscarinic receptor antagonists such as atropine produce a much stronger pupillary dilation, adrenergic agonists are useful because they cause mydriasis without paralyzing the ciliary muscle (cycloplegia). Even greater mydriasis can be obtained if a combination of a muscarinic receptor–blocking drug and an adrenergic agonist drug is used. Phenylephrine and hydroxyamphetamine are the principal adrenergic agonists used to produce mydriasis.

The mechanisms for the reduction in intraocular pressure by adrenergic agonist drugs are not well elucidated, but several of these drugs appear to reduce the production and enhance the outflow of aqueous humor and are useful in treating wide-angle glaucoma. These drugs include the nonselective adrenergic agents epinephrine and dipivefrin (a prodrug of epinephrine), and the α_2-adrenergic receptor–selective agonists apraclonidine and brimonidine. A discussion of the treatment of glaucoma is presented in Chapter 8.

Treatment of Allergic States

Adrenergic agonists, especially epinephrine, are especially useful in reversing the effects of histamine and other mediators associated with allergic reactions. Unlike the antihistamines, adrenergic agonists are physiologic antagonists, producing responses opposite to the acute effects produced by histamine and associated autacoids. For acute allergic reactions such as urticaria, subcutaneous injection of 0.3 to 0.5 ml of 1 : 1000 epinephrine should be adequate. Fulminating disturbances such as anaphylactic shock require a faster absorption of epinephrine than provided by subcutaneous injection, especially if circulation is impaired. Intramuscular (intralingual) injection of 0.4 to 0.6 ml of 1 : 1000 epinephrine or, if the patient has previously been prepared for intravenous injections, slow intravenous administration of 1 : 10,000 epinephrine is recommended. With this latter route of administration, there is a considerable risk of precipitating serious cardiac arrhythmias and ventricular fibrillation. Because of the rapid metabolism of epinephrine, reinjection at intervals of 5 to 15 minutes may be required. Subcutaneous administration generally provides the longest duration of action, and intravenous injection provides the shortest.

Central Nervous System Stimulation

For many years, selected adrenergic agonists have been used clinically because of their ability to produce stimulation of certain functions of the CNS that result in increased alertness and attention span and decreased sense of fatigue. Another potentially therapeutic effect of these agents is stimulation of the lateral hypothalamus and satiation of the food drive. The principal sympathomimetic drugs that cross the blood-brain barrier are ephedrine, amphetamines, mephentermine, and methylphenidate. Because of the history of abuse of amphetaminelike drugs, their procurement and use are strictly controlled by various state and federal statutes.

A major accepted use of amphetamine and related drugs is for the management of children with attention deficit–hyperactivity disorder. The use of CNS stimulants, along with psychotherapy and family counseling, has provided remarkable relief from the restlessness, brief attention span, and impulsiveness that mark this disorder. Methylphenidate has been used most often for the pharmacologic treatment of attention deficit–hyperactivity disorder. Unfortunately, it has a relatively brief duration of action (3 to 5 hours), requiring a second dose which often must be administered by teachers or day-care providers. Alternative agents that have gained wider use in recent years include extended duration formulations of methylphenidate or the combination of amphetamine and dextroamphetamine.[16] Another clinical use of adrenergic CNS stimulants is for the treatment of narcolepsy, a disorder characterized by uncontrollable attacks of sleep in the daytime. Modafinil, a nonadrenergic CNS stimulant, is an alternative therapy with a different adverse effects profile (e.g., higher incidence of headache, less cardiovascular stimulation).

A clinical application that has drawn considerable attention is the pharmacologic suppression of hunger in short-term adjuvant therapy in weight loss programs. Among the drugs that produce anorexia are the amphetamines, diethylpropion, phentermine, and ephedrine. Some states restrict the use of amphetamines for weight loss because these drugs have a relatively high potential for abuse. Ephedrine is not approved for weight loss but is a common component of oral herbal products *(ephedra, ma huang)* and dietary supplements that have been promoted to increase energy and decrease weight. In its first formal action against an herbal remedy, the Food and Drug Administration recently banned the use of ephedra alkaloids, including ephedrine, in these products.

A limitation to the therapeutic use of these classic sympathomimetic anorexic drugs is that they also produce undesired effects, including CNS stimulation, insomnia, anxiety, nervousness, gastrointestinal disturbances, cardiovascular stimulation, and the development of psychologic dependence. These drugs are also generally without long-term benefit if not accompanied by stringent caloric restrictions. In fact, they are often taken to make a rigid diet seem more acceptable. They are contraindicated in patients taking MAO inhibitors and those with hypertension, cardiac arrhythmias, thyrotoxicosis, or other severe cardiovascular disease.

Treatment of Hypertension

As mentioned earlier and discussed in Chapter 28, four centrally acting α_2-adrenergic receptor selective agonists are used for the treatment of hypertension: clonidine, guanabenz, guanfacine, and methyldopa. They act on central α_2 receptors that are involved in the autonomic regulation of the cardiovascular system. Activation of inhibitory neurons in the brain causes peripheral vasodilation by inhibiting sympathetic outflow from the CNS and decreasing cardiac output through enhanced vagal tone and decreased sympathetic tone. In general, these drugs do not reduce sympathetic tone as much as do peripherally acting inhibitors of the sympathetic nervous system or its receptors (see Chapter 7).

THERAPEUTIC USES IN DENTISTRY

Vasoconstrictors are widely used in conjunction with local anesthetic solutions. The vasoconstrictor most commonly used in dentistry is *l*-epinephrine, with levonordefrin (the *l* isomer of nordefrin) being used less frequently, usually with mepivacaine.

Table 6-3 lists the concentrations and amounts of adrenergic vasoconstrictors contained in commercially available dental local anesthetic cartridges. The concentration listed for levonordefrin is considered approximately equivalent in clinical effectiveness to 1:100,000 epinephrine, as judged by prolongation of dental anesthesia. The maximum recommended strength of the vasoconstrictor is 1:100,000 epinephrine equivalency for routine nerve block anesthesia. When local tissue hemostasis is required for surgical procedures, such as periodontal surgery, the dentist may additionally choose to infiltrate the area with local anesthetic solution containing up to 1:50,000 epinephrine, but repeated injections of 2% lidocaine with 1:50,000 epinephrine may cause tissue necrosis and microscarring.[2]

Vasoconstrictors serve several useful purposes when used with local anesthetic solutions. First, they prolong the duration of local anesthesia severalfold and may improve the frequency of successful nerve block.[23] Table 6-4 illustrates the effect of vasoconstrictors on duration of local anesthesia. Second, toxicity of the local anesthetic may be minimized by delaying and reducing the peak blood concentration of the anesthetic agent.[7] Third, when anesthetic solutions are given by infiltration, vasoconstrictors tend to reduce blood loss associated with surgical procedures (see Chapter 16).

Local anesthesia with vasoconstrictors has been implicated, however, with ischemic conditions of the pulp and alveolar bone, the latter being associated with an increased incidence of osteitis after extractions.[5] Furthermore, local tissue damage at the site of injection is related to or accentuated by the presence of vasoconstrictor adrenergic agonists.

An important issue related to potential toxicity is the systemic effects of vasoconstrictors after intraoral injection. A related question often faced by the dentist is whether to administer a vasoconstrictor-containing local anesthetic solution to a patient with cardiovascular disease. A traditional opinion held that vasoconstrictors contained in dental anesthetic cartridges produced little, if any, clinically significant systemic effects. Some older reports recommend that cardiac patients be given local anesthetics with vasoconstrictors if needed for adequate anesthesia because the benefits of satisfactory pain control were greater than the risks of small amounts of vasoconstrictor.[32] The validity of this statement depends on the level of stress on the patient and the amount, rate, and manner in which the epinephrine-containing solution is injected.

In the last three decades, numerous well-controlled studies have shown that even the small amounts of vasoconstrictor used in dentistry significantly increase resting plasma catecholamine concentrations and alter some measures of

Table 6-3

Concentrations and Amounts of Adrenergic Vasoconstrictors in Dental Local Anesthetic Cartridges

VASOCONSTRICTOR	DILUTION	AMOUNT PER DENTAL CARTRIDGE (μg/1.8 ml)
Epinephrine hydrochloride	1:200,000	9
Epinephrine hydrochloride	1:100,000	18
Epinephrine hydrochloride	1:50,000	36
Levonordefrin hydrochloride	1:20,000	90

cardiac function (e.g., increase stroke volume).[20,24,29,43] As illustrated in Figure 6-5, intraoral injection of lidocaine with 1:100,000 epinephrine for removal of impacted third molars resulted in significantly increased circulating epinephrine compared with patients injected with a local anesthetic without vasoconstrictor.[44] Although large therapeutic dosages were used in this study, injection of even a single cartridge of local anesthetic with 1:100,000 epinephrine can result in a temporary doubling of the plasma epinephrine concentration.[47] It is often assumed that the amount of epinephrine released from the adrenal medulla during acute stress greatly exceeds that contained in local anesthetic cartridges. However, with clinically achievable doses, as shown in Figure 6-5, the stress-induced increase in epinephrine concentration in the "no epinephrine" group was only a small fraction (approximately 14%) of that obtained after intraoral injection of lidocaine with 1:100,000 epinephrine.

With these developments in mind, a joint report of the American Heart Association and American Dental Association concluded that "vasoconstrictor agents should be used in local anesthesia solutions during dental practice only when it is clear that the procedure will be shortened or the analgesia

Table • 6-4

Effect of Epinephrine on the Duration of Local Anesthesia

LOCAL ANESTHETIC	VASOCONSTRICTOR	DURATION MEAN (min)	DURATION MAXIMUM (min)
Lidocaine 2%	None	44	100
Lidocaine 2%	Epinephrine 1:1,000,000	57	130
Lidocaine 2%	Epinephrine 1:750,000	67	145
Lidocaine 2%	Epinephrine 1:250,000	90	175
Lidocaine 2%	Epinephrine 1:50,000	88	210

Data were obtained by oral surgeons from patients undergoing exodontia. The mean and maximum duration of anesthesia was judged by luxation of the tooth and by the use of probes for soft tissue effects. All injections were inferior alveolar nerve blocks; 24 patients were included in each group.
Adapted from Keesling GG, Hinds EC: Optimal concentrations of epinephrine in lidocaine solutions, *J Am Dent Assoc* 66:337-340, 1963.

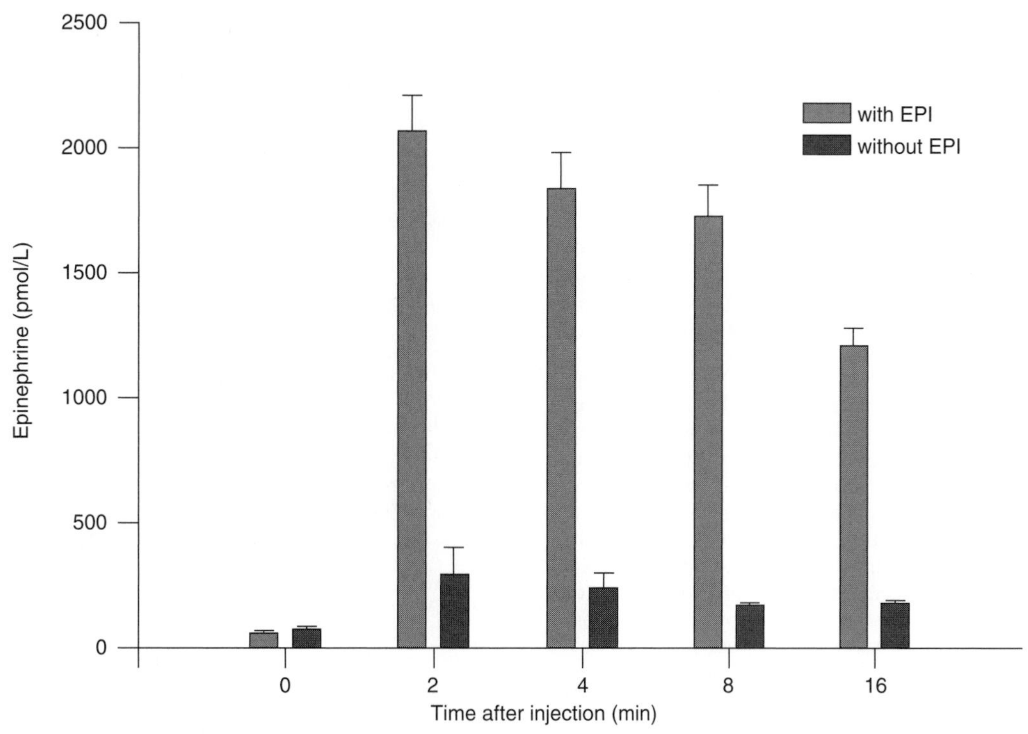

Fig. 6-5 Effect of intraoral local anesthetic injections on plasma epinephrine. Unsedated oral surgery patients ($n = 26$) were injected with either 14.4 ml of 2% lidocaine with 1:100,000 epinephrine (*with EPI,* 144 μg epinephrine total dose) or 3% mepivacaine without vasoconstrictor (*without EPI*) under randomized, double-blind conditions. *Brackets* indicate the standard error. (Adapted from Troullos ES, Hargreaves KM, Goldstein DS, et al: Epinephrine suppresses stress-induced increases in plasma immunoreactive β-endorphin in humans, *J Clin Endocrinol Metab* 69:546-551, 1989.)

rendered more profound," that "extreme care should be taken to avoid intravascular injection," and that "the minimum possible amount of vasoconstrictor should be used."[21] More recent reports support this recommendation (see General References). Moreover, an alternative is available; effective local anesthetic preparations without vasoconstrictor agents (e.g., 3% mepivacaine) have been shown to provide clinically effective local anesthesia, especially for nerve block procedures (see Chapter 16).

It is often necessary to produce gingival retraction for operative procedures on teeth and for making impressions. Besides astringents such as zinc and aluminum salts, cotton cord impregnated with racemic (both *d* and *l* isomers) epinephrine, containing up to 1.0 mg of drug per inch of cord, is commercially available. Racemic epinephrine has approximately half the potency of *l*-epinephrine because *d*-epinephrine has approximately one fifteenth the activity of *l*-epinephrine.

Whether these large amounts of epinephrine present a hazard to the normal patient as well as to patients with cardiovascular disease depends on several factors. Both experimental and clinical studies indicate a relatively high absorption of the vasoconstrictor if the epithelium is abraded or the vasculature is exposed, which is common in extensive restorative procedures. Systemic absorption is marked by signs of anxiety, elevated blood pressure, increased heart rate, and occasional arrhythmias. These effects can be extremely serious in a patient with cardiovascular disease or in one who is taking medication that reduces the uptake or otherwise enhances the activity of adrenergic agents. Because of this concern, epinephrine-impregnated retraction cord is used much less often than other types of retraction cord.

Various products are available to control capillary bleeding occurring with surgical procedures on gingival tissues. Epinephrine hydrochloride (1 : 1000) and phenylephrine (1 : 100) are most common. More concentrated solutions have occasionally been advocated, but their use can only heighten the risk of cardiovascular problems without producing any significant increased effectiveness in reducing hemorrhage.

ADVERSE EFFECTS

Almost all adverse effects of the adrenergic agonists are dose related. Toxic reactions can result from the administration of too large a dose, accidental intravascular injection, impaired uptake of the drug, a heightened sensitivity or number of adrenergic receptors, or therapeutic doses given to a patient with preexisting cardiovascular disease. Relatively small amounts of epinephrine can cause potentially grave effects in the highly susceptible patient. In general, however, serious complications may be expected with doses of epinephrine greater than 0.5 mg, and fatalities are likely to occur with doses of 4 mg or more, although one patient is reported to have survived an injection of 30 mg.[45] Correct dosage calculations, careful reading of labels, and a complete medical history can help reduce accidents. Reviews of the literature indicate that reported adverse reactions attributable to vasoconstrictors used with local anesthetics in dentistry are rare.[6,45]

Most serious of the toxic effects of epinephrine are cardiac disturbances, with increased stimulation of the heart leading to myocardial ischemia, possibly heart attack, and arrhythmias, including ventricular fibrillation. Patients with a history of uncontrolled hyperthyroidism, hypertension, or angina pectoris are particularly susceptible. If epinephrine is administered to a patient who is taking a nonselective β-adrenergic receptor blocking drug such as propranolol (see Chapter 7), unopposed α-receptor stimulation may cause excessive vasoconstriction. The increase in blood pressure from rapid parenteral administration can be severe enough to result in hypertensive crisis, which can cause cardiac disturbances or a cerebrovascular accident.[10] Drugs with primarily α-adrenergic receptor stimulation can cause excessive vasoconstriction in overdose. Local tissue necrosis may result from any vasoconstrictor injected into a region where ischemia is likely, such as the digits of the hands or feet.

CNS reactions to classic sympathomimetic drugs include nervousness, excitability, insomnia, dizziness, and tremors. Long-term use of amphetamines can lead to psychotic symptoms. The most common side effects of the centrally acting α_2-agonist antihypertensive agents are dizziness, drowsiness, and xerostomia. The xerostomia appears to be most severe with clonidine and guanabenz. Constipation, sexual dysfunction, CNS disturbances, bradycardia, and excessive hypotension have also been reported. A particularly troubling adverse effect is rebound hypertension of serious proportions if these drugs are withdrawn abruptly.

Unique to methyldopa is the occurrence of drug-induced hepatitis, with a fever that may reach alarming levels (105° F). Withdrawal of the drug usually allows liver function to return to normal. This reaction has been shown to be related to the transformation of methyldopa to reactive compounds that combine covalently with cellular macromolecules.[9] Other adverse effects of methyldopa include parkinsonian signs, hyperprolactinemia, and hemolytic anemia.

Adrenergic Agonists

Nonproprietary (generic) name	*Proprietary (trade) name*
Ophthalmic products	
Mydriatics	
Hydroxyamphetamine	Paredrine
Phenylephrine	Neo-Synephrine
Decongestants	
Naphazoline	Naphcon
Phenylephrine	Neo-Synephrine
Tetrahydrozoline	Visine
Antiglaucoma agents (see Chapter 8)	
Respiratory tract products	
Nasal decongestants	
Ephedrine	Pretz-D
Epinephrine	Adrenalin
Naphazoline	Privine
Oxymetazoline	Afrin
Phenylephrine	Neo-Synephrine
Propylhexedrine	Benzedrex
Pseudoephedrine	Sudafed
Tetrahydrozoline	Tyzine
Xylometazoline	Otrivin
Cold remedies	
These preparations consist of antihistamines, analgesics, cough suppressants, other drugs, and one of the following adrenergic agonists:	

Nonproprietary (generic) name	*Proprietary (trade) name*
Phenylephrine	In Dristan Multi-Symptom Nasal Decongestant
Pseudoephedrine	In Sudafed Multi-Symptom Cold & Cough
Bronchodilators	
Albuterol	Proventil, Ventolin, in Combivent
Bitolterol	Tornalate
Ephedrine	Primatene Tablets
Epinephrine	Adrenalin
Ethylnorepinephrine	Bronkephrine
Formoterol	Foradil
Isoetharine	Bronkosol
Isoproterenol	Isuprel
Levalbuterol	Xopenex
Metaproterenol	Alupent
Pirbuterol	Maxair
Salmeterol	Serevent
Terbutaline	Brethine, Bricanyl
Cardiovascular system products	
Vasoconstrictors and cardiac stimulants	
Dobutamine	Dobutrex
Dopamine	Intropin
Ephedrine	—
Epinephrine	Adrenalin
Isoproterenol	Isuprel
Levonordefrin	Neo-Cobefrin
Mephentermine	Wyamine
Metaraminol	Aramine
Methoxamine	Vasoxyl
Midodrine	ProAmatine
Norepinephrine	Levophed
Phenylephrine	Neo-Synephrine
Antihypertensive agents	
Clonidine	Catapres
Fenoldopam	Corlopam
Guanabenz	Wytensin
Guanfacine	Tenex
Methyldopa	Aldomet
Methyldopate	—
CNS stimulants and anorexiants	
Amphetamine	In Adderall
Benzphetamine	Didrex
Dexmethylphenidate	Focalin
Dextroamphetamine	Dexadrine, in Adderall
Diethylpropion	Tenuate
Methamphetamine	Desoxyn
Methylphenidate	Methylin, Ritalin
Pemoline	Cylert
Phendimetrazine	Bontril, Plegine
Phentermine	Adipex-P, Fastin
Sibutramine	Meridia
Miscellaneous products	
Ritodrine	Yutopar

CITED REFERENCES

1. Arnold A, McAuliff JP, Colella DF, et al: The β_2-receptor mediated glycogenolytic responses to catecholamines in the dog, *Arch Int Pharmacodyn Ther* 176:451-457, 1968.
2. Benoit PW: Microscarring in skeletal muscle after repeated exposures to lidocaine with epinephrine, *J Oral Surg* 36:530-533, 1978.
3. Braun H: Über einige neue örtliche Änasthetica (Stovain, Alypin, Novacain), *Deutsche Med Wochens* 31:1667-1671, 1905.
4. Bylund DB, Eikenberg DC, Hieble JP, et al: International Union of Pharmacology nomenclature of adrenoceptors, *Pharmacol Rev* 46:121-136, 1994.
5. Calhoun NR: Dry socket and other postoperative complications, *Dent Clin North Am* 15:337-348, 1971.
6. Campbell RL: Cardiovascular effects of epinephrine overdose: case report, *Anesth Prog* 24:190-193, 1977.
7. Cannell H, Walters H, Beckett AH, et al: Circulating levels of lignocaine after perioral injections, *Br Dent J* 138: 87-93, 1975.
8. Drugs used in extrapyramidal movement disorders, *Drug evaluations annual 1995,* Chicago, 1995, American Medical Association.
9. Dybing E, Nelson SD, Mitchell JR, et al: Oxidation of α-methyldopa and other catechols by cytochrome P-450-generated superoxide anion: possible mechanism of methyldopa hepatitis, *Mol Pharmacol* 12:911-920, 1976.
10. Foster CA, Aston SJ: Propranolol-epinephrine interaction: a potential disaster, *Plast Reconstr Surg* 72:74-78, 1983.
11. Fuller RW, Roush BW: Substrate-selective and tissue-selective inhibition of monoamine oxidase, *Arch Int Pharmacodyn Ther* 198:270-276, 1972.
12. Funakoshi Y, Iwai S, Kaneda H, et al: Hemodynamic effects of locally applied epinephrine used with various general anesthetic techniques, *J Oral Surg* 35:713-718, 1977.
13. Gerke DC, Ahrns B, Frewin DB, et al: The effect of local anaesthetics on the neural uptake of catecholamines in isolated arteries—a histochemical study, *Aust J Exp Biol Med Sci* 54:601-604, 1976.
14. Gingrich JA, Caron MG: Recent advances in the molecular biology of dopamine receptors, *Annu Rev Neurosci* 16:299-321, 1993.
15. Goldberg LI, Kohli JD: Peripheral dopamine receptors: classification based on potency series and specific antagonism, *Trends Pharmacol Sci* 4:64-66, 1983.
16. Greenhill LL: Pharmacologic treatment of attention deficit hyperactivity disorder, *Psychiatr Clin North Am* 15:1-27, 1992.
17. Guanfacine for hypertension, *Med Lett Drugs Ther* 29: 49-50, 1987.
18. Hanbauer I: Regulation of tyrosine hydroxylase in carotid body, *Adv Biochem Psychopharmacol* 16:275-280, 1977.
19. Hieble JP, Bylund DB, Clarke DE, et al: International Union of Pharmacology. X. Recommendation for nomenclature of α_1-adrenoceptors: consensus update, *Pharmacol Rev* 47:267-270, 1995.
20. Jastak JT, Yagiela JA: Vasoconstrictors and local anesthesia: a review and rationale for use, *J Am Dent Assoc* 107:623-630, 1983.
21. Kaplan EL, ed: *Cardiovascular disease in dental practice,* Dallas, 1986, American Heart Association.

22. Katz RL, Epstein RA: The interaction of anesthetic agents and adrenergic drugs to produce cardiac arrhythmias, *Anesthesiology* 29:763-784, 1968.
23. Keesling GR, Hinds EC: Optimal concentration of epinephrine in lidocaine solutions, *J Am Dent Assoc* 66:337-340, 1963.
24. Knoll-Köhler E, Frie A, Becker J, et al: Changes in plasma epinephrine concentration after dental infiltration anesthesia with different doses of epinephrine, *J Dent Res* 68:1098-1101, 1989.
25. Kopin IJ: Monoamine oxidase and catecholamine metabolism, *J Neural Transm Suppl* 41:57-67, 1994.
26. Kopin IJ: Catecholamine metabolism: basic aspects and clinical significance, *Pharmacol Rev* 37:333-364, 1985.
27. Lal H, Fielding S: Clonidine in the treatment of narcotic addiction, *Trends Pharmacol Sci* 4:70-71, 1983.
28. Leier CV: Current status of non-digitalis positive inotropic drugs, *Am J Cardiol* 69:120G-129G, 1992.
29. Lipp M, Dick W, Daublander M, et al: Exogenous and endogenous plasma levels of epinephrine during dental treatment under local anesthesia, *Reg Anesth* 18:6-12, 1993.
30. Lomasney JW, Cotecchia S, Lefkowitz RT, et al: Molecular biology of α-adrenergic receptors: implications for further classification and structure-function relationships, *Biochem Biophys Acta* 1095:127-139, 1991.
31. Malta E, McPherson GA, Raper C: Selective β_1-adrenoceptor agonists—fact or fiction? *Trends Pharmacol Sci* 6:400-403, 1985.
32. Management of dental problems in patients with cardiovascular disease, Council on Dental Therapeutics, American Dental Association and American Heart Association joint report, *J Am Dent Assoc* 68:333-342, 1964.
33. Michel MC, Kenny B, Schwinn DA: Classification of α_1-adrenoceptor subtypes, *Naunyn Schmiedebergs Arch Pharmacol* 352:1-10, 1995.
34. Minneman KP, Theroux TL, Hollinger S, et al: Selectivity of agonists for cloned α_1-adrenergic receptor subtypes, *Mol Pharmacol* 46:929-936, 1994.
35. Murphy MB, Elliott WJ: Dopamine and dopamine receptor agonists in cardiovascular therapy, *Crit Care Med* 18:S14-S18, 1990.
36. Nelson HS: β-Adrenergic bronchodilators, *N Engl J Med* 333:499-507, 1995.
37. Piascik MT, Perez DM: α_1-Adrenergic receptors: new insights and directions, *J Pharmacol Exp Ther* 298: 403-410, 2001.
38. Priori SG, Napolitano C, Schwartz PJ: Cardiac receptor activation and arrhythmogenesis, *Eur Heart J* 14(suppl E):20-26, 1993.
39. Rabe KF, Jorres R, Nowark D, et al: Comparison of the effects of salmeterol and formoterol on airway tone and responsiveness over 24 hours in bronchial asthma, *Am Rev Respir Dis* 147:1436-1441, 1993.
40. Ruffolo RR, Jr, Nichols AJ, Stadel JM, et al: Pharmacologic and therapeutic applications of α_2-adrenoceptor subtypes, *Annu Rev Pharmacol Toxicol* 33:243-279, 1993.
41. Sibley DR, Monsma FJ, Jr: Molecular biology of dopamine receptors, *Trends Pharmacol Sci* 13:61-69, 1992.
42. Strader CD, Candetore MR, Hill WS, et al: Identification of two serine residues involved in agonist activation of the β-adrenergic receptor, *J Biol Chem* 264:13572-13578, 1989.
43. Trollops ES, Goldstein DS, Hargreaves KM, et al: Plasma epinephrine levels and cardiovascular response to high administered doses of epinephrine contained in local anesthesia, *Anesth Prog* 34:10-13, 1987.
44. Troullos ES, Hargreaves KM, Goldstein DS, et al: Epinephrine suppresses stress-induced increases in plasma immunoreactive β-endorphin in humans, *J Clin Endocrinol Metab* 69:546-551, 1989.
45. Verrill PJ: Adverse reactions to local anaesthetics and vasoconstrictor drugs, *Practitioner* 214:380-387, 1975.
46. Wilhelmi BJ, Blackwell SJ, Miller JH, et al: Do not use epinephrine in digital blocks: myth or truth? *Plast Reconstr Surg* 107:393-397, 2001.
47. Yagiela JA: Local anesthetics, *Anesth Prog* 38:128-141, 1991.

General References

Cardiovascular effects of epinephrine in hypertensive dental patients. *Summary, Evidence Report/Technology Assessment: Number 48. AHRQ Publication Number 02-E005*, Rockville, MD, 2002, Agency for Healthcare Research and Quality, http://www.ahrq.gov/clinic/epcsums/ephypsum.htm.

Cooper JR, Bloom FE, Roth RH: *The biochemical basis of neuropharmacology*, ed 8, New York, 2003, Oxford University Press.

Jowett NI, Cabot LB: Patients with cardiac disease: considerations for the dental practitioner, *Br Dent J* 189:297-302, 2000.

Nestler EJ, Hyman SE, Malenka RC: *Molecular neuropharmacology: a foundation for clinical neuroscience*, New York, 2001, McGraw-Hill.

Ruffolo RR, Jr, Hieble JP: Alpha-adrenoceptors, *Pharmacol Ther* 61:1-64, 1994.

Wong J: Adjuncts to local anesthesia: separating fact from fiction, *J Can Dent Assoc* 67:391-397, 2001.

CHAPTER • 7

Adrenergic Blocking Drugs

Michael T. Piascik and Peter W. Abel

Our understanding of the mechanisms of transmission in the sympathetic nervous system has increased significantly as a result of a better understanding of the actions of drugs, an increased appreciation of receptors and the second messenger pathways used by them, and extensive investigation of important diseases such as congestive heart failure, coronary artery disease, and hypertension. The consequence of this work has been the development of a large number of new pharmacologic agents possessing increasingly selective mechanisms of action. Chapter 5 includes a discussion of the theoretical mechanisms by which drugs produce effects on the autonomic nervous system (see Table 5-3). The drugs presented in this chapter all interfere with sympathetic nervous system transmission. Despite having diverse mechanisms of action, these drugs are collectively referred to as *adrenergic blocking drugs* or *sympatholytics.* Most but not all adrenergic blocking drugs are competitive antagonists of either α- or β-adrenergic receptors (adrenoceptors). As a result, these agents block the actions of the endogenous neurotransmitters epinephrine and norepinephrine as well as exogenously administered adrenergic agonists and therefore are also called *adrenergic receptor blockers.* In addition, several agents are known collectively as *adrenergic neuron–blocking drugs.* They act on nerve terminals to produce their sympatholytic effects. A third group of agents with sympatholytic activity includes drugs that are actually agonists at α_2-adrenergic receptors in key brain nuclei controlling cardiovascular function (see Chapter 6). These drugs reduce blood pressure by decreasing the outflow of sympathetic nervous system transmission to cardiovascular effectors.

HISTORY

Evidence that drugs could be used to antagonize the actions of other pharmacologic agents was obtained shortly after the isolation and synthesis of epinephrine. In 1906, Dale and associates noticed that certain alkaloids isolated from ergot, produced by a fungus disease of rye grain, blocked the ability of epinephrine to increase systemic arterial blood pressure.[9] Indeed, after an injection of ergotoxine (a mixture of ergot alkaloids), a hypotensive effect was observed in response to epinephrine treatment; it was aptly named by Dale the "epinephrine reversal" response.[9] These early studies also provided the first example of selective antagonism by showing that ergot derivatives were capable of blocking some, but not all, of the actions of epinephrine. This idea of selective antagonism remains an important aspect of drug development and use.

The pioneering work of Ahlquist[1] in defining the α- and β-adrenergic receptors provided the framework necessary to classify more systematically antagonists of sympathetic nervous system function. Nickerson and Goodman reported in 1947 the development of dibenamine, an agent capable of irreversibly blocking the α-adrenergic receptor, which inhibited certain responses to exogenous epinephrine and to adrenergic nerve stimulation.[20] Selective blockade of α-adrenergic receptors by ergotoxine also explained the epinephrine reversal described by Dale.[9] Phentolamine and related imidazolines were early examples of nonselective, competitive antagonists at α-adrenergic receptors. Selective antagonists of both the α_1- and α_2-adrenergic receptors have now been developed. Dichloroisoproterenol was the first β-adrenergic receptor blocker developed. The first clinically useful β blocker introduced was propranolol, which blocks both β_1- and β_2-adrenergic receptors. Selective β_1 antagonists were then discovered. We now know that there are at least nine adrenergic receptors (α_{1A}, α_{1B}, α_{1D}, α_{2A}, α_{2B}, α_{2C}, β_1, β_2, and β_3). Increasingly selective antagonists against each of these receptors are being developed with the goal of obtaining drugs capable of specifically interfering with the receptor involved in a pathophysiologic condition without blockade of other receptors that could lead to unwanted side effects.

In addition to effects on adrenergic receptors, it was found that sympathetic nervous system transmission could also be altered by actions directly on the nerve terminal. The drug bretylium, for example, interferes with the release of norepinephrine in response to nerve stimulation.[4] Other drugs were also developed that interfere with neuronal function at the level of the nerve terminal. Reserpine, for example, depletes the norepinephrine stored in these nerve terminals.[5] However, these adrenergic neuron–blocking drugs are not as effective as the selective receptor antagonists and are associated with many more unpleasant side effects.

NONSELECTIVE α-ADRENERGIC RECEPTOR ANTAGONISTS

The nonselective α-adrenergic receptor blocking drugs prevent the action of adrenergic transmitters and sympathomimetic agonists at all α-adrenergic receptors. Although a fairly large number of drugs exhibit some α-blocking activity, only the imidazolines and haloalkylamines are classified and used clinically as nonselective α-adrenoceptor antagonists. As discussed in Chapter 5, α_1-adrenergic receptors are located predominantly on the postjunctional membranes of glands and smooth muscle. The α_1-adrenergic receptors associated with smooth muscle of both arteries and veins play an important role in promoting vasoconstriction and in the regulation of systemic arterial blood pressure and blood flow. α_1-Adrenergic receptors are also important in regulating the tone of nonvascular smooth muscle, such as in the neck of the urinary bladder and capsule of the prostate. The α_2-adrenergic receptors are found on the prejunctional neuronal membrane, where they play an autoregulatory role in inhibiting norepinephrine release. They are also located postjunctionally on the membranes of pancreatic islet cells, smooth muscle, and blood platelets.[16]

Imidazolines

Analogues of the imidazoline adrenergic amines were among the first synthetic adrenergic blocking agents to be identified. Phentolamine is the only compound from this class that is still clinically available. It is a competitive antagonist at both α_1- and α_2-adrenergic receptors. It also evokes histamine release, acts as a cholinomimetic, and blocks 5-hydroxytryptamine (serotonin, 5-HT) receptors. Therapeutically, doses sufficient to achieve adrenergic blockade produce side effects attributable to these other actions.

A complication can arise from the relatively nonselective nature of phentolamine. By blocking prejunctional α_2 receptors, it interferes with the negative feedback mechanism (autoregulation) that normally limits the amount of norepinephrine released. Lack of autoregulation leads to excessive transmitter release, which may produce a significant degree of cardiac acceleration.[26,28]

Currently, phentolamine has very limited therapeutic applications. It has been used to control acute episodes of hypertension during anesthesia and in the preoperative and intraoperative management of patients with pheochromocytoma. It has also been used in clonidine withdrawal and in the treatment of hypertensive crises resulting from the interaction of monoamine oxidase (MAO) inhibitors and sympathomimetic amines.

β-Haloalkylamines

Phenoxybenzamine (Figure 7-1) is the only currently used member of this class of drugs. It is a potent noncompetitive antagonist at α_1- and α_2-adrenergic receptors. Phenoxybenzamine initially binds reversibly to the receptors and then undergoes a chemical reaction that allows the drug to become covalently bound. The initial binding is governed by the same chemical binding forces described in Chapter 1. During the development of the blockade, the presence of an agonist, or even a competitive α-blocking drug, will decrease the blocking activity of phenoxybenzamine by competing for the α-adrenergic receptors. However, once the block has developed completely, usually in approximately an hour, no agonist can successfully compete for the receptor because phenoxybenzamine will have formed a stable covalent bond with the receptor. This stage of the block is referred to as *irreversible* or *nonequilibrium* and has a half-life of about 24 hours, with effects persisting for several days. Like phentolamine, phenoxybenzamine is nonselective and therefore blocks the prejunctional α_2 receptors responsible for regulating the release of norepinephrine. Its adverse effects are largely predicated on its long-lasting, insurmountable blockade of α receptors. However, in high doses, phenoxybenzamine also inhibits responses to histamine, acetylcholine, and 5-HT and blocks transporter systems responsible for the tissue uptake of norepinephrine.

It was originally hoped that phenoxybenzamine would prove to be a useful antihypertensive. Unfortunately, many nonspecific effects and troublesome side effects have significantly restricted its therapeutic application. Phenoxybenzamine is used in the long-term therapy of pheochromocytoma in preparation for surgery or in patients who are judged to be unsuited for surgery. On rare occasions it has been used to relax the bladder sphincter of patients with motor paralysis of the bladder or obstruction caused by prostatic hyperplasia.

Most of the adverse effects of phenoxybenzamine are shared by other α-receptor antagonists; however, they are often more intense and prolonged with phenoxybenzamine because of the irreversible nature of the receptor block. The lowering of blood pressure caused by blockade of postjunctional α_1 and α_2 receptors, coupled with the inhibition of regulatory prejunctional α_2 receptors and possibly norepinephrine reuptake, results in prominent compensatory reflex activity, especially increased cardiac excitability, contractility, rate, and output. Orthostatic hypotension commonly results from the loss of control over the capacitance vessels (veins); exaggerated sensitivity to hypovolemia and the hypotensive influences of other drugs is also a common outcome. Symptoms of tachycardia, dizziness, headache, and syncope are all typical. Abdominal distress and diarrhea caused by uncompensated parasympathetic activity are added problems, as are the minor irritants of nasal stuffiness and miosis. In addition, inhibition of ejaculation has made compliance among male patients extremely poor. It is not surprising that the symptoms of therapy with phenoxybenzamine can seem worse than those of the disease this drug is used to treat.

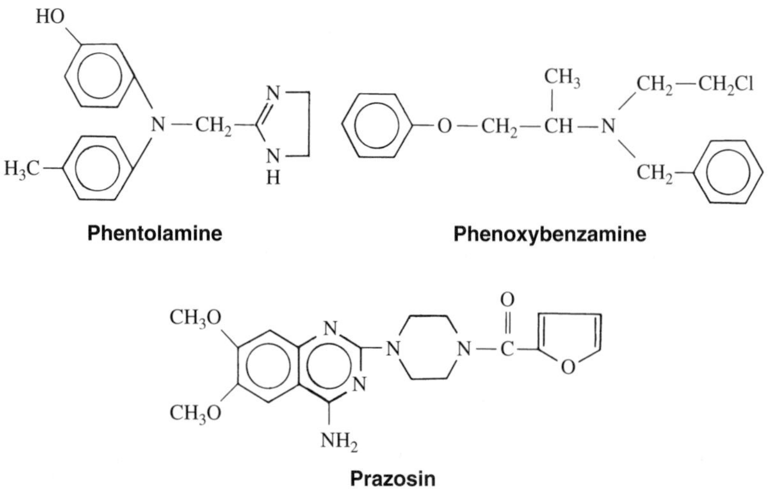

Phentolamine

Phenoxybenzamine

Prazosin

Fig. 7-1 Structural formulas of three α-adrenergic receptor–blocking agents. Prazosin is selective for α_1 receptors.

SELECTIVE α_1-ADRENERGIC RECEPTOR ANTAGONISTS

Prazosin and Analogues

Drugs such as phenoxybenzamine and phentolamine, the first antagonists of the α_1-adrenergic receptor, were not suitable as antihypertensive agents, presumably because they also block the α_2-adrenergic receptor. The disadvantages associated with the nonselective blockade of α receptors inspired a search for agents with receptor selectivity.

The first therapeutically useful α_1-adrenergic receptor blocker developed was prazosin (see Figure 7-1).[3,18] Terazosin and doxazosin are structural analogues that were subsequently introduced. Although these agents differ in pharmacokinetic properties, their mechanism of action is the same. The α_1-adrenergic receptor antagonists prevent the action of sympathetic neurotransmitters and exogenously administered agonists at α_1-adrenergic receptors on effector organs. Prazosin and related compounds have essentially equal affinity for all three subtypes (α_{1A}, α_{1B}, and α_{1D}) of the α_1-adrenergic receptor.

As a result of blocking smooth muscle α_1-adrenergic receptors, prazosin dilates both arterioles and veins. Each of these actions contributes to the hypotension seen with this drug. Blockade of arterial smooth muscle produces hypotension by reducing peripheral resistance. The venodilation resulting from blocked venous α_1-adrenergic receptors decreases cardiac preload. Compared with the nonselective α-receptor antagonists, prazosin causes less tachycardia, a smaller increase in cardiac output, and less renin release.[3]

Absorption, fate, and excretion

Prazosin is variably absorbed, with 40% to 70% of an oral dose becoming systemically bioavailable. A large percentage of circulating drug in the plasma is bound to α_1-acid glycoprotein. The plasma half-life is approximately 2 to 3 hours, requiring dosing two to three times per day. Most of the drug is demethylated and conjugated in the liver. Some prazosin metabolites are pharmacologically active and contribute to its therapeutic effect. Metabolites are excreted in the bile.

Terazosin is almost completely absorbed after oral administration and thus has a higher bioavailability than prazosin. It is also highly bound to plasma proteins. With a half-life of approximately 12 hours, the drug can be administered once a day. It is extensively metabolized in the liver, with both active and inactive metabolites formed. Approximately 60% of the drug is eliminated in the bile and 40% in the urine.

The systemic bioavailability of doxazosin is between 60% and 70% after oral administration. Like the other members of this class of compounds, doxazosin circulates highly bound to plasma proteins, is extensively metabolized, and is excreted in the bile and urine. Its half-life ranges from 10 to 20 hours, giving it an extended duration of action.

Therapeutic uses

Prazosin, terazosin, and doxazosin can be used in monotherapy for the treatment of hypertension (see Chapter 28). Terazosin and doxazosin, which are given once a day, may have advantages over prazosin, which requires administration at least twice daily. Otherwise, the clinical effects of terazosin and doxazosin are similar to those of prazosin. Although prazosin and analogues can alleviate the signs and symptoms of congestive heart failure (because of a reduction in preload and afterload), they have not been shown to increase survival in patients with congestive heart failure.[19,22] These drugs do not have adverse effects on lipids or cholesterol and may be particularly useful in treating patients with hyperlipidemia.[7,17] Prazosin and its analogues are also effective in treating benign prostatic hyperplasia caused by the blocking of the α_1-adrenergic receptors associated with smooth muscle of the bladder neck and prostate. This action reduces the pressure on the urethra and improves urine flow. Terazosin and doxazosin, because of their longer plasma half-lives, may be preferred over prazosin for this indication.[7,17]

Adverse effects

Prazosin and related α_1-adrenergic receptor antagonists may cause a so-called "first-dose" effect, characterized by orthostatic hypotension and syncope within 30 to 90 minutes of the first dose. The reason for this effect is not clear, but a short-lived central inhibition of sympathetic tone may be a contributing factor. Therapy with prazosin should be instituted initially with small doses, followed by a gradual dosage increase over time. Prazosin may cause fluid retention and edema; thus it may be necessary to give a diuretic simultaneously. Other adverse effects include dry mouth, dizziness, headache, nasal stuffiness, and fatigue.

Tamsulosin

Tamsulosin represents the first clinically available antagonist that blocks a specific subset of the α_1-adrenergic receptors, specifically the α_{1A} and α_{1D} subtypes. The α_{1A}-adrenergic receptor has been shown to mediate the contraction of human prostatic smooth muscle.[25] Because tamsulosin has a relatively high affinity for the α_{1A}-adrenergic receptor, it is effectively used to treat benign prostatic hyperplasia. The selectivity of this compound for the prostate is reflected in the fact that there is little decrease in blood pressure after therapeutic doses of the drug. Tamsulosin is well absorbed after oral administration and circulates tightly bound to plasma proteins. It is extensively metabolized in the liver and excreted as inactive conjugation products in the urine. Tamsulosin is less likely to cause orthostatic hypotension and syncope than are other α_1-selective antagonists.[7,17] Other adverse effects include amblyopia, nasal stuffiness, and skin rash.

β-ADRENERGIC RECEPTOR ANTAGONISTS

The β-adrenergic receptor antagonists, also called *β-adrenergic receptor blockers*, represent an important and versatile class of drugs widely used in cardiovascular therapeutics. The β blockers are also used to treat a number of noncardiovascular disease states. Several of the β blockers are among the most widely prescribed medicines in the United States.

β-Adrenergic receptors are currently categorized into three subtypes: β_1, β_2, and β_3. The physiologic role of the β_3 receptor is not as well defined as are those of the β_1- and β_2-adrenergic receptors.[15,29] Although β_3-adrenergic receptors have been shown to regulate cardiac function and vasodilation in some species, a major research effort has been made regarding the antiobesity actions of these receptors.[15,29] Activation of the β_3-adrenergic receptor has been shown to stimulate lipolysis, and a number of β_3-receptor–selective agonists have been developed and are effective in rodent models of obesity. Thus far none of the selective β_3-receptor agonists has been shown to be effective in stimulating weight loss in human beings.[15,29]

Propranolol was the first β-blocking drug to be approved in the United States and is considered the prototype for this class of compounds. This drug is a competitive antagonist at both β_1- and β_2-adrenergic receptors and is therefore referred to as a *nonselective β blocker.* The beneficial effects of propranolol and other nonselective β blockers are attributable to the blockade of the β_1-adrenergic receptor. As discussed below, blockade of the β_2-adrenergic receptor is associated with undesirable effects on the airways, vascular smooth muscle, and endocrine function. Metoprolol, the first selective

β_1-receptor antagonist, and its successors atenolol, acebutolol, and esmolol, have attracted considerable attention because of their relative freedom from the unwanted effects of β_2-adrenergic receptor blockade. It should be noted that this β_1 selectivity is relative with existing agents and that these drugs lose much of their selectivity at higher doses. Presently, both nonselective and selective β_1 blockers are used clinically. Certain β blockers have weak partial agonistic properties; this is referred to as *intrinsic sympathomimetic activity (ISA)*. The value of such drugs is discussed below. The pharmacodynamic and pharmacokinetic properties of propranolol and other selected β blockers are summarized in Table 7-1.

Chemistry

As exemplified by the first β blocker, dichloroisoproterenol, halogen substitution of the catechol hydroxyl groups of the β agonist isoproterenol results in a partial agonistic activity at the β receptor. As illustrated in Figure 7-2, the currently available β-blocking drugs all possess an ethylamino moiety similar to that seen in β-adrenergic receptor agonists attached through a methoxy linkage to a variant ring structure. β_1 Selectivity is conferred by a benzene ring with a large substitution in the para position.

Pharmacologic Effects

The pharmacologic effects of the β blockers occur as a result of preventing binding and subsequent receptor activation by epinephrine, norepinephrine, and exogenously administered adrenergic agonists in tissues regulated by β-adrenergic receptors.

Drugs that do not have ISA decrease resting heart rate, plasma renin activity, and cardiac output. Because of their partial agonist activity, drugs with ISA, such as pindolol, do not depress resting cardiac output or plasma renin activity to the degree seen with other β blockers. However, increases in these parameters will be small because of the low intrinsic activity of pindolol-like drugs. In situations of high sympathetic nervous system activity, β blockers with ISA will antagonize the ability of neuronally released epinephrine and norepinephrine (agonists with high intrinsic activity) to increase heart rate, contractility, and renin secretion. Under these conditions, epinephrine and norepinephrine must compete for binding with drugs that have much less intrinsic activity.

Several of the β blockers can exert a local anesthetic effect in the heart. This activity derives from the blockade of Na^+ channels and results in disruption of electrical impulse propagation in the heart. This activity is also referred to as *membrane-stabilizing activity* (see Table 7-1). Membrane-stabilizing activity is especially strong with propranolol. Blockade of Na^+ channels is a property of local anesthetic compounds and many antiarrhythmic agents (see Chapters 16 and 24). However, in the case of β blockers, the blockade of Na^+ channels requires higher blood concentrations than those necessary for receptor blockade.[8] Thus, in toxic doses, propranolol can exert effects similar to certain antiarrhythmic drugs such as quinidine.[10] These effects include a decrease in the slope of the upstroke of the action potential (phase 0) and an increase in the refractory period in ischemic ventricular tissue.

Effects on the cardiovascular system

The major regulatory β-adrenergic receptor in the human myocardium is the β_1 receptor. β_2- and β_3-adrenergic receptors are also expressed in the human heart; however, their contribution to cardiac performance in the normal myocardium is not entirely known.[15,29] As typified by propranolol, the prototype for this class of drugs, β blockers decrease the force and rate of myocardial contraction. A major site of action for the negative chronotropic effects of the β blockers is the β_1-adrenergic receptor associated with the sinoatrial (SA) node. β blockers can also inhibit β_1-receptor–mediated responses of the atrioventricular (AV) node and the His-Purkinje system. This results in a decrease in SA nodal firing rate, slowed conduction, and a decrease in automaticity. These actions contribute to the antiarrhythmic efficacy of the β blockers. The decrease in contractile force occurs largely as a result of β_1-adrenergic receptor blockade associated with ventricular (the major site of action) and atrial muscle. Collectively, these changes result in a decrease in cardiac output. The negative inotropic and chronotropic actions lessen the oxygen consumption of the heart and contribute to the usefulness of the β blockers in treating ischemic heart disease. The effects of the β blockers are most pronounced under conditions of heightened sympathetic activity, when there are significant amounts of circulating and neuronally released catecholamines.

β Blockers do not reduce blood pressure in normotensive patients; however, they are highly effective in reducing blood pressure in hypertensive patients. Propranolol lowers blood pressure equally in both the supine and standing positions, with no orthostatic hypotension. This attribute was discovered serendipitously while β blockers were being used to treat angina pectoris. Since that time, propranolol and other β blockers, alone or in combination with other drugs, have gained status as important agents in the treatment of hypertension. Although the mechanism by which the β blockers lower blood pressure is not completely understood, certain facts are known. The reduction in blood pressure is associated only with the *l* isomer, which has a much higher affinity for β-adrenergic receptors than does the *d* isomer. When propranolol is first administered to a patient, cardiac output decreases and peripheral resistance increases. The latter effect may result from β_2-receptor blockade in the vasculature or from a baroreceptor-mediated increase in sympathetic tone. However, with continued therapy, peripheral resistance also decreases. Propranolol causes a lowering of plasma renin concentrations by blocking renal β_1-adrenergic receptors involved in renin secretion. The reduction in plasma renin activity eventually leads to a reduction in angiotensin II concentrations and aldosterone secretion. Other mechanisms that appear to contribute to the reduction in blood pressure include a decrease in heart rate, cardiac output, central nervous system (CNS) sympathetic outflow,[14] and an alteration in baroreceptor responsiveness.

Effects on smooth muscle

By blocking the β_2-adrenergic receptors associated with airway smooth muscle, propranolol and other nonselective β blockers prevent sympathetic stimulation of bronchiolar smooth muscle while leaving parasympathetic activity and other bronchoconstrictive influences unchecked. This imbalance can lead to a marked increase in airway resistance in patients with bronchospastic disorders such as asthma, chronic bronchitis, and emphysema. Indeed, propranolol and other nonselective β blockers are contraindicated in patients with bronchospastic disease. This limitation was a major impetus for development of selective β_1-receptor–blocking drugs. In a similar fashion, nonselective β blockers can also exacerbate peripheral vascular disease by blocking vasodilatory β_2-adrenergic receptors on vascular smooth muscle.

Gastrointestinal tract effects

Like other adrenergic blocking agents, propranolol tends to produce a relative preponderance of parasympathetic activity in the gastrointestinal tract. The net effect is related to the amount of sympathetic activity that is blocked, but it is usually of little importance.

Table 7-1

Comparison of β-Adrenergic Receptor Blocking Drugs

DRUG	POTENCY OF BLOCKADE (PROPRANOLOL = 1)	MEMBRANE-STABILIZING ACTIVITY	INTRINSIC SYMPATHOMIMETIC ACTIVITY	ORAL BIOAVAILABILITY (%)	HALF-LIFE (HR)	ROUTE OF ELIMINATION	LIPOPHILICITY	DOSING FREQUENCY (TIMES/DAY)	THERAPEUTIC INDICATIONS
Nonselective ($\beta_1 + \beta_2$)									
Nadolol	1.0	0	0	30	10 to 24	Renal	Low	1	Angina pectoris Hypertension
Pindolol	6.0	+	++	80	3 to 4	Hepatic/renal	Moderate	1 to 2	Hypertension
Propranolol	1.0	++	0	30	3 to 5	Hepatic	High	2 to 3	Angina pectoris Arrhythmias Hypertension Hypertrophic subaortic stenosis Migraine prophylaxis Myocardial infarction Pheochromocytoma
Timolol	6.0	0	0	50	3 to 5	Hepatic/renal	Moderate	1 to 2	Hypertension Migraine prophylaxis Myocardial infarction Glaucoma
Selective (β_1)									
Acebutolol	0.3	+	+	40	3 to 4	Hepatic/renal/nonrenal	Moderate	2 to 3	Hypertension Ventricular arrhythmias
Atenolol	1.0	0	0	50	6 to 9	Renal	Low	1 to 1	Angina pectoris Hypertension Myocardial infarction
Esmolol*	0.02	0	0	—	0.15	Red blood cell esterase		—	Supraventricular tachycardias Noncompensatory tachycardias
Metoprolol	1.0	—	0	40	3 to 7	Hepatic/renal	Moderate	2 to 3	Angina pectoris Hypertension Myocardial infarction

*Has a very brief duration of action and is given only intravenously.

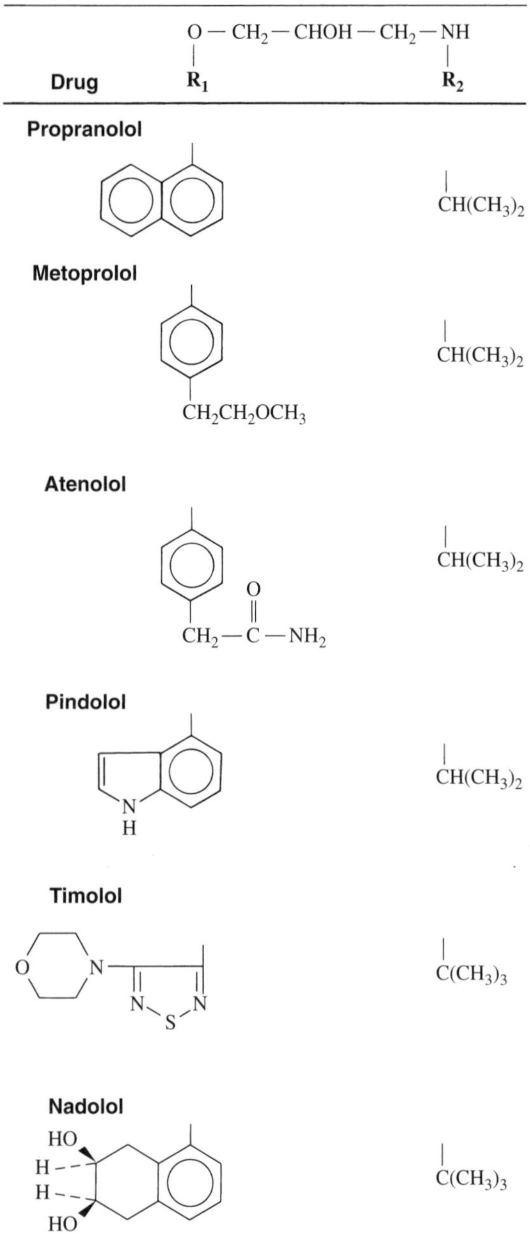

$O-CH_2-CHOH-CH_2-NH$

Drug	R_1	R_2
Propranolol		$CH(CH_3)_2$
Metoprolol	$CH_2CH_2OCH_3$	$CH(CH_3)_2$
Atenolol	$CH_2-C(=O)-NH_2$	$CH(CH_3)_2$
Pindolol	N H	$CH(CH_3)_2$
Timolol	O N N S N	$C(CH_3)_3$
Nadolol	HO H H HO	$C(CH_3)_3$

Fig. 7-2 Structural formulas of some β-adrenoceptor–blocking agents. All the drugs share a similar side chain, differing only in the terminal hydrocarbon group *(R_2)*. Considerable variation exists in the ring structures *(R_1)*.

Metabolic effects

Propranolol blocks the β_2-adrenergic receptors responsible for initiating glycogenolysis in the liver and in skeletal muscle. Hypoglycemia may result from this action but is rare in the nondiabetic person. The release of fatty acids from adipocytes by epinephrine is mediated by β_1- or β_3-adrenergic receptors. β-Adrenergic antagonists blunt this release. Nevertheless, β blockers increase triglyceride concentrations and decrease high-density lipoprotein titers.

Ocular effects

While the antihypertensive effects of the β blockers were being studied, investigators noticed that intraocular pressure in patients with open-angle glaucoma was reduced.[32] β Blockers decrease the production of aqueous humor and as a result decrease intraocular pressure. Thus these agents are useful in treating glaucoma and ocular hypertension. The pharmacotherapy of glaucoma is discussed in Chapter 8.

Central nervous system effects

The versatility of the β blockers is reflected in the fact that they can by used to treat a variety of disorders that have CNS involvement. These include migraine headache, tremor associated with anxiety (stage fright), and benign essential tremor. Reduction of tremors is also mediated by blocking β_2-adrenergic receptors in skeletal muscle.

As is described below, the β-blocking drugs can cause a variety of side effects related to their CNS activity. Theoretically, the most hydrophilic β blockers (e.g., nadolol and atenolol) should have the least access to the CNS and be associated with the lowest occurrence of such CNS effects; studies of atenolol tend to confirm this relationship.[30]

Absorption, Fate, and Excretion

Most clinically approved β blockers are available in oral dosage forms. Esmolol, a selective β_1-receptor antagonist with a very brief duration of action, is given only intravenously to treat hypertension acutely and to control ventricular rate in patients with supraventricular tachyarrhythmias. Levobunolol and metipranolol are available only in solutions suitable for ophthalmic use. Key features of the pharmacokinetic properties of selected β blockers are provided in Table 7-1.

In its first pass through the liver, approximately 50% of propranolol is metabolized. The first-pass extraction can vary widely among patients, thus necessitating individualized dosing regimens. Peak plasma concentrations of propranolol occur approximately 90 minutes after oral administration, with as much as 90% of the drug bound to plasma proteins. The half-life after oral administration is 3 to 5 hours; intravenous administration results in a half-life of 1.5 to 2 hours.[21] Nadolol is unique among currently available drugs because it has an elimination half-life of up to 24 hours. The bioavailability of propranolol and metoprolol may be significantly improved if the drugs are taken after a high-protein meal, presumably because the protein reduces the first-pass metabolism of the drugs. To minimize variation in drug effects, the dosing schedule should be consistent regarding meals.

Metabolism of propranolol occurs almost exclusively in the liver, with oxidative reactions involving both the benzene ring and the side chain. One metabolite, 4-hydroxypropranolol, is as active as the parent compound.[6] Less than 5% of the administered drug is excreted intact in the urine. As noted in Table 7-1, most of the other β-blocking drugs are excreted more extensively by the kidney than is propranolol.

Therapeutic Uses

A brief discussion of the important therapeutic uses of the β blockers is provided below. Individual indications are also covered in greater detail in other sections of this text, including Chapters 24 to 26 and 28.

Hypertension

The β blockers are major drugs used in the treatment of hypertension. Numerous studies have shown these agents to be safe and effective at decreasing the morbidity and mortality associated with elevated blood pressure. The β blockers can be used as monotherapy to control hypertension or used in combination with other drugs, such as diuretics, to produce a more vigorous hypotensive action. Many of the side effects associated with the use of other hypertensives, such as Na^+ and water retention or the development of tolerance, do not occur with the β blockers. The effects of the β blockers on triglyceride levels and glucose metabolism (see above) may limit their use in patients with hyperlipidemia and diabetes. The only systemic β blockers not approved for use in hypertension are esmolol and sotalol.

Ischemic heart disease

β Blockers are widely used to prevent angina pectoris associated with atherosclerotic coronary artery disease. In this condition, there is an imbalance between the oxygen demand of the myocardium and the ability of the partially occluded coronary arteries to deliver oxygen-rich blood to the myocardial muscle. This leads to cardiac ischemia and development of the characteristic chest pain of angina pectoris. Two of the major determinants of myocardial oxygen consumption, the force and rate of contraction, are decreased by the β blockers. Thus cardiac ischemia and associated angina pectoris are reduced.

Post–myocardial infarction

The favorable action on cardiac work and on myocardial oxygen consumption is the reason the β blockers are used after myocardial infarction. These drugs can limit the likelihood and reduce the severity of reinfarction. The antiarrhythmic activity of the β blockers may also contribute to reducing mortality rates after myocardial infarction.

Congestive heart failure

In patients with left ventricular dysfunction, a variety of sympathetically mediated reflexes are activated that ultimately contribute to the signs and symptoms of congestive heart failure. These sympathetic reflex responses include increases in circulating catecholamines, angiotensin II formation, and peripheral vascular resistance; activation of hypertrophic growth responses; and activation of myocardial β-adrenergic receptors. These activities further impair cardiac performance. Thus the disease process sets in motion a vicious cycle that further compromises ventricular performance (see Chapter 25). Numerous recent clinical studies have shown that the β blockers decrease the morbidity and mortality rates of congestive heart failure.[13,22] These drugs act at several levels to interrupt the sympathetic nervous system contribution to heart failure. The β_1-adrenergic receptor–mediated increase in renin secretion is blocked, thus decreasing circulating levels of angiotensin II. Angiotensin II not only has the ability to increase peripheral vascular resistance and promote Na^+ and water retention, but it is also a positive signal for hypertrophic growth. In heart failure, chronic activation of the sympathetic nervous system leads to the desensitization and downregulation of the myocardial β_1-adrenergic receptor. The downregulation of this signaling pathway, a pathway vital to producing increases in contractile force, also contributes to contractile dysfunction and the development of heart failure. Blocking β_1-adrenergic receptors prevents chronic receptor stimulation and the associated downregulation of the β_1-adrenergic receptor signaling pathway. Thus β blockers may actually promote the upregulation of β_1-adrenergic receptor signaling in heart failure. Bisoprolol, carvedilol, and metoprolol have been shown to decrease mortality and morbidity rates associated with congestive heart failure.[13]

Treatment of arrhythmias

The β blockers can be used to treat a variety of supraventricular tachyarrhythmias, including atrial flutter and atrial fibrillation. In treating sinus tachycardia, the major site of action is the SA node, whereas the AV node is the site of action in atrial flutter and fibrillation. In these conditions, the slowing of conduction and increased refractory period protect the ventricle from the excessive stimulation caused by the arrhythmia. Sotalol has antiarrhythmic properties not shared by other β blockers and can be used to treat life-threatening ventricular arrhythmias. Acebutolol can be used to treat premature ventricular contractions. Esmolol has a short plasma half-life, which makes it useful in the acute management of supraventricular tachyarrhythmias.

Other uses

The β blockers can be used to treat pheochromocytoma (administered with an α-adrenergic receptor–blocking drug), thyrotoxicosis, migraine headache (prophylaxis only), glaucoma, hypertrophic subaortic stenosis, stage fright, and tremors and to prevent bleeding episodes associated with esophageal varices. Propranolol has the largest number of approved uses among the β blockers. Timolol, metoprolol, nadolol, and atenolol can be used to treat migraine headaches. Levobunolol and metipranolol are used exclusively as ophthalmics.

Adverse Effects

Many of the adverse effects of the β blockers (Table 7-2) are logical extensions of their pharmacologic effects, which are caused by blockade of β-adrenergic receptors. These effects are most prominently seen on the heart, smooth muscle, brain, and organs that mediate metabolic responses.[27]

Effects on the heart

As an extension of their actions on SA and AV nodal function, β blockers can induce bradycardia and AV block. The abrupt withdrawal of propranolol has been linked to attacks of angina pectoris, myocardial infarction, and sudden death, especially in patients with angina. The chronic blockade of the β-adrenergic receptor may induce β-receptor supersensitivity that contributes to a rebound exacerbation of these clinical problems.[2] For this reason, withdrawal from β-blocking drugs should be done slowly, over a period of 1 to 2 weeks. In patients with moderate to severe congestive heart failure, β blockers can precipitate bradyarrhythmias, AV nodal conduction abnormalities, severe ventricular dysfunction, and cardiac failure. The risk is higher in patients with preexisting cardiac disease and in patients who take the β blocker with cardiac glycosides or other drugs that also slow pacemaker activity and impair AV nodal conduction velocity. A reduction in myocardial contractility is especially great when β blockers are combined with drugs such as verapamil.

Effects on smooth muscle

Because of the blockade of β_2 receptors in blood vessels, nonselective β blockers tend to cause a reduction in the vasodilator response of the vasculature. This effect is of little consequence in most patients, even though cold hands and feet may result. However, in patients with peripheral vascular disease, such as Raynaud's disease, worsening of the condition is likely, and β blockers, especially nonselective ones, are therefore contraindicated in such patients.

Bronchospasm resulting from blockade of β_2 receptors is apt to occur in patients with chronic obstructive airway diseases such as asthma, chronic bronchitis, and emphysema. Drugs selective for β_1 receptors have less effect on bronchial smooth muscle than do the nonselective blockers. Nevertheless, the risk of bronchoconstriction with these drugs is still present because of their limited selectivity for the β_1 receptor.

Metabolic effects

In the diabetic patient taking hypoglycemic drugs, the compensatory sympathetic stimulation and epinephrine release resulting from lowered blood glucose concentrations may be blocked in patients receiving β blockers.[24] A common warning sign of hypoglycemia to the diabetic patient is an increase in heart rate. Because this action is mediated by the β_1-adrenergic receptor, this early sign of hypoglycemia is blunted by all β blockers.

Table • 7-2

Major Adverse Effects of Drugs That Suppress the Activity of the Sympathetic Nervous System or Inhibit Adrenergic Receptors

	RECEPTOR-BLOCKING DRUGS			PREJUNCTIONAL ADRENERGIC NEURON INHIBITORS			SELECTIVE α_2-ADRENERGIC RECEPTOR AGONISTS ACTING ON THE CNS	
ADVERSE EFFECT	NONSELECTIVE α-RECEPTOR–BLOCKING DRUGS	SELECTIVE α_1-RECEPTOR–BLOCKING DRUGS	β-RECEPTOR–BLOCKING DRUGS	RESERPINE	GUANETHIDINE	MAO INHIBITORS	METHYLDOPA	CLONIDINE
CNS Effects								
Depression		+	+	+++	+		+	+
Drowsiness			++	+++		++	++	+++
Dreams/insomnia			++	++		++		
Cardiovascular Effects								
Orthostatic hypotension	+++	++ (first dose)		+	+++	+++	+	+
Heart rate	↑		↓		⟶	↑	↓	↓
General Autonomic Effects								
Diarrhea	++	+		+++	+++		++	Constipation
Nasal stuffiness	++	+		+++	+	+	++	
Xerostomia		+		+++		+	++	+++
Asthma			++					
Fluid retention				++	+++		++	++
Special Reactions			**Heart failure, angina withdrawal reaction**	**Enhanced adrenergic amine response**	**Enhanced adrenergic amine response**	**Hypertensive crisis with chemicals that release catecholamines**	**Positive Coombs' test, hemolytic anemia, hepatitis**	**Withdrawal reaction**

+, Rare; ++, occasional; +++, common; ↑, increase; ↓, decrease; ⟶, arrhythmia.

Central nervous system effects
Patients receiving β blockers may experience CNS depression, weakness, fatigue, sleep disturbance, depression, insomnia, nightmares, hallucinations, and dizziness.

DRUGS WITH COMBINED α- AND β-ADRENERGIC RECEPTOR ANTAGONIST ACTIVITY

Labetalol
Labetalol is an unusual drug in that it combines nonselective β-blocking properties with α_1-adrenergic blocking activity. It is five to seven times more potent at blocking β-adrenergic receptors compared with α_1 receptors. These properties are the result of the different receptor-blocking characteristics of the four isomers that make up the drug formulation. Because of actions at β- and α_1-adrenergic receptors, labetalol decreases blood pressure. The drug also has some direct vasodilatory properties, because at least one isomer is a partial agonist at β_2 receptors and at least one isomer may have vasodilator properties independent of adrenergic receptors. Administration of labetalol will lead to a decrease in peripheral vascular resistance and occasionally orthostatic hypotension; however, the use of labetalol is usually not associated with decreased cardiac output, severe bradycardia, or congestive heart failure. Labetalol can be used orally in the long-term treatment of hypertension or administered intravenously for the treatment of hypertensive emergencies (see Chapter 28). It exhibits near complete oral absorption. However, extensive first-pass metabolism significantly decreases the amount of drug that reaches the systemic circulation. The adverse effects seen with labetalol are predictable considering the drug is a nonspecific β blocker as well as an α_1-receptor blocker. Orthostatic hypotension and syncope can occur. Untoward reactions associated with β-receptor blockade include bradycardia and AV block, complications in diabetic patients, airway dysfunction, sedation, fatigue, and other CNS manifestations.

Carvedilol
Carvedilol, a racemic mixture of two isomers, is the second drug to be marketed with both α_1- and β-blocking activities. In contrast to labetalol, carvedilol is without ISA. Carvedilol is also much more selective for β-adrenergic receptors than is labetalol. Initially approved for use as an antihypertensive (because of the ability to block α_1 and β receptors), recent studies have shown that carvedilol decreases the risk of morbidity and mortality associated with congestive heart failure.[13] The pharmacologic actions that make carvedilol useful in treating heart failure are probably the result of blockade of α_1- and β-adrenergic receptors. The beneficial effects of β-receptor blockade in heart failure have been previously discussed. The vasodilatory actions of carvedilol that occur as a result of α_1-receptor blockade decrease peripheral resistance and, as a result, the workload of the heart. There is also evidence that carvedilol exerts antioxidant activity and acts as a free radical scavenger, which could provide benefit in patients with heart failure.[12] Like labetalol, carvedilol is metabolized in the liver and undergoes extensive first-pass metabolism. The adverse effects of carvedilol are similar to those observed with labetalol.

DRUGS THAT REDUCE CNS SYMPATHETIC OUTFLOW

Several drugs, including methyldopa, clonidine, guanabenz, and guanfacine, inhibit sympathetic outflow through actions within the CNS. These drugs are actually α_2-adrenergic agonists and are discussed in Chapter 6. They interfere with sympathetic nervous system activity by stimulating regulatory α_2 receptors in the CNS. Some of the major adverse effects of these drugs are summarized in Table 7-2; their use in the treatment of hypertension is covered in Chapter 28.

ADRENERGIC NEURON–BLOCKING DRUGS

The category of adrenergic neuron–blocking drugs encompasses a wide variety of drugs having diverse mechanisms of action. The net effect of these drugs is to reduce activity of the sympathetic nerve terminal. These drugs are mainly of historic interest and have limited therapeutic use today.

Metyrosine
Metyrosine (α-methyl-L-tyrosine) competitively inhibits tyrosine hydroxylase, the rate-limiting enzyme in the synthesis of norepinephrine, preventing the formation of dihydroxyphenylalanine from tyrosine and ultimately the synthesis of norepinephrine in the CNS and the periphery.[11] Metyrosine is used to inhibit catecholamine biosynthesis in the treatment of pheochromocytoma. Adverse effects include sedation, Parkinson-like tremors, anxiety, and crystalluria.

Reserpine
Reserpine depletes monoamines from neuronal storage vesicles, both in the periphery and in the CNS, by binding to the vesicles and inhibiting the vesicular uptake pump. This action results in a loss of neurotransmitter from the vesicle and indirectly prevents the final synthesis of the neurotransmitter in the vesicle.[5] Monoamines present in the cytoplasm are metabolized by MAO. Although the sympatholytic action described below occurs as a result of depleting epinephrine and norepinephrine, reserpine can also decrease neuronal stores of dopamine and 5-HT. The binding of reserpine with the vesicular amine-concentrating mechanism is quite permanent, and its effect lasts considerably longer than its plasma half-life would indicate. Clinically, a reduction in stored catecholamines of 70% or greater is required to impair sympathetic nerve transmission. Depletion of catecholamines from the adrenal medulla is slower and less complete than for nerve terminals. As a result of depleting catecholamines, reserpine decreases systemic arterial blood pressure by reducing peripheral vascular resistance and cardiac output. Reserpine was developed in the 1950s as an antihypertensive; however, the drug was only modestly effective and is rarely used today. Reserpine easily penetrates the blood-brain barrier and exerts prominent CNS effects resulting from the depletion of monoamines such as norepinephrine, dopamine, and 5-HT. Troubling side effects include sedation, interference with sleep patterns, insomnia, and depression.

Guanethidine, Bretylium, and Guanadrel
Guanethidine, bretylium, and guanadrel (Figure 7-3) share the ability to inhibit the function of adrenergic neurons of the sympathetic nervous system. An identifying characteristic of these adrenergic neuron–blocking drugs is their ability to prevent the release of norepinephrine that occurs after activation of sympathetic nerves. Bretylium was the first drug shown to uncouple the excitation-release mechanism linking the nerve action potential with the junctional release of norepinephrine. Long-term administration of guanethidine allows it to accumulate in the vesicles, where it replaces norepinephrine to the extent that catecholamine depletion results. The major indication for guanethidine and guanadrel is in the treatment of hypertension; however, these agents are not widely used for this purpose. Bretylium was used to treat certain ventricular arrhythmias but is no longer available in the United States.

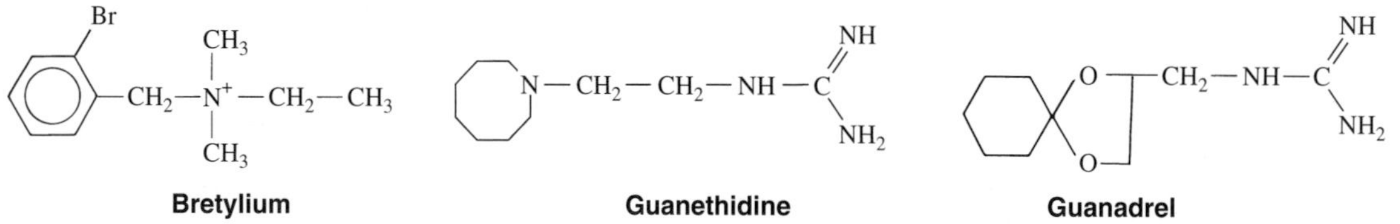

Bretylium **Guanethidine** **Guanadrel**

Fig. 7-3 Structural formulas of bretylium, guanethidine, and guanadrel.

Orthostatic hypotension is common with these agents. Na^+ and water retention occurs with guanadrel and guanethidine, and this effect may require therapy with a thiazide diuretic. Other side effects, such as diarrhea, failure to ejaculate, and a feeling of weakness, are also quite common with guanethidine and guanadrel. These drugs also tend to depress myocardial contractility by reducing sympathetic tone.

Monoamine Oxidase Inhibitors

Paradoxic as it may seem, MAO inhibitors—drugs capable of inhibiting the intracellular enzyme responsible for the inactivation of norepinephrine—cause a lowering of blood pressure. One such drug, pargyline, was specifically marketed for the treatment of essential hypertension. Other drugs, phenelzine and tranylcypromine, are used to treat depression. They are discussed in Chapter 12. The exact antihypertensive mechanism of action is not understood. The risks of pargyline therapy in the treatment of hypertension outweigh its benefits, and its use as an antihypertensive drug is rare. The most frequent adverse effects are those associated with other adrenergic neuron–blocking drugs and with ganglionic blocking drugs: orthostatic hypotension, dizziness, weakness, xerostomia, and syncope. Tremors and hallucinations have also been reported. Difficulties in micturition and ejaculation are also experienced. Most serious is the hypertensive crisis that can occur after eating or drinking foodstuffs containing substantial amounts of tyramine. Aged cheese, liver, beer, and wines are among the most common of these tyramine-containing foods. Hypertension is the result of three factors: (1) the metabolism of tyramine by MAO that would normally take place in the gastrointestinal tract is blocked by the MAO inhibitors; (2) tyramine is an indirect-acting amine and causes release of neurotransmitter from the cytoplasmic pool of adrenergic nerve endings; and (3) large amounts of the transmitter accumulate in the cytoplasmic pool of adrenergic nerve endings as a result of the inhibition of MAO. In addition to the typical symptoms of acute hypertension (throbbing headache, flushing, and hyperpyrexia), cerebral vascular accidents and occasionally deaths have occurred.[23] The use of drugs that release catecholamines should be scrupulously avoided with MAO inhibitors. Thus guanethidine, guanadrel, reserpine, amphetamines, and drugs with mixed sympathomimetic actions such as ephedrine and mephentermine are absolutely contraindicated. Methyldopa and levodopa are also contraindicated because they are metabolized to active catecholamines. MAO inhibitors can inhibit other oxidative enzymes throughout the body, including those in the liver. Thus MAO inhibitors prolong the action of a number of drugs. The use of the analgesic meperidine is contraindicated in patients taking MAO inhibitors because a syndrome of CNS excitation, hyperthermia, and convulsions may result. Opioid analgesics unrelated to meperidine (e.g., morphine) are not contraindicated in the presence of pargyline but should be used cautiously because MAO inhibitors tend to increase the CNS depression from a number of opioid analgesics and sedatives.

IMPLICATIONS FOR DENTISTRY

Many of the drugs discussed in this chapter are widely used to treat hypertension, ischemic heart disease, congestive heart failure, and cardiac rhythm disturbances. This usage has important implications in the practice of dentistry and signals a need for the dentist to pay heed to the potential risks associated with these conditions and the therapeutic agents used to manage them.

Physical Implications

A consideration for patients being treated with adrenergic blocking drugs is the patient's position during and after dental procedures. Suddenly standing upright after being in a supine position in the dental chair is apt to cause syncope. This problem is particularly true for the antihypertensive drugs more prone to cause orthostatic hypotension (e.g., α_1-adrenergic receptor–blocking drugs, drugs with combined α- and β-receptor–blocking activity, and adrenergic neuron–blocking agents). Accidents ranging from chipped teeth and restorations to fractured mandibles and worse have resulted from falls. Contemporary practice standards require the monitoring of blood pressure in dental patients. Such monitoring is particularly important in hypertensive patients.

Drug Interactions

Because nonselective β blockers block β_2-adrenergic receptor–mediated vasodilation, there is a risk of a hypertensive episode after administration of local anesthetic agents that contain vasoconstrictors or the use of epinephrine-impregnated retraction cords.[31] In this situation, the vasoconstrictor actions of epinephrine at α-adrenergic receptors are not opposed by the vasodilatory actions of β_2-adrenergic receptors, resulting in an exaggerated increase in blood pressure that could be deleterious in patients with hypertension or ischemic heart disease.

Clonidine and the other selective α_2-adrenergic receptor agonists are among the drugs that cause xerostomia. This effect also occurs with reserpine and, less frequently, with α-adrenergic receptor antagonists. The use of these drugs may result in clinical symptoms related to dry mouth, such as difficulty in swallowing and speech. Long-term use of xerostomia-causing drugs is associated with a higher incidence of oral candidiasis and dental caries. The use of β-adrenergic receptor blockers is likely to alter the composition of salivary proteins. The effects of these changes have not been fully explored; however, there is a concern that they could adversely influence oral health. The effect of drugs that alter the function of adrenergic nerve endings on salivary proteins is also not well explored.

Patients taking MAO inhibitors must not be given drugs that have indirect sympathomimetic activity or are inactivated by MAO. Phenylephrine has been used in the past as a vasoconstrictor in local anesthetic solutions. Because it causes even a minor release of norepinephrine from adrenergic nerves and is subject to metabolism by MAO, phenylephrine must be

Adrenergic Blocking Agents

Nonproprietary (generic) name	Proprietary (trade) name
α-Adrenergic blocking agents (selectivity)	
Alfuzosin (α_1)	Uroxatral
Doxazosin (α_1)	Cardura
Phenoxybenzamine (α_1, α_2)	Dibenzyline
Phentolamine (α_1, α_2)	Regitine
Prazosin (α_1)	Minipress
Terazosin (α_1)	Hytrin
Tolazoline (α_1, α_2)*	Priscoline
Tamsulosin (α_{1A})	Flomax
β-Adrenergic blocking agents (selectivity)	
Acebutolol (β_1)	Sectral
Atenolol (β_1)	Tenormin
Betaxolol (β_1)	Betoptic, Kerlone
Bisoprolol (β_1)	Zebeta
Carteolol (β_1, β_2)	Cartrol
Esmolol (β_1)	Brevibloc
Levobunolol (β_1, β_2)	AKBeta, Betagan
Metipranolol (β_1, β_2)	OptiPranolol
Metoprolol (β_1)	Lopressor, Toprol XL
Nadolol (β_1, β_2)	Corgard
Penbutolol (β_1, β_2)	Levatol
Pindolol (β_1, β_2)	Visken
Propranolol (β_1, β_2)	Inderal
Sotalol (β_1, β_2)	Betapace
Timolol (β_1, β_2)	Blocadren
Combined α- and β-adrenergic blocking agents	
Carvedilol (β_1, β_2, α_1)	Coreg
Labetalol (β_1, β_2, α_1)	Trandate, Normodyne
Neuronal blocking agents	
Bretylium*	Bretylol
Guanadrel	Hylorel
Guanethidine	Ismelin
Metyrosine	Demser
Reserpine	—

*Not currently available in the United States.

avoided in patients taking MAO inhibitors. Epinephrine and levonordefrin, which are currently the vasoconstrictors used in local anesthetic solutions, are not contraindicated because they are direct agonists and are largely inactivated by catechol-O-methyltransferase. Nonetheless, in patients taking MAO inhibitors, the avoidance of hemostatic preparations containing high concentrations of epinephrine is recommended.

Opioids and other CNS depressants should be used cautiously and usually at lower doses in patients who are taking MAO inhibitors. Meperidine is absolutely contraindicated. The dentist should reinforce the physician's instructions to the patient about dietary restrictions and contraindications of several drugs for patients taking MAO inhibitors.

For the drugs reserpine, guanadrel, and guanethidine, a condition resembling denervation supersensitivity may be clinically evident; the intensity of the response to exogenous amines may be significantly increased as a result. This increased sensitivity does not usually contraindicate the use of vasoconstrictors in local anesthetic solutions; however, caution must be exercised to avoid accidental intravenous injection and giving high amounts of vasoconstrictor. The use of adrenergic hemostatic agents, as found in certain gingival retraction cords, is best avoided.

CITED REFERENCES

1. Ahlquist RP: A study of adrenotropic receptors, *Am J Physiol* 153:586-600, 1948.
2. Alderman EL, Coltart DJ, Wettach GE, et al: Coronary artery syndromes after sudden propranolol withdrawal, *Ann Intern Med* 81:625-627, 1974.
3. Brogden RN, Heel RC, Speight TM, et al: Prazosin: a review of its pharmacological properties and therapeutic efficacy in hypertension, *Drugs* 14:163-197, 1977.
4. Cass R, Spriggs TLB: Tissue amine levels and sympathetic blockade after guanethidine and bretylium, *Br J Pharmacol* 17:442-450, 1961.
5. Chidsey CA, Braunwald E, Morrow AG, et al: Myocardial norepinephrine concentration in man: effects of reserpine and of congestive heart failure, *N Engl J Med* 269:653-658, 1963.
6. Cleaveland CR, Shand DG: Effect of route of administration on the relationship between adrenergic blockade and plasma propranolol level, *Clin Pharmacol Ther* 13:181-185, 1972.
7. Clifford GM, Farmer RD: Medical therapy for benign prostatic hyperplasia: a review of the literature, *Eur Urol* 38:2-19, 2000.
8. Coltart DJ, Gibson DG, Shand DG: Plasma propranolol levels associated with suppression of ventricular ectopic beats, *Br Med J* 1:490-491, 1971.
9. Dale HH: On some physiological actions of ergot, *J Physiol* (London) 34:163-206, 1906.
10. Davis LD, Temte JV: Effects of propranolol on the transmembrane potentials of ventricular muscle and Purkinje fibers of the dog, *Circ Res* 22:661-677, 1968.
11. Engelman K, Horwitz D, Jequier E, et al: Biochemical and pharmacologic effects of α-methyltyrosine in man, *J Clin Invest* 47:577-594, 1968.
12. Feuerstein G, Yue TL, Ma X, et al: Novel mechanisms in the treatment of heart failure: inhibition of oxygen radicals and apoptosis by carvedilol, *Prog Cardiovasc Dis* 41:17-24, 1998.
13. Frantz RP: Beta blockade in patients with congestive heart failure, *Postgrad Med* 108(3):103-106, 109-110, 116-118, 2000.
14. Garvey HL, Ram N: Comparative antihypertensive effects and tissue distribution of beta adrenergic blocking drugs, *J Pharmacol Exp Ther* 194:220-233, 1975.
15. Gauthier C, Langin D, Balligand JL: β_3-adrenoceptors in the cardiovascular system, *Trends Pharmacol Sci* 21:426-431, 2000.
16. Hoffman BB, Lefkowitz RJ: Alpha-adrenergic receptor subtypes, *N Engl J Med* 302:1390-1396, 1980.

17. Kirby RS: Clinical pharmacology of α_1-adrenoceptor antagonists, *Eur Urol* 36(suppl 1):48-53, 1999.
18. Massingham R, Hayden ML: A comparison of the effects of prazosin and hydralazine on blood pressure, heart rate and plasma renin activity in conscious renal hypertensive dogs, *Eur J Pharmacol* 30:121-124, 1975.
19. Messerli FH, Grossman E: Doxazosin arm of the ALLHAT study discontinued: how equal are antihypertensive drugs? Antihypertensive and lipid lowering treatment to prevent heart attack trial, *Curr Hypertens Rep* 2:241-242, 2000.
20. Nickerson M, Goodman LS: Pharmacological properties of a new adrenergic blocking agent: N, N-dibenzylchloroethylamine (Dibenamine), *J Pharmacol Exp Ther* 89:167-185, 1947.
21. Nies AS, Shand DG: Clinical pharmacology of propranolol, *Circulation* 52:6-15, 1975.
22. Packer M: Therapeutic options in the management of chronic heart failure. Is there a drug of first choice? *Circulation* 79:198-204, 1989.
23. Pettinger WA, Oates JA: Supersensitivity to tyramine during monoamine oxidase inhibition in man: mechanism at the level of the adrenergic neuron, *Clin Pharmacol Ther* 9:341-344, 1968.
24. Podolsky S, Pattavina CG: Hyperosmolar nonketotic diabetic coma: a complication of propranolol therapy, *Metabolism* 22:685-693, 1973.
25. Schwinn DA, Price RR: Molecular pharmacology of human α_1-adrenergic receptors: unique features of the α_{1a}-subtype, *Eur Urol* 36(suppl 1):7-10, 1999.
26. Starke K: Presynaptic α-autoreceptors, *Rev Physiol Biochem Pharmacol* 107:73-146, 1987.
27. Stephen SA: Unwanted effects of propranolol, *Am J Cardiol* 18:463-472, 1966.
28. Stokes GS, Oates HF: Prazosin: new alpha-adrenergic blocking agent in the treatment of hypertension, *Cardiovasc Med* 3:41-57, 1978.
29. Strosberg AD: Structure and function of the β_3-adrenergic receptor, *Annu Rev Pharmacol Toxicol* 37:421-450, 1997.
30. Westerlund A: Central nervous system side-effects with hydrophilic and lipophilic β-blockers, *Eur J Clin Pharmacol* 28(suppl):73-76, 1985.
31. Yagiela JA: Adverse drug interactions in dental practice: interactions associated with vasoconstrictors. Part V of a series, *J Am Dent Assoc* 130:701-709, 1999.
32. Zimmerman TJ, Kaufman HE: Timolol. A β-adrenergic blocking agent for the treatment of glaucoma, *Arch Ophthalmol* 95:601-604, 1977.

General References

Bristow MR: Pathophysiologic and pharmacologic rationales for clinical management of chronic heart failure with beta-blocking agents, *Am J Cardiol* 71:12C-22C, 1993.

Emilien G, Maloteaux J-M: Current therapeutic uses and potential of β-adrenoceptor agonists and antagonists, *Eur J Clin Pharmacol* 53:389-404, 1998.

Glick M: New guidelines for the prevention, detection, evaluation and treatment of high blood pressure, *J Am Dent Assoc* 129:1588-1594, 1998.

Houston MC: Alpha$_1$-blocker combination therapy for hypertension, *Postgrad Med* 104(3):167-170, 176-178, 181-182, 1998.

Jønler M, Riehmann M, Bruskewitz RC: Benign prostatic hyperplasia. Current pharmacological treatment, *Drugs* 47:66-81, 1994.

Jowett NI, Cabot LB: Patients with cardiac disease: considerations for the dental practitioner, *Br Dent J* 189:297-302, 2000.

McDevitt DG: Comparison of pharmacokinetic properties of beta-adrenoceptor blocking drugs, *Eur Heart J* 8(suppl M):9-14, 1987.

Moore PA, Gage TW, Hersh EV, et al: Adverse drug interactions in dental practice: professional and educational implications, *J Am Dent Assoc* 130:47-54, 1999.

Muzyka BC, Glick M: The hypertensive dental patient, *J Am Dent Assoc* 128:1109-1120, 1997.

Prichard BN, Graham BR, Cruickshank JM: New approaches to the uses of beta blocking drugs in hypertension, *J Hum Hypertens* 14(Suppl 1):S63-S68, 2000.

van Zwieten PA: The renaissance of centrally acting antihypertensive drugs, *J Hypertens* 17(suppl 3):S15-S21, 1999.

Which beta-blocker? *Med Lett Drugs Ther* 43:9-11, 2001.

CHAPTER • 8

Cholinergic Drugs

Frank J. Dowd

Cholinergic drugs are agents that mimic the actions of the endogenous neurotransmitter acetylcholine (ACh). As described in Chapter 5, ACh is the primary neurotransmitter released from the nerve terminals of the preganglionic fibers of the parasympathetic and sympathetic nervous systems, the postganglionic fibers of the parasympathetic nervous system (which include most of the postganglionic cholinergic neurons), and some postganglionic fibers of the sympathetic nervous system. ACh is also the primary neurotransmitter released from somatic efferents innervating skeletal muscle and from certain central nervous system (CNS) neurons.

Most cholinergic, or *cholinomimetic,* agonists produce parasympathetic responses by stimulating muscarinic receptors located on tissues innervated by the postganglionic fibers of the parasympathetic nervous system. These drugs are often referred to as *muscarinic* or *parasympathomimetic* agonists. Some cholinergic agonists produce a nonselective stimulation of the parasympathetic and sympathetic branches of the autonomic nervous system by activating ganglionic nicotinic receptors located on the cell bodies of postganglionic fibers. In addition, some cholinergic agonists excite skeletal muscle by activating a separate group of nicotinic receptors located on the motor endplate of the neuromuscular junction. Those synapses in the CNS that contain nicotinic and muscarinic receptors can be stimulated by cholinomimetic agonists capable of penetrating the blood-brain barrier.

Drugs that inhibit the hydrolysis of ACh by the enzyme acetylcholinesterase (AChE) produce their cholinomimetic effects indirectly. These *anticholinesterases* prolong the effective life of ACh released at neuroeffector junctions. As a group, the anticholinesterases are less selective in effect than many direct-acting cholinomimetics, and they are largely without activity in denervated tissues. Nevertheless, their dependence on ACh release confers the potential advantage of retaining neural control over their effects.

CHOLINOMIMETIC AGONISTS

The cholinomimetic agonists directly stimulate cholinergic receptors, muscarinic or nicotinic or both, to cause a pharmacologic response in an effector. These cholinergic drugs are classified into two groups on the basis of their origin and chemical composition: choline esters, which include ACh and its synthetic congeners, and the naturally occurring alkaloids and their congeners, including muscarine, pilocarpine, cevimeline, and nicotine. With few exceptions (e.g., nicotine), all these agents exert prominent parasympathomimetic effects.

Chemistry and Classification

Choline esters

The history of the discovery of ACh and its identification is covered in Chapter 5. In 1909, Hunt synthesized the acetyl ester of choline, and earlier Hunt and Taveau reported on the pharmacology of a number of synthetic congeners of ACh.[25] Interest in the choline esters arose, in part, out of the hope that some of these compounds would have a longer duration of action than ACh and, at the same time, a greater degree of selectivity. This goal has only partially been realized, and in general ACh and related drugs are either not used therapeutically or used only in selected instances. The structures of ACh and the three principal synthetic esters of choline, namely methacholine, carbachol, and bethanechol, are shown in Figure 8-1. Succinylcholine, a diacetylcholine derivative with selective nicotinic receptor effects in skeletal muscle, is discussed in Chapter 10.

Natural alkaloids and congeners

Several alkaloids obtained from various plants possess direct cholinomimetic activity. Muscarine, the prototype muscarinic agonist, is present during certain times of the year in the mushroom *Amanita muscaria* and is especially prominent in several *Inocybe* and *Clitocybe* species. Although a quaternary ammonium compound (Figure 8-2), muscarine has a rapid onset of action after oral ingestion and produces physiologic responses characteristic of profound parasympathetic nervous system stimulation. In severe poisoning, cardiovascular collapse may occur. Pilocarpine is found in the leaves of the South American shrub *Pilocarpus jaborandi.* It is also a selective muscarinic receptor agonist. Pilocarpine remains in the armamentarium for a few specific uses and has a specific dental indication. Cevimeline, a synthetic agent, is similar in pharmacology to pilocarpine. Arecoline is the primary alkaloid of betel nuts. It is a euphoretic and stimulates both muscarinic and ganglionic nicotinic receptors. Nicotine, an alkaloid found in tobacco leaves *(Nicotiana tabacum),* is important historically as the prototype nicotinic receptor agonist. In the form of cigarettes, nicotine is the most commonly used cholinergic agonist, and it is responsible for the physical dependence associated with smoking. The sole therapeutic use of nicotine, as an adjunct in tobacco cessation programs, is reviewed in Chapter 10. Commercially, nicotine finds application as an insecticide.

Mechanism of Action

Direct-acting cholinomimetic drugs produce their effects by binding to and stimulating muscarinic and nicotinic receptors. As noted previously, these receptors are located in junctional regions of both the peripheral nervous system and the CNS.

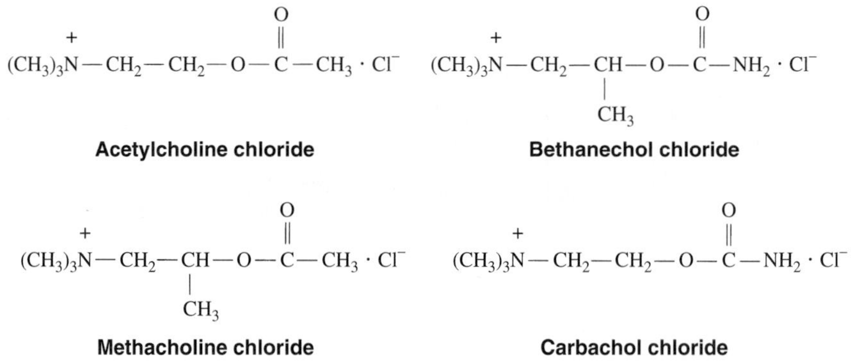

$(CH_3)_3\overset{+}{N}-CH_2-CH_2-O-\overset{O}{\overset{\|}{C}}-CH_3 \cdot Cl^-$

Acetylcholine chloride

$(CH_3)_3\overset{+}{N}-CH_2-\underset{CH_3}{\underset{|}{CH}}-O-\overset{O}{\overset{\|}{C}}-NH_2 \cdot Cl^-$

Bethanechol chloride

$(CH_3)_3\overset{+}{N}-CH_2-\underset{CH_3}{\underset{|}{CH}}-O-\overset{O}{\overset{\|}{C}}-CH_3 \cdot Cl^-$

Methacholine chloride

$(CH_3)_3\overset{+}{N}-CH_2-CH_2-O-\overset{O}{\overset{\|}{C}}-NH_2 \cdot Cl^-$

Carbachol chloride

Fig. 8-1 Structural formulas of ACh and three congeners.

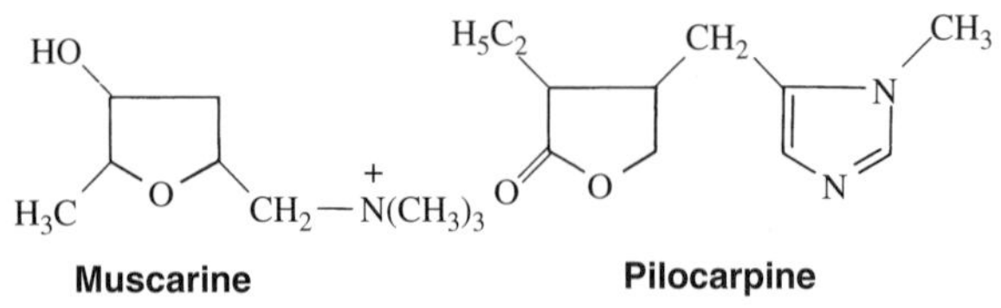

HO, H_3C, O, $CH_2-\overset{+}{N}(CH_3)_3$

Muscarine

H_5C_2, CH_2, CH_3, N, N, O, O

Pilocarpine

Fig. 8-2 Structural formulas of muscarine and pilocarpine.

ACh is capable of stimulating both muscarinic and nicotinic receptors when administered systemically; however, although muscarinic responses are produced by low doses of ACh, effects on ganglionic and somatomotor transmission require increasingly higher doses. The choline ester bethanechol and the plant alkaloid muscarine both produce a relatively selective activation of muscarinic receptors located on autonomic effector tissues (especially in smooth muscle and glandular tissues) and on the cell bodies of unique populations of CNS neurons. Although these muscarinic agonists produce qualitatively similar responses in different organ systems, they vary in their relative potencies in evoking these reactions.

Parasympathomimetic responses to cholinergic drugs are mediated by the stimulation of several populations of muscarinic receptors. Receptor-ligand studies with the investigational agents McN-A-343 (a muscarinic receptor agonist) and pirenzepine (a muscarinic antagonist) initially provided evidence for at least two different muscarinic receptors. Both of these compounds show greater affinity for muscarinic receptors located in sympathetic ganglia and on certain neurons in the cerebral cortex than for muscarinic receptors located on cardiac muscle, smooth muscle, and most secretory glands. Subsequent molecular biology studies and the synthesis of more selective receptor agonists and antagonists have complicated the situation even further. A total of five muscarinic receptor proteins (m_1 through m_5, corresponding to the pharmacologically identified receptors M_1 through M_5) have been produced from cloned muscarinic receptor genes, and it has been established that multiple receptor subtypes can coexist in the same organ or tissue. The exact distribution of these receptors and their functional properties are currently areas of active investigation, but a few general concepts have emerged.[54] In the periphery, the M_1 receptor appears to be localized in ganglia, some exocrine gland cells, and the enterochromaffin cells of the stomach (see Chapter 33). The M_2 receptor is the primary subtype found in the heart and is also present, along with the M_4 receptor, in the lung. The M_3 receptor is widely distributed and is most prominent in glandular tissue. Although a peripheral distribution of the M_5 receptor has not been identified, it is expressed, as are the other subtypes, in discrete regions of the CNS.

Muscarinic receptors belong to a large family of plasma membrane receptors whose basic structure consists of seven helical segments spanning the membrane and joined by alternating intracellular and extracellular peptide bridges (see Chapter 1). Although the hydrophobic helical segments, which form the ligand binding site, demonstrate considerable structural homology among the muscarinic receptor subtypes, the third intracellular loop, joining helices V and VI, is highly divergent. Biochemical studies suggest that this loop is of primary importance in the coupling between receptor binding and intracellular action.

Stimulation of muscarinic receptors initiates a cascade of intracellular events that ultimately leads to the observed pharmacologic effects. Evidence to date suggests that all muscarinic receptor subtypes regulate the activity of G proteins (see Chapter 5). The G proteins modulate intracellular processes by influencing "second messenger" systems. Agonist-induced activation of M_1, M_3, or M_5 receptors stimulates the enzyme phospholipase C, which then produces Ca^{++}-dependent phosphorylation of specific cellular regulatory proteins. The stimulation of M_2 or M_4 receptors inhibits the activity of adenylyl cyclase, thus lowering the intracellular concentration of cyclic adenosine 3′,5′-monophosphate. In the heart, this outcome of M_2 receptor activation results in increased K^+ efflux and hyperpolarization of cardiac atrial fibers. The activation of M_2 receptors on the intact vascular endothelium produces a profound vasodilation by stimulating the production and release of nitric oxide, an important endothelium-derived relaxing factor (Figure 8-3).[17,26] Nitric oxide stimulates guanylyl cyclase located in vascular smooth muscle, which in turn catalyzes the formation of cyclic guanosine 3′,5′-monophosphate. This cyclic nucleotide reduces intracellular Ca^{++} concentrations, leading to vascular smooth muscle relaxation and vasodilation.

The systemic administration of high doses of ACh activates nicotinic receptors located on the cell bodies of postganglionic nerve fibers of the autonomic nervous system (N_N receptors) and nicotinic receptors located in the neuromuscular junction (N_M receptors). As described in Chapter 5, nicotinic receptors are composed of five glycoprotein subunits forming a rosette around a central channel spanning the plasma membrane. The α subunits (see also Figure 1-2)

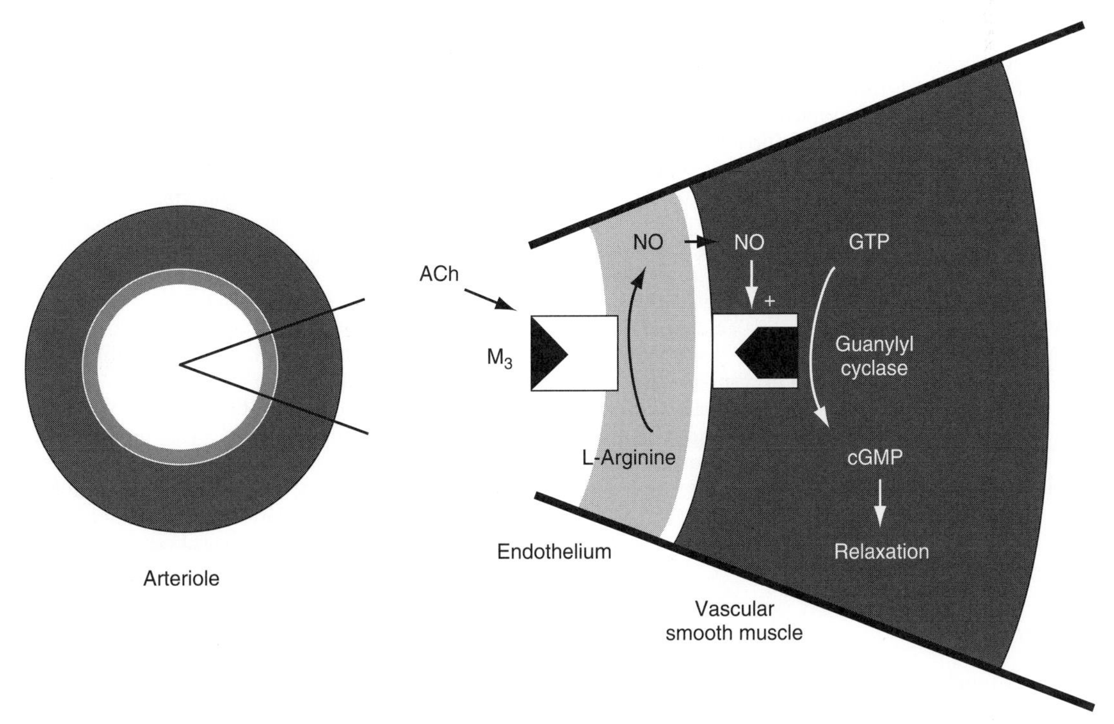

Fig. 8-3 Mechanism of vascular relaxation by muscarinic receptor agonists. The muscarinic agent *ACh* binds to its receptor *(M_3)* on the intact vascular endothelium. Newly synthesized nitric oxide *(NO)* diffuses into the vascular smooth muscle, where it stimulates the formation of cyclic guanosine 3′,5′-monophosphate *(cGMP)* from guanosine triphosphate *(GTP)*.

contain the ACh-binding sites. When stimulated by ACh, nicotine, or another nicotinic receptor agonist, a conformational change in the protein occurs, allowing Na^+ and, to a lesser extent, Ca^{++} ions to move down their respective concentration gradients. The net ionic movement depolarizes the postganglionic cell body or muscle endplate. Prolonged stimulation of nicotinic receptors with ACh or nicotine results in a phenomenon referred to as "depolarization blockade," in which responses to further stimulation are attenuated and then lost (see Chapter 10).

Pharmacologic Effects

The pharmacologic effects produced by direct-acting cholinergic drugs vary according to the receptors they stimulate, their distribution throughout the body, and their mode of inactivation. The duration of action of ACh and its congeners is determined by their susceptibility to hydrolysis by AChE and pseudocholinesterase. Methacholine, with some susceptibility only to AChE, has a longer duration of action than ACh. Bethanechol, carbachol, cevimeline, and the natural alkaloids are not affected by the cholinesterases at all and therefore have even greater durations.

Currently available agents exhibit significantly different affinities for muscarinic and nicotinic sites, so that carbachol has more pronounced nicotinic effects than does ACh, and bethanechol, muscarine, pilocarpine, and cevimeline have very few nicotinic properties. Differences in effect are also noted regarding various target tissues. Thus bethanechol and carbachol are very effective stimulants of the gastrointestinal and urinary tracts, whereas ACh and methacholine exert more prominent cardiovascular effects. Some of the limitations of injected ACh arise because the drug is so quickly metabolized that it gains little access to tissues that are not well perfused.

Peripheral muscarinic effects

Cholinergic agonists that stimulate muscarinic receptors produce end-organ responses that mimic parasympathetic nervous system stimulation. Table 5-1 outlines several of the physiologic responses produced by direct electrical stimulation of parasympathetic nerves. The following listing of the specific muscarinic effects of the cholinergic drugs is limited to those actions that have some therapeutic application or toxicologic importance, and it is emphasized once more that not all of the cholinergic drugs possess all these actions.

Eye

Muscarinic receptor agonists activate the sphincter muscle of the iris and produce constriction of the pupil (miosis). At the same time, there is contraction of the ciliary muscle, so that the eye is fixed for near vision. Intraocular pressure is decreased, particularly if the tension was elevated initially. There may also be a transient hyperemia of the conjunctiva.

Heart

Direct cardiac effects are similar to those associated with vagal stimulation. The heart rate is decreased by drug-induced slowing of the spontaneous depolarization of the sinoatrial node (negative chronotropic effect). There is also a decrease in the force of contraction (negative inotropic effect) of atrial and, to a much lesser extent, ventricular muscle. While the effective refractory period is shortened in atrial muscle, the refractory period in the atrioventricular node and conducting system of the heart is increased, and conduction is slowed.

These direct effects on the heart are subject to autonomic modification. For example, a baroreceptor-mediated increase in sympathetic nervous system activity may occur if the muscarinic drug produces a significant fall in blood pressure. In a patient receiving the muscarinic blocking drug atropine, a dose of a cholinergic drug great enough to activate nicotinic receptors in autonomic ganglia and the adrenal gland will promote the release of catecholamines and result in cardiac stimulation.

Vascular smooth muscle
Muscarinic receptor agonists produce a generalized vasodilation that causes a fall in blood pressure. All vascular beds are affected, which is consistent with pharmacologic evidence that all parts of the vasculature, including pulpal blood vessels, are supplied with muscarinic receptors. The physiologic significance of these receptors is still in doubt, however, in part because much of the vasculature receives no parasympathetic innervation. In the absence of an administered drug, it is likely that vasodilation in local tissues occurs most often in response to autoregulatory factors, such as high carbon dioxide concentrations, low oxygen concentrations, and an acidic pH, and not to stimulation of cholinergic nerves. ACh produced and released locally may facilitate vasodilation in response to local blood flow increases. As noted previously, muscarinic receptor agonists produce their vasodilatory effects by inducing the vascular endothelium to release nitric oxide into the surrounding vascular smooth muscle, where it produces muscle relaxation.[17,26]

Bronchial smooth muscle
The smooth muscle of the bronchioles is constricted by muscarinic receptor agonists.

Gastrointestinal smooth muscle
Motility, peristaltic contractions, amplitude of contraction, and tone are all increased by muscarinic receptor agonists. Conversely, sphincter muscles are relaxed.

Secretory glands
All glands that are innervated by cholinergic fibers are potentially stimulated by cholinergic drugs. These include the salivary, lacrimal, bronchial, sweat, gastric, intestinal, and pancreatic glands. It should be noted again that the secretion by sweat glands is controlled by sympathetic nerves, which in this case have cholinergic postganglionic fibers.

Urinary tract
Muscarinic receptor agonists stimulate contraction of the detrusor muscle, which results in decreased bladder capacity and opening of the urethral orifice in the fundus of the bladder. (Micturition is then permitted by voluntary relaxation of the urethral sphincter.) Peristaltic activity in ureteral smooth muscle may also be stimulated.

Peripheral nicotinic effects
Several cholinomimetic drugs can stimulate nicotinic receptors. Nicotinic receptor agonists have varying effects at different nicotinic sites, and these effects are related to the structure of the molecule,[3,4] the dosage of the drug, and the location and type of nicotinic receptor activated. As noted earlier, there are at least two major kinds of peripheral nicotinic receptors: those on ganglia (N_N) and those in skeletal muscle (N_M). Although exogenous ACh at low doses stimulates muscarinic receptors rather selectively, in substantially higher doses it stimulates N_N receptors and, by close intraarterial injection of high doses, N_M receptors. Several ACh congeners, such as methacholine, and, to an even greater extent, carbachol, have nicotinic properties at therapeutic doses. There is evidence that carbachol not only occupies the postsynaptic cholinergic receptor but also causes the release of ACh from nerve terminals in certain locations by activating presynaptic nicotinic receptors.[42,52] Muscarinic effects are then obtained indirectly through increased ACh release at parasympathetic ganglia and muscarinic neuroeffector sites. Although pilocarpine is essentially muscarinic in action, it has been reported to produce ganglionic stimulation in high doses.

Stimulation of autonomic ganglia leads to a mixture of parasympathetic and sympathetic effects. Because these effects often oppose each other, the resultant outcome is often difficult to predict. In the case of ACh and carbachol, which also exert prominent muscarinic activity, parasympathetic effects predominate. The pharmacology of nicotine, which is devoid of direct muscarinic properties, is reviewed in Chapter 10. None of these agents produces clinically useful skeletal muscle stimulation.

Central nervous system effects
As previously mentioned, there are both muscarinic and nicotinic receptors in the CNS. ACh, the choline esters, and the cholinomimetic alkaloids are all known to evoke CNS actions when applied directly to brain tissue. Central cholinergic systems have been implicated in central regulation of most physiologic systems (i.e., cardiovascular, respiratory, gastrointestinal, and somatomotor systems) and influence cognition and emotion. The observation that cholinergic agonists affect so many functions indicates that cholinergic receptors play an important role in central neurotransmission. In the intact individual, however, many cholinergic agents are excluded from the CNS because of their quaternary ammonium constituents. The fact that these drugs may still produce behavioral arousal responses is probably the result of their peripheral influences, which lead to changes in sensory inputs conducted to the brain by visceral afferent fibers.

Absorption, Fate, and Excretion
All the above cholinergic receptor agonists are absorbed after administration by both oral and parenteral routes, although the absorption of the quaternary ammonium compounds from the gastrointestinal tract is likely to be unpredictable. Parenteral administration of the choline esters must be carried out with extreme caution because of the profound effects they may have on cholinergic effectors. ACh is rapidly destroyed by AChE and pseudocholinesterase and exerts an effect measured in seconds if given by bolus intravenous injection. Methacholine, more slowly metabolized than ACh by AChE and immune to pseudocholinesterase, is therefore longer in duration of action. Carbachol and bethanechol are, for all practical purposes, not affected by the cholinesterases, so they have a much longer duration of action and the potential for producing widespread and prolonged cholinergic effects.

Pilocarpine is well absorbed after oral, subcutaneous, or topical administration. It also gains ready access to the CNS, and it is well distributed through the tissues and organs of the body. A large fraction is excreted unchanged by the kidneys. Cevimeline is also well absorbed after oral administration, with peak blood concentrations occurring in 1.5 to 2 hours. Most of the drug is metabolized to sulfoxides and glucuronic acid conjugates, with an elimination half-life of about 5 hours.

Adverse Effects
In general, adverse reactions to the cholinomimetic drugs are predictable consequences of the stimulation of cholinergic receptors. Patients with increased risk of adverse responses include those with asthma, cardiovascular disease, and peptic ulcer. Untoward reactions may include a response profile that many autonomic pharmacologists refer to as the SLUD response (*s*alivation, *l*acrimation, *u*rination, and *d*efecation). In addition to the SLUD response, muscarinic receptor agonists can produce bronchospasm, hypotension, and arrhythmias. Hypertensive responses to pilocarpine and cevimeline may occur with parenteral injection of large doses; this seemingly atypical effect is the result of sympathetic ganglionic stimulation caused by activation of excitatory muscarinic receptors

on postganglionic neurons. Intravenous and intramuscular injection is generally avoided because of the increased possibility for producing cardiopulmonary reactions; toxic reactions in general are reduced by the restricted and often topical use of these agents.

The mushrooms *Amanita pantherina* and *A. muscaria* contain muscarine but in amounts that are probably too small to account for the symptoms of poisoning that result from their ingestion. On the other hand, the mushroom *Inocybe lateraria*, with a much higher muscarine content, produces signs and symptoms of intoxication that resemble those produced by muscarine. These include profuse salivation and sweating; miosis; bradycardia; severe abdominal pain with vomiting, cramps, and diarrhea; and respiratory difficulties arising from the constriction of bronchial muscle and increased secretion in the respiratory tract. The onset of poisoning is rapid, and treatment consists of the administration of atropine in large quantities, gastric lavage, and appropriate supportive measures. Recovery usually takes place in 1 or 2 days. In many cases of mushroom poisoning, there are delayed symptoms, including violent emesis and diarrhea and damage to parenchymatous organs (principally the liver), which are not amenable to atropine treatment and are produced by a group of cyclopeptide toxins from the mushroom that inhibit the synthesis of messenger ribonucleic acid.[2]

ANTICHOLINESTERASES

Anticholinesterases are drugs that stimulate cholinergic transmission indirectly by inhibiting the enzyme AChE, which hydrolyzes and inactivates ACh in the synaptic clefts of the autonomic nervous system, the CNS, and the neuromuscular junction of the somatic nervous system. Agents in this class derive their pharmacologic effects from their ability to prolong the life of ACh at receptor sites. These cholinesterase inhibitors are sometimes referred to as *indirect-acting* cholinergic drugs.

Anticholinesterases can be subclassified as either *reversible* or *irreversible* cholinesterase inhibitors. Reversible inhibitors (e.g., edrophonium, neostigmine, and physostigmine) temporarily inactivate the enzyme by forming noncovalent associations with the enzyme or covalent bonds that are readily hydrolyzed. Irreversible cholinesterase inhibitors (organophosphates) inactivate the enzyme by forming a permanent covalent bond with the enzyme.

Physostigmine, or eserine, the earliest known anticholinesterase, has a colorful history. An alkaloid, it is derived from a bean, or nut, known as the Calabar, ordeal, or Esére bean, and it was used in witchcraft trials by certain native tribes in West Africa. The bean was brought to England by a British medical officer stationed in Calabar in the mid-1800s, and its pharmacologic properties were investigated in a number of laboratories, including those of Fraser, who studied its toxicity in the 1860s and noted that its actions were antagonized by atropine.[39] As early as 1877, physostigmine was used for the treatment of glaucoma, which remains one of its principal uses today. In 1914, noting the extreme brevity of the action of ACh, Dale[7] suggested that an enzyme capable of destroying ACh must exist in the body, and in 1930 it was found that physostigmine could prevent the rapid destruction of ACh.[11]

By the 1930s, the chemical structure of physostigmine had been elucidated,[1,47] a series of synthetic analogues had been synthesized, and several researchers had reported independently that the derivative neostigmine was effective in the treatment of myasthenia gravis.[41,53] Until the basic mechanism of neurohumoral transmission was elucidated, however, it was not understood that these drugs acted therapeutically as anticholinesterases.

The first organophosphate anticholinesterase was actually synthesized in 1854, before physostigmine was known, by de Clermont, who made and tasted tetraethyl pyrophosphate (and survived to record the fact). Modern interest in these compounds did not begin, though, until 1932 when Lange and von Krueger[30] synthesized some compounds with a phosphorofluoride linkage and gave a remarkable description of the pharmacologic properties of this group of chemicals. Lange believed that these compounds would prove useful as insecticides, and he offered them to the I.G. Farben Company in Germany. It was some years before this company took an active interest, but they soon realized the potential of these compounds as chemical warfare agents. The manufacture of nerve gas began in Germany in 1940. Related investigations were being carried out in England at the same time, and in the United States diisopropyl fluorophosphate was being studied during World War II. (This agent has been given the official name of *isoflurophate.*) Two compounds developed by the Germans, tabun and sarin, are among the most toxic nerve gases known. Of the thousands of organophosphates that have been tested, several dozen are widely available as insecticides, and a number of others have military implications as lethal nerve gases.[20]

Chemistry and Classification

Reversible anticholinesterases include the truly reversible nonester quaternary ammonium compounds and the esters of carbamic acid, which react covalently with the enzyme surface. The carbamoylated enzyme is regenerated by hydrolysis in about 30 minutes; the continued presence of the anticholinesterase yields a duration of action of several hours. The reversible anticholinesterases may be classified as simple quaternary ammonium compounds (edrophonium) or carbamate ester derivatives, including tertiary amines (physostigmine), quaternary amines (neostigmine), and bisquaternary amines (ambenonium). Three representative reversible anticholinesterases are shown in Figure 8-4.

Irreversible anticholinesterases are organophosphates that result in a phosphorylated enzyme not significantly regenerated by hydrolysis. They have limited therapeutic value but are of great toxicologic significance. Four examples include (1) isoflurophate, the best known and studied compound of this class; (2) malathion, a widely used insecticide; (3) echothiophate, one of the first compounds in this class to have a therapeutic application; and (4) tabun, one of the most potent and toxic nerve gases. Structures of several irreversible anticholinesterases are given in Figure 8-5. The anticholinesterases are classified according to their use in Table 8-1.

Mechanism of Action

In Chapter 5 it is pointed out that AChE hydrolyzes ACh with great rapidity, that the enzyme is localized in the region of the receptor, and that it acts most efficiently when ACh is present in low concentrations. There is also a nonspecific plasma cholinesterase, or pseudocholinesterase (butyrylcholinesterase), that has a greater affinity for butyric esters than for acetyl esters and is more effective when the concentration of ACh and other esters is high.[39]

AChE is composed of protein units that have an individual molecular weight of 70,000 daltons. The enzyme exists in synaptic plasma membranes in the form of simple oligomers (single units, dimers, and tetramers). A much larger configuration, present in the outer basal lamina of the synapse (and especially evident in the neuromuscular junction), has tetramers of the catalytic unit attached to a collagen-like

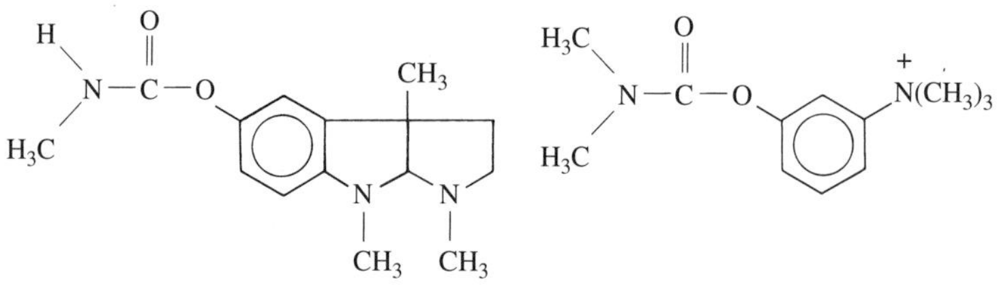

Physostigmine

Neostigmine

Fig. 8-4 Representative reversible anticholinesterases.

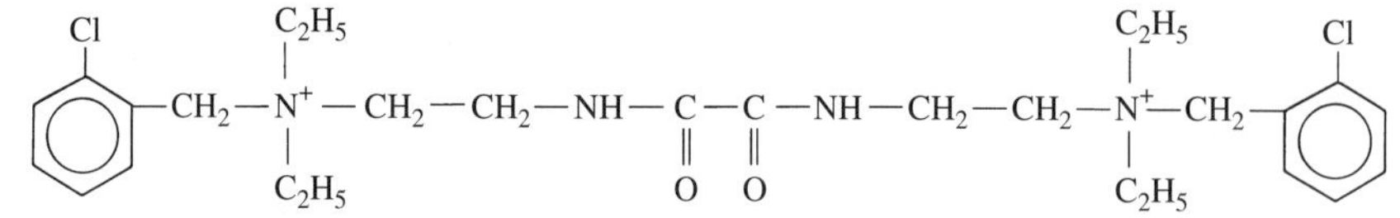

Ambenonium

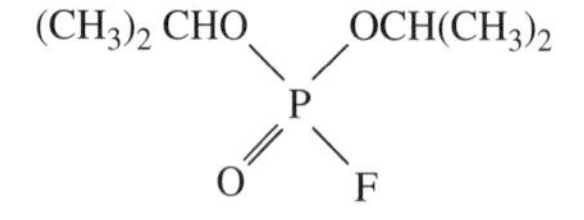

Isoflurophate

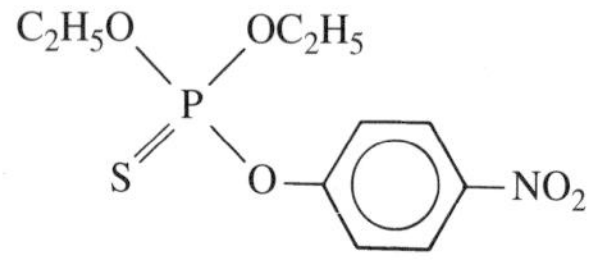

Parathion

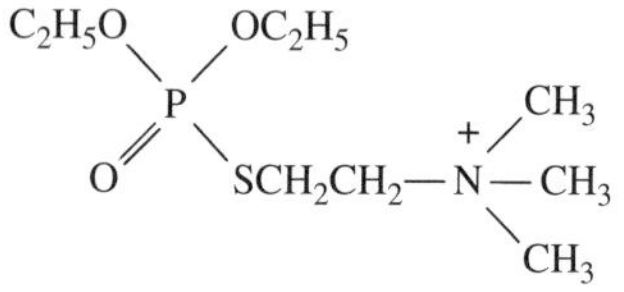

Echothiophate

Fig. 8-5 Representative irreversible anticholinesterases.

Table • 8-1

Some Anticholinesterases and Their Uses

USE	DRUGS
Treatment of glaucoma	Demecarium, echothiophate, physostigmine
Treatment of myasthenia gravis	Ambenonium, edrophonium*, neostigmine, pyridostigmine
Treatment of Alzheimer's disease	Donepezil, rivastigmine, tacrine
Reversal of nondepolarizing muscle relaxants	Edrophonium, neostigmine, pyridostigmine
Nerve gas	Sarin, soman, tabun
Insecticides (organophosphates)	Malathion, paraoxon, parathion
Insecticides (carbamates)	Aldicarb, carbaryl, propoxur

*Diagnostic purposes only.

structure through disulfide linkages to yield a filament 50 nm in length and weighing 10^6 daltons.[35]

The ACh molecule reacts with the enzyme AChE at two primary sites; these sites are shown, with ACh and several anticholinesterases, in Figure 8-6. AChE is depicted as having a choline-binding site, to which the quaternary ammonium portion of the ACh molecule is attracted, and an esteratic site, with an affinity for the ester portion of the molecule.[49] It is at the esteratic site that the ACh molecule is split, leaving the acetylated enzyme, which is rapidly regenerated by combination with water. The organophosphate anticholinesterases have an affinity chiefly for the esteratic site of the AChE molecule. They produce a very stable covalent attachment; indeed, there is virtually no hydrolysis with many of these compounds, and cholinesterase activity remains depressed until new enzyme is synthesized. Because enzyme turnover may take several weeks, the organophosphates are referred to as *irreversible* in action. The anticholinesterase agents that enjoy the greatest therapeutic use are those drugs, like neostigmine and physostigmine, that interact strongly with both binding sites of the receptor. As with the organophosphates, attachment of such drugs to the serine residue at the esteratic site is achieved by a covalent linkage. This bond is subject to hydrolysis, however, and these drugs are categorized as *reversible* cholinesterase inhibitors. The simplest quaternary anticholinesterase, edrophonium (see Figure 8-6), binds AChE in a noncovalent manner. Its inhibition is rapidly reversible, making it useful for situations requiring a short duration of

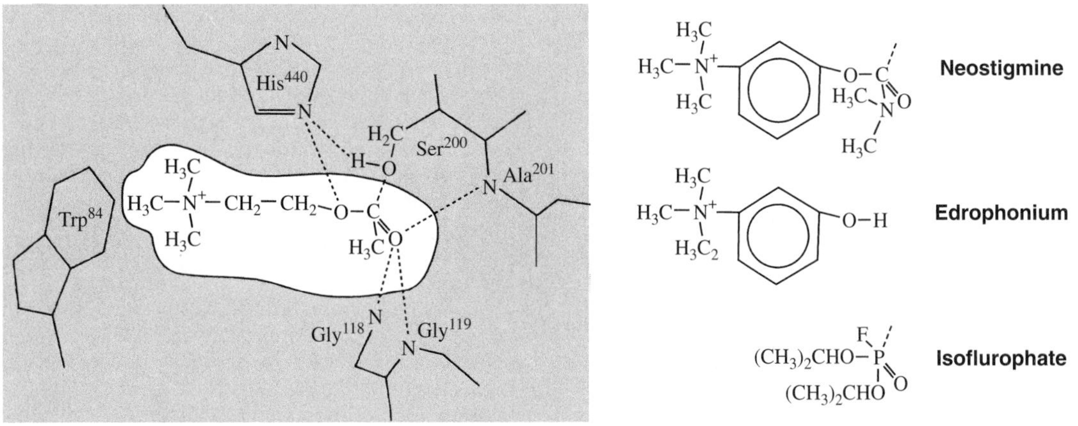

Fig. 8-6 Interaction between ACh and three anticholinesterases with AChE. The positive charge of the quaternary ammonium group of ACh is attracted to the choline-binding site of AChE by the π electrons of surrounding aromatic amino acids, including the tryptophan *(Trp*[84]*)* shown in the illustration. Hydrophobic interactions strengthen the binding of the choline moiety. A covalent attachment occurs with the serine *(Ser*[200]*)* residue at the esteratic site. As a result, choline is split off and the enzyme is briefly acetylated before spontaneous hydrolysis frees the enzyme. Nitrogen from nearby amino acids participates in this process by forming hydrogen bonds with the acetate group. Neostigmine mimics ACh in its binding to AChE; however, the carbamoyl group is not as easily removed from the esteratic site. Edrophonium binds primarily to the choline-binding site but also participates in a hydrogen bond with the histidine *(His*[440]*)* nitrogen of the esteratic site. The organophosphate isoflurophate reacts only at the esteratic site, where it creates a stable covalent bond. (Adapted from Sussman JL, Harel M, Frolow F, et al: Atomic structure of acetylcholinesterase from *Torpedo californica:* a prototypic acetylcholine-binding protein, *Science* 253:872-879, 1991.)

action, such as for diagnostic purposes. The terms *reversible* and *irreversible,* it should be noted, connote differences in duration of effect, not necessarily in site of attachment.

The anticholinesterases, whether reversible or irreversible, owe their pharmacologic effects chiefly to the fact that they prolong the life of ACh at sites where it is a mediator. Thus their actions are often identical with those of ACh, although much more prolonged and, in most cases, completely dependent on the presence of endogenous ACh in the area of the effector. For this reason, most of the anticholinesterases are ineffective in denervated organs. Exceptions to this generalization are the quaternary ammonium compounds such as neostigmine and pyridostigmine and the bisquaternary amine ambenonium that have direct actions on cholinergic sites, either stimulating the effectors or blocking transmission. Neostigmine, for example, is capable of direct stimulation of the neuromuscular junction and is effective on denervated skeletal muscle. Its pharmacology is therefore the result of a combination of anticholinesterase and cholinomimetic properties.

Pharmacologic Effects

The cholinesterase inhibitors produce muscarinic effects similar to those elicited by the direct-acting cholinergic agonists (described above and outlined in Chapter 5). These effects are mediated by increasing the concentration of ACh at the autonomic neuroeffector junction and skeletal muscle neuromuscular junction. The activity of the anticholinesterases is greatest for those organs that receive more or less continuous cholinergic nerve stimulation. As a result, their effects are seen first in the smooth muscles of various ocular structures, the gastrointestinal tract, and the urinary bladder.

An important disparity in action between anticholinesterases and direct-acting muscarinic drugs is that the former do not cause significant muscarinic receptor–mediated vasodilation because many blood vessels receive no parasympathetic innervation, and thus no ACh is available to be protected against hydrolysis. Instead, vascular effects of high doses of anticholinesterases are largely mediated through their effects on autonomic ganglia and on medullary vasomotor centers. (The latter case occurs primarily with physostigmine, which is not permanently charged and can penetrate the blood-brain barrier.) Cholinesterase inhibitors stimulate, and in high doses subsequently block, both N_N and N_M receptors indirectly by increasing the synaptic concentrations of ACh at ganglionic and neuromuscular sites. Hypotensive responses can then arise from blockade of sympathetic ganglia. Quaternary cholinesterase inhibitors such as neostigmine are also able to directly stimulate N_M receptors and, to a lesser extent, N_N receptors.

As is the case with cholinomimetic alkaloids, the anticholinesterases are also known to evoke CNS actions. The CNS effects that are seen in anticholinesterase poisoning—confusion, ataxia, respiratory abnormalities, convulsions, coma, and death from respiratory paralysis—provide powerful evidence that cholinergic receptors play an important role in central neurotransmission. As pointed out in Chapter 5, there are both muscarinic and nicotinic receptors in the CNS; to which subtypes these receptors belong is not currently known. As already mentioned, quaternary ammonium compounds penetrate biologic membranes poorly, so anticholinesterases that contain a quaternary ammonium group (such as neostigmine or edrophonium) are poorly absorbed after oral administration and do not readily pass through the blood-brain barrier. Predictably, they are quite effective at skeletal neuromuscular junctions but have no CNS effects.

Absorption, Fate, and Excretion

Physostigmine is readily absorbed after oral, subcutaneous, and topical administration, and it is destroyed principally through hydrolysis at the ester linkage by plasma esterases, including pseudocholinesterase. The other reversible cholinesterases listed in this chapter, such as neostigmine and pyridostigmine, are quaternary ammonium compounds, which means that they pass through biologic membranes with difficulty. Some of these compounds are broken down by esterases or hepatic microsomal enzymes. Both they and their metabolites appear in the urine.

The organophosphate anticholinesterases, with the exception of echothiophate, are highly lipid soluble, and they are rapidly absorbed from the gastrointestinal tract, the skin and mucous membranes, and the lungs. These characteristics explain their potential toxicity when used as aerosols, dusts, vapors, or liquids. Most of the organophosphates are metabolized by A-esterases (paraoxonases) in the plasma and liver and by microsomal oxidation; for a few drugs, enzymatic transformation results in a more toxic product than the original compound.[37] In the case of isoflurophate, approximately 80% of the drug is metabolized and excreted in the urine and feces during the first 24 hours, and approximately 20% remains protein bound in the tissues for a prolonged period.

Adverse Effects

In human beings, intoxication from anticholinesterases has resulted from overdosage with drugs used in the treatment of myasthenia gravis (MG) and from exposure to toxic amounts of organophosphate in insecticides or chemical warfare agents.[20] Organophosphate insecticides have gained wide use in many countries, and thousands of cases of poisoning are attributable to these compounds, especially parathion. Most of the organophosphates are volatile liquids at ordinary temperatures and are highly lipid soluble. They are readily absorbed through the skin, the respiratory tract, the gastrointestinal tract, and the eyes. The symptomatology of anticholinesterase poisoning reflects the role of ACh as a neuromediator at muscarinic and nicotinic receptors located both peripherally and in the CNS. In high doses, the reversible anticholinesterases can produce the same symptoms as the irreversible anticholinesterases; the chief difference between these two groups lies in the ready access to the circulation and the longer duration of action of the irreversible anticholinesterases.

The first signs and symptoms to appear, especially after local exposure through aerosols, vapor, or dust, are an intense miosis, an inability to accommodate for far vision, severe rhinorrhea, and a frontal headache attributable to ciliary muscle spasm. The respiratory tract is also affected very soon after exposure. In addition to the watery nasal discharge, there is nasal hyperemia, a sensation of tightness in the chest, probably because of bronchoconstriction, and increased bronchial secretion. Audible wheezing may follow, related to both the bronchoconstriction and the hypersecretion. Laryngospasm may occur because of the secretory activity, which triggers a reflex spasm of laryngeal muscle. In fact, respiration can be severely and very rapidly compromised. Other manifestations of muscarinic stimulation include such gastrointestinal effects as salivation, anorexia, nausea, vomiting, severe cramps, diarrhea, and even involuntary defecation. There is also sweating, lacrimation, bradycardia, urinary frequency, and involuntary micturition.

With the onset of muscarinic effects, various nicotinic effects also become apparent. The affected individual shows easy fatigability and generalized weakness, especially on exertion. Involuntary muscle twitching, fasciculations, and muscle cramps follow; then generalized muscle weakness, including the muscles of respiration, increases in severity. Respiratory movements become more shallow and rapid, and respiratory failure may take place in a matter of minutes unless artificial respiration is instituted. It should be remembered that respiration is also greatly hampered by the constriction of the airway and the intense secretory activity in the respiratory tract. Sympathetic ganglia may be stimulated and later blocked in moderate to severe intoxication, but this usually does not pose a life-threatening problem. Finally, there are outstanding CNS manifestations that start with tension, restlessness, and jitteriness and progress to confusion and ataxia, coma, disappearance of reflexes, Cheyne-Stokes respirations, and finally generalized convulsions. The cause of death is respiratory failure resulting from paralysis of the muscles of respiration, central depression of respiration, and airway obstruction. Box 8-1 summarizes the signs of poisoning with the anticholinesterases according to muscarinic, nicotinic, and CNS effects.

The treatment of acute intoxication with an organophosphate should include the following actions:

1. Remove the victim from the source of contamination, or remove the organophosphate-containing contaminant.
2. Administer atropine in very large doses. Atropine does not relieve the neuromuscular blockade produced by these agents, but it does alleviate the effects of excessive

Box • 8-1

Some Manifestations of Overdosage with Anticholinesterases

MUSCARINIC EFFECTS (PERIPHERAL)	NICOTINIC EFFECTS* (PERIPHERAL)	CNS EFFECTS
Miosis, frontal headache (brow ache), conjunctival hyperemia, blurred vision	Muscular weakness, twitching, fasciculations	Restlessness, giddiness, tension, anxiety, nausea
Rhinorrhea, nasal hyperemia	Tachycardia	Tremors, electroencephalographic changes
Lacrimation, salivation, sweating	Elevation or depression of blood pressure	Confusion, ataxia, convulsions
Increased bronchial secretions, tightness of chest, bronchoconstriction, wheezing	Death from respiratory failure	Depression of respiratory and circulatory centers, cyanosis, coma, respiratory and circulatory collapse
Anorexia, nausea, vomiting, cramps, diarrhea, involuntary defecation		Death from respiratory failure
Urinary urgency, involuntary micturition		
Bradycardia, hypotension		

* Nicotinic effects include both stimulation and inhibition of synaptic or junctional transmission.

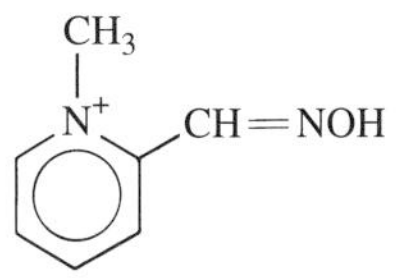

CH_3 / N^+ / $CH{=}NOH$

Fig. 8-7 Structural formula of pralidoxime.

muscarinic receptor stimulation, including many of the CNS manifestations of poisoning. Repeated, often very large doses may be required.
3. Maintain the airway and administer artificial respiration.
4. Inject a benzodiazepine such as diazepam if atropine fails to relieve the convulsions.
5. Administer pralidoxime. This drug is one of several oximes that were synthesized in the 1950s as cholinesterase reactivators.

Once the mechanism of organophosphate poisoning was fully understood, it became possible to conceptualize a molecule that could reverse the inhibition of AChE. It was reasoned that by attaching a nucleophilic group to a cationic quaternary nitrogen group at a proper atomic distance, the phosphorus group of the alkyl phosphate would be attacked and would be removed from AChE in a displacement reaction. It was further reasoned that the cationic group of this ideal molecule would be attracted to the choline-binding site and the nucleophilic atom would be directed toward the phosphorus atom.[55] A number of compounds were synthesized, and one of the most potent was pralidoxime, the structure of which is shown in Figure 8-7. Intravenous administration of the oximes produces a remarkably rapid reactivation of the AChE at neuromuscular junctions in which transmission has failed as a result of poisoning with irreversible anticholinesterases. The reactivation occurs within minutes, but the effect of the oximes is much less dramatic at muscarinic sites and, with few exceptions, negligible in the CNS because many of the reactivators are quaternary compounds and cannot pass the blood-brain barrier. Also, the oximes are most effective when given immediately after exposure to the organophosphate, because a process of "aging" of the phosphorylated AChE complex makes the enzyme resistant to reactivation. Therapeutic use of pralidoxime and its congeners is reserved for cases of intoxication with the irreversible anticholinesterases.

In some instances of organophosphate poisoning, the acute cholinergic phase may be followed by delayed peripheral neuropathy. Two types have been described. One appears 2 to 5 weeks after exposure to the organophosphate and involves phosphorylation and inhibition of an enzyme called *neurotoxic esterase.* The second neuropathy, called an *intermediate syndrome,* has been reported in approximately 10% of patients recently treated for organophosphate poisoning and appears 24 to 96 hours after exposure.[45] This condition, which is unresponsive to atropine and pralidoxime, involves the proximal limb muscles, neck flexors, certain cranial nerves, and the muscles of respiration. These patients require respiratory support, and several have died of respiratory failure. It is theorized that the intermediate syndrome may be caused by contamination of the organophosphate or an interaction of the organophosphate with some other pesticides.

GENERAL THERAPEUTIC USES

ACh itself has had very little therapeutic application because of the extreme brevity of its action. The synthesis of congeners has solved the duration problem and in addition resulted in drugs with more selective actions. Although these compounds have limited use in contemporary therapeutics, the choline esters and the alkaloid pilocarpine are still used for some important purposes, as are the reversible anticholinesterases. The irreversible anticholinesterases are principally used as laboratory tools, as insecticides, and therapeutically for ophthalmologic purposes.

Glaucoma

Glaucoma is the name given to a group of diseases characterized by an elevation of intraocular pressure (IOP), a progressive atrophy of the optic disk, and a gradual loss in the field of vision. The aqueous humor is produced in the ciliary epithelium, passes into the posterior chamber, and then through the pupil into the anterior chamber. It leaves the eye by two pathways in the anterior chamber angle. In the first, the aqueous humor passes through the trabecular meshwork across the inner wall of Schlemm's canal and then into the venous circulation. In the second route, called the *uveoscleral pathway,* aqueous humor flows across the iris and anterior face of the ciliary muscle and ultimately exits through the sclera. Most forms of glaucoma result from an interference with the drainage from the trabecular meshwork or from closure of the angle by the iris.

Glaucoma is classified as primary, secondary, or congenital, based on characteristics and etiology. Of the primary types, open-angle (wide-angle, chronic simple) glaucoma and narrow-angle (angle-closure, acute congestive) glaucoma are the most common. In open-angle glaucoma, outflow resistance is elevated because there is a disturbance in the trabecular meshwork that may represent an exaggeration of normal aging.[14] The disease is slowly progressive, chronic, and often insidious because irrevocable damage can be done to the visual apparatus before symptoms develop. Narrow-angle glaucoma is usually, as its other name *acute congestive glaucoma* suggests, a medical emergency, triggered by an acute elevation of IOP, usually because iris-lens contact has obstructed the outflow of aqueous humor from the posterior to the anterior chamber. The secondary glaucoma types are associated with various systemic or ocular diseases, trauma, or drugs.

Therapy in glaucoma is directed at stimulating the musculature of the iris and ciliary body, increasing the facility of outflow of aqueous humor, reducing its formation, or extracting liquid from the eye. Although historically the cholinergic agents (in this application called *miotics*) have been the initial and principal drugs used in the treatment of chronic open-angle glaucoma, a number of other drugs (Table 8-2) are currently used, either alone or in conjunction with the cholinergic miotics.[24,38] There is also interest in the use of cannabinoids in the treatment of glaucoma because of the beneficial effects on glaucoma from cannabinoid receptor agonists.

Pilocarpine is the miotic most commonly used for initial and maintenance therapy in primary open-angle glaucoma and other chronic forms of glaucoma. Like other cholinergic drugs, it lowers IOP by decreasing resistance to aqueous humor outflow and is usually effective without adjunctive medication. It is available for topical administration in various solutions, combined with physostigmine or epinephrine, in a long-acting gel formulation, or in a drug-delivery system that is placed in the cul-de-sac of the eye and provides sustained delivery of the drug over a period of approximately 7 days. Carbachol, a slightly longer-acting drug, is also used in chronic open-angle glaucoma, especially when intolerance or resistance to pilocarpine has developed. Physostigmine is quite effective in the short- and long-term maintenance of open-angle glaucoma, secondary glaucoma, and acute congestive glaucoma. Its effects last from 12 to 36 hours, and, like pilocarpine and carbachol, it is classified as a short-acting miotic.

Table • 8-2

Some Drugs Used in the Treatment of Glaucoma

CLASS	DRUGS
Cholinergic Receptor Agonists	Carbachol, pilocarpine
Anticholinesterases	
Short-acting	Physostigmine
Long-acting	Demecarium, echothiophate
Adrenergic Receptor Agonists	
α And β agonist	Epinephrine
Prodrug	Dipivefrin
α_2 Agonist	Apraclonidine, brimonidine
β-Adrenergic Receptor Antagonists	
Nonselective	Carteolol, levobunolol, metipranolol, timolol
β_1 Selective	Betaxolol
Other Drugs	
Prostaglandin $F_{2\alpha}$ analogues	Bimatoprost, latanoprost, travoprost, unoprostone
Carbonic anhydrase inhibitors	Acetazolamide, brinzolamide, dorzolamide
Osmotic agents	Glycerin, isosorbide, mannitol
Combination products	Dorzolamide and timolol; pilocarpine and epinephrine

The long-acting miotics—the anticholinesterases demecarium, echothiophate, and isoflurophate—are used for patients with chronic open-angle glaucoma who are refractory to the short-acting miotics and the other conventionally used drugs. These agents are quite potent and are administered in the lowest possible concentrations. Long-term administration (6 months or more) has been associated with the development of cataracts and, rarely, retinal detachment. These adverse effects clearly limit their usefulness in the long-term therapy of glaucoma.

Xerostomia

Xerostomia can occur at any age but it is most often seen in the elderly population. However, xerostomia is not inevitable with aging. In fact, age-related decreases in salivary gland production are not the reason many older people have dry mouth. Dry mouth may result from several causes, including radiation to the salivary glands, therapy with antineoplastic agents, disease (e.g., Sjögren's syndrome), and treatment with a variety of drugs more common in the older population. Saliva serves several functions in protecting the oral cavity.[13,32] Adequate saliva volume is required for cleaning the teeth and cleansing the oral cavity. Buffers in saliva reduce the effect of acids. Proteins, including mucins, aid in mineralization of dental enamel; reduce wear on the teeth by providing lubrication; have antibacterial, antiviral, and antifungal properties; and provide growth factors for tissue repair.[9,32] It is clear that reduced salivary flow rate, which is a major (but not the only) cause of the perception of dry mouth, is a risk factor for oral disease. Xerostomia can be insupportably uncomfortable and is known to be associated with increased caries; oral pain; increased oral infection; and difficulty speaking, chewing, and swallowing.[32-34] Both pilocarpine and cevimeline have been approved for the treatment of xerostomia in subjects with functional salivary gland tissue.[15]

A 5- to 10-mg dose of pilocarpine elicits significant increases in parotid, submandibular, and sublingual secretion, with maximal flow rates being achieved in 30 minutes and a return to basal rates in approximately 3 hours.[16] The drug is usually given three times daily. The saliva-stimulating effect depends on residual salivary gland function. Generally, at these doses, there is no significant effect on blood pressure, heart rate, or cardiac function. Sweating is a common side effect; chills, nausea, and dizziness have also been reported.[27] Cevimeline is a selective M_1 and M_3 muscarinic receptor agonist also used for the treatment of xerostomia. Because of its receptor preference, this drug is reported to have fewer adverse effects than pilocarpine; however, clinical studies have not been carried out to confirm this claim. It is administered at a dose of 30 mg three times daily. The dentist must carefully determine whether muscarinic receptor agonists should be used to treat dry mouth. Therapy for xerostomia must not compromise other therapy the patient may be receiving. Moreover, risk factors for muscarinic receptor agonists need to be considered.

Oral fluids, including saliva substitutes, may be added for the relief of dry mouth and should be substituted for pilocarpine and cevimeline if the drugs are not well tolerated, in patients with uncontrolled asthma, and where there is a complete loss of salivary function.

Reversal of Neuromuscular Block

The use of reversible anticholinesterases to terminate the neuromuscular block of curarelike drugs in general anesthesia is covered in Chapter 10.

Myasthenia Gravis

MG is a disease characterized by weakness and easy fatigability of the skeletal muscles, particularly ocular and oropharyngeal muscles, and by marked variations in severity of symptoms even in the course of a single day. It is thought that there are approximately 30,000 cases in the United States, with two peaks of age incidence: in the twenties for women and in the fifties for men. Approximately 10% of patients die from the disease. There is also a neonatal form of MG that tends to be transient. Although the disease was described more than 300 years ago, the underlying mechanisms and suitable treatment were unclear until two investigators, Remen in 1932[41] and Walker in 1934,[53] unknown to each other, administered neostigmine to patients with MG and reported relief of symptoms.

The typical patient with MG initially has ocular complaints—double vision and/or ptosis—and difficulty in chewing and swallowing. Later, dyspnea and other respiratory problems may arise. Approximately 10% of myasthenic patients have a tumor of the thymus, and approximately 75% have some abnormality of the thymus. At least 30% of patients with an enlarged thymus have a remission of myasthenic symptoms after thymectomy. Since the work of Remen and Walker, it has been accepted that the defect in MG is probably at the neuromuscular junction, and one of the early findings was that the synaptic vesicles of the myasthenic patient appeared to contain less than normal amounts of ACh. Other investigators showed that although synaptic vesicle diameter is unaltered, the mean nerve terminal area and the postsynaptic membrane are abnormally simple, with clefts that are sparse, shallow, wide, or absent.[44] The favorable response of some patients to thymectomy and certain features of the muscle response in MG have led to the hypothesis that the condition results from an autoimmune phenomenon, an idea that was given a solid basis by the demonstration in rabbits that injection of highly purified receptor protein from the electric eel results in the production of a precipitating antibody specific for the ACh receptor (AChR).[40] Later it was shown that rats immunized with eel electroplax AChR protein develop a myastheniälike syndrome and that, as a result of such immunization, AChRs degenerate.[28] A similar alteration of AChRs was induced in mice by the injection of immunoglobulin from myasthenic patients[46,51] whose blood had been shown to contain receptor-binding antibodies. Experimental autoimmune MG is characterized, then, by simplified postsynaptic membrane structures, high concentrations of anti-AChR antibodies in the serum, binding of antibodies to most AChR in the muscle, and reduction of the AChR content to approximately 30% of normal.

MG is currently viewed as an autoimmune disorder in which there is continuous production of antibody to the AChR at the neuromuscular junction.[10] The primary defect in MG is loss of AChR through accelerated destruction of receptors and without a concomitant increase in rate of synthesis, and by complement-mediated focal lysis of the postsynaptic membrane.

Treatment for MG is now fairly standardized. Diagnosis is made on the basis of an elevated titer of AChR antibodies or an improvement in muscle strength after the intravenous or intramuscular injection of edrophonium, a short-acting anticholinesterase. After a positive diagnosis, four methods of treatment are available. In the first, one of three reversible anticholinesterases (neostigmine, pyridostigmine, or ambenonium) is used to enhance neuromuscular transmission. Thymectomy constitutes a second therapeutic alternative and is especially indicated in patients with thymomas. Plasmapheresis to remove offending antibodies is an effective, albeit temporary, third modality. Finally, immunosuppression has proved to be a very successful fourth therapeutic approach. Adrenal corticosteroids (e.g., prednisone or, for the hospitalized patient, adrenocorticotropic hormone) and azathioprine have provided relief in a substantial percentage of cases. Cyclosporine was also effective in a number of patients whose condition could not be adequately controlled with anticholinesterases.[5]

Treatment with immunosuppressive drugs is attended by undesirable side effects. With azathioprine, toxic effects on the gastrointestinal and hematologic systems are most common, with prominent nausea, vomiting, and abdominal discomfort in the first months. Cyclosporine use is associated with nephrotoxicity, as well as transient diarrhea, gingival pain, nausea, and headaches.

Therapy with an anticholinesterase is likely to be complicated by side effects resulting from the accumulation of ACh at cholinergic receptor sites. Some of these effects are characteristically muscarinic—abdominal cramps, diarrhea, sweating, salivation, lacrimation—and can be well controlled by the administration of atropine and related drugs. Other side effects, such as muscle fasciculations and CNS symptoms, are not controllable by the muscarinic blocking drugs and may be warning signs of an impending cholinergic crisis, which results from overdosage with the anticholinesterases. Cholinergic crisis is characterized by muscle weakness, particularly of the respiratory muscles, resulting from persistent depolarization of the neuromuscular junction. Cholinergic crisis closely resembles myasthenic crisis, the latter of which may come about because of inadequate medication, and it is urgently necessary in such patients to determine quickly which of the two conditions exists. This can be done by giving, with great caution and with resuscitation equipment immediately available, a very low dose of edrophonium. If the symptoms are relieved, the problem is myasthenic weakness; if muscle strength decreases, cholinergic crisis is established.

Antidote for Atropine Poisoning

All the cholinergic drugs with muscarinic properties should theoretically be useful in antagonizing the effects of atropine, but the most effective drugs for this purpose are the anticholinesterases, and the drug of choice is physostigmine. When the diagnosis of atropine poisoning is confirmed, physostigmine is administered intravenously, and it rapidly relieves the delirium and coma.[43] Neostigmine and other quaternary ammonium compounds are of limited use because they are incapable of counteracting the CNS effects of atropine.

A number of psychotropic agents (e.g., tricyclic antidepressants, phenothiazines, and antihistamines) share to varying degrees the antimuscarinic effects of atropine. Particularly when used in combination (for intravenous sedation or for other reasons), these agents may induce a central anticholinergic syndrome consisting of confusion, delirium, hallucination, and psychotic behavior. Intravenous physostigmine in doses of 0.5 to 2 mg is effective in reversing this syndrome. Inasmuch as the duration of action of parenteral physostigmine is 1 to 2 hours, repeated administrations may be necessary to avoid recurrence of the syndrome.

Paralytic Ileus and Bladder Atony

After abdominal and pelvic surgery, there is often a failure of normal peristalsis that leads to postoperative abdominal distention and discomfort. Neostigmine has been used to advantage in the treatment of this condition, as has bethanechol, which is preferred to other choline esters because of its reduced cardiac effect.

Bladder atony also follows surgery and sometimes parturition. It leads to urinary retention and is treated with bethanechol, neostigmine, or sometimes pilocarpine.

Senile Dementias of the Alzheimer Type

Alzheimer's disease and related senile dementias are progressive neuropsychiatric diseases and represent the fourth major cause of death in the developed world. Alzheimer's disease is manifested by memory loss and usually terminates in death from some debilitating condition in approximately a decade. Although the cause of Alzheimer's disease remains an active area of investigation, the dementia appears to be a form of amyloid encephalopathy resulting from the deposition of the protein β-amyloid in selective regions of the CNS.[22,23] The deposition of this protein causes the formation of neuritic plaques, neuronal cell death, and loss of several different neurotransmitters important in cognition and memory. One central neurochemical affected by Alzheimer's disease, especially early in the course of the illness, is ACh.

Deficits in ACh and in choline acetyltransferase, the enzyme responsible for the formation of ACh from choline and acetyl coenzyme A, have been identified in the brains of Alzheimer's patients.[6,8] The identification of these deficiencies suggested a treatment strategy for Alzheimer's disease analogous to that used in the pharmacologic therapy of Parkinson's disease, namely, replacement of the missing (in this case cholinergic) agonist.[18,19] In fact, early experiments with physostigmine showed some transient, if variable, improvement.[50] The AChE inhibitors that are used to treat Alzheimer's disease easily penetrate the blood-brain barrier. Tacrine, a longer-acting reversible anticholinesterase is approved for palliative treatment of mild to moderate forms of Alzheimer's disease. Potential benefits of tacrine therapy include improved memory, cognition, and general affect. The long-term oral administration of this drug to patients in the middle and late stages of Alzheimer's disease has provided mixed results, with some studies reporting improvement[12,29,48] and others finding no significant benefit compared with placebo or no treatment.[31,36] Tacrine is also capable of producing significant, although reversible, hepatotoxicity at therapeutic doses. Donepezil, a newer piperidine anticholinesterase indicated for patients with Alzheimer's disease, appears to be better tolerated than tacrine. Rivastigmine and galantamine are the latest AChE inhibitors used to treat Alzheimer's disease.[21,56]

The use of direct-acting cholinomimetics in Alzheimer's disease has been largely discouraging. However, acetyl-L-carnitine, a structural analogue of ACh, has shown promise in decreasing the signs and symptoms of the dementia and possibly slowing the disease's progression. In addition to increasing cholinergic transmission, acetyl-L-carnitine may act as an antioxidant.

Other Uses

Methacholine inhalation is sometimes used as a challenge test for the diagnosis of bronchial asthma, and edrophonium has been given intravenously to abort attacks of paroxysmal atrial tachycardia. However, both approaches have undesirable adverse potentials (bronchoconstriction and bradycardia, respectively) and are indicated only when more established diagnostic or therapeutic approaches have been exhausted.

THERAPEUTIC USES IN DENTISTRY

All the cholinomimetic drugs that have an affinity for muscarinic sites are capable of stimulating salivation. Xerostomia is a common problem encountered by dentists in patients with Sjögren's syndrome, those who have had head and neck radiation, and those undergoing treatment involving drugs that produce dry mouth. Pilocarpine may be useful in stimulating salivary flow when there is functional salivary gland tissue present. The drug is usually taken at doses of 5 or 10 mg three times a day, 30 minutes before each meal. Cevimeline is given at doses of 30 mg three times daily.

As mentioned previously, physostigmine may be of value in treating certain adverse reactions to antimuscarinic drugs used for intravenous sedation.

Cholinergic Drugs

Nonproprietary (generic) name	*Proprietary (trade) name*
Cholinomimetics	
Acetylcholine	Miochol-E
Bethanechol	Urecholine
Carbachol	Miostat, Isopto Carbachol
Cevimeline	Evoxac
Methacholine	Provocholine
Pilocarpine hydrochloride	Pilocar, Pilocel, Salagen
Pilocarpine nitrate*	P.V. Carpine Liquifilm
Pilocarpine ocular therapeutic system	Ocusert Pilo-20, Ocusert Pilo-40
Pilocarpine and epinephrine	E-Pilo-1, P_2E_1
Pilocarpine and physostigmine	Isopto P-ES
Anticholinesterases	
Ambenonium	Mytelase
Demecarium	Humorsol
Donepezil	Aricept
Echothiophate	Phospholine
Edrophonium	Tensilon, Reversol
Galantamine	Reminyl
Isoflurophate*	Floropryl
Neostigmine	Prostigmine
Physostigmine	Eserine Sulfate, Isopto Eserine
Physostigmine salicylate	Antilirium
Pyridostigmine	Mestinon
Rivastigmine	Exelon
Tacrine	Cognex
Cholinesterase reactivator	
Pralidoxime	Protopam

* Not currently available in the United States.

CITED REFERENCES

1. Aeschlimann JA, Reinert M: Pharmacological action of some analogues of physostigmine, *J Pharmacol Exp Ther* 43:413-444, 1931.
2. Ammirati JF, Traquair JA, Morgen PA: *Poisonous mushrooms of the northern United States and Canada*, Markham, Ontario, 1985, Fitzhenry & Whiteside.
3. Beers WH, Reich E: Structure and activity of acetylcholine, *Nature* 228:917-922, 1970.
4. Chothia C: Interaction of acetylcholine with different cholinergic nerve receptors, *Nature* 225:36-38, 1970.
5. Ciafaloni E, Nikhar NK, Massey JM, et al: Retrospective analysis of the use of cyclosporine in myasthenia gravis, *Neurology* 55:448-450, 2000.
6. Coyle JT, Price DL, DeLong MR: Alzheimer's disease: a disorder of cortical cholinergic innervation, *Science* 219: 1184-1190, 1983.
7. Dale HH: The action of certain esters and ethers of choline, and their relation to muscarine, *J Pharmacol Exp Ther* 6:147-190, 1914.

8. Davies P, Maloney AJF: Selective loss of central cholinergic neurons in Alzheimer's disease, *Lancet* 2:1403, 1976.
9. Dowd FJ: Saliva and dental caries, *Dent Clin North Am* 43:579-597, 1999.
10. Drachman DB: Myasthenia gravis, *N Engl J Med* 330: 1797-1810, 1994.
11. Engelhardt E, Loewi O: Fermentative Azetylcholinspaltung im Blut und ihre Hemmung durch Physostigmine, *Naunyn Schmiedebergs Arch Pharmacol* 150:1-13, 1930.
12. Farlow M, Gracon SI, Hershey SA, et al: A controlled trial of tacrine in Alzheimer's disease. The Tacrine Study Group, *JAMA* 268:2523-2529, 1992.
13. Featherstone JD: Science and practice of caries prevention, *J Am Dent Assoc* 131:887-899, 2000.
14. Fine BS, Yanoff M, Stone RA: A clinicopathologic study of four cases of primary open-angle glaucoma compared to normal eyes, *Am J Ophthalmol* 91:88-105, 1981.
15. Fox PC, Atkinson JC, Macynski AA, et al: Pilocarpine treatment of salivary gland hypofunction and dry mouth (xerostomia), *Arch Intern Med* 151:1149-1152, 1991.
16. Fox PC, van-der-Ven PF, Baum BJ, et al: Pilocarpine for the treatment of xerostomia associated with salivary gland dysfunction, *Oral Surg Oral Med Oral Pathol* 61:243-248, 1986.
17. Furchgott RF: Endothelium-derived relaxing factor: discovery, early studies, and identification as nitric oxide, *Biosci Rep* 19:235-251, 1999.
18. Giacobini E: Cholinesterase inhibitors: from the Calabar bean to Alzheimer's therapy. In Giacobini E, ed: *Cholinesterases and cholinesterase inhibitors,* London, 2000, Martin Dubitz.
19. Grantham C, Geerts H: The rationale behind cholinergic drug treatment for dementia related to cerebrovascular disease, *J Neurol Sci* 203-204:131-136, 2002.
20. Grob D: Anticholinesterase intoxication in man and its treatment. In Koelle GB, ed: *Cholinesterases and anticholinesterases. Handbuch der Experimentellen Pharmakologie,* vol 15, Berlin, 1963, Springer-Verlag.
21. Grutzendler J, Morris JC: Cholinesterase inhibitors for Alzheimer's disease, *Drugs* 61:41-52, 2001.
22. Hardy J, Allsop D: Amyloid deposition as the central event in the aetiology of Alzheimer's disease, *Trends Pharmacol Sci* 12:383-388, 1991.
23. Harkany T, Penke B, Luiten PG: β-Amyloid excitotoxicity in rat magnocellular nucleus basalis. Effect of cortical deafferentation of cerebral blood flow regulation and implications for Alzheimer's disease, *Ann NY Acad Sci* 903:374-386, 2000.
24. Hoyng PG, van Beek LM: Pharmacological therapy for glaucoma: a review, *Drugs* 59:411-434, 2000.
25. Hunt R, Taveau RdeM: On the physiological action of certain choline derivatives and new methods for detecting choline, *Br Med J* 2:1788-1791, 1906.
26. Ignarro LJ, Cirino G, Casini A, et al: Nitric oxide as a signaling molecule in the vascular system: an overview, *J Cardiovasc Pharmacol* 34:879-886, 1999.
27. Johnson JT, Ferretti GA, Nethery WJ, et al: Oral pilocarpine for post-irradiation xerostomia in patients with head and neck cancer, *N Engl J Med* 329:390-395, 1993.
28. Kao I, Drachman DB: Myasthenic immunoglobulin accelerates acetylcholine receptor degradation, *Science* 196: 527-529, 1977.
29. Knapp MJ, Knopman DS, Soloman PR, et al: A 30-week randomized controlled trial of high-dose tacrine in patients with Alzheimer's disease. The Tacrine Study Group, *JAMA* 271:985-991, 1994.
30. Lange W, von Krueger G: Über Ester der Monofluorphosphorsäure, *Bericht Deutschen Keramischen Gesellschaft* 65:598-1601, 1932.
31. Maltby N, Broe GA, Creasey H, et al: Efficacy of tacrine and lecithin in mild to moderate Alzheimer's disease: double blind trial, *Br Med J* 308:879-883, 1994.
32. Mandel ID: The role of saliva in maintaining oral homeostasis, *J Am Dent Assoc* 119:298-304, 1989.
33. Mandel ID: A contemporary view of salivary research, *Crit Rev Oral Biol Med* 4:599-604, 1993.
34. Mandel ID, Wotman S: The salivary secretions in health and disease, *Oral Sci Rev* 8:25-47, 1976.
35. Massoulié J, Bon S: The molecular forms of cholinesterase and acetylcholinesterase in vertebrates, *Annu Rev Neurosci* 5:57-106, 1982.
36. Molloy DW, Guyatt GH, Wilson DB, et al: Effect of tetrahydroaminoacridine on cognition, function and behaviour in Alzheimer's disease, *Can Med Assoc J* 144: 29-34, 1991.
37. Mounter LA: Metabolism of organophosphorus anticholinesterase agents. In Koelle GB, ed: *Cholinesterases and anticholinesterases. Handbuch der Experimentellen Pharmakologie,* vol 15, Berlin, 1963, Springer-Verlag.
38. Novack GD, O'Donnell MJ, Molloy DW: New glaucoma medications in the geriatric population: efficacy and safety, *J Am Geriatr Soc* 50:956-962, 2002.
39. Paton WDM: Anticholinesterases. In *Lectures on the scientific basis of medicine,* vol 3, London, 1955, Athlone Press, University of London.
40. Patrick J, Lindstrom J: Autoimmune response to acetylcholine receptor, *Science* 180:871-872, 1973.
41. Remen L: Zur Pathogenese und Therapie der Myasthenia gravis pseudoparalytic, *Deutsche Z Nervenheilkunde* 128:66-78, 1932.
42. Renshaw RR, Green D, Ziff M: A basis for the acetylcholine action of choline derivatives, *J Pharmacol Exp Ther* 62:430-448, 1938.
43. Rumack BH: Anticholinergic poisoning: treatment with physostigmine, *Pediatrics* 52:449-451, 1973.
44. Santa T, Engel AG, Lambert EH: Histometric study of neuromuscular junction ultrastructure, *Neurology* 22:71-82, 1972.
45. Senanayake N, Karalliedde L: Neurotoxic effects of organophosphorus insecticides: an intermediate syndrome, *N Engl J Med* 316:761-763, 1987.
46. Stanley EF, Drachman DB: Effect of myasthenic immunoglobulin on acetylcholine receptors of intact mammalian neuromuscular junction, *Science* 200:1285-1287, 1978.
47. Stedman E, Barger G: Physostigmine (eserine). Part III, *J Chem Soc Perkin Transactions 1: Organic Bio-organic Chem* 127:247-258, 1925.
48. Summers WK, Majovski, LV, Marsh GM, et al: Oral tetrahydroaminoacridine in long-term treatment of senile dementia, Alzheimer type, *N Engl J Med* 315:1241-1245, 1986.

49. Sussman JL, Harel M, Frolow F, et al: Atomic structure of acetylcholinesterase from *Torpedo californica:* a prototypic acetylcholine-binding protein, *Science* 253:872-879, 1991.
50. Thal LJ, Fuld PA, Masur DM, et al: Oral physostigmine and lecithin improve memory in Alzheimer's disease, *Psychopharmacol Bull* 19:454-456, 1983.
51. Toyka KV, Drachman DB, Griffin DE, et al: Myasthenia gravis: study of humoral immune mechanisms by passive transfer to mice, *N Engl J Med* 296:125-131, 1977.
52. Volle RL, Koelle GB: The physiological role of acetylcholinesterase (AChE) in sympathetic ganglia, *J Pharmacol Exp Ther* 133:223-240, 1961.
53. Walker MB: Case showing the effect of prostigmine on myasthenia gravis, *Proc R Soc Lond [Biol]* 28:759-761, 1935.
54. Wess J: Molecular basis of muscarinic acetylcholine receptor function, *Trends Pharmacol Sci* 14:308-313, 1993.
55. Wilson IB: Acetylcholinesterase. XI. Reversibility of tetraethyl pyrophosphate inhibition, *J Biol Chem* 190:111-117, 1951.
56. Wolfson C, Oremus M, Shukla V, et al: Donepezil and rivastigmine in the treatment of Alzheimer's disease: a best-evidence synthesis of the published data on their efficacy and cost-effectiveness, *Clin Ther* 24:862-866, 2002.

General References

Birdsall NJM, Buckley NJ, Caulfield MP, et al: Muscarinic acetylcholine receptors. In *The IUPHAR compendium of receptor characterization and classification,* London, 1998, IUPHAR Media.

Massoulie J: Molecular forms and anchoring of acetylcholinesterase. In Giacobini E, ed: *Cholinesterase and cholinesterase inhibitors,* London, 2000, Martin Dunitz.

CHAPTER • 9

Antimuscarinic Drugs

Frank J. Dowd

A variety of drugs can interfere with the transmission of nerve impulses at cholinergic junctions. As shown in Table 5-2, some drugs prevent the uptake of choline by the nerve terminal or the release of acetylcholine (ACh) from the terminal; other drugs block at ganglia or, by a competitive or depolarizing form of blockade, at neuromuscular junctions. The drugs in this chapter block responses in muscarinic receptors and are essentially without effect, except at inordinately high doses, at nicotinic receptors. Hence, these drugs are known as *antimuscarinic* or *muscarinic receptor–blocking drugs;* the term *anticholinergic,* although often used for this class of drugs, should not be used to imply that they act at all cholinergic sites. They are also termed *atropine-like* because of their derivation from, or relation to, the oldest and best known member of the group. Because peripheral muscarinic receptors are the primary targets of ACh released by postganglionic cholinergic neurons, the effects achieved by the antimuscarinic drugs are chiefly on the smooth muscle, cardiac muscle, and glands that are innervated by these neurons.

The antimuscarinic drugs have a colorful, even sinister, history. The natural alkaloids are derived from a number of plants, including *Atropa belladonna* (deadly nightshade), *Datura stramonium*, also known as jimsonweed or Jamestown weed, *Hyoscyamus niger* (henbane), and mandragora, among others. Datura was used in India in ancient times; in fact, its name comes from the Sanskrit. These drugs are mentioned in the Ebers papyrus (circa 1550 BC), in the Greek herbal of Dioscorides, and by Galen.[2] In Western civilization, the drugs were used by professional poisoners in the Middle Ages for slow poisoning because of the obscure symptoms and the slow course of illness. The Swedish botanist Linné named the shrub *Atropa belladonna* after Atropos, one of the three Fates, who cuts the thread of life. The term *belladonna* comes from the Italian "beautiful woman" and is so named because instillation of one of these drugs into the eyes was said to make women more attractive.[11] Atropine, scopolamine, and related natural chemicals are therefore also referred to as *belladonna alkaloids.*

CHEMISTRY AND CLASSIFICATION

Antimuscarinic drugs fall into four categories:

1. Naturally occurring belladonna alkaloids—atropine and scopolamine—which are organic esters. Atropine and scopolamine are composed of an aromatic acid (tropic acid) and a complex organic base (tropine or scopine, respectively). Atropine is a racemic mixture of *d*- and *l*-hyoscyamine; the *l* isomer is the active form and is often used separately.
2. Semisynthetic derivatives, such as homatropine, which is produced by combining tropine with mandelic acid, and the quaternary ammonium derivatives of atropine, scopolamine, and homatropine (atropine methylnitrate, methscopolamine bromide, and homatropine methylbromide, respectively).
3. Synthetic quaternary ammonium compounds, such as methantheline, propantheline, and ipratropium.
4. Synthetic antimuscarinic drugs that are not quaternary ammonium compounds, such as benztropine, trihexyphenidyl, and cyclopentolate.

An example of each of these types is shown in Table 9-1.

MECHANISM OF ACTION

The antimuscarinic drugs, whether the naturally occurring alkaloids or the semisynthetic or synthetic derivatives, are competitive antagonists of ACh at muscarinic receptors. They have an affinity for muscarinic receptor sites but lack intrinsic activity.[3] Thus they occupy the receptor sites and prevent access of ACh, creating a blockade that is reversible by increasing the amount of ACh in the area of the receptor, as would occur after the administration of an anticholinesterase drug. Because atropine can antagonize the muscarinic effects of the anticholinesterases and vice versa, each drug can be used as an antidote for the other in case of poisoning. In effect, the antimuscarinic drugs are capable of blocking responses to parasympathetic nerve stimulation, to sympathetic nerve stimulation of thermoregulatory sweat glands, to ACh protected from hydrolysis by anticholinesterases, and to direct-acting muscarinic agents, although their capability for inhibiting the latter two is greater than for the first two.

Several explanations have been offered for why atropine is more effective in blocking the pharmacologic effects produced by muscarinic receptor agonists than in blocking physiologic responses evoked by parasympathetic nervous system stimulation. One possibility is that ACh released into the restricted environs of a junctional cleft may overwhelm the antagonist by the high, although temporary, concentrations achieved. A second possibility is that the antimuscarinic drugs facilitate ACh release from cholinergic neurons by blocking presynaptic muscarinic receptors that serve to limit evoked ACh release. A third explanation arises from the fact that physiologic responses to parasympathetic nervous system stimulation are mediated by several neurotransmitters in addition to ACh. Direct electrical stimulation of the parasympathetic nervous system causes the release of ACh and several other neurotransmitters from the postganglionic nerve terminal.[18] For example, both ACh and vasoactive intestinal peptide

Table • 9-1

Chemical Structures of Representatives of the Four Classes of Antimuscarinic Drugs

TYPE OF COMPOUND	EXAMPLE	CHEMICAL STRUCTURE
Naturally occurring alkaloid	Atropine	
Semisynthetic derivative of alkaloid	Methscopolamine	
Synthetic quaternary ammonium compound	Propantheline	
Synthetic but not quaternary ammonium compound	Benztropine	

Table • 9-2

The Relative Effects of Atropine and Scopolamine on Various Effectors

	IRIS	CILIARY BODY	SECRETION: SALIVA, SWEAT, BRONCHIAL	BRONCHIAL MUSCLE	GASTROINTESTINAL MUSCLE	HEART	CNS
Atropine	+	+	+	++	++	++	+
Scopolamine	++	++	++	+	+	+	++

are released from postganglionic autonomic fibers innervating skeletal muscle blood vessels, sweat glands, and salivary glands.[20,21] The release of these substances is frequency dependent, with higher frequency stimulation producing vasoactive intestinal peptide release. High-frequency parasympathetic nervous system stimulation produces both vasodilatory and secretory responses that are only partially blocked by muscarinic receptor antagonists.[13]

Although atropine is a highly effective antagonist at all muscarinic receptors, evidence has accumulated that there are five muscarinic subtypes, M_1 to M_5, each with different affinities for certain muscarinic agonists and antagonists, different anatomic distributions, and different second messenger signaling mechanisms (see Chapters 5 and 8). The relatively selective affinity of the tricyclic benzodiazepine pirenzepine for M_1 and M_4 versus M_2 and M_3 receptors gives it stronger antimuscarinic properties in certain sites (e.g., corpus striatum, cerebral cortex, and enterochromaffin cells) over others (e.g., heart and ileum).[6] Available outside of the United States, pirenzepine was the first clinically useful selective muscarinic receptor antagonist. Tolterodine, a synthetic agent unrelated chemically to other antimuscarinics, is moderately selective against the M_3 receptor and now available for treatment of urinary incontinence in adults. The characterization of different muscarinic receptor subtypes continues to provide an impetus for development of selective antagonists.

PHARMACOLOGIC EFFECTS

Therapeutic doses of the antimuscarinic drugs produce effects attributable to the blockade of peripheral muscarinic receptors and similar receptors in the central nervous system (CNS) located within the medulla and higher cerebral centers. In the discussion that follows, the principal review is of atropine and scopolamine, which have always been considered the prototypes for this class of drugs, but it must be emphasized that (1) atropine and scopolamine differ in the relative intensity of their antimuscarinic effects on specific organs (Table 9-2); (2) there is a difference in the susceptibility of various

Table • 9-3

Order of Susceptibility of Effectors to Increasing Doses of Antimuscarinic Agents

RESPONSE	DOSE
Secretion (saliva, sweat, bronchial)	Low
Mydriasis, cycloplegia, tachycardia	↓
Loss of parasympathetic control of urinary bladder and gastrointestinal smooth muscle	↓
Inhibition of gastric secretion	High

Table • 9-4

Onset and Duration of Cycloplegia Induced by Some Topical Antimuscarinic Drugs

DRUG	ONSET (min)	DURATION
Atropine	30 to 40	6 days or longer
Scopolamine	20 to 30	3 to 6 days
Homatropine	40 to 60	36 to 48 hours
Cyclopentolate	25 to 75	6 to 24 hours
Tropicamide	20 to 35	2 to 6 hours

effectors to antimuscarinic agents in general (Table 9-3); (3) because of differences in chemical structure, some antimuscarinic drugs pass readily into the CNS, whereas others do not; (4) there are some major differences among antimuscarinic drugs in the onset and duration of their actions (Table 9-4); and (5) muscarinic receptor subtypes have differing affinities for specific antimuscarinic drugs.

Peripheral Nervous System Actions

The antimuscarinic drugs possess both peripheral and CNS actions, but the nature and intensity of these vary with the individual drug and the dose administered. Most peripheral effects are caused by an interruption of parasympathetic impulses to a given effector; where there is sympathetic innervation, this means that the effector is under the control of the sympathetic nervous system only, which often exerts opposing effects. The pharmacologic effects observed depend in large part on the existing activity of postganglionic cholinergic neurons. Thus inhibition of sweating and hyperthermia are likely to be observed on a hot day, but no effect on thermoregulation is apparent in a cold environment. In general, atropinelike drugs block the salivation, lacrimation, urination, and defecation response to cholinergic drugs described in Chapter 8 and the hypotensive and bradycardic effects of muscarinic receptor stimulation. The effects of antimuscarinic agents on specific tissues are described below.

Eye

Atropinelike drugs block muscarinic receptors in the sphincter of the iris and in the ciliary muscle, leading, respectively, to dilation of the pupil (mydriasis) and paralysis of accommodation (cycloplegia). Photophobia and fixation of the lens occurs for far vision, and thus vision for near objects is blurred. Intraocular pressure is not significantly affected except in the case of narrow-angle (or angle-closure) glaucoma, for which administration of these drugs may cause a dangerous rise in intraocular pressure. The onset and duration of the mydriatic and cycloplegic effects differ, as shown for cycloplegia in Table 9-4, and to some extent the choice of an agent for an ophthalmologic procedure will be influenced by these differences.

Respiratory tract

After administration of antimuscarinic drugs, the bronchial smooth muscle is left under the sole control of the sympathetic nervous system and is therefore relaxed. This relaxation of the smooth muscle decreases airway resistance. Sometimes there is an increase in respiratory minute volume resulting from an increase in the physiologic dead space and medullary stimulation. The bronchoconstriction caused by muscarinic agonists, sulfur dioxide, and certain other bronchial spasmogens is easily reversed by atropine, but that caused by histamine, 5-hydroxytryptamine, and the leukotrienes is resistant.

Secretion of all glands in the nose, mouth, pharynx, and respiratory tree is inhibited. This suppression of secretory activity in the respiratory tract is the underlying reason for the effectiveness of atropine and scopolamine in preventing laryngospasm during general anesthesia[12]; these agents are not capable of directly blocking contraction of the laryngeal muscle.

Salivary glands

Parasympathetically mediated salivary secretion is abolished in a dose-dependent manner, whereas salivary gland vasodilation is much less affected. The mouth and throat become unpleasantly dry, to the point that speech and swallowing may become difficult. Dry mouth or xerostomia can lead to any one of a number of adverse effects on the oral cavity (see Chapter 8).

Gastrointestinal tract

Although the antimuscarinic drugs are quite effective in preventing the expected motor and secretory responses of the gastrointestinal tract to administered cholinergic drugs, their effects on vagal stimulation are more ambiguous. Antimuscarinic drugs have a marked inhibitory effect on motility throughout the gastrointestinal tract. Thus interference with the normal parasympathetic impulses to the gastrointestinal tract, as would occur with the antimuscarinic drugs and the ganglionic blocking agents, will cause a profound decrease in the tone of gastrointestinal smooth muscle as well as in the frequency and amplitude of peristaltic contractions. Regarding secretion, gastric secretory activity in human beings is inhibited only at very high doses of the belladonna alkaloids, when essentially all other parasympathetic function has been blocked and the patient has an extremely dry mouth, blurred vision, an increased heart rate, and marked inhibition of gastrointestinal motility. At these high doses, atropine reduces gastric acidity, pepsin secretion, and total gastric secretion. The fact that the gastrointestinal tract, particularly the secretory apparatus, is resistant to the belladonna alkaloids and the fact that the therapeutic use of these drugs as antiulcer and antispasmodic drugs has been disappointing underscore the finding that transmitters in addition to ACh are involved in the regulation of secretion and motor activity in the gastrointestinal tract (see Chapter 33). Two of these transmitters are adenosine triphosphate and histamine. It should be noted that at high doses atropine has antihistaminic (H_1) activity, and the antihistamine diphenhydramine has marked antimuscarinic activity, one manifestation of which is xerostomia.

Cardiovascular system

The effects of antimuscarinic drugs differ according to the dose administered and whether the subject is in the erect or recumbent position. With oral doses used to limit salivation (e.g., 0.4 to 0.6 mg of atropine or scopolamine in adults), mild bradycardia often results. At these low doses, a selective blockade of prejunctional muscarinic receptors augments ACh release from postganglionic parasympathetic fibers innervating the heart. In most cases, however, the heart rate increases significantly in human beings given more than 0.4 mg intravenously or 1.0 mg orally. In the standing or upright patient, there is little or no change in cardiac output.[28] As is shown in Table 9-2, doses of scopolamine that cause mydriasis rarely cause tachycardia, whereas atropine administered systemically in doses sufficient to have ocular effects will inevitably accelerate the heart.

Genitourinary tract

The ureters and the urinary bladder (detrusor muscle) are relaxed by atropine. The sphincter and trigone muscles are contracted by atropine. Together these changes in the bladder cause urinary retention in human beings. This retention is particularly likely in the presence of prostatic hypertrophy.

Body temperature

The belladonna alkaloids suppress sweating because the sweat glands (other than the apocrine sweat glands as found on the palms of the hand) are innervated by cholinergic fibers of the sympathetic nervous system. The receptors at the neuroeffector sites in the sweat glands are therefore muscarinic. The rise in body temperature that can follow the administration of large doses of atropine or scopolamine may have a CNS component, but the primary cause is the peripheral inhibition of sweating. It is also the most serious and life-threatening result of an overdose of one of these drugs.

Central Nervous System Effects

CNS effects are produced only by those antimuscarinic drugs that can penetrate the blood-brain barrier. The quaternary amines, such as methscopolamine and propantheline, therefore have no effect on the CNS.

Medulla and higher cerebral centers

Both scopolamine and atropine produce complex effects on the CNS. With conventional therapeutic doses of atropine, there is direct stimulation of the CNS, which is generally manifested only as a mild stimulation of respiratory centers located in the vagal nuclei of the medulla. At therapeutic doses, scopolamine usually produces effects ranging from decreased psychologic efficiency to drowsiness, sedation, euphoria, and amnesia, but it can also cause excitement, restlessness, hallucinations, and delirium. Atropine is much less active in this respect than scopolamine.

Antitremor activity

The belladonna alkaloids were first used in the treatment of Parkinson's disease in the mid-1800s, long before their mechanism of action was understood and before the biochemical nature of the defect of parkinsonism had been elucidated. Their effectiveness in suppressing tremor was later suggested to result from a "central atropine-ACh antagonism," and more recently it has become apparent that the striatum is the site of cholinergic systems that in parkinsonism are released from an inhibitory balance mediated by dopamine (see Chapter 15).

Vestibular function

The belladonna alkaloids have since ancient times been the basis of various remedies to treat motion sickness.[23] Scopolamine is more effective than atropine, and it probably acts on vestibular end organs, the cortex, or both.[7]

ABSORPTION, FATE, AND EXCRETION

The belladonna alkaloids and their tertiary derivatives and analogues are readily absorbed from all parts of the gastrointestinal tract except the stomach, as would be expected with alkaloids that form acid salts. Absorption is more rapid from subcutaneous tissue or muscle than it is from the gastrointestinal tract. The drugs are distributed throughout the body, including the CNS. The fate of most of these drugs in human beings is not well studied, but the kidneys provide the main route for excretion of atropine in changed and unchanged form. Within 24 hours, 27% to 94% of a dose of labeled atropine is excreted, and very little is excreted after 24 hours. A third of the atropine appears as unchanged atropine and the remainder as a metabolite of uncertain identity.[19] Rabbits possess a genetically determined enzyme, atropinesterase, that explains their singular ability to tolerate large doses of atropine.[5] Various idiosyncratic responses or variations in sensitivity to one or another of the actions of these drugs are not uncommon. Young people show a high incidence of idiosyncratic responses; persons with Down syndrome are more sensitive to the mydriatic effects,[4] whereas African Americans develop more exaggerated tachycardia.[11]

Antimuscarinics with a quaternary ammonium structure are incompletely absorbed after oral ingestion and are often given by nonenteral routes. These drugs are largely excluded from the CNS.

GENERAL THERAPEUTIC USES

The therapeutic uses of the antimuscarinic drugs are all based on the pharmacologic effects, peripheral and central, already discussed. However, as should be clear, it is difficult to obtain a high degree of selectivity in the organ or organs to be affected because the antimuscarinic drugs tend to affect many muscarinic sites. Certain drugs, however, are more effective and therefore potentially more useful in a particular therapeutic role than others. It should also be noted that the quaternary ammonium compounds, two of which are shown in Table 9-1, differ from atropine and scopolamine in a number of important respects. Two important differences are (1) they do not readily pass the blood-brain barrier because they are ionized at physiologic pH, and thus they have no effect on the CNS, and (2) they have greater ganglionic blocking properties than do the nonquaternary compounds. This latter point may explain why orthostatic hypotension and impotence are sometimes encountered in patients being treated with these drugs. It has been claimed that these synthetic compounds possess a greater selectivity for the gastrointestinal tract than do the other antimuscarinic drugs and that they are therefore preferred agents for the treatment of gastrointestinal disorders because they cause fewer side effects. Although it has been difficult to demonstrate that these synthetic compounds do, in fact, have fewer muscarinic side effects and are at the same time more selective for the gastrointestinal tract, it has been shown in patients with duodenal ulcer that low doses of propantheline are as effective as near-toxic doses of that drug in inhibiting food-stimulated gastric secretion.[14] Furthermore, it was shown in the same experiment that when the low dose of propantheline was given with a conventional dose of the H_2-receptor antagonist cimetidine, the inhibitory effect on gastric secretion was significantly enhanced (see Chapter 33).

Ophthalmology

By local administration of antimuscarinic drugs, it is possible to produce mydriasis and cycloplegia of very long duration (atropine), medium duration (scopolamine), and very short duration (tropicamide). Mydriasis is necessary for a thorough examination of the retina and optic disk; cycloplegia is necessary for measurement of the refractive powers of the lens. Mydriasis can be produced alternately with miosis for the purpose of breaking up adhesions that may have developed between the lens and the iris. The topical use of these drugs is strongly contraindicated in patients with a predisposition to narrow-angle glaucoma, and although systemic anticholinergic drugs are usually safe for patients with open-angle glaucoma, they may precipitate a first attack of acute angle-closure glaucoma. Homatropine, cyclopentolate, and tropicamide are the major mydriatics used. The duration of effects ranges from 1 to 3 days for homatropine to 6 hours for tropicamide.

Respiratory Tract

Belladonna alkaloids were once commonly used for the treatment of bronchial asthma, but liabilities, including limited effectiveness and a tendency to inhibit secretions, which often led to the retention of a viscid residuum further obstructing airflow, resulted in their abandonment as soon as replacement therapies became available. Subsequently, the quaternary ammonium compound ipratropium was marketed in aerosol form for the treatment of chronic obstructive pulmonary disease.[9] It is highly effective for patients with chronic bronchitis and has been used in acute asthma and status asthmaticus in patients unresponsive to β_2-adrenergic receptor agonists, although it is considered a secondary drug in the treatment of acute asthma.[10] The inhalation route limits systemic side effects and avoids inhibition of bronchial secretion. As an antimuscarinic drug, ipratropium is unique in its preservation of ciliary motility in the bronchial mucosa, an important benefit in preventing the formation of mucous plugs.[27] Tiotropium is a drug similar in action to ipratropium. It also is given by inhalation but has a longer duration of action than ipratropium and can be administered once a day.[25]

The ability of atropinelike drugs to suppress secretion throughout the respiratory tract is advantageous during the administration of general anesthesia because these drugs produce a dry field, lessen the danger of pulmonary aspiration, and help prevent laryngospasm.[11]

Salivary Secretion

The antimuscarinic drugs are widely used to diminish salivary secretion before surgery, particularly oral surgical procedures. The use of atropine for this purpose provides a dry oral cavity and diminishes the salivary response to irritating anesthetic gases. Atropine is occasionally used to reduce excessive salivary secretion in heavy metal poisoning and parkinsonism.

Gastrointestinal Tract

The antimuscarinic drugs have been used extensively as antispasmodics, as antiulcer therapy, and for a variety of disorders characterized by the term *spasticity.* Although their use is often attended by symptomatic relief, they have proved of questionable benefit in the treatment of peptic ulcer, severe dysenteric illnesses, and so-called spasticity syndromes. It has become popular to substitute the synthetic quaternary ammonium compounds for the naturally occurring alkaloids for these therapeutic goals on the questionable basis that side effects would be less severe with the synthetic compounds. As shown in Table 9-3, it is clear that if reduction in intestinal peristalsis is a therapeutic aim with this kind of drug, then tachycardia, blurring of vision, and dryness of mouth must be accepted as inevitable accompaniments. The more selective drug pirenzepine has been found to suppress both resting and stimulated acid and pepsin secretion without producing as many effects on the heart, bladder, or ocular structures, all locations where receptors other than M_1 muscarinic receptors predominate.

Cardiovascular System

The application of the antimuscarinic drugs to the treatment of cardiovascular disorders is limited. They can be used during anesthesia and surgery to prevent vagal reflexes, in cases of myocardial infarction in which there is excessive vagal tone causing sinus or nodal bradycardia, in cases of a hyperactive carotid sinus reflex producing bradycardia and syncope, and in certain cases of digitalis-induced heart block. Several other forms of heart block are also amenable to atropine.

Genitourinary Tract

The belladonna alkaloids have been used to treat a variety of urologic disorders, including renal colic (usually in combination with opioids), nocturnal enuresis, and overactive bladder associated with urge incontinence and urinary frequency. Inasmuch as the bladder is less susceptible than some other tissues to the action of muscarinic drugs (see Table 9-3), these drugs have not proved very useful in the treatment of these disorders. Drugs that also have direct relaxant effects on smooth muscle, such as flavoxate and oxybutynin, are preferred for symptomatic relief of dysuria, urgency, and incontinence associated with inflammatory or neurogenic conditions. Tolterodine and propiverine are additional antimuscarinic drugs used to treat these conditions. They appear to have some selectivity for the urinary bladder.[8] Tricyclic antidepressants are currently the drugs of choice for nocturnal enuresis in children; surgery is generally indicated for adults who suffer from nocturnal enuresis without daytime incontinence.

Preanesthetic Medication

Preanesthetic medication constitutes a major use for the belladonna alkaloids. Scopolamine in particular provides the CNS effects of euphoria, amnesia, and sedation, as well as the inhibition of salivary and other secretions and the protection that this inhibition furnishes against laryngospasm.[11] Many of the newer inhalation anesthetics do not have the irritating properties that former anesthetics such as ether had, so the need for suppression of respiratory and salivary secretions is not as great as it was in the past.

Central Nervous System

Part of the rationale for the use of scopolamine as a preanesthetic medication is that it has outstanding CNS effects. Other uses for the central effects of the antimuscarinic drugs are to prevent motion sickness and to treat Ménière's disease and parkinsonism. Scopolamine is the drug most frequently chosen for the first two purposes and, in fact, is the most effective single agent for severe, brief motion sickness when given prophylactically. It is not particularly effective in preventing nausea and vomiting from most other causes, such as radiation sickness. Scopolamine has been prepared in a transdermal system for the prevention of motion sickness. The system is a flexible disk with an adhesive surface that, when placed on the skin behind the ear, delivers 1 mg of scopolamine over a period of 3 days. An effective concentration of the drug in the blood is achieved in about 4 hours. Delivered transdermally, the usual effects of cholinergic blockade are minimized, although there is occasional dryness of the mouth and drowsiness.[26] In Parkinson's disease, discussed in Chapter 15, the anticholinergics are the oldest drugs used for this condition and are still considered useful in the early stages of the disease and in combined therapy with levodopa and other antiparkinsonian drugs. The anticholinergic drugs favored for this purpose are the nonquaternary synthetic compounds that gain ready access to the brain and have greater CNS effects than peripheral nervous system effects. These drugs include benztropine, biperiden, trihexyphenidyl, and such antihistamines as diphenhydramine (see Chapter 15).

Antidote to Anticholinesterases

Toxicity from anticholinesterases may result from their use in the treatment of myasthenia gravis (particularly in the early phase of therapy when the patient is not as tolerant to the muscarinic effects of these drugs) or from exposure to one of the organophosphate insecticides or anticholinesterase nerve gases. These anticholinesterases typically produce a spectrum of peripheral muscarinic and nicotinic effects as well as CNS effects. Atropine is effective in antagonizing all the effects at muscarinic sites and thus will relieve the hypersecretion of salivary, lacrimal, and respiratory glands; bronchoconstriction; gastrointestinal symptoms; sweating; various other manifestations of muscarinic stimulation; and some CNS actions. It does not interfere with the desired effects of anticholinesterases at neuromuscular junctions when these drugs are being used for myasthenia gravis or to reverse neuromuscular blockade induced by curarelike agents (see Chapter 10); it also does not prevent the neuromuscular stimulation, followed by respiratory failure, characteristic of excessive nicotinic stimulation. For the treatment of acute toxicity with anticholinesterases, very large doses of atropine are used; for the treatment of milder symptoms of muscarinic stimulation, as in the treatment of myasthenia gravis, much lower doses suffice.[16]

Antidote to Poisoning by Mushrooms Containing Muscarine

As stated in Chapter 8, the mushroom *Inocybe lateraria* is poisonous because of its high content of the alkaloid muscarine. Atropine is a specific antagonist.

ADVERSE EFFECTS

Atropine and related drugs, despite wide availability, have produced relatively few fatal cases of poisoning. In fact, atropine has a large margin of safety in adults, as has been demonstrated in cases in which massive doses were used in so-called atropine toxicity therapy for schizophrenia.[15] Most of the reported fatalities have involved children who accidentally ingested eye drops or other medicines that contained atropine or scopolamine. Children are more susceptible to hyperthermia and other toxic effects of atropine; dosages therefore need to be carefully controlled. The colloquialism "hot as a hare, red as a beet, dry as a bone, blind as a bat, and mad as a hatter" vividly conveys the symptoms of atropine intoxication, which are predictable extensions of the pharmacologic effects of this group of drugs. Present are dryness of the mouth, extreme thirst, a burning sensation in the throat, and difficulty in swallowing; dilation of the pupils and cycloplegia with severe impairment of vision and photophobia; flushing of the skin, vasodilation of skin vessels, absence of sweating, and a rise in body temperature in warm environments to 105° F or more; urinary retention; and derangements of CNS activity. Toxic CNS effects of atropine and homatropine in children include ataxia that becomes so severe that the patients are unable to sit or stand unassisted; a dysarthric quality of speech; restlessness with constant muttering, shouting, and singing; great confusion; visual hallucinations; and violent, aggressive, and maniacal behavior.[1,17] Mild toxic reactions may subside in a few hours; most patients require a day or more for complete recovery. Therapy for atropine poisoning involves physostigmine, which is useful in raising the amount of ACh in the vicinity of the receptors and acts rapidly to terminate the atropine blockade. The antianxiety drugs such as diazepam may be used to control CNS excitation. Therapy also includes supportive care.

Topical use of antimuscarinic drugs in the eye is absolutely contraindicated in cases of suspected or diagnosed glaucoma. Systemic doses of anticholinergic drugs can be used in patients with open-angle glaucoma but not in patients with narrow-angle glaucoma. As previously mentioned, use of these drugs may precipitate the first attack of acute intraocular hypertension. In prostatic hypertrophy, anticholinergic drugs may cause urinary retention.

DRUG INTERACTIONS

The anticholinergic effect of the atropinelike drugs is potentiated by antihistamines (which particularly accentuate the xerostomia), the tuberculostatic drug isoniazid, monoamine oxidase inhibitors, and tricyclic antidepressants. The phenothiazines tend to potentiate the CNS effects of the antimuscarinic drugs. When atropine is given in the presence of propranolol, it is likely to antagonize the slowing of the heart and the increased duration of the atrioventricular nodal refractory period for which propranolol may have been prescribed to achieve; it may also block the vagal actions of the digitalis glycosides.

THERAPEUTIC USES IN DENTISTRY

The principal use of the anticholinergic drugs in dentistry is to decrease the flow of saliva during dental procedures. Small doses given orally or parenterally approximately 30 minutes to 2 hours before the procedure are effective, but the drug may also produce side effects that may be objectionable to some patients. The same dose may also be used to diminish salivary flow in heavy metal poisoning. Atropine is often selected because it is well absorbed, but scopolamine can be used if sedation is a desired side effect. Table 9-5 lists some preparations and oral dosages used in dentistry.

Table • 9-5

Preparations and Oral Dosages Used in Dentistry

DRUG	DOSE	TIME OF ADMINISTRATION*
Atropine sulfate	0.4 to 1 mg	1 to 2 hours
Belladonna tincture	0.6 to 1 ml	2.5 to 3 hours
Glycopyrrolate	1 to 2 mg	30 to 45 minutes
Propantheline bromide	15 to 30 mg	30 to 45 minutes
Scopolamine hydrobromide	0.4 to 0.8 mg	30 to 60 minutes

*Time before the procedure when the drug is administered.

Atropine and glycopyrrolate are frequently used in the oral surgery setting as intraoperative antisialagogues. They are administered intravenously in doses of 0.4 to 0.6 mg and 0.1 to 0.2 mg, respectively. Because it is a quaternary amine, glycopyrrolate has fewer CNS effects than the belladonna alkaloids. Compared with atropine, it is a more selective antisialagogue and less likely to promote tachycardia in conventional doses.[22,24] During general anesthesia, the anticholinergics will also diminish secretions in the respiratory tract, thus lessening the likelihood of laryngospasm, and help prevent reflex vagal slowing of the heart.

IMPLICATIONS FOR DENTISTRY

Not only do dentists occasionally have reason to use antimuscarinic drugs, but dentists often encounter patients who are taking them for any one of the reasons enumerated. The most characteristic effects of these drugs that concern dentists are xerostomia and the discomfort that this brings to the patient as well as the deterioration in oral health. Small doses of pilocarpine will often be effective in stimulating salivary flow; however, this strategy is complicated by the fact that the pilocarpine may also counter the therapeutic benefit being achieved by the antimuscarinic drug. In these cases, for the treatment of xerostomia, most dentists therefore advise their patients to drink water, suck on noncariogenic lemon drops, irrigate the mouth with saliva substitutes, and pay scrupulous attention to oral hygiene. If there is progressive deterioration in oral health, consultation with the patient's physician may be helpful in identifying suitable therapeutic alternatives with reduced xerostomia.

Antimuscarinic Drugs

Nonproprietary (generic) name	*Proprietary (trade) name*
Naturally occurring alkaloids	
Atropine	Atropisol, Sal-Tropine
Belladonna (tincture and extract)	—
l-Hyoscyamine	Levsin
Levorotatory alkaloids of belladonna	In Bellamine
Scopolamine	Isopto Hyoscine, Scopace
Scopolamine (transdermal therapeutic system)	Transderm Scōp
Semisynthetic derivatives	
Atropine methylnitrate*	—
Homatropine	Isopto Homatropine
Methscopolamine	Pamine
Synthetic quaternary ammonium compounds	
Anisotropine*	Valpin 50
Clidinium	Quarzan
Glycopyrrolate	Robinul
Hexocyclium*	Tral Filmtabs
Ipratropium	Atrovent
Isopropamide*	Darbid
Mepenzolate	Cantil
Methantheline*	Banthine
Propantheline	Pro-Banthine
Tiotropium*	Spiriva
Tridihexethyl*	Pathilon
Synthetic nonquaternary ammonium compounds	
Benztropine	Cogentin
Biperiden	Akineton
Cyclopentolate	Cyclogyl, in Cyclomydril
Dicyclomine	Bentyl, Byclomine
Flavoxate	Urispas
Oxybutynin	Ditropan
Procyclidine	Kemadrin
Propiverine*	Detrunorm
Tolterodine	Detrol
Trihexyphenidyl	Artane
Tropicamide	Mydriacyl, Tropicacyl
Tricyclic benzodiazepine	
Pirenzepine*	Gastrozepine

* Not currently available in the United States.

CITED REFERENCES

1. Alexander E, Jr, Morris DP, Eslick RL: Atropine poisoning: report of a case, with recovery after the ingestion of one gram, *N Engl J Med* 234:258-259, 1946.
2. Ambache N: The use and limitations of atropine for pharmacological studies on autonomic effectors, *Pharmacol Rev* 7:467-494, 1955.
3. Ariëns EJ: Affinity and intrinsic activity in the theory of competitive inhibition. Part 1. Problems and theory, *Arch Int Pharmacodyn Ther* 99:32-49, 1954.
4. Berg JM, Brandon MWG, Kirman BH: Atropine in mongolism, *Lancet* 2:441-442, 1959.
5. Bernheim F, Bernheim MLC: The hydrolysis of homatropine and atropine by various tissues, *J Pharmacol Exp Ther* 64:209-216, 1938.
6. Bianchi Porro G, Petrillo M: Pirenzepine in the treatment of peptic ulcer disease: review and commentary, *Scand J Gastroenterol* 17(suppl 72):229-235, 1982.
7. Brand JJ, Whittingham P: Intramuscular hyoscine in control of motion sickness, *Lancet* 2:232-234, 1970.
8. Chapple CR: Muscarinic receptor antagonists in the treatment of overactive bladder, *Urology* 55:33-46, 2000.
9. Cockcroft DW: Pharmacologic therapy for asthma: overview and historical perspective, *J Clin Pharmacol* 39:216-222, 1999.
10. Easton PA, Jadue C, Dhingra S, et al: A comparison of the bronchodilating effects of a beta-2 adrenergic agent (albuterol) and an anticholinergic agent (ipratropium bromide), given by aerosol alone or in sequence, *N Engl J Med* 315:735-739, 1986.
11. Eger EI II: Atropine, scopolamine, and related compounds, *Anesthesiology* 23:365-383, 1962.
12. Eger EI II, Kraft ID, Keasling HH: A comparison of atropine, or scopolamine, plus pentobarbital, meperidine, or morphine as pediatric preanesthetic medications, *Anesthesiology* 22:962-969, 1961.
13. Fazekas A, Gazelius B, Edwall B, et al: VIP and noncholinergic vasodilation in rabbit submandibular gland, *Peptides* 8:13-20, 1987.

14. Feldman M, Richardson CT, Peterson WL, et al: Effect of low-dose propantheline on food-stimulated gastric acid secretion: comparison with an "optimal effective dose" and interaction with cimetidine, *N Engl J Med* 297:1427-1430, 1977.
15. Forrer GD: Symposium on atropine toxicity therapy: history and future research, *J Nerv Ment Dis* 124:256-259, 1956.
16. Grob D: Anticholinesterase intoxication in man and its treatment. In Koelle GB, ed: *Cholinesterases and anticholinesterases. Handbuch der Experimentellen Pharmakologie,* vol 15, Berlin, 1963, Springer-Verlag.
17. Hoefnagel D: Toxic effects of atropine and homatropine eyedrops in children, *N Engl J Med* 264:168-171, 1961.
18. Hökfelt T, Bean A, Ceccatelli S, et al: Neuropeptides and classical transmitters. Localization and interaction, *Arzneimittelforschung* 42:196-201, 1992.
19. Kalser SC: The fate of atropine in man, *Ann NY Acad Sci* 179:667-683, 1971.
20. Lindh B, Lundberg JM, Hökfelt T: NPY-, galanin-, VIP/PHI-, CGRP-, and substance P-immunoreactive neuronal subpopulations in cat autonomic and sensory ganglia and their projections, *Cell Tissue Res* 256:259-273, 1989.
21. Lundberg JM, Hökfelt T, Schultzberg M, et al: Occurrence of vasoactive intestinal polypeptide (VIP)-like immunoreactivity in certain cholinergic neurons of the cat: evidence from combined immunohistochemistry and acetylcholinesterase staining, *Neuroscience* 4:1539-1559, 1979.
22. Meyers EF, Tomeldan SA: Glycopyrrolate compared with atropine in prevention of the oculocardiac reflex during eye-muscle surgery, *Anesthesiology* 51:350-352, 1979.
23. Nishiike S, Takeda N, Uno A, et al: Cholinergic influence on vestibular stimulation-induced locus coeruleus inhibition in rats, *Acta Otolaryngol* 120:404-409, 2000.
24. Odura KA: Glycopyrrolate methylbromide. Comparison with atropine sulfate in anaesthesia, *Can Anaesth Soc J* 22:466-473, 1975.
25. Panning CA, DeBisschop M: Tiotropium: an inhaled, long-acting anticholinergic drug for chronic obstructive pulmonary disease, *Pharmacotherapy* 23:183-189, 2003.
26. Price NM, Schmitt LG, McGuire J, et al: Transdermal scopolamine in the prevention of motion sickness at sea, *Clin Pharmacol Ther* 29:414-419, 1981.
27. van Noord JA, Bantje TA, Eland ME, et al: A randomized controlled comparison of tiotropium and ipratropium in the treatment of chronic obstructive pulmonary disease. The Dutch Tiotropium Study Group, *Thorax* 55:289-294, 2000.
28. Weissler AM, Leonard JJ, Warren JV: Effects of posture and atropine on the cardiac output, *J Clin Invest* 36:1656-1662, 1957.

General References

Adler CHI, Ahlskog JE: *Parkinson's disease and movement disorders: diagnosis and treatment guidelines for the practicing physician*, Totowa NJ, 2000, Humana Press.

Ali-Melkkila A, Kanto J, Iisalo E: Pharmacokinetics and related pharmacodynamics of anticholinergic drugs, *Acta Anaesthesiol Scand* 37:633-642, 1993.

Lucas-Meunier E, Fossier P, Baux G, et al: Cholinergic modulation of the cortical neuronal network, *Pflugers Arch* 446:17-29, 2003.

Mesulam MM, Guillozet A, Shaw P, et al: Acetylcholinesterase knockouts establish central cholinergic pathways and can use butyrylcholinesterase to hydrolyze acetylcholine, *Neuroscience* 110:627-639, 2002.

CHAPTER • 10

Drugs Affecting Nicotinic Receptors

Joel D. Schiff

Early in the sixteenth century, Spanish explorers of the New World encountered a plant extract used by South American natives to poison the tips of their hunting arrows. This extract, known as *curare,* was brought back to Europe, and its lethal action was quickly found to depend on muscular paralysis. Further understanding of the actions of curare did not come for many years.

In 1856, Claude Bernard[8] reported that the site of action of curare was the junction between nerve and muscle. He found that although curare blocked neuromuscular transmission, it did not impede conduction of impulses along the motor nerve or contraction of a directly stimulated muscle. The active substance used by Bernard in his studies, *d*-tubocurarine, was subsequently purified, and in 1942 it was administered for the first time to a patient undergoing surgery for appendicitis to relax the abdominal musculature.[28] Tubocurarine and other drugs that block neuromuscular transmission have since found widespread acceptance for their ability to produce muscular flaccidity and are frequently administered as adjuncts to general anesthesia during surgery.[9]

In 1889, Langley showed that nicotine could "paralyze" transmission at autonomic ganglia, and in 1905 he demonstrated that nicotine could stimulate muscle when applied to the motor endplate and that curare could block this effect.[40] These findings led to the adoption of the term *nicotinic* to refer to the receptors present at both autonomic ganglia and the neuromuscular junction.

Thus the discovery of curare led to developments in two somewhat different directions: to drugs that affect transmission at nicotinic cholinergic receptors and to drugs that interfere with the mechanisms of skeletal muscle contraction. These two topics are the subjects of this chapter.

GANGLIONIC TRANSMISSION

Nicotinic receptors play a crucial role in the transmission of autonomic impulses across the ganglionic synapse. As described in Chapter 5, acetylcholine (ACh) is the primary neurotransmitter at both sympathetic and parasympathetic ganglia, where it is released by preganglionic neurons and stimulates postganglionic neurons by activating nicotinic N_N receptors. Although it is sometimes convenient to think of autonomic ganglia as simple relay stations between the central nervous system (CNS) and effector tissues, the existence of other receptors and neurotransmitters within the ganglia indicates that some modulation of the primary nervous inputs may occur. It is also evident that transmission is not the same in sympathetic and parasympathetic ganglia even though N_N receptors are the primary receptors in both cases.

A variety of pharmacologic and electrophysiologic studies on sympathetic ganglia have led to models of ganglionic transmission that involve at least four classes of receptors: cholinergic nicotinic, cholinergic muscarinic, α-adrenergic, and peptidergic.[24,38] Muscarinic and peptidergic receptors mediate, respectively, slow and late slow excitatory postsynaptic potentials, which appear to facilitate the transmission of high-frequency impulses through the primary nicotinic receptor pathway. Catecholamine-containing (dopamine or norepinephrine) interneurons have been proposed for sympathetic ganglia[27,35] but are not found in parasympathetic ganglia.[55] As shown in Figure 10-1, these interneurons may be stimulated by preganglionic muscarinic activity to release catecholamines that hyperpolarize the postganglionic neuron.[27] This inhibitory postsynaptic potential, which may represent a simple membrane permeability change or be mediated by cyclic adenosine 3′,5′-monophosphate,[44] may serve to impose an upper limit on the action potential frequency through the primary transmission pathway, but it is not known to what extent this effect is physiologically significant.

Despite these uncertainties, two facts remain clear: (1) the autonomic ganglia contain neuronal components that are not protected by a structure analogous to the blood-brain barrier, which means that they are affected by many drugs and chemicals that never gain access to central synapses; and (2) ACh is the primary transmitter of the ganglionic synapse, and any drug that interferes with the synthesis, release, or inactivation of ACh or with its interaction with the nicotinic receptor has the capacity to interfere with ganglionic transmission.

GANGLIONIC BLOCKERS

Between 1895 and 1926 a number of compounds having the generic structure shown in Table 10-1 and termed *methonium compounds* were synthesized. In 1915, Burn and Dale[11] described the ganglionic blocking action of tetraethylammonium (TEA). In the 1940s an entire series of diiodide and dibromide derivatives of these methonium compounds were synthesized, and in 1946, Acheson and Moe[1] published a systematic and extensive pharmacologic study of TEA. Interest in these drugs arose because they could be used as pharmacologic tools for exploring various aspects of autonomic pharmacology and because, at least at first, they offered the promise of being useful therapeutic agents in the treatment of hypertension, peptic ulcers, and other diseases that seemed to have an autonomic component and that had not yet yielded to therapeutic measures then available.

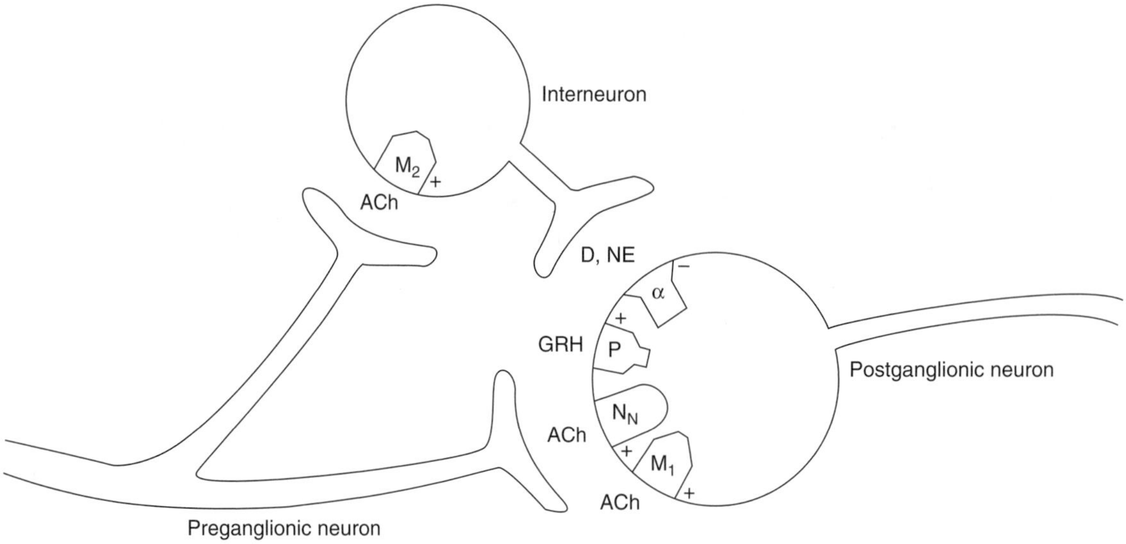

Fig. 10-1 Synaptic connections in the mammalian superior cervical ganglion. The principal pathway involves nicotinic receptor transmission *(N_N)* sensitive to conventional ganglionic blocking drugs. Muscarinic receptors (M_l and M_2), sensitive to atropine blockade, respectively support and inhibit depolarization of the postganglionic neuron. As shown, a catecholamine-containing interneuron may participate in causing inhibition. Corelease of peptides such as gonadotropin-releasing hormone *(GRH)* produces long-lasting facilitation of transmission. *D,* Dopamine; *NE,* norepinephrine; *α,* α-adrenergic receptor; *P,* peptidergic receptor.

Table • 10-1

Some Nondepolarizing Ganglionic Blocking Agents

AGENT	CHEMICAL STRUCTURE
Methonium compounds	$(CH_3)_3N^+—(CH_2)_n—^+N(CH_3)_3$
Hexamethonium	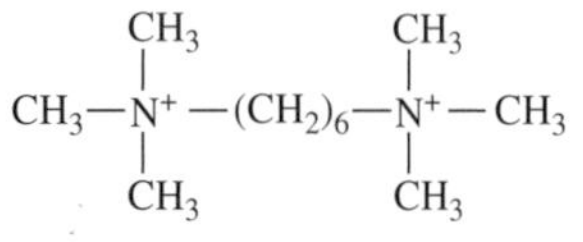
Trimethaphan	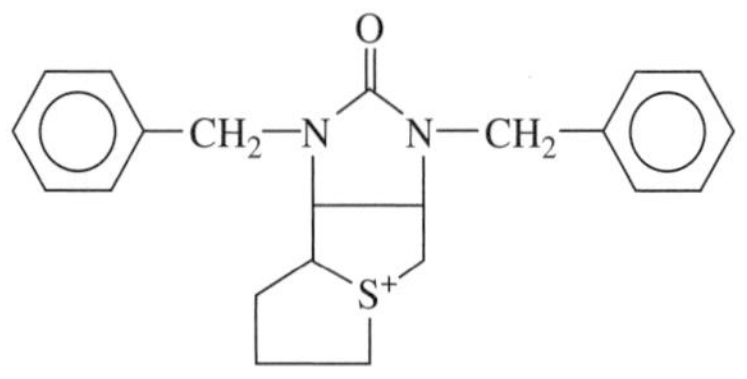
Mecamylamine	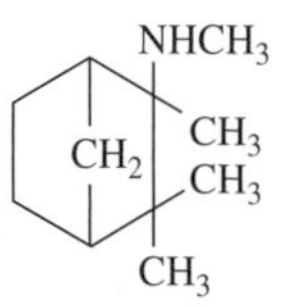

Classification

Ganglionic blocking agents can be classified on the basis of their chemical structure or mechanism of action. One scheme[56] divides these drugs into three groups:

1. Depolarizing drugs, such as nicotine and dimethylphenylpiperazinium, which produce initial stimulation and varying degrees of subsequent block through a mechanism analogous to that of succinylcholine (see below). At higher doses, these agents can stimulate and block other cholinergic receptors, such as those at the neuromuscular junction and in the CNS.
2. Competitive drugs, such as trimethaphan and TEA, which interfere with the binding of ACh to the nicotinic receptor.
3. Noncompetitive agents, such as hexamethonium and mecamylamine, a secondary amine. Hexamethonium interferes with ganglionic transmission[30] by blocking ion channels that have been opened by ACh, whereas mecamylamine appears to share properties associated with both hexamethonium and the competitive blocking agents.[57]

Pharmacologic Effects

This section is restricted to a discussion of the pharmacology of the competitive and noncompetitive nondepolarizing blocking agents because clinically used ganglionic blockers belong to these two groups. Nicotine is discussed separately regarding its ganglionic stimulating properties and its use in tobacco cessation programs.

All the ganglionic blocking drugs, irrespective of their structure or their mechanism of action, have the same basic pharmacology, although a number of them have additional actions at sites other than ganglionic receptors. An ideal ganglionic blocking agent would be a compound that interferes only with ganglionic transmission, blocks without previous excitation, and does not influence the release of transmitter.[47] Hexamethonium is a prototype agent that meets these criteria.

The pharmacology of the ganglionic blocking drugs is predictable because all ganglia, parasympathetic and sympathetic, are blocked by most of the available agents. However, it is important to realize that ganglia are not equally sensitive to the blocking drugs and some effects are easier to block than others. The effects of ganglionic agents are profoundly influenced by the background tone; that is, the effect of blocking a ganglion is proportional to the rate of nerve transmission through that ganglion at any given time. If vascular tone is high, as it would be in a standing individual, the ganglionic blocking agents will produce a profound fall in blood pressure, much greater than they would in a recumbent individual, in whom vascular tone would be lower. Finally, as is shown in Table 10-2, because these drugs block both sympathetic and

Table • 10-2

Usual Predominance of Sympathetic or Parasympathetic Tone at Various Effector Sites, with Consequent Effects of Autonomic Ganglionic Blockade

SITE	PREDOMINANT TONE	EFFECT OF GANGLIONIC BLOCKADE
Arterioles	Sympathetic (adrenergic)	Vasodilation, increased peripheral blood flow, hypotension
Veins	Sympathetic (adrenergic)	Vasodilation, peripheral pooling of blood, decreased venous return, decreased cardiac output
Heart	Parasympathetic (cholinergic)	Tachycardia
Iris	Parasympathetic (cholinergic)	Mydriasis
Ciliary muscle	Parasympathetic (cholinergic)	Cycloplegia
Gastrointestinal tract	Parasympathetic (cholinergic)	Reduced tone and motility, constipation, decreased gastric and pancreatic secretions
Urinary bladder	Parasympathetic (cholinergic)	Urinary retention
Salivary glands	Parasympathetic (cholinergic)	Xerostomia
Sweat glands	Sympathetic (cholinergic)	Anhidrosis

From Hardman JG, Limbird LE, Gilman AG, eds: *Goodman & Gillman's The pharmacological basis of therapeutics*, ed 10, New York, 2001, McGraw-Hill, p. 211.

parasympathetic actions, the direction and magnitude of their effects are related to which autonomic division provides the dominant baseline control for a given organ.

Eye

Parasympathetic neurons play a dominant role in the maintenance of pupillary diameter and activity in the ciliary muscle. Blockade of autonomic ganglia, therefore, leads to partial, but not maximal, dilation of the pupil and to paralysis of accommodation.

Respiratory tract

There is inhibition of secretory activity in the respiratory tract and slight bronchial relaxation, but ganglionic blocking drugs do not directly affect respiration.

Salivary glands

The salivary glands are predominantly under the control of the parasympathetic nervous system. Thus ganglionic blockade results in marked xerostomia.

Gastrointestinal tract

The volume and acidity of gastric secretions that occur spontaneously are strongly inhibited by the ganglionic blocking agents, but there is little effect on secretion induced by histamine.[36] Vagal stimulation is inhibited, and marked inhibition of motility occurs throughout the gastrointestinal tract, leading to paralytic ileus and causing constipation. On the other hand, sympathetically maintained sphincter tone is also lost, and so the constipation may alternate with diarrhea.

Cardiovascular system

Ganglionic blocking drugs cause a fall in blood pressure that depends on posture. Normotensive recumbent subjects show the least change; the most prominent alteration in blood pressure occurs in sitting or standing subjects for the obvious reason that vascular reflexes play an important role in the maintenance of blood pressure in these circumstances. The blood pressure may fall by 35%. Changes in heart rate depend on the existing vagal tone, but generally cardiac rate rises slightly in human beings. Cardiac output, on the other hand, tends to drop, mainly because of poor venous return and pooling of blood in the extremities. Localized blood flow alterations depend on the location of the vascular bed. In the skin, there is an increase in blood flow that manifests itself as a rise in surface temperature and a pinkness of the skin. The effects on coronary, pulmonary, muscle, renal, cerebral, and splanchnic circulation are inconsistent because, although vascular resistance may drop in some of these organs, the reduced cardiac output may not permit a concomitant increase in blood flow.

Urinary tract

The parasympathetic component of the efferent arm of the spinal reflex normally responsible for micturition is blocked. As a result, distention of the bladder does not trigger the voiding response, and urinary retention develops because of incomplete bladder emptying.

Sweat glands

Sympathetic stimulation of the eccrine sweat glands is inhibited, so the skin becomes dry as well as warm and flushed from the vasodilation of skin blood vessels.

Central nervous system

In therapeutic doses, the cationic blocking drugs, including hexamethonium and its congeners, do not gain ready access to the CNS, and they usually have no direct CNS effects. Mecamylamine and other secondary and tertiary amine–blocking agents have been reported to produce such effects as tremor, choreiform movements, mental aberrations, and convulsions.[23]

Absorption, Fate, and Excretion

Quaternary ammonium compounds are poorly absorbed when administered by the oral route because they have a low membrane permeability at any pH. For ganglionic blocking agents, this is an academic question because only one drug, mecamylamine (a secondary amine), is available in an oral formulation, and it is seldom used because of its numerous side effects. Trimethaphan is administered by intravenous drip; it has a rapid onset and short duration of action.

General Therapeutic Uses

Trimethaphan has been used as an adjunct during anesthesia to produce controlled hypotension, although this can frequently be accomplished by simply deepening anesthesia.

Controlled hypotension can be useful during certain surgical procedures (e.g., plastic, vascular, oral) when a reduction in bleeding is desirable. Trimethaphan has also been used in hypertensive emergencies and acute dissecting aortic aneurysm, but other drugs (e.g., sodium nitroprusside) are preferred agents.[17,37] Mecamylamine is available for the treatment of hypertension refractory to other agents.

Adverse Effects

As is true of other autonomic drugs, toxicity from the ganglionic blocking agents is an extension of their known pharmacologic effects. Some of these effects are annoying but bearable: xerostomia, blurring of vision, and constipation. Other side effects, such as orthostatic hypotension, urinary hesitancy, and sexual impotence, present more severe problems, but, because considerable tolerance to these effects may develop, they may seem less problematic as time goes on. However, the ganglionic blocking agents can produce peripheral circulatory collapse with cerebral and coronary insufficiency as well as paralytic ileus and complete urinary retention, and these toxic liabilities of the drugs are the major reason for their gradual abandonment in the treatment of hypertension.

Drug Interactions

Mecamylamine, the only ganglionic blocking agent used to any extent for the ambulatory patient, is potentiated by a variety of drugs, including alcohol, general anesthetics, several diuretics (thiazides, chlorthalidone, and furosemide), antacids, and other antihypertensives. Sympathomimetic drugs administered to a patient taking mecamylamine will produce exaggerated effects, possibly because of upregulation of adrenergic receptors and blockade of opposing parasympathetic activity. The significance of this interaction for the dental patient receiving a local anesthetic with epinephrine has not been described.

Implications for Dentistry

The ganglionic blocking agents are no longer in wide use with ambulatory patients; thus patients with problems stemming from ganglionic blockade that might ordinarily prove troublesome to the dentist, such as xerostomia and orthostatic hypotension, are not likely to be encountered.

NICOTINE

Nicotine, as indicated in Chapter 8, is the principal psychoactive ingredient in tobacco products. As a selective depolarizing drug at nicotinic receptors, this alkaloid stimulates transmission at autonomic ganglia and at nicotinic synapses in the CNS. It also activates a variety of sensory fibers equipped with nicotinic receptors, including mechanoreceptors in the lung, skin, mesentery, and tongue; nociceptive nerve endings; and chemoreceptors in the carotid body and aortic arch. Stimulation of nicotinic receptors in skeletal muscle is easily demonstrated in the laboratory, but it is not evident normally in human beings because initial stimulation is soon followed by inhibition at these nicotinic sites.

An important feature of nicotinic receptors is their tendency to become desensitized (i.e., unresponsive) on continuous exposure to agonists (e.g., succinylcholine, as described later). Thus the actions of nicotine are highly time and concentration dependent, and complex patterns of stimulation and depression are observed. The heart rate, for instance, may be increased by stimulation of sympathetic ganglia and the adrenal medulla and/or by inhibition of vagal transmission in the heart. Conversely, blockade of sympathetic transmission to the heart and stimulation of parasympathetic transmission can cause bradycardia. The heart rate may also be affected by central influences and by actions at peripheral sensory sites.

In general, usual amounts of nicotine absorbed during cigarette smoking cause mild cardiovascular stimulation, increased gastrointestinal activity, and CNS stimulation accompanied in regular users by a feeling of well-being and decreased irritability. With long-term use, tolerance and physical dependence occur.

Acute overdose of nicotine causes nausea and vomiting, abdominal pain, dizziness and confusion, and muscular weakness. If untreated, death may ensue from cardiopulmonary collapse. Nevertheless, the primary health issues regarding nicotine stem from the chronic use of tobacco products. An increased incidence of cancer and cardiovascular and pulmonary disease has been well documented.[54] In dentistry, tobacco use has been linked to oropharyngeal carcinoma, leukoplakia, acute and chronic periodontal disease, delayed wound healing, halitosis, and tooth staining.[14]

The only therapeutic use of nicotine is as an adjunct in tobacco cessation programs. Nicotine is administered in a multiplicity of forms (Table 10-3) to maintain pharmacologic concentrations of the alkaloid and prevent tobacco cessation from triggering an acute withdrawal syndrome, which includes irritability, anxiety, sleep disturbances, and cognitive impairment. It also dissociates the self-administration of nicotine from the social, tactile, and oral and olfactory components of tobacco smoking, thereby weakening the psychologic link between satisfaction of the nicotine craving and the physical actions of tobacco use. The nicotine dose is reduced in a stepwise fashion over a period of several months, during which time the patient ideally receives continued counseling and motivational assistance to remain abstinent. Because of the deleterious effects of smoking and smokeless tobacco on oral health, the dentist is encouraged to participate actively in helping patients quit tobacco use.[14] Such participation may include procedures to promote fresh breath and tooth bleaching to remove tobacco stains from teeth, which may provide additional positive psychologic feedback to encourage abstinence from tobacco use.

NEUROMUSCULAR TRANSMISSION

Nervous control of skeletal muscle contraction is mediated by ACh. In response to a motor neuron action potential, ACh is released from the terminal region of the nerve fiber. The transmitter then diffuses across the junctional cleft and binds with the nicotinic receptor on the postjunctional membrane (endplate) of the muscle fiber. The N_M receptor has two binding sites for cationic ligands, and the binding of two molecules of ACh to the receptor brings about an increase in the cation permeability of the endplate membrane and a consequent depolarization (excitatory endplate potential) of the junctional region of the muscle fiber. Under normal conditions, the depolarization is sufficient to trigger an action potential in the electrically excitable muscle fiber membrane, and muscular contraction follows.[33] Figure 10-2 shows the physiologic events that occur in a nerve, neuromuscular junction, and skeletal muscle and lead to contraction of muscle and indicates points along the pathway at which drugs can block these events.

NEUROMUSCULAR JUNCTION BLOCKERS

Neuromuscular blocking drugs interfere with the ability of ACh to evoke endplate depolarization at the nicotinic N_M receptor. They are generally separated into two groups according to whether they themselves bring about endplate

Table • 10-3

Nicotine-Containing Smoking Deterrents

PRODUCT	PROPRIETARY (TRADE) NAME	NICOTINE CONTENT PER DOSE FORM (mg)	DAILY NICOTINE DOSE (mg)	DURATION*
Nicotine inhalation system	Nicotrol Inhaler	4 (delivered)	As needed	Up to 24 weeks
Nicotine polacrilex gum	Nicorette	2	≤48	Up to 12 weeks
	Nicorette DS	4	≤96	Up to 12 weeks
Nicotine polacrilex lozenge	Commit	2 and 4	≤80	10 to 12 weeks
Nicotine transdermal system (skin patch)	Habitrol	52.5	21	3 to 4 weeks
		35	14	3 to 4 weeks
		17.5	7	3 to 4 weeks
	NicoDerm CQ	114	21	6 weeks
		76	14	2 weeks
		38	7	2 weeks
	Nicotrol	24.9	15†	6 weeks
		16.6	10†	2 weeks
		8.3	5†	2 weeks
	ProStep	30	22	4 weeks
		15	11	4 weeks
Nicotine nasal spray	Nicotrol NS	0.5‡	40	Up to 12 weeks

*For the gum, lozenge, and inhalation dosage forms, the number of units used per day is gradually decreased, beginning after 6 to 12 weeks of therapy. The transdermal systems use a sequential schedule, beginning with the strongest patch.
†Patch is worn 16 hours a day.
‡Dose per actuation; one spray in each nostril (1 mg) is the recommended dose.

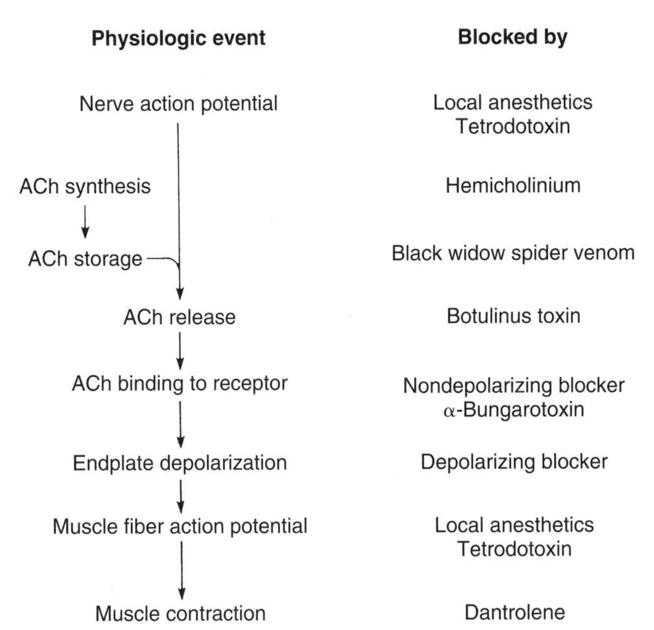

Fig. 10-2 Physiologic events that occur in a motor nerve, neuromuscular junction, and skeletal muscle, leading to contraction of the muscle, and drugs that can block these events.

depolarization in the course of their action. As will be seen, the depolarizing and the nondepolarizing blocking agents differ in the mechanisms through which they produce neuromuscular blockade.

Nondepolarizing Agents

The nondepolarizing, or competitive, neuromuscular blocking drugs include tubocurarine (*d*-tubocurarine), metocurine (dimethyl-*d*-tubocurarine), and several other benzylisoquinolines (e.g., atracurium and rocuronium); steroids such as pancuronium and vecuronium; and a few unrelated drugs (e.g., gallamine). Tubocurarine, rocuronium, and vecuronium are monoquaternary amines with a second nitrogen that is partially ionized at physiologic pH; the other drugs are bisquaternary compounds (except for gallamine, which is a trisquaternary ether). Commonly, these drugs incorporate two cationic nitrogen sites into a relatively rigid molecular structure (Figure 10-3).

Although tubocurarine has the longest history of use and can be thought of as the prototype of this category of drugs, it and metocurine and gallamine are currently used only infrequently because of their tendency to evoke undesirable side effects. Congeners with more selective neuromuscular blocking effects are preferred.[53]

All these drugs act by occupying the endplate N_M receptor sites of the muscle fiber, thus blocking access to these sites by ACh. The drugs themselves do not cause endplate depolarization.[16] Inhibition of neuromuscular transmission is essentially competitive, with the blocking agent and ACh competing for receptor sites on the muscle fiber.[50] By interfering with nervous excitation of muscle without themselves producing any excitation, the nondepolarizing blocking agents cause flaccid paralysis. Because of the very large safety margin in neuromuscular transmission, which results from the sixfold to tenfold excess of ACh released from the motor neuron terminal and from the large number of postjunctional receptor sites, at least 50% of the ACh receptors must normally be blocked to produce any clinically apparent effect on muscle function.

Depolarizing Agents

As with most of the nondepolarizing blockers, succinylcholine, the major depolarizing agent, is a bisquaternary compound. However, unlike the nondepolarizing agents, succinylcholine is a much smaller molecule, composed simply of

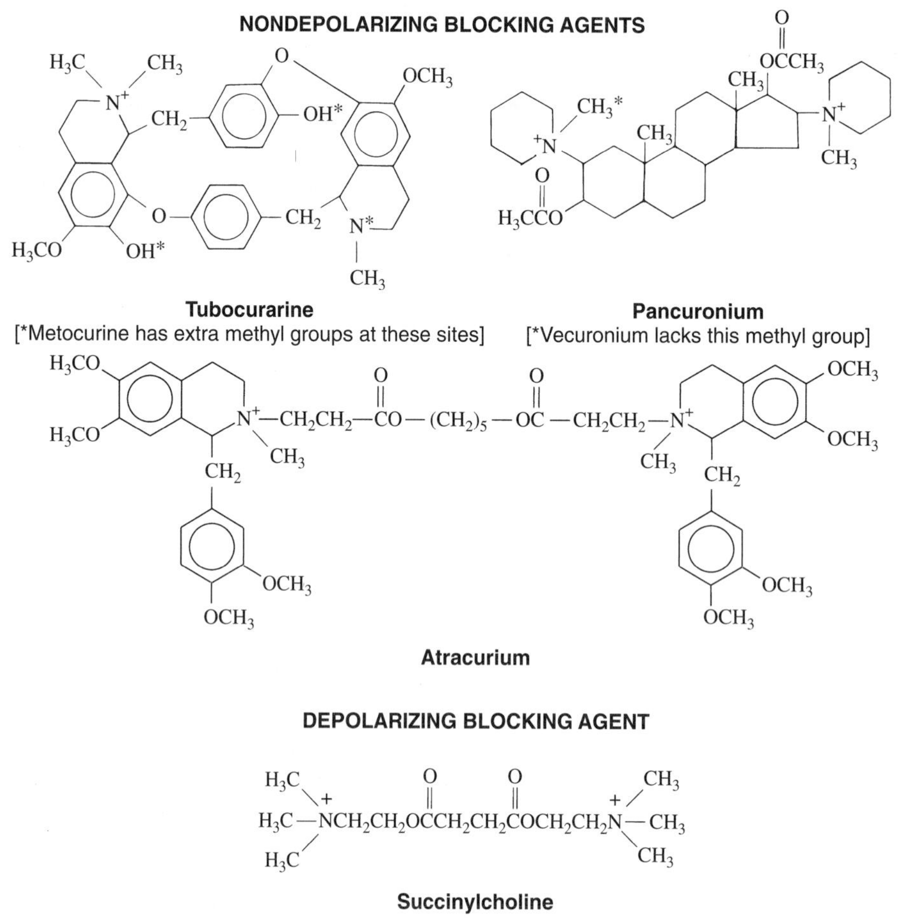

NONDEPOLARIZING BLOCKING AGENTS

Tubocurarine
[*Metocurine has extra methyl groups at these sites]

Pancuronium
[*Vecuronium lacks this methyl group]

Atracurium

DEPOLARIZING BLOCKING AGENT

Succinylcholine

Fig. 10-3 Structural formulas of some neuromuscular blocking agents.

two ACh molecules attached at the acetyl ends. Thus succinylcholine has a flexible chain linkage between its cationic moieties.

Succinylcholine acts by binding to the cholinergic receptor at the muscle endplate. As the class name suggests, the initial effect of the binding of this agent is a depolarization of the muscle fiber. During the early phase of its action, there is a period of excitation during which the sensitivity of the muscle to ACh is actually increased. Indeed, it is common for the drug-induced depolarization to be great enough to trigger action potentials and fasciculations (i.e., spontaneous twitching) in the muscle fibers.

The depolarization produced by the blocking agent gradually diminishes, but the endplate membrane potential does not completely return to its resting level. After the transient excitation, and during the period in which endplate depolarization is still prominent, neuromuscular transmission is blocked in what is referred to as a phase 1 block. Here, continued depolarization of the motor endplate traps surrounding voltage-gated Na^+ channels in an inactivated state (see Chapter 16 for a discussion of Na^+ channel states) refractory to further stimulation until the membrane potential is restored to normal. Recovery from this form of neuromuscular paralysis occurs quickly after cessation of succinylcholine administration. With continued drug infusion, however, the endplate slowly repolarizes despite the presence of succinylcholine, and there is a gradual transition to a longer-lasting phase 2, or desensitization, block. Recovery in this situation is delayed beyond the removal of the depolarizing agent.

A number of theories have been proposed to account for the endplate receptor desensitization in the phase 2 blockade produced by the depolarizing agents. It should be noted that a similar receptor desensitization occurs under laboratory conditions when the presence of ACh is prolonged at the neuromuscular junction by exposure to anticholinesterase or by continuous perfusion with the transmitter.[5] Thus the loss of the depolarizing ability of ACh may be considered a form of drug tachyphylaxis, and a valid explanation for the actions of the depolarizing blocking agents may also account for this more general phenomenon. One currently accepted model for desensitization blockade of the endplate receptor is a modification of that originally proposed by Katz and Thesleff in 1957.[34] This scheme (Figure 10-4) is, to be sure, an oversimplification of the true situation in that detailed kinetic studies have indicated the existence of multiple active and inactive conformations.[21]

Pharmacologic Effects

The major pharmacologic actions of the neuromuscular blocking agents are on the motor endplate of skeletal muscle, and all the therapeutic applications of these drugs stem from those actions. Nevertheless, the neuromuscular blocking agents affect a number of other body systems. Some of the more important of these actions on other sites must be considered when choosing blocking drugs to administer and observing additional precautions in their use.

An ideal neuromuscular blocker would be rapid in onset, consistent in duration of action (even in patients with advanced renal and/or hepatic disease), and readily reversible in effect. It would be a nondepolarizing drug so that it would not cause muscle fasciculations; it would be free of autonomic and cardiovascular effects; and it would not liberate histamine

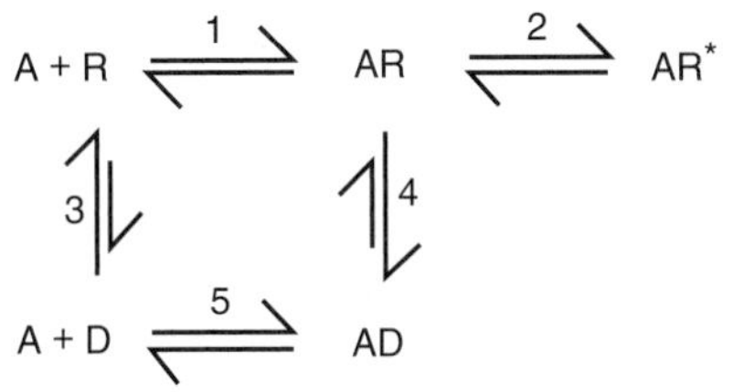

$$A + R \underset{}{\overset{1}{\rightleftharpoons}} AR \underset{}{\overset{2}{\rightleftharpoons}} AR^*$$
$$3 \updownarrow \qquad \updownarrow 4$$
$$A + D \underset{}{\overset{5}{\rightleftharpoons}} AD$$

Fig. 10-4 Scheme for desensitization blockade of endplate receptors. A two-state model in which reactions *1*, *2*, and *5* are assumed to be in relatively rapid equilibrium, whereas equilibrium of reactions *3* and *4* is reached more slowly. *A* is the ligand, which may be ACh or a depolarizing blocking drug; *R* and *D* are, respectively, the active and desensitized states of the receptor; and *AR** is the open-channel conformation. The equilibrium constant of reaction 3 very likely favors the conversion of D to R, but that of reaction 4 favors the formation of *AD* from AR. Thus a depolarizing blocker such as succinylcholine, which has a greater affinity for D than for R, will tend to drive reaction 5 to the right, depleting D, which shifts equilibrium 3 downward and depletes the pool of R; as a result, ACh is less effective as an agonist. On the other hand, in the continuous presence of ACh, reactions 1 and 4 tend to run to the right and downward, respectively, and most receptors end up inactivated to the AD state; this produces tachyphylaxis (see text). (Modified from Katz B, Thesleff S: A study of the "desensitization" produced by ACh at the motor endplate, *J Physiol* (London) 138:63-80, 1957.)

from muscle or other tissues. Additionally it would not induce tachyphylaxis, so that prolonged blockade could be maintained without the need to increase the dosage over time. None of the existing neuromuscular blocking agents fulfills all these expectations; however, cisatracurium, vecuronium, doxacurium, and pipecuronium are notable for their relative lack of effects other than neuromuscular blockade (Table 10-4).[7,58]

Neuromuscular junction

On slow intravenous infusion, neuromuscular blocking agents, both depolarizing and nondepolarizing, first affect the facial muscles and then the other muscles of the head and neck. In the conscious subject, this action produces diplopia, dysarthria, and dysphagia; because of dysphagia, secretions accumulate in the throat, and breathing becomes difficult. In addition, there is an uncomfortable sensation of warmth. As the blockade progresses, the small muscles of the hands and body are affected. Paralysis of the intercostal muscles forces breathing to become entirely diaphragmatic. Finally, complete flaccid paralysis, including paralysis of all respiratory muscles, occurs.

This sequence of effects occurs when maximal doses of neuromuscular blocking agents are administered slowly; lower doses may produce only the earlier manifestations and spare the respiratory muscles from becoming paralyzed. In addition, there is some evidence that succinylcholine preferentially blocks transmission in white muscles, such as those of the limb musculature, with less effect on the slower red muscles, including those of respiration.

Rapid intravenous injection of full paralyzing doses produces a different temporal pattern of blockade. In this situation, the upper airway muscles (larynx, tongue, jaw) and the diaphragm are blocked before peripheral muscles, such as the adductor of the thumb. The respiratory muscles also recover much more quickly. The faster onset in this case may result from increased blood flow or higher temperature in these muscles; the faster recovery is in keeping with the differential sensitivity to neuromuscular blockade already described.

Central nervous system

None of the neuromuscular blocking drugs described here has any apparent influence on the CNS. The reason for this is the inability of these compounds, all of which are permanent cations with low lipid solubility, to cross the blood-brain barrier.

It should be emphasized that neuromuscular blockade does not provide anesthesia or analgesia but can make it

Table • 10-4

Pharmacologic Properties of Neuromuscular Receptor–Blocking Agents

DRUG	ONSET (min)	GANGLIONIC BLOCKADE	HISTAMINE RELEASE	VAGAL BLOCKADE
Ultrashort-Acting				
Succinylcholine	0.5 to 1	–	+	–
Short-Acting				
Mivacurium	2 to 2.5	0	+	0
Intermediate-Acting				
Atracurium	2 to 2.5	0	+	0
Cisatracurium	2.5 to 3	0	0	0
Rocuronium	1 to 1.5	0	0	+
Vecuronium	2.5 to 3	0	0	0
Long-Acting				
Doxacurium	4 to 5	0	0	0
Gallamine	2 to 3	0	0	+++
Metocurine	3 to 4.5	+	+	0
Pancuronium	2 to 3	0	0	++
Pipecuronium	2.5 to 3	0	0	0
Tubocurarine	3 to 5	++	++	0

+++, Strong; *++*, moderate; *+*, slight; *–*, opposite effect (i.e., stimulation of ganglionic and vagal transmission); *0*, no effect.

impossible for a patient to show outward signs of pain. Therefore, when these drugs are used as adjuncts to general anesthesia, the depth of the anesthesia must be monitored closely.

Autonomic nervous system

Because of their selectivity for the N_M receptors of the muscle endplate, the neuromuscular blocking drugs as a group have no major influence on the autonomic nervous system. However, individual drugs of this category do exert certain specific autonomic influences (see Table 10-4).

Pancuronium and especially gallamine can increase the heart rate, in part by inhibiting vagal activity and by increasing norepinephrine release in the heart. Succinylcholine causes a transient bradycardia as it is administered, probably through a vagomimetic action on the muscarinic receptors of the heart.[26] After administration of succinylcholine, there is a longer period of tachycardia that seems to be the result of muscarinic receptor stimulation of sympathetic ganglia.

Histamine release

Several neuromuscular blocking agents, most prominently tubocurarine, cause the release of histamine from mast cells into the circulation (see Table 10-4).[2] Thus these drugs are capable of producing the histamine-mediated effects of hypotension, edema, bronchospasm, and increased salivary flow. The last two actions may introduce complications during performance of controlled respiration and can be prevented by prior administration of antihistamines. Histamine-related effects can be minimized by avoiding rapid intravenous injection. Neuromuscular blocking drugs with a steroid nucleus (pancuronium, pipecuronium, rocuronium, vecuronium) are free of this side effect; doxacurium and cisatracurium are the first benzylisoquinolines without this clinical liability.[19]

Cardiovascular system

Although none of the neuromuscular blocking drugs has any direct effect on vascular tone, all can produce hypotension by a combination of indirect actions. The release of histamine, as described earlier, causes edema and vasodilation. The loss of skeletal muscle tone as a result of neuromuscular blockade eliminates the skeletal muscle pumping action on the veins of the extremities; hence, there is pooling of blood in the veins of the legs, and a concomitant reduction in venous return to the heart. In addition to these physiologic effects on the circulation, another factor of consequence is the use of assisted or controlled ventilation during the period of muscular paralysis. The increased intrathoracic pressure produced by the respirator during its positive-pressure phase further reduces venous return to the heart. In this respect, alternating positive- and negative-pressure respirators are less problematic than are intermittent positive-pressure devices because of the increased venous return in the negative-pressure phase of the former.

These causes of hypotension can be treated by positioning the patient with the lower extremities elevated slightly above the heart and by administering isotonic fluids intravenously, possibly in combination with sympathomimetic vasoconstrictors.

Absorption, Fate, and Excretion

Neuromuscular blocking agents are generally administered intravenously. Intramuscular administration is somewhat effective for most of the agents discussed and may be used in treating some pediatric patients in whom intravenous injection might present difficulties, but this route does not offer the precision of control or the rapidity of onset of action afforded by the intravenous route. The drugs discussed in this chapter are ineffective when given orally. This was known to be the case for tubocurarine by South American hunters, who readily ate prey felled by arrows laden with the drug.

All the clinically useful blocking agents show their effects within a few minutes after administration (see Table 10-4). Succinylcholine provides intubating conditions (vocal cord relaxation) within 30 to 60 seconds after intravenous injection and gives its maximal effect within 2 minutes. Recovery is apparent after 5 to 10 minutes. The nondepolarizing blockers exhibit slower onsets and longer durations of action. However, rocuronium has been found to produce intubating conditions almost as rapidly as succinylcholine in children, and mivacurium, a short-acting agent, has a clinical duration of action of only 15 to 20 minutes after an intubating dose, so these drugs offer nondepolarizing alternatives to succinylcholine for tracheal intubation and other brief procedures. Comparative durations for intermediate- and long-acting blockers (as classified in Table 10-4) are 30 to 90 minutes and 60 to 150 minutes, respectively.[3] With any of the drugs, blockade may be prolonged either by repeated injection or continuous intravenous infusion.

Succinylcholine and mivacurium are both hydrolyzed by plasma pseudocholinesterase, which explains their relatively brief durations of action. Mivacurium is broken down to inactive metabolites, whereas succinylcholine is first converted to succinylmonocholine, a much weaker depolarizing blocking agent, and then to succinic acid and choline. It is possible to inhibit the plasma pseudocholinesterase with hexafluorenium, after which the action of succinylcholine is prolonged much longer.

It should be noted that in some individuals with atypical plasma cholinesterase, succinylcholine and mivacurium will persist in the body for at least 30 minutes. Such patients can be identified before drug administration by a cholinesterase activity assay. Purified cholinesterase has been injected intravenously before treatment to obtain a neuromuscular blockade of short duration in these patients.[25]

The long-acting neuromuscular blockers are to a large extent excreted unchanged by the kidneys[12]; thus their actions are greatly prolonged in patients with renal insufficiency, and they are largely contraindicated in such persons. The intermediate-acting drugs are eliminated in both the urine and bile. Vecuronium, for example, is partially metabolized by the liver; one of its metabolites, the 3-deacetyl derivative, is about 80% as potent as the parent compound. Some of the parent drug and most of the metabolites are excreted by the biliary-fecal route. Vecuronium is suitable for use in patients with renal insufficiency, but it is contraindicated in those with cirrhosis.[58] Atracurium is noteworthy in that it is hydrolyzed by nonspecific esterases and degraded nonenzymatically by a process known as Hofmann elimination. This later process converts the quaternary nitrogens to the tertiary form, cleaving the molecule and yielding laudanosine, a metabolite with CNS stimulatory properties in high concentrations. Because atracurium is almost completely inactivated by metabolism, it is useful in patients with reduced renal function. Thus it is usable irrespective of the adequacy of hepatic and renal function.[4] Cisatracurium, one of the 10 stereoisomers of atracurium, is largely inactivated by Hofmann elimination.

General Therapeutic Uses

Since the first clinical use of tubocurarine in 1942,[28] several applications for the neuromuscular blocking agents have gained wide acceptance.[20,22] These are described below.

Endotracheal intubation

To secure a patent, protected airway, an endotracheal tube is often inserted in patients receiving general anesthesia or those who are otherwise unconscious and/or in need of respiratory assistance. Succinylcholine has long been the drug of choice because of its fast onset of action. Rocuronium is the first nondepolarizing blocker to approach the rapidity of onset of succinylcholine.

Surgery

Neuromuscular blocking agents, most commonly the intermediate-acting competitive blockers, are frequently used as adjuncts to general anesthesia during surgical procedures. The most common indication under this heading is to relax the abdominal wall musculature during abdominal surgery. This application is especially useful in procedures such as appendectomy, in which the underlying condition has produced reflex splinting of these muscles. During brain or cerebrovascular surgery in which the patient is sedated but conscious, neuromuscular blockade is needed to suppress cough and sneeze reflexes so that the field of operation may remain immobilized.

Tetanus

In mild cases of tetanus, the patient is generally able to sustain respiration except during intermittent spasms. Here, neuromuscular blocking agents are administered to reduce the severity of these spasms. In severe cases of tetanus, in which the rigor of the patient extends to the respiratory musculature, blocking drugs are administered to induce flaccidity so that artificially assisted respiration may be used.

Electroconvulsive therapy

In the treatment of depressive illness with electroconvulsive therapy, the therapeutic result is a consequence of the electrical stimulation of the CNS; the massive muscle spasm that accompanies such treatment is of no therapeutic benefit and has the potential for producing bodily injury. Neuromuscular blockade is therefore induced by injection of succinylcholine before the electrical stimulation of the brain. Succinylcholine is used here because of its short duration of action and lack of residual side effects, although mivacurium is a nondepolarizing alternative.

Other uses

Succinylcholine is used to produce a short-lived muscular relaxation to permit a number of brief nonsurgical manipulations, such as bronchoscopy. In cases of laryngospasm, succinylcholine may be needed to relax the vocal cords and permit ventilation.

Short-acting nondepolarizing blockers facilitate the setting of fractures of extremities or the mandible. Despite the fact that only a brief blockade is needed for such a procedure, succinylcholine is unsuitable because the fasciculations it causes may compound the fracture-associated injury.

Nondepolarizing neuromuscular blockers are sometimes used in the intensive care unit to facilitate the mechanical ventilation of patients. As this use is associated with a wide range of problems, including deep venous thrombosis, unrecognized inadequate sedation or analgesia, and prolonged paralysis after stopping the agent, this use should be minimized whenever possible.

Applications in Dentistry

Dental practice holds few indications for the use of neuromuscular blocking agents. Among the situations in which use of these drugs might be appropriate are mandibular fractures, when muscle relaxation is needed to permit manipulation of bone fragments, and trismus, when no more conservative means exist to permit mouth opening for diagnosis and treatment. In addition, succinylcholine or a relatively short-acting nondepolarizing blocker is used to aid the insertion of an endotracheal tube when the use of general anesthesia makes intubation appropriate. Indeed, in any office where general anesthesia is used, succinylcholine should always be available to treat otherwise intractable laryngospasm.

Adverse Effects

The major threat of overdosage with neuromuscular blocking agents is death from respiratory failure. Certainly, when any neuromuscular blocking drug is administered, the practitioner must be prepared for the loss of respiratory function and have equipment immediately available for assisted or controlled respiration. In cases of respiratory arrest, ventilation must be maintained with external devices, generally with an endotracheal tube. Paralysis from nondepolarizing agents may be reversed to some extent through administration of an anticholinesterase (e.g., neostigmine), generally accompanied by an antimuscarinic drug (e.g., atropine) to prevent excessive muscarinic receptor–mediated sequelae to the anticholinesterase. The use of an anticholinesterase to reverse the phase 2 block of succinylcholine is also possible; however, with nondepolarizing drugs available with a wide range of durations of action, there should be no need for patient exposure to succinylcholine for a period long enough to produce a phase 2 block.

Arrhythmogenic effects of the neuromuscular blocking drugs stem from their ability to influence autonomic transmission in the ganglia and heart. Of the commonly used drugs, pancuronium is notable for its tendency to increase heart rate. Conversely, transient bradycardia is a known feature of succinylcholine, especially in small children. After a second dose of succinylcholine, bradycardia is more pronounced, and cardiac asystole has been reported. Arrhythmias have also resulted from the tendency of succinylcholine to cause hyperkalemia, especially in burn patients and individuals with certain neuromuscular deficits. Sudden death may occur in children with undiagnosed muscular dystrophy. Hypotension and responses to drug-evoked histamine release have been previously reviewed.

Succinylcholine, as the only depolarizing neuromuscular blocker in clinical use, initially stimulates muscle contraction. Muscle pain is a common result, especially in ambulatory patients. Masseter spasm occurs in up to 1% of children and may complicate endotracheal intubation. In rare individuals, masseter spasm is an indicator of malignant hyperthermia, which is discussed in the section on dantrolene.

Drug Interactions

Many different classes of drugs are capable of interacting, either positively or antagonistically, with the neuromuscular blocking agents (Table 10-5). The following sections describe the actions of drugs likely to be administered in conjunction with neuromuscular blockers and their effects on the activities of the blocking agents.

Anticholinesterases

Inhibitors of acetylcholinesterase, by blocking the enzymatic hydrolysis of ACh at the motor endplate, increase the amount of transmitter available at the receptor sites. These drugs antagonize the blockade produced by the nondepolarizing blocking agents, which act by competing with ACh for occupancy of receptor binding sites. Their effect when administered in conjunction with succinylcholine is more complex; after a brief period of antagonism, during which the blockade is reduced, they act to intensify the neuromuscular blockade by further desensitizing the receptors to transmitter. Organophosphates such as echothiophate inhibit plasma cholinesterase as well as acetylcholinesterase. Therefore systemic absorption of organophosphates will prolong the action of succinylcholine and mivacurium as well as reduce the effects of the nondepolarizing blockers in general.

Table • 10-5

Effect of Various Agents on the Depth of Blockade Produced by Nondepolarizing and Depolarizing Blocking Agents

AGENT	NONDEPOLARIZING BLOCKER	SUCCINYLCHOLINE
Nondepolarizing blocker	+	–
Succinylcholine	–, +	+
Anticholinesterase	–	+
Hexafluorenium	0*	+
Halothane, isoflurane	+	+
Aminoglycosides	+	+
Phenytoin, carbamazepine (long-term use)	–	0
Magnesium salts	+	+
Reduced temperature	–	+

* May intensify the blockade by mivacurium.
+, Intensification of the blockade; *–*, reversal or lessening of the blockade; *0*, no major effect.

Neostigmine and pyridostigmine, but not edrophonium, also inhibit plasma cholinesterase.

Hexafluorenium, which specifically inhibits plasma pseudocholinesterase without affecting the endplate acetylcholinesterase, prolongs the presence of succinylcholine in the circulation. This action both extends the duration of the neuromuscular blockade by succinylcholine, and presumably mivacurium, and decreases the dose necessary to obtain that blockade. In addition to its inhibitory effect on plasma cholinesterase, hexafluorenium is itself a weak nondepolarizing neuromuscular blocker and as such may slightly potentiate the blockade induced by other nondepolarizing blockers.

General anesthetics

Anesthetics that stabilize excitable membranes, most prominently ether and the halogenated inhalation agents, tend to interact positively with the nondepolarizing blocking agents. When ether was used for general anesthesia, doses of tubocurarine had to be reduced by 50% or more.[46] A similar reduction is necessary with isoflurane and pancuronium, but a more modest interaction occurs with sevoflurane and vecuronium.

Antibiotics

Some antibiotics, such as the aminoglycosides, reduce the amount of ACh released by the motor nerve terminal in response to an action potential and thus augment the muscle relaxation caused by nondepolarizing neuromuscular blocking drugs.[6,18,52] Succinylcholine is also potentiated. Other antibiotics that may lower dosage requirements for the neuromuscular blockers include the tetracyclines, clindamycin, and the polymyxins.

Sympathomimetics

Catecholamines and other sympathomimetic agents may increase the amount of ACh released from the motor neuron and thereby antagonize the blockade produced by nondepolarizing blocking agents.[39]

Lithium

Lithium salts, used for the prophylaxis and treatment of manic-depressive illness, can slow the onset of neuromuscular blockade caused by succinylcholine but not that caused by the competitive blockers. Lithium also intensifies the blockade by pancuronium but not that by tubocurarine or succinylcholine, and it prolongs the effect of succinylcholine and pancuronium but not that of tubocurarine.[31]

Neuromuscular blocking agents

Administration of a nondepolarizing blocking agent to a patient under the influence of the same drug or a different nondepolarizing blocking drug augments the blockade. This augmentation is usually additive; however, some combinations, such as pancuronium and metocurine, demonstrate supraadditive effects.[59] This drug interaction is used clinically; a small "priming" dose of one nondepolarizing blocker may be given to hasten the onset of the subsequent paralyzing dose of another.

Administration of a second dose of succinylcholine to a patient already treated with the drug may lighten the blockade for a brief interval, which would correspond to the period of early transient fasciculation that follows administration of any of the depolarizing drugs. However, the ultimate effect of the second dose is augmentation of the neuromuscular blockade. Some tachyphylaxis occurs, however, to repeated administrations.

Combinations of depolarizing and nondepolarizing neuromuscular blocking drugs are generally antagonistic and therefore have little clinical value. Use has been made of this antagonism, however, in the administration of a low dose of nondepolarizing blocker before paralyzing the patient with succinylcholine. In this case, the nondepolarizing agent prevents the fasciculations normally caused by succinylcholine. It is also a frequent practice to use succinylcholine to induce a rapid blockade for tracheal intubation before the production of a long-term blockade with a nondepolarizing agent. Here, the short lifetime of succinylcholine in the body effectively prevents any significant antagonism between the two drugs.[22] Interestingly, subsequent administration of the nondepolarizing drug generally gives evidence of enhanced neuromuscular blockade.

OTHER AGENTS AFFECTING NEUROMUSCULAR TRANSMISSION

A number of substances, both synthetic and of biologic origin, have been found to act by affecting one or more of the processes involved in normal neuromuscular transmission. Although clinical applications have not yet been found for all of these drugs, it should be recalled that nearly a century elapsed between Bernard's discovery of the site of action of curare and the first use of that drug in surgery. As the mechanisms of action of each of the following drugs become more completely known, it is possible that useful applications for some or all of them will be found.

Hemicholinium

Most of the choline produced by the enzymatic hydrolysis of ACh is returned to the motor nerve terminal by a specific transport system and is then used in the synthesis of new transmitter.[49] Hemicholinium, by blocking the neuronal uptake of choline, interferes with the synthesis of ACh and thus acts to deplete the nerve terminal of this substance.[42] The resulting blockade of neuromuscular transmission is gradual in onset but is accelerated by increased motor neuron activity. Because hemicholinium inhibits choline transport in all peripheral cholinergic nerves, it affects transmission at all cholinergic synapses and junctions. Hemicholinium has no clinical applications at present.

Botulinum Toxin

The toxin produced by *Clostridium botulinum* acts on the motor nerve terminal to prevent the release of ACh in response to the arrival of an axonal action potential.[10] The toxin interferes with the influx of extracellular Ca^{++} into the nerve terminal[51]; Ca^{++} influx during the action potential is necessary for ACh release.[49] Therefore botulinum toxin affects all peripheral cholinergic nerves.

Botulinum toxin is used in ophthalmology in the treatment of strabismus and certain ocular deviations (tropias). The toxin, applied focally, can produce long-lasting (weeks to months) paralysis of an excessively contracting extraocular muscle, and the hope is that, as function gradually recovers, CNS adaptation will maintain the correction. The toxin is also used to relieve severe blepharospasm. It is injected into the orbicularis oculi, where it blocks spasmodic contractions for up to 3 months. The treatment can then be repeated indefinitely.[60] Another serologically distinct form of botulinum toxin is used for certain types of skeletal muscle dystonias, such as cervical dystonias. In a cosmetic application, botulinum toxin is used to inhibit activity of certain facial muscles, such as those of the forehead, whose contractions cause skin wrinkling.

α-Bungarotoxin

α-Bungarotoxin isolated from the venom of the banded krait, as well as the similar if not identical neurotoxin from the venom of the cobra, is capable of binding avidly to the cholinergic receptor proteins of the muscle endplate.[13,41] The toxin does not cause endplate depolarization, and its effect, although essentially irreversible, is similar to that of the nondepolarizing blocking agents. The ability of radiolabeled α-bungarotoxin to bind stoichiometrically with skeletal muscle nicotinic receptors makes it possible to locate and count receptor sites; this has provided a useful technique for research on a number of subjects ranging from denervation supersensitivity to myasthenia gravis.

Tetrodotoxin

Tetrodotoxin, found in a number of tissues of the puffer fish, or fugu, prevents the propagation of both peripheral axon and skeletal muscle action potentials by interfering with electrically activated Na^{+} conductance. Saxitoxin, which is produced by certain strains of dinoflagellates and has been implicated in the occasional contamination of shellfish that consume these organisms, has a similar effect on Na^{+} channels. The mechanism of action of these toxins is similar to that of local anesthetics, but their potencies are a millionfold greater, and they act for up to a day or more after a single exposure.

Dantrolene

Dantrolene (Figure 10-5) is an agent that acts within the skeletal muscle fiber rather than on the neuromuscular junction. Its site of action is the sarcoplasmic reticulum, where it inhibits the depolarization-induced release of Ca^{++} from the cisternae of the sarcoplasmic reticulum into the cytoplasm,

O_2N—(C₆H₄)—(furan)—CH=N—N(hydantoin: C=O, NH, C=O)

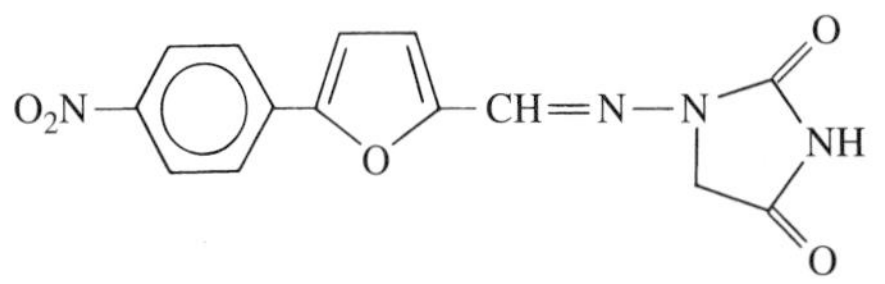

Fig. 10-5 Structural formula of dantrolene.

thus interfering with excitation-contraction coupling.[45] The principal therapeutic applications of dantrolene are for the relief of spasticity associated with upper motor neuron disorders and for the prophylaxis and treatment of malignant hyperthermia (MH).[29,32]

Spastic movements, clonus, and rigidities that result from stroke or cerebral palsy are often relieved by dantrolene[15]; the spasticity of multiple sclerosis is relieved to a lesser extent, possibly because the lesions of this condition are more widespread.[48] On the other hand, dantrolene is strongly contraindicated in amyotrophic lateral sclerosis because the muscular weakness associated with this condition, when exacerbated by the drug (see below), can lead to respiratory difficulty.[48]

MH is a genetically transmitted condition in which there is an apparent reduction in the threshold for Ca^{++} release from the sarcoplasmic reticulum of skeletal muscle, often because of a mutation in the ryanodine receptor that forms the Ca^{++}-release channel.[43] Under normal conditions, Ca^{++} is released from the sarcoplasmic reticulum in response to an all-or-none action potential propagating down the transverse tubular system. Because there are no partial depolarizations physiologically, the actual threshold for Ca^{++} release by the sarcoplasmic reticulum is unimportant. However, a depolarizing neuromuscular blocking drug does produce such a partial depolarization of the muscle fiber membrane. Thus succinylcholine and the volatile general anesthetics such as halothane or isoflurane, which may also lower the release threshold, can trigger an attack of MH in which the increased release of Ca^{++} into muscle cytoplasm causes contracture and an enormous acceleration of the cellular metabolism of muscle; the latter generates heat (body temperature can rise by 1° C every 5 minutes and reach 43° C), carbon dioxide (arterial tensions more than 100 mm Hg), and lactic acid (arterial blood pH below 7.0). The hyperthermia, hypoxemia, and acidosis, in turn, cause muscle edema and structural damage.[29] In addition, the hyperthermia and resultant sympathetic reflex response increase heart metabolism fivefold to eightfold and can lead to arrhythmias. Before dantrolene, attacks of MH were frequently (70%) fatal. Dantrolene, by blocking the precipitating event, the release of Ca^{++} from the sarcoplasmic reticulum, can prevent or halt an attack of MH and has reduced the mortality rate to less than 10%.[29]

Side effects of dantrolene include muscle weakness and hepatotoxicity. The muscle weakness, which is simply an extension of the drug's therapeutic action, generally does not appear at dosages used for treatment of spastic movements, although doses high enough to produce this effect are sometimes needed to achieve symptom remission. Doses of dantrolene that produce muscle weakness are sometimes used in prophylaxis of MH before surgery on patients with a familial history of the condition.

Hepatotoxicity of varying degrees has been reported in approximately 1% of patients taking dantrolene for 60 days or longer. Accordingly, hepatic function should be monitored during long-term therapy with dantrolene.[48] Furthermore, the minimal effective dose should be used.

Dantrolene is effective when administered either intravenously or orally; in the latter case, approximately 20% is absorbed, largely through the small intestine.[48] Metabolism of dantrolene takes place in the liver, largely by 5-hydroxylation of the hydantoin moiety.

Agents Affecting Nicotinic Receptor Transmission

Nonproprietary (generic) name	*Proprietary (trade) name*
Ganglionic blocking agents	
Hexamethonium*	—
Mecamylamine	Inversine
Trimethaphan*	Arfonad
Ganglionic stimulating agents	
Nicotine	See Table 10-3
Neuromuscular blockers	
Nondepolarizing	
Alcuronium*	Alloferin
Atracurium	Tracrium
Cisatracurium	Nimbex
Doxacurium	Nuromax
Gallamine*	Flaxedil
Metocurine*	Metubine
Mivacurium	Mivacron
Pancuronium	Pavulon
Pipecuronium	Arduan
Rocuronium	Zemuron
Tubocurarine	—
Vecuronium	Norcuron
Depolarizing	
Succinylcholine	Anectine, Quelicin
Miscellaneous agents	
Botulinum toxin type A	Botox
Botulinum toxin type B	Myobloc
Dantrolene	Dantrium
Hexafluorenium*	Mylaxen

* Not currently available in the United States.

Cited References

1. Acheson GH, Moe GK: The action of tetraethylammonium ion on the mammalian circulation, *J Pharmacol Exp Ther* 87:220-236, 1946.
2. Alam M, Anrep GV, Barsoum GS, et al: Liberation of histamine from the skeletal muscle by curare, *J Physiol* (London) 95:148-158, 1939.
3. Atherton DP, Hunter JM: Clinical pharmacokinetics of the newer neuromuscular blocking drugs, *Clin Pharmacokinet* 36:169-189, 1999.
4. Atracurium—a novel muscle relaxant, *Drug Ther Bull* 23:51-52, 1985.
5. Axelsson J, Thesleff S: The "desensitizing" effect of acetylcholine on the mammalian motor endplate, *Acta Physiol Scand* 43:15-26, 1958.
6. Barnett A, Ackermann E: Neuromuscular blocking activity of gentamicin in cats and mice, *Arch Int Pharmacodyn Ther* 181:109-117, 1969.
7. Basta SJ, Savarese JJ, Ali HA, et al: Clinical pharmacology of doxacurium chloride: a new long-acting nondepolarizing muscle relaxant, *Anesthesiology* 69:478-486, 1988.
8. Bernard C: Analyse physiologique des propriétés des systèmes musculaire et nerveux au moyer du curare, *Compt Rend Soc de Biol. Section D: Sciences Naturelles* (Paris) 43:825-829, 1856.
9. Booij LHDJ: The history of neuromuscular blocking agents, *Curr Anaesth Crit Care* 11:27-33, 2000.
10. Burgen ASV, Dickens F, Zatmen LJ: The action of botulinum toxin on the neuro-muscular junction, *Physiol* (London) 109:10-24, 1949.
11. Burn JH, Dale HH: The action of certain quaternary ammonium bases, *J Pharmacol Exp Ther* 6:417-438, 1915.
12. Chagas C: The fate of curare during curarization. In de Reuck AVS, ed: *Curare and curare-like agents,* Boston 1962, Little, Brown.
13. Chang CC, Lee CY: Isolation of neurotoxins from the venom of *Bungarus multicinctus* and their modes of neuromuscular blocking action, *Arch Int Pharmacodyn Ther* 144:241-257, 1963.
14. Crews KM, Johnson L, Nichols M: Patient management in a tobacco-cessation program in the dental practice, *Compend Contin Educ Dent* 15:1142-1155, 1994.
15. Dantrolene sodium for treatment of spasticity, *Med Lett Drugs Ther* 16:61-62, 1974.
16. del Castillo J, Katz B: A study of curare action with an electrical micromethod, *Proc R Soc Lond [Biol]* 146:339-356, 1957.
17. Drugs for hypertensive emergencies, *Med Lett Drugs Ther* 29:18-20, 1987.
18. Enomoto K-I, Maeno T: Presynaptic effects of 4-aminopyridine and streptomycin on the neuromuscular junction, *Eur J Pharmacol* 76:1-8, 1981.
19. Faulds D, Clissold SP: Doxacurium. A review of its pharmacology and clinical potential in anaesthesia, *Drugs* 42:673-689, 1991.
20. Feldman SA: *Muscle relaxants,* Philadelphia, 1973, WB Saunders.
21. Feltz A, Trautmann A: Desensitization at the frog neuromuscular junction: a biphasic process, *J Physiol* (London) 322:257-272, 1982.
22. Foldes FF: The choice and mode of administration of relaxants. In Foldes FF, ed: *Muscle relaxants,* Philadelphia, 1966, FA Davis.
23. Freis ED: Clinical uses of ganglionic blocking agents in the treatment of hypertension and a comparison of different blocking agents. In Moyer J, ed: *Hypertension,* Philadelphia, 1959, WB Saunders.
24. Gibbins IL, Jobling P, Messenger JP, et al: Neuronal morphology and the synaptic organisation of sympathetic ganglia, *J Auton Nerv Syst* 81:104-109, 2000.
25. Goedde HW, Altland K: Suxamethonium sensitivity, *Ann NY Acad Sci* 179:695-703, 1971.
26. Graf K, Strom G, Wahlin A: Circulatory effects of succinylcholine in man, *Acta Anesthesiol Scand* 114(suppl):1-48, 1963.
27. Greengard P, Kebabian JW: Role of cyclic AMP in synaptic transmission in the mammalian peripheral nervous system, *Fed Proc* 33:1059-1067, 1974.

28. Griffith HR, Johnson GE: The use of curare in general anesthesia, *Anesthesiology* 3:418-420, 1942.
29. Gronert GA: Malignant hyperthermia, *Anesthesiology* 53:395-423, 1980.
30. Gurney AM, Rang HP: The channel-blocking action of methonium compounds on rat submandibular ganglion cells, *Br J Pharmacol* 82:623-642, 1984.
31. Hill GE, Wong KC, Hodges MR: Lithium carbonate and neuromuscular blocking agents, *Anesthesiology* 46:122-126, 1977.
32. Hopkins PM: Malignant hyperthermia: advances in clinical management and diagnosis, *Br J Anaesth* 85:118-128, 2000.
33. Hubbard JI: Microphysiology of vertebrate neuromuscular transmission, *Physiol Rev* 53:674-723, 1973.
34. Katz B, Thesleff S: A study of the "desensitization" produced by acetylcholine at the motor end-plate, *J Physiol* (London) 138:63-80, 1957.
35. Kawai Y: Noradrenergic synaptic transmission in the superior cervical ganglion, *Kaibogaku Zasshi* 74:167-173, 1999.
36. Kay AW, Smith AN: Effect of hexamethonium iodide on gastric secretion and motility, *Br Med J* 1:460-463, 1950.
37. Koch-Weser J: Hypertensive emergencies, *N Engl J Med* 290:211-214, 1974.
38. Koketsu K, Akasu T: Modulation of nicotinic transmission by endogenous substances in sympathetic ganglia. In Kalsner S, ed: *Trends in autonomic pharmacology,* vol 3, London, 1985, Taylor & Francis.
39. Kuba K: Effects of catecholamines on the neuromuscular junction in the rat diaphragm, *J Physiol* (London) 211:551-570, 1970.
40. Langley JN: On the reaction of cells and of nerve endings to certain poisons chiefly as regards the reaction of striated muscle to nicotine and to curari, *J Physiol* (London) 33:374-413, 1905.
41. Lester HA: Blockade of acetylcholine receptors by cobra toxin: electrophysiological studies, *Mol Pharmacol* 6:623-631, 1972.
42. MacIntosh FC: Effect of HC-3 on acetylcholine turnover, *Fed Proc* 20:562-568, 1961.
43. MacLennan DH, Phillips MS: Malignant hyperthermia, *Science* 256:789-794, 1992.
44. McAfee DA, Henon BK, Whiting GJ, et al: The action of cAMP and catecholamines in mammalian sympathetic ganglia, *Fed Proc* 39:2997-3002, 1980.
45. Morgan KG, Bryant SH: The mechanism of action of dantrolene sodium, *J Pharmacol Exp Ther* 201:138-147, 1977.
46. Ngai SH: Action of general anesthetics in producing muscle relaxation: interaction of anesthetics with relaxants. In Katz RL, ed: *Muscle relaxants,* New York, 1975, American Elsevier.
47. Paton WDM, Zaimis EJ: The methonium compounds, *Pharmacol Rev* 4:219-253, 1952.
48. Pinder RM, Brogden RN, Speight TM, et al: Dantrolene sodium: a review of its pharmacological properties and therapeutic efficacy in spasticity, *Drugs* 13:3-23, 1977.
49. Potter LT: Synthesis, storage and release of (14C) acetylcholine in isolated rat diaphragm muscles, *J Physiol* (London) 206:145-166, 1970.
50. Shaker N, Eldefrawi AT, Aguayo LG, et al: Interactions of *d*-tubocurarine with the nicotinic acetylcholine receptor/channel molecule, *J Pharmacol Exp Ther* 220:172-177, 1982.
51. Simpson LL: Ionic requirements for the neuromuscular blocking action of botulinum toxin: implications with regard to synaptic transmission, *Neuropharmacology* 10:673-684, 1971.
52. Singh YN, Marshall IG, Harvey AL: The mechanisms of the muscle paralysing actions of antibiotics, and their interaction with neuromuscular blocking agents, *Rev Drug Metab Drug Interact* 3:129-153, 1980.
53. Sparr HJ, Beaufort TM, Fuchs-Buder T: Newer neuromuscular blocking drugs: how do they compare with established agents? *Drugs* 61:919-942, 2001.
54. Surgeon General: *The health consequences of smoking. Nicotine addiction,* Office of Smoking and Health, Department of Health and Human Services Publication No. (CDC) 88-8406, Washington, DC, 1988, US Government Printing Office.
55. Suzuki T, Volle RL: Nicotinic, muscarinic, and adrenergic receptors in a parasympathetic ganglion, *J Pharmacol Exp Ther* 211:252-256, 1979.
56. van Rossum JM: Classification and molecular pharmacology of ganglionic blocking agents. Part I, *Int J Neuropharmacol* 1:97-110, 1962.
57. van Rossum JM: Classification and molecular pharmacology of ganglionic blocking agents. Part II, *Int J Neuropharmacol* 1:403-421, 1962.
58. Vecuronium, *Med Lett Drugs Ther* 26:102, 1984.
59. Waud BE, Waud DR: Interaction among agents that block end-plate depolarization competitively, *Anesthesiology* 63:4-15, 1985.
60. Wirtschafter JD, Rubenfeld M: Botulinum toxin injections for treatment of blepharospasm and hemifacial spasm, *Int Ophthalmol Clin* 31:117-132, 1991.

General References

Bevan DR: Fifty years of muscle relaxants, *Acta Anaesthesiol Scand Suppl* 106:2-6, 1995.

Birmingham AT: Fifth WDM Paton Memorial Lecture, *Br J Pharmacol* 128:1685-1689, 1999.

Bowman WC: *Pharmacology of neuromuscular function,* ed 2, Boston, 1990, Butterworth.

Kharkevich DA, ed: *New neuromuscular blocking agents. Handbook of experimental pharmacology,* vol 79, Berlin, 1986, Springer-Verlag.

Savarese JJ, Caldwell JE, Lien CA, et al: Pharmacology of muscle relaxants and their antagonists. In Miller RD, ed: *Anesthesia,* ed 5, New York, 2000, Churchill Livingstone.

Volle RL, Hancock JC: Transmission in sympathetic ganglia, *Fed Proc* 29:1913-1918, 1970.

CHAPTER • 11

Introduction to Central Nervous System Drugs

Kenneth M. Hargreaves, Douglass L. Jackson, and Mark T. Roszkowski

An overview of neuropharmacology indicates that drugs that alter neurotransmitter synthesis, release, receptors, signal transduction pathways, or termination mechanisms are likely to have considerable impact on neuronal activity. An understanding of these fundamental mechanisms permits appreciation of the therapeutic actions and side-effect profiles of many of the central nervous system (CNS) drugs. The interested student is encouraged to seek several excellent reviews in this area.[3,4,8,11] The pharmacology of specific CNS drugs is examined in greater detail in Chapters 12 through 21 and Chapter 23.

The CNS consists of the brain and spinal cord. Through mechanisms still incompletely understood, the CNS integrates sensory information from the external and internal environments, maintains homeostasis through visceral and somatic secretory and motor activity, and generates memory, thoughts, and emotions. Many common diseases have their origins in CNS dysfunction, including Alzheimer's disease, epilepsy, stroke, anxiety, psychoses, movement disorders, mental impairment, and some forms of chronic pain. In addition, the therapeutic and/or side effects of many drugs arise from alterations in CNS activity. Approximately 20% of the most frequently prescribed medications have their principal sites of action within the CNS (e.g., opioid-containing analgesics, benzodiazepines such as alprazolam, antidepressants such as sertraline and fluoxetine, and sleep aids such as zolpidem), and it is virtually certain that every practicing dentist will perform dental treatment on patients taking these drugs. This chapter reviews the anatomic, cellular, and biochemical organization of the CNS from the perspective of drug actions in the CNS. Table 11-1 lists examples of drugs that act on the CNS to produce their therapeutic effects.

ANATOMIC ORGANIZATION OF THE CENTRAL NERVOUS SYSTEM

Several excellent texts are available that provide comprehensive descriptions of the organizational structure and pharmacology of the CNS.[3,4,8,11,12] Accordingly, the following section reviews only those key structural elements of the CNS most pertinent to understanding drug actions and effects.

Cerebral Cortex

Anatomy

The cerebral cortex consists of two hemispheres with deeply enfolded grooves termed *gyri*. The extensive folding of the cerebral cortex increases its surface area. The major divisions of the cortex are the somatosensory cortex (which processes sensory information), motor cortex (which initiates and coordinates somatic muscle activity), association cortex, and visual and auditory areas. These cortical regions are involved with voluntary movement and integration of sensation, consciousness, abstract thought, memory, and learning.

A primary organizational feature of the cerebral cortex is its arrangement as a series of densely packed columns of interconnected cells. The columnar organization of the cerebral cortex is probably a major factor in the integration of neural activity that occurs in the structure. Each column is approximately 0.5 to 1 mm in diameter and includes 10,000 to 50,000 interconnected neurons. The classic studies by Penfield determined the somatic representation of the human body surface on the sensory cortex (the "sensory homunculus").[14] These studies indicated that approximately 75% of the sensory cortex processes afferent input from orofacial structures, including the lips, jaws, tongue, and teeth. This predominant cerebral processing of orofacial sensation may contribute to the aversive anxiety that many patients have during the course of dental care.

Pharmacology

Drugs that alter cerebral cortical activity include general anesthetics, antianxiety drugs, sedative-hypnotics, antidepressants, and antipsychotics. As detailed below (and in subsequent chapters), the sites of action and the precise biochemical mechanisms for many of these drugs are still incompletely understood. The clinical consequence, however, of a reduction in cortical activity is generally sedation or unconsciousness. For example, administration of the inhalation anesthetic halothane reduces cerebral activity in the frontal cortex during the induction of general anesthesia.[5]

Limbic System

Anatomy

The limbic system, another major organizational component of the CNS, is composed of the amygdala, septum, hippocampus, hypothalamus, olfactory lobes, basal ganglia, and portions of the thalamus. These interrelated structures act to coordinate affective (i.e., emotional) sensations with motor, visceral, and endocrine functions. In addition, many behavioral functions ascribed to the limbic system are linked functionally to the reticular formation.

Pharmacology

Many drugs act, in part, by modifying activity of the limbic system. For example, benzodiazepines act at several discrete sites within this system to potentiate the effects of the neurotransmitter γ-aminobutyric acid (GABA), resulting in a reduction of anxiety and the development of sedation (Table 11-1).[16] Benzodiazepines also reduce seizure activity. Endoge-

Table • 11-1

Selected Drug Actions in the CNS

DRUG CLASS	EXAMPLE DRUG	MAJOR SITE(S) OF ACTION*	MECHANISM†	PHARMACOLOGIC EFFECT
Drugs Commonly Used in Dentistry				
Opioids	Morphine	PAG/medulla/spinal cord	Presynaptic inhibition	Analgesia
Benzodiazepines	Diazepam	Limbic system/cerebral cortex	GABA potentiation	Anxiety reduction/sedation
Local anesthetics	Lidocaine	Nonselective	Na^+-channel blockade	Convulsions
Other Commonly Used Drugs				
Antihypertensives	Clonidine	Medulla	α_2-Adrenoceptor stimulation	Reduced sympathetic activity
Inhalation anesthetics	Isoflurane	Reticular formation, etc.	Ion-channel blockade	General anesthesia
Antiparkinson agents	Levodopa	Basal ganglia	Increased dopamine synthesis	Reduced motor symptoms
Antipsychotics	Haloperidol	Limbic system/reticular formation	Dopamine receptor antagonism	Control of schizophrenia

*Several of these drugs have more than one site of action in the CNS.
†Drugs may exert different mechanisms through activation of multiple receptors (see text).
GABA, γ-Aminobutyric acid; *PAG*, periaqueductal gray matter.

nous ligands for the benzodiazepine receptor may be involved in the pathogenesis of epilepsy because epileptic patients have a significant reduction in benzodiazepine receptors.[15] If administered in excess, local anesthetics such as lidocaine may induce seizure activity. This toxic reaction is mediated by activity within the CNS.

A major hypothesis for some forms of mental dysfunction (e.g., schizophrenia) proposes an excess in dopaminergic activity. Several antipsychotic drugs are dopamine receptor antagonists and are thought to act at various sites in the limbic system and reticular formation. The clinical consequence of dopamine receptor blockade in these patients is the amelioration of psychotic behavior. On the other hand, Parkinson's disease is associated with a chronic reduction of dopamine activity in the basal ganglia complex of the limbic system. This disease is commonly managed by the administration of drugs such as levodopa (L-dihydroxyphenylalanine, the amino acid precursor to dopamine) that increase dopamine activity.

Many drugs have a site of action in the hypothalamus and related structures. For example, the estrogens contained in many birth control formulations act, in part, by inhibiting release of the hypothalamic gonadotropin-releasing hormone and thus luteinizing hormone and follicle-stimulating hormone, thereby preventing ovulation. In addition, alcohol-induced diuresis results from inhibition of the release of antidiuretic hormone (also known as *vasopressin*). The clinical disease caused by chronically diminished release or activity of antidiuretic hormone is known as *diabetes insipidus.*

Midbrain and Brainstem

Anatomy

The midbrain and brainstem regions consist of the mesencephalon, pons, medulla, reticular activating system, and most of the cranial nerve nuclei, including the trigeminal nuclei. This region acts to process sensory information from the viscera, coordinate visceral (i.e., cardiovascular, pulmonary, and gastrointestinal) systems, and integrate various reflexes (such as swallowing and vomiting). In addition, the reticular activating system is implicated in the maintenance of arousal and development of sleep. The reticular activating system is sensitive to many drugs, including most CNS depressants.[2]

Pharmacology

Several drugs have major sites of action within midbrain structures. Opioids such as morphine produce much of their analgesia by activating opioid receptors located in the periaqueductal gray region, locus ceruleus, and nucleus raphe magnus. Atropine can increase the respiratory rate by an action on vagal nuclei in the medulla. In addition, the antihypertensive drug clonidine is an α_2-adrenergic receptor agonist whose therapeutic effect, in part, results from activating medullary receptors that inhibit sympathetic outflow.

Not all drug effects in the CNS are considered therapeutic. For example, opioid-induced emesis is caused by activation of receptors located in the chemoreceptor trigger zone of the medulla. This side effect is especially prominent in ambulatory patients, whose walking increases activity in the vestibular system. This interaction between drug effect and neural input is the rationale for instructing patients in acute pain receiving opioid analgesics to avoid excessive motion and thereby minimize nausea and vomiting.

Spinal Cord

The spinal cord is involved with the processing and modulation of general sensory information (e.g., touch, heat, cold, pressure, and pain), somatic motor activity, and skeletal and visceral reflexes. A number of drugs are thought to activate spinal cord mechanisms. For example, opioids produce analgesia, in part, by stimulating receptors located in the spinal dorsal horn. (An analogous site of action for opioid inhibition of trigeminal pain involves interaction with receptors located in the medullary dorsal horn, as mentioned in Chapter 20.) This site of action is the basis for the administration of opioids through epidural catheters to elicit spinal analgesia. In addition, the epidural administration of local anesthetics such as bupivacaine is commonly used for the production of regional anesthesia in surgical and obstetric procedures. Moreover, recent studies suggest that the nonsteroidal antiinflammatory drugs produce analgesia after intrathecal injection, suggesting that these drugs have both peripheral and central sites of action.

Blood-Brain Barrier

The CNS is isolated from the rest of the body by the blood-brain barrier. Endothelial cells of the brain capillary system are modified by numerous tight junctions and are surrounded with extensive perivascular astrocytic processes. These modifications prevent the free diffusion of many substances into the CNS. Lipid solubility is a key factor in dictating the CNS actions of many drugs. Drugs that are highly lipophilic (e.g., thiopental, diazepam, and heroin) easily cross the blood-brain barrier and have a rapid onset of action. In contrast, hydrophilic drugs (e.g., dopamine and some antibiotics) do not cross the blood-brain barrier, minimizing their therapeutic effects in the CNS. The blood-brain barrier is incompletely developed at the time of birth, and thus many drugs administered to neonates achieve relatively greater concentrations in the CNS than occur in older children or adults.[10]

SYNAPTIC ORGANIZATION OF THE CENTRAL NERVOUS SYSTEM

Information Encoding

Communication within the CNS incorporates both digital and analog encoding.[4,11] The digital encoding consists of the frequency of action potential depolarizations that are conveyed along the plasma membrane of the neuron. The major pharmacologic intervention of this form of signal encoding is the use of drugs that block ion channels, thereby preventing the initiation and conduction of action potentials. The blockade of Na^+ channels by local anesthetics is a primary example. This CNS effect is the basis for many of the toxic effects of local anesthetics (e.g., sedation, convulsions).

The analog form of neuronal communication occurs at the synapse (Figure 11-1), where diffusible chemicals contained in synaptic vesicles or gases (e.g., nitric oxide) are released from the presynaptic neuron to activate receptors located on the postsynaptic neuron. A variable (or analog) response at the postsynaptic membrane occurs because a variable number of vesicles may be released. Factors that alter the number of vesicles released include the frequency of action potential depolarizations that arrive at the presynaptic membrane, its preexisting membrane potential, and its metabolic status. Stimulation of presynaptic receptors that augment or inhibit neurotransmitter release and activation of postsynaptic receptors by other neurochemicals also promote graded responses. In addition to chemically mediated signals, direct electrical signaling between cells is possible (e.g., by gap junctions), but this form of communication is currently of minor importance to pharmacotherapy and will not be discussed further.

Chemical communication between neurons is well suited for mediating either inhibitory or excitatory signals and permits flexible neuronal processing in response to environments that are constantly changing. Another important quality of chemical transmission is the potential for amplification of the signal from a single presynaptic cell to a large number of postsynaptic neurons by extensive axonal synaptic connections.

In contrast to the relatively meager number of drugs that modulate digital neuronal encoding, numerous drugs modulate analog encoding. Indeed, most CNS drugs with a known mechanism of action appear to act primarily by altering synaptic activity. This list includes most receptor agonists and antagonists, enzyme inhibitors, and drugs that alter the reuptake of neurotransmitters. Before exploring the pharmacologic actions of CNS drugs, it is important to understand the physiologic system of chemical communication between neurons, including neurotransmitters, their synthesis, release into the extracellular space, actions on target cells, and termination of effects.

Organizational Features of the Synapse

A schematic representation of chemical communication is presented in Figure 11-1. Because the cell body contains all the intracellular organelles necessary for protein synthesis (nucleus, ribosomes, endoplasmic reticulum, and Golgi apparatus), microtubular transport plays an important role in carrying newly synthesized proteins (e.g., enzymes, neuropeptides, and receptors) to the nerve terminals. Accordingly, drugs that block microtubular transport, such as colchicine, could play an important role in the inhibition of neuronal function. Presynaptic modification of synaptic activity is a major form of neuronal signal processing. Presynaptic terminals may inhibit or facilitate synaptic activity by altering the membrane potential. Opioids are thought to act, at least in part, through a presynaptic mechanism. Activation of opioid receptors may hyperpolarize the neuronal membrane, thereby inhibiting release of neurotransmitter across the synapse. Additional sites for pharmacologic manipulation include the synthesis, release, action, and inactivation of various neurotransmitters. These mechanisms are considered in further detail in the following section.

BIOCHEMICAL ORGANIZATION OF THE CENTRAL NERVOUS SYSTEM

Neurotransmitters

Several criteria must generally be fulfilled for a substance to be considered a neurotransmitter.[4,11] For instance, the substance must be synthesized in the presynaptic nerve, stored in synaptic vesicles, released by nerve stimulation, and rapidly inactivated. In addition, exogenous application of the substance should produce the same effects as does endogenous release. By some estimates, nearly 100 substances have partially or completely fulfilled these criteria. They can be classified, on the basis of their chemical structure, as amino acids, small organic compounds, large organic complexes, lipids, small peptides, and gases. Within the CNS, acetylcholine (ACh), monoamines, amino acids, peptides, and purines represent the main classes of chemicals involved in neuronal signaling. Some important CNS neurotransmitters and some important receptor subtypes are listed in Table 11-2.

Acetylcholine

After the discovery that ACh acts as a peripheral neurotransmitter, considerable research has elucidated its role as a CNS neurotransmitter. Cholinergic neurons are now thought to innervate motor neurons of the ventral spinal cord as well as form projection and local circuit neurons in the cerebral cortex, limbic system, and thalamus. Both muscarinic and neuronal nicotinic receptor subtypes have been identified in the CNS. ACh is thought to modulate arousal, respiration, motor activity, pain, vertigo, and memory. Many cholinergic agonists have prominent CNS effects. Antimuscarinic drugs are often used as adjunctive therapy in the management of Parkinson's disease or as a prophylactic treatment to prevent motion sickness. The anticholinesterase physostigmine is used to manage certain acute delirium reactions. Several other anticholinesterases (including donepezil, tacrine, and ri-

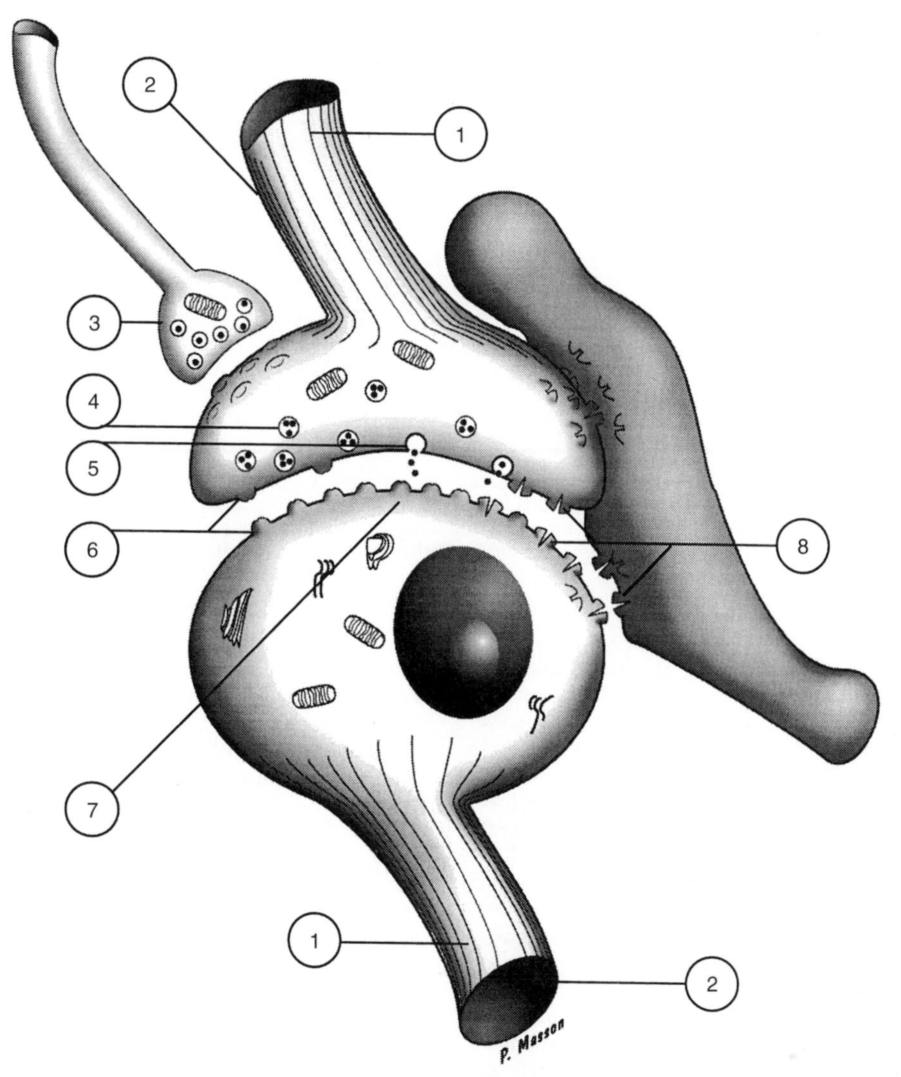

Fig. 11-1 The major elements involved in synaptic communication, including several sites of drug action. *1*, Microtubules are involved in transporting proteins synthesized in the cell body; drugs such as colchicine can disrupt microtubular transport. *2*, The neuronal membrane potential is normally negative with respect to the extracellular surface. Depolarization is a major form of digital communication and can be blocked by local anesthetics. *3*, Presynaptic neuronal processes can inhibit or facilitate activity of presynaptic neurons. Many drugs, such as opioids, may act in part by presynaptic inhibition. *4*, The synthesis or storage of neurotransmitters can be altered by a number of drugs (e.g., levodopa, which serves as a dopamine precursor). *5*, The secretion of neurotransmitters is the major component of analog signaling. Drugs such as amphetamine acutely increase release of norepinephrine from a cytoplasmic source. *6*, Receptors can exist on presynaptic and postsynaptic membranes and can be affected by either agonists or antagonists. *7*, Signal transduction mechanisms mediate receptor events and can be classified as either metabotropic or ionotropic in nature. Drugs such as the methylxanthines (e.g., caffeine) can increase intracellular cyclic adenosine 3′,5′-monophosphate concentrations by inhibiting phosphodiesterase. *8*, Neurotransmitters are inactivated by either metabolic mechanisms or by uptake into either neurons or glia. Drugs can alter synaptic activity by inhibiting reuptake (e.g., tricyclic antidepressants inhibit reuptake of norepinephrine and 5-hydroxytryptamine) or by inhibiting degradation (e.g., physostigmine, which blocks the metabolism of acetylcholine by acetylcholinesterase).

vastigmine) have been approved to improve memory in early phases of Alzheimer's disease.

Monoamines

The monoamines, otherwise known as the biogenic amines, constitute a major class of neurotransmitters. Dopamine, norepinephrine, epinephrine, 5-hydroxytryptamine (5-HT), and histamine are the primary members of this class. Dopamine is a major CNS neurotransmitter, functioning in areas of motor control, behavior, mood, and perception. Dopamine constitutes more than 50% of the total CNS content of catecholamines. The importance of this neurotransmitter is also demonstrated in its critical role in such debilitating CNS diseases as Parkinson's disease, Huntington's disease, and schizophrenia. A by-product of illicit opioid manufacture known as MPTP (1-methyl-4-phenyl-1,2,5,6-tetrahydropyridine) has been shown to produce a parkinsonlike syndrome in addicts by causing selective destruction of nigrostriatal dopaminergic neurons (see Chapter 15).[9]

Norepinephrine is the next most common catecholamine (approximately 30% of total CNS catecholamines) and is a neurotransmitter of brainstem neurons within the locus ceruleus, with projections to the cortex, cerebellum, and spinal cord. In addition, norepinephrine is the neurotransmitter of

Table • 11-2

Some Important CNS Transmitters and Their Receptor and Signaling Characteristics

TRANSMITTER	RECEPTOR SUBTYPE	SIGNALING MECHANISM	EFFECTOR MECHANISM
5-HT (serotonin)	$5HT_{1A}$	$G_{i/o}$ protein	↓cAMP, ↑K^+ conductance
	$5HT_{2A}$	$G_{q/11}$ protein	↓K^+ conductance
Dopamine	D_1	G_s protein	↑cAMP
	D_2	$G_{i/o}$ protein	↓cAMP, ↑K^+ conductance
GABA	$GABA_A$	Ion channel	↑Cl^- conductance
	$GABA_B$	$G_{i/o}$ protein	↑K^+, ↓Ca^{++} conductances*
Glutamate-aspartate	NMDA	Ion channel	↑K^+, ↑Na^+, ↑Ca^{++} conductances
	AMPA	Ion channel	↑K^+, ↑Na^+ conductances
Glycine		Ion channel	↑Cl^- conductance

*Responses vary depending on tissue.
Peptide and purine neurotransmitters and their receptors are not listed. ACh, norepinephrine, and histamine receptors are discussed extensively in other chapters. Only some receptor subtypes are listed for 5-HT, dopamine, and glutamate-aspartate. *AMPA*, α-Amino-3-hydroxy-5-methyl-4-isoxazole propionate; *cAMP*, cyclic adenosine 3′, 5′-monophosphate; *GABA*, γ-aminobutyric acid; *5-HT*, 5-hydroxytryptamine; *NMDA*, N-methyl-D-aspartate.

postganglionic neurons of the sympathetic nervous system. Norepinephrine is thought to modulate affective disorders, learning, reward, sleep, and pain perception.

In contrast to dopamine and norepinephrine, concentrations of epinephrine in the CNS are quite low (approximately 5% to 17% of the norepinephrine content) and are localized primarily in cell bodies of the reticular formation. The precise roles of epinephrine in the CNS are still under active investigation.

Neurons containing 5-HT are found primarily near the midline raphe nuclei of the brainstem and project to the cortex, cerebellum, and spinal cord. 5-HT is thought to modulate sleep, pain, and affective states. Neurochemical evidence also reveals a concentration of histamine in the hypothalamus and histamine-binding sites in various brain regions. Blockade of these binding sites is thought to account for the drowsiness experienced by many people who take antihistamines such as diphenhydramine and hydroxyzine.

Amino acids

An additional major class of neurotransmitters consists of single amino acids.[7,8] Research on the neurotransmitter roles of amino acids has been difficult to interpret because these substances are integral components of general intermediary metabolism and are present in numerous cell types. However, a number of studies now support the proposition that amino acids are quantitatively the major neurotransmitters in the CNS. These amino acids can be divided into those that are excitatory, capable of depolarizing neurons (glutamic acid, aspartic acid, cysteic acid, and homocysteic acid), and those that are inhibitory, capable of hyperpolarizing neurons (GABA, glycine, taurine, and β-alanine).

Glutamate is found in high concentrations within the brain and has been shown to have potent excitatory effects. Current evidence indicates that this excitatory amino acid has possible roles in learning, pain, and neuronal toxicity. Studies conducted in experimental animals suggest that glutamate receptor antagonists protect against neuronal death and may have therapeutic potential for reducing neuronal damage in stroke victims.[13] Certain drugs that block excitatory amino acid transmission have been shown to have antiparkinson activity in some experimental settings. CNS-acting drugs such as the dissociative anesthetic ketamine are known to affect glutamate neurotransmission by binding to a site on the N-methyl-D-aspartate receptor and impeding the flow of Ca^{++} through the channel of the receptor.

GABA and glycine are believed to be the major inhibitory neurotransmitters in the CNS. GABA is found in high concentrations in the mammalian brain and spinal cord. When GABA binds to the $GABA_A$ receptor, the result is hyperpolarization of the postsynaptic neuron, mediated by the inward flow of Cl^-. Antianxiety drugs such as benzodiazepines are thought to function as facilitators of GABAergic transmission in the CNS by increasing the affinity of GABA for its receptor and by increasing effective coupling of the $GABA_A$ receptor to the Cl^- channel.[4,16] Glycine is thought to function primarily in the spinal cord, the lower brainstem, and perhaps the retina. High concentrations of glycine are found in the ventral horn of the spinal cord, suggesting an inhibitory function on the interneurons and motor neurons in this region. Convulsions induced by the administration of strychnine are thought to occur because of inhibition of glycine receptors.

Neuropeptides

A large number of pharmacologically active peptides have been found in neurons. These peptides are capable of causing excitation as well as inhibition when applied to target tissues. Many neuropeptides are classified into distinct families that share a common amino acid sequence. The opioid peptides constitute an important example. This neuropeptide family includes the endomorphins, endorphins, enkephalins, and dynorphins. With the exception of the endomorphins, members of this family with opioid activity contain the amino acid sequence tyrosine-glycine-glycine-phenylalanine (Tyr-Gly-Gly-Phe).[6]

Peptides differ from the small molecular weight neurotransmitters in several regards. The primary difference is demonstrated in their synthesis. Unlike the small molecular weight transmitters, which can be synthesized anywhere within the neuron by cytoplasmic enzymes, peptides depend on mechanisms concentrated in the cell body (e.g., transcription, translation, posttranslational processing). Posttranslational processing involves splitting of the precursor protein into smaller peptides. It is not uncommon for a single precursor molecule to yield multiple copies of the active peptide (e.g., proenkephalin) or even several different active peptides (e.g., proopiomelanocortin).[1] In addition, alternative splitting of the precursor may occur in different tissues, in which the precursor may be cleaved in different locations, yielding completely different peptides with totally unrelated functions. This response is tissue specific and driven by different splicing enzymes.

The neuroactive peptides leave the Golgi apparatus in secretory vesicles that also contain enzymes capable of converting peptides to the final active form. These vesicles are transported to the nerve terminal by axonal transport mechanisms and are then released in response to action potentials. The phenomenon of co-localization of such neurotransmitters as monoamines and ACh with neuropeptides and adenosine triphosphate (ATP) is common, with each chemical exerting a slightly different effect on the target tissue provided that receptors exist for each mediator.

Purines

ATP, found in purinergic nerves or co-localized with catecholamines or ACh, may act as a neurotransmitter and may modulate the effect of other neurotransmitters. Adenosine also appears to act as an inhibitory neurotransmitter.

RELEASE OF NEUROTRANSMITTER

The release of neurotransmitter from the neuron is mediated by action potentials. To briefly review this mechanism, membrane depolarization activates voltage-gated Na^+ channels, allowing an influx of Na^+ into the presynaptic cell. The resulting depolarization of the presynaptic terminus activates voltage-gated Ca^{++} channels that are hypothesized to exist in greater abundance at the nerve terminal. This Ca^{++} current is known as the *secretory potential* and initiates mechanisms leading to the release of transmitter from the presynaptic neuron during membrane depolarization.[11] Repolarization of the nerve terminal occurs as the Na^+ channels become inactivated and K^+ channels open, leading to an efflux of K^+ out of the presynaptic cell.

Research indicates that there is a clustering of synaptic vesicles at the nerve terminal. The number of vesicles at this site of the neuron is much greater than that in other areas of the cell. The vesicles aggregate adjacent to areas of presynaptic membrane thickening known as *dense bars.* This region of the nerve terminal is termed the *active zone* because it is the site where the neurotransmitter is actually released from the synaptic vesicles by exocytosis. In response to an action potential, synaptic vesicles fuse with the presynaptic membrane, releasing their contents into the extracellular space of the synapse. The actual mechanics of neurotransmitter release occurs in stages. Synaptic vesicles must first dock with the plasma membrane. After docking, a priming reaction occurs that prepares the vesicle to fuse with the plasma membrane when an action potential is present at the terminal. With the arrival of the action potential and the subsequent increase in Ca^{++} in the terminal, the vesicle fuses with the plasma membrane and releases the vesicle contents into the synapse. The events leading to the fusion of synaptic vesicles to the plasma membrane occur very quickly (within a fraction of a millisecond) and depend on the presence of a Ca^{++} influx. A number of important molecules have been implicated in the process of vesicle docking and fusion. Synaptobrevin, syntaxin, and SNAP-25 are three molecules that are integral to the process and are collectively referred to as the *SNARE complex.* Equally important to the process are guanosine triphosphate–binding proteins such as rab3 that regulate the fusion process. Ca^{++} concentrations in the nerve terminal also evoke the release of vesicles anchored to the cytoskeletal processes in the nerve terminal. The release of these vesicles allows them to move toward the active zone, increasing the probability of their fusion with the plasma membrane and the subsequent release of their contents. Changes in the duration of the action potential and the pattern of firing of the action potentials can alter the amount of intracellular Ca^{++} and affect the number and type of vesicles released.

The process described previously is representative of the mechanism for the release of the small clear vesicles that primarily contain the low molecular weight neurotransmitters.[13] The larger dense core vesicles, which contain the monoamines and peptides, are thought to be released by essentially similar mechanisms but with different proteins for vesicle docking and fusion. The mechanisms for the release of the contents of the dense core vesicles, however, still depend on the influx of Ca^{++}. Additionally, some of the neurons that release monoamines and peptides do not possess active zones, and the transmitter substances are released at nonspecialized sites of the presynaptic membrane.

RECEPTOR BINDING AND SIGNAL TRANSDUCTION

The various types of receptors for neurotransmitters, hormones, and drugs that act on the CNS are discussed in the broader context of general receptor pharmacology in Chapter 1. Table 11-2 identifies several neurotransmitters and receptors that are uniquely or closely associated with the CNS.

TERMINATION OF NEUROTRANSMITTER EFFECT

Termination of the neurotransmitter signal is important for efficient functioning of the signaling process. If the neurotransmitter were to remain at the synapse and continue to bind to its receptor, new signals could not get through. Desensitization of the receptor would also result from continued exposure to the neurotransmitter. Three mechanisms are involved in signal termination: uptake of the neurotransmitter back into the presynaptic neuron, enzymatic degradation of the neurotransmitter, and diffusion out of the synapse.

Reuptake

Reuptake of the neurotransmitter into the presynaptic cell is the most important mechanism for terminating the effects of catecholamines and 5-HT. The existence of high-affinity uptake systems has been demonstrated for norepinephrine as well as other monoamines and some of the excitatory amino acids. These uptake mechanisms are selective for specific neurotransmitters and rely on carrier or transporter proteins that span the plasma membrane. The transporters depend on the exchange of ions (primarily Na^+) or the hydrolysis of ATP to drive the system. Many antidepressants function by inhibiting the uptake of neurotransmitters such as norepinephrine and 5-HT, leaving a greater concentration of transmitter at the synapse and prolonging its duration of action. Blockade of this uptake mechanism is also responsible for the effects seen with cocaine administration. Cocaine is a powerful inhibitor of the uptake of norepinephrine and dopamine from the synaptic cleft. Augmentation of dopaminergic transmission in the nucleus accumbens region of the brain has been linked to the euphoria produced by cocaine. A similar increase in synaptic concentrations of norepinephrine over long periods results in several cardiovascular side effects seen with cocaine abuse, namely dysrhythmia and hypertension. The danger of administering exogenous catecholamines to the person intoxicated with cocaine should be readily apparent.

Enzymatic Degradation

Enzymatic degradation is an efficient method for terminating the effect of neurotransmitters such as ACh and ATP. The enzymes involved in metabolizing ACh and ATP are found primarily on the extracellular face of the plasma membrane of the postsynaptic neuron. The degradation of ACh by extracellular acetylcholinesterase in the synaptic cleft is a prototypic example of the regulation of transmitter effect. Anticholinesterases (e.g., physostigmine) are used clinically to inhibit this degradation, thereby increasing the amount of ACh present within the synaptic cleft. Enzymes for metabolizing many other neurotransmitters are found in neurons. Enzymatic inactivation occurs after the neurotransmitter is taken up into the neuron, usually the presynaptic neuron. The intracellular regulation of neurotransmitter concentrations is tightly controlled and compartmentalized, as is demonstrated by the monoamine oxidase system. This enzyme is found on the surface of mitochondria and degrades catecholamines and 5-HT in the cytoplasmic pool (see Figure 5-5). The monoamine oxidase inhibitors used to treat depression (e.g., isocarboxazid) function by blocking the degradation of the monoamines within the presynaptic neuron, resulting in an increase in the amount of cytoplasmic monoamines. This effect then leads to chronic adaptive receptor changes, which are discussed in Chapter 12.

Diffusion

Diffusion and removal by bulk flow are the simplest methods of terminating the neurotransmitter effect. The kinetics of diffusion depend on the concentration gradient of the neurotransmitter through the synaptic cleft and the affinity of the ligand for its receptor. Diffusion occurs at all synapses to some degree; its relative importance in terminating neurotransmitter action is inversely related to the combined influence of local metabolism and reuptake.

Cited References

1. Akil H, Watson SJ, Young E, et al: Endogenous opioids: biology and function, *Annu Rev Neurosci* 7:223-255, 1984.
2. Bimar J, Bellville JW: Arousal reactions during anesthesia in man, *Anesthesiology* 47:449-454, 1977.
3. Carpenter MB, Sutin J: *Human neuroanatomy,* ed 8, Baltimore, 1983, Williams & Wilkins.
4. Cooper JR, Bloom FE, Roth RH: *The biochemical basis of neuropharmacology,* ed 7, New York, 1996, Oxford University Press.
5. Cooper JR, Meyer EM: Possible mechanisms involved in the release or modulation of release of neuroactive agents, *Neurochem Int* 6:419-427, 1984.
6. Cox BM: Endogenous opioid peptides: a guide to structures and terminology, *Life Sci* 31:1645-1658, 1982.
7. Fagg GE, Foster AC: Amino acid neurotransmitters and their pathways in the mammalian central nervous system, *Neuroscience* 9:701-719, 1983.
8. Kandel ER, Shwartz JH, Jessell TM, eds: *Principles of neural science,* ed 4, New York, 2000, McGraw-Hill.
9. Langston JW: MPTP neurotoxicity: an overview and characterization of phases of toxicity, *Life Sci* 36:201-206, 1985.
10. Levine RR: *Pharmacology: drug actions and reactions,* ed 6, Boston, 2000, Little, Brown.
11. Levitan IB, Kaczmarek LK: *The neuron: cell and molecular biology,* ed 3, New York, 2002, Oxford University Press.
12. Liebman M: *Neuroanatomy made easy and understandable,* ed 4, Rockville, MD, 1991, Aspen.
13. Meldrum B: Possible therapeutic applications of antagonists of excitatory amino acid neurotransmitters, *Clin Sci* (London) 68:113-122, 1985.
14. Penfield W, Rasmussen T: *The cerebral cortex of man; a clinical study of localization of function,* New York, 1950, Macmillan.
15. Savic I, Widen L, Thorell JO, et al: Cortical benzodiazepine receptor binding in patients with generalized and partial epilepsy, *Epilepsia* 31:724-730, 1990.
16. Sieghart W: $GABA_A$ receptors: ligand-gated Cl^- ion channels modulated by multiple drug-binding sites, *Trends Pharmacol Sci* 13:446-450, 1992.

General References

2002 Receptor and ion channel nomenclature supplement, *Trends Pharmacol Sci* 23(suppl):1-73, 2002.

Alberts B, Bray D, Lewis J, et al: *Molecular biology of the cell,* ed 4, New York, 2002, Garland.

Nestler E, Hyman S, Malenka R: *Molecular basis of neuropharmacology: a foundation for clinical neuroscience,* New York, 2001, McGraw Hill.

Shepherd GM: *Neurobiology,* ed 3, New York, 1994, Oxford University Press.

Snyder SH: Drug and neurotransmitter receptors in the brain, *Science* 224:22-31, 1984.

Strange PG: *Brain biochemistry and brain disorders,* Oxford, 1992, Oxford University Press.

CHAPTER • 12

Psychopharmacology: Antipsychotic and Antidepressant Drugs*

Vahn A. Lewis

According to the National Institutes of Mental Health, 20% of the population will have a diagnosable mental disorder in their lifetime.[30] There are many types of mental disorders, as classified in the *Diagnostic and Statistical Manual of Mental Disorders (DSM-IV)* of the American Psychiatric Association.[11] Schizophrenia, which afflicts 0.5% to 1% of the population, is the most severe of the psychiatric disorders, and disturbances of mood (affective disorders) are the most common. Approximately 10% to 25% of women and 5% to 12% of men will have at least one major depressive episode during their lifetimes. Schizophrenia and the affective disorders are episodic and progressive disorders. Although appropriate treatment tends to improve the course of a disorder, it rarely produces a cure. The psychotherapeutic drugs have contributed much to our understanding of mental illness and have reduced hospital bed occupancy by mental patients to a tenth of what it was before their use. Pharmacotherapy has permitted persons who would otherwise have been hospitalized long term to be more integrated into society. The Surgeon General's report on mental health has indicated that more people could benefit from treatment with psychotropic agents than are currently being treated.[30] Thus, in daily practice, the dentist can expect to treat persons taking psychotherapeutic agents for a variety of mental disorders. These agents may contribute to oral pathology or become a factor when rendering dental care.[15]

Brain imaging, molecular biology, and genetic studies promise to improve the understanding of psychotic disorders. Results from such research have identified changes that may relate to the pathology of these conditions. Key findings include the observation of genetic, structural, and functional changes in schizophrenia, bipolar disorder, and depression. There are still inconsistencies between the symptoms and observable signs that continue to challenge our understanding and treatment of psychiatric disorders. Difficulties in categorizing these illnesses can result in inconsistent treatment outcomes. Many of these difficulties are based on our limited knowledge of the biochemical processes involved.

Psychotic states such as schizophrenia are treated therapeutically with antipsychotic drugs, sometimes also referred to as *neuroleptics;* depression is treated therapeutically with antidepressant drugs, and manic-depressive illness (bipolar disorder) is treated with lithium salts and some anticonvulsant drugs. The neuroses (e.g., anxiety), which are less severe psychiatric disorders, are treated with antianxiety agents and are covered separately (see Chapter 13). Selective serotonin reuptake inhibitor (SSRI) antidepressants are also effective in treaing several anxiety disorders, including obsessive-compulsive disorder, panic disorder, posttraumatic stress disorder, and social anxiety disorder. These drugs may be referred to as *delayed action antianxiety agents.* Sympathomimetic stimulants are effective treatments for attention deficit–hyperactivity disorders and narcolepsy, and they are discussed elsewhere (see Chapter 6). Because of the perceived stigma associated with psychiatric illness, or the effects of the psychotropic drugs themselves, patients may forget or be reluctant to discuss their disorder with dentists or to provide complete information regarding its treatment.

The term *major tranquilizer* is sometimes used for the antipsychotic drugs and *minor tranquilizer* for the antianxiety drugs. The use of these terms should be discontinued because they imply that the two groups of drugs have similar mechanisms of action, differing only in degree of activity or efficacy, which is not the case.

MAJOR PSYCHIATRIC DISORDERS

Schizophrenia

In schizophrenia, the patient's ability to function is markedly impaired because of disturbances in thought processes. These disturbances increase the likelihood of adverse social outcomes such as unemployment, poverty, social isolation, and suicide.[4]

Schizophrenic patients have positive and/or negative symptoms and memory disorders. Positive symptoms include hallucinations (false perceptions), delusions (false beliefs), and agitation. Negative symptoms include interpersonal withdrawal, loss of drive, and flattened affect (restricted range of emotions). There is disagreement regarding whether these symptoms represent different disease states or variable presentations of the same illness. Nonetheless, positive symptoms respond more favorably to the antipsychotics that were developed first (typical or "classic" antipsychotics), whereas negative symptoms are better correlated with demonstrable structural abnormalities in the brain and may be more responsive to newer "atypical" antipsychotic drugs (see below). Schizophrenic patients also have subtle changes in process planning and memory, but these continue to be resistant to treatment.

Neither the etiology nor the pathogenesis of schizophrenia is known. Current thinking suggests that a genetic predisposition and early injury (in utero or early childhood) may set the stage for neurodevelopmental changes that ultimately manifest as behavioral difficulties later in life (often in early adulthood) and that may be triggered by a stressful lifetime event.[30] For the disease to manifest itself, the effect of several

* The authors wish to recognize Dr. Leslie Felpel for her past contributions to this chapter. See the Acknowledgments.

cumulative factors likely combine to result in the clinical disorder.[4]

Dopamine hypothesis

The classic "dopamine hypothesis" for schizophrenia, which suggests that schizophrenia is caused by hyperactivity of central dopamine pathways, has been a dominant theme since the early 1960s. The hypothesis was based primarily on indirect pharmacologic evidence. For example, all the known antipsychotics are dopamine antagonists in a variety of experimental conditions, and agents that release dopamine (e.g., amphetamine) can induce an acute psychotic state similar to schizophrenia. On the other hand, the hypothesis does not explain why the therapeutic effect of the antipsychotics takes several weeks to develop, although dopamine blockade is known to occur within hours, or why some schizophrenic persons are refractory to antipsychotics and why some drugs that affect neurotransmitters other than dopamine have antipsychotic activity.

The role of dopamine in schizophrenia has been further complicated by the identification and cloning of several dopamine receptor subtypes and the discovery that other neurochemicals, either independently or by regulating dopamine, may be involved in the disease process. Thus, although hyperactive dopaminergic neural pathways offer a simple and attractive mechanism to explain schizophrenia, clearly we are far from understanding the disease. It is justified to assume, however, that the parkinsonlike motor disturbances, which are common side effects of the antipsychotics, result from blockade of dopamine transmission in the basal ganglia (Table 12-1). Five dopaminergic cell groups are considered important either for the therapeutic actions of antipsychotic drugs or for side effects of the antipsychotic agents. These dopamine cell groups and their proposed relation to activity are summarized in Table 12-2.

Other neurotransmitters

Other neurotransmitters have been implicated in psychotic behavior and are of some interest regarding the cause of psychotic symptoms. Phencyclidine-induced psychosis is proposed to be an even better model for schizophrenia than the dopamine hypothesis. The predominant action of phencyclidine is thought to be blockade of N-methyl-D-aspartate–type glutamate (glutamatergic) receptors. The hallucinogens lyser-

Table • 12-1

Summary of Therapeutic and Adverse Effects Associated with Some Receptors Bound by Common Antipsychotic and Antidepressant Drugs

RECEPTOR OR PROCESS BLOCKED	THERAPEUTIC EFFECT OF BLOCK	ADVERSE EFFECTS RESULTING FROM BLOCKADE OF RECEPTOR OR PROTEIN
Histamine (H_1)	Sedation, anxiolysis, antiallergy effect	CNS depression, hypotension, dry mouth, weight gain
Muscarinic	Reduction of extrapyramidal side effects	Dry mouth, blurred vision, sinus tachycardia, constipation, urinary retention, memory dysfunction
Adrenoceptor		
α_1-Adrenergic		Memory dysfunction, postural (orthostatic) hypotension, reflex tachycardia, epinephrine reversal, dizziness, dry mouth, weight gain, priapism
α_2-Adrenergic	Blockade of presynaptic autoregulation, increasing CNS 5-HT and NE	Priapism
Dopamine (D_2)	Amelioration of the positive signs and symptoms of psychosis	Extrapyramidal movement disorders, sexual dysfunction, dry mouth, weight gain
5-HT uptake	Reversal of depression	Gastrointestinal disturbance, sexual dysfunction, activating effects, dry mouth
NE uptake	Reversal of depression	Dry mouth, urinary retention, erectile dysfunction, CNS stimulation, tremor, proconvulsant
Dopamine reuptake	Antidepressant effect (?)	Psychomotor activation, psychosis, proconvulsant action (?), dependence

5-HT, 5-Hydroxytryptamine; *NE*, norepinephrine.

Table • 12-2

Dopaminergic Cell Groups and Their Relationship to Actions and Side Effects of Antipsychotic Drugs

CELL GROUP	RELATIONSHIP/ACTION
Mesolimbic and mesocortical	Considered the major therapeutic targets for antipsychotics
Nigrostriatal	Essential for motor function, related to the motor side effects of antipsychotics
Tuberoinfundibular	Regulation of hormones, especially inhibition of prolactin secretion; thought to mediate side effects such as galactorrhea and infertility
Chemoreceptor trigger zone	Receptors thought to mediate the antiemetic actions of antidopaminergic drugs
Medullary-periventricular	May mediate the actions of antidopaminergic drugs on appetite

gic acid diethylamide and mescaline can induce hallucinations and delusions and are thought to produce their actions through 5-hydroxytryptamine type 2 (5-HT_2) receptors.[2] Anticholinergics, cannabinoids, and sigma receptor agonists are other drugs that can induce psychosislike reactions.

Anatomic changes

It has been difficult to establish what area of the brain is involved in the pathologic process leading to schizophrenia, but numerous neuronal pathways exist in the prefrontal and frontal cortex, amygdala, hippocampus, nucleus accumbens, ventral basal ganglia, and limbic cortex that contain dopamine (see Table 12-2). These same areas are involved in mood and thought processes. Dopamine may act as a regulator or modulator of the function of the other neurotransmitter systems. If dysfunction of dopaminergic systems were to occur, it is reasonable to expect that alterations in mood, personality, and thought processes would follow. However, whether dopamine changes are the cause or the result of schizophrenia is unclear.

Genetic and developmental vulnerability

There is evidence for a genetic predisposition to schizophrenia. If both parents are schizophrenic, 46% of the children are likely to become schizophrenic; if one parent is schizophrenic, 18% of the children show the disorder, compared with 1% of the general population. The possibility of early (in utero or childhood) stresses such as infection, exposure to toxic elements, winter birth, starvation, migration travel, or radiation have been correlated to increased vulnerability to the disease.

Affective Disorders

The affective illnesses are expressed as dysregulations of mood. There are many types of affective disorders categorized in the DSM-IV, but for purposes of this discussion it is sufficient to consider only depression and mania. Most people have had reactive, or secondary depression with feelings of sadness or grief associated with a personal loss.[11] In normal circumstances, such reactions are related to specific causes, are not incapacitating, and are generally short lived (1 to 2 weeks). In contrast, for the mentally ill patient depression is a severe, disabling disorder characterized by reclusiveness and nonverbalization that may last for extended periods of time (2 to 5 weeks). The patient is sad or blue most of the day, gains little pleasure from activities, and may have other signs such as weight loss, irritability, insomnia, feelings of guilt, agitation, or difficulty concentrating.[11] A serious consequence of depression is an increased risk of suicide. Depression is also a risk factor for higher morbidity in other diseases such as myocardial infarction and coronary artery disease. This kind of depression is called *primary, endogenous, unipolar,* or *major depressive disorder (MDD)*. A variant of depression is seasonal affective disorder (SAD), which is triggered by changes in seasons and can respond to treatment with intense lights.[11]

Unipolar depression tends to be more common in women, but the risk of suicide is greatest in elderly men. Triggering factors for depression in women and men overlap, but women tend to be more strongly affected by interpersonal factors whereas men tend to be more greatly affected by legal problems and job loss. In women, the factors of poor relations with parents, early marriage, incomplete education, divorce, and financial difficulties can contribute to repeated stressful life events (cycle of adversity). The incidence of mood disorders in women is greatest at times of life when shifts of ovarian hormones occur. Thus a higher incidence of depression can occur at the beginning of menstruation, after childbirth, and in the perimenopausal period. Depression may be more likely during the progesterone-dominated components of the menstrual cycle. Estrogens tend to be antidepressant and facilitate neuronal repair. A genetic risk is evident for the mood disorders but thus far not clearly understood. Concordance rates for mood disorders are 46% in monozygotic twins and 20% for dizygotic twins.

Persons with mania exhibit a distinct period of abnormally elevated, expansive, or irritable mood, sometimes requiring hospitalization. Three or more of the following symptoms also suggest a manic episode: (1) inflated self-esteem, (2) decreased need for sleep, (3) talkativeness, (4) flight of ideas, (5) distractibility, (6) increased goal-directed activity, and (7) excessive interest in pleasure.

Manic individuals may also have alternating periods of severe depression, in which case the disorder may be referred to as *bipolar (manic-depressive) illness.* The incidence of bipolar disorder may be as high as 5% of the population and 45% of community mental health patients.[3] Three forms of bipolar disorder have been distinguished. Bipolar I involves cycles of mania and depression; bipolar II involves cycles of hypomania and depression. Hypomania is a less severe form of mania that does not have psychotic features (e.g., hallucinations). Bipolar III is mania associated with the use of antidepressants. Bipolar II patients only rarely convert to bipolar I, and bipolar II disorder may have the highest risk for suicide.

There is great interest in identifying the underlying brain processes that may help explain depression. However, heterogeneity in the expression and causes of depression has made this process challenging. Both environmental and genetic factors have a role. Environmental factors (stresses) may act as triggers for depressive episodes by altering the release of mineralocorticoids and glucocorticoids, which under some conditions can predispose to brain damage. Depressive episodes tend to increase the likelihood of further depressive episodes, a phenomenon referred to as *kindling.* Individuals who also have a genetic predisposition for depression act as though they are "prekindled." Their episodes of depression are less related to precipitating stressful causes, are more serious, and are more often seen in younger patients. Late-onset depressions are less related to genetics or stresses and may involve damage in subcortical white and gray matter from disease states such as arteriosclerosis or Parkinson's disease.

Although bipolar disorder shares some characteristics with unipolar depression, there are several important differences: the treatment is different from unipolar depression; bipolar disorder has a stronger genetic involvement; and bipolar disorder is thought to have somewhat greater observable brain structural changes. Currently, treatment is aimed at the manic phase first, which is treated with lithium salts and anticonvulsants. In addition, these agents may exert a neuroprotective effect and can reduce the extent of brain structural changes occurring in bipolar disease.

Monoamine hypothesis

As in the case of schizophrenia, various theories have been offered to explain the cause of affective disorders, again with attention focusing on putative neurotransmitters. The classic monoamine hypothesis (also called the *biogenic amine hypothesis* or simply *amine hypothesis*) of affective disorders proposes that depression results from a deficiency of norepinephrine (NE), 5-HT, or both at central synaptic sites. Although little evidence exists that directly substantiates this hypothesis, it is indirectly supported by the fact that most of the antidepressant drugs increase synaptic concentrations of one or more monoamines, either by blocking the reuptake of monoamine into the presynaptic nerve terminal or by preventing its catabolism by the enzyme monoamine oxidase (MAO) in the nerve terminal after reuptake.

Although these findings are consistent with the monoamine hypothesis of affective disorders, there are several discrepancies. One of the findings most difficult to reconcile with the monoamine hypothesis is that the blockade of amine reuptake by antidepressants and of amine metabolism by MAO inhibitors (MAOIs) can be demonstrated almost immediately after drug administration, yet full therapeutic effects are not observed until the drugs have been taken continuously for several weeks. In addition, some antidepressants, such as mirtazapine, do not have a significant effect on either monoamine reuptake or MAOI activity. Moreover, cocaine, which blocks the reuptake of amines, is not effective as an antidepressant. Because of these and other findings, new possibilities have been investigated to explain the action of antidepressants. Attention is focusing on presynaptic and postsynaptic structural mechanisms as evidence mounts that the reuptake inhibitors, MAOIs, atypical antidepressants, and even electroconvulsive therapy all produce consistent changes in the relative density or sensitivity of certain receptor processes. Clearly, the classic monoamine hypothesis is too limited and will need to be modified in accordance with new research findings. Changes in biochemistry of 5-HT, NE, dopamine, acetylcholine, glutamate, γ-aminobutyric acid (GABA), corticosteroids, ovarian hormones, substance P, and omega-3 fatty acids have been demonstrated.[40]

Historic Development of Antipsychotic and Antidepressant Drugs

Most of the psychotherapeutic properties of the psychoactive drugs were discovered by accident. In 1950, while attempting to develop antihistaminic agents, the Rhône-Pauline Laboratories in France synthesized the phenothiazine chlorpromazine (Figure 12-1). The unusual neuroleptic property of chlorpromazine was noted, and the drug was used to treat schizophrenic patients in 1952. The discovery of chlorpromazine and other phenothiazines made possible the outpatient treatment of psychotic disorders.

A characteristic of many antipsychotic drugs is interference with multiple neurotransmitter systems. In addition to blocking dopaminergic receptors, many can block α-adrenergic and serotonergic receptors and thereby alter functions of cells such as ion channel activity. These drugs have a number of side effects that can be related to these multiple receptor actions (see Table 12-1). The next phase of development focused on drugs with selective drug receptor binding. However, in the case of antipsychotic drugs, action at multiple receptor types may provide therapeutic advantages. The current challenge is to identify which combination of actions is most beneficial.

The antidepressant properties of the MAOIs were discovered when it was observed that isoniazid, an antituberculosis drug, produced a euphoric state in patients and was found to be an MAOI. The tricyclic antidepressants (TCAs) were synthesized in an attempt to produce more specific antipsychotic agents (note in Figures 12-1 and 12-5 the chemical similarity of the TCAs and the phenothiazines). However, it was soon recognized that imipramine, a prototypic TCA, was more beneficial in treating depression than in treating schizophrenia. There are two forms of MAO, MAO-A treating present in catecholamine neurons and MAO-B found in 5-HT–containing neurons and astrocytes. Selective antidepressant MAOIs inhibit the MAO-A form.

The TCAs were the mainstay for treating depression for many years. However, their use has been limited by the wide number of side effects resulting from their actions on many nontherapeutic receptor sites. Efforts to develop better agents have been rewarded with a newer class of drugs, the SSRIs, with fewer adverse effects than TCAs and fewer drug interactions than MAOIs. These drugs have revolutionized the use of antidepressant medication.

St. John's wort is a botanical remedy with a long history of use for depression. It is now thought that the active principle is the compound hyperforin (instead of hypericin as had been believed).[10]

Although the psychoactive properties of lithium salts were noted as early as 1949,[7] it was not until 1970 that lithium carbonate was developed and widely recognized as an effective treatment for manic-depressive illness. Recent studies have focused on a possible neural protective role for lithium salts. Carbamazepine and valproic acid were first investigated for treatment of mania (bipolar disorder) in the early 1980s, and since that time their use has been increasing.

ANTIPSYCHOTIC DRUGS

The principal drugs effective in the treatment of schizophrenia are dopaminergic receptor antagonists. Five dopamine receptors (D_1 through D_5) have been cloned. Some of these receptors express extra long or short variants. The possibility that each of these receptors may subserve a different physiologic function illustrates the complexity of the dopaminergic system. D_1 and D_5 have similar actions and often increase cyclic 3′,5′-adenosine monophosphate synthesis, whereas D_2, D_3, and D_4 are thought to decrease cyclic 3′,5′-adenosine monophosphate synthesis. Interest has now focused on the relative specificity and affinity of the antipsychotic agents for each of the dopamine receptors. For example, both the older typical antipsychotics (e.g., phenothiazines) and the atypical agents (e.g., clozapine) are dopamine antagonists. Clinical potency as an antipsychotic drug relates most closely to blocking D_2 receptors (Table 12-3). However, the affinity of clozapine for the D_1 and D_4 receptors relative to D_2 is proportionally greater than that of the older agents. It is interesting to note that in postmortem brain samples from schizophrenic patients there is an increase in the number of D_2 receptors, but not D_1 receptors.

Although there is little doubt that dopamine is involved in schizophrenia, other neurotransmitter systems may also play a crucial role in this disease. In addition to dopamine, neurotransmitters such as NE, 5-HT, glutamate, glycine, and GABA have been implicated in schizophrenia, suggesting that this is a very complex and multifaceted illness and that many mechanisms may be involved in the disease process.[2] Preliminary gene chip microarray analysis has demonstrated changes in signal transduction, transcription, and metabolic enzymes

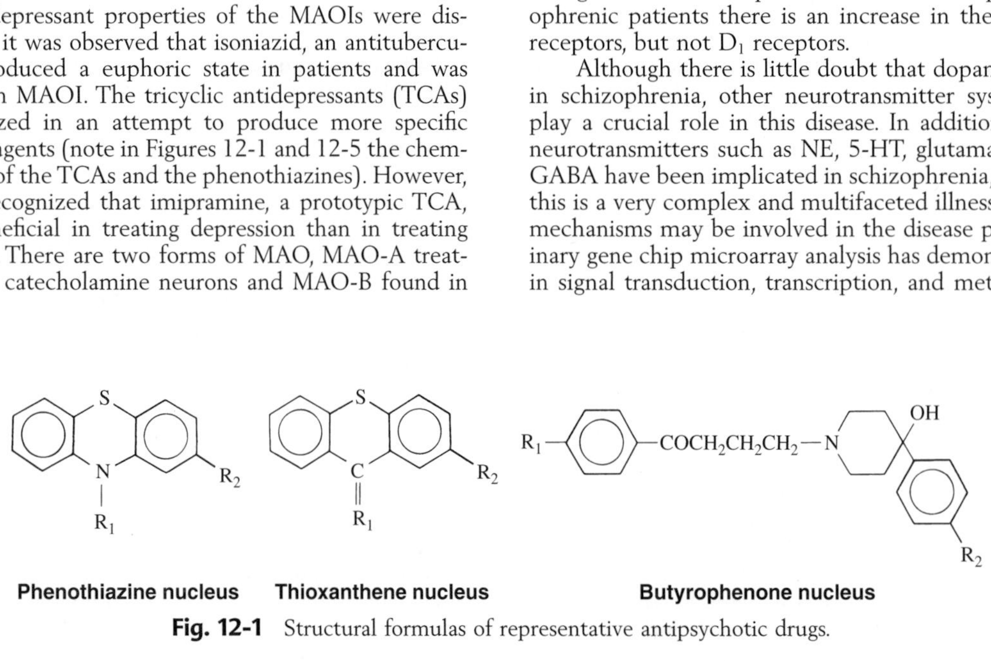

Phenothiazine nucleus   Thioxanthene nucleus   Butyrophenone nucleus

Fig. 12-1 Structural formulas of representative antipsychotic drugs.

Table • 12-3

Comparison of Relative Receptor Antagonist Affinities of Typical and Atypical Antipsychotic Drugs

DRUG	AFFINITY ORDER						
Chlorpromazine	$\alpha_1 \geq$	5-HT_2>	**D_2**>	D_1>	M>	α_2	
Haloperidol	sigma =	**D_2**>	$D_1 = D_4$	α_1>	5-HT_2		
Clozapine	M>	5-$HT_{2,6,7}$ =	H_1 =	α_1 =	α_2 =	D_4>	D_1
Olanzapine	5-HT_2>	M_1>	α_1 =	**D_2** =	H_1>	D_1	
Risperidone	5-HT_{2A}>	**D_2** =	α_1 =	α_2>>	M		
Quetiapine	α_1 =	H_1 =	**D_2** =	5-HT_2>	D_1		
Ziprasidone	5-HT_{2A} =	5-HT_{1A} (agonist)>	**D_2**>	α_1>	H_1		
Aripiprazole	**D_2** (partial agonist)>	5-HT_{1A} (partial agonist)>	5-HT_{2A}>>	5-HT_{2C}>	D_4>	α_1>	H_1

The relative affinity for D_2 receptors is shown. Binding to other receptors has also been reported for some of the other drugs.
=, Equal to the following receptor type; >, greater than the following receptor type; >>, much greater than the following receptor type; *α*, α-adrenergic; *D*, dopaminergic; *M*, muscarinic; *H*, histaminergic.
D_2 receptors are **bolded** for emphasis.

associated with altered regulation of certain genes in schizophrenia.

Chemistry and Structure-Activity Relationships

Of the several classes of antipsychotics, some are closely related structurally, others share a stereochemical resemblance, and still others appear to be chemically unrelated. The term *typical antipsychotic* is used for drugs that improve chiefly positive symptoms, whereas *atypical psychotic* is used for agents that cause fewer extrapyramidal side effects or improve both positive and negative symptoms.

Phenothiazines and thioxanthenes

The basic ring structure of the phenothiazines is illustrated in Figure 12-1. Substitutions at R_1 divide the phenothiazine antipsychotics into three major groups. One group, represented by chlorpromazine, has an aliphatic chain at C_1. Compounds such as chlorpromazine with three carbons in the chain ($—CH_2—CH_2—CH_2—N(CH_3)_2$) have antipsychotic properties, whereas those with only two carbons, such as promethazine, are usually more antihistaminic or anticholinergic in nature and possess little antipsychotic effects. A second group, represented by thioridazine, has a piperidine ring at R_1. These phenothiazines are usually less sedating than the aliphatic agents but more sedating than the next group. A third group, represented by prochlorperazine, contains a piperazine ring at R_1. Drugs in this group are the most potent of the three as antipsychotic agents but are also the most likely to produce extrapyramidal side effects. In all three groups, drugs with antipsychotic activity have a nitrogen on the side chain (or side ring) separated from the nitrogen of the phenothiazine nucleus by three carbons.

Substitutions at the R_2 position can increase the potency of a given antipsychotic. Promazine, which lacks a substituent group at R_2, is made much more potent when a chlorine atom is placed at the R_2 position, resulting in chlorpromazine. Increasing the number of halogen atoms at R_2 (e.g., trifluoperazine) increases the antipsychotic potency to an even greater extent. Minor structural changes, such as the addition of a chlorine atom adjacent to R_2 on the phenothiazine ring, can result in compounds devoid of antipsychotic activity. Obviously, the clinical effectiveness of these drugs depends on highly specific molecular properties.

The thioxanthene antipsychotics, represented by thiothixene, are closely related to the phenothiazines and are formed when the nitrogen of the central ring is replaced by a carbon atom.

Butyrophenones

The butyrophenone antipsychotics are not chemically related to the phenothiazines but contain a stereochemically related nucleus (see Figure 12-1). The only butyrophenone antipsychotic available in this country is haloperidol. Droperidol, another butyrophenone, is marketed as an antipsychotic in some countries but is used in the United States primarily to reduce nausea and vomiting associated with anesthesia and surgery.

Dihydroindolones

The structure of molindone is shown in Figure 12-2. This compound is not structurally related to the phenothiazines, thioxanthenes, or butyrophenones. The pharmacologic and clinical profile of molindone very closely resembles that of the piperazine group of phenothiazines. Ziprasidone, another dihydroindolone, is pharmacologically an atypical antipsychotic and is discussed below.

Dibenzoxazepines

Loxapine (see Figure 12-2) is the only dibenzoxazepine available in the United States. The structure of this compound is interesting in that it contains seven members in its central ring and therefore resembles a tricyclic antidepressant. However, loxapine does not appear to have antidepressant activity. Like molindone, this drug has a clinical and pharmacologic profile similar to that of the piperazine phenothiazines.

Diphenylbutylpiperidines

Pimozide, a diphenylbutylpiperidine derivative, is a modified butyrophenone in which a keto group in the side chain has been replaced with a 4-fluorophenyl moiety. Pimozide is a selective dopamine D_2 antagonist that has antipsychotic properties and typical parkinsonlike side effects. The Food and Drug Administration (FDA) approved pimozide for the treatment of Tourette's syndrome, a condition characterized by phonic and motor tics, but it has been used in Europe to treat schizophrenia. Penfluridol, another diphenylbutylpiperidine, is undergoing clinical trials in the United States for the treatment of Tourette's syndrome. Both these agents have long half-lives.

Dibenzodiazepines

Clozapine (Figure 12-3) is the only dibenzodiazepine available in the United States. Its chemical structure closely resembles that of loxapine, but unlike loxapine it is classified as an atypical antipsychotic in light of its low risk for producing

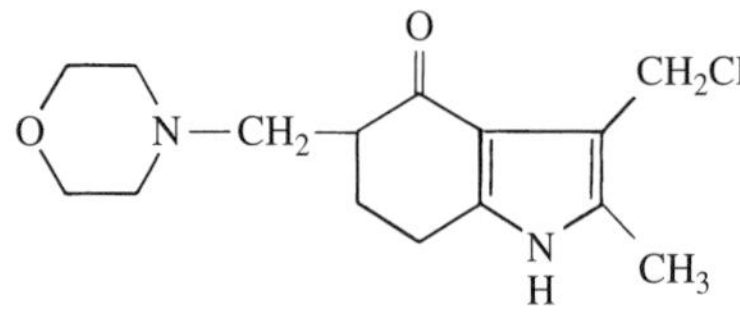

Molindone

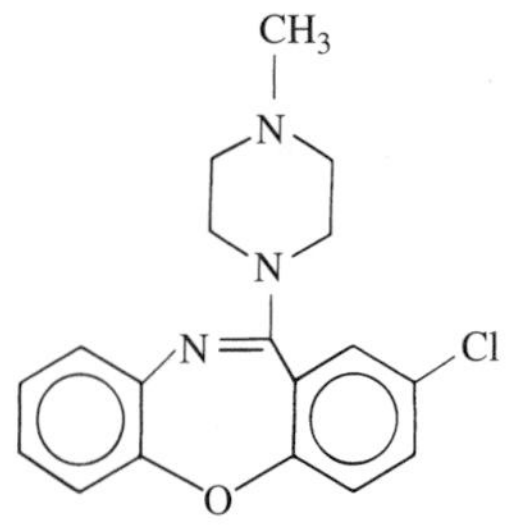

Loxapine

Fig. 12-2 Structural formulas of molindone and loxapine.

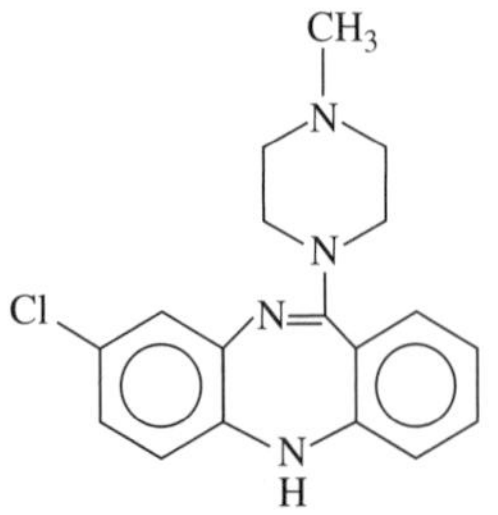

Fig. 12-3 Structural formula of clozapine.

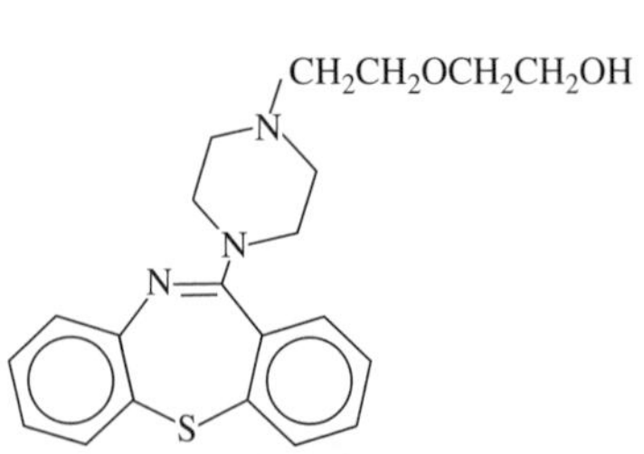

Quetiapine

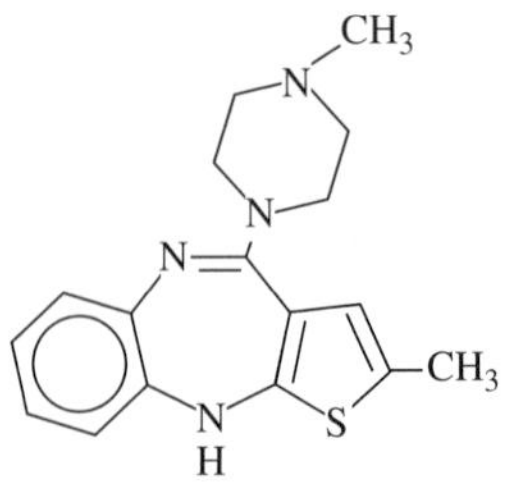

Olanzapine

Fig. 12-4 Structural formulas of quetiapine and olanzapine.

extrapyramidal side effects. Clozapine is reported to improve both positive and negative symptoms of schizophrenia and may reverse the progression of schizophrenic symptoms. Clozapine also has muscarinic, $5\text{-}HT_{2,6,7}$, α_1-adrenergic, and D_1, D_2, and D_4 receptor–blocking properties. Unfortunately, clozapine use can be accompanied by significant toxicity, especially agranulocytosis, seizures, and hypotension. Myocarditis and cardiomyopathy may rarely occur.

Thienobenzodiazepines

Olanzapine (Figure 12-4) is an atypical antipsychotic approved for clinical use. Its inhibitory actions at monoamine synapses are similar to those of clozapine except that olanzapine has a higher affinity for D_2 receptors (see Table 12-3). It is associated with fewer adverse effects than clozapine, particularly agranulocytosis.

Benzisoxazoles

Risperidone is a neuroleptic agent that combines activity against both D_2 and $5\text{-}HT_2$ receptors. This addition to the antipsychotic armamentarium provides therapeutic effects similar to haloperidol, but in low doses it is considered to be atypical because of its relative freedom from extrapyramidal effects.

Other drugs expressing atypical antipsychotic activity

Several new atypical antipsychotic agents representing a new structural class of antipsychotic agent have been marketed. Quetiapine (a dibenzothiazepine) (see Figure 12-4) is effective for both positive and negative symptoms. Sertindole (a fluorophenylindole) is similar in its pharmacology to olanzapine but has been withdrawn over concerns that it produced long QT syndrome. Ziprasidone (a dihydroindolone) has actions similar to those of risperidone. Ziprasidone also carries warnings for inducing long QT syndrome. Aripiprazole is a dihydrocarbostyril derivative with a unique spectrum of action. Aripiprazole has been found to act as a partial agonist at D_2, D_3, and $5\text{-}HT_{1A}$ receptors. It is reported to produce minimal side effects commonly associated with antipsychotic drugs.

Miscellaneous antipsychotics

Experimental drugs that show the greatest potential for clinical use are those that are highly selective for various receptors or are selective for receptors in specific areas of the brain. Thus the benzamide derivatives sulpride, remoxipride, and amisulpride may preferentially block D_2 receptors in the mesolimbic system rather than the striatum, which may account for their clinical effectiveness yet low incidence of extrapyramidal side effects. Sulpride has been available for use as an antipsychotic in Europe for several years but is still in clinical trials in this country. A number of drugs are being used as antipsychotics even though their primary indication is for other conditions, and still others are not currently approved for use in the United States.

The benzodiazepines are primarily used as antianxiety and hypnotic drugs, but recently the clinical indications for this drug group have been expanded to include some psychotic disorders. Diazepam, chlordiazepoxide, alprazolam, clonazepam, and lorazepam have all found clinical usefulness in the treatment of schizophrenia, schizoaffective disorders, assaultiveness, agitation, and delirium. The benzodiazepines appear to have marginal antipsychotic properties when used alone and may be most useful as adjuncts to standard antipsychotic agents.

Ondansetron, a $5\text{-}HT_3$ receptor antagonist used to treat chemically induced nausea, is also undergoing clinical investigation as an antipsychotic agent.

Pharmacologic Effects

Chlorpromazine is a classic typical antipsychotic drug. Typical antipsychotics include phenothiazines, thioxanthenes, haloperidol, molindone, loxapine, and pimozide. They have similar neuropharmacologic properties and adverse effects. However, the adverse effects vary in their frequency and severity depending on the drug group. The prototype for the atypical antipsychotics is clozapine. It is too early to know whether all the atypical antipsychotic agents share all the advantages that have been proposed for clozapine.

Antipsychotic effects

Although the precise mechanism of action of the antipsychotic drugs is not known, they all share the ability to block dopamine receptors in the brain. For typical antipsychotic agents the dose required to alleviate positive symptoms of psychosis is most closely related to affinity of the drug for blocking the D_2 receptor.

There are several dopaminergic pathways in the central nervous system (CNS) (see Table 12-2) that, when antagonized by the antipsychotics, can explain both their therapeutic efficacy and some of their side effects. The antipsychotic action may be ascribed to blockade of the mesolimbic/mesocortical tract, which plays an important role in behavior, arousal, cognitive function, communication, and psychologic responses. Extrapyramidal motor dysfunction results from blockade of the nigrostriatal pathway, and endocrine disorders (amenorrhea, dysmenorrhea) result from the blockade of the hypothalamic-adenohypophyseal system. Two effects of antipsychotics may relate to blockade of dopamine receptors in the brainstem. Blockade of dopamine receptors in the medullary chemoreceptor trigger zone is thought to contribute to the antiemetic actions of antipsychotic drugs. Blockade of dopamine receptors in the medulla or brainstem may also play a role in appetite regulation. (There are also dopamine interneurons in the olfactory bulb and retina, but no clinical action has been ascribed to their inhibition thus far.)

Atypical antipsychotic agents appear to be more effective for the negative symptoms of schizophrenia and tend to produce fewer extrapyramidal side effects. In addition, these drugs (e.g., clozapine) appear to be more effective in treating patients with schizophrenia resistant to other drugs. Exactly why they are better is not known. Whereas the typical antipsychotics block nearly all central dopamine pathways, the atypical antipsychotic clozapine may selectively block mesolimbic and mesocortical dopaminergic pathways. This selectivity may explain both its effectiveness in the treatment of schizophrenia and the relative absence of extrapyramidal and endocrine side effects.

Several hypotheses are proposed for this selectivity. The first relates the action of these drugs to binding of specific dopamine receptors. Clozapine has a stronger binding to D_1 and D_4 receptors than do the classic antipsychotics. D_4 receptors are enriched in the mesolimbic parts of the brain. However, some studies have suggested that selective D_4 receptor blockade does not confer atypical properties. Other atypical and classic antipsychotics have significant affinity for the D_3 receptor. The D_3 receptor is also found to be enriched in the mesolimbic brain. The affinity of antipsychotic drugs for the D_3 receptor, however, is generally less than that for the D_2 receptor, and the contribution of the D_3 receptor to schizophrenia is also difficult to assess.

A second hypothesis is that other receptor types, in combination with dopamine blockade, may contribute to clozapine's atypical profile. Clozapine has a variety of effects on 5-HT receptors. For example, clozapine is a potent 5-HT_{2A} antagonist, with an affinity greater than that for D_2 receptors. This binding is thought to contribute to clozapine's ability to relieve the negative symptoms of schizophrenia. It may also contribute to the reduction in extrapyramidal side effects. Clozapine additionally causes downregulation of 5-HT_2 receptors. 5-HT has a widespread distribution in limbic areas of the brain and is known to modulate dopamine function. Limited affinity for D_2 receptors and greater blockade of 5-HT_2 receptors are common findings for newer agents characterized as atypical antipsychotic drugs. Clozapine also binds to muscarinic receptors, which may help reduce extrapyramidal side effects, to histaminergic receptors, which may help reduce anxiety, and to α-adrenergic receptors, which may lower blood pressure.

A third hypothesis is that by blocking only a fraction of the D_2 receptors a drug will have an atypical spectrum. Patients with Parkinson's disease do not exhibit typical extrapyramidal side effects until approximately 80% of the dopamine neurons in the striatum are damaged. If an antipsychotic agent is effective in reducing psychotic symptoms at doses that occupy less than 70% to 80% of the dopamine receptors, then it would produce fewer extrapyramidal side effects.

A fourth (but related) hypothesis is that partial dopamine agonists may produce a limited dopaminergic tone to avoid typical side effects but still prevent excessive receptor activation by occupying and competing with endogenously released dopamine that promote psychotic symptoms. Aripiprazole is the only example of this kind of agent currently available.

Finally, a fifth hypothesis for atypical antipsychotic action states that the newer agents may rapidly dissociate from the D_2 receptor, which accounts for their atypical effects.

The potent anticholinergic activity of clozapine, the 5-HT_{2A} receptor–blocking effect, and the limited occupation of D_2 receptors (less than 60%) at therapeutic doses may all contribute to its atypical profile. Olanzapine and risperidone have lower D_2 receptor binding and higher 5-HT_2 receptor binding and are also relatively free of dyskinesias.[22] Quetiapine has a therapeutic effect and a side effect profile similar to olanzapine. Aripiprazole is a partial agonist at D_2, D_3, and 5-HT_{1A} receptors and an antagonist at 5-HT_2 receptors.

Sedative actions

Phenothiazines and related antipsychotics produce sedation on initial administration, but tolerance develops in 1 to 4 weeks, so the patient becomes progressively more alert as treatment continues. Sedation is the most commonly reported side effect of clozapine. Fortunately, tolerance does not seem to develop to the antipsychotic action of these drugs. Unlike sedatives such as barbiturates, chlorpromazine does not depress the reticular formation. However, it does raise the threshold for incoming sensory stimuli at the level of the reticular formation, so that the output of the reticular formation in response to sensory stimuli is depressed. Because schizophrenia may in part be a result of continual "flooding" of the brain by afferent input, reduction of this input by antipsychotics may, in part, explain their clinical efficacy.

Extrapyramidal effects

The extrapyramidal side effects produced by the antipsychotic drugs include acute dystonias, a parkinsonlike syndrome, akathisia, and tardive dyskinesia. The different types of phenothiazines produce varying degrees of extrapyramidal side effects; in descending order of most to least potent are the piperazines, aliphatics, and piperidines. These compounds follow the reverse ranking order regarding their anticholinergic potency, which may explain why fluphenazine and haloperidol, weak anticholinergics, commonly produce extrapyramidal side effects, whereas thioridazine, a more potent anticholinergic drug, produces fewer motor disturbances. More recently, the role of 5-HT_2 receptors in reducing extrapyramidal systems and dystonias has been considered. As can be seen in Table 12-3, chlorpromazine is a more potent inhibitor of 5-HT_2 than it is for the muscarinic receptor. In addition, many newer antipsychotic drugs having atypical properties also block 5-HT_2 receptors. Molindone and loxapine are similar to chlorpromazine in their potential for causing extrapyramidal reactions. Haloperidol may have some unique effects on motor function. It is metabolized to a potentially neurotoxic metabolite, which may slowly poison the dopaminergic cells in the substantia nigra, inducing Parkinson's disease. Haloperidol also blocks sigma receptors. Sigma receptors in the red nucleus have been shown to participate in the generation of dystonias (oculogyric crisis and torticollis) associated with neuroleptic use. This observation may be particularly important for facial dystonias because sigma receptors are also expressed in cranial nerve nuclei.

Antiparkinson drugs (see Chapter 15) may be used to antagonize certain antipsychotic-induced motor disturbances, but levodopa is not helpful in this regard. Because dopamine receptors are blocked by the antipsychotic drugs, levodopa, the precursor of dopamine, is less effective than are the anticholinergics, antihistamines, and amantadine, which act through other mechanisms. Greater emphasis is currently being placed on using lower doses of antipsychotic drugs or using atypical antipsychotic drugs to reduce motor side effects.

Tardive dyskinesia is an extrapyramidal disorder that appears after long-term antipsychotic therapy. Most of the extrapyramidal side effects of the antipsychotic drugs occur during drug administration and disappear when the agent is withdrawn, but tardive dyskinesia develops after prolonged use and may be irreversible. This condition is thought to reflect the development of supersensitive dopamine receptors in the basal ganglia in response to their chronic blockade. Tardive dyskinesia has been estimated to occur in as many as 15% to 20% of patients receiving long-term typical antipsychotic drug therapy. Tardive dyskinesia consists of abnormal, rapid, and alternating movements of the tongue (thrusting) and perioral areas, facial grimacing, tics, nose twitching, and other abnormal movements. It sometimes involves the extremities and torso and may become severe enough to disrupt eating and breathing patterns. Unlike other extrapyramidal side effects, tardive dyskinesia does not necessarily regress on reduction of the dose or withdrawal of the drug. In fact, this side effect is frequently not seen until the antipsychotic drug is either withdrawn or reduced in dosage. The only consistently effective treatment for tardive dyskinesia has been increasing the dose of the antipsychotic that caused it in the first place. Obviously, such a procedure leads to a vicious cycle and a serious therapeutic dilemma. Typical antipsychotics cause this side effect. Clonazepam may be helpful in mild cases, whereas botulinum toxin may allow control of overactive muscle groups.[41] Atypical agents such as clozapine and risperidone seem to have a reduced liability for tardive dyskinesia; however, long-term experience is not yet available. The low incidence of extrapyramidal side effects and the apparent absence of tardive dyskinesia are additional reasons for the interest in clozapine and other atypical drugs.

Seizure threshold

Most of the antipsychotics, including clozapine, lower the seizure threshold. The incidence of antipsychotic-induced seizures is approximately 1% but nearly 7% in epileptic patients who receive antipsychotics. The convulsion is usually of the generalized tonic-clonic type. Chlorpromazine is more likely to cause this effect than fluphenazine, thiothixene, or molindone. The lowering of the seizure threshold appears to be inversely related to the antipsychotic potency of the drug and may depend on the particular dopamine receptor blocked (D_1 versus D_2) or possibly on the blockade of sigma receptors or changes in receptor sensitivity associated with chronic dosing. Seizures are more likely in patients with a history of seizures or under conditions where seizures are more likely, such as during withdrawal of sedative-hypnotic drugs.

Other central nervous system actions

Although medullary respiratory centers can be depressed by chlorpromazine, therapeutically active doses normally elicit little or no effect. However, if a sedative-hypnotic, antianxiety, or opioid drug is given to a patient receiving antipsychotic medication, summation of the depressant effects may result in clinically evident respiratory depression. Antipsychotics, including clozapine, may disrupt thermoregulation by an action on the hypothalamus. Either hypothermia or hyperthermia may occur, depending on the ambient temperature.

Antiemetic action

Chlorpromazine is an effective antiemetic and was at one time commonly used for this purpose. (Neuroleptics that are still used to treat nausea include prochlorperazine and droperidol.) The antiemetic action is exerted on the chemoreceptor trigger zone rather than the vomiting center. Hence, motion sickness is less responsive to dopamine antagonists than to anticholinergics and antihistamines.

Endocrine system

Endocrine system alterations result, in part, from actions on the hypothalamus. Most of the endocrine effects of antipsychotics are related to disturbances in the secretion of pituitary hormones. Particularly prominent is hyperprolactinemia elicited by blockade of dopamine receptors. Stimulation of dopamine receptors in the adenohypophysis normally inhibits prolactin release. Chlorpromazine may cause lactation and amenorrhea or delay ovulation and menstruation in women and gynecomastia and impotence or decreased libido in men. The urinary excretion of estrogens, progestins, and 17-hydroxycorticoids is decreased by chlorpromazine. Both diuretic and antidiuretic effects have been demonstrated in animals and human beings, although a weak diuresis seems to be the predominant effect in human beings. The relative lack of effect of clozapine on dopamine receptors of the anterior pituitary accounts for its mild endocrine side effects.

Autonomic nervous system

The following side effects of the phenothiazines may result from their antimuscarinic properties: blurring of vision; constipation; and decreased sweating, salivation, gastric secretion, and intestinal tone. Phenothiazines also have antihistaminic, antitryptaminergic, and antiadrenergic properties that further complicate the overall pattern of their CNS and peripheral activities. Dry mouth associated with a series of neuroleptics was found to correlate significantly with their blocking potency at α_1-adrenergic, H_1-histaminergic, and D_1-dopaminergic receptors.[38] The autonomic effects of haloperidol, molindone, and loxapine are similar, although weaker, than those of the phenothiazines. Clozapine has significant anticholinergic properties, yet a commonly reported side effect is hypersalivation. Often this phenomenon is most prominent during sleep; the mechanism responsible for it is unknown. Although the autonomic effects of antipsychotics can be annoying, tolerance usually develops to these reactions.

Cardiovascular system

Orthostatic hypotension is a result of both CNS and peripheral (α-adrenergic receptor blocking) actions of antipsychotics (see Table 12-1), whereas tachycardia and increased coronary blood flow derive from central compensatory cardiovascular reflexes. The aliphatic and piperidine phenothiazines and clozapine are the most likely, and the piperazines the least likely, to cause orthostatic hypotension (Table 12-4). In the emergency treatment of phenothiazine-induced vasomotor

Table • 12-4

Principal Side Effects of the Antipsychotic Drugs

ANTIPSYCHOTIC AGENT	APPROXIMATE EQUIVALENT DOSE (mg)	SEDATION	EXTRAPYRAMIDAL SYMPTOMS	ANTICHOLINERGIC EFFECTS	ORTHOSTATIC HYPOTENSION	WEIGHT GAIN	PROLONGED QT/TdP
Conventional (Typical) Agents							
Phenothiazines (aliphatic)							
Chlorpromazine	100	+++	++	++	+++	++	+
Triflupromazine	25	+++	++	+++	++	ND	ND
Piperazines							
Fluphenazine	2	+	+++	+	+	0/+	ND
Perphenazine	10	++	++	+	+	ND	ND
Prochlorperazine	15	++	+++	+	+	ND	ND
Trifluoperazine	5	+	+++	+	+	ND	ND
Piperidines							
Mesoridazine	50	+++	+	+++	++	+++	+
Thioridazine	100	+++	+	+++	+++	+++	++
Thioxanthene							
Thiothixene	4	+	+++	+	++	ND	ND
Butyrophenones							
Haloperidol	2	+	+++	+	+	+	+
Droperidol*	2.5	++	ND	ND	++	ND	++
Diphenylbutylpiperidine							
Pimozide	1	++	+++	++	+	ND	+
Dihydroindolones							
Molindone	10	++	++	+	+	0	ND
Ziprasidone	20	+	+	+	+	0/+	+
Dibenzoxazepine							
Loxapine	15	+	++	+	+	ND	ND
Novel (Atypical) Agents							
Dibenzodiazepine							
Clozapine	50	+++	+	+++	++	++++	+
Thienobenzodiazepine							
Olanzapine	5	+++	+	+++	++	++++	+
Dibenzothiazepine							
Quetiapine	50	++	+	0	++	++	+
Benzisoxazole							
Risperidone	2	+	+ to ++	0	+	++	+
Dihydrocarbostyril							
Aripiprazole	15	0/+	0/+	0/–	0/+	0/+	0/–

Level and risk for each adverse effect is indicated by the number of + signs.
*Not used to treat psychosis in the United States.
TdP, Torsades de pointes; *ND,* no data.

collapse, epinephrine is contraindicated because the α-adrenergic receptor–blocking action of the phenothiazines may cause "epinephrine reversal" and an even greater reduction in blood pressure. NE or phenylephrine, both of which lack significant β_2-adrenergic receptor stimulation, is preferred in these circumstances. Chlorpromazine has a direct depressant effect on the heart, as well as an antiarrhythmic action, that may be caused in part by its local anesthetic effect. Vascular reflexes mediated by vasomotor centers of the brainstem are depressed by chlorpromazine. Haloperidol rarely causes pronounced hypotensive effects, but tachycardia is a common side effect. Many antipsychotic and antidepressant agents have been found to cause or exacerbate the condition known as *long QT syndrome* (see Chapter 24). This syndrome is associated with increased likelihood of the arrhythmia *torsades de pointes*, which is potentially fatal. The condition is often produced by decreasing the function of cardiac K^+ channels responsible for cardiac repolarization (see Chapter 24). Phenothiazines, butyrophenones, pimozide, thioridazine, mesoridazine, and several atypical antipsychotic agents have been implicated (see Table 12-4). Clozapine is also known to block D_4 receptors, which are abundant in the heart. This action may contribute to the cardiovascular risk seen with clozapine.

Absorption, Fate, and Excretion

Metabolism of antipsychotic drugs is complex.[36] Most agents are metabolized by the P450 isoforms CYP2D6 or CYP3A4.[13] Other isoforms may also participate (1A2, 2B6, 2C9), and flavin monoxygenases also contribute in the liver and in the brain (Table 12-5). Olanzapine is of interest because it is primarily glucuronidated and may possess advantages when oxidative metabolism is reduced. The P450 isoforms CYP2D6 and CYP1A2 are known to have genetic polymorphisms, and preliminary investigations suggest that patients who are poor metabolizers may have more antipsychotic toxicity than normal metabolizers. Although metabolites for many antipsychotic drugs are active, their antipsychotic effects are usually not as potent as those of the parent compounds. Moreover, the plasma half-lives of the antipsychotic drugs are not true indicators of their long durations of action. For example, half-lives for the phenothiazines range from 20 to 40 hours, yet the lipid solubilities of the drugs and their metabolites allow them to remain in tissues for prolonged periods of time.

Adverse Effects

The most troublesome side effects of the antipsychotic agents, particularly the phenothiazines and butyrophenones, are the extrapyramidal disorders consisting of tremor, akathisia, dystonia, bradykinesia, and dyskinesia. Therapy may have to be terminated in patients exhibiting pronounced and intractable motor disturbances. Use of atypical agents may help reduce this problem. However, the use of an anticholinergic drug, antihistamine, or amantadine can alleviate parkinsonlike symptoms and less readily the motor restlessness of akathisia without compromising antipsychotic therapy. Acute dystonic reactions (torticollis, facial grimacing, oculogyric crisis) are also treated with centrally acting antihistamines and antimuscarinic drugs such as diphenhydramine and benztropine.

Tardive dyskinesia is a problematic neurologic disorder because of its disabling effect and resistance to pharmacologic management. The adverse effect is irreversible or only slowly reversible. The low incidence of extrapyramidal responses to clozapine and atypical agents has given new hope that these disturbing side effects of the antipsychotics can be separated from their therapeutic effect.

Other adverse effects may also be serious enough to necessitate adjustment of the dosage or withdrawal of the medication. These reactions may be manifested as cholestatic jaundice, blood dyscrasias, or dermatologic responses. The latter may take the form of contact dermatitis, urticaria, or photosensitivity.

Clozapine can produce some serious adverse reactions. It was initially withdrawn from the market because it was discovered to cause agranulocytosis in approximately 1% of the patient population. The drug was reintroduced with the provision that all patients receiving it be continually monitored for hematologic changes. Clozapine is also associated with a higher incidence of seizures than are the other antipsychotic drugs.[17] Orthostatic hypotension and cardiovascular and respiratory collapse have also been documented. Some predisposing factors have been proposed. Excessive sedation and respiratory collapse may be associated with concomitant use of depressant agents, including benzodiazepines. Epinephrine reversal (caused by α-adrenergic receptor blockade by clozapine) can contribute to declines in blood pressure. These toxicities may be more likely during rapid changes in blood concentrations, which may occur from adjustment of drug dosing or the use of other drugs that may displace clozapine from binding sites or alter the metabolism of clozapine.

Normally, less severe side effects of the antipsychotics include orthostatic hypotension and syncope, xerostomia, nasal stuffiness, urinary retention, constipation, and alterations in body temperature (usually hypothermia). In prolonged, high-dose therapy with the phenothiazines, a blue-gray pigmentation may occasionally occur in skin exposed to direct sunlight.

A potentially debilitating gain in weight has been observed with schizophrenic patients taking antipsychotic agents. This side effect is of increased concern for patients taking the newer atypical agents.[8] Nearly all the antipsychotics cause a gain in weight (see Table 12-4). Although this is rarely a severe side effect, it frequently leads to noncompliance. Clozapine and olanzapine may be the most likely, and molindone and ziprasidone the least likely, to cause this effect.[28] The

Table • 12-5

Metabolism of Selected Antipsychotic Drugs

	1A2	2B	2C9	2C19	2D6	3A4	FMO
Chlorpromazine	S				S	S	S
Haloperidol					S, Inh	S	
Thioridazine					S, Inh		
Pimozide						S	
Clozapine	S, Ind	Ind	Inh	S, Inh	S	S, Ind	S
Risperidone					S	S	
Olanzapine*	S				S		S
Quetiapine						S	
Ziprasidone						S	
Aripiprazole					S	S	

Column headings refer to specific enzymes involved in drug metabolism.
*Primarily glucuronidated.
FMO, Flavin monoxygenases; *S*, substrate; *Inh*, inhibitor; *Ind*, inducer; *PM*, poor metabolizer.
Data from Flockhart DA: *Cytochrome P450 drug interaction table,* Indiana University, Department of Medicine, Division of Clinical Pharmacology, http://medicine.iupui.edu/flockhart/table.htm, 2003.

Table • 12-6

Interactions of Antipsychotic Drugs with Other Drugs*

DENTAL DRUG OR OVER-THE-COUNTER DRUG	POSSIBLE RESPONSE WHEN COMBINED WITH ANTIPSYCHOTIC DRUG
Promethazine	CNS depression
Barbiturates	CNS depression
Benzodiazepines	Cardiovascular and respiratory collapse with clozapine
General anesthetics (inhalation and intravenous)	CNS depression (especially respiratory depression)
Ethanol	CNS depression
Opioid analgesics	CNS depression, respiratory depression (especially with meperidine), miosis
Antihistamines	CNS depression, anticholinergic effect
Epinephrine	Epinephrine reversal, orthostatic hypotension
Anticholinergics	Anticholinergic toxicity: arrhythmias, hallucinations, gastrointestinal inhibition
Metabolic inhibitors (erythromycin, clarithromycin)	Elevation of antipsychotic blood concentrations
Protein-bound drugs	Displacement of clozapine might result in adverse reactions

*Primarily the phenothiazines, thioxanthenes, butyrophenones, molindone, and loxapine.

cause of the weight gain is unknown but may be associated with the blockade of histamine or dopamine receptors.

A rare but sometimes fatal idiosyncratic effect, usually associated with potent antipsychotics such as haloperidol and fluphenazine, is the neuroleptic malignant syndrome (NMS). It is characterized by sustained and widespread muscular contractions, fluctuating levels of consciousness, autonomic abnormalities, and fever. Treatment for NMS includes immediate withdrawal of the drug and supportive measures. Some benefit may be gained from the skeletal muscle relaxant dantrolene. Bromocriptine, a dopaminergic agonist, may also be helpful. Physical cooling to reduce fever may be necessary. It is generally believed that the risk of developing NMS with clozapine is low, but some cases have been reported. Drug interactions for antipsychotic drugs are summarized in Table 12-6.

The partial agonist antipsychotic aripiprazole is reported to have a low incidence of many of the side effects associated with typical antipsychotic drugs, including reduced extrapyramidal effects, reduced release of prolactin, minimal weight gain, and little effect on the QT interval.

General Therapeutic Uses

Currently, the antipsychotic drugs are primarily used for the treatment of psychotic states. However, the wide variety of pharmacologic effects of the phenothiazines has led to their use as antiemetics, preoperative medications to relax and calm the patient, antihistamines, and antihelmintics (in veterinary preparations). Antipsychotics may be used to control the manic phase of bipolar disorder. Other applications of the phenothiazines include the control of hallucinations associated with acute alcohol withdrawal and the treatment of intractable hiccough. As mentioned previously, pimozide finds special application in the treatment of Tourette's syndrome.

Because of the perceived reduced side effects and improved efficacy of the atypical antipsychotic drugs, an expansion of indications for these agents can be anticipated. A number of new indications for these drugs in children have been proposed, including autism, disruptive disorder, juvenile treatment-resistant schizophrenia, and pervasive developmental disorder of childhood. Additional indications in adult patients include borderline personality disorder, delusional disorder, first-episode schizophrenia, mood disorders with psychotic features, obsessive-compulsive disorder, polydipsia syndrome, schizoaffective disorders, and personality problems. Finally, increased use in the elderly is likely, with the main indication being dementia. There are few controlled studies to support these indications, except for the use of olanzapine for the treatment of acute mania.

Although dose requirements of antipsychotic drugs for most patients usually fall within a relatively narrow spectrum, dosage may vary considerably. Adjustments in dose are frequently made depending on the patient's clinical response and side effects. Effective plasma concentrations vary widely among patients, and their determination is not very helpful. As a rule, treatment with the antipsychotic agents is uninterrupted and indefinite in duration.

Long-acting depot antipsychotic preparations, such as fluphenazine enanthate, fluphenazine decanoate, and haloperidol decanoate, are convenient in patients for whom compliance is a problem. These injectable forms are effective for a period of 2 to 3 weeks once therapeutic blood concentrations are obtained and stabilized. A reduced total drug dose is frequently possible because problems with absorption from the gastrointestinal tract are bypassed. In general, depot forms are safe for younger patients in good physical condition. A disadvantage to this mode of administration is that the drug cannot be withdrawn if side effects occur, and therapeutic levels are sometimes difficult to stabilize.

Antipsychotics such as the phenothiazines, thioxanthenes, and butyrophenones were for decades the drugs of choice in the treatment of schizophrenia. Olanzapine, quetiapine, and possibly low doses of risperidone are now the preferred agents and are of particular use in cases of schizophrenia refractory to older antipsychotics or when administration of other antipsychotics results in unacceptable adverse effects. Because molindone and ziprasidone result in less weight gain than other agents, they may have application when weight gain is a special concern. Clozapine is considered to be a second-line drug primarily because of its propensity to cause agranulocytosis.

Implications for Dentistry

Because many people in the United States will at some point in their lives receive pharmacotherapy for mental illness, the dentist will inevitably encounter these patients in practice. Many patients will be receiving more than one drug for their condition, and they may be taking a variety of other drugs (e.g., alcohol, cough remedies, aspirin, dietary supplements) that may not be revealed in a medical history questionnaire.

Many antipsychotics can add to the depressant effects of sedative-hypnotics, antianxiety agents, anesthetics, or opioid analgesics used in the course of dental treatment. Chlorpromazine is known to potentiate the effects of general anesthetics and the respiratory depressant response to opioids (see Table 12-6). The cardiac effects of thioridazine can be potentiated by hydroxyzine, and other antihistamines may pose similar concerns. Both the antipsychotic and antihistaminic drugs have substantial antimuscarinic activity and may also contribute to the long QT syndrome.

Tardive dyskinesia has important implications in dentistry because the facial musculature is prominently involved in the disorder. The abnormal movements of tardive dyskinesia often start in the orofacial musculature, particularly the tongue, which alternately protrudes, retracts, and undergoes a rolling movement. Because the orofacial muscles are primarily affected in the early development of tardive dyskinesia, the patient often believes that the dentist can correct the problem.

Unfortunately, persons who require treatment with the phenothiazine antipsychotics usually take these drugs for a long period of time, if not for life. Prolonged phenothiazine use can sometimes cause a reduction in leukocyte count, which rarely predisposes the patient to infection, and frequent oral candidiasis. Clozapine's tendency to cause agranulocytosis is a factor that can lead to serious susceptibility to infection.

The reduced salivary flow caused by the antipsychotics can result in xerostomia and an increased incidence of dental caries. On the other hand, clozapine-induced hypersalivation may be problematic for some clinical procedures.[37] The patient should be forewarned that this condition is likely to be most pronounced at night.

ANTIDEPRESSANTS

Numerous mechanisms are responsible for the actions of the known antidepressant drugs (Table 12-7). Most of the clinically used antidepressants increase the synaptic concentrations of 5-HT and/or NE in the brain, and this relation has given support to the monoamine hypothesis of affective disorders.[9] The increase in neurotransmitters can be measured in a few hours from the time that the medications are administered.

Studies of diets deficient in tryptophan, the precursor amino acid for 5-HT, have found that depressed patients taking SSRIs have a return of symptoms of depression within a few hours after eating a tryptophan-deficient diet. Women seem to be somewhat more sensitive to tryptophan restriction. Tryptophan restriction does not reverse the effects of NE-selective antidepressants, however. Selective inhibition of NE synthesis with metyrosine triggers symptoms of depression in patients treated with a NE reuptake–blocking antidepressant and in untreated patients with latent depression. Patients responding to SSRIs do not exhibit depressive symptoms when taking metyrosine. Normal patients do not show depression symptoms after either tryptophan depletion or metyrosine treatment. Altogether these studies suggest 5-HT, NE, or both monoamines may play a role in depression; the predominant factor may vary in different patients.

A significant challenge to the monoamine hypothesis, however, is the time required for full antidepressant activity to be expressed, which may vary from 2 to 8 weeks in clinical practice. This time lag is long enough for considerable rearrangement of cellular structure to occur. Part of this delay may simply be related to the pharmacokinetics of the antidepressants, which have half-lives averaging 24 hours. Thus to reach plasma equilibrium the drugs will need, on average, to be taken for at least 4 to 5 days. However, this certainly does not explain the entire delay. The action of antidepressants is closely linked to the neurotransmitters 5-HT and NE. Information on 5-HT in the CNS is particularly instructive about mechanisms of antidepressant action. The raphe nuclei contain the bulk of the 5-HT–synthesizing neurons in the brain, and these project to wide areas of the brain (Table 12-8).[27] In the awake animal, raphe 5-HT–containing neurons are generally tonically active with a firing rate of approximately 5 Hz, which is maintained by depolarizing Ca^{++} and hyperpolarizing K^+ currents. These cells may also respond to phasic activity such as loud sounds. Afferent inputs to the 5-HT cells include tonic excitatory input from catecholamines (NE from the locus ceruleus [LC] and dopamine from the ventral tegmental area) and phasic excitatory glutamate inputs. Noradrenergic input is thought to activate excitatory α_1 receptors on the raphe 5-HT neurons. Extracellular 5-HT is also present and may originate from raphe collateral feedback or possibly from a nonsynaptic source, which might be "leakage" from 5-HT neurons themselves.[33] A GABA inhibitory afferent input is also known.

Table • 12-7

Some Mechanisms of Antidepressant Drugs

MECHANISM	DRUG EXAMPLES
Block 5-HT reuptake	TCAs, most second- and third-generation drugs, SSRIs
Block NE reuptake	TCAs, most second- and third-generation drugs
Inhibit MAO	MAOIs, St. John's wort*
Block presynaptic autoreceptors	Mirtazapine
Block dopamine reuptake	Bupropion
Block Na^+ gradients needed for many neurotransmitter reuptake transports	St. John's wort
Neuroprotective actions	SSRIs, anticonvulsants
Facilitate GABA	Alprazolam
Hormone adjustment	Estrogens, levothyroxine

*Only at high doses.

Table • 12-8

Key Serotonergic Pathways in the Action of SSRIs

MIDBRAIN (RAPHE) PROJECTION TO:	POSSIBLE SSRI EFFECT	SIGNS OF DYSREGULATION
Prefrontal cortex	Relief of depression	Depression
Hippocampus, limbic cortex	Alleviation of panic disorder	Anhedonia, anxiety, panic, sexual dysfunctions
Basal ganglia	Alleviation of obsessive-compulsive disorder	Agitation; extrapyramidal side effects, including akathisia, parkinsonlike tremor, and rigidity
Hypothalamus	Alleviation of eating disorder	Bulimia and binge-eating disorders, prolactin dysregulation
Spinal cord (pontine-medullary cell bodies)	Sexual dysfunction	Inhibited ejaculation and orgasm

A current hypothesis to explain some of the therapeutic delay follows. Antidepressant drugs produce an increased serotonergic tone in the raphe nuclei. However, because of abundant presynaptic autoregulatory receptors (autoreceptors), the release of 5-HT is acutely "turned off" in the raphe nuclei. With continued exposure to the antidepressant drugs, the autoreceptors desensitize or downregulate, allowing increased 5-HT release at the synaptic terminals ("turned on"). This increased release may then lead to a downregulation of some terminal field postsynaptic 5-HT receptors. In the brainstem, the raphe nucleus is known to reciprocally innervate the LC and may also reciprocally innervate dopaminergic areas such as the ventral tegmental area and cortex. These innervations hint at additional layers of control and interaction. Additionally, the delay in onset of antidepressant action suggests that some form of cellular remodeling may occur.

NE has long been suspected to have involvement with depression. A large amount of the NE in the brain is found in the LC, whose neurons project as far as the forebrain. The LC neurons respond to a variety of phasic external stimuli and stress-related stimuli (fight or flight) but also participate in tonic brain states, including the sleep-wake cycle and arousal. The LC may be involved in mediating anxiety, depression, panic attacks, and posttraumatic stress disorder. Although a number of peptides can alter the activity of the LC, one of the most interesting influences may be the increased LC firing rate induced by corticotropin-releasing hormone (which may mediate the involvement of corticosteroids in the response to stressful conditions).

NE actions are mediated by several receptor types (α_1, α_2, and β_1 adrenoceptors) (see Chapter 6). Changes in noradrenergic systems that are linked to depression include alterations in α_2-receptor number and function in the brain and platelets of depressed patients and decreased cell counts and tyrosine hydroxylase in the LC of suicide victims. Clonidine, an α_2 agonist, can increase the release of growth hormone and thyroid-stimulating hormone in normal patients. In depressed patients, the magnitude of these hormone responses is reduced to approximately 50% of control subjects. The clonidine test may identify the depressive trait.

Long-term antidepressant use reduces postsynaptic β adrenoceptors in the brain without significantly affecting postsynaptic α_1 adrenoceptors. This change apparently happens because the increases in synaptic NE resulting from presynaptic effects of antidepressants (downregulation of autoregulatory α_2 adrenoceptors) are able to affect adrenoceptors differently (β adrenoceptors downregulate and α_1 adrenoceptors do not). Exactly how these changes benefit the depressed patient is still being investigated; however, the increase in synaptic NE coupled with a change in postsynaptic adrenoceptor profile is likely to be the basis for the therapeutic effects of antidepressant drugs. TCAs, SSRIs, and electroconvulsive therapy all lead to similar changes. The effect of the antidepressant drugs on 5-HT dynamics is analogous to that on NE dynamics. Therefore the mechanism by which antidepressants act seems to depend on differential changes among various receptors and receptor-signaling processes. Although this hypothesis is useful for explaining the actions of several classes of antidepressant drugs, it is not a complete explanation for the actions of all antidepressants.

Efforts to speed up the onset of action of antidepressants based on some of these finding are being investigated. Strategies have included attempts to block somatodendritic 5-HT_{1A} autoreceptors with pindolol (a clinically available β blocker that coincidentally blocks 5-HT_{1A} receptors),[5] and use of antidepressants that block α_2- or β-adrenergic receptors. Currently, only a few studies have reported efficacy with these approaches.[6] Sleep deprivation has also been found to produce a rapid, but temporary, reversal of depression and the depression of bipolar disorder. Not all patients respond, however. There have been attempts to prolong the beneficial effect by using bright light therapy. These observations have so far defied explanation.

The TCAs and the MAOIs, sometimes referred to as *first-generation antidepressants,* share a number of characteristics: they are effective in a broad spectrum of depressive syndromes (although 20% to 30% of patients remain unresponsive to pharmacotherapy); they have a delayed onset of therapeutic effect; and they have troublesome side effects.

Newer drugs (second- and third-generation antidepressants) such as amoxapine, maprotiline, bupropion, trazodone, nefazodone, and mirtazapine were introduced to overcome the disadvantages of first-generation compounds. This heterogeneous group of agents share antidepressant efficacy but vary in their particular actions, which are listed in Box 12-1.

An important addition to the pharmacologic armamentarium for the treatment of depression is the class of drugs called *SSRIs.* As the group name implies, these drugs have greater pharmacologic selectivity than the TCAs and therefore have the potential for therapeutic effectiveness with fewer side effects. The SSRIs also require 2 to 3 weeks before therapeutic efficacy is noted. The first drug of this class approved for use in the United States was fluoxetine. Fluoxetine quickly became a very popular drug because it is effective in major depression and refractory depression. It also has fewer side effects compared with previous drugs. The more recently approved SSRIs—sertraline, fluvoxamine, paroxetine, and citalopram—exhibit a similar pharmacologic profile, differing from fluoxetine primarily in their pharmacokinetic properties. Because of the relative safety of these agents, investigations of their efficacy in a wide array of behavioral disorders have lead to broadened indications for their use. SSRIs may be more beneficial in women and TCAs more beneficial in men.

Venlafaxine and reboxetine are selective agents that block NE and 5-HT reuptake; St. John's wort has a unique action blocking the reuptake of 5-HT, NE, dopamine, GABA, glycine, and glutamate, but with no known receptor-blocking actions.

Tricyclic Antidepressants

Chemistry and structure-activity relationships

A relatively small modification of the phenothiazine ring structure resulted in an entirely new group of drugs, the TCAs. The name of these compounds is derived from the triple-ring structure consisting of two benzene moieties connected through a seven-membered ring (Figure 12-5).

The prototype for the TCAs is imipramine, a dibenzazepine derivative. Structural analogues of imipramine include the dibenzocycloheptadienes, in which a carbon atom is substituted for the nitrogen of the central ring, and the dibenzoxepines, in which an oxygen atom replaces one of the methylene groups of the center ring of the dibenzocycloheptadiene molecule. A prototype drug for the dibenzocycloheptadienes is amitriptyline, and for the dibenzoxepines, doxepin.

Substitutions at R (see Figure 12-5) usually consist of aminopropyl groups that may be either dimethyl or monomethyl amino derivatives. Compounds such as imipramine, amitriptyline, and doxepin have two methyl moieties on the nitrogen atom of the side chain and are tertiary amines. Desipramine, nortriptyline, and protriptyline have one methyl group and are secondary amines.

Box • 12-1

Actions of Antidepressant Drugs

Drugs that Inhibit Reuptake of NE and 5-HT with Similar Potencies (20-Fold Difference or Less)

- Amitriptyline
- Amoxapine*
- Clomipramine
- Desipramine
- Doxepin
- Imipramine
- Nefazodone
- Nortriptyline
- Protriptyline

Drugs that Inhibit 5-HT Reuptake with Greater Potency (>50-Fold More Than NE Reuptake)

- Citalopram
- Fluoxetine
- Fluvoxamine
- Paroxetine
- Sertraline
- Trazodone†
- Venlafaxine†

Drug that Inhibits NE Reuptake with Greater Potency (Approximately 500-Fold More Than 5-HT Reuptake)

- Maprotiline

Drugs that Have Little Effect on Either 5-HT or NE Uptake

- Bupropion
- Mirtazapine

*Also blocks dopamine uptake.
†Not classified as an SSRI.

Pharmacologic effects

Like the antipsychotic drugs, the TCAs have therapeutically useful effects on the CNS and a variety of side effects. Common properties of these agents are blockade of 5-HT and/or NE reuptake, histaminergic receptors, muscarinic receptors, and α_1-adrenergic receptors as well as a local anesthetic action.

Central Nervous System When administered to a normal individual, the TCAs initially produce drowsiness, lethargy, and often an increased feeling of anxiety. With continued administration, the individual may have thought disorders and become increasingly confused. Conversely, after the TCAs have been administered for approximately 2 to 3 weeks to depressed patients, they become less confused and have an elevation of mood. Untoward CNS effects include dizziness, lightheadedness, and even delirium and hallucinations.

All the TCAs seem to have in common the ability to inhibit the reuptake of NE or 5-HT or both into central presynaptic nerve terminals. Normally most of the transmitter is recycled into the presynaptic terminal, stored, and made available for reuse (see Chapter 11). TCAs, by blocking this reuptake, increase the concentrations of NE and/or 5-HT at critical central synapses. This increase in concentration of these biogenic amines leads to the receptor changes discussed above and an antidepressant effect.

Autonomic Nervous System The TCAs are more potent anticholinergics than are their phenothiazine analogues. Thus dry mouth, constipation, urinary retention, and ophthalmologic changes (blurred vision and mydriasis) are commonly observed, especially with the tertiary amines. Paradoxically, excessive sweating is also reported, although in a large overdose the skin is dry. Sexual dysfunction (including loss of libido, impaired erection and ejaculation, and anorgasmy) is an additional side effect that may lead to patient noncompliance. Peripheral cholinergic and α-adrenergic blockade have been associated with sexual dysfunction. Excess serotonergic

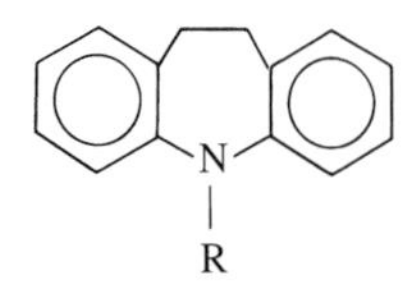

Dibenzazepine

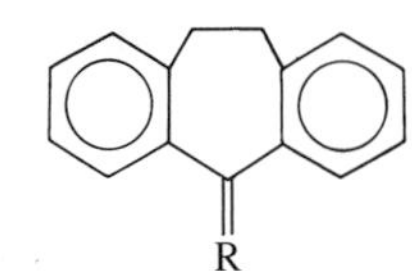

Dibenzocycloheptadiene

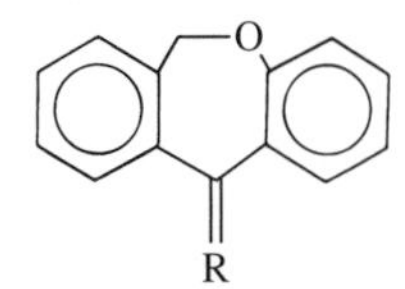

Dibenzoxepine

Fig. 12-5 Structural formulas of the tricyclic rings of the dibenzazepine, dibenzocycloheptadiene, and dibenzoxepine antidepressants.

tone at some 5-HT receptors may also be responsible for the sexual side effects of these agents (see Table 12-1).

Cardiovascular System The TCAs can cause hypotension and compensatory tachycardia. Tricyclics affect the heart in a manner similar to the class I antiarrhythmics such as quinidine and procainamide.[16] Prolongation of the QT interval, flattening of the T wave, and various arrhythmias have been reported. Postural hypotension, particularly in the elderly, is not uncommon, probably because of α_1-adrenergic receptor blockade. Because tricyclics block the reuptake of catecholamines, they can increase the response to endogenously released catecholamines or directly acting sympathomimetic drugs that are actively transported into adrenergic nerve terminals.

Absorption, fate, and excretion

The TCAs are readily absorbed from the gastrointestinal tract. The drugs are distributed throughout the body and are tightly bound to plasma and tissue proteins. Many pharmacologically active metabolites are formed in the liver by microsomal oxidation reactions, including N-demethylation. Subsequent glucuronidation inactivates the agents and promotes their excretion. Approximately two thirds of a single dose is eliminated in the urine and one third in the feces over the course of several days. TCAs are metabolized by several isoforms of P450, with particular involvement of CYP1A2, CYP2C19, CYP2D6, and CYP3A4.[13]

Adverse effects

The TCAs may initially cause insomnia and restlessness or feelings of fatigue and weakness (Table 12-9), but tolerance develops to these effects. Although these agents do not elicit the extrapyramidal side effects of the antipsychotic agents, mild tremor may sometimes occur. In some persons, tics, ataxia, and incoordination have been reported. The anticholinergic effects cause dryness of the mouth, mydriasis, and urinary retention and may also contribute to cardiovascular disturbances. Amitriptyline is one of the most potent anticholinergic TCAs; it is about one eighth as potent as atropine.

Acute overdosage, sometimes self-inflicted by the suicidal patient, presents a potentially life-threatening situation and is characterized by CNS excitation and depression, anticholinergic effects, and cardiovascular complications. Life-threatening cardiac arrhythmias are a potential consequence of acute overdose. Even in conventional doses, the incidence of sudden death from myocardial infarction or ventricular arrhythmias is increased in patients with cardiac disease. Several TCAs produce long QT syndrome, which can lead to *torsades de pointes*. Fatalities have also occurred in children with no apparent preexisting cardiac defect. Blood dyscrasias, skin rashes, photosensitization, and cholestatic jaundice, many of which are manifestations of allergic reactions, have been reported but are less frequent than with the phenothiazines. TCAs may also increase the risk for seizures, with clomipramine among the most likely to produce this effect. The likelihood of seizures is directly related to the dose taken and a history of previous seizure disorders.[34]

Adverse drug interactions are another potential problem for the antidepressant-treated patient. Coadministration of the TCAs with MAOIs may cause anxiety, vomiting, tremor, convulsions, coma, and death. The tricyclics may also obtund the antihypertensive action of guanethidine and the sympathomimetic action of amphetamine and tyramine by preventing their uptake into nerve terminals. The effects of clonidine (an α_2 agonist) are also inhibited. Drug interactions that the dentist must consider are discussed below and similar to those listed in Table 12-6.

Monoamine Oxidase Inhibitors

The MAOIs include many chemically unrelated compounds that share the ability to antagonize the action of MAO, the enzyme responsible for the metabolic degradation of the naturally occurring monoamines epinephrine, NE, dopamine, and 5-HT. Some of these inhibitors, such as tranylcypromine, are structurally related to amphetamine.

Pharmacologic effects

Like the TCAs, the MAOIs increase the concentration of NE and 5-HT in the CNS. By preventing the catabolic action of MAO, the MAOIs allow the buildup of monoamines in the presynaptic nerve terminals (see Chapters 6 and 11). This effect apparently leads to adaptive changes in receptors similar to the changes seen with the TCAs. Although these effects are compatible with the monoamine hypothesis of depression, it should be noted that the MAOIs are not specific for MAO because they affect other enzymes and have nonenzymatic actions as well. We do not have a clear understanding of the mechanism of the antidepressant action of this group of drugs. However, the existence of at least two forms of MAO (MAO-A and MAO-B) in the brain and selective inhibitors of MAO-A and MAO-B suggest that selective inhibition of specific forms of MAO will be of potential use in the future. Moclobemide and brofaromine, selective inhibitors of MAO-A, are effective antidepressants; unlike most other MAOIs, they are reversible inhibitors of MAO and have a number of advantages because of their selectivity and shorter duration of action.

The MAOIs are generally considered to be less effective and to have more serious side effects and drug interactions than the TCAs. However, these drugs are making a comeback with the discovery that they are effective for atypical depression and that in some of the early studies inappropriate dosages were used. Similar to the SSRIs, the MAOIs also have antiobsessional, antipanic, and anxiolytic effects. Nevertheless, a number of precautions, particularly regarding drug interactions and dietary restrictions, must be observed with the clinical use of these compounds.

The most prominent autonomic effects of the MAOIs are exerted on the cardiovascular system. Hypotension occurs because of reduced NE release from peripheral adrenergic nerves (except in the presence of indirectly acting sympathomimetic drugs). Tachycardia, dry mouth, sweating, hot flashes, diarrhea, constipation, difficulty in micturition, and impotence may also occur. The MAOIs antagonize transmission of nerve impulses through autonomic ganglia, and evidence suggests that sympathetic ganglia are the more severely affected.

Absorption, fate, and excretion

The MAOIs are rapidly absorbed from the gastrointestinal tract. The metabolic fate of the MAOIs is not fully known, but the drugs are apparently rapidly metabolized and excreted. The long duration of effect (weeks) results from an irreversible inactivation of MAO and can be of concern when adding new therapies after an MAOI has been discontinued.

Adverse effects

Most of the original MAOIs have been withdrawn from the market because of their serious side effects. An important adverse reaction to the remaining MAOIs (and a major problem with the original drugs) is hepatotoxicity. The MAOIs may also cause orthostatic hypotension and, in overdosage, central excitatory manifestations of insomnia, agitation, hyperreflexia, and convulsions.

Drug interactions are of particular concern with the MAOIs because they are likely to be serious and potentially fatal. Among the drugs with which the MAOIs interact are

Table • 12-9

Major Adverse Effects of Antidepressant Drugs

DRUG	ANTICHOLINERGIC	SEDATION	ORTHOSTATIC HYPOTENSION	PROLONGED QT	SEXUAL DYSFUNCTION	WEIGHT GAIN OR LOSS
Tricyclics—Tertiary Amines						
Amitriptyline	++++	++++	+++	TdP	+	++
Clomipramine	+++	++	++	+		+
Doxepin	++	+++	+++	+	+	++
Imipramine	++	++	+++	+	+	++
Trimipramine	++	+++	++	ND		++
Tricyclics—Secondary Amines						
Amoxapine	+++	++	+	ND		+
Desipramine	+	+	+	+	+	+
Nortriptyline	++	++	+	+	+	+
Protriptyline	+++	+	+	ND		+
Second- and Third-Generation Agents						
Maprotiline	++	++	+	ND		+
Mirtazapine	++	+++	++	TdP	0	++
Trazodone	+	++++	++	+	0	+, –
Nefazodone	0/+	++	+		0	0, +
Bupropion	++	0/+		+/0	0	+, –
SSRIs						
Fluoxetine	0/+	0/+	0/+	+	++	+, –
Paroxetine	0	0/+	0	+/0	++	+, –
Sertraline	0	0/+	0	+/0	++	+, –
Fluvoxamine	0/+	0/+	0	+	++	+, –
Citalopram	0/+	0/+	0/+	+/0	+	+, –
Venlafaxine*	0	0	0	+	++	0, –
MAOIs						
Tranylcypromine	+	+	0			+
Phenelzine	+	+	+			+

Severity of adverse effects is indicated by the number of + signs.
*May induce hypertension; not classified as an SSRI.
TdP, Torsades de pointes resulting from prolonged QT; *ND,* no data.

the TCAs and the SSRIs, other classes of antidepressants, opioid analgesics (especially meperidine), alcohol and other CNS depressants, indirect-acting or mixed-acting sympathomimetics such as amphetamine or ephedrine, sympathomimetics metabolized predominantly by MAO such as phenylephrine (commonly used in over-the-counter preparations as a nasal decongestant), and monoamine precursors such as levodopa.

In addition to drug interactions, acute hypertensive crises have been precipitated by the ingestion of foods containing naturally occurring pressor amines, such as tyramine, that release NE from nerve endings. Patients treated with MAOIs have elevated stores of NE available for release. In addition, ingested tyramine, which is normally metabolized by enteric and hepatic MAO, reaches the systemic circulation in increased amounts. Foods containing sympathomimetic amines that should be avoided include aged cheeses (especially cheddar and Swiss), fermented alcoholic beverages (particularly Chianti wine), canned fish products, snails, liver, nuts, broad beans, citrus fruits, coffee, and almost any product made with yeast. Hypertensive crises precipitated by such foods are characterized by severe headaches, often localized in the occipital region, and fever. This type of drug interaction will probably become less important as more selective or reversible MAOIs are developed. The reversible and selective MAO-A inhibitor moclobemide has been reported to produce less of this "cheese effect."

The MAOIs are contraindicated with the SSRIs. This combination may precipitate the "serotonin syndrome," which consists of hyperthermia, facial flushing, dizziness, confusion, headache, sweating, fever, rigidity, myoclonus or tremor, respiratory disturbances, gastrointestinal upset, and mental status changes from delirium to coma. This drug interaction may occur even several weeks after termination of fluoxetine because of its slow elimination from the body (half-life up to 250 hours for active metabolites of SSRIs).

Second- and Third-Generation Antidepressants

The second- and third-generation antidepressants (or atypical antidepressants) include a diverse array of drugs. Amoxapine (Figure 12-6), a dibenzoxazepine resembling the TCAs in chemical structure, is the N-demethylated metabolite of the antipsychotic loxapine. Amoxapine shares many properties with the atypical antipsychotic agents and has been shown to have both atypical antipsychotic and antidepressant effects, making it useful for patients with both psychotic and mood disturbances. Maprotiline is related to the tricyclics but contains a tetracyclic ring structure (see Figure 12-6). Trazodone and nefazodone (see Figure 12-6) are triazole derivatives, trazodone being noted for having 5-HT_2 blocking activity in addition to its reuptake-blocking action. Bupropion, an aminoketone, is structurally dissimilar to all other antidepressants (Figure 12-7). Bupropion is a weak reuptake inhibitor of dopamine and 5-HT as well as a weak α_2-adrenergic receptor blocker. Mirtazapine (see Figure 12-7), a piperazinoazepine, is similar to the TCAs in general effects but is reported to block several additional receptors (α_2-adrenergic, 5-HT_2, 5-HT_3). There has been some interest in using these agents as adjunct therapy to SSRIs. Venlafaxine (see Figure 12-7) acts selectively on 5-HT reuptake at low doses but blocks NE reuptake at higher doses. Reboxetine is relatively selective for NE reuptake.

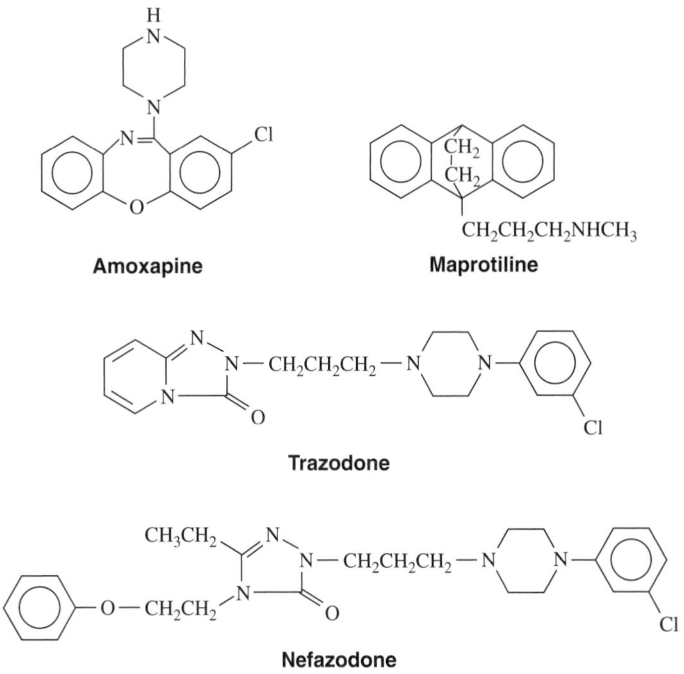

Pharmacologic effects

These compounds differ significantly in their selectivity of action on monoamine uptake and neurotransmitter receptors. Amoxapine resembles the secondary amine TCAs in pharmacologic activity, but it also blocks dopamine and 5-HT_{2A} receptors, accounting for its atypical antipsychotic effect. Differences in potency in inhibiting 5-HT and NE transport are summarized in Box 12-1. Venlafaxine acts selectively on 5-HT reuptake at therapeutic doses.[42] Venlafaxine has little effect at muscarinic and α-adrenergic receptors (see Table 12-9). Differences between venlafaxine and the SSRIs are only seen at higher doses.

Reboxetine is approximately eight times more potent at blocking NE reuptake than 5-HT reuptake; it blocks other receptors to a minimal degree. It has been called an *NE reuptake inhibitor*[24] even though its selectively (NE versus 5-HT) is relatively low (see Box 12-1 for ranges of selectivity). Side effects include dry mouth, insomnia, blurred vision, sweating, and constipation. Studies of the effect of reboxetine on autonomic function have indicated that it tends to increase heart rate and can also induce a dose-related increase in systolic blood pressure. This drug can also reduce salivary secretion to approximately one half of control.[31] An open-design study found reboxetine useful for reducing sleepiness in narcolepsy.[26] Reboxetine has not been approved for use in the United States by the FDA. A related drug, atomoxetine, has been approved for use in the treatment of attention deficit–hyperactivity disorder. Both drugs are structurally similar to fluoxetine.

Absorption, fate, and excretion

All the second-generation agents are well absorbed from the oral route. Peak concentrations of the drugs are reached in approximately 1 to 3 hours. Amoxapine is almost completely metabolized (one hydroxylated metabolite retains pharmacologic activity) and excreted in the urine over several days. Several active metabolites of trazodone are formed, and 70%

Amoxapine

Maprotiline

Trazodone

Nefazodone

Fig. 12-6 Structural formulas of amoxapine, maprotiline, trazodone, and nefazadone.

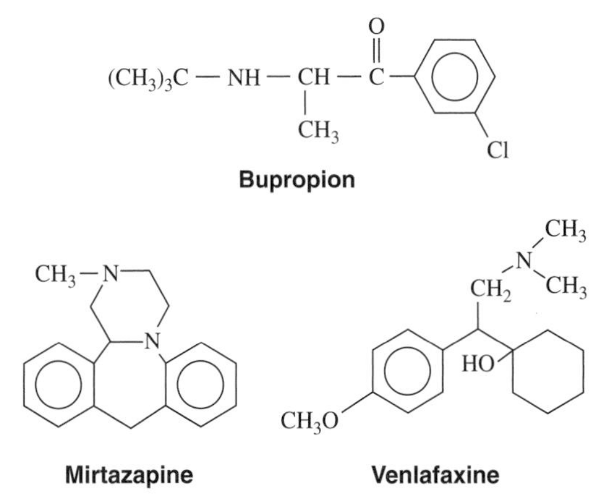

Fig. 12-7 Structural formulas of bupropion, mirtazapine, and venlafaxine

to 75% of an ingested dose is excreted in the urine within 72 hours after administration. The metabolite *m*-chlorophenylpiperazine, a 5-HT_2 agonist, is metabolized by CYP2D6 and is therefore more likely to accumulate if CYP2D6 activity is low or inhibited. Bupropion also yields two active metabolites (including hydroxybupropion) that may accumulate and contribute to antidepressant activity by acting on NE reuptake. Peak action is seen in 3 hours, with a half-life of approximately 21 hours. Bupropion is metabolized by CYP2B6, which may cause the drug to have an important drug interaction profile. Smoking does not alter its kinetics. Nearly 80% of an orally administered dose is excreted as inactive metabolites in the urine. Mirtazapine is metabolized to several metabolites by several P450 isozymes and is primarily excreted in the urine (75%). Venlafaxine is metabolized to an

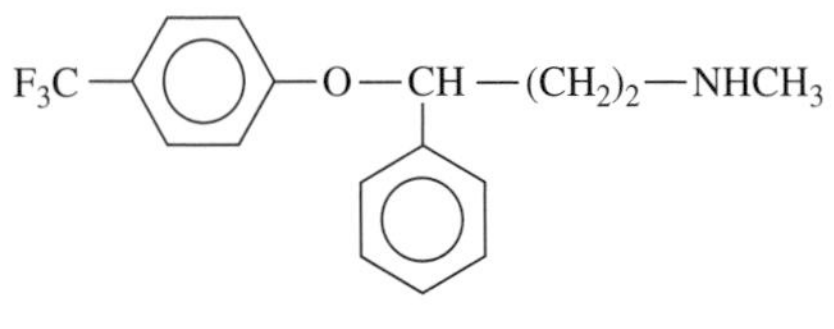

Fluoxetine

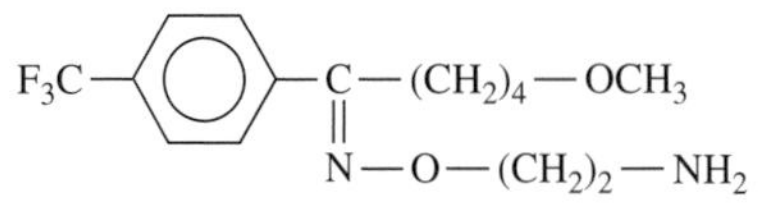

Fluvoxamine

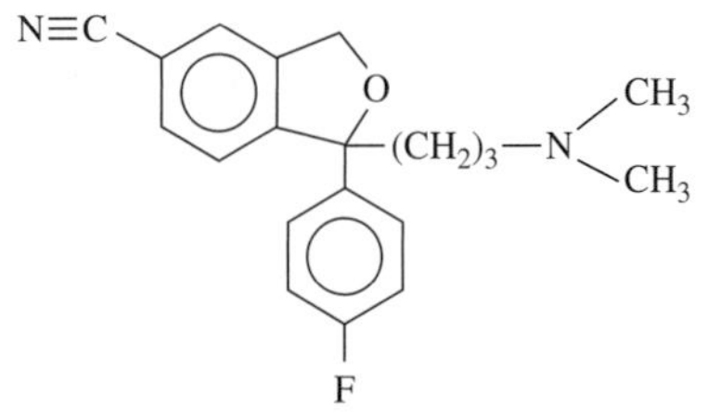

Citalopram

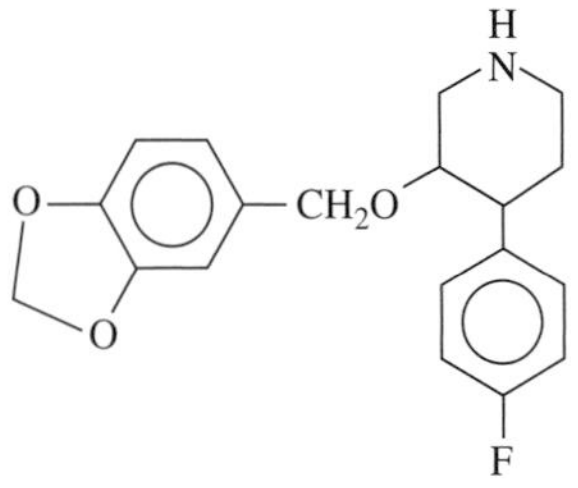

Paroxetine

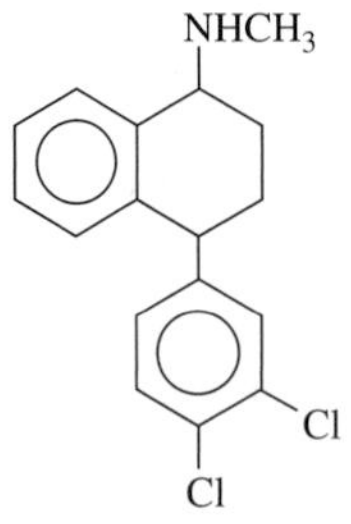

Sertraline

Fig. 12-8 Structural formulas of the SSRIs fluoxetine, fluvoxamine, paroxetine, sertraline, and citalopram.

active metabolite, O-desmethyl venlafaxine, and is eliminated by both renal and hepatic routes. The elimination half-life is approximately 5 hours. The antihistamine diphenhydramine has been found to inhibit the metabolism of venlafaxine.

Adverse effects

Amoxapine, maprotiline, trazodone, mirtazapine, and nefazodone share common side effects such as sedation, antimuscarinic and cardiovascular effects, and skin rashes (see Table 12-9). The incidence and severity of these reactions, however, vary considerably among the drugs. Amoxapine, for instance, is approximately equal to the tricyclics in cardiotoxicity, whereas maprotiline has less effect on the heart and, unlike the TCAs, causes a slight bradycardia and a fall in blood pressure. Bupropion has minimal cardiovascular effects and only infrequently produces orthostatic hypotension. Venlafaxine can cause dose-related hypertensive effects, QT interval prolongation, insomnia, nausea and vomiting, xerostomia, mydriasis, and sexual side effects. It may also increase the likelihood of seizures.

Each of the second- and third-generation agents has some unique side effects that can limit clinical usefulness. Amoxapine, because of its antidopaminergic activity, produces extrapyramidal side effects and can increase prolactin secretion as well as cause amenorrhea, gynecomastia, and galactorrhea. Trazodone sometimes produces persistent priapism requiring surgical detumescence, which can result in permanent impotence. Priapism may be related to α_1- and α_2-adrenergic receptor blockade or 5-HT_{2C} receptor stimulation (by *m*-chlorophenylpiperazine).

Maprotiline and bupropion may trigger seizure activity. Drugs that block the reuptake of catecholamines seem to have a higher incidence of seizures. Bupropion is especially likely to cause convulsions. In fact, bupropion was withdrawn from the market after its initial introduction because of seizures; it was reintroduced at lower recommended doses. Bupropion is contraindicated in patients with epilepsy and in patients who have had bulimia or anorexia nervosa because of an increased risk of seizures in these patients. This drug is marketed (for different purposes) under two trade names, Wellbutrin and Zyban, so patients should not accidentally be given both because of dose-related increased risk for seizures. Other side effects of bupropion include headache and dry mouth, tremor, insomnia, and the possible induction of psychosis. Less commonly it generates rashes or even erythema multiforme (Stevens-Johnson syndrome).

Nefazodone and some of its metabolites are potent inhibitors of CYP3A4. As such, nefazodone is capable of blocking the metabolism of numerous drugs. Mirtazapine has been associated with agranulocytosis and seizures developing in a few patients. It should not be given with MAOIs. Weight gain is a common side effect of antidepressants and, in many instances, contributes to noncompliance (see Table 12-9). Mirtazapine and maprotiline, along with the TCAs doxepin, trimipramine, and amitriptyline, are among the most potent blockers of histamine receptors, producing marked sedation and weight gain. The second- and third-generation antidepressants produce fewer sexual dysfunctional side effects compared with the TCAs or SSRIs.

Levodopa and MAOIs increase bupropion toxicity. Ritonavir, an antiviral agent metabolized by CYP2B6, increases bupropion actions. Also of note is that carbamazepine reduces bupropion blood concentrations.

Selective Serotonin Reuptake Inhibitors

Fluoxetine, fluvoxamine, sertraline, paroxetine, citalopram, and escitalopram (Figure 12-8) are the SSRIs currently approved for use in the United States.

Pharmacologic effects

The selectivity of these drugs for 5-HT provides a theoretical basis for both greater specificity in various depressive states and fewer side effects, and to a significant extent this has been realized clinically. By selectively inhibiting 5-HT reuptake, these drugs cause downregulation of presynaptic inhibitory 5-$HT_{1B/D}$ autoreceptors, which in turn facilitates 5-HT transmission. This leads to postsynaptic changes analogous to those seen with TCAs. As for the TCAs, the SSRIs have also been reported to cause downregulation of central β-adrenergic receptors, but this is not a consistent finding. Nevertheless, it again illustrates the complexity of depression and the pharmacologic similarities of effective antidepressants.

Several serotonergic pathways account for a variety of effects of the SSRIs (see Table 12-8). SSRIs have been found useful for other psychiatric disorders in which 5-HT is thought to play a role, such as obsessive-compulsive disorders, panic disorders, a variety of eating disorders, migraine, social phobia, posttraumatic stress disorder, generalized anxiety disorder, social anxiety disorder, and premenstrual distress disorder.

Absorption, fate, and excretion

The major difference among the SSRIs is their pharmacokinetic profile. The elimination half-life of fluoxetine is approximately 45 hours compared with 26 hours for sertraline, 21 hours for paroxetine, and 14 hours for fluvoxamine. In general these drugs are metabolized by CYP2D6 and CYP3A4 isozymes. Fluoxetine is metabolized to norfluoxetine, an active metabolite with an extended half-life (7 days) that is also an inhibitor of both CYP2D6 and CYP3A4. Paroxetine has active metabolites that contribute to its pharmacologic effect, whereas the metabolites of sertraline and fluvoxamine are inactive. The long half-lives of these compounds, particularly fluoxetine, become clinically relevant when considering drug interactions.

Adverse effects

Compared with the TCAs, the SSRIs have minimal anticholinergic effects and considerably fewer cardiotoxic and hypotensive effects and produce less sedation and less lethality in overdosage. Because they have only mild anticholinergic effects, the SSRIs may be especially useful in the elderly.

Side effects have been categorized as early onset or late onset (Box 12-2). The most prominent early side effect of the SSRIs is gastrointestinal upset (diarrhea, nausea, vomiting); tolerance to this effect develops over a period of 4 to 6 weeks. Patients may also have anxiety, agitation, and sleep disturbances. Tolerance to sleep disturbances may not occur. Late-onset side effects include weight gain, sexual dysfunction (such as anorgasmy and decreased libido), asthenia (weakness), and drug withdrawal symptoms. The intensity of the long-term side effects varies among the SSRIs. Sexual dysfunction is more common with sertraline than fluoxetine.

There have been some reports of dose-related motor side effects, including akathisia, dystonia, dyskinesia, tardive dyskinesia, parkinsonism, and bruxism.[12] $5\text{-HT}_{1\text{-}4}$ receptors are located in the basal ganglia or related structures and may participate in regulating dopamine release. Hyponatremia has been reported in elderly patients, which may reflect the effect of 5-HT on mineralocorticoid function.

Reports of fluoxetine-induced suicidal contemplation have been given widespread coverage in the media, but this problem has never been confirmed in controlled studies. Recently, the FDA has opened an investigation of suicide in patients after additional reports that other SSRIs may increase the risk of adolescent suicide in the absence of antidepressant efficacy. At this time the literature reports similar annual suicide rates in treated and placebo groups (about 0.1% to 0.5%). One reviewer has proposed a possible doubling of risk by SSRIs based on reanalysis of previously performed drug studies. In the absence of better information, efforts at patient education and patient monitoring might help manage this potential risk.

Drug interactions

The potential for a life-threatening drug interaction (5-HT syndrome) exists with the SSRIs and the MAOIs. An interaction of this nature would be particularly problematic clinically when switching from fluoxetine to an MAOI because of the long duration of action of fluoxetine. A number of drug interactions are possible because certain SSRIs compete with other drugs for metabolism by the CYP2D6 or CYP3A4 isozymes. Thus drugs such as cimetidine can interfere with the metabolism of fluoxetine, and fluoxetine can impair the biotransformation of drugs such as propranolol and carbamazepine. Fluoxetine decreases the metabolism of TCAs when used in combination and significantly prolongs their half-life. Increased bleeding has been reported in patients taking warfarin, but this problem is not necessarily associated with inhibition of warfarin metabolism.

Box • 12-2

Side Effects of SSRIs

Early Onset, Transient

Nausea
Anxiety
Agitation
Sleep disturbance/insomnia

Late Onset

Weight gain
Asthenia
Sexual dysfunction
Withdrawal syndrome

St. John's Wort

St. John's wort, a traditional herbal remedy, is helpful for treating mild to moderate depression. In ancient Greece and Rome, St. John's wort *(Hypericum perforatum)* was placed above icons for its mystical powers (*hyper* means above, *eikon* means icon). *St. John* may refer to the flowering time of the plant around June 24, St. John's day. The drug is available as an herbal preparation from health food stores and pharmacies in the United States and outsells fluoxetine in Germany.

St. John's wort has many biologically active components, including hypericin, hyperforin, and some flavinoids.[10] Commercially available capsules contain approximately 3% to 5% hyperforin and 0.3% hypericin. It has only recently been understood that hyperforin may be the most active constituent, so labeling may still refer to hypericin as the active agent.

St. John's wort blocks the reuptake of 5-HT, NE, dopamine, GABA, and glycine with approximately equal potency, a unique therapeutic property. These neurotransmitter symporters use the Na^+ gradient produced by the Na^+, K^+–adenosine triphosphatase pump to transport neurotransmitters into the cell. Once a neurotransmitter is in the cell, proton-dependent antiporters pump it into the synaptic vesicles. Hyperforin may reduce the Na^+ gradient on which the symporters depend, thereby decreasing neurotransmitter uptake.[10]

St. John's wort reaches peak plasma concentrations in approximately 4 hours and has a half-life of approximately 9 hours. There is disagreement as to the relative clinical effectiveness of St. John's wort, despite evidence of an antidepressant action. Commonly noted side effects include gastrointestinal upset, fatigue, dizziness, dry mouth (but less than with other antidepressants), and restlessness. The drug seems to be relatively free of the typical autonomic side effects associated with TCAs. A rare, but possibly dose-related toxicity, is phototoxicity. Cows that eat too much St. John's wort can get severe phototoxic blisters attributed to hypericin. The eye may be susceptible to increased cataract formation because of a related effect.

Drug interactions are of possible concern with St. John's wort and can result from multiple mechanisms. St. John's wort can activate the pregnane X receptor, a member of the steroid/thyroid family of gene promoters that increases CYP3A4 transcription.[10] This induction is thought to be caused by hyperforin. On the other hand, St. John's wort can inhibit certain cytochrome P450 enzymes. Another mechanism for drug interactions is the induction of intestinal P-glycoprotein, which may reduce absorption of other drugs such as cyclosporine and indinavir. Drug interactions may involve other antidepressants that elevate brain biogenic amines. St. John's wort can also block MAO-A and MAO-B, but this is thought to occur only at higher than therapeutic doses. Drug interactions with cyclosporine, oral contraceptives, warfarin, indinavir, digoxin, nefazodone, sertraline, and paroxetine have been reported.

Potential Antidepressants and Antidepressant Potentiators

Benzodiazepines, although not approved for use as antidepressants, are increasingly being prescribed for affective disorders. Alprazolam, a triazolobenzodiazepine marketed as an antianxiety agent, appears to have definite antidepressant properties. It is rather commonly used for the treatment of mild cases of depression and for panic attacks. Clonazepam, an anticonvulsant, is also sometimes used in the treatment of panic attacks (see Chapter 13), and lorazepam, an antianxiety drug, may be effective against mania. The response of panic attacks to benzodiazepines suggests that doses higher than those recommended for anxiety are required. Benzodiazepines are less effective than the TCAs in severely depressed patients. The disinhibitory effect of the benzodiazepines can provoke paradoxic aggression and suicide attempts in some patients.

Buspirone, a partial 5-HT_{1A} agonist and an effective antianxiety agent (see Chapter 13), is being evaluated for the treatment of depression. Other drugs of this class under investigation for relief of depression and anxiety are gepirone and ipsapirone. Clinical trials indicate that gepirone possesses both antianxiety and antidepressant activity.

Ovarian hormones can induce biochemical changes in the brain. Estrogen can alter 5-HT, acetylcholine, and catecholamine function, whereas progesterone may alter function at GABA receptors.[39] These effects can lead to changes in both mood and memory. In some cases, mood disorders in women can be treated with steroidal hormones. In other cases, steroidal hormones may be useful adjuncts that improve the efficacy of traditional antidepressants.[39]

Drugs such as lithium salts, usually associated with the treatment of bipolar disorder, are sometimes used in unipolar depression when conventional therapy is insufficient.

Thyroid replacement therapy may enhance antidepressant therapy in as many as 50% of patients.[21] Thyroid hormone can affect the function of catecholamines. Thyroxine is converted to triiodothyronine in the cells of the LC. In the cortex, triiodothyronine may be released as a cotransmitter with NE.[21]

Many antidepressant drugs are investigational only or have been approved for use outside the United States. These compounds vary in mechanism of action, side effects, and efficacy. The diversity of the chemical structures and pharmacologic activities of antidepressant drugs suggests that clinical depression is caused by a variety of biochemical alterations. Although this implication poses a therapeutic dilemma clinically, it is encouraging that such an impressive array of new and effective antidepressants is being developed and evaluated for therapeutic use. In the long run, these drugs are likely to provide enhanced medical care and a better understanding of the underlying causes of depression.

General Therapeutic Uses

Antidepressants are primarily indicated for the treatment of depression. The clinician is confronted with a variety of treatments but relatively few absolute indicators of which approach is ideal for each patient. Psychotherapy can be provided as initial therapy and is frequently beneficial; however, it usually takes longer than drug treatment to be effective. A combination of drugs and psychotherapy may be more effective than either treatment alone. Drug selection is ideally based on efficacy, side effects, and cost. Patients may be started on an SSRI (fewer side effects) or on a TCA or other antidepressant if some factor favoring its use over an SSRI is identified. If the patient responds, no further adjustment is necessary. If the patient responds partially or not at all, then a different class of drug can be tried. If treatment is still unsatisfactory, combination therapy with antidepressants of different classes may be effective. If all these fail, a trial of electroconvulsive therapy may prove beneficial. Other therapies such as antipsychotic agents, vagal stimulation therapy, and transcranial magnetic stimulation may be tried in extremely resistant cases.

The TCAs are used in the treatment of chronic pain, which is a common codiagnosis in the depressed patient. Although analgesia may result from their antidepressant effect, a direct analgesic action is suggested by the fact that analgesia can be obtained in patients free of depressive illness and at lower doses than those required for relief of depression. Common types of chronic pain syndromes possibly amenable to the TCAs include headache, diabetic neuropathy, neuralgias, postherpetic neuralgia, arthritis, and atypical facial pain (see below). TCAs should be used with special caution in the elderly because of the possible exacerbation of cardiovascular disease. In patients older than 50 years, initial doses should be one third of the normal recommended dose, with increases made gradually over a 7- to 14-day period.

The FDA recognizes additional indications for several of these agents. Amitriptyline is indicated for delusions, doxepin for alcoholism, and desipramine for attention deficit–hyperactivity disorder. Imipramine may be prescribed for the management of nocturnal enuresis in older children and incontinence in adults. Although effective, no mechanism has yet been demonstrated for these indications[20]; however, their clinical efficacy is greater than that of anticholinergic agents.

Second- and third-generation antidepressants may have advantages in some patients. Trazodone, because of its sedative property, is useful in agitated depression and in depressed patients who have insomnia. Trazodone, nefazodone, and bupropion may also be of special use in the elderly because these drugs have mild cardiovascular and anticholinergic side effects. However, trazodone has been associated with ventricular dysrhythmias in some patients with cardiac disease. Most second- and third-generation antidepressants produce less sexual dysfunction than do the SSRIs. Nefazodone is indicated for panic disorder and posttraumatic stress disorder. Amoxapine may have special use in psychotic depression, where its activity as a dopamine antagonist may prove beneficial.

Bupropion, like the SSRIs, has very low potential for causing sedation and is therefore useful when daytime alertness is desired. Bupropion is used for smoking cessation[19] and may be successful in up to 44% of patients. (Nicotine formulations are also used for smoking cessation, whereas clonidine and nortriptyline are second-line treatments.) Bupropion is available in regular and extended-release dosage forms and is effective in doses from 200 to 450 mg/day in divided doses. Treatment is usually continued for 7 to 12 weeks. Other uses for bupropion include attention deficit–hyperactivity disorder and posttraumatic stress disorder.

The MAOIs may be particularly effective in the treatment of atypical affective disorders (e.g., depression with hysteria), panic attacks, depression coupled with somatic anxiety, and patients whose conditions are refractory to the other antidepressants. They have, however, been largely replaced by safer, more effective drugs. Moclobemide, a reversible MAO-A–selective drug, produces fewer side effects than the older MAOIs.

The SSRIs are currently the most commonly prescribed antidepressants. Clinical trials and case reports also suggest that these drugs may be useful in the treatment of obsessive-compulsive disorders (the FDA has approved fluoxetine and paroxetine), bulimia (fluoxetine), panic disorders (paroxetine and sertraline), social phobia (paroxetine), and poststroke depression (citalopram). Posttraumatic stress disorder may also be an indication. To date, these drugs have been found to be effective antidepressants while producing fewer side effects than previous agents. Depression associated with other medical illness or surgery is not uncommon. This depression may contribute to adverse treatment responses. The SSRIs are effective for treatment of depression in patients with myocardial infarction, diabetes, and Parkinson's disease.

SSRIs are generally less effective in chronic pain syndromes than are drugs that block both NE and 5-HT uptake, although SSRIs may be effective in diabetic neuropathy (citalopram) and migraine pain (paroxetine).

As with the antipsychotics, antidepressants must be administered over a long period and are often continued for several weeks after clinical remission to guard against relapse. Several weeks to 2 months of continuous drug administration are usually necessary before therapeutic effects are noted. This slow onset in effect may be related to alterations in brain neurochemistry or receptors. Drug treatment should continue for at least 6 months. If the patient has had more than one previous depressive episode, treatment should be continued for at least 2 years, and in some cases indefinitely. Although it has been claimed that some of the newer agents have a more rapid onset of action than the TCAs, this assertion has yet to be consistently confirmed in clinical studies. Like other antidepressants, SSRIs may precipitate mania, especially in the bipolar patient.

Implications for Dentistry]

Untreated depression has been correlated with a number of intraoral changes that may predispose the depressed patient to dental or oral disease. Some of the factors involved include reduced salivary flow, preference for carbohydrates (possibly because of decreased brain 5-HT), higher oral lactobacillus counts, and decreased motivation and interest in oral health maintenance.[15] Depressed patients may be more likely to have periodontitis. Chronic facial pain, burning sensations in the mouth, and temporomandibular joint disorders may be associated with depression.

All the drugs used to treat depression have been reported to produce varying degrees of xerostomia and may increase the likelihood for dental caries. Estimates of degree of dry mouth vary widely in the literature for the same drug. The reasons for this variability may include differences in dosage, duration of therapy, and underlying physical status among patients. Although antimuscarinic action has been a principal explanation for dry mouth, other drug actions may also contribute. Thus changes in salivary function can reflect actions of drugs on the salivary glands, the cardiovascular system, immune function, or the CNS centers controlling these functions. The relative likelihood of xerostomia is much greater with the TCAs than with the other antidepressants. Other common oral side effects of antidepressants include altered taste sensation, stomatitis, and glossitis.[15]

Tricyclic antidepressants

The anticholinergic side effects of the TCAs have important dental implications. Reduced salivary flow increases the risk of dental caries, oral candidiasis, and oral functional abnormalities.[44] Three quarters of patients taking imipramine may report dry mouth compared with one third of patients taking the SSRI sertraline.

Anticholinergic agents should not be administered with the TCAs because additive effects can result in toxic reactions (confusion, agitation, hyperthermia, tachycardia, urinary retention). The use of antianxiety agents, barbiturates, and other sedatives should be carefully controlled in patients receiving TCAs because of additive depressant effects on the CNS. The duration of action of barbiturates may be prolonged by the TCAs, but the long-term use of barbiturates can reduce half-lives of the TCAs by microsomal enzyme induction. Propoxyphene, which has been reported to interfere with several P450 isozymes, may inhibit the metabolism of TCAs and increase their half-lives.

Like the antipsychotic agents, the risk of long QT syndrome and *torsades de pointes* is increased by many antidepressants so adding other agents that increase this risk should be avoided. These include several of the macrolide (erythromycin, clarithromycin) and fluoroquinolone (moxifloxacin, gatifloxacin) antibiotics, imidazole antifungal agents (ketoconazole, itraconazole), antihistamines, and cholinergic agonists.

Because of the cardiotoxic effects of the TCAs and their potentiation of adrenergic drugs, high doses or accidental intravascular injection of local anesthetic solutions may precipitate arrhythmias and hypertension. The use of TCAs, however, is not a contraindication for the use of epinephrine with local anesthetics as long as care is taken not to inject the vasoconstrictor intravenously or in large doses.

Abrupt termination of an antidepressant may lead to withdrawal symptoms. Such patients may exhibit hypersensitivity to touch and pain and may have paresthesias, headache, and muscle spasms.

Monoamine oxidase inhibitors

Various drug interactions involve MAOIs, particularly the irreversible nonselective type. Perhaps those most relevant for the practicing dentist may be the prolongation and enhancement of the CNS effects of the opioid analgesics, barbiturates, and other CNS depressants. MAOIs given in conjunction with meperidine cause potentially fatal reactions, including hyperthermia, excitement, and seizures, in addition to reactions that resemble an opioid overdose. This interaction requires that meperidine not be used concurrently with the MAOIs or for several weeks after therapy with MAOIs has ceased. Other opioids, which are not similar chemically to meperidine, may be used with caution.

Hypotension can develop with the concomitant use of general anesthetics and MAOIs. It is prudent to discontinue the use of MAOIs for 2 weeks before surgery. Neither epinephrine nor levonordefrin is potentiated by inhibition of MAO activity.

Second- and third-generation antidepressants

Although these generations of antidepressants may have fewer side effects than the TCAs, their anticholinergic and sedative properties should be kept in mind.[15] Bupropion is exceptional in that central stimulation is more likely than sedation. This side effect may aggravate the condition of an already nervous patient. The drug is reported to produce dry mouth in approximately 25% of patients who use it, including patients in smoking cessation programs. The dentist should recognize that bupropion, although generally safe, occasionally can produce severe reactions such as seizures or severe reactions such as Stevens-Johnson syndrome. The drug should be avoided in patients who pose a risk for these reactions. Long-term success rates in smoking cessation programs, even with pharmacotherapy, are low.

Amoxapine can cause extrapyramidal side effects that can affect prosthodontic care. Drug interactions involving amoxapine and maprotiline are similar to those involving the first-generation TCAs. Mirtazapine has some potential for drug interactions. Because of its ability to block H_1 histamine receptors, it tends to be sedating and could produce additive sedative effects with other CNS depressants.

Selective serotonin reuptake inhibitors

The high incidence of gastrointestinal disturbances, particularly nausea and vomiting, during initial treatment with the SSRIs can pose clinical problems. Postponement of clinical procedures to a later date may be advisable because tolerance develops to these side effects. Fluoxetine (or its metabolite norfluoxetine) prolongs the duration of action of certain benzodiazepines, probably by decreasing their metabolism. This inhibition may lead to protracted sedation, especially in light of the long half-lives of fluoxetine and its active metabolite. The interaction is most pronounced with benzodiazepines (alprazolam, midazolam, and triazolam) that are metabolized by CYP3A4-catalyzed α hydroxylation on the triazolo ring of these drugs.

Atypical facial pain

Amitriptyline and other antidepressants are among the more commonly used drugs for facial pain, including atypical facial pain and facial arthromyalgia (Costen's syndrome and temporomandibular joint dysfunction syndrome). Drug responses vary from patient to patient. Although effective doses are somewhat lower than those required for the treatment of depression, the same delayed onset to effect (several weeks) has been reported. Similar results have been obtained with dothiepin, an investigational thio derivative of amitriptyline. Dothiepin may have analgesic efficacy for treating idiopathic fibromyalgia, rheumatoid arthritis, and atypical facial pain.

ANTIMANICS

Manic disorder or bipolar disorder presents as a unique diagnostic condition. A genetic component is suspected. Numerous biochemical pathways appear to be altered in manic or bipolar patients, both in the brain and blood elements. Elevated concentrations of Ca^{++} have been observed in brain cells, platelets, and lymphocytes. Brain mitochondrial function and intracellular pH are decreased, choline/creatine-phosphocreatine ratios are higher than normal, and phosphocreatine and N-acetylaspartate concentrations are decreased in specific brain regions. These results indicate possible neuronal damage and impaired function. Abnormalities on several chromosomes are suspected, and there is an increased maternal transmission rate with several mutations of mitochondrial DNA associated with increased risk of the disorder.

Lithium salts are important for treating mania, but Li^+ alone may be inadequate treatment for half of patients exhibiting bipolar disorder.[35] In addition to lif's antimanic effects, evidence suggests lif may also exert neuroprotective actions that may be prophylactic in unipolar and bipolar disorders and possibly in neural degenerative disorders such as Alzheimer's disease.[32] Other agents can be used to control manic patients temporarily while Li^+ therapy is being instituted and to treat individuals for whom Li^+ alone proves ineffective. Antipsychotic drugs, both typical and atypical types, are used in 85% of patients during initiation of therapy.[43] Interest has been directed toward the use of established anticonvulsants (valproate and carbamazepine), several new anticonvulsants,[35] omega-3 fatty acids,[40] Ca^{++}-channel blockers, thyroid-stimulating hormone, and thyroid hormone as adjunctive agents in the treatment of bipolar disorder. Ultimately, a variety of drugs is available if needed.

Lithium Salts

Li^+ was observed to be effective for mania by Cade (1949) but was not generally embraced until the late 1960s.

Pharmacologic effects

The mechanism of action of Li^+ is not established. Many changes resulting from Li^+ administration have been documented. These include effects on plasma membrane cation channels, plasma membrane ion pumps, and exchange systems, as well as positive and negative effects on neuronal release of various neurotransmitters.

Although the mechanism of action of Li^+ remains unresolved, two effects of Li^+ offer likely explanations for the therapeutic and possibly adverse effects (Figure 12-9). The first is the inhibitory effect of the ion on phosphomonoesterases involved in inositol signaling pathways. Li^+ inhibits phosphoinositide metabolism by inhibiting inositol monophosphatase, the enzyme responsible for converting inositol monophosphate to inositol. Li^+ also inhibits inositol polyphosphate-1-phosphatase, which catalyzes the 1-dephosphorylation of certain inositol bis- and polyphosphates. Li^+ might therefore inhibit the effect of neurotransmitters that use signaling pathways involving inositol trisphosphate. The effect of inhibiting this pathway could be the depletion of inositol, which in turn would deplete phosphatidylinositol bisphosphate. This effect would reduce signaling through receptors whose signaling involves the use of phosphatidylinositol bisphosphate as a substrate for the formation of inositol trisphosphate and diacylglycerol.

A second effect that may play an important role in the action of Li^+ is inhibition of glycogen synthase kinase-3β (GSK-3β). This inhibition can affect at least two intracellular signaling cascades: activation of β-catenin and increased glycogen synthesis.[1,32] By inhibiting GSK-3β, Li^+ acts like the endogenous inhibitor of GSK-3β, which stimulates cell receptors linked to GSK-3β (see Figure 12-9). This results in changes in cell-cell interaction, axonal remodeling, and signaling in neurons. By inhibiting GSK-3β, Li^+ also acts like insulin, which stimulates glycogen synthesis (GSK-3β inhibits glycogen synthase).[32]

Clinically, Li^+ alleviates the manifestations of mania over a course of 1 to 2 weeks. Sleep and appetite disturbances abate, and swings in mood are prevented. Li^+ has little effect on mood in patients who do not have mania. Li^+ may provide a prophylactic action against future manic attacks. Patients who stop taking Li^+ may not respond as well to subsequent Li^+ treatment trials, possibly because of progression of the neurodegenerative process.

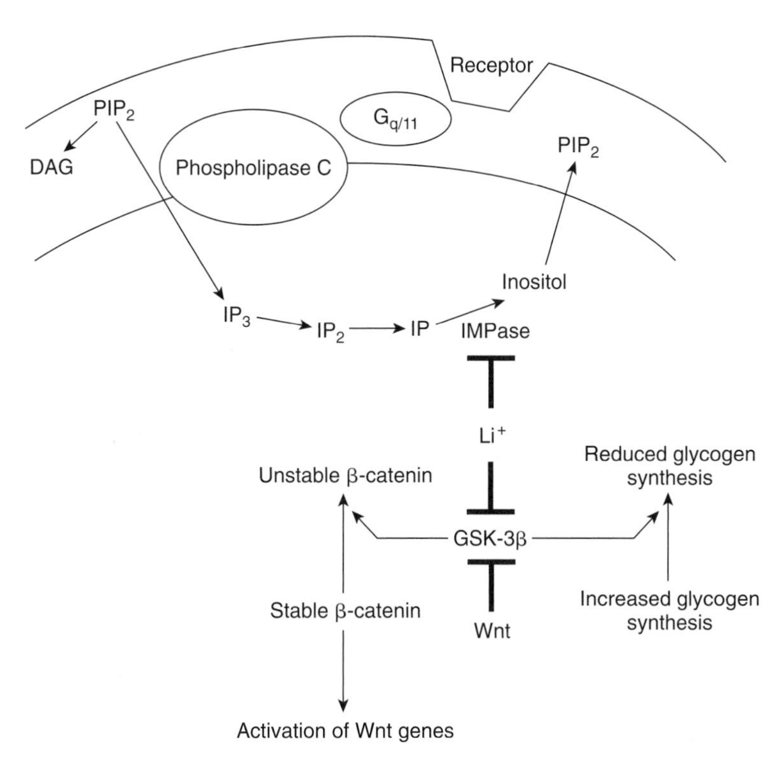

Fig. 12-9 Two mechanisms by which Li^+ may mediate its pharmacologic effects. Li^+ inhibits both inositol monophosphatase *(IMPase)* and glycogen synthase kinase-3β (*GSK-3β*). By the first mechanism, Li^+ inhibits signaling through the inositol pathway by depleting phosphatidylinositol bisphosphate *(PIP_2)*. The result of this depletion is the inability to produce sufficient inositol-1,4,5 trisphosphate *(IP_3)*. By the second mechanism, Li^+ stabilizes β-catenin, leading to changes in neuronal function such as receptor signaling and remodeling. In addition, glycogen synthesis is promoted by Li^+. *Wnt,* A glycoprotein that inhibits GSK-3β; *DAG,* diacylglycerol; *IP,* inositol monophosphate; *IP_2,* inositol bisphosphate.

Li^+ does not have anticonvulsant actions. In fact, when a lithium salt is given in combination with pilocarpine, a severe form of continuous seizures can occur.[18]

Absorption, fate, and excretion

Li^+ is readily absorbed from the gastrointestinal tract. The cation eventually equilibrates throughout the total body water; no particular affinity for the brain or a specific organ has been detected. Excretion of Li^+ is primarily through the kidney, and reduced kidney function is associated with greater Li^+ toxicity if blood concentrations are not carefully monitored.

Adverse effects

Some of the most common side effects of lithium salts (gastrointestinal irritation, fine hand tremor, muscular weakness, polyuria, thirst, sleepiness, and a sluggish feeling) are often associated with initial therapy and usually fade within 1 to 2 weeks. Thirst, polyuria, and hand tremor may occasionally continue for several months or even years. Severe intoxication results in vomiting, diarrhea, unconsciousness, and convulsions. Most adverse effects of Li^+ have been found to correlate very closely with serum Li^+ concentrations. The therapeutic index for Li^+ is low, and plasma titers of Li^+ must be carefully monitored to ensure therapeutic effectiveness and avoid toxicity.

Li^+ inhibits the renal response to antidiuretic hormone and may cause nephrogenic diabetes insipidus. This is the basis for the thirst and polyuria associated with the drug. Renal effects are usually moderate and reversible. Thiazides and other diuretics reduce renal excretion of Li^+. Dosages of Li^+ therefore may need to be reduced during concurrent therapy with a diuretic. Na^+ depletion leads to reduced excretion of Li^+ and a higher risk of toxicity. Therefore any situation, such as a Na^+-restricted diet or sweating, that tends to reduce the Na^+ load may increase Li^+ toxicity. Patients must be warned not to begin a Na^+-restricted diet without medical surveillance. Cardiovascular disease, renal disease, or severe dehydration can also increase the risk of toxicity from Li^+.

Li^+ may cause hypotension and cardiac arrhythmias. If Li^+ produces electrocardiographic changes, the changes are not usually significant if concentrations remain in the therapeutic range. Li^+ can also induce hypothyroidism in as many as 20% to 40% of patients.[25] This can be managed with thyroid replacement therapy. In some cases of Li^+-resistant mania, increasing thyroxin concentrations to 150% of normal may overcome the resistance. With continued Li^+ therapy, approximately 4% of patients develop diffuse, nontoxic goiters. Patients may have elevated plasma Ca^{++}, which may be related to increased renal Ca^{++} reabsorption. Li^+, however, inhibits the effect of parathyroid hormone on osteoclasts, and parathyroid hormone levels may increase. Li^+ may cause a number of dermatologic side effects and alopecia.

Teratogenic effects, such as cleft palate and deformities of the ear and eye, as well as cardiac defects are associated with Li^+ administration during the first trimester of pregnancy.

Simple and convenient methods for measuring Li^+ have been sought that do not involve taking blood samples. One such method has been the use of salivary measurements to predict serum concentrations. Li^+ concentrations in saliva are higher than those in the plasma because the ion is actively secreted into saliva. Although the saliva/plasma Li^+ ratio varies considerably from patient to patient, within a single patient its variability is low. Thus there is some promise that saliva sampling may be of benefit in Li^+ monitoring.

General therapeutic uses

Lithium salts are used for the treatment of mania and as chronic treatment of manic-depressive illness. Initial high (therapeutic) doses are often adjusted downward to maintenance levels, which may partially explain the initial feelings of tiredness. Even so, the delay of onset is such that 7 to 10 days are required before the antimanic effects are noted, and a short course of antipsychotic medication is normally required in cases of fully developed mania. Frequent measurements of Li^+ are required to maintain proper plasma concentrations and are particularly important as a guard against toxicity.

Implications for dentistry

Patients with bipolar disease may have substantial dental pathology. These patients have a greater risk for poor oral hygiene, accumulations of supragingival and subgingival calculus, extensive dental caries, and numerous missing teeth.[14,15] Hyposalivation from the disease is common (approximately 71%), which may be associated with dental caries.

Nonsteroidal antiinflammatory analgesics may decrease the renal excretion of Li^+ and lead to toxic plasma concentrations after several days of combined therapy. Although drugs such as piroxicam and indomethacin most readily cause this drug interaction, it is most likely to occur with formulations of ibuprofen, naproxen, and related drugs that are available over the counter and likely to be taken without professional supervision. Interestingly, aspirin and sulindac do not seem to potentiate Li^+ toxicity. The combination of Li^+ and pilocarpine must be avoided because of the risk of seizures.

Patients taking Li^+ frequently have a metallic taste that can alter the palatability of food. Most patients taking Li^+ have salivary gland dysfunction and a resultant decrease in salivary flow.[29] Polydipsia is common because of Li^+-induced diuresis and xerostomia. In early phases of Li^+ therapy, facial spasm and transient facial paralysis, especially of the lower jaw, have occurred. On the other hand, facial pains associated with cluster headaches may respond to treatment with Li^+.

Other Antimania Drugs

Approximately 50% of patients who have mania do not respond to Li^+. Characteristics common to many Li^+-refractory patients include severe mania mixed with either psychotic episodes or anxiety and a history of rapid cycling. Antipsychotic agents are frequently used to help control the florid excitation and delusions early in treatment and the atypical antipsychotic olanzapine has recently been approved for this use. Carbamazepine, an anticonvulsant discussed in Chapter 14, may be effective in some refractory cases. Carbamazepine has been reserved for those who do not respond to conventional therapy. Surprisingly, patients who seem to respond most favorably to carbamazepine are those who have severe forms of the disease. A Li^+/carbamazepine combination is sometimes effective in patients who are refractory to either drug alone. Carbamazepine may also be effective as a prophylactic agent. Valproic acid is another anticonvulsant that finds clinical usefulness for the treatment of mania refractory to Li^+ and carbamazepine.

Newer anticonvulsant medications such as lamotrigine, gabapentin, and topiramate are being evaluated as adjuncts and have been called *mood stabilizers* when used in this context.[23] The benzodiazepines clonazepam and lorazepam, when used in combination with haloperidol, are helpful in calming the severely manic patient until Li^+ administration achieves a therapeutic concentration. This combination often permits adequate control without excessive doses of either the antipsychotic or the benzodiazepine. Ca^{++}-channel blockers such as verapamil have proved helpful in some cases of Li^+-refractory mania, but more studies are required to assess their overall usefulness. Like Li^+, verapamil is not a depressant and therefore is of little use for the initial treatment of the severely manic patient. Consistent with the monoamine hypothesis of affective disorders, clonidine, an α_2-adrenergic receptor agonist that decreases NE release, may be an effective antimania drug in some cases. Omega-3 fatty acid treatment of bipolar disorder is under study.[40]

Antipsychotic Drugs

Nonproprietary (generic) name	*Proprietary (trade) name*
Phenothiazines	
Acetophenazine*	Tindal
Chlorpromazine	Thorazine
Fluphenazine	Prolixin
Mesoridazine	Serentil
Perphenazine	Trilafon
Prochlorperazine	Compazine
Promazine*	Sparine
Thioridazine	Mellaril
Trifluoperazine	Stelazine
Triflupromazine*	Vesprin
Thioxanthenes	
Chlorprothixene*	Taractan
Thiothixene	Navane
Butyrophenone	
Haloperidol	Haldol
Dibenzoxazepine	
Loxapine	Loxitane
Diphenylbutylpiperidine	
Pimozide	Orap
Dibenzodiazepine	
Clozapine	Clozaril
Benzisoxazole	
Risperidone	Risperdal
Thienobenzodiazepine	
Olanzapine	Zyprexa
Dihydroindolones	
Ziprasidone	Zeldox
Molindone	Moban
Dibenzothiazepine	
Quetiapine	Seroquel
Dihydrocarbostyril	
Aripiprazole	Abilify

Antidepressant Drugs—cont'd

Nonproprietary (generic) name	*Proprietary (trade) name*
Tricyclics	
Amitriptyline	Elavil, Endep
Clomipramine	Anafranil
Desipramine	Norpramin
Doxepin	Adapin, Sinequan
Dothiepin*	Prothiaden
Imipramine	Tofranil
Nortriptyline	Aventyl, Pamelor
Protriptyline	Vivactil
Trimipramine	Surmontil
MAO inhibitors	
Phenelzine	Nardil
Isocarboxazid	Marplan
Tranylcypromine	Parnate
Second- and third-generation	
Amoxapine†	Asendin
Maprotiline	Ludiomil
Trazodone	Desyrel
Nefazodone	Serzone
Bupropion	Wellbutrin, Zyban
Mirtazapine	Remeron
Reboxetine*	Vestra
SSRIs	
Fluoxetine	Prozac
Fluvoxamine	Luvox
Paroxetine	Paxil
Sertraline	Zoloft
Citalopram	Celexa
Escitalopram	Lexapro
Venlafaxine‡	Effexor
Antimanics	
Carbamazepine	Tegretol
Lithium carbonate	Eskalith, Lithobid
Lithium citrate	Cibalith-S
Valproic acid (and derivatives)	Depakene, Depakote

*Not currently available in the United States.
†Amoxapine is listed separately from the other tricyclics because it is a second-generation or atypical antidepressant.
‡Not classified as an SSRI but is selective for 5-HT transport at therapeutic doses.

Cited References

1. Ackenheil M: Neurotransmitters and signal transduction processes in bipolar affective disorders: a synopsis, *J Affect Disord* 62:101-111, 2001.
2. Aghajanian GK, Marek GJ: Serotonin model of schizophrenia: emerging role of glutamate mechanisms, *Brain Res Rev* 31:302-312, 2000.
3. Akiskal HS, Bourgeois ML, Angst J, et al: Re-evaluating the prevalence of and diagnostic composition within the broad clinical spectrum of bipolar disorders, *J Affect Disord* 59(suppl 1):S5-S30, 2000.
4. Andreasen NC: Schizophrenia: the fundamental questions, *Brain Res Rev* 31:106-112, 2000.
5. Artigas F, Celada P, Laruelle M, et al: How does pindolol improve antidepressant action? *Trends Pharmacol Sci* 22:224-228, 2001.
6. Blier P: Possible neurobiological mechanism underlying faster onset of antidepressant action, *J Clin Psychiatry* 62(suppl 4):7-11, 2001.
7. Cade JFJ: Lif salts in the treatment of psychotic excitement, *Med J Aust* 2:349-352, 1949.
8. Casey DE, Zorn SH: The pharmacology of weight gain with antipsychotics, *J Clin Psychiatry* 62(suppl 7):4-10, 2000.
9. Charney DS: Monoamine dysfunction and the pathophysiology and treatment of depression, *J Clin Psychiatry* 59(suppl 14):11-14, 1998.
10. Di Carlo G, Borrelli F, Ernst E, et al: St John's wort: Prozac from the plant kingdom, *Trends Pharmacol Sci* 22:292-297, 2001.
11. *Diagnostic and statistical manual of mental disorders*, ed 4 (DSM-IV), Washington, DC, 1994, American Psychiatric Association.
12. Ellison JM, Stanziani P: SSRI-associated nocturnal bruxism in four patients, *J Clin Psychiatry* 54:432-434, 1993.
13. Flockhart DA: *Cytochrome P450 drug interaction table*, Indiana University, Department of Medicine, Division of Clinical Medicine, http://medicine.iupui.edu/flockhart/table.htm, accessed October 31, 2003.
14. Friedlander AH, Birch NJ: Dental conditions in patients with bipolar disorder on long-term lif maintenance therapy, *Spec Care Dentist* 10:148-151, 1990.
15. Friedlander AH, Mahler ME: Major depressive disorder. Psychopathology, medical management and dental implications, *J Am Dent Assoc* 132:629-638, 2001.
16. Glassman AH: Cardiovascular effects of antidepressant drugs: updated, *Int Clin Psychopharmacol* 13(suppl 5):S25-S30, 1998.
17. Haller E, Binder RL: Clozapine and seizures, *Am J Psychiatry* 147:1069-1071, 1990.
18. Honchar MP, Olney JW, Sherman WR: Systemic cholinergic agents induce seizures and brain damage in lif-treated rats, *Science* 220:323-325, 1983.
19. Hughes JR, Stead LF, Lancaster T: Antidepressants for smoking cessation (Cochrane Review), In *Cochrane Library*, ed 2, 2001, Oxford.
20. Hunsballe JM, Djurhuus JC: Clinical options for imipramine in the management of urinary incontinence, *Urol Res* 29:118-125, 2001.
21. Joffe RT, Sokolov ST: Thyroid hormone treatment in primary unipolar depression: a review, *Int J Neuropsychopharmacol* 3:143-147, 2000.
22. Kapur S, Zipursky RB, Remington G, et al: 5-HT_2 and D_2 receptor occupancy of olanzapine in schizophrenia: a PET investigation, *Am J Psychiatry* 155:921-928, 1998.
23. Keck PE, Jr, Mendlwicz J, Calabrese JR, et al: A review of randomized, controlled clinical trials in acute mania, *J Affect Disord* 59(suppl 1):S31-S37, 2000.
24. Kent JM: SNaRIs, NaSSAs, and NaRIs: new agents for the treatment of depression, *Lancet* 355:911-918, 2000.
25. Kusalic M, Engelsmann F: Effect of lif maintenance therapy on thyroid and parathyroid function, *J Psychiatr Neurosci* 24:227-233, 1999.

26. Larrosa O, de la Llave Y, Bario S, et al: Stimulant and anticataleptic effects of reboxetine in patients with narcolepsy: a pilot study, *Sleep* 24:282-285, 2001.
27. Lesch KP: Serotonergic gene expression and depression: implications for developing novel antidepressants, *J Affect Disord* 62:57-76, 2001.
28. Lieberman JA, Kane JM, Johns CA: Clozapine: guidelines for clinical management, *J Clin Psychiatry* 50:329-338, 1989.
29. Markitziu A, Shani J, Avni J: Salivary gland function in patients on chronic lif treatment, *Oral Surg Oral Med Oral Pathol* 66:551-557, 1988.
30. *Mental health: a report of the Surgeon General*, US Public Health Service, http://www.surgeongeneral.gov/library/mentalhealth/home.html, 1999.
31. Penttila J, Syvalahti E, Hinkka S, et al: The effects of amitriptyline, citalopram and reboxetine on autonomic nervous system. A randomized placebo-controlled study on healthy volunteers, *Psychopharmacology* (Berlin) 154:343-349, 2001.
32. Phiel CJ, Klein PS: Molecular targets of lif action, *Ann Rev Pharmacol Toxicol* 41:789-813, 2001.
33. Pineyro G, Blier P: Autoregulation of serotonin neurons: role in antidepressant drug actions, *Pharmacol Rev* 51:533-591, 1999.
34. Pisani F, Spina E, Oteri G: Antidepressant drugs and seizure susceptibility: from in vitro data to clinical practice, *Epilepsia* 40(suppl 10):S48-S56, 1999.
35. Post RM, Frye MA, Denicoff KD, et al: Emerging trends in the treatment of rapid cycling bipolar disorder: a selected review, *Bipolar Disord* 2:305-315, 2000.
36. Prior TI, Chue PS, Tibbo P, et al: Drug metabolism of atypical antipsychotics, *Eur Neuropsychopharmacol* 9:301-309, 1999.
37. Rogers DP, Shramko JK: Therapeutic options in the treatment of clozapine-induced sialorrhea, *Pharmacotherapy* 20:1092-1095, 2000.
38. Sekine Y, Rikihisa T, Ogata H, et al: Correlations between in vitro affinity of antipsychotics to various central neurotransmitter receptors and clinical incidence of their adverse drug reactions, *Eur J Clin Pharmacol* 55:583-587, 1999.
39. Stahl SM: Basic psychopharmacology of antidepressants, part 2: estrogen as an adjunct to antidepressant treatment, *J Clin Psychiatry* 59(suppl 4):15-24, 1998.
40. Stoll AL, Severus WE, Freeman MP, et al: Omega 3 fatty acids in bipolar disorder: a preliminary double-blind, placebo-controlled trial, *Arch Gen Psychiatry* 56:407-412, 1999.
41. Tarsy D: Tardive dyskinesia, *Curr Treat Options Neurol* 2:205-214, 2000.
42. Tatsumi M, Groshan K, Blakely RD, et al: Pharmacological profile of antidepressants and related compounds at human monoamine transporters, *Eur J Pharmacol* 340:249-258, 1997.
43. Tohen M, Zhang F, Taylor CC, et al: A meta-analysis of the use of typical antipsychotic agents in bipolar disorder, *J Affect Disord* 65:85-93, 2001.
44. Valdez IH, Fox PC: Diagnosis and management of salivary dysfunction, *Crit Rev Oral Biol Med* 4:271-277, 1993.

General References

Bloom FE, Kupfer DJ, eds: *Psychopharmacology: the fourth generation of progress*, New York, 1995, Raven Press.

Buckley PF: New dimensions in the pharmacologic treatment of schizophrenia and related psychoses, *J Clin Pharmacol* 37:363-378, 1997.

Drugs for psychiatric disorders, *Med Lett Drugs Ther* 39:33-40, 1997.

Frazer A: Pharmacology of antidepressants, *J Clin Psychopharmacol* 17(suppl 1):2S-18S, 1997.

Hales RE, Yudofsky SC, eds: *The American Psychiatric Publishing textbook of clinical psychiatry*, ed 4, Washington, DC, 2003, American Psychiatric Publishing.

Holsboer F: Stress, hypercortisolism and corticosteroid receptors in depression: implications for therapy, *J Affect Disord* 62:77-91, 2001.

McDaniel KD: Clinical pharmacology of monoamine oxidase inhibitors, *Clin Neuropharmacol* 9:207-234, 1986.

Richelson E: Pharmacology of antidepressants, *Mayo Clin Proc* 76:511-527, 2001.

Schatzberg AF, Nemeroff CB, eds: *The American Psychiatric Publishing textbook of psychopharmacology*, Washington, DC, 2004, ed 3, American Psychiatric Publishing.

Whooley MA, Simon GE: Managing depression in medical outpatients, *New Engl J Med* 343:1942-1950, 2000.

CHAPTER • 13

Sedative-Hypnotics, Antianxiety Drugs, and Centrally Acting Muscle Relaxants*

Paul A. Moore

The drugs discussed in this chapter have the common pharmacologic characteristic of being central nervous system (CNS) depressants and are capable of inducing a variety of clinical responses. These responses include anxiety relief, sedative-hypnotic effects, and centrally acting muscle relaxation. Although all such drugs induce CNS impairment, drugs in certain categories have some degree of selectivity that determines their therapeutic indications in medical and dental practice. However, the ability of these agents to selectively induce sedation, hypnosis, anxiolysis, or muscle relaxation is limited, and significant overlap in the clinical indications for these drugs occurs. Pharmacokinetic differences as well as differences in mechanisms of action often distinguish these agents. The multiple actions and uses of these agents are also apparent in other chapters of this text that address the anticonvulsants (see Chapter 14), the general anesthetic agents (see Chapter 18), and the antihistamines (see Chapter 22).

The drugs discussed in this chapter can be viewed as having dose-dependent CNS-depressing effects progressing through anxiolysis, sedation, hypnosis, anesthesia, and ultimately death if the dose is sufficiently high. As anxiolytics, these drugs reduce the anxiety response; as sedatives, they produce relaxation, calmness, and decreased motor activity without loss of consciousness. As hypnotics, they induce drowsiness and a depressed state of consciousness that resembles natural sleep, with decreased motor activity and impaired sensory responsiveness. As anesthetics, these drugs cause a state of unconsciousness from which the patient is unable to be aroused. Not all sedative-hypnotics are readily capable of inducing anesthesia, nor can all CNS depressants be used as sedative-hypnotics. For example, the general anesthetic agents easily induce unconsciousness and are not suitable as sedative-hypnotics on an outpatient basis.

Insomnia is the salient feature of the nearly 90 different forms of sleep disorders.[10] Epidemiologic studies report that insomnia is widespread, affecting as much as one third of the population. Insomnia is more prevalent among women than men and is more common in the elderly than in the young. Nearly half of all Americans over the age of 65 years experience sleep disorders.[35]

Fifty years ago barbiturates were the most commonly prescribed sedative-hypnotics. Today they have been almost entirely replaced by benzodiazepine receptor agonists. One advantage of the benzodiazepines and related drugs over the barbiturates is their wider margin of safety. Additional advantages include a slower development of tolerance and physical dependence, minimal induction of hepatic enzyme activity, and generally fewer drug interactions.

Anxiety is one of the most common of the psychiatric disorders. In the United States, approximately 8% of the population will have an anxiety disorder during any given 6-month period. Although most people have certain periods and degrees of anxiety, it is only when anxiety begins to interfere with daily life that pharmacotherapy is indicated. Similarly, pharmacotherapy should be considered when situational anxiety, such as might be experienced by a patient in anticipation of an operative or diagnostic procedure, is judged to be sufficient to compromise satisfactory clinical care.

According to the *Diagnostic and Statistical Manual of Mental Disorders (DSM-IV)* of the American Psychiatric Association,[9] the anxiety disorders comprise various acute and chronic anxiety and phobic states. Specific anxiety disorders include panic disorder with or without agoraphobia, agoraphobia without panic disorder, generalized anxiety disorder, obsessive-compulsive disorder, acute stress disorder, posttraumatic stress disorder, social phobia, specific (simple) phobia, substance-induced anxiety disorder, and anxiety resulting from a general medical condition. The major emphasis in this chapter will be on drugs effective against anxiety as a symptom rather than as a specific disorder. Although the antianxiety drugs find application for treatment of anxiety disorders in general, other drugs, including the tricyclic antidepressants, monoamine oxidase (MAO) inhibitors, and selective serotonin reuptake inhibitors, are used in the pharmacotherapy of panic disorders, phobic disorders, and obsessive-compulsive disorders. These latter agents are discussed in detail in Chapter 12.

Nearly all CNS depressants, including ethanol, chloral hydrate, opioids, and barbiturates, can be used as antianxiety agents, but nonselective CNS sedation accounts for their antianxiety effect. The first drug that appeared to have some selectivity as an antianxiety agent was meprobamate. Originally developed and marketed as a skeletal muscle relaxant in the early 1950s, meprobamate soon became more widely used as an antianxiety agent. The popularity of meprobamate declined rapidly with the introduction of the benzodiazepines in the 1960s. The benzodiazepines became extremely popular drugs because they were found to be anxioselective and to be relatively safe even after overt overdose. Nonetheless, sedation is a prominent side effect of the benzodiazepines, and additive CNS depression occurs if other CNS depressants are used concurrently. Thus their anxiolytic selectivity is best described in relative rather than absolute terms. The possibility that antianxiety and CNS depressant properties are pharmacologically distinguishable has been raised again with the intro-

* The authors with to recognize Dr. Leslie Felpel for her past contributions to this chapter. See the Acknowledgments.

duction of buspirone, an azapirone derivative, which is an effective antianxiety agent with little or no sedative properties and causes very little additional depression when used with CNS depressants.

Antianxiety agents are referred to by several names: *anxiolytics, sedatives,* or *minor tranquilizers.* The terms *minor* and *major tranquilizers* should be avoided because the antianxiety agents and the antipsychotic drugs have entirely different mechanisms of action and their behavioral effects are dissimilar.

The usefulness and effectiveness of any given antianxiety agent varies depending on the patient, the clinical surroundings, the "chairside" manner of the dentist, the route of administration, and the properties of the chosen drug. Knowledge of the pharmacologic characteristics of the various antianxiety agents is crucial for selecting the proper drug, avoiding drug interactions, and obtaining the desired therapeutic response with minimal adverse side effects.

BENZODIAZEPINES

The benzodiazepines rank as one of the most widely used drug classes in the history of medicine because of their high selectivity and margin of safety. There have been literally thousands of benzodiazepine derivatives synthesized, and more than 100 of these have been tested for clinical activity. Currently there are several dozen benzodiazepines being marketed throughout the world.

Diazepam was the most frequently prescribed drug in the United States during the 1970s and remained among the 10 most frequently prescribed drugs for nearly two decades. Alprazolam is the most frequently prescribed benzodiazepine today. Surveys indicate that approximately 15% of adults in the United States take one of the benzodiazepines at least once a year. In fact, members of the medical community and the lay press have suggested that the benzodiazepines are overused and that they frequently serve either as a substitute for the practitioner's time or as a placebo for a population increasingly unwilling to accept a mild state of unhappiness. In response to this problem, manufacturers' prescribing information warns practitioners that benzodiazepines should not be prescribed for longer than 4 months without a careful reassessment of the patient's status and that they should not be prescribed for the stress of everyday life. In an attempt to decrease illegal use and inappropriate prescribing of benzodiazepines, the state of New York required that prescriptions for benzodiazepines be written as for schedule II drugs (see Chapter 55). This action effectively reduced the number of prescriptions written for the benzodiazepines, but surveys showed that the older CNS depressants (barbiturates, meprobamate), which are less selective, more dangerous, and have greater abuse liability, were then prescribed more frequently.[64] Other reports suggest that most benzodiazepines are used appropriately, and are abused primarily by individuals with a prior history of drug abuse.[46,66] Some also believe that a number of patients who truly need anxiety relief may be denied benzodiazepines because of the bad publicity associated with their use and concern about the potential for habituation and drug abuse. Obviously, medical opinion is divided regarding the use of benzodiazepines.

Chemistry and Structure-Activity Relationships

The basic structure of the pharmacologically active 1,4-benzodiazepines is shown in Table 13-1. All the benzodiazepines currently available in the United States are derived

Table • 13-1

Chemical Structures of Various Benzodiazepines

R_1 R_2 9 N 2 8 R_3 4 5 N R_7 6 R_2'

SUBSTITUENT GROUPS

DRUG	R_1	R_2	R_3	R_7	R_2'
Alprazolam	See Figure 13-1				
Chlordiazepoxide	See Figure 13-1				
Clonazepam	—H	=O	—H	$—NO_2$	—Cl
Clorazepate	—H	=O	—COOH	—Cl	—H
Diazepam	$—CH_3$	=O	—H	—Cl	—H
Estazolam	See Figure 13-1				
Flurazepam	$—CH_2CH_2N(C_2H_5)_2$	=O	—H	—Cl	—F
Halazepam	$—CH_2CF_3$	=O	—H	—Cl	—H
Lorazepam	—H	=O	—OH	—Cl	—Cl
Midazolam	See Figure 13-1				
Oxazepam	—H	=O	—OH	—Cl	—H
Prazepam	$—CH_2—$◁	=O	—H	—Cl	—H
Quazepam	$—CH_2CF_3$	=S	—H	—Cl	—F
Temazepam	$—CH_3$	=O	—OH	—Cl	—H
Triazolam	See Figure 13-1				

from this molecule, to which are added various substituent groups. Slight modifications of the basic structure have produced the triazolobenzodiazepines (alprazolam and triazolam) and imidazobenzodiazepines (e.g., midazolam). These compounds, along with chlordiazepoxide, the first benzodiazepine marketed in the United States, are shown in Figure 13-1. Rearrangement of the nitrogen atom from the 4 to the 5 position of the seven-member ring yields the 1,5-benzodiazepines. No 1,5-benzodiazepines are yet approved for use in the United States, but they have antianxiety, sedative, and anticonvulsant activity. All benzodiazepines with psychopharmacologic activity have an electronegative group at R_7. A chlorine atom appears to confer optimal activity, whereas bromo and nitro substitutions are only weakly anxiolytic. However, a nitro moiety at R_7 enhances antiseizure properties, as illustrated by clonazepam, which is used as an anticonvulsant. Hydrogen or methyl groups at R_7 significantly reduce pharmacologic activity. Substitution at position 5 with any group other than a phenyl ring also reduces activity. Halogenation at R_2' increases potency; larger alkyl substitutions decrease it. Substitution on the nitrogen at R_1 with a methyl group enhances activity, as do methyl or hydrogen groups at R_3. A biosynthetic pathway for the in vivo formation of diazepam-like benzodiazepines has been proposed.[6] Whether synthesis occurs naturally is unknown, but, surprisingly, benzodiazepines are found in a variety of foods.[65]

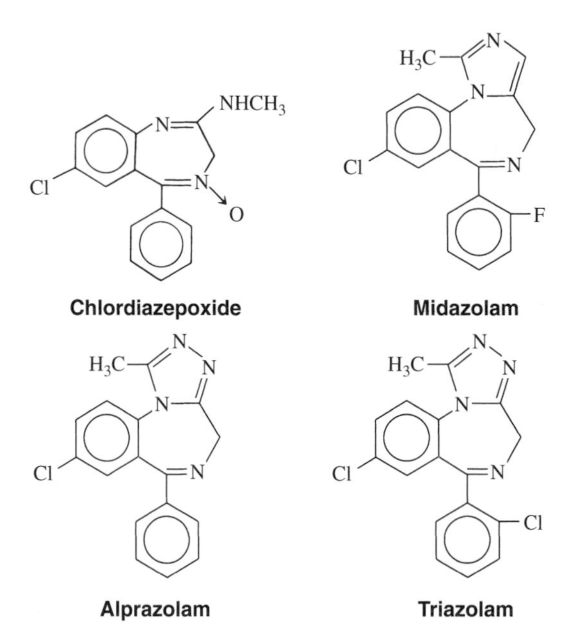

Fig. 13-1 Structural formulas of chlordiazepoxide, the first benzodiazepine used clinically; midazolam, an imidazobenzodiazepine; and the triazolobenzodiazepines alprazolam and triazolam. Triazolam is derived from alprazolam by the addition of a chlorine atom on the ortho position of the phenyl group. Estazolam is formed from alprazolam by removal of the methyl group of the triazolo ring (not shown).

Mechanism of Action

Perhaps the most exciting and significant advance in the understanding of anxiety and the mechanism of action of the benzodiazepines occurred with the discovery of specific benzodiazepine binding sites in the brain and the understanding that these were in some way linked to the inhibitory neurotransmitter γ-aminobutyric acid (GABA). As shown schematically in Figure 13-2, when the GABA receptor is activated, the Cl^- channel opens, allowing Cl^- influx, membrane hyperpolarization, and neuronal inhibition. Benzodiazepines, by interacting at high-affinity benzodiazepine binding sites on the GABA receptor complex, facilitate GABA action. Thus, while devoid of direct GABA-mimetic effects, benzodiazepines increase inhibitory neurotransmission resulting from GABA. Although the exact mechanism by which benzodiazepines accomplish their effect is not fully delineated, it is known that they increase the frequency at which Cl^- channels open in response to GABA.[55] Thus GABA inhibition (chiefly postsynaptic inhibition) is enhanced by the benzodiazepines, and any transmitter system modulated by this inhibitory drive is inhibited to a greater extent in the presence of the benzodiazepines.

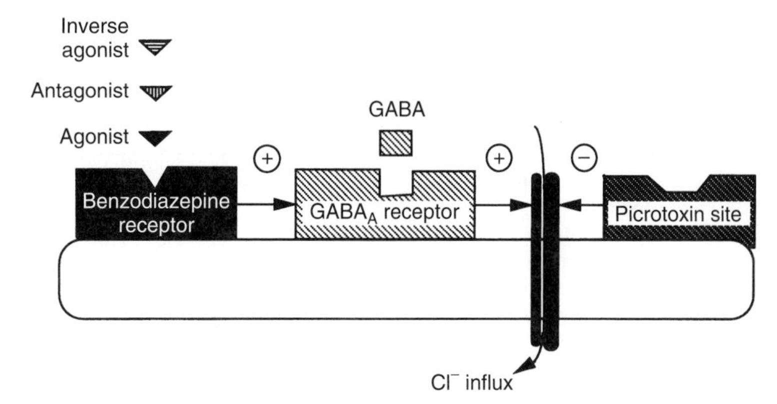

Fig. 13-2 A schematic of the *$GABA_A$ receptor* complex illustrating the sites of action of benzodiazepine agonists, antagonists, and *GABA*. The *benzodiazepine receptor* is coupled to the $GABA_A$ receptor so that its activation facilitates (denoted by the + symbol) the action of GABA on the Cl^- ionophore. Increased *Cl^- influx* leads to hyperpolarization (i.e., inhibition) of the neuron. Benzodiazepine antagonists inhibit the binding of benzodiazepines. Inverse agonists inhibit the constitutive activity of the benzodiazepine–$GABA_A$ receptor complex by binding to the benzodiazepine receptor. Also illustrated is the *picrotoxin site*, that, when acted on by picrotoxin, antagonizes (– symbol) the influx of Cl^- and can lead to convulsions. (Adapted from Dubovsky SL: Generalized anxiety disorder: new concepts and psychopharmacologic therapies, *J Clin Psychiatry* 51(suppl 1):3-10, 1990.)

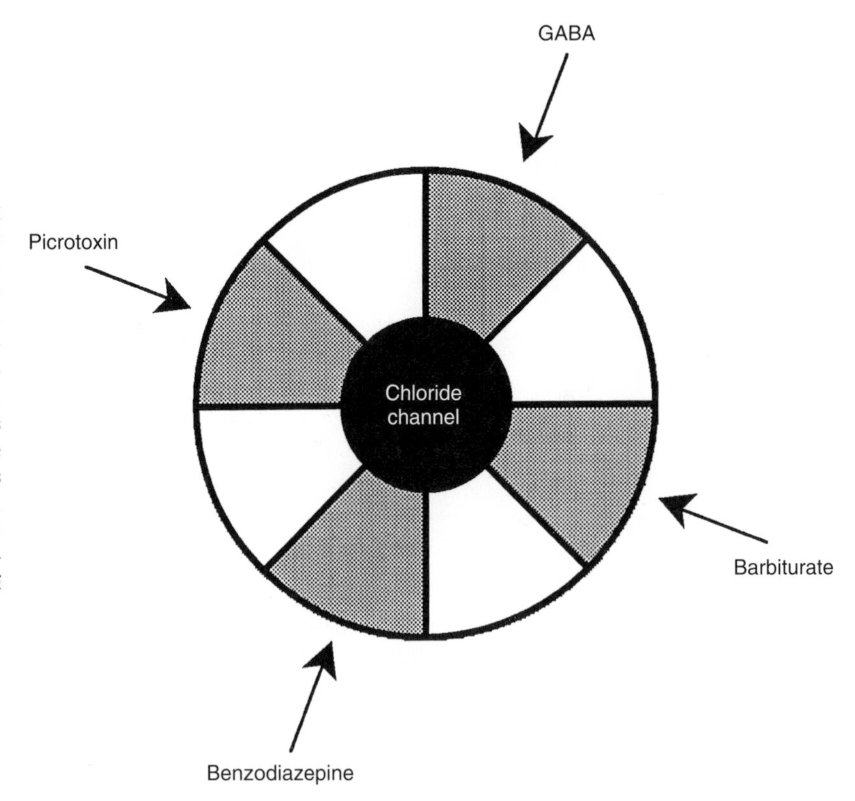

Fig. 13-3 The arrangement of allosteric binding domains on the $GABA_A$ receptor complex. The complex is composed of five unique subunits. Multiple receptor subtypes are possible on the basis of different combinations of the subunits. Binding sites for picrotoxin (a convulsant), barbiturates, GABA, and benzodiazepines are presented for illustrative purposes. In addition, distinct binding sites for other chemical agents have been identified (shown as blank areas). The figure does not identify which receptor subunits are involved in the binding of each drug. (Adapted from Sieghart W: $GABA_A$ receptors: ligand-gated Cl^- ion channels modulated by multiple drug-binding sites, *Trends Pharmacol Sci* 13:446-450, 1992.)

Benzodiazepine receptors are found in the brains of all mammalian species as well as birds, amphibians, reptiles, and higher fishes. Benzodiazepine receptors are linked to a specific GABA receptor subtype, the $GABA_A$ receptor (see Figure 13-2). Figure 13-3 gives further details on binding domains associated with the $GABA_A$ receptor. Historically, GABA receptors have been classified into two subtypes: the Cl^- channel–linked $GABA_A$ receptors and the G protein–linked $GABA_B$ receptors. Benzodiazepine-sensitive $GABA_A$ receptors are activated by GABA agonists, such as muscimol (a hallucinogen), and blocked by GABA antagonists, such as picrotoxin and bicuculline (both convulsants).[69] $GABA_B$ receptors are benzodiazepine and bicuculline insensitive and are activated by baclofen, a centrally acting muscle relaxant.

The benzodiazepine receptor—along with the $GABA_A$ receptor, a barbiturate receptor, the Cl^- channel, and binding domains for other drugs—forms a single macromolecular complex. Like GABA receptors, benzodiazepine receptors are heterogeneous; there are at least three types: type 1 (BZ_1), type 2 (BZ_2), and the "peripheral type" benzodiazepine receptor. The presence of BZ_1 and BZ_2 receptor types is apparently determined by the subunit composition of the $GABA_A$ macromolecular complex. The BZ_1 receptor may be linked to sleep, whereas the BZ_2 receptor may be linked to cognition and motor function. High-affinity benzodiazepine binding sites are found on specific subunits of the $GABA_A$ receptor complex, which, as shown in Figure 13-4, is a pentamer composed of several glycoprotein subunits (α, β, γ). This organization is analogous to that of the nicotinic receptor. As illustrated in Figure 13-4, which depicts the most common form of $GABA_A$ receptor complex in the rat brain, a γ subunit is necessary (but not sufficient) for benzodiazepine binding and pharmacologic effects.[51] Cloning experiments have demonstrated that there are multiple subtypes of α, β, and γ subunits,[27] which provide a basis for GABA receptor heterogeneity.[12,44] This heterogeneity of receptor subunits may offer an explanation for the diverse pharmacologic effects (antianxiety, anticonvulsant, sedative, and skeletal muscle relaxant) of the benzodiazepines.

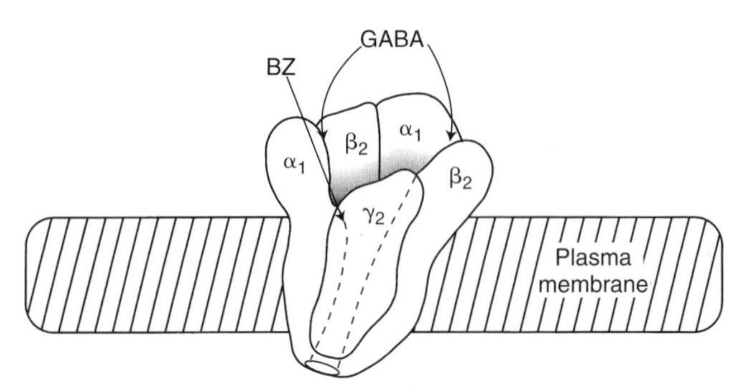

Fig. 13-4 A structural model of the GABA-benzodiazepine receptor complex. The arrangement of the subunits (α, β, γ) forms the Cl^- channel. GABA binding sites are illustrated at the two analogous interfaces between the α and β subunits. The BZ binding site is associated with the interface of the α and γ subunits. (Adapted from Zorumski CF, Isenberg KE: Insights into the structure and function of GABA-benzodiazepine receptors: ion channels and psychiatry, *Am J Psychiatry* 148:162-173, 1991.)

Determination of the molecular basis of receptor heterogeneity may eventually facilitate the development of benzodiazepines with a greater degree of selectivity in producing each of these effects. At present, none of the clinically available antianxiety benzodiazepines shows selectivity for either BZ_1 or BZ_2 receptors, although the hypnotic benzodiazepine quazepam is likely selective for the BZ_1 receptor.[45] Zolpidem and zaleplon, two nonbenzodiazepines selective for the BZ_1 receptor, are discussed later in this chapter.

The heterogeneous nature of $GABA_A$ receptors may explain some of the differences in clinical profile between the benzodiazepines and the barbiturates. The barbiturates increase the duration (but not the frequency) of opening of Cl^- channels activated by GABA, and in high concentrations promote Cl^- conductance even in the absence of GABA. Variations of $GABA_A$ receptor responses to benzodiazepines and barbiturates in specific CNS areas may be another factor contributing to their respective pharmacologic profiles.

The benzodiazepine-insensitive $GABA_B$ receptors coupled to G proteins are associated with a decrease in Ca^{++} conductance and an increase in K^+ conductance and therefore could be expected to cause pharmacologic effects when stimulated or antagonized. $GABA_B$ receptors are less widely distributed than $GABA_A$ receptors but are found in high concentrations in the cerebral cortex and cerebellum. Subtypes of $GABA_B$ receptors may exist. $GABA_B$ receptors have not been as extensively studied as $GABA_A$ receptors, but they may participate in blood pressure regulation[56] and offer a potential site for therapeutic drug action.

The existence of subclasses of benzodiazepine receptors suggests that some agents, with specific activity for individual receptor subtypes, may be more selective than others in terms of their pharmacologic profile. Whether this selectivity results in significant clinical differences is an open question.[13] Quazepam, a long-acting benzodiazepine hypnotic, produces sedation but appears to have little ataxic effect and may cause less tolerance than other benzodiazepines. Autoradiographic studies have demonstrated selective binding of quazepam to BZ_1 receptors,[26] which may account for sedation with minimal muscle relaxant effects. Of all currently available benzodiazepines, only quazepam, one of its active metabolites (1-oxoquazepam), and possibly the antianxiety agent halazepam have selectivity for the BZ_1 receptor subtype. These benzodiazepines differ chemically from other benzodiazepines by having a trifluoroethyl substituent (see Table 13-1), which may be responsible for BZ_1 selectivity. However, selective activity at the BZ_1 receptor has not been associated with any special clinical benefit of quazepam, compared with other benzodiazepines, for treating insomnia.

Another potential site for pharmacotherapy is found on "peripheral" benzodiazepine receptors. Peripheral benzodiazepine binding sites, which can be pharmacologically differentiated from central BZ_1 and BZ_2 receptors, have been found not only in the periphery (kidney, lung) but also in the brain. In the CNS, they are most prevalent on glial cells. The functions of peripheral benzodiazepine receptors are under active investigation.

Although the pharmacologic actions of the benzodiazepines are closely tied to GABA receptors, a number of other neurotransmitters, including glycine, norepinephrine, and 5-hydroxytryptamine (5-HT), have been suggested as playing a role in their action. In fact, an interaction between GABA and 5-HT has been demonstrated experimentally with diazepam and tryptaminergic anxiolytics.[30] This finding is interesting in light of the suggested mechanism of action of the nonsedating antianxiety agent buspirone (see below), a $5\text{-}HT_{1A}$ partial agonist.

Pharmacologic Effects

The most important pharmacologic effects of the benzodiazepines are on the CNS. The benzodiazepines have clinically useful antianxiety, sedative-hypnotic, amnestic, anticonvulsant, and skeletal muscle relaxant properties. At one time the benzodiazepines were thought to differ pharmacologically only in terms of their pharmacokinetics. Although differences in pharmacokinetic properties explain many of their clinical differences, certain benzodiazepines appear to have unique properties. For example, alprazolam has documented antidepressant and antipanic properties, and diazepam may be more selective as a skeletal muscle relaxant than other benzodiazepines. Diazepam is, in fact, the only benzodiazepine approved for the treatment of skeletal muscle spasm and spasticity of central origin.

Central nervous system

Many of the gross CNS effects of the benzodiazepines are similar to those of such older sedative-hypnotics as the barbiturates. All the benzodiazepines produce a dose-dependent depression of the CNS. Drowsiness and sedation are common manifestations of this central depressant action and may be considered a side effect in some instances and therapeutically useful in others. Some benzodiazepines, such as flurazepam and temazepam, are marketed specifically as hypnotic agents. Although the hypnotic benzodiazepines are probably no more specific in promoting sleep than are the antianxiety benzodiazepines, differences in their pharmacokinetics may make a given benzodiazepine more suitable as either a hypnotic or an antianxiety agent.

Although it is difficult clinically to differentiate the CNS effects of the benzodiazepines from those of other sedative-hypnotics, there are certain experimental animal models that indicate the benzodiazepines have selective antianxiety properties. For example, normally vicious macaque monkeys and rats made highly irritable by lesions placed in the septal area of the brain are tamed and calmed by the benzodiazepines. The doses required to produce these effects are one tenth of those that cause ataxia and somnolence. Barbiturates also tame these animals, but the doses required invariably produce incoordination and drowsiness. In addition to behavioral investigations, numerous studies have examined the effects of benzodiazepines on the electrical activity of areas of the brain that are associated with emotion and behavior. In these studies, evidence again suggests a somewhat more selective antianxiety action of the benzodiazepines compared with the barbiturates. For example, unlike the barbiturates, the benzodiazepines depress the limbic system (an area of the brain associated with emotion and behavior) at doses lower than those that depress the reticular formation and cerebral cortex. The selective effects of benzodiazepines on the limbic system correlate with taming in experimental animals and anxiety relief in human beings. Experimentally, neurons in the hippocampus (a major structure of the limbic system) are depressed by the benzodiazepines. Although these studies are interesting, their significance is not clear because the causes, mechanisms, and neural structures involved in anxiety are not fully understood.

Certain benzodiazepines in clinical doses can induce anterograde amnesia, which means that memory of events occurring for a period of time after drug administration is not retained.[11] This effect is useful therapeutically when multiple procedures, such as burn wound debridement, must be performed; it has toxicologic and even criminal implications when it interferes with daily living or is used to commit date rape.

Muscle relaxation and antiseizure activity represent additional CNS effects of the benzodiazepines. These effects are discussed, respectively, later in this chapter and in Chapter 14.

Cardiovascular system

In the healthy adult, normal therapeutic doses of the benzodiazepines cause few alterations in cardiac output or blood pressure. Greater than normal doses decrease blood pressure, cardiac output, and stroke volume in both normal subjects and patients with cardiac disease, but these effects are usually not clinically significant. The benzodiazepines are often prescribed for cardiac patients in whom anxiety contributes to their symptoms.

Respiratory system

As is true of any sedative drug, the benzodiazepines are respiratory depressants. In normal doses the benzodiazepines have little effect on respiration in the healthy person. However, there have been reports of benzodiazepine-induced respiratory failure in patients with pulmonary disease. The benzodiazepines may cause additive respiratory depressant effects with other CNS depressant drugs. Poor suckling, hypothermia, and a need for ventilatory assistance have been reported in the neonate if the mother has received intravenous lorazepam shortly before delivery. Midazolam, used primarily for intravenous sedation and for the induction of anesthesia, can cause respiratory depression and apnea. Clinically significant respiratory depression may occur if an opioid is used in combination with midazolam.[11]

Absorption, Fate, and Excretion

The pharmacokinetics of individual benzodiazepines differ, and therefore there is a wide range in speed of onset and duration of action among these compounds. The benzodiazepines frequently are classified according to their elimination half-life, as illustrated in Table 13-2; however, the elimination half-life of a given drug is only one factor affecting its clinical profile. The rates of drug absorption and tissue distribution and redistribution are often important factors in determining onset and duration of clinical effects after short-term administration. Additionally, there is a wide variation in drug half-lives among patients.

After oral administration, most of the benzodiazepines are rapidly absorbed and highly bound to plasma protein. Lorazepam, oxazepam, prazepam, and temazepam are more slowly absorbed. Peak blood concentrations are generally obtained in 1 to 3 hours. However, the lipid solubility of these compounds differs significantly, so that a highly lipid-soluble drug such as diazepam exerts its effect more rapidly, whereas lorazepam, which is less lipid soluble, has a slower onset of action even after systemic absorption. Diazepam also accumulates in body fat because of its lipophilic properties, and it is slowly eliminated from these stores. This characteristic partially accounts for the prolonged half-life of diazepam, which can range from 1 day to as many as 4 days.

Many of the benzodiazepines are converted to pharmacologically active metabolites that have long half-lives (Figure 13-5). Clorazepate and prazepam are nearly completely converted (in the stomach and liver, respectively) to the long-acting metabolite desmethyldiazepam (nordazepam) before they enter the systemic circulation. Desmethyldiazepam is a metabolite of many other benzodiazepines, including chlordiazepoxide, diazepam, and halazepam. Flurazepam is also converted to active metabolites in its first pass through the liver. In general, the products of phase I metabolism are eventually conjugated with glucuronic acid and thereby inactivated and excreted in the urine and feces. Because the half-lives of the different active metabolites vary considerably, the overall duration of the pharmacologic effect of benzodiazepines also varies considerably. Oxazepam and lorazepam are not converted to active metabolites but are directly conjugated and excreted. These drugs are therefore eliminated fairly rapidly and may be especially useful in patients who have a deficiency in hepatic microsomal enzymes resulting from liver disease or other reasons. Alprazolam and triazolam, containing a fused triazolo ring, undergo α-hydroxylation on the methyl group of the ring. This reaction (also referred to as *1′-hydroxylation*) and the subsequent conversion to the glucuronide occur rapidly in the case of triazolam and account for the short duration of action of the drug. Alprazolam and triazolam also undergo 4-hydroxylation of the benzodiazepine ring and then conjugation to the glucuronide. Midazolam, which contains a fused imidazo ring, is quickly metabolized in a similar manner. Midazolam has a rapid onset of action, a high metabolic clearance, a rapid rate of elimination, and a short duration of action. Termination of CNS activity is a result of peripheral redistribution and metabolic transformation. It is converted into

Table • 13-2

Classification of Benzodiazepines on the Basis of Elimination Half-Life after Oral Administration

DRUG	TIME TO PEAK PLASMA CONCENTRATION (hr)	ELIMINATION HALF-LIFE (hr)	MAJOR ACTIVE METABOLITES
Short- to Intermediate-Acting			
Alprazolam	1-2	12-15	α-Hydroxyalprazolam
Estazolam	2	10-24	None
Lorazepam	1-6	10-18	None
Midazolam	0.2-1	2-5	α-Hydroxymidazolam
Oxazepam	1-4	5-15	None
Temazepam	2-3	10-20	None
Triazolam	1-2	1.5-5	α-Hydroxytriazolam
Long-Acting			
Chlordiazepoxide	0.5-4	5-30	Desmethylchlordiazepoxide Demoxepam Desmethyldiazepam
Clorazepate*	1-2	30-100	Desmethyldiazepam
Diazepam	0.5-2	30-60	Desmethyldiazepam
Flurazepam*	0.5-1	50-100	N-Desalkylflurazepam
Halazepam	1-3	14	Desmethyldiazepam
Prazepam*	2.5-6	30-100	Desmethyldiazepam
Quazepam	2	40	2-Oxo-quazepam N-Desalkylflurazepam

*Does not reach the circulation as the parent drug in clinically significant amounts. Values reflect the primary metabolite.

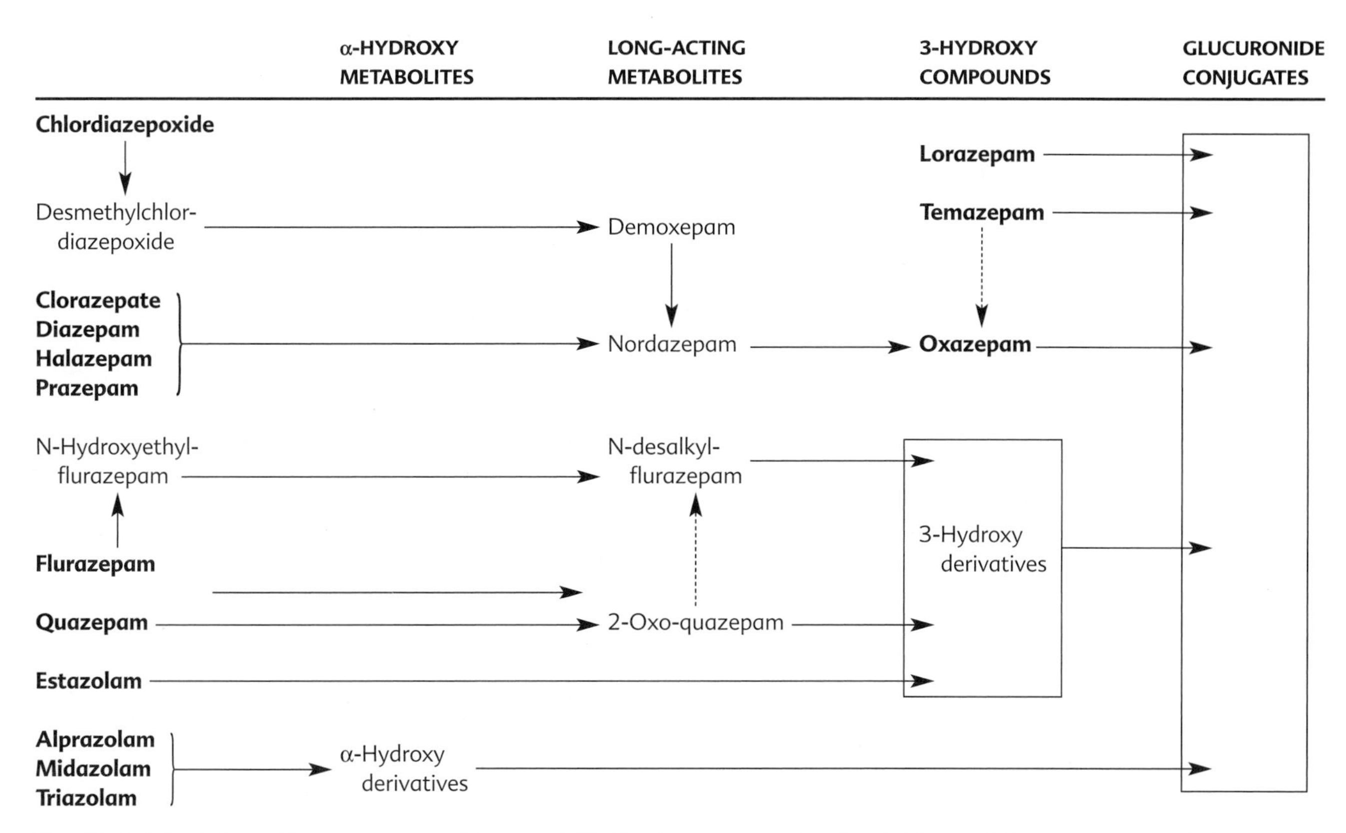

Fig. 13-5 Metabolism of benzodiazepines. Drugs available for clinical use are listed in bold type. With the exception of the prodrugs clorazepate and prazepam, only the glucuronide conjugates are inactive.

several metabolites that have little pharmacologic activity; however, because of extensive first-pass metabolism, the α-hydroxy (or 1′-hydroxy) metabolite may contribute to the sedative effect when midazolam is given orally to children.

Many benzodiazepines are biotransformed to long-acting metabolites. These metabolites are the cause of hangover the next day after initial drug use, and they accumulate with repeated administration. An active metabolite of both flurazepam and quazepam, N-desalkylflurazepam, which accounts for some of the activity of quazepam and nearly all the activity of flurazepam, has an elimination half-life of 50 to 100 hours. In sleep laboratory studies, it has been shown that flurazepam does not reach full effectiveness until the second or third consecutive night of intake. Quazepam decreases sleep latency and facilitates sleep maintenance after a single dose.

Temazepam has a half-life of about 13 hours, and only a very small amount of oxazepam is formed as a metabolite; estazolam has a similar half-life and forms no clinically active metabolites. Triazolam, with a mean half-life of 2.9 hours, is converted to metabolites that, although active, are rapidly eliminated. Because of their short durations of action, temazepam and triazolam do not generally accumulate even with repeated nightly use. Indeed, triazolam is indicated for patients who have difficulty falling asleep but who stay asleep once sleep ensues.

Adverse Effects and Drug Interactions

The most common side effect of the benzodiazepines is drowsiness. This may not necessarily be an unwanted reaction, but rather a therapeutic benefit in anxiety states that cause insomnia. Other signs and symptoms of dose-dependent CNS depression include ataxia, incoordination, dysarthria, confusion, apathy, muscle weakness, dizziness, and somnolence. The elderly (older than 65 years) appear to be particularly susceptible, and persons with a history of alcohol or barbiturate abuse particularly resistant, to the gross CNS depressant properties of the benzodiazepines.

The elderly and the young occasionally respond to the benzodiazepines with excitement rather than depression. Excitatory CNS effects may include an increased incidence of nightmares, hyperactivity, insomnia, irritability, agitation, and even rage and hostility. Because these responses are unlike what would be expected of a CNS depressant, they have been termed *paradoxic reactions.* A paradoxic decrease in seizure threshold, particularly in patients with grand mal epilepsy, has also been observed, even though diazepam, for instance, is used in acute treatment of *status epilepticus.* These unusual occurrences of what appears to be a CNS excitatory action may be a disinhibitory effect similar to that observed with alcohol.

The benzodiazepines cause changes in normal sleep patterns. Patients seem to adapt fairly quickly to the nonspecific CNS depression of the benzodiazepines. Nonetheless, daytime sedation after a nighttime dose, referred to as "hangover," is a common side effect, especially of the long-acting benzodiazepines. This residual effect may be beneficial in some cases but undesirable in others.

Adverse effects of the benzodiazepines other than those referable to their CNS depressant actions are usually more irritating than life threatening. Allergic reactions to the benzodiazepines usually manifest as relatively minor skin rashes. Because injectable formulations of diazepam contain propylene glycol and ethyl alcohol solvents, intramuscular and intravenous administration can cause local pain, phlebitis, and thrombosis. Phlebitis is more likely to occur if a vein in the hand or wrist is used and may be more common after repeated injections, especially in heavy smokers, the elderly, and women taking oral contraceptives. A more severe complication arises if the injection has been inadvertently made into an artery. In such a case, the patient usually reports pain that radiates distally, and ischemic changes are noted in the digits. This reaction can occur up to 3 days after the injection and in the worst case could lead to gangrene, necessitating amputation. If an intraarterial injection is made, it has been suggested that the needle be left in place and the artery flushed with a vasodilator such as papaverine or procaine.[43] With the introduction of the water-soluble benzodiazepine midazolam, the occurrence of venous complications and pain at the injection site has diminished.

Tolerance and psychologic dependence develop rather frequently with the benzodiazepines, but true physical dependence is less common. Nevertheless, the abuse potential of the benzodiazepines should not be ignored. Tolerance to the sedative-hypnotic effects of the benzodiazepines is slower to develop with the longer-acting agents. In cases of physical dependence, the severity of withdrawal depends on the dose of the drug being used and the drug's half-life. Rapid discontinuation of the benzodiazepines, especially the short-acting compounds, can lead to symptoms of withdrawal. Often these symptoms are nearly identical to those for which treatment was initiated, including anxiety, irritability, insomnia, and fatigue. The symptoms become more severe with high doses and prolonged treatment. Withdrawal can be minimized by reducing the dosage very gradually (10% or less per day over a course of 10 to 14 days) or by the use of longer-acting compounds. Fortunately, withdrawal from lower doses is usually not life threatening, and symptoms last no longer than 2 weeks. Withdrawal from high doses may be life threatening because of the accompanying convulsions. Mechanisms involved in the development of tolerance are unknown, but the long-term administration of benzodiazepines to animals causes downregulation of benzodiazepine receptors,[34] which could be a contributing factor. Diazepam has been particularly popular as a drug of abuse. Because of the strong binding of diazepam to tissue constituents, it is not rapidly removed by dialysis or diuresis in patients with acute overdose. Flumazenil, a benzodiazepine antagonist described below, can reverse benzodiazepine overdose if drug ingestion is limited to benzodiazepines and not multiple depressant drugs. However, flumazenil can precipitate withdrawal in benzodiazepine-dependent patients.

Some of the short-acting benzodiazepines are especially prone to elicit amnesia; triazolam also causes confusional states and delusions. Because of the prominence of these adverse CNS effects, the United States and several European countries have removed the 0.5-mg tablet form of triazolam from the market. The Food and Drug Administration (FDA) also approved labeling for triazolam that recommended use only for short-term (7 to 10 days) treatment of insomnia, emphasized the need to monitor patients for bizarre behavioral side effects, and set new limits on the maximum dosage. Triazolam is abused more frequently than either temazepam or flurazepam, probably because of its more rapid absorption.

Despite these problems, one of the major advantages of the benzodiazepines compared with other sedatives is their high margin of safety. Death is rare in cases of overdose and is usually the result of a combination of drugs (especially alcohol) with the benzodiazepines. The few deaths associated with the use of a benzodiazepine alone have primarily involved either geriatric patients, very young children, or suicides.

Benzodiazepines cross the placental barrier. During the first trimester, long-term use of these drugs has been associated with increased fetal malformations, including cleft lip and cleft palate in human beings. There is no clear estimate of the risk following single-dose use. It is generally agreed, however, that these drugs should be avoided during pregnancy.[37] The frequent use of benzodiazepines during late pregnancy may lead to withdrawal in the neonate. Large doses of benzodiazepines given to the mother during labor and delivery may result in respiratory depression, hypotonia, and hypothermia in the infant.

Drug interactions associated with anxiolytic and sedative drugs used in dentistry are listed in Table 13-3. The therapeutic index for benzodiazepines is normally so large that wide ranges of dosing recommendations and blood concentrations do not significantly affect their safety and efficacy. Plasma concentrations after a given dose may normally vary such that a minor shift in elimination from drug interactions is unlikely to result in an overdose. For example, in healthy subjects taking no other medications, plasma concentrations 3 hours following a single 15-mg dose of diazepam have been reported to range from 20 to 260 μg/ml.[32] A drug interaction that causes a 20% increase in diazepam plasma concentrations is unlikely to have significant toxicity. Most healthy patients can tolerate small variations in a drug's absorption or metabolism that are caused by coadministration of another drug. On the other hand, combining sedatives is problematic. The combination of ethanol with a benzodiazepine remains an important source of serious toxicity.[58]

Rifampin induces metabolic enzymes in the gut and liver responsible for the metabolism of diazepam, midazolam, and triazolam. Reduction in the bioavailability of midazolam as great as 96% has been reported.[2] Triazolam is so rapidly and completely metabolized in the gut that peak plasma concentrations are only 12% of normal.[63] This interaction is one of the most pronounced alterations in drug kinetics ever reported. The almost complete loss of triazolam bioavailability and subsequent efficacy is quite significant and warrants use of an alternative anxiolytic such as oral oxazepam, nitrous oxide inhalation, or an intravenous agent. The anticonvulsant carbamazepine can also induce hepatic enzymes for the oxidative metabolism of benzodiazepines such as alprazolam, triazolam, and midazolam.[3] Decreased benzodiazepine plasma concentrations and greatly reduced sedative effects after oral administration of these agents may occur. This interaction may be important in medicine because of loss of seizure control. A loss of sedative efficacy in dentistry may also occur. Benzodiazepines that are metabolized solely through glucuronidation, such as oxazepam, are suitable alternative agents for sedation in these situations.

The Ca^{++} channel blockers verapamil and diltiazem have been shown to inhibit the CYP3A isozymes required for the metabolism of triazolam and midazolam. In controlled clinical trials, a 2-day regimen of these drugs decreased the metabolism and increased the bioavailability of midazolam and triazolam administered orally. Peak blood concentrations were increased as much as two- to three-fold and were associated with increased sedation and performance deficits.[1] Avoidance of this combination is recommended, particularly in elderly populations known to be sensitive to benzodiazepines.

Cimetidine also inhibits the oxidative metabolism of certain benzodiazepines, such as triazolam and alprazolam. Half-life increases of 30% to 63% have been reported.[17] Metabolism of diazepam may also be delayed. An increased and prolonged level of sedation after oral administration may occur because of the decreased first-pass metabolism.[47]

Table • 13-3

Adverse Drug Interactions: Anxiolytics and Sedative-Hypnotics

ADVERSE DRUG INTERACTION (SPECIFIC EXAMPLES)	CLINICAL IMPLICATIONS
Anxiolytics and Sedative-Hypnotics with:	
Other anxiolytics and sedative-hypnotics, alcohol, opioids, antipsychotics, antidepressants, centrally acting muscle relaxants, local and general anesthetics, and other CNS depressants	In combination, CNS depression summates with anxiolytics and sedatives; loss of consciousness, respiratory depression, and death are possible complications.
Benzodiazepines with:	
Carbamazepine, rifampin	Increased rate of metabolism reduces the bioavailability of several benzodiazepines.
Cimetidine, diltiazem, verapamil, erythromycin, clarithromycin, protease inhibitors (indinavir, nelfinavir, ritonavir), some azole antimycotics (itraconazole, ketoconazole), and some antidepressants (fluoxetine, fluvoxamine, trazodone)	Decreased rate of metabolism increases the bioavailability of some benzodiazepines and significantly augments and prolongs their effects.
Chloral Hydrate with:	
Alcohol	Each drug limits the metabolism of the other; depression is greater than additive.
Warfarin	Competition for plasma protein binding causes a temporary increase in the anticoagulant effect.
Furosemide	Rare reports of diaphoresis, tachycardia, and hypertension.
Barbiturates with:	
Valproic acid and phenobarbital	Elimination of barbiturates is decreased; prolonged and enhanced sedation is reported.
Warfarin	Bleeding risk increases when long-term barbiturate therapy is discontinued. Anticoagulant effect of warfarin is reduced with concurrent therapy with phenobarbital.

Benzodiazepines that are metabolized directly to the glucuronide conjugate (e.g., oxazepam) are not affected. Similarly, the antimicrobials erythromycin and clarithromycin, as well as the azole antifungals ketoconazole and itraconazole, are potential inhibitors of the hepatic isozymes required for oxidative metabolism of these benzodiazepines. By decreasing the first-pass effect and improving bioavailability, triazolam blood concentrations may increase three-fold.[62] The antiviral agents indinavir, nelfinavir, and ritonavir inhibit hepatic oxidative enzymes required for metabolism of many benzodiazepines. Although this reaction has not been reported after dental therapy, it could potentially cause oversedation and respiratory depression.

Inverse Agonists and Antagonists

Although the benzodiazepines produce their pharmacologic effects by acting on benzodiazepine receptors to facilitate GABAergic transmission, there are compounds that act at the same benzodiazepine receptor sites but yield pharmacologic effects opposite to those of the benzodiazepines (see Figure 13-2). Such substances are known as *inverse benzodiazepine agonists*. These drugs promote anxiety and convulsions.

As described in Chapter 1, an inverse agonist can inhibit the action of both a conventional agonist and a receptor that is constitutively active (i.e., active without agonist). Thus an inverse agonist is said to have negative intrinsic activity, whereas a pure antagonist, which blocks the binding of other drugs to the receptor without altering constitutive receptor activity, has an intrinsic activity of zero. Two conformations may exist for the benzodiazepine receptor, with only one conformation promoting the binding of GABA. The inverse agonist may promote the conformation that does not bind GABA.

Inverse agonists are of clinical interest because, if they exist endogenously, excessive release or hyperactivity of such ligands could explain pathologic anxiety. The β-carboline n-butyl-β-carboline-3-carboxylate is a synthetic compound that can act as an inverse agonist.[14] More important therapeutically are the pure antagonists. These compounds have the potential to reverse the effects of both benzodiazepines and inverse agonists; they have no intrinsic activity of their own yet do not reverse constitutive benzodiazepine receptor activity. Flumazenil (Figure 13-6) is currently the only benzodiazepine receptor antagonist approved by the FDA.

Flumazenil finds clinical application in managing benzodiazepine overdose and in hastening recovery from benzodiazepine sedation or anesthesia after diagnostic procedures or minor surgery. Although certain precautions must be observed, flumazenil may allow for a shorter monitoring period after surgery and earlier discharge of the patient.[19] Flumazenil has been used successfully in reversing benzodiazepine-induced coma, but whether it should be given routinely to comatose patients when the coma is of unknown cause is not clear. The routine use of flumazenil is not

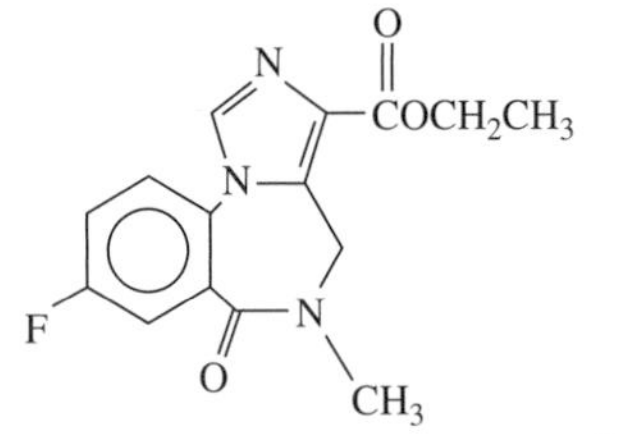

Fig. 13-6 Structural formula of flumazenil.

recommended in cases of mixed drug overdose, airway obstruction, or seizure disorders. Flumazenil may increase the risk of cardiac arrhythmias and seizures in patients who have overdosed with tricyclic antidepressants.[20] Ventricular arrhythmias have also been precipitated by flumazenil in patients with chloral hydrate overdose.[50]

Flumazenil administered intravenously can generally reverse benzodiazepine-induced sedation in 1 to 2 minutes. Reversal of benzodiazepine sedation by flumazenil may last for several hours. However, in a study in which patients were sedated with midazolam before dental extraction, flumazenil significantly improved patient assessment regarding state of alertness compared with placebo controls (Figure 13-7) only for the first 30 minutes.[7] It is therefore important to note that the duration of action of flumazenil (elimination half-life of 45 to 75 minutes) is likely to be shorter than that of a benzodiazepine agonist. Other studies have also noted that the duration of action of flumazenil is shorter than that of midazolam and that sedation and respiratory depression may recur.[19] Flumazenil is therefore not a substitute for careful postoperative monitoring.

Another cautionary note is the possibility of flumazenil precipitating withdrawal in patients who are dependent on the benzodiazepines. Signs of benzodiazepine withdrawal include flushes, agitation, tremor, and seizures. Resedation with a benzodiazepine or barbiturate may be required in these circumstances. Although some studies suggest the amnesia from the benzodiazepines is reversed by flumazenil, this is not consistently observed.[8]

General Therapeutic Uses

Obviously not everyone requires pharmacotherapy for anxiety, fear, and apprehension; anxious states are often brought on by a series of events that eventually pass, allowing the anxiety to subside. Only when anxiety becomes chronic, or when it interferes with the person's functioning, is pharmacotherapy indicated. It should be remembered that benzodiazepines and other antianxiety agents are not curative but merely treat the symptoms of anxiety. The patient then copes more effectively with the situation or responds more favorably to psychotherapy or other pharmacotherapy. Approximately 35% of patients with a generalized anxiety disorder show marked improvement with benzodiazepines; 40% are moderately improved, and 25% remain unresponsive.[14] These antianxiety agents are useful in the treatment of acute anxiety resulting from transient stress, whether environmental, physical, or psychologic in origin. For the treatment of long-standing anxiety, benzodiazepines should ideally be used only with appropriate psychotherapy. Sometimes benzodiazepines are prescribed inappropriately and with too little supervision. Despite concerns about the abuse potential of the benzodiazepines, which can be a very real problem, patients who have no prior history of drug abuse are unlikely to be at risk. Table 13-4 lists benzodiazepines and other drugs used for the management of acute anxiety.

Although capable of selectively relieving anxiety, benzodiazepines are also CNS depressants capable of producing sedation and hypnosis. Some of the benzodiazepines, namely flurazepam, temazepam, triazolam, estazolam, and quazepam, are promoted specifically as hypnotics rather than as antianxiety agents. Whether a benzodiazepine is used primarily as an antianxiety agent or a hypnotic depends on a subtle interplay of the drug's pharmacodynamic properties, its pharmacokinetic characteristics, and the manufacturer's marketing strategy.

During natural sleep, human beings cycle through several stages of sleep ranging from the deepest stage, categorized as

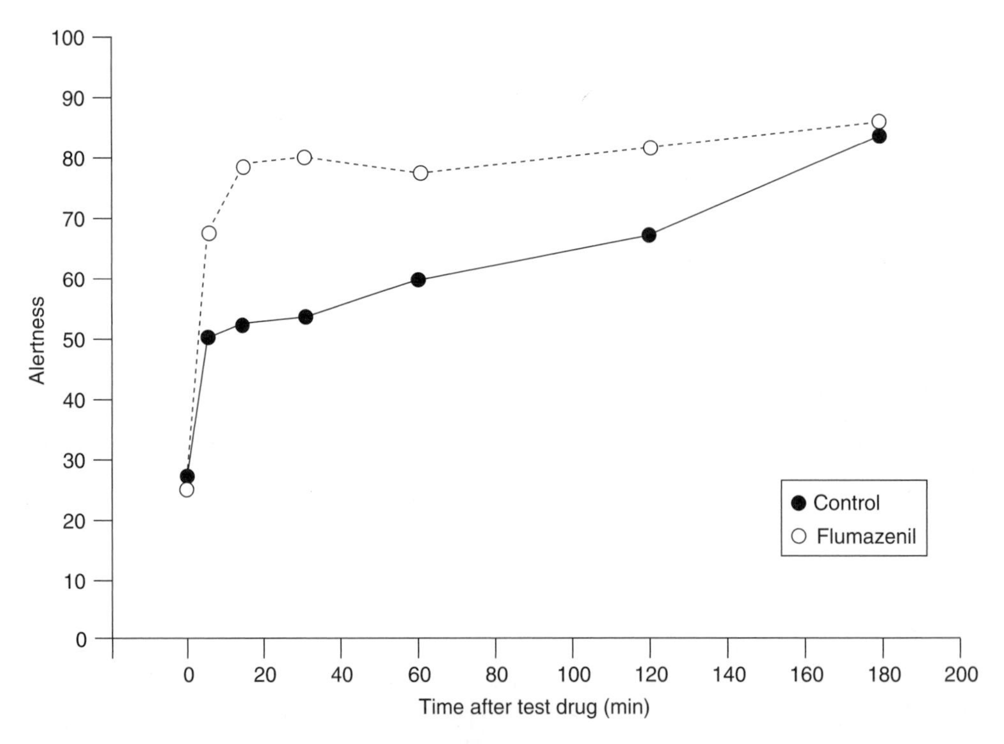

Fig. 13-7 Reversal of midazolam sedation by flumazenil in patients undergoing a surgical dental extraction. Flumazenil or placebo was administered after intravenous midazolam and dental extraction. Differences between flumazenil and control groups were significant at the $p < 0.05$ level for the 5-, 15-, and 30-minute time periods. The *dashed line* represents the flumazenil group; the *solid line* represents the placebo group. (Adapted from Clark MS, Lindenmuth JE, Jafek BW, et al: Reversal of central benzodiazepine effects by intravenous flumazenil, *Anesth Prog* 38:12-16, 1991.)

Table • 13-4

Preparations for the Treatment of Anxiety

DRUG	USUAL DOSE* (mg)	ROUTE OF ADMINISTRATION
Alprazolam	0.75-4.0 (adult)	Oral
	0.5-0.75 (elderly)	Oral
Clorazepate	15-60 (adult)	Oral
	7.5-15 (elderly)	Oral
Chlordiazepoxide	15-100 (adult)	Oral
	50-100 (adult)	IM, IV
	10-20 (elderly)	Oral
Diazepam	4-40 (adult)	Oral
	2-20 (adult)	IM, IV
	2-5 (elderly)	Oral
	0.3-0.6 mg/kg (children)	Oral
Halazepam	60-160 (adult)	Oral
	20-40 (elderly)	Oral
Lorazepam	1.5-10 (adult)	Oral
	1-2 (elderly)	Oral
	2-4 (adult)	IM, IV
Midazolam	2-10 (adult)	IM, IV
	0.25-1 mg/kg up to 20 mg (children)	Oral
Oxazepam	30-120 (adult)	Oral
	30-60 (elderly)	Oral
Prazepam	20-60 (adult)	Oral
	10-15 (elderly)	Oral
Triazolam	0.25-0.5 (adult)	Oral
	0.125 (elderly)	Oral
Hydroxyzine (hydrochloride and pamoate salts)†	200-600 (adult)	Oral
	25-100 (adult)	IM
	0.5-0.7 mg/kg (children)	Oral
	12.5-50 (children >6 years)	Oral
	0.6-1.1 mg/kg (children)	IM
Meprobamate	1200-2400 (adult)	Oral
	100-200 (children 6 to 12 years)	Oral

*Oral adult and elderly doses represent daily amounts given in divided doses (except triazolam). Parenteral, children, and triazolam doses reflect single administration.

†The pamoate salt is reported to be converted to the hydrochloride salt in the stomach, with a resultant prolonged effect, but there is no experimental evidence to support this claim.

stage IV, to the most active form, known as *rapid eye movement (REM) sleep.* Benzodiazepines used as hypnotics increase stage II sleep at the expense of stages I, III, and IV and REM sleep. The significance of these changes is unknown, but a goal of the pharmacotherapy of insomnia is to achieve a normal sleep pattern. The sedative-hypnotic benzodiazepines may have an advantage over the barbiturates with regard to REM sleep. For instance, low doses of temazepam and flurazepam may leave REM sleep unaffected, and triazolam has such a short duration of effect that an early loss of REM cycles may be made up later in the same sleep period. On the other hand, slow-wave sleep (as in stage IV) is now recognized as the most important restorative phase of sleep, and benzodiazepine suppression of slow-wave sleep may be equally problematic with long-term administration as are the effects of barbiturates on REM sleep.

Because hypnotics are most commonly used for the treatment of patients who have difficulty falling asleep, rapid absorption is essential. Most of the hypnotic benzodiazepines are rapidly absorbed after oral administration, and various dosage forms have been formulated to hasten absorption.

Discontinuation of a benzodiazepine after long-term administration can lead to a pronounced withdrawal phenomenon and rebound insomnia in which the duration of sleep is reduced and its quality affected.[49] Because this temporary effect can cause patients to assume that the drug is still needed for satisfactory sleep, they should be made aware of the possibility of rebound insomnia if therapy is abruptly terminated. Actually, rebound insomnia need not be an automatic consequence of drug abstinence. Withdrawal symptoms and rebound insomnia can be minimized with longer-acting benzodiazepines because of the gradual decline of their active metabolites over time.[26]

In addition to relief of anxiety and insomnia, benzodiazepines are useful for a number of other conditions. They are generally accepted as major drugs for the treatment of alcohol withdrawal. Clonazepam has been approved as an anticonvulsant for several types of epilepsy, and diazepam, midazolam, and lorazepam are major drugs for the control of status epilepticus (see Chapter 14). Intravenous diazepam and midazolam are also used in the control of seizures caused by local anesthetics. The skeletal muscle relaxant properties of diazepam have led to its successful use in the treatment of tetanus and for the relief of the spasticity associated with cerebral palsy. Diazepam has been widely used as an adjunct in general anesthesia, but midazolam is now more popular (see Chapter 18). Benzodiazepines (especially alprazolam) find some use in the treatment of depression because of their rapid onset, their antianxiety properties (which are often desirable in depression), and their low potential for lethal overdose. In general, the benzodiazepines are more useful for reactive or neurotic depression, in which anxiety and insomnia are major components, than for severe depression.

ZOLPIDEM AND ZALEPLON

Zolpidem is a novel short-acting hypnotic having an imidazopyridine structure (Figure 13-8). Zaleplon is a pharmacologically similar drug that belongs to the pyrazolopyridine class of compounds. Although unrelated chemically to the benzodiazepines, both drugs are selective agonists at central BZ_1 receptor sites. This selectivity may dictate why they exert little skeletal muscle relaxation or anticonvulsant activity.[68] They have little effect on REM sleep and appear to induce a physiologic pattern of slow-wave sleep. Rebound insomnia at recommended doses, if it occurs, is mild. The drugs are particularly interesting because they establish that the benzodiazepine structure is not an absolute requirement for a compound to act as a benzodiazepine receptor agonist.

Zolpidem and zaleplon have the advantage of being very rapidly absorbed after oral administration, with clinically demonstrable effects occurring in 15 to 20 minutes. Zolpidem has a half-life of approximately 2.5 hours and is metabolized in the liver to inactive metabolites. Zaleplon is similar except its half-life is about 1 hour. Adverse effects include dizziness, drowsiness, and gastrointestinal symptoms. Increases in hepatic enzymes in the plasma suggest that these drugs may not be suitable for patients with liver disease. Conversely, zolpidem is a sedative-hypnotic of choice for pregnant women (FDA pregnancy category B). Also in contrast to the benzodiazepines, neither zolpidem nor zaleplon is contraindicated in patients with a history of narrow-angle glaucoma. Flumazenil effectively reverses the CNS depression produced by the selective BZ_1 receptor agonists. These properties collectively help explain why these two drugs are now the most commonly prescribed sedative-hypnotics in the United States.

BARBITURATES

Chemistry and Structure-Activity Relationships

The basic chemical structure of all barbiturates is barbiturate acid (Figure 13-9). Barbituric acid, formed by the condensation of urea and malonic acid, lacks CNS-depressant activity. To obtain barbiturates that have CNS-depressant properties, both hydrogens at C_5 must be replaced by organic groups. Depending on the substituents added, three types of barbiturates are formed (Table 13-5). In the first group, substitutions are made only at C_5, yielding a large variety of drugs. The addition of a phenyl group at C_5 results in a drug with antiepileptic activity. If the side chain on C_5 reaches eight carbon atoms, the drug becomes more toxic and assumes convulsant properties. When alkyl groups are substituted at N_3, the N-

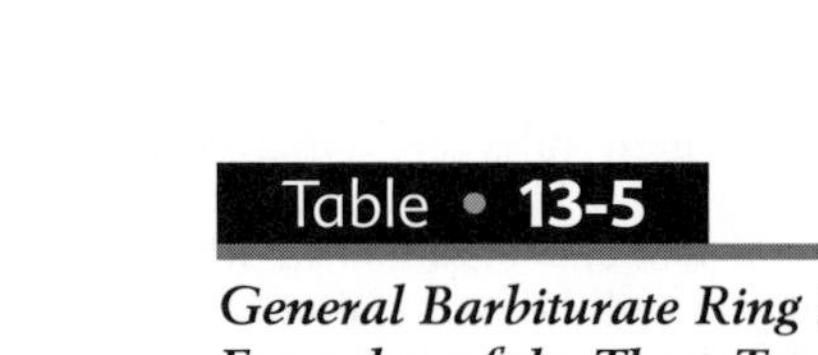

Zolpidem

Fig. 13-8 Structural formula of zolpidem.

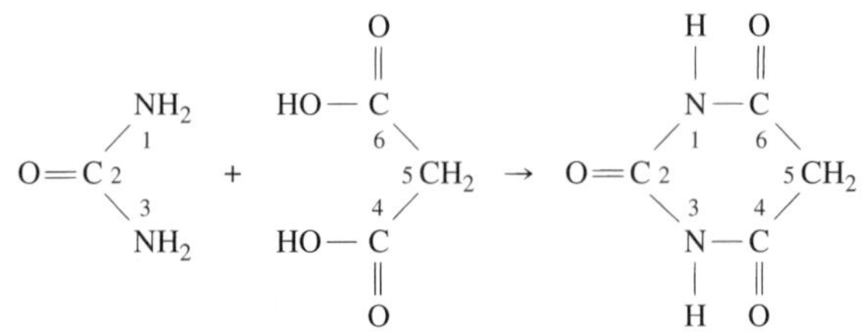

Urea Malonic acid Barbituric acid

Fig. 13-9 Chemical formulation of barbituric acid.

Table • 13-5

General Barbiturate Ring Structure with Examples of the Chemical Formulas of the Three Types of Barbiturates

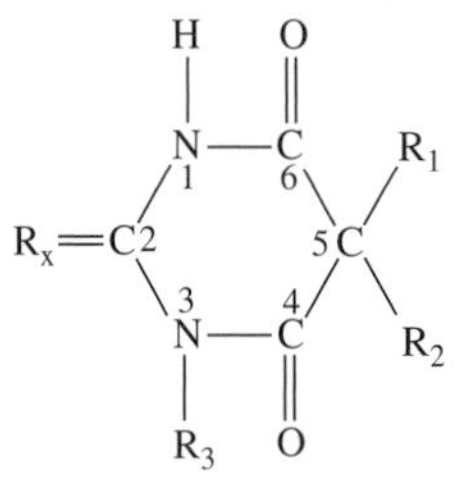

GENERIC NAME	TYPE	R_1	R_2	R_3	R_x
Pentobarbital	Oxybarbiturate	Ethyl	1-Methylbutyl	H	O
Mephobarbital	N-alkylbarbiturate	Ethyl	Phenyl	CH_3	O
Thiopental	Thiobarbiturate	Ethyl	1-Methylbutyl	H	S

alkylbarbiturates are formed. The only N-alkylbarbiturates used clinically are the N-methyl derivatives (mephobarbital and methohexital).

A third class of barbiturates is formed when the oxygen at C_2 of the barbiturate nucleus is replaced with a sulfur atom. Technically, the sulfur-substituted drugs are not true barbiturates because, by definition, barbiturates require oxygen at C_2. The sulfur-substituted barbiturates are commonly referred to as *thiobarbiturates,* whereas the true barbiturates are sometimes called *oxybarbiturates.* Thiopental and thiamylal are examples of thiobarbiturates.

The clinical properties of barbiturates vary considerably depending on the lipid/aqueous partition coefficient. As lipid solubility of the barbiturate increases, hypnotic activity increases, the onset time decreases, and the duration of action decreases. With their extreme lipid solubility, thiopental and thiamylal have an extremely short duration of action and are commonly used as intravenous anesthetics (see Chapters 18 and 48).

Mechanism of Action

The mechanism by which the barbiturates exert their CNS-depressant effect is not completely established, but many pharmacologic effects bear striking similarities to those of the benzodiazepines. Barbiturates enhance GABA binding and increase the duration of GABA-activated Cl^- channel opening by acting at specific barbiturate binding sites on the $GABA_A$ receptor complex (see Figure 13-3), leading to hyperpolarization and decreased neuronal firing.[31,49] Barbiturates thus modulate GABA receptor function to prolong both presynaptic and postsynaptic inhibition. Although the benzodiazepines increase the frequency (as opposed to increasing the duration) of Cl^- channel opening, the end result (increased inhibition) is similar for the two groups of compounds. Their similar therapeutic and pharmacologic properties are therefore not surprising. At high concentrations, barbiturates also appear to act directly on the Cl^- channel, not requiring the presence of GABA. A third action of the barbiturates is inhibition of a specific subset of glutamate receptors. These latter two actions are not shared by the benzodiazepines and may help explain the lower margin of safety and steeper dose-response relationship for the barbiturates compared with the benzodiazepines.

Pharmacologic Effects

The primary pharmacologic effects of the barbiturates involve the brain and spinal cord, the cardiovascular system, and the respiratory system.

Central nervous system

As with all sedative-hypnotics, the barbiturates depress the CNS to varying degrees, ranging from mild sedation to respiratory arrest and death. Many factors contribute to the level of depression attained: the specific drug, dose, and route of administration; the patient's initial behavioral state; and the environmental surroundings at the time of administration. It has long been known that the physical environment and the psychological state of the patient influence the effectiveness of sedatives and hypnotics. Thus a barbiturate taken at home before retiring for the evening is more likely to produce the desired sedative or hypnotic effect than the same drug taken at a rock concert.

The behavioral effects of the barbiturates indicative of general CNS depression include diminished psychologic performance and responsiveness to external stimuli. Subjectively, the patient experiences relaxation, a feeling of well-being, and drowsiness. Coincident with these subjective feelings, the electroencephalogram (EEG) displays an increase in fast activity (25 to 35 Hz) referred to as *barbiturate activation.* As the dose increases and the patient goes to sleep, an increase in high-amplitude slow waves (2 to 8 Hz) similar to those observed during natural sleep occurs. These high-amplitude slow waves frequently occur in bursts called *spindles.* Occasional periods of electrical silence occur as toxic doses are approached.

The EEG patterns recorded after the administration of barbiturates are similar to those observed during natural sleep, but there are important differences. Barbiturates decrease the time spent in REM sleep. REM sleep is the period in which vivid dreaming occurs; it is also believed to be involved in the consolidation of learning. A person deprived of REM sleep will "make up" the loss by increasing the time spent in REM sleep at a subsequent time. A typical pattern would be an increase in the frequency and duration of REM sleep subsequent to the cessation of barbiturate therapy, leading to "restless sleep." The individual may then find it difficult to have a good night's sleep for several nights without readministration of a sedative-hypnotic. Thus a vicious cycle may be started. With the exception of moderate doses of certain benzodiazepine receptor agonists, all sedative-hypnotics significantly reduce REM sleep.

Although the barbiturates appear to depress all levels of the CNS, the reticular formation—a complex network of neurons, nuclei, and neural pathways that extends throughout the brainstem—is particularly sensitive to the depressant action of some barbiturates. The reticular formation and its rostral thalamocortical projections are referred to collectively as the *ascending reticular activating system (ARAS).* The importance of the ARAS in the modulation of sleep and wakefulness has long been known. Stimulation of appropriate areas of the reticular formation in a sleeping animal causes behavioral arousal and converts the EEG from a characteristic sleep pattern to that of an awake animal. If the appropriate area of the ARAS is experimentally destroyed, the EEG pattern becomes that of a drowsy or sleeping animal.

Cardiovascular system

At sedative doses, barbiturates do not affect the cardiovascular system. At hypnotic doses, they produce mild hypotension and a decrease in heart rate. Progressive depression of the cardiovascular system develops as the dose of barbiturates is increased beyond the hypnotic range.

Respiratory system

Sedative doses of barbiturates have little effect on respiration, but as doses are increased, the barbiturates become progressive respiratory depressants. Medullary respiratory centers are depressed by toxic concentrations of barbiturates, and eventually even the carotid arch and aortic body receptors are depressed. These depressant effects are most apparent with multiple drug regimens used for intravenous sedation and anesthesia.[11,36] The barbiturates increase respiratory reflex activity, such as cough, hiccough, sneezes, and laryngospasm, which complicates their use in anesthesia.

Absorption, Fate, and Excretion

The barbiturates are generally available as sodium salts, which are completely absorbed from the gastrointestinal tract and distributed to nearly all tissues of the body. One of the most important factors determining barbiturate distribution to the brain is lipid solubility. Thiopental, which is highly lipid soluble, readily crosses the blood-brain barrier and, when administered intravenously, attains high concentrations in the CNS in seconds. The high blood flow to the brain also contributes significantly to the entry of thiopental. The placental barrier is equally permeable to the barbiturates, and severe respiratory depression can occur in the fetus if a barbiturate is used during delivery.

Barbiturates such as phenobarbital that are relatively lipid insoluble penetrate the blood-brain barrier slowly. Thus phenobarbital, even if it is administered intravenously, may require up to 15 minutes to produce maximal CNS depression. With oral administration of phenobarbital, sedative effects begin after approximately 1 hour.

Phenobarbital is metabolized by the liver, but 25% to 50% is eliminated unchanged in the urine. Most other barbiturates are transformed completely by the liver to inactive metabolites, which are then excreted by the kidney. The primary mechanism by which the CNS effects of the barbiturates are terminated after a single administration is redistribution from the brain to muscle and other body tissues. Subsequent storage of the barbiturates occurs primarily in body fat. From this depot, the drugs are slowly released, metabolized, and excreted; this slow turnover of drug accounts for the prolonged depressant effect, or hangover, after general anesthesia with thiopental and after sedation with pentobarbital or phenobarbital. On repeated administration, redistribution becomes increasingly less important, and eventually the duration of effect is essentially determined by the elimination half-life.

Long-term use of the barbiturates causes an increase in liver microsomal enzyme activity that results from increased synthesis of enzyme. Increased enzyme activity facilitates the rate of metabolism of many drugs, including the barbiturates themselves, and gives rise to a number of drug interactions (see Table 13-3).

The duration of action of the various barbiturates serves as a useful criterion for classification, as illustrated in Table 13-6. As mentioned previously, the onset and duration of action of the barbiturates are inversely related to the agents' respective lipid solubilities.

Adverse Effects and Drug Interactions

The principal toxic reactions associated with the use of the barbiturates result from their effects on the CNS (particularly when combined with other CNS depressants), their abuse potential (see Chapter 51), and their ability to induce hepatic microsomal enzymes.

Because barbiturates are CNS depressants, at high doses they can depress respiration and should not be administered to patients whose respiration is already compromised. Additionally, the intravenously administered anesthetic barbiturates increase the incidence of respiratory complications such as laryngospasm, coughing, sneezing, and hiccough. Confusion, somnolence, and impaired psychomotor performance are other possible undesired consequences of CNS depression. As is the case with benzodiazepines, a number of unusual behavioral reactions have been attributed to the barbiturates. Such reactions include attitudinal depression, agitated toxic psychosis, manic behavior, increased anxiety, hostility, and rage. Careful evaluation reveals that the incidence of these paradoxic responses is very small. In many cases, the response may be predictable if the patient has a history of poor impulse control or aggressive and destructive behavior.

Combining two or more CNS depressant drugs is known to produce increased levels of CNS depression. This summation reaction is the basis for many useful drug combinations in dental therapeutics, such as multidrug intravenous sedation in adults and oral sedation in children.[11,39,40,54] The popularity of "balanced anesthesia" used for general anesthesia is based on the appreciation that CNS depressants have additive effects, and premedication with an opioid such as morphine and the addition of nitrous oxide will permit a significant reduction in the concentration of the primary anesthetic gas required for surgical procedures. The use of combinations of CNS drugs also increases the risk of unexpected oversedation and respiratory depression, particularly if opioids are included in the regimen.[11,39]

Because of the possible severe consequences that may occur with the combination of CNS depressants, dentists routinely inform patients to restrict alcohol consumption after general anesthesia or sedation. This additive drug interaction has been demonstrated in healthy young adults after general anesthesia with thiopental.[28] When 0.7 g/kg of alcohol was administered to these subjects 4 hours after thiopental, performance on psychomotor tests was impaired more than when alcohol alone had been used. This summation reaction has also been demonstrated for oral diazepam[29] and sedative antihistamines such as diphenhydramine and promethazine. Alcohol consumption after sedation therapy can cause severe drowsiness and significantly impair psychomotor performance, including driving skills, and therefore must be restricted.

Some medically compromised patients may have reduced activities of drug-metabolizing enzymes because of hepatic disease, age (both very young and very old), or genetic factors, and thus an exaggerated depressant response to a given regimen of sedative-hypnotics may be anticipated. Some drugs, such as valproic acid, reduce the hepatic clearance of the barbiturates, leading to an enhanced response (see Table 13-3). On the other hand, a number of drug interactions with the barbiturates arise from the ability of these agents to induce hepatic microsomal enzyme activity. Because the dentist administers sedative-hypnotics to patients as single doses or for short regimens, this reaction should not be a problem unless the patient is taking the drugs long term. If hepatic microsomal enzyme activity has been elevated, the effectiveness of warfarin and other drugs metabolized by this enzyme system will be decreased. Many potentially dangerous drug interactions may be prevented simply by obtaining an accurate medical history, keeping a continuous record of drugs (both prescribed and self-administered) taken by the patient, and consulting with the patient's physician when the patient's clinical status or drug history is uncertain.[36]

Barbiturates augment porphyrin synthesis and are therefore strictly contraindicated in patients with acute intermittent porphyria, hereditary coproporphyria, or porphyria variegata. Barbiturates increase the concentration of δ-aminolevulinic acid synthase, the initial enzyme in the synthesis of porphyrin rings found in hemoglobin and other proteins. Because these forms of porphyria are caused by

Table • 13-6

Classification of Barbiturates According to Duration of Action

	ONSET OF EFFECT	DURATION OF EFFECT
Long-acting	1-3 hr*	10 hr
Phenobarbital		
Short- to intermediate-acting	30-60 min*	3-8 hr
Amobarbital		
Pentobarbital		
Secobarbital		
Ultrashort-acting	Immediate†	15-30 min‡
Thiopental		

*Oral administration.
†Intravenous administration.
‡After single intravenous dose.

defective enzymes involved in heme synthesis, blockade of the synthetic pathway downstream from δ-aminolevulinic acid causes porphyrin precursors to build up, leading to an acute exacerbation of the disease.

General Therapeutic Uses

The indications for barbiturates reflect their durations of action and selective effects of some drugs. The long-acting agent phenobarbital is used to manage tonic-clonic seizures and other types of convulsive disorders. Short- and intermediate-acting drugs can be prescribed for sedative-hypnotic purposes, although they are much less commonly used since the advent of the benzodiazepines. Short- and ultrashort-acting barbiturates are administered as intravenous sedatives and anesthetics.

CHLORAL HYDRATE AND OTHER SEDATIVE-HYPNOTICS

Various drugs of diverse chemical structure, including chloral hydrate, paraldehyde, ethchlorvynol, glutethimide, and methyprylon, have sedative-hypnotic properties. Except for chloral hydrate, these agents have few clinical indications in dentistry. Physicians occasionally prescribe these agents, and the dentist should recognize that all depress the CNS.

Pharmacologic Effects

Chloral hydrate, one of the oldest nonbarbiturate sedative-hypnotics, continues to have dental applications. It is available in a liquid preparation that is convenient for the sedation of uncooperative children. In fact, chloral hydrate is a commonly used sedative in children for painless technical procedures such as diagnostic imaging. Similarly, chloral hydrate is a popular sedative-hypnotic in pediatric dentistry. Although its overall safety record is considered acceptable, the therapeutic index of the drug is actually very small. In addition, severe laryngospasm with cardiorespiratory arrest after aspiration of orally administered chloral hydrate in liquid form has been reported.[22] Chloral hydrate is commonly used in combination with other drugs, such as nitrous oxide, hydroxyzine, and promethazine. These agents are useful in augmenting the sedative effect of chloral hydrate and, in the case of promethazine, in relieving the nausea and vomiting produced by chloral hydrate.[24] Because of the drug's low therapeutic index, it is imperative that dose calculations be based on weight when it is used for pediatric sedation.[38] Chloral hydrate has minimal effects on REM sleep, although a dose-dependent depression may occur with higher doses. The drug has been successfully used for the treatment of alcohol withdrawal, but the benzodiazepines are now preferred.

Absorption, Fate, and Excretion

Chloral hydrate is well absorbed after oral or rectal administration and is rapidly converted by the liver to trichloroethanol, which is responsible for the CNS-depressant properties of the parent compound (Figure 13-10). Plasma concentrations of chloral hydrate are nearly undetectable after administration. Trichloroethanol is conjugated with glucuronic acid and excreted in the urine. Trichloroethanol has a half-life of 4 to 12 hours. A portion of chloral hydrate and trichloroethanol is metabolized to di- and trichloroacetic acid. When administered long term, chloral hydrate can induce liver enzyme activity and compete for plasma protein binding sites, giving rise to several drug interactions (see below).[36]

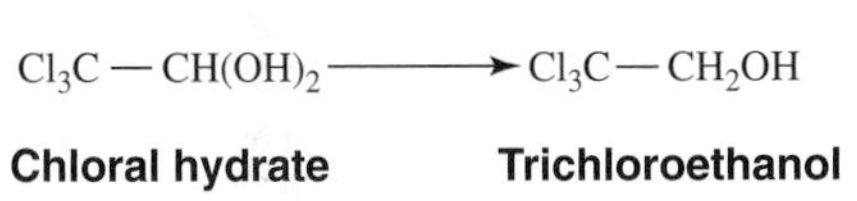

$$Cl_3C-CH(OH)_2 \longrightarrow Cl_3C-CH_2OH$$

Chloral hydrate **Trichloroethanol**

Fig. 13-10 Structural formulas of chloral hydrate and its active metabolite trichloroethanol.

Adverse Effects and Drug Interactions

Choral hydrate has only minor cardiovascular effects in conventional doses. However, as the dose is increased beyond the therapeutic range, cardiovascular depression may occur. Chloral hydrate can precipitate cardiac arrhythmias in the sensitized heart as well as in the apparently healthy heart, and it may have been responsible for the reported death of a patient undergoing third molar extractions.[25] Chloral hydrate and trichloroethanol have chemical structures (see Figure 13-9) that resemble halothane, an anesthetic known to sensitize the myocardium to adrenergic amines. Trichloroacetic acid may also be cardiotoxic. The respiratory effects of sedative doses of chloral hydrate and the other nonbarbiturates are minimal but become more severe as the dose is increased.

Chloral hydrate has been implicated in a variety of drug interactions (see Table 13-4). As one might expect, chloral hydrate produces increased CNS depression when administered with other sedatives. The therapeutic advantage of this drug interaction is that it allows practitioners to decrease the dose of both CNS depressants and therefore limit the side effects of the individual drugs. For example, the reduced dosage requirement for chloral hydrate when combined with the sedative antiemetic promethazine has been shown to appreciably decrease the incidence of nausea and vomiting.[24] Similarly, the use of nitrous oxide in combination with chloral hydrate will deepen the level of sedation. This therapeutic advantage may be lost when nitrous oxide is used in combination with higher doses of chloral hydrate because the CNS depression may be increased to such an extent that the child's protective reflexes become compromised.[40]

Beyond the expected summation of CNS depressant effects, the combination of chloral hydrate with alcohol is thought to produce a potentiation drug interaction through an alteration of alcohol metabolism. Chloral hydrate and its primary metabolite, trichloroethanol, competitively inhibit alcohol-metabolizing dehydrogenases, thereby elevating alcohol blood concentrations (see Table 13-3). This combination, known as a "Mickey Finn" or "knock-out drops," can induce severe alcohol intoxication with stupor, coma, or death. The interaction is significant because it induces greater than additive effects and may result in a potentially life-threatening CNS depression. However, the dental indications for chloral hydrate are almost exclusively in pediatric sedation, and alcohol is usually not a concomitantly administered drug.

Chloral hydrate has been implicated in modifying responses to the oral anticoagulants dicumarol and warfarin. Another metabolite of chloral hydrate, trichloroacetic acid, may increase free warfarin plasma concentrations by interfering with its protein binding (normally 98% to 99%). The possible result is a transient and usually small hypoprothrombinemia. Although caution is indicated, these interactions may be clinically insignificant, particularly with single-dose therapy of chloral hydrate.[36,61] Sedation with benzodiazepine regimens is a recommended alternative.

An unusual interaction characterized by transient diaphoresis, hot flashes, variable blood pressure, and tachycardia has been reported with chloral hydrate and the diuretic furosemide (see Table 13-3).[42] The mechanism is not well understood but may relate to enhanced sensitivity to a chloral hydrate metabolite. Although rarely reported, this is a moderately severe reaction and can occur when furosemide is administered within a day of chloral hydrate.

Chloral hydrate and trichloroethanol can be detected in maternal milk within 15 minutes and for as long as 24 hours after administration. Peak concentrations in milk are sufficient to sedate the infant. A potential caution concerning the widespread use of chloral hydrate in infants and children is that chloral hydrate, trichloroethanol, and trichloroacetic acid are all metabolites of trichloroethylene,[52] an industrial solvent, environmental contaminant, and carcinogen. Chloral hydrate is also a mutagen and can cause chromosomal damage. Although no indication of human toxicity has been found with therapeutic uses of chloral hydrate, these concerns have decreased the popularity of chloral hydrate for use in pediatric dentistry.

ANTIHISTAMINES

A common side effect of the first-generation H_1 antihistamines is drowsiness and sedation. This response is probably caused by receptor antagonism of histamine neurotransmitter receptors within the CNS. Antihistamines such as hydroxyzine, a piperazine derivative, and promethazine, a phenothiazine derivative, have proved to be useful adjuncts in sedation regimens (see Chapter 48). Part of their popularity relates to their ability to augment the sedative effects of other sedative-hypnotics and to reduce the incidence of nausea and vomiting. Similarly, the ethanolamine antihistamine diphenhydramine, although used primarily for the management of allergic reactions, is also marketed as an over-the-counter agent to treat motion sickness and insomnia.

The chemical structure of hydroxyzine, the most popular antihistamine used for its sedative effects, is shown in Figure 13-11. Hydroxyzine's depression of CNS activity appears to be primarily subcortical. Bronchodilator, peripheral antihistaminic, antiemetic, and analgesic properties have also been clinically demonstrated.

Pharmacologic Effects

All the first-generation H_1 antihistamines produce mild CNS depression. These drugs also have prominent and sometimes beneficial anticholinergic, antihistaminic, and antiemetic properties. The only side effects that may be of concern with these compounds at therapeutic doses are drowsiness and dry mouth. Additive effects occur if these drugs are used in conjunction with other CNS depressants.

Hydroxyzine has a very slight depressant effect on the cardiovascular and respiratory systems. Like other antihistamines, hydroxyzine has antiarrhythmic properties and may cause bronchodilation. Hydroxyzine appears to have a slight analgesic effect and, when combined with morphine, produces greater analgesia than morphine alone. Hydroxyzine is helpful in diminishing the emetic effects of opioids, but the hydroxyzine-opioid combination produces significant drowsiness. When used as an adjunct to anesthesia, hydroxyzine has been reported to potentiate significantly the effects of barbiturates as well as opioids such as meperidine; reduction of total doses of these CNS depressant drugs is indicated.

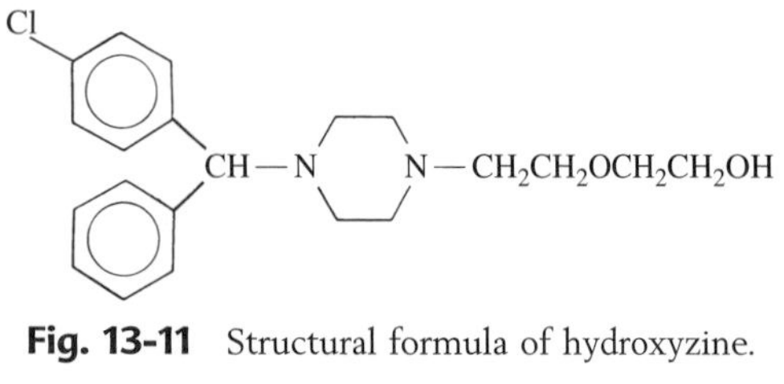

Cl

CH—N N—$CH_2CH_2OCH_2CH_2OH$

Fig. 13-11 Structural formula of hydroxyzine.

Absorption, Fate, and Excretion

Hydroxyzine is rapidly absorbed from the gastrointestinal tract, and pharmacologic effects may begin within 15 to 30 minutes. Peak concentrations are achieved in 1 to 3 hours. The metabolic fate of hydroxyzine includes hepatic conversion to the lipid-soluble derivative norchlorcyclizine and the water-soluble hydroxyzine N-oxide. Hydroxyzine N-oxide is excreted rapidly, whereas norchlorcyclizine is excreted slowly and tends to accumulate in the body. The second-generation antihistamine cetirizine is an active carboxylated metabolite and contributes to the clinical effect. The terminal elimination half-life for hydroxyzine is approximately 1 day in adults but considerably shorter in children.

Adverse Effects and Drug Interactions

Hydroxyzine is generally considered to have low toxicity. The CNS depressant effect of hydroxyzine summates with that of other CNS depressants. There are indications that norchlorcyclizine may be dangerous to the fetus, but such an effect has been demonstrated experimentally only at doses 50 to 100 times those considered to be therapeutic. Parenteral hydroxyzine is available for intramuscular injection only. Tissue necrosis is associated with subcutaneous or intraarterial injections, and hemolysis may occur after intravenous administration.

GENERAL THERAPEUTIC USES OF SEDATIVE-HYPNOTICS

The use of barbiturate sedative hypnotics to relieve fear and anxiety during dental procedures has been supplanted by the benzodiazepines. Chloral hydrate and the antihistamine sedatives are still used in pediatric dentistry.[41] Agents that are useful as sedative-hypnotics are listed in Table 13-7. Barbiturates, particularly the ultrashort-acting agents, are useful in anesthesia and intravenous conscious sedation to deepen CNS depression for brief periods. These therapeutic indications for the sedative hypnotic agents are discussed further in Chapters 18 and 48.

When prescribing sedative-hypnotics for sleep disorders, three categories of insomnia must be considered: long-term, short-term, and transient. The role of sedative-hypnotics in the treatment of long-term insomnia is controversial. Various medical and psychiatric conditions as well as drug dependence and abuse contribute to long-term insomnia. Obviously, in these situations the primary goal of therapy must be directed to correcting the underlying medical condition, with the sedative-hypnotics serving as temporary adjuncts. Short-term insomnia is often associated with emotional reactions to a serious medical illness or stress from family or employment problems. Because this kind of insomnia may last for several weeks, intermittent use of sedative-hypnotic agents may be appropriate. Transient insomnia occurs in persons who normally do not have insomnia but whose sleep is adversely affected as a result of acute stress or alterations in their environment. This kind of insomnia is most often encountered in dentistry because of a patient's apprehension regarding scheduled procedures. The sedative-hypnotics are administered in dentistry to relax and calm the anxious patient as well as to facilitate sleep preoperatively.

Evidence from sleep laboratories has shed new light on the physiologic roles and mechanisms of sleep and has invalidated some faulty, ill-conceived ideas about sleep. For example, not every individual requires 8 hours of sleep; many persons who think they have insomnia really do not; sleep patterns, even in the normal individual, sometimes fluctuate; and psychological therapy often is more rational and beneficial than drugs. It is recommended, therefore, that insomnia be

Table • 13-7

Preparations and Doses of Some Sedative-Hypnotics

		ADULT DOSE (mg)	
	ROUTE OF ADMINISTRATION	SEDATION	HYPNOSIS
Barbiturates*			
Pentobarbital	O, R, IM, IV	§	100
Secobarbital	O, R, IM, IV	§	100-200
Benzodiazepines			
Clorazepate	O	7.5-15	15-30
Diazepam†	O, IM, IV	2-10	10
Flurazepam	O	15	15-30
Lorazepam	O, IM, IV	1-3	2-4
Quazepam	O	7.5-30	7.5-30
Temazepam	O	7.5-15	15-30
Triazolam	O	0.125-0.25	0.125-0.5
Chloral Derivatives			
Chloral hydrate‡	O, R		500-1000
Selective $GABA_A$ Receptor Agonists			
Zaleplon	O	§	5-20
Zolpidem	O	§	5-10

O, Oral; *R*, rectal; *IM*, intramuscular; *IV*, intravenous.
*Dose for children for preoperative sedation, 2 mg/kg.
†Dose for children for preoperative sedation, 0.04 to 0.6 mg/kg.
‡Dose for children for preoperative sedation, 50 mg/kg up to 1000 mg.
§Rarely or never used as a daytime sedative.

approached not by automatically prescribing a sedative-hypnotic drug. Rather, a careful assessment of the type, cause, and severity of the insomnia should first be made. Temporary and rational use of a sedative-hypnotic may then be indicated.

AZASPIRODECANEDIONES

Buspirone (Figure 13-12), an azaspirone (short for azaspirodecanedione) derivative structurally unrelated to the benzodiazepines, represents a unique class of antianxiety agents. Buspirone has antianxiety effects that are therapeutically equivalent to those of diazepam, but it lacks the more prominent CNS depressant effects as well as the anticonvulsant and muscle relaxant properties of the benzodiazepines. In addition, buspirone does not augment the sedative effect of ethyl alcohol or other sedatives and has little effect on psychomotor or cognitive function. Physical dependence does not occur; neither does withdrawal at abrupt cessation. This drug has a more anxiolytic-selective profile than the benzodiazepines, thus representing a major advance in antianxiety therapy and a useful alternative to the benzodiazepines.

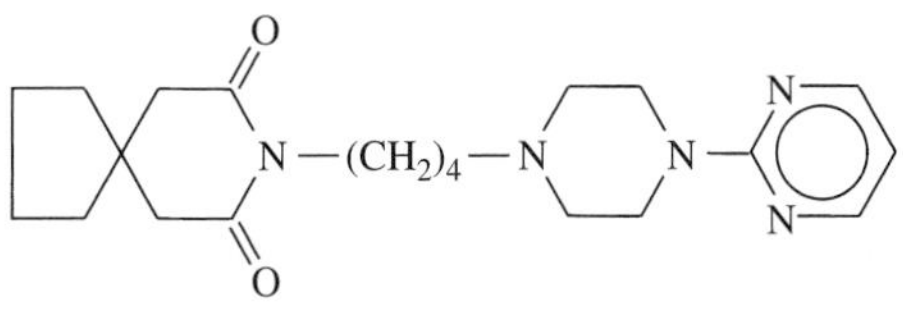

Fig. 13-12 Structural formula of buspirone.

Although the mechanism of antianxiety action of buspirone is unknown, it appears to diminish serotonergic tone. Buspirone is a partial $5\text{-}HT_{1A}$ agonist at both presynaptic $5\text{-}HT_{1A}$ autoregulatory receptors, which results in decreased 5-HT synthesis and release, and at postsynaptic $5\text{-}HT_{1A}$ receptors, which diminishes the effects of 5-HT.[67] Studies have demonstrated dense labeling by radiolabeled buspirone of limbic structures (amygdala, hippocampus, entorhinal cortex) that have high affinity for $5\text{-}HT_{1A}$ ligands. Furthermore, in animal studies, neurotoxins that selectively destroy tryptaminergic systems abolish the activity of buspirone.[15] There is, therefore, good evidence for a tryptaminergic mechanism for the anxiolytic action of buspirone.[21] However, although buspirone does not bind to the GABA-benzodiazepine receptor complex, the benzodiazepine antagonist flumazenil can block the antianxiety effect of ipsapirone,[30] a buspirone derivative, suggesting an interaction between benzodiazepine and tryptaminergic systems.

Peak plasma concentrations of buspirone are reached in less than 1 hour, but this may vary from patient to patient. Buspirone is extensively metabolized, with both active and inactive metabolites excreted in the urine and feces. The elimination half-life ranges from 2 to 8 hours.

Adverse effects of buspirone, such as headache, dizziness, nervousness, paresthesia, and gastrointestinal upset, are similar to those of the benzodiazepines but milder. Buspirone does not appear to produce additive sedative effects with the concomitant use of ethanol, a major advantage over the benzodiazepines. Additionally, buspirone does not seem to produce significant CNS depression, which may offer a major clinical advantage for those patients who, because of their employment, cannot afford an impairment in psychomotor skills. The abrupt withdrawal of buspirone is not associated with rebound anxiety or withdrawal symptoms. In fact, there have been reports that patients taking long-term diazepam who are quickly switched to buspirone may exhibit signs of increased anxiety and withdrawal because buspirone does not suppress benzodiazepine withdrawal or show cross-tolerance with the benzodiazepines. Switching a patient who is currently taking long-term benzodiazepines to buspirone is accomplished by initiating low doses of buspirone and gradually tapering the dosage of benzodiazepine. Another problem associated with the use of buspirone is the long delay (1 to 3 weeks) to onset of clinical effects. This limits its usefulness in clinical dentistry.

CENTRALLY ACTING MUSCLE RELAXANTS

Propanediol and Glycerol Derivatives

This group of drugs includes several traditional agents, most of which are used as centrally acting muscle relaxants. They have, however, many effects in common with the benzodiazepines.

Meprobamate, a propanediol carbamate, was considered the agent of choice for the treatment of anxiety in the mid-1950s. However, with the discovery of the addictive properties of this compound and the introduction of the benzodiazepines, its popularity declined rapidly. The pharmacologic profile of meprobamate differs little from the barbiturates, although its antianxiety effects are demonstrable at doses that do not markedly diminish motor or intellectual performance. The site and mechanism of action of meprobamate are not known. Meprobamate depresses polysynaptic pathways more effectively than monosynaptic pathways, thus forming the basis for its classification as an interneuronal blocking agent.

Meprobamate is rapidly absorbed from the gastrointestinal tract and reaches a peak plasma concentration in 2 to 3 hours. The half-life of a single dose of meprobamate is approximately 7 to 15 hours. Like the barbiturates, meprobamate induces hepatic microsomal enzyme activity, but this induction appears to be more selective with meprobamate, and it may not induce its own metabolism. Indeed, the half-life of meprobamate may be as long as 48 hours with long-term therapy.

The CNS depressant properties of meprobamate account for most of its troublesome side effects: somnolence, dizziness, ataxia, and confusion. Allergic reactions consisting of skin eruptions, bronchospasm, hypotension, anuria, and fever have been observed. There have also been reports of blood dyscrasias (aplastic anemia, leukopenia, and agranulocytosis). Toxic doses result in marked respiratory and cardiovascular depression. Perhaps the most serious limitation of meprobamate is the development of physical and psychologic dependence. Withdrawal symptoms (insomnia, restlessness, tremor, and anxiety) are common when the drug is suddenly withdrawn from patients who have received 2 g or more per day for many weeks.

Mephenesin, chlorphenesin, methocarbamol, and carisoprodol are used primarily as centrally acting skeletal muscle relaxants. In 1945 the muscle relaxant effects of aryl-glycerol esters in experimental animals were observed, and, after evaluation of several analogues, mephenesin was introduced for clinical use in 1948. Mephenesin proved to be of limited usefulness because of its short duration of action. Methocarbamol and chlorphenesin have a more prolonged duration of action because of slow metabolic transformation and excretion. Mephenesin and similar drugs have also been shown to reduce polysynaptic spinal reflexes in experimental animals. In human beings, these drugs act as mild sedatives and are used primarily to reduce abnormal muscle activity. Nevertheless, these and other centrally acting muscle relaxants are never used at doses that could cause flaccid paralysis of voluntary muscles.

Centrally acting muscle relaxants should be clearly distinguished from several other classes of drugs that can reduce muscular activity through peripheral mechanisms. The neuromuscular blocking agents, such as tubocurarine and succinylcholine, act by blocking transmission at the neuromuscular junction. Dantrolene, a peripherally acting muscle relaxant, blocks excitation-contraction coupling in skeletal muscle. Curare-like drugs, succinylcholine, and dantrolene have very specific indications for their muscle relaxant properties (see Chapter 10).

Chemistry and structure-activity relationships

The chemical structures of meprobamate, mephenesin, and carisoprodol are shown in Figure 13-13. Meprobamate and carisoprodol are dicarbamate esters of propanediol, which have additional substituents to increase their potency and absorption.

Pharmacologic effects

Table 13-9 compares some pharmacologic characteristics of various classes of drugs discussed in this chapter. Qualitatively, centrally acting muscle relaxants, sedative-hypnotics, and antianxiety drugs are similar pharmacologically, whereas the antihistamines produce sedation that is qualitatively different.

The centrally acting muscle relaxants, of which mephenesin can be taken as the prototype, cause relaxation of voluntary muscle through depression of the CNS. These depressant effects have not been associated with an action on any specific transmitter system or neurologic circuit. Rather, alteration of the excitability of neural membranes in general may be involved. Although early investigations emphasized depression of spinal interneurons as the mechanism of action, these agents generally reduce neural activity in a variety of brain structures, including the brainstem, thalamus, and basal ganglia. Furthermore, certain agents that do not produce muscle relaxation also show some preferential depression of polysynaptic reflexes; thus depression of interneurons is not an identifying characteristic of this class. At progressively larger doses, sedation, hypnosis, unconsciousness, and death occur. Elevation of the convulsant threshold can be demonstrated. The drugs are used orally.

The cardiovascular effects of sedative doses of the centrally acting muscle relaxants of the mephenesin type are minimal. Adequate cardiovascular performance is usually maintained at doses higher than those that produce respiratory depression. However, the problems of shock and renal failure can complicate recovery from toxic doses of the agents.

Miscellaneous Drugs Affecting Skeletal Muscle

Significantly different from the glycerol and propanediol derivatives, orphenadrine (see Figure 13-13) is an analogue of the antihistamine diphenhydramine. The pharmacologic profile of orphenadrine, an antihistamine, differs from that of compounds similar to mephenesin. Conventional antihistamines, in addition to blocking histamine receptors, are frequently anticholinergic and produce drowsiness and sedation. This sedation is of a different character from that produced by mephenesinlike drugs; increasing the dose of an antihistamine leads to hallucinations, delusions, and convulsions. Nevertheless, because the dose-response curve for antihistamines is rather flat, these drugs have been considered

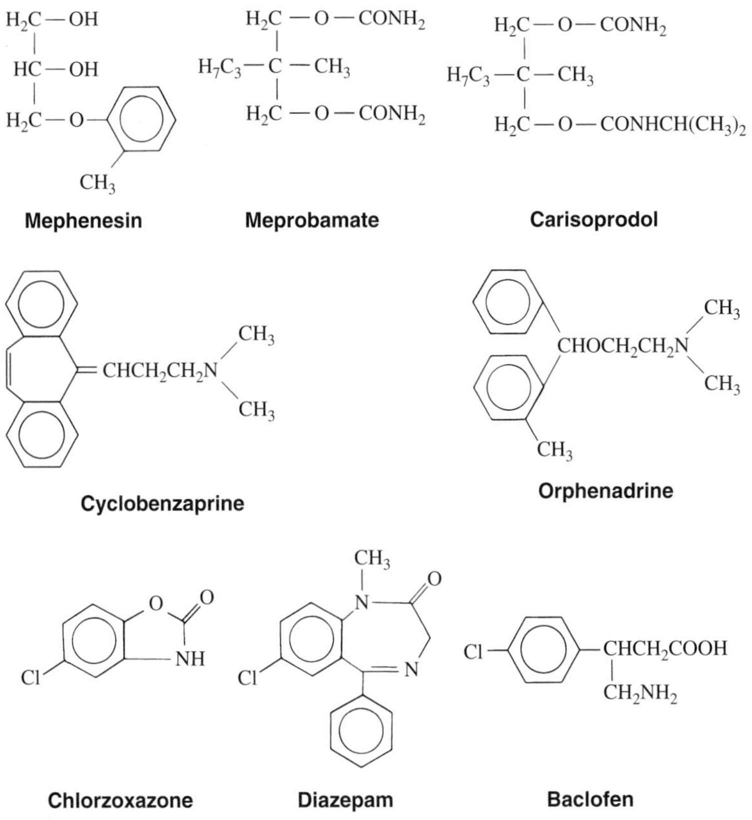

Mephenesin

Meprobamate

Carisoprodol

Cyclobenzaprine

Orphenadrine

Chlorzoxazone

Diazepam

Baclofen

Fig. 13-13 Structural formulas of some centrally acting muscle relaxants.

Table • 13-8

Pharmacologic Comparison of Centrally Acting Muscle Relaxants, Sedative-Hypnotics, Antianxiety Drugs, and Antihistamines

PHARMACOLOGIC PROPERTIES	CENTRALLY ACTING MUSCLE RELAXANTS (PROTOTYPE MEPHENESIN)	SEDATIVE-HYPNOTICS (PROTOTYPE PHENOBARBITAL)	ANTIANXIETY DRUGS (PROTOTYPE DIAZEPAM)	ANTIHISTAMINES (PROTOTYPE DIPHENHYDRAMINE)
Anticholinergic properties	No	No	Mild	Yes
Antihistaminic properties	No	No	No	Yes
Paradoxic low-dose excitement	Yes	Yes	Yes	No
Ataxia	Yes	Yes	Yes	No
Anesthesia	Yes	Yes	Variable	No
Arousal at high doses	Difficult	Difficult	Difficult	Easy
Lethal effect	Respiratory depression	Respiratory depression	Respiratory depression	Convulsions
Convulsant threshold	Raised	Raised	Raised	Lowered
Dependence liability	Yes, but usually mild	Yes	Yes, but usually mild	No

relatively safe and have been widely used in over-the-counter sleep aids for this reason. Physical dependence liability is also minimal. Orphenadrine has been used primarily as an adjunct in the treatment of Parkinson's disease. Compared with the mephenesin group of drugs, no special advantage has been demonstrated for orphenadrine as a muscle relaxant.

Cyclobenzaprine (see Figure 13-13), a structural and pharmacologic analogue of the tricyclic antidepressants, is used for the short-term (2 to 3 weeks) treatment of muscle spasm associated with acute painful musculoskeletal conditions. One hypothesis for its mechanism of action is that it increases brainstem norepinephrine-mediated inhibition of ventral motor neurons of the spinal cord. Its effectiveness is similar to that of diazepam, but it produces more xerostomia, drowsiness, tachycardia, and dizziness. Many tricyclic antidepressants have significant antihistaminic effects, and the general pharmacologic properties of cyclobenzaprine are similar to those shown in Table 13-8 for the antihistamines. Metaxalone and chlorzoxazone (see Figure 13-13) are heterocyclic carbamates that demonstrate muscle-relaxing properties.

The α_2-adrenergic receptor agonist tizanidine is a centrally acting muscle relaxant used for spasticity states, especially multiple sclerosis and spasticity arising from spinal cord injury. Within the spinal cord, the medullary locus ceruleus, and the substantia nigra, α_2 receptors have been shown to contribute to its action.[57,59] It is interesting that other centrally acting muscle relaxants, namely midazolam and baclofen, also depress spinal reflexes when applied directly to the substantia nigra.[59] Tizanidine is similar to clonidine, an α_2 agonist used to lower blood pressure and to treat certain kinds of drug withdrawal.

Baclofen has been shown to stimulate $GABA_B$ receptors, which are G protein–linked receptors and are not coupled to Cl^- channels in the nerve membrane.[5] These $GABA_B$ receptors may inhibit motor tone by reducing the release of excitatory amino acid transmitters, reducing Ca^{++} conductance, and increasing K^+ conductance. Blocking the receptor sites for excitatory amino acid transmitters may be a mechanism of action applicable to other centrally acting muscle relaxants. Baclofen, the *p*-chlorophenyl analogue of GABA, is recommended in multiple sclerosis or traumatic spinal cord injury for the relief of spasticity. Baclofen is also used to treat trigeminal neuralgia.

Although a considerable number of agents are available as centrally acting muscle relaxants, the most commonly used drug for many muscle spasms is diazepam or another long-acting benzodiazepine. The benzodiazepines are thought to act primarily within the CNS, where they increase the response to GABA at $GABA_A$ receptor sites. Benzodiazepines, although they tend to have more sedative properties than some of the drugs used almost exclusively as centrally acting muscle relaxants, have a favorable clinical profile compared with the latter agents because of their relatively strong muscle-relaxing properties and relatively low toxic and physical dependence liabilities.[49]

Adverse Effects

Muscle relaxants are generally used at sedative doses, and these drugs have limited effectiveness in the treatment of muscle spasms. Data obtained from experimental animals compare the relative safety of some commonly prescribed muscle relaxants (Table 13-9). The therapeutic index for muscle relaxation as well as other effects is many times greater for benzodiazepines than for barbiturates. The other clinically useful muscle relaxants have therapeutic indexes between these extremes.

Tolerance and physical dependence develop with the long-term administration of muscle relaxants, but, in general, withdrawal is mild although qualitatively similar to that seen with other CNS depressant drugs. Side effects associated with centrally acting muscle relaxants are primarily related to effects on the CNS: drowsiness, dizziness, headache, blurred vision, ataxia, lethargy, paradoxic excitement, and nystagmus. Gastrointestinal symptoms such as vomiting, heartburn, nausea, anorexia, and abdominal distress have been reported. Allergic reactions may also occur and include skin rash, pruritus, and fever. Cyclobenzaprine has some additional side effects that stem from its actions on the autonomic nervous system. Because it has substantial anticholinergic properties, its use should be especially avoided in certain conditions (e.g., narrow-angle glaucoma, prostatic hypertrophy). Because of its effect on norepinephrine reuptake, cyclobenzaprine may also be contraindicated in patients for whom increased sympathetic activity is to be avoided (e.g., in persons with hyperthyroidism or recovering from a myocardial infarction). A report of a manic episode after cyclobenzaprine use in a patient with a history of psychosis suggests that cyclobenzaprine should also be avoided in such patients.[4]

Baclofen can cause drowsiness, ataxia, and confusion, which may be especially troublesome in the elderly. Acute toxicity may lead to respiratory depression and seizures. Sudden withdrawal from therapeutic doses is associated with a high risk of hallucinations and tachycardia. Cessation of therapy should involve tapering the doses over several days.

Drug interactions with the centrally acting muscle relaxants are of several kinds. First, these drugs augment the depressant actions of each other and of the opioids, other sedatives (including ethanol),[58] antianxiety drugs, antihistamines, and antidepressants.[36] Second, drug interactions can occur when these agents induce drug- and hormone-metabolizing enzymes of the liver. Although the degree of enzyme induction varies substantially among the various sedatives, caution should be used in patients taking anticoagulants and in those with porphyria. Third, increased skeletal muscle relaxation should be expected when the centrally acting muscle relaxants are given with drugs whose primary pharmacologic activity is neuromuscular blockade (e.g., succinylcholine) or with drugs that have such an activity as a side effect (e.g., the aminoglycosides or volatile general anesthetics). Fourth, cyclobenzaprine should not be given to patients taking MAO inhibitors or guanethidine and related drugs. (Barbiturates, benzodiazepines, and other sedatives should be used with considerable caution with MAO inhibitors.) Fifth, because the muscle relaxant actions of diazepam are partially reversed by aminophylline,[60] patients being treated with diazepam should avoid the use of xanthine-containing foods.

General Therapeutic Uses

Centrally acting muscle relaxants are used medically as adjuncts to rest, physical therapy, and other measures for the relief of discomfort associated with acute, painful musculoskeletal conditions. They have been promoted for use in

Table • 13-9

Comparison of the Ataxic and Lethal Doses of Central Depressant Drugs in Mice

AGENT	LD_{50} (mg/kg)	ATAXIA ED_{50} (mg/kg)	THERAPEUTIC INDEX
Phenobarbital	242	120	2.0
Mephenesin	610	178	3.4
Meprobamate	800	235	3.4
Carisoprodol	980	165	5.9
Chlordiazepoxide	720	100	7.2
Diazepam	620	30	20.7

skeletal muscle spasms of local origin, multiple sclerosis, cerebral palsy, sprains, strains, fibrositis, rheumatoid spondylitis, bursitis, the urethral syndrome, and arthritis. Drugs such as salicylates and adrenal corticosteroids may be used concomitantly. Longer-acting nonsteroidal antiinflammatory agents are perceived as having an advantage in many of these disorders.

Certain conditions of skeletal muscle, such as muscle spasm or trismus, are believed to be the result of dysfunctional output patterns from the motor areas of the CNS to skeletal muscle. Drugs that could prevent or lessen these neurotropic influences on voluntary muscle would be helpful in physical medicine and dentistry. The centrally acting muscle relaxants, which overlap pharmacologically with the antianxiety drugs, represent a diverse group of drugs whose pharmacologic effects include diminished output of nerve impulses to voluntary muscle. Benzodiazepines are sometimes used to alleviate abnormal muscle contractions by depressing polysynaptic CNS pathways, including polysynaptic spinal reflexes. Some newer benzodiazepine partial agonists have a minimum amount of muscle relaxant activity.[16] Thus full agonist agents such as diazepam should be used if muscle relaxation is desired.

β-ADRENERGIC RECEPTOR–BLOCKING DRUGS

The β-adrenergic receptor–blocking agent propranolol is not approved for the treatment of anxiety, but it is effective in decreasing the peripheral autonomic symptoms of anxiety (e.g., tremor, tachycardia, palpitation). Propranolol may be used for healthy patients who have disabling situational anxiety, or it may be combined with a benzodiazepine in patients who have the somatic manifestations of anxiety. Propranolol has gained some popularity with performing actors and musicians in preventing "stage fright." It is not appropriate or effective for the treatment of chronic anxiety.

IMPLICATIONS FOR DENTISTRY

Drugs Used as Sedative-Hypnotics

There is little difference between the dental and medical uses of the sedative-hypnotics. Whether used by the dentist or physician, the common desired therapeutic response is sedation or hypnosis. Additional therapeutic applications for the sedative-hypnotics are also discussed in detail in Chapters 14 (anticonvulsant drugs), 18 (general anesthetics), and 48 (management of fear and anxiety).

As a class, the benzodiazepines are very safe and highly effective agents for producing sedation and sleep.

Zolpidem and zaleplon appear to offer advantages similar to those described for the benzodiazepines: they are well tolerated, have a high margin of safety and a shallow dose-response profile. In addition, their rapid onset of action makes it possible for the patient to take the drugs immediately before bedtime.

Despite the declining use of barbiturates, they can occasionally be helpful in dentistry. Barbiturates are effective and relatively inexpensive. A wide range in duration of effect can be attained depending on the drug and dose prescribed. The problems frequently associated with long-term use of barbiturates, such as tolerance and drug interactions, do not generally apply to their short-term use. However, the barbiturates are contraindicated in pregnancy and latent porphyria (as described previously).

With the exception of the benzodiazepines and the pharmacologically related benzodiazepine receptor agonists, the nonbarbiturate sedative-hypnotics offer little advantage over the barbiturates. Although antihistamines are not considered to cause physical dependence, most of the nonbarbiturate nonbenzodiazepine sedative-hypnotics have abuse potential, cause dependence, depress the CNS, and may be more troublesome than the barbiturates in overdose. Because of these limitations, few nonbarbiturate/nonbenzodiazepine sedative-hypnotics are used in dentistry. The primary exceptions are chloral hydrate, which is still used for sedation in young children, and the antihistamines hydroxyzine, diphenhydramine, and promethazine.

Chloral hydrate may be an appropriate sedative-hypnotic for patients allergic to, or intolerant of, the barbiturates or benzodiazepines. The onset and duration of action of chloral hydrate are approximately the same as those of the short- and intermediate-acting barbiturates. Chloral hydrate is frequently used to sedate children, although the impression that it is a safe agent is thrown into question by reports of fatalities, near-fatalities, and the carcinogenic potential previously described. Transient, partial blockage of the airway as a result of depressing the mandible in patients treated with a combination of chloral hydrate, nitrous oxide, and promethazine has been described, emphasizing the importance of careful monitoring of the patient with such combinations.[24,38] Chloral hydrate has an unpleasant taste, which is masked in commercially available syrups and elixirs or when mixed in orange juice.

The use of nonbarbiturate sedatives other than those already described is not warranted for dental practice because they offer no significant advantages. The clinician is best advised to recognize the names of the nonbarbiturate sedative-hypnotics and to be aware of the potential for drug interactions with other CNS depressants. In addition, the use of any of the hypnotic drugs for insomnia should be limited to short-term treatment at the lowest effective dose. An ongoing FDA program encourages physicians and dentists to restrict the prescribing of hypnotics and advises that the underlying cause of insomnia be sought and treated by nonpharmacologic means, if possible. Preparations and doses for clinically useful sedative-hypnotics are listed in Table 13-8. These doses should be used only as guidelines because each patient has different requirements and dosages should be individualized.

Many of the problems associated with the sedative-hypnotics, such as tolerance to sedative effects, addiction, abuse, rebound sleep disturbances, and the induction of hepatic microsomal enzyme activity, result from long-term use. Fortunately, the sedative-hypnotic drugs are indicated only for short-term use in dentistry; thus many of the usual factors limiting their use are not pertinent. This assertion is not to imply that problems do not arise with the administration of sedative-hypnotics in dental practice, but only that they are minimized. For example, although overdose with the sedative-hypnotics would be unlikely with the amount of drug required for most dental situations, a potential problem exists if the patient combines the prescribed sedative-hypnotic with other CNS depressants, such as alcohol. It is the responsibility of the clinician to ensure that the patient is made cognizant of the danger of combining other CNS depressants, particularly alcohol, with these drugs.

Certain patients require special precautions. The elderly are at special risk for impaired cognitive and motor function after the administration of a sedative-hypnotic. Patients with impaired liver function also fall into this category. Patients with sleep apnea, which is more common among the obese and elderly (especially men), should be treated cautiously because any hypnotic may exacerbate this condition. A complete medical history, including input from a spouse, might alert the practitioner to the possibility of such complications. The use of sedative-hypnotics is generally contraindicated in the pregnant patient, especially during the first trimester. Because patients with a history of drug abuse are at a higher risk of becoming dependent on the sedative-hypnotics, the minimally effective dose should be prescribed and only when absolutely necessary.

Although the barbiturates produce significant depression of the CNS, even to the point of unconsciousness, it should be noted that they are not analgesics. In fact, the patient receiving sedative doses may exhibit increased responsiveness to painful stimuli. When pain is present or evoked, the patient may become aroused, agitated, and delirious. Obviously, if pain is a contributing factor to either anxiety or insomnia, an analgesic is required to obtain sedation or hypnosis.

Drugs Used to Treat Anxiety

The antianxiety agents are important in dentistry for the premedication of the apprehensive adult patient, the patient exhibiting mild neurosis, and the uncooperative child. Antianxiety agents, particularly intravenous midazolam and diazepam, are used as adjuncts to local anesthesia. An example of the effectiveness of intravenous diazepam in the relief of intraoperative anxiety in a patient population undergoing surgical removal of impacted third molars is illustrated in Figure 13-14. Although intravenous sedation with diazepam usually lasts approximately 45 minutes, the duration of anxiety relief may be as long as 3 hours.[23] Midazolam and diazepam cause anterograde amnesia so that patients often cannot recall the procedures performed. Both drugs also depress the gag reflex and are major drugs for the treatment of seizures induced by local anesthetic overdose.

Midazolam has become very popular as a preoperative sedative because it is prepared in a water-soluble form and produces little irritation on injection. In contrast to diazepam, residual CNS depression and anxiety relief extending beyond the period of clinical recovery are not commonly observed when midazolam is administered as a single agent. For clinicians using midazolam, it is important to note that the manufacturer's original dosage recommendations were excessive for some patients and that small initial doses should be injected slowly while carefully observing the patient. By the same token, careful observation of the patient is absolutely mandatory in attempting to reverse benzodiazepine-induced sedation with flumazenil. Careful attention must be paid to the manufacturer's recommended dose, time interval of administration, and prolonged patient monitoring time.

Perhaps one of the more perplexing questions for the practicing dentist is which oral benzodiazepine to choose from the ever-expanding list. There is little doubt of the clinical effectiveness of these drugs in a variety of dental procedures,[18,54] but there are no unusual characteristics associated with any one benzodiazepine that would make it clearly superior to the others. Essentially, any benzodiazepine is suitable as an antianxiety agent if the pharmacokinetics of that drug are kept in mind. The major decision to be made in the treatment of the anxious patient is therefore not which drug to use but rather when to administer it. Although there is no simple rule of thumb, the pharmacokinetic characteristics of individual compounds to a large extent dictate the optimal dose schedule. Oxazepam and lorazepam are potentially useful drugs in patients with liver disease because they are converted to inactive glucuronides, and the conjugation reaction is often affected less by hepatic disease than are other steps in drug metabolism. Although buspirone offers many advantages for the treatment of anxiety, its usefulness in dentistry is limited by its delayed onset of effect. Other azaspirones currently undergoing clinical trials may offer anxiety relief with a short onset time.

The primary concern of the dentist in using an antianxiety agent should be excessive CNS depression. CNS depression may result from the antianxiety agent alone or its combination with other CNS depressants that the dentist may plan to give or that the patient may already have taken. The antianxiety agents summate with the anesthetics, antipsychotics, antidepressants, opioid analgesics, and sedative-hypnotics. Alcohol may markedly increase the CNS depressant effects of benzodiazepines. If CNS depressant drugs are used for deep sedation and general anesthesia in the dental clinic, suction and monitoring equipment, emergency drugs, and a means to deliver oxygen under positive pressure must be readily available. Obviously, the practitioner should have appropriate advanced training in anesthesia techniques. The

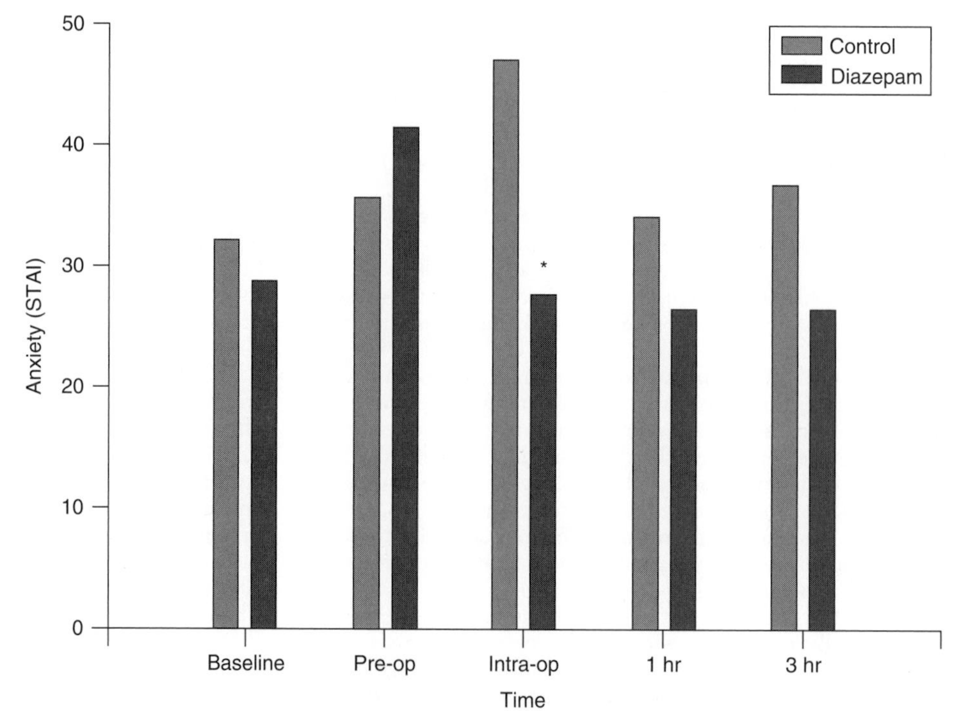

Fig. 13-14 Effects of placebo and diazepam on reported anxiety with a state-trait anxiety index *(STAI)* in patients undergoing surgical removal of impacted third molars. Patients were treated with placebo solution or diazepam (0.3 mg/kg) 5 minutes before surgery. All patients also received standard local anesthesia with 2% lidocaine containing 1:100,000 epinephrine. Anxiety was assessed before ingestion and before, during, and after surgery. *, Significantly different from control ($p < 0.01$). (Adapted from Hargreaves KM, Dionne RA, Mueller GP, et al: Naloxone, fentanyl, and diazepam modify plasma beta-endorphin levels during surgery, *Clin Pharmacol Ther* 40:165-171, 1986.)

benzodiazepine antagonist flumazenil offers the opportunity to reverse benzodiazepine-induced sedation after dental procedures,[8,18,19] thus hastening postoperative patient recovery. Flumazenil is also a rapidly acting antidote for benzodiazepine intoxication. The possibility of resedation and recurrence of respiratory depression because of its short half-life has been described. Certainly, the best practice in the use of benzodiazepines is to limit their administration so that an emergency antidote is never required.

The patient should be reminded that antihistamines, even the small amounts contained in over-the-counter preparations promoted as cold remedies or for insomnia, may add to the CNS depressant effect of the antianxiety agents. Because of benzodiazepine-induced psychomotor impairment, the dentist should caution patients on the hazards of driving an automobile or operating potentially dangerous machinery for up to 24 hours after drug administration.

A great number of factors influence the choice of an antianxiety drug. This chapter has covered some of the more important ones that the dentist should consider when making a selection. The therapeutic use of drugs for anxiety relief in dentistry is further reviewed in Chapter 48. In practice, the dentist should become familiar and comfortable with a limited number of antianxiety drugs and select from these according to the drugs' pharmacokinetics, the particular treatment to be rendered, and the needs of the patient. The obvious potential for the development of more specific antianxiety agents should serve as a stimulus for the practicing dentist to stay current in the field of antianxiety medication. Knowledge of the pharmacologic profile of the existing drugs may also prevent the dentist from being misled by dubious claims of specificity for newly introduced agents.

Table 13-4 lists preparations and doses recommended for anxiety control. The doses indicated should be viewed only as guidelines; each patient requires individualized treatment, and the minimum effective dose should be administered.

Drugs Used as Centrally Acting Muscle Relaxants

Although the indications are limited, centrally acting muscle relaxants may be valuable therapeutic agents for some dental procedures.[53] Diazepam is generally preferred because of its good muscle-relaxing properties, prolonged action, and safety. It has been found to reduce postprocedural trismus and may be used as an adjunct for treating muscle spasms of the head and neck, as in temporomandibular disorders. However, the causes of temporomandibular pain are complex, involving multiple interacting factors such as patient anxiety, muscle spasms, occlusal problems, and joint dysfunction. The effectiveness of therapy with centrally acting muscle relaxants is greater if anxiety or muscle spasm primarily causes the dysfunction. Because the relationship between CNS activity and peripheral muscle tone is complex, it is unlikely that the centrally acting muscle relaxants will produce either consistent or predictable results. There are still few double-blind studies that demonstrate the benefit of such treatment; what is clear from such studies is that the incidence of improvement from placebos is high. The use of centrally acting muscle relaxants should be monitored carefully, and long-term therapy beyond a few weeks is generally not indicated.

Although combinations of centrally acting muscle relaxants and peripherally analgesic drugs may be valuable, fixed-dose combinations often provide suboptimal doses of the analgesic drug (see Chapter 47). Prescribing full therapeutic doses of each agent is warranted if the use of a combination is indicated. In addition, better results have been obtained from longer-acting agents on a once- or twice-daily dosing schedule. The interaction between sensory and motor systems suggests that a multiple drug treatment approach could be useful. The idea that hyperalgesia produces a significant increase of noxious sensory afferent input from injured muscle has been documented.[33] The decrease in peripheral sensory thresholds produced by hyperalgesia is the result of many different inflammatory compounds, which implies that antiinflammatory drugs of some kind may be useful by reducing the inflammation. Also, the concept of extensive convergence of afferents from skin, muscle, joints, and other tissues onto brain sensory nuclei, which can result in decreased sensory thresholds and increased referred pain, has also been documented.[48] The use of analgesics to reduce peripheral and spinal (or trigeminal) hyperalgesia, and centrally acting muscle relaxants to reduce brain excitation, may help to reduce muscle spasm. This may explain why analgesics combined with muscle relaxants can sometimes produce a better effect than either one given alone. It should be noted that centrally acting muscle relaxants in general are not the primary treatment for every type of facial pain. Trigeminal neuralgia (tic douloureux), for instance, requires specific therapies (see Chapter 23).

Drugs Used as Antianxiety Agents

Nonproprietary (generic) name	*Proprietary (trade) name*
Benzodiazepines	
Alprazolam	Xanax
Chlordiazepoxide	Librium
Clorazepate	Tranxene
Diazepam	Valium
Halazepam*	Paxipam
Lorazepam	Ativan
Midazolam	Versed
Oxazepam	Serax
Prazepam*	Centrax
Triazolam	Halcion
Azaspirodecanediones	
Buspirone	BuSpar
Propanediol carbamates	
Meprobamate	Miltown, Equanil
Chlormezanone*	Trancopal

*Not currently available in the United States.

Drugs Used as Sedative-Hypnotics

Nonproprietary (generic) name	*Proprietary (trade) name*
Barbiturates	
Amobarbital	Amytal
Aprobarbital*	Alurate
Butabarbital	Butisol
Butalbital	in Fiorinal
Mephobarbital	Mebaral
Pentobarbital	Nembutal
Phenobarbital	Luminal
Secobarbital	Seconal

Continued

Drugs Used as Sedative-Hypnotics—cont'd

Nonproprietary (generic) name	*Proprietary (trade) name*
Benzodiazepines	
Estazolam	ProSom
Flurazepam	Dalmane
Quazepam	Doral
Temazepam	Restoril
Triazolam	Halcion
Antihistamines	
Hydroxyzine hydrochloride	Atarax
Hydroxyzine pamoate	Vistaril
Promethazine	Phenergan
Diphenhydramine	Benadryl, Nytol
Others	
Acetylcarbromal	Paxarel
Chloral hydrate	Aquachloral Supprettes
Ethchlorvynol*	Placidyl
Glutethimide*	Doriden
Methyprylon*	Noludar
Paraldehyde*	Paral
Zaleplon	Sonata
Zolpidem	Ambien

*Not currently available in the United States.

Drugs Used Primarily as Muscle Relaxants

Nonproprietary (generic) name	*Proprietary (trade) name*
Benzodiazepines	
Diazepam	Valium
Miscellaneous	
Baclofen	Lioresal
Carisoprodol	Soma
Chlorphenesin	Maolate
Chlorzoxazone	Paraflex
Cyclobenzaprine	Flexeril
Mephenesin*	—
Meprobamate	Miltonin, Equanil
Metaxalone	Skelaxin
Methocarbamol	Robaxin
Orphenadrine	Norflex
Tizanidine	Zanaflex

*Not currently available in the United States.

Cited References

1. Backman JT, Olkkola KT, Aranko K, et al: Dose of midazolam should be reduced during diltiazem and verapamil treatments, *Br J Clin Pharmacol* 37:221-225, 1994.
2. Backman JT, Olkkola KT, Neuvonen PJ: Rifampin drastically reduces plasma concentrations and effects of oral midazolam, *Clin Pharmacol Ther* 59:7-13, 1996.
3. Backman JT, Olkkola KT, Ojala M, et al: Concentrations and effects of oral midazolam are greatly reduced in patients treated with carbamazepine or phenytoin, *Epilepsia* 37:253-257, 1996.
4. Beeber AR, Manring JM, Jr: Psychosis following cyclobenzaprine use, *J Clin Psychiatry* 44:151-152, 1983.
5. Bowery NG: $GABA_B$ receptor pharmacology, *Annu Rev Pharmacol Toxicol* 33:109-147, 1993.
6. Bringmann G: A first biosynthetic proposal for the in vivo formation of naturally occurring diazepam-like 1,4-benzodiazepines, *J Neural Transm* 88:77-82, 1992.
7. Clark MS, Lindenmuth JE, Jafek BW, et al: Reversal of central benzodiazepine effects by intravenous flumazenil, *Anesth Prog* 38:12-16, 1991.
8. Curran HV, Birch B: Differentiating the sedative, psychomotor and amnesic effects of benzodiazepines: a study with midazolam and the benzodiazepine antagonist, flumazenil, *Psychopharmacology* 103:519-523, 1991.
9. *Diagnostic and statistical manual of mental disorders,* ed 4 (DSM-IV), Washington, DC, 1994, American Psychiatric Association.
10. Diagnostic Classification Steering Committee of the American Sleep Disorders Association: *The international classification of sleep disorders: diagnostic and coding manual,* Rochester, MN, 1990, American Sleep Disorders Association.
11. Dionne RA, Yagiela JA, Moore PA, et al: Comparing efficacy and safety of four intravenous sedation regimens in dental outpatients, *J Am Dent Assoc* 132:740-751, 2001.
12. Doble A: New insights into the mechanism of action of hypnotics, *J Psychopharmacol* 13(4 suppl 1):S11-S20, 1999.
13. Doble A, Martin IL: Multiple benzodiazepine receptors: no reason for anxiety, *Trends Pharmacol Sci* 13:76-81, 1992.
14. Dubovsky SL: Generalized anxiety disorder: new concepts and psychopharmacologic therapies, *J Clin Psychiatry* 51(suppl):3-10, 1990.
15. Eison AS, Eison MS, Stanley M: Serotonergic mechanisms in the behavioral effects of buspirone and gepirone, *Pharmacol Biochem Behav* 24:701-707, 1986.
16. Facklam M, Schoch P, Bonetti EP, et al: Relationship between benzodiazepine receptor occupancy and functional effects in vivo of four ligands of differing intrinsic efficacies, *J Pharmacol Exp Ther* 261:1113-1121, 1992.
17. Fee JPH, Collier PS, Howard PJ, et al: Cimetidine and ranitidine increase midazolam bioavailability, *Clin Pharm Ther* 41:80-84, 1987.
18. Finder RL, Moore PA: Benzodiazepines for intravenous conscious sedation: agonists and antagonists, *Compendium* 14:972, 974, 976-980, 1993.
19. Finder RL, Moore PA, Close JM: Flumazenil reversal of conscious sedation induced with intravenous fentanyl and diazepam, *Anesth Prog* 42:11-16, 1995.
20. Geller E, Crome P, Schaller MD, et al: Risks and benefits of therapy with flumazenil (Anexate) in mixed drug intoxications, *Eur Neurol* 31:241-250, 1991.
21. Gorman JM: New molecular targets for antianxiety interventions, *J Clin Psychiatry* 64(suppl 3):28-35, 2003.
22. Granoff DM, McDaniel DB, Borkowf SP: Cardiorespiratory arrest following aspiration of chloral hydrate, *Am J Dis Child* 122:170-171, 1971.

23. Hargreaves KM, Dionne RA, Mueller GP, et al: Naloxone, fentanyl, and diazepam modify plasma beta-endorphin levels during surgery, *Clin Pharmacol Ther* 40:165-171, 1986.
24. Houpt MI, Weiss NJ, Koenigsberg SR, et al: Comparison of chloral hydrate with and without promethazine in the sedation of young children, *Pediatr Dent* 7:41-46, 1985.
25. Jastak JT, Pallasch T: Death after chloral hydrate sedation: report of case, *J Am Dent Assoc* 116:345-348, 1988.
26. Kales A, Bixler EO, Vela-Bueno A, et al: Comparison of short and long half-life benzodiazepine hypnotics: triazolam and quazepam, *Clin Pharmacol Ther* 40:378-386, 1986.
27. Levitan ES, Schofield PR, Burt DR, et al: Structural and functional basis for $GABA_A$ receptor heterogeneity, *Nature* 335:76-79, 1988.
28. Lichtor JL, Zacny JP, Coalson DW, et al: The interaction between alcohol and residual effects of thiopental anesthesia, *Anesthesiology* 79:28-35, 1993.
29. Linnoila M, Mattila MJ: Drug interaction on psychomotor skills related to driving: diazepam and alcohol, *Eur J Clin Pharmacol* 5:186-194, 1973.
30. Lopez-Rubalcava C, Saldivar A, Fernandez-Guasti A: Interaction of GABA and serotonin in the anxiolytic action of diazepam and serotonergic anxiolytics, *Pharmacol Biochem Behav* 43:433-440, 1992.
31. MacDonald RL, Olsen RW: $GABA_A$ receptor channels, *Annu Rev Neurosci* 17:569-602, 1994.
32. Mandelli M, Tognoni G, Garattini S: Clinical pharmacokinetics of diazepam, *Clin Pharmacokin* 3:72-91, 1978.
33. Mense S: Physiology of nociception in muscles, *Adv Pain Res Ther* 17:67-85, 1990.
34. Miller LG, Greenblatt DJ, Barnhill JG, et al: Chronic benzodiazepine administration. I. Tolerance is associated with benzodiazepine receptor downregulation and decreased γ-aminobutyric $acid_A$ receptor function, *J Pharmacol Exp Ther* 246:170-176, 1988.
35. Monjan AA: Sleep disorders of older people: report of a consensus conference, *Hosp Community Psychiatry* 41:743-744, 1990.
36. Moore PA: Adverse drug interactions in dental practice: interactions associated with local anesthetics, sedatives and anxiolytics. Part IV of a series, *J Am Dent Assoc* 130:541-554, 1999.
37. Moore PA: Selecting drugs for the pregnant dental patient, *J Am Dent Assoc* 129:1281-1286, 1998.
38. Moore PA: Therapeutic assessments of chloral hydrate premedication for pediatric dentistry, *Anesth Prog* 31:191-196, 1984.
39. Moore PA, Finder RL, Jackson DL: Multidrug intravenous sedation: determinants of the sedative dose of midazolam, *Oral Surg Oral Med Oral Pathol Oral Radiol Endod* 84:5-10, 1997.
40. Moore PA, Mickey EA, Hargreaves JA, et al: Sedation in pediatric dentistry: a practical assessment procedure, *J Am Dent Assoc* 109:564-569, 1984.
41. Moore PA, Studen-Pavlovich D: Pharmacosedation for pediatric patients. In Fonseca RJ, ed: *Oral and maxillofacial surgery*, vol 1, Philadelphia, 2000, WB Saunders.
42. Pevonka MP, Yost RL, Marks RG, et al: Interaction of chloral hydrate and furosemide: a controlled retrospective study, *Drug Intel Clin Pharm* 11:332-335, 1977.
43. Rees M, Dormandy J: Accidental intra-arterial injection of diazepam, *Br Med J* 281:289-290, 1980.
44. Rudolph U, Crestani F, Mohler H: GABA(A) receptor subtypes: dissecting their pharmacological functions, *Trends Pharmacol Sci* 22:188-194, 2001.
45. Rush CR, Ali JA: A follow-up study of the acute behavioral effects of benzodiazepine-receptor ligands in humans: comparison of quazepam and triazolam, *Exp Clin Psychopharmacol* 7:257-265, 1999.
46. Salzman C: The APA Task Force report on benzodiazepine dependence, toxicity, and abuse, *Am J Psychiatry* 148:151-152, 1991.
47. Sanders LD, Whitehead C, Gildersleve CD, et al: Interaction of H_2-receptor antagonists and benzodiazepine sedation. A double-blind placebo-controlled investigation of the effects of cimetidine and ranitidine on recovery after intravenous midazolam, *Anaesthesia* 48:286-292, 1993.
48. Sessle BJ: Central nervous system mechanism of muscular pain, *Adv Pain Res Ther* 17:87-105, 1990.
49. Shader RI, Greenblatt DJ: Use of benzodiazepines in anxiety disorders, *N Engl J Med* 328:1398-1405, 1993.
50. Short TG, Maling T, Galletly DC: Ventricular arrhythmia precipitated by flumazenil, *Br Med J* 296:1070-1071, 1988.
51. Smith AJ, Simpson PB: Methodological approaches for the study of $GABA_A$ receptor pharmacology and functional responses, *Anal Bioanal Chem* 377:843-851, 2003.
52. Smith MT: Chloral hydrate warning, *Science* 250:359, 1990.
53. Stanko JR: Review of oral skeletal muscle relaxants for the craniomandibular disorder (CMD) practitioner, *Cranio* 8:234-243, 1990.
54. Stopperich PS, Moore PA, Finder RL, et al: Oral triazolam pretreatment for intravenous sedation, *Anesth Prog* 40:117-121, 1993.
55. Study RE, Barker JL: Cellular mechanisms of benzodiazepine action, *JAMA* 247:2147-2151, 1982.
56. Sved AF, Tsukamoto K: Tonic stimulation of $GABA_B$ receptors in the nucleus tractus solitarius modulates the baroreceptor reflex, *Brain Res* 592:37-43, 1992.
57. Takahashi T, Koyama N: Effects of tizanidine, a central muscle relaxant, upon spinal reflexes [in Japanese], *Masui* 41:751-765, 1992.
58. Tanaka E: Toxicological interactions between alcohol and benzodiazepines, *J Toxicol Clin Toxicol* 40:69-75, 2002.
59. Turski L, Klockgether T, Schwarz M, et al: Substantia nigra: a site of action of muscle relaxant drugs, *Ann Neurol* 28:341-348, 1990.
60. Turski L, Schwarz M, Turski WA, et al: Effect of aminophylline on muscle relaxant action of diazepam and phenobarbitone in genetically spastic rats: further evidence for a purinergic mechanism in the action of diazepam, *Eur J Pharmacol* 103:99-105, 1984.
61. Udall JA: Warfarin-chloral hydrate interaction: pharmacological activity and clinical significance, *Ann Intern Med* 81:341-344, 1974.
62. Varhe A, Olkkola KT, Neuvonen PJ: Oral triazolam is potentially hazardous to patients receiving systemic antimycotics ketoconazole or itraconazole, *Clin Pharm Ther* 56:601-607, 1994.

63. Villikka K, Kivisto KT, Backman JT, et al: Triazolam is ineffective in patients taking rifampin, *Clin Pharm Ther* 61:8-14, 1997.
64. Weintraub M, Singh S, Byrne L, et al: Consequences of the 1989 New York State triplicate benzodiazepine prescription regulations, *JAMA* 266:2392-2397, 1991.
65. Wildmann J: Increase of natural benzodiazepines in wheat and potato during germination, *Biochem Biophys Res Commun* 157:1436-1443, 1988.
66. Woods JH, Katz JL, Winger G: Use and abuse of benzodiazepines. Issues relevant to prescribing, *JAMA* 260:3476-3480, 1988.
67. Yocca FD: Neurochemistry and neurophysiology of buspirone and gepirone: interactions at presynaptic and postsynaptic 5-HT_{1A} receptors, *J Clin Psychopharmacol* 10(3 suppl):6S-12S, 1990.
68. Zolpidem for insomnia, *Med Lett Drugs Ther* 35:35-36, 1993.
69. Zorumski CF, Isenberg KE: Insights into the structure and function of GABA-benzodiazepine receptors: ion channels and psychiatry, *Am J Psychiatry* 148:162-173, 1991.

General References

Alger BE, Möhler H, eds: *Pharmacology of GABA and glycine neurotransmission. Handbook of experimental pharmacology,* vol 150, New York, 2001, Springer.

Biggio G, Costa E, eds: GABA and benzodiazepine receptor subtypes: molecular biology, pharmacology, and clinical aspects. In *Advances in biochemical psychopharmacology,* vol 46, New York, 1990, Raven Press.

Halbreich U, Montgomery SA: *Pharmacotherapy for mood, anxiety, and cognition disorders,* Washington, DC, 2000, American Psychiatric Press.

McKim WA: *Drugs and behavior: an introduction to behavioral pharmacology,* ed 5, Upper Saddle River, NJ, 2003, Prentice Hall.

Olsen RW, Venter JC: *Benzodiazepine/GABA receptors and chloride channels: structural and functional properties,* New York, 1986, Alan R. Liss.

Raffa RB: Thermodynamics of benzodiazepine receptor interactions. In Raffa RB, ed: *Drug receptor thermodynamics: introduction and applications,* Chichester, England, 2001, John Wiley & Sons.

Smith MC, Riskin BJ: The clinical use of barbiturates in neurological disorders, *Drugs* 42:365-378, 1991.

Trimble MR, Hindmarch I: *Benzodiazepines,* Philadelphia, 2000, Wrightson Biomedical.

CHAPTER • 14

Anticonvulsants*

Vahn A. Lewis

Epilepsy comprises a group of disorders characterized by the periodic and abnormal discharge of nervous tissue. Violent involuntary muscle contractions, or *convulsions,* are characteristic of most forms of epilepsy, and the epileptic attack, accompanied in most cases by convulsions, is called a *seizure.* The abnormal neuronal discharge causes electroencephalographic (EEG) disturbances, abnormal metabolism indicated by positron emission tomography (PET) or single photon emission computed tomography, and accompanying anatomic derangements that can be imaged by computed tomography or magnetic resonance imaging. Various epileptic syndromes exist, each defined by such factors as cause, seizure type, age of onset, and clinical manifestations. Convulsions can have many causes and therefore constitute evidence of an underlying neurologic disorder, not a disease per se. The signs and symptoms of these syndromes frequently overlap, and differential diagnosis of the form of epilepsy is sometimes difficult.

CLASSIFICATION OF EPILEPTIC DISORDERS

The classification proposed in 1989 by the Commission on Classification and Terminology of the International League Against Epilepsy[3] is necessarily complex because of the variable characteristics of many epileptic syndromes. A simplified approach more suited to this discussion limits consideration to the seizures themselves (Table 14-1). Seizure patterns are broadly divided into two major groups: (1) partial seizures, in which convulsions begin in a localized region of the brain, involve restricted areas of the body, are initially unilateral, and yield EEG recordings of rhythmic activity that is restricted at least initially to one hemisphere; and (2) generalized seizures, with convulsions often involving the entire body and EEG recordings having characteristic bilateral patterns.

Generalized Seizures

The most common type of generalized seizure is *tonic-clonic* (grand mal), which has a sudden onset (sometimes preceded by an aura, a brain sensation recognized by the patient), beginning with the so-called epileptic cry caused by the forcing of air through the tonically contracted muscles of the larynx. This cry is followed by a loss of consciousness, loss of postural tone, and tonic-clonic contraction of skeletal muscles. Autonomic responses commonly include sweating, loss of sphincter control (often resulting in urination and defecation), pupillary dilation, and loss of light reflexes. The EEG pattern displays bilateral, synchronous high-voltage polyspike activity. Injury may occur as a result of the uncontrolled movements or loss of postural tone. Tongue biting and fracturing of teeth may result from the powerful contraction of the muscles of mastication. After the tonic-clonic contractions, the patient usually awakens, is confused and lethargic, and goes to sleep for approximately 30 minutes. On reawakening, the patient is again lethargic, confused, disoriented, and often has headache and muscle ache. Fortunately, grand mal epilepsy is often responsive to pharmacotherapy.

A second common form of generalized seizure is the *absence* seizure, which characteristically occurs in childhood. There are several varieties of absence seizures. The most common form (petit mal) is characterized by an abrupt but very short (5 to 10 seconds) loss of consciousness, often with minor muscular twitching (commonly restricted to the eyelids and face), and a 3-Hz spike-and-wave EEG pattern but no loss of postural control. Severe cases may involve hundreds of seizures per day. The term *absence* is appropriate because of the brief loss of consciousness and the vacant stare of the patient during a seizure. Like tonic-clonic seizures, absence seizures are often responsive to pharmacotherapy.

Uncommon types of generalized seizures include (1) *myoclonic,* characterized by sudden, brief, and violent spasms of one or more muscles or muscle groups; and (2) *atonic,* characterized by a sudden and brief loss of muscle tone. These varieties are usually associated with diffuse and severe progressive diseases of the brain and are often refractory to drug treatment. Rarely seizures are precipitated by triggers, such as catamenial seizures (associated with menstruation) or reflex seizures, which can be triggered by tones, visual stimulation (e.g., video games, flashing lights), or touching.

Generalized seizures occurring in the form of repeated or continuous attacks are referred to as *status epilepticus.* Tonic-clonic status epilepticus is rare but life threatening. Status epilepticus may develop in patients with convulsive disorders, with acute disease affecting the brain (meningitis, encephalitis, toxemia of pregnancy, uremia, acute electrolyte imbalances), after abrupt withdrawal of depressant or anticonvulsant medication (barbiturates, benzodiazepines, opioids), or rarely after local anesthetic administration. Status epilepticus can occur in the absence of a prior history of seizures. The drugs most widely used to treat status epilepticus are the intravenous benzodiazepines (i.e., lorazepam, diazepam, midazolam), phenytoin or fosphenytoin, and phenobarbital.[35,49] Because large doses of these drugs are usually required, there is the danger of respiratory depression and respiratory arrest, especially with phenobarbital. In refractory status epilepticus, the patient may have to undergo general anesthesia. An anesthetic dose of pentobarbital or propofol is

*The authors wish to recognize Dr. Leslie Felpel for her past contributions to this chapter. See the Acknowledgments.

Table • 14-1

Classification of Epileptic Seizures

CLASSIFICATION	CLINICAL ASPECTS
I. Partial (focal, local) seizures	Involves one side of brain at onset
A. Simple partial seizures (e.g., Jacksonian)	Consciousness not impaired; specific or localized motor, sensory
B. Complex partial seizures (e.g., psychomotor, temporal lobe)	Consciousness impaired, automatisms, autonomic or psychologic signs or symptoms; patients may report aura beforehand
C. Partial seizures evolving to generalized seizures	See generalized seizures; patients may report aura beforehand
II. Generalized seizures	Involve both sides of brain at onset
A. Tonic-clonic seizures (grand mal)	Consciousness is lost; bilateral sharp tonic contraction of muscles, generalized from onset, is followed by clonic contractions; patient may report aura before seizure
B. Absence seizures (e.g., petit mal)	Consciousness impaired, postural muscles not impaired, EEG spike and slow wave complexes at approximately 3 Hz
C. Myoclonic seizures	Sudden, brief contractions of individual muscles or groups producing shocklike spasms in muscles of face, trunk, and extremities
D. Clonic seizures	Repetitive clonic jerking (alternating contractions of opposing muscles)
E. Tonic seizures	Violent muscular contraction (simultaneous contraction of flexors and extensors) with limbs in strained position
F. Atonic seizures (astatic)	Sudden loss of muscle tone, consciousness sometimes lost, patients sustain fall injuries
III. Unclassified seizures	Cannot be classified because of insufficient data or atypical pattern of seizure

Adapted from Commission on Classification and Terminology of the International League Against Epilepsy, *Epilepsia* 22:489-501, 1981.

effective and has a more rapid onset than phenobarbital. Grand mal status epilepticus is best treated in a hospital setting.

Partial Seizures

The partial epilepsy syndromes are divided into three broad categories. The first type, called *simple partial seizure,* is characterized by seizures limited to certain muscles or involving specific sensory changes, psychic symptoms, or autonomic activity. The seizure may remain localized or it may spread to contiguous brain tissue, causing progressive symptoms as the wave of depolarization "marches" along the cerebral cortex. This latter seizure type is referred to as *Jacksonian epilepsy,* after John Hughlings Jackson, who first described the phenomenon. The motor version begins with contraction of an isolated muscle, followed by the gradual involvement of other muscles. Jacksonian sensory epilepsy, on the other hand, gives rise to sensations from various areas of the body. By definition, however, the affected individual remains conscious.

A second type of partial seizure, known as *complex partial seizure,* usually originates in the temporal or frontal lobe but spreads to broader areas, frequently in a bilateral pattern. Consciousness is impaired, flashbacks or psychoticlike behavior may occur, and autonomic dysregulation and automatisms (involuntary, repetitive, and coordinated movements) are common.

A third type of partial seizure is one that progresses to a generalized attack. The initial inciting seizure may be simple or complex. The final clinical result depends on the type of generalized seizure that is triggered. Partial seizures are more refractory to drugs than are the common generalized seizures.

Secondary Seizures

Seizures may be caused by a fundamental disorder in the ability of the brain to regulate excitation because of genetic causes or abnormal development. However, seizures may also occur as a symptom of another medical condition. Seizures in an otherwise normal individual may be precipitated by inhibition of the respiratory chain (anoxia, metabolic poisons), hyperbaric oxygen, intoxication, fever, cerebral infection or inflammation, traumatic brain injury, repeated electrical brain stimulation, drug use, systemic administration of local anesthetics, overdose of stimulant or antidepressant drugs, or withdrawal of depressant drugs (e.g., alcohol, barbiturates, opioids). These seizures may resolve after resolution of the underlying cause or may continue if the insult or seizures have resulted in brain injury.

PATHOPHYSIOLOGY

The pathophysiologic characteristics of the epilepsies are not well understood. Idiopathic epilepsy has a primary genetic basis, with some influence of environmental factors.[25] The various types of epilepsies share many features but also differ in many respects. The fact that many anticonvulsant drugs are selective for specific seizure types[13] suggests that the origin and progression of all seizures are not identical. Several hypotheses have been proposed to explain why seizures occur. Not surprisingly, these hypotheses focus on defects in (1) ionic conductance of the neuronal membrane, including Na^+, Ca^{++}, K^+, Cl^-, and H^+; (2) inhibitory neuronal circuits, especially those involving the inhibitory neurotransmitter γ-aminobutyric acid (GABA); (3) excitatory mechanisms, especially those involving the excitatory neurotransmitter glutamate; (4) altered synaptic function; and (5) other processes supporting presynaptic or postsynaptic function, such as other neurotransmitters with modulatory roles, peptides, hormones, growth factors, second messengers, nuclear changes, glial function, and gap junctional function.

Different brain structures may participate as seizure sources. The cortex is often involved. In complex partial epilepsy, unusual activity in the temporal lobe and limbic structures is found. For absence seizures, changes in the thalamus and basal ganglia appear to be important. Audiogenic seizures seem to involve the mesencephalon and basal ganglia. In otherwise normal brains, seizures can sometimes be initiated by repeated electrical stimulations, a phenomenon called *kindling.*

Seizures may be triggered by a variety of causes. Epilepsy may result when a genetic predisposition or environmental factor triggers a seizure, which is followed by additional processes such as seizure-induced neuronal death and abnormal postseizure tissue repair. Repeated seizures can produce cumulative damage. By studying patients, animal models of epilepsy, and the mechanism of action of the anticonvulsant drugs, new ideas for therapy are developed. Individual anticonvulsants often have more than one possible pharmacologic action that may explain their anticonvulsant effect.

ANTICONVULSANT THERAPY

Anticonvulsants control but do not cure epilepsy. They may play a neuroprotective role, though, by limiting cumulative pathology resulting from the seizures. The primary objective of anticonvulsant therapy is to suppress seizures while causing minimal impairment of central nervous system (CNS) function or other deleterious side effects. With the currently available anticonvulsants, significant seizure control can be obtained in 70% to 80% of cases. Many patients with epilepsy have to take medication for life to ensure control of seizures.

Drugs are described as having characteristic spectra for treating the various forms of seizures (Figure 14-1). Prescribing antiepileptic drugs for conditions outside their spectra may lead to problems beyond simple therapeutic failure. In particular, absence seizures can be exacerbated by many of the drugs used to treat tonic-clonic seizures. Some children "outgrow" absence epilepsy but have a tendency to develop other forms of epilepsy in later years. The discovery of valproic acid, which can control many forms of epilepsy, was a major breakthrough for those patients in whom absence seizures convert to tonic-clonic seizures. The careful withdrawal of anticonvulsant therapy in children with a history of tonic-clonic epilepsy, but who have been seizure free for several years, is sometimes successful. Finally, adults whose seizures were few in number before initiation of treatment and are well controlled with a single anticonvulsant may be weaned after 2 years of therapy with a reasonable expectation (more than 50%) of avoiding relapse.

Phenobarbital, introduced in 1912, was the first drug used extensively to treat seizures. Between 1938 and 1960, numerous anticonvulsant agents were introduced, including the hydantoins, succinimides, and primidone. However, the field languished after the passage of the Kefauver-Harris Amendments (1962), which required proof of efficacy and safety. Still, between 1960 and 1992 several novel anticonvulsants were introduced (e.g., carbamazepine, valproic acid, clonazepam, clorazepate). With the passages of the Expedited Drug Approval Act and Prescription Drug User Fee Act in 1992, the approval process was facilitated, and 10 agents have been introduced (with several more currently in clinical trials). Many of these drugs have been approved as adjunctive agents for use with earlier drugs in the treatment of "partial onset seizures"; these indications have broadened with increased experience in their use. Typically about 50% of patients respond to traditional agents, and between 20% and 40% of the remainder respond to the addition of a supplemental agent. The drugs used to treat epilepsy and their proposed mechanisms of action and current indications are summarized in Table 14-2.

Because anticonvulsants are often taken for prolonged periods, the likelihood of detecting and documenting side

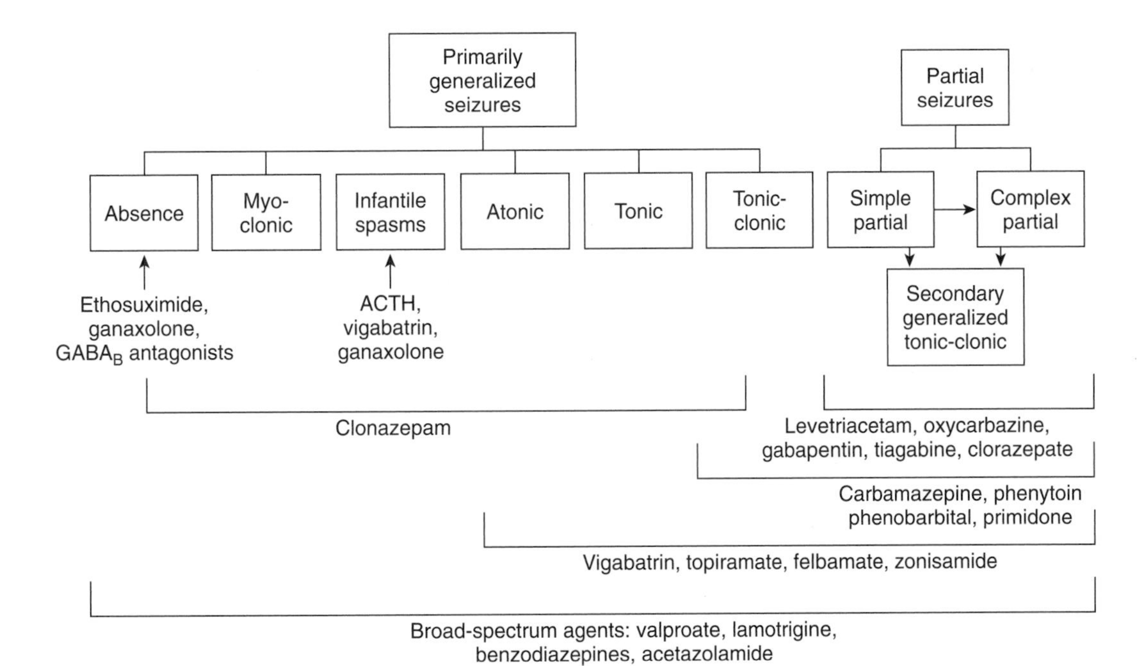

Fig. 14-1 Therapeutic spectra of anticonvulsant drugs. Anticonvulsant agents need to be matched to the convulsive disorder being treated. Phenytoin, phenobarbital, carbamazepine, oxycarbazine, vigabatrin, gabapentin, and tiagabine are not effective in, but can aggravate, absence and myoclonic seizures. Benzodiazepines and acetazolamide have broad spectrums, but tolerance develops to their actions, so they cannot be used for maintenance therapy.

Table • 14-2

Mechanisms of Action and Uses for Anticonvulsant Drugs

DRUG	ION CHANNEL INHIBITION		INCREASED GABA EFFECT	DECREASED EXCITATORY AMINO ACID EFFECT	USES*			COMMENTS
	Na^+	Ca^{++}			SEIZURE TYPE	ABSENCE	OTHER	
Hydantoins								
Phenytoin	x		x	x	TC, CP, SE		NP, rarely cardiac arrhythmias	Prompt and extended-dose forms
Fosphenytoin	x		x	x	SE			IM and IV form for injection
Ethotoin	x		x	x	TC, CP			
Mephenytoin	x		x	x	TC, CP, JM			
Iminostilbenes								
Carbamazepine	x		x	x (?)	TC, CP		BI, NP other	
Oxcarbazepine	x				P-AJ			Prodrug; action similar to carbamazepine
Barbiturates								
Phenobarbital			x	AK[‡]	TC, CF, SE		LA, F	
Primidone			x	AK[‡]	TC, CP, focal			
Mephobarbital			x	AK[‡]				
Carboxylic Acid								
Valproic acid	x	x	x (?)	x (?)	TC	x	BI, NP, F, migraine	First broad-spectrum anticonvulsant
Succinimides								
Ethosuximide		x				x		
Methsuximide		x				x		
Phensuximide		x				x		
Oxazolidinediones								
Trimethadione		x				x		Rarely used because of serious toxicity
Benzodiazepines								
Lorazepam			x	x (?)	SE		LA	
Clonazepam			x	x (?)	CP (?)	x	AK	
Clorazepate			x	x (?)	P			
Diazepam			x	x (?)	SE		LA	
Midazolam			x	x (?)	SE		F	May be effective after buccal administration but can reduce respiration rate
Carbonic Hydrase Inhibitors								
Acetazolamide[†]						x	CT	Rapid tolerance
Newer Agents								
Lamotrigine	x			x (?)	P-AJ, LG		NP	Restricted LG use in children <16 years

Table • 14-2

Mechanisms of Action and Uses for Anticonvulsant Drugs—cont'd

DRUG	ION CHANNEL INHIBITION		INCREASED GABA EFFECT	DECREASED EXCITATORY AMINO ACID EFFECT	USES*			COMMENTS
	Na^+	Ca^{++}			SEIZURE TYPE	ABSENCE	OTHER	
Phenytoin	x		x	x	TC, CP, SE		NP, rarely	Prompt and
Gabapentin		x	x		P		NP	May be useful for neuropathic pain
Vigabatrin			x		P-AJ, CP, LG, WS			Irreversible GABA transaminase inhibitor
Felbamate	x		x	x	P-AJ, LG			Use limited by toxicity
Tiagabine			x		P-AJ			Blocks GABA reuptake
Topiramate	x		x	AK[‡]	P-AJ			Unique monosaccharide structure
Zonisamide	x	x	x		P-AJ			Sulfonamide-like structure, some antidepressant-like action and carbonic anhydrase action
Levetiracetam					P-AJ			Synaptic inhibitor

AJ, Adjunctive use; *AK*, akinetic; *BI*, bipolar disorder; *CF*, corticofocal; *CP*, complex partial psychomotor; *CT*, catamenial; *F*, febrile; *IM*, impulse disorder; *JM*, Jacksonian motor; *LA*, local anesthetic-induced seizures; *LG*, Lennox-Gastaut syndrome (children); *NP*, trigeminal neuralgia, diabetic neuropathy, or postherpetic neuropathy; *P*, partial seizures; *SE*, status epilepticus; *TC*, tonic-clonic; *WS*, West's syndrome (children).

*Several anticonvulsants are being used to treat bipolar disorder, neuralgia (and chronic pain), and impulse control disorders. They may be referred to by the term *mood stabilizers.*

†Derived from the sulfonamides.

‡α-Amino-3-hydroxy-5-methyl-4-isoxazole propionate (AMPA) or kainate glutamate process inhibition.

effects and adverse reactions is greater than for agents used for shorter periods. Anticonvulsants may have long lists of potential adverse reactions, but the incidence of many of these reactions is low. Adverse reactions can result from the direct action of the drug, such as dizziness, drowsiness, and ataxia. These dose-related reactions are common but not usually dangerous. Reported adverse reactions may also include withdrawal phenomena, which make the reactions appear paradoxic. Some reactions reflect manifestations of allergic reactions, which may be as mild as a rash or as serious as life-threatening Stevens-Johnson syndrome. Other adverse reactions are detected by standard blood tests. These range from benign elevation of liver enzymes to serious hepatic failure.

Several antiepileptic drugs can alter liver enzyme function. A cluster of adverse reactions and drug interactions can result from induction of hepatic enzymes, which may alter the metabolism of (1) the inducing anticonvulsant agent; (2) other drugs, altering their half-lives or toxicity; (3) vitamins (folate, vitamins D or K), which can produce vitamin deficiency disorders such as megaloblastic anemia, decreased bone density, fetal toxicity, or bleeding disorders; and (4) hormones (thyroid hormone or birth control pills). Drug effects on liver microsomal enzyme activity are summarized in Box 14-1. Carbamazepine, phenobarbital, phenytoin, and primidone are well-documented induction agents for both the oxidative cytochrome P450 pathway and for phase II synthetic or conjugation elimination pathways (including uridine diphosphate glucuronosyltransferase [UGT]) and in some cases for P-glycoprotein, which may play a role in multiple drug resistance and poor seizure control. Phenobarbital, phenytoin, carbamazepine, felbamate, lamotrigine, gabapentin, and topiramate bind to P-glycoproteins that appear to facilitate their elimination from the brain. Lamotrigine selectively inhibits UGT. Valproate and topiramate may inhibit oxidative enzymes, prolonging the actions of other drugs. Oxcarbazepine and phenytoin may also inhibit some liver enzymes, as shown in Box 14-1.

Additional adverse reactions associated with anticonvulsant drugs include gingival overgrowth, aplastic anemia, hepatotoxicity, renal stones, visual disturbances, and fevers. These may represent pharmacogenomic processes or poorly understood aspects of their pharmacologic features in susceptible patients. Sometimes the reaction is manifested as teratogenicity or cancer; these delayed toxicities are dose independent but host dependent. Recent studies have found new evidence that anticonvulsant drug use contributes to an increased incidence of birth defects.[18] Behavioral, neurologic, and psychiatric reactions are not uncommon and can occur with several of the anticonvulsants. Drugs that facilitate GABA or inhibit glutamate pathways may be more likely to induce amnesia.

Anticonvulsant drugs can paradoxically promote seizure activity or precipitate new seizure types. Carbamazepine, for instance, can increase absence and other seizures. Other

Box • 14-1

Adverse Effect of Antiepileptic Drugs on Liver Microsomal Enzymes

Drugs That Can Induce Liver Microsomal Enzymes

Phenobarbital
Phenytoin
Carbamazepine
Oxcarbazepine
Lamotrigine

Drugs That Can Inhibit Liver Microsomal Enzymes

Oxcarbazepine*
Topiramate
Valproic acid
Phenytoin*

*Inhibition and induction have both been reported. This is possible because different cytochrome P450 enzyme classes are involved in each effect.

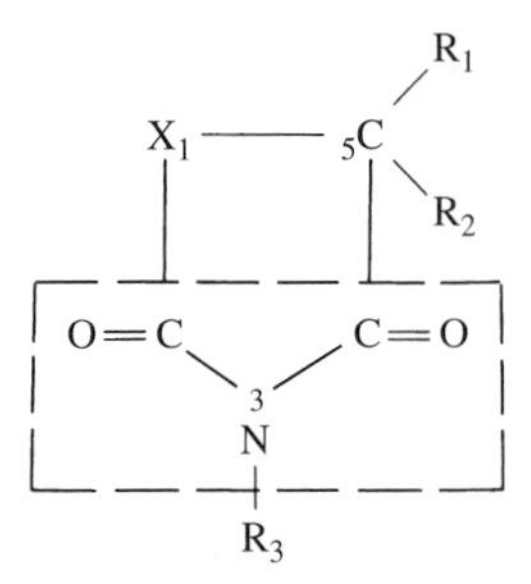

Fig. 14-2 Basic ring structure common to classic anticonvulsants.

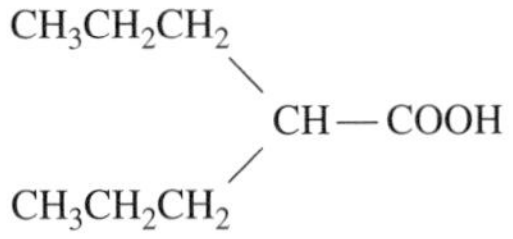

$CH_3CH_2CH_2$
CH—COOH
$CH_3CH_2CH_2$

Fig. 14-3 Structural formula of valproic acid.

N
O=C—NH_2
Carbamazepine

O
10
N
O=C—NH_2
Oxcarbazepine

Fig. 14-4 Structural formulas of carbamazepine and oxcarbazepine.

anticonvulsants that may exacerbate seizures include phenytoin, phenobarbital, vigabatrin, oxycarbazine, lamotrigine, gabapentin, felbamate, and tiagabine.[13] Increased seizure frequency is more likely in patients with severe seizure disorders. A number of studies have shown that the substantia nigra pars reticulata may be involved in absence (and other) seizure genesis.[32]

Newer agents are expected to have more favorable safety profiles based on their different mechanisms of action and their lessened interaction with the microsomal drug metabolizing system.[6] However, a full understanding of the clinical toxicology of drugs can take years to develop. In the case of vigabatrin, early reports about the drug can be found in the 1970s, yet the first report of patients commonly (30% or more) developing irreversible visual field defects was published in 1997.[17] Gabapentin was found to have a low side effect profile in evaluation trials but is now being used at doses that are many times greater than were typically studied. Experts have noted that much of what is known about the new anticonvulsant drugs has been derived from manufacturer-sponsored trials.[6] Differences in studied patient populations, dosages used, and the end points reported make clinically meaningful comparisons problematic; larger comparison studies by independent groups are still needed.[9]

Table • 14-3

Classes of Anticonvulsants According to Substitution at Position X_1 of the Chemical Structure (see Figure 14-2)

ANTICONVULSANT	SUBSTITUTION
Barbiturates	—CO—NH—
Hydantoins	—NH—
Succinimides	—CH_2—

CHEMISTRY AND STRUCTURE-ACTIVITY RELATIONSHIPS

Figure 14-2 shows the common structure present in all the clinically effective anticonvulsants developed before 1960. Substitution at position 1 of the ring results in the various classes of anticonvulsants indicated in Table 14-3.

A phenyl ring at R_1 or R_2, such as appears in phenytoin, is a highly desirable though not crucial substituent for protection against tonic-clonic epilepsy. An alkyl substituent at R_1 or R_2, such as appears in ethosuximide, is desirable (but again not crucial) for control of absence seizures. A great deal of detailed structure activity information was obtained to identify opportunities for developing improved agents. However, recent discoveries have included several agents with unrelated structures. Valproic acid, for instance, is N-dipropylacetic acid (Figure 14-3), a simple branched-chain carboxylic acid, and carbamazepine (Figure 14-4) is chemically related to the tricyclic antidepressants and is used in the treatment of certain affective disorders (see Chapter 12).

HYDANTOINS

Phenytoin (diphenylhydantoin) is one of the first drugs to be discovered through an organized scientific search for a therapeutically effective compound. Introduced in 1938, phenytoin was immediately recognized as a breakthrough in anticonvulsant therapy because it suppressed seizures without causing as much sedative effect as phenobarbital. Phenytoin has served as an effective anticonvulsant against tonic-clonic and

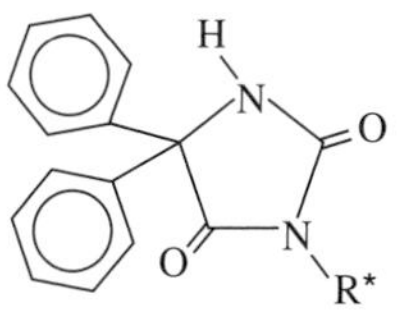

Phenytoin R* = H

Fosphenytoin R* = $-OPO_3^{--} + 2\,Na^+$

Fig. 14-5 Structural formulas of phenytoin and fosphenytoin.

partial seizures as well as an important pharmacologic tool that has increased our understanding of the underlying mechanisms responsible for epileptic syndromes. Mephenytoin and ethotoin are hydantoins related to phenytoin but are now rarely used. Fosphenytoin, the newest hydantoin, is a phosphorylated prodrug that is rapidly converted to phenytoin by endogenous phosphatase enzymes. It is water soluble and is better tolerated by parenteral administration. The structures of phenytoin and fosphenytoin are shown in Figure 14-5.

Pharmacologic Effects

Although the mechanism of action responsible for the anticonvulsant effect of phenytoin is not established, many of its known pharmacologic properties may contribute to it. In neurophysiologic studies, phenytoin prevents the spread of abnormal neuronal depolarization from the epileptic focus to surrounding normal neuronal populations, yet spontaneous discharge at the focus is not depressed. Additionally, phenytoin suppresses the duration of neuronal afterdischarge. Phenytoin may reduce the spread of neuronal activity and afterdischarge by blocking posttetanic potentiation, a phenomenon in which synaptic transmission is enhanced as a result of repetitive presynaptic activation (as would occur at an abnormally firing epileptic focus).

The major site of action of phenytoin appears to be at the Na^+ channel, and various actions have been demonstrated at this site. However, the only mechanism evident at concentrations equivalent to therapeutic plasma concentrations (10 to 20 μg/ml) is a reduction in sustained high-frequency neuronal firing caused by phenytoin binding reversibly to inactivated Na^+ channels.[26] Phenytoin thus delays the neuronal recovery process whereby Na^+ channels cycle from the refractory, inactivated state to the responsive, closed configuration, which is required before an action potential can once again be generated. Phenytoin binding to inactivated Na^+ channels is frequency and voltage dependent, so that it becomes greater as neuronal depolarization and firing frequency increase. These properties are ideally suited for anticonvulsant activity because high-frequency neuronal discharge is characteristic of the epileptic disorders. High extracellular K^+, typically found during seizures, also increases the effectiveness of phenytoin. Furthermore, normal (slower) neuronal activity is relatively unaffected by phenytoin, which may explain its minimal sedative effects. At slightly greater than therapeutic concentrations, phenytoin interferes with Ca^{++} channels and the interaction of Ca^{++} and calmodulin,[8] which in turn disrupts Ca^{++}-dependent phosphorylation of proteins necessary for neurotransmitter release from presynaptic nerve terminals. There are also some reports of phenytoin facilitating GABA or inhibiting glutamate processes.[7] Phenytoin has also been found to alter the metabolism of some growth factors, which could play a role in neuroprotective actions of the drug (see below).

In summary, although many mechanisms have been demonstrated for phenytoin, prolonging Na^+ channel inactivation is the most compelling explanation for its anticonvulsant effect. This action is one of the few that occur at therapeutic concentrations, and the characteristics of this mechanism are ideally suited for anticonvulsant activity.

Absorption, Fate, and Excretion

Phenytoin is absorbed slowly from the gastrointestinal tract. The absorption rate varies with the individual, but differences in formulation of the dosage unit account for much of this fluctuation. The Food and Drug Administration (FDA) requires that phenytoin capsules be labeled as "extended" or "prompt" depending on their absorption rate. An extended-action capsule has slow absorption, with peak blood concentrations obtained in 4 to 12 hours. A prompt-action capsule has rapid absorption, with peak concentrations occurring in 1.5 to 3 hours. Because noncompliance is a major problem in anticonvulsant therapy, it is sometimes advisable to administer the total daily dose of phenytoin at one time. Once-a-day administration is not appropriate for suspensions of phenytoin (commonly used for children) because plasma concentrations may reach toxic values. Changing from one dosage form or manufacturer to another has led to suboptimal plasma concentrations from differences in bioavailability.

Phenytoin given by intravenous injection can produce thrombophlebitis, arrhythmia, and hypotension. These side effects are largely caused by the vehicle needed to solubilize phenytoin for injection. Intramuscular injection of phenytoin may precipitate in the muscle, cause pain, and be poorly absorbed. Fosphenytoin is a water-soluble analogue that may be given intravenously or intramuscularly. After intramuscular administration, it produces much less pain and is absorbed rapidly.[35]

Phenytoin is highly protein bound (90%), which may play a role in interactions with drugs that compete for plasma protein binding sites. Phenytoin is inactivated in the liver to its primary metabolite, the parahydroxyphenyl derivative. Phenytoin can induce drug metabolizing enzymes, including CYP3A4 and UGT. After conjugation with glucuronic acid, phenytoin and its metabolites are eliminated in the urine. Phenytoin removal from the brain may be facilitated by P-glycoproteins and multiple drug resistance–associated proteins, which may be induced in epileptic tissue. Phenytoin is also excreted by the salivary glands, which may be a contributing factor in producing gingival overgrowth (hyperplasia, see below). With peak concentrations seen at 3 to 12 hours, the elimination half-life of phenytoin (and fosphenytoin) generally varies from 6 to 24 hours. Near the effective dose, however, phenytoin often exhibits capacity-limited metabolism because the enzymes responsible for its metabolism are readily saturated. The drug's half-life can become longer, and, if blood concentrations are increased beyond the saturation threshold, rapid drug accumulation may increase the likelihood of toxic reactions.

Adverse Effects

Ataxia, nystagmus, incoordination, and unsteadiness occur with phenytoin overdose. These sequelae may result from phenytoin-induced changes on Purkinje cells of the cerebellum (such changes may also be caused by repeated seizures). Drowsiness, lethargy, diplopia, confusion, and (rarely) hallucinations are other manifestations of phenytoin toxicity. Phenytoin in usual doses has little detrimental effect on the cardiovascular system; however, it can cause cardiovascular collapse, irreversible coma, and death if administered in massive intravenous doses.

Phenytoin causes gingival overgrowth in approximately 10% to 30% of all patients. Gingival overgrowth is usually more severe in children, for whom its incidence may be as high as 50%. The primary mechanism responsible for this side effect is not known. Several hypotheses have been proposed involving inflammation, bacterial plaque, the presence of teeth or dental implants, gingival fibroblast phenotype, epithelial growth factor, collagenase activation, folic acid deficiency, Na^+/Ca^{++} flux, and perhaps salivary delivery of phenytoin into the mouth.[1] It has recently been observed that phenytoin increases platelet-derived growth factor B (PDGF-B) and its mRNA from macrophages that are thought to induce gingival fibroblast proliferation and local angiogenesis.[20] The result is an increase in fibroblast cell growth with increased interstitial ground substance.[38] Other drugs that induce gingival overgrowth include the immunosuppressant cyclosporine A and the dihydropyridine Ca^{++} channel–blocking drugs. Figure 14-6 represents a possible model of gingival overgrowth. Phenytoin may also cause numerous other side effects as summarized in Table 14-4. Phenytoin interferes with the metabolic activation of vitamins D and K and the absorption of Ca^{++}. Although the resultant effect on bone metabolism is usually subclinical, overt cases of rickets and osteomalacia have been observed.[14] Vitamin D or K supplements may prevent these conditions.[19,34] Vitamin K modulates the synthesis of osteocalcin and matrix Gla proteins, which in turn influence Ca^{++} metabolism in bone. Children born to mothers who have received phenytoin (often in combination with phenobarbital, carbamazepine, or valproic acid) throughout their pregnancy are at increased risk of congenital malformation.[18] The most common anomalies are cleft lip, cleft palate, and congenital heart disease. These developmental defects, as well as a delay in psychomotor development, prenatal and postnatal growth deficiencies, impaired intellectual performance, and genitourinary and skeletal deformations, are collectively referred to as the *fetal hydantoin syndrome.* Although none of the well-studied anticonvulsants is completely devoid of teratogenic potential, animal data suggest that, of the older drugs, carbamazepine and phenobarbital may be the safer anticonvulsants to use in pregnancy.[47]

BARBITURATES

Phenobarbital is one of the oldest, least expensive, least toxic, and most effective anticonvulsants available. Because of its sedative effect and the introduction of newer drugs, the use of phenobarbital for treating epileptic disorders has waned. Phenobarbital offers an appreciable spectrum of anticonvulsant activity because of its effectiveness against many tonic-clonic and partial seizures.

Barbiturates other than phenobarbital are occasionally used for the treatment of epilepsy. Mephobarbital is less sedating than phenobarbital, although its anticonvulsant properties result largely from its metabolic conversion to phenobarbital. Primidone, a deoxybarbiturate relative of phenobarbital, is used for generalized and partial seizures, particularly those refractory to other drugs. The use of primidone is somewhat limited because of its marked sedative properties immediately after administration.

Pharmacologic Effects

The barbiturates are CNS depressants and exert a marked inhibitory effect on repetitive neuronal activity in CNS pathways. Like phenytoin, phenobarbital limits the spread of seizure discharge, but it also raises the threshold for activation of epileptic foci. As discussed in Chapter 13 (which also covers the general pharmacology of these drugs), the barbiturates enhance the binding of GABA to postsynaptic $GABA_A$ receptors and increase the time that GABA-activated Cl^- channels are open. They also activate Cl^- channels independently of GABA. Inhibition of the excitatory effects of glutamate may also be a major antiepileptic mechanism. Other mechanisms appear to play lesser roles. Barbiturates block the transcellular transport of Na^+ and K^+, which could explain their membrane-stabilizing properties. Like phenytoin, barbiturates interfere with Ca^{++} channels and inhibit Ca^{++} entry into presynaptic nerve terminals.

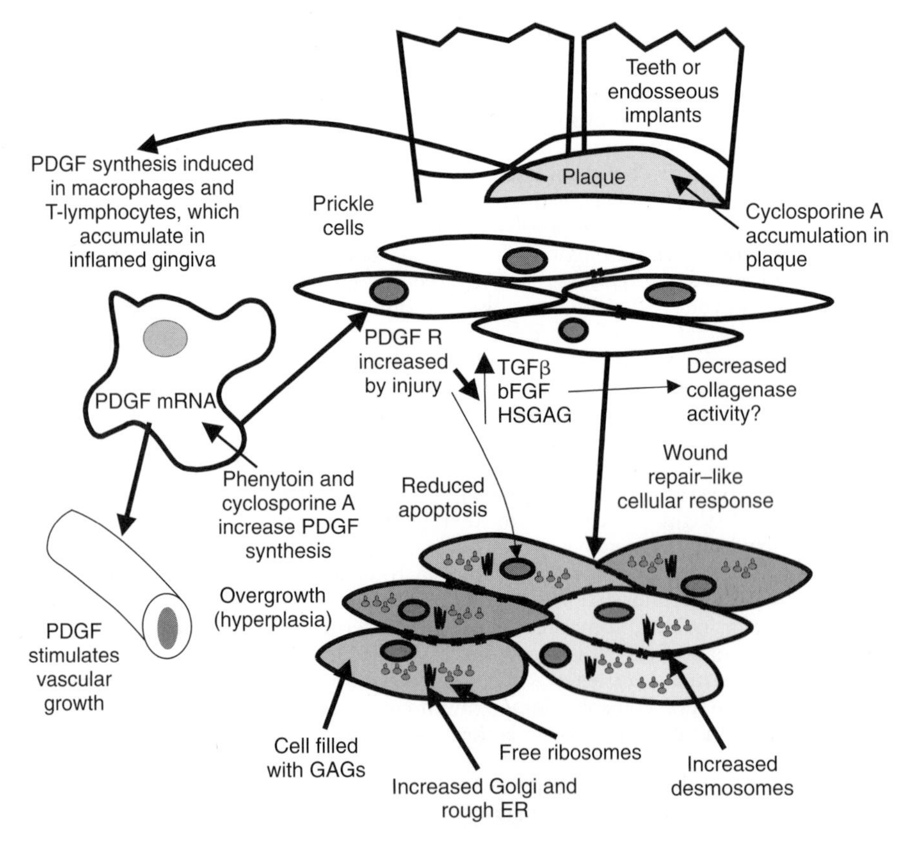

Fig. 14-6 The effect of *phenytoin and cyclosporine A* on gingival overgrowth. Predisposing factors include the presence of teeth or implants, inflammation, and overgrowth-inducing drugs. Phenytoin increases by sixfold *PDGF mRNA* in reparative/proliferative macrophages.[38] PDGF is thought to increase both angiogenesis and wound repair. Increases in fibroblastic growth factors, such as transforming growth factor β *(TGFβ)* and basic fibroblast growth factor *(bFGF)*, and production of heparin sulfate glycosaminoglycan *(HSGAG)* are induced by PDGF acting on its receptors *(R)*. *Prickle cells* in the gingiva become filled with glycosaminoglycans *(GAGs)*, rough endoplasmic reticulum *(ER)*, and *ribosomes* and their connective *desmosomes* proliferate *(bottom)*.

Table • 14-4

Some Adverse Reactions Reported for Anticonvulsant Drugs

DRUG	ADVERSE REACTIONS
Phenytoin and fosphenytoin	Gingival hyperplasia, hirsutism, megaloblastic anemia, osteomalacia, sedation, ataxia, gastrointestinal disturbances, behavioral changes
Carbamazepine and oxcarbazepine	Sedation, weakness, ataxia, diplopia, gastrointestinal disturbances, skin rash, behavioral changes, aplastic anemia (rare)
Phenobarbital	Sedation, weakness, ataxia, reduced cognition, respiratory depression, blood dyscrasias, megaloblastic anemia, osteomalacia, drug dependence
Valproic acid	Sedation, weakness, ataxia, gastrointestinal disturbances, weight gain, hepatic toxicity (especially in children <2 years), spina bifida if given during pregnancy, visual disturbances, pancreatitis, hyperammonemia
Ethosuximide	Sedation, weakness, gastrointestinal disturbances, ataxia, behavioral changes, lupus erythematosus (rare)
Diazepam	Sedation, weakness, nystagmus, ataxia, drug dependence, drug tolerance
Lorazepam	Same as diazepam
Midazolam	Same as diazepam
Chlorazepate	Same as diazepam
Clonazepam	Same as diazepam
Gabapentin	Sedation, weakness, ataxia, rash, tremor
Lamotrigine	Sedation, weakness, ataxia, diplopia, rash, headache, gastrointestinal disturbances, Stevens-Johnson syndrome (1% of children)
Topiramate	Sedation, weakness, ataxia, visual disturbances, paresthesias, kidney stones, breast pain
Tiagabine	Sedation, weakness, ataxia, gastrointestinal disturbances, tremor
Vigabatrin	Sedation, weakness, ataxia, psychotic reactions, visual disturbances, blood dyscrasias
Zonisamide	Sedation, weakness, ataxia, gastrointestinal disturbances, skin rashes, Stevens-Johnson syndrome, renal tubule acidosis, renal stones
Levetiracetam	Sedation, weakness, ataxia, behavioral changes, withdrawal reactions

Absorption, Fate, and Excretion

Phenobarbital is completely but slowly absorbed from the gastrointestinal tract. About half of the drug is bound to plasma protein. Approximately 30% of phenobarbital is excreted unchanged in the urine, and the rest is inactivated by the liver. Phenobarbital is a substrate for several cytochrome P450 isozymes. As discussed in Chapter 2, phenobarbital can also induce CYP2A, CYP2B, CYP2C, CYP3A, and CYP6A isoforms, reduced nicotinamide adenine dinucleotide cytochrome P450 reductase, UGT,[46] P-glycoproteins, and multiple drug resistance–associated proteins (see Chapter 2). The plasma half-life of phenobarbital ranges between 50 and 140 hours. Because of its long half-life, very small fluctuations in plasma concentrations occur over a 24-hour period. Primidone is metabolized to phenobarbital (which can be detected in the plasma in approximately 24 to 48 hours) and phenylethylmalonamide, which also has anticonvulsant properties and is measurable in plasma within 1 to 2 hours and has a 10- to 18-hour half-life.

Adverse Effects

The major adverse effects of phenobarbital are covered in Chapter 13. The most common initial effect of phenobarbital and the other barbiturates is sedation. (A paradoxic excitatory reaction may sometimes occur in children and the elderly.) Tolerance usually develops to the sedative effect. Like phenytoin, phenobarbital has been reported to cause megaloblastic anemia and osteomalacia, which have been successfully treated with folic acid and vitamins D and K, respectively. Phenobarbital appears to be relatively free of teratogenic effects, but when phenobarbital is given with phenytoin (a commonly used combination), teratogenicity appears to increase.

The most common side effects of primidone are primarily a result of its CNS depressant properties. Complications include sedation, dizziness, ataxia, and nystagmus. Various blood dyscrasias and rashes similar to those described for phenytoin can occur.

CARBAMAZEPINE

Carbamazepine is an iminostilbene derivative (see Figure 14-4) closely related chemically to the tricyclic antidepressants. It differs from the tricyclic antidepressant imipramine by the presence of a double bond in the central ring and a shorter side chain. Carbamazepine is a major anticonvulsant drug and is highly effective against tonic-clonic and partial seizures. It also lacks dysmorphic side effects (gingival hypertrophy, acne, hirsutism) common to phenytoin. Like phenytoin, carbamazepine is indicated for the treatment of trigeminal neuralgia; in fact, carbamazepine has been the most commonly used drug for this disorder. Carbamazepine is also effective for other neuropathic pains such as glossopharyngeal neuralgia, postherpetic neuralgia, diabetic neuropathy, causalgia, and hemifacial spasm, but it is not a typical analgesic because it is ineffective for other types of pain. As discussed in Chapter 12, carbamazepine is sometimes effective in the treatment or prophylaxis of affective disorders.

A keto analogue, oxcarbazepine, has a therapeutic profile similar to carbamazepine. It may have fewer side effects than carbamazepine and is well tolerated. Oxcarbazepine is a prodrug, requiring metabolic reduction to the 10-hydroxy metabolite before it becomes active.

Pharmacologic Effects

Like phenytoin, carbamazepine reduces experimentally induced sustained high-frequency neuronal firing at doses that produce clinically relevant plasma concentrations.[30] This effect, like that of phenytoin, appears to result from carbamazepine binding to inactivated Na^+ channels, thus slowing neuronal recovery after activation. This action has been confirmed by using neurophysiologic techniques such as cell membrane voltage clamping. Carbamazepine also reduces Ca^{++} and Na^+ flux across the neuronal membrane. As with other anticonvulsants, various mechanisms may contribute to its anticonvulsant effect. Nevertheless, limitation of sustained repetitive neuronal firing offers the most likely explanation for the drug's antiepileptic properties. Because of its structural similarity to antidepressants, effects on monamine reuptake function might be expected, but these effects, if any, appear to be minor.

Absorption, Fate, and Excretion

Carbamazepine is absorbed slowly, reaching peak plasma concentrations in 4 to 8 hours. It is distributed throughout the body; highest concentrations occur in the liver, kidneys, and brain. The drug is transported out of the brain by P-glycoproteins and multiple drug resistance–associated proteins. Carbamazepine is metabolized by cytochrome P450 3A4 and can also induce CYP3A4 and UGT, leading to drug interactions and a significant reduction in its own half-life, which is 25 to 65 hours initially and 12 to 17 hours after long-term administration. CYP3A4 inhibitors (e.g., erythromycin) can increase the duration of action of carbamazepine. At least one metabolite of carbamazepine, carbamazepine-10,11-epoxide, has anticonvulsant properties and is relatively stable. Carbamazepine is inactivated by further oxidation and conjugation before being excreted in the urine.

The carbamazepine analogue oxcarbazepine (see Figure 14-4) is rapidly converted to the 10-hydroxy metabolite, which exerts peak activity from 3 to 13 hours and has a 9-hour half-life. Oxcarbazepine is a mild CYP3A4 inducer and, like carbamazepine, can accelerate the metabolism of several drugs, including oral contraceptives.

Adverse Effects

The most common signs and symptoms of overdose with carbamazepine include dizziness, diplopia, drowsiness, headache, ataxia, and slurred speech. Convulsions may be precipitated by acute intoxication with carbamazepine, and it exacerbates absence and myoclonic seizures. Various types of involuntary motor activity in the elderly have been reported, and hallucinations have occurred. Skin rashes have been reported. If leukopenia occurs, it is usually mild. Other hematologic reactions to carbamazepine are rare but sometimes life threatening. Aplastic anemia is of particular concern, and agranulocytosis has also occurred.

VALPROIC ACID

Valproic acid (dipropylacetic acid), approved by the FDA in 1978, is a broad-spectrum anticonvulsant particularly effective against absence seizures but also useful for other generalized forms of epilepsy (e.g., tonic-clonic, myoclonic) and partial seizures. Interest has focused on valproic acid because it has a simple chemical structure (see Figure 14-3) unrelated to that of traditional anticonvulsant drugs and was the first drug effective against both absence and tonic-clonic seizures.

Pharmacologic Effects

Like phenytoin and carbamazepine, valproic acid reduces sustained high-frequency neuronal firing at therapeutic doses.[26] Valproic acid appears to bind to a different site on the Na^+ channel than does phenytoin, yet the final result is similar. As discussed for phenytoin, inhibition of Na^+ channels represents a plausible action because the drug effect is frequency and voltage dependent, thus becoming more prominent at increasing rates of neuronal depolarization.

Experimental studies have shown that supertherapeutic doses of valproic acid increase brain GABA concentrations by interfering with enzymes involved with GABA. Valproic acid is a weak inhibitor of GABA transaminase, the first enzyme in the catabolic pathway, and a more potent inhibitor of succinic semialdehyde dehydrogenase, the next enzyme in the pathway. Valproic acid may also increase brain GABA by stimulating glutamic acid decarboxylase, the major synthetic enzyme for GABA. Other research has found an association between valproate anticonvulsant activity and reductions of the excitatory neurotransmitter aspartate in the brain.[26]

The salutary effect of valproic acid on absence seizures is most likely associated with the drug's ability to inhibit Ca^{++} influx through T-type Ca^{++} channels. This mechanism is discussed below in the section on the succinimides. In addition to seizures, valproic acid is approved for the treatment of bipolar disorder, and its divalproex extended-release form for the prevention of migraine headaches.

Absorption, Fate, and Excretion

Valproic acid is completely absorbed from the gastrointestinal tract and is highly bound to plasma proteins. The absorption rate depends on the formulation (capsules, tablets, or syrup); food may delay absorption. Divalproex sodium, a combination of valproic acid and its sodium salt, is supplied in capsules that are designed to be opened and sprinkled on soft food. This product is a convenient dosage form for children and geriatric patients.

Valproic acid crosses membrane barriers and is found in the fetus, milk, liver, kidney, and brain. It also accumulates in growing bone. Valproic acid is thought to enter the brain through a saturable process and brain concentrations can be increased by blocking the multiple drug resistance–associated protein with probenecid. Valproic acid undergoes complex oxidation and conjugation before excretion in the urine. It inhibits its own metabolism and that of other drugs, such as phenobarbital. This effect can contribute to drug accumulation and drug interactions. Valproic acid inhibits the metabolism of some substrates metabolized by CYP3A4. The half-life of valproic acid is approximately 5 to 20 hours, with peak blood concentrations at 1 to 4 hours.

Adverse Effects

The most common manifestations of valproic acid toxicity are appetite disturbances, indigestion, heartburn, nausea, and weight change. Fortunately, the gastrointestinal reactions are usually temporary. Tremor is also a common adverse effect, especially at higher doses. Valproic acid can cause fatal hepatic dysfunction, and children are particularly susceptible. The likelihood of this apparently idiosyncratic effect decreases with age, being most common in children younger than 2 years and uncommon after 10 years. Irreversible hepatotoxicity appears to be caused by a toxic metabolite (2-n-propyl-4-pentenoic acid). Because its production is known to be increased by enzyme-inducing anticonvulsants, combined therapy of valproic acid and such anticonvulsants puts the patient at increased risk of liver damage. More commonly, valproic acid may cause a reversible hepatotoxicity that is dose dependent. Another serious toxicity associated with valproate is life-threatening pancreatitis. This can occur in children or adults and may follow a rapid course. This reaction may occur any time when taking the medication. Presenting signs include abdominal pain, nausea, vomiting, and/or anorexia. If pancreatitis is diagnosed the drug should be stopped. Other serious side effects, such as neurologic and hematologic toxicity, are rare. High doses of valproic acid may cause platelet disorders, leading to bruising of the skin and, occasionally, gingival bleeding. However, platelet dysfunction usually is not severe, and the patient is asymptomatic. Valproic acid is associated with neural tube defects, and its use during pregnancy results in a significantly higher risk of spina bifida.

SUCCINIMIDES

Ethosuximide is a major drug for the treatment of absence seizures. The use of related succinimides (methsuximide, phensuximide) is restricted to patients refractory to ethosuximide because these agents are less effective and/or more toxic. Another agent, the oxazolidinedione trimethadione, has also been used in absence seizures but is rarely used today because of its toxicity.

Pharmacologic Effects

Ethosuximide prevents absence seizures in approximately 50% of patients and reduces their frequency in another 40% to 45%. The mechanism of action of ethosuximide is not firmly established; however, its administration leads to a dose-dependent inhibition of low-threshold Ca^{++} currents carried by T-type Ca^{++} channels.[5] Low-threshold Ca^{++} currents are an important factor in oscillatory behavior of thalamic neurons, and the thalamus is known to play an important role in generating the 3-Hz spike-and-wave rhythms that characterize petit mal epilepsy. This effect occurs at clinical concentrations and is the best explanation yet proposed for the mechanism of action of drugs effective against absence seizures.

Absorption, Fate, and Excretion

The succinimides are absorbed from the gastrointestinal tract, metabolized in the liver (by CYP3A4), and excreted as metabolites in the urine. The plasma half-life of ethosuximide is approximately 30 hours in children and 45 to 60 hours in adults. Ethosuximide passes membrane barriers rapidly and thus appears in cerebrospinal fluid, milk, saliva, and fetal tissues. Salivary titers accurately reflect plasma concentrations and may be useful to monitor blood levels.[42]

Adverse Effects

The succinimides commonly cause gastrointestinal distress, headache, dizziness, and skin rash. More serious reactions have been reported but are rare, especially with ethosuximide. Nevertheless, blood counts are recommended at no greater than monthly intervals, because potentially fatal bone marrow depression may occur. Patients with hematopoietic toxicity may exhibit fever, sore throat, and coagulopathy, as indicated by oral and cutaneous petechiae. Ethosuximide is less teratogenic than alternative drugs for absence seizures and is therefore preferred in pregnancy.[47]

DRUGS AFFECTING GABA TRANSMISSION

GABAergic mechanisms appear to contribute to seizure susceptibility in a number of animal models of epilepsy. Impaired GABAergic function can be demonstrated in rats, mice, gerbils, and baboons genetically prone to epilepsy. Although faulty GABAergic mechanisms have not been convincingly demonstrated in human beings, cerebrospinal fluid concentrations of GABA are reduced in epileptic patients, and surgically removed epileptic brain tissue exhibits decreased GABAergic activity. Drugs that are antagonists at $GABA_A$ receptors (bicuculline, picrotoxin) are potent convulsants, whereas drugs that facilitate GABAergic mechanisms (benzodiazepines) are anticonvulsants. Flumazenil, a benzodiazepine receptor antagonist, has been reported to precipitate seizures in patients who have an elevated seizure risk, are taking anticonvulsant benzodiazepines or tricyclic antidepressants,[43] or received midazolam to treat local anesthetic toxicity.[51] Abnormal flumazenil binding, imaged with PET, is used to target abnormal epileptogenic tissue for surgical removal.[22] Furthermore, inverse agonists at the benzodiazepine receptors can also act as convulsants because they reduce the contribution of constitutively active (active without agonist) benzodiazepine receptors. This effect leads to decreased Cl^- channel conductance, resulting in depolarization.

Similar to other neurotransmitter pathways, the $GABA_A$ receptor system has multiple sites that may lend themselves to pharmacologic control (Figure 14-7).[2] Presynaptically, neurotransmitter synthesis, storage, and release mechanisms may be targeted. Additionally there are GABA reuptake transporters, autoreceptors, and catabolic enzymes found presynaptically. Some GABAergic neurons contain cotransmitters such as enkephalin or substance P. Postsynaptically, multiple forms of $GABA_A$ receptors (ligand-gated ion channels) are found. The ligand-gated ion channel can be composed of a variety of component isoforms. At this time six α, four β, three γ, three ρ, and individual δ, ε, π, and θ subunit isoforms have been identified. Each ion channel is a mixture of five of these subunits, with the most predominant isoform being two α_1, two β_2, and one γ_2. Some changes in the ion channel composition have been seen in epileptic brain.[4] A postsynaptic machinery for controlling the numbers and types of receptors has been described, and there are postsynaptic second messenger processes and receptor phosphorylation.[27] Cooperative relationships may exist between GABA receptors and other receptor types that produce adaptive changes.[2] These processes may include the basis for developing tolerance to the actions of some antiepileptic drugs. In addition, GABA uptake proteins and metabolic enzymes may also be found in glial cells and some perineural structures.[2] GABA also acts through $GABA_B$ receptors (metabotropic receptors; see Chapter 13).

Benzodiazepines

Most of the benzodiazepine agonists have anticonvulsant properties. The pharmacologic profiles of these drugs and the mechanisms by which they facilitate GABAergic transmission are discussed in detail in Chapter 13. Diazepam, clonazepam, clorazepate, midazolam, and lorazepam are the principal benzodiazepines used clinically in the United States as anticonvulsants. Midazolam, clonazepam, and lorazepam have higher affinities for the benzodiazepine receptor and may be more effective anticonvulsants.[37] Diazepam is effective in terminating the life-threatening continual convulsion of status epilepticus and for the treatment of local anesthetic-induced seizures. Intravenous lorazepam (0.1 mg/kg) was found to be more effective than phenytoin alone (18 mg/kg) for the treatment of generalized status epilepticus[49] and successfully treated a greater percentage of patients than diazepam. Intravenous midazolam has also been found to be effective in the treatment of status epilepticus and local anesthetic excitotoxicity, and its use by the buccal route is being explored.[16,54] Clonazepam is generally effective for absence seizures and childhood myoclonic epilepsy and is sometimes effective for complex partial seizures and reflex epilepsies (photosensitive epilepsy). Clorazepate is indicated as adjunctive therapy in the management of partial seizures.

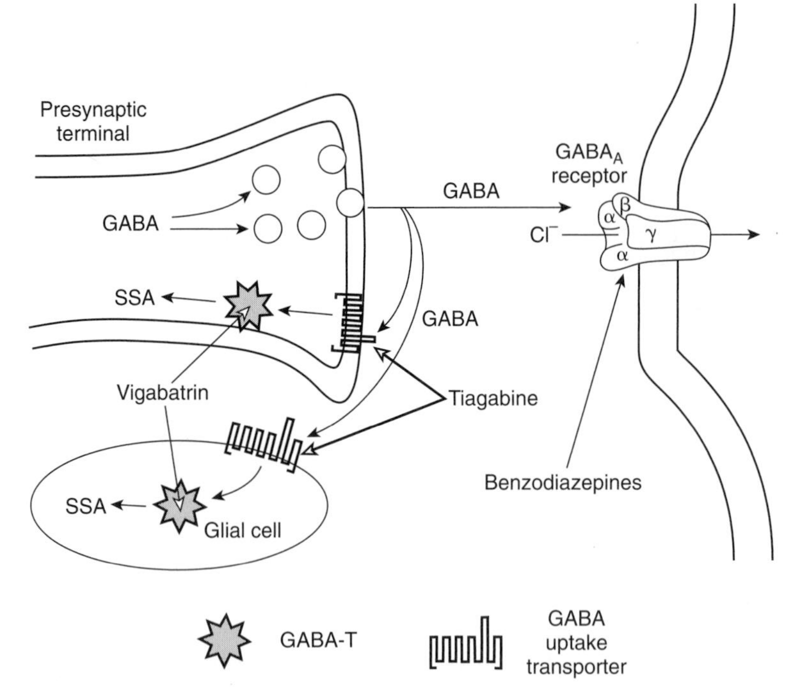

Fig. 14-7 Proposed sites of actions for drugs acting at the GABA synapse. *GABA* inhibits the postsynaptic neuron by acting on a receptor *($GABA_A$)* on the Cl^- channel. *Benzodiazepines* act to facilitate the action of GABA postsynaptically by interacting with a separate site on the Cl^- channel. The action of GABA can be terminated by reuptake or catabolism. GABA is taken back into the presynaptic nerve terminals and glial cells by a Na^+-driven symporter protein. *Tiagabine* blocks this *GABA transporter*. GABA α-oxoglutarate transaminase *(GABA-T)* terminates the action of GABA by converting it to succinic semialdehyde. *Vigabatrin* inhibits GABA-T.

Like phenytoin, the benzodiazepines prevent the spread of the seizure discharge but have little effect on neuronal firing at the seizure focus. The anticonvulsant effect of the benzodiazepines is thought to be exerted through modification of GABA-mediated systems, as is the case for their antianxiety effect. However, different receptor subtypes might be involved. Both $GABA_A$ and $GABA_B$ mechanisms are believed to be involved in absence seizures.[44]

The absorption, fate, and excretion of the benzodiazepines are discussed in Chapter 13. There are no differences in these properties when these drugs are used as anticonvulsants compared with when they are used as antianxiety agents. Desmethyldiazepam, the major metabolite of both clorazepate and diazepam, has anticonvulsant properties. Although the benzodiazepines are useful adjuncts to the conventional anticonvulsants for seizure prophylaxis, patients appear to develop tolerance to their antiseizure effect rather quickly. The benzodiazepines may find their greatest clinical usefulness in short-term therapy, such as when anticonvulsant medication is being changed or for emergency treatment.

The predictable adverse effects of drowsiness, dizziness, ataxia, nystagmus, dysarthria, and hypotonia occur with all benzodiazepines. Respiratory depression can be an issue when intravenous agents are used. Serious side effects are very rare. The administration of clonazepam occasionally precipitates a different variety of seizure from the one being treated. The teratogenic potential of the benzodiazepines is discussed in Chapter 13. There is little evidence that clonazepam is teratogenic, but it is recommended that use of the compound during pregnancy be limited to those cases in which the clinical situation warrants the risk.

Nitrazepam, used primarily as a hypnotic, is prescribed in some countries as an anticonvulsant, particularly for the treatment of infantile spasms (see neurosteroids below). Nitrazepam is not available in the United States nor are the 1,5-benzodiazepines, including clobazam. They have anticonvulsant properties and adverse effects similar to the 1,4-benzodiazepines.

Vigabatrin

The inhibitory effect of GABA may be increased by mechanisms other than facilitating its action, as occurs with the benzodiazepines. For example, inhibition of enzymes responsible for the catabolism of GABA results in increased brain concentrations of GABA.[50] Vigabatrin (γ-vinyl GABA, Figure 14-8) is an irreversible inhibitor of the enzyme GABA transaminase. Vigabatrin is considered an adjunctive anticonvulsant and is effective for drug-refractory epilepsy. It is more effective for simple and complex partial seizures than for generalized seizures. The drug is rapidly absorbed by the oral route, reaching peak blood concentrations in 0.75 to 2 hours. It does not bind appreciably to plasma protein. Vigabatrin has no active metabolites and is excreted by the kidneys. Its plasma half-life ranges from 4 to 7 hours, but irreversible inhibition of GABA transaminase lasts for several days after the drug is cleared, thus prolonging the antiepileptic effect. Adverse effects of vigabatrin include sedation, fatigue, weight gain, amnesia,[11] and visual field defects, which include hemi or concentric field contractions and may be related to retinal damage produced by edema. The defects may be more common in men and seem to be related to the total drug exposure.[17] They persist after drug withdrawal. Psychosis may also infrequently occur.

Tiagabine

Tiagabine (see Figure 14-8), approved in 1996 as an adjunct for refractory complex epilepsy, is a nipecotic acid derivative that inhibits GABA uptake. Tiagabine is readily absorbed, with a peak blood concentration reached in 45 minutes. This drug is metabolized in the liver by CYP3A4 and possibly CYP1A2, 2C19, and 2D6 to inactive 5-oxo metabolites and is also glucuronidated. Tiagabine has a half life of 7 to 9 hours. Side effects include dizziness, fatigue, sleepiness, nausea, tremor, and difficulty concentrating.

Neurosteroids

In addition to its receptor for benzodiazepines, the $GABA_A$ receptor complex has a separate binding site for steroid

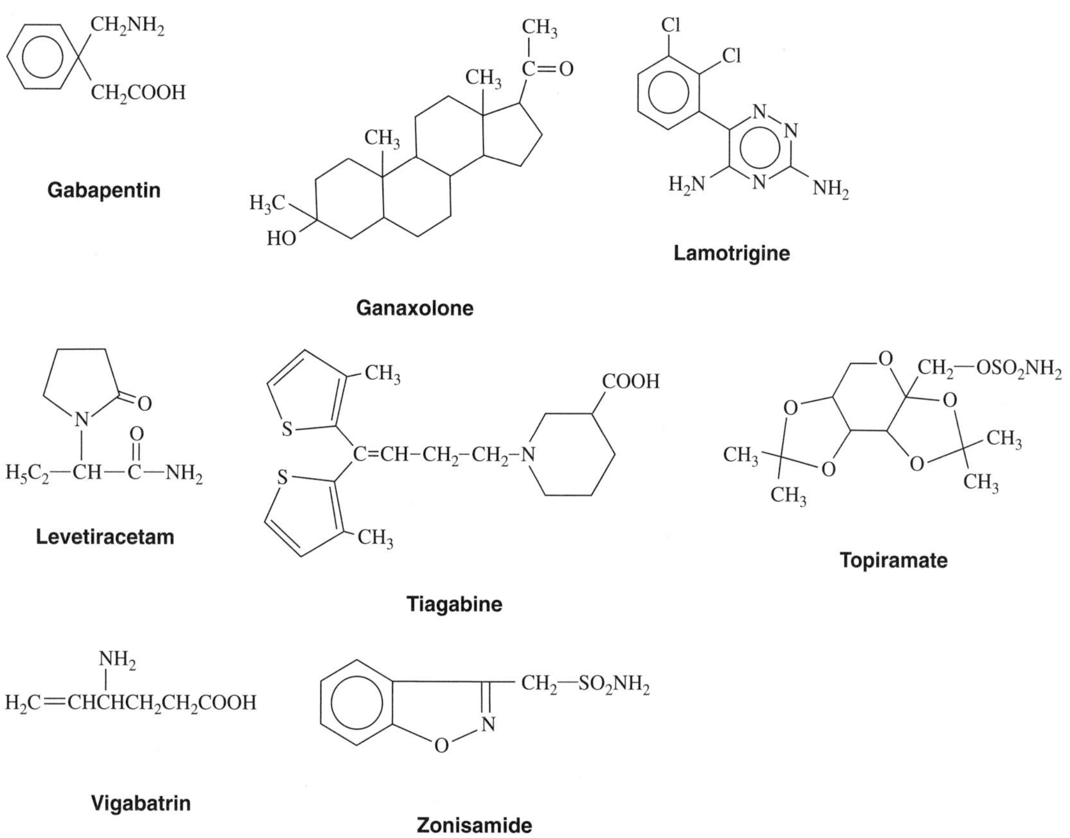

Gabapentin

Ganaxolone

Lamotrigine

Levetiracetam

Tiagabine

Topiramate

Vigabatrin

Zonisamide

Fig. 14-8 Structural formulas of newer antiepileptic drugs.

molecules. Steroid hormones in general are thought to act through steroid nuclear binding proteins that modify DNA translation in the cell nucleus. However, some steroids, such as allopregnenolone, also act on these cell surface receptors to facilitate the action of GABA on the $GABA_A$ receptor of the Cl^- ion channel.

Infantile spasm with a "chaotic" EEG is a serious epileptic condition of early life that is refractory to most anticonvulsants and has a poor prognosis. Historically, it has been effectively treated with adrenocorticotropic hormone. Recent studies have shown that vigabatrin and the neurosteroid ganaxolone[24] are also effective for this condition. Ganaxolone (see Figure 14-8) is a pregnenolone derivative without progestational hormonal activity. It exerts anticonvulsant activity against complex partial seizures, has an anticonvulsant spectrum that suggests usefulness in absence seizures, and is anticonvulsant in an animal model of catamenial epilepsy.[36] It is thought to act on selective $GABA_A$ component isoforms. Other newer anticonvulsant drugs that are being evaluated for treatment of infantile spasms include topiramate, lamotrigine, and zonisamide.[53]

GABAmimetic Agents

Drugs that successfully mimic GABA in the CNS include progabide, a GABA agonist available in Europe. Progabide is effective in rodent models and some human forms of epilepsy, but it can cause serious adverse effects. Despite its toxicity, progabide has been used to treat simple and complex partial and generalized tonic-clonic, atonic, and myoclonic seizures in patients refractory to other anticonvulsants. GABA agonists in general have a lack of specificity and, theoretically, could result in GABA receptor downregulation.

MISCELLANEOUS ANTICONVULSANTS

Gabapentin and Related Drugs

Gabapentin (see Figure 14-8) is a GABA analogue specifically designed to cross the blood-brain barrier. It is effective as an adjunct for patients with refractory partial seizures. Surprisingly, gabapentin does not interact with GABA receptors, uptake, or metabolism. It may influence synthesis or release of GABA and increases GABA concentrations in certain regions of the brain. Gabapentin also binds to an L-type Ca^{++} channel subunit, $\alpha 2\delta$. It inhibits depolarizing high-voltage–activating Ca^{++} channel currents at therapeutic concentrations.[45] Analogues that bind more tightly to the $\alpha 2\delta$ subunit appear to be more potent anticonvulsants for partial seizures. Gabapentin is not effective in the treatment of absence seizures[31] but has proved useful in the treatment of chronic pain conditions such as postherpetic neuralgia, diabetic neuropathy, trigeminal neuralgia, and pain associated with multiple sclerosis.[10,29] It is worth noting that the Ca^{++} channel $\alpha 2\delta$ subunit is upregulated in peripheral nerves with chronic nerve injury.[28] The drug is used orally and has saturable absorption. Elevations of the dose do not produce equivalent increases in blood concentration. It is not bound to plasma protein, is excreted almost entirely by the kidneys, and has a plasma half-life of 4 to 7 hours. The drug is generally well tolerated. Adverse effects include fatigue, dizziness, headache, nausea, and ataxia.[11]

Felbamate

In 1993 the FDA approved felbamate, a meprobamate derivative, for use in refractory partial seizures and as adjunctive therapy in children for seizures associated with

Lennox-Gastaut syndrome, a disease resistant to most antiepileptic drugs. Shortly thereafter, felbamate was linked to aplastic anemia and acute hepatic failure, and an advisory by the FDA recommended against its use except in cases in which withdrawal or avoidance of the drug represented a serious risk for the patient.

Lamotrigine

Lamotrigine (see Figure 14-8) is a phenyltriazine derivative that inhibits Na^+ influx in rapidly firing neurons. The drug has also been shown to inhibit the release of glutamate from the cortex of rat brain.[50] Lamotrigine exerts anticonvulsant effects in several experimental models of epilepsy and in patients with partial and generalized tonic-clonic seizures. The drug is used orally and is well absorbed from the gastrointestinal tract. The plasma half-life is approximately 24 hours, but induction of liver microsomal enzymes by such drugs as phenobarbital, phenytoin, and carbamazepine may decrease the half-life to approximately 12 hours. Conversely, valproic acid may increase the half-life of lamotrigine up to 60 hours by inhibiting its metabolism. Lamotrigine usually has mild side effects, including ataxia, dizziness, diplopia, and rash.[11] Stevens-Johnson syndrome has been reported in 0.8% to 2% of young children using the drug,[9] and the drug is only approved for treatment of Lennox-Gastaut syndrome in children younger than 16 years. Lamotrigine binds to melanin and may accumulate in the eyes and other tissues containing melanin. No adverse consequences of this binding have been reported.

Carbonic Anhydrase Inhibitors

Acetazolamide and other carbonic anhydrase inhibitors are primarily effective against absence seizures but are also useful for the control of seizures that have a tendency to recur at a specific time of the menstrual cycle (catamenial epilepsy). However, tolerance develops rapidly so the carbonic anhydrase inhibitors are primarily used as adjunctive agents. The diuretic and natriuretic effects of acetazolamide are well known. By inhibiting carbonic anhydrase (located in glial cells), carbon dioxide is allowed to accumulate in the brain, which can decrease intracellular Na^+ and increase intracellular K^+. This ionic shift results in neuronal hyperpolarization and decreased excitability, which is thought to block the spread of seizure discharge.

Topiramate

Topiramate (see Figure 14-8) is a broad-spectrum anticonvulsant currently approved for partial-onset seizures. The drug exerts multiple actions, including frequency-dependent blockade of Na^+ channels, benzodiazepine-like potentiation of GABA activity, and inhibition of kainate receptors for glutamate. Absorption after oral ingestion is rapid; an elimination half-life of approximately 20 hours permits twice-daily dosing. It may specifically inhibit CYP2C19.[12] Topiramate is reported to be more effective than several of the newer anticonvulsants; however, it also produced more side effects.[6] This may reflect the dosages used to evaluate the drug rather than absolute efficacy. CNS depression is the most common side effect. Topiramate can compromise short-term memory function.

Zonisamide

Zonisamide (see Figure 14-8) was developed in Japan and is now available in the United States. Zonisamide is structurally related to the sulfonamides. It is completely absorbed, with peak concentrations occurring in 4 to 6 hours. Primarily metabolized by CYP3A4, blood concentrations may vary if inducing antiepileptic drugs are used concurrently. Zonisamide may act by multiple mechanisms, including blocking of Na^+ and T-type Ca^{++} channels; the drug binds to the $GABA_A$ channel but does not alter Cl^- currents. Zonisamide facilitates dopaminergic and serotonergic transmission. The drug also is a weak carbonic anhydrase inhibitor. Zonisamide was studied as adjunctive therapy for the treatment of partial-onset seizures and found to improve therapy. Since it is a sulfonamide, it can produce a number of allergic reactions in patients who are sensitive to sulfonamides. These reactions include skin rashes (Stevens-Johnson syndrome), epidermal necrolysis, and agranulocytosis. The incidence of these events is very low. Other unusual side effects include a propensity to produce renal acidification[21] and renal stones and, rarely, dehydration and hyperthermia in children during hot weather.

Levetiracetam

Levetiracetam (see Figure 14-8) is a pyrrolidine derivative that is rapidly absorbed (1 hour to peak) after oral administration and is less than 10% bound to plasma proteins. Steady state is reached in 2 days with twice daily dosing. The half-life is approximately 7 hours, and the drug is metabolized by a non-cytochrome P450 route and is eliminated by renal excretion. The drug has a unique anticonvulsant profile; it is effective in some common tests predictive of efficacy in partial seizures but not in other tests. Its mechanism is unknown, but it binds stereoselectively to synaptic plasma membranes in the brain. Levetiracetam was evaluated as adjunct therapy for adult partial-onset seizures and found to reduce seizures in a dose-dependent manner. Typical side effects included somnolence and fatigue, coordination difficulties, and behavioral problems. Most of the side effects were reported in the first month of therapy. This drug should be terminated gradually to avoid withdrawal reactions. Drug interactions with this agent seem to be minimal.

Magnesium Salts

Although not used in treating epilepsy, magnesium sulfate is used to prevent or control convulsions of eclampsia and severe preeclampsia of pregnancy. The drug acts on the CNS to decrease excitability and also acts to reduce activity at the neuromuscular junction. Its mechanism of action is not well defined. In addition, magnesium reduces cardiac and smooth muscle activity and lowers blood pressure, which is of benefit in eclampsia and preeclampsia.

Experimental Drugs

Although many seizures can be controlled with anticonvulsant medication, approximately 20% remain resistant to treatment. Recognizing this need, the Epilepsy Branch of the National Institute of Neurological Disorders and Stroke began clinical trials in 1968 of a number of drugs, including those already approved for other uses in the United States. Carbamazepine, clonazepam, valproic acid, and clorazepate were made available between 1974 and 1981 as a result of these efforts. Further government, industrial, and academic support for anticonvulsant drug research resulted in the creation of a formal government program, the National Anticonvulsant Drug Development Program and Antiepileptic Screening Project, which has introduced a series of potential anticonvulsant drugs. Significant advances in understanding the synthesis and regulation of receptors, ion channels, drug elimination mechanisms, and other components of cells have revealed many new opportunities for intervention.

One approach involves excitatory neuronal mechanisms. Abnormal distribution patterns of excitatory amino acid receptors have been demonstrated in the hippocampus and parahippocampal gyrus of human beings with temporal lobe epilepsy. Thus a novel anticonvulsant strategy is to decrease excitatory neurotransmitter drive. Evidence exists that classic anticonvulsants may have this ability. For example, phenytoin, carbamazepine, benzodiazepines, and lamotrigine may decrease the synaptic release of excitatory amino acids.

There are several excitatory amino acid antagonists. Their variety stems not only from the fact that both competitive and noncompetitive antagonists exist, but also because there are both metabotropic glutamate receptors (which modulate intracellular second messengers) and three major classes of glutamate-gated ion-channel receptors (N-methyl-D-aspartate [NMDA], kainate, and α-amino-3-hydroxy-5-methyl-4-isoxazole propionate). These receptors are all stimulated by glutamate but can be distinguished according to their preferred agonists and antagonists. The phosphonic acid derivatives 2-amino-5-phosphonovaleric acid (AP5) and 2-amino-7-phosphonoheptanoic acid (AP7) are competitive NMDA antagonists that are potent anticonvulsants in experimental epilepsy models. Because AP5 and AP7 are restricted by the blood-brain barrier, derivatives of AP5 and AP7 have been developed to enter the CNS more effectively. Side effects (impairment of learning and memory, behavioral changes) may limit the use of these compounds. Noncompetitive NMDA antagonists (e.g., phencyclidine) are effective anticonvulsants, but side effects (hallucinations, ataxia, altered sensory perception, interference with memory, and behavioral disturbances) are prominent. Despite their problems, NMDA antagonists are effective in preventing the development of seizure kindling. This characteristic could be extremely important for the prevention of seizures (and epilepsy) after severe head trauma. Although a baseline level of excitatory neuronal activity presumably is required for normal physiologic activity, overactivity may lead to neurotoxicity. The excitotoxic effect of glutamate is well known, and data suggest that nitric oxide, a highly reactive local hormone, may be the agent responsible for glutamate-induced cell death. An excitotoxic effect may play a role in epilepsy.

Novel approaches to anticonvulsant therapy may include other endogenous compounds. Adenosine, inosine, hypoxanthine, β-endorphin and other endogenous opioids, somatostatin, cholecystokinin, neuropeptide Y, and prostaglandins have been investigated.

NONPHARMACOLOGIC TREATMENTS

Surgical treatment of seizure disorders is possible when the focus is localized and located in nonessential brain tissue. Removal of poorly healed and abnormally functioning brain tissue can produce "cures." This procedure is performed with growing success because of the availability of improved EEG and diagnostic imaging techniques (PET, single-photon emission computed tomography, magnetic resonance imaging).

A nonpharmacologic approach to the treatment of seizures has resulted from studies demonstrating that stimulation (by implanted pulse generators) of the vagus nerve blocks experimentally induced seizures in rats, dogs, and primates. This experimental technique has recently been extended to human beings.[52] Vagal stimulation has obvious implications regarding cholinergic drugs.

Another approach for the treatment of childhood epilepsy is the ketogenic diet. A ketogenic diet is high in fats and low in carbohydrates and proteins. These diets must be carefully controlled but have been found effective in some patients. It is unknown how the ketogenic diet results in a decreased incidence of seizures.

GENERAL THERAPEUTIC USE

The goal of anticonvulsant therapy is to obtain complete control of epileptic seizures with the fewest drugs and at the least toxic and lowest possible dose. Approximately 80% of all patients can be seizure free if drug plasma concentrations are properly monitored and the appropriate dose adjustments are made. Initial anticonvulsant therapy sometimes necessitates frequent alterations in dose and a trial-and-error approach until the seizure responds to a specific anticonvulsant. Even after seizures are initially controlled, the continued administration of anticonvulsant drugs may lead to the development of tolerance. The addition of other anticonvulsants again necessitates dosage adjustments. Anticonvulsant therapy is not static, routine, and completely predictable, but rather subject to a variety of ever-changing factors.

Febrile seizures, induced by high fevers, are the most frequent seizures in children. Propensity for these seizures may have a genetic basis, be related to particular diseases (influenza), or be caused by immaturity of CNS excitation control. Children with febrile seizures rarely develop other seizure disorders or continue to have seizures. Short-term treatment with diazepam, phenobarbital, or intranasal midazolam has been used. In some patients in whom febrile seizures are recurrent, prophylactic phenobarbital or diazepam may be prescribed to prevent seizures in future fevers. Rarely, patients may need longer-term continuous phenobarbital or valproic acid treatment.

Although anticonvulsant medications have substantial toxic potential, uncontrolled seizures also carry important risks. Repeated seizures can result in loss of memory and mental function. For several of the newer anticonvulsants that facilitate GABA or inhibit excitatory amino acid function, there is the potential for additional drug-induced compromise of memory function.

Anticonvulsants can be of value in treating patients with a variety of chronic pain problems. Neuropathic pain results from abnormalities in nerve fiber conduction, such as neuralgia, causalgia, and phantom pain. Beneficial actions of anticonvulsants may be related to blockade of Na^+ and Ca^{++} channels, activation of GABAergic transmission, and inhibition of NMDA and other glutamate receptors. Agents that have proved effective in these conditions include carbamazepine, phenytoin, sodium valproate, gabapentin, and clonazepam.[10]

Traditional anticonvulsants (carbamazepine and valproic acid) and "mood stabilizers" (a synonym used in psychiatry for some of the newer anticonvulsants) are sometimes valuable adjuncts in treating the manic phase of bipolar disorder.[23] Other anticonvulsant drugs may also be of use; however, in one study adjunctive gabapentin was no more effective than placebo.[33]

IMPLICATIONS FOR DENTISTRY

Dentists should expect to be confronted at some time by a seizing patient in the dental office. It is extremely helpful if an emergency plan has been previously developed and practiced before having to deal with convulsions clinically. One of the best ways to manage seizures is to prevent them. Appointments should be planned for times when the epileptic patient will have high blood concentrations of anticonvulsant medication. The dentist should verify that the patient has taken his or her medications before the appointment. Careful attention to local anesthetic doses and avoiding accidental intravascular injections by practicing aspiration before administration are helpful. If the patient's seizure is of the reflexive type, avoiding the triggering stimuli is important. Ask the patient before treatment if he or she is aware of any triggering stimuli. Finally, attention to the patient's fear and apprehension can limit the risk of inciting an attack.

Some patients will sense the onset of seizure activity in the form of auras. If a patient reports an aura, the dentist should prepare for a seizure by removing all instruments from the patient's mouth and pulling back trays or other objects from which the patient might sustain injury. The patient should be placed in the supine position. If no seizure occurs, the patient can determine when to proceed. If the patient does have a seizure, the dentist must protect the patient from injury and falls. No attempt should be made to open the patient's mouth during a tonic-clonic seizure because this can induce more injuries than will usually occur if the patient is left alone. Seizures will generally end in 2 to 5 minutes, after which the patient will be disoriented or fall asleep for 30 or more minutes. If the patient is snoring or appears to have an obstructed airway, the head, neck, and jaw should be positioned to ensure a clear airway.

If a second seizure occurs it may indicate status epilepticus. Seizures induced by local anesthetic overdoses tend to be prolonged and may require anticonvulsant treatment. Animal experiments suggest that benzodiazepines and phenobarbital are highly effective for treating local anesthetic–induced seizures, whereas carbamazepine, phenytoin, and valproate may increase seizure activity.[39] Emergency medical services should be called if the seizure recurs or is prolonged or if respiration is compromised. Patients may need supportive care after a seizure, which would include treatment of any wounds that may have occurred and dealing with incontinence.

In most cases, seizures are brief and self-limiting. However, there may be occasions when pharmacotherapy will be required. Part of the dentist's emergency plan should include a properly stocked emergency cart and staff trained in the use of the medications. Anticonvulsant medications should ideally be administered by the intravenous route. However, this is not always possible in the dental office. New products have improved this situation. Midazolam has been tried and found effective in the treatment of status seizures and can be administered intravenously or intramuscularly.[16,54] Seizure control is almost immediate with intravenous administration. Midazolam has also been administered by the buccal route for prolonged seizures.[40,41] The buccal route would be natural in the dental office. A rectal gel dosage form of diazepam (Diastat) is available that can produce anticonvulsant blood concentrations in approximately 15 minutes. This product has been formulated for use by lay people for the emergency treatment of seizures at home and thus simplifies emergency treatment if an intravenous line is not available. The disadvantage of this approach is that many are uncomfortable with the route of administration.

Because diazepam and midazolam have relatively short durations of action, the use of a longer-acting agent such as lorazepam, phenytoin, or phenobarbital may be needed in the hospital to provide prolonged seizure control. Fosphenytoin may have some advantages over traditional agents. Fosphenytoin at 15 to 20 mg/kg phenytoin equivalents is tolerated better and can be effective 10 to 60 minutes after intramuscular injection into the gluteus maximus.[35] The volume of fosphenytoin to achieve this dose can range from 20 to 40 ml, which should be divided into smaller volumes and then administered bilaterally. Care should be taken to avoid injections into the sciatic nerve or inferior gluteal vessels.

As described in this chapter, patients receiving anticonvulsants are subject to a variety of adverse effects. Common or significant adverse effects that are pertinent for the everyday practice of dentistry should be noted. For example, most of the anticonvulsant drugs produce some degree of CNS depression. The clinician should therefore be aware of the additive effect of other CNS depressants, such as local and general anesthetics, antianxiety agents, antidepressants, and the opioid analgesics. Some of the newer agents may also interfere with memory. Therefore patients should receive written treatment instructions, which should also be provided to appropriate guardians if prudent. Blood dyscrasias are rare but serious side effects seen with most of the anticonvulsant agents; they may increase the patient's susceptibility to infection. Aplastic anemia may manifest as increased gingival bleeding, whereas agranulocytosis may be identified by pharyngitis or oral mucosal lesions. The fact that some anticonvulsants alter mineral metabolism should be considered when confronted with anomalies in tooth development or advanced bone loss. Several of the anticonvulsants can produce teratogenic effects. The defects produced can involve the facial and oral structures. Practitioners should be alert for new drug-related adverse effects and report them to the FDA Medwatch program.

Several side effects specific to individual anticonvulsant agents are clinically relevant to dentistry. Phenytoin-induced gingival overgrowth is a well-known example. Overgrowth most commonly occurs in the anterior mandibular region, especially in the case of "mouth breathers," and develops to the greatest extent in the interdental papillae between the incisors. Edentulous areas of the alveolar mucosa do not undergo hypertrophy or do so to a lesser extent than other areas. Whatever the mechanism, phenytoin-induced overgrowth may totally or partially obscure the crowns of teeth, which obviously hampers mastication and oral hygiene, is aesthetically unpleasant, and necessitates periodic resection. Because of the angiogenesis induced, the gingival tissue is quite vascular; thus surgery by cautery or laser is often preferred. The rate of development of gingival overgrowth can be diminished by proper oral hygiene.

An interesting proposal is to use phenytoin to enhance wound healing. Considerable evidence exists that this procedure holds promise.[48] There is interest in applying modern knowledge of growth factors to aid in the healing of periodontitis and other oral wounds. Because phenytoin is widely available and relatively inexpensive, it might be helpful in some cases. Research in this area is clearly needed.

Anticonvulsants may increase hepatic microsomal enzyme activity, which can reduce the blood concentration of other drugs metabolized by the same enzyme system. Of relevance to dentistry is the effect of enzyme induction on antibiotics (e.g., tetracycline) and other agents (midazolam, triazolam) used in clinical practice. Drugs that inhibit CYP3A4 (e.g., erythromycin) can lead to unexpected elevations of anticonvulsant drugs and potential toxicity. The microsomal enzyme–inducing anticonvulsants can reduce the effectiveness of oral contraceptives. Valproic acid can inhibit CYP3A4 drug metabolism. It can also inhibit platelet aggregation, so increased monitoring of patient use of aspirin or nonsteroidal antiinflammatory drugs may be warranted.

Some short-term effects directly involve the mouth. For instance, carbamazepine-induced taste disorders have been reported, but these apparently subside with time.[15] Xerostomia has also been reported. Primidone is known to cause the unusual side effect of localized gingival pain. This response has led patients and dentists to assume erroneously that the pain is of pathologic rather than pharmacologic origin. Clonazepam has been reported to produce hypersalivation in some patients. A complete medical history is therefore essential for proper dental treatment.

It is often recommended that the patient with epilepsy be treated somewhat cautiously to reduce emotional upset and help prevent the precipitation of a seizure. Except when seizures are not well controlled, individuals with epilepsy need not be handled differently from other patients. Indeed, because of the lingering stigma associated with epilepsy, these patients may be reluctant to reveal their disease. A seizure disorder may only be ascertained by the clinician who is alert to subtle clues offered by anticonvulsant-induced side effects and by careful questioning of the patient.

Anticonvulsants may be used in the treatment of chronic orofacial pain problems such as trigeminal neuralgia or burning mouth syndrome. Carbamazepine has been the first-choice drug for the treatment of trigeminal neuralgia. Some patients will also respond to other anticonvulsants. Burning mouth syndrome is currently a treatment challenge and may involve pathologic and psychologic components. Current treatments include clonazepam, capsaicin, and antidepressant therapy.

Finally, saliva offers a readily available and potentially useful tool for monitoring concentrations of several antiepileptic drugs. Saliva/plasma correlations have been described for carbamazepine, phenobarbital, phenytoin, and ethosuximide.[42]

Anticonvulsants

Nonproprietary (generic) name	*Proprietary (trade) name*
Hydantoins	
Ethotoin	Peganone
Fosphenytoin	Cerebyx
Mephenytoin*	Mesantoin
Phenytoin	Dilantin
Barbiturates	
Mephobarbital	Mebaral
Phenobarbital	Luminal
Primidone†	Mysoline
Succinimides	
Ethosuximide	Zarontin
Methsuximide	Celontin
Phensuximide*	Milontin
Oxazolidinediones	
Paramethadione*	Paradione
Trimethadione*	Tridione
Benzodiazepines	
Clobazam*	Frisium
Clonazepam	Klonopin
Clorazepate	Tranxene, Gen-Xene
Diazepam	Valium, Diastat
Midazolam	Versed
Nitrazepam*	Mogadon
Lorazepam	Ativan
Others	
Acetazolamide	Diamox
Carbamazepine	Tegretol
Felbamate‡	Felbatol
Gabapentin	Neurontin
Lamotrigine	Lamictal
Levetiracetam	Keppra
Oxcarbazepine	Trileptal
Tiagabine	Gabatril
Topiramate	Topamax
Valproic acid	Depakene, Depakote§
Vigabatrin*	Sabril
Zonisamide	Zonegran
Phenacemide*	Phenurone

*Not currently available in the United States.
†Not a true barbiturate.
‡Restricted use.
§Divalproex, a stable compound of valproic acid, and sodium valproate.

CITED REFERENCES

1. Brown RS, Beaver WT, Bottomly WK: On the mechanism of drug-induced gingival hyperplasia, *J Oral Pathol Med* 20:201-209, 1991.
2. Cherubini E, Conti F: Generating diversity at GABAergic synapses, *Trends Neurosci* 24:155-162, 2001.
3. Commission on Classification and Terminology of the International League Against Epilepsy: Proposal for revised classification of epilepsies and epileptic syndromes, *Epilepsia* 30:389-399, 1989.
4. Coulter DA: Epilepsy-associated plasticity in γ-aminobutyric acid receptor expression, function and inhibitory synaptic properties, *Int Rev Neurobiol* 45:237-252, 2001.
5. Coulter DA, Huguenard JR, Prince DA: Characterization of ethosuximide reduction of low-threshold calcium current in thalamic neurons, *Ann Neurol* 25:582-593, 1989.
6. Cramer JA, Fisher R, Ben-Menachem E, et al: New antiepileptic drugs: comparison of key clinical trials, *Epilepsia* 40:590-600, 1999.
7. Cunningham MO, Dhillon A, Wood SJ, et al: Reciprocal modulation of glutamate and GABA release may underlie the anticonvulsant effect of phenytoin, *Neuroscience* 95:343-351, 2000.
8. DeLorenzo RJ: Phenytoin: calcium- and calmodulin-dependent protein phosphorylation and neurotransmitter release, *Adv Neurol* 27:399-414, 1980.
9. Devinsky O, Cramer J: Safety and efficacy of standard and new antiepileptic drugs, *Neurology* 55(suppl 3):S5-S10, 2000.
10. Drugs for pain, *Med Lett Drugs Ther* 42:73-78, 2000.
11. Fisher RS: Emerging antiepileptic drugs, *Neurology* 43(suppl 5):S12-S20, 1993.
12. French JA, Gidal BE: Antiepileptic drug interactions, *Epilepsia* 41(suppl 8):S30-S36, 2000.
13. Genton P: When antiepileptic drugs aggravate epilepsy, *Brain Dev* 22:75-80, 2000.
14. Hahn TJ, Hendin BA, Scharp CR, et al: Serum 25-hydroxycalciferol levels and bone mass in children on chronic anticonvulsant therapy, *N Engl J Med* 292:550-554, 1975.
15. Halbreich U: Tegretol dependency and diversion of the sense of taste, *Isr Ann Psychiatry Related Disciplines* 12:328-332, 1974.
16. Hanley DF, Jr, Pozo M: Treatment of status epilepticus with midazolam in the critical care setting, *Int J Clin Pract* 54:30-35, 2000.
17. Hardus P, Verduin WM, Englesman M, et al: Visual field loss associated with vigabatrin: quantification and relation to dosage, *Epilepsia* 42:262-267, 2001.

18. Holmes LB, Harvey EA, Coull BA, et al: The teratogenicity of anticonvulsant drugs, *N Engl J Med* 344:1132-1138, 2001.

19. Howe AM, Lipson AH, Sheffield LJ, et al: Prenatal exposure to phenytoin, facial development, and possible role for vitamin K, *Am J Med Genet* 58:238-244, 1995.

20. Iacopino AM, Doxey D, Cutler CW, et al: Phenytoin and cyclosporine A specifically regulate macrophage phenotype and expression of platelet-derived growth factor and interleukin-1 in vitro and in vivo: possible molecular mechanism of drug-induced gingival hyperplasia, *J Periodontol* 68:73-83, 1997.

21. Inoue T, Kira R, Kaku Y, et al: Renal tubular acidosis associated with zonisamide therapy, *Epilepsia* 41:1642-1644, 2000.

22. Juhasz C, Chugani DC, Muzik O, et al: Relationship of flumazenil and glucose PET abnormalities to neocortical epilepsy surgery outcome, *Neurology* 56:1650-1658, 2001.

23. Keck PE, Mendlwicz J, Calabrese JR, et al: A review of randomized, controlled clinical trials in acute mania, *J Affect Disord* 59(suppl 1):S31-S37, 2000.

24. Kerrigan JF, Shields WD, Nelson TY, et al: Ganaxolone for treating intractable infantile spasms: a multicenter open-label, add-on trial, *Epilepsy Res* 42:133-139, 2000.

25. Kjeldsen MJ, Kyvik KO, Christensen K, et al: Genetic and environmental factors in epilepsy: a population-based study of 11,900 Danish twin pairs, *Epilepsy Res* 44:167-178, 2001.

26. Kwan P, Sills GJ, Brodie MJ: The mechanisms of action of commonly used antiepileptic drugs, *Pharmacol Ther* 90:21-34, 2001.

27. Lin Y-F, Angelotti TP, Dudek EM, et al: Enhancement of recombinant $\alpha 1\beta 1\gamma 2L$ γ-aminobutyric $acid_A$ receptor whole-cell currents by protein kinase C is mediated through phosphorylation of both $\beta 1$ and $\gamma 2L$ subunits, *Mol Pharmacol* 50:185-195, 1996.

28. Luo ZD, Chaplan SR, Higuera ES, et al: Upregulation of dorsal root ganglion $\alpha_2\delta$ calcium channel subunit and its correlation with allodynia in spinal nerve-injured rats, *J Neurosci* 21:1868-1875, 2001.

29. Mao J, Chen LL: Gabapentin in pain management, *Anesth Analg* 91:680-707, 2000.

30. McLean MJ, Macdonald RL: Carbamazepine and 10, 11-epoxycarbamazepine produce use- and voltage-dependent limitation of rapidly firing action potentials of mouse central neurons in cell culture, *J Pharmacol Exp Ther* 238:727-738, 1986.

31. Morris GL: Gabapentin, *Epilepsia* 40(suppl 5):S63-S70, 1999.

32. Moshe SL, Garant DS, Sperber EF, et al: Ontogeny and topography of seizure regulation by the substantia nigra, *Brain Dev* 17(suppl):61-72, 1995.

33. Pande AC, Crockatt JG, Janney CA, et al: Gabapentin in bipolar disorder: a placebo-controlled trial of adjunctive therapy. Gabapentin Bipolar Disorder Study Group, *Bipolar Disord* 2(3 pt 2):249-255, 2000.

34. Pedrera JD, Canal ML, Carvajal J, et al: Influence of vitamin D administration on bone ultrasound measurement in patients on anticonvulsant therapy, *Eur J Clin Invest* 30:895-899, 2000.

35. Pryor FM, Gidal B, Ramsay RE, et al: Fosphenytoin: pharmacokinetics and tolerance of intramuscular loading doses, *Epilepsia* 42:245-250, 2001.

36. Reddy DS, Rogawski MA: Enhanced anticonvulsant activity of ganaxolone after neurosteroid withdrawal in a rat model of catamenial epilepsy, *J Pharmacol Exp Ther* 294:909-915, 2000.

37. Rey E, Treluyer JM, Pons G: Pharmacokinetic optimization of benzodiazepine therapy for acute seizures. Focus on delivery routes, *Clin Pharmacokinet* 36:409-424, 1999.

38. Saito K, Mori S, Iwakura M, et al: Immunohistochemical localization of transforming growth factor β, basic fibroblast growth factor and heparan sulfate glycosaminoglycan in gingival hyperplasia induced by nifedipine and phenytoin, *J Periodontal Res* 31:545-555, 1996.

39. Sawaki K, Ohno K, Miyamoto K, et al: Effects of anticonvulsants on local anaesthetic-induced neurotoxicity in rats, *Pharmacol Toxicol* 86:59-62, 2000.

40. Scott RC, Besag FM, Boyd SG, et al: Buccal absorption of midazolam: pharmacokinetics and EEG pharmacodynamics, *Epilepsia* 39:290-294, 1998.

41. Scott RC, Besag FM, Neville BG: Buccal midazolam and rectal diazepam for treatment of prolonged seizures in childhood and adolescence: a randomized trial, *Lancet* 353:623-626, 1999.

42. Siegel IA: The role of saliva in drug monitoring, *Ann NY Acad Sci* 694:86-90, 1993.

43. Spivey WH: Flumazenil and seizures: analysis of 43 cases, *Clin Ther* 14:292-305, 1992.

44. Staak R, Pape H-C: Contribution of $GABA_A$ and $GABA_B$ receptors to thalamic neuronal activity during spontaneous absence seizures in rats, *J Neurosci* 21:1378-1384, 2001.

45. Stefani A, Spadoni F, Giacomini P, et al: The effects of gabapentin on different ligand- and voltage-gated currents in isolated cortical neurons, *Epilepsy Res* 43:239-248, 2001.

46. Sueyoshi T, Negishi M: Phenobarbital response elements of cytochrome P450 genes and nuclear receptors, *Annu Rev Pharmacol Toxicol* 41:123-143, 2001.

47. Sullivan FM, McElhatton PR: A comparison of the teratogenic activity of the antiepileptic drugs carbamazepine, clonazepam, ethosuximide, phenobarbital, phenytoin, and primidone in mice, *Toxicol Appl Pharmacol* 40:365-378, 1977.

48. Talas G, Brown RA, McGrouther DA: Role of phenytoin in wound healing—a wound pharmacology perspective, *Biochem Pharmacol* 57:1085-1094, 1999.

49. Treiman DM, Meyers PD, Walton NY, et al: A comparison of four treatments for generalized convulsive status epilepticus. Veterans Affairs Status Epilepticus Cooperative Study Group, *N Engl J Med* 339:792-798, 1998.

50. Upton N: Mechanisms of action of new antiepileptic drugs: rational design and serendipitous findings, *Trends Pharmacol Sci* 15:456-463, 1994.

51. Watanabe S, Satumae T, Takeshima R, et al: Opisthotonos after flumazenil administered to antagonize midazolam previously administered to treat developing local anesthetic toxicity, *Anesth Analg* 86:677-678, 1998.

52. Wilder BJ, ed: Vagus nerve stimulation for the control of epilepsy, *Epilepsia* 31(suppl 2):S1-S60, 1990.

53. Wong M, Trevathan E: Infantile spasms, *Pediatr Neurol* 24:89-98, 2001.

54. Yoshikawa H, Yamazaki S, Abe T, et al: Midazolam as a first-line agent for status epilepticus in children, *Brain Dev* 22:239-242, 2000.

General References

Brodie MJ, Dichter MA: Drug therapy: antiepileptic drugs, *N Engl J Med* 334:168-175, 1996.

Davis KL, Martin E, Turko IV, et al: Novel effects of nitric oxide, *Annu Rev Pharmacol Toxicol* 41:203-236, 2001.

Löscher W, Potschka H: Role of multidrug transporters in pharmacoresistance to antiepileptic drugs, *J Pharmacol Exp Therap* 301:7-14, 2002.

Lowenstein DH: Seizures and epilepsy. In Braunwald E, Fauci AS, Kasper DL, et al, eds: *Harrison's Principles of internal medicine,* ed 15, New York, 2001, McGraw-Hill.

Meldrum B, Chapman A: Epileptic seizures and epilepsy, In Siegel GJ, et al, eds: *Basic neurochemistry: molecular, cellular and medical aspects,* ed 6, New York, 1999, Lippincott-Raven.

Porter RJ, Chadwick D, eds: *The epilepsies 2,* Boston, 1997, Butterworth-Heinemann.

Walker MC, Sander JW: New anti-epileptic drugs, *Exp Opin Investig Drugs* 8:1497-1510, 1999.

Willmore LJ: Clinical pharmacology of new antiepileptic drugs, *Neurology* 55(suppl 3): S17-S24, 2000.

Wong IC, Lhatoo SD: Adverse reactions to new anticonvulsant drugs, *Drug Saf* 23:35-56, 2000.

Xue H: Identification of major phylogenetic branches of inhibitory ligand-gated channel receptors, *J Mol Evol* 47:323-333, 1998.

CHAPTER • 15

Antiparkinson Drugs*

Vahn A. Lewis

Parkinson's disease, first clearly described in 1817 by James Parkinson, is a chronic, progressive, degenerative disease of the central nervous system (CNS). The disease rarely occurs before the age of 40 years but affects approximately 1% of the population older than 50 years. As a rule, Parkinson's disease has an insidious onset, beginning with mild signs such as slight unilateral weakness of the hand, mild tremor, and subtle changes in speech and writing. Symptoms of depression may develop,[2] and there is decreased fluorodopa uptake in positron emission tomography (PET) imaging studies.[8] The essential signs of clinical parkinsonism are resting tremor, rigidity, bradykinesia, and postural instability. In some patients motor "freezing" may occur when negotiating doorways or stairs. Abnormalities of posture and balance—which impair righting reflexes, equilibrium adjustments, and locomotion—contribute to the disability. Control of respiratory muscles and the larynx is impaired, so that breathing capacity is reduced, and the voice develops a monotonous quality. The patient may have a variety of ill-defined sensory symptoms consisting of numbness, tingling, abnormal temperature sensation, and visual disturbances. Sleep disturbances, including increased daytime sleepiness, abnormal rapid eye movement (REM) sleep, and increased motor activity during REM sleep, have been identified.[18] A little discussed sensory abnormality of Parkinson's disease is loss of olfaction for particular odors (e.g., gasoline, banana, pineapple, smoke, cinnamon).[10] This loss appears before any motor abnormality develops and may have implications as a biologic "marker" for the disease. Disorders of the autonomic nervous system, such as orthostatic hypotension, urinary retention or incontinence, and excessive sweating, are common. Drooling commonly occurs and is mainly caused by difficulty in swallowing (dysphagia) rather than excessive salivation. Dysphagia may be severe and can result in death by asphyxia, aspiration, or pneumonia.

Although Parkinson indicated that the senses and intellect were "uninjured" in parkinsonism, the disease is associated with mental slowing that can be reversed with treatment. In addition, the incidence of dementia is approximately three times greater in patients with Parkinson's disease than in age-matched control subjects, and clinical depression is a frequent aspect of the disease. Approximately 30% of patients report hallucinations or delusions.

Parkinson's disease may be primary, secondary, or Parkinson's plus. The primary or idiopathic form is the typical late-onset disorder with motor signs and a poorly understood cause. Some cases of primary Parkinson's disease may have a genetic contribution, and candidate loci have been identified on chromosomes 2, 4, 6, and 12.[36,41] Secondary Parkinson's is preceded by cerebral infections (syphilis, influenza), toxic chemicals (e.g., carbon monoxide, manganese, pesticides, welding-related fumes), cerebral hypoxia (vascular defects), traumatic brain injury, or antipsychotic drugs. The best-documented infectious source was the influenza epidemic of the late 1910s, which contributed to a delayed epidemic of cases as the patients aged. Parkinson's plus disorders are a group of maladies in which the signs and symptoms of Parkinson's disease contribute to a larger disorder (e.g., multiple system atrophy). In many cases, the exact cause of the parkinsonism is unknown.

The degenerative progression of Parkinson's disease proceeds at irregular rates in different patients. A subclinical form of the disorder may exist for many years before the patient becomes symptomatic. Noninvasive dopamine receptor brain-mapping studies suggest that a 60% to 80% loss of dopaminergic neurons occurs before clinical signs become evident.[5] The overt symptoms generally progress over a period of 10 to 20 years, ultimately terminating in severe invalidism. Life expectancy is reduced because of the usual complications associated with long-term invalidism. There is growing interest in developing neuroprotective treatments that might be useful before these debilitating changes occur.

NEUROBIOLOGY AND PATHOPHYSIOLOGY

Although the actual cause of Parkinson's disease remains undetermined, tremendous advances have been made in our understanding of the neuropathology of parkinsonism, the central control of movement, and the role of neurotransmitters in motor control and extrapyramidal function.

Motor function in the spinal cord and trigeminal nucleus is directly controlled by motor regions of the cerebral cortex. A model of basal ganglia function is shown in Figure 15-1. Motor activity in the cerebral cortex is stimulated by thalamocortical input, which is modulated by many factors, including sensory feedback, memory readout, and emotional response.[11] The basal ganglia modulate the thalamocortical processing through a γ-aminobutyric acid (GABA)–mediated inhibitory input derived from the substantia nigra pars reticulata and the internal part of the globus pallidus, nuclei whose functions appear to be similar and for this discussion will be referred to as the *basal ganglia thalamic inhibitor (BGTI)*. The output of the BGTI is influenced by two pathways within the basal ganglia, the direct and indirect. The direct pathway generally inhibits the BGTI and thus disinhibits the thalamic drive and increases motor activity. The indirect pathway involving excitatory input from the subthalamic nucleus,

*The authors wish to recognize Dr. Leslie Felpel for her past contributions to this chapter. See the Acknowledgments.

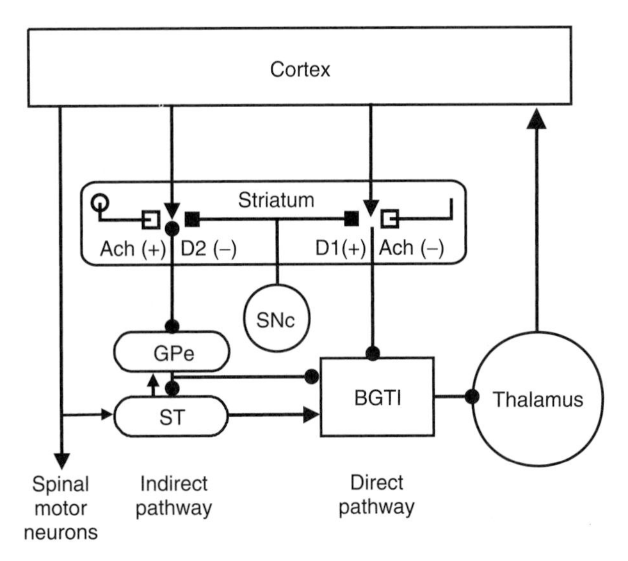

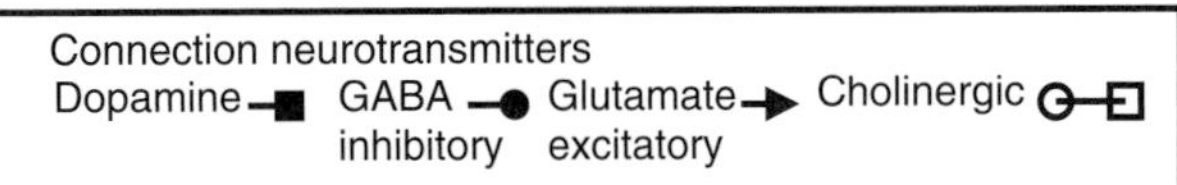

Fig. 15-1 Movement controlled by the cortex under the influence of the *thalamus* and basal ganglia. The thalamus relays excitatory input to the cortex. Glutamatergic cortical fibers project to the striatum, activation. GABAergic neurons. The GABAergic output from the basal ganglia is funneled through the *BGTI*, which exerts an inhibitory action on the thalamus. By the direct pathway, cortical input inhibits the BGTI and disinhibits the thalamus output. The indirect pathway, involving the alobus palldos externa (*Gpe*) and the subthalamic nucleus (*ST*), is complex but generally leads to an increase in inhibitory output from the BGTI. Excitatory D_1 dopamine receptors are believed to modulate the output of the direct pathway while inhibitory D_2 receptors modulate the output of the indirect pathway. Dopamine neuron cell bodies are located in the *SNc*. Acetylcholine is found in large interneurons within the striatum and opposes the effects of dopamine.

inhibits movement by facilitating BGTI outflow. Dopamine from the substantia nigra pars compacta (SNc) innervates both the direct and indirect pathways in the striatum. However, in the direct pathway it acts on D_1 receptors, which increase GABA inhibition of the BGTI. In the indirect pathway, dopamine acts on D_2 receptors, which inhibit GABA outflow to the indirect pathway. The large cholinergic striatal interneurons tend to oppose the actions of dopaminergic neurons. In the case of Parkinson's disease, a loss of dopamine neurons from the SNc leads to dysregulation of the indirect pathway by the subthalamic nucleus, producing activation of the BGTI and inhibition of movement (bradykinesia or akinesia). Parallel thalamocortico-basal ganglia circuits are proposed, each subserving a different function but converging onto the BGTI and then returning to the thalamus. Damage anywhere in this loop may result in localized motor abnormalities such as dystonias. The tremor associated with Parkinson's disease has been more difficult to explain. Recent research has suggested that the interaction between the subthalamic nucleus and the external segment of the globus pallidus may be one source of tremor.[33] Others suggest a role for the thalamus in tremor generation.

A dramatic upsurge of interest in environmental factors as a cause for Parkinson's disease occurred when several young drug abusers developed severe parkinsonian symptoms after self-administering a drug that they thought was a heroin analogue. The compound, 1-methyl-4-phenyl-1,2,3,6-tetrahydropyridine (MPTP), was a byproduct of a faulty synthesis of the meperidine like analgesic alphaprodine. Later work established that the chemical causing the toxicity was actually 1-methyl-4-phenylpyridinium (MPP+), a metabolite of MPTP. MPP+ toxicity stems from its transportation into cells by catecholamine reuptake transporters and subsequent interference with mitochondrial energy production. Environmental causes of Parkinson's are suspected, and various pyridines are present in the environment as insecticides, herbicides, and contaminants. Recently, the insecticide rotenone (structurally related to MPP+) has been found to produce a parkinsonlike syndrome in rats.[3] Although MPP+ does not duplicate the clinical condition of Parkinson's disease, it selectively destroys dopamine neurons in the substantia nigra and replicates many of the neuropathologic features of the disease. The antipsychotic agent haloperidol is metabolized to a pyridinium metabolite that increases oxidative damage in experimental animals.[4] For neural mitochondrial respiratory complexes, complex 1 has been found to be most prone to functional compromise.[7] However, Parkinson's patients may have deficiencies in other mitochondrial complexes as well.[17]

DOPAMINE REPLACEMENT AS A BASIS FOR THERAPY

In the 1960s, investigators discovered high concentrations of dopamine in two areas of the extrapyramidal system: the striatum and the SNc. Patients with Parkinson's disease were found to have low concentrations of dopamine in these areas. The drug reserpine was known to reduce catecholamines and produce characteristic Parkinson's disease–like effects (extrapyramidal signs). Levodopa (L-3,4-dihydroxyphenylalanine, the precursor of dopamine) was shown to reverse reserpine-induced bradykinesia, and a link between dopamine and extrapyramidal motor function was established.

The clinical effectiveness of intravenously administered levodopa on Parkinson's disease was soon discovered, but its oral effectiveness was limited. Much of the drug (97% to 99%) is metabolized to dopamine before gaining access to the CNS, which led to adverse side effects such as nausea, vomiting, and cardiovascular problems.

Carbidopa, a dopa-decarboxylase inhibitor, prevents much of the peripheral metabolism of levodopa (Figure 15-2). Carbidopa does not cross the blood-brain barrier, so it does not inhibit the CNS synthesis of dopamine from levodopa. Systemically administered levodopa is transported into the brain through the blood-brain barrier by a saturable amino acid transporter. Thus combining levodopa with carbidopa permits the use of lower doses of levodopa with greater effectiveness in parkinsonism compared with levodopa alone. It has been found that catechol-O-methyltransferase (COMT) may become upregulated in patients taking carbidopa. This discovery has prompted the development of COMT inhibitors to inhibit further the peripheral metabolism of levodopa.

NEUROPROTECTION

Neuroprotective strategies for the treatment of Parkinson's disease have evolved from theories regarding the cause of the disease. The free radical hypothesis is based on the concept that free radicals, generated from oxidative reactions, react with membrane lipids and cause lipid peroxidation, cell injury, and subsequent cell death. Mitochondrial damage and inhibition of oxidative phosphorylation also occur as a result of free radical attack. Figure 15-3 illustrates the relationship between dopamine metabolism and the generation of reactive oxygen species. In addition, the damaged neurons may also lose

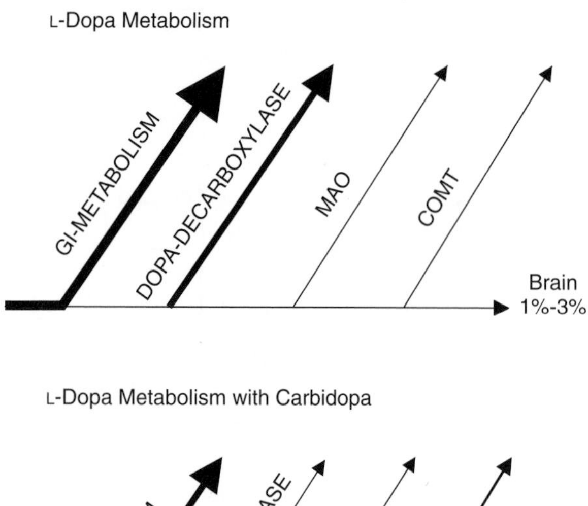

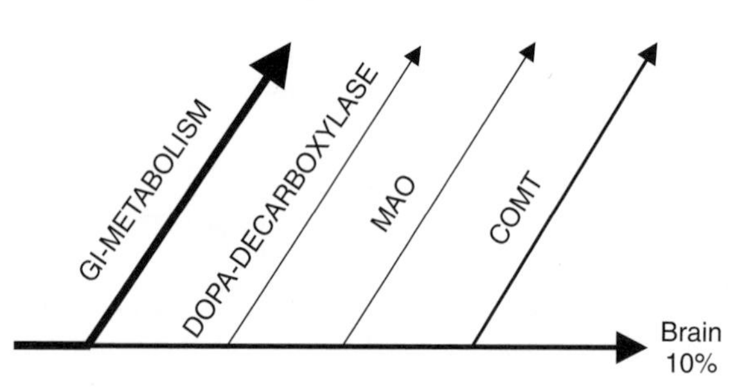

Fig. 15-2 Levodopa (*L-popa*) metabolism alone and with a dopa-decarboxylase inhibitor. Levodopa can be eliminated by several mechanisms before it reaches the brain. Substantial elimination occurs in the gastrointestinal (GI) traced and peripheral tissues. *Carbidopa* reduces levodopa metabolism outside the brain. A higher percentage (10% versus 1% to 3%) of the dose of levodopa gets to the brain when administered with carbidopa. To further reduce metabolism of dopamine, *COMT* inhibitors may be added; these drugs also reduce 3-O-methyldopa competition for levodopa transport into the brain. *MAO*, Monoamine oxidase.

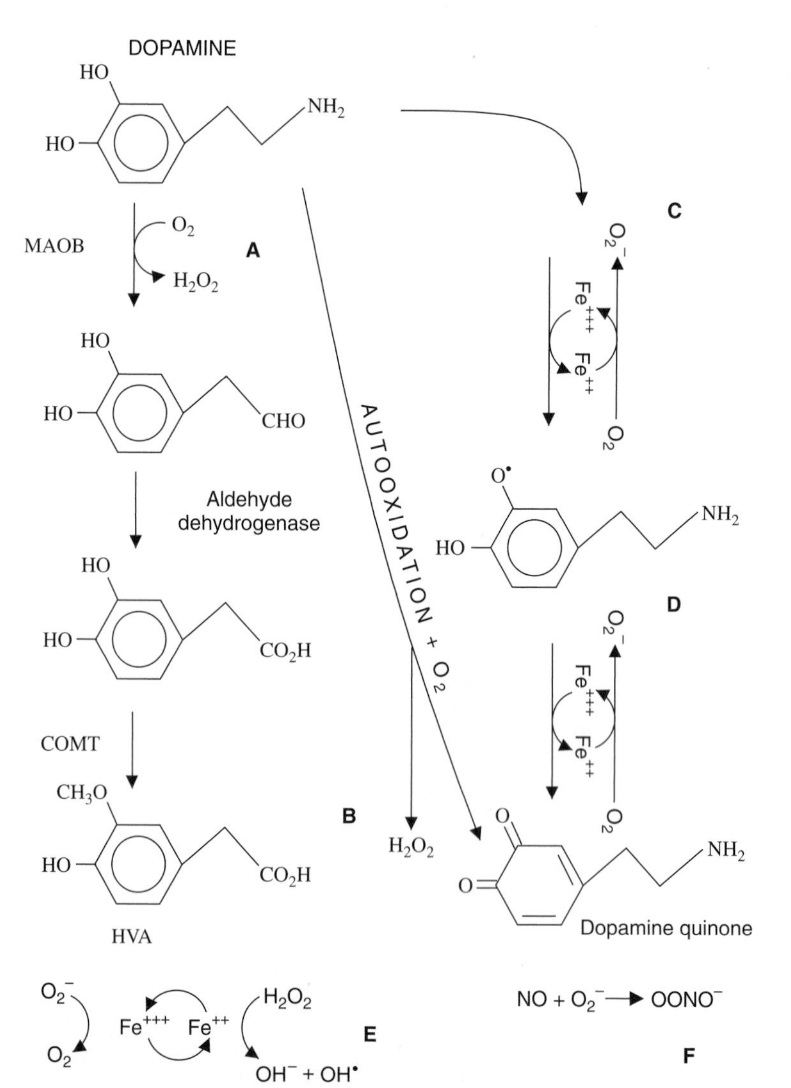

Fig. 15-3 Dopamine metabolism and the oxidative challenge to the SNc. Metabolism of dopamine can generate hydrogen peroxide *(H_2O_2)* at steps *A* and *B*. In the presence of *Fe^{++}* (pathologically elevated in the substantia nigra of patients with Parkinson's disease), increased generation of reactive hydroxy ions *(OH^-)*, superoxide species *(O_2^-)*, and free radicals occurs (*C, D,* and *E*). Finally, additional reactions may occur between these active oxygen species and nitric oxide to generate toxic peroxynitrite free radicals *($OONO^-$) (F)*. Dysregulation of these reactions may lead to oxidative damage in dopaminergic nerves. *HVA*, Homovanillic acid.

resistance to the toxic effects of the afferent excitatory neurotransmitter glutamate (afferents from the cortex, pedunculopontine nucleus, and subthalamic nucleus),[23] whose toxicity is mediated by excessive Ca^{++} flux and nitric oxide synthesis (Figure 15-4). In the most severe case these reactions can lead to apoptosis and cell death.

The brain is usually protected from damage caused by free radicals because it contains protective substances (e.g., glutathione, ascorbic acid, melatonin, vitamin E) and enzymes (e.g., glutathione peroxidase, superoxide dismutase) that prevent their buildup. The SNc of parkinsonian patients has reduced concentrations of both glutathione and glutathione peroxidase. This decrease may be one of the earliest events in the disorder and can by itself decrease mitochondrial complex 1 function.[21]

In addition to cell death in the SNc, patients with Parkinson's disease may develop neuronal inclusion bodies, or Lewy bodies, and neurofibrillary tangles, made of amyloidlike protein. Recent advances in the understanding of intracellular protein synthesis point to failure of removal or repair of irregular proteins as contributing to the development of the amyloid filled cells of Parkinson's disease. α-Synuclein, a protein found in synaptic membranes,[22] accumulates in the Lewy bodies of Parkinson's patients. In recent experiments, mutant α-synuclein was artificially expressed in fruit flies, which induced symptoms similar to Parkinson's disease in the flies.[13] Other abnormal proteins, such as parkin, have been identified in families with early-onset familial Parkinson's disease.[36]

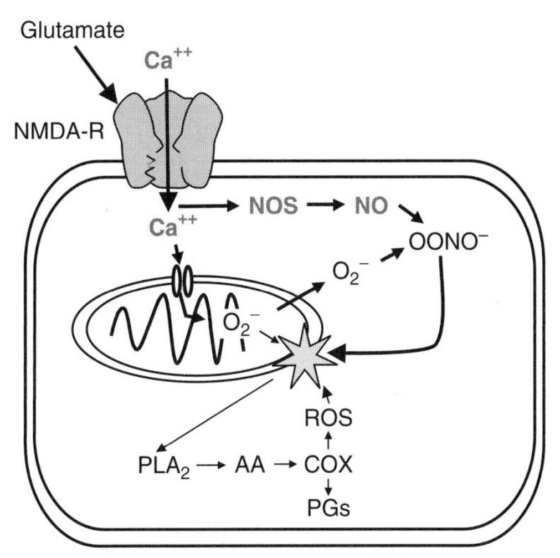

Fig. 15-4 Ca^{++}-mediated oxidative stress in nerves with glutamate (or glutamatergic) receptors. Activation of N-methy-D-asparate (NMDA) receptors (*NMDA-R*, one type of glutamate receptor) permits Ca^{++} currents to enter the cell. Intracellular Ca^{++} is normally reduced by sequestration in mitochondria and endoplasmic reticulum (not shown). Excess Ca^{++} stimulates nitric oxide synthtase *(NOS)*, which catalyzes the synthesis of nitric oxide *(NO)*. Excessive Ca^{++} currents are thought to compromise the function of mitochondria and permit the generation of free radicals and superoxide *(O_2^-)*, which can react with nitric oxide to produce the toxic peroxynitrite radical *($OONO^-$)*, which in turn can damage the mitochondria and cell membranes. Damaged membranes can be further metabolized by phospholipase A_2 *(PLA_2)*, producing arachidonic acid *(AA)*, a substrate for cyclooxygenase *(COX)*. Additional reactive oxygen species *(ROS)* are generated in the synthesis of prostaglandins *(PGs)* from arachidonic acid. These reactions may contribute to the sensitivity of the SNc neurons to premature cell death.

Scavenger drugs such as vitamin E have been administered experimentally, albeit so far without much success. The monoamine oxidase (MAO)-B inhibitor selegiline offers a potential, but as yet unproved, neuroprotective action by inhibiting the intraneuronal breakdown of dopamine. The pituitary hormone melatonin has antioxidant and proglutathione actions and has been found to be protective in the MPP+ model. An understanding of why Parkinson's disease continues to progress (perhaps deficient growth factors or vascular problems) may offer the possibility of better control or cures.

DRUG THERAPY FOR PARKINSON'S DISEASE

Table 15-1 presents an overview of the drugs used in the treatment of Parkinson's disease. Before the discovery of levodopa, the standard drugs for the treatment of Parkinson's disease were the antimuscarinic agents. Antimuscarinic drugs may be effective antiparkinson agents because they restore the dopaminergic/cholinergic balance that is upset when the dopaminergic nigrostriatal pathway degenerates (see Figure 15-1).

The classic dopaminergic/cholinergic imbalance concept of Parkinson's disease explains a variety of clinical and pharmacologic responses, but clinical parkinsonism is more complicated than an imbalance between two neurotransmitters. There are many other neurotransmitters in the basal ganglia, including norepinephrine, 5-hydroxytryptamine (5-HT), GABA, adenosine, and glutamate. Peptides such as enkephalins (indirect pathway) and substance P (direct pathway) coexist with GABA in some striatal efferent neurons. Although the role of these substances in Parkinson's disease is unknown, they offer possible pharmacologic approaches for therapy. There are occasional reports of parkinsonism being exacerbated or improved by agents acting at these other receptor systems.

Adding to this complexity is the discovery of several neurotransmitter receptor subtypes. Dopamine D_2, D_3, and D_4 receptors are thought to be more important than D_1 and D_5 receptors for antiparkinson effectiveness, but stimulation of both groups of receptors appears to be involved in the therapeutic efficacy of levodopa.[12] The fact that the cardinal symptoms of Parkinson's disease (tremor, rigidity, bradykinesia, and postural instability) do not respond uniformly to the antiparkinson drugs raises the possibility that these symptoms may be associated with other receptors, including muscarinic (M_1 and M_2) and nicotinic receptors, which may serve different functions in the basal ganglia.

Drugs Affecting Dopaminergic Transmission

Various drugs effective in Parkinson's disease promote dopaminergic receptor stimulation in the striatum. All stages of dopaminergic transmission, from the synthesis of dopamine to its release, binding to receptors, and termination of activity, are susceptible to pharmacologic modulation.

Levodopa

Levodopa (Figure 15-5) is a neutral amino acid formed from L-tyrosine, and it is a precursor of the endogenous catecholamines, including dopamine and norepinephrine. The major metabolic fate of levodopa is decarboxylation to dopamine by aromatic L-amino acid decarboxylase, commonly referred to as *dopa decarboxylase.*

Pharmacologic effects The central and peripheral nervous system actions of levodopa are thought to result from its conversion to dopamine. In practice, levodopa is almost always given with a decarboxylase inhibitor to increase the

Table • 15-1

Overview of Drugs and Procedures Used in the Treatment of Parkinson's Disease

DRUG OR PROCEDURE	PURPOSE	COMMENTS
Levodopa	Transported into brain then converted to dopamine	Natural precursor to dopamine; side effects include nausea, vomiting, dystonias, and postural hypotension
Carbidopa (with levodopa)	Blocks metabolism of levodopa in peripheral circulation	Reduces dose of levodopa and thereby its peripheral side effects
Tolcapone, entacapone	Nitrocatechol COMT inhibitors; help spare levodopa from peripheral metabolism and competition for brain amino acid transporters	Tolcapone may induce hepatic failure; possible drug interactions between COMT inhibitors and dental drugs
Selegiline (also called deprenyl)	Blocks MAO-B; may reduce synthesis of active oxygen metabolites; may only provide symptomatic relief	Possibly delays the progression of Parkinson's disease; drug interactions with meperidine, tricyclic antidepressants, and SSRIs
Dopamine Receptor Agonists		
Bromocriptine, pergolide, lisuride, ergoline, apomorphine, pramipexole (D_2, D_3), ropinirole (D_2, D_3)	Act directly on dopaminergic receptors; newer agents used to initiate therapy; also used in off cycles or when presynaptic dopaminergic neurons loss is great	Use limited by postural hypotension, nausea, and sedation; may contribute to confusion, hallucinations, psychosis, and livedo reticularis
Anticholinergics (Antimuscarinic)		
Trihexyphenidyl, benztropine, biperiden, procyclidine, diphenhydramine	Balance CNS dopamine/acetylcholine ratios	Can cause dry mouth, constipation, urinary retention, triggering of acute-angle glaucoma, impaired memory, and hallucinations
Amantadine	Increases release of dopamine; blocks dopamine reuptake and NMDA receptors	Originally used as an antiviral agent
Antidepressants		
Trazodone, paroxetine, tricyclic antidepressants	Used to treat depression associated with disease	Antidepressants may worsen Parkinson's symptoms in some patients
Clozapine or atypical antipsychotic agents	May be useful in treating levodopa-induced psychosis	Hematologic toxicity (especially with clozapine) but minimal parkinsonian side effects
Procedures		
Globus pallidus stimulation	Used to relieve essential tremor	Commercial stimulator unit has been marketed
Surgical lesions for Parkinson's disease	Unilateral stereotaxic lesions are introduced to control levodopa dystonias as well as parkinsonism tremor, rigidity, or bradykinesia	Some risk of stroke, paralysis, and visual field defects
Fetal transplants, stem cells, special cell culture implants	Used to replace dopamine cells	More effective in younger patients

SSRIs, Selective serotonin reuptake inhibitors.

percentage of levodopa delivered to the CNS and to reduce toxicity from levodopa.

Central Nervous System Because Parkinson's disease is characterized by a dopamine deficiency, the obvious therapeutic strategy would be to restore dopamine concentrations to normal. However, dopamine does not cross the blood-brain barrier and thus is not effective when administered systemically. The immediate amino acid precursor of dopamine, levodopa, is readily transported into the brain and is decarboxylated to dopamine in nigrostriatal neurons. The newly synthesized dopamine is sequestered in vesicles in the neuron terminals in the striatum, where it is available for release. Despite this seemingly physiologic approach, levodopa is not curative. Postmortem examinations of the brains of parkinsonian patients indicate that morphologic changes in

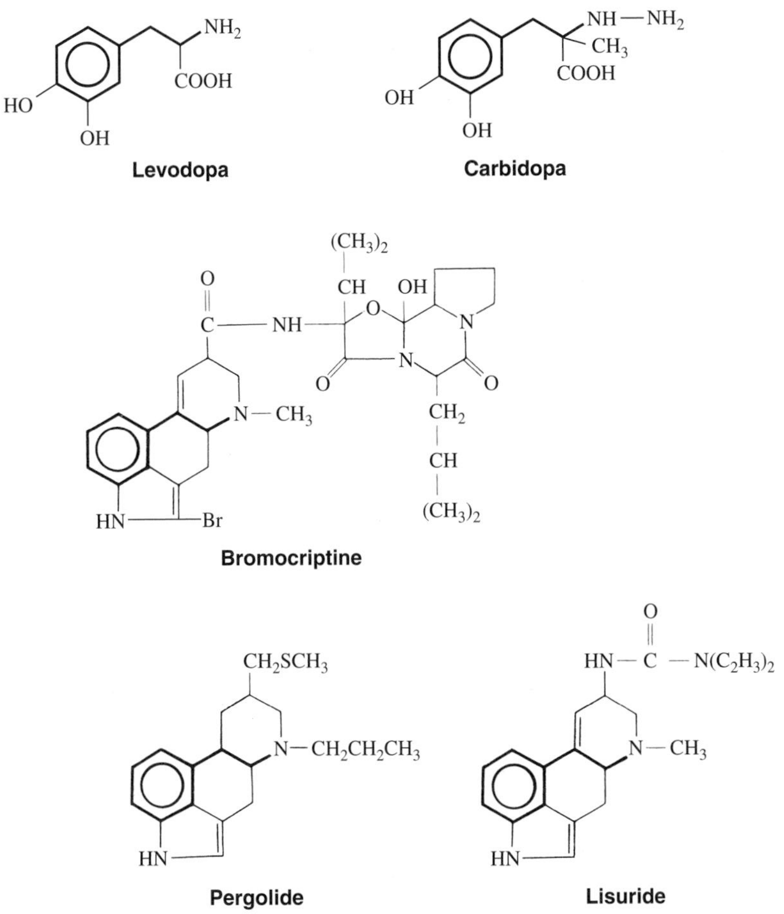

Levodopa

Carbidopa

Bromocriptine

Pergolide

Lisuride

Fig. 15-5 Structural formulas of some dopamine-related drugs used in the treatment of Parkinson's disease. The dopamine backbone contained within these structures is emphasized.

the CNS are similar regardless of whether patients are treated with levodopa.

A beneficial response to levodopa is obtained in approximately 75% of patients. Signs of parkinsonism, including tremor, bradykinesia, and rigidity, are typically well controlled, but the clinical efficacy decreases with time.

Patients receiving long-term levodopa therapy commonly experience a "wearing-off" effect, which refers to an apparent decrease in the length of time that a given dose of levodopa exerts its therapeutic effect. Another complication of long-term levodopa therapy is the "on-off" phenomenon. The patient has periods in which the levodopa is effective in reducing parkinsonian symptoms but where abnormal involuntary movements (AIMs) occur as levodopa side effects. AIMs may take the form of dyskinesias, which may correlate with the maximum plasma concentration of levodopa (peak-dose dyskinesia), or of dystonias, which are not strictly related to plasma concentrations of levodopa. This "on" state alternates with an "off" state in which there is a lack of therapeutic response to the drug, characterized by rigidity and akinesia. Oscillations in performance are so disabling and troublesome that, in an attempt to control them, patients may increase their total dose of levodopa to the point of abuse, thereby suffering the consequences of severe AIMs.[28]

The mechanisms responsible for these unusual responses are unknown but may relate to variations in drug absorption or receptor changes. Loss of dopaminergic input (denervation) to the striatum would be expected to increase the sensitivity of postsynaptic dopamine receptors (denervation supersensitivity) to dopamine. D_1 receptor–stimulated adenylyl cyclase activity is increased by both denervation and by chronic levodopa.[6] Despite this, neither D_1 nor D_2 receptors are increased in the postmortem brain tissue of these individuals.[5,16] Receptor desensitization may play a role in the diminishing response to levodopa as well as in the on-off effect. Support for this concept is provided by the observation that withdrawal of levodopa for 2 to 3 weeks (drug holiday) may permit its reinstitution at a greatly reduced dose and with less therapeutic fluctuation.[9] In summary, levodopa-induced dyskinesias are a common problem, and a variety of factors may be involved in their generation. Current efforts to minimize abnormal movements are focusing on variables such as dose, dosing schedules, prolonged-release dose forms, and the degree of D_1 and D_2 receptor activation caused by dopaminergic agents. The development of receptor-selective agents should clarify the role of receptors in therapy and drug-induced dyskinesia.

All clinical manifestations of parkinsonism respond in some degree to levodopa therapy. Tremor is less responsive to levodopa than is rigidity or bradykinesia, but abnormalities of posture, equilibrium, and locomotion all improve with treatment.

Whereas levodopa initially improves the mental status of the parkinsonian patient, a progressive dementia may still occur. Levodopa-induced behavioral changes are dose dependent and subside with dose reduction, but parkinsonian symptoms then worsen. Atypical antipsychotic agents such as clozapine and olanzapine[20] may be preferred for treating levodopa-induced psychosis because they are effective and have a reduced potential for extrapyramidal side effects.[4] Ondansetron, a 5-HT_3 receptor antagonist (used as an antiemetic agent), has been found to diminish levodopa-induced visual hallucinations and psychotic symptoms.[42]

Cardiovascular System A moderate degree of tachycardia and hypotension may occur with levodopa therapy. These effects are caused by dopamine formed by the metabolism of levodopa outside the CNS. Dopamine may also be responsible for the increased incidence of arrhythmia and hypertension reported with levodopa therapy, but age-related coronary heart disease is also likely to contribute. The incidence of levodopa-induced sinus tachycardia and atrial and ventricular extrasystoles is low and can be reduced further with the addition of a peripherally acting decarboxylase inhibitor (carbidopa). Severe hypertension from levodopa is much more likely to result from a drug interaction with one of the nonselective MAO inhibitors compared with MAO-B–selective inhibitors.

Gastrointestinal Tract Levodopa is rapidly converted to dopamine in the gastrointestinal tract and elsewhere. The dopamine produced causes significant nausea and other gastrointestinal disturbances. These effects are minimized by the coadministration of a decarboxylase inhibitor.

Absorption, fate, and excretion Levodopa is absorbed from the gastrointestinal tract, but approximately 95% of the drug is converted to dopamine in the small intestine and liver. As little as 1% of orally administered levodopa reaches the brain. When the drug is combined with a peripherally acting decarboxylase inhibitor, the dose of levodopa can be greatly reduced, much as 80%. The enzymes MAO and COMT found in the nervous system and various tissues further metabolize dopamine, and inactive metabolites are excreted in the urine. A diminished response to levodopa may occur when it is taken with a meal high in protein because other amino acids compete with levodopa for saturable carrier transport systems both in the gut and in the CNS. Protein-restricted diets are therefore sometimes advocated.[34]

Adverse effects Initially, most patients treated with levodopa experience nausea, vomiting, and orthostatic hypotension. Fortunately, tolerance develops to these side effects, reducing the need for therapeutic intervention. These symptoms are greatly reduced if a decarboxylase inhibitor is given concurrently. The most perplexing and perhaps most disabling toxic effect of levodopa is the appearance of AIMs. These movements are often restricted initially to the orofacial muscles and include abnormal mouth movements, protrusion and retraction of the tongue, chewing motions, facial grimacing, and abnormal movements of the head. The limb and trunk musculature may be involved with continued treatment. Unfortunately, AIMs often occur at dosages of levodopa that are just at the threshold for control of the parkinsonian symptoms. Although they are relieved somewhat by a reduction in levodopa dose, this strategy results in increased parkinsonian symptoms.

On initial therapy, levodopa often produces anxiety, insomnia, nightmares, and nervousness. More serious psychiatric side effects occur in a small proportion of patients and can result in delirium, depression, and psychotic states.

Levodopa combined with decarboxylase inhibitors

Aromatic L-amino acid decarboxylase is responsible for the enzymatic decarboxylation of levodopa to dopamine. Carbidopa is one of the commonly used decarboxylase inhibitors. The decarboxylase inhibitors do not penetrate the blood-brain barrier and therefore only inhibit the peripheral conversion of levodopa to dopamine, including the conversion that takes place in the intestinal lumen (see Figure 15-2). Carbidopa allows up to an 80% decrease in the dosage of levodopa necessary to control parkinsonian symptoms. Unfortunately, the AIMs, particularly those of the orofacial muscles, are not significantly diminished by the administration of carbidopa with levodopa, and, in fact, there are indications that they become more frequent and start earlier. There also appears to be little difference between the mental disturbances produced by levodopa alone and those produced by this drug combination. Carbidopa is relatively nontoxic but is inactive as an antiparkinson drug in the absence of levodopa. The levodopa-carbidopa combination is not recommended in pregnancy or in patients younger than 18 years. Carbidopa is available as a single agent or formulated with levodopa in a fixed ratio of 10 mg/100 mg and 25 mg/100 mg (carbidopa/levodopa). Packaged alone (but used in combination with levodopa), carbidopa is useful for patients who require either greater or lesser amounts of the drug than is provided in the standard ratios.

Catechol-O-methyltransferase inhibitors

MAO and COMT are the two major catabolic enzymes for catecholamines. Therapeutic block of dopamine decarboxylase with carbidopa can induce an increased metabolism of levodopa by COMT to 3-O-methyldopa. This loss of levodopa and greater competition by 3-O-methyldopa for levodopa transporters reduce the effectiveness of levodopa treatment. The nitrocatechols tolcapone and entacapone (Figure 15-6) reversibly inhibit COMT and enhance or extend the effect of levodopa in patients who have advanced or fluctuating Parkinson's disease. Typically, the levodopa dose can be reduced by approximately 30% when a COMT inhibitor is added.

Tolcapone is administered three times a day and inhibits both peripheral and central COMT. It is absorbed in 2 hours, is highly protein bound, and is extensively glucuronidated to an inactive metabolite. Tolcapone has been occasionally associated with severe hepatotoxicity and death. Therefore patients using this agent need to be carefully selected and need to have their hepatic function monitored. Entacapone is a peripherally acting drug and is also administered in conjunction with the levodopa-carbidopa combination. Entacapone is approximately 35% absorbed and extensively protein bound (98%). Entacapone is isomerized and then glucuronidated and eliminated in the bile (90%). Its half-life (1 to 2 hours) is similar to that of levodopa.

The main adverse effects of the COMT inhibitors are related to increased dopaminergic effects such as dyskinesia,

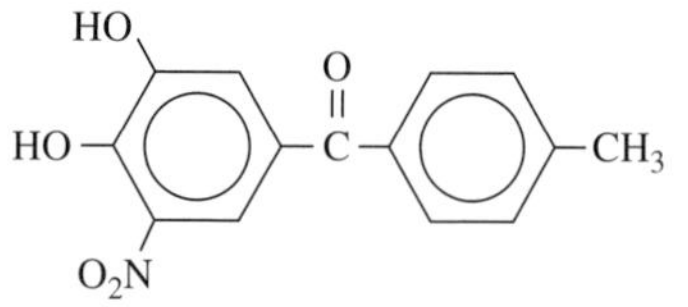

Tolcapone

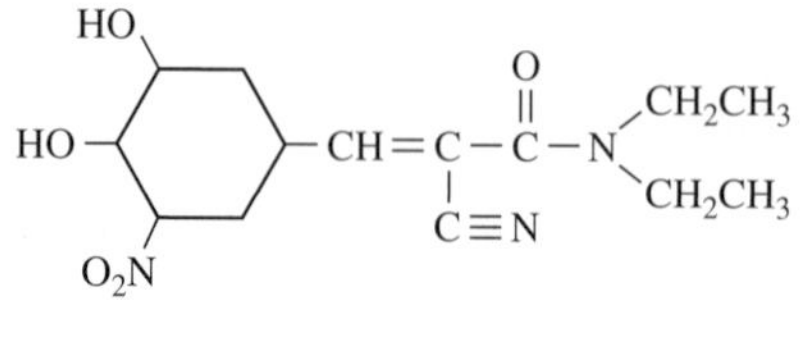

Entacapone

Fig. 15-6 Structural formulas of the nitrocatechol COMT inhibitors tolcapone and entacapone.

hallucinations, orthostatic hypotension, sleep disorders, and gastrointestinal side effects (e.g., nausea, vomiting). Reduction of the levodopa dose may be required to minimize these side effects.

Drug interactions of concern with COMT inhibitors include the catecholamines (e.g., epinephrine), drugs that interfere with biliary excretion (including ampicillin and erythromycin), drugs with sedative actions (anxiolytics, sedative antihistamines, barbiturates, opioid agonists, antipsychotics, and many tricyclic antidepressants), and nonselective MAO inhibitors.

Direct dopamine receptor agonists

The discovery of dopamine receptor subtypes, recognition of the limits of levodopa therapy, and advances in knowledge of the neurochemistry of normal and parkinsonism-altered nerve pathways have stimulated the search for dopamine agonists for the treatment of Parkinson's disease. Because these agents act directly on postsynaptic dopamine receptors, they complement levodopa. These drugs offer several advantages over levodopa: they (1) do not require metabolic conversion to an active compound; (2) do not require the presence of nigrostriatal neurons or nerve impulses for their activity; (3) have longer durations of action than levodopa with fewer on-off changes; (4) are more selective than levodopa on specific subpopulations of dopamine receptors; and (5) are less likely to generate damaging free radicals.

Bromocriptine, pergolide, and lisuride are amine ergot derivatives that share a common dopaminelike substructure, as shown in Figure 15-5. These agents may be used alone or in combination with levodopa-carbidopa. Efficacy tends to decline as the disease progresses.

Bromocriptine is the oldest and best studied of this group of drugs. It is a potent D_2 receptor agonist and a weak D_1 antagonist. When combined with levodopa therapy, it may alleviate the on-off phenomenon and can be useful in patients who are unresponsive to levodopa-carbidopa. Patients placed on bromocriptine cannot stop taking levodopa-carbidopa because a dramatic increase in parkinsonian symptoms would otherwise occur. This finding suggests that activation of both D_2 and D_1 receptors are required for full therapeutic benefit.[40] Pergolide is a potent D_1, D_2, and D_3 receptor agonist. As a result of its prolonged action, pergolide may decrease levodopa-induced dyskinesias and increase the "on" time after the patient begins on-off fluctuations. A third ergot derivative, lisuride, is more potent than bromocriptine. Lisuride is primarily a D_2 receptor agonist, but it is a 5-HT receptor agonist as well.

Adverse effects of these amine ergot agents are similar and include AIMs, mental changes (confusion and psychosis), nausea, vomiting, hiccough, and orthostatic hypotension. Rare side effects include pleural or retropleural fibrosis and livedo reticularis, a reddish skin eruption of the lower extremities. The adverse effects are generally reversible on withdrawal of the drug. In some patients, pergolide may cause hallucinations, cardiac arrhythmias, hepatotoxicity, worsened dyskinesias, and sudden episodes of "freezing" and somnolence. Lisuride appears to also cause somnolence and greater psychiatric changes than bromocriptine, which may result from its tryptaminergic properties. Lisuride is not available in the United States.

Pramipexole and ropinirole are two new, nonergot-derived dopamine receptor agonists at D_2, D_3, and D_4 receptors (Figure 15-7). Their antiparkinsonian effect is thought to be caused by activity at the D_2 receptor but may also include a neuroprotective component. These agents can be used as initial monotherapy (reduced risk of dyskinesia compared with levodopa)[37] or as an adjunct to levodopa therapy to smooth out its fluctuating propensity (on-off phenomena).

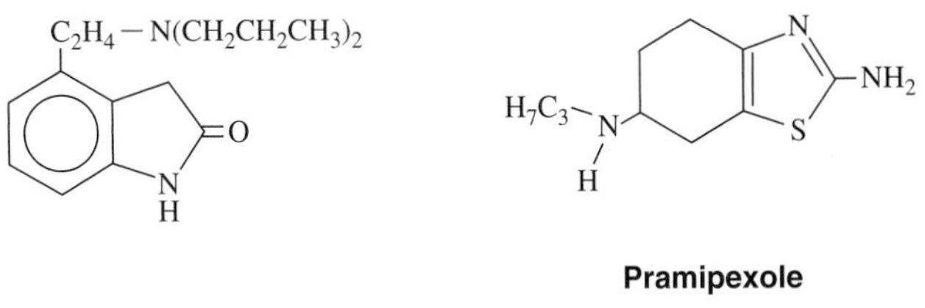

$C_2H_4-N(CH_2CH_2CH_3)_2$

Ropinirole

Pramipexole

Fig. 15-7 Structural formulas of ropinirole and pramipexole.

Pramipexole is cleared primarily by renal excretion (96%), whereas ropinirole is metabolized mainly by the cytochrome P450 1A2 isoform. Ciprofloxacin can inhibit CYP1A2 and significantly increase ropinirole blood concentrations.

Several side effects have been noted with these drugs. Postural hypotension and peripheral edema can occur. Asthenia, fatigue, and somnolence are reported. Some patients, usually older patients with more severe disease, have daytime sleepiness and have fallen asleep during daytime activities, including driving.[31] Insomnia and hallucinations have also been reported. Motor side effects include dyskinesias and extrapyramidal reactions. The gastrointestinal side effects of nausea and constipation have been reported.

Direct-acting dopamine agonists alone may begin to lose their clinical effectiveness after 1 or 2 years. Switching to a different dopamine agonist when one begins to fail sometimes restores clinical efficacy. Side effects of the dopamine agonists are similar to those of levodopa. Dopamine agonists have typically been used as adjuncts in antiparkinson therapy. In combination with levodopa-carbidopa they allow reduction in the levodopa dose, which may diminish on-off responses and other side effects. Most clinical trials with dopamine agonists have been conducted on patients who are either taking other antiparkinson drugs or whose conditions are refractory to conventional treatments. The fact that any of these patients respond to the dopamine agonists at all is encouraging.

Apomorphine has been recognized as a direct dopamine agonist since 1951. However, it has been rarely used clinically. It has been rediscovered as an agent to reverse off periods; subcutaneous injection may be more efficacious than oral therapy for this indication.[35]

Miscellaneous drugs

Amantadine The antiparkinson effects of amantadine, an antiviral agent, were discovered when the drug was used to treat a viral infection in a patient who had Parkinson's disease. The mechanism of action of amantadine is not known. It has been proposed that the drug (1) prevents dopamine reuptake and facilitates the release of dopamine, (2) has weak anticholinergic properties, and (3) blocks the glutamate N-methyl-D-aspartate (NMDA) receptor, which could contribute to reducing excitation-induced neurotoxicity and dyskinesias.[39] Several amantadine analogues are being tested for antiparkinson activity.

Amantadine is usually prescribed in combination with levodopa-carbidopa because an additive effect has been demonstrated when these drugs are used together. When given alone, its efficacy diminishes after several weeks. Amantadine is probably best used (1) alone at the early stages of Parkinson's disease, when symptoms are troublesome but not severe; (2) alone for the management of patients who do not respond well to levodopa; or (3) in combination with levodopa-carbidopa when a more beneficial response is required.

Approximately 80% to 90% of amantadine is excreted unchanged in the urine, and thus accumulation occurs in patients with impaired renal function. This accumulation may lead to the toxic manifestations of confusion, hallucinations, toxic psychosis, convulsions, and coma. Like the direct-acting dopamine agonists, amantadine may cause livedo reticularis of the lower extremities. More common side effects include anorexia, insomnia, nausea, vomiting, dizziness, AIMs, lightheadedness, edema, and sweating. These side effects are not severe and are further limited by the development of tolerance.

Selegiline Selegiline is a selective irreversible inhibitor of MAO-B, the major MAO enzyme in the striatum.[30] Because MAO-A is not inhibited, peripheral catecholamine metabolism is little affected. The rationale for using a selective MAO-B inhibitor is to elevate brain dopamine concentrations while causing little or no effect on norepinephrine or 5-HT. Selegiline is effective as adjunct therapy to levodopa-carbidopa in slowing the progression of parkinsonian symptoms. It has recently been evaluated as monotherapy in early-stage Parkinson's disease, and it improves motor function[19] and reduces freezing.[14] Selegiline is metabolized to amphetamine and methamphetamine in the brain and liver. Very often patients report that they feel better after selegiline therapy, possibly because of an amphetaminelike action. Recent studies appear to confirm selegiline's efficacy; however, its benefits decline as the disease progresses. Selegiline's inhibition of dopamine metabolism may contribute to its putative neuroprotective effect.

Adverse effects of selegiline include nausea, dry mouth, confusion, occasional visual hallucinations, dizziness, headache, and insomnia, especially at higher doses. The combined use of selegiline at high doses and levodopa results in an increased incidence of dyskinesia and psychoses. This effect may result from the formation of toxic quantities of amphetamine. Selegiline does not potentiate the pressor response to tyramine and is devoid of interaction with various foods that contain sympathomimetic amines. Nevertheless, it interacts adversely with meperidine, tricyclic antidepressants, and the selective serotonin reuptake inhibitors.

Antioxidants Selegiline (also known as deprenyl) and tocopherol formed the basis of the DATATOP (Deprenyl and Tocopherol Antioxidant Therapy of Parkinsonism) study,[32] a large clinical project designed to test the effectiveness of selegiline and antioxidants in Parkinson's disease. The results of studies with tocopherol have shown no significant benefit either alone or with selegiline.[32]

Drugs with Antimuscarinic Activity

Both muscarinic and nicotinic receptors are found in the striatum; however, to date most successful therapeutic interventions involving acetylcholine neurotransmission are associated with antimuscarinic drug treatment. Antimuscarinic drugs act to restore the dopaminergic/cholinergic balance by antagonizing the action of acetylcholine, and they may also inhibit dopamine uptake. The antimuscarinic drugs are not highly effective antiparkinson agents, but, surprisingly, tremor often responds better to these drugs than to levodopa-carbidopa.

The antimuscarinic drugs produce sedation and, in high doses, can elicit visual hallucinations and changes in mood. Trihexyphenidyl has been reported to have abuse potential, and parkinsonian patients may "fake" parkinsonian signs to obtain the drug. Toxic doses of the antimuscarinics can cause severe mental disturbances, including excitement, confusion, hallucinations, delirium, depression, coma, and medullary paralysis. Because of muscarinic receptor blockade, these drugs may produce xerostomia; increase intraocular pressure; and cause tachycardia, palpitation, arrhythmias, urinary retention, constipation, and tachypnea.

Muscarinic receptor antagonists are effective in the treatment of neuroleptic-induced extrapyramidal reactions. Formerly many psychiatrists advocated the coadministration of the anticholinergic agents with neuroleptic drugs as a prophylactic measure to minimize extrapyramidal side effects. There is controversy regarding this practice because the antiparkinson drugs may worsen tardive dyskinesia, induce delirium or psychosis, lower the plasma concentration of the neuroleptic agent, and cause other adverse effects. At present, the coadministration of an antiparkinson agent with a neuroleptic is generally reserved for persons who have treatable motor side effects.

Newer Antiparkinson Drugs

Although not new drugs, the β-adrenergic receptor blockers propranolol and nadolol and the benzodiazepine clonazepam are finding a new use in the treatment of parkinsonian tremor. The fact that nadolol is excluded from entry into the brain suggests that peripheral β-adrenergic receptors have a role in parkinsonian tremor. Because brain norepinephrine release may also be decreased in parkinsonism, L-threo-3,4-dihydroxyphenylserine, a norepinephrine precursor transported into the brain, has been used with some success to reduce depression in the Parkinson's plus multiple system atrophy disorder. Clonazepam may be effective in treating some aspects of Parkinson's disease, presumably because of its GABAergic activity. Although baclofen and other $GABA_B$ agonists have not been effective in Parkinson's disease, the known and prominent GABAergic pathways of the basal ganglia suggest that manipulation of GABAergic transmission might be a valid approach to the treatment of this disease.

Blockade of glutamatergic transmission with excitatory amino acid antagonists is a new approach to antiparkinson therapy. The effectiveness of these agents in experimental Parkinson's disease is encouraging and may offer another therapeutic modality if the side effects of the drugs can be minimized. Interestingly, both amantadine and the anticholinergic drugs used to treat parkinsonism have NMDA receptor antagonist activity. A glutamate-dopamine balance may exist in the basal ganglia that can be improved with glutamate antagonists. These agents may also be neuroprotective.

General Therapeutic Uses

There can be little doubt that the combination of levodopa and carbidopa is the most effective antiparkinson treatment available to date. However, because of the serious side effects associated with levodopa therapy and its limited period of effectiveness, other drugs and drug combinations are commonly used. Some physicians now prefer to initiate therapy with selegiline or a selective dopamine agonist (ropinirole or pramipexole) and add levodopa-carbidopa when the disease begins to create functional disabilities. However, because these drugs are expensive, other physicians initiate therapy with the anticholinergic drugs. When the disease is judged to be moderate, levodopa-carbidopa is added. As the disease progresses, adjunctive agents, such as the dopamine agonists and amantadine, may be added to the regimen. There is still a strong interest in drugs that may provide a neuroprotective effect and reduce progression of the disease.

Levodopa therapy, even with carbidopa, has several limitations. Levodopa-induced dyskinesias are the rule rather than the exception, but often these are not seriously disturbing to the patient. The fluctuations in responsiveness of parkinsonian symptoms to levodopa and the progressively greater severity of these oscillations are distressing, however, as is the progressive deterioration of mental function. Finally, the continual use of levodopa often results in unresponsiveness to the drug. It is at this stage that drug holidays are attempted and adjunctive agents added.[9]

Although antiparkinson therapy, in particular levodopa-carbidopa, has improved the quality of life for the patient with Parkinson's disease, life expectancy has not been significantly prolonged. This limitation further illustrates the slow, persistent degenerative process occurring in the brain, a deterioration apparently not responsive to current treatment.

SURGICAL THERAPY

Advances in brain imaging techniques have resulted in improvements of surgical approaches to the treatment of Parkinson's disease. Ablation of the globus pallidus or thalamus or stimulation of the thalamus, globus pallidus, and subthalamic nucleus can reduce motor disturbances in Parkinson's patients.[29] It is not always predictable before surgery whether ablation or stimulation will be effective. The presumed effect of surgery is to reduce excessive excitatory neuronal activity or to increase inhibitory tone by stimulation. Efferent pathways of the subthalamic nucleus appear to be excitatory and mediated by glutamate, as are corticosubthalamic pathways. Accordingly, studies have now shown that agents that inhibit excitatory amino acid transmission block experimentally induced parkinsonism.[24,25]

Another approach to the treatment of Parkinson's disease involves the grafting of small pieces of fetal brain tissue or the patient's own adrenal medullary tissue (chromaffin autograft) into the caudate nucleus or putamen.[27] These tissues release catecholamines, primarily epinephrine and norepinephrine, but in the absence of adrenocortical influences, the synthesis of epinephrine slows and the dopamine/norepinephrine ratio increases. A suggested advantage of such grafts is that they could also release growth factors, which may be deficient in Parkinson's patients. These patients show initial improvement, but long-term results have not been overwhelmingly positive. A number of patients in the United States have undergone this operation, and their clinical course is being closely followed. Some patients continue to improve for as long as 5 years.[27] There is also interest in developing dopamine-releasing cells from mesencephalon cells by using stem cell–culturing techniques.

Finally, brain stimulation in the globus pallidus or subthalamic nucleus can reduce tremor associated with parkinsonism. Deep brain electrodes must be surgically placed, and the patient has a battery-powered neurostimulator implanted near the collarbone.

DRUGS USED FOR OTHER MOVEMENT DISORDERS

Several disorders less common than Parkinson's disease also cause movement disabilities. These diseases include Huntington's disease (Huntington's chorea), Gilles de la Tourette's syndrome (Tourette's syndrome), Wilson's disease, and dystonic syndromes. Although these movement disorders are more refractory to pharmacotherapy than is Parkinson's disease, some drugs are beneficial and have furthered our understanding of the role of the basal ganglia in motor control.

Huntington's disease, probably the best known of these disorders, is characterized by choreic hyperkinesias and dementia. Huntington's disease is caused by a genetic error in the huntingtin gene and subsequent abnormal synthesis of a huntingtin protein that contains excess polyglutamine repeats.[38] The pathologic change in Huntington's disease is degeneration of GABAergic neurons in the striatum. The strategy followed in parkinsonism of "replacing" the missing neurotransmitter has not proved effective in Huntington's disease inasmuch as GABA receptor agonists and various inhibitors of GABA catabolism have been clinically disappointing. Adjusting the dopamine/acetylcholine balance by antagonizing dopamine is more effective. Thus the antipsychotic drugs, which are potent dopamine antagonists, may be useful for certain chorea symptoms. A dopamine-depleting drug, tetrabenazine, has also been useful in Huntington's disease. In advanced stages of the disease, pharmacotherapy is without effect.

Tourette's syndrome, characterized by phonic and motor tics and complex mannerisms, is responsive to haloperidol, fluphenazine, and pimozide. However, the effectiveness of these compounds is short lived. Many novel approaches are being investigated, including a variety of atypical antipsychotic agents. The dopamine receptor agonist pergolide has been found to be effective and well tolerated.[15] In addition, some beneficial results have been reported with clonidine, an α_2-adrenergic receptor agonist.[26]

Wilson's disease, an inherited disorder of copper metabolism, is characterized by damage to the liver, a characteristic brown stain at the edge of the cornea, and a variety of motor disorders, including akinesia, rigidity, and dystonia. Wilson's disease can generally be managed by chelating excess copper with penicillamine. However, if treatment is begun late in the course of the disease, penicillamine may not control the neurologic symptoms. At this point, levodopa and the anticholinergic antiparkinson drugs are useful.

Many common dystonic syndromes, such as torsion dystonia and spasmodic torticollis, are largely refractory to pharmacotherapy. Low doses of levodopa and high doses of bromocriptine and lisuride have mild beneficial effects, especially in young patients. High doses of antimuscarinic antiparkinson agents are also somewhat helpful, again in the young, probably because these patients can better tolerate the side effects. Botulinum toxin A, which inhibits the release of acetylcholine from cholinergic neurons, may be useful in treating certain dystonias. Botulinum toxin A and antimuscarinic drugs are both useful for treating focal dystonias. Because of the effectiveness of antimuscarinic agents and drugs that interrupt cholinergic transmission, it has been suggested that cholinergic hyperactivity might be responsible for the dystonias, but the underlying pathology and cause of these syndromes remain unknown.

IMPLICATIONS FOR DENTISTRY

Parkinson's Disease

Patients with untreated Parkinson's disease face a number of potential challenges to maintaining adequate oral health. These patients may have a low salivary rate and xerostomia caused by their treatment. In addition, they may experience nausea and vomiting more frequently than other patients, with possible adverse effects on tooth enamel. Parkinson's patients have difficulty in sustaining repetitive motions, such as those used for tooth brushing or flossing. Electric tooth brushes can help circumvent some of the problem, although a patient with motor freezing may still have difficulty and need assistance. Oral tremor can also make oral health care challenging for the dentist, and prosthetic restoration may pose additional challenges because of the presence of uncontrolled oral movements.

Parkinsonian patients may react slowly to pain and thus not provide rapid feedback about progressive tissue damage. They have difficulty maintaining postural stability and normal walking gait and may be more prone to falling; therefore some assistance entering and leaving the office should be considered. In addition to motor freezing, these patients may have difficulty comprehending or remembering prolonged instructions; therefore written or taped treatment plans and medication instructions should be provided to the patient and responsible accompanying parties. Orthostatic hypotension can be present, so patients should be allowed to change position slowly and stabilize their blood pressure. During a procedure, consideration should be given to the patient's difficulty with swallowing. Aggressive saliva control and not tipping the patient too far back in the dental chair can be helpful.

Levodopa

It has been recommended that patients be scheduled for treatment within 60 to 90 minutes of the patient's levodopa dosage to reduce their disability during treatment. For some patients this may lead to a higher incidence of dyskinesias during the visit because of pulsatile exposure of the brain to elevated dopamine at the peak of the absorption curve.[9] Facial movements induced by levodopa may cause a number of dental problems, including inflammation, damage to oral structures, movement of anterior teeth (because of tongue thrusting), and difficulty in wearing and retaining dentures. Dyskinesias can become so severe that they interfere with swallowing, speech, and respiration.

Orofacial motor impairment of Parkinson's disease may be different from motor impairment in the extremities and may not respond to pharmacotherapy in the same manner. There is also evidence suggesting that the tongue is the most severely impaired of all orofacial musculature in Parkinson's disease.[1] Levodopa can cause dysgeusia, or alteration in the sensation of taste, possibly explained by the loss of olfaction. This reaction is not seen when levodopa is combined with a decarboxylase inhibitor.

Tolerance usually develops to levodopa-induced orthostatic hypotension. Nonetheless the patient still sometimes has episodes of hypotension, perhaps more frequently after dosage adjustments. Orthostatic hypotension can be a particular problem for the dentist because of the reclining position of the patient during dental care. If orthostatic hypotension persists, lowering the levodopa dosage may be required to control it.

A number of drug interactions involving levodopa are of potential concern to the dentist. It is believed by some investigators that levodopa sensitizes the heart to epinephrine-induced arrhythmias. The mechanism responsible for this effect is unknown, but the excitatory action of levodopa on the heart may result from an action of dopamine on cardiac β_1-adrenergic receptors. Although some practitioners believe that this interaction provides a valid contraindication for the use of local anesthetics with vasoconstrictors in patients taking levodopa, the clinical significance of these interactions is not established. The use of phenothiazines (including promethazine), hydroxyzine, and metoclopramide as antinauseants should be discouraged for patients undergoing levodopa therapy. Such agents can exacerbate the motor irregularities of Parkinson's disease because of their dopamine receptor–blocking properties. A peripheral dopamine antagonist, domperidone, is a useful antinauseant, but it is not currently available in the United States. Analgesics may be used with levodopa, but if general anesthesia is required, consultation with the patient's physician is recommended. Pyridoxine (vitamin B_6), which is present in over-the-counter multivitamin preparations, antagonizes the antiparkinson effect of levodopa because it enhances levodopa's conversion to dopamine in the periphery. Fortunately, this antagonism does not occur when a peripheral decarboxylase inhibitor is coadministered with levodopa.

Levodopa and anticholinergic drugs can induce hallucinations. Addition of adjunctive agents such as carbidopa elevate dopamine in the CNS and contribute to this adverse effect.

Dopaminergic agonists, amantadine, and selegiline

Side effects of these drugs are generally related to their effect of stimulating (directly or indirectly) dopaminergic receptors. If a patient has recently been started on any of these medications, transient nausea and vomiting may occur. A patient scheduled for dental work at this time is more susceptible to gagging, nausea, and vomiting. Because of hypotension on initial therapy, the same precautions described for levodopa apply. Dopamine agonists can cause oral dyskinesia similar to those produced by levodopa. The new dopamine agonists ropinirole and pramipexole may induce daytime sleepiness in some patients; caution should be used if sedative or opioid therapy is planned.

Catechol-O-methyltransferase inhibitors

These agents have the potential to cause drug interactions such as tachycardia, an increase in blood pressure, or arrhythmias with vasoconstrictors, and increased sedative effects with antianxiety drugs, sedating antihistamines, opioid analgesics, and other drugs with CNS depressant properties. Several antibiotics (e.g., ampicillin, erythromycin) used by dentists can reduce the elimination of entacapone. Because the COMT inhibitors have only been available for a short time, it is not known how clinically significant these interactions may be.

Anticholinergic agents

The patient taking antimuscarinic agents may have typical antimuscarinic side effects. Xerostomia may increase the incidence of caries, impair swallowing, increase the likelihood of soft tissue disease in the oral cavity, and even make speech difficult. Drugs with which the antiparkinson anticholinergics might summate include the antihistamines, tricyclic antidepressants, and other drugs with antimuscarinic effects. Adverse reactions and drug interactions involving the antimuscarinic drugs are discussed further in Chapter 9.

Antiparkinson Drugs and Drugs for Other Movement Disorders

Nonproprietary (generic) name	*Proprietary (trade) name*
Anticholinergics	
Benztropine	Cogentin
Biperiden	Akineton
Procyclidine	Kemadrin
Trihexyphenidyl	Artane, Trihexy-2
Other drugs with anticholinergic activity	
Diphenhydramine	Benadryl
Ethopropazine*	Parsidol
Dopamine precursor and decarboxylase inhibitors	
Carbidopa	Lodosyn
Levodopa	Dopar, Larodopa
Levodopa + benserazide*	Madopar
Levodopa + carbidopa	Sinemet
Levodopa + carbidopa + entacapone	Stalevo

Antiparkinson Drugs and Drugs for Other Movement Disorders—cont'd

Nonproprietary (generic) name	*Proprietary (trade) name*
Dopamine receptor agonists	
Bromocriptine	Parlodel
Pergolide	Permax
Pramipexole	Mirapex
Ropinirole	Requip
Other antiparkinson drugs	
Amantadine	Symmetrel
Entacapone	Comtan
Selegiline (L-deprenyl)	Eldepryl
Tolcapone	Tasmar

*Not currently available in the United States.

Some Drugs for Other Movement Disorders

Nonproprietary (generic) name	*Proprietary (trade) name*
Clonidine	Catapres
Fluphenazine	Prolixin
Gabapentin	Neurontin
Haloperidol	Haldol
Nadolol	Corgard
Pimozide	Orap
Primidone	Mysoline
Propranolol	Inderal
Tetrabenazine*	Nitoman

*Not currently available in the United States.

CITED REFERENCES

1. Abbs JH, Hartman DE, Vishwanat B: Orofacial motor control impairment in Parkinson's disease, *Neurology* 37:394-398, 1987.
2. Becker G, Muller A, Braune S, et al: Early diagnosis of Parkinson's disease, *J Neurol* 249(suppl 3):III/40-48, 2002.
3. Betarbet R, Sherer TB, MacKenzie G, et al: Chronic systemic pesticide exposure reproduces features of Parkinson's disease, *Nat Neurosci* 3:1301-1306, 2000.
4. Bloomquist J, King E, Wright A, et al: 1-Methyl-4-phenylpyridinium-like neurotoxicity of a pyridinium metabolite derived from haloperidol: cell culture and neurotransmitter uptake studies, *J Pharmacol Exp Ther* 270:822-830, 1994.
5. Brooks DJ: PET studies and motor complications in Parkinson's disease, *Trends Neurosci* 23(10 suppl):S101-S108, 2000.
6. Cash R, Raisman R, Ploska A, et al: Dopamine D-1 receptor and cyclic AMP-dependent phosphorylation in Parkinson's disease, *J Neurochem* 49:1075-1083, 1987.
7. Davey GP, Peuchen S, Clark JB: Energy thresholds in brain mitochondria. Potential involvement in neurodegeneration, *J Biol Chem* 273:12753-12757, 1998.
8. DeKosky ST, Marek K: Looking backward to move forward: early detection of neurodegenerative disorders, *Science* 302:830-834, 2003.
9. Direnfeld L, Spero L, Marotta J, et al: The L-dopa on-off effect in Parkinson disease: treatment by transient drug withdrawal and dopamine receptor resensitization, *Ann Neurol* 4:573-575, 1978.
10. Double KL, Rowe DB, Hayes M, et al: Identifying the pattern of olfactory deficits in Parkinson disease using the brief smell identification test, *Arch Neurol* 60:545-549, 2003.
11. Doya K: Complementary roles of basal ganglia and cerebellum in learning and motor control, *Curr Opin Neurobiol* 10:732-739, 2000.
12. Emilien G, Maloteaux JM, Geurts M, et al: Dopamine receptors—physiological understanding to therapeutic intervention potential, *Pharmacol Ther* 84:133-156, 1999.
13. Feany MB, Bender WW: A *Drosophila* model of Parkinson's disease, *Nature* 404:394-398, 2000.
14. Giladi N, McDermott MP, Fahn S, et al: Freezing of gait in PD: prospective assessment in the DATATOP cohort, *Neurology* 56:1712-1721, 2001.
15. Gilbert DL, Sethuraman G, Sine L, et al: Tourette's syndrome improvement with pergolide in a randomized, double-blind, crossover trial, *Neurology* 54:1310-1405, 2000.
16. Guttman M, Seeman P, Reynolds GP, et al: Dopamine D_2 receptor density remains constant in treated Parkinson's disease, *Ann Neurol* 19:487-492, 1986.
17. Haas RH, Nasirian F, Nakano K, et al: Low platelet mitochondrial complex I and complex II/III activity in early untreated Parkinson's disease, *Ann Neurol* 37:714-722, 1995.
18. Henderson JM, Lu Y, Wang S, et al: Olfactory deficits and sleep disturbances in Parkinson's disease: a case-control survey, *J Neurol Neurosurg Psychiatry* 74:956-958, 2003.
19. Hocherman S, Levin G, Giladi N, et al: Deprenyl monotherapy improves visuo-motor control in early parkinsonism, *J Neural Transm* 52:63-69, 1998.
20. Jankovic J: Complications and limitations of drug therapy for Parkinson's disease, *Neurology* 55(suppl 6):S2-S6, 2000.
21. Jha N, Jurma O, Lalli G, et al: Glutathione depletion in PC12 results in selective inhibition of mitochondrial complex I activity. Implications for Parkinson's disease, *J Biol Chem* 275:26096-26101, 2000.
22. Kim TD, Paik SR, Yang CH, et al: Structural changes in α-synuclein affect its chaperone-like activity in vitro, *Protein Sci* 9:2489-2496, 2000.
23. Kitai ST, Shepard PD, Callaway JC, et al: Afferent modulation of dopamine neuron firing patterns, *Curr Opin Neurobiol* 9:690-697, 1999.
24. Klockgether T, Turski L: NMDA antagonists potentiate antiparkinsonian actions of L-dopa in monoamine-depleted rats, *Ann Neurol* 28:539-546, 1990.
25. Klockgether T, Turski L, Honore T, et al: The AMPA receptor antagonist NBQX has antiparkinsonian effects in monoamine-depleted rats and MPTP-treated monkeys, *Ann Neurol* 30:717-723, 1991.
26. Leckman JF, Hardin MT, Riddle MA, et al: Clonidine treatment of Gilles de la Tourette's syndrome, *Arch Gen Psychiatry* 48:324-328,1991.

27. Lopez-Lozano JJ, Bravo G, Brera B, et al: Long-term improvement in patients with severe Parkinson's disease after implantation of fetal ventral mesencephalic tissue in a cavity of the caudate nucleus: 5-year follow up in 10 patients: Clinica Puerta de Hierro Neural Transplantation Group, *J Neurosurg* 86:931-942, 1997.
28. Nausieda PA: Sinemet "abusers," *Clin Neuropharmacol* 8:318-327, 1985.
29. Obeso JA, Rodriguez MC, Gorospe A, et al: Surgical treatment of Parkinson's disease, *Baillieres Clin Neurol* 6:125-145, 1997.
30. Olanow CW: MAO-B inhibitors in Parkinson's disease, *Adv Neurol* 60:666-671, 1993.
31. Pal S, Bhattacharya KF, Agapito C, et al: A study of excessive daytime sleepiness and its clinical significance in three groups of Parkinson's disease patients taking pramipexole, cabergoline, and levodopa mono and combination therapy, *J Neural Transm* 108:71-77, 2001.
32. Parkinson Study Group: Effects of tocopherol and deprenyl on the progression of disability in early Parkinson's disease, *N Engl J Med* 328:176-183, 1993.
33. Perkel DJ, Farries MA: Complementary "bottom-up" and "top-down" approaches to basal ganglia function, *Curr Opin Neurobiol* 10:725-731, 2000.
34. Pincus JH, Barry K: Protein redistribution diet restores motor function in patients with dopa-resistant "off" periods, *Neurology* 38:481-483, 1988.
35. Poewe W, Wenning GK: Apomorphine: an underutilized therapy for Parkinson's disease, *Mov Disord* 15:789-794, 2000.
36. Polymeropoulos MH: Genetics of Parkinson's disease, *Ann N Y Acad Sci* 920:28-32, 2000.
37. Rascol O, Brooks DJ, Korczyn AD, et al: A five-year study of the incidence of dyskinesia in patients with early Parkinson's disease who were treated with ropinirole or levodopa. 056 Study Group, *N Engl J Med* 342:1484-1491, 2000.
38. Sawa A, Tomoda T, Bae B-I: Mechanisms of neuronal cell death in Huntington's disease, *Cytogenet Genome Res* 100:287-295, 2003.
39. Stoof JC, Booij J, Drukarch B: Amantadine as N-methyl-D-aspartic acid receptor antagonist: new possibilities for therapeutic applications? *Clin Neurol Neurosurg* 94(suppl):S4-S6, 1992.
40. Walters JR, Bergstrom DA, Carlson JH, et al: D_1 dopamine receptor activation required for postsynaptic expression of D_2 agonist effects, *Science* 236:719-722, 1987.
41. Zimprich A, Muller-Myhsok B, Farrer M, et al: The PARK8 locus in autosomal dominant parkinsonism: confirmation of linkage and further delineation of the disease-containing interval, *Am J Hum Genet* 74:11-19, 2004.
42. Zoldan J, Friedberg G, Weizman A, et al: Ondansetron, a 5-HT_3 antagonist for visual hallucinations and paranoid delusional disorder associated with chronic L-DOPA therapy in advanced Parkinson's disease, *Adv Neurol* 69:541-544, 1996.

General References

Adler CH, Ahlskog JE, eds: *Parkinson's disease and movement disorders: diagnosis and treatment guidelines for the practicing physician*, Totowa, NJ, 2000, Humana Press.

Alexander RE, Gage TW: Parkinson's disease: an update for dentists, *Gen Dent* 48:572-582, 2000.

Davis KL, Martin E, Turko IV, et al: Novel effects of nitric oxide, *Annu Rev Pharmacol Toxicol* 41:203-236, 2001.

Jankovic J, Hallett M: *Therapy with botulinum toxin*, New York, 1994, Marcel Dekker.

Kaneko S, Hikida T, Watanabe D, et al: Synaptic integration mediated by striatal cholinergic interneurons in basal ganglia function, *Science* 289:633-637, 2000.

Koller WC, Paulson G, eds: *Therapy of Parkinson's disease*, ed 2, New York, 1995, Marcel Dekker.

Mouradian MM, Chase TM: Improved dopaminergic therapy of Parkinson's disease. In Marsden CD, Fahn S, eds: *Movement disorders 3*, Oxford, 1994, Butterworth-Heinemann.

Wallace KB, Starkov AA: Mitochondrial targets of drug toxicity, *Annu Rev Pharmacol Toxicol* 40:353-388, 2000.

CHAPTER • 16

Local Anesthetics

John A. Yagiela

Local anesthetics are agents that reversibly block nerve conduction when applied to a circumscribed area of the body. Although numerous substances of diverse chemical structure are capable of producing local anesthesia, most drugs of proven clinical usefulness (identified by the suffix *-caine*) share a fundamental configuration with the first true local anesthetic, cocaine.

For centuries, natives of the Peruvian highlands have relied on the leaves of the coca bush to prevent hunger, relieve fatigue, and uplift the spirit. European interest in the psychotropic properties of *Erythroxylon coca* led to the isolation of cocaine by Niemann in 1859 and to a study of its pharmacology by von Anrep in 1880. Although both men reported on the local anesthetic action of cocaine, credit for its introduction into medicine belongs to Carl Koller, a Viennese physician. In 1884, Koller was familiarized with the physiologic effects of cocaine by Sigmund Freud. Koller recognized the drug's great clinical significance and quickly demonstrated its pain-relieving action in several ophthalmologic procedures. The benefits of cocaine were widely appreciated; within a year, local anesthesia had been successfully administered for a variety of medical and dental operations.

Knowledge of cocaine's potential for adverse reactions soon followed its general acceptance as a local anesthetic. Several deaths attributed to acute cocainization testified to the drug's low therapeutic index. The abuse liability of cocaine was dramatically illustrated by the self-addiction of William Halsted, a pioneer in regional nerve blockade. A chemical search for safer, nonaddicting local anesthetics was instituted by Einhorn and his associates in 1892, culminating 13 years later in the synthesis of procaine. Since then, numerous improvements in the manufacture of local anesthetic solutions have been made, and many useful agents have been introduced into clinical practice. However, because no drug is currently devoid of potentially serious toxicity, the search for new and better local anesthetics continues.

CHEMISTRY AND CLASSIFICATION

Certain physicochemical characteristics are required of a drug intended for clinical use as a local anesthetic. One obvious prerequisite is that the agent must depress nerve conduction. Because an axon whose cytoplasmic contents have been completely removed can still transmit action potentials, a drug must be able to interact directly with the axolemma to exert local anesthetic activity. A second important consideration is that the agent must have both lipophilic and hydrophilic properties to be effective by parenteral injection. Lipid solubility is essential for penetration of the various anatomic barriers existing between an administered drug and its site of action, including the nerve sheath. Water solubility ensures that, once injected in an effective concentration, a drug will not precipitate on exposure to interstitial fluid. These requirements have placed important structural limitations on the clinically useful local anesthetics.

Structure-Activity Relationships

The typical local anesthetic molecule can be divided into three parts: an aromatic group, an intermediate chain, and a secondary or tertiary amino terminus (Figure 16-1). All three components are important determinants of a drug's local anesthetic activity. The aromatic residue confers lipophilic properties on the molecule, whereas the amino group furnishes water solubility. The intermediate portion is significant in two respects. First, it provides the necessary spatial separation between the lipophilic and hydrophilic ends of the local anesthetic. Second, the chemical link between the central hydrocarbon chain and the aromatic moiety serves as a suitable basis for classification of most local anesthetics into two groups, the esters (—COO—) and the amides (—NHCO—). This distinction is useful because there are marked differences in allergenicity and metabolism between the two drug categories.

Minor modifications of any portion of the local anesthetic molecule can significantly influence drug action. For example, the addition of a chlorine atom to the ortho position on the benzene ring of procaine yields chloroprocaine, a more lipophilic local anesthetic four times as potent as the parent compound yet half as toxic when injected subcutaneously. Table 16-1 lists several important physicochemical properties of local anesthetics and how they correlate with clinical activity.

Influence of pH

By virtue of the substituted amino group, most local anesthetics are weak bases with a negative logarithm of the acid ionization constant (pK_a) ranging from 7.5 to 9.0. A local anesthetic intended for injection is usually prepared in salt form by the addition of hydrochloric acid. Not only is water solubility improved, but stability in aqueous media is also increased. Once injected, the acidic local anesthetic solution is quickly neutralized by tissue fluid buffers, and a fraction of the cationic form is converted to the nonionized base. As determined by the Henderson-Hasselbalch equation (Figure 16-2), the percentage of drug converted depends primarily on the local anesthetic pK_a and the tissue pH. Because only the base form can diffuse rapidly into the nerve, drugs with a high pK_a tend to be slower in onset than similar agents with more

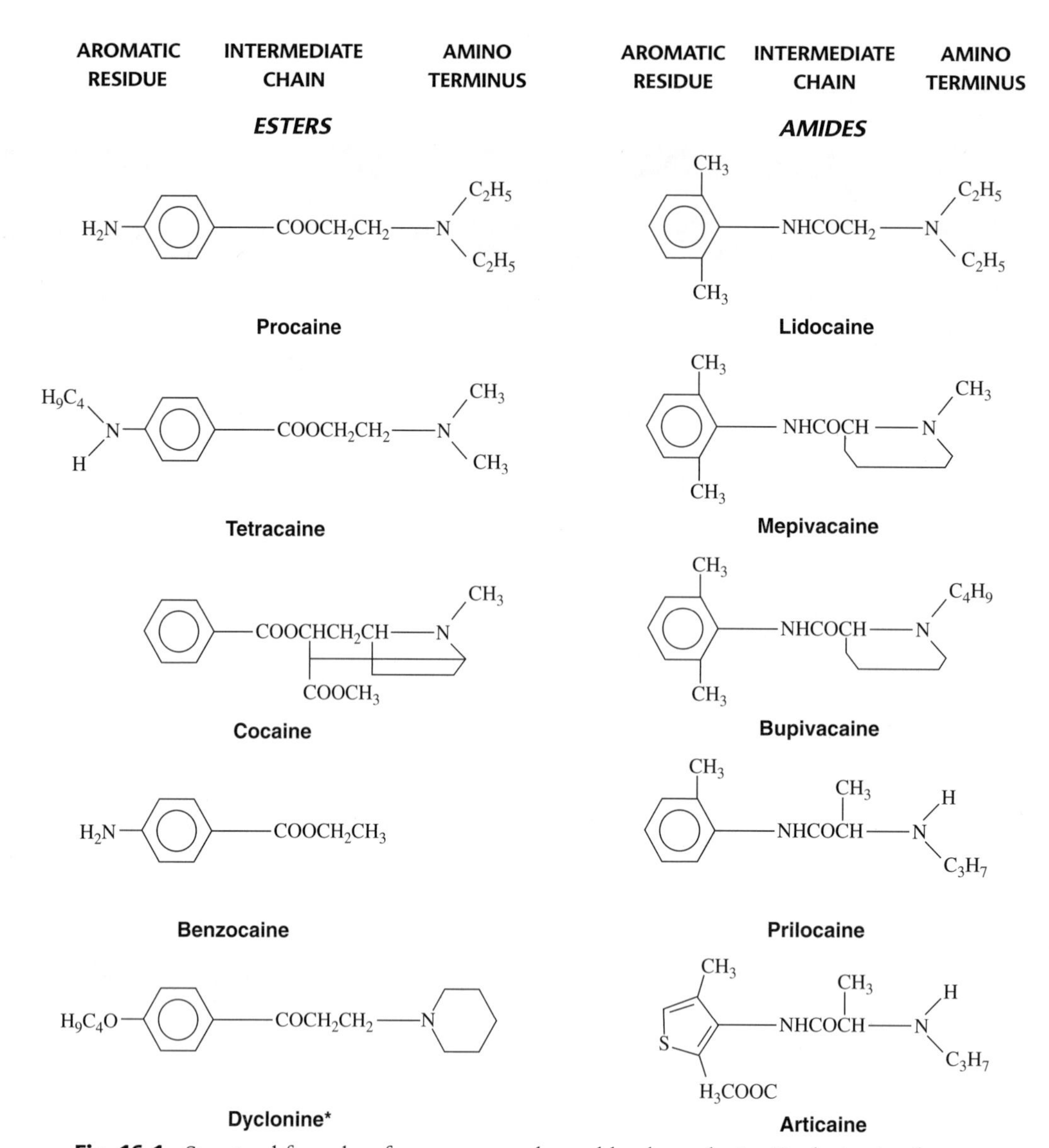

Fig. 16-1 Structural formulas of some commonly used local anesthetics. Dyclonine is a ketone.

favorable dissociation constants. Tissue acidity may also impede the development of local anesthesia. Products of inflammation can lower the pH of the affected tissue and limit formation of the free base. Ionic entrapment of the local anesthetic in the extracellular space delays the onset of local anesthesia and may also render effective nerve blockade impossible.

Numerous attempts have been made to augment local anesthesia by capitalizing on the influence of pH. Alkalization should theoretically increase local anesthetic activity by promoting tissue penetration and nerve uptake. Indeed, many topical agents are marketed in the base form to improve diffusion across epithelial barriers. Although it has been shown experimentally that alkalization of local anesthetic solutions just before use enhances nerve blockade, practical considerations have limited routine clinical application. Even so, extracellular fluid has in most instances sufficient buffering capacity to negate differences in local anesthetic pH soon after injection. An alternative approach to modifying drug distribution is through the addition of carbon dioxide. Carbonation of a local anesthetic solution can increase the rate of onset and sometimes the depth of anesthesia. It has been suggested that the hydrocarbonate salt of the local anesthetic penetrates membranes more rapidly than does the conventional formulation and that the injected carbon dioxide diffusing into the nerve trunk lowers the internal pH and concentrates local anesthetic molecules by ion trapping.[51] There is also evidence that carbon dioxide may potentiate local anesthetic activity by a direct effect on the nerve membrane.[13,18] Although promising, carbonated local anesthetic solutions are not available in the United States, and a study of carbonated lidocaine used for mandibular anesthesia failed to reveal any significant benefit compared with lidocaine hydrochloride.[21]

MECHANISM OF ACTION

Local anesthetics block the sensation of pain by interfering with the propagation of peripheral nerve impulses. Both the generation and the conduction of action potentials are inhibited. Electrophysiologic data indicate that local anesthetics do

Table • 16-1

Physicochemical Correlates of Local Anesthetic Activity

DRUG	OCTANOL/BUFFER DISTRIBUTION COEFFICIENT*	ANESTHETIC POTENCY (TONIC BLOCK)	DURATION OF ANESTHESIA	MOLECULAR WEIGHT	PHASIC BLOCK†	pKa*	RATE OF ONSET
Procaine	3	Low	Short	236	Moderate	8.9	Moderate
Articaine‡	17	Moderate	Moderate	284	Moderate	7.8	Fast
Mepivacaine	42	Moderate	Moderate	246	Moderate	7.7	Fast
Prilocaine	55	Moderate	Moderate	220	Low	7.8	Fast
Lidocaine	110	Moderate	Moderate	234	Moderate	7.8	Fast
Ropivacaine	186	High	High	274	Moderate	8.1	Moderate
Bupivacaine	560	High	High	288	High	8.1	Moderate
Tetracaine	541	High	High	264	Moderate	8.4	Moderate

*Measurements made at 36° C, except for prilocaine and ropivacaine, which are extrapolated from values taken at 25° C. (Data from Strichartz GR, Sanchez V, Arthur GR, et al: Fundamental properties of local anesthetics: II. Measured octanol/buffer partition coefficients and pK_a values of clinically used drugs, *Anesth Analg* 71:158-170, 1990.)
†Relative tendency to cause phasic (use-dependent) block in peripheral nerve. (Data from Courtney KR: Structure-activity relations for frequency-dependent sodium channel block in nerve by local anesthetics, *J Pharmacol Exp Ther* 213:114-119, 1980.)
‡Data from *Mosby's drug consult 2003*, St Louis, 2003, Mosby.

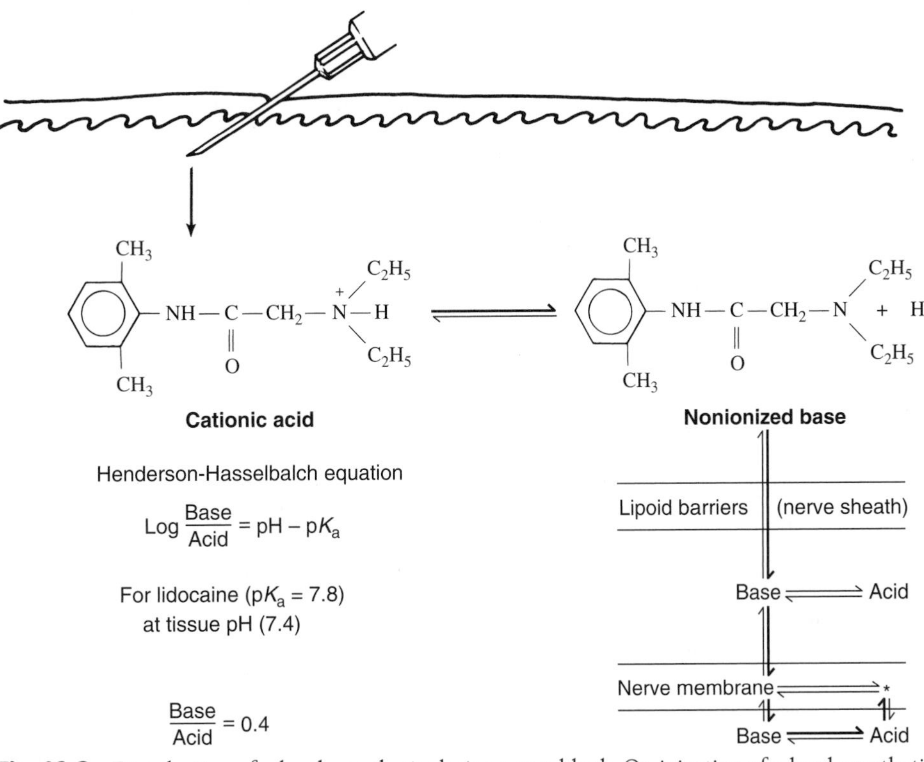

Fig. 16-2 Distribution of a local anesthetic during nerve block. On injection of a local anesthetic solution, a portion of the cationic acid is converted to the free base. Calculated for lidocaine is the base/acid ratio in the extracellular fluid at equilibrium. *Dark arrows* depict the major pathway followed by a local anesthetic in reaching its site of action *(asterisk)* within the nerve membrane. Although the acid form is presumed responsible for most of the blocking activity, the contribution of the nonionized base (*light arrows* within the axolemma) must not be overlooked.

not significantly alter the normal resting potential of the nerve membrane—instead they impair certain dynamic responses to nerve stimulation.

Effects on Ionic Permeability

The quiescent nerve membrane is relatively impermeable to Na^+. Excitation of the axolemma by an appropriate stimulus, however, temporarily increases Na^+ conductance and causes the nerve cell to become less electronegative regarding the outside. If the transmembrane potential is sufficiently depressed, a critical threshold is reached at which the depolarization becomes self-generating. A marked increase in Na^+ permeability induces a rapid influx of Na^+ through Na^+-selective channels traversing the nerve membrane. The inward Na^+ current creates an action potential of approximately +40 mV, which is then propagated down the nerve. The action potential is quite transient at any given segment of membrane; loss of Na^+ permeability (inactivation of the Na^+ channels) and an outward flow of K^+ (in nonmyelinated axons) quickly repolarize the membrane. These events are reviewed in Figure 16-3.

Local anesthetics interfere with nerve transmission by blocking the influence of stimulation on Na^+ conductance.[75] A developing local anesthetic block is characterized by a progressive reduction in the rate and degree of depolarization and a slowing of conduction. When depolarization is retarded so that repolarization processes develop before the threshold potential can be reached, nerve conduction fails.[1]

Site of Action

Several sites exist within the nerve membrane where drugs could potentially interfere with Na^+ permeability. It was argued, for example, that local anesthetics could interact with membrane lipids to impair Na^+ channel function, just as has long been proposed for general anesthetics (see Chapter 17). By disrupting the organization of these lipids, local anesthetics may prevent the physical accommodations necessary for channel gating.[81] Although this explanation might account for the ability of local anesthetics to impede the functioning of membrane-bound proteins besides the Na^+ channel, such as other ion channels, autonomic receptor systems, and various enzymes,[17] it does not readily account for the fact that stereoisomers of local anesthetics exhibit differential blocking potencies,[83] and it cannot explain certain other features of local anesthetic action, such as use-dependent block or the effects of permanently charged local anesthetics (both described later).

In recent years, evidence has accumulated that conventional local anesthetics interact directly with the Na^+ channel to inhibit nerve conduction. The Na^+ channel is composed of several subunits. The α subunit is the largest component (260,000 daltons) and forms the actual channel. As depicted in Figure 16-4, the α subunit consists of four homologous domains (I to IV), each containing six helical segments (S1 to S6) that traverse the plasma membrane.[19] Collectively, the four S4 segments of each domain constitute the "activation gate," which is the portion of the channel protein that moves in response to a depolarizing stimulus and opens the channel. Each S4 segment contains positively charged amino acid residues, specifically arginine and lysine, at every third position of the α helix. In the "helical screw model" of activation,[20] depolarization causes the outward rotation of the S4 segments, which can be detected experimentally as the small gating current that precedes the action potential. Local anesthetic blockade of the Na^+ channel is characterized by a reduction in the peptide movements responsible for the gating current.[54] Lidocaine, for example, tends to trap the S4 segment of domain III in the external, depolarized configura-

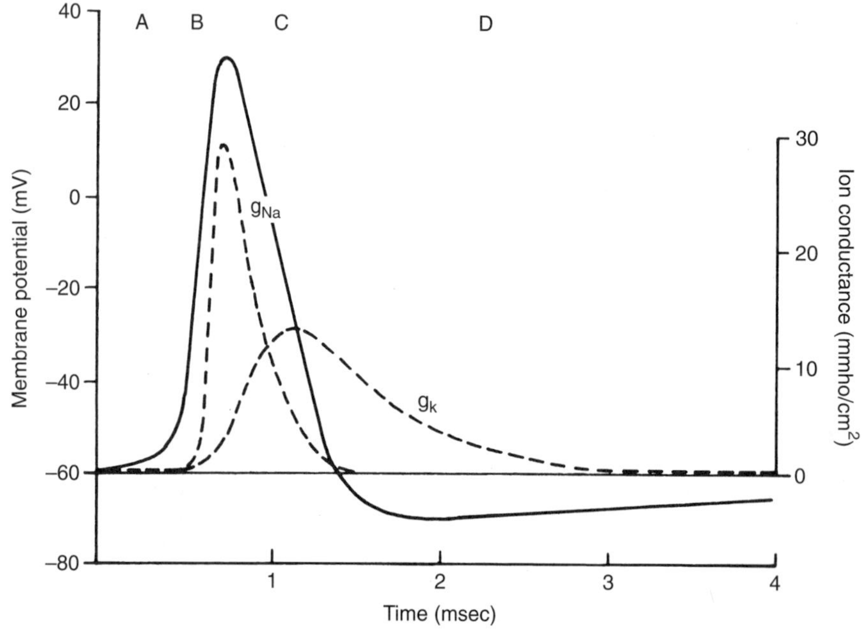

Fig. 16-3 The action potential. *Dashed lines* indicate the Na^+ (g_{Na}) and K^+ (g_K) conductance changes responsible for membrane depolarization and recovery. *A*, Resting state; Na^+ channels are in the resting (closed) configuration. *B*, Depolarization phase; Na^+ channels open. C, Repolarization phase; Na^+ channels become inactivated (closed) and the nerve refractory to stimulation. *D*, Recovery phase; Na^+ channels convert from the inactivated to the resting state, and the nerve regains the ability to conduct action potentials.

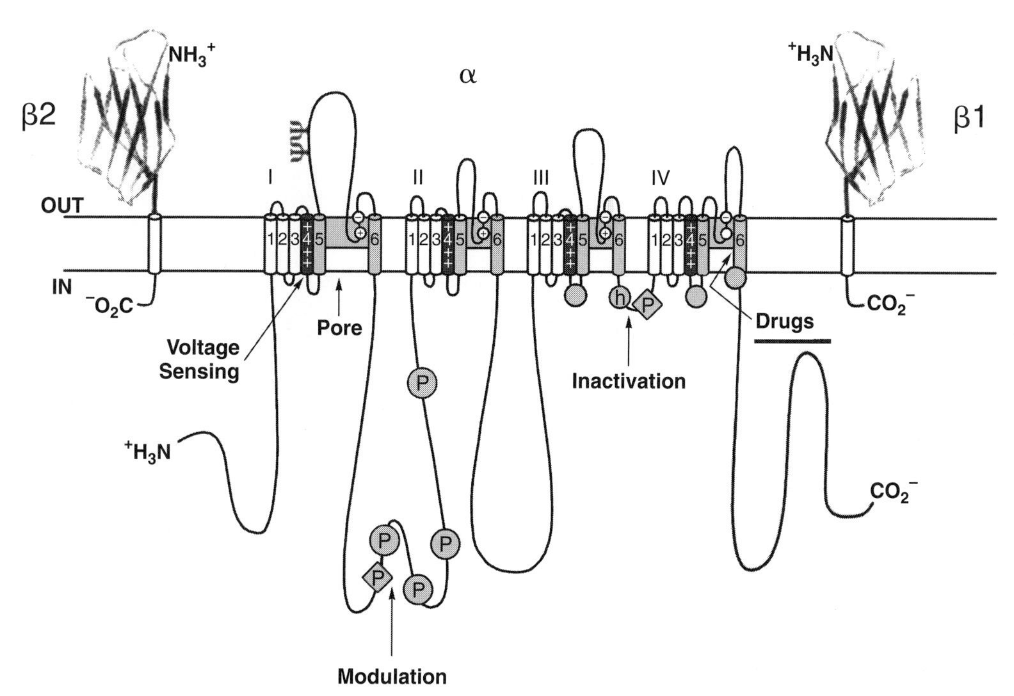

Fig. 16-4 Functional structure of the Na^+ channel (linear representation). The four primary domains of the α subunit are indicated by Roman numerals, with the six helical segments (designated S1 through S6, *left to right*) of each domain shown spanning the membrane. A portion of each of the S5-S6 linkages lines the outer portion of the pore and confers ion selectivity to the channel. The inner portion is lined by the S6 helices. Outward rotation of the positively charged S4 cylinders and coupled movements of the S6 segments open the pore. Concurrently, portions of the S4-S5 linkages of domains III and IV, which help form the inner mouth of the channel, and the S6 segment of domain IV create a receptor *(unlettered circles)* for the intracellular loop between domains III and IV, which constitutes the h gate (ⓗ). Binding of the h gate to its receptor inactivates the channel within about 1 ms. Each *P* indicates a phosphorylation site for protein kinase A *(circles)* and protein kinase C *(diamonds)*. Phosphorylation of the h gate slows inactivation; phosphorylation of other sites reduces channel activation. The Ψ symbols indicate glycosylation sites. The β subunits ($β_1$ and $β_2$) stabilize the α subunit in the nerve membrane. (From Catterall WA: From ionic currents to molecular mechanisms: the structure and function of voltage-gated sodium channels, *Neuron* 26:13-25, 2000.)

tion and to retard movements of the S4 segment of domain IV.[71]

If the active site for local anesthetics resides within the Na^+ channel, access becomes an important issue. In this regard, studies with permanently charged local anesthetics have proved enlightening.[42] Conversion of the amino terminus of certain local anesthetics (e.g., lidocaine) to the quaternary form (e.g., QX-314) yields permanently charged cations largely incapable of crossing the nerve membrane. Although ineffective when applied externally to the axolemma, these experimental compounds demonstrate full blocking activity on internal administration. They gain access to the receptor by traveling up an aqueous route within the Na^+ channel, which must be open or at least partially activated to permit their entry from the cytoplasm. Lipophilic molecules, such as benzocaine or the uncharged form of lidocaine, can reach the channel and receptor site by traversing a hydrophobic route, which may include the membrane lipid as well as hydrophobic portions of the Na^+ channel.

Ragsdale et al[61] reported that specific mutations of the S6 segment of domain IV of the Na^+ channel greatly alter local anesthetic blockade. Replacement of the phenylalanine amino acid midway down the S6 helix with an alanine residue reduced by 99% the apparent binding affinity of the local anesthetic etidocaine to open and inactivated channels. A similar, although smaller, effect occurred when the tyrosine located 11 Å and two turns inward on the same side of the S6 helix was replaced with alanine. Because these aromatic amino acids can interact with local anesthetics through hydrophobic and π electron interactions, and their spatial separation conforms to the length of the typical local anesthetic molecule (10 to 15 Å), they may identify and be part of the local anesthetic receptor site. Subsequent mutation studies have demonstrated specific amino acid residues on the S6 segments of domains I and III that also appear to form part of the receptor site (Figure 16-5).[91]

As previously mentioned, local anesthetics block nerve conduction by preventing the gating mechanism that underlies cycling of the Na^+ channel. Other actions that could contribute to nerve blockade include a physical occlusion of the channel, an allosterically mediated change in channel conformation, or a distortion of the local electrical field. Figure 16-6 depicts possible interactions of local anesthetics with the Na^+ channel as it cycles through its primary configurations in response to a depolarizing stimulus.

Use-Dependent Block

Conventional local anesthetics inhibit high-frequency trains of impulses more readily than they do single action potentials. This phenomenon, variously referred to as *use-* or *frequency-dependent* conduction block, *phasic* or *transitional* block, or *Wedensky inhibition*, was long ignored by neuroscientists, perhaps because it was believed to be a nonspecific response

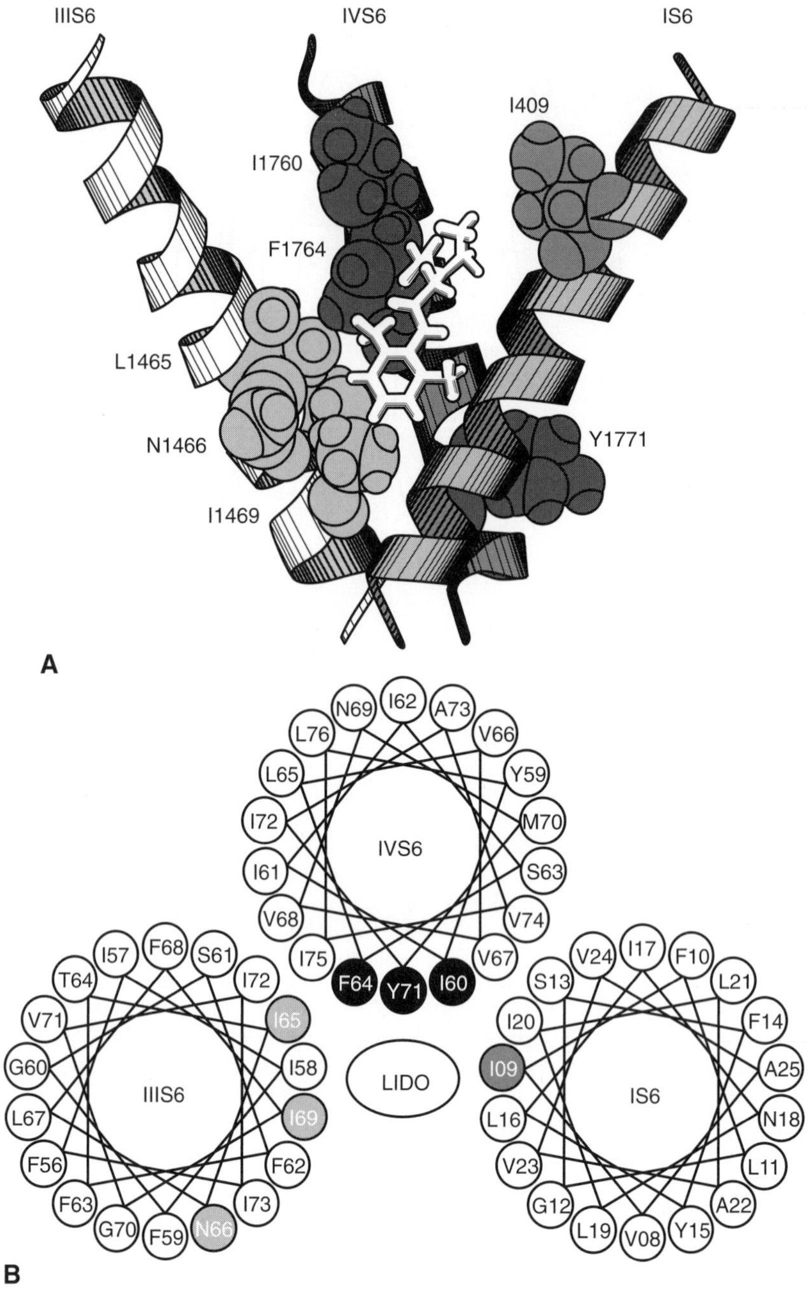

Fig. 16-5 Proposed local anesthetic binding to transmembrane segments *IS6, IIIS6,* and *IVS6.* **A,** Three-dimensional model. The local anesthetic lidocaine is shown in stick representation; amino acid residues important to local anesthetic binding are shown in space-filling representation. For each amino acid illustrated, the letter identifies the amino acid present (*F,* phenylalanine; *I,* isoleucine; *L,* leucine; *N,* asparagine; *Y,* tyrosine), and the number indicates its position on the α subunit polypeptide. One isoleucine *(I1760)* does not bind lidocaine per se but blocks its potential exit through a hydrophilic pathway. **B,** α-Helical representation showing the axial positions of the amino acids *(solid circles)* whose mutation causes reduction in the affinity of lidocaine *(Lido)* for the inactivated Na^+ channel. (Adapted from Yarov-Yarovoy V, McPhee JC, Idsvoog D, et al: Roles of amino acid residues in transmembrane segments IS6 and IIS6 of the Na^+ channel α subunit in voltage-dependent gating and drug block, *J Biol Chem* 277:35393-35401, 2002.)

to overstimulation of the nerve. Since the early 1970s, however, use-dependent block has come to be recognized as an important pharmacologic attribute of local anesthetics and one vital to the elucidation of their interaction with the Na^+ channel.

As previously mentioned, quaternary derivatives of local anesthetics retain nerve-blocking activity when they are injected intraaxonally but are ineffective by external administration. Because these drugs can reach their site of action within the Na^+ channel only when the channel is open to the cytoplasm, repetitive stimulation of the nerve should increase exposure of the receptor site to the anesthetic—and therefore lead to increasing drug action—until a steady state is established between the bound drug within the channel and the free drug in the axoplasm. A similar although less extensive use dependency could be anticipated for lidocaine and related drugs that are partially ionized at physiologic pH.

Numerous studies have proved that high-frequency stimulation increases the magnitude of channel blockade by local anesthetics as well as the rate at which it occurs, and that, within certain limits, the degree of axonal block is strongly and continuously dependent on the stimulus rate irrespective of equilibration time. For example, a concentration of lidocaine that reduces maximally a compound action potential by 40% at a stimulation rate of 1 Hz causes a depression of 80% after 15 seconds at 40 Hz.[12] These results, as embodied in the modulated receptor hypothesis of local anesthesia, suggest that stimulation of the nerve membrane not only exposes the site of action to local anesthetic cations, but it also increases temporarily the affinity of the channel receptor for them.

As originally proposed by Hille,[42] the modulated receptor hypothesis holds that local anesthetics, both the charged and neutral forms, bind preferentially to open and inactivated Na^+ channels. The binding reciprocally tends to stabilize the channels in the inactivated state. If stimulations are sufficiently infrequent, time is available after each depolarization for the slower than normal transition from inactivated to resting channels to take place. This conversion then reduces

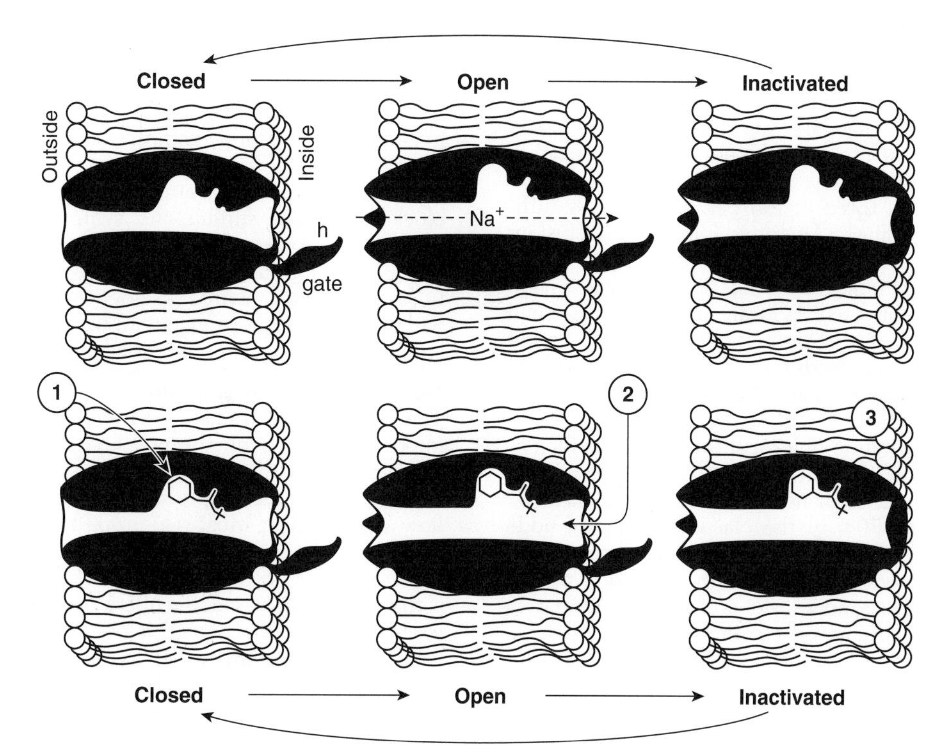

Fig. 16-6 Na^+ channel cycling and local anesthetic blockade. The top row illustrates the major transformations of the Na^+ channel during an action potential; the bottom row depicts the binding of local anesthetics to specific channel receptors. *1,* Uncharged anesthetic molecules can reach the active site within the channel through a hydrophobic route and may therefore bind to channels in any configuration. *2,* Local anesthetic cations are restricted to a hydrophilic pathway and therefore depend on channel activation for exposing the receptor to the drug. *3,* Inactivation traps charged local anesthetics within the channel, and local anesthetic binding stabilizes the inactivated configuration.

local anesthetic binding and permits a net diffusion of neutral anesthetic molecules out of the channels. The remaining anesthetic bound to closed channels provides a basal or tonic block. Repeated stimuli do not allow for full recovery between depolarizations; anesthetic binding remains enhanced, Na^+ channels in the inactive configuration accumulate, and use-dependent block ensues. Subsequent refinements to the modulated receptor hypothesis include discoveries that the increased affinity state of the receptor caused by depolarization of the membrane is not necessarily synonymous with the open or inactivated forms of the channel but may include closed but partially activated channels[76] and that charged anesthetic molecules may gain access to or egress from this receptor without the necessity for complete opening of the channel.[92]

Marked differences in use dependency have been recorded for various local anesthetics. Benzocaine and related nonionized compounds show little phasic block and then only at very high stimulus rates. Conventional local anesthetics exhibit an approximate tenfold range in frequency dependence, with phasic block becoming clinically significant at 2.5 Hz for lidocaine and at 0.5 Hz for bupivacaine.[23] Permanently charged local anesthetic derivatives develop use-dependent blocks with stimulus rates as low as 2.4 per minute (0.04 Hz).[92] Basic knowledge gained by the study of use dependency is increasingly being applied to clinical questions involving local anesthetic efficacy and toxicity and to related classes of drugs, such as various antiarrhythmic and anticonvulsant agents, that also exhibit phasic block. Ultimately, new drugs and modes of therapy will arise from the pharmaceutical exploitation of this phenomenon.

Differential Nerve Block

Clinically, neurons vary according to fiber size and type in their susceptibility to local anesthetics. Autonomic functions subserved by preganglionic B and postganglionic C fibers are readily disrupted by local anesthetics, whereas motor control dependent on larger A fibers is not. Sensory neurons are quite heterogeneous in size and exhibit a wide range of sensitivity. Modalities listed in increasing order of resistance to conduction block include the sensations of pain, cold, warmth, touch, and deep pressure. In general, the more susceptible a fiber is to a local anesthetic agent, the faster it is blocked and the longer it takes to recover.

Critical length

The clinical observations already described (and best seen after spinal or epidural anesthesia) should not be construed as proof that large myelinated axons are inherently more resistant to local anesthetics than are smaller fibers. A careful study of individual axons by Franz and Perry[33] revealed that the minimum blocking concentration of procaine is not directly related to fiber diameter. A differential block, in which small C and A fibers were affected but larger A fibers were not, could be obtained, but only when the length of compound nerve exposed to procaine was restricted in length. On the basis of these findings, the authors concluded that differential sensitivities of fibers of unequal diameter result from variations in the "critical length" that must be exposed to a local anesthetic for conduction to fail. In myelinated nerves, for instance, action potentials are propagated from one node of Ranvier to the next in a saltatory fashion, with a safety factor sufficient to require at least three consecutive nodes to be completely blocked before impulse transmission is interrupted. Because internodal distance tends to be directly related to fiber diameter, small neurons may appear to be more sensitive clinically than large fibers to conduction block. As a local anesthetic diffuses into the nerve trunk, it reaches an effective concentration over a length required to inhibit small axons (i.e., block three nodes) before it spreads sufficiently to block large fibers. Anatomic barriers to diffusion, nonuniform distribution of drug, or the use of a minimal amount of local anesthetic may even preclude some large axons from ever being affected. As local anesthesia fades, small neurons are the last to recover because circumscribed areas of drug concentrations adequate for their inhibition remain along the nerve after the more substantial areas required for large axons have broken up.

When the concentration of local anesthetic is insufficient to block three adjacent nodes completely, anesthesia may still occur if a larger series of nodes is partially blocked.[32,62] As long as more than 70% of the Na^+ channels in a node are inhibited, the resulting action potential at that node is reduced in size. Progressive declines in the action potentials of partially blocked nodes along the axon ultimately result in failure of conduction if a sufficient length of nerve is exposed to the drug. As shown in Figure 16-7, smaller neurons are again more readily blocked because of the shorter length required for exposure of the requisite number of nodes.[62]

The critical length hypothesis may also be applied to unmyelinated axons as a group. Differences in modes of impulse transmission, however, preclude direct comparisons based on fiber size between myelinated and unmyelinated axons. Smaller in diameter, C fibers nevertheless have approximately the same apparent critical length as do small myelinated axons.

Use-dependent block

In addition to anatomic and physiologic variables, the pattern of impulse traffic normally carried in situ by the different nerve fibers may contribute greatly to a differential nerve block.[67] Noxious stimuli and sympathetic nervous system transmissions are encoded in rapid bursts of impulses, whereas motor function usually involves low-frequency discharges. Local anesthetics whose use-dependent characteristics fall within this frequency range tend to block pain sensations and autonomic responses preferentially.

Peripheral nerve organization

The location of various axons within a nerve trunk has an important bearing on the rate and sometimes the depth of local anesthesia. In major nerve blocks, the epineurium (nerve sheath) prevents the spread of anesthetic solution by bulk flow, and the drug must rely on diffusion to reach the axons within the nerve. Diffusion takes considerable time with nerves that are 1 mm in diameter or greater, and the net result is that the outer, or mantle, fibers are blocked well before the inner core fibers have been exposed to an effective concentration of drug. Removal of the agent by the bloodstream, particularly by intraneuronal blood vessels, may prevent anesthesia of core fibers altogether. In general, the more proximal tissues supplied by a nerve are more readily affected by local anesthetics because the axons that serve them are located peripherally. Moreover, the nonuniform distribution of various fiber types within a particular nerve may lead to differential blockade of sensory, motor, and autonomic axons innervating a given structure.

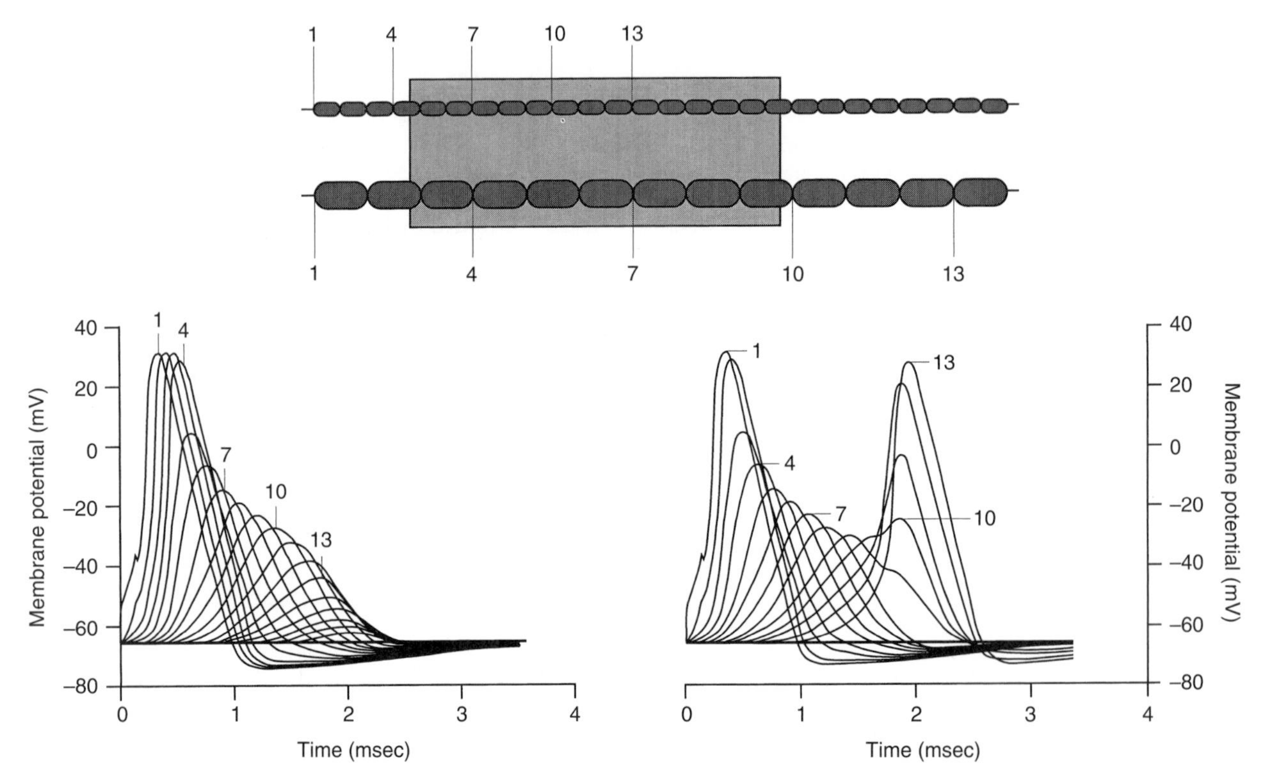

Fig. 16-7 Differential nerve block. Two adjacent myelinated axons, differing in diameter and internodal distance by a factor of two, are exposed to a local anesthetic *(gray zone)*. Impulses arising from successive nodes of the small axon are plotted on the *left*. Exposure of 14 nodes to a specific concentration of local anesthetic causes conduction to fail. Identical exposure of the larger axon *(right)* results in seven nodes being affected, an insufficient number to prevent conduction at this local anesthetic concentration. (Adapted from Raymond SA, Thalhammer JG, Strichartz GR: Axonal excitability: endogenous and exogenous modulation. In Dimitrijevic, Wall PD, Lindblom U, eds: *Altered sensation and pain*, Basel, Switzerland, 1990, Karger.)

Local anesthetic selectivity
Local anesthetics vary somewhat in their relative inherent ability to block sensory versus motor fibers. The best clinical example of this form of differential block involves bupivacaine and etidocaine. Both these drugs are highly lipid-soluble agents capable of producing prolonged nerve blockade. However, bupivacaine can elicit sensory anesthesia at one third the concentration required for motor blockade, whereas etidocaine shows no selectivity of effect whatsoever.[72] Because maintenance of uterine muscle contractility is important in childbirth, bupivacaine is the preferred agent for epidural anesthesia during labor and delivery.

The mechanism behind such differential effects of local anesthetics has not been elucidated. One possibility relates to the drugs' relative tendency to block specific K^+ channels. A local anesthetic (presumably etidocaine) with a strong ability to block voltage-gated K^+ channels important in reversing neuronal depolarization might be expected to work against itself in nonmyelinated axons subserving the perception of pain, where inhibition of K^+ efflux would give Na^+ influx a better chance of reaching threshold and propagating the action potential. On the other hand, a relatively strong bupivacaine blockade of K^+ *influx* through channels that control the resting membrane potential would result in partial membrane depolarization and a potentiation of Na^+ channel inactivation and local anesthetic blockade.[47]

Inflammation
The failure to obtain satisfactory clinical pain relief in inflamed tissues is a well-known, undesirable form of differential nerve block. Clinically, this phenomenon is encountered in the patient with profound local anesthesia except in the specific area requiring treatment. If inflammation lowers the pH at the injection site, then, as described previously, diffusion of the drug into the axolemma would be impaired. There is some evidence, however, that the buffering capacity of inflamed tissues is not always reduced[60] and that other reasons for local anesthetic failure must exist.

Increased blood flow and decreased catecholamine effectiveness in inflamed tissues may speed removal of the local anesthetic from the injection site. Inflammatory exudates may also inhibit local anesthesia directly by enhancing nerve conduction.[16] Alteration of Na^+ channel number or function (through modulation of the α subunit, as indicated in Figure 16-3, or the β subunits, which influence Na^+ channel gating[40]) may account for this effect, as could the release of neuromediators and other substances, such as prostaglandin E_1, kinins, adenine nucleotides, and substance P, which increase the responsiveness of free nerve endings to noxious stimuli.

PHARMACOLOGIC EFFECTS

Although primarily used to depress peripheral nerve conduction, local anesthetics are not selective and may interfere with impulse transmission in any excitable tissue. Most prominent of the systemic effects of local anesthetics are those related to the cardiovascular and central nervous systems, but virtually any organ dependent on nervous or muscular activity may be affected. Local anesthetics may also influence a variety of tissues through actions unrelated to specific disturbances in Na^+ conductance.

Central Nervous System
Local anesthetics readily pass from the peripheral circulation into the brain. Because central nervous system (CNS) neurons are particularly sensitive to local anesthetics, blood concentrations incapable of altering peripheral nervous activity may profoundly influence CNS function.

Sensitive psychomotor tests and subjective reports of mild drowsiness indicate that systemic effects caused by local anesthetics can occur in plasma concentrations that are achieved in dental patients.[5] Analgesic and anticonvulsant effects also occur in subtoxic concentrations.

Initial signs and symptoms of a toxic effect are often excitatory in nature and consist of a feeling of lightheadedness and dizziness, followed by visual and auditory disturbances, apprehension, disorientation, and localized involuntary muscular activity. Depressant responses such as slurred speech, drowsiness, and unconsciousness may also occur and are especially prominent with certain drugs (e.g., lidocaine). As higher blood concentrations of drug are attained, muscular fasciculations and tremors intensify and develop into generalized tonic-clonic convulsions. On termination, seizure activity is often succeeded by a state of CNS depression identical to general anesthesia. With excessively large doses, respiratory impairment becomes manifest; if untreated, death by asphyxiation may ensue.

The CNS excitation sometimes observed after local anesthesia is intriguing because the sole action ascribed to these agents is one of depression. Indeed, studies involving the topical application of local anesthetics to exposed cortical or spinal cord neurons document that the only direct effect of procaine and related drugs is to inhibit electrical activity.[25] The apparent stimulation observed clinically may be explained on the basis that inhibitory cortical neurons or synapses are highly susceptible to transmission block. Initial disruption of these pathways results in a disinhibition of excitatory neurons, manifested clinically as stimulation. Electroencephalographic studies indicate that local anesthetic seizures begin in the amygdala.[35,70] Disinhibition of this part of the limbic system allows high-voltage discharges to occur, which then spread throughout the brain. (Recent findings that local anesthetics can block a family of K^+ channels whose inhibition increases neuronal excitability raises the possibility that CNS stimulation and cardiac arrhythmias may arise in part from direct neuronal excitation.[47])

Cardiovascular System
Local anesthetics can exert a variety of effects on the cardiovascular system. Some influences are beneficial and serve as a basis for the use of selected agents in the treatment of cardiac arrhythmias; others are not and merely serve to accentuate systemic toxicity. In almost all instances, however, the observed effect results from the interplay of direct actions of local anesthetics on the myocardium and peripheral vasculature and CNS actions indirectly mediated through the autonomic nervous system.

Myocardium
At nontoxic concentrations, local anesthetics differ somewhat in their electrophysiologic influences on the heart. Whereas lidocaine shortens the action potential duration and the effective refractory period in Purkinje fibers, procaine acts in the opposite direction. Both drugs, however, increase the effective refractory period relative to the action potential duration and decrease cardiac automaticity, especially in ectopic pacemakers.

Presumably because of their ability to block Ca^{++} channels and evoked Ca^{++} release from the sarcoplasmic reticulum and to reduce myofibrillar responsiveness to available Ca^{++}, local anesthetics depress myocardial contractility in a dose-dependent manner.[52] With conventional doses of lidocaine, this effect is minor, and sympathetic reflexes and direct vascular effects produce a compensatory increase in peripheral resistance, which prevents a fall in blood pressure. Through a centrally mediated disinhibition of sympathetic nervous activity, heart rate and arterial blood pressure may actually become elevated coincident with CNS excitation. Conversely, mepivacaine has been reported in moderate doses to decrease peripheral vascular resistance and increase cardiac output,[46] which suggests that local anesthetics may exert dissimilar patterns of direct and indirect effects on the heart at subtoxic blood concentrations.

Local anesthetics in doses toxic to the heart are qualitatively similar in action. Membrane excitability and conduction velocity are depressed throughout the heart. Sinus bradycardia and impairment of myocardial contractility contribute to a reduction in cardiac output. These effects are magnified by hypoxia, but, even if respiration is supported artificially, circulatory collapse will occur after excessively large doses.

Reports in human beings suggest, and experiments in several species confirm, that bupivacaine and certain other highly lipophilic local anesthetics are relatively cardiotoxic compared with less lipophilic congeners. In particular, serious ventricular arrhythmias and cardiovascular collapse are more likely to occur, and resuscitation is more problematic. One explanation for these observations involves use-dependent blockade.[23] As indicated in Table 16-2, bupivacaine has a high molecular weight for a local anesthetic; that, coupled with its lipophilic tendency and perhaps its high pK_a, enables the drug to exert a strong phasic block at normal heart rates. Inhibition of K^+ and Ca^{++} channels may also contribute to the arrhythmogenic potential of bupivacaine in toxic concentrations.

Peripheral vasculature

The effects of local anesthetics on blood vessels are complex and dose dependent.[4,10] Dilute solutions enhance spontaneous myogenic contractions and peripheral resistance in certain vascular beds, presumably by increasing the cytoplasmic concentration of Ca^{++} within smooth muscle fibers. Coincidentally, local anesthetics reduce vascular tone related to autonomic function by diminishing neurotransmitter release and smooth muscle responsiveness. Subconvulsive doses of local anesthetics exert minor influences on the peripheral vasculature as a whole. Toxic blood concentrations may cause arteriolar dilation and profound hypotension.

The net effect on any vasculature bed depends on the local anesthetic, its concentration, and the existing sympathetic tone in the tissue. Local anesthetics listed in decreasing potential for causing vasodilation include bupivacaine, procaine, lidocaine, prilocaine, mepivacaine, and cocaine. With the possible exception of cocaine, local anesthetics used clinically inhibit both myogenic activity and autonomic tone and cause vasodilation in the area of injection.

Miscellaneous Effects

Aside from their influences on cardiovascular and CNS function, local anesthetics in concentrations compatible with life exert few systemic effects. Transmission at the neuromuscular junction and at autonomic ganglia may be affected, but intraarterial administration is usually required for these effects to be observed in vivo. A variety of smooth muscle actions and antibacterial, antihistaminic, and antimuscarinic effects have also been reported,[26] and local anesthetics have been shown to influence the metabolism of arachidonic acid and to inhibit platelet aggregation.[14]

In tissue culture, local anesthetics can disrupt numerous cellular functions: locomotion, endocytosis, exocytosis, axonal transport, cell fusion, and maintenance of normal morphology. These effects have been ascribed to disturbances of the cytoskeleton (microtubules and microfilaments). Various Ca^{++}- and calmodulin-dependent enzymatic activities and membrane transport systems are also susceptible to local anesthetic influences.[82] The toxicologic and therapeutic implications of these actions remain to be determined.

Vasoconstrictor Effects

Vasoconstrictors are often added to local anesthetic solutions to impede systemic absorption of the anesthetic agent (see Chapter 6). Epinephrine in concentrations of 4 to 20 μg/ml (1 : 250,000 to 1 : 50,000) is most commonly used for this purpose, but other sympathomimetic amines, including levonordefrin, norepinephrine, and phenylephrine, are or have been used. Localization of the anesthetic solution in the area of injection by epinephrine is often highly beneficial. The duration of local anesthesia may be prolonged several times, and even the success rate and intensity of nerve block may be improved. Systemic toxicity may be reduced because less anesthetic may be needed, and drug metabolism is more likely to keep pace with drug absorption. During surgery, hemostasis afforded by the infiltration of a local anesthetic solution containing epinephrine may also be advantageous.

Normally, sympathomimetic drugs included in anesthetic formulations produce no pharmacologic effects of clinical consequence other than localized arteriolar constriction. Low doses of epinephrine, such as those contained in one or two dental cartridges of lidocaine with 1 : 100,000 epinephrine (18 to 36 μg), decrease total peripheral resistance by 20% to 30%, but a commensurate rise in cardiac output supported by increases in stroke volume and/or heart rate leaves the mean blood pressure unchanged. Injudicious dosage, accidental intravascular injection, or adverse drug interactions, however, may promote clinically noticeable effects on the CNS and sympathetic nervous system. Heart rate and systolic blood pressure may be elevated by epinephrine, causing uncomfortable palpitation and pain in the chest. Restlessness and apprehension similar to the effects produced by local anesthetics may also occur. Phenylephrine, a relatively pure α-adrenergic agonist, avoids most of the direct cardiac stimulation associated with epinephrine, but it may significantly elevate systolic and diastolic pressures and reflexively slow the heart for an extended period. Other sympathomimetics, such as norepinephrine and levonordefrin, are somewhat intermediate in their systemic effects.

As a guideline for cardiac patients, the New York Heart Association recommended in 1955 that the amount of epinephrine administered during any one session not exceed 200 μg (equivalent to 20 ml of a 1 : 100,000 epinephrine solution).[74] Current evidence indicates that this amount is excessive for patients with compromised cardiovascular systems and that more restrictive guidelines are indicated (see Chapter 6). Several studies have shown that the intraoral injection of 20 μg of epinephrine effectively doubles the preoperative plasma concentration and that higher doses produce proportionately greater elevations.[80] At doses approaching 200 μg, the resulting epinephrine titers can surpass those associated with heavy exercise, surgery, and pheochromocytoma.[24,27] Increases in cardiac work become significant, and myocardial ischemia and cardiac arrhythmias are more likely to occur.

ABSORPTION, FATE, AND EXCRETION

Pharmacokinetic considerations regarding local anesthetics are vital because the balance between a local anesthetic's uptake into the systemic circulation and its removal through redistribution, metabolism, and excretion determines in large measure the drug's toxic potential.

Absorption

The rate of absorption depends on several factors, including the dosage and pharmacologic profile of the drug used, the presence of a vasoconstrictor agent, and the nature of the administration site. Obviously, the more drug that is injected the higher its resultant blood concentration will be. Less obvious are the qualitative influences of the anesthetic solution and how these interact with the site of administration. Drugs with potent vasodilating properties, such as procaine and lidocaine, may significantly enhance their own uptake, particularly when injected into a highly vascular space. Inclusion of epinephrine or another vasoconstrictor is especially important in these instances. Drugs that are not strong vasodilators, such as mepivacaine and prilocaine, do not markedly accentuate their own absorption and do not require as much vasoconstrictor to limit uptake.

Absorption after topical application varies widely. Although intact skin and keratinized mucosa are relatively impermeable, local anesthetics are readily absorbed from most mucosal surfaces. Instillation of tetracaine into the pyriform fossa, for instance, results in a peak plasma concentration one third to one half that obtained after rapid intravenous infusion. By comparison, absorption of lidocaine from the tracheobronchial tree is much slower. Regardless of the site of application, sympathomimetic agents are ineffective topically in delaying absorption. Uptake may be minimized, however, by using local anesthetics prepared in the form of an ointment or gel instead of an aqueous spray.

Distribution

On entering the circulation, a local anesthetic is partially (5% to 95%) bound by plasma proteins, α_1-acid glycoprotein in particular (and albumin to a much lesser extent), and red blood cells. Plasma protein binding is directly correlated with the hydrophobicity of the local anesthetic.[79] Because the concentration of α_1-acid glycoprotein is influenced by many factors (see Chapter 2), the fractional binding of local anesthetics differs among individuals and within the same individual at different times. Factors that depress binding acutely include respiratory acidosis and possibly the coadministration of other basic drugs.

After distribution throughout the intravascular space, the unbound drug is free to diffuse into the various tissues of the body. So-called barriers to diffusion are relatively ineffective against local anesthetics. In addition to entering the CNS, these drugs readily cross the placenta and occasionally may induce severe cardiac depression in the fetus.

Distribution to peripheral tissues is a major means for the removal of amide and slowly metabolized ester local anesthetics from the bloodstream and for keeping their plasma concentrations below the toxic range. By virtue of the pulmonary circulation, the lung plays a unique role in this process when a local anesthetic is injected intravascularly.[45] Initially, up to 90% of the drug may be taken up by the lung. Although most of the agent back-diffuses into the bloodstream within the first minute after injection, the evanescent buffering action of the lung can nevertheless reduce the peak arterial blood concentration by a factor of three.

Metabolism and Excretion

The metabolic fate of a particular agent largely depends on the chemical linkage between the aromatic residue and the rest of the molecule. Ester drugs are inactivated by hydrolysis. Derivatives of *p*-aminobenzoic acid (e.g., procaine and tetracaine) are preferentially metabolized in the plasma by pseudocholinesterase; the ratio between plasma and liver hydrolysis with other esters is somewhat variable. Products of hydrolytic cleavage may undergo further biotransformation in the liver before being eliminated in the urine. The half-life for the hydrolysis of procaine is normally less than 1 minute, and less than 2% of the drug is excreted unchanged by the kidneys.

Metabolism of amide drugs primarily occurs in the liver. The initial reaction is usually N-dealkylation of the tertiary amino terminus, principally by CYP3A4 and CYP1A2.[56,84] The resultant secondary amine of most amides is susceptible to hydrolysis by hepatic amidase activity, but conjugation, hydroxylation, and/or further dealkylation may also occur. Hepatic blood flow appears to be the rate-limiting factor governing metabolism of lidocaine and some other amides; elimination half-lives range from 1.5 to 3.5 hours. Inactivation of prilocaine, a secondary amine, is unusual because dealkylation is not required before hydrolysis can take place, which may explain why almost half of its metabolism is extrahepatic. Articaine is also atypical in that it is inactivated in the plasma (90%) and liver (10%) by hydrolysis of an ester side chain required for local anesthetic activity. With a metabolic half-life of approximately 25 minutes, articaine is removed from the circulation faster than are other injected amides.

Some local anesthetic metabolites retain significant pharmacologic activity and may contribute to drug toxicity. Much of the sedative effect of lidocaine, for example, has been attributed to its de-ethylated metabolites monoethylglycinexylidide and glycinexylidide.[77] As with ester compounds, minimal amounts (1% to 20%) of administered amides appear in the urine as unmetabolized compounds.

Differences in biotransformation of the various local anesthetics are at times clinically relevant. Individuals with certain genetically based defects in pseudocholinesterase activity are unusually sensitive to procaine and other esters (but not articaine); conventional doses of these drugs may occasionally lead to toxic reactions. Alternatively, severe hepatic disease or reduced hepatic blood flow may produce systemic intolerance to lidocaine and presumably other local anesthetics dependent on adequate liver function for their metabolism.

ADVERSE EFFECTS

Modern local anesthetic solutions are quite safe when used by competent personnel. Nevertheless, a substantial amount of literature describing various adverse reactions attests to the potential toxicity of these agents, particularly when they are used in a cavalier manner.

Systemic Toxicity

Most toxic effects of a serious nature are related to excessive blood concentrations caused by inadvertent intravascular injection or the administration of large quantities of drug. Convulsions, respiratory arrest, and cardiovascular collapse represent the greatest hazards to health. Such reactions can usually be prevented by observing three precautions: (1) administer the smallest dose that will provide effective anesthesia; (2) use proper injection techniques, including aspiration; and (3) use a vasoconstrictor-containing solution when not contraindicated by patient history or operative need. If an adverse response occurs despite these procedures, immediate therapy must be administered. The patient should be placed in the supine position, and oxygen should be given. This procedure is often all that is needed for mild toxic reactions, epinephrine responses, or syncopal attacks.

Convulsions are usually self-limiting and require no treatment other than supporting ventilation and protecting the patient from bodily harm. Pharmacologic intervention is necessary, however, when seizures are so intense or prolonged that hypoxia threatens to ensue. The most satisfactory method of seizure control for the dentist is the intravenous administration of a rapidly acting benzodiazepine.[53] Experimental evidence and clinical experience indicate that intravenous diazepam (0.1 to 0.3 mg/kg) or midazolam (0.03 to

0.1 mg/kg) can eliminate local anesthetic convulsions without producing significant effects on ventilation or circulation. Small intravenous doses of a rapidly acting barbiturate (e.g., thiopental) may also terminate local anesthetic seizures, but they tend to potentiate the postconvulsive depressant phase of local anesthetic toxicity. Succinylcholine, a neuromuscular blocker without CNS depressant action, is sometimes used in refractory cases. However, neuromuscular blockade treats only the outward manifestations of a convulsion; electrical disturbances within the CNS progress unimpeded. An immediate ability to institute artificial ventilation is a mandatory prerequisite for its use because the drug paralyzes the muscles of respiration.

Various agents have been used in attempts to prevent seizures. Most anticonvulsants examined have been disappointing in this regard, but diazepam has been shown in cats to double the median convulsant dose of lidocaine without causing undesirable CNS disturbances.[28] Midazolam appears to provide a similar benefit, and consequently either drug is a premedication of choice when the administration of a large quantity of local anesthetic is anticipated. Some drugs once commonly used for preoperative sedation, including meperidine and promethazine, may actually increase the likelihood of local anesthetic convulsions.

Treatment of most severe toxic reactions is symptomatic and consists of reversing respiratory and circulatory disruptions as they occur. Because most deaths attributed to local anesthetics are related to tissue anoxia, support of ventilation is of paramount importance. Arterial hypotension is controlled by the coadministration of intravenous fluids and sympathomimetic agents. Cardiopulmonary resuscitative techniques are necessary when cardiac function is disrupted.

Local Tissue Responses

Commercially available local anesthetics are relatively nonirritating to tissues. Many reactions described in the past were caused not by local anesthetics but by metallic or alcoholic contaminants that gained access to the solutions during or after manufacture. Local anesthetic concentrations able to damage peripheral nerves usually far exceed those required for transmission blockade. Accidental intraneural injection, however, may lead to nerve damage from the combination of undiluted local anesthetic, strong hydrostatic pressure, and direct physical injury. High-concentration agents, namely 4% solutions of prilocaine or articaine, are significantly more likely to cause long-lasting or permanent nerve injury when administered for inferior alveolar nerve block.[39] Exposure of unsheathed neurons to these concentrations results in an irreversible increase in intracellular Ca^{++} and necrotic cell death.[44]

Conventional anesthetic preparations may induce focal necrosis in skeletal muscle tissue approximating the injection site.[90] The damage occurs rapidly after a single administration and is completely reversed in a matter of several weeks. Local anesthetics may also impede cell motility, depress collagen synthesis, and delay wound healing in certain circumstances.

Tissue responses to injected local anesthetic preparations are usually caused or augmented by vasoconstrictor additives. Epinephrine creates tissue hypoxia by reducing local blood flow while simultaneously increasing oxygen consumption. Although tissue injury may be induced by any of the sympathomimetics currently used, norepinephrine is particularly apt to cause ischemic necrosis. The injection of local anesthetic with a vasoconstrictor has been described as especially hazardous in areas supplied by terminal arteries (e.g., nose, digits, and penis). However, one recent study found no tissue injury after digital block by lidocaine with epinephrine.[85] In dentistry, tissue irritation may result in an increased incidence of postanesthetic pain at the injection site in patients receiving local anesthetic formulations containing vasoconstrictors.

Idiosyncratic Reactions

In rare instances, patients have had toxic reactions to small amounts of local anesthetic. Some of these reactions may represent an abnormal susceptibility to the local anesthetic.[37] Most often, however, these responses are anxiety related, associated with the vasoconstrictor, or the result of inadvertent intravascular injection. Regarding the latter possibility, it has been accidentally determined that the convulsant dose of lidocaine in human beings is only 10 mg when the drug is injected into the vertebral artery.[48]

Amide local anesthetics were once thought by some authorities to be causative agents for malignant hyperthermia (MH). This conclusion was based on a few anecdotal cases of supposed MH and on the ability of lidocainelike drugs to potentiate contracture of skeletal muscle in various experimental situations. Direct evidence indicates, however, that no injectable local anesthetic is a triggering agent. For example, lidocaine has no effect on porcine MH, and it has not caused problems when used for local anesthesia in patients with a history of MH.[86] Amide local anesthetics are safe for routine dental use in MH-susceptible patients, and lidocaine may be used for the treatment of ventricular arrhythmias during an acute episode of MH.

Allergic Phenomena

Local anesthetics rarely cause allergic reactions; however, when one does occur, an ester derivative of *p*-aminobenzoic acid is usually involved. Methylparaben, a preservative used in certain local anesthetic preparations (but not in dental cartridges), may also serve on occasion as an antigenic stimulant. Historically, most documented cases of allergy—in the form of contact dermatitis—occurred in dentists and other health professionals exposed to ester agents on a regular basis. Urticarial eruptions, erythematous rashes, and other dermatologic responses represent typical manifestations of local anesthetic allergy in patients and are regularly treated with antihistamines. Anaphylactic responses of a serious nature require epinephrine.

Since 1976, evidence has accumulated that certain persons, mostly asthmatic patients, are intolerant of sulfites, including the bisulfite and metabisulfite preservatives used in local anesthetic solutions with vasoconstrictors. Although the original case report[58] appears to have had an immunologic basis, subsequent findings suggest that most affected persons are hyperreactive to sulfites that are inhaled or ingested but not injected. These reactions are more properly classified as idiosyncratic and do not contraindicate the use of sulfite-containing local anesthetics, except perhaps in some patients with steroid-dependent asthma. Isolated case reports of bisulfite allergy occurring after the intraoral administration of local anesthesia constitute the rare absolute contraindication.[66]

Despite the low incidence of verifiable allergy to local anesthetic solutions in patients, a relatively high percentage of persons have medical histories of presumptive local anesthetic hypersensitivity. Many of these cases undoubtedly represent anxiety or toxic reactions misdiagnosed as immunologic in origin. Such mistakes are particularly apparent when amides are concerned because most investigations have shown these compounds to be virtually nonallergenic.[6] When a single agent is involved, substitution with another local anesthetic is the simplest method of resolving the problem if consideration is given to the fact that esters may exhibit cross-allergenicity with each other and with methylparaben. Drug selection becomes more difficult when a patient has an allergy to all conventional agents. Diphenhydramine (1% with 1 : 100,000 epinephrine) and other antihistamines have been used with some success in such instances, but their overall suitability as local anesthetics is limited. An alternative approach is to screen for drug allergy. Although sensitivity testing methods are generally somewhat unreliable and may be potentially dangerous, a regimen of intracutaneous injections graduating to full challenge tests in a supervised medical setting has proved useful in identifying local anesthetic formulations that can be used safely.[29]

Use During Pregnancy

Local anesthetics are generally regarded as safe for use throughout pregnancy, and retrospective studies of women receiving local anesthesia for emergency procedures in the first trimester have supported this view. Animal studies are also largely negative, although bupivacaine has been shown to cause fetal death at five times the maximum recommended human dose. The Food and Drug Administration has classified lidocaine and prilocaine in pregnancy risk category B and articaine, mepivacaine, and bupivacaine in category C (see Chapter 3).

The possibility has been raised that local anesthetics may affect behavioral development in offspring. Injection at midgestation of a single intramuscular dose of local anesthetic equivalent to the maximum recommended human dose was found to produce developmental delays and behavioral deficits in rats.[73] These results have not been verified in primates but remain sobering in the face of an estimate that 23% of all children are exposed to local anesthetics sometime in utero.

DRUG INTERACTIONS

Because of their influences on excitable membranes, local anesthetics are potentially capable of interacting with a wide spectrum of therapeutic agents. For example, the CNS-depressant effects of local anesthetics summate with those of the general anesthetics, barbiturates, and opioid analgesics, yielding interactions with both therapeutic and toxicologic significance. Lidocaine combined with another antiarrhythmic drug may generate profound disturbances in cardiac automaticity and conduction, far in excess of what either compound would have caused if given alone. Although feeble by itself, the neuromuscular blocking activity of local anesthetics has been used to advantage in preventing succinylcholine-induced fasciculations and in reducing the dose of succinylcholine required during surgery for adequate muscle relaxation. Elucidation of the role of CYP3A4 and CYP1A2 enzymes in the metabolism of amide local anesthetics has led to the discovery that inhibitors of these enzymes, such as erythromycin and fluvoxamine, respectively, can modestly increase plasma concentrations of lidocaine and related agents.[56]

In coronary care units, where large doses of lidocaine may be infused intravenously to treat ventricular arrhythmias, the coadministration of cimetidine,[43,64] a histamine H_2-receptor blocker, or propranolol,[8] a β-adrenoceptor antagonist, has led to lidocaine toxicity. Both agents appear to inhibit the oxidation of lidocaine directly; propranolol also reduces hepatic blood flow and thus delivery of the local anesthetic to the liver.

A unique interaction may occur between certain esters and the sulfonamides. Procaine and several other local anesthetics (benzocaine, tetracaine) are metabolized to yield *p*-aminobenzoic acid. The antibacterial action of sulfonamides is competitively antagonized by this metabolite.

Although the potential for interactions involving local anesthetics is great, clinical manifestations appear infrequently outside the hospital and then only when very large doses are used or when unusual patient factors are present. Much more likely to occur are interactions between various drugs and the vasoconstrictors used during local anesthesia. Epinephrine, for example, may generate ventricular arrhythmias during halothane anesthesia. Similarly, catecholamines can induce undesirable changes in cardiac action and blood pressure in patients taking tricyclic antidepressants, cocaine, nonselective β-adrenergic blockers, digoxin, inhibitors of catechol-O-methyltransferase, or adrenergic neuron–blocking drugs (e.g., guanethidine). Compounds with prominent α-adrenoceptor–blocking activity, such as the phenothiazine and butyrophenone antipsychotics, may lead to hypotension if coadministered in large doses with epinephrine.

Despite statements to the contrary in local anesthetic product information approved by the Food and Drug Administration, local anesthetics containing epinephrine may be used without special reservation in patients taking monoamine oxidase (MAO) inhibitors.[55] Exogenous catecholamines are mostly degraded by the enzyme catechol-O-methyltransferase; inhibition of MAO has little impact on their respective metabolic fates[7] or cardiovascular actions.[11] Of the vasoconstrictors used with local anesthetics, only phenylephrine is contraindicated with concomitant MAO therapy.

Certainly the most important interaction featuring vasoconstrictors is the intended one—inhibition of local anesthetic uptake from the injection site. Animal data suggest, however, that this is not the only interaction that can occur involving the anesthetic agent and its vasoconstrictor partner. Acute lethality studies document that epinephrine potentiates the toxicity of several local anesthetics administered intravenously.[2,88] By protecting against local anesthetic depression of blood pressure, the vasoconstrictor allows a greater than normal fraction of anesthetic to reach the brain and spinal cord.[89] It is not known if this interaction occurs in human beings.

Largely because of the cardiovascular stimulation associated with the sympathomimetic amines, attention has been focused on noncatecholamine alternatives for vasoconstriction. Of these, several analogues of the antidiuretic hormone vasopressin have proved suitable, and one, felypressin (2-phenylalanine-8-lysine vasopressin), is in widespread use in Europe and elsewhere as a vasoconstrictor for local anesthesia. Although felypressin is not quite as effective as epinephrine and cannot be relied on for surgical hemostasis, it avoids the drug interaction problems of the catecholamines. Local toxicity is also reduced because felypressin does not stimulate tissue oxygen consumption. Local anesthetics with felypressin are not available in the United States.

GENERAL THERAPEUTIC USES

Local anesthetics are widely used for the relief of pain. By obviating the necessity of general anesthesia, these drugs have been instrumental in reducing the mortality and morbidity rates associated with a variety of operative procedures. They also render valuable, although less conspicuous, service by obtunding the pain of sunburn, toothache, and other mundane afflictions. In addition, local anesthetics are increasingly being used for purposes unrelated to pain control.

Techniques of Anesthesia

The onset, quality, extent, and duration of local anesthesia vary markedly with the technique of administration used. As might be expected, no single agent is capable of performing all the clinical duties local anesthetics are expected to fulfill.

Surface application

Local anesthetics are prepared for topical use in several different forms. Aqueous solutions and sprays are especially suited for coverage of large surfaces; anesthesia of small areas is often best accomplished with an ointment or viscous gel. Although penetration of the intact epidermis is insignificant, uptake by injured skin or by mucous membranes can be rapid. Topical activities are often not related to efficacies determined for other administration sites; tetracaine and lidocaine are useful topical agents as single agents, whereas mepivacaine, prilocaine, and procaine are not. Benzocaine, ineffective parenterally, is well adapted for surface anesthesia because of its slow systemic absorption and relative safety.

Infiltration and nerve block

Inhibition of transmission in circumscribed portions of the peripheral nervous system is accomplished by the techniques of infiltration and nerve block. Infiltration anesthesia is performed by injecting a local anesthetic into the area to be anesthetized. In this manner, the nerve endings exposed to the anesthetic solution are quickly rendered unresponsive. Nerve block is produced by depositing a local anesthetic solution close to the appropriate nerve trunk but proximal to the intended area of anesthesia. After a certain latency period required for penetration of the local anesthetic into the nerve interior, sensations will be lost in all tissues innervated by the distal portion of the affected nerve. Although infiltrations and single nerve blocks usually anesthetize discrete areas, compound injections (e.g., brachial plexus or sciatic-femoral blocks) may affect large segments of the body, including whole limbs. All the many local anesthetics suitable for infiltration are also useful for nerve blockade.

Spinal anesthesia

Deposition of a local anesthetic solution in the subarachnoid space can be used to produce surgical anesthesia in all structures of the body below the diaphragm. Injection is ordinarily made inferior to the first lumbar vertebra to avoid possible injury to the spinal cord. Once introduced, the drug mixes with the cerebrospinal fluid and begins to spread throughout the subarachnoid space. The extent of cephalad diffusion of the local anesthetic, and therefore the level of anesthesia obtained, is governed by several factors: the dose, specific gravity, and volume of local anesthetic solution administered; the size and position of the spinal canal; and the degree of cerebrospinal fluid mixing imposed by the rate of injection and by movements of the patient. Tetracaine, lidocaine, and bupivacaine are most commonly used for spinal anesthesia in the United States, but numerous other agents are also used.

Epidural block

Local anesthetic infusion into the potential space between the dura mater and the connective tissue lining of the vertebral canal provides an effective alternative to subarachnoid anesthesia. Patient resistance to epidural injection is less of a problem, and the neurologic difficulties sometimes encountered after spinal block are avoided. Epidural anesthesia is comparatively slow in onset, however, and requires considerably more total drug than does its subarachnoid counterpart. The level of anesthesia is also less predictable and more difficult to control. Bupivacaine, ropivacaine, and lidocaine are especially popular for epidural anesthesia, but virtually any local anesthetic available for nerve blockade may be used.

Intravascular injection

Local anesthetics are sometimes introduced directly into a blood vessel to effect short-term regional analgesia. One popular technique consists of injecting an anesthetic solution (e.g., 0.5% lidocaine) intravenously into a limb previously exsanguinated by elevation or with an Esmarch bandage. Isolation of the local anesthetic solution from the systemic circulation is accomplished by placing a pneumatic tourniquet proximal to the injection site. Egress of the local anesthetic from the vascular compartment to peripheral tissues is so rapid that releasing the tourniquet as soon as 5 minutes after injection does not result in toxic blood concentrations. Other techniques that use intravascular local anesthetics have also been practiced on occasion. For example, lidocaine may be mixed with irritating drugs in an attempt to alleviate the pain associated with their intravascular injection.

Treatment of Cardiac Arrhythmias

Lidocaine, procainamide (the amide congener of procaine), and several local anesthetic–like drugs (e.g., tocainide and mexiletine) have established roles in the therapeutic management of cardiac arrhythmias, especially of ventricular origin. The antiarrhythmic properties of these agents are discussed in Chapter 24.

Other Uses

Local anesthetics are sometimes administered intravenously to produce or to supplement general anesthesia. As an adjunctive agent, lidocaine has been used to prevent postoperative muscle pain caused by succinylcholine and to depress airway reflexes and sympathetic nervous system responses during endotracheal intubation and extubation and other procedures affecting the bronchial tree. Local anesthetics have also been used, with mixed success, to treat protracted cough and laryngospasm and as intravenous analgesic and anticonvulsant medications. An adhesive patch containing 5% lidocaine is now approved for relief of postherpetic neuralgia.[65] Finally, the antiinflammatory effect of lidocaine has been used to manage postoperative paralytic ileus.[63]

USES IN DENTISTRY

It would be difficult to overstate the profound influence of local anesthesia on the practice of dentistry. Many of the complex restorative procedures routinely performed on conscious patients would be inconceivable without effective pain control. By eliminating most nociceptive sensations associated with dental care, local anesthetics improve patient acceptance of dental treatment and, as a result, contribute significantly to oral health. Because local anesthetics are so frequently used and, for many practitioners, represent the only drugs administered parenterally, the toxicity as well as efficacy of these agents is of particular interest and concern.

Safety in Dentistry

Without question, local anesthesia is often considerably safer in dentistry than in medicine. Dosages used for infiltration and nerve block in the oral cavity are often less than one tenth those used for compound nerve block or for epidural injection. Recipients of dental anesthesia are usually in better systemic health than some medical patients requiring surgery and usually undergo only minor operative stress. Reports, nevertheless, occasionally appear describing instances of death from local anesthesia in dental practice.

Statistics related to local anesthetic toxicity in dentistry are meager and subject to error. Mortality figures range from 1 death in 1.4 million local anesthetic administrations[68] to 1 in 45 million.[69] These values are open to question. It is possible that some deaths from local anesthetics go unreported and that others are mistakenly identified as myocardial infarctions, cerebrovascular accidents, or the like. It is also quite likely that some deaths imputed to local anesthetics are caused by procedural stress or are merely accidents of time and place and are not causally related to drug administration at all. Tabulations of nonfatal adverse reactions directly attributable to local anesthetics are limited, but in one of the largest and best controlled investigations, Persson[57] recorded adverse effects in 2.5% of 2960 patients given one to two cartridges of various anesthetic agents. Because most of the complications observed—pallor, unrest, sweating, fatigue, palpitation, nausea, and fainting—are common manifestations of acute anxiety, it is evident that many adverse effects ascribed to local anesthesia are actually generated by the process of injection and not by the drugs themselves.

Most nonpsychogenic systemic reactions in adult patients probably arise from accidental intravascular injections. In view of the small amount of drug (e.g., less than 100 mg of lidocaine) routinely administered for most procedures, toxic overdosage seems unlikely; allergic responses are also considered rare, particularly with the amide drugs in current use. Aspiration tests indicate that the needle is placed inside a blood vessel in approximately 3% of all injections and much more frequently during blockade of the inferior alveolar and posterior superior alveolar nerves. Negative aspiration, unfortunately, does not guarantee that the needle lumen is outside the vessel; using improper aspiration force or placing the lumen against a vessel's intimal lining can prevent blood from entering the anesthetic cartridge.

In view of the fact that lidocaine is routinely given intravenously in quantities that exceed the amount in a dental cartridge without producing toxic manifestations in cardiac patients, it has been proposed that local anesthetics injected intraarterially within the oral cavity may gain direct access to the CNS by passing regressively down the branches and trunk of the external carotid artery and into the internal carotid artery.[3] This hypothesis would seemingly account for adverse reactions associated with relatively small amounts of drug; however, studies in rats have shown that internal carotid injections are actually less toxic than intravenous administrations.[88] The explanation for this finding is that the circle of Willis is not patent physiologically in the normal brain, thus precluding drug entry into the medulla where it can depress respiration. It is possible that toxic reactions in dentistry might only occur in patients with an abnormal cerebral circulation, but a more plausible explanation is that intravenous injection of even the small amounts of drug in a single dental cartridge can cause adverse responses in sensitive persons, particularly if the drug is given rapidly and a vasoconstrictor is present in the solution.

Notwithstanding the previous discussion, there are two situations in which the chances for toxic overdose assume real proportions: local anesthesia in small children, and administration of large doses during deep sedation or light general anesthesia. Maximum dosage limits are quickly reached in young patients. For instance, the use of two cartridges of 3% mepivacaine exceeds the maximum recommended dose for a 15-kg child, and inattention to such limits has needlessly resulted in fatalities.[9,41] The combination of CNS depression, possible respiratory acidosis, and a tendency to perform dental procedures in multiple quadrants increases the risk of systemic toxicity in both adults and children receiving sedation or anesthesia. When overdoses of sedative, analgesic, and local anesthetic agents are given together, fatal outcomes are to be expected.[36]

Drug Selection

Selection of a local anesthetic for dental application must include considerations of efficiency, safety, and individual patient and operative needs. That such factors are difficult to evaluate is illustrated by the diversity of results obtained in various clinical trials. One of the few areas of agreement is that the introduction of the amide lidocaine in 1948 marked a significant advance over the ester preparations then available. Indeed, 2% lidocaine hydrochloride with 1 : 100,000 epinephrine remains a standard dental anesthetic for routine use.

Besides lidocaine, four additional amides are available in dental cartridges that possess similar advantages in stability, nonallergenicity, and efficacy over the ester agents (Table 16-2). Mepivacaine, introduced in 1957, is generally equivalent to lidocaine in its pharmacologic profile. Two distinctive features of mepivacaine are its topical ineffectiveness and its use as a 3% solution without a vasoconstrictor. Prilocaine,

Table • 16-2

Comparison of Local Anesthetics Used in Dentistry

PREPARATION CONTENTS	PROPRIETARY (TRADE) NAME	MAXIMUM DOSE*		DURATION OF ANESTHESIA (SOFT TISSUE)	
		(mg/kg)	(mg)	MAXILLARY INFILTRATION (min)	INFERIOR ALVEOLAR BLOCK (min)
2% Lidocaine hydrochloride; 1 : 100,000 epinephrine	Xylocaine with epinephrine	7	500	170	190
2% Lidocaine	Xylocaine	4.5	300	40†	100†
2% Mepivacaine hydrochloride; 1 : 20,000 levonordefrin	Scandonest 2%	6.6	400	130	185
3% Mepivacaine hydrochloride	Carbocaine	6.6	400	90	165
4% Prilocaine hydrochloride; 1 : 200,000 epinephrine	Citanest Forte	8	600	140	220
4% Prilocaine hydrochloride	Citanest	8	600	105	190
0.5% Bupivacaine hydrochloride; 1 : 200,000 epinephrine	Marcaine with epinephrine	—	90	340	440
4% Articaine hydrochloride; 1 : 100,000 epinephrine	Septocaine	7	—	190	230

*The maximum dose is the smaller of the two values (e.g., 7 mg/kg lidocaine up to a maximum dose of 500 mg).
†Lidocaine without epinephrine produces unreliable pulpal anesthesia.

used clinically for the first time in 1960, is a less potent and less toxic alternative to lidocaine. Like mepivacaine, it is not used topically as a single agent but is effective for dental application without epinephrine. Articaine, the only thiophene-based amide local anesthetic, was first tested in human beings in 1970 and is now available for dental use in the United States as well as in Canada and Europe. An issue of current interest is whether the marketed formulation of 4% articaine with 1 : 100,000 epinephrine is equivalent or superior to other amide preparations.[38,87] Although no properly controlled clinical study has demonstrated increased efficacy, many dentists believe articaine increases the likelihood of obtaining adequate pain relief in cases in which other agents have failed.[50] Bupivacaine, used initially in 1963 but not marketed in a dental cartridge until 1983, is slightly slower in onset than the other amides but is equally efficacious and has a much longer duration of action, making it well suited for providing postoperative pain relief in oral surgery. The bupivacaine preparation intended for dental use is a 0.5% solution with 1 : 200,000 epinephrine.

One significant dissimilarity among the amide preparations concerns the presence or absence of a vasoconstrictor additive. Local anesthetic formulations without epinephrine-like drugs are particularly useful when sympathomimetic amines are contraindicated. Plain solutions are additionally promoted on the basis of a shorter duration of action. Although it is true that soft tissue anesthesia is comparatively brief after maxillary infiltration with 3% mepivacaine or 4% prilocaine (both without vasoconstrictor), differences in duration of mandibular injections are trivial (see Table 16-3). Because the period of pulpal anesthesia is often 20% to 25% that of soft tissue anesthesia, the limited maxillary duration of these agents is sometimes disadvantageous. For instance, 4% prilocaine, which compares favorably with 2% lidocaine with epinephrine in both onset and depth of anesthesia, fails approximately one fifth of the time to provide adequate pain relief toward the end of restorative procedures averaging 25 minutes in length.[15]

The use of local anesthetics without vasoconstrictors in pediatric dentistry deserves special comment. It is sometimes said that the shorter duration of soft tissue symptoms with plain local anesthetic solutions should reduce the incidence of self-inflicted tongue, cheek, and lip trauma. Such claims are dubious because blockade of the lingual, inferior alveolar, and buccal nerves that supply most of the tissues at risk is not significantly shortened by these preparations. Furthermore, no studies relating a reduction in traumatic cheilitis to the use of plain solutions have been reported. Consideration of systemic toxicity should actually limit the pedodontic use of local anesthetics without vasoconstrictors.[22] Because the safety margin of local anesthetics is quite low in small children, it is advisable to use a preparation containing a vasoconstrictor if not doing so would result in more total drug being administered.

Other than amide compounds being advocated over esters, it is difficult to suggest a particular local anesthetic for routine dental application. Certainly, if a proposed treatment requires a considerable volume of drug or necessitates a relatively prolonged operation, formulations such as lidocaine with epinephrine are indicated. Small volumes of lidocaine with 1 : 50,000 epinephrine can be advantageous when surgical hemostasis is desired. Articaine with epinephrine may be considered for situations in which the drug's short metabolic half-life and possible increased efficacy may prove advantageous. Bupivacaine with epinephrine would be a good choice for nerve block if a truly extended effect is desired. A plain local anesthetic solution might be more appropriate, however, for short procedures involving the maxillary arch.

When special patient factors or operative needs are not present, drug selection is best founded on the respective anesthetic efficacies and potential toxicities of the agents available. Because no local anesthetic preparation has emerged that is definitely superior to the rest in affording pain relief, use of any particular drug should be dictated largely by its relative likelihood of avoiding untoward responses. Estimates of systemic toxicity of local anesthetics as used in dentistry have not been published. Accepting that serious adverse reactions in most patients are caused by intravascular injections, one could predict by considering just the local anesthetic moieties involved that a 3% mepivacaine solution would be 50% more toxic than an equal volume of 2% mepivacaine with levonordefrin.[22] As described previously, however, some evidence suggests that sympathomimetic amines may potentiate the intravascular toxicity of concomitantly administered local anesthetics, making conclusions at this point impossible. Until definitive information about the intravascular toxic potentials of the various local anesthetic formulations becomes available, the recommendation of any single preparation for general use over all the others cannot be made.

PREPARATIONS AND DOSAGE

Agents for Parenteral Administration

Local anesthetics intended for injection within the oral cavity are supplied in 1.8-ml (1.7-ml for articaine) single-dose cartridges. Pyrogen-free distilled water with sodium chloride added for osmotic balance serves as the local anesthetic vehicle. Local anesthetic solutions range in pH from less than 3.0 to more than 6.0; generally, preparations with vasoconstrictors are adjusted to a lower pH than are plain formulations to enhance stability of the sympathomimetic amine constituents. Citric acid and sodium metabisulfite or an equivalent antioxidant are also included to help prevent vasoconstrictor breakdown. Some local anesthetics contain methylparaben. Useful for its antimicrobial action in multidose vials, methylparaben serves no purpose in dental cartridges, and its incorporation has been discontinued in the United States. Currently available local anesthetics marketed for dentistry in the United States and Canada are discussed below.

Lidocaine hydrochloride

Lidocaine is an aminoethylamide derivative of xylidine. It is several times more potent and toxic than procaine and provides local anesthesia that is by comparison more prompt, more extensive, and longer lasting. The administration of 2% lidocaine hydrochloride with 1 : 100,000 epinephrine is most suitable for routine dental use, but the drug is also available as a plain solution and with 1 : 50,000 epinephrine. Although 2% lidocaine with vasoconstrictor provides satisfactory dental anesthesia in normal circumstances, it has sometimes proved ineffective in rendering extremely sensitive teeth completely pain free. A concentrated solution of 5% lidocaine with 1 : 80,000 epinephrine has been shown to produce effective anesthesia in most instances when conventional local anesthetic preparations have failed.[31] Lidocaine is the only amide marketed as a single agent for topical anesthesia in dentistry. Formulations of lidocaine hydrochloride include a 2% gel, a 2% viscous solution, a 4% solution, and in Canada a 10% topical spray. Lidocaine base is marketed in a 2.5% and 5% ointment and solution and a 10% aerosol spray. A mucosal adherent patch 2 cm long by 1 cm wide and containing 46.1 mg of lidocaine is also available.

Mepivacaine hydrochloride

Mepivacaine is an amide product of xylidine and N-methylpipecolic acid. Similar in many respects to lidocaine, mepivacaine hydrochloride is marketed in a 2% concentration with 1 : 20,000 levonordefrin and as a 3% solution without vasoconstrictor. In contrast to some ester local anesthetics, cross-allergenicity is rare between mepivacaine and related agents.

Prilocaine hydrochloride

Unlike other amide anesthetics, prilocaine is a secondary amino derivative of toluidine. Somewhat less potent than lidocaine, prilocaine hydrochloride is marketed as a 4% solution with and without 1 : 200,000 epinephrine. Because the systemic toxicity of prilocaine is approximately half that of lidocaine, toxic effects on a milliliter basis are essentially equal. Instances of cyanosis observed after large doses of prilocaine (greater than 400 mg) result from its metabolic breakdown to *o*-toluidine, an inducer of methemoglobin.

Articaine hydrochloride

Articaine is unique among the amides in that it is based on a thiophene ring structure. Marketed in the United States in a 4% concentration with 1 : 100,000 epinephrine (and with 1 : 200,000 epinephrine in Canada), articaine has become a popular agent for routine use in dentistry. The relatively rapid hydrolysis of the ester side chain helps reduce toxicity associated with slow absorption from the injection site; conversely, the high concentration of the agent may accentuate the danger of intravascular injection and the risk of nerve damage in the immediate area of injection.

Bupivacaine hydrochloride

Bupivacaine is a homologue of mepivacaine rendered highly lipid soluble by replacement of the N-methyl group with a butyl chain. Bupivacaine is approximately four times as potent and as toxic as mepivacaine; it also has a slightly higher pK_a and a slower onset of action. For dentistry, 0.5% bupivacaine hydrochloride is available with 1 : 200,000 epinephrine. Clinical trials indicate that bupivacaine with epinephrine given for nerve block produces operative anesthesia several times longer than that afforded by other drugs.[49,59] Additionally, the formulation provides postoperative analgesia averaging 8 hours in the mandible and 5 hours in the maxilla. Bupivacaine is less effective and shorter acting than lidocaine (both with epinephrine), however, for pulpal anesthesia after maxillary supraperiosteal injection. Bupivacaine is so lipid soluble that the agent is largely absorbed by the mucosal tissues, leaving little free drug to diffuse into bone.

Agents Limited to Surface Application

Topical anesthetics are used in the oral cavity for a variety of purposes. Formulations marketed as pressurized sprays produce widespread surface anesthesia appropriate for making impressions or intraoral radiographs. Such preparations are potentially hazardous, however, and only products with metered valve dispensers to help prevent inadvertent overdose should be used. Topical liquids, which avoid the possibility of aerosol inspiration, may also be used for anesthetic coverage of large surface areas. Nonaqueous topical preparations are suitable for most other procedures. Common local anesthetic vehicles include lanolin, petrolatum, sodium carboxymethylcellulose, and polyethylene glycol.

Benzocaine

Benzocaine is a derivative of procaine in which the amino terminus is lacking. Poorly soluble in aqueous fluid, benzocaine tends to remain at the site of application and is not readily absorbed into the systemic circulation. Because of its low toxic potential, benzocaine is especially useful for anesthesia of large surface areas within the oral cavity. Benzocaine is not totally innocuous, however; cases of methemoglobinemia have been reported after the administration of very large doses to small children. Benzocaine is available in a variety of preparations; a 20% concentration in the form of an aerosol spray, gel, ointment, paste, and solution is most commonly advocated for intraoral use. A mucosal gel patch (containing 36 mg per 2 cm long by 1 cm wide patch) is also available.

Tetracaine hydrochloride

Tetracaine is an ester derivative of *p*-aminobenzoic acid in which a butyl chain replaces one of the hydrogens on the *p*-amino group. The drug has approximately 10 times the toxicity and potency of procaine. It is no longer available for injection in dentistry, but for surface application it is most commonly marketed as a 2% hydrochloride salt in combination with 14% benzocaine and 2% butamben in an aerosol spray, solution, gel, and ointment under the proprietary name Cetacaine. Tetracaine is one of the most effective topical anesthetics, but the drug's toxic potential after surface application should dictate caution in its use.

Dyclonine hydrochloride

Dyclonine is unusual in that it has a ketone linkage between the aromatic moiety and the rest of the anesthetic molecule. Available in lozenge form for topical use, dyclonine hydrochloride is not administered by injection because of its propensity for producing tissue irritation. Dyclonine may be used in patients allergic to derivatives of *p*-aminobenzoic acid.

Chlorobutanol

Chlorobutanol is a weak local anesthetic usually used with other agents. The drug is used primarily in obtundent dressings to relieve acute pulpitis and postextraction wound pain.

Cocaine hydrochloride

Cocaine, the first anesthetic used in dentistry and medicine, is a naturally occurring benzoic acid ester. The pharmacologic characteristics of cocaine are unique among the local anesthetics in that the drug inhibits the uptake of catecholamines by adrenergic nerve terminals. Cocaine therefore potentiates the action of endogenously released and exogenously administered sympathomimetic amines. As a result, cocaine may cause pupillary mydriasis, vascular constriction, and other manifestations of sympathetic nervous system activity. Cocaine is also a powerful CNS stimulant and a popular drug of abuse (see Chapter 51). Restricted to therapeutic applications where its vasoconstricting property is of special benefit (as in intranasal surgery), cocaine has no place in the routine practice of dentistry.

Lidocaine/prilocaine

Marketed under the acronym of EMLA, a eutectic mixture of 2.5% lidocaine and 2.5% prilocaine is available in the form of a cream for topical anesthesia of the skin. When placed under an occlusive dressing for 1 hour, EMLA obtunds the pain of venipuncture and finds special use in young children and other patients intolerant of needle insertion. Although this formulation is not intended for topical anesthesia of the oral cavity (and tastes bad and has poor physical characteristics for intraoral use), several investigations have proved its superiority over other topical anesthetics in relieving pain associated with manipulation of oral tissues. For instance, EMLA significantly relieved the discomfort of palatal injections after a 5-minute application[78] and allowed deeper probing of the gingival sulcus without discomfort than did 5% topical lidocaine.[30]

An intraoral preparation with the same active ingredients of EMLA has been marketed with the trade name of Oraqix. A low-viscosity fluid at room temperature, the anesthetic mixture becomes an elastic gel after being applied to the gingival sulcus to provide local anesthesia for periodontal scaling and root planing.[34]

Local Anesthetics

Nonproprietary (generic) name	Proprietary (trade) name
Agents for parenteral administration	
Articaine	Septocaine, Astracaine,* Astracaine Forte,* Ultracaine D-S,* Ultracaine Forte D-S*
Bupivacaine	Marcaine, Sensorcaine
Chloroprocaine	Nesacaine
Etidocaine*	Duranest
Levobupivacaine	Chirocaine
Lidocaine	Xylocaine, Lignospan, Lignospan Forte, Octocaine
Mepivacaine	Carbocaine, Arestocaine, Isocaine, Polocaine, Scandonest
Prilocaine	Citanest, Citanest Forte
Procaine	Novocain
Ropivacaine	Naropin
Tetracaine	Pontocaine
Agents limited to surface application	
Benzocaine	Americaine, Gingicaine, Hurricaine, Topicale, in Cetacaine
Butamben	Butesin Picrate, in Cetacaine
Cocaine	—
Dibucaine	Nupercainal
Dyclonine	in Sucrets
Lidocaine/prilocaine	EMLA, Oraqix
Pramoxine	Prax, Tronothane
Proparacaine	Alcaine, Ophthaine

*Not currently available in the United States.

CITED REFERENCES

1. Adriani J, Naraghi M: The pharmacologic principles of regional pain relief, *Annu Rev Pharmacol Toxicol* 17:223-242, 1977.
2. Åkerman B: Effects of felypressin (Octopressin®) on the acute toxicity of local anesthetics, *Acta Pharmacol Toxicol* 27:318-330, 1969.
3. Aldrete JA, Narang R, Sada T, et al: Reverse carotid blood flow—a possible explanation for some reactions to local anesthetics, *J Am Dent Assoc* 94:1142-1145, 1977.
4. Altura BM, Altura BT: Effects of local anesthetics, antihistamines, and glucocorticoids on peripheral blood flow and vascular smooth muscle, *Anesthesiology* 41:197-214, 1974.
5. Armstrong PJ, Morrison LM, Noble D, et al: Effects of I.V. lignocaine on psychological performance and subjective state in healthy volunteers, *Br J Anaesth* 67:532-538, 1992.
6. Arora S, Aldrete JA: Investigation of possible allergy to local anesthetic drugs: correlation of intradermal with intramuscular injections, *Anesthesiol Rev* 3:13-16, 1976.
7. Axelrod J: Metabolism of epinephrine and other sympathomimetic amines, *Physiol Rev* 39:751-776, 1959.
8. Bax NDS, Tucker GT, Lennard MS, et al: The impairment of lignocaine clearance by propranolol—major contribution from enzyme inhibition, *Br J Clin Pharmacol* 19:597-603, 1985.
9. Berquist HC: The danger of mepivacaine 3% toxicity in children, *J Calif Dent Assoc* 3:13, 1975.
10. Blair MR: Cardiovascular pharmacology of local anesthetics, *Br J Anaesth* 47:247-252, 1975.
11. Boakes AJ, Laurence DR, Teoh PC, et al: Interactions between sympathomimetic amines and antidepressant agents in man, *Br Med J* 1:311-315, 1973.
12. Bokesch PM, Post C, Strichartz G: Structure-activity relationship of lidocaine homologs producing tonic and frequency-dependent impulse blockade in nerve, *J Pharmacol Exp Ther* 237:773-781, 1986.
13. Bokesch PM, Raymond SA, Strichartz G: Dependence of lidocaine potency on pH and PCO_2, *Anesth Analg* 66:9-17, 1987.
14. Borg T, Modig J: Potential anti-thrombotic effects of local anaesthetics due to their inhibition of platelet aggregation, *Acta Anaesthesiol Scand* 29:739-742, 1985.
15. Brown G, Ward NL: Prilocaine and lignocaine plus adrenaline, *Br Dent J* 126:557-562, 1969.
16. Brown RD: The failure of local anaesthesia in acute inflammation: some recent concepts, *Br Dent J* 151:47-51, 1981.
17. Butterworth JF IV, Strichartz GR: Molecular mechanisms of local anesthesia: a review, *Anesthesiology* 72:711-734, 1990.
18. Catchlove RFH: Potentiation of two different local anaesthetics by carbon dioxide, *Br J Anaesth* 45:471-474, 1973.
19. Catterall WA: From ionic currents to molecular mechanisms: the structure and function of voltage-gated sodium channels, *Neuron* 26:13-25, 2000.
20. Catterall WA: Structure and function of voltage-sensitive ion channels, *Science* 242:50-61, 1988.
21. Chaney MA, Kerby R, Reader A, et al: An evaluation of lidocaine hydrocarbonate compared with lidocaine hydrochloride for inferior alveolar nerve block, *Anesth Prog* 38:212-216, 1991.
22. Chin KL, Yagiela JA, Quinn CL, et al: Serum mepivacaine concentrations after intraoral injection in young children, *J Calif Dent Assoc* 31:757-764, 2003.
23. Clarkson CW, Hondeghem LM: Mechanism for bupivacaine depression of cardiac conduction: fast block of sodium channels during the action potential with slow recovery from block during diastole, *Anesthesiology* 62:396-405, 1985.
24. Cotton BR, Henderson HP, Achola KJ, et al: Changes in plasma catecholamine concentrations following infiltration with large volumes of local anaesthetic solution containing adrenaline, *Br J Anaesth* 58:593-597, 1986.
25. Covino BG: Local anesthesia, *N Engl J Med* 286:975-983, 1972.
26. Covino BG, Vassallo HG: *Local anesthetics—mechanisms of action and clinical use,* New York, 1976, Grune & Stratton.

27. Cryer PE: Physiology and pathophysiology of the human sympathoadrenal neuroendocrine system, *N Engl J Med* 303:436-444, 1980.
28. de Jong RH, Heavner JE: Local anesthetic seizure prevention: diazepam versus pentobarbital, *Anesthesiology* 36:449-457, 1972.
29. deShazo RD, Nelson HS: An approach to the patient with a history of local anesthetic hypersensitivity: experience with 90 patients, *J Allergy Clin Immunol* 63:387-394, 1979.
30. Donaldson D, Meechan JG: A comparison of the effects of EMLA® cream and topical 5% lidocaine on discomfort during gingival probing, *Anesth Prog* 42:7-10, 1995.
31. Eldridge DJ, Rood JP: A double-blind trial of 5 per cent lignocaine, *Br Dent J* 142:129-130, 1977.
32. Fink BR: Mechanisms of differential axial blockade in epidural and subarachnoid anesthesia, *Anesthesiology* 70:851-858, 1989.
33. Franz DN, Perry RS: Mechanisms for differential block among single myelinated and nonmyelinated axons by procaine, *J Physiol* (London) 236:193-210, 1974.
34. Friskopp J, Nilsson M, Isacsson G: The anesthetic onset and duration of a new lidocaine/prilocaine gel intra-pocket anesthetic (Oraqix®) for periodontal scaling/root planing, *J Clin Periodontol* 28:453-458, 2001.
35. Garfield JM, Gugino L: Central effects of local anesthetic agents. In Strichartz GR, ed: *Local anesthetics. Handbook of experimental pharmacology,* vol 81, Berlin, 1987, Springer-Verlag.
36. Goodson JM, Moore PA: Life-threatening reactions after pedodontic sedation: an assessment of narcotic, local anesthetic, and antiemetic drug interaction, *J Am Dent Assoc* 107:239-245, 1983.
37. Grenadier E, Alpan G, Keidar S, et al: Respiratory and cardiac arrest after the administration of lidocaine into the central nervous system, *Eur Heart J* 2:235-237, 1981.
38. Haas DA, Harper DG, Saso MA, et al: Lack of differential effect by Ultracaine™ (articaine) and Citanest™ (prilocaine) in infiltration anesthesia, *J Can Dent Assoc* 57:217-223, 1991.
39. Haas DA, Lennon D: A 21 year retrospective study of reports of paresthesia following local anesthetic administration, *J Can Dent Assoc* 61:319-320, 323-326, 329-330, 1995.
40. Hanlon MR, Wallace BA: Structure and function of voltage-dependent ion channel regulatory β subunits, *Biochemistry* 41:2886-2894, 2002.
41. Hersh EV, Helpin ML, Evans OB: Local anesthetic mortality: report of case, *ASDC J Dent Child* 58:489-491, 1991.
42. Hille B: Local anesthetics: hydrophilic and hydrophobic pathways for the drug-receptor reaction, *J Gen Physiol* 69:497-515, 1977.
43. Jackson JE, Bentley JB, Glass SJ, et al: Effects of histamine-2 receptor blockade on lidocaine kinetics, *Clin Pharmacol Ther* 37:544-548, 1985.
44. Johnson ME, Saenz JA, DaSilva AD, et al: Effect of local anesthetic on neuronal cytoplasmic calcium and plasma membrane lysis (necrosis) in a cell culture model, *Anesthesiology* 97:1466-1477, 2002.
45. Jorfeldt L, Lewis DH, Löfström JB, et al: Lung uptake of lidocaine in healthy volunteers, *Acta Anaesthesiol Scand* 23:567-574, 1979.
46. Jorfeldt L, Löfström B, Pernow B, et al: The effect of local anaesthetics on the central circulation and respiration in man and dog, *Acta Anaesthesiol Scand* 12:153-169, 1986.
47. Kindler CH, Paul M, Zou H, et al: Amide local anesthetics potently inhibit the human tandem pore domain background K^+ channel TASK-2 (KCNK5), *J Pharmacol Exp Ther* 306:84-92, 2003.
48. Kozody R, Ready LB, Barsa JE, et al: Dose requirement of local anaesthetic to produce grand mal seizure during stellate ganglion block, *Can Anaesth Soc J* 29:489-491, 1982.
49. Laskin JL, Wallace WR, de Leo B: Use of bupivacaine hydrochloride in oral surgery—a clinical study, *J Oral Surg* 35:25-29, 1977.
50. Malamed SF, Gagnon S, Leblanc D: Efficacy of articaine: a new amide local anesthetic, *J Am Dent Assoc* 131:635-642, 2000.
51. Martin R, Lamarche Y, Tétreault L: Effects of carbon dioxide and epinephrine on serum levels of lidocaine after epidural anaesthesia, *Can Anaesth Soc J* 28:224-227, 1981.
52. Mio Y, Fukuda N, Kusakari Y, et al: Bupivacaine attenuates contractility by decreasing sensitivity of myofilaments to Ca^{2+} in rat ventricular muscle, *Anesthesiology* 97:1168-1177, 2002.
53. Munson ES, Wagman IH: Diazepam treatment of local anesthetic-induced seizures, *Anesthesiology* 37:523-528, 1972.
54. Neumcke B, Schwarz W, St. Adampfli R: Block of Na channels in the membrane of myelinated nerve by benzocaine, *Pflügers Archiv* 390:230-236, 1981.
55. Newcomb GM: Contraindications to the use of catecholamine vasoconstrictors in dental local analgesics, *NZ Dent J* 69:25-30, 1973.
56. Orlando R, Piccoli P, De Martin S, et al: Effect of the CYP3A4 inhibitor erythromycin on the pharmacokinetics of lignocaine and its pharmacologically active metabolites in subjects with normal and impaired liver function, *Br J Clin Pharmacol* 55:86-93, 2003.
57. Persson G: General side effects of local dental anaesthesia, *Acta Odontol Scand Suppl* 53:1-140, 1969.
58. Prenner BM, Stevens JJ: Anaphylaxis after ingestion of sodium bisulfite, *Ann Allergy* 37:180-182, 1976.
59. Pricco DF: An evaluation of bupivacaine for regional nerve block in oral surgery, *J Oral Surg* 35:126-129, 1977.
60. Punnia-Moorthy A: Buffering capacity of normal and inflamed tissues following the injection of local anaesthetic solutions, *Br J Anaesth* 61:154-159, 1988.
61. Ragsdale DS, McPhee JC, Scheuer T, et al: Molecular determinants of state-dependent block of Na^+ channels by local anesthetics, *Science* 265:1724-1728, 1994.
62. Raymond SA, Steffensen SC, Gugino LD, et al: The role of length of nerve exposed to local anesthetics in impulse blocking action, *Anesth Analg* 68:563-570, 1989.
63. Rimbäck G, Cassuto J, Tollesson P-O: Treatment of postoperative paralytic ileus by intravenous lidocaine infusion, *Anesth Analg* 70:414-419, 1990.
64. Roberts RK, Heath CA, Johnson RF, et al: Effect of H_2-receptor antagonists on steady-state extraction of indocyanine green and lidocaine by the perfused rat liver, *J Lab Clin Med* 107:112-117, 1986.
65. Rowbotham MC, Davies PS, Verkempinck C, et al: Lidocaine patch: double-blind controlled study of a new treatment method for post-herpetic neuralgia, *Pain* 65:39-44, 1996.

66. Schwartz HJ, Sher TH: Bisulfite sensitivity manifesting as allergy to local dental anesthesia, *J Allergy Clin Immunol* 75:525-527, 1985.

67. Scurlock JE, Meymaris E, Gregus J: The clinical character of local anesthetics: a function of frequency-dependent conduction block, *Acta Anaesthesiol Scand* 22:601-608, 1978.

68. Seldin HM: Survey of anesthetic fatalities in oral surgery and a review of the etiological factors in anesthetic deaths, *J Am Dent Soc Anesthesiol* 5:5-12, 1958.

69. Seldin HM, Recant BS: The safety of anesthesia in the dental office, *J Oral Surg* 13:199-208, 1955.

70. Seo N, Oshima E, Stevens J, et al: The tetraphasic action of lidocaine on CNS electrical activity and behavior in cats, *Anesthesiology* 57:451-457, 1982.

71. Sheets MF, Hanck DA: Molecular action of lidocaine on the voltage sensors of sodium channels, *J Gen Physiol* 121:163-175, 2003.

72. Sinclair CJ, Scott DB: Comparison of bupivacaine and etidocaine in extradural blockade, *Br J Anaesth* 56:147-153, 1984.

73. Smith RF, Wharton GG, Kurtz SL, et al: Behavioral effects of mid-pregnancy administration of lidocaine and mepivacaine in the rat, *Neurobehav Toxicol Teratol* 8:61-68, 1986.

74. Special Committee of the New York Heart Association, Inc: Use of epinephrine in connection with procaine in dental procedures, *J Am Dent Assoc* 50:108, 1955.

75. Strichartz G: Molecular mechanisms of nerve block by local anesthetics, *Anesthesiology* 45:421-441, 1976.

76. Strichartz GR, Ritchie JM: The action of local anesthetics on ion channels of excitable tissues. In Strichartz GR, ed: *Local anesthetics. Handbook of experimental pharmacology,* vol 81, Berlin, 1987, Springer-Verlag.

77. Strong JM, Parker M, Atkinson AJ: Identification of glycinexylidide in patients treated with intravenous lidocaine, *Clin Pharmacol Ther* 14:67-72, 1973.

78. Svensson P, Petersen JK: Anesthetic effect of EMLA occluded with orahesive oral bandages on oral mucosa. A placebo-controlled study, *Anesth Prog* 39:79-82, 1992.

79. Taheri S, Cogswell LP III, Gent A, et al: Hydrophobic and ionic factors in the binding of local anesthetics to the major variant of human α_1-acid glycoprotein, *J Pharmacol Exp Ther* 304:71-80, 2003.

80. Troullos ES, Goldstein DS, Hargreaves KM, et al: Plasma epinephrine levels and cardiovascular response to high administered doses of epinephrine contained in local anesthesia, *Anesth Prog* 34:10-13, 1987.

81. Trudell JR: A unitary theory of anesthesia based on lateral phase separations in nerve membranes, *Anesthesiology* 46:5-10, 1977.

82. Volpi M, Sha'afi RI, Epstein PM, et al: Local anesthetics, mepacrine, and propranolol are antagonists of calmodulin, *Proc Natl Acad Sci USA* 78:795-799, 1981.

83. Wang GK: Binding affinity and stereoselectivity of local anesthetics in single batrachotoxin-activated Na^+ channels, *J Gen Physiol* 96:1105-1127, 1990.

84. Wang J-S, Backman JT, Taavitsainen P, et al: Involvement of CYP1A2 and CYP3A4 in lidocaine N-deethylation and 3-hydroxylation in humans, *Drug Metab Dispos* 28:959-965, 2000.

85. Wilhelmi BJ, Blackwell SJ, Miller JH, et al: Do not use epinephrine in digital blocks: myth or truth? *Plast Reconstr Surg* 107:393-397, 2001.

86. Wingard DW, Bobko S: Failure of lidocaine to trigger porcine malignant hyperthermia, *Anesth Analg* 58:99-103, 1979.

87. Winther JE, Nathalang B: Effectivity of a new local analgesic Hoe 40 045, *Scand J Dent Res* 80:272-278, 1972.

88. Yagiela JA: Intravascular lidocaine toxicity: influence of epinephrine and route of administration, *Anesth Prog* 32:57-61, 1985.

89. Yagiela JA: Vasoconstrictors: their role in local anesthetic toxicity, *J Jpn Dent Soc Anesthesiol* 21:261-278, 1993.

90. Yagiela JA, Benoit PW, Buoncristiani RD, et al: Comparison of myotoxic effects of lidocaine with epinephrine in rats and humans, *Anesth Analg* 60:471-480, 1981.

91. Yarov-Yarovoy V, McPhee JC, Idsvoog D, et al: Roles of amino acid residues in transmembrane segments IS6 and IIS6 of the Na^+ channel α subunit in voltage-dependent gating and drug block, *J Biol Chem* 277:35393-35401, 2002.

92. Yeh JZ, Tanguy J: Na channel activation gate modulates slow recovery from use-dependent block by local anesthetics in squid giant axons, *Biophys J* 47:685-694, 1985.

General References

Berde CB, Strichartz GR: Local anesthetics. In Miller RD, ed: *Anesthesia,* ed 5, New York, 2000, Churchill Livingstone.

Cousins MJ, Bridenbaugh PO, eds: *Neural blockade in clinical anesthesia and management of pain,* ed 3, Philadelphia, 1998, Lippincott-Raven.

Covino BG, Vassallo HG: *Local anesthetics—mechanisms of action and clinical use,* New York, 1976, Grune & Stratton.

Liu SS, Hodgson PS: Local anesthetics. In Barash PG, Cullen BF, Stoelting RK, eds: *Clinical anesthesia,* ed 4, Philadelphia, 2001, Lippincott Williams & Wilkins.

Strichartz GR, ed: *Local anesthetics. Handbook of experimental pharmacology,* vol 81, Berlin, 1987, Springer-Verlag.

CHAPTER • 17

Principles of General Anesthesia

John A. Yagiela and Daniel A. Haas

HISTORY

The pioneering use of anesthetics is credited to two dentists: Horace Wells and his one-time pupil and partner, William T.G. Morton, who practiced dentistry in New England in the early 1800s. Their achievements were preceded by the contributions of many others and came at a time when still others were carrying out experiments that would lead them to compete for recognition as the discoverers of anesthesia.

The history of anesthesia is no doubt as old as humankind itself, for surely since the dawn of time people have sought ways to alleviate pain. Records spanning thousands of years make it clear that patients about to undergo painful procedures have had recourse to prayer, magic, the intervention of witch doctors and medicine men, techniques such as compression of nerves and blood vessels, and various plant products such as opium, mandragora, and cocaine. It was not until the eighteenth and early nineteenth centuries, however, that modern anesthesiology had its beginnings. The development of physics and chemistry led to the discovery of elements and simple molecules, including a number of gases. Joseph Priestley, an English scientist, is credited with the discovery of carbon dioxide, oxygen, and, in 1772, nitrous oxide. Although he thought oxygen might have some medical use, Priestley was unaware of the anesthetic properties of nitrous oxide. In 1795, Humphry Davy, a 17-year-old surgeon's assistant in England who later became a distinguished scientist himself, began experiments with nitrous oxide. He inhaled the gas and used it on one occasion to relieve the pain of his erupting third molar (although at this time nitrous oxide was still considered to be extremely poisonous). He noted in his published studies of nitrous oxide the giddiness, pleasurable sensations, relaxation of muscles, and diminution of pain that were produced by inhalation of the gas. In 1799, Davy constructed the first machine for the storage and inhalation of nitrous oxide.

The development of anesthesia was carried further by Michael Faraday, Davy's student, who in 1818 noted the anesthetic properties of diethyl ether (then known as "sweet vitriol"), and by Henry Hills Hickman, an English surgeon who carried out painless surgery on laboratory animals with carbon dioxide gas as the anesthetic. In 1824, Hickman published a pamphlet, "A Letter on Suspended Animation," in which he suggested that patients could be made unconscious before surgery.

In the United States in the early 1800s, there was both scientific and popular interest in ether and nitrous oxide. Itinerant entertainers who called themselves professors went about delivering lectures on these substances and demonstrating their effects. One of the earliest of these demonstrations was conducted in 1824 by Joseph Dorfeuille, a museum director from Cincinnati, who gave nitrous oxide to a dozen spectators. "Laughing gas" parties and "ether frolics" became common among medical students, and, because of his experiences at such an ether party, one medical student, William E. Clarke, administered ether from a towel to a young woman having a tooth extracted in Rochester, New York. This use of ether in 1842 is the first on record.

Crawford W. Long, a Georgia physician who had been trained at the University of Pennsylvania Medical School, had attended ether frolics while a student, and, later in 1842, he used ether when he removed two small tumors from the neck of James Venable, a friend who had previously experienced the effects of inhaling ether. Thus credit for the first use of ether in a nondental procedure belongs to Dr. Long. His anesthetic fee, also the first on record, was $2. Because Long wanted to include observations of the effects of ether in major surgical procedures, he did not publish reports of his pioneering use of ether until 1849, 3 years after the accounts of Morton's use of ether had appeared. A letter from Long written in 1844 suggests that he was visited by a dentist and a surgeon from Boston, that the dentist was Morton or Wells, and that it was from Long that they learned the technique of administering ether during surgery.

On December 10, 1844, Horace Wells attended a demonstration, staged by Gardner Quincy Colton in Hartford, Connecticut, of the effects of "laughing gas." One subject who volunteered to take the gas injured himself in the leg. Wells noticed that he was unaware of his injury and apparently had no pain until the effects of the gas wore off. The next day, Wells persuaded Dr. John Riggs, a prominent Hartford dentist, to remove one of his own teeth while under nitrous oxide anesthesia administered by "Professor" Colton. Wells claimed that he felt no more than a pinprick. Wells then obtained permission to demonstrate his technique before a class at the Harvard Medical School and administered nitrous oxide to a student, who proceeded to scream loudly while his tooth was being removed. The boy later said he had felt no pain. Discouraged by the apparent failure of his demonstration and by the hostile reception that followed, Wells became ill and was unable to practice dentistry on a regular basis. He nevertheless continued to administer nitrous oxide, with mixed success, for both dental and medical operations until several weeks before his untimely death in January 1848. Wells also experimented with ether as early as 1845 and with chloroform once its anesthetic effect became known (in November 1847). Wells became deranged by overexposure to chloroform and committed suicide while in jail for having accosted a prostitute. Nitrous oxide was abandoned after his death until 1863, when Colton reintroduced its use for dental extractions.

William T.G. Morton of Boston, a former student and partner of Wells, had begun to use ether topically for its local numbing effect on his denture patients. With the help of his chemistry professor at Harvard, Charles T. Jackson, Morton refined his technique and successfully administered anesthesia to a patient for the extraction of a molar tooth. Convinced of the importance of his discovery, he obtained an invitation to demonstrate his technique for Dr. John C. Warren, a surgeon at Massachusetts General Hospital. There, on October 16, 1846, Morton prepared a young patient for the surgical removal of a large mandibular tumor. To Morton is credited the discovery of anesthesia and the custom of saying, "Doctor, your patient is now ready."

Morton was anxious to patent the substance he called "Letheon," but several physicians from the Massachusetts General Hospital thought it unsuitable to patent a medical discovery and indicated that they would not continue to use it if its chemical nature remained a secret. Morton then offered to make known the nature of the substance and to serve as an anesthetist at various hospitals. He abandoned his medical studies and his dental practice and became the first professional anesthetist. In 1846, Oliver Wendell Holmes addressed a letter to Morton suggesting that the term *anesthesia* be given to the state produced by ether and that the agent itself be called an *anesthetic*.

Following Morton's demonstration in Boston, the use of anesthesia spread rapidly despite opposition from various groups, many of whom still believed that there was something spiritually ennobling about pain, particularly the pain of childbirth. In 1847, Sir James Young Simpson first used ether in his obstetric practice and in the same year successfully delivered a child with chloroform. Later, when Queen Victoria was delivered of her seventh child while under chloroform anesthesia, most ecclesiastic opposition was stilled.

No new agents were added until the 1920s and 1930s, when ethylene, cyclopropane, and divinyl ether were introduced. Since the early 1950s, a series of halogenated agents containing fluorine have been introduced clinically and have essentially replaced other inhalation agents except nitrous oxide.

Intravenous agents, mainly the thiobarbiturates (e.g., thiopental), became popular in the late 1930s. Other ultrashort-acting barbiturates were added to the list and were supplemented in the late 1960s by ketamine and the neuroleptanalgesic combination of droperidol-fentanyl. Additional newer intravenous anesthetics include etomidate, midazolam, and propofol.

Neuromuscular blocking drugs were added to the practice of anesthesia in 1942 with the introduction of curare to facilitate endotracheal intubation and relaxation of muscles for abdominal surgery. Opioid anesthesia, in which morphine and subsequently fentanyl and its congeners found use as principal agents in obtunding autonomic responses to surgical stimulation, originated with cardiac surgery in the late 1950s.

Finally, it is interesting to note that the use of nitrous oxide by dentists has exhibited a cyclic pattern of popularity every 25 to 30 years since Wells first used it. Nitrous oxide, as a sedative agent, is currently enjoying an extended fifth cycle; with the development of new technologies and practices, its use has apparently stabilized.

COMMON TERMS

Consciousness is the mental state in which the person is capable of a rational response to commands and has all protective reflexes intact, including the ability to maintain a patent airway.

Sedation describes a state of partial or complete awareness of the environment but with a significant reduction of anxiety and restlessness. As described in Chapter 48, two levels of sedation have been defined: *conscious sedation*, in which the patient retains protective airway reflexes and responsiveness to light physical stimulation and/or verbal command, and *deep sedation*, in which protective reflexes and responsiveness to nonnoxious stimuli may be obtunded.

Analgesia refers to a reduced perception of and responsiveness to noxious stimuli (i.e., stimuli that are described as painful) but without amnesia or loss of consciousness. Other modes of sensory perception remain intact (e.g., vision and hearing).

Amnesia refers to a loss of memory of the surgical experience, although the patient may be aware of the environment during surgery.

Anxiolysis indicates a selective reduction or elimination of fear and apprehension produced without amnesia or loss of consciousness.

Induction is that phase of anesthesia beginning with the administration of anesthetic and continuing until the desired level of patient unresponsiveness is reached.

Unconsciousness is the state in which the patient is no longer aware of the environment and does not respond to familiar stimuli such as calling the patient's name.

Unresponsiveness refers to a loss of reaction to sensory stimuli, both noxious and nonnoxious.

Muscle relaxation is a reduction or loss of CNS regulation of skeletal muscle tone and reflexes that produces a state of flaccid paralysis and unresponsiveness of muscle to stretching and surgical cutting.

Surgical anesthesia is the state of unconsciousness, unresponsiveness, anxiolysis, amnesia, analgesia, and muscle relaxation that allows the goals of surgery to be accomplished.

Maintenance is the process of keeping a patient in surgical anesthesia.

Recovery is the phase of anesthesia beginning when surgery is complete and the delivery of the anesthetic is terminated and ending when the anesthetic has been eliminated from the body.

Emergence delimits the stage of recovery during which the patient is regaining consciousness.

Minimum alveolar concentration (MAC) is used for quantifying the potency of inhalation anesthetic agents. MAC, as defined by Eger et al,[11] is the alveolar concentration of anesthetic at which 50% of patients do not respond to a standard surgical stimulus.

GOALS OF ANESTHESIA

General anesthesia may be defined as "a drug-induced reversible depression of the central nervous system (CNS) resulting in the loss of response to and perception of all external stimuli."[13] In practice, this simple definition is inadequate because it neglects the contributions of unconsciousness, amnesia, immobility, and autonomic stability to the anesthetic state and the fact that general anesthetics differ significantly in the effects they achieve.

A complete anesthetic is one that produces unconsciousness, amnesia, analgesia, and muscle relaxation by itself without eliciting undue homeostatic disturbances in the patient. An example of such a complete anesthetic is diethyl ether (or simply ether). Although there are other complete anesthetics, the tendency in modern anesthesiology is to use a combination of drugs to take advantage of the best properties of each and to minimize unwanted side effects. Among the agents that may be used preoperatively are the antimuscarinic drugs to minimize salivation, laryngospasm, and reflex bradycardia and various analgesics and CNS depressants to provide preoperative pain relief, sedation, and amnesia. Drugs that are used during the administration of general anesthesia in addition to the primary anesthetic include nitrous oxide, which lessens the total required dose of anesthetic and increases analgesia, drugs that paralyze skeletal muscle, and, if necessary, drugs that help maintain cardiovascular stability and renal function.

The primary goals of general anesthesia are to preserve the life of the patient, to provide the operator with an adequate surgical field, and to obtund pain. Ideally, a general anesthetic should (1) provide a smooth and rapid induction; (2) produce a state of unconsciousness or unresponsiveness; (3) produce a state of amnesia; (4) maintain essential physiologic functions while blocking reflexes that might lead to bronchospasm, salivation, and arrhythmias; (5) produce skeletal muscle relaxation, but preferably not of the respiratory muscles, through the blockade of various efferent impulses; (6) block the conscious perception of sensory stimuli so that there is adequate analgesia to perform the procedure; and (7) provide a smooth, rapid, and uneventful emergence and recovery with no long-lasting adverse effects.

The goals of anesthesia for general surgery also apply to dental surgery, but there are some important differences. Most dental patients are outpatients; in many dental procedures, particularly those not involving extensive oral surgery, the procedures are usually not as traumatic as those of general surgery, and it is neither necessary nor desirable to render the patient unconscious. Although general anesthesia is occasionally used for dental patients, specific techniques have been developed for producing conscious sedation in dental patients, as is described in Chapter 48.

THEORIES OF ANESTHETIC ACTION

Since the introduction of general anesthetics, efforts have been directed toward discovering the mechanism of action of these agents. Our incomplete knowledge of the structure and behavior of membrane constituents; neurotransmitters and neurologic circuits; and behavioral states relevant to clinical anesthesia such as consciousness, sleep, pain, and anxiety makes elucidation of the mechanism extremely difficult. Theories have been advanced for each of the above-mentioned functions, however, and are summarized in the following sections.

Membrane Molecular Theories

Membrane molecular theories attempt to describe the action of the extremely diverse chemicals known to be general anesthetics by their ability to perturb the molecular structure and function of biologic membranes. Most anesthetic agents appear to be rather indiscriminate in affecting biophysical properties of cellular and subcellular membranes, and for many years it was generally agreed that there are no specific receptors for general anesthetics (and thus no direct antagonists) as there are for neurotransmitters. In this setting, a universal mechanism of action of general anesthesia based on the physicochemical properties of anesthetic agents was a likely possibility.

Correlates of anesthetic potency

Various theories of general anesthesia began to appear shortly after the landmark demonstration of ether-induced insensibility by Morton; however, the first important observation was made independently by Meyer in 1899 and Overton in 1901, who emphasized the correspondence between the lipid solubility of an agent and its anesthetic potency (Figure 17-1). The Meyer-Overton theory in essence states that anesthesia begins when any chemical substance has attained a certain molar concentration in the hydrophobic phase of the cell membrane. When olive oil is used to represent the hydrophobic medium, this concentration is approximately 50 mmol/L. Experiments with different lipid media indicate that the best fit between solubility and anesthetic potency is obtained with lipids that are amphophilic (i.e., they have both polar and nonpolar attributes) and can serve as hydrogen bond acceptors. These characteristics are descriptive of membrane phospholipids and cholesterol.

In 1954, Mullins,[38] in his critical volume hypothesis, modified the original theory to include consideration of the volume of the hydrophobic region occupied by the anesthetic agent. He reasoned that large molecules would have greater effects on the membrane than would smaller molecules. Indeed, the correlation between anesthetic potency and a function of both lipid solubility and molecular size may be somewhat better than the correlation between anesthetic potency and lipid solubility alone.

Plasma membrane involvement

Numerous investigators have sought to link the notion of a critical number or volume of anesthetic molecules with plasma membrane disturbances that could result in general anesthesia. Variations in proposed theories include the nature of the constituents most directly affected by the anesthetic: lipids, proteins (including lipoproteins), or water.

Lipids In years past, most attention was directed at the lipid bilayer of the plasma membrane, specifically the ability of anesthetics to cause membrane expansion, lipid fluidization, or lateral phase separation. With each of these effects, it is postulated that, as a result of the alteration in the lipid bilayer, the neuronal membrane becomes unable to facilitate the changes in protein configuration that are required for such essential steps in the transmission of nerve impulses as ion gating, synaptic transmitter release, and binding of the transmitter to the receptor.[51]

The membrane expansion theory is a natural outgrowth of the critical volume hypothesis. It simply holds that the

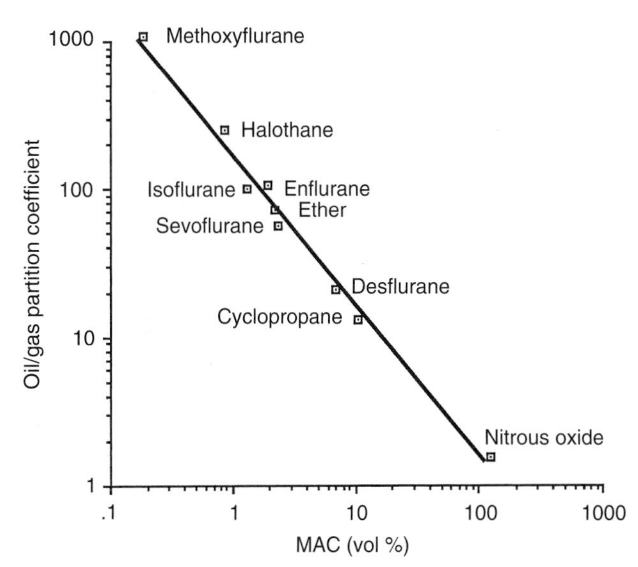

Fig. 17-1 Linear correlation between anesthetic potency and lipid solubility. Potency is indicated by the MAC and lipid solubility by the olive oil/gas partition coefficient.

absorption of anesthetic molecules by the lipid phase causes the membrane to expand, thus preventing important intrinsic membrane constituents from functioning properly.[46] Measurements indicate that the expansion associated with general anesthesia is approximately 0.4%. Fluidization, or disordering, of lipids by anesthetic agents was noted in studies of lipid bilayers prepared with phospholipid and cholesterol to mimic cell membranes.[46] Parallel shifts in measures of lipid fluidization and the activity of membrane-bound enzymes suggested that this perturbation of the normal lipid structure may result in functional changes sufficient to disrupt nerve transmission. The lateral phase separation theory was based on the idea that membrane lipids exist in two states: a high-volume, disordered sol state and a compact, ordered gel state.[51] The ability of lipids to convert from the sol to the gel configuration, or to be compressed laterally within the membrane, was thought to accommodate conformational changes that need to occur for the opening of ion channels. Several lines of evidence indicate that anesthetics inhibit phase transition and increase the proportion of lipid in the liquid (sol) form.[35]

These lipid perturbation theories were supported by the finding that hyperbaric pressures[36,46] and certain convulsant drugs[7] antagonize anesthesia, presumably by reversing membrane expansion or reestablishing order. However, it is now understood that pressure or drug reversal of anesthesia arises from a physiologic antagonism of anesthetic action brought on by independent neurologic stimulation. Moreover, different anesthetics are affected differently by the same pressure, including chloral hydrate, whose anesthetic effect is immune to pressure reversal. Evidence has also mounted to cast doubt on membrane expansion or lipid perturbation per se as a cause of anesthesia. Direct measurements of the expansion of lipid bilayers and red cell membranes in response to anesthetic concentrations of ethanol and halothane yield values that are effectively insignificant,[15] and other measurements have shown nonanesthetic long-chain alcohols to cause membrane expansion similar to that of inhalation anesthetics.[53] Regarding fluidization or sol-gel transformations, changes equivalent to those associated with anesthesia can be attained by temperature elevations less than 1° C.[52]

Calculations based on the Meyer-Overton relationship argue in general against a significant effect of anesthetic drugs on membrane lipids. At concentrations sufficient to produce surgical anesthesia, there is only approximately 1 molecule of drug in the membrane for every 60 to 80 molecules of the much larger lipid constituents. Therefore, unless anesthetic molecules are distributed unevenly in the membrane (e.g., concentrated in lipids adjacent to ion channels) or the lipid phase serves as a barrier to the diffusion of anesthetic agents (i.e., limiting access of anesthetics to their effector site) or as a reservoir for them (i.e., retaining anesthetic molecules where they have direct access to their effector sites), it is unlikely that membrane lipids play a major role in the mechanism of anesthesia.

Proteins Membrane proteins constitute a second hydrophobic environment with which anesthetic molecules may interact. The theory that membrane proteins are the targets of anesthetic action is attractive for several reasons. First, it is consistent with the mode of action of most drugs that influence the CNS. Second, allosteric regulation of a protein by the binding of even a single small molecule can have pronounced effects on protein function. Third, it can best explain differences in action among the various anesthetics by assuming that these agents exert different effects on the same protein or influence different proteins altogether.

Although technical difficulties have long inhibited direct examination of anesthetic drug interactions with membrane proteins, the firefly enzyme luciferase has provided a good model for study.[16] Luciferase is a water-soluble protein that produces light when activated by its substrate, luciferin. For a wide variety of agents, anesthetic potency correlates directly with the ability to inhibit luciferin binding and prevent light emission. Moreover, certain nonanesthetic alcohols have no effect. The binding site on the enzyme is amphophilic in nature and capable of accepting a hydrogen bond. Several other proteins, including hemoglobin and cholinergic receptors, also bind anesthetic drugs and undergo conformational changes as a result.[31] A number of potential sites exist for direct anesthetic interactions with proteins: hydrophobic regions within globular or folded polypeptides, between polypeptides joined in an oligomeric structure, and at the protein-lipid or protein-water interface.

The synthesis of a water-soluble four-α-helix protein bundle similar in structure to peptides forming ligand-gated ion channels has allowed characterization of direct anesthetic-protein interactions.[25] A hydrophobic cavity within the bundle binds halothane best when the cavity is lined with methionine and aromatic acid residues. In turn, halothane binding stabilizes the protein in a conformation that putatively promotes anesthesia.

A close correspondence between the anesthetic potencies of stereoisomers of halothane and isoflurane and their ability to perturb ion channel function provides strong evidence that these membrane proteins are the immediate target for general anesthetic action.[17] In fact, it is now firmly established that certain classes of general anesthetics inhibit or activate specific ligand-gated ion channels in clinically relevant concentrations. For example, binding studies indicate a specific active site for volatile anesthetics on nicotinic receptors.[10,33] Moreover, specific mutations on the M_2 domains of the nicotinic receptor, which correspond to the α-helix segments that form the aqueous pore of the receptor's ion channel, enhance the blocking action of anesthetics such as isoflurane and alcohols such as octanol.[14] It is postulated that hydrophobic general anesthetic agents bind at a discrete site in the vicinity of the mutation loci. The more polar alcohols gain access to the same site preferentially after channel opening, suggesting that the binding site is within the channel itself. Inhibition of nicotinic receptors in skeletal muscle probably contributes to the ability of volatile anesthetics to enhance muscle relaxation. Actions at neuronal nicotinic receptors promote such effects as amnesia, hyperalgesia, and excitation observed at subanesthetic concentrations of volatile anesthetics and barbiturates.

The γ-aminobutyric $acid_A$ ($GABA_A$) receptor has been implicated in the CNS-depressant effect of most anesthetic drugs.[13,48] Specific binding sites for benzodiazepines, barbiturates and other intravenous anesthetics, and volatile anesthetics have been described.[13] Stimulation of these receptor sites increases the activity of GABA at its own separate site; many agents other than benzodiazepines can also open the $GABA_A$ Cl^- channel in the absence of GABA. Hyperpolarization of the affected neuron inhibits neuronal activity. Glycine receptors constitute another group of inhibitory receptors that are activated by at least some general anesthetics (inhalation anesthetics, alcohols, thiopental, and propofol) in clinically relevant concentrations.

Excitatory receptors blocked by specific anesthetic agents include the N-methyl-D-aspartate (NMDA), kainate, and α-amino-3-hydroxy-5-methyl-4-isoxazole propionate (AMPA) receptors. Ketamine[59] and nitrous oxide[24] selectively inhibit NMDA receptors, whereas barbiturates block AMPA and kainate receptors.[13]

In addition to ligand-gated ion channels, several other proteins involved in signal transduction may contribute to general anesthesia. An important example is the α_2-adrenergic receptor effector system. Stimulation of this G protein–coupled receptor (GPCR) by the selective α_2 agonists clonidine and dexmedetomidine significantly potentiates the anesthetic potency of halothane.[34] Similar potentiation can be obtained by drugs that stimulate opioid receptors or block nitric oxide synthase.[26] A unique family of anesthetic-activated K^+ channels have been discovered.[13] These channels are responsive to intracellular second messengers and may regulate background neuronal excitability. Recently, demonstration of a blocking action of halothane on the GPCR rhodopsin underscores the possibility that similar interactions with other GPCRs may support the effects of inhalation anesthetics on consciousness, nociception, and various autonomic effects observed during general anesthesia.[22]

Lastly, general anesthetics may exert some influences through effects on voltage-gated ion channels. Although most voltage-gated channels require supraanesthetic concentrations to be significantly affected, several types of Ca^{++} channels are inhibited by clinical concentrations of drugs and may contribute an inhibitory effect on neurotransmitter release.

Water Theories in which anesthesia is caused by directly altering the properties of water have not withstood experimental scrutiny. However, it remains possible for water-membrane interactions to play a role in general anesthesia. Anesthetic agents, by dehydrating the membrane surface and making it more hydrophobic, may inhibit the flow of hydrated ions necessary for synaptic or nerve transmission.[53]

Other sites

Several investigators have raised the possibility that mitochondria and synaptic vesicles may be targets of general anesthetics. Certain anesthetics have been shown to impair the ability of synaptosomes (isolated nerve terminals) to sequester and retain catecholamine neurotransmitters and of mitochondria to produce adenosine triphosphate and to take up Ca^{++}. Although the latter effect has been used to explain the finding that anesthetics hyperpolarize cells in direct relation to their anesthetic potency,[40] a lack of correlation between catecholamine influences and general anesthesia, coupled with the failure of adenosine triphosphate concentrations in the brain to fall during anesthesia, argues against a primary role for these other sites in producing anesthesia. Nevertheless, demonstration of altered responses to volatile anesthetics in nematodes (*Caenorhabditis elegans*) expressing mutated proteins responsible for synaptic exocytosis promotes the likelihood for a site of action involving synaptic fusion.[42]

Neurophysiologic Theories

Membrane molecular theories may provide a fundamental explanation of the pharmacodynamic actions of general anesthetics, but they are not useful in describing the selective changes in consciousness, pain perception, and muscle relaxation observed clinically. Therefore much research has been directed toward determining the neurologic sites and pathways affected by the various anesthetics. A first step to unraveling these more complex issues is to identify the component of the neuronal circuit most affected by anesthetic action. Studies of the sympathetic nervous system have conclusively demonstrated that synaptic transmission is much more susceptible to anesthetic block than is axonal conduction.[31] Nevertheless, this finding does not rule out an axonal contribution to general anesthesia. Anesthetic agents in clinical concentrations can diminish the amplitude of the action potential, which then may impair synaptic transmission prejunctionally by reducing the evoked release of neurotransmitter. Conduction block is strongest at branch points of small-diameter axons and becomes even more prominent as the frequency of nerve transmission increases.

Evidence in favor of a direct presynaptic site of action includes some observations that anesthetics depress excitatory neuroeffector responses to prejunctional nerve stimulation but not to iontophoretic application of the appropriate neurotransmitter.[27] Release of epinephrine and norepinephrine from chromaffin cells by K^+ or acetylcholine has also been reported to be reduced by a variety of anesthetics.[43] The most likely mechanism of action for this effect is a depression of Ca^{++} influx through presynaptic voltage-gated Ca^{++} channels or interference with the proteins involved in vesicle docking and neurotransmitter release.

A postsynaptic action at specific sites in the CNS is supported by decreased responses to directly applied stimulatory neurotransmitters such as acetylcholine, aspartate, and glutamate. At the neuromuscular junction, general anesthetics appear to reduce the sensitivity of the motor endplate to acetylcholine by increasing the closing rate of ion channels opened by nicotinic receptor activation and by increasing receptor desensitization. Conversely, numerous anesthetics increase transmission at inhibitory synapses by increasing activation of GABA receptors and Cl^- conductance. In addition, inhalation anesthetics and some intravenous agents may affect a different set of GABA receptors and activate an inhibitory K^+ current.[28]

A crucial unknown in the study of general anesthesia is the site at which unconsciousness is produced. Areas in the CNS that have been implicated in this primary anesthetic action include the dorsal lamina of the spinal cord (substantia gelatinosa), the reticular system (including the midbrain reticular formation), sensory relay nuclei of the thalamus, and cortical areas.

Beginning with the studies of French et al,[18] much attention has been directed toward the role of the mesencephalic reticular activating formation. This system, which receives a variety of nonspecific sensory inputs, is a major center supporting consciousness and alertness of higher brain centers. As the activity of the system is depressed, the ascending influences on the limbic system and cortical structures are reduced, and unconsciousness ensues. Interestingly, gross lesions that abolish the arousal effect of the reticular formation as recorded on the electroencephalogram may leave the animal behaviorally awake. This complex of neurons may also respond quite differently to various anesthetics.[6,8] Whereas barbiturates, ether, and halothane cause depression of spontaneous electrical activity, enflurane may briefly enhance it, and ketamine alters the pattern of firing.[27,37] All agents, however, appear to block neuronal responses in the reticular formation to sensory input.

General anesthetics in clinically relevant concentrations may also exert direct effects on various nuclei of the thalamus, the hippocampus, the olfactory cortex, and various circuits in the cerebral cortex. Most reactions are consistent with the inhibition of excitatory neuronal pathways and/or facilitation of inhibitory influences. However, as with the reticular formation, net excitatory reactions also occur depending on the anesthetic administered and region studied.

Numerous investigators have argued for a central role of thalamocortical-corticothalamic loop circuits in maintaining consciousness. As illustrated in Figure 17-2, these circuits are tonically active in the conscious state.[2] Direct sensory input and excitatory stimuli arising from the reticular activating system help maintain this activity. Loss of depolarizing stimuli (e.g., reduced glutamate receptor stimulation) and/or increased inhibitory stimuli (e.g., GABA receptor activation) hyperpolarize the thalamocortical neurons and block the tonic circuit activity, resulting in unconsciousness.

Because of its role in modulating pain, the spinal cord has been studied as a possible site of anesthetic action.[30,49] Investigators have shown that the analgesic action of nitrous oxide involves the laminar structures (substantia gelatinosa) of the dorsal horns, often referred to as the gateway for

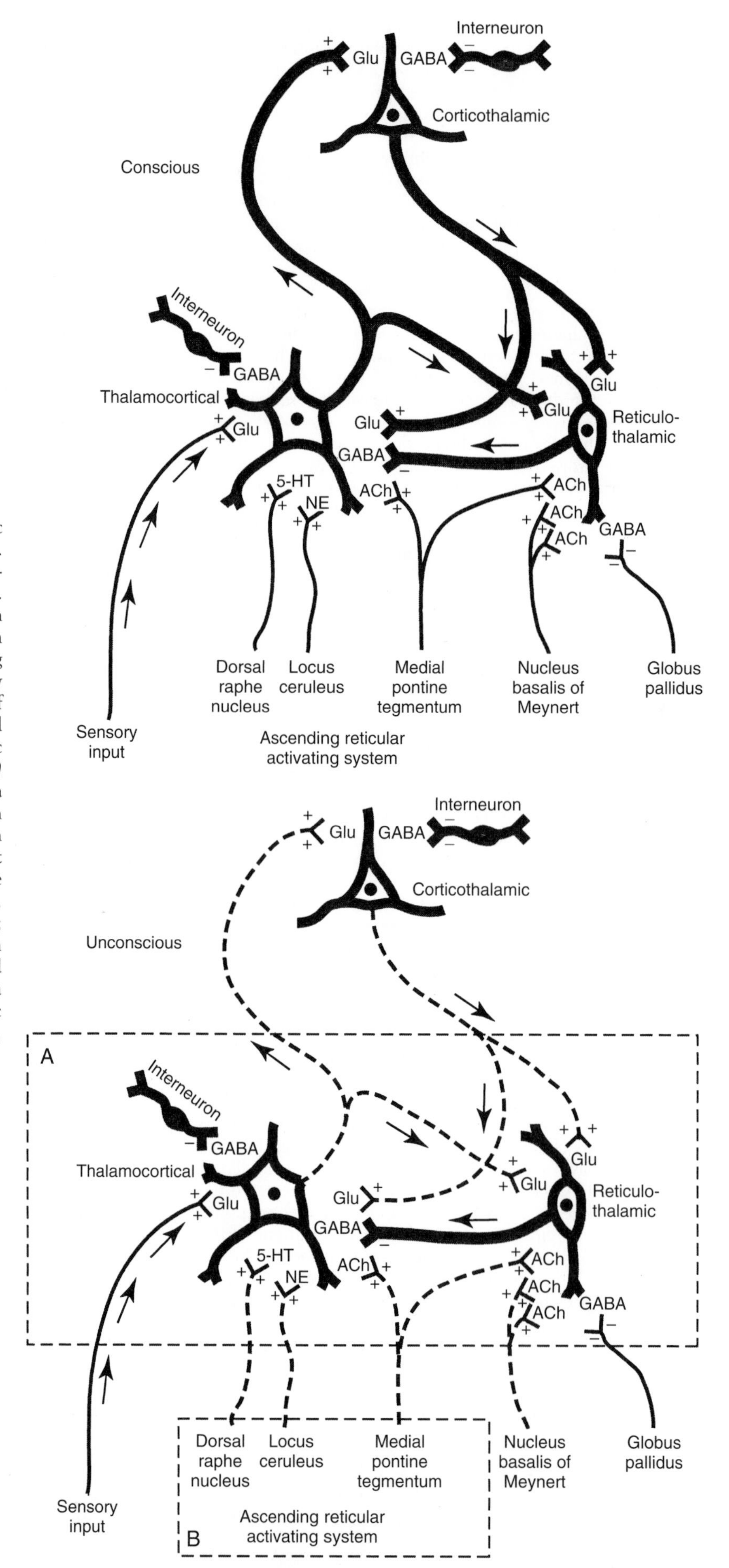

Fig. 17-2 A neuroanatomic/neurophysiologic model of anesthetic-induced unconsciousness. The key cellular players are the thalamocortical, corticothalamic, and reticulothalamic cells. *Top,* The system during consciousness, when sensory information can be processed through the thalamus. *Bottom,* The system during anesthetic-induced unconsciousness. Sensory information processing is blocked at the level of the thalamus secondary to thalamocortical hyperpolarization. The thalamus/thalamic reticular area *(A)* and the midbrain region *(B)* specifically suppressed by inhalation anesthesia in human beings are outlined. Anesthetics in general cause thalamocortical hyperpolarization through many mechanisms, including direct hyperpolarization, GABA agonism, glutamate antagonism, and cholinergic antagonism. *ACh,* Acetylcholine; *5-HT,* 5-hydroxytryptamine; *Glut,* glutamate; *NE,* norepinephrine. (From Alkire MT, Haier RJ, Fallon JH: Toward a unified theory of narcosis: brain imaging evidence for a thalamocortical switch as the neurophysiologic basis of anesthetic-induced unconsciousness, *Conscious Cogn* 9:370-386, 2000.)

nociceptive impulses into the CNS.[9] The similarity of analgesia produced by opioids, nitrous oxide, and ketamine suggests a common mode of action.[3,56] Cross-tolerance to the analgesic effect of morphine and nitrous oxide, as well as the ability to block nitrous oxide analgesia with the opioid antagonist naloxone, indicates that nitrous oxide may release endogenous morphinelike substances.[60] That the endogenous opioid system cannot be invoked as a mechanism of anesthesia generally is demonstrated by the failure of naloxone to block the analgesic action of several anesthetics and the anesthetic action of nitrous oxide (as well as other drugs).[32,47]

Recent research has demonstrated that both α_1- and α_2-adrenergic receptor activation is involved in the analgesic action of nitrous oxide. Indeed, blockade of either α_1 receptors by prazosin or α_2 receptors by yohimbine negates the analgesic effect of nitrous oxide in animals.[41] A possible sequence of events underlying nitrous oxide (and ketamine) analgesia is as follows: (1) nitrous oxide inhibition of NMDA receptors[24]; (2) release of endogenous opioid neurotransmitters[60]; (3) activation of descending norepinephrine pathways[62]; (3) activation of α-adrenergic receptors in the spinal cord[41]; and (4) inhibition of the classical nociceptive pathways. The analgesic action of isoflurane and clonidine may also be explained by their ability to stimulate α_2 receptors.[29]

Behavioral Manifestations of Anesthesia

Progressive depression

In 1920, Guedel[19] divided the course of ether anesthesia into a sequence of four stages and further subdivided the third, or surgical, stage into four planes (Figure 17-3). Each of these stages and planes represented a progressive and deepening depression of the CNS. In modern anesthesiology, these observations are no longer used in their entirety because the anesthetic signs are obscured by the presence of other drugs used before and during the anesthetic period and because different anesthetics create different patterns of responses. Nevertheless, Guedel's scheme is useful in describing some of the effects caused by various anesthetic drugs. The classic stages of anesthesia, as described by Guedel, are stage I, analgesia; stage II, delirium; stage III, surgical anesthesia (planes 1, 2, 3, and 4); and stage IV, medullary paralysis.

Stage I starts with the beginning of anesthetic administration and ends with the loss of consciousness. The patient is unresponsive to mild pain-provoking stimuli and is able to respond to verbal commands. This stage is followed by delirium in stage II, during which uncontrolled movements, retching, and laryngospasm can occur. It is desirable to traverse this stage rapidly; propofol or thiopental is often given intravenously to bypass this stage and induce anesthesia immediately. Stage III has been subdivided, as indicated previously, into four planes in order of increasing depth of anesthesia by using a variety of indexes, including the diameter of the pupil; loss of ocular, oropharyngeal, and other reflexes; muscle relaxation; depth and regularity of respiration; and separation of the thoracic and abdominal (diaphragmatic) phases of respiration. Stage IV begins with the disappearance of the purely diaphragmatic respiration of stage III plane 4 and ends with complete respiratory and circulatory collapse, culminating in death if the anesthetic is not discontinued and the patient given support for the cardiopulmonary systems.

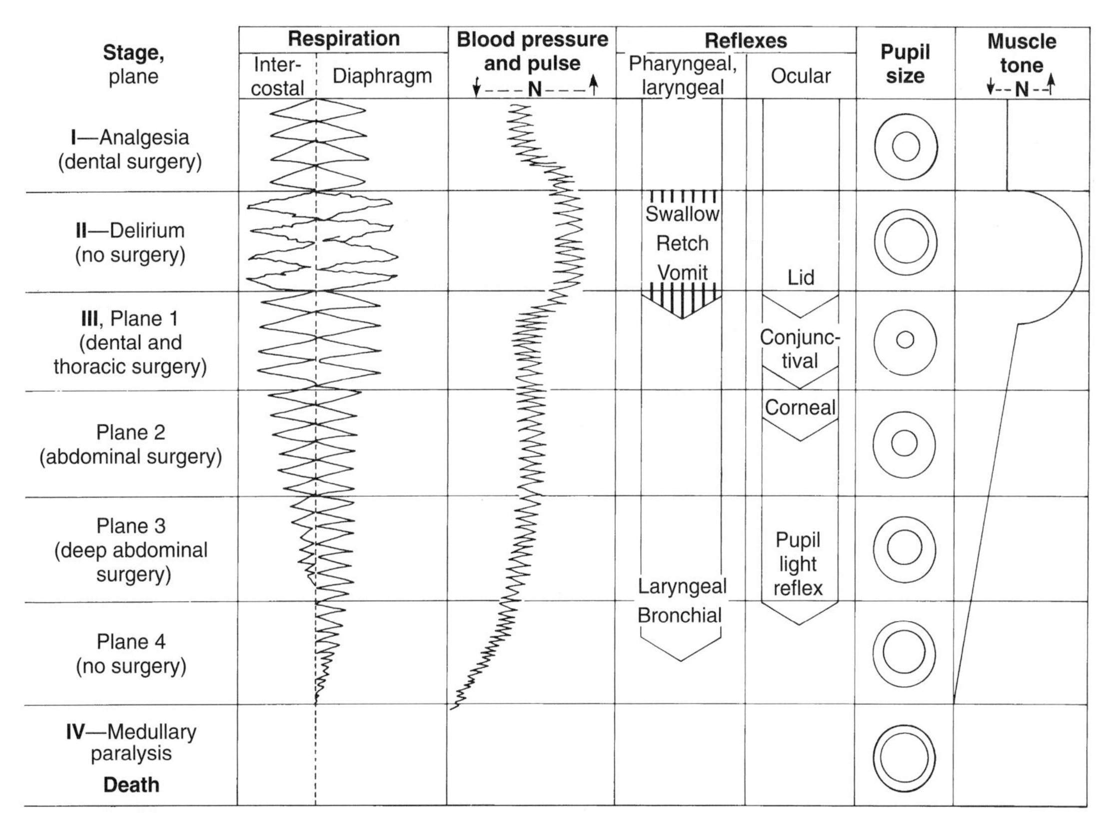

Fig. 17-3 Guedel's scheme of progressive CNS depression produced by the anesthetic ether. Changes in physiologic functions are shown for the different stages and planes of Guedel's classification. Examples of surgery that can be performed at these anesthetic levels are given in *parentheses*.

The recovery from general anesthesia is the reverse of the process of induction. The patient progressively regains reflexes, and a short period of excitement similar to that previously encountered during stage II may occur, followed by emergence to consciousness with residual analgesia.

Whereas the stages of anesthesia can be useful in a descriptive sense, the further subdivision of the surgical stage into planes is no longer useful. Anesthetic agents currently used do not produce the same pattern of concentration-dependent changes in autonomic, motor, and reflex activity observed with ether, and many adjunctive drugs used during anesthesia tend to obscure these same signs. For instance, muscular relaxation can hardly be used to gauge the depth of anesthesia if a neuromuscular blocking agent has been administered, and the arterial blood pressure cannot be useful if an adrenergic amine has been given to prevent hypotension. Nevertheless, indexes of autonomic function, such as progressive lowering of blood pressure and alterations in heart rate, can be valuable guides to the patient's status during anesthesia in the absence of medications that specifically obscure these functions.

In modern anesthesiology, the depth of anesthesia is to some extent determined by the needs of surgery. Because there is a diversity of purposes in surgery, along with a variety of types of anesthetic agents, an assessment of the desirable depth of anesthesia is made for each type of procedure. For example, if the procedure necessitates a bloodless field, as in plastic surgery, halothane may be used for its hypotensive properties. The end point of anesthesia becomes the production of hypotension, and other indexes of depth, such as respiratory movements, have little direct bearing on the choice of anesthetic depth for the surgical procedure.

The effects of anesthetic agents depend on both the degree of sensory input and the dose of the anesthetic used. After surgical stimulation, the respiratory and cardiovascular systems tend to be less depressed, and the patient can appear to be in a lighter plane of anesthesia than the injected dose or inspired concentration would indicate.

Selective depression

In general, the volatile anesthetic agents follow Guedel's scheme of progressive anesthesia. Certain discrepancies noted with these agents as well as experience with injectable drugs (e.g., ketamine), however, make clear the fact that surgical anesthesia is not synonymous with generalized CNS depression.[57] A quantitative autoradiographic analysis of brain glucose metabolism graphically demonstrates this point.[21] Whereas thiopental reduced metabolic activity throughout the rat brain in vivo, etomidate selectively depressed the forebrain, and ketamine had a mixed effect, inhibiting some areas but more strongly stimulating others, such as the hippocampus. This work and complementary neurophysiologic investigations[58] indicate that amnesia and a loss of responsiveness to painful stimuli can occur with or without comprehensive CNS depression. In the latter case, the psychomotor unresponsiveness of surgical anesthesia apparently devolves from a functional disorganization of the activated neurons' interactions with one another. Although motor output may be enhanced, as demonstrated by muscular rigidity, coordinated motor activity is gone, resulting in an unresponsive surgical patient.

UPTAKE AND DISTRIBUTION OF INHALATION ANESTHETICS

The depth of anesthesia produced by an inhalation anesthetic depends on the concentration of the anesthetic agent in the brain. The speed of induction and the speed of recovery follow the rate at which the concentration of the agent changes in the brain. During induction, the gas must move from the anesthetic apparatus to the pulmonary alveoli, from the alveoli to the blood, and from the blood to the brain. On termination of anesthesia, the inhaled gas moves in the opposite direction across the same interfaces. The principal force governing this movement of anesthetic gas is the diffusion or concentration gradient, and the behavior of the gases as they move from one compartment to another across biologic interfaces is defined by two gas laws. *Dalton's law* deals with the partial pressure (or tension) of gases and states that in a mixture the partial pressure of each component gas is directly related to its concentration in the mixture. *Henry's law* describes the solubility of gases in liquids and states that the quantity that will dissolve in a liquid is proportional to the partial pressure of that gas in direct contact with the liquid.

The partition coefficient is an expression of the relative solubility of a substance in two immiscible phases. When applied to anesthetic gases, it compares the relative amount of gas dissolved in one phase when one part is present in the other phase. Thus the blood/gas partition coefficient of 2.5 for halothane indicates that 2.5 parts of halothane are dissolved in blood for every part contained in an equal volume of alveolar air. These relationships are shown schematically in Figure 17-4.

As was mentioned earlier, during induction the various compartments of the body are brought into equilibrium regarding the inhaled anesthetic gas. When equilibrium is reached, the tensions of the anesthetic gas in the inspired air, alveolar air, arterial blood, body tissues, and mixed venous blood will be equal, but the concentrations will vary in concert with the relative solubility of the agent in each compartment. The speed with which equilibrium is achieved is influenced by a number of variables, and each of these is considered below, particularly regarding how it affects the alveolar concentration.

The alveolar concentration of an inhalation anesthetic is of pivotal importance to the onset of anesthesia. Because the

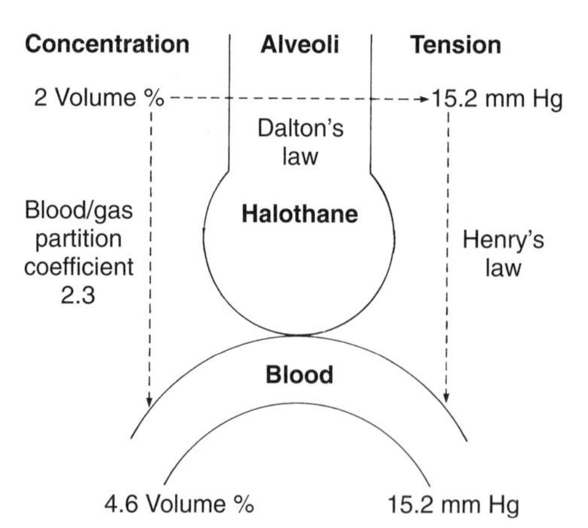

Fig. 17-4 Effect of the blood/gas partition coefficient and the tension (partial pressure) exerted by halothane, 2% (by volume), in the inspired air. Across the top of the diagram is the statement of Dalton's law that 2% (by volume) of halothane will exert 15.2 mm Hg pressure (0.02×760 mm Hg = 15.2 mm Hg) at 1 atmosphere pressure. Application of Henry's law indicates that, at equilibrium, the tension of the gas in the inspired air will equal the tension of the gas in the blood *(right)*, but the concentration dissolved in the blood will be the product of the concentration in the air and the blood/gas partition coefficient (2% [by volume] $\times$ 2.5 = 5.0% [by volume], *left*).

brain is extremely well perfused, the tension of an inhaled anesthetic in the brain closely follows that of the arterial blood, which itself is equilibrated with the alveolar tension as the blood passes through the pulmonary microvasculature. Within broad limits, anything that increases delivery of anesthetic to the alveoli, and thus *increases* its partial pressure, will *hasten* anesthesia, and anything that enhances its removal from the lungs—in other words, anything that increases overall systemic uptake—will *lower* its alveolar partial pressure and *delay* anesthesia. Mathematically, the factors governing the alveolar concentration (F_A) of an anesthetic gas during induction can be approximated as follows:

$$\Delta F_A \approx (F_i - F_A) \times V_A - \lambda \times Q \times (P_A - P_V)/P_B$$

where ΔF_A is the change in alveolar concentration, F_i the inspired concentration, V_A the minute alveolar ventilation, λ the blood/gas partition coefficient, Q the cardiac output, P_A and P_V the arterial and venous tensions, respectively, and P_B the barometric pressure. The function $(P_A - P_V)/P_B$ represents the gradient for diffusion and approaches zero as the body becomes equilibrated with the inspired gas. At that point, $\Delta F_A = 0$ and $F_i = F_A$.

Concentration in Inspired Air

The greater the concentration of the anesthetic gas in the inspired air, the more rapid will be the induction. This inspired tension normally is not held constant during induction. With irritating agents such as isoflurane, the tension is raised slowly. With sevoflurane, which is nonirritating, or in situations in which acceleration of the speed of induction is desired, the concentration at the outset may be two to three times what it will be during the maintenance phase of anesthetic administration. This technique, sometimes referred to as *overpressurization*, is analogous to administering a loading dose of drug, as is discussed in Chapter 2.

Ventilation Rate and Depth

The greater the ventilation of the lungs, the more anesthetic is delivered to the alveoli and thence to the brain, resulting in a more rapid induction. This factor is most significant during the initial phase of induction when the air of the lungs is mixing with, and being replaced by, the inspired gases. As the primary physiologic variable influencing the delivery of anesthetic to the lung, it is also important in replacing gas removed from the alveoli by the pulmonary circulation. In this regard, alveolar ventilation is of less importance with insoluble agents such as nitrous oxide and desflurane, which achieve high (near equilibrium) blood tensions rapidly, than it is with the more soluble drugs such as halothane, which equilibrate with the blood more slowly. In patients who are breathing spontaneously, high concentrations of inhalation anesthetics can decrease anesthetic uptake by inhibiting ventilatory drive. This action can help protect against overmedication during induction when overpressurization is being used.

Concentration and Second Gas Effects

The *concentration effect* occurs when nitrous oxide, a relatively nonpotent anesthetic, is administered in high concentrations (e.g., 75%) during induction of general anesthesia. Initially, nitrous oxide is taken up rapidly by the pulmonary circulation. This uptake would create a vacuum in the lungs were it not for the fact that fresh gas flows into the alveoli to replace the absorbed nitrous oxide. The net result is that alveolar ventilation is effectively increased, and the alveolar concentration rises more rapidly than would otherwise be the case.

With potent drugs given in lower concentrations (e.g., 2% to 5%), the concentration effect is negligible. However, if the anesthetic is administered along with nitrous oxide, then it too will be delivered to the alveoli in increased amounts as gas rushes inward to replace the nitrous oxide absorbed by pulmonary blood. This phenomenon is called the *second gas effect*. Oxygen delivery to the lungs is also enhanced during induction of anesthesia by the second gas effect when nitrous oxide is administered in high concentrations.

Solubility in Blood

Blood solubility is a major factor in the rate of induction of anesthesia. Solubility is generally expressed as the blood/gas partition coefficient, which, as previously mentioned, is the ratio of the concentration of the anesthetic gas in arterial blood to that in the alveolar air at 37° C at a time when the partial pressures in the two compartments are the same. The anesthetic gases are generally divided into three groups: agents of low solubility in blood (desflurane, nitrous oxide), those of intermediate solubility (e.g., halothane, isoflurane), and those of high solubility (methoxyflurane, ether). The blood/gas partition coefficients for the respective anesthetics are shown in Table 17-1. If an agent is poorly soluble in blood, as is true of nitrous oxide and desflurane, only a small percentage of it will be removed from the alveolar air before an equilibrium

Table • 17-1

Some Properties of Inhalation Anesthetics

ANESTHETIC	BLOOD/GAS PARTITION COEFFICIENT*	BRAIN/BLOOD PARTITION COEFFICIENT	FAT/BLOOD PARTITION COEFFICIENT	MAC (%)†
Desflurane	0.45	1.3	27	6
Nitrous oxide	0.47	1.1	2.3	104
Sevoflurane	0.65	1.7	48	2.05
Isoflurane	1.4	1.6	45	1.15
Enflurane	1.8	1.4	36	1.68
Halothane	2.5	1.9	51	0.75
Ether	12	1.1	3.7	1.92
Methoxyflurane	13	1.4	38	0.16

*All coefficients are taken at 37° C.
†*MAC* is defined as that alveolar concentration (in volume %) of a gas necessary to prevent a skeletal muscle response to a standard surgical stimulus in 50% of patients.

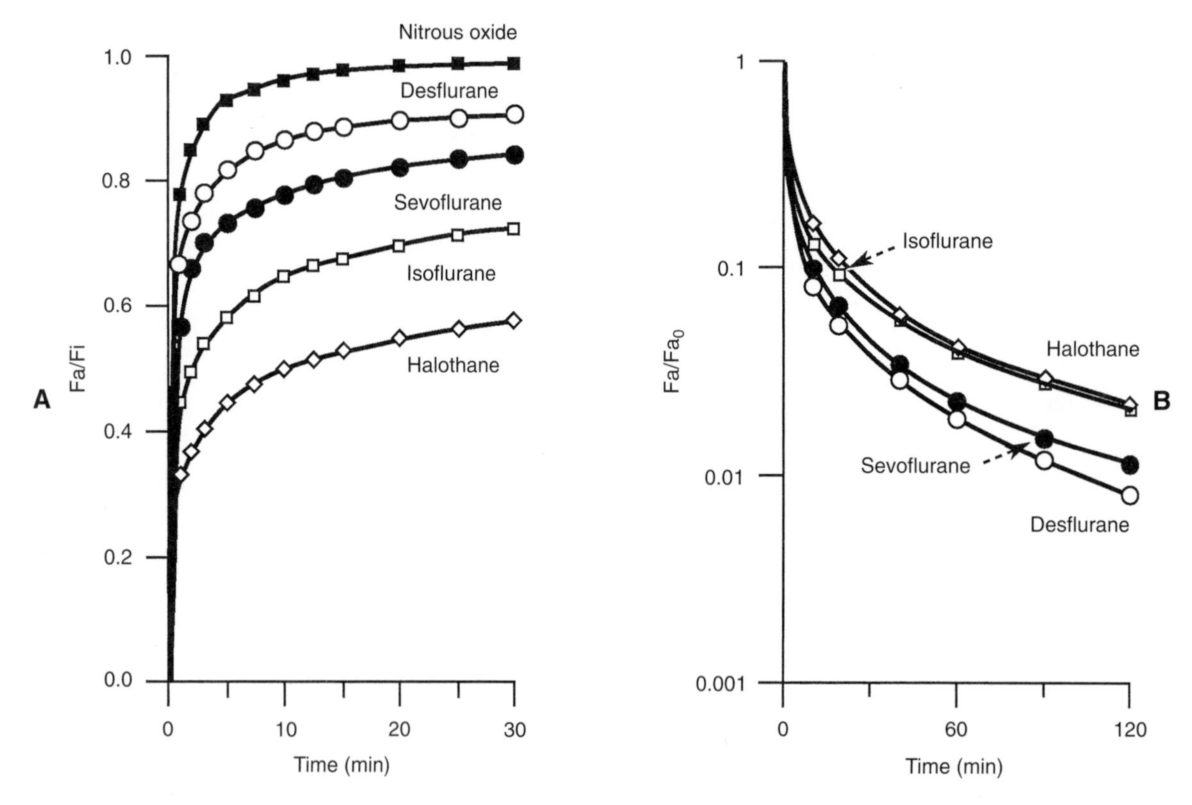

Fig. 17-5 Rate of change of alveolar anesthetic tension during induction (**A**) and recovery (**B**). For induction, the ratio of the alveolar tension *(Fa)* to the inspired tension *(Fi)* is plotted against the time of drug administration. For recovery, the ratio of Fa to the Fa at the end of drug administration *(Fa_0)* is plotted against the time after termination of anesthesia. (Adapted from Yasuda N, Lockhart SH, Eger EI II, et al: Comparison of kinetics of sevoflurane and isoflurane in humans, *Anesth Analg* 72:316-324, 1991.)

between arterial blood and alveolar air is reached. Thus the attainment of anesthetic concentrations in the brain will be rapid and the induction phase short. With agents of very high blood solubility, such as ether, large fractions of gas will be removed from the alveolar air, and relatively large amounts will have to be delivered from the inspired air. Therefore the alveolar tension will rise slowly, and induction will be similarly slow. Agents of intermediate solubility obviously will have an induction time somewhat slower than that of nitrous oxide and somewhat faster than that of ether. The rate of change of alveolar tension for some common anesthetic agents during both induction and emergence is shown in Figure 17-5.

Inasmuch as recovery or emergence is essentially a reversal of the process of induction, those anesthetics that are insoluble in blood will leave the blood very rapidly after the anesthetic gas is removed from the inspired air, and recovery will be very rapid. Conversely, recovery is slow with ether. High solubility is not completely disadvantageous, however, because transient fluctuations of the anesthetic's concentration in the inspired air during maintenance will have little effect on the depth of anesthesia.

Cardiac Output and Blood Flow

Cardiac output influences anesthetic uptake in opposite ways. On the one hand, if the cardiac output is very high, it will remove large quantities of gas from the alveoli and lower the alveolar tension, thereby delaying the achievement of equilibrium between inspired air and arterial blood. On the other hand, a high cardiac output will deliver a greater amount of anesthetic to the tissues as a whole, thereby hastening the rate at which the body comes to equilibrium with the arterial blood. Because the brain follows the arterial partial pressure of anesthetics closely, increasing total cardiac output generally slows the induction of general anesthesia.

The tissue uptake of an anesthetic agent depends on the blood flow, the arterial gas tension, and the blood/tissue coefficient, which varies according to the amount of lipid present. As shown in Table 17-1, halothane is 1.9 times as concentrated in the brain and 51 times as concentrated in fat as it is in blood. Muscle tissue has an affinity for anesthetic agents similar to that of blood, and the ratio is approximately 1 : 1. Lipids have a high affinity for anesthetic agents, and fatty tissues therefore act as a reservoir for anesthetic gases.

The uptake of anesthetic gases proceeds sequentially into three main compartments of the body, based on differences in vascularity and lipid content of the tissues. Initially, the most active compartment is the vessel-rich group (VRG), consisting of the heart, liver, kidneys, lungs, and brain. As previously stated, equilibration between blood and brain is usually very rapid because the brain receives a large share of the cardiac output and because the brain/blood coefficient is relatively low (see Table 17-1). Nitrous oxide is initially absorbed into the VRG compartment at a rate of up to 1 L/min for the first 10 to 15 minutes. The uptake drops to less than 0.5 L/min over the next 1 to 1½ hours, during which time the anesthetic fills the muscle compartment. If anesthetic administration is continued beyond this time, the uptake rate drops still further (to less than 0.1 L/min) until the fat group of tissues is equilibrated. The sequence of halothane uptake is similar to that of nitrous oxide, except that considerably more time is needed for equilibration of each compartment.

In patients who are mechanically ventilated, high concentrations of anesthetic may hasten anesthesia by inhibiting cardiac output. During induction, this effect increases the danger of overmedication when overpressurization is being used.

ELIMINATION AND METABOLISM OF ANESTHETIC GASES

The same factors that determine the uptake of anesthetic gas and the rate of induction are also important during the elimination phase. This process is initiated by the removal of the gas from the inspired air mixture, so that the inspired air tension of anesthetic gas falls to zero. When this happens, the anesthetic begins to diffuse from the blood through the alveoli, and as the blood tension falls, there is a fall in tissue tension. The less soluble the agent, the more completely and quickly the anesthetic is removed from the blood and tissues and the more rapid is the recovery.

Although Figure 17-5 would seem to suggest that recovery is a near mirror image of induction, several important differences do exist. For instance, the delivery of anesthetic to the lungs is not under the control of the clinician but is a function of the cardiopulmonary status of the patient. Also, a number of differences arise because anesthesia is normally terminated well before equilibrium with the inspired gas is attained in the various tissue compartments, at least for anesthetics other than nitrous oxide. Often muscle and fat continue to absorb anesthetic from blood and the VRG for some time after administration has ceased. A possible outcome of this redistribution is a relatively rapid recovery from short anesthetic courses. Nevertheless, the high fat/blood partition coefficients of most agents indicate that anesthetic retention may last for many hours and that recovery from prolonged anesthesia can be delayed. A final disparity between induction and recovery is the influence of metabolism. It was long believed that inhalation anesthetics were eliminated through the lungs without any metabolic transformation. It is now recognized, however, that most agents are biotransformed in the liver, some quite extensively. From 20% to 40% of administered halothane is metabolized in human beings to trifluoroacetic acid, Cl^-, and Br^-.[50] Because the enzymes responsible for this metabolism are capacity limited, this percentage may increase during the recovery phase, hastening emergence from anesthesia. Approximately 50% of methoxyflurane is metabolized, resulting in plasma F^- concentrations that can cause nephrotoxicity, severely limiting the use of this drug.[61]

CHEMICAL PROPERTIES OF INHALATION ANESTHETICS

The wide diversity of chemical substances capable of producing the anesthetic state precludes any uniform statements regarding their chemical properties. Although a number of drugs can produce general anesthesia, the volatile liquids or gases are often preferred because the administration by inhalation permits rapid and precise control of the dose.

None of the current halogenated anesthetics or the obsolete agents chloroform and trichloroethylene present a flammability or explosion hazard under normal circumstances. Ether, however, is flammable and explosive. Cyclopropane, a three-carbon cyclic hydrocarbon, is a highly explosive gas. The only inorganic anesthetic in use, nitrous oxide, is not flammable but will support combustion of other substances.

Other chemical reactions besides fire and explosion can occur with anesthetic agents. Chloroform in the presence of high temperature or flame will be converted to phosgene, an extremely toxic, irritating gas. Trichloroethylene is decomposed by soda lime used to absorb carbon dioxide in closed systems; the resultant product is both toxic and explosive. Sevoflurane also breaks down on exposure to carbon dioxide absorbents, yielding fluoromethyl-2,2-difluoro-1-(trifluoromethyl)vinyl ether, more simply known as *compound A*. Although there is little evidence of human toxicity, some question remains regarding prolonged exposure to high concentrations of compound A. Ether, when exposed to air (oxygen) and light, forms peroxides that lower the ignition temperature for the anesthetic. Brass and aluminum are subject to corrosion when exposed to halothane and water. Finally, the volatile inhalation agents are absorbed in soda lime and in the rubber or plastic connections used in the administration system and are difficult to leach out of the anesthetic circuit.

PHARMACOLOGIC EFFECTS OF INHALATION ANESTHETICS

The pharmacology of individual anesthetic agents is covered in Chapter 18. Included here for discussion are the major effects common to inhalation anesthetics in general.

Cardiovascular System

All inhalation agents depress myocardial contractility; the extent is related to the potency of the particular agent used, its concentration, and the duration of anesthesia. As a group, the halogenated anesthetics are the worst offenders in affecting contractility as well as in sensitizing the automaticity and conducting properties of the myocardium to norepinephrine and epinephrine. Cardiac rates are variably influenced, and the anesthetic effects are often masked by the preoperative administration of atropine or glycopyrrolate, both of which block activity of the vagus nerve. Agents that can directly excite the discharge of the sympathoadrenal axis are ether, nitrous oxide, cyclopropane, desflurane, and possibly isoflurane. Other agents may indirectly cause discharge by depressing respiration or arterial blood pressure. Baroreceptor function, as measured by a change in heart rate in response to a vasoactive drug, is generally depressed.

Inhalation agents tend to decrease peripheral vascular resistance, although nitrous oxide may increase it mildly and the effect of halothane is mild in concentrations up to 3 MAC. When it was in widespread use, cyclopropane was preferred for patients in shock states because of its minimal effect on vascular smooth muscle. Isoflurane, on the other hand, strongly relaxes vascular smooth muscle, producing a hypotension that can be useful in procedures such as surgical repair of an intracranial aneurysm.

Respiration

The effect of most anesthetics on the respiratory centers in the brain is depression; the amount of respiratory depression is related to the type and amount or concentration of anesthetic used. Respiratory depression with inhalation anesthetics, measured by decreased medullary responsiveness to carbon dioxide tensions, is associated with a progressive decline in tidal volume. This effect is accompanied by a pronounced increase in respiratory rate. The most sensitive component of respiration to inhalation anesthetics is the ventilatory response to hypoxemia. Peripheral chemoreceptors that normally respond to low oxygen tensions are strongly inhibited by concentrations as low as 0.1 MAC and become completely inoperative during general anesthesia.

Hypercarbia resulting from depressed ventilatory exchange excites the sympathoadrenal system, thereby causing a release of catecholamines. When breathing is impaired, increased oxygen tensions or mechanical respiratory assistance may be necessary.

Liver

Liver function tests indicate that almost all inhalation anesthetic agents cause some alterations in hepatic function. In most cases the effects are reversible and not serious. Halothane, however, has been associated with serious hepatic necrosis, especially if the patient has had prior anesthesia with halothane or has preexisting liver disease. There is evidence that a reactive metabolite, trifluoroacetyl chloride, combines with hepatic proteins to form antigens that can trigger a fulminant allergic reaction.[23]

Kidney

General anesthetics depress glomerular filtration and urine output by reducing renal blood flow. Fortunately, these alterations in renal function are transitory and readily reversible. The release of F^- from certain halogenated anesthetics (especially methoxyflurane) has occasionally produced serious renal damage.

Skeletal Muscle

Although most general anesthetics produce muscle relaxation by their actions on spinal cord and brainstem motor reflex centers, the volatile anesthetic agents have an additional effect on the neuromuscular junction. Ether is most prominent in this respect and can produce sufficient muscle relaxation by itself for surgical procedures. Even agents with a lesser degree of action, such as enflurane and isoflurane, can decrease the dose of a neuromuscular blocker by up to 65%. Cholinesterase inhibition by neostigmine does not antagonize this effect as it does for such nondepolarizing blocking agents as tubocurarine and vecuronium.

ADMINISTRATION OF ANESTHETIC GASES

Various delivery systems have been used since the inception of anesthesia, and these range from simple techniques such as the open-drop method on a face mask or nose cone to anesthetic machines that incorporate a considerable number of technical devices. Figure 17-6 illustrates the major components of modern delivery systems, including the nonrebreathing system used for nitrous oxide administration in dentistry, and the circle system commonly used in the hospi-

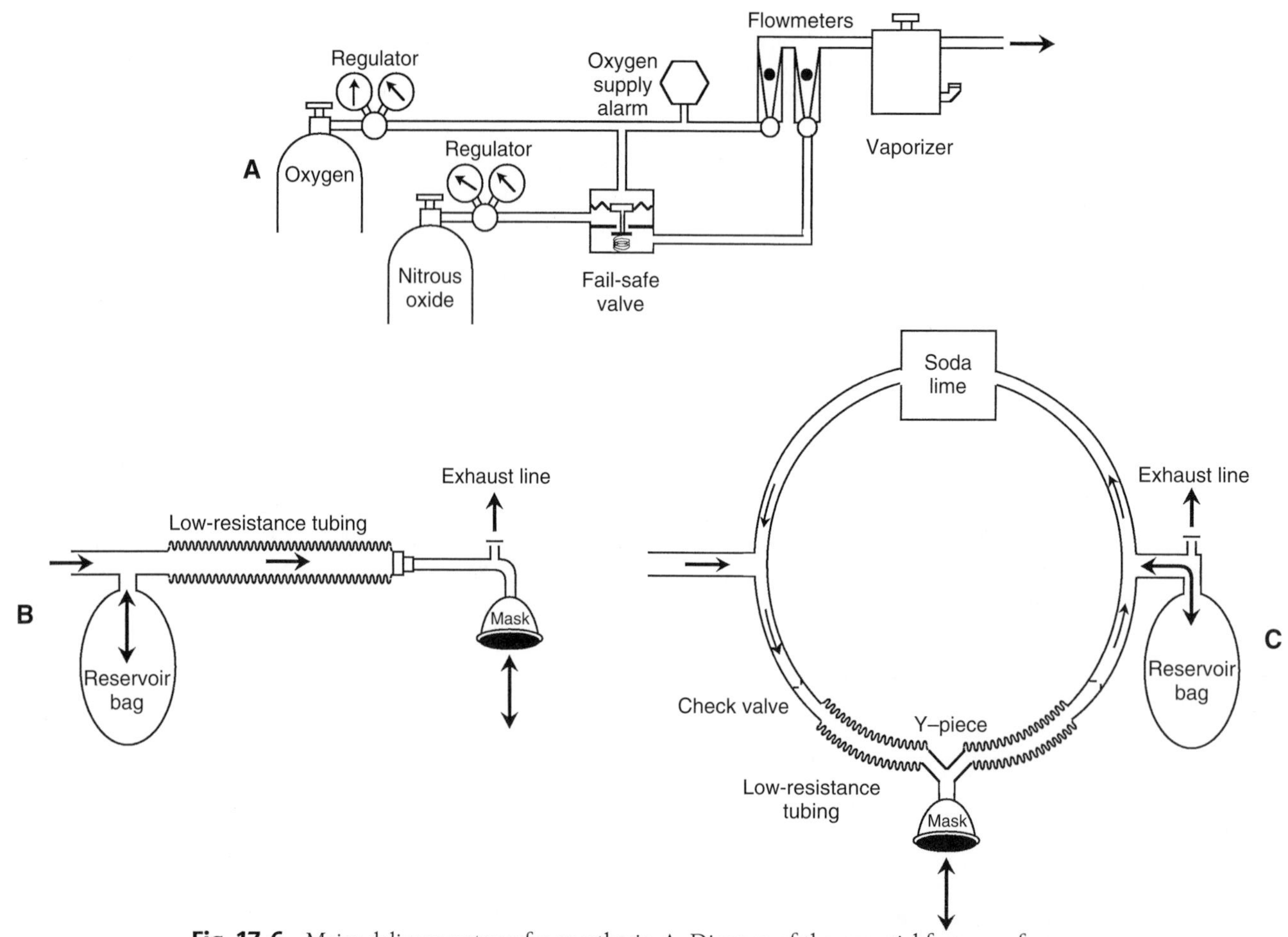

Fig. 17-6 Major delivery systems for anesthesia. **A,** Diagram of the essential features of an anesthesia machine. A dedicated nitrous oxide-oxygen machine lacks the vaporizer. **B,** Mapleson A (or Magill) anesthetic circuit. Rebreathing of exhaled gas in the spontaneously ventilating patient does not occur if the fresh gas flow is at least 100% of the minute ventilation. **C,** Circle system anesthetic circuit. Partial or full rebreathing is made possible by the removal of exhaled carbon dioxide (as with soda lime).

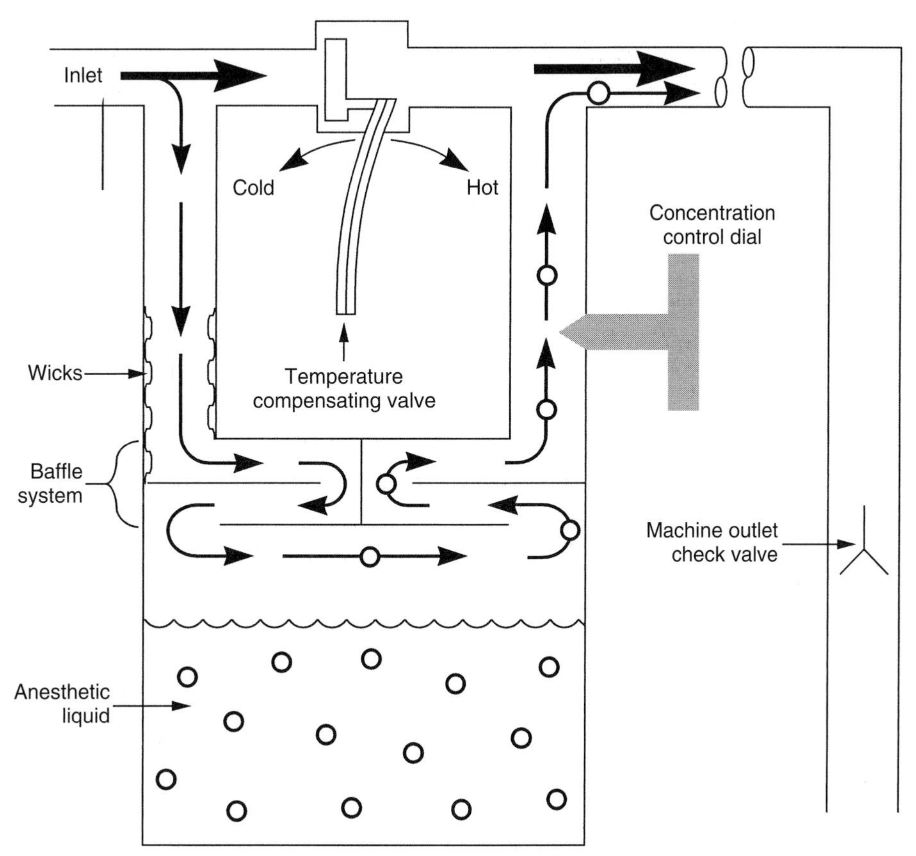

Fig. 17-7 Temperature-compensated, variable-bypass vaporizer. (Redrawn from Andrews JJ, Brockwell RC: Delivery systems for inhaled anesthetics. In Barash PG, Cullen BF, Stoelting RK, eds: *Clinical anesthesia*, ed 4, Philadelphia, 2001, Lippincott Williams & Wilkins.)

tal in which the patient rebreathes at least a portion of the exhaled gas.

Anesthesia delivery systems incorporate the following features: (1) gases, including oxygen, stored in either local tanks or a central delivery system; (2) regulators to control the pressure of gases delivered; (3) safety systems that warn of dangerous pressures and shut off flow if oxygen delivery is interrupted; (4) mixing valves (adjustable flowmeters) to regulate the percentages of gases; (5) vaporizers to volatilize anesthetic liquids; (6) carbon dioxide absorber system (not required for nonrebreathing systems); (7) reservoir bag, ventilator, or both; (8) assorted tubing and one-way valve systems; (9) face mask, laryngeal mask, or endotracheal tube; and (10) exhaust line.

Central to the administration of volatile general anesthetics is the temperature-compensated, variable-bypass vaporizer (Figure 17-7). This device provides the simple selection of anesthetic concentration because it automatically compensates for changes in total gas flow and for changes in the ambient temperature. In the case of desflurane, which volatilizes at 23° C, the vaporizer must be heated to ensure adequate, controlled delivery.

Several considerations in the administration of anesthetic gases in modern anesthesiology should be mentioned. First, whereas some older agents (e.g., ether and cyclopropane) were highly effective, certain deficits caused their abandonment in favor of newer agents, such as isoflurane, which do not share the same problems. In particular, the explosive character of cyclopropane has caused its use to be banned. Second, some of the newer agents, such as desflurane, are expensive, so closed systems for their administration are favored. Third, retrospective surveys and animal studies have provided evidence that operating room personnel (surgeons, anesthesiologists, nurses) and dentists who use nitrous oxide in their offices may be adversely affected by trace amounts of anesthetics in the operatory. Specifically, exposed health care workers reported a higher incidence of hepatic, renal, and neurologic disorders; increased congenital malformations in children born to exposed women; and increased spontaneous abortions in exposed women and wives of exposed men.[4,5] Animal studies indicate that nitrous oxide is the agent of major concern and that the threshold concentration of nitrous oxide for producing a biologic response is approximately 500 to 1000 ppm.[54] Although retrospective studies that used examination of public health registries in Sweden[12] and in Finland[20] could find no link between working in an operating room (and/or being exposed to anesthetic gases) and increased risk of miscarriage or congenital malformation, Rowland et al have linked reproductive toxicity in dental assistants to nitrous oxide exposure of more than 3 to 5 hours per week.[44,45] Most authorities therefore favor rebreathing systems in conjunction with scavenger exhaust systems and ventilation systems that remove leaked anesthetic gases from the vicinity of the patient.[1,55] Because many dentists function as both anesthetist and surgeon, the nonrebreathing flow machine is most commonly used. Its simplicity of operation and compatibility with conscious sedation, however, has the major disadvantage of exposing operatory personnel to high concentrations of anesthetic gases (i.e., nitrous oxide) unless a concerted effort is made to minimize pollution, as is outlined in Box 17-1. The National Institute for Occupational Safety and Health has prepared a monograph to assist dentists in minimizing exposure to nitrous oxide in the workplace.[39]

Box • 17-1

Steps To Reduce Nitrous Oxide Exposure

Facility and Equipment Preparation

- Purchase scavenging nitrous oxide delivery systems with air sweeper capabilities.
- Check plumbing for leaks by pressure retention of closed system.
- Check all fittings for leaks with disclosing solution or nitrous oxide analyzer.
- Ensure exhaust system vents to the outside away from air intake.
- Maximize room air circulation.
- Consider use of a local exhaust system.

Daily Use

- Adjust vacuum setting to manufacturer's maximum recommended value.
- Place hood on nose before administering nitrous oxide.
- Adjust flow to patient's minute respiratory volume.
- Instruct patient to exhale through nose.
- Instruct patient not to talk.
- Consider using rubber dam.
- Use suction when mouth is open.
- Administer 100% oxygen for 3 to 5 minutes before removing hood.

Monitoring

- Inspect delivery apparatus each day of use.
- Periodically monitor exposure by passive dosimetry or nitrous oxide analyzer.
- Record monitoring results.

CITED REFERENCES

1. Adams D, Allen GD, Scaramella J: Modifying nitrous oxide analgesia circuits to reduce pollution in the dental operatory, *Anesth Prog* 23:176-180, 1976.
2. Alkire MT, Haier RJ, Fallon JH: Toward a unified theory of narcosis: brain imaging evidence for a thalamocortical switch as the neurophysiologic basis of anesthetic-induced unconsciousness, *Conscious Cogn* 9:370-386, 2000.
3. Berkowitz BA, Finck AD, Ngai SH: Nitrous oxide analgesia: reversal by naloxone and development of tolerance, *J Pharmacol Exp Ther* 203:539-547, 1977.
4. Chenoweth MB: Inhalation anesthetics, *Fed Proc* 37:2501-2503, 1978.
5. Cohen EN, Gift HC, Brown BW, et al: Occupational disease in dentistry and chronic exposure to trace anesthetic gases, *J Am Dent Assoc* 101:21-31, 1980.
6. Cohen PJ: The reticular activating system revisited, *Anesthesiology* 39:1-2, 1973.
7. Cohen S, Goldschmid A, Shtacher G, et al: The inhalation convulsants: a pharmacodynamic approach, *Mol Pharmacol* 11:379-385, 1975.
8. Darbinjan TM, Golovchinsky VB, Plehotkina SI: The effects of anesthetics on reticular and cortical activity, *Anesthesiology* 34:219-229, 1971.
9. de Jong RH, Robles R, Morikawa K-I: Actions of halothane and nitrous oxide on dorsal horn neurons ("the spinal gate"), *Anesthesiology* 31:205-212, 1969.
10. Dilger JP, Vidal AM, Mody HI, et al: Evidence for direct actions of general anesthetics on an ion channel protein. A new look at a unified mechanism of action, *Anesthesiology* 81:431-442, 1994.
11. Eger EI II, Brandstater B, Saidman LJ, et al: Equipotent alveolar concentrations of methoxyflurane, halothane, diethyl ether, fluroxene, cyclopropane, xenon, and nitrous oxide in the dog, *Anesthesiology* 26:771-777, 1965.
12. Ericson HA, Kallen AJB: Hospitalization for miscarriage and delivery outcome among Swedish nurses working in operating rooms 1973-1978, *Anesth Analg* 64:981-988, 1985.
13. Evers AS: Cellular and molecular mechanisms of anesthesia. In Barash PG, Cullen BF, Stoelting RK, eds: *Clinical anesthesia*, ed 4, Philadelphia, 2001, Lippincott Williams & Wilkins.
14. Forman SA, Miller KW, Yellen G: A discrete site for general anesthetics on a postsynaptic receptor, *Mol Pharmacol* 48:574-581, 1995.
15. Franks NP, Lieb WR: Is membrane expansion relevant to anaesthesia? *Nature* 292:248-251, 1981.
16. Franks NP, Lieb WR: Mechanisms of general anesthesia, *Environ Health Perspect* 87:199-205, 1990.
17. Franks NP, Lieb WR: Molecular and cellular mechanisms of general anaesthesia, *Nature* 367:607-614, 1994.
18. French JD, Verzeano M, Magoun HW: A neural basis of the anesthetic state, *Arch Neurol Psychiatry* 69:519-529, 1953.
19. Guedel AE: *Inhalation anesthesia: a fundamental guide*, New York, 1937, Macmillan.
20. Hemminki K, Kyyronen P, Lindbohm M-L: Spontaneous abortions and malformations in the offspring of nurses exposed to anaesthetic gases, cytostatic drugs, and other potential hazards in hospitals, based on registered information of outcome, *J Epidemiol Commun Health* 39:141-147, 1985.
21. Hibbard LS, McGlone JS, Davis DW, et al: Three-dimensional representation and analysis of brain energy metabolism, *Science* 236:1641-1646, 1987.
22. Ishizawa Y, Pikdikiti R, Liebman PA, et al: G protein–coupled receptors as direct targets of inhaled anesthetics, *Mol Pharmacol* 61:945-952, 2002.
23. Isner RJ, Brown BR, Jr: Clinical pharmacology and applications of inhalational anesthetic agents. In Bowdle TA, Horita A, Kharasch ED, eds: *The pharmacologic basis of anesthesiology*, New York, 1994, Churchill Livingstone.
24. Jevtovic-Todorovic V, Todorovic SM, Mennerick S, et al: Nitrous oxide (laughing gas) is an NMDA antagonist, neuroprotectant and neurotoxin, *Nat Med* 4:460-463, 1998.
25. Johansson JS, Scharf D, Davies LA, et al: A designed four-α-helix bundle that binds the volatile general anesthetic halothane with high affinity, *Biophys J* 78:982-993, 2000.
26. Johns RA, Moscicki JC, DiFazio CA: Nitric oxide synthase inhibitor dose-dependently and reversibly reduces the threshold for halothane anesthesia, *Anesthesiology* 77:779-784, 1992.

27. Julien RM, Kavan EM: Electrographic studies of a new volatile anesthetic agent: enflurane (Ethrane), *J Pharmacol Exp Ther* 183:393-403, 1972.

28. Kendig JJ: Neuronal basis of the anaesthetic state. In Nunn JF, Utting JE, Brown BR, Jr, eds: *General anaesthesia*, ed 5, London, 1989, Butterworths.

29. Kingery WS, Agashe GS, Guo TZ, et al: Isoflurane and nociception: spinal α_{2A} adrenoceptors mediate antinociception while supraspinal α_1 adrenoceptors mediate pronociception, *Anesthesiology* 96:367-374, 2002.

30. Kitahata LM, Kosaka Y, Taub A, et al: Lamina-specific suppression of dorsal-horn unit activity by morphine sulfate, *Anesthesiology* 41:39-48, 1974.

31. Koblin DD: Mechanisms of action. In Miller RD, ed: *Anesthesia*, ed 5, New York, 2000, Churchill Livingstone.

32. Levine LL, Winter PM, Nemoto EM, et al: Naloxone does not antagonize the analgesic effects of inhalation anesthetics, *Anesth Analg* 65:330-332, 1986.

33. Lin L, Koblin DD, Wang HH: Saturable binding of anesthetics to nicotinic acetylcholine receptors: a possible mechanism of anesthetic action, *Ann NY Acad Sci* 625:628-644, 1991.

34. Maze M, Regan JW: Role of signal transduction in anesthetic action: α_2 adrenergic agonists, *Ann NY Acad Sci* 625:409-422, 1991.

35. Miller KW: General anaesthetics. In Feldman SA, Scurr CF, Paton W, eds: *Drugs in anaesthesia: mechanisms of action*, London, 1987, Edward Arnold.

36. Miller KW: Inert gas narcosis, the high pressure neurological syndrome, and the critical volume hypothesis, *Science* 185:867-869, 1974.

37. Mori K, Winters WD, Spooner CE: Comparison of reticular and cochlear multiple unit activity with auditory evoked responses during various stages induced by anesthetic agents, *Electroencephalogr Clin Neurophysiol* 24:242-248, 1968.

38. Mullins LJ: Some physical mechanisms in narcosis, *Chem Rev* 54:289-323, 1954.

39. National Institute for Occupational Safety and Health: *Hazard controls, HC3: control of nitrous oxide in dental operatories* (series title: DHHS Publication No. [NIOSH] 96-107), Cincinnati, 1996, US Department of Health and Human Services, Public Health Service, Centers for Disease Control and Prevention, National Institute for Occupational Safety and Health.

40. Nicoll RA, Madison DV: General anesthetics hyperpolarize neurons in the vertebrate central nervous system, *Science* 217:1055-1057, 1982.

41. Orii R, Ohashi Y, Guo T, et al: Evidence for the involvement of spinal cord α_1 adrenoceptors in nitrous oxide-induced antinociceptive effects in Fischer rats, *Anesthesiology* 97:458-465, 2002.

42. Perouansky M, Hemmings HC, Jr: Presynaptic actions of general anesthetics. In Antognini JE, Carstens EE, Raines DE, eds: *Neural mechanisms of anesthesia*, Totowa, NJ, 2003, Humana.

43. Pocock G, Richards CD: Cellular mechanisms of general anaesthesia, *Br J Anaesth* 6:116-128, 1991.

44. Rowland AS, Baird DD, Shore DL, et al: Nitrous oxide and spontaneous abortion in female dental assistants, *Am J Epidemiol* 141:531-538, 1995.

45. Rowland AS, Baird DD, Weinberg CR, et al: Reduced fertility among women employed as dental assistants exposed to high levels of nitrous oxide, *N Engl J Med* 327:993-997, 1992.

46. Seeman P: Anesthetics and pressure reversal of anesthesia: expansion and recompression of membrane proteins, lipids, and water, *Anesthesiology* 47:1-3, 1977.

47. Smith RA, Wilson M, Miller KW: Naloxone has no effect on nitrous oxide anesthesia, *Anesthesiology* 49:6-8, 1978.

48. Tanelian DL, Kosek P, Mody I, et al: The role of the $GABA_A$ receptor/chloride channel complex in anesthesia, *Anesthesiology* 78:757-776, 1993.

49. Taub A, Kitahata LM: Modulation of spinal-cord function by anesthesia, *Anesthesiology* 43:383-385, 1975.

50. Tinker JH, Gandolfi AJ, Van Dyke RA: Elevation of plasma bromide levels in patients following halothane anesthesia: time correlation with total halothane dosage, *Anesthesiology* 44:194-196, 1976.

51. Trudell JR: A unitary theory of anesthesia based on lateral phase separations in nerve membranes, *Anesthesiology* 46:5-10, 1977.

52. Trudell JR: Biophysical concepts in molecular mechanisms of anesthesia. In Fink BR, ed: *Molecular mechanisms of anesthesia. Progress in anesthesiology*, vol 2, New York, 1980, Raven Press.

53. Ueda I, Kamaya H: Molecular mechanisms of anesthesia, *Anesth Analg* 63:929-945, 1984.

54. Vieira E, Cleaton-Jones P, Moyes D: Effects of low intermittent concentrations of nitrous oxide on the developing rat fetus, *Br J Anaesth* 55:67-69, 1983.

55. Whitcher C, Zimmerman DC, Piziali RL: Control of occupational exposure to nitrous oxide in the oral surgery office, *J Oral Surg* 36:431-440, 1978.

56. White PF, Way WL, Trevor AJ: Ketamine—its pharmacology and therapeutic uses, *Anesthesiology* 56:119-136, 1982.

57. Winters WD: Effects of drugs on the electrical activity of the brain: anesthetics, *Annu Rev Pharmacol Toxicol* 16:413-426, 1976.

58. Winters WD, Ferrar-Allado T, Guzman-Flores C, et al: The cataleptic state induced by ketamine: a review of the neuropharmacology of anesthesia, *Neuropharmacology* 11:303-315, 1972.

59. Yamamura T, Harada K, Okamura A, et al: Is the site of action of ketamine anesthesia the N-methyl-D-aspartate receptor? *Anesthesiology* 72:704-710, 1990.

60. Yang JC, Clark WC, Ngai SH: Antagonism of nitrous oxide analgesia by naloxone in man, *Anesthesiology* 52:414-417, 1980.

61. Yoshimura N, Holaday DA, Fiserova-Bergerova V: Metabolism of methoxyflurane in man, *Anesthesiology* 44:372-379, 1976.

62. Zhang C, Davies MF, Guo T-Z, et al: The analgesic action of nitrous oxide is dependent on the release of norepinephrine in the dorsal horn of the spinal cord, *Anesthesiology* 91:1401-1407, 1999.

General References

Antognini JE, Carstens EE, Raines DE, eds: *Neural mechanisms of anesthesia,* Totowa, NJ, 2003, Humana.

Barash PG, Cullen BF, Stoelting RK, eds: *Clinical anesthesia,* ed 4, Philadelphia, 2001, Lippincott Williams & Wilkins.

Davis AB: The development of anesthesia, *Am Sci* 70:522-528, 1982.

Frost EAM: *Essays on the history of anesthesia,* Georgetown, CT, 1985, McMahon.

Longnecker DE, Murphy FL, eds: *Dripps/Eckenhoff/Vandam Introduction to anesthesia,* ed 9, Philadelphia, 1997, Saunders.

Miller RD, ed: *Anesthesia,* ed 5, New York, 2000, Churchill Livingstone.

Wolfe RJ, Menczer LF, eds: *I awaken to glory,* Canton, MA, 1994, Science History Publications/USA.

CHAPTER • 18

Agents Used in General Anesthesia, Deep Sedation, and Conscious Sedation

Daniel A. Haas and John A. Yagiela

Compounds of diverse chemical structure, including elemental gases, halogenated hydrocarbons, simple alcohols, aromatic agents, steroids, and other drugs that affect the central nervous system (CNS), can induce general anesthesia. General anesthetics are available as gases, volatile liquids, and solutions suitable for parenteral injection. When administered in lower doses, many of these same drugs may cause clinically useful sedation. This chapter describes the pharmacologic features of drugs used in general anesthesia, deep sedation, and conscious sedation. The application of these agents in dentistry, in particular for conscious sedation, is reviewed in Chapter 48.

INHALATION AGENTS

Gases and volatile liquids are the oldest known anesthetic agents and have been the most widely used. Today the only commonly used gas is nitrous oxide. Although general anesthetic agents administered by inhalation are often divided into gases and volatile liquids, there are few differences between these two classes of substances other than boiling point (Table 18-1) and solubility in various tissues (see Table 17-1). Regarding boiling point, which determines the vapor pressure of the gaseous phase, liquids need vaporizers, which are special devices used to produce and maintain an adequate amount of anesthetic in the inspired air. However, because tissue solubility (i.e., solubility in brain membranes) is normally greater with the volatile liquids, a smaller concentration of volatile agent is therefore required to produce general anesthesia. It has been suggested that an ideal inhalation anesthetic should possess a number of characteristics, as outlined in Box 18-1.[51,58]

Nitrous Oxide

Nitrous oxide is arguably the oldest general anesthetic (see Chapter 17 for a historic review of the discovery of anesthesia) and the only gaseous anesthetic still in use. Nitrous oxide is also the only inorganic substance used clinically as an anesthetic. Several features unique to nitrous oxide include a minimum alveolar concentration (MAC) greater than 100%, strong analgesic properties in subanesthetic concentrations, and minimal relaxation of skeletal muscle.

Physical and chemical properties

Nitrous oxide is a colorless, nonirritating gas with a pleasant, mild odor and taste. The structural formula is shown in Figure 18-1. Its blood/gas partition coefficient of 0.47 means that it is poorly soluble in blood. It is nonflammable but can support combustion in the absence of oxygen. It is available in pressurized steel cylinders as a liquid in equilibrium with its gas phase. As the nitrous oxide gas is delivered from the cylinder, liquid nitrous oxide spontaneously vaporizes to replace the lost gas phase. Cylinder pressure is maintained unaltered by this process until all the liquid has vaporized, at which point approximately three fourths of the contents have been released. This vaporization process requires heat, which is provided from the cylinder and the air around it, causing the tank to become cold.

Anesthetic properties

Because of its very low solubility in blood, a state of equilibrium between the alveolar and arterial tensions is quickly reached; thus induction and awakening occur very rapidly. Its primary disadvantage as a general anesthetic is its lack of potency, as reflected by its high MAC of approximately 105%. (A concentration more than the 100% value obtainable at ambient conditions is achieved by placing the subject in a hyperbaric chamber.) Nitrous oxide is incapable of producing full surgical anesthesia by itself (outside of a hyperbaric chamber) when given with adequate amounts of oxygen, and it is most commonly used as a supplement to volatile anesthetics. To ensure adequate oxygenation of the patient, nitrous oxide is normally not used at a concentration greater than 70%. When it is administered with other anesthetic agents, the maintenance concentration normally used is 50% to 70%. In dentistry, nitrous oxide is often administered in subanesthetic concentrations of 20% to 50% to provide conscious sedation and analgesia. Concentrations above this range may impair the patient's ability to maintain consciousness and lead to a greater incidence of adverse effects, such as nausea or dysphoria. At a 40% concentration, there is good hard and soft tissue analgesia. Awareness of sensory input is reduced, with the exception that sounds may seem louder and qualitatively different.[113]

When nitrous oxide is used with a more potent agent, it is possible to lower the concentration of the other drug and still achieve a more rapid induction and a shorter recovery period. This phenomenon is a reflection of the fact that the MAC of the rapidly acting nitrous oxide is additive with that of other, slower-acting inhalation anesthetics. For instance, the addition of 70% nitrous oxide, which is approximately 0.6 MAC, reduces the MAC of halothane from 0.75% to 0.29%, the MAC of enflurane from 1.68% to 0.6%, and the MAC of isoflurane from 1.15% to 0.5%, each approximately a 60% reduction. In addition, the concentration and second gas effects described in Chapter 17 can help hasten the onset of anesthesia.

Cardiovascular effects In contrast to the volatile anesthetics in current use, nitrous oxide does not usually produce

Table • 18-1

Physical Properties of Inhalation Anesthetics

AGENT	MOLECULAR WEIGHT	BOILING POINT (°C [1 atm])	VAPOR PRESSURE (mm Hg [20° C])
Nitrous oxide	44.0	–88.5	38,000 (gas)
Desflurane	168.0	22.8	669
Ether	74.1	34.6	440
Isoflurane	184.5	48.5	250
Halothane	197.4	50.2	243
Enflurane	184.5	56.5	175
Sevoflurane	200.0	58.6	157
Methoxyflurane	165.0	105	22.5

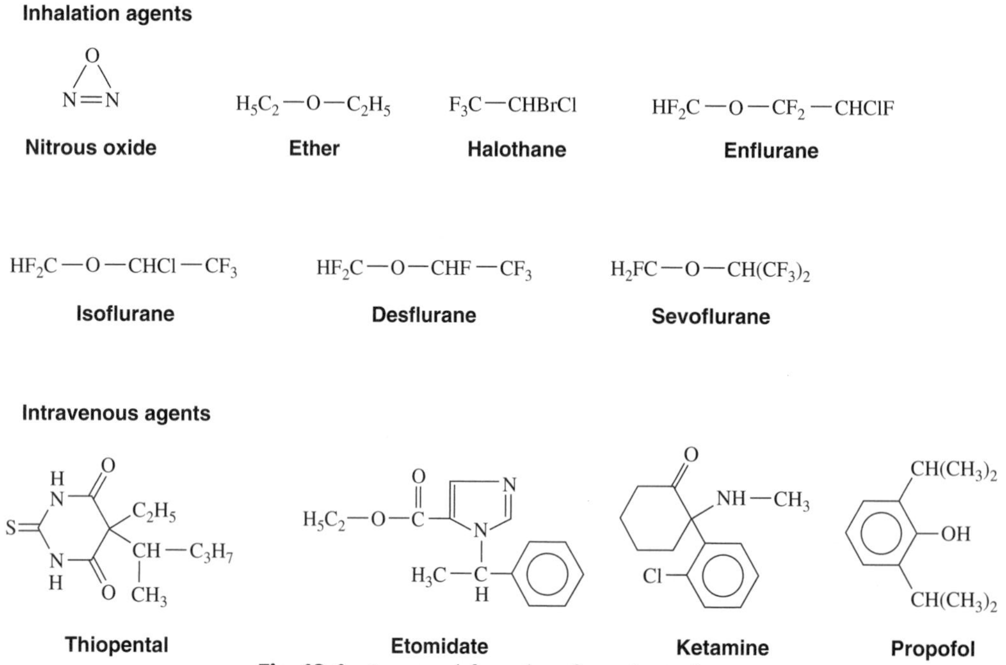

Inhalation agents

Nitrous oxide (N=N with O)

$H_5C_2—O—C_2H_5$ **Ether**

$F_3C—CHBrCl$ **Halothane**

$HF_2C—O—CF_2—CHClF$ **Enflurane**

$HF_2C—O—CHCl—CF_3$ **Isoflurane**

$HF_2C—O—CHF—CF_3$ **Desflurane**

$H_2FC—O—CH(CF_3)_2$ **Sevoflurane**

Intravenous agents

Thiopental (S, N, H, O, C_2H_5, $CH—C_3H_7$, CH_3)

Etomidate ($H_5C_2—O—C$, O, N, N, $H_3C—C$, H)

Ketamine (O, $NH—CH_3$, Cl)

Propofol ($CH(CH_3)_2$, OH, $CH(CH_3)_2$)

Fig. 18-1 Structural formulas of anesthetic drugs.

Box • 18-1

Ideal Characteristics of an Inhalation Agent

- Stable in light, alkali, and soda lime
- Nonflammable
- Highly potent, allowing use with high concentrations of oxygen
- Low solubility in blood to allow rapid induction and rapid recovery
- No or minimal biotransformation
- No toxicity
- Nonirritating to the respiratory mucosa
- Minimal cardiovascular and respiratory effects

any clinically significant cardiovascular effects. It has a weak and dose-dependent myocardial depressant effect as well as a mild sympathomimetic effect.[53] These opposing influences tend to cancel each other, leading to no change in cardiac output. Patients at increased risk of the cardiodepressant effects of nitrous oxide include those with chronic hypertension, left ventricular failure, and advanced atherosclerotic disease.

Respiratory effects Nitrous oxide is not a strong respiratory depressant (Figure 18-2), but it will decrease tidal volume and increase respiratory rate. Even so, there is likely to be less respiratory depression than would be caused by an equal depth of anesthesia induced by a single potent anesthetic drug. Although nitrous oxide has little effect on respiration in normal individuals, whose ventilation is regulated by the arterial carbon dioxide tension ($PaCO_2$), patients with severe chronic obstructive pulmonary disease whose ventilatory drive depends on the arterial oxygen tension may become severely hypoxic on exposure to even sedative concentrations of anesthetic.[123] Even if hypoxemia is prevented by the high concentration of oxygen that is being coadministered (which by itself blunts the hypoxic drive for respiration), hypoventilation and respiratory acidosis are likely outcomes.

Elimination Nitrous oxide is eliminated unchanged in the exhaled gas. However, 0.004% undergoes reductive metabolism to nitrogen in the gastrointestinal tract.

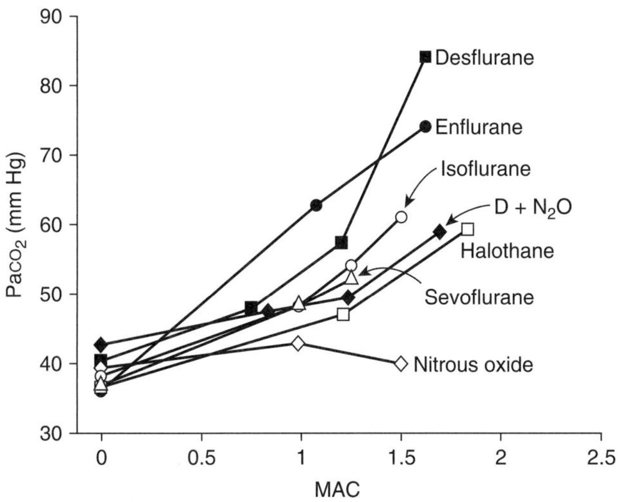

Fig. 18-2 Arterial carbon dioxide tension ($PaCO_2$) in spontaneously breathing volunteers as a function of the MAC. (Adapted from Eger EI II: Isoflurane: a review, *Anesthesiology* 55:559-576, 1981; Lockhart SH, Rampil IJ, Yasuda N, et al: Depression of ventilation by desflurane in humans, *Anesthesiology* 74:484-488, 1991; and Doi M, Ikeda K: Respiratory effects of sevoflurane, *Anesth Analg* 66:241-244, 1987.)

Adverse effects

When used for conscious sedation, nitrous oxide usually provides a feeling of relaxation, along with the possible symptoms of body warmth, tingling of the hands and feet, circumoral numbness, auditory effects, and euphoria. As the dose increases, the patient is more likely to develop adverse symptoms such as dysphoria and nausea.[30,32] Some patients may develop acute tolerance to these effects.[89]

For general anesthesia, high concentrations are used, and because its solubility in blood greatly exceeds that of nitrogen, nitrous oxide increases the volume of any enclosed air pocket in the body. There are several situations in which this property can be problematic, as with a pneumothorax or lung bullae, injection of air into the ventricles during a pneumoencephalogram, an obstructed bowel, a blocked eustachian tube (with potential damage to the tympanic membrane), or after eye surgery that uses intraocular gases. With respect to vitreoretinal surgery, such as the surgical repair of retinal detachments and macular holes, perfluoropropane or sulfurhexafluoride is introduced within the eye to act as a tamponading agent. These gases may persist in the eye for up to 3 months. Administration of general anesthesia during this interval has led to case reports of irreversible loss of vision.[41,117,124] Although not confirmed by clinical trials,[10] these case reports suggest that nitrous oxide should be avoided in patients who have had vitreoretinal surgery with intraocular gas infusion in the past 3 months.

High concentrations of nitrous oxide may also result in a considerable accumulation of dissolved gas within the body, and when the administration is stopped, large volumes of nitrous oxide diffuse from the blood into the lung alveoli, diluting oxygen. This temporary reduction in the amount of alveolar oxygen is termed *diffusion hypoxia* and can be prevented by administering 100% oxygen for 3 to 5 minutes after the cessation of nitrous oxide.

Nitrous oxide is not acutely toxic, but it can affect DNA synthesis by inducing changes in folate and amino acid metabolism. Its administration leads to an increase in homocysteine and the dietary form of folate[38] in the plasma and impaired metabolism of histidine.[64] Nitrous oxide oxidizes the cobalt atom in vitamin B_{12}, which renders inactive the vitamin B_{12}-dependent enzyme methionine synthase. Methionine synthase is required to form the essential amino acid methionine (from homocysteine) and to transform folate to the active form; the enzyme has been shown to be inactivated in vivo by even brief exposures to nitrous oxide.[28,65] This inactivation increases with the nitrous oxide exposure.[63,96] Methionine deficiency is believed to be associated with degenerative nervous system changes. It has been suggested that preoperative administration of methionine may counteract some of the adverse effects of nitrous oxide on the hematologic and nervous systems,[17] and methionine has been used in the treatment of nitrous oxide–induced neuropathy.[108]

Continuous inhalation of nitrous oxide can result in altered hematopoiesis depending on the concentration and duration of exposure. Patients exposed to 50% nitrous oxide for as little as 6 hours begin to show evidence of impaired thymidylate metabolism; hematopoietic changes suggestive of pernicious anemia occur after 24 hours of continuous inhalation.[1] Intermittent exposures have a cumulative effect if spaced more frequently than once every 3 to 4 days.[85] These findings have limited the use of nitrous oxide as an analgesic agent for extended use and for procedures that must be repeated often, such as debridement of burned skin.

Similar to other mood-altering drugs, nitrous oxide may be abused by individuals with access to the drug, including those in the dental profession. This abuse is associated with myeloneuropathic changes indicative of a pernicious anemia–like syndrome: numbness and paresthesia, muscular weakness and incoordination, altered spinal reflexes, impotence, and shooting sensations on flexion of the neck (Lhermitte's sign).[71]

Nitrous oxide has been shown to inhibit the release of luteinizing hormone–releasing hormone by the hypothalamus, which theoretically may impair fertility.[69,70] Potential reproductive toxicity has also been proposed to be caused by the sympathomimetic effects of nitrous oxide leading to vasoconstriction and hence diminished uterine blood flow.[42] However, clinical use in pregnant women carries no apparent increased risk to the fetus over other acceptable forms of pain control.[25,77] Long-term exposure has been strongly implicated in other reproductive abnormalities such as spontaneous abortion[19] and impaired fertility,[95] but these effects have not been substantiated by any controlled prospective study.

The possibility that long-term exposure to trace concentrations of nitrous oxide may be a health hazard to dental office and operating room personnel is discussed in Chapter 17.[19] An early report of inhaled concentrations as low as 50 ppm over a 2-hour span causing impairment in audiovisual performance tasks[13] has not been reproduced.[21,106] Nevertheless, this finding prompted the National Institute for Occupational Safety and Health to recommend 25 ppm as a maximum permissible time-weighted exposure limit per anesthetic administration for all health care workers. This level may not be achievable with existing scavenging systems.[122] As discussed in Chapter 17, the issue of controlling waste anesthetic gas in the workplace continues to evolve.

Therapeutic uses

Nitrous oxide is one of the most widely used inhalation anesthetics and continues to play a major role in the delivery of general anesthesia.[36] It is valuable in reducing the concentration of volatile anesthetics during inhalation anesthesia and as a component in "balanced anesthesia."* Historically, nitrous

**Balanced anesthesia* is a term used to describe a concept in which combinations of drugs are used to produce general anesthesia, with each drug chosen for a specific effect. In this context, nitrous oxide might be selected for its analgesic and anesthetic actions, a benzodiazepine for amnesia, a neuromuscular blocking drug for muscle relaxation, and an opioid for additional analgesia and hemodynamic stability.

oxide was first used for dental surgery, but with the advent of local anesthetics, it was replaced as the drug of choice for providing pain control sufficient for most dental procedures. Since the late 1950s, there has been an upsurge in the use of nitrous oxide, not to provide dental anesthesia but to provide relief from anxiety in the form of conscious sedation. In this role, it is often the agent of first choice. Its therapeutic application in dentistry is described in Chapter 48.

Ether

Ether (diethyl ether) was the most widely used volatile anesthetic in the century that followed the first successful demonstration of general anesthesia in 1846. As described in Chapter 17, the sequential effects of ether inhalation were the basis for Guedel's stages of anesthesia. Ether has been superseded by newer inhalation agents and is rarely used as a general anesthetic in North America. A brief description is included because of its historic importance.

Ether is both flammable and explosive and is an irritating liquid with a pungent odor. This last property, combined with a blood/gas partition coefficient of 12.1, makes its induction and recovery periods slow and unpleasant. Ether's advantages are its ability to produce good analgesia and muscle relaxation and to maintain respiration and circulation, its relative freedom from myocardial sensitization and organ toxicity, and its ease of administration. The drug's main disadvantages are its flammability and explosive potential, slow induction, slow recovery, irritation to the upper airway causing copious mucus secretion, and prominent emetic properties.

Halothane

Halothane has been one of the most widely used anesthetics since its introduction into clinical anesthesia in 1956 in the United Kingdom and in 1958 in the United States. Although its use has declined with the introduction of newer volatile agents, it is still a standard with which other inhalation anesthetics are compared.

Physical and chemical properties

Halothane is a halogenated hydrocarbon; it is nonflammable, has a characteristic sweet odor, and is available in brown glass bottles with thymol added to maintain chemical stability. Its physical and solubility properties are summarized in Tables 17-1 and 18-1.

Anesthetic properties

Table 18-2 compares the pharmacologic properties of halothane with other inhalation anesthetics. With a MAC of 0.75%, halothane is a potent general anesthetic that can be administered with excess amounts of oxygen. With its blood/gas partition coefficient of 2.5, the induction time of halothane is faster than that of older drugs such as ether, but slower than that of nitrous oxide and the newer volatile agents currently in use. Halothane has poor analgesic properties, and even at surgical anesthetic levels the unconscious patient may respond to a noxious stimulus with increased motor activity and alteration of autonomic parameters. For this reason, halothane is most often used with nitrous oxide and/or an opioid analgesic. Because halothane produces incomplete

Table • 18-2

Pharmacologic Properties of Inhalation Anesthetics

ATTRIBUTE OR EFFECT	NITROUS OXIDE	HALOTHANE	ENFLURANE	ISOFLURANE	DESFLURANE	SEVOFLURANE
Analgesia	Good	Poor	Moderate	Moderate	Moderate	Moderate
Muscle relaxation	None	Moderate	Good	Good	Good	Moderate
Heart rate	May increase	Unchanged	Increased	Increased	Increased	Unchanged
Myocardial depression	Mild	Marked	Marked	Moderate	Moderate	Moderate
Cardiac output	Unchanged	Decreased	Decreased	Unchanged	Unchanged	Decreased
Vascular resistance	Unchanged	Slightly decreased	Decreased	Decreased	Decreased	Decreased
Blood pressure	Unchanged	Decreased	Decreased	Decreased	Decreased	Decreased
Arrhythmogenic potential	None	High	Moderate	Low	Low	Low
Respiratory depression	Mild	Moderate	Marked	Moderate to marked	Marked	Moderate to marked
Respiratory rate	Slightly increased	Increased	Increased	Increased	Increased	Increased
Tidal volume	Decreased	Decreased	Decreased	Decreased	Decreased	Decreased
Bronchi	No effect	Dilation	Dilation	Dilation	Brief constriction	Dilation
Airway irritation	None	Mild	Mild to moderate	Moderate	Marked	Mild
Electroencephalographic activity	No effect	Depressed	Stimulated	Depressed	Depressed	Depressed
Renal function	No effect	Decreased	Decreased	Decreased	Decreased	Decreased
Biotransformation	None*	20% to 40%	2% to 10%	0.2%	0.02%	2% to 3%
Hepatotoxicity	None	Reported	Rare	Rare	Rare	None

*Enteric bacteria metabolize small amounts (≤0.004%) of nitrous oxide.

muscle relaxation, it is also often combined with neuromuscular blocking agents.

Cardiovascular effects Halothane decreases the mean arterial blood pressure, primarily as a result of decreased cardiac output, and at 1 MAC it falls by 25% (Figure 18-3). The decrease in cardiac output is greater than that found with equipotent amounts of isoflurane. Halothane, like other volatile general anesthetics, has a direct, significant, and dose-dependent depressant effect on myocardial contractility and, to a lesser degree, on vascular smooth muscle.[97] The negative inotropic effect is attributed to a decrease in the influx of Ca^{++} through the slow channels of the sarcolemma, a decrease in Ca^{++} accumulation in the sarcoplasmic reticulum, and a decrease in Ca^{++} sensitivity of contractile proteins.

Halothane exerts a direct negative chronotropic effect at the sinoatrial node as a result of reduced cardiac sympathetic activity and vagal predominance. This depression leads to a slowing of the heart rate and possible junctional rhythms. Halothane also depresses the baroreceptor reflex and therefore suppresses the expected increase in heart rate caused by hypotension.[5] Halothane is a vasodilator; the peripheral systemic vascular resistance may be decreased, especially in patients with high sympathetic tone (e.g., those with congestive heart disease or hypertension).

There is no stimulation of sympathoadrenal discharge with halothane and no increase in plasma catecholamines. However, halothane sensitizes the myocardium to catecholamines, which can predispose to cardiac dysrhythmias,[8] and this effect may be further potentiated by thiopental or hypercarbia. Dysrhythmias can occur as a result of catecholamines released endogenously in response to an elevated $PaCO_2$ or surgical stress, or after the injection of pressor agents given to augment blood pressure. Of direct relevance to dentistry is the use of epinephrine as the vasoconstrictor in local anesthetics and gingival retraction cords. For submucosal administration, it is recommended to limit exogenous epinephrine administration to 1 μg/kg if halothane is used with thiopental and 2 μg/kg if used alone.[18] Avoidance of hypoxia, hypercarbia, and electrolyte abnormalities also reduces the likelihood of this adverse event.

Respiratory effects Halothane induces a dose-dependent depression of respiration. At light anesthetic levels, breathing becomes shallow and rapid, and the $PaCO_2$ is maintained at a concentration 25% higher than normal (see Figure 18-2). Tidal volume decreases. As with all inhalation anesthetics, the ventilatory response to carbon dioxide is diminished, and controlled ventilation is frequently necessary in deeper planes of anesthesia. Halothane virtually eliminates the respiratory stimulant effect of hypoxia at concentrations as low as 0.1 MAC. Halothane is an effective bronchodilator, which is of benefit in the asthmatic patient.

Other effects Halothane depresses the cerebral metabolic rate. Intracranial pressure increases, as does cerebral blood flow. The production of cerebrospinal fluid is decreased, but so too is its absorption. Halothane relaxes uterine smooth muscle. Halothane also causes a dose-dependent decrease in renal blood flow and glomerular filtration, which is thought to parallel the decrease in cardiac output.

Metabolism A significant portion (≥20%) of the administered halothane is biotransformed in the liver, primarily by oxidation by the cytochrome P450 microsomal oxidase system.[15,26,83] Reduction accounts for up to 2% of the

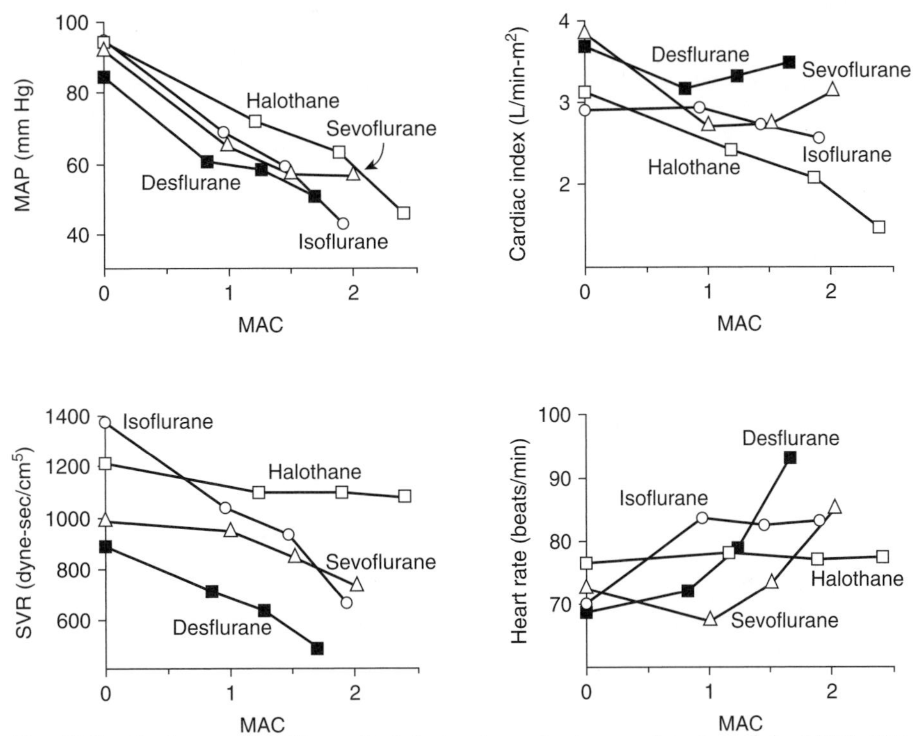

Fig. 18-3 Cardiovascular effects of inhalational anesthetics as a function of the MAC. *SVR*, Systemic vascular resistance; *HR*, heart rate; *MAP*, mean arterial blood pressure. (Adapted from Weiskopf RB, Cahalan MK, Eger EI II, et al: Cardiovascular actions of desflurane in normocarbic volunteers, *Anesth Analg* 73:143-156, 1991; and Malan TP, Jr, DiNardo JA, Isner RJ, et al: Cardiovascular effects of sevoflurane compared with those of isoflurane in volunteers, *Anesthesiology* 83:918-928, 1995.)

metabolism. Thus alveolar excretion and hepatic metabolism are both important in the elimination of halothane. The metabolites include trifluoroacetic acid, which may be responsible for toxic effects in the liver (as described below), as well as Cl^- and Br^-.

Adverse effects

Halothane has been associated with delayed hepatotoxicity, which may present as one of two syndromes.[33,37] The first is a mild, self-limited form of liver dysfunction that may occur after an initial exposure and has an incidence approximating 20%. This disturbance, usually recognized by an increase of liver enzymes in the plasma, may result from a direct effect of the drug or its metabolites. It may be exacerbated by liver hypoxia, as it is strongly associated with impaired hepatocyte oxygenation, either because of preexisting liver disease, hypoxemia, or decreased hepatic blood flow. The second syndrome, known as *halothane hepatitis,* is characterized by the development of massive hepatic failure with a high mortality rate. This latter syndrome has an incidence approximating 1 : 35,000 and is associated with repeated exposure to halothane. The clinical features of halothane hepatitis include gastrointestinal upset, jaundice, fever, rash, eosinophilia, and serum autoantibodies.[5,90] This more fulminant form may be caused by an immunologic mechanism. It is presumed that oxidative metabolism of halothane leads to a reactive trifluoroacetyl halide metabolite. This metabolite induces antigenic changes to hepatic microsomal proteins, producing neoantigens and subsequent autoantibodies. Because of this syndrome, halothane is contraindicated in patients who have previously been exposed to halothane within a short period or who have shown signs of liver toxicity on previous exposure to halothane or related anesthetics,[37,93] as well as for any abdominal surgery likely to decrease the alveolar ventilation or liver blood flow.

Malignant hyperthermia is a rare adverse effect of general anesthesia involving halothane, other volatile anesthetic agents, and the neuromuscular blocking drug succinylcholine. In the United States, the incidence of malignant hyperthermia is 1 : 50,000 in adults and 1 : 15,000 in children. It is a genetic disorder of multifactorial etiology. It is associated with central core disease; Duchenne's muscular dystrophy; King-Denborough syndrome; other myopathies; and musculoskeletal congenital defects such as cleft palate, scoliosis, clubfoot, ptosis, strabismus, cryptorchidism, and congenital hernias.[12,109]

An acute crisis of malignant hyperthermia is a hypercatabolic reaction that often manifests initially as masseter or generalized muscle rigidity; other early signs include elevation of oxygen use and carbon dioxide production, tachypnea, and tachycardia. Cardiovascular instability, cardiac dysrhythmias, electrolyte disturbances, and elevation in temperature are other classic signs. The body temperature, often unaffected early in an acute attack, progressively increases to alarming and sometimes fatal levels. The elevated heat production, associated with increased Ca^{++} concentrations in the myoplasm and hypermetabolic activity of skeletal muscle, is responsible for the hyperthermia.[48]

Immediately on recognition, all triggering agents should be discontinued and hyperventilation with 100% oxygen instituted. Dantrolene, an inhibitor of Ca^{++} transport (see Chapter 10), should be administered intravenously as soon as possible because this drug provides lifesaving, definitive treatment.[47] Dantrolene should be administered as a bolus intravenously at a dose of 2 to 3 mg/kg and then titrated in response to the patient's clinical condition. If present, metabolic acidosis should be treated, as well as any dysrhythmias and electrolyte disturbances. Cooling in the form of cold intravenous solutions, packing the patient in ice, and ice water lavage of body cavities should be performed to increase heat loss and lower body temperature. Effective treatment rendered quickly after prompt recognition of malignant hyperthermia has reduced its mortality rate from 70% to less than 10%.

Therapeutic uses

Halothane was one of the most widely used general anesthetics in the two decades after its clinical introduction. Although its use has diminished with the introduction of newer inhalation and intravenous agents, halothane is still often selected when a child is to be induced by inhalation because it does not have a strong odor and is nonirritating to the respiratory tract. Its primary drawback is its potential hepatotoxicity.

Enflurane

Physical and chemical properties

Enflurane is a halogenated methyl ethyl ether introduced into clinical use in the United States in 1972. It is chemically stable and nonflammable, is available in brown glass bottles, and has an "ethereal" odor. Its blood/gas partition coefficient of 1.8 makes it less soluble in blood than halothane.

Anesthetic properties

Enflurane is less potent than halothane. In general, however, the clinical anesthesia with enflurane resembles that produced by halothane.

Cardiovascular effects Enflurane is similar to halothane in its depressant effects on blood pressure and myocardial contractility. The reduction in systemic vascular resistance is greater than that found with halothane but less than that with isoflurane. Because enflurane does not completely block baroreceptor-mediated reflexes, the heart rate may increase. Enflurane is less likely to trigger catecholamine-induced dysrhythmias than is halothane, but it is not as reliable in this regard as is isoflurane.

Respiratory effects Of all the inhalation agents in current use, enflurane is the most respiratory depressant at low anesthetic concentrations (see Figure 18-2). Hypercarbia associated with spontaneous respiration is such that mechanical ventilation is normally used. This attribute, plus its pungent odor, negates the theoretical advantage over halothane in its speed of induction of anesthesia. Enflurane is similar to halothane in promoting bronchial dilation and is safe for use in asthmatic patients. On the other hand, enflurane may be mildly irritating to the airway because it causes a modest stimulation of salivary and tracheobronchial secretions.

Other effects Enflurane induces less cerebral vasodilation but greater depression of the cerebral metabolic rate than does halothane. There is increased cerebrospinal fluid production and increased resistance to reabsorption. One qualitative difference between enflurane and halothane is that enflurane produces high-voltage discharges on the electroencephalogram. This excitatory response can progress to a state in which seizures with involuntary motor movements and frank convulsions occur.[59] High inspired tensions of enflurane and overventilation-induced hypocarbia promote seizure activity. However, enflurane does not increase seizure activity in patients with epilepsy and, in fact, increases the seizure threshold to such stimuli as electroconvulsant shock and CNS stimulants.

Metabolism Enflurane is biotransformed slowly by the hepatic mixed function oxidase system. It is estimated that anywhere from 2% to 10% of the inhaled dose is metabolized. Hepatotoxicity has not been clearly associated with enflurane, although both the mild and the severe forms described previously for halothane have been reported,[11] with an estimated incidence of 1 : 800,000. Because metabolism of enflurane can lead to an oxidative halide metabolite and subsequent severe hepatitis by the same immune-mediated mechanism as occurs with halothane, there may be cross-sensitivity between the two agents. A byproduct of enflurane metabolism is F^-, which does not normally reach nephrotoxic concentrations, except after prolonged administration (more than 10 MAC hours).[78] Because of the availability of alternative agents that do not release F^-, it may be best to avoid enflurane use in patients with renal failure.

Therapeutic uses

Enflurane is used as a general anesthetic for maintenance of anesthesia in adult patients. It is not considered to be as hepatotoxic as is halothane, probably because of the decreased magnitude of biotransformation, and it is much less likely in most patients to sensitize the heart to the dysrhythmogenic action of catecholamines. Halothane is preferred, however, when spontaneous ventilation and mask induction of anesthesia are contemplated, as may be the case in general anesthesia for pediatric dental patients.

Isoflurane

After its release in the United States in 1981, isoflurane became the most widely used volatile anesthetic. An isomer of enflurane, isoflurane combines the desirable properties of enflurane with less respiratory depression and hepatic metabolism. Although the newer, less soluble volatile anesthetics have made inroads in its use, isoflurane remains an anesthetic of choice for many purposes.

Physical and chemical properties

The blood/gas partition coefficient of 1.4 for isoflurane results in a more rapid onset of action compared with halothane and enflurane. Isoflurane is nonflammable and is marketed in brown glass bottles. The stability and chemical characteristics of isoflurane are similar to those of enflurane, but the vapor is more pungent.

Anesthetic properties

Isoflurane may be thought of as a moderately improved and more potent (MAC of 1.15%) version of enflurane. Induction should theoretically be rapid with isoflurane, but it is somewhat limited by its pungent odor, which, if induction is allowed to proceed too rapidly, leads to breath holding, laryngospasm, and coughing. This problem is usually overcome by inducing the patient with an intravenous agent. Isoflurane, like enflurane, is sufficiently potent to provide muscle relaxation adequate for any surgical procedure, but neuromuscular blocking agents are normally used instead of the high concentrations of anesthetic needed to secure muscle relaxation. As with other potent inhalation anesthetics, isoflurane increases the action of the nondepolarizing neuromuscular blocking drugs.

Cardiovascular effects Similar to all volatile anesthetics, isoflurane produces a dose-dependent depression of myocardial contractility, although it is considerably less than that seen with halothane or enflurane. Isoflurane also causes coronary vasodilation, mostly at the distal (resistance) arterioles.[88] Although this effect may be beneficial, it may also lead to "coronary steal" in patients with ischemic heart disease, in which blood flow is redistributed from myocardial tissues supplied by atherosclerotic arteries to areas with healthy coronary vessels. Coronary steal develops only when the coronary perfusion pressure is decreased, is more likely to occur with excessive tachycardia, and is most probably not a special concern with isoflurane. Cardiac output is well maintained with isoflurane (see Figure 18-3), even though stroke volume is decreased, by virtue of an increase in the heart rate, demonstrating isoflurane's greater preservation of baroreceptor reflexes. Arterial blood pressure declines are similar to those produced by halothane and enflurane, however, because of the relatively greater vasodilator effect of isoflurane. Isoflurane does not sensitize the heart to dysrhythmias; indeed, the permissible injected dose of epinephrine during isoflurane anesthesia is three times that with halothane.

Respiratory effects Respiratory depression, intermediate between that of halothane and enflurane (see Figure 18-2), manifests as a decreased ventilatory response to hypercapnia and a complete loss of sensitivity to hypoxia. Isoflurane increases respiratory rate only up to 1 MAC. It bronchodilates similarly to halothane.

Other effects Isoflurane depresses cerebral metabolism in a manner similar to enflurane. It is a less powerful cerebral vasodilator than either enflurane or halothane and causes little change in the cerebrospinal fluid pressure. Isoflurane does not significantly alter cerebrospinal fluid production. All these effects intracranially are beneficial in neurosurgery. Anesthesia with isoflurane is not usually associated with epileptiform electroencephalographic activity.

Metabolism In contrast to halothane and enflurane, biotransformation of isoflurane is negligible (0.2% or less). This finding suggests that it is neither nephrotoxic nor hepatotoxic, a conclusion supported by observations that repeated and prolonged exposures to isoflurane have not caused hepatorenal injury in animals. It is biotransformed by the same enzymatic pathway as are halothane and enflurane. Although there are a few case reports of hepatic necrosis after isoflurane administration,[16,46] it is currently believed that isoflurane is highly unlikely to be responsible for postoperative hepatotoxicity.[90]

Therapeutic uses

Isoflurane is a suitable drug whenever a potent inhalation anesthetic is to be administered, except when a mask induction of anesthesia is contemplated. In pediatric patients, induction with isoflurane is more likely than halothane to elicit coughing, salivation, and laryngospasm.[79] These effects can be prevented by prior administration of an intravenous induction agent. Isoflurane has a number of advantages: it is chemically stable, nonflammable, and potent; induction is rapid and muscle relaxation adequate; and it is not dysrhythmogenic or toxic to the kidneys or liver. On the other hand, isoflurane does depress the cardiovascular and respiratory systems. It is also contraindicated in patients with a history of malignant hyperthermia.

Desflurane

Desflurane, approved for clinical use in 1992, is the first volatile anesthetic agent whose blood/gas partition coefficient (0.45) compares favorably with that of nitrous oxide (0.47). The theoretic advantages desflurane should have regarding rapid induction and recovery of anesthesia are partially offset by the drug's tendency to irritate the airway during induction. Nevertheless, the agent is particularly suited for ambulatory anesthesia and is commonly being used for other situations in which an inhalation anesthetic is indicated and the increased cost of the agent is offset by the faster recovery of the patient.

Physical and chemical properties

Desflurane is chemically very similar to isoflurane, with only a single substitution of fluorine for a chlorine atom (see Figure 18-1). Desflurane shows marked chemical stability, possibly because of the additional fluorine, which provides resistance to breakdown in soda lime and to biotransformation. The anesthetic has a high vapor pressure of 664 mm Hg at 20° C, becomes a gas (vapor pressure 760 mm Hg) at 23° C, and is not flammable at concentrations less than 17%. The low potency and high volatility of desflurane requires the use of a heated vaporizer to enable the delivery of this agent.[14]

Anesthetic properties

The low solubility of desflurane in blood results in rapid onset, recovery, and adjustment of anesthetic depth, similar to that found with nitrous oxide.[35,125] A propensity to cause breath holding, coughing, and laryngospasm during mask induction, however, precludes its routine use as a primary induction agent.

With a MAC of 6.0% (in middle-aged adults), desflurane is less potent than the other volatile agents. Its physiologic effects, however, are similar to those induced by isoflurane. The systemic vascular resistance, mean arterial blood pressure, and stroke volume are reduced, but the cardiac output is maintained by a progressive increase in heart rate.[118] As shown in Figure 18-3, significant increases in heart rate occur as the anesthetic concentration exceeds 1.25 MAC. Similar to isoflurane, desflurane may possibly cause coronary steal.[34] There is no sensitization of the myocardium to catecholamines. Desflurane causes a dose-related decrease in tidal volume and, despite an increase in the respiratory rate, a significant depression of minute ventilation. As with other halogenated ethers, respiratory depression is reduced if desflurane is used with nitrous oxide for anesthesia (see Figure 18-2).

Desflurane is contraindicated in patients susceptible to malignant hyperthermia because it can trigger the syndrome in the swine model and has been linked to malignant hyperthermia in the clinical setting. Because desflurane is notable for having minimal biotransformation, it has a very low likelihood for causing serious hepatic toxicity.[62]

Therapeutic uses

Despite its favorable blood/gas partition coefficient, desflurane is not indicated for the induction of anesthesia, especially in pediatric patients and patients with heart disease. Once anesthesia has been achieved with other agents, desflurane may be administered for maintenance purposes. Then desflurane permits a more rapid control over the depth of anesthesia than other inhalation agents and a more rapid recovery, allowing for a more precise duration of general anesthesia.

Sevoflurane

First synthesized in the United States in 1968, sevoflurane has been widely used in Japan since 1990. It became available for clinical use in the United States in 1995. A pleasant odor, lack of airway irritation, and rapid onset of action make sevoflurane an attractive alternative to halothane for mask induction of anesthesia.

Physical and chemical properties

Sevoflurane is characterized by a low blood/gas partition coefficient (0.65) and chemical stability under normal storage conditions. A potential drawback is the agent's reactivity to chemicals (e.g., soda lime) used as carbon dioxide absorbents.

Anesthetic properties

As would be expected, the low solubility of sevoflurane results in rapid onset, recovery, and adjustment of anesthetic depth. Similar to the other volatile agents in current use, sevoflurane is relatively potent, with a MAC of 2%. Sevoflurane undergoes oxidative defluorination by the hepatic enzyme CYP2E1. This same enzyme may also be responsible for the degradation of isoflurane, enflurane, and possibly desflurane.[34] The degree of biotransformation is approximately 2% to 3%, with plasma inorganic F^- concentrations similar to those previously found in patients with renal dysfunction after methoxyflurane anesthesia. However, plasma F^- declines much more rapidly with sevoflurane, and there is no evidence of nephrotoxicity in human beings.[20,43,58] Sevoflurane is not believed to be hepatotoxic because it is not broken down to yield the trifluoroacetyl halide metabolite.

The cardiovascular effects induced by sevoflurane are intermediate between those of halothane and isoflurane.[34,50] At 1 MAC, sevoflurane causes a decrease in cardiac output, peripheral vascular resistance, and arterial blood pressure. Above 1 MAC, further decreases in peripheral vascular resistance and myocardial contractility are partially offset by an increase in heart rate. Sevoflurane does not sensitize the myocardium to catecholamines. There is a decrease in alveolar ventilation similar to that observed with isoflurane.

Therapeutic uses

Sevoflurane has the advantages of a rapid onset, good control over the depth of anesthesia, and a rapid recovery, as previously noted for desflurane. One important advantage of sevoflurane over desflurane is that it is much less irritating to the respiratory tract, which, combined with its rapid induction and maintenance of heart rate, makes it an attractive alternative to halothane for induction of anesthesia in children.[54,84,98] A potential drawback is that it breaks down in soda lime to compound A,[111,127] thereby greatly limiting its potential use in low-flow systems with conventional carbon dioxide absorbers. This problem can be circumvented by avoiding low gas flows (less than 2 L/min) or by using specific carbon dioxide absorbents without this characteristic.

Methoxyflurane

Methoxyflurane is a halogenated ether similar to enflurane. With a MAC of 0.16, it is very potent, and the blood/gas partition coefficient is high, so that induction is very slow. This prolonged induction period necessitates methoxyflurane being used only as a maintenance agent after induction is accomplished by one of the intravenous agents. The anesthetic action of methoxyflurane is similar to that of halothane, except that there is less respiratory depression and more muscle relaxation and analgesia. The major reason for methoxyflurane's relative disuse is that it is biotransformed to a large extent, from 50% to 75%. Plasma F^- concentrations become elevated to a degree that can produce renal failure with prolonged use.[126] Specifically, a vasopressin-resistant diabetes insipidus may result. Although still available, methoxyflurane is rarely used today because of this nephrotoxic potential and the availability of superior inhalation agents.

INTRAVENOUS AGENTS

Intravenous agents are used widely in anesthesiology. Historically, their primary role was as induction agents for inhalation general anesthesia, for which they were usually administered as a single dose. In recent years, they have also become commonly used for maintenance in the technique known as *total intravenous anesthesia* and for various modes of sedation, as described in Chapter 48. Total intravenous anesthesia has increased in popularity because of the introduction of drugs combining rapid redistribution with shorter elimination half-lives and because of increasing concern regarding occupational exposure to inhalation agents. For this technique, the drugs are ideally administered by continuous infusion, with intermittent boluses as needed to rapidly adjust the anesthetic depth.

The primary advantage of intravenous agents is their rapid distribution into the vessel-rich group of tissues, which

Box 18-2

Characteristics of an Ideal Intravenous Anesthetic Agent

PHYSICAL PROPERTIES	PHARMACOKINETIC PROPERTIES	PHARMACODYNAMIC PROPERTIES
Soluble in water	Rapid onset of action	Reliable induction of anesthesia
Stable in solution	Ability to titrate	Anxiolytic at subanesthetic doses
Stable to light exposure	Predictable duration of effect	Analgesic at subanesthetic doses
Absence of pain on injection	Short duration of effect	Amnestic at subanesthetic doses
No local irritation	Short elimination half-life	Minimal respiratory effects
Long shelf life	Rapid recovery	Minimal cardiovascular effects
	Rapid biotransformation	No effects on other systems
	Inactive metabolites	High therapeutic index
	Nontoxic metabolites	Small interindividual variation
		No allergy

includes the brain. The rapid uptake into the CNS, in turn, facilitates a rapid onset of action. The high lipid solubility of these drugs allows for a smooth and rapid induction. For most intravenous anesthetics, the termination of effect depends largely on redistribution of the drug out of the brain. Metabolic inactivation generally assumes a more central role when the agent is administered over an extended period of time. With the exception of the benzodiazepines, these drugs can easily induce anesthesia, at which time maintenance may be carried out by either inhalation agents or by continued infusion of the intravenous drug. Usual advantages over the inhalation drugs are their superior ability at induction, less cardiovascular depression, and lack of operatory air pollution. Suggested ideal properties for an intravenous anesthetic drug are listed in Box 18-2.[49,120]

Although the short-acting and ultrashort-acting barbiturates were once widely used to produce all modes of anesthesia and sedation, drugs from other classes are now used more frequently. These agents include various combinations of antianxiety or antipsychotic drugs, opioids, and anesthetics such as propofol and ketamine. The relatively short action of most of these drugs and their relative freedom from emetic properties (opioids and ketamine excepted) make their use especially suited for sedation or general anesthesia in dentistry. The basic pharmacologic features of many intravenous agents are presented elsewhere in this book, and a more complete discussion of their use in the control of fear and anxiety for the dental patient is provided in Chapter 48.

Barbiturates

The ultrashort-acting barbiturates were the first drugs used as intravenous anesthetics. Much of what is known about intravenous anesthesia was developed through their use. The barbiturates available for this purpose include thiopental, methohexital, and thiamylal.

Thiopental

Thiopental, the thiobarbiturate analogue of pentobarbital, is the most commonly used intravenous barbiturate in medicine and is prototypical of the group. Its molecular structure is depicted in Figure 18-1. Thiopental, a weak acid (pK_a 7.4), is available as the sodium salt. When reconstituted for injection, the solution is buffered to a pH of 10 to 11. Once injected, the alkalinity is neutralized, and approximately half the drug converts to the highly lipophilic free acid. Thiopental is primarily an induction agent, although it may also be used for maintenance in relatively short surgical procedures or to treat seizures or elevated intracranial pressure. Induction is smooth and rapid, with the patient losing consciousness within seconds after a rapid bolus intravenous injection. Generally, however, induction is accomplished by administering the drug over a 30-second period, after which inhalation anesthesia is then initiated. After a single dose, the patient regains consciousness in 10 to 20 minutes. Repeated doses required for extended anesthesia may cause cumulative effects and a prolonged recovery period (see Figure 2-15). It is approximately 80% bound to plasma proteins.

Because of their high lipid solubility, the ultrashort-acting barbiturates have the ability to penetrate all tissues after injection. The amount of drug entering a given tissue primarily depends on the regional blood flow. How this property influences tissue uptake is illustrated in Figure 2-7. The vessel-rich group of tissues, which includes the brain, receives the highest proportion of the cardiac output relative to tissue mass and hence attains the highest concentration of thiopental. Later, as the agent is redistributed to the more poorly perfused tissues, such as muscle and then fat, a progressive decline in the blood and brain concentrations occurs. With a redistributional half-life of 4.6 to 8.5 minutes, the concentration of thiopental in the CNS diminishes from the peak value at 1 minute to less than 10% at 30 minutes. Thiopental is biotransformed in the liver to inactive products; only 1% is eliminated unchanged by the kidney. The mean metabolic half-life in adults is 11.6 hours but may exceed 24 hours in obese patients and in late pregnancy.[55]

Cardiovascular effects Induction doses in the normovolemic patient will decrease blood pressure by 10 to 20 mm Hg, followed by a reflex increase in heart rate of 15 to 20 beats/min. Selective venodilation is largely responsible for the hypotension inasmuch as total peripheral resistance remains unchanged and myocardial depression is relatively modest. After high doses, there is a more marked depressant effect on the cardiovascular system, which lowers blood pressure and may alter the redistribution pattern of the drug. Profound hypotension and even cardiac arrest may occur during induction of anesthesia in the hypovolemic or septic patient. Extra caution with the elderly is warranted to avoid cardiovascular collapse. Intraoperatively, heart rate and blood pressure may increase as a result of painful stimuli, in part because the barbiturates are hyperalgesic. Thiopental is not inherently dysrhythmogenic.

Respiratory effects Respiratory depression occurs in a dose-dependent manner and accounts for the major toxic effects of the barbiturates. Tidal volume is decreased, respiratory rate is usually depressed, and patients are predisposed to apnea, especially if other respiratory depressants are coadministered. Coughing, laryngospasm, and bronchospasm may develop as a result of irritation from premature manipulation of the airway or insertion of the endotracheal tube. Histamine release and increased sensitivity of the pharynx to stimulation may contribute to these adverse effects, although barbiturates are considered to be safe in asthmatics.

Other effects Thiopental is hyperalgesic at subanesthetic doses and may necessitate concurrent use of an analgesic. Cerebral blood flow is decreased as a result of a reduction in mean arterial pressure. Cerebral metabolic rate and intracranial pressure are decreased as well. Thiopental is an anticonvulsant.

Therapeutic use The usual induction doses approximate 4 mg/kg for adults and 6 mg/kg in infants. Thiopental is irritating to tissue, so care must be taken to prevent intraarterial injection or extravasation, either of which may result in tissue necrosis. Both the high alkalinity of the solution and the chemical nature of the drug itself are responsible for this effect. Intraarterial injection may cause intense vasospasm. As with all barbiturates, thiopental is contraindicated in patients with certain forms of porphyria (the acute intermittent, variegate, and hereditary coproporphyria types).[57] The drug should be used cautiously in the elderly and in patients with acute asthma, congestive heart failure, and shock states. Although thiopental is able to induce the synthesis of several important microsomal enzymes, it is unlikely that single induction doses will result in clinically significant drug interactions.

Methohexital

Methohexital, a methylated barbiturate, is used less commonly than thiopental for the induction of general anesthesia in hospital operating rooms but is used more widely for anesthesia in dentistry. The two drugs are similar except that methohexital is 2.5 times more potent, has shorter half-lives of distribution and elimination, and hence has a shorter duration of action. The sleep time after a single dose is 5 to 7 minutes, and the mean elimination half-life is 3.9 hours. Methohexital is biotransformed only in the liver, with a clearance rate three times greater than that of thiopental.[55] Excitatory phenomena such as hiccoughs, spontaneous movements, and seizures occur more frequently than with other barbiturates used clinically. These excitatory phenomena represent the primary disadvantage of methohexital. Methohexital does not induce histamine release. Although it is more likely than thiopental to cause pain on intravenous injection, methohexital is much less damaging after intraarterial injection or extravasation into local tissues. Its primary advantage is the rapid recovery and lower cumulative effect compared with thiopental, making it more suitable for outpatient procedures, which are often performed in dentistry. Methohexital also is much more stable when reconstituted; a 1% solution can be stored at room temperature and used for 6 weeks (versus 1 week for thiopental when refrigerated). The use of methohexital has diminished since the introduction of propofol, described below.

Thiamylal

Thiamylal is the thio derivative of secobarbital. It is similar to thiopental except that it is slightly more potent and shorter acting.

Propofol

Propofol (2,6-diisopropylphenol) is unrelated to any other general anesthetic. Its structure is illustrated in Figure 18-1. Propofol is formulated in an oil-in-water emulsion containing soybean oil, glycerol, and egg lecithin. Clinically, the pharmacokinetic properties of propofol include a rapid onset of action, an initial distributional half-life of 1 to 8 minutes—which results in an extremely short duration of action—and a terminal elimination half-life reportedly as short as 3 hours. It is extensively conjugated in the liver to inactive glucuronide and sulfate metabolites, with less than 0.3% of an administered dose appearing in the urine as the unchanged drug. Propofol's extensive plasma (98%) and tissue protein binding contributes, in part, to an enormous steady-state volume of distribution of 2 to 12 L/kg.[107] The clearance of propofol exceeds the hepatic blood flow, implying that continued tissue uptake and extrahepatic metabolism are factors in its removal from the blood.[101] After a continuous 10-day infusion of propofol that produces tissue saturation, the volume of distribution approaches 60 L/kg with a metabolic half-life of 1 to 3 days. After bolus administration, the plasma concentrations of propofol and thiopental are similar initially, but propofol subsequently disappears from the bloodstream more rapidly.[107]

Cardiovascular effects

Propofol can depress mean arterial pressures by 20% to 30% without eliciting a reflex increase in heart rate. This finding may be attributed to the drug's ability to decrease myocardial contractility, dilate the peripheral vasculature, depress baroreflex activity, and possibly inhibit the sympathetic nervous system.[100] Effects on cardiac output vary, depending on the $PaCO_2$. Clinically, these hemodynamic effects are transient and rarely require pharmacologic correction.[56] The cardiovascular effects are well tolerated in healthy patients, but significant hypotension may ensue in the elderly, hypovolemic patients, or those with limited cardiac reserve.[107]

Respiratory effects

Apnea is the most significant respiratory effect of propofol, with a reported incidence varying from 22% to 45% after an induction dose. Other respiratory effects include decreased sensitivity to carbon dioxide, decreased laryngeal reflexes, and decreased functional residual capacity. Propofol does not release histamine and therefore should be safe for use in asthmatics.

Other effects

Propofol decreases cerebral blood flow, cerebral metabolic rate and oxygen consumption, and intracranial pressure. Although it is believed to have anticonvulsant properties,[7] there are reports of grand mal seizures, opisthotonus, and unusual muscle activity with propofol,[39,99] and the drug should therefore be administered with caution to epileptic patients. The most common adverse reaction is pain on injection, which is noted more frequently when propofol is administered in the small veins on the dorsum of the hand. The incidence of pain may be reduced by using larger veins (e.g., antecubital veins), diluting the drug with a rapidly flowing intravenous line, or mixing the drug with lidocaine. Propofol is associated with less postoperative nausea and vomiting compared with inhalation anesthetics, and it even has antiemetic properties in doses as low as 10 to 20 mg.[107] Furthermore, propofol may have antipruritic properties.[7] There is no analgesic effect.

Therapeutic use

Propofol's major advantage is its extremely rapid recovery in patients.[2] In addition to induction, propofol can be used for maintenance of general anesthesia or for conscious sedation.

The dose for induction is 2 to 2.5 mg/kg. For total intravenous anesthesia, a maintenance infusion rate of 50 to 300 μg/kg per minute is recommended, depending on the age and health of the patient. If used alone, a dose of 25 to 75 μg/kg per minute should maintain conscious sedation in healthy adults after an initial infusion of 100 to 150 μg/kg per minute for 3 to 5 minutes. Doses must be reduced in the elderly and the debilitated and when propofol is used with other CNS depressants. An allergy to any of the emulsion constituents (e.g., soybeans) contraindicates the use of propofol. Because the soybean vehicle is an excellent bacterial culture medium, strict antiseptic technique should be used when administering propofol, and any unused portion should be discarded after 6 hours.

Infusion of propofol is also used long term in intensive care units to provide sedation. A rare syndrome has been described when propofol is administered in high doses (more than 4 mg/kg per hour) for long durations (at least 48 hours). This potentially fatal "propofol infusion syndrome" involves only critically ill patients,[60] primarily children.[9] The main features of this syndrome include acidosis, bradyarrhythmia, and rhabdomyolysis of cardiac and skeletal muscle, signs that mimic mitochondrial myopathies.[121] The use of propofol in lower doses or shorter durations has not been associated with these outcomes.

Ketamine

Ketamine, a relative of the psychedelic drug phencyclidine ("angel dust"), produces a unique state known as *dissociative anesthesia* that is characterized by profound analgesia, amnesia, and catalepsy.[120] This excitatory state is quite different from that seen after administration of the other general anesthetic agents previously discussed.[82] It has been suggested that this dissociative state is a result of a functional and electrophysiologic dissociation between the thalamoneocortical and limbic systems.[22] In this state, it is believed that the brain fails to transduce correctly afferent impulses because of disruption in normal communications between the sensory cortex and the association areas. The result resembles catalepsy, in which the eyes may remain open with slow nystagmus and intact corneal and pupillary reflexes.[80] Most protective reflexes are maintained. Varying degrees of skeletal muscle hypertonus may be present, along with nonpurposeful skeletal muscle movements that are independent of surgical stimulation. The molecular structure of ketamine is shown in Figure 18-1.

Ketamine is an antagonist of the N-methyl-D-aspartate class of glutamate receptors, and it is suggested that this action is the mechanism for its anesthetic and behavioral effects.[66] N-methyl-D-aspartate inhibition produces catalepsy, consistent with the effect of ketamine administration. Ketamine produces profound analgesia, which appears to be at least partially mediated by μ opioid receptors.[105,116] It has also been shown to interact with sigma/phencyclidine binding sites,[104] which may mediate the dysphoria that can be induced.

The onset of action and peak plasma concentrations have been reported to occur within 1 minute after intravenous administration, 5 to 15 minutes after intramuscular injection, and 30 minutes after oral ingestion.[31,45] The distributional half-life ranges from 11 to 16 minutes and the elimination half-life from 2 to 3 hours. Ketamine is highly lipid soluble and little bound to plasma protein (12%), which facilitates rapid transfer across the blood-brain barrier. The duration of anesthesia is about 5 to 10 minutes after a bolus intravenous infusion and 10 to 20 minutes after intramuscular injection.

Ketamine is metabolized in the liver into multiple products, including norketamine, which has an anesthetic potency approximately one third that of ketamine. Norketamine is then hydroxylated and conjugated, yielding water-soluble compounds that are excreted in urine. A small amount (4%) is excreted unchanged. Because of a high first-pass effect, oral administration results in increased concentrations of norketamine, which could theoretically prolong the anesthetic action.

Cardiovascular effects

Ketamine differs from most anesthetic agents in that, in the normal patient, it appears to stimulate the cardiovascular system, producing increases in heart rate, cardiac output, and blood pressure.[49,81] The mechanism for this effect is not well understood because ketamine has been shown to depress myocardial contractility directly[4] as well as enhance vasodilation. Ketamine's induction of central sympathetic stimulation or its ability to increase circulating catecholamine concentrations usually overrides the negative inotropism.[74] Its ability to maintain arterial blood pressure is useful in hypovolemic patients and those in cardiogenic shock. Caution should be used when ketamine is administered to critically ill patients or those who have chemical- or trauma-induced sympathectomy, in which case it may lead to myocardial depression and even cardiovascular collapse. Ketamine increases pulmonary vascular resistance and may exacerbate pulmonary hypertension or cor pulmonale.

The sympathomimetic and cardiovascular-stimulating effects contraindicate the use of ketamine in patients in whom an elevation of blood pressure or heart rate should be avoided, such as those with a cerebrovascular accident, significant hypertension, or advanced ischemic heart disease.[92]

Respiratory effects

Compared with other anesthetic agents, ketamine appears to be unique in its ability to maintain functional residual capacity on induction of anesthesia,[103] thereby decreasing the chances of intraoperative hypoxemia.[44,115] During ketamine anesthesia in spontaneously breathing patients, the minute ventilation may be maintained at the same level as in the awake state.[114] Ventilatory responses to hypercarbia and airway reflexes appear to be preserved. Ketamine has other beneficial effects on the respiratory apparatus, including increased lung compliance and decreased airway resistance. Ketamine is reported to be safe for the asthmatic patient because it causes bronchodilation and does not induce histamine release.[87,94,110] However, ketamine is a potent stimulator of salivary and tracheobronchial secretions, and therefore antimuscarinics are often administered concurrently.

Other effects

In doses less than those used to induce general anesthesia, ketamine may produce sedation, analgesia, and amnesia. Excitatory activity in both the thalamus and limbic systems, without clinical evidence of seizure activity, has been recorded. This electrical activity does not seem to spread to the cortex, and ketamine has been demonstrated to have anticonvulsant properties.[40,91] Ketamine strongly dilates cerebral blood vessels, increasing cerebral blood flow by 60% to 80%,[27,112] which, in turn, increases intracranial pressure in patients with compromised intracranial compliance.[102]

Emergence phenomena have been the most frequently reported adverse effects of ketamine. These reactions are described as a feeling of floating, vivid dreams, hallucinations, and delirium.[119] They have a reported incidence ranging from less than 5% to greater than 30%.[61,68,73,119] The incidence is related to the dose and rate of drug administration and is reduced when benzodiazepines are administered concomitantly.[67] The frequency of emergence delirium is less in children than in adults.

Therapeutic use

Ketamine may be administered by the intravenous, intramuscular, oral, and rectal routes. Induction of anesthesia may be achieved typically by an intravenous dose of 1 to 2 mg/kg or intramuscularly at a dose of 4 to 6 mg/kg. Intramuscular injection may be necessary when a patient is unable to cooperate. Anesthesia can be maintained by repeated injections or by using a continuous infusion, the latter in a dose of 15 to 90 μg/kg per minute. Smaller doses or infusion rates are useful for sedation and analgesia. Ketamine is safe for use in malignant hyperthermia patients, although it may induce some signs (e.g., muscle rigidity, tachycardia) that mimic the early stages of a crisis.

Etomidate

Etomidate, a carboxylated imidazole derivative, is chemically and pharmacologically unrelated to other intravenous anesthetics. Its pharmacokinetic profile, however, is similar to that of thiopental. Onset of anesthesia is rapid, and the duration of action is brief after conventional doses.

Etomidate is believed to modulate the action of the inhibitory neurotransmitter γ-aminobutyric acid on γ-aminobutyric $acid_A$ receptors. Both the amplitude and duration of inhibitory currents are increased. Etomidate has the advantages over thiopental of causing only mild respiratory depression and little effect on the cardiovascular system. Induction doses of 0.3 mg/kg elicit a mild (15%) drop in total peripheral resistance, which is mirrored by similar decrements in cardiac output and myocardial oxygen consumption. Coronary blood flow is mildly increased. Several significant liabilities, however, limit the use of etomidate. The drug inhibits adrenocorticosteroid synthesis; causes severe pain on injection in up to 50% of patients; and is associated with a relatively high incidence of nausea and vomiting, thrombophlebitis, involuntary myoclonic movements, hypertonus, and hiccough. These adverse events have greatly limited the clinical application of this drug for general anesthesia to that small group of patients who require the cardiovascular stability afforded by etomidate. There is essentially no indication for etomidate in dental anesthesia.

Benzodiazepines

Benzodiazepines have enjoyed widespread use as either adjuncts to general anesthesia, induction agents in patients with serious cardiovascular abnormalities, or agents for either deep or conscious sedation. Their pharmacologic advantages have given them a major role in the management of fear and anxiety in dentistry (see Chapter 48). As described in Chapter 13, all benzodiazepines are capable, in varying degree, of producing anxiolysis, sedation, anterograde amnesia, skeletal muscle relaxation, and anticonvulsant activity. There is minimal depression of the cardiovascular and respiratory systems when they are administered alone in therapeutic doses, reflecting the fact that benzodiazepines have a wide safety margin in the absence of interacting drugs. These agents are useful for their ability to attenuate the stress response and associated catecholamine release.[29] Although all benzodiazepines share similar pharmacodynamic effects, they are differentiated by their pharmacokinetic characteristics. The agents commonly used in anesthesia and dentistry are diazepam, midazolam, triazolam, and lorazepam. Although rarely used alone for general anesthesia because they lack analgesic properties and may be insufficient to induce or maintain general anesthesia in some patients, benzodiazepines are routinely used with other agents in balanced anesthesia for their superior sedative and amnestic effects and relative freedom from cardiovascular depression.

Diazepam

Diazepam, the prototypic benzodiazepine, has had a long and successful history of use as an agent for conscious sedation when administered either orally or intravenously. However, it is currently being superseded by other oral and parenteral benzodiazepines considered to have superior properties. Diazepam is classified as a long-acting agent, with an elimination half-life that increases from 20 to 70 hours in rough concert with the patient's age. A high lipid solubility means that diazepam is taken up by adipose tissue, which may cause postanesthesia drowsiness as the drug is slowly released from fat. Nevertheless, the drug is relatively short acting when used in a single dose. Indeed, the duration of effect of an intravenous injection of diazepam is approximately 1 hour, similar to that of the short-acting midazolam. Diazepam has a rapid onset of action (less than 1 minute intravenously), with a distributional half-life of 10 to 15 minutes. Peak plasma concentrations are achieved in 30 to 120 minutes when the drug is given orally. Intramuscular administration does not significantly improve absorption. Diazepam is not water soluble and is generally solubilized in the United States with propylene glycol, which predisposes to phlebitis when the formulation is administered intravenously into small-caliber veins. Propylene glycol also contributes to the delayed and variable absorption from intramuscular sites. An emulsion of diazepam in soybean oil, glycerol, and various lipids is now available that minimizes these problems.

Although efficacious, diazepam's drawbacks are the long elimination half-life, active metabolites, and common formulation in an irritating vehicle for parenteral administration. For induction of general anesthesia, intravenous doses of 0.3 to 0.5 mg/kg are appropriate.

Midazolam

Midazolam, the first water-soluble benzodiazepine, is prepared in an aqueous vehicle buffered to a pH of 3.5. Below a pH of 4 the benzodiazepine ring is open, making the molecule highly polar. Above pH 4, as is found physiologically, the ring closes, making midazolam very lipid soluble and leading to a rapid onset of action. This pharmaceutical sleight of hand eliminates the problem of thrombophlebitis on intravenous administration and also improves uptake after intramuscular administration, both important advantages over diazepam. Midazolam is biotransformed into metabolites with no significant activity, another advantage over diazepam. Midazolam is classified as a short-acting agent because its elimination half-life is approximately 1.7 to 2.6 hours in young adults. Cimetidine, erythromycin, and other CYP3A4 enzyme inhibitors may slow hepatic biotransformation, resulting in higher than expected midazolam concentrations in the plasma. Of special interest to dentistry, interactions between oral midazolam and erythromycin leading to oversedation have been reported.[52,86] For induction of general anesthesia, the usual dose is 0.2 mg/kg.

Lorazepam

Lorazepam is classified as an intermediate-acting benzodiazepine, but its effects after a single administration last considerably longer than for other benzodiazepines used in anesthesia. The drug is most useful as an oral or parenteral premedicant, where its slow onset of action is not a significant problem. The usual induction dose is 0.1 mg/kg.

Triazolam

Triazolam has effective anxiolytic, hypnotic, and amnestic properties, with a rapid onset of action after oral use that peaks within 2 hours. The drug has a short elimination half-life of 1.5 to 5.5 hours, and it is converted into inactive metabolites. CYP3A4 inhibitors may block hepatic biotransformation, resulting in higher than expected plasma concentrations. Triazolam is only available for oral use.

Opioids

The opioid analgesics play a major role in facilitating the delivery of general anesthesia and sedation, primarily as adjuncts used in combination with other agents. They also have a role as regional analgesics when administered as part of an epidural or spinal anesthetic. As described in more detail in Chapter 20, all opioids share the properties of analgesia, sedation, mood alteration, and the potential for tolerance, physical dependence, and addiction. Their antitussive effect may be of value in the immediate postoperative period or for procedures such as bronchoscopy. Nausea and vomiting are common adverse effects and are characteristically exacerbated if the patient is ambulatory. Opioids decrease the MAC of inhalation anesthetics.

An important action is respiratory depression caused by a dose-dependent decrease in the response of the medullary respiratory center to carbon dioxide. High doses can totally block spontaneous respiration without necessarily inducing unconsciousness. In susceptible patients, this effect may be seen in low to medium doses. Clinically, the respiratory depression manifests as a decrease in the breathing rate, with an overall decrease in minute ventilation and a compensatory increase in tidal volume. The $PaCO_2$ is elevated in a dose-dependent manner. Because of these respiratory effects, administration of opioids to patients with respiratory disorders, such as chronic obstructive pulmonary disease, must be done with extreme caution.

Specific sedation techniques with opioids are discussed in more detail in Chapter 48. Opioid doses should be reduced in the elderly, in patients with preexisting respiratory disease, and in those with significant hepatic disease. Several drugs, most notably sufentanil, may be used as primary agents for cardiac anesthesia. Their cardiac stability is attributable to a lack of negative inotropic effects. The anesthetic properties of individual opioids used for anesthesia and sedation follow.

Morphine

Morphine, the prototypic opioid analgesic, has been widely used as an adjunct to general anesthesia. Peak action after intravenous administration takes 15 to 20 minutes (Table 18-3). This delay reflects morphine's relatively poor lipid solubility and limited ability to cross the blood-brain barrier.

Cardiovascular effects Morphine exerts little direct effect on cardiovascular function. This discovery led to morphine's use for a time as a primary anesthetic for patients with significant cardiovascular disease. High doses, such as 1 mg/kg, however, significantly decrease systemic vascular resistance and mean arterial pressure, predisposing the patient to orthostatic hypotension. Hypotension may result from morphine-induced histamine release, bradycardia, or a sympatholytic action. Bradycardia is believed to be caused by stimulation of the vagal nuclei in the brainstem. There may also be a direct depressant effect at the sinoatrial node of the heart. The hypotensive actions of morphine lead to an increased requirement for fluid administration. In combination with nitrous oxide, morphine administration can result in cardiovascular depression, decreased cardiac output, and hypotension.

Respiratory effects The maximum respiratory depression from morphine occurs approximately 30 minutes after intravenous injection. Increased intracranial pressure may also result because of hypercarbia, and morphine should not be used in patients in whom this is a concern, as with an intracranial lesion or traumatic head injury.

Other effects Emesis is a result of direct stimulation of the chemoreceptor trigger zone. There is also decreased gastrointestinal motility and increased secretions (which contributes to the direct emetic effect). Sphincter tone is increased, which in the case of the sphincter of Oddi can lead to increased bile pressure and epigastric distress that may mimic anginal pain.

Therapeutic use When used as an adjunct to general anesthesia, the recommended dose of morphine is 0.1 mg/kg. Morphine has been administered by a number of techniques, including high doses with oxygen or as a supplement to inhalation agents, to obtain profound analgesia. Precautions apply to asthmatic patients because of the histamine release and cough suppression. The same is relevant to patients with a history of chronic obstructive pulmonary disease or other causes of decreased respiratory reserve. As with the administration of all opioids, the severely ill or elderly patient is more susceptible to the depressant effects of morphine. Chest wall rigidity has been reported and tends to occur when morphine is administered rapidly and if combined with nitrous oxide.

Meperidine

For many years, meperidine was the most widely used opioid for outpatient sedation and anesthesia in dentistry. This synthetic opioid has approximately one tenth the potency of

Table • 18-3

Comparison of Opioids Used for Sedation/Anesthesia

DRUG (PROPRIETARY [TRADE] NAME)	EQUIPOTENT DOSE (mg)	TIME TO PEAK ANALGESIC EFFECT (min)	DURATION OF ANALGESIA	PROTEIN BINDING (%)	ELIMINATION HALF-LIFE (hr)
Morphine	10	20	4 to 5 hr	30	2 to 3
Meperidine (Demerol)	80	5 to 7	2 to 4 hr	60	2.5 to 4
Fentanyl (Sublimaze)	0.1	3 to 5	30 to 60 min	85	3 to 4
Alfentanil (Alfenta)	0.7	1 to 2	10 to 15 min	92	1 to 2
Sufentanil (Sufenta)	0.015	3 to 5	15 to 30 min	93	2 to 3
Remifentanil (Ultiva)	0.05	1 to 2	5 to 10 min	70	0.1
Pentazocine (Talwin)	60	15 to 30	2 to 3 hr	65	2 to 3
Nalbuphine (Nubain)	10	30	3 to 4 hr	50	2 to 5
Butorphanol (Stadol)	2	30	2 to 4 hr	80	2.5 to 4

morphine and is characterized by having atropinelike properties in addition to its opioid agonist effects. The vagolytic actions may result in a decrease in upper respiratory tract secretions and an increase in heart rate, although these effects are minimal in the usual doses administered for sedation. At equianalgesic doses, meperidine has the same effects as does morphine, except that it differs from morphine in having a shorter duration of action, more complex biotransformation, and greater lipid solubility. Meperidine has a high hepatic extraction ratio, leading to a strong first-pass effect if the drug is administered orally.

Cardiovascular effects of meperidine administration include hypotension caused by a direct negative inotropism, decreased systemic vascular resistance, and decreased venous return. Orthostatic hypotension is commonly seen because of interference with compensatory sympathetic reflexes. As with morphine, meperidine is contraindicated when histamine release or increased intracranial pressure is undesirable and when decreased respiratory reserve exists.

Meperidine is biotransformed into a number of metabolites. One of them, normeperidine, has a long elimination half-life, can accumulate, and has been associated with CNS toxicity. The adverse reaction manifests as excitation, including agitation, seizures, and hallucinations, particularly in patients with hepatic and renal disease.

Exaggerated toxic responses to meperidine are especially likely in patients concurrently taking monoamine oxidase inhibitors (MAOIs) or amphetamines. Potential interactions between meperidine and amphetamines include increased risk of hypotension, possibly leading to cardiovascular collapse, severe respiratory depression, and convulsions. Potential interactions between meperidine and MAOIs can be similar but are particularly characterized by unpredictable excitatory effects such as seizures, delirium, rigidity, coma, and hypertension leading to cardiovascular collapse. Meperidine is absolutely contraindicated in patients having taken an MAOI within the past 3 weeks.

Fentanyl

The synthetic opioid agonist fentanyl is approximately 100 times as potent as morphine and is characterized by a rapid onset and short duration of action after a single dose. It is most commonly administered intravenously but may be given intramuscularly, transmucosally in the oral cavity, and, for chronic pain, transdermally. Fentanyl's high lipid solubility contributes to its rapid onset because it readily crosses the blood-brain barrier. It also contributes to rapid redistribution and significant accumulation in peripheral tissues. The subsequent slow release of fentanyl from muscle and fat lengthens the terminal half-life to beyond that of morphine. (See Figure 2-15 for an illustration of the influence of infusion duration on the plasma half-life of fentanyl.) Histamine is not released, which makes it preferable in patients predisposed to bronchospasm.

Intravenous doses of less than 10 μg/kg can be given as an adjunct to volatile agents in general anesthesia to minimize cardiovascular responses to specific stimuli such as pain, anxiety, or endotracheal intubation. Doses in the range of 50 to 150 μg/kg have been used alone to produce general anesthesia. These large doses are used because of the hemodynamic stability as a result of the lack of direct myocardial depression, absence of histamine release, and suppression of stress responses to surgery. Rapid administration of fentanyl is associated with bradycardia, an event more common in children. It is a potent respiratory depressant, but this lasts only 5 to 15 minutes if doses less than 100 μg are given. Chest wall rigidity has been reported but is unlikely to occur if fentanyl is administered at a rate of 1 μg/kg per minute or less. The incidence of nausea is reported to be less than with morphine or meperidine.

Alfentanil

An analogue of fentanyl, alfentanil is 5 to 10 times less potent and is characterized by a very rapid elimination half-life. This property contributes to a duration of action that is much shorter than that of fentanyl after prolonged infusion. Alfentanil has an especially rapid onset of action because of its low pK_a (most of the drug is uncharged at plasma pH). The drug can be used for both induction of anesthesia after bolus administration and maintenance by infusion. For bolus administration, recovery will be more rapid than with fentanyl or sufentanil, whereas no significant differences occur with short infusions. Because alfentanil is not prone to significant accumulation after continuous infusion, it is an opioid of choice for total intravenous anesthesia in the outpatient setting.

Sufentanil

Sufentanil is 5 to 10 times as potent as fentanyl and has a more rapid recovery after prolonged intravenous infusion. It is more lipid soluble than fentanyl but has a smaller volume of distribution and a shorter elimination half-life. Cardiovascular effects are similar to those found with fentanyl; however, sufentanil produces better hemodynamic stability during cardiac anesthesia and exhibits a somewhat more favorable ratio of analgesia to respiratory depression. Histamine is not released. High doses of sufentanil may reduce the dose of neuromuscular blocker required. As with fentanyl and alfentanil, sufentanil can be used for both induction of anesthesia after bolus administration and maintenance by infusion.

Remifentanil

Remifentanil is a relatively new opioid agonist used as an adjunct in general anesthesia. It is structurally unique in that it contains ester linkages. The drug is almost always given by intravenous infusion, because less controlled administration results in unstable effects and easily leads to chest wall rigidity and/or respiratory depression. Compared with fentanyl, remifentanil demonstrates a more rapid onset and offset of action. The ultrashort duration of action is not from redistribution of the drug but because of its unique metabolic inactivation by nonspecific esterases in the plasma and tissue. One of the most notable characteristics of remifentanil is its invariant context-sensitive half-life, which approximates 6 minutes regardless of the duration of infusion.

Opioid agonist-antagonists

Opioid agonist-antagonists are sometimes used for anesthesia and sedation in lieu of pure opioid agonists. Although the analgesic and respiratory depressant effects of the agonist-antagonists are similar to those of morphine and other agonists in conventional doses, a ceiling effect occurs as the dose is increased. Thus these drugs are not indicated as replacements for high-dose opioids as used in open-heart surgery. Pentazocine, butorphanol, and nalbuphine have all been administered for outpatient sedation procedures.

Pentazocine depresses myocardial contractility, but myocardial oxygen demand is greater than normal because of increases in peripheral resistance, systolic blood pressure, and plasma catecholamines. Although the antagonist action of pentazocine is weak, it is sufficient to precipitate opioid withdrawal reactions in physically dependent individuals. Adverse reactions include a potential for psychotomimetic effects, such as disorientation, confusion, depression, hallucinations, and dysphoria. Doses that produce sedation have also been associated with diaphoresis and dizziness. Butorphanol shares many of the cardiovascular and psychotomimetic side effects of pentazocine, although it is less likely to precipitate withdrawal in an opioid-dependent individual. Nalbuphine is a strong μ receptor antagonist, but it does not increase blood pressure or heart rate, which makes it the agonist-antagonist of choice in patients with cardiac disease.

α_2-Adrenergic Agonists

A relatively recent consideration for intravenous anesthesia is the use of α_2 agonists. These agents have been used in veterinary practice as anesthetic adjuncts for a number of years. In human beings, these drugs have been primarily indicated as antihypertensives and are described in detail in Chapters 6 and 28. Clonidine, the prototype for this group, has an α_2/α_1 selectivity of 200 : 1. Other α_2 agonists include methyldopa (10 : 1 selectivity) and dexmedetomidine (1300 : 1 selectivity). Stimulation of α_2 receptors affects numerous systems. In the CNS, α_2 agonists induce sedation, probably through stimulation within the locus ceruleus, and analgesia through stimulation within the spinal cord as well as the locus ceruleus.[24,76] For inhalation anesthesia, clonidine has been shown to decrease the MAC of halothane in dogs by up to 50%.[6] Clinically, α_2 agonists reduce the required dose of sufentanil, fentanyl, isoflurane, and droperidol.

Dexmedetomidine is used as a sedative agent in the adult intensive care unit setting. It is a short-acting agent that needs to be administered by intravenous infusion. Administration is usually initiated with a loading infusion of 1 μg/kg for the first 10 minutes, followed by a maintenance infusion of 0.2 to 0.7 μg/kg per hour.

Other Agents Used for Conscious Sedation

A number of drugs described elsewhere in this book have application in conscious sedation. They are summarized below, and details of their application in conscious sedation are included in Chapter 48.

Antihistamines

A number of H_1 antagonists possess sedative, antiemetic, and anticholinergic properties, which make them beneficial for use in conscious sedation. Promethazine, for instance, is a phenothiazine antihistamine used for conscious sedation, particularly of the pediatric patient. It has an onset of action of 15 to 60 minutes after oral ingestion, 20 minutes after rectal administration, and 20 minutes after intramuscular injection. The sedative effect lasts 2 to 8 hours.

There have been several reports of death after convulsive seizures when the combination of promethazine, an opioid, and a local anesthetic has been administered. These outcomes may have been caused by a lowering of the convulsive threshold or by respiratory depression in an overly sedated and undermonitored patient. Nevertheless, they emphasize the need for reduced doses when CNS depressants are administered together. Other side effects include extrapyramidal reactions, exaggerated effects in the elderly, and an intensification of side effects in patients taking MAOIs.

Hydroxyzine is another antihistamine with clinically useful anxiolytic and antiemetic properties. It is rapidly absorbed, with an onset of action of 15 to 30 minutes, a terminal half-life of 20 to 25 hours, and a duration of 4 to 6 hours. It may be administered either orally or intramuscularly. Hydroxyzine is relatively free of toxic effects, but anticholinergic side effects such as xerostomia may occur.

Alcohols

Chloral hydrate has been widely used as a sedative agent in pediatric dentistry and for minor procedures such as diagnostic imaging.[23] The drug appears to have a margin of safety similar to the barbiturates. It is well absorbed; peak effects occur in approximately 1 hour; the duration of action ranges from 4 to 8 hours; and it has an elimination half-time of 8 to 10 hours. Chloral hydrate is biotransformed into the active metabolite trichloroethanol, which is primarily responsible for its effects. It can cause nausea and vomiting as well as diarrhea and has the potential for cardiac dysrhythmogenicity in higher doses. Deep sedation may be induced if other CNS depressants, including nitrous oxide, are coadministered.[72]

Chloral hydrate is contraindicated in patients with marked hepatic impairment, severe renal disease, gastritis or gastric ulcers, severe cardiac disease, or acute intermittent porphyria. At a recommended dose of 50 mg/kg up to a maximum of 1 g, chloral hydrate is approximately as effective as diazepam for oral sedation in children.[3] Larger doses are more effective; however, the level of CNS depression is also beyond that of conscious sedation, and complete recovery can take more than 24 hours in sensitive patients.[75] Reduced doses must be used if chloral hydrate is combined with another sedative.

Antimuscarinic drugs

Scopolamine, like atropine, is generally used as a premedication for its antimuscarinic properties, usually in combination with an opioid or a barbiturate. However, it can also be used to produce conscious sedation with marked amnesia. Scopolamine has no analgesic properties and may produce excitation and delirium in a painful situation.

ANESTHETIC ADJUVANTS AND PREMEDICATION

Numerous drugs may be used for premedication or as anesthetic adjuvants. The pharmacologic features of the neuromuscular blocking agents, which are frequently used during anesthesia to provide greater muscle relaxation, are discussed in Chapter 10. Many of the sedatives, analgesics, antihistamines, and antimuscarinics previously mentioned in this chapter and covered elsewhere in the book are administered to the patient minutes to several hours before anesthesia and surgery. Commonly used drugs for premedication are listed in Table 18-4.

The indications for premedication include relief of anxiety; induction of sedation, analgesia, and amnesia; vagal blockade; reduction of secretions in the upper respiratory tract; and prevention of nausea and vomiting. Premedicants are also used to decrease the acidity and volume of gastric secretions. Finally, they are administered to reduce the dose of general anesthetic agent needed for a smooth induction.

An effective method of alleviating preoperative anxiety is the preoperative visit by the anesthesiologist, which allows information to be given to the patient as well as permits questions to be answered. The following classes of drugs, whose pharmacologic features are described elsewhere in this text, are routinely used as adjuncts to the careful psychologic preparation of the patient.

Opioid analgesics offer analgesia, euphoria, and sedation. Complicating problems can be respiratory depression, nausea and vomiting, gastric retention, and reduced sympathetic tone. Benzodiazepines provide a reduction in anxiety without significant effects on respiration or cardiovascular function. They are also effective in providing amnesia and sedation.

The antimuscarinics atropine, glycopyrrolate, and scopolamine may be used as premedicants to block vagal reflexes and inhibit salivation and respiratory tract secretion. They may also oppose the bradyarrhythmias that may accompany the use of other drugs in anesthesia, such as succinylcholine. Scopolamine also has central effects leading to sedation and amnesia. Glycopyrrolate does not cross the blood-brain barrier, is a more efficacious antisialagogue than atropine, and is less likely to induce tachycardia.

Both H_1 and H_2 antihistamines may be given for premedication. The H_1 antagonists, such as hydroxyzine or promethazine, offer antiemetic effects as well as some sedation. The H_2 antagonists, such as cimetidine or ranitidine, decrease gastric secretion and acidity. These effects are important in certain patients because general anesthesia eliminates the usual protective reflexes that prevent aspiration after regurgitation of stomach contents. The dopaminergic antago-

Table • 18-4

Agents Used for Premedication in General Anesthesia

DRUG (PROPRIETARY [TRADE] NAME)	ADULT DOSE (mg)	ROUTE OF ADMINISTRATION	INDICATIONS
Antimuscarinics			
Atropine	0.5	IV, IM	Secretion decrease, vagal blockade
Scopolamine	0.3	IV	Secretion decrease, sedation, amnesia
Glycopyrrolate (Robinul)	0.2	IV, IM	Secretion decrease
Antihistamines			
Hydroxyzine (Atarax, Vistaril)	25 to 100	Oral	Anxiolysis, sedation, antiemetic effect
Promethazine (Phenergan)	25 to 50	IM, IV	Sedation, antiemetic effect
Ranitidine (Zantac)	150	Oral	Aspiration prophylaxis
Benzodiazepines			
Diazepam (Valium)	5 to 20	Oral, IV	Anxiolysis, sedation, amnesia
Lorazepam (Ativan)	0.5 to 4	Oral, IV	Anxiolysis, sedation, amnesia
Midazolam (Versed)	2 to 5	IM, IV*	Anxiolysis, sedation, amnesia
Triazolam (Halcion)	0.125 to 0.5	Oral	Anxiolysis, sedation, amnesia
Neuroleptics			
Droperidol (Inapsine)	0.25 to 2.5	IM, IV	Sedation, antiemetic effect
Prochlorperazine (Compazine)	5 to 10	IM	Antiemetic effect
Opioids			
Morphine	5 to 10	IM	Sedation, analgesia
Meperidine (Demerol)	50 to 100	IM	Sedation, analgesia

*Midazolam is also administered orally and intranasally to children.

nist metoclopramide is also sometimes administered to increase gastric emptying.

Postoperative nausea and vomiting are common adverse events after general anesthesia. To improve comfort and safety, patients who are predisposed to nausea and vomiting may be given one of a wide variety of antiemetics, which include the dopamine antagonists droperidol and prochlorperazine, anticholinergics/antihistamines such as scopolamine and hydroxyzine, the adrenocorticosteroid dexamethasone, and the 5-hydroxytryptamine antagonists, including ondansetron and dolasetron.

CITED REFERENCES

1. Amess JA, Burman JF, Rees GM, et al: Megaloblastic haemopoiesis in patients receiving nitrous oxide, *Lancet* 2:339-342, 1978.
2. Apfelbaum JL, Grasela TH, Hug CC, Jr, et al: The initial clinical experience of 1819 physicians in maintaining anesthesia with propofol: characteristics associated with prolonged time to awakening, *Anesth Analg* 77:S10-S14, 1993.
3. Badalaty MM, Houpt MI, Koenigsberg SR, et al: A comparison of chloral hydrate and diazepam sedation in young children, *Pediatr Dent* 12:33-37, 1990.
4. Balfors E, Haggmark S, Nyhman H, et al: Droperidol inhibits the effects of intravenous ketamine on central hemodynamics and myocardial oxygen consumption in patients with generalized atherosclerotic disease, *Anesth Analg* 62:193-197, 1983.
5. Berthoud MC, Reilly CS: Adverse effects of general anaesthetics, *Drug Saf* 7:434-459, 1992.
6. Bloor BC, Flacke WE: Reduction in halothane anesthetic requirement by clonidine, an alpha-adrenergic agonist, *Anesth Analg* 61:741-745, 1982.
7. Borgeat A, Wilder-Smith OHG, Suter PM: The nonhypnotic therapeutic applications of propofol, *Anesthesiology* 80:642-656, 1994.
8. Bosnjak ZJ, Turner LA: Halothane, catecholamines, and cardiac conduction: anything new? *Anesth Analg* 72:1-4, 1991.
9. Bray RJ: Propofol infusion syndrome in children, *Pediatr Anaesth* 8:491-499, 1998.
10. Briggs M, Wong D, Groenewald C, et al: The effect of anaesthesia on the intraocular volume of the C3F8 gas bubble, *Eye* 11:47-52, 1997.
11. Brown BR, Jr, Gandolfi AJ: Adverse effects of volatile anaesthetics, *Br J Anaesth* 59:14-23, 1987.
12. Brownell AKW: Malignant hyperthermia: relationship to other diseases, *Br J Anaesth* 60:303-308, 1988.
13. Bruce DL, Bach MJ: Effects of trace anaesthetic gases on behavioural performance of volunteers, *Br J Anaesth* 48:871-876, 1976.
14. Caldwell JE: Desflurane: clinical pharmacokinetics and pharmacodynamics, *Clin Pharmacokinet* 27:6-18, 1994.
15. Carpenter RL, Eger EI II, Johnson BH, et al: The extent of metabolism of inhaled anesthetics in humans, *Anesthesiology* 65:201-205, 1986.

Agents Used in General Anesthesia, Deep Sedation, and Conscious Sedation

Nonproprietary (generic) name	*Proprietary (trade) name*
Inhalation agents	
Gases	
Cyclopropane*	—
Nitrous oxide	—
Ethylene*	—
Volatile liquids	
Desflurane	Suprane
Enflurane	Ethrane
Ether*	—
Halothane	Fluothane
Isoflurane	Forane
Methoxyflurane†	Penthrane
Sevoflurane	Ultane
Injectable agents	
Barbiturates	
Methohexital	Brevital
Thiamylal	Surital
Thiopental	Pentothal
Alkylphenol	
Propofol	Diprivan
Carboxyimidazole	
Etomidate	Amidate
Benzodiazepines	
Diazepam	Valium, Dizac
Lorazepam	Ativan
Midazolam	Versed
Opioids	
See Table 18-3	
Arylcycloalkylamine	
Ketamine	Ketalar
Others	
See Table 18-4	

*Not currently available in the United States.
†Generally considered obsolete and not recommended for use.

16. Carrigan TW, Straughen WJ: A report of hepatic necrosis and death following isoflurane anesthesia, *Anesthesiology* 67:581-583, 1987.
17. Christensen B, Guttormsen AB, Schneede J, et al: Preoperative methionine loading enhances restoration of the cobalamin-dependent enzyme methionine synthase after nitrous oxide anesthesia, *Anesthesiology* 80:1046-1056, 1994.
18. Christensen LQ, Bonde J, Kampmann JP: Drug interactions with inhalational anaesthetics, *Acta Anaesthesiol Scand* 37:231-244, 1993.
19. Cohen EN, Brown BW, Wu ML, et al: Occupational disease in dentistry and chronic exposure to trace anesthetic gases, *J Am Dent Assoc* 101:21-31, 1980.
20. Conzen PF, Kharasch ED, Czerner SF, et al: Low-flow sevoflurane compared with low-flow isoflurane anesthesia in patients with stable renal insufficiency, *Anesthesiology* 97:578-584, 2002.
21. Cook TL, Smith M, Starkweather JA, et al: Behavioral effects of trace and subanesthetic halothane and nitrous oxide in man, *Anesthesiology* 49:419-424, 1978.
22. Corssen G, Miyasaka M, Domino EF: Changing concepts in pain control during surgery: dissociative anesthesia with CI-581. A progress report, *Anesth Analg* 47:746-759, 1968.
23. Coté CJ: Sedation for the pediatric patient. A review, *Pediatr Clin North Am* 41:31-58, 1994.
24. Coursin DB, Coursin DB, Maccioli GA: Dexmedetomidine, *Curr Opin Crit Care* 7:221-226, 2001.
25. Crawford JS, Lewis M: Nitrous oxide in early human pregnancy, *Anaesthesia* 41:900-905, 1986.
26. Dale O, Brown BR, Jr: Clinical pharmacokinetics of the inhalational anaesthetics, *Clin Pharmacokinet* 12:145-167, 1987.
27. Dawson B, Michenfelder JD, Theye RA: Effects of ketamine on canine cerebral blood flow and metabolism: modification by prior administration of thiopental, *Anesth Analg* 50:443-447, 1971.
28. Deacon R, Lumb M, Perry J, et al: Selective inactivation of vitamin B_{12} in rats by nitrous oxide, *Lancet* 2:1023-1024, 1978.
29. Dionne RA, Goldstein DS, Wirdzek PR: Effects of diazepam premedication and epinephrine-containing local anesthetic on cardiovascular and plasma catecholamine responses to oral surgery, *Anesth Analg* 63:640-646, 1984.
30. Dohrn CS, Lichtor JL, Finn RS, et al: Subjective and psychomotor effects of nitrous oxide in healthy volunteers, *Behav Pharmacol* 3:19-30, 1992.
31. Domino EF, Domino SE, Smith RE, et al: Ketamine kinetics in unmedicated and diazepam-premedicated subjects, *Clin Pharmacol Ther* 36:645-653, 1984.
32. Dwyer R, Bennett HL, Eger EI II, et al: Effects of isoflurane and nitrous oxide in subanesthetic concentrations on memory and responsiveness in volunteers, *Anesthesiology* 77:888-898, 1992.
33. Dykes MHM: Is halothane hepatitis chronic active hepatitis? *Anesthesiology* 46:233-235, 1977.
34. Eger EI II: New inhaled anesthetics, *Anesthesiology* 80:906-922, 1994.
35. Eger EI II: The clinical use of desflurane, *Yale J Biol Med* 66:491-500, 1993.
36. Eger EI II, Lampe GH, Wauk LZ, et al: Clinical pharmacology of nitrous oxide—an argument for its continued use, *Anesth Analg* 71:575-585, 1990.
37. Elliott RH, Strunin L: Hepatotoxicity of volatile anaesthetics, *Br J Anaesth* 70:339-348, 1993.
38. Ermens AAM, Refsum H, Rupreht J, et al: Monitoring cobalamin inactivation during nitrous oxide anesthesia by determination of homocysteine and folate in plasma and urine, *Clin Pharmacol Ther* 49:385-393, 1991.
39. Finley GA, MacManus B, Sampson SE, et al: Delayed seizures following sedation with propofol, *Can J Anaesth* 40:863-865, 1993.

40. Fisher MM: Use of ketamine hydrochloride in the treatment of convulsions, *Anaesth Intensive Care* 2:266-268, 1974.
41. Fu AD, McDonald HR, Eliott D, et al: Complications of general anesthesia using nitrous oxide in eyes with preexisting gas bubbles, *Retina* 22:569-574, 2002.
42. Fujinaga M, Baden JM, Suto A, et al: Preventive effects of phenoxybenzamine on nitrous oxide–induced reproductive toxicity in Sprague-Dawley rats, *Teratology* 43:151-157, 1991.
43. Gentz BA, Malan TP, Jr: Renal toxicity with sevoflurane: a storm in a teacup? *Drugs* 61:2155-2162, 2001.
44. Gooding JM, Dimick AR, Tavakoli M, et al: A physiologic analysis of cardiopulmonary responses to ketamine anesthesia in noncardiac patients, *Anesth Analg* 56:813-816, 1977.
45. Grant IS, Nimmo WS, Clements JA: Pharmacokinetics and analgesic effects of i.m. and oral ketamine, *Br J Anaesth* 53:805-810, 1981.
46. Gregoire S, Smiley RK: Acute hepatitis in a patient with mild factor IX deficiency after anaesthesia with isoflurane, *Can Med Assoc J* 135:645-646, 1986.
47. Gronert GA, Milde JH, Theye RA: Dantrolene in porcine malignant hyperthermia, *Anesthesiology* 44:488-495, 1976.
48. Gronert GA, Milde JH, Theye RA: Role of sympathetic activity in porcine malignant hyperthermia, *Anesthesiology* 47:411-415, 1977.
49. Haas DA, Harper DG: Ketamine: a review of its pharmacologic properties and use in ambulatory anesthesia, *Anesth Prog* 39:61-68, 1992.
50. Harkin CP, Pagel PS, Kersten JR, et al: Direct negative inotropic and lusitropic effects of sevoflurane, *Anesthesiology* 81:156-167, 1994.
51. Heijke S, Smith G: Quest for the ideal inhalation anaesthetic agent, *Br J Anaesth* 64:3-6, 1990.
52. Hiller A, Olkkola KT, Isohanni P, et al: Unconsciousness associated with midazolam and erythromycin, *Br J Anaesth* 65:826-828, 1990.
53. Hohner P, Reiz S: Nitrous oxide and the cardiovascular system, *Acta Anaesthesiol Scand* 38:763-766, 1994.
54. Holzki J, Kretz FJ: Changing aspects of sevoflurane in paediatric anaesthesia: 1975-1999, *Paediatr Anaesth* 9:283-286, 1999.
55. Hudson RJ, Stanski DR, Burch PG: Pharmacokinetics of methohexital and thiopental in surgical patients, *Anesthesiology* 59:215-219, 1983.
56. Hug CC, Jr, McLeskey CH, Nahrwold ML, et al: Hemodynamic effects of propofol: data from over 25,000 patients, *Anesth Analg* 77:S21-S29, 1993.
57. Jensen NF, Fiddler DS, Striepe V: Anesthetic considerations in porphyrias, *Anesth Analg* 80:591-599, 1995.
58. Jones RM: Desflurane and sevoflurane: inhalation anaesthetics for this decade? *Br J Anaesth* 65:527-536, 1990.
59. Julien RM, Kavan EM: Electrographic studies of a new volatile anesthetic agent: enflurane (Ethrane), *J Pharmacol Exp Ther* 183:393-403, 1972.
60. Kang TM: Propofol infusion syndrome in critically ill patients, *Ann Pharmacother* 36:1453-1456, 2002.
61. Knox JW, Bovill JG, Clarke RS, et al: Clinical studies of induction agents. XXXVI: ketamine, *Br J Anaesth* 42:875-885, 1970.
62. Koblin DD: Characteristics and implications of desflurane metabolism and toxicity, *Anesth Analg* 75:S10-S16, 1992.
63. Koblin DD, Tomerson BW: Dimethylthiourea, a hydroxyl radical scavenger, impedes the inactivation of methionine synthase by nitrous oxide in mice, *Br J Anaesth* 64:214-223, 1990.
64. Koblin DD, Tomerson BW, Waldman FM, et al: Effect of nitrous oxide on folate and vitamin B_{12} metabolism in patients, *Anesth Analg* 71:610-617, 1990.
65. Koblin DD, Waskell L, Watson JE, et al: Nitrous oxide inactivates methionine synthetase in human liver, *Anesth Analg* 61:75-78, 1982.
66. Koek W, Woods JH, Winger GD: MK-801, a proposed noncompetitive antagonist of excitatory amino acid neurotransmission, produces phencyclidine-like behavioral effects in pigeons, rats and rhesus monkeys, *J Pharmacol Exp Ther* 245:969-974, 1988.
67. Kothary SP, Zsigmond EK: A double-blind study of the effective antihallucinatory doses of diazepam prior to ketamine anesthesia, *Clin Pharmacol Ther* 21:108-109, 1977.
68. Krestow M: The effect of post-anaesthetic dreaming on patient acceptance of ketamine anaesthesia: a comparison with thiopentone-nitrous oxide anaesthesia, *Can Anaesth Soc J* 21:385-389, 1974.
69. Kugel G, Letelier C, Zive MA, et al: Nitrous oxide and infertility, *Anesth Prog* 37:176-180, 1990.
70. Kugel G, Zive M, Agarwal RK, et al: Effect of nitrous oxide on the concentrations of opioid peptides, substance P, and LHRH in the brain and β-endorphin in the pituitary, *Anesth Prog* 38:206-211, 1991.
71. Layzer RB, Fishman RA, Schafer JA: Neuropathy following abuse of nitrous oxide, *Neurology* 28:504-506, 1978.
72. Litman RS, Kottra JA, Verga KA, et al: Chloral hydrate sedation: the additive sedative and respiratory depressant effects of nitrous oxide, *Anesth Analg* 86:724-728, 1998.
73. Little B, Chang T, Chucot L, et al: Study of ketamine as an obstetric anesthetic agent, *Am J Obstet Gynecol* 113:247-260, 1972.
74. Lundy PM, Lockwood PA, Thompson G, et al: Differential effects of ketamine isomers on neuronal and extraneuronal catecholamine uptake mechanisms, *Anesthesiology* 64:359-363, 1986.
75. Malviya S, Voepel-Lewis T, Prochaska G, et al: Prolonged recovery and delayed side effects of sedation for diagnostic imaging studies in children, *Pediatrics* 105:E42, 2000.
76. Maze M, Tranquilli W: Alpha-2 adrenoceptor agonists: defining the role in clinical anesthesia, *Anesthesiology* 74:581-605, 1991.
77. Mazze RI: Nitrous oxide during pregnancy, *Anaesthesia* 41:897-899, 1986.
78. Mazze RI, Calverley RK, Smith NT: Inorganic fluoride nephrotoxicity: prolonged enflurane and halothane anesthesia in volunteers, *Anesthesiology* 46:265-271, 1977.
79. McAteer PM, Carter JA, Cooper GM, et al: Comparison of isoflurane and halothane in outpatient paediatric dental anaesthesia, *Br J Anaesth* 58:390-393, 1986.
80. Miyasaka M, Domino EF: Neural mechanisms of ketamine-induced anesthesia, *Int J Neuropharmacol* 7:557-573, 1968.

81. Morel DR, Forster A, Gemperle M: Noninvasive evaluation of breathing pattern and thoraco-abdominal motion following the infusion of ketamine or droperidol in humans, *Anesthesiology* 65:392-398, 1986.

82. Mori K, Kawamata M, Miyajima S, et al: The effects of several anesthetic agents on the neuronal reactive properties of thalamic relay nuclei in the cat, *Anesthesiology* 36:550-557, 1972.

83. Mukai S, Morior M, Fujii K, et al: Volatile metabolites of halothane in the rabbit, *Anesthesiology* 47:248-251, 1977.

84. Naito Y, Tamai S, Shingu K, et al: Comparison between sevoflurane and halothane for paediatric ambulatory anaesthesia, *Br J Anaesth* 67:387-389, 1991.

85. Nunn JF, Sharer NM, Gorchein A, et al: Megaloblastic haemopoiesis after multiple short-term exposure to nitrous oxide, *Lancet* 1:1379-1381, 1982.

86. Olkkola KT, Aranko K, Luurila H, et al: A potentially hazardous interaction between erythromycin and midazolam, *Clin Pharmacol Ther* 53:298-305, 1993.

87. Park GR, Manara AR, Mendel L, et al: Ketamine infusion. Its use as a sedative, inotrope and bronchodilator in a critically ill patient, *Anaesthesia* 42:980-983, 1987.

88. Priebe H-J: Coronary circulation and factors affecting coronary "steal," *Eur J Anaesthesiol* 8:177-195, 1991.

89. Ramsay DS, Brown AC, Woods SC: Acute tolerance to nitrous oxide in humans, *Pain* 51:367-373, 1992.

90. Ray DC, Drummond GB: Halothane hepatitis, *Br J Anaesth* 67:84-99, 1991.

91. Reder BS, Trapp LD, Troutman KC: Ketamine suppression of chemically induced convulsions in the two-day-old white leghorn cockerel, *Anesth Analg* 59:406-409, 1980.

92. Reves JG, Lell WA, McCracken LE, Jr, et al: Comparison of morphine and ketamine anesthetic techniques for coronary surgery: a randomized study, *South Med J* 71:33-36, 1978.

93. Reynolds ES, Moslen MT: Halothane hepatotoxicity: enhancement by polychlorinated biphenyl pretreatment, *Anesthesiology* 47:19-27, 1977.

94. Rock MJ, Reyes de la Rocha S, L'Hommedieu CS, et al: Use of ketamine in asthmatic children to treat respiratory failure refractory to conventional therapy, *Crit Care Med* 14:514-516, 1986.

95. Rowland AS, Baird DD, Weinberg CR, et al: Reduced fertility among women employed as dental assistants exposed to high levels of nitrous oxide, *N Engl J Med* 327:993-997, 1992.

96. Royston BD, Nunn JF, Weinbren HK, et al: Rate of inactivation of human and rodent hepatic methionine synthase by nitrous oxide, *Anesthesiology* 68:213-216, 1988.

97. Rusy BF, Komai H: Anesthetic depression of myocardial contractility: a review of possible mechanisms, *Anesthesiology* 67:745-766, 1987.

98. Sarner JB, Levine M, Davis PJ, et al: Clinical characteristics of sevoflurane in children. A comparison with halothane, *Anesthesiology* 82:38-46, 1995.

99. Saunders PRI, Harris MNE: Opisthotonus and other unusual neurological sequelae after outpatient anaesthesia, *Anaesthesia* 45:552-557, 1990.

100. Searle NR, Sahab P: Propofol in patients with cardiac disease, *Can J Anaesth* 40:730-747, 1993.

101. Shafer SL: Advances in propofol pharmacokinetics and pharmacodynamics, *J Clin Anesth* 5(6 suppl 1):14S-21S, 1993.

102. Shapiro HM, Wyte SR, Harris AB: Ketamine anaesthesia in patients with intracranial pathology, *Br J Anaesth* 44:1200-1204, 1972.

103. Shulman D, Beardsmore CS, Aronson HB, et al: The effect of ketamine on the functional residual capacity in young children, *Anesthesiology* 62:551-556, 1985.

104. Sircar R, Nichtenhauser R, Ieni JR, et al: Characterization and autoradiographic visualization of (++)-[3H]SKF10,047 binding in rat and mouse brain: further evidence for phencyclidine/"sigma opiate" receptor commonality, *J Pharmacol Exp Ther* 237:681-688, 1986.

105. Smith DJ, Bouchal RL, deSanctis CA, et al: Properties of the interaction between ketamine and opiate binding sites in vivo and in vitro, *Neuropharmacology* 26:1253-1260, 1987.

106. Smith G, Shirley AW: Failure to demonstrate effect of trace concentrations of nitrous oxide and halothane on psychomotor performance, *Br J Anaesth* 49:65-70, 1977.

107. Smith I, White PF, Nathanson M, et al: Propofol. An update on its clinical use, *Anesthesiology* 81:1005-1043, 1994.

108. Stacy CB, Di Rocco A, Gould RJ: Methionine in the treatment of nitrous-oxide–induced neuropathy and myeloneuropathy, *J Neurol* 239:401-403, 1992.

109. Strazis KP, Fox AW: Malignant hyperthermia: a review of published cases, *Anesth Analg* 77:297-304, 1993.

110. Strube PJ, Hallam PL: Ketamine by continuous infusion in status asthmaticus, *Anaesthesia* 41:1017-1019, 1986.

111. Strum DP, Johnson BH, Eger EI II: Stability of sevoflurane in soda lime, *Anesthesiology* 67:779-781, 1987.

112. Takeshita H, Okuda Y, Sari A: The effects of ketamine on cerebral circulation and metabolism in man, *Anesthesiology* 36:69-75, 1972.

113. Tekavec MM: Nitrous oxide sedation with auditory modification, *Anesth Prog* 23:181-186, 1976.

114. Tokics L, Strandberg A, Brismar B, et al: Computerized tomography of the chest and gas exchange measurements during ketamine anaesthesia, *Acta Anaesthesiol Scand* 31:684-692, 1987.

115. Tweed WA, Minuck M, Mymin D: Circulatory responses to ketamine anesthesia, *Anesthesiology* 37:613-619, 1972.

116. Vaupel DB: Naltrexone fails to antagonize the sigma effects of PCP and SKF 10,047 in the dog, *Eur J Pharmacol* 92:269-274, 1983.

117. Vote GJ, Hart RH, Worsley DR, et al: Visual loss after use of nitrous oxide gas with general anesthetic in patients with intraocular gas still persistent up to 30 days after vitrectomy, *Anesthesiology* 97:1305-1308, 2002.

118. Warltier DC, Pagel PS: Cardiovascular and respiratory actions of desflurane: is desflurane different from isoflurane? *Anesth Analg* 75:S17-S31, 1992.

119. White PF, Ham J, Way WL, et al: Pharmacology of ketamine isomers in surgical patients, *Anesthesiology* 52:231-239, 1980.

120. White PF, Way WL, Trevor AJ: Ketamine—its pharmacology and therapeutic uses, *Anesthesiology* 56:119-136, 1982.

121. Wolf A, Weir P, Segar P, et al: Impaired fatty acid oxidation in propofol infusion syndrome, *Lancet* 357:606-607, 2001.

122. Wood C, Ewen A, Goresky G, et al: Exposure of operating room personnel to nitrous oxide during paediatric anaesthesia, *Can J Anaesth* 39:682-686, 1992.

123. Yacoub O, Doell D, Kryger MH, et al: Depression of hypoxic ventilatory response by nitrous oxide, *Anesthesiology* 45:385-389, 1976.

124. Yang YF, Herbert L, Ruschen H, et al: Nitrous oxide anaesthesia in the presence of intraocular gas can cause irreversible blindness, *Br Med J* 325:532-533, 2002.

125. Yasuda N, Lockhart SH, Eger EI II, et al: Kinetics of desflurane, isoflurane, and halothane in humans, *Anesthesiology* 74:489-498, 1991.

126. Yoshimura N, Holaday DA, Fiserova-Bergerova V: Metabolism of methoxyflurane in man, *Anesthesiology* 44:372-379, 1976.

127. Young CJ, Apfelbaum JL: A comparative review of the newer inhalational anaesthetics, *CNS Drugs* 10:257-310, 1998.

General References

Barash PG, Cullen BF, Stoelting RK, eds: *Clinical anesthesia*, ed 4, Philadelphia, 2001, Lippincott Williams & Wilkins.

Evers AS, Crowder CM: General anesthetics. In Hardman JG, Limbird LE, Gilman AG, eds: *Goodman & Gilman's The pharmacological basis of therapeutics*, ed 10, New York, 2001, McGraw-Hill.

Miller RD, ed: *Anesthesia*, ed 5, New York, 2000, Churchill Livingstone.

USP dispensing information, vol 1, Drug information for the health care professional, ed 23, Greenwood Village, CO, 2003, MICROMEDEX Thomson Healthcare.

CHAPTER • 19

Introduction to Antinociceptive Drugs

Hyungsuk Kim and Raymond A. Dionne

Pain has always been a barrier to dentistry, serving as a continuing motivation for the use of drugs to prevent, block, or attenuate pain in the perioperative period. Despite the efficacy of local anesthesia, many procedures can result in substantial postoperative discomfort and edema, thus limiting mouth opening for several days. Poorly controlled pain in the perioperative period also contributes to anxiety about future dental therapy, leading to postponed or canceled appointments.[2,7,13] Effective control of orofacial pain facilitates the delivery of care, lowers anxiety about dentistry, and may even improve dental health by promoting preventive and routine dentistry as an alternative to general neglect with episodic care for acute problems. Emerging basic and clinical studies have demonstrated that the effective use of antinociceptive drugs to attenuate perioperative pain is an effective approach to prevent the development of hyperalgesia manifesting as increased pain hours to days after a procedure. The availability of safe and effective antinociceptive drugs now permits effective prevention and management of perioperative pain for the mutual benefit of the patient and the dental practitioner.

The multiplicity of pain mechanisms and the difficulty of separating nociceptive processing from physiologic pain perception represent significant barriers to improving pain therapy. In addition to the molecular events associated with tissue injury, inflammation, the development of sensitization, and activation of ascending and descending pathways, it is now recognized that gender and genetic factors also contribute to individual variation in pain perception, processing, and the evaluation of nociceptive input. Because of this mechanistic complexity, use of analgesic drugs in fixed doses that have been validated in a relatively homogenous patient sample may not result in effective therapy when used in a patient population with wide genetic diversity in pain processing and drug metabolism. Although individual variation in the human pain experience is traditionally explained by a variety of factors such as cultural or psychologic influences, recent studies in animal and human pain models demonstrate phenotypic differences in pain sensitivity that may result from genetic factors.[19,20,36] This genetic variation among patients, along with other sources of variation, provides a physiologic rationale for individualizing pain treatment.

The management of chronic pain has a long history of therapeutic misadventure, including the misuse of drugs for symptomatic relief of chronic orofacial pain. There is still no generally accepted agreement on the cause of chronic orofacial pain; its natural history; the need for aggressive treatment; and the effectiveness, safety, and indications for most clinical practices. Differences of opinion on these issues are often fostered by a lack of appreciation of the difference between clinical observations, which may form the basis for therapeutic innovation, and the need to verify the efficacy and safety of treatments in studies that control for factors that can mimic clinical success. Drug classes for the treatment of pain associated with temporomandibular disorders range from short-term treatment with nonsteroidal antiinflammatory drugs (NSAIDs) and muscle relaxants for pain of presumed muscular origin to long-term administration of antidepressants and anticonvulsants for less well-characterized pain (see Chapter 23). The management of pain associated with temporomandibular disorders rests on the same principles that apply to the use of all drugs: demonstrated efficacy for the indication, an acceptable incidence of adverse reactions for the condition being treated, and safety when used in large numbers of patients for prolonged periods.

Increasing numbers of elderly people in the population raise the prevalence of age-related painful conditions such as osteoarthritis or various neuropathies. Improvements in the management of cancer increase life expectancy but are accompanied by a rise in the cumulative incidence of cancer-related pain as well as painful conditions associated with cancer treatment (e.g., chemotherapy, radiotherapy, surgery). In these patients with a complicated history, currently available analgesic modalities are often not helpful or effective. In spite of astonishing advancements in our understanding of the neurobiology of pain, pain continues to produce severe distress, dominating and disrupting the lives of many patients from lack of adequate pain relief or the consequences of its treatment.

PATHWAYS OF OROFACIAL PAIN

Pain Transduction and Transmission in the Periphery

Noxious stimuli, which can produce tissue damage, are detected by the terminal endings of two major classes of nociceptive (pain-detecting) afferent nerve fibers (Figure 19-1). These nociceptors are distributed throughout the skin, oral mucosa, and tooth pulp. The Aδ fibers are fast-conducting, lightly myelinated neurons responding primarily to noxious mechanical stimuli. Aδ fibers are thought to mediate the initial sensation of pain, which has a sharp perceptual quality. The second group of nociceptive fibers are the C fibers, slowly conducting unmyelinated neurons that respond to thermal, mechanical, and chemical stimuli. The C fibers likely mediate secondary pain, which occurs after the initial sharp, pricking pain and is generally described as having a dull, aching, or burning perceptual quality. There are approximately three to five times more C fibers than Aδ fibers.[23] Other classes of

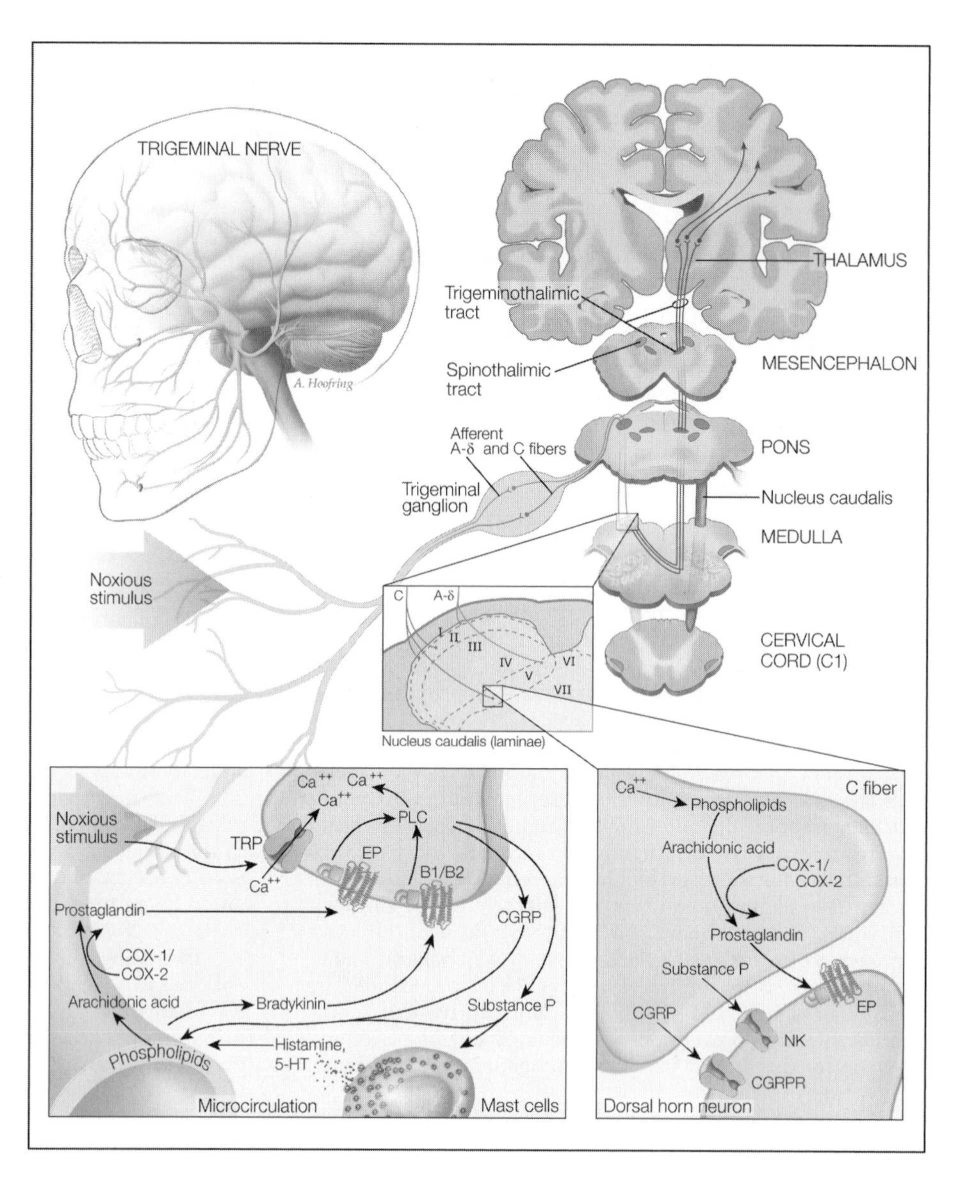

Fig. 19-1 Diagram of trigeminal nociceptive pathways. After a noxious stimulus is applied in the orofacial region, multiple chemical mediators are released from damaged cells and from local nerve terminals and inflammatory cells *(lower left)*. Some mediators act on their receptors and directly activate nociceptors, evoking pain. Others act together to produce a sensitization of the nervous system. Small A-δ and C afferents synapse with nociceptive-specific trigeminothalamic neurons in the nucleus caudalis *(center)*. By the released neurotransmitters from the primary afferents *(lower right)*, trigeminothalamic neurons are activated, and noxious information is transmitted directly to the thalamus and ultimately to the cerebral cortex.

cutaneous fibers have been described but are not as well characterized.

The detection of noxious stimuli in the orofacial region and the encoding of pain are conveyed primarily by nerves of the trigeminal system. The trigeminal nerve, or fifth cranial nerve, is the largest of the cranial nerves; its three branches (ophthalmic, maxillary, and mandibular) innervate most of the face and anterior scalp. The trigeminal nerve also innervates the mucous membranes and gingivae of the mouth; the teeth and jaws; the anterior two thirds of the tongue; the nasopharynx, nasal cavities, and sinuses; and a portion of the meninges. The facial (seventh cranial) nerve encodes pain from the skin of the mastoid region and the external auditory meatus; most of the sensory function of this nerve, however, is involved in taste sensation. The glossopharyngeal (ninth cranial) nerve innervates the back of the tongue, the tonsillar region, tympanic cavity, and antrum as well as oronasal portions of the pharynx. The vagus (tenth cranial) nerve innervates the larynx and parts of the pharynx, ear, and external auditory meatus. These cranial nerves provide the peripheral innervation necessary for the detection of orofacial and dental pain.[16]

Pain Modulation in the Brainstem

The Aδ and C fibers from the orofacial region transmit nociceptive signals primarily by the branches of the trigeminal nerve to the trigeminal nucleus caudalis; noxious information from additional regions is conveyed by other cranial nerves. Most clinical and laboratory data indicate that the nucleus caudalis is the principal brainstem relay site for trigeminal nociceptive information.[27] The nucleus caudalis is located in the medulla; its laminated structure, types of cells, and function in processing pain signals are similar to the area on the dorsal aspect of the spinal cord known as the *dorsal horn*. As previously stated, the small-diameter afferents carrying nociceptive information from the various craniofacial tissues predominantly terminate in I, II, and V lamina of the nucleus caudalis. By contrast, primary afferent A fibers conducting low-threshold mechanosensitive (tactile) information terminate primarily in the most rostral components of the trigeminal brainstem complex and in laminae III to VI of the nucleus caudalis. Recent studies have also revealed increases in immunocytochemical markers of neuronal activity in caudalis neurons after noxious stimulation of craniofacial tissues.[27]

Additionally, many studies using microelectrode recording have shown that many neurons in the nucleus caudalis are activated by cutaneous nociceptive input in craniofacial region. For these reasons, the nucleus caudalis has been termed the *medullary dorsal horn*.[28]

The medullary and spinal dorsal horns contain four major components related to the processing of noxious stimuli: central terminals of afferent fibers, local circuit neurons, projection neurons, and descending neurons. The first component, primary nociceptive afferents (Aδ and C fibers), enter the medullary dorsal horn by the trigeminal tract. Nerves that enter the spinal dorsal horn traverse the lateral aspect of the tract of Lissauer. For both medullary and the spinal dorsal horns, Aδ and C fibers terminate mainly in laminae I, IIa, and V. The primary nociceptive afferents transmit information by the synaptic release of neuropeptides (e.g., substance P, calcitonin gene–related peptide [CGRP]) and amino acids (e.g., glutamate).

The second component of the dorsal horn—the local circuit neurons—consists of two major subtypes, the islet cell and the stalked cell. The islet cell is found throughout lamina II and is thought to be an inhibitory interneuron possibly using γ-aminobutyric acid (GABA) or enkephalin as neurotransmitters. Stalked cells are found primarily at the junction between lamina I and II and have been proposed to be excitatory interneurons conveying nociceptive output from primary afferents to projection neurons located in lamina I. The local circuit neurons play a crucial role in conveying and modulating nociceptive signals from the primary afferents to the projection neurons.

Projection neurons constitute the third component of the dorsal horn. Their function, and that of the descending neurons, is described later. Both projection neurons and local circuit neurons can be divided into two major classes: wide dynamic range and nociceptive-specific neurons. The wide dynamic range neurons are activated by weak mechanical stimuli but respond maximally to intense and potentially tissue-damaging stimuli. In contrast, nociceptive-specific neurons respond only to intense noxious forms of mechanical, thermal, or chemical stimuli.

Pain Perception and Modulation by the Cerebral Cortex

Two major projections carrying noxious information from the medullary and spinal dorsal horns, respectively, are the trigeminothalamic tract and the spinothalamic tract. These tracts are composed of axons from the wide dynamic range and nociceptive neurons. These axons cross to the contralateral side of the medulla or spinal cord and ascend rostrally to the thalamus. From the thalamus, additional neurons convey this information to the cerebral cortex (see Figure 19-1).

Axonal collaterals of the trigeminothalamic and spinothalamic tracts terminate in the rostral medullary reticular formation and the periaqueductal gray. The projection and local circuit neurons encode information about the location, intensity, duration, and the type of noxious input.

The fourth component of the dorsal horn is composed of the terminal endings of descending neurons. These neurons form an important component of the endogenous pain modulatory system. Because the cerebral cortex is an important center for integrating all perceptual modalities together with higher functions, such as expectation and recall of previous events, it is not surprising that the cortex is involved in pain perception and response. Evidence suggests that the cerebral cortex is involved with the sensory discriminative aspect of pain and may also activate the endogenous analgesic system and thus represents its most rostral component.[16]

PERIPHERAL MECHANISMS OF PAIN AND ANALGESIC DRUG ACTIONS

Activation of Nociceptors

Most noxious stimuli are transduced into electrical activity at the peripheral terminals of Aδ and C fibers by specific receptors or ion channels sensitive to heat, mechanical stimuli, protons, or cold. Ligand-gated channels expressed on nociceptive neurons include excitatory amino acid receptors, GABA receptors, nicotinic acetylcholine receptors, serotonergic (tryptaminergic or 5-hydroxytryptamine) receptors, and adenosine triphosphate P2X receptors. These receptors permit primary nociceptive neurons to respond to a wide range of mediators.[22]

Among the hundreds of channels that modulate the passage of charged ions across cell membranes, Ca^{++} channels are particularly important in cellular homeostasis and activity, and the surface of each cell holds thousands of channels that precisely control the timing and entry of Ca^{++}. Small conformational changes cause these channels to open, allowing more than 10 million ions per second to flow through each channel. The opening of Ca^{++} channels is the crucial link between cell depolarization and Ca^{++} entry, which can result in local intracellular Ca^{++} concentrations as great as 100 μmol/L. The subsequent binding of Ca^{++} to intracellular molecules can lead to many significant responses, including triggering of neurotransmitter release, the activation of second messenger systems, and Ca^{++} spikes (action potentials in which the depolarizing current is carried predominantly by Ca^{++}).[22]

Transient receptor potential (TRP) channels are the vanguard of sensory systems, responding to temperature, touch, pain, osmolarity, and other stimuli. TRPV1, also known as the *vanilloid receptor 1*, is a Ca^{++}-permeable channel that is opened by heat (>43° C) and decreased pH. TRPV1 contributes to acute thermal nociception and hyperalgesia after tissue injury. TRPV2, which is 50% identical to TRPV1 in primary structure, may mediate high-threshold (>52° C) noxious heat sensation, perhaps through lightly myelinated Aδ nociceptors. The ankyrinlike protein with transmembrane domains 1 channel is a Ca^{++}-permeable, nonselective channel distinguished by approximately14 amino-terminal ankyrin repeats. It is activated by noxious cold temperature (<15° C) but bears little similarity to the menthol-sensitive TRPV8 channel. It is found in a subset of nociceptive sensory dorsal root ganglion neurons in the company of capsaicin-sensitive TRPV1 channels.[3]

Activation of nociceptors is not the only way to trigger pain. After peripheral tissue injury or damage to the nervous system, low-threshold sensory fibers, which normally only produce innocuous sensations such as light touch, can begin to produce pain, a very substantial change in the normal functional specificity of the sensory system. Although this pain obviously no longer represents the presence of a damaging external stimulus, to the individual it feels that the pain arises in the periphery from a noxious stimulus. With inflammation, components of the "inflammatory soup" such as bradykinin or prostaglandins bind to G protein–coupled receptors and induce activation of protein kinases A and C in nociceptor peripheral terminals, which then phosphorylate ion channels and receptors. As a result, the threshold for activation of transducer receptors such as TRPV1 is reduced.

One of the best established pronociceptive substances derived from nerve endings is substance P. Substance P causes vasodilation and extravasation of plasma proteins from capillaries, which contribute to the edema associated with inflammation and to the generation of bradykinin from kininogen. Because the neurokinin-1 receptor is the major receptor for substance P, neurogenic inflammation is markedly attenuated by receptor antagonists specific for this receptor. Another putative mediator of neurogenic inflammation is CGRP, which produces vascular leakage and vasodilation leading to inflammation and tenderness. Immune cells may be involved in inflammatory pain, cancer pain, and pain after nerve injury. They are activated both in the periphery and within the central nervous system (CNS) in response to tissue damage, inflammation, or mechanical nerve lesions. The immune reaction may increase nociception through the release of cytokines, but granulocytes and monocytes can also promote analgesia by secreting β-endorphin and enkephalin.

Inflammatory Pain

Inflammation represents a complex series of physiologic reactions required for normal healing after physical injury or infection. Mediators formed during the evolution of the inflammatory process contribute to the genesis of acute pain by stimulating or sensitizing primary afferent neurons by peripheral and central mechanisms. The biochemical composition of the local environment of inflamed tissue is complex. Protons, cytokines, prostanoids, leukotrienes, neuropeptides, histamine, bradykinin, and free radicals are ingredients of the inflammatory soup that defines the biochemical environment of inflamed tissue. Although each of these molecular species may directly or indirectly contribute to inflammation, inflammatory pain probably results from an interplay of neuronal signals generated by inflammatory mediators, resulting in synergistic biochemical interactions with primary afferent neurons.

If a particular biochemical in the inflammatory soup is a primary contributor to the genesis of inflammatory pain, drugs that block its actions or synthesis should provide significant analgesia. Agents that block the actions of histamine or substance P and the synthesis of bradykinin or prostaglandins all possess analgesic activity in animal models of inflammation. In addition, combinations of these agents can exert additive effects, consistent with the view that the total composition of the inflammatory soup governs the genesis and maintenance of inflammatory pain.

Analgesic Mechanisms Acting Primarily in the Periphery

Pharmacologic management of pain can be accomplished by blocking either the nociceptive input at the receptor or the nociceptive impulse along the peripheral nerve. As previously mentioned, various biochemicals at inflammatory sites affect nociceptive input by direct or indirect mechanisms. For example, prostaglandins, especially PGE_2, sensitize nociceptive nerve endings and thereby potentiate the actions of other inflammatory mediators such as bradykinin. Sensitization of peripheral nociceptors is minimized in the absence of PGE_2, and pain sensations are thus attenuated. Therefore drugs designed to block prostaglandin synthesis or function should be effective analgesics for some inflammatory pains.

Aspirinlike drugs, which include aspirin, acetaminophen, and NSAIDs, exert their actions in damaged tissue. These drugs inhibit generation of the pain signal and accompanying sensitization at the nerve ending through blockade of prostaglandin synthesis.[11,12] In addition, NSAIDs have been reported to possess moderate efficacy for inhibiting postoperative edema.[33] However, there appears to be a maximal effect, or ceiling effect, beyond which additional increments of drugs do not produce significantly greater analgesia. This ceiling effect probably reflects the contribution of other inflammatory mediators that are unaffected by aspirinlike drugs.

The physiologic mechanism for the synthesis of prostaglandins is the activation of phospholipase A_2 and cyclooxygenase during the process of tissue damage (e.g., during surgery). This information has an important practical application—pretreating patients with NSAIDs before surgery. The rationale for this therapy is the blockade of enzymes before the initiation of tissue damage. Although the advantages of pretreatment have been most clearly established for ibuprofen,[17] several other drugs, including flurbiprofen, have been demonstrated to reduce pain. Pretreating patients with ibuprofen delays the onset and reduces the magnitude of postoperative pain. This therapeutic strategy emphasizes how clinicians can improve patient care by knowledge of pain physiology.[16]

Inhibition of prostaglandin synthesis can also be accomplished by administering glucocorticoids. This group of steroids has very potent antiinflammatory activity. Glucocorticoids inhibit all phases of inflammation, including capillary dilation, migration of leukocytes, and phagocytosis. Steroids have been demonstrated to activate synthesis of a protein inhibitor of phospholipase A_2 called *lipocortin*.[21] Blockade of arachidonic acid formation by inhibiting phospholipase A_2 is an early step in the cascade and thus prevents formation of both cyclooxygenase and lipoxygenase end products. In addition, glucocorticoids induce the synthesis of angiotensin-converting enzyme, a peptidase that degrades bradykinin and decreases the capillary permeability, probably from the increased synthesis of peptides promoting vascular stability or the reduced release of proteolytic enzymes.[9] These multiple mechanisms for the suppression of inflammatory mediators probably account for the impressive antiinflammatory efficacy of steroids. Another approach to peripheral pain management is to block the nociceptive impulse as it moves along the nerve axon. Local anesthetics prevent the propagation of action potentials in peripheral nerves by interfering with Na^+ channel permeability. Nociceptive Aδ and C fibers are very susceptible to blockade by local anesthetics. Local anesthetics with increased potency and prolonged duration of action have been developed on the basis of their enhanced physicochemical properties, such as increased lipid solubility and greater protein binding. Thus, sustained blockade of Aδ and C fibers can result in prolonged suppression of postoperative pain.

Many studies indicate that the immune system can interact with peripheral sensory nerve endings to inhibit pain within inflamed tissue. In contrast to the traditional view that opioid antinociception is mediated exclusively within the CNS, peripheral opioid receptors have been discovered and shown to mediate analgesic effects when activated by locally applied opioid agonists.[31] Opioid receptors are present on peripheral sensory nerves and are upregulated during the development of inflammation. Their endogenous ligands—opioid peptides—are expressed in resident immune cells within peripheral inflamed tissue. These findings have led to the concept that endogenous opioid peptides can be secreted from immunocytes, occupy opioid receptors on sensory nerves, and produce analgesia by inhibiting either the excitability of these nerves or the release of excitatory, proinflammatory neuropeptides.[32] It appears that peripheral opioid receptors can modulate sensory nerve impulses in a way similar to spinal presynaptic opioid receptors. The local application of exogenous opioids[8] or enzyme inhibitors preventing the degradation of endogenous opioid peptides may provide a new approach to pain management by producing analgesia without central side effects.

CENTRAL MECHANISMS OF PAIN AND ANALGESIC DRUG ACTIONS

Neurotransmitters Involved in Nociceptive Signaling

The central endings of trigeminal nociceptive primary afferents within the nucleus caudalis contain certain excitatory amino acids (e.g., glutamate) and neuropeptides (e.g., substance P, CGRP) that transmit the nociceptive signals to the second-order trigeminal neurons. In lamina II, the axons of most substantia gelatinosa neurons arborize locally within the trigeminal brainstem complex and release neuromodulatory substances such as enkephalin or GABA. The substantia gelatinosa receives a mix of inputs from other areas in the brain as well as craniofacial afferent input, and it is one of the main sites where peripheral afferents and brain centers modulate somatosensory transmission.[28] Glutamate is a particularly important excitatory neurotransmitter in trigeminal nociceptive mechanisms.[10] It is released from the central endings of trigeminal nociceptive afferents and activates caudalis nociceptive neurons. This process involves two different ionotropic receptors for glutamate—N-methyl-D-aspartate (NMDA) and α-amino-3-hydroxy-5-methyl-4-isoxazole propionic acid receptors—as well as metabotropic receptors.

Substance P and the neurokinin-1 receptor are also concentrated in afferent endings in the superficial and deep laminae of the nucleus caudalis, where the nociceptive neurons predominate. Noxious craniofacial stimulation is reported to result in the release of substance P within the nucleus caudalis, presumably from the nociceptive afferent terminals within the substantia gelatinosa, and the released substance P acts through neurokinin receptors to produce a long-latency and sustained excitation of the nociceptive neurons.

Central Convergence of Neurons Signaling Pain

Many nociceptive and wide dynamic range neurons can be excited by stimulation of cutaneous or mucosal receptive fields and seem to play an important role in the localization, detection, and discrimination of superficial noxious stimuli. These same neurons can also be excited by peripheral afferents from other tissues such as cerebral blood vessels, tooth pulp, the temporomandibular joint (TMJ), or muscle. The extensive convergent afferent input patterns are particularly characteristic of nociceptive-specific and wide dynamic range neurons in the nucleus caudalis. The presence of a cutaneous as well as a deep receptive field for most of these neurons may explain the poor localization of deep pain and contribute to the spread and referral of pain typical of deep pain conditions involving the TMJ and associated musculature. The poor localization of pain and the frequent occurrence of pain referral with toothache and headache may also be related to analogous convergence patterns from tooth pulp and cerebrovascular afferents onto the nociceptive neurons.

Development of Central Sensitization

The convergence of afferent input may also contribute to central neuronal changes that can be induced by inflammation or injury of peripheral tissues or nerves. Several chemicals released from the peripheral tissue or primary afferent nerve endings by tissue injury or inflammation can increase the excitability of peripheral nociceptors. This in turn produces a barrage of nociceptive primary afferent input into the CNS. Peripheral nerve damage or lesions can also increase nociceptive afferent input. Whatever the cause, this nociceptive afferent barrage can lead to prolonged functional alterations in the nucleus caudalis (and spinal dorsal horn) collectively termed *central sensitization*. For example, the nociceptive afferent activity caused by damage or inflammation of tooth pulp, TMJ, or muscle induces spontaneous activity, receptive field expansion, lowering of the activation threshold, and enhancement of responses of caudalis nociceptive-specific and wide dynamic range neurons that may include a gradually augmenting response to a series of repeated noxious stimuli.[28]

These alterations indicate that the afferent inputs and brainstem circuitry are not "hard-wired" but reflect neuroplastic changes in the receptive fields and response properties of the nociceptive neurons. The changes are thought to result, at least in part, from the unmasking and increased efficacy of the extensive convergent afferent input to the nociceptive neurons noted above. The neurons' responses to this input are enhanced and their receptive fields enlarged, reflecting a greater number of more effective input. It appears that this central sensitization is produced by a cascade of events that starts with the nociceptive afferent barrage causing the release centrally of a number of chemical mediators such as substance P (mentioned previously). These substances prolong neuronal depolarization and increase the excitability of the nociceptive neurons by actions at glutamate receptors and G protein–coupled receptors. Activation of these receptors is associated with removal of the voltage-dependent Mg^{++} block of the NMDA receptor, the entry of Ca^{++} into the neurons, phosphorylation of the NMDA receptor, and a change in neuronal kinetics. These changes may also involve other ionotropic and metabotropic excitatory amino acid receptors, neurotrophins, and kinases involved in the phosphorylation of receptors. A loss of central inhibitory processes may contribute to the increased neuronal excitability that is characteristic of central sensitization.[4]

The increased central excitatory state depends on peripheral nociceptive afferent input for its initiation but may not fully depend on peripheral afferent drive for its maintenance. Central sensitization can last for days or even weeks and is thought to contribute to persistent pain and to the spontaneous pain and tenderness that characterize many clinical cases of injury or inflammation. Central sensitization can explain the hyperalgesia that is a feature of many persistent pain conditions, by virtue of the increase in excitability to Aδ- and C-fiber nociceptive input that it produces in central nociceptive neurons. It also may enhance low-threshold mechanosensitive afferent input (which is not normally associated with pain) to respond as nociceptive neurons after peripheral injury or inflammation, and thus could contribute to the allodynia that is often associated with pain conditions. Peripheral sensitization can also contribute to hyperalgesia and allodynia by increasing the excitability and decreasing the activation threshold of primary afferents. Thus many pain conditions may involve a mixture of peripheral and central sensitization phenomena.[28]

Central Effects of Opioid Drugs

Traditional pharmacologic pain management usually involves the administration of opioid analgesics. Parenteral opioid analgesics are the standard care for severe pain in hospitalized patients. The profound analgesic efficacy of opioid drugs results from their ability to mimic the actions of the family of endogenous opioid peptides. Because endogenous opioids and their receptors are present at all levels of the endogenous analgesic system, opioid drugs can activate this system to suppress the transmission of nociceptive signals at the medullary and spinal dorsal horns. Unfortunately, the oral efficacy of most opioid drugs is very poor. An additional problem with opioids is their propensity to cause nausea in ambulatory patients. Thus the opioids for most orofacial pain are limited to an adjunctive role. In general, the combination of an aspirinlike drug with an opioid increases analgesia at the cost of an increased incidence of side effects.[16]

Three opioid receptor classes are generally recognized, and experimental observations indicate that a common mechanism of opioid action is the cellular inhibition of neuronal activity. Although the opioid inhibitory effects may be cell dependent, accumulating evidence suggests a link to the receptor-mediated suppression of voltage-gated Ca^{++} channels, the activation of inwardly rectifying K^{+} channels, and the inhibition of adenylyl cyclase activity. However, opioid effects in sensory neurons are both inhibitory and excitatory, and opioids can suppress a Na^+-dependent inward current. High levels of endogenous opioid peptides and opioid receptors are found within the periaqueductal gray, rostral ventral medulla, and dorsal horn, and neurons in these areas can be activated by opioids. Because opioid receptors generally produce inhibitory effects on neuronal firing, the ability of endogenous opioid peptides or opioid drugs to activate neurons within these brain regions depends on an anatomic arrangement in which opioid receptors inhibit GABAergic (inhibitory) interneurons. Neurons of the rostral ventral medulla that project to the dorsal horn activate enkephalinergic interneurons that are located in the dorsal horn.[22]

GABA is present in highly diverse inhibitory interneurons and projection neurons throughout the brain. The wide-ranging and ubiquitous role of GABA as an inhibitory transmitter is supported by evidence linking numerous neuropsychiatric disorders with altered GABA function and the degradation of GABAergic neurons. In the past, the action of GABA on its receptors was considered to be solely inhibitory, on the basis of observation that GABA receptor activation moves the membrane potential of a cell away from action potential threshold. However, the role of GABA is more complex. During development, GABA may also function as an excitatory transmitter causing neuronal depolarization.

Analgesic Actions of Antidepressant Drugs

Descending noradrenergic projections from the locus ceruleus or from related noradrenergic nuclei in the dorsal pons inhibit dorsal horn neurons and thereby contribute to descending analgesia. The role of norepinephrine in descending analgesia may explain the analgesic effects of tricyclic antidepressants, including those of selective norepinephrine reuptake inhibitors, which are often effective in the treatment of neuropathic pain. Although many individuals with chronic neuropathic pain have depression, the analgesic effects of these agents are clearly independent of their antidepressant effects, because the analgesic effects occur at lower doses and after shorter periods of treatment.

MOLECULAR-GENETIC INFLUENCES ON PAIN AND ANALGESIC DRUG ACTIONS

Progress is being made in discerning the molecular and cellular mechanisms that operate in sensory pathways to generate those neural signals that we ultimately interpret as pain.[26] It is now possible to assess entire pathways that might be relevant to disease or to drug responses at the DNA, mRNA, and protein levels. With the advanced knowledge of molecular and cellular mechanisms and technologies, it is likely that most people in the future will be given prescription drugs to treat common diseases or to reduce the risk of adverse reactions on the basis of their genetic information.[14]

Mendelian traits exist when a single mutation at a locus results in large, often discrete phenotypic effects. Unlike Mendelian traits, pain is one of the complex traits in which many genes are involved, each with usually a small effect. For traits like individual differences in pain sensitivity, variations are generally not attributable to different alleles at a single locus. Rather, many different genes, each with allelic variations, contribute to the total observed variability in a trait, with no particular gene having a singly large effect. Thus an individual phenotype results from the sum total of the effects of all the numerous contributing loci.[25] Remarkably little is known about the genetic architecture underlying pain. With the human genome sequence completion, new opportunities are being presented for unraveling the complex genetic basis of non-Mendelian disorders on the basis of large-scale genome-wide studies.

Sensory input in human beings is filtered through an individual's genetic composition as well as through prior learning, current physiologic status, idiosyncratic appraisals, expectations, current mood state, and the sociocultural environment.[34] These influences manifest as variability in pain sensitivity, perception, and tolerance. However, the relative contribution and interaction of these many factors to individual variations in pain is currently unknown. Moderate heritability estimates combined with findings that specific polymorphisms in human beings are linked to responses to painful stimuli[18,29,36] may be sufficient evidence to support a genetic contribution to pain sensitivity. However, the lack of concordance between pain sensitivities suggests that there is not one "global" insensitive- or sensitive-pain phenotype.

Adverse reactions to prescription drugs cause at least 100,000 deaths each year in the United States and are responsible for more than 10% of hospital admissions in some European countries.[1] Study of pharmacogenetics that relate heritability to individual variation in drug response might lead to associations between genotype and analgesic drug response that have prognostic value. For example, we might be able to use genetic predictors to avoid adverse effects or select which of several alternative drugs will have the highest efficacy. Initial studies have already been started for analgesics including cyclooxygenase inhibitors and opioidlike drugs.[1,24,30,35] Truly personalized analgesic medication remains a distant goal. It is unlikely that genome-wide single nucleotide polymorphism profiles will provide the basis for the genetic personalization of medicines in the near future. To overcome the gap between the far advanced neurobiologic knowledge of pain and the lack of success in clinical pain therapy, greater effort needs to be directed to the discovery of targets for new analgesics.

THERAPEUTIC STRATEGIES FOR USING ANTINOCICEPTIVE DRUGS

Pain Prevention

Interfering with nociceptive input into the CNS, especially in the perioperative period, also interferes with processes that contribute to the development of central sensitization. The consequence of central sensitization is that innocuous sensations may be interpreted as painful (central hyperalgesia) and persist long after the initiating stimulus has ended. This phenomenon and the related process of sensitization of nociceptors are probably additive and contribute to both the intensity and duration of pain postoperatively. Recognition of the possible clinical importance of the development of central sensitization has led to attempts to block its development and thus minimize postoperative pain and lower analgesic use during recovery. The ability to lower analgesic use is particularly desirable in ambulatory patients who are much more sensitive to the adverse effects of opioid drugs. Decreasing pain and adverse drug effects makes the postoperative period less unpleasant and also enhances return to normal function and likely lowers apprehension about future clinical procedures.

Translating these observations and hypotheses into the management of pain in the dental environment can be readily achieved with currently available drugs. The use of either an NSAID or a long-acting local anesthetic before a dental procedure results in less pain during the first 4 to 8 hours postoperatively[5,6] and appears to attenuate pain intensity over the first 2 to 3 days thereafter.[15] The administration of an NSAID before pain onset suppresses the release of inflammatory mediators such as prostaglandins that contribute to the sensitization of peripheral nociceptors. Patients have a much slower onset and less intense pain postoperatively after NSAID pretreatment, thereby lessening nociceptive input and the development of central sensitization as well. The combination of NSAID pretreatment and the use of a long-acting local anesthetic greatly reduces pain after oral surgery, such that many patients report little pain in the first 6 to 7 hours postoperatively and reduced pain at 24 and 48 hours compared with standard treatment.

Pain Management

NSAIDs such as ibuprofen are among the most widely used drugs for dental pain and are generally more efficacious than aspirin, acetaminophen, or codeine in most studies, presumably because of the inflammatory cause of most dental pain and the prominent antiinflammatory effects of the NSAIDs. When possible, NSAID therapy is preferable for ambulatory patients who generally have a high incidence of side effects when given an opioid. NSAIDs also modestly suppress swelling after surgical procedures, providing additional therapeutic benefit without the potential liabilities of administering steroids. These considerations and the vast clinical experience gained through 25 years of clinical experience with ibuprofen make NSAIDs the drug class of choice for dental pain for patients who do not have any contraindications to its use.

Limitations to orally administered NSAIDs for dental pain include delayed onset when compared with an injectable opioid, the inability to relieve severe pain consistently, and an apparent lack of effectiveness when given repeatedly for chronic pain. For patients who do not receive satisfactory relief from an NSAID alone, combining it with an opioid may provide additive analgesia but will also be accompanied by more frequent side effects. Chapters 20 and 21 review, respectively, the pharmacology of the opioids and NSAIDs, and the clinical use of these agents for acute pain is discussed in Chapter 47.

Cited References

1. Abbott A: With your genes? Take one of these, three times a day, *Nature* 425:760-762, 2003.
2. Berggren U, Meynert G: Dental fear and avoidance: causes, symptoms, and consequences, *J Am Dent Assoc* 109:247-251, 1984.
3. Clapham DE: TRP channels as cellular sensors, *Nature* 426:517-524, 2003.
4. Dickenson A: Pharmacology of pain transmission and control. In Campbell JN, ed: *Pain 1996—an updated review. Refresher course syllabus,* Seattle, 1996, IASP Press.
5. Dionne RA, Campbell RA, Cooper SA, et al: Suppression of postoperative pain by preoperative administration of ibuprofen in comparison to placebo, acetaminophen, and acetaminophen plus codeine, *J Clin Pharmacol* 23:37-43, 1983.
6. Dionne RA, Cooper SA: Evaluation of preoperative ibuprofen for postoperative pain after removal of third molars, *Oral Surg Oral Med Oral Pathol* 45:851-856, 1978.
7. Dionne RA, Gordon SM, McCullagh LM, et al: Assessing the need for anesthesia and sedation in the general population, *J Am Dent Assoc* 129:167-173, 1998.
8. Dionne RA, Lepinski AM, Gordon SM, et al: Analgesic effects of peripherally administered opioids in clinical models of acute and chronic inflammation, *Clin Pharmacol Ther* 70:66-73, 2001.
9. Di Rosa M, Calignano A, Carnuccio R, et al: Multiple control of inflammation by glucocorticoids, *Agents Actions* 17:284-289, 1986.
10. Dubner R, Basbaum A: Spinal dorsal horn plasticity following tissue or nerve injury. In Wall RD, Melzack R, eds: *Textbook of pain*, London, 1994, Churchill Livingstone.
11. Ferreira SH, Moncada S, Vane JR: Prostaglandins and the mechanism of analgesia produced by aspirin-like drugs, *Br J Pharmacol* 49:86-97, 1973.
12. Flower RJ, Blackwell GJ: Anti-inflammatory steroids induce biosynthesis of a phospholipase A_2 inhibitor which prevents prostaglandin generation, *Nature* 278:456-459, 1979.
13. Gatchel RJ, Ingersoll BD, Bowman L, et al: The prevalence of dental fear and avoidance: a recent survey study, *J Am Dent Assoc* 107:609-610, 1983.
14. Goldstein DB, Tate SK, Sisodiya SM: Pharmacogenetics goes genomic, *Nat Rev Genet* 4:937-947, 2003.
15. Gordon SM, Brahim JS, Dubner R, et al: Attenuation of pain in a randomized trial by suppression of peripheral nociceptive activity in the immediate postoperative period, *Anesth Analg* 95:1351-1357, 2002.
16. Hargreaves KM, Milam SB: Mechanisms of orofacial pain and analgesia. In Dionne RA, Phero JC, Becker DE, eds: *Management of pain and anxiety in the dental office*, ed 2, Philadelphia, WB Saunders, 2002.
17. Jackson DL, Moore PA, Hargreaves KM: Preoperative nonsteroidal anti-inflammatory medication for the prevention of postoperative dental pain, *J Am Dent Assoc* 119:641-647, 1989.
18. Kim HS, Neubert JK, Iadarola MJ, et al: Genetic influence on pain sensitivity in humans: evidence of heritability related to single nucleotide polymorphisms (SNPs) in opioid receptor genes. In Dostrovsky JO, Carr DB, Koltzenburg M, eds: *Proceedings of the 10th World Congress on Pain*, vol 24, Seattle, 2003, IASP Press.
19. Krishinaraju RK, Kim H, Neubert JK, et al: *Use of classification and regression tree (CART) analysis for study of genetic contributions to experimental pain in humans,* Society for Neuroscience Abstract 2003, Program No. 694.2.
20. Mogil JS, Wilson SG, Chester EJ, et al: The melanocortin-1 receptor gene mediates female-specific mechanisms of analgesia in mice and humans, *Proc Natl Acad Sci USA* 100:4867-4872, 2003.
21. Munck A, Guyre PM, Holbrook NJ: Physiological functions of glucocorticoids in stress and their relation to pharmacological actions, *Endocr Rev* 5:25-44, 1984.
22. Nestler EJ, Hyman SE, Malenka RC, eds: *Molecular neuropharmacology: a foundation for clinical neuroscience,* New York, 2001, McGraw-Hill.
23. Ochoa J, Mair WG: The normal sural nerve in man. I. Ultrastructure and numbers of fibres and cells, *Acta Neuropathol* (Berlin) 13:197-216, 1969.
24. Papafili A, Hill MR, Brull DJ, et al: Common promoter variant in cyclooxygenase-2 represses gene expression: evidence of role in acute-phase inflammatory response, *Arterioscler Thromb Vasc Biol* 22:1631-1636, 2002.
25. Risch NJ: Searching for genetic determinants in the new millennium, *Nature* 405:847-856, 2000.
26. Scholz J, Woolf CJ: Can we conquer pain? *Nat Neurosci* 5(suppl):1062-1067, 2002.

27. Sessle BJ: Acute and chronic craniofacial pain: brainstem mechanisms of nociceptive transmission and neuroplasticity, and their clinical correlates, *Crit Rev Oral Biol Med* 11:57-91, 2000.
28. Sessle BJ, Iwata K: Central nociceptive pathways. In Lund JP, Lavigne GJ, Dubner R, et al, eds: *Orofacial pain: from basic science to clinical management. The transfer of knowledge in pain research to education,* Chicago, 2001, Quintessence.
29. Solovieva S, Leino-Arjas P, Saarela J, et al: Possible association of interleukin 1 gene locus polymorphisms with low back pain, *Pain* 2004. In press.
30. Stamer UM, Lehnen K, Hothker F, et al: Impact of CYP2D6 genotype on postoperative tramadol analgesia, *Pain* 105:231-238, 2003.
31. Stein C, Hassan AH, Lehrberger K, et al: A. Local analgesic effect of endogenous opioid peptides, *Lancet* 342:321-324, 1993.
32. Stein C, Schäfer M, Cabot PJ, et al: Opioids and inflammation. In Borsook D, ed: *Molecular neurobiology of pain,* vol 9, Seattle, 1997, IASP Press.
33. Troullos ES, Hargreaves KM, Butler DP, et al: Comparison of nonsteroidal anti-inflammatory drugs, ibuprofen and flurbiprofen, with methylprednisolone and placebo for acute pain, swelling, and trismus, *J Oral Maxillofac Surg* 48:945-952, 1990.
34. Turk DC: Remember the distinction between malignant and benign pain? Well, forget it, *Clin J Pain* 18:75-76, 2002.
35. Ulrich CM, Bigler J, Sibert J, et al: Cyclooxygenase 1 *(COX1)* polymorphisms in African-American and Caucasian populations, *Hum Mutat* 20:409-410, 2002.
36. Zubieta JK, Heitzeg MM, Smith YR, et al: COMT $val^{158}met$ genotype affects μ-opioid neurotransmitter responses to a pain stressor, *Science* 299:1240-1243, 2003.

CHAPTER • 20

Opioid Analgesics and Antagonists

Gerald F. Gebhart

Opioids are primarily used for the relief of pain and consequently find widespread application in dentistry. Opioids also possess therapeutically useful antitussive (cough suppressant) and constipating effects in addition to several undesirable effects, including respiratory depression, urinary retention, sedation, nausea and vomiting, and unwanted constipation. Repeated use of opioids for control of pain can lead to analgesic tolerance as well as physical and sometimes psychologic dependence. These shortcomings notwithstanding, no other drugs are more efficacious as analgesics than opioids. Three groups of opioid compounds are discussed in this chapter: pure agonists, those that in the same molecule possess agonist and antagonist properties, and pure antagonists. Drugs that are pure agonists and those that are mixed agonist-antagonists are used principally for relief of pain; the pure antagonists prevent or reverse the effects of pure agonists and mixed agonist-antagonists and are used principally to reverse opioid intoxication.

OPIOID ANALGESICS

Morphine, the prototypic opioid analgesic, and codeine are both natural phenanthrene alkaloids contained in opium, which is derived from the poppy plant *Papaver somniferum*. The unripe seed capsules of the plant are incised and the milky exudate is collected, dried, and powdered. Opium powder contains 5% to 20% morphine and 0.5% to 2.5% codeine, depending on the source, as well as many other alkaloids. None of the other alkaloids is therapeutically useful in pain control; one constituent, papaverine, has been used as a smooth muscle relaxant.

The first documented descriptions of *Papaver somniferum* appear in approximately 1550 BC in the Ebers papyrus of ancient Egypt.[26] Later, in the third century BC, writings of the Greek philosopher Theophrastus contained references to poppy juice. The active analgesic and constipative principle of the poppy plant, though, was not isolated and the drug was not named (after Morpheus, the Greek god of sleep) until 1806, when Sertürner first isolated morphine from opium and described its properties. In addition to morphine and codeine, currently available opioid analgesics are either semisynthetic congeners of morphine (e.g., hydromorphone, oxymorphone, hydrocodone, and oxycodone) or are entirely synthetic (e.g., meperidine, fentanyl, methadone, and propoxyphene).

Basis of Opioid Action

The mechanisms by which opioids act at specific central nervous system (CNS) and peripheral sites to produce their effects are fairly well understood. In the early 1970s, binding sites in the CNS were discovered that stereospecifically, saturably, and reversibly combined with opioids.[28] These receptors were later demonstrated to be the natural effectors of opioid action; that is, specific pharmacologic effects were produced by binding of opioids to these receptors. The discovery of opioid receptors naturally raised questions about their biologic significance and spurred research that led to the discovery of endogenous opioid peptides. Subsequently, several families of endogenous opioid peptides, as well as a number of opioid receptors, have been characterized.

Endogenous opioid peptides

There are four families of endogenous opioid peptides: endomorphins, endorphins, enkephalins, and dynorphins. Figure 20-1 illustrates their biologic derivations and structural relationships. The pentapeptide enkephalins—methionine-enkephalin (met-enkephalin) and leucine-enkephalin (leu-enkephalin)—were the first endogenous opioids to be discovered.[10] These peptides were subsequently demonstrated to be potent opioid receptor agonists in the same biologic systems in which morphine is active. Initially, the enkephalins were thought to be derived from a larger 91-amino acid peptide, β-lipotropin, but it is now clear that β-lipotropin gives rise to a separate group of opioid peptides, the endorphins (see below).

Endomorphin-1 and endomorphin-2 are newly discovered endogenous opioid peptides.[33] Both are short tetrapeptides (NH_2-Tyr-Pro-Trp/Phe-Phe-$CONH_2$) and structurally distinct from the other opioid peptides (see below). The endomorphins have been localized to areas in the CNS associated with pain processing (e.g., spinal dorsal horn, trigeminal nucleus, midbrain periaqueductal gray) and in the endings of sensory neurons that terminate in the spinal dorsal horn. Whereas the genes for the endorphins, enkephalins, and dynorphins are known, the gene for the endomorphins has yet to be isolated.

The precursor of the enkephalins, proenkephalin, is present in both the CNS and the adrenal medulla. Although proenkephalin in the brain is similar, if not identical, to proenkephalin in the adrenal medulla, processing of the large precursor polypeptide differs in the two locations. In the brain, cleavage of proenkephalin is generally more complete, and free enkephalins are the predominant products (four copies of met-enkephalin, one copy of leu-enkephalin, and one copy each of a heptapeptide and an octapeptide). In the adrenal medulla, large enkephalin-containing polypeptides predominate.

Prodynorphin is the common precursor for several larger opioid peptides, three dynorphins and two neoendorphins, all of which share with the enkephalins the same N-terminal

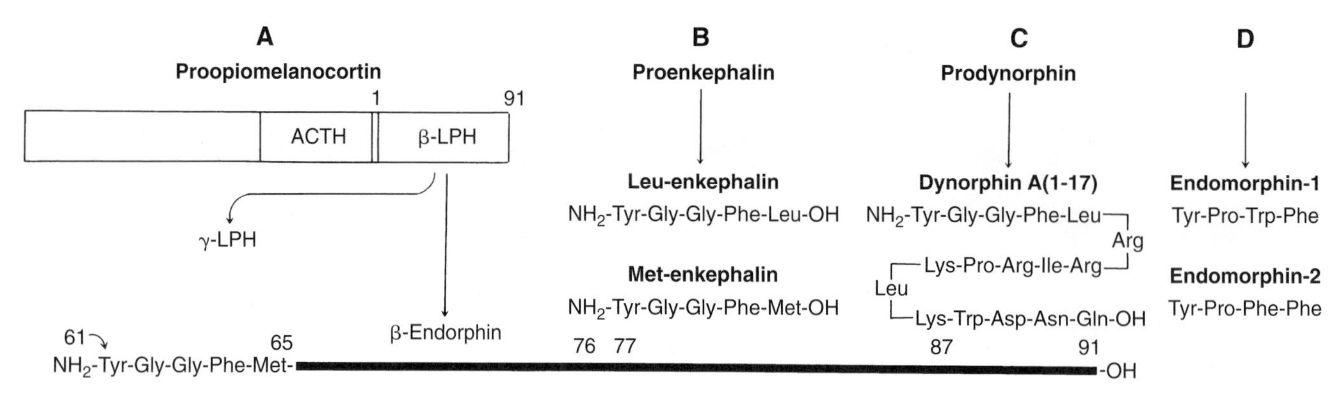

Fig. 20-1 Derivations and structures of endogenous opioids. **A,** Endorphins. Proteolysis products of the pituitary hormone β-lipotropin *(β-LPH)*, endorphins are ultimately derived from the precursor molecule proopiomelanocortin. Other peptides of biologic importance obtained from proopiomelanocortin include adrenocorticotropin *(ACTH)*, γ-lipotropin *(γ-LPH)*, and several melanotropins (not shown). The initial amino acid sequence of β-endorphin is shown (at bottom left) to illustrate its structural relationship to the enkephalins and dynorphins; the numbers refer to amino acid residues of β-LPH. **B,** Enkephalins. In addition to met- and leu-enkephalins, proenkephalin may give rise to at least two other biologically active molecules, a heptapeptide and an octapeptide, both of which contain met-enkephalin as part of their structure. **C,** Dynorphins. A common precursor, prodynorphin, yields several dynorphins, including dynorphin A(1-17) (illustrated above), dynorphin A(1-8), dynorphin B(1-13), and at least two other peptides: α-neoendorphin and β-neoendorphin. **D,** Endomorphins. The precursor for these two endogenous opioid peptides is not known.

amino acid sequence: NH_2-Tyr-Gly-Gly-Phe-Met or Leu. The products of prodynorphin are often found in association with the enkephalins within the CNS.

The endorphins are a group of endogenous peptides that are larger in size and are distributed differently in the CNS than the endomorphins, enkephalins, or dynorphins. The precursor for the endorphins, proopiomelanocortin, gives rise to several important hormones, including adrenocorticotropic hormone and β-lipotropin, which in turn are further processed to form biologically active products. The most important opioid derived from β-lipotropin is β-endorphin, the 30-amino acid carboxy terminal sequence of β-lipotropin. Shorter cleavage products of β-endorphin, such as α-endorphin and γ-endorphin, have been isolated from the pituitary, but their function is uncertain.

Sites in the CNS where opioid peptides are located differ for the different peptides, confirming that they are involved in different functions. It is a mistaken impression that all opioid peptides in all locations are involved in the modulation of pain. Neurons containing endomorphins are not as widely distributed in the CNS as neurons containing other opioid peptides, but endomorphins are located in pain processing areas where they are considered to function as neurotransmitters that act at opioid receptors. Neurons containing enkephalins are widely distributed throughout the brain (e.g., striatum, limbic system, midbrain, and medulla) and the spinal cord where they, too, are considered to function principally as neurotransmitters.[15] Prodynorphin-derived peptides are abundant in the pituitary, hypothalamus, midbrain, and striatum. Differential processing of proenkephalin and prodynorphin in various brain areas leads to different products having different functions. The endomorphins, enkephalins, and dynorphins are stored in nerve terminals and are quickly destroyed by peptidases (aminopeptidase N [EC 3.4.11.2] and neutral endopeptidase [EC 3.4.24.11]) when released. β-Endorphin is present in high concentrations in the intermediate lobe of the pituitary and in neurons in the mediobasal hypothalamus, whose axons terminate in the amygdala, periaqueductal gray matter, and brainstem. β-Endorphin coexists with adrenocorticotropic hormone in pituitary secretory granules, and both peptides can be released simultaneously. Thus β-endorphin is believed to function more as a neurohormone than as a neurotransmitter, mediating diverse autonomic and psychologic responses to pain and stress.

Opioid receptors

Three opioid receptors have been cloned: mu (μ), kappa (κ), and delta (δ) (Table 20-1).[12,24] They share considerable structural homology (approximately 60% to 65%), contain seven membrane-spanning α-helical segments, and are coupled to transducing G proteins (Figure 20-2). G proteins couple opioid receptors to intracellular effectors and exist as heterotrimers; there is both structural and functional diversity in the three G protein subunits. Each heterotrimer consists of an α subunit isoform (of which there are at least 18) and a dimer of β-γ subunits (which also exist in multiple isoforms) that in turn link with specific (and potentially diverse, given the numbers of isoform combinations that are possible) effector systems. Specifically, opioid receptors couple in this way with adenylyl cyclase and ion channels to reduce neurotransmitter release (see below).

The amino acid sequences of the three opioid receptors are most homologous in the transmembrane domains and intracellular loops; the sequences share little homology in the extracellular loops and N- and C-termini. Each receptor is distributed differently in the CNS, peripheral nervous system, and smooth muscle of the gastrointestinal tract. A receptor with high sequence homology to the three cloned opioid receptors, termed *ORL-1* (for opioid-receptor–like, an "orphan" receptor), has been discovered.[14,25] Despite its structural similarity to opioid receptors, opioids do *not* bind to ORL-1 with high affinity. A heptadecapeptide termed *orphanin FQ* (or nociceptin), which is structurally similar to the endogenous opioid peptide dynorphin, appears to be the endogenous ligand for ORL-1 (which has been renamed the *N/OFQ receptor,* or *NOP*). Nociceptin, however, does not act at any of the three cloned opioid receptors, and the nociceptin–NOP ligand–receptor complex may instead function to facilitate pain at some sites. Another heptadecapeptide, termed *nocistatin,* is also derived from the same gene that gives rise to nociceptin. Nocistatin is reported to "block" the effects of nociceptin, but nocistatin does not displace nociceptin from its receptor (ORL-1),[19] indicating that the opposing effects of nocistatin are produced at a yet to be discovered receptor.[34]

The μ receptor is the site at which all the currently available pure agonists act to produce analgesia. Morphine and other similar pure agonists have greatest affinity for μ receptors in the CNS and peripheral nervous system and lower affinity for δ and κ receptors. Among the endogenous opioid

Table • 20-1

Characterization of Opioid Receptors and Their Ligands

	RECEPTOR SUBTYPE		
	μ	κ	δ
Proprietary CNS distribution*	Cerebral cortex Striatum Hippocampus Dorsal horn Midbrain	Cerebral cortex Striatum Hippocampus Dorsal horn Midbrain	Cerebral cortex Striatum Hippocampus Dorsal horn Amygdala
Pharmacologic functions	Analgesia Sedation Miosis Euphoria Constipation Respiratory depression Pruritus	Analgesia Sedation Miosis Dysphoria Micturition Diuresis Hallucinations	Analgesia Emotion/reward Seizures (?)
Prototypic ligands	Morphine Methadone	Dynorphin A Ethylketocyclazocine	Enkephalins Deltorphin II
Effects of Binding			
Morphine	Ag	Ag (weak)	—
Etorphine	Ag	Ag	Ag
Buprenorphine	Pag	Ant	?
Butorphanol	Pag (weak)	Ag	?
Pentazocine	Ant (weak)	Ag	—
Nalbuphine	Ant	Ag	—
Naloxone	Ant	Ant	Ant (weak)

*Opioid receptors are also present in the autonomic nervous system, peripheral nerves, and the gastrointestinal tract, where they can mediate effects on heart rate, nociception, and gastrointestinal motility.
Ag, Agonist; *Pag*, partial agonist; *Ant*, antagonist.

peptides, the endomorphins have the highest affinity for the μ receptor; β-endorphin and the enkephalins also exert some of their effects at μ receptors. Two subtypes of μ receptor have been characterized by pharmacologic means: μ_1, which is associated with supraspinal analgesia, and μ_2, which subserves spinal analgesia, respiratory depression, and gastrointestinal actions. Similarly, pharmacologic studies have implied the existence of two subtypes of δ receptor, at which the endogenous enkephalins are considered to be the prototypic agonists, although the enkephalins also interact with μ receptors. The δ receptor is also involved in analgesia, both spinal and supraspinal, and in causing, along with μ receptors, opioid reinforcement (see Chapter 51). Dynorphins, representing the third class of endogenous opioid peptides, are thought to be the natural ligands for the κ receptor, of which three subtypes have been characterized pharmacologically. Two κ receptors mediate spinal (κ_1) and supraspinal (κ_3) analgesia and are principally responsible for the analgesic effects of the mixed agonist-antagonist group of opioid analgesics currently available. Neither the endogenous opioids nor clinically available drugs bind selectively to specific opioid receptors. Thus, although morphine and other pure agonists preferentially bind at μ receptors, they can produce effects at δ- and κ-opioid receptors as well, particularly as the dosage is increased.

Despite pharmacologic evidence for the existence of multiple subtypes of opioid receptors, only one of each opioid receptor has been cloned. There is no evidence at present for the existence of genes other than those that give rise to the already cloned μ, δ, and κ receptors. It is possible that not all opioid receptor genes have been cloned, but molecular mechanisms and other factors most likely explain the pharmacologic diversity of effects produced by various ligands at opioid receptors. For example, receptor isoforms may be produced by alternative splicing in the coding regions of the three cloned opioid receptors.[4] Variant mRNAs have been reported for all three opioid receptors, although their expression is typically very low and it is not clear that splice variants can be distinguished pharmacologically. It seems more likely that other mechanisms (e.g., posttranslational regulation, variable activation of receptors by different ligands, receptor dimerization, intracellular interactions with proteins associated with different effectors, etc.) explain the pharmacologic diversity of opioid receptor subtypes. Moreover, many G protein–coupled receptors exist as dimers (two receptors linked) and heterodimerization of δ and κ receptors, for example, could result in a complex pharmacologic profile.

The sigma (σ) receptor, initially considered to be an opioid receptor, is now known to mediate the dysphoric and psychotomimetic effects of opioids, as well as those of phencyclidine, a nonopioid hallucinogen. This phencyclidine receptor has been identified as an inhibitory component of the N-methyl-D-aspartate receptor complex, which modulates opioid tolerance and dependence.

Physiologic functions

Much remains to be learned about the physiologic roles of the endomorphins, enkephalins, dynorphins, and endorphins. It is established that enkephalins, present principally in local

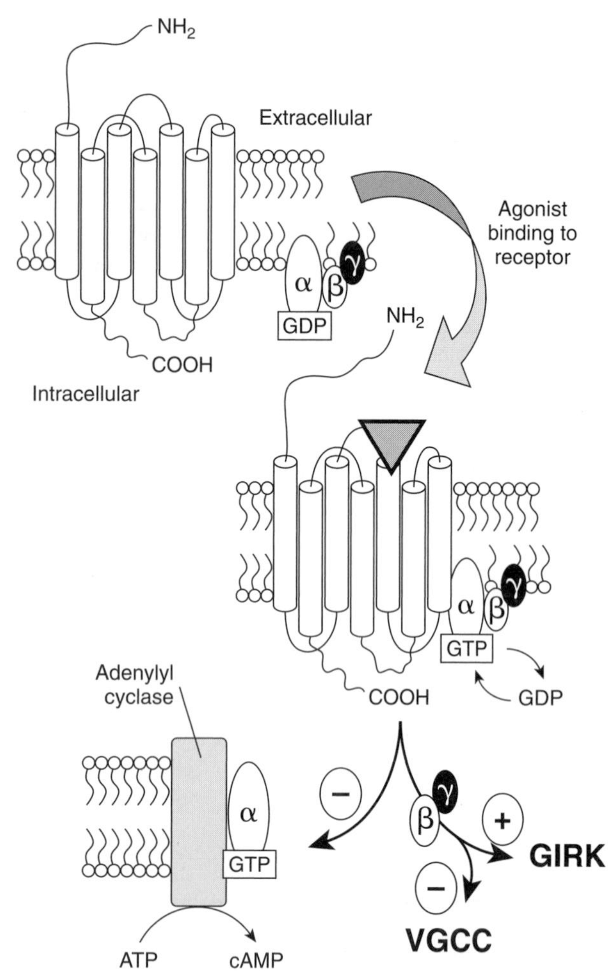

Fig. 20-2 Diagram of a G protein–coupled opioid receptor. Opioids bind within the hydrophobic membrane-spanning domains of the receptor. Opioid agonist effects at the receptor are mediated by G proteins, an α subunit associated with guanosine diphosphate *(GDP)*, and a β-γ dimer. When an opioid agonist binds, the conformation of the receptor is changed as the membrane-associated G proteins assemble with the receptor. GDP is exchanged with guanosine triphosphate and this activated G-α complex negatively regulates adenylyl cyclase. The β-γ dimer activates conductance in a G protein inwardly rectifying K^+ *(GIRK)* channel and inhibits voltage-gated Ca^{++} channels *(VGCC)* in the cell membrane. (See Chapters 1 and 5 for more details on signal transduction.) *ATP,* Adenosine triphosphate; *cAMP,* cyclic 3′5′–adenosine monophosphate.

circuits or interneurons in the CNS, have an inhibitory effect on other cells. For example, endogenous opioids tonically modulate the secretion of gonadotropins from the pituitary. When the opioid receptor antagonist naloxone is administered to normal subjects, the plasma concentrations of luteinizing hormone and follicle-stimulating hormone are increased because naloxone releases hypothalamic neurons from a tonic endogenous opioid inhibition.

Considerable attention has been given to the notion that endogenous opioid peptides tonically modulate nociception (pain). One would expect occupation of opioid receptors by naloxone to prevent any action by endogenous opioid peptides and thus lower the response threshold for pain if endogenous opioids tonically modulated nociception. A number of studies have shown that the administration of naloxone to normal human volunteers does not affect their resting pain thresholds or responses to experimental pain stimuli. In other situations, however, naloxone has been reported to attenuate the analgesic effects of acupuncture and of placebo administration after minor oral surgery and to be *hyper*algesic in human beings after major surgery.[23] From these and other findings,[5] it would appear that endogenous antinociceptive opioid systems are normally quiescent but can become physiologically active and affect pain processing when significant pain or stress is present.

Sites and mechanism of action

Among the many effects of opioids, analgesia has been most thoroughly studied. We now know that opioids acting at opioid receptors in the periphery and at both spinal and supraspinal sites can produce clinically effective analgesia. Knowledge of the central sites of opioid action came first; documentation of direct peripheral analgesic actions of opioids is relatively recent.[29]

Early investigators attempted to determine the central locus of morphine's analgesic action by administering morphine directly into selected brain sites. These studies succeeded in identifying an area of the brainstem surrounding the cerebral aqueduct as a site important to morphine analgesia. Corollary studies found that electrical stimulation of this same area in the midbrain in animals and human beings produced a potent and long-lasting analgesia mediated in part by endogenous opioids.[8] Morphine and other opioid agonists acting at this site produce analgesia by engaging a descending system of pain inhibition.[5] As illustrated in Figure 20-3, information about pain from nociceptors, that is, peripheral receptors in skin, muscle, joints, and viscera that respond to pain-producing stimuli, can be influenced at the first central synapse (spinal or medullary dorsal horn) by this descending system of pain inhibition. It is important to appreciate two features of this pain-modulating system: the descending pathway from the midbrain is indirect (there is a synaptic relay in the medulla and/or the dorsolateral pons) and, although engaged by an opioid acting at opioid receptors in the midbrain, the neurotransmitters in the spinal cord or medullary dorsal horn that ultimately inhibit pain transmission are nonopioids such as 5-hydroxytryptamine (5-HT, serotonin) and norepinephrine.[5]

A second means by which morphine and other opioid agonists modulate pain is by acting at opioid receptors in the brain at sites not associated with activation of the descending pain inhibitory system. Actions of opioids at these brain sites do not affect the response threshold to a painful stimulus, but rather influence the interpretation of and emotional reaction to the stimulus.[23] This so-called motivational-affective component of the response to pain is discussed later in this chapter.

A final means by which morphine and other opioid agonists produce analgesia is by acting at opioid receptors located on the peripheral and central terminals of nociceptors. Opioid receptors are located on the terminals of these specialized nerve fibers, typically Aδ and C fibers, which connect the periphery directly with the CNS. Analgesic effects of opioids can thus be produced by direct administration of an opioid into a joint or, more commonly, the epidural or intrathecal space.[32]

Opioids thus can act at several sites, each of which can contribute independently to the analgesia produced. Obviously, when given systemically, opioids have access to all potential sites of action, and the analgesia produced is likely a product of peripheral, spinal, and supraspinal interactions with opioid receptors. This knowledge can be used to improve pain control and limit the incidence and/or severity of undesirable opioid effects. For example, because pain modulation descending from the brainstem is mediated in the spinal cord by norepinephrine and 5-HT, the direct effects of an opioid given into the epidural space can be enhanced by epidural

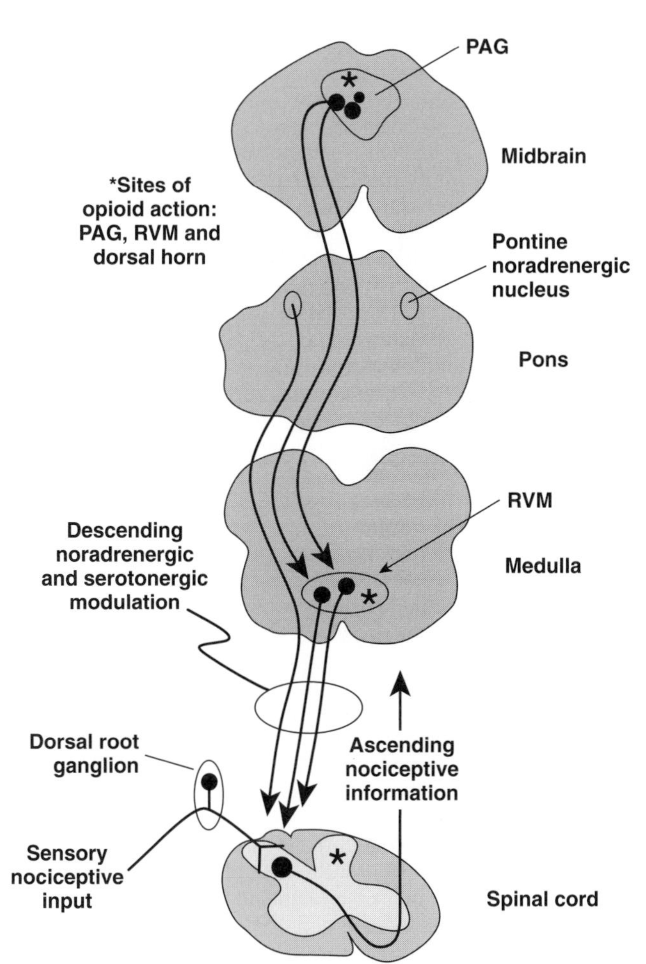

Fig. 20-3 Descending pain-modulating pathways from the brainstem to the spinal cord. Descending influences, whether activated in the midbrain periaqueductal gray *(PAG)* or rostroventral medial medulla *(RVM)* by endogenous or exogenous opioids (*) or stimulation, are mediated at the level of the spinal cord by noradrenergic and serotonergic receptors.

administration of an α-adrenoceptor agonist such as clonidine.[17] Tricyclic antidepressants, which block the reuptake of norepinephrine and 5-HT, are also effective adjuvants (although it should be appreciated that antidepressants such as amitriptyline also possess analgesic efficacy unrelated to their effects on monoamine reuptake). This strategy allows reduction of the dose of opioid without compromising the analgesia produced. By requiring less opioid for adequate pain control, undesirable opioid effects, such as urinary retention, respiratory depression, sedation, and development of analgesic tolerance, can be reduced. It has also been documented that administration of very low doses of morphine directly into the knee joint after arthroscopic knee surgery can control postoperative pain.[29]

The mechanisms by which opioids produce their effects are best established for direct actions at opioid receptors located on neurons. Actions commonly produced at all three opioid receptors include inhibition of adenylyl cyclase, inhibition of Ca^{++} conductance, activation of a potassium conductance, and inhibition of neurotransmitter release (see Figure 20-2). Acute inhibition of adenylyl cyclase by an opioid leads to a decrease in intracellular cyclic 3′,5′-adenosine monophosphate, decreasing an inward, nonselective cation current and thus decreasing cell excitability. All three opioid receptors also activate a G protein inwardly rectifying K^+ conductance and inhibit voltage-activated Ca^{++} currents, both events mediated by G protein β-γ subunits. Because Ca^{++} influx is required for the stimulus-secretion coupling of neurotransmitter release, opioids decrease the release of neurotransmitters such as substance P and glutamate from nociceptor terminals and thus attenuate the transmission of nociceptive information at the first central synapse. Because opioids activate this G protein–rectifying K^+ conductance, they produce a relative hyperpolarization of neurons, making them relatively more difficult to excite.

Morphine

The structure of morphine is shown in Figure 20-4. Morphine is the prototypic opioid analgesic (pure agonist) and the one about which most is known. Morphine is widely used for pain control and can be given by virtually any route of administration. All opioid analgesics share with morphine the ability to produce analgesia, respiratory depression, constipation, gastrointestinal spasm, and physical dependence; none has yet been demonstrated to be significantly different from or superior to morphine regarding its important pharmacologic features. The incidence of untoward effects (e.g., respiratory depression) and the intensity of action of pure agonists are qualitatively similar and differ little when compared at doses that produce equivalent analgesia. Consequently, morphine is discussed in greater detail than other opioid analgesics, and what is stated for morphine applies in general to other pure agonists. Significant differences that do exist between morphine and other opioids are introduced as each individual agent is discussed.

Central pharmacologic effects

The CNS effects of morphine are a combination of stimulation and depression and include analgesia, drowsiness, euphoria-dysphoria, respiratory depression, suppression of the cough reflex, pupillary constriction, suppression of the secretion of some (luteinizing hormone) and enhancement of other (prolactin) pituitary hormones, and initial stimulation of the medullary chemoreceptor trigger zone for emesis followed by depression of vomiting.

Analgesia The analgesia produced by morphine and other pure agonists occurs without loss of consciousness. When opioids are administered for relief of pain (or for a cough or diarrhea), it must be appreciated that they provide only symptomatic relief without alleviation of the cause of the pain (or cough or diarrhea). The analgesia produced by opioid analgesics is dose-dependent and selective in that other sensory modalities (e.g., vision, audition) are unaffected at therapeutic doses. The standard parenteral analgesic dose of morphine, 10 mg/70 kg of body weight, is considered a

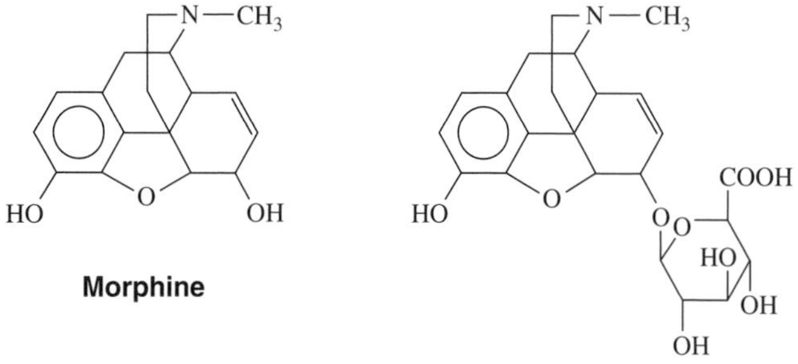

Morphine

Morphine-6-glucuronide

Fig. 20-4 Structural formulas of morphine and its active metabolite morphine-6-glucuronide.

therapeutic dose for relief of moderate to severe pain. Because pain is a highly subjective and personal experience, however, adequate pain relief is best achieved by titrating the dose to the needs of the patient.

As already discussed, the sites of opioid-produced analgesia include the periphery and both spinal and supraspinal brain areas. It is generally accepted that opioid-induced analgesia involves both the sensory-discriminative and motivational-affective components of pain. The sensory-discriminative component of pain is associated with identification and localization of the source of pain, whereas the motivational-affective component of pain is related to one's reaction to pain.[25] Pain is not a simple sensation associated with a single pain pathway from the periphery to the cortex, but rather is a complex experience that can be influenced by the environment in which the pain arises; prior experience and expectation; attention and anxiety; and other societal, emotional, and cognitive contributions. Accordingly, the nociceptive component of pain may not be as much affected by opioid analgesics as is the reaction to pain. A common report from patients after receiving an opioid for relief of pain is that the pain is still present but that it is not discomforting. Thus clinical impressions and patients' reports suggest a prominent action by opioid analgesics on the motivational-affective component of pain, presumably resulting from opioid actions at opioid receptors within the limbic system of the brain.

An additional significant feature of opioid analgesics is that they are generally more effective against continuous, dull, aching pain than against sharp, intermittent pain. Neuropathic pain, such as trigeminal neuralgia or peripheral nerve injury, is less responsive to opioids than is nociceptive pain. It is also known that sensitivity to pain and the ability to clear morphine decrease with age, whereas the elimination half-life of morphine increases with age; thus the pain relief provided by morphine typically increases with age.[11,20]

Respiratory depression Morphine and its congeners depress respiration in a dose-related fashion. Respiratory depression represents the principal undesirable, potentially life-threatening effect of opioids as a group. The opioids are capable of depressing both the tidal volume and the rate of respiration. In human beings, morphine decreases the response of brainstem respiratory centers to the carbon dioxide tension of the blood. It also significantly depresses pontine and medullary centers that regulate respiratory frequency.[1] Thus irregular rhythms and periodic breathing are not uncommon after toxic doses of morphine or its congeners, and the normal respiratory rate of 16 to 18 breaths/min may be reduced to as low as 3 to 4 breaths/min. All currently available opioid analgesics are capable of depressing respiration in a manner similar to that of morphine when administered in doses that produce equal analgesia.

Cough suppression Morphine and other pure agonists are effective antitussives; codeine, for example, is widely used in cough preparations for this purpose. Morphine itself, however, is not commonly used as a cough suppressant. The opioids exert their antitussive effect by depressing an area in the brainstem. Although the brainstem sites for the respiratory depressant and antitussive effects of opioids are anatomically close, there is no apparent relationship between opioid depression of one or the other, because several nonanalgesic, nonrespiratory-depressant opioid analogues (e.g., dextromethorphan) are effective antitussives. In addition, suppression of the cough reflex occurs at opioid doses lower than those required to produce an analgesic effect or to depress respiration.

Pupillary reaction At therapeutic doses, morphine and most of its congeners produce pupillary constriction (miosis) in human beings. The emphasis on human beings is significant because in some other species, such as cats, in which opioids exert primarily an excitatory effect, the pupils are dilated by morphine. The miosis produced by opioids results from a central effect mediated by the oculomotor nerve and not from a direct action on the circular or radial muscles of the iris of the eye. Although tolerance to opioids has not yet been discussed, it is appropriate to indicate here that tolerance to the pupillary-constricting effect of morphine and some other opioids does not develop to any appreciable extent. Consequently, long-term users of morphine and heroin, for example, continue to have constricted pupils, although they likely will have developed tolerance to many other opioid effects.

Nausea and vomiting Opioids directly stimulate the chemoreceptor trigger zone in the medulla and can produce emesis. Opioids are commonly given before, during, and after surgery, and nausea and vomiting are obviously undesirable. However, after the initial period of stimulation, opioids will depress the brainstem medullary center for vomiting. This subsequent depression occurs at therapeutic concentrations and is virtually total; other opioid analgesics or emesis-inducing agents administered during this time are generally ineffective in causing emesis. There is also apparently a vestibular component to the nausea produced by morphine and its congeners because nausea occurs more frequently in ambulatory than in recumbent patients.

Peripheral pharmacologic effects

Morphine exerts important influences on smooth muscle tone that have both therapeutic and toxic implications. The drug also affects gastrointestinal activity by reducing glandular secretions.

Gastrointestinal tract The use of opium for relief of diarrhea and dysentery antedated by centuries the use of opium for relief of pain. Indeed, opioids exert significant effects on smooth muscle all along the gastrointestinal tract. The overall action of morphine and its congeners is constipating, an effect that is useful therapeutically. Opioid analgesics, acting principally at opioid receptors in the gastrointestinal tract, but also at opioid receptors in the CNS,[30] increase smooth muscle tone and decrease propulsive motility throughout the gastrointestinal tract. In the large intestine, muscle spasms can result from the marked increase in muscle tone and nonpropulsive muscle contractions. Spasm of the smooth muscle of the biliary tract, which can be very painful, can also occur after the administration of therapeutic doses of morphine and related drugs.

Morphine and other pure agonists delay gastric emptying. In addition, gastric acid secretion is usually depressed, and pancreatic, biliary, and intestinal secretions are routinely depressed by opioid administration as well. Inhibition of intestinal hypersecretion is an important contributor to the beneficial effect of morphine in the treatment of diarrhea.

Other smooth muscle Morphine and other pure agonists also increase muscle tone in smooth muscle of organs other than those of the gastrointestinal tract, such as the ureters, urinary bladder, uterus, and bronchioles, but at therapeutic doses the effect of opioids on these muscles is generally unremarkable. Urinary retention, characterized by urgency and increased tone of the bladder sphincter, is common after all routes of opioid administration. In addition to effects on tone and contractility of smooth muscle, opioids also possess antidiuretic effects. Although opioids increase uterine tone, they do not generally influence the duration of labor. Likewise in the bronchial musculature, opioids administered at usual therapeutic doses do not produce significant bronchoconstriction, even though they may aggravate an asthmatic condition or precipitate an asthmatic attack resulting in part from histamine release.

In large doses, opioid effects on all these smooth muscles may be significant. Contraction of the ureter will contribute to cessation of urine flow; increased uterine tone will significantly prolong labor and may increase neonatal morbidity rates; and bronchoconstriction will occur.

Cardiovascular system The effects of morphine and other pure agonists on blood pressure, heart rate, and cardiac work are generally minor at analgesic doses. The vasomotor center of the medulla is relatively unaffected by opioid analgesics, and blood pressure is maintained near normal even after intoxicating doses of opioids. The fall in blood pressure observed during acute opioid intoxication is primarily caused by hypoxia that results from opioid-induced respiratory depression.

Morphine and a number of other opioid analgesics release histamine and produce some vasodilation of the peripheral vasculature, often resulting in an overall sensation of warmth accompanied occasionally by itching of the face and nose. There also appears to be a poorly understood contribution by the CNS to peripheral vasodilation. The resultant fall in peripheral resistance is the primary cause of the orthostatic hypotension and fainting that occur occasionally in some recumbent patients when the head-up position is suddenly assumed. Opioids have no direct effect on the vasculature and circulation of the brain, but cerebral vasodilation is not an uncommon consequence of opioid administration. Cerebral vasodilation is considered to be a consequence of the respiratory depression produced by morphine and its congeners and the subsequent retention of carbon dioxide in the blood. The result is an increase in cerebrospinal fluid pressure, which requires that opioids be used cautiously in cases of cranial trauma and head injury, where cerebrospinal fluid pressure may already be elevated. Morphine is also occasionally used in the treatment of pulmonary edema, where it is quite effective. The mechanism by which morphine exerts this beneficial action is unclear, but morphine appears to inhibit adrenergic tone centrally, promoting redistribution of blood to the periphery and reducing pressure in the pulmonary veins and capillaries without causing concomitant reduction of systemic arterial pressure.

Peripheral analgesia An increasingly important peripheral action of opioids, namely analgesia, is now appreciated.[29] As indicated earlier in this chapter, opioid receptors are located on both the central and peripheral terminals of nociceptors. When tissue is insulted and inflamed, peripheral opioid receptors upregulate (increase in number or are inserted into peripheral nociceptor terminals in greater number). This event is presumably part of the normal response to tissue insult where endogenous opioid peptides contained in monocytic cells or lymphocytes, attracted to the site of tissue insult, are released to modulate pain associated with the tissue insult. Therapeutically, the upregulation of opioid receptors can be taken advantage of by application of exogenous opioid agonists directly to the site of insult (e.g., intraarticular injection of morphine, topical application of μ-opioid receptor agonists).

Acute opioid intoxication

Death from acute intoxication by an opioid analgesic is the result of profound, direct respiratory depression. The cardinal signs of acute opioid intoxication (overdose) represent an extension of the pharmacologic features of these drugs: stupor, constricted pupils, and depressed respiration. As the severity of intoxication increases, coma ensues and the blood pressure, initially maintained near normal, steadily falls if the hypoxia associated with the respiratory depression is unaltered. Measures must be instituted to support respiration in cases of intoxication; pupillary dilation and shock, both caused by persistent hypoxia, precede death in the absence of alteration in the respiratory status of the intoxicated person.

The essential principle of treatment of acute opioid intoxication is restoration of adequate ventilation. This is most rapidly and dramatically achieved by administration of an opioid receptor antagonist (e.g., naloxone), but in the absence of immediately effective opioid receptor antagonism, a patent airway must be established and efficient pulmonary gas exchange restored, by artificial respiration if necessary. Restoration of adequate pulmonary ventilation prevents the hypoxic cardiovascular sequelae of opioid intoxication. Although opioid antagonists have not yet been discussed, it is important to interject two notes of caution regarding their use in cases of opioid intoxication. First, the duration of action of naloxone, the standard opioid receptor antagonist, is shorter than that of most opioid analgesics (which, moreover, have been given or taken in excess). Consequently, the opioid-intoxicated person typically requires continued monitoring and readministration of additional naloxone as necessary. Second, administration of an opioid receptor antagonist to an acutely intoxicated, opioid-dependent person can precipitate a withdrawal syndrome that cannot readily be attenuated during the period of action of the antagonist.

Tolerance and dependence

Tolerance is a decreased effect of drug as a consequence of prior administration of that drug. Accordingly, increasingly greater doses of drug must be administered over time to produce an effect equivalent to that produced on initial administration. Tolerance does not develop uniformly to all opioid effects. In general, tolerance develops to the depressant effects of opioids but not to the stimulant effects. Thus tolerance develops to opioid-induced analgesia, euphoria, drowsiness, and respiratory depression but not, to any appreciable extent, to opioid effects on the gastrointestinal tract or the pupil.

In the therapeutic setting, the initial indication that tolerance has developed is generally reflected in a shortened duration or reduced analgesic effect. The rate at which tolerance develops is a function of the dose and the frequency of administration, as well as perhaps other, nonpharmacologic factors. Patients treated for 5 to 7 or more days will exhibit tolerance to the analgesic (and other) effects of opioids. In general, the greater the opioid dose and the shorter the interval between doses, the more rapid is the development of tolerance. Tolerance, in fact, can develop to such an extent that the lethal dose of the opioid is increased significantly. However, for any individual there always exists an opioid dose capable of producing death by respiratory depression regardless of the extent to which tolerance has developed.

Tolerance becomes apparent during repeated drug administration, whereas dependence is apparent only in the absence of drug. Dependence can be physical or psychologic. *Physical dependence,* as defined by the American Society of Addiction Medicine, is a state of physiologic adaptation that is manifested by a drug class–specific withdrawal syndrome that can be produced by abrupt cessation of the drug, rapid dose reduction, decreasing blood content of the drug, and/or administration of an antagonist. Just as the rate of development of tolerance to opioids is dose related, so too is the development of physical dependence. The greater the opioid dose and the longer the duration of administration, the greater the degree of physical dependence and the more intense is the withdrawal syndrome. The mechanisms underlying the development of tolerance to and physical dependence on opioids are not fully understood. Tolerance and physical dependence develop concurrently, but apparently by different mechanisms.

G protein–coupled receptors, including opioid receptors, are internalized after being bound by an agonist. Internalization is a multistep process in which opioid receptors are uncoupled from their heterotrimeric G proteins, phosphorylated by a receptor kinase, and targeted for endocytosis by clathrin-coated pits. Once in the intracellular endosomal compartment, opioid receptors can be recycled for reinsertion into the cell membrane or degraded, which can result in receptor downregulation (a reduction in the number of receptors). This acute desensitization is common to virtually all G protein–coupled receptors and occurs rapidly (seconds to minutes) after occupation of a receptor by its agonist. Tolerance represents longer-term desensitization and downregulation of receptor-effector coupling by mechanisms not yet fully understood. Physical dependence results from adaptations at cellular, synaptic, and system levels that in some ways are analogous to adaptive processes better understood as nervous system plasticity in the context of learning and memory (i.e., long-term potentiation). The underlying cellular and synaptic mechanisms that contribute to the development of opioid physical dependence, however, are not known.

Psychologic dependence is more difficult to define and measure. Psychologic dependence contributes more to drug-seeking behavior than does physical dependence and thus contributes significantly to addiction. As defined by the American Society of Addiction Medicine, *addiction* is the extreme of compulsive drug use and is characterized by continued use, impaired control over drug use, and craving despite harm. It should be clear that physical dependence can exist in the absence of psychologic dependence, and it is therefore inappropriate to identify as "addicted" a person who becomes physically dependent after repeated opioid administration during hospitalization. All three phenomena—tolerance, physical dependence, and psychologic dependence—are reversible, although psychologic dependence provides a strong drive to drug abuse. It is now well documented that drugs that release or prolong the actions of the monoamine neurotransmitter dopamine in the mesocortical or mesolimbic systems potently activate endogenous reward pathways in the brain. Although the commonly abused drugs are structurally and pharmacologically heterogenous (e.g., nicotine, alcohol, opioids, cannabinoids, cocaine), they all possess the ability to activate the mesocorticolimbic system, a brain network important to initiating and maintaining drug craving.

Opioid analgesics are often rated in terms of "dependence liability" to indicate those opioids considered to be more likely to produce significant physical dependence than others (Table 20-2). It is not clear how significant the differences are among opioid analgesics when they are compared at equianalgesic doses given by the same route of administration and at appropriate intervals. However, when opioid analgesics are compared in terms of how they are generally used therapeutically, differences in dependence liability are apparent. For example, morphine has a greater dependence liability than codeine when both are used in traditional therapeutic modes (i.e., morphine given parenterally for moderate to severe pain and codeine given orally for mild to moderate pain).

There exists on the part of health professionals and patients alike concern about the use of opioids for pain control, particularly in cases of persistent pain. This so-called "opiophobia" is a reaction to fear of dose escalation (caused by the development of tolerance) and subsequent physical dependence (erroneously termed "addiction") associated with treatment for pain that lasts more than a few days. Most of our knowledge about analgesic tolerance and physical dependence derives from studies that use models of acute pain or repeated dosing with opioids in the absence of persistent pain. Recent clinical investigations and observations in chronic pain patients have led to modification of our views on the potential importance of analgesic tolerance and physical dependence to adequate pain control.[21,31] It has been found, for example, that dose escalation for pain control is usually required only at the start of therapy (i.e., when titrating the dose to provide adequate analgesia) and that dose requirements tend to stabilize thereafter for long periods of time.

Absorption, fate, and excretion

Morphine in particular and most opioids in general are not nearly as effective when given orally as when given parenterally in the same dose. For morphine, oral administration for relief of pain is approximately one third to one sixth as potent as the same dose given parenterally. Because absorption of morphine is good after oral administration, most of the difference in effect between the oral and parenteral routes is caused by metabolic inactivation during morphine's first pass through the liver. The primary pathway for the metabolism of morphine is conjugation with glucuronic acid, and the principal metabolite is morphine-3-glucuronide (approximately 55% of the administered dose). Morphine is also glucuronidated at the 6 position (approximately 10% of the administered dose; see Figure 20-4). Interestingly, morphine-6-glucuronide has a high affinity for the μ receptor and is a potent and efficacious analgesic, especially when injected to bypass the blood-brain barrier.[6,22] Because it accumulates in the bloodstream, morphine-6-glucuronide may be largely responsible for the analgesic effects of morphine administered on a long-term basis.

Most of the conjugated morphine is eliminated from the body by glomerular filtration; only small amounts of free morphine are found in the urine. Some morphine glucuronide also appears in the bile, and a small percentage is eventually excreted in the feces. Morphine does not generally accumulate in tissues; the total excretion of an administered dose is usually approximately 90% complete in the first 24 hours.

Although morphine is subject to significant first-pass metabolism after its oral administration, it is widely used orally for the management of chronic pain (e.g., management of cancer pain). The oral dose of morphine in liquid form can range from less than 10 mg every 4 hours to 2500 mg every 4 hours; most patients require no more than 200 mg per day. Morphine is also available for oral use in controlled-release tablets to produce longer-lasting analgesia (e.g., 12 hours). Regarding the wide dose ranges reported necessary for pain control in cases of chronic pain, it must first be appreciated that chronic pain is controlled by titration of the dose to prevent pain breakthrough and, second, that analgesic tolerance is likely present or will develop. Accordingly, dosages of morphine required to manage chronic pain can be quite high. In terminally ill patients, there should be no concern about the development of physical dependence.

General therapeutic uses

Pain is a common symptom that initiates a visit to a dentist or physician. Moreover, pain is almost always present after invasive procedures or surgery. Morphine and other pure agonist opioid analgesics are the most efficacious analgesic drugs known and are without peer in their ability to control pain. As emphasized earlier, these drugs provide only symptomatic relief of pain without influencing its underlying cause. The opioids, when administered at therapeutic doses to produce analgesia, also produce a drowsiness from which the patient is generally easily aroused, as well as a tranquilization. There is without doubt a significant antianxiety or sedating

Table • 20-2

Comparison of Opioid Analgesics

NONPROPRIETARY (GENERIC) NAME	PROPRIETARY (TRADE) NAME	USUAL THERAPEUTIC DOSE (mg)	ROUTE OF ADMINISTRATION	DURATION (hr)	DEPENDENCE LIABILITY
Alfentanil	Alfenta	0.5 to 2*	IV	0.5	High
Buprenorphine†	Buprenex	0.3 to 0.6	IM, IV	4 to 6	Low
Butorphanol†	Stadol	1 to 4	IM	3 to 4	Low
		0.5 to 2	IV	2 to 4	Low
		1 to 2	Nasal	3 to 4	Low
Codeine	—	30 to 60	Oral	4 to 6	Low to moderate
Dezocine†	Delgan	5 to 20	IM	3 to 6	Low
		2.5 to 10	IV	2 to 4	Low
Fentanyl	Sublimaze	0.05 to 0.1	IM	1.0 to 1.5	High
		0.05 to 0.1*	IV	0.5 to 1.0	High
Heroin‡	—	3 to 5	IM	3 to 4	High
Hydrocodone	Dicodid	5 to 10	Oral	4 to 6	Moderate
Hydromorphone	Dilaudid	1 to 4	IM, SC	4 to 6	High
		2 to 4	Oral	4 to 6	High
Levorphanol	Levo-Dromoran	2 to 3	SC, oral	4 to 5	High
Meperidine	Demerol	50 to 150	IM, SC	3 to 4	High
		50 to 150	Oral§	3 to 4	Moderate
Methadone	Dolophine	2.5 to 10	IM, SC	3 to 5	Moderate
		5 to 15	Oral	4 to 6	Moderate
Morphine	—	10 to 15	IM, SC	4 to 5	High
		20 to 60	Oral	3 to 5	Moderate
Nalbuphine†	Nubain	10	IM, IV, SC	3 to 6	Low
Oxycodone	In Percodan	5 to 10	Oral	4 to 5	High
Oxymorphone	Numorphan	1 to 1.5	IM, SC	4 to 6	High
		0.5	IV	4 to 6	High
Pentazocine†	Talwin	30	IM, IV, SC	3 to 4	Low
	Talwin NX	50	Oral	3 to 4	Low
Propoxyphene	Darvon	32 to 65	Oral§	4 to 6	Low to moderate
Sufentanil	Sufenta	0.01 to 0.025*	IV	0.5 to 1.0	High
Tramadol	Ultram	50 to 100	Oral	4 to 6	Low

Estimates of duration and dependence liability are based on information in the literature and are not definitive.
*Larger doses may be used for general anesthesia.
†Mixed agonist-antagonist.
‡Heroin is a Schedule I drug and therefore not available for routine clinical use.
§The efficacy of oral meperidine and propoxyphene is a matter of controversy.
IM, Intramuscular; *IV*, intravenous; *SC*, subcutaneous.

component in the analgesic effect of opioids. Thus, although nausea and vomiting, respiratory depression, constipation, and tolerance and physical dependence can be drawbacks to their use, opioids undeniably produce an important combination of desirable effects (e.g., analgesia and sedation) in the patient with pain.

Aside from their application for pain relief, opioids can be useful in inducing sleep, provided that sleeplessness is caused by pain or coughing. Opioid analgesics should not be used for nighttime sedation in the absence of coughing or pain. Morphine is also effective in the treatment of pulmonary edema. The use of morphine and other opioids in anesthesia is discussed at the end of this section.

Codeine

Codeine, like morphine, is a naturally occurring alkaloid present in opium powder. It differs from morphine only in that a methoxy substitution (—OCH_3) replaces the hydroxyl group at position 3 of the molecule (Figure 20-5). This relatively subtle structural change provides codeine with significant oral effectiveness. In fact, codeine is primarily used as an orally administered analgesic and antitussive. Like morphine, codeine is metabolized primarily by the liver and is excreted chiefly in the urine, largely in inactive forms. Additionally, a small percentage (approximately 10%) of codeine is demethylated at position 3 to form morphine, and both free and conjugated morphine are found in small quantities in the urine after therapeutic doses of codeine. This conversion, plus the fact that codeine itself binds poorly to the μ receptor, has led to consideration of codeine as a prodrug insofar as its analgesic action is concerned.

As with all opioid analgesics, the analgesic and antitussive actions of codeine (as well as its respiratory depressant and sedative effects) are central in origin. Codeine is frequently classified as a weak or mild opioid analgesic. That codeine is a mild analgesic incapable of providing an analgesic effect equivalent to morphine is an erroneous, but widely held, impression. Morphine as an analgesic is about 12 times more potent than codeine when both drugs are administered intramuscularly. This ratio simply means that approximately

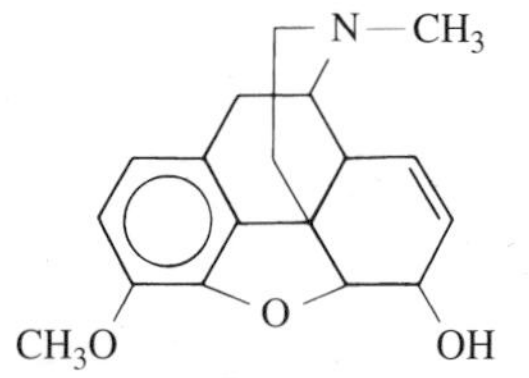

Fig. 20-5 Structural formula of codeine.

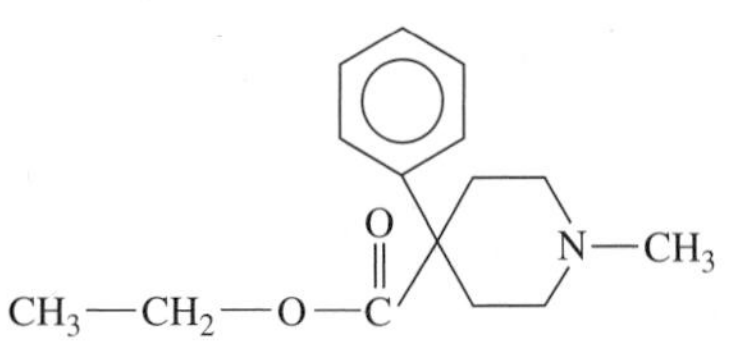

Fig. 20-6 Structural formula of meperidine.

120 mg of codeine is required to produce an analgesic effect equivalent to 10 mg of morphine. At the present time, however, doses of codeine in excess of 60 mg (orally) are not commonly used and, moreover, are not officially recognized as generally safe and effective by the Food and Drug Administration. Consequently, the impression remains that codeine has limited analgesic efficacy and that a dose of 60 mg of codeine represents an "analgesic ceiling" above which increasing doses will not provide greater analgesic effect. This widely held belief, although supported by legal regulation, is not consistent with clinical evaluations regarding codeine's analgesic efficacy.[9]

The recommended analgesic dose of codeine is 30 to 60 mg orally; the recommended antitussive dose is 15 to 20 mg orally. At these doses, the side effects of codeine are relatively few and generally insignificant; nausea, constipation, dizziness, and sedation are the effects most frequently observed. At greater doses, the incidence of nausea and vomiting is increased, a particularly undesirable effect in persons who have undergone dental surgery. Among the opioids, codeine is especially suitable for relief of pain in the ambulatory person because it is orally effective; can provide significant analgesia and relief of dull, continuous pain; and can be taken for relatively long periods of time with little or no risk of physical dependence. For example, a dose of 60 mg of codeine taken three to four times daily over a period of 6 to 8 weeks is not associated with the development of significant physical dependence. Tolerance will, however, develop to the analgesic effect of codeine over time, and it is likely that the dose will have to be gradually increased. Codeine's demonstrated analgesic usefulness in some situations that show little or limited response to nonopioid analgesics makes codeine a useful drug for certain pain states. It should be noted, however, that dental pain associated with inflammation should not be treated with codeine alone because neither codeine nor any of the other opioids has antiinflammatory properties. Rather, aspirin or another nonsteroidal antiinflammatory drug alone or in combination with codeine is appropriate for cases of dental pain involving or arising from inflammation.

Dihydrocodeine, Oxycodone, and Hydrocodone

Dihydrocodeine (contained in Synalgos DC), oxycodone (contained in Percodan), and hydrocodone (contained in Vicodin) are phenanthrene opioids similar in structure to morphine and codeine. Like codeine, these drugs have a methoxy substitution (—OCH_3) for the hydroxy group at position 3 of the basic morphine molecule. Thus they have good oral efficacy and are primarily used as oral analgesics. They do not differ significantly from morphine in terms of their important pharmacology. Oxycodone is approximately equipotent with morphine when given parenterally; it is only used in oral preparations, however. An oral dose of 5 mg of oxycodone is approximately equivalent to 30 to 60 mg of codeine. A controlled-release preparation of oxycodone (OxyContin) has been the subject of recent controversy because of abuse potential and toxicity. The abuse potential for this form of oxycodone appears to be caused, at least in part, by the higher net quantity of the drug present in the controlled-release formulation. Hydrocodone has roughly half the potency of oxycodone; as an antitussive, it is approximately 2.5 times more potent than codeine. The usual analgesic dose of dihydrocodeine is half that of codeine.

Meperidine

Meperidine is a synthetic phenylpiperidine analgesic drug that is structurally dissimilar to morphine (Figure 20-6). Meperidine was initially developed as an atropinelike drug but was subsequently discovered to possess significant analgesic efficacy. In 1939, it was introduced as an analgesic, sedative, and antispasmodic drug effective against most types of pain and supposedly free of many of morphine's undesirable properties. Over time, however, it has become clear that meperidine does not significantly differ from morphine in its important pharmacology, and in therapeutic doses (80 to 100 mg parenterally) it produces analgesia, sedation, and respiratory depression as well as the other CNS actions common to the opioids as a class. Meperidine is approximately one eighth to one tenth as potent as morphine; when given parenterally at equianalgesic doses, the degree of sedation and respiratory depression is the same for both drugs. Because it retains some atropinelike action, pupillary constriction is somewhat less with meperidine, as is the incidence of spasm of the biliary tract. Like other opioid analgesics, however, meperidine can be spasmogenic to the smooth muscle of the gastrointestinal tract but differs from other opioids in that it is generally not considered to be of value in the treatment of diarrhea. A meperidine congener, diphenoxylate (contained in Lomotil), is widely used for that purpose.

Meperidine, more than other pure agonists, is used as an analgesic in labor and delivery. Its peak analgesic effect after parenteral administration occurs soon and its duration of action is short (3 to 4 hours). Maternally administered meperidine can produce neonatal respiratory depression, and the content of normeperidine, an active metabolite, in fetal blood increases over time; studies, however, have not reported additional neonatal risks when meperidine was used.[13]

Meperidine is often mistakenly considered to be a useful oral analgesic drug at approximately the same dose given parenterally (50 to 100 mg). Its oral effectiveness, however, is approximately one fourth of its parenteral effectiveness; thus approximately four times the dose of meperidine must be administered orally to produce analgesia equivalent to that achieved with parenteral meperidine. The duration of action of meperidine is shorter than that of morphine, necessitating more frequent administration of meperidine for relief of continuing pain. Acute intoxication associated with meperidine also differs from that with morphine in that CNS excitation, produced by the normeperidine metabolite and manifested as tremors and convulsions, can occur instead of the stupor and coma typically associated with morphine intoxication.

Finally, it is important to note that meperidine is commonly abused by health professionals who mistakenly believe that meperidine has a lower dependence liability and is easier to stop using than morphine. In fact, meperidine dependence has been widely documented since the drug was first introduced, and it should be appreciated that meperidine has significant abuse potential.

Alphaprodine

Alphaprodine is a phenylpiperidine opioid similar in structure and pharmacology to meperidine. The drug was first used clinically in 1949 and subsequently became a popular premedicant in obstetrics and in pediatric dentistry. It was withdrawn from the market in 1986 because of concerns by the manufacturer about liability. The submucosal administration of alphaprodine gained wide use in pediatric dentistry because it was easy to administer by this route, had a rapid onset and a relatively short duration of action, and was effective in sedating anxious, uncooperative children. Tragically, the occasional use of excessive doses of alphaprodine (and of local anesthetics) coupled with improper monitoring techniques and ineffective emergency responses proved too often to be a lethal combination.[18] The fact that fatalities have occurred when other opioids were used in similar circumstances indicates that the clinical failure of alphaprodine is more attributable to how it was used rather than to any inherent shortcoming of the drug itself.

Methadone

Methadone is a synthetic pure agonist opioid analgesic qualitatively similar in its pharmacology to other opioids. The diphenylheptane structure of methadone is shown in Figure 20-7; although it does not resemble morphine, methadone is induced by steric factors to assume the configuration that apparently is required for agonist interaction with μ-opioid receptors. Methadone is approximately equipotent to morphine and, aside from methadone's greater oral efficacy, differs little from morphine. Methadone, like morphine, produces analgesia, sedation, respiratory depression, miosis, and antitussive effects, as well as subjective effects similar to those of morphine. It also is constipating and can cause biliary tract spasm. It is well absorbed from the gastrointestinal tract and eventually becomes localized in the lung, kidney, and liver, where it undergoes extensive biotransformation. The major metabolites of methadone are excreted in the urine and in the bile, along with small quantities of unchanged drug.

Because methadone is a potent, orally effective analgesic agent, its use as a replacement for heroin in the treatment of opioid addiction previously was restricted by law. Methadone possesses a combination of properties that make its use in maintenance programs superior to other opioids. As already indicated, methadone has significant oral efficacy. Although its duration of action is similar to that of morphine after a single administration, methadone exhibits a persistent effect when given repeatedly. Thus methadone's duration of action is effectively increased, permitting single daily dosage to suppress withdrawal symptoms in opioid-dependent persons.

The term *blockade* unfortunately was used when the use of methadone in maintenance programs for heroin addicts was initially reported. Blockade of the effects of heroin and a disappearance of "drug hunger" in heroin addicts after the administration of relatively high doses of methadone were claimed. This use, however, is misleading because it promotes the interpretation that methadone's action is equivalent to receptor antagonism, thus endowing methadone with a pharmacologic property it does not possess. Methadone is not an opioid receptor antagonist; it is a pure agonist, as are the other opioids discussed in this section. The use of methadone (or any other opioid agonist) in maintenance programs relates to cross-tolerance and cross-dependence and not to some unique ability of methadone to "block" heroin's effects. Cross-tolerance among opioids means that if a person has become tolerant to the effects of one opioid (heroin, for example), he or she will also exhibit tolerance to the effects of other opioids. When cross-dependence exists, a person physically dependent on one opioid can be switched to a different opioid to prevent the expression of withdrawal symptoms. These are general statements of principles that apply to the opioids as a class because the μ receptor is the principal receptor at which these agonists act. In practice, because there are differences among opioid agonists, cross-tolerance and cross-dependence are not complete. As used in maintenance programs, methadone simply represents the substitution of one opioid for another, and methadone is used rather than other opioids primarily because it can be given orally and has an extended duration of action.

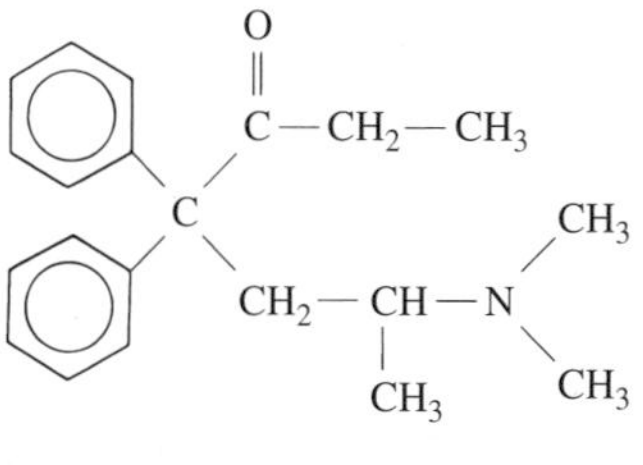

Fig. 20-7 Structural formula of methadone.

Propoxyphene

Propoxyphene is a synthetic opioid analgesic structurally related to methadone. Propoxyphene was initially introduced and legally classified as a "nonnarcotic" analgesic. Currently, it is listed in Schedule IV of the Controlled Substances Act of 1970, whereas codeine, the opioid with which propoxyphene is usually compared, is listed in Schedule II. It has been amply demonstrated that propoxyphene is subject to abuse and that physical dependence does develop during high-dose, long-term use. Overall, propoxyphene's dependence liability is estimated to be slightly less than that of codeine.

Despite the foregoing, there is considerable doubt about the analgesic efficacy of propoxyphene. Undeniably, propoxyphene produces CNS effects that appear qualitatively similar to those of codeine and other opioids. However, it is not generally agreed that analgesia is one of those central actions, at least at the doses commonly used. Critical review of the published literature on propoxyphene leads to the conclusion that the drug is no more efficacious an analgesic than aspirin and perhaps is even inferior to aspirin for relief of pain.[16] Nevertheless, propoxyphene is widely used as an analgesic, and it is claimed that approximately 65 mg of propoxyphene hydrochloride or 100 mg of propoxyphene napsylate is equivalent in analgesic efficacy to 65 mg of codeine. The currently recognized use of propoxyphene is for treatment of mild to moderate pain, and propoxyphene is often prescribed in place of codeine, apparently because of unjustified overconcern regarding codeine's dependence liability. Acute intoxication with propoxyphene can produce respiratory and CNS depression, confusion, hallucinations, and occasionally convulsions. Like meperidine, a demethylated metabolite of propoxyphene, norpropoxyphene, is a CNS stimulant.

Fentanyl and Congeners

Fentanyl, alfentanil, sufentanil, and remifentanil are 4-anilopiperidines (Figure 20-8). They are potent analgesics with relatively short durations of action used often as intravenous supplements during general anesthesia with inhalation or intravenous anesthetic drugs or as the principal component of balanced anesthesia (e.g., with nitrous oxide and a neuromuscular blocking drug), especially for cardiac surgery. The primary advantage of these more potent opioids is the cardiovascular stability they provide during surgery.[2]

Analgesic anesthesia with morphine dates to the turn of the 20th century, when morphine was combined with scopolamine for surgery. Meperidine and alphaprodine were subsequently tested because of the incomplete amnesia, histamine

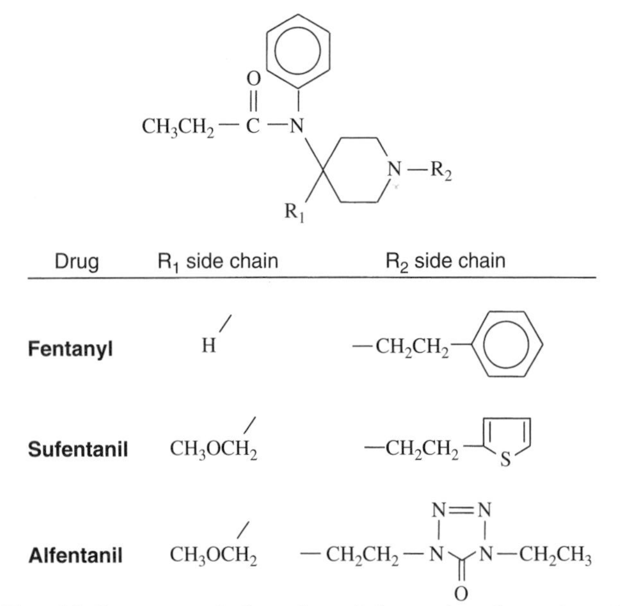

Drug	R_1 side chain	R_2 side chain
Fentanyl	H	$-CH_2CH_2-$(phenyl)
Sufentanil	CH_3OCH_2	$-CH_2CH_2-$(thienyl, S)
Alfentanil	CH_3OCH_2	$-CH_2CH_2-N$(N=N, C=O)$N-CH_2CH_3$

Fig. 20-8 Structural formulas of fentanyl, sufentanil, and alfentanil.

release, hypotension, and postoperative respiratory depression associated with the high doses of morphine that were required during surgery. Meperidine and alphaprodine, however, presented other disadvantages (e.g., poor cardiovascular stability) and have since been replaced by fentanyl and its congeners, all of which are more effective than morphine in reducing the endocrine and metabolic responses to surgery and maintaining cardiovascular stability.

Although these newer agents have found widespread application in current anesthetic practice, particularly for cardiac surgery, they are not without limitations. The most serious disadvantage associated with opioids used as analgesic anesthetics is that they are not anesthetics and their use is associated with a high incidence of signs of inadequate anesthesia (e.g., sweating, pupillary dilation, or opening of the eyes during surgery). Use of the term *anesthetic* to describe the pharmacologic characteristics of these agents is inappropriate. In addition, awareness during surgery and inadequate amnesia after surgery are not uncommon. Other disadvantages include hypertension after sternotomy (which can result in myocardial ischemia and infarction), bradycardia (which can be prevented by pretreatment with atropine), respiratory depression, and muscle rigidity, particularly of the abdominal and thoracic cavities. Thus, although these opioids provide improved cardiovascular stability during induction and throughout an operation, the "anesthesia" produced may be incomplete.

Fentanyl is much more lipid soluble than morphine, which largely accounts for its more rapid onset and shorter duration of action; fentanyl is also 80 to 100 times more potent than morphine. The speed of onset allows fentanyl to play a role in the induction of anesthesia. Sufentanil is 5 to 10 times more potent than fentanyl, whereas alfentanil is somewhat less potent than fentanyl. Like fentanyl, these drugs are rapidly acting when given parenterally and have short durations of action. Because of its rapid onset and short duration of action even after repeated administrations, alfentanil has become a drug of choice for outpatient anesthesia. Remifentanil, the newest of the anesthetic opioids, is quickly broken down in the bloodstream and tissues by esterases. It has the shortest duration of action of all 4-anilopiperidine opioids and may play a special role in brief procedures when a temporary analgesic effect is desired.

In addition to its use in cardiac surgery, fentanyl is currently available in two unique dosage forms for pain control. Because fentanyl is lipophilic, it is available as an adherent skin patch for transdermal delivery of drug. This formulation, used principally for treatment of chronic pain (e.g., cancer pain), provides continuous drug delivery in therapeutic concentrations with reduced incidence of constipation and nausea.[3,7] Patients with chronic pain often have what is termed "breakthrough pain" while taking opioids for pain control. Fentanyl formulated as a lollipop is available for rapid onset (sublingual absorption) analgesia to control episodes of breakthrough pain.

Other Opioids

A number of opioid analgesics, some listed in Table 20-2, have not been discussed because they offer no therapeutic advantage over morphine or codeine and for the most part are not widely used. New opioid analgesics continue to be developed, particularly those with mixed agonist-antagonist properties (see below), and it is likely that some of these will find clinical application.

MIXED AGONIST-ANTAGONISTS AND OPIOID RECEPTOR ANTAGONISTS

Drugs possessing both agonist and antagonist efficacy were first synthesized 100 years ago. They possessed predominant antagonist effects (e.g., nalorphine) and were initially used to reverse or block the effects of pure opioid agonists. Today, naloxone and naltrexone, both of which are pure opioid receptor antagonists, have supplanted the use of nalorphine, a mixed agonist-antagonist used for years as an opioid receptor antagonist to reverse acute opioid intoxication. Naloxone is used almost exclusively to reverse the effects of opioid agonists (e.g., in acute opioid intoxication); naltrexone finds application in the maintenance of detoxified opioid abusers.

The number of mixed agonist-antagonists has grown since the early 1950s because it was hoped that such drugs would be potent analgesics devoid of dependence and abuse liability. Chemical manipulation of the opioid structure produces compounds with varying agonist and antagonist properties. It was anticipated that the correct combination of such properties would yield a potent and efficacious analgesic drug that would not be abused. It was quickly learned, however, that drugs having both agonist and antagonist properties were often unsuitable for clinical use as analgesics because of undesirable dysphoric side effects. Furthermore, the opioid receptor–blocking aspect of their pharmacologic profile does not prevent their abuse or free these drugs from tolerance and dependence. In carefully controlled studies in animals, mixed agonist-antagonists have been established to possess reinforcing properties that lead to self-administration. In this respect, the mixed agonist-antagonists are like pure opioid agonists (e.g., morphine), although they clearly have less reinforcing efficacy than do the pure opioid agonists. Tolerance will develop to the agonist but not antagonist effects of these drugs. Subjects who repeatedly use mixed agonist-antagonists may become physically dependent, just as can occur with repeated use of morphine and other pure opioid agonists, although the withdrawal symptoms differ somewhat from those produced by morphinelike agonists.

Naloxone and Naltrexone

Naloxone (Figure 20-9) and naltrexone are the only opioid receptor antagonists currently available that are essentially devoid of opioid agonist effects. In addition to antagonizing

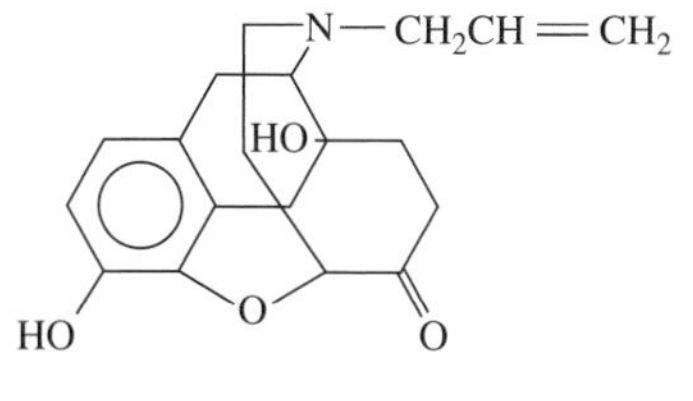

Fig. 20-9 Structural formula of naloxone.

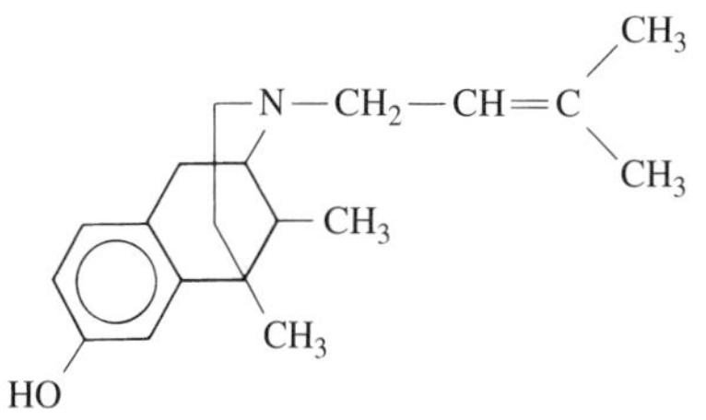

Fig. 20-10 Structural formula of pentazocine.

the effects of opioids, these drugs can block the agonist actions of most mixed agonist-antagonists. This is an important point because the respiratory depression produced by pentazocine, a mixed agonist-antagonist, is reversible by naloxone and naltrexone but not by other mixed agonist-antagonist drugs used as analgesics. Accordingly, the principal use of the pure opioid receptor antagonists is in the treatment of acute opioid intoxication. These pure opioid antagonists are specific and will rapidly improve ventilation. It must be appreciated, however, that these antagonists are not general respiratory stimulants. Conversely, they will not further embarrass respiration if administered to persons with respiratory depression produced by other drugs (e.g., barbiturates and alcohol). In fact, the lack of response to naloxone or naltrexone in a case of respiratory depression of unknown cause would be highly suggestive of nonopioid drug intoxication.

Naloxone, which is not effective when given orally, has an almost immediate onset and a relatively short duration of action (between 1 and 4 hours) when given parenterally. This means that additional doses may be required at 20- to 60-minute intervals, especially if naloxone is being used to reverse intoxication by a long-acting opioid agonist. Naltrexone differs from naloxone in that it is effective orally and has a remarkably long duration of action. A single oral dose can suppress the effects of opioid agonists for 48 to 72 hours. These attributes suggest that naltrexone may be of use in the maintenance of an opioid-free state in detoxified, formerly opioid-dependent persons. Indeed, a single daily administration of the drug can effectively block the action of 25 mg of heroin injected intravenously 24 hours after the last dose of naltrexone. Naltrexone may also prove useful in treating morphine overdose because it might obviate the need to monitor the patient for a relapse of respiratory depression.

Mixed Agonist-Antagonists

Pentazocine

Pentazocine is an agonist at κ opioid receptors and a partial agonist or weak antagonist at μ receptors. A benzomorphan derivative, pentazocine is structurally related to morphine (Figure 20-10), but it has an allyl-like substitution on the nitrogen of the piperidine ring (as do many of the opioid receptor antagonists). Pentazocine is an early product of continuing efforts to develop efficacious opioid analgesics with little or no dependence liability or abuse potential. Pentazocine was initially promoted as being free of dependence liability, but like other mixed agonist-antagonist and pure agonist opioids, it produces its major effects on the CNS and gastrointestinal tract and induces morphinelike subjective effects and euphoria. Thus physical and psychologic dependence can develop to pentazocine, and the drug has been widely abused. Pentazocine tablets for oral use were crushed and self-administered intravenously, often in combination with the antihistamine tripelennamine, to produce a euphoric effect. To prevent this use of pentazocine in the United States, the opioid receptor antagonist naloxone (0.5 mg) was added to the formulation, and the proprietary name of the drug was changed to Talwin NX. Because naloxone has little effect when taken orally, use of pentazocine as directed produces the desired analgesia. When subverted to intravenous use, however, the amount of naloxone present in the formulation is sufficient to antagonize completely the CNS effects of pentazocine. Unlike codeine (or other pure agonists), pentazocine will not suppress withdrawal symptoms in persons dependent on other opioids, but neither can it antagonize morphine-induced respiratory depression. Pentazocine, however, can precipitate signs of withdrawal in an opioid-dependent person because of its residual antagonist activity at μ receptors.

Pentazocine is well absorbed from the gastrointestinal tract. It is metabolized primarily in the liver to glucuronide conjugates, although small quantities of free pentazocine are excreted in the urine. It is approximately one third as potent an analgesic as morphine when given intramuscularly. As used orally, generally in place of codeine, approximately 50 mg of pentazocine is considered equivalent to 60 mg of codeine for relief of pain. Pentazocine's ability to relieve pain at greater doses is not comparable to that of the pure opioid agonists. In general, the maximal analgesic effect of mixed agonist-antagonist analgesics is less than that of morphine or other pure opioid agonists. At therapeutic doses, pentazocine exhibits effects on the CNS and gastrointestinal tract that are qualitatively similar to those of other opioids (e.g., dizziness, nausea, and sedation as well as analgesia). Unlike most other opioids, however, pentazocine can increase both heart rate and blood pressure. In toxic doses, it produces both dysphoric effects and characteristic opioidlike respiratory depression, although the respiratory depression does not increase proportionately with increasing doses as it does for the pure opioid agonists.

Butorphanol, buprenorphine, and nalbuphine

Butorphanol, buprenorphine, and nalbuphine are other examples of drugs with a mixture of opioid agonist and antagonist properties. The major thrust in developing compounds having predominant effects at the κ-opioid receptor was the belief that such drugs would retain significant analgesic activity but would be devoid of the respiratory depression and dependence liability associated with morphinelike drugs whose prominent analgesic and respiratory depressant effects are produced at the μ-opioid receptor. This effort has been partially successful. Although at therapeutic doses they cause respiratory depression equivalent to that produced by 10 mg of morphine, the depression does not increase proportionately with increasing doses. Unfortunately, neither does the analgesia.

Butorphanol is a morphinan derivative approximately four to six times more potent than morphine as an analgesic. Butorphanol is an agonist at κ-opioid receptors and a weak partial agonist at the μ receptor. The drug is unlikely to precipitate withdrawal symptoms in opioid-dependent persons, but it shows no cross-dependence either. As an analgesic substitute for morphine, butorphanol has a low abuse potential, and respiratory depression tends to plateau beyond therapeutic doses. Butorphanol has been tested as an analgesic anesthetic (like the pure agonist fentanyl), but because it has a tendency, like pentazocine, to increase cardiac work, it is not well suited for this application. Another limitation of butorphanol is the possibility of dysphoric side effects. Butorphanol is subject to significant first-pass metabolism; approximately 80% of an oral dose is metabolized initially, and bioavailability after oral administration is accordingly low.

Buprenorphine is a strong partial agonist at the μ-opioid receptor and is 25 to 50 times more potent an analgesic than morphine. It is unlike other agonist-antagonists in that it is a potent κ receptor antagonist and has fewer psychotomimetic effects than pentazocine or butorphanol. Its agonistic effects are qualitatively similar to those of morphine, and buprenorphine produces a physical dependence described by former addicts as morphinelike. However, administration of buprenorphine to an opioid-dependent person can precipitate an immediate abstinence syndrome, even as it can relieve withdrawal symptoms caused by prior opioid withholding. These conflicting observations are explained by the fact that buprenorphine is a partial agonist at μ receptors. Thus it mimics the effects of morphine in drug-free patients but antagonizes pure agonists on coadministration.

Nalbuphine is structurally related to naloxone, but is equipotent with regular analgesic doses of morphine. It is distinguished from other available mixed agonist-antagonists in having a pronounced antagonist action at the μ receptor. Nalbuphine is an agonist at κ-opioid receptors but produces few dysphoric reactions. Because of its unique blend of agonistic and antagonistic efficacy, nalbuphine has been used to reverse respiratory depression produced by other opioids without causing a loss of analgesia. Such use finds its greatest application in debilitated surgical patients for whom the abrupt loss of pain relief caused by naloxone reversal can be life threatening. Also beneficial in this setting is the fact that nalbuphine produces minimal myocardial depression. Nevertheless, opioid reversal even with nalbuphine is potentially dangerous in the patient at risk of heart attack. Nalbuphine should also not be considered a replacement for naloxone for treatment of drug overdose in other settings.

Dezocine

Dezocine, an aminotetralin derivative, is a μ receptor antagonist and a κ receptor agonist. The drug may increase the cardiac index and pulmonary vascular resistance but lowers peripheral vascular resistance and is generally benign to the heart. In conventional doses, the potency and duration of action of dezocine are similar to those of morphine.

Novel Compounds

Tramadol is an aminocyclohexanol derivative. It and an O-demethylated metabolite are weak μ receptor agonists, the metabolite being more potent. Tramadol also inhibits the reuptake of norepinephrine and 5-HT, which may contribute to the analgesic effect of the drug. Thus the analgesia caused by tramadol is only partially reversed by naloxone. As a perioperative analgesic, tramadol can relieve moderate to severe pain and is generally well tolerated.[27] The most common adverse effects include nausea, vomiting, and drowsiness; effects on respiratory or cardiovascular parameters are not clinically relevant at recommended doses in adults or children. Seizures have been reported for tramadol. The drug is used orally and has a terminal half-life of approximately 7 hours.

USE OF OPIOIDS IN THE CONTROL OF PAIN

A full discussion of the differentiating features of acute and chronic pain is beyond the scope of this chapter, but some comment is required to better understand the use of opioids in the clinical management of pain. Both the opioid agonists and mixed agonist-antagonists can be used satisfactorily as analgesics for the relief of acute pain. The long-term use of opioids in clinical pain states, however, raises questions regarding the choice of opioid, the route of administration, and the role played by the development of tolerance and physical dependence in therapy.[21,31] The use of mixed agonist-antagonists in chronic pain management is limited. Escalating doses of pentazocine and related drugs are associated with undesirable psychotomimetic effects. More importantly, the antagonistic properties of mixed agonist-antagonists at the μ receptor restrict the ability to switch between pure agonists and mixed agonist-antagonists for the control of pain.

Heroin was initially considered the drug of choice for management of cancer pain, but it has been clearly established that heroin offers no therapeutic advantage over morphine. Indeed, heroin is a prodrug that is metabolized to morphine. Although morphine's bioavailability is limited because of first-pass metabolism, the dose can be adjusted for successful pain control by oral administration in liquid or sustained-release tablet form. Methadone is a useful alternative to morphine, but because its plasma half-life averages 24 hours, methadone will accumulate with repeated dosing, and greater care is required with its use.

Oral administration is generally considered optimal for the treatment of chronic pain, but epidural, intrathecal, and intravenous routes of administration are also used, more recently in situations of patient-controlled analgesia. Although an exaggerated fear of "addicting" patients exists, as well as a sense that allowing patients to self-administer opioids for the control of pain will lead to uncontrolled use, studies indicate that the total amount of opioid that is self-administered by patient-controlled analgesic methods is usually no more and often less than that given conventionally by health professionals.

It requires reemphasis that the fear of addiction held by health professionals and patients often limits adequate opioid dosing for the control of pain. Physical dependence will undeniably develop with repeated opioid administration, but evidence that psychologic dependence and opioid abuse are a consequence of long-term medical use of opioids is virtually nonexistent.

USES IN DENTISTRY

Opioids used in dentistry are primarily those available for oral administration, such as codeine, hydrocodone, oxycodone, and pentazocine. In addition, morphine, meperidine, and fentanyl are used parenterally (as described in Chapter 47). Although these drugs all possess therapeutically useful actions in addition to analgesia, they are used in dentistry exclusively for pain relief. It should be recognized, however, that pain of dental origin frequently arises from or is accompanied by inflammation. Because opioids are not antiinflammatory, nonopioid analgesic drugs with antiinflammatory efficacy (e.g., aspirin, ibuprofen) are often the first choice for relief of pain. Opioids are particularly useful when additional pain control is required. Combinations of opioids with aspirin or acetaminophen, for example, are commonly used and are rational because different, complementary central and peripheral mechanisms of pain relief are invoked. It should be appreciated, however, that whereas aspirin and ibuprofen have antiinflammatory efficacy, acetaminophen is not antiinflammatory and thus is not a good choice when it is desired to reduce both inflammation and pain.

Among the opioids available for use in dentistry, codeine, hydrocodone, and oxycodone are the most common. As previously indicated, the analgesic efficacy of propoxyphene is somewhat controversial, as is that of meperidine given orally in conventional doses.

IMPLICATIONS FOR DENTISTRY

The opioid analgesics are, of course, subject to abuse, and both significant physical and psychologic dependence can develop. The pharmacologic and sociologic aspects of opioids are discussed in Chapter 51. Additional implications for dentistry relate to the possible interactions of opioids with other drugs that dentists may prescribe or that patients may be taking for medical reasons. Drug interactions with orally administered opioids are not common or not usually of great clinical importance when they do occur. There are, however, recognized interactions between opioids and CNS depressants, neuroleptics, tricyclic antidepressants, monoamine oxidase inhibitors, local anesthetics, and oral anticoagulants that can be clinically significant, particularly if opioids are given parenterally.

In general, the coadministration of CNS depressants produces summation of effects and occasionally a greater than anticipated depression (i.e., supraadditive effect). Opioids and phenothiazines (e.g., chlorpromazine) are known to produce at least additive CNS depression, including respiratory depression. Moreover, this combination may also produce a greater incidence of orthostatic hypotension than either drug administered alone. Increased hypotension has also been reported with combinations of opioids and tricyclic antidepressants. When combinations of opioids and other CNS depressants are used in dentistry, the drugs are commonly given by intravenous infusion, and the effects can be titrated to the desired level. When used orally, doses should have a sufficient margin of safety to avoid dose-dependent toxicity. Thus the clinical significance of these interactions, particularly at the doses of opioids used orally in dentistry, is uncertain.

The coadministration of local anesthetics and parenteral opioid analgesics is a common and generally safe practice. However, large doses of these classes of drugs display supraadditive toxicity. It is likely that respiratory acidosis caused by an opioid can increase the entry of a local anesthetic into the CNS.

Interaction of opioids with oral anticoagulants has been reported to result in an enhanced response to the latter, but the clinical significance has not been established, and it is not likely that short-term opioid administration has an appreciable effect on the patient's response to oral anticoagulants.

A well-documented interaction of meperidine and monoamine oxidase inhibitors results in severe and immediate reactions that include excitation, rigidity, hypertension, and sometimes death. Chemically unrelated opioids are not likely to cause a similarly violent reaction.

Opioid Analgesics and Antagonists

Nonproprietary (generic) name	*Proprietary (trade) name*
Agonist analgesics	
Alfentanil	Alfenta
Alphaprodine*	Nisentil
Codeine†	—
Dihydrocodeine	Synalgos DC
Fentanyl	Sublimaze
Fentanyl transdermal system	Duragesic
Fentanyl transmucosal system	Fentanyl Oralet
Hydrocodone†	Dicodid
Hydromorphone	Dilaudid
Levomethadyl	ORLAAM
Levorphanol	Levo-Dromoran
Meperidine	Demerol
Methadone	Dolophine
Morphine	—
Opium	Pantopon, Paregoric
Oxycodone	Oxycontin; in Percodan
Oxymorphone	Numorphan
Propoxyphene	Darvon
Remifentanil	Ultiva
Sufentanil	Sufenta
Mixed agonist-antagonist analgesics	
Buprenorphine	Buprenex
Butorphanol	Stadol
Dezocine	Dalgan
Nalbuphine	Nubain
Pentazocine	Talwin; in Talwin NX
Antagonists	
Naloxone	Narcan; in Talwin NX
Naltrexone	Revia
Others	
Methotrimeprazine	Levoprome
Tramadol	Ultram

*Not currently available in the United States.
†Also used as antitussives or cough suppressants.

CITED REFERENCES

1. Borison HL: Central nervous system respiratory depressants—narcotic analgesics, *Pharmacol Ther [B]* 3:227-237, 1977.
2. Bovill JG, Sebel PS, Stanley TH: Opioid analgesics in anesthesia: with special reference to their use in cardiovascular anesthesia, *Anesthesiology* 61:731-755, 1984.
3. Donner B, Zenz M, Strumpf M, et al: Long-term treatment of cancer pain with transdermal fentanyl, *J Pain Symptom Manage* 15:168-175, 1998.
4. Gavériaux-Ruff C, Peluso J, Befort K, et al: Detection of opioid receptor mRNA by RT-PCR reveals alternative splicing for the δ- and κ-opioid receptors, *Mol Brain Res* 48:298-304, 1997.
5. Gebhart GF, Proudfit HK: Descending modulation of pain processing. In Hunt S, Koltzenburg M, eds: *The neurobiology of pain,* Oxford, 2004, Oxford University Press.
6. Grace D, Fee JP: A comparison of intrathecal morphine-6-glucuronide and intrathecal morphine sulfate as analgesics for total hip replacement, *Anesth Analg* 83:1055-1059, 1996.
7. Grond S, Zech D, Lehman KA, et al: Transdermal fentanyl in the long-term treatment of cancer pain: a prospective study of 50 patients with advanced cancer of the gastrointestinal tract or the head and neck region, *Pain* 69:191-198, 1997.
8. Hosobuchi Y, Adams JE, Linchitz R: Pain relief by electrical stimulation of the central gray matter in humans and its reversal by naloxone, *Science* 197:183-186, 1977.
9. Houde RW, Wallenstein SL, Beaver WT: Clinical measurement of pain. In deStevens G, ed: *Analgetics,* New York, 1965, Academic Press.

10. Hughes J: Isolation of an endogenous compound from the brain with pharmacological properties similar to morphine, *Brain Res* 88:295-308, 1975.
11. Kaiko RF, Wallenstein SL, Rogers AG, et al: Narcotics in the elderly, *Med Clin North Am* 66:1079-1089, 1982.
12. Kieffer BL: Molecular aspects of opioid receptors. In Dickenson AH, Besson J-MR, eds: *The pharmacology of pain. Handbook of experimental pharmacology,* vol 130, Berlin, 1997, Springer.
13. Marcus MME, Gogarten W, Van Aken H: Opioids in obstetrics. In Stein C, ed: *Opioids in pain control,* Cambridge, 1999, Cambridge University Press.
14. Meunier JC, Mollereau C, Toll L, et al: Isolation and structure of the endogenous agonist of opioid receptor-like ORL-1 receptor, *Nature* 377:532-535, 1995.
15. Miller RJ: Peptides as neurotransmitters: focus on the enkephalins and endorphins, *Pharmacol Ther* 12:73-108, 1981.
16. Miller RR, Feingold A, Paxinos J: Propoxyphene hydrochloride. A critical review, *JAMA* 213:996-1006, 1970.
17. Mogensen T, Eliasen K, Ejlersen E, et al: Epidural clonidine enhances postoperative analgesia from a combined low-dose epidural bupivacaine and morphine regimen, *Anesth Analg* 75:607-610, 1992.
18. Moore PA, Goodson JM: Risk appraisal of narcotic sedation for children, *Anesth Prog* 32:129-139, 1985.
19. Okuda-Ashitaka E, Ito S: Nocistatin: a novel neuropeptide encoded by the gene for the nociceptin/orphanin FQ precursor, *Peptides* 21:1101-1109, 2000.
20. Owen JA, Sitar DS, Berger L, et al: Age-related morphine kinetics, *Clin Pharmacol Ther* 34:364-368, 1983.
21. Portenoy RK: Tolerance to opioid analgesics: clinical aspects, *Cancer Surv* 21:49-65, 1994.
22. Portenoy RK, Thaler HT, Inturrisi CE, et al: The metabolite morphine-6-glucuronide contributes to the analgesia produced by morphine infusion in patients with pain and normal renal function, *Clin Pharmacol Ther* 51:422-431, 1992.
23. Price DD: *Psychological mechanisms of pain and analgesia. Progress in pain research and management,* vol 15, Seattle, 1999, IASP Press.
24. Raynor K, Kong H, Chen Y, et al: Pharmacological characterization of the cloned kappa-, delta-, and mu-opioid receptors, *Mol Pharmacol* 45:330-334, 1994.
25. Reinscheid RK, Nothacker HP, Bourson A, et al: Orophanin FQ: a neuropeptide that activates an opioid-like G protein–coupled receptor, *Science* 270:792-794, 1995.
26. Sapira JD: Speculations concerning opium abuse and world history, *Perspect Biol Med* 18:379-398, 1975.
27. Scott LJ, Perry CM: Tramadol: a review of its use in perioperative pain, *Drugs* 60:139-176, 2000.
28. Simon EJ: The opiate receptors, *Neurochem Res* 1:3-28, 1976.
29. Stein C, Cabot PJ, Schafer M: Peripheral opioid analgesia: mechanisms and clinical implications. In Stein C, ed: *Opioids in pain control,* Cambridge, 1999, Cambridge University Press.
30. Thorn SE, Wattwil M, Lindberg G, et al: Systemic and central effects of morphine on gastroduodenal motility, *Acta Anesthesthesiol Scand* 40:177-186, 1996.
31. Twycross RG: Opioids, In Wall PD, Melzack R, eds: *Textbook of pain,* London, 1999, Churchill Livingstone.
32. Yaksh TL: The spinal actions of opioids. In Hertz A, ed: *Opioids II. Handbook of experimental pharmacology,* vol 104, Berlin, 1993, Springer-Verlag.
33. Zadina JE, Hackler L, Ge L, et al: A potent and selective endogenous agonist for the μ-opiate receptor, *Nature* 386:499-502, 1997.
34. Zeilhofer, HU, Reinscheid RK, Okuda-Ashitaka E: Nociceptin, nocistatin and pain. In Dostrovsky, JO, Carr DB, Koltzenburg M, eds: *Proceedings of the 10th World Congress on Pain. Progress in pain research and management,* vol 24, Seattle, 2003, IASP Press.

GENERAL REFERENCES

Dickenson AH, Besson J-MR, eds: *The pharmacology of pain. Handbook of experimental pharmacology,* vol 130, Berlin, 1997, Springer.

Dostrovsky J, Carr DB, Koltzenburg M, eds: *Proceedings of the 10th World Congress on Pain,* Seattle, 2003, IASP Press.

Peptides 21:891-1154, 2000. (issue devoted to nociceptin/orphanin FQ/ORL-1 receptor system)

Reisine T: Opiate receptors, *Neuropharmacology* 34:463-472, 1995.

Stein C, ed: *Opioids in pain control,* Cambridge, 1999, Cambridge University Press.

Taylor DA, Fleming WA: Unifying perspectives of the mechanisms underlying the development of tolerance and physical dependence to opioids, *J Pharmacol Exp Ther* 297:11-18, 2001.

Williams JT, Christie MJ, Manzoni O: Cellular and synaptic adaptations mediating opioid dependence, *Physiol Rev* 81:299-343, 2001.

Zakrezewska JM, Harrison SD, eds: *Assessment and management of orofacial pain. Pain research and clinical management,* vol 14, Amsterdam, 2002, Elsevier.

CHAPTER • 21

Nonopioid Analgesics, Nonsteroidal Antiinflammatory Drugs, and Antirheumatic and Antigout Drugs

Paul J. Desjardins, Elliot V. Hersh, Clarence L. Trummel, and Stephen A. Cooper

Nonopioid analgesics, nonsteroidal antiinflammatory drugs (NSAIDs), and agents used in the control of rheumatoid arthritis and gout represent a diverse group of chemical compounds whose mechanism of action typically involves the inhibition of one or more components of the inflammatory response. Acute pain, such as typically accompanies inflammatory insults resulting from a variety of dental surgical procedures, can often be controlled by the use of the nonopioid analgesic acetaminophen or NSAIDs such as ibuprofen. In addition, the NSAIDs play an important role in the symptomatic relief of the inflammation and pain that accompany arthritis. However, they do not eliminate or reduce the underlying causes of the arthritic disease, and joint damage can continue to progress despite the long-term use of these drugs.

Disease-modifying antirheumatic drugs play a major role in the management of rheumatoid arthritis. They represent a group of chemically unrelated agents that have additional uses in medicine, ranging from the treatment of malaria and cancer to the prevention of transplanted organ rejection. In some instances, these agents can slow and arrest some of the pathologic changes seen in rheumatoid arthritis. Unfortunately, they are fraught with serious adverse effects, and many patients cannot tolerate their long-term use.

CAUSE OF INFLAMMATION

Inflammation typically represents the response to tissue injury and includes products of activated mast calls, leukocytes, and platelets; prostaglandins (PGs); leukotrienes; and complement-derived products. The clinical features of inflammation include tumor (edema), rubor (redness), calor (heat), dolor (pain), and loss of function.

Although inflammation is often thought of as only a pathologic event, it serves a normal homeostatic function. In the case of tissue injury from minor trauma or a dental surgical procedure, the inflammatory process results in a series of well-regulated humoral and cellular events leading to localization of injury, removal of noxious agents, repair of physical damage, and restitution of function in the injured tissue. In patients unable to mount a competent inflammatory response, such as those with agranulocytosis induced by some cancer chemotherapeutic drug regimens (see Chapter 42), the results are often fulminant infection and death.

The inflammatory response is, of course, not always beneficial to the host. If it becomes excessive or chronic, as is the case with rheumatoid arthritis, it may result in the progressive destruction of joint tissue and a whole host of untoward systemic effects. Only now are drugs being developed with relatively favorable therapeutic indexes that show promise in halting some of the destructive inflammatory events of chronic rheumatic diseases.

Inflammation can be divided into three phases: acute inflammation, subacute inflammation, and chronic inflammation. In acute inflammation, small preformed inflammatory mediators such as histamine are released, causing vasodilation and increased capillary permeability. In the subacute stage, inflammatory cells migrate and invade the site. PGs, leukotrienes, platelet-activating factor (PAF), and cytokines also play major roles. The third, or chronic, stage of inflammation involves the lymphocytic phase of injury cleansing and repair. Cytokines, especially interleukins and tumor necrosis factor α (TNF-α), are prominent in this stage. In reality these phases are not distinct entities. For example, components of the subacute phase participate in the acute inflammatory process, and acute inflammatory mediators are present in chronic inflammatory disorders such as arthritis. Even so, this classification still offers a useful way to categorize this highly complex process. The following section briefly reviews some of the key mediators of the inflammatory process. A more complete list of inflammatory mediators is provided in Table 21-1.

Tissue Mediators

Histamine

Histamine is the first mediator for which a role in the inflammatory process was clearly established. This vasoactive amine is formed by decarboxylation of histidine and is widely distributed in the body. Although some free histamine exists in tissues, most is stored in mast cell and basophil granules in a physiologically inactive form. (For a more complete discussion, see Chapter 22.) A variety of physical and chemical stimuli, such as antigens, complement fragments, or simple mechanical trauma, can cause extrusion of the granules and release of active histamine into the extracellular fluid. One of the most characteristic actions of histamine is dilation of vessels of the microcirculation and a marked, but transient, increase in the permeability of capillaries and postcapillary venules. These vascular changes are similar to those that occur in tissue after injuries of all sorts. The evidence that histamine released from the ubiquitous mast cell is responsible for the initial permeability changes seen in an inflammatory response is extensive. For example, the histamine content of tissue fluid at the site of injury rises within minutes after the insult and then falls. Concurrent with these changes, mast cells in the area of damage are found to be degranulated. Furthermore, it has been shown that prior depletion of tissue histamine stores by various means or pretreatment with classic antihistamines will reduce the initial vascular response to injury.[81] However,

Table • 21-1

Classification of Some Endogenous Mediators of Inflammation

MAJOR GROUPS	MAJOR MEDIATORS
Tissue	
Lymphocyte products	MCP-1
	GM-CSF
	Other chemoactive factors
	Interferon γ
	Interleukins
	Skin reactive factor
Macrophage products	Interleukin-1
	Interferon γ
	TNF-α
	PAF
Mast cell products	Histamine
	Cytokines
	TNF-α
	Leukotrienes
	Prostaglandin D_2
	PAF
Eosinophil products	Lysosomal enzymes
	Major basic protein
	Other cationic proteins
	Leukotrienes
	PAF
Others	Reactive metabolites of oxygen
	Endogenous pyrogens from leukocytes
	Leukocytosis factors
Plasma	
Kinin system	Bradykinin
Complement system	C3 fragments
	C5 fragments
	$\overline{\text{C5b67}}$ complex
	Membrane attack complex
Clotting system	Fibrinopeptides
	Fibrin degradation products

MCP-1, Monocyte chemoattractive protein-1; *GM-CSF,* granulocyte-macrophage colony-stimulating factor; *PAF,* platelet-activating factor.

it should be noted that inhibition of initial histamine-dependent events does not block the further development of the inflammatory response.

In patients with chronic inflammation caused by rheumatoid arthritis, increased concentrations and penetration depth of mast cells in synovial tissue are found, possibly related to the expression of stem cell factor by synovial fibroblasts. However, astemizole, a potent antihistamine, does not affect the clinical course of this disease.[113] Thus the role played by histamine in inflammation is early, transient, and nonessential for subsequent events that may lead to lasting tissue alterations.

Antihistamines have little use as general antiinflammatory agents. In certain situations, such as immediate allergic reactions, large amounts of histamine are released locally or systemically from sensitized mast cells and basophils as a consequence of antigen-antibody reactions. In these instances, antihistamines that block the H_1 receptor are useful in reducing symptoms attributable to histamine. As is discussed in Chapter 22, antihistamines that block the action of histamine at the H_2 receptor have a supporting role in the management of anaphylaxis.

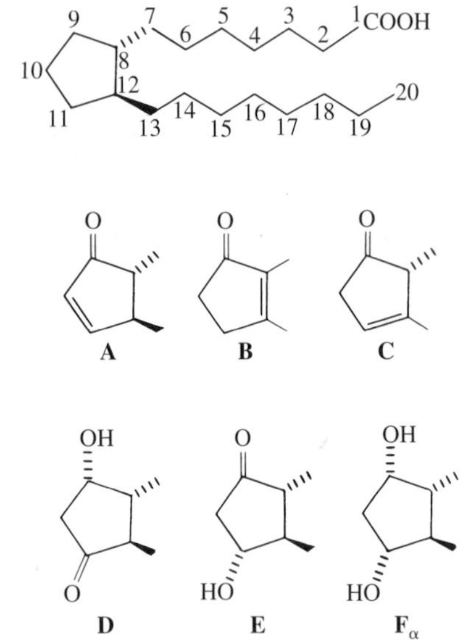

Fig. 21-1 Molecular structure of prostaglandins (PGs). At *top* is the structure of prostanoic acid, a hypothetical compound of which the PGs can be considered analogues. At *bottom* are the basic ring structures of PG groups *A* through *F.*

Prostaglandins

The PGs are a unique family of closely related acidic lipids found in all tissues. The basic structure of all PGs is a prostanoic acid skeleton composed of a 20-carbon polyunsaturated fatty acid with a five-member ring at C8 through C12 (Figure 21-1). Like the leukotrienes described below, PGs are derived from arachidonic acid and similar 20-carbon polyunsaturated fatty acids that are liberated from the cell membranes of local tissues by the action of acylhydrolases, principally phospholipase A_2, and, in platelets, diacylglycerol lipase. Inflammatory cells, including human monocytes and mast cells, also have the ability to generate PGs. Although there are multiple oxygenation products derived from arachidonic acid, the PG molecules all contain a five-membered carbon ring. The alphabetical PG nomenclature (A-F) is based on the structure of this cyclopentane ring. For example, PGE and PGF_{α} differ only in the presence of a ketone or hydroxyl group at C9. Also in the nomenclature the subscript 1 indicates the presence of a double bond at C13 to C14 (PGE_1), 2 indicates the presence of an additional double bond at C5 to C6 (PGE_2), and 3 would indicate the presence of a third double bond at C17 to C18 (PGE_3).

One of the key events in the acute inflammatory process is the liberation of arachidonic acid from damaged cell membranes upon exposure to phospholipase A_2 (Figure 21-2).[43] This step can be inhibited indirectly by a powerful group of antiinflammatory agents known as *glucocorticoids,* which are described in detail in Chapter 35. From this point, the oxidative metabolism of arachidonic acid can proceed along two divergent pathways. One pathway uses the enzyme cyclooxygenase (COX), also known as *PG endoperoxide synthase,* whereas the second uses the enzyme lipoxygenase. Virtually all cells in the body, with the exception of red blood cells, contain the COX enzyme, whereas lipoxygenase appears to

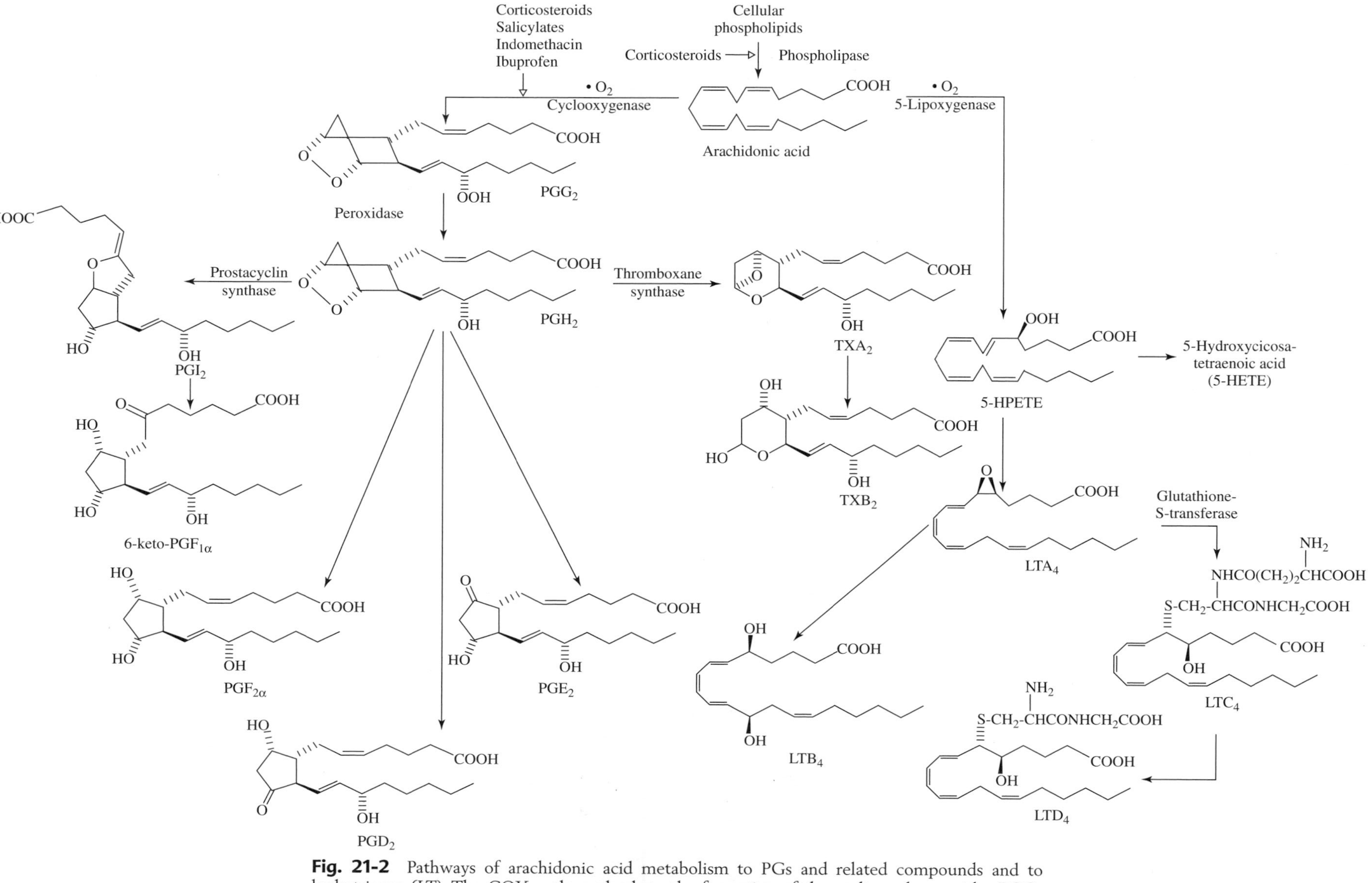

Fig. 21-2 Pathways of arachidonic acid metabolism to PGs and related compounds and to leukotrienes *(LT)*. The COX pathway leads to the formation of the cyclic endoperoxides PGG_2 and PGH_2 and subsequently to prostacyclin *(PGI_2)*, thromboxane *(TX)*, or the stable PGs *(E_2, $F_{2\alpha}$, and D_2)*. The lipoxygenase pathway yields 5-hydroperoxyeicosatetraenoic acid *(5-HPETE)* and subsequently leukotrienes A_4, B_4, C_4, and D_4. The *open arrows* indicate the metabolic steps that are inhibited by corticosteroids or nonsteroidal antiinflammatory agents such as aspirin and ibuprofen. Not shown are leukotrienes E_4 and F_4 and other lipoxygenase pathways.

be limited to inflammatory cells (neutrophils, mast cells, eosinophils, and macrophages).

COX catalyses the transformation of arachidonic acid to the short-lived cyclic endoperoxide PGG_2. PGG_2 is then converted to PGH_2 by peroxidation, which is an additional function of COX. Unstable and potentially tissue-toxic oxygen radicals can be liberated by this process. From this point, PGH_2 is converted to the stable PGs E_2 and $F_{2\alpha}$, thromboxanes, or prostacyclin (PGI_2) by appropriate enzymes.

It is now well established that COX exists in two isoforms. Both are 72-kd proteins but differ in terms of their sequence homology (approximately 60%) and their genomic regulation.[36,122,123] COX-1 is regarded as the constitutive or housekeeping isoform and is the major isoform found in healthy tissues. It is always present in a number of tissues, including the central nervous system (CNS), gastric mucosa, platelets, and kidneys.[27] In the gastric mucosa, COX-1 plays a major role in the synthesis of PGs involved in the formation of the mucous protective barrier (so-called cytoprotection) against stomach acid. In platelets, COX-1 is the key enzyme involved in thromboxane production and its subsequent platelet aggregatory properties necessary for proper hemostasis. COX-2 is, for the most part, an inducible isoform upregulated by such products as cytokines, growth factors, and mitogens in human monocytes, macrophages, endothelial cells, chondrocytes, synoviocytes, and osteoblasts.[27] It is associated with elevated concentrations of PGs during inflammation, pain, and fever. Figure 21-3 illustrates some of the physiologic roles of the COX isoforms. Although initially it was hoped the COX-2 products only participated in inflammatory and other pathologic processes, it is now known that oxidation products of the COX-2 isoform help regulate some normal physiologic processes, including the maintenance of adequate water and Na^+ excretion by the kidneys.

PGs and the other active metabolites of the intermediate endoperoxides (e.g., PGI_2 and thromboxane A_2 [TXA_2]) exert a multitude of effects in almost every biologic process examined so far. These processes include smooth muscle contraction and relaxation, vascular permeability, renal electrolyte and water transport, gastrointestinal and pancreatic secretion, various central and autonomic nervous system functions, release of hormones (e.g., growth hormone, steroids, and gonadotropins), luteolysis and parturition, lipolysis, bone resorption, and platelet aggregation. Not only are the affected processes diverse and the effects complex, but the different PGs and related molecules also sometimes appear to have antagonistic actions. For example, PGE_2 and PGI_2 in general

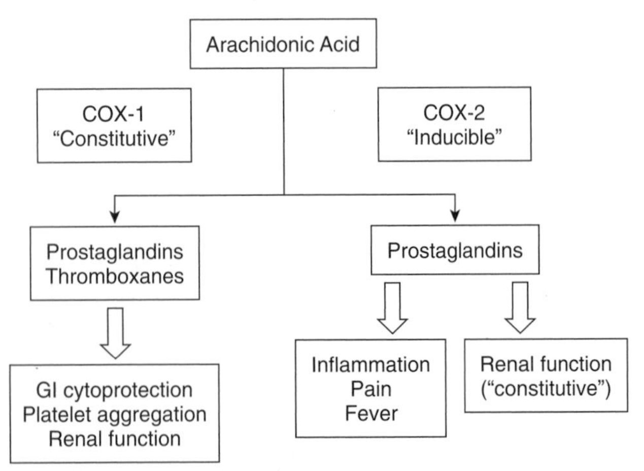

Fig. 21-3 Some physiological roles of the COX isoforms. Renal function is influenced by both COX isoforms.

cause vasodilation and inhibit platelet aggregation, whereas TXA_2 causes vasoconstriction and induces platelet aggregation. The effects of $PGF_{2\alpha}$ on vascular tone depend on the vascular bed. Qualitative and quantitative differences in response to the PGs exist among mammalian species, further complicating elucidation of the biologic roles of these substances. It is thus axiomatic that generalizations about the actions of PGs and related compounds are misleading; the response to a given agent must be considered in the context of the particular tissue involved, the assay system used, and the species of experimental animal.

There is abundant evidence that PGs and the intermediate endoperoxides are mediators of inflammation.[31,87] Arachidonic acid and other fatty acid precursors of PGs present in the membrane phospholipid of cells can be released by hydrolase enzymes activated by direct cellular damage or by any nondestructive perturbation of the membrane, whether physical, chemical, hormonal, or neurohumoral. PG synthesis can then ensue as shown in Figure 21-2. In acute inflammatory reactions, PGs appear in fluids and exudates later (2 to 12 hours after injury) than some other mediators, such as histamine and bradykinin. PGs are being formed, then, at a time when tissue damage and disintegration are more prominent. It is possible that some of the PG content found in sites of inflammation is derived from infiltrating neutrophils and macrophages because these cells are capable of PG synthesis.[1]

Once released in tissue, PGs may contribute to the inflammatory response in multiple ways. The evidence that they do so can be summarized as follows[31]: (1) PGs are found in experimentally or naturally produced inflammatory fluids; (2) neutrophils and macrophages produce PGs during phagocytosis; (3) PGI_2 and PGE_2 injected intradermally are potent inducers of vasodilation as well as of increased vascular permeability, an effect that is greatly augmented by the presence of histamine or 5-hydroxytryptamine and may last for several hours; (4) minute amounts of PGI_2 and PGE_2 injected intradermally markedly increase the pain sensitivity to other mediators, such as bradykinin and histamine; (5) PGE_2 is pyrogenic when injected into the cerebral ventricles or anterior hypothalamus, suggesting a mediator function; (6) a severe disabling arthritis is produced in animals by injecting PGs into the knee joint, and rheumatoid synovial cells produce PGs in culture; and (7) certain antiinflammatory drugs that are potent inhibitors of PG synthesis reduce experimentally produced inflammation.

Although PGs stimulate certain inflammatory events, they inhibit or modulate others. The fact that PGs inhibit the proliferation and release of certain inflammatory mediators from neutrophils and activated lymphocytes and the fact that some effects of PGE_2 are opposed by $PGF_{2\alpha}$ provide evidence of a modulating function.

The precise roles of PGs in the inflammatory process are far from established, but these unique compounds clearly have the potential to act as mediators, modulators, or both. If both functions are involved, PGs could occupy a central regulatory position. A balance between enhancement and suppression of inflammatory events could be achieved by local regulation of PG metabolism, because in some systems PGs have been shown to be either stimulatory or inhibitory depending on their concentration. Altering the relative concentrations of PGE and PGF could provide an additional means of balance because different PGs have diverse and occasionally antagonistic actions in the same system (e.g., PGE_2 causes bronchodilation whereas $PGF_{2\alpha}$ causes bronchoconstriction).

Leukotrienes

The term *slow-reacting substance* (SRS) was first applied to a lipid-soluble material produced by treatment of lung tissue with cobra venom. This material was characterized by its production of a slow, prolonged contraction of a smooth muscle preparation in contrast to the rapid and transient action of histamine. A chemically and biologically similar material was subsequently found in the lungs of sensitized guinea pigs challenged with specific antigen in vitro.[125] This material was designated as the *SRS of anaphylaxis* (SRS-A) to distinguish it from SRSs produced by nonimmunologic mechanisms. Studies of the biologic properties of SRS-A indicated that it might be an important mediator of anaphylactic and other immediate allergic reactions. SRS-A can be found in most tissues, especially in the lung, after appropriate antigenic challenge. It is released along with histamine and other active products from mast cells.

Although SRS-A was known for some time to be an acidic, sulfur-containing lipid of low molecular weight, elucidation of its exact structure and biosynthesis was delayed until intensive study of the metabolism of arachidonic acid showed that SRS-A belonged to a class of compounds known as *leukotrienes*.[83,110] The leukotrienes are formed by the conversion of arachidonic acid to noncyclized, 20-carbon carboxylic acids with one or two oxygen substitutes and three conjugated double bonds (see Figure 21-2). The critical step in the biosynthetic pathway is generation of a 5,6-epoxide of arachidonic acid (leukotriene A_4) by the combined actions of 5-lipoxygenase and leukotriene A synthase. Leukotriene A_4 may be converted to leukotriene B_4 by a hydrolase enzyme or, alternatively, to leukotriene C_4 by the addition of glutathione. Removal of glutamate from leukotriene C_4 generates leukotriene D_4. These lipid-peptide derivatives appear to account for all the biologic activity of SRSs found in immediate allergic reactions. Leukotrienes C_4 and D_4 constitute SRS-A. However, asthmatic reactions may also involve other leukotrienes. The ability of cells to produce leukotrienes appears to be limited to the lung, leukocytes, blood vessels, and epicardium. In contrast, all cells except erythrocytes can convert arachidonic acid to PGs and related compounds by the action of COX.

Leukotrienes C_4 and D_4 are potent in vivo and in vitro constrictors of bronchial smooth muscle in the guinea pig. Both compounds have similar effects in human bronchial muscle preparations, in which they are approximately 1000 times more potent than histamine. Because these leukotrienes also increase vascular permeability, it seems likely that either one or both play a role in the bronchial constriction and mucosal edema of asthma. Leukotriene B_4 can enhance chemotactic and chemokinetic responses in human neutrophils, monocytes, and eosinophils.[48] These findings suggest that leukotrienes may be involved in localized inflammatory processes as well as in asthma. Drugs that block leukotriene receptors or inhibit leukotriene synthesis by blocking the enzyme lipoxygenase are used in the treatment of asthma (see Chapter 32).

Lysosomal products

The lysosomes of neutrophils contain a variety of enzymatic and nonenzymatic factors that play important roles in the manifestations and sequelae of inflammatory reactions (Box 21-1). During phagocytosis of bacteria or foreign material by neutrophils, the contents of lysosomes are released into the extracellular environment. They are also released on lysis of the cell. Cationic proteins from lysosomes contribute to the inflammatory process by triggering mast cell degranulation, which in turn leads to increased vascular permeability. Other lysosomal enzymes may contribute to the inflammatory response in several ways. First, several of these enzymes have the potential to damage host tissues. Thus collagen, elastin, mucopolysaccharides, basement membrane, and other structural elements may be degraded. Second, lysosomal proteases cause the production of kininlike substances from plasma kininogen and can generate chemotactic factors for neutrophils from complement, as described in a later section. Leukotrienes and PAF are also released by neutrophils. Neutrophils thus may play a central role in perpetuating the inflammatory response by their dual ability to cause tissue damage and to elaborate specific mediators of inflammation. Another source of lysosomal factors, especially in chronic inflammatory lesions, may be the mononuclear phagocyte, or macrophage, the lysosomes of which contain substances similar to those of the neutrophil.[1] These substances are released into the extracellular environment on activation of macrophages by a variety of soluble factors, such as leukotriene B_4, C5a complement factor, and PAF, and during the process of phagocytosis of bacteria or other particulate matter.

Box 21-1

Factors in the Neutrophil with Inflammatory Potential

Tissue-damaging enzymes	Elastase Cathepsins B and G Collagenase Other proteases
Microbicidal enzymes	Myeloperoxidase Lysozyme
Permeability factors	Leukotrienes PAF Leukokinin-forming enzyme Basic peptides
Leukotactic factors	Leukotrienes PAF C5-cleaving enzyme Basic peptides (chemotactic for monocytes)

Lymphocyte products

Delayed allergic reactions may be involved in some inflammatory processes, especially those of a chronic nature in which there is a persistent antigenic stimulus (e.g., in tuberculosis). These reactions are mediated by factors called *cytokines* (*lymphokines* if derived from lymphocytes), which are produced by sensitized thymus-dependent lymphocytes, or T cells, after specific antigenic challenge. Although many putative cytokines have been described in recent years, their role in inflammatory reactions with an immune component is not firmly established. Some of the better studied cytokines that may function in inflammation-related events are (1) interleukins that stimulate the function of T cells and bursa-dependent lymphocytes (B cells); (2) monocyte chemoattractive protein-1, which promotes accumulation of monocytes; (3) granulocyte/macrophage colony-stimulating factor; (4) other chemotactic factors that are specific attractants for neutrophils, macrophages, basophils, and eosinophils; (5) interferon α, which has both antiviral and macrophage activation properties; and (6) skin reactive factor, which mimics a delayed allergic reaction when injected into normal skin (i.e., it causes increased vascular permeability and migration of mononuclear cells).

Macrophage products
Like lymphocytes, macrophages appear to be little involved in acute inflammatory responses but do play a very prominent role in chronic inflammation and are crucial in the immune response. In addition to their phagocytic activity, macrophages have a major secretory function in established inflammatory lesions. Secretory products include the constituents of lysosomes (see above), reactive metabolites of oxygen, interferon α, interleukin-1 (IL-1), and TNF-α. The latter two substances are crucial mediators of the complex interplay between macrophages and lymphocytes, which in large measure determines the course and eventual outcome of an inflammatory process. IL-1 is produced by macrophages exposed to bacterial, viral, and fungal products; antigens; or macrophage activation factor. It may have several roles, but chief among these seems to be the stimulation of differentiation of a pre–T-lymphocyte population to T cells capable of responding to an antigen processed and presented by macrophages. Another mediator of inflammation produced by macrophages and other cells is PAF. PAF is a closely related family of substances derived from phosphatidylcholine generated in the metabolism of arachidonic acid. It is also synthesized in other cells, including mast cells and eosinophils. Platelets also contain PAF. PAF initiates a variety of actions, including platelet activation, vasodilation, vascular permeability, neutrophil chemotaxis, and discharge of lysosomal enzymes. It also contributes to allergic and inflammatory responses.

Mast cell products
Mast cells release a number of inflammatory mediators in addition to histamine, including cytokines (e.g., TNF-α), leukotrienes, PGD_2, and PAF. Mast cells can become activated by immunoglobulin (Ig) E antibodies that bind to the plasma membrane and sensitize the mast cell to specific allergens. Several allergic reactions, including allergic asthma, involve this mechanism. Basophils have many of the same characteristics as mast cells.

Eosinophil products
Eosinophils release a number of enzymes and toxins that can lead to tissue destruction. For instance, major basic protein is a toxic substance that can cause tissue damage as well as destruction of parasites. Eosinophils also release leukotrienes and PAF.

Plasma Mediators
Kinins
The term *kinins* refers primarily to two small peptides that are similar in structure and actions: bradykinin and lysylbradykinin (or kallidin). Bradykinin can be considered the prototype. It is a linear nonapeptide with a molecular weight of 1060 d. As with the release of histamine, almost any process causing tissue injury can trigger the series of events leading to the production of bradykinin. Bradykinin exists in plasma as an inactive precursor (kininogen) and is released in a cascade of reactions beginning with activation of Hageman factor (clotting factor XII). Hageman factor can be activated by exposure to a host of substances, including cartilage, collagen, basement membrane, sodium urate crystals, proteolytic enzymes, and bacterial lipopolysaccharides. Hageman factor in turn activates an enzyme called *prekallikrein* to yield kallikrein. Kallikrein then cleaves bradykinin from kininogen, an α_2-globulin precursor. (In addition, activated Hageman factor triggers both the clotting cascade by activating factor XI and the fibrinolytic system by activating plasminogen proactivator, ultimately yielding plasmin.) Kinins may also be produced extravascularly from tissue kininogen. After release, bradykinin is rapidly metabolized by enzymes present in both plasma and tissues.

Bradykinin has striking pharmacologic effects in human beings and animals. It is a potent but transient vasodilator of both arteries and veins by a direct action on smooth muscle. Intradermal injection of bradykinin causes marked increases in vascular permeability; in this regard, it is more potent than histamine on a molar basis. Bradykinin applied to a blister base or injected intradermally or intraarterially in human beings evokes sharp pain. Experimental pain can also be produced by a bradykininlike substance isolated from human blister fluid and from synovial fluid obtained from acutely inflamed joints. In extraction sockets, local concentrations of immunoreactive bradykinin as well as PGs rise in patients after the removal of impacted third molar teeth.[108,131] All these phenomena implicate bradykinin in various aspects of acute inflammatory reactions, including acute pain.

Complement system
The complement system plays an important role in the inflammatory process. In human beings, this system consists of at least 20 component proteins that react in a fixed sequence (Figure 21-4). An immune complex on a cell surface activates the first component, C1, and a cascade of events results in the formation of a complex that leads to membrane damage and cell lysis.

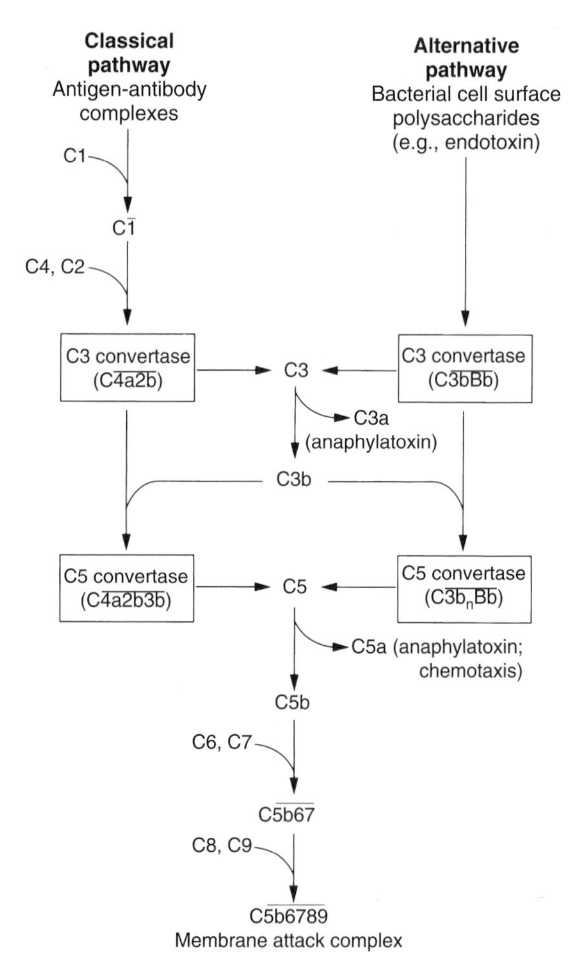

Fig. 21-4 The complement cascade. The classic and alternate pathways of complement activation are shown. Activated components are designated by a *horizontal bar* above the component number (e.g., $\overline{C5b67}$). The steps by which bacterial polysaccharides interact with several plasma proteins (B, D, and properdin) to generate the C3 convertase of the alternate pathway, $\overline{C3bBb}$, are not shown.

This so-called classic pathway of complement activation can be initiated by most antigen-antibody complexes and by such nonimmune factors as trypsin and plasmin. Other substances, such as complex polysaccharides, aggregated IgA, and bacterial endotoxin, may trigger an alternate pathway in which the first component to be activated is C3, followed then by the usual components in the activation scheme.

In addition to the direct cellular damage cited above, certain fragments produced during the cascade of complement activation have biologic properties of importance. Two of them (C3a and C5a) cause increased vascular permeability by inducing the release of histamine from mast cells. These substances are therefore referred to as *anaphylatoxins* and have been implicated in anaphylaxis and other allergic reactions. The C5a anaphylatoxin is also a potent chemotactic factor. Neutrophils, monocytes, and eosinophils exhibit directed locomotion in response to it. Enhancement of phagocytosis and release of lysosomal enzymes have been attributed to other components of the activation scheme.

Complement fragments can be produced by mechanisms extrinsic to the complement system (e.g., by plasmin, trypsin, and bacterial proteases). This action suggests that complement fragments may participate in tissue injury and in the subsequent inflammatory response without classic or alternative complement activation.

Nitric oxide

Nitric oxide is another inflammatory mediator. Its role in controlling vasomotor tone is also well established. Nitric oxide produces hyperalgesia, and the enzyme responsible for its synthesis, nitric oxide synthase, is a potential target for future antiinflammatory drugs. Like COX, nitric oxide synthase exist in two forms: a constitutive form and an inducible form.[137] The latter is thought to be involved in inflammatory reactions, although its role at this point is not defined.

NONSTEROIDAL ANTIINFLAMMATORY DRUGS (NSAIDs)

The NSAIDs include some of the most frequently taken medications. Because these agents share a common mechanism of action, they exert qualitatively similar therapeutic and toxic effects. For the treatment of pain and inflammation that accompany a variety of dental surgical procedures, the short-term use (typically 1 week or less) of NSAIDs has generally proved to be highly efficacious and safe. Compared with opioid-combination drugs (described later in this chapter), they lack a variety of undesirable CNS depressant effects that contribute to the relatively high incidence of drowsiness, dizziness, and nausea commonly seen with opioid-containing entities. This favorable efficacy and safety profile has led the Food and Drug Administration (FDA) to approve three NSAIDs (ibuprofen, naproxen sodium, and ketoprofen) in addition to aspirin for over-the-counter (OTC) use. It is important to note that the use of these drugs under OTC package insert guidelines mandates no more than 10 days of consecutive dosing for pain and only 3 days for fever, plus absolute maximums on both single and daily doses that are lower than the prescription use of these drugs.[66]

When treating chronic inflammatory conditions such as rheumatoid arthritis, the duration of NSAID therapy is typically measured in months or years, and the daily doses required to control the arthritic symptoms are often twofold to threefold higher than that required to control acute pain. This type of therapy leads to a greatly increased incidence of both minor and major side effects, requiring more vigilant monitoring of these patients.

The recent development of NSAIDs that are selective or specific COX-2 inhibitors appears to offer a safety advantage regarding some of the more serious adverse effects seen with chronic NSAID therapy, specifically gastrointestinal ulcers, perforations, and bleeds.[10,116] The appropriate role of COX-2 inhibitors in the management of acute postoperative dental pain is currently being defined.[95]

Salicylates

The salicylates are among the oldest known drugs. Hippocrates recommended the consumption of the juices of the poplar and willow bark some 2400 years ago, which later were discovered to contain salicin (a glycoside of salicylic alcohol), for the treatment of the pain of childbirth. In 60 AD, Discorides reported that a boiled extract of willow bark could be used to treat a variety of maladies, including corns, gout, and earache. In a 1763 report to the Royal Society in London, The Reverend Edward Stone made one of the earliest references to the antipyretic effect of willow bark extracts. The active principle of willow and poplar preparations, salicylic acid, was first extracted in 1835 from natural sources and later prepared by chemical synthesis. Kolbe was credited with the first full-scale commercial synthesis of salicylic acid and its derivative sodium salicylate. In 1853, Charles Frederich von Gerhardt became the first to synthesize aspirin (acetylsalicylic acid) by treating sodium salicylate with acetyl chloride. Despite the untoward gastrointestinal effects of large doses of salicylic acid and sodium salicylate, the development of salicylates culminated in the introduction of aspirin into medicine in 1899 by Heinrich Dresser of the Bayer Company of Germany. The popularity of aspirin was immediate, and today it remains one of the most consumed drugs in the world.

Several additional salicylates have also been marketed. Choline salicylate, magnesium salicylate, and their combination product are ion complexes of salicylate. Salsalate is an ester composed of two salicylate molecules, which are freed as the molecule is hydrolyzed. These salicylate formulations are said to have fewer gastrointestinal side effects than aspirin. However, because released salicylate is the active moiety of all these drugs, the rest of their pharmacology is quite similar to aspirin. The structure of aspirin and some of the related salicylates are shown in Figure 21-5. Aspirin may be considered a prototype of the NSAIDs and is the standard of reference against which these agents are compared and evaluated.

Mechanism of action

The efficacy of salicylates and all related NSAIDs as analgesic, antiinflammatory, and antipyretic agents results from their ability to inhibit COX activity, thereby preventing the synthesis and release of COX products, most prominently the PGs. All salicylates and, in fact, almost all the currently available NSAIDs with the exception of the newly marketed COX-2 inhibitors inhibit both COX-1 and COX-2. The majority of these nonselective COX-inhibiting NSAIDs, including aspirin, are more potent or at least equipotent inhibitors of COX-1,[107,137] which accounts for some of the more important adverse effects of these drugs. Figure 21-6 displays the relative COX-2 versus COX-1 selectivity of some representative NSAIDs. As shown in this figure, aspirin is approximately a hundred-fold more selective inhibitor of COX-1 than COX-2. It should be noted that the published COX selectivities of individual drugs vary with the assay system being used.

Aspirin uniquely inactivates COX by irreversibly acetylating the enzyme. Acetylation occurs on serine 530 of COX-1.[85] A comparable serine on COX-2, serine 516, is also acetylated by aspirin. The later modification not only inhibits PG production during inflammation but also enables COX-2 to produce 15-hydroxyeicosatetraenoic acid.[78,103] This

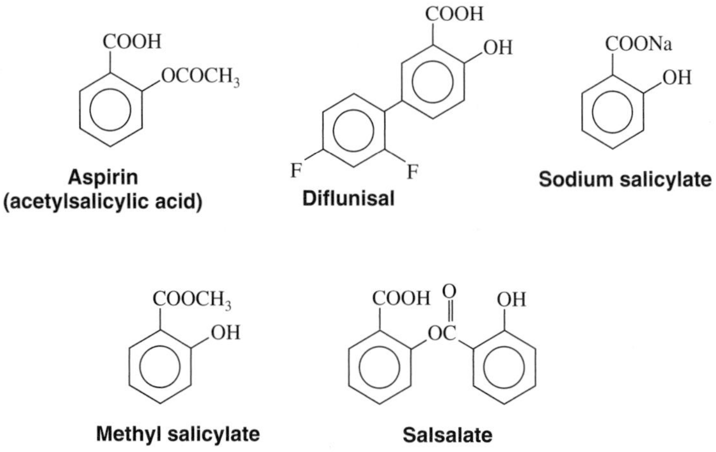

Aspirin (acetylsalicylic acid)

Diflunisal

Sodium salicylate

Methyl salicylate

Salsalate

Fig. 21-5 Structural formulas of aspirin and other salicylates.

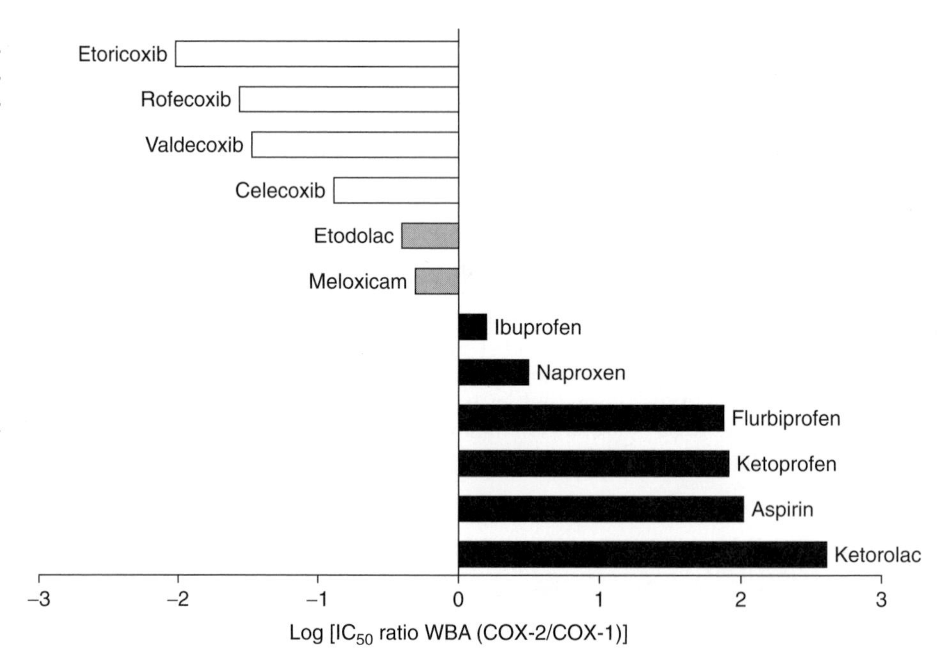

Fig. 21-6 The ratio of the log of inhibitory concentrations *(IC)* of various NSAIDs needed to block 50% of COX-2 activity versus 50% of COX-1 activity in the whole blood assay *(WBA)*. The *zero line* indicates equipotency. Bars on the *right* represent drugs with greater selectivity for COX-1, whereas those on the *left* represent drugs with greater selectivity for COX-2. (Adapted from Riendau D, Percival MD, Brideau C, et al: Etoricoxib (MK-0663): preclinical profile and comparison with other agents that selectively inhibit cyclooxygenase-2, *J Pharmacol Exp Ther* 296:558-566, 2001; Warner TD, Guiliano F, Vojnovic I, et al: Nonsteroid drug selectivities for cyclo-oxygenase-1 rather than cyclo-oxygenase-2 are associated with human gastrointestinal toxicity: a full in vitro analysis, *Proc Natl Acad Sci* 96:7563-7568, 1999.)

Table • 21-2

Antiinflammatory and COX Inhibitory Activity of Some NSAIDs Compared with Acetaminophen

DRUG	INHIBITION OF PG SYNTHESIS (IC_{50}, μM)	REDUCTION OF CARRAGEENIN-INDUCED RAT PAW EDEMA (ED_{50}, moles/kg)	PEAK PLASMA CONCENTRATION (μmol/L)	PLASMA-PROTEIN BINDING (%)
Indomethacin	0.17	0.017	5.0	90
Phenylbutazone	7.25	0.325	230 to 500	98
Aspirin	37.0	0.833	280 to 300	50 to 80
Acetaminophen	660.0	Inactive	350	25

Adapted from Arrigoni-Martelli E: *Inflammation and antiinflammatories*, New York, 1977, Spectrum Publications.
ED_{50}, Median effective dose; *IC_{50}*, median inhibitory concentration.

metabolite may be associated with certain adverse effects. Other salicylates and NSAIDs do not acetylate COX but are reversible competitive inhibitors of the enzyme. Because PGs are not stored, but rather are synthesized immediately before release, the reduction of PG concentrations by NSAIDs can be observed rather quickly.

The potency of the salicylates as inhibitors of PG synthesis in vitro correlates well with their ability to alleviate carrageenin-induced inflammation in animals (Table 21-2). In human beings, antiinflammatory doses of aspirin (3 g daily), sodium salicylate (3 g daily), or indomethacin (100 mg daily) reduce the output of PG metabolites in the urine by more than 75%, indicating a close correlation of the inhibition of COX with antiinflammatory effects.[59] Although inhibition by COX is the major mechanism of action of the NSAIDs, participation in other antiinflammatory mechanisms may occur and account for some of the variation in clinical response seen with these drugs. Salicylates may inhibit cell migration and some functions of neutrophils. A reduced production of rheumatoid factor may also occur by stimulation of suppressor T-cell activity. Other mechanisms contributing to antiinflammatory effects may include reduced capillary permeability, reduced antibody production, and alterations in connective tissue synthesis. The relative potencies against COX-1 and COX-2 also account for important differences among various NSAIDs.

Inhibition of PG synthesis at the site of injury or inflammation can explain at least some of the analgesic effect of aspirin. Although PGs themselves do not appear to cause pain when injected locally, PGE_2 and $PGF_{2\alpha}$ do sensitize pain receptors to other mediators such as histamine and bradykinin. In this connection, it is interesting that aspirin and related drugs can prevent the writhing response elicited by bradykinin but not that produced by PGs. This finding is explained by the fact that the salicylates, indeed all NSAIDs, inhibit the synthesis of PGs induced by bradykinin but not the binding of PGs to their receptors. Animal experimentation has revealed that NSAIDs also have central analgesic actions, which may involve the inhibition of COX or other unknown mechanisms at the level of the spinal dorsal horn or at higher levels of the CNS.[86,91] The antipyretic effect of aspirin and similar drugs is also mediated by the reduction of PGE_2 synthesis as a result of inhibition of COX.

General therapeutic effects

Aspirin has clinically useful analgesic, antipyretic, antiinflammatory, and antiplatelet effects. The analgesic effect sought and attained with aspirin is probably caused in many cases by its antiinflammatory actions, a fact not usually appreciated by its users. In addition to their widespread use for the symptomatic relief of acute pain and fever, salicylates (most commonly aspirin) are drugs of major importance in the treatment of numerous chronic inflammatory diseases. In the section that follows, some of the major therapeutic uses of aspirin are considered.

Acute Pain It is difficult to separate the analgesic and antiinflammatory effects of NSAIDs because the majority of painful conditions have an inflammatory component. There is little doubt that the cascade of reactions leading to the formation of PGs is integrally involved with the inflammatory response and that aspirin's efficacy in treating inflammation and pain is closely related to its inhibition of PG synthesis. By using microdialysis techniques, it has been demonstrated that after dental surgery the analgesic effects of NSAIDs correlate with a local reduction in PG synthesis.[101,108] Nevertheless, several observations suggest that the analgesic and antiinflammatory effects of NSAIDs may occur by different mechanisms. First, there is a different time course for the onset of analgesic and antiinflammatory effects. Clinically significant analgesia usually occurs within 1 hour of drug administration, whereas antiinflammatory effects sometimes take several days or weeks to reach maximum levels because chronic inflammatory processes may be occurring that cannot be quickly reversed by inhibiting PG production. Also, the maximum human analgesic effect usually occurs at lower doses than do the antirheumatic and other antiinflammatory effects.

Aspirin is an effective analgesic for almost any type of acute dental pain. Double-blind, controlled studies of the relief of pain after the surgical extraction of third molars have demonstrated that 650 mg of aspirin is substantially more effective than 60 mg of codeine in relieving postoperative pain (Figure 21-7).[22] In fact, most controlled clinical studies have established that, regardless of the cause of the pain, aspirin (650 mg) provides equal or greater pain relief than codeine in standard doses (60 mg).[7] Aspirin, as well as other NSAIDs and acetaminophen, has what is known as a ceiling or plateau effect in the treatment of acute pain. In other words, there is a dose-response for pain relief up to 650 to 1000 mg of aspirin, but increasing the dose beyond these amounts does not further enhance the analgesic effect but does increase the likelihood for toxic effects.

Rheumatic Fever One of the early uses of salicylates was in the treatment of rheumatic fever. Aspirin markedly reduces the acute inflammatory components of the disease, such as fever, joint pain, swelling, and immobility. However, the salicylates do not affect other aspects of the disease, such as the proliferative reaction in the myocardium leading to scarring, and they do not alter the progression of the disease. Although antiinflammatory drugs, including corticosteroids (see Chapter 35), may be used to reduce inflammation, antibiotic therapy is the major therapeutic strategy.

Rheumatoid Arthritis Rheumatoid arthritis is a chronic systemic disease of unknown origin. Several tissues and organs may be involved, but in most patients the chief clinical and pathologic features result from chronic inflammation of synovial membranes. Irreversible joint injury (subluxation, loss of motion, or ankylosis) results from formation of chronic granulation tissue that causes erosions of articular cartilage, subchondral bone, ligaments, and tendons. Extraarticular manifestations such as subcutaneous or subperiosteal nodules of granulation tissue, peripheral neuropathy, and chronic skin ulcers occur to a variable extent and appear to result from generalized focal vasculitis.

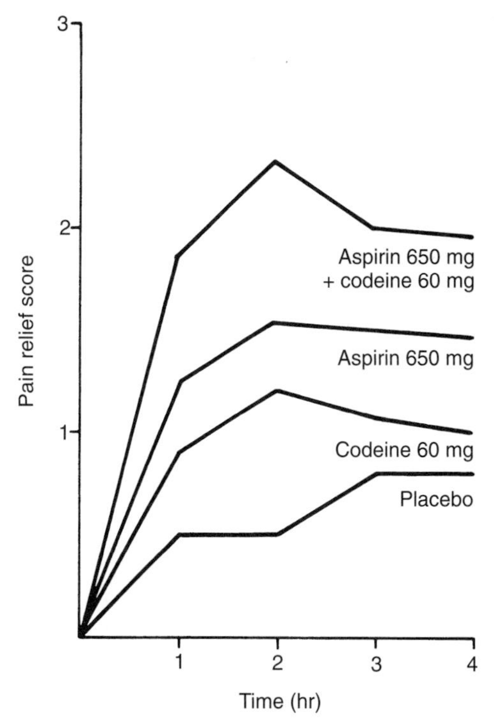

Fig. 21-7 Time-effect curves for placebo, aspirin, codeine, and an aspirin-codeine combination. The mean pain relief scores are plotted against time in hours. (Adapted from Cooper SA, Engel L, Lador M, et al: Analgesic efficacy of an ibuprofen-codeine combination, *Pharmacotherapy* 2:162-167, 1982.)

The cause of the inflammatory response in rheumatoid arthritis is obscure, but the inflammatory events result largely from an autoimmune reaction. Rheumatoid arthritis is considered an autoimmune disease with many contributing factors. Lymphocytes that have become activated produce TNF-α and IL-1. These cytokines lead to the release of other inflammatory mediators, such as the PGs. Antiimmunoglobulins, referred to as the *rheumatoid factor* and found in rheumatoid synovial fluid, can form complexes with IgG. These complexes may activate complement, which in turn triggers a number of inflammatory phenomena in the joint tissues, including histamine release, production of factors chemotactic for neutrophils and mononuclear cells, cell membrane damage, and PG synthesis. The antigen-antibody complexes also activate antigen-presenting cells, which in turn stimulate T cells, leading to the further release of cytokines. Both neutrophils and macrophages accumulate in the synovial fluid and are found to contain aggregated IgG, rheumatoid factor, complement fragments, and fibrin; these substances are apparently acquired by phagocytosis. Lysosomal materials are released that amplify the inflammatory reaction and may directly damage tissues. Cytokines produced by the lymphocytic cell infiltrate may also help propagate the reaction and participate in tissue destruction.

Salicylates (usually as aspirin) are still widely used in the clinical management of rheumatoid arthritis. The majority of cases of rheumatoid arthritis can be controlled with salicylates alone (or with another NSAID).[124] Salicylates produce a measurable reduction of inflammation in the joints and associated tissues, a lessening of symptoms, and improved mobility. Salicylates may also reduce neutrophil activity in addition to inhibiting PG synthesis. Clinical observation suggests that salicylate therapy can diminish or delay the development of crippling. This benefit is probably not a direct effect of the drug on the progression of the disease but relates more to reduction of pain and subsequent facilitation of mobility. In addition to salicylates, the basic therapeutic regimen in rheumatoid arthritis includes rest, physical measures (primarily heat), and exercise. When salicylate therapy is not effective or is not well tolerated, other drugs can be used. These include NSAIDs such as ibuprofen and naproxen, corticosteroids, and disease-modifying antirheumatic drugs, including gold compounds, sulfasalazine, penicillamine, antimalarials, methotrexate, azathioprine, cyclosporine, and leflunomide.

In rheumatoid arthritis, salicylates are given in doses sufficient to control the symptoms, often 3 to 6 g/day. The degree of suppression of inflammation increases with the plasma salicylate concentration even beyond the point of toxicity. Thus patients with severe arthritis will tolerate tinnitus and other mild toxic manifestations to obtain the antiinflammatory effects gained by high plasma titers of salicylate. A regular dose interval to maintain constant effective blood concentrations is important. Evaluation of drug therapy in rheumatoid patients may be complicated by the spontaneous remissions and exacerbations characteristic of this disease.

Other inflammatory diseases Aspirin is a commonly used antiinflammatory agent in various other inflammatory diseases, including juvenile rheumatoid arthritis, ankylosing spondylitis, psoriatic arthritis, Reiter's syndrome, and degenerative joint disease (osteoarthritis). The arthralgia and fever of mild lupus erythematosus may be alleviated by aspirin. Acute episodes of inflammation in isolated joints, tendons, or bursae caused by trauma are also best treated with aspirin given in full doses immediately after the injury.

Fever Fever is typically a symptom of a disease process, usually a viral or bacterial infection brought about by both exogenous (microbial products) and endogenous pyrogens.[29,128] It is believed that exogenous pyrogens stimulate host cells to produce endogenous pyrogens, of which IL-1 has been the best characterized.[40,128] IL-1 is thought to act on the anterior hypothalamus, generating the local release of PGs.[40,127] Injection of PGs into the brain of various animal species is known to raise body temperature.[42] The PGs and possibly other non-PG endogenous pyrogens elevate the thermal set point of the body so that it retains the ability to closely regulate its temperature but at a higher temperature than normal.[29,128]

By inhibiting the synthesis of PGs in the hypothalamus, aspirin, other NSAIDs, and acetaminophen are thought to reduce the thermal set point toward normal. In addition, the fall in body temperature also involves the ability of aspirin and other antipyretics to induce a vasodilation of superficial blood vessels. Because of its association with Reye's syndrome, aspirin is no longer recommended to treat most febrile episodes in children.

Prophylaxis against platelet aggregation The correlation between the ability of aspirinlike compounds to simultaneously inhibit platelet aggregation and the production of PGs has been known for 30 years.[121] Aspirin inhibits the synthesis of TXA_2 by irreversible acetylation of the COX enzyme in platelets.[61,109] Lacking a nucleus, platelets cannot generate new enzyme, and the ability of affected platelets to produce TXA_2 is permanently blunted during their 10-day lifetimes. The majority of platelet COX acetylation may occur presystemically as platelets pass through gut capillaries before the hydrolysis of aspirin to salicylate (a weak inhibitor of COX) in the gut and the liver.[105] This possibility may partially explain the relative lack of effect of low-dose aspirin on the antiaggregatory PGI_2 molecule produced by the systemic vascular endothelium. The fact that endothelial cells, by possessing a nucleus, can generate new COX enzyme after aspirin administration may also contribute to the relatively selective and complete block of TXA_2 synthesis over PGI_2. This relatively selective block of TXA_2 synthesis in platelets provides the rationale for using long-term low-dose aspirin therapy to prevent myocardial infarction (MI) and occlusive stroke in at-risk patients. Other salicylates and NSAIDs are either much weaker or only reversibly inhibit COX in platelets and thus have limited therapeutically beneficial antiplatelet effects.

The FDA published a set of indications for aspirin prophylaxis that include definitive dosing guidelines for each condition (Table 21-3).[33] Vascular indications include the reduction of death or nonfatal stroke in patients who have had ischemic strokes or transient ischemic attacks; reduction of vascular mortality in patients with acute MI; reduction of combined risk of death and nonfatal MI in patients with previous MI or unstable angina; and reduction of the combined risk of MI and sudden death in patients with chronic stable angina. The recommended daily dose for all these indications is low (≤325 mg/day) compared with the analgesic and antiinflammatory uses of the drug. In addition, aspirin is indicated for patients who have undergone revascularization procedures, including coronary artery bypass grafting, percutaneous transluminal coronary angioplasty, and carotid endarterectomy, when there are preexisting conditions for which aspirin is already indicated.

Absorption, fate, and excretion

When aspirin is taken orally, it is rapidly absorbed from the stomach and small intestine. Aspirin is a weak acid, with a pK_a of approximately 3.5, which favors its absorption in the stomach. However, most absorption takes place in the small intestine because of its much larger surface area. The rate-limiting steps in the absorption of aspirin are the disintegration and dissolution of the tablet. These two steps can be greatly influenced by the manufacturing process, which determines such factors as particle size and compression of the tablet. Buffering the tablet increases the rate of dissolution, but the fastest absorption is obtained when aspirin is dissolved in hot water before ingestion. Other factors, such as gastric emptying time, gastric contents, and level of autonomic activity of the patient, may also influence the rate of absorption.[80,82]

Aspirin has a 15-minute half-life. It is quickly metabolized by gastric and plasma esterases to salicylate ion (Figure 21-8). Although some aspirin becomes bound to plasma proteins, 80% to 90% of the salicylate ion is bound for a short time, principally to albumin. Salicylate is distributed throughout most body fluids and tissues. It can be isolated from spinal, peritoneal, and synovial fluids, saliva, breast milk, and sweat. Salicylate freely crosses the placenta from mother to fetus.

The elimination half-life of sodium salicylate is 2 to 3 hours after a single analgesic dose. The liver is the main site of biotransformation, and conjugation is the primary route. Because the metabolism of salicylate is capacity limited, large repeated doses or single toxic ingestions result in plasma half-lives of 5 to 30 hours. The three primary products of salicylate conjugation are salicyluric acid (the glycine conjugate), the ether or phenolic glucuronide, and the acyl or ester glucuronide. A small portion, less than 1%, is oxidized to gentisic acid (see Figure 21-8). Free salicylate and the salicylate metabolites are excreted both by glomerular filtration and by active proximal tubular secretion in the kidney. In normal human beings, approximately 10% of ingested salicylate appears unchanged in the urine; however, this fraction may fall to 2% or rise to 30% with urinary acidosis or alkalosis, respectively. Furthermore, a higher percentage of free salicylate is excreted at higher doses because the liver is not able to maintain the same percentage of metabolism at higher doses of salicylates.

Adverse effects

The severity of side effects that can accompany aspirin ingestion depends on the overall health of the patient, the length of dosing, and the total daily intake of drug. When used under OTC package insert guidelines (for no more than 10 days and no more than 4 g/day), the majority of reported side effects are more annoying than serious, with dyspepsia and nausea occurring in up to 10% of patients. In addition, occult bleeding (hidden amounts of blood in the stool), which is usually less than 10 ml/day, develops in more than 70% of patients ingesting the drug. The bleeding is thought to originate from both direct capillary and mucosal damage as aspirin disintegrates in contact with gastric tissues and from the ability of

Table • 21-3

Antiplatelet Indications and Dosing Guidelines for Aspirin

INDICATIONS	RECOMMENDED DAILY DOSE	DURATION OF THERAPY
Vascular Indications		
Ischemic stroke and TIA	50 to 325 mg	Indefinitely
Suspected acute MI	160 to 162.5 mg taken as soon as infarction is suspected, then once daily	For 30 days after infarction (after 30 days, consider further treatment if previous MI)
Prevention of recurrent MI	75 to 325 mg	Indefinitely
Unstable angina pectoris	75 to 325 mg	Indefinitely
Chronic stable angina pectoris	75 to 325 mg	Indefinitely
Revascularization Procedures in Select Patients		
CABG	325 mg starting 6 hours after procedure	1 year
PTCA	325 mg 2 hours before surgery; maintenance therapy: 160 to 325 mg	Indefinitely
Carotid endarterectomy	80 to 650 mg twice daily started before surgery	Indefinitely

CAGB, Coronary artery bypass grafting; *PTCA*, percutaneous transluminal coronary angioplasty; *TIA*, transient ischemic attack.

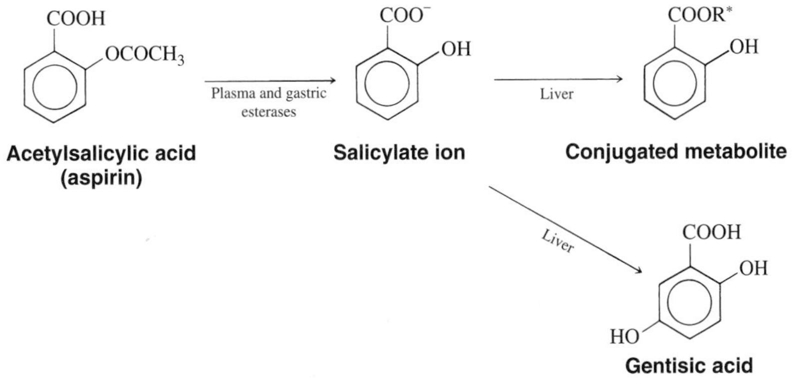

COOH, $OCOCH_3$ — Acetylsalicylic acid (aspirin) → Plasma and gastric esterases → COO^-, OH — Salicylate ion → Liver → $COOR^*$, OH — Conjugated metabolite

Salicylate ion → Liver → COOH, OH, HO — Gentisic acid

Fig. 21-8 Metabolic fate of aspirin. **R*, Glycine or glucuronate. (The phenolic glucuronide metabolite is not shown.) The glycine conjugate is called *salicyluric acid.*

aspirin to inhibit COX-1, which interferes with cytoprotective mechanisms and platelet aggregation. Although this occult bleeding is usually of little clinical significance, aspirin and, in fact, all related NSAIDs are contraindicated in patients with active gastrointestinal ulcers because their ingestion may lead to sudden, potentially fatal gastrointestinal hemorrhage.

With more long-term, high-dose regimens of aspirin and other nonselective NSAIDs used in the treatment of various inflammatory disorders, the inhibition of COX-1 leads to several common and predictable effects, the occurrence of which varies with each drug. The inhibition of PGI_2 and PGE_2 synthesis and the resulting loss of their protective effects on the gastric mucosa lead to a significant increase in gastrointestinal problems, the most serious of which include significant gastric bleeding, symptomatic peptic ulcers, and gastrointestinal perforations and obstructions. The incidence of these more serious events ranges from 3% to 5% of patients per year. Even long-term low-dose (81 mg/day) aspirin therapy is associated with an increased risk of serious gastrointestinal events, at a rate of 0.1% to 0.2% of patients per year.[104] This increase in gastrointestinal complications has led experts to question the widespread use of low-dose aspirin therapy in patients without significant cardiovascular or cerebrovascular risks. The nonaspirin salicylates generally elicit fewer adverse effects in the gastrointestinal tract but cannot be used for platelet antiaggregatory therapy. Most other NSAIDs have some antiplatelet effect based on inhibition of the production of TXA_2, but the effects are not as pronounced as with aspirin because aspirin is an irreversible inhibitor of COX.

The antiplatelet effects of aspirin can lead to pronounced increases in bleeding time. As previously discussed, this effect is long lasting compared with other NSAIDs because aspirin irreversibly acetylates COX in the nonnucleated platelet. Even a single dose of aspirin can increase the bleeding time for several days. A theoretical concern is the fact that this prolongation of bleeding time can promote intraoperative and postoperative hemorrhage in dental surgical patients. Although the risk/benefit ratio of discontinuing chronic cardioprotective low-dose aspirin therapy before dental surgery remains a contentious area of debate, from a medicolegal standpoint it should not be done without the approval of the patient's physician. The remote but real chance of a patient suffering an MI or occlusive stroke shortly after a dental practitioner interrupts low-dose aspirin therapy dictates medical consultation. In addition, once a clot is established, aspirin therapy may be reinstituted.

The adverse effects of aspirin and other NSAIDs on the kidney are well known. Normal renal function is partly dependent on PG synthesis. It is believed that both COX-1 and COX-2 are important in producing PGs involved in reducing water and Na^+ reabsorption at the ascending loop of Henle and maintaining proper dilation of the renal vasculature.[11] With NSAID therapy, dose-dependent water and Na^+ retention manifested by peripheral edema, elevation in blood pressure, and rarely congestive heart failure are thought to follow the inhibition of PGE_2 synthesis. Renal artery vasoconstriction, possibly causing acute renal ischemia and kidney failure, is ascribed to an inhibition of PGI_2 synthesis. Acute renal failure is more likely to develop in patients with preexisting renal insufficiency, congestive heart failure, or dehydration because the renal arterioles are more dependent on PGs to maintain normal perfusion of the glomeruli.[98] Acute renal failure is also more likely when NSAIDs are given concurrently with an angiotensin-converting enzyme (ACE) inhibitor because the lack of angiotensin II weakens reactive constriction of the efferent arteriole, a normal protective response for maintaining glomerular filtration in patients with reduced renal blood flow. The NSAIDs are likewise responsible for chronic renal toxicity, commonly known as *analgesic-associated nephropathy.* This disorder sometimes occurs with long-term use of high doses of NSAIDs and is characterized by papillary necrosis and chronic interstitial nephritis. The mechanism may be related to the acute ischemic response described above, but the cause has not been definitely established. It is estimated that serious renal problems requiring hospitalization occurs in 0.5% to 1.0% of long-term NSAID users.

The use of aspirin in children with viral infections has been associated with Reye's syndrome.[68] First described in 1963, Reye's syndrome is an acute childhood illness that produces metabolic encephalopathy and liver disease.[106] Typically, the children are recovering from influenza or varicella when the acute encephalopathic symptoms of lethargy, agitation, delirium, and seizures appear. Without aggressive supportive treatment, the disease progresses to deep coma, brainstem dysfunction, and, in 80% to 90% of cases, death.[68] Even with heroic treatment, the mortality rate can exceed 30%, and survivors can be left with permanent brain damage. Clinical reviews and case-controlled studies performed in the 1970s and 1980s reported a strong association between the development of Reye's syndrome and the ingestion of aspirin in children and teenagers with viral infections.[69,84,139] Aspirin and related salicylates are thus contraindicated for the treatment of flulike symptoms, chicken pox, gastroenteritis, and, in the opinion of most pediatricians, any febrile respiratory condition in children or teenagers.

Toxicity caused by aspirin overdose is common. Its symptoms and severity depend on the dose. Chronic toxicity caused by salicylates results in a syndrome termed *salicylism,* which is characterized by tinnitus, nausea, vomiting, headache, hyperventilation, and mental confusion. Aspirin holds the dubious distinction of being one of the more frequently used drugs for attempted suicide. The drug is commonly involved in accidental poisoning, especially in children, because it is found in almost every household and proper precautions for its storage are often neglected. Serious clinical manifestations of acute aspirin overdose typically occur at doses greater than 6 to 10 g in adults or when intake exceeds 150 to 200 mg/kg of body weight. The cardinal signs and symptoms of acute aspirin overdose include nausea, vomiting, tinnitus, hyperthermia, and hyperventilation. Hyperventilation arises in part from a direct stimulation of respiratory centers in the brain and from a compensatory increase in respiration in response to excessive carbon dioxide produced by large doses of aspirin partially uncoupling oxidative phosphorylation. This uncoupling also accounts for the paradoxic (because therapeutic doses of aspirin are used for antipyresis) increase in body temperature.[12] The hyperventilation eventually can lead to respiratory alkalosis, which may be followed by a combined respiratory and metabolic acidosis accompanied by dehydration. Acidosis is more prominent as the level of overdose increases. Acidosis is also more likely to occur in children and infants. Impaired vision, hallucinations, delirium, and other CNS effects may be evident, and the situation is considered life threatening.

The treatment of aspirin overdose is primarily palliative and supportive. Chronic toxicity usually is treated simply by withholding the drug temporarily and then reinstituting therapy at lower doses. Acute toxicity often requires respiratory support, gastric lavage, maintenance of electrolyte balance (e.g., K^+ replacement if necessary), maintenance of plasma pH, and alkalinization of the urine with intravenous bicarbonate. Alkalinization of the urine increases the percentage of ionized salicylate in the glomerular filtrate. Salicylate reabsorption is reduced, and renal clearance is increased up to fourfold. The carbonic anhydrase inhibitor acetazolamide may also be used to promote urinary alkalinization.

Allergic reactions to aspirin can also occur. Many patients, however, confuse side effects such as nausea or tinnitus with true allergic responses manifested by skin rashes, hives, angioedema, or anaphylaxis. Patients with a history of skin eruptions caused by aspirin ingestion should be cautioned to avoid all proprietary compounds containing aspirin or any salicylate to avoid more serious anaphylactic reactions.

Intolerance to salicylates can occur, with symptoms ranging from rhinitis to severe asthma. This reaction does not appear to be immune mediated even though it resembles drug allergy in clinical presentation. Aspirin intolerance is more common in patients with preexisting asthma or nasal polyps. The incidence of this reaction in asthmatic patients has been reported to be as high as 20%. Patients with a history of asthma, allergic disorders, or nasal polyps should be questioned to be sure that they can tolerate aspirin and other NSAIDs. The bronchoconstriction may be caused by a shift in the arachidonic acid cascade when the COX enzyme is blocked. This inhibition prevents arachidonate metabolism from producing bronchodilating PGs, primarily PGE_2.[132] The lipoxygenase pathway then predominates and produces leukotrienes that constrict bronchioles in sensitive persons, mimicking the asthmatic attack.[14,28] Other manifestations of aspirin intolerance include urticaria (hives) and angioedema. Switching from aspirin to another salicylate or even another NSAID does not prevent the reaction; acetaminophen is the only antipyretic analgesic that may be used safely in patients with aspirin intolerance.

Contraindications and precautions

Aspirin is contraindicated in a number of medical conditions (Table 21-4). Serious internal bleeding can result from the ingestion of aspirin by a patient with an ulcer. Patients with compromised liver function should use aspirin cautiously because, when used on a long-term basis, aspirin raises the prothrombin time, which could aggravate bleeding problems. Low doses of aspirin can increase plasma urate concentrations and exacerbate gouty arthritis as a result of competition between salicylate and uric acid at the active secretion sites in the proximal tubule of the kidney or by an increase in uric acid reabsorption. High doses of aspirin may either raise or lower plasma glucose concentrations by stimulating epinephrine and glucocorticoid release or by depleting liver glycogen, respectively. Salicylates may also increase insulin secretion because PGE_2 inhibits insulin secretion.[54] Asthma patients, patients with nasal polyps, and those with chronic allergic disorders (e.g., urticaria) should use aspirin cautiously because, as previously mentioned, as many as 20% of these patients have reported intolerance to aspirin, other salicylate drugs, and other NSAIDs. Of course, aspirin is contraindicated in patients with aspirin intolerance or true salicylate allergy.

Aspirin is not absolutely contraindicated in pregnancy, but it should be used with caution. In the third trimester, aspirin tends to prolong labor by inhibiting the synthesis of PGs involved in initiating uterine contractions. Aspirin has also been reported to increase blood loss at the time of delivery and may cause premature closure of the ductus arteriosus in the fetus. Some evidence also suggests that, in very high doses, aspirin can have teratogenic effects.

A number of drug interactions may involve aspirin (Table 21-5). Because of its effects on blood glucose, aspirin can interact adversely with insulin or oral hypoglycemic agents, causing unpredictable changes in blood glucose concentrations. Furthermore, aspirin and other salicylates compete with oral hypoglycemic drugs for binding sites on plasma proteins. This interaction theoretically leads to higher amounts of unbound oral hypoglycemic in the plasma and an enhanced hypoglycemic effect. Internal bleeding may occur if aspirin, which causes gastrointestinal irritation and inhibition of platelet aggregation, is used in conjunction with anticoagulants such as warfarin and heparin. In addition, warfarin can be displaced from plasma proteins by aspirin. As with the oral hypoglemic drugs, this competition for binding is more of a theoretical concern than a practical issue (as discussed in Chapter 2). Another potentially dangerous drug combination

Table • 21-4

Contraindications to the Use of Aspirin and Other Salicylates

DISEASE STATE	POSSIBLE ADVERSE EFFECT OF ASPIRIN
Ulcer	Internal bleeding, possible hemorrhaging
Asthma	Asthmatic attack resembling an allergic reaction
Diabetes	High doses may cause hyperglycemia or hypoglycemia
Gout	Low doses increase plasma urate; high doses lower plasma urate
Influenza	Reye's syndrome in children
Hypocoagulation states	Excessive bleeding

Table • 21-5

Some Drug Interactions Involving Aspirin

DRUG	POSSIBLE INTERACTION WITH ASPIRIN
Warfarin	Internal bleeding, possible hemorrhaging
Heparin	Internal bleeding, possible hemorrhaging
Insulin	Aspirin may cause hyperglycemia or enhancement of hypoglycemic effect
Sulfonylureas (oral hypoglycemic agents)	Enhancement of hypoglycemic effect
Phenytoin	Increased free plasma concentration of phenytoin, valproic acid
Methotrexate	Increased free plasma concentration of methotrexate
Ethanol	Internal bleeding, possible hemorrhaging
Probenecid, sulfinpyrazone	Decreased uricosuric effect, reappearance of gout
ACE inhibitors, β-adrenergic blockers, diuretics	Loss of antihypertensive effect

is aspirin and alcohol because alcohol sensitizes the gastric mucosa to aspirin. Aspirin and other NSAIDs also increase the toxicity of methotrexate and valproic acid and can decrease the effect of certain antihypertensive drugs (e.g., β-adrenoceptor blockers, diuretics, and ACE inhibitors). However, long-term low doses of aspirin used for antiplatelet therapy appear not to interact with antihypertensive drugs.[104]

Diflunisal

Diflunisal is a difluorophenyl derivative of salicylic acid (see Figure 21-5) with antiinflammatory, analgesic, and antipyretic activity. Although structurally related to salicylates, diflunisal is not hydrolyzed in vivo to salicylate and therefore is unique among the salicylates. Like other salicylates, diflunisal blocks the synthesis of PGs by inhibiting COX. Diflunisal is approximately tenfold more potent than aspirin in suppressing PG formation in rats.

The drug is well absorbed after oral administration, with peak blood concentrations occurring in 2 to 3 hours. It is highly bound to plasma protein. Diflunisal has a long plasma half-life (8 to 12 hours versus 2.5 hours for salicylate), which permits dosing intervals of up to 12 hours. The drug is excreted in the urine, with two soluble glucuronide conjugates accounting for approximately 90% of the administered dose.

Diflunisal is indicated for the treatment of mild to moderate pain and for osteoarthritis and rheumatoid arthritis. In postoperative dental pain, 500 to 1000 mg of diflunisal produces greater analgesia than does aspirin or acetaminophen (both 650 mg), and peak effects are comparable to those obtainable with fixed combinations containing optimal doses of opioids.[45,47] Because diflunisal has an extended duration of action and a relatively slow onset of action in acute pain models, the recommended dosage regimen is a 1000 mg loading dose followed by 500 mg every 8 to 12 hours. The effectiveness of diflunisal in osteoarthritis appears to be comparable to that of aspirin.

In terms of adverse effects, diflunisal qualitatively resembles aspirin. Effects on the gastrointestinal tract range from nausea and epigastric pain to peptic ulcer and gastrointestinal bleeding. However, diflunisal is less problematic in this respect than aspirin. Platelet function and bleeding time are affected in a dose-related fashion but to a lesser degree than with aspirin because diflunisal is a competitive, reversible inhibitor of COX. Like aspirin, diflunisal prolongs the prothrombin time in patients receiving oral anticoagulants, perhaps by competitive displacement of coumarins from protein binding sites. Diflunisal does not penetrate the blood-brain barrier as well as does aspirin, and diflunisal therefore causes fewer CNS effects, including tinnitus. For this same reason, it is not used as an antipyretic.

Other NSAIDs

Many NSAIDs unrelated to the salicylates are now available. They all inhibit COX, but they vary in their relative potencies against COX-1 and COX-2.[107,140] Some NSAIDs may have other antiinflammatory actions in addition to inhibiting COX.[100] A number of these NSAIDs have been evaluated in postoperative dental pain and have been found to be superior to optimal doses of either aspirin or acetaminophen in terms of peak analgesic effect and duration of effect. For more long-term use, as in the treatment of rheumatoid arthritis, the choice of an NSAID for therapy is largely empiric and often based on what drug is best tolerated and best relieves symptoms in the individual patient. Most of these drugs are arylalkanoic or heteroarylalkanoic acid derivatives and will be discussed according to their chemical classification. The newly developed COX-2 inhibitors will be discussed separately.

Propionic acid derivatives

Among the NSAIDs, the substituted phenylpropionic acid derivatives constitute the largest group of aspirin alternatives (Figure 21-9). In addition to their antiinflammatory indications in treating the symptoms of rheumatoid arthritis, osteoarthritis, and degenerative joint disease, ibuprofen, naproxen, ketoprofen, and fenoprofen are also approved as analgesic agents. The short-term use of ibuprofen, naproxen, and ketoprofen is available without a prescription for relief of headache, fever, dysmenorrhea, and mild to moderate musculoskeletal and postoperative pain. In patients with rheumatoid arthritis, the propionic acid derivatives and other NSAIDs reduce joint swelling, pain, and morning stiffness, and they improve mobility as measured by an increase in walking time.

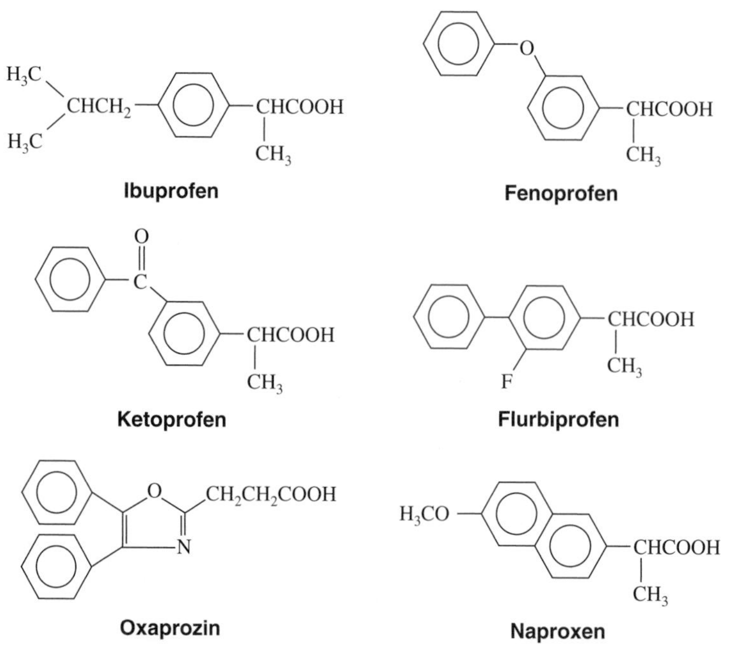

Ibuprofen

Fenoprofen

Ketoprofen

Flurbiprofen

Oxaprozin

Naproxen

Fig. 21-9 Structural formulas of some propionic acid derivatives.

When used in patients treated with corticosteroids, these agents may permit reduction of the steroid dose.

Like aspirin and other NSAIDs, these drugs inhibit PG synthesis by nonselective inhibition of COX. Their ability to inhibit COX, and thereby prevent the effect of PGs on uterine smooth muscle, makes them useful in the treatment of dysmenorrhea. Although they share a common pharmacologic profile, some unique characteristics exist among individual drugs. Naproxen, for example, appears to be especially effective in reducing leukocyte activity in inflammation, and ketoprofen appears to prevent lysosomal enzyme release by stabilizing the membranes of lysosomes.

Because the propionic acid derivatives as a group are less likely than aspirin to cause gastrointestinal or bleeding disturbances, they have increasingly been used in place of aspirin. However, with the emergence of the specific COX-2 inhibitors celecoxib and rofecoxib, their place in the forefront of antiarthritic therapy is being severely challenged.

The propionic acid NSAIDs are almost completely absorbed from the gastrointestinal tract. The rate of absorption is generally rapid but can be altered for some drugs by the presence of food in the stomach. Peak blood concentrations are reached in 1 to 4 hours. All these agents are highly bound (>90%) to plasma proteins; they are theoretically capable of interfering with the binding of other drugs such as phenytoin or the sulfonamides. The drugs are variably metabolized and conjugated, and they are then largely excreted in the urine. Ibuprofen, fenoprofen, and ketoprofen have short plasma half-lives (1 to 4 hours), whereas naproxen has a plasma half-life of approximately 15 hours, which allows less frequent dosing. Flurbiprofen has an intermediate half-life of approximately 6 hours; the half-life of oxaprozin is approximately 50 hours.

A brief overview of some of the individual drugs follows, with an emphasis on the analgesic use of these drugs in patients with postsurgical dental pain.

Ibuprofen Ibuprofen was the first single-entity oral analgesic to be approved by the FDA that showed a greater peak analgesic effect than 650 mg of aspirin.[17,25] It is also available as a nonprescription drug. The recommended prescription analgesic dose of ibuprofen is 400 mg every 4 to 6 hours. When used OTC without a health professional's guidance, the maximum daily dose should not exceed 1200 mg. In one study, a 400-mg dose of ibuprofen was more effective than a combination of 650 mg aspirin with 60 mg codeine (Figure 21-10).[22] In another study, an ibuprofen liquigel formulation containing 200 mg of solubilized potassium ibuprofen displayed greater peak analgesic effects and a longer duration of action than 1000 mg of acetaminophen.[65] Doses of ibuprofen larger than 400 mg have not demonstrated enhanced analgesic efficacy in nonrheumatic pain. Preoperative or immediately postoperative ibuprofen can delay the onset and lessen the severity of postoperative pain.[35,135,138] Such treatment may be particularly useful when there is a high likelihood of moderate to severe postoperative discomfort. For rheumatic pain and inflammation, doses of ibuprofen can range from 1200 mg to 3600 mg daily. Ibuprofen is widely used as an antipyretic and is second to acetaminophen as the most used antipyretic in the pediatric population. Dosages for antipyresis are based on the child's age and body weight.

Ibuprofen is a weak organic acid and is highly (approximately 99%) bound to plasma albumin. It is extensively metabolized and then excreted as the metabolites or their conjugates in the urine, with an elimination half-life of approximately 2 hours.

Naproxen Naproxen is approved for a variety of inflammatory conditions and for the relief of pain. It is the only NSAID manufactured as the active (S) enantiomer. It is available as both the free acid and as the sodium salt, the latter of which is more rapidly absorbed from the gastrointestinal tract and is the preferred form for analgesic use. The sodium salt of naproxen at a 220-mg dose is available over the counter (OTC) with a maximum recommended daily dose of 660 mg. Naproxen sodium by prescription can be taken at a dose of up to 1375 mg/day. In one study of postsurgical dental pain, a 220-mg dose of naproxen sodium was equivalent in analgesic efficacy and duration to 200 mg ibuprofen.[75] In two other studies, 440 mg of naproxen sodium was superior to 1000 mg acetaminophen in peak analgesia and duration and equivalent in efficacy to 400 mg ibuprofen.[50,74] At doses between 440 mg and 550 mg, naproxen sodium displays a duration of action of between 8 and 12 hours, which is the recommended dosing interval. This extended duration of action is explained by its relatively long half-life of approximately 15 hours. Naproxen is somewhat more irritating to the gastrointestinal tract than ibuprofen.[66] The drug is partially metabolized, and its clearance is almost entirely renal. Like ibuprofen, naproxen is highly bound to plasma albumin.

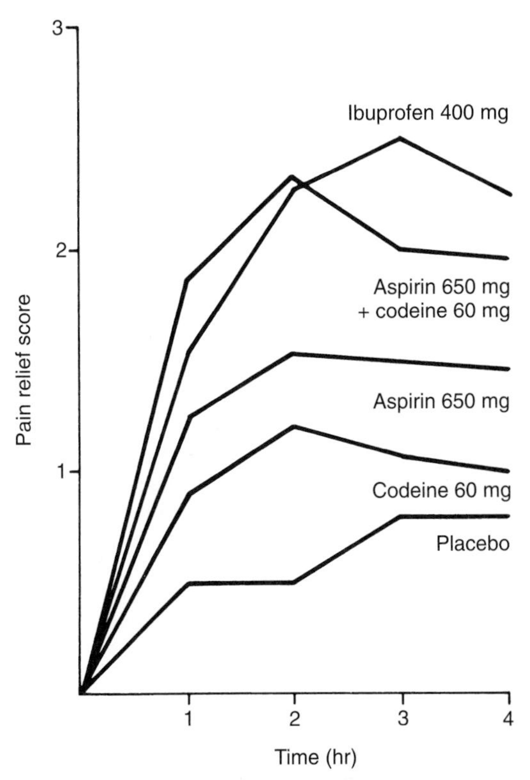

Fig. 21-10 Time-effect curves for placebo, codeine, aspirin, aspirin plus codeine, and ibuprofen. Mean pain relief scores are plotted against time in hours. (Adapted from Cooper SA, Engel L, Lador M, et al: Analgesic efficacy of an ibuprofen-codeine combination, *Pharmacotherapy* 2:162-167, 1982.)

Fenoprofen Fenoprofen is marketed with both analgesic and antiinflammatory indications. The recommended dose of 200 mg every 4 to 6 hours is likely to be superior to 650 mg of aspirin. As with the other propionic acid derivatives, fenoprofen is extensively (approximately 99%) and reversibly protein bound. It has a mean plasma half-life of approximately 2.5 hours in healthy adults. Most of the drug is excreted by the kidney as hydroxylated and conjugated metabolites.[57]

Ketoprofen Ketoprofen is an FDA-approved analgesic that is also effective for the symptomatic management of rheumatoid arthritis, osteoarthritis, and dysmenorrhea. Like the other propionic acid derivatives, it inhibits PG synthesis. However, ketoprofen has also been shown to inhibit leukotriene synthesis in at least two in vitro cell culture systems. In addition, ketoprofen stabilizes lysosomal membranes and has an antibradykinin effect. It is more potent than ibuprofen, with 25 to 50 mg about equally effective for mild to moderate pain as 400 mg of ibuprofen. In one dental pain study, 100 mg of ketoprofen was significantly more effective than 400 mg of ibuprofen, although this represents an unapproved analgesic dose of ketoprofen (Figure 21-11).[19]

Although approved OTC at a 12.5-mg dose, ketoprofen has been reported to be more irritating to the gastrointestinal tract than aspirin.[66] Ketoprofen is extensively bound to plasma proteins (approximately 99%), and it has an elimination half-life of 2 to 4 hours in young adults and middle-aged subjects. It is conjugated with glucuronic acid in the liver and excreted by the kidney. For nonarthritic pain, doses of 25 to 50 mg three or four times daily are usually sufficient. For arthritic pain, daily doses may approach 300 mg.

Flurbiprofen Flurbiprofen offers no unique advantages over ibuprofen. However, it is much more potent, with 50 to 100 mg of flurbiprofen being equal in effectiveness to 400 mg ibuprofen.[90] Although approved by the FDA as an antiarthritic drug, flurbiprofen does not possess an analgesic indication. Of particular interest to periodontists is that flurbiprofen (in addition to some other NSAIDs) taken on a long-term basis has been shown to slow the progression of alveolar bone resorption in different experimental models of periodontal disease.[70,143,144]

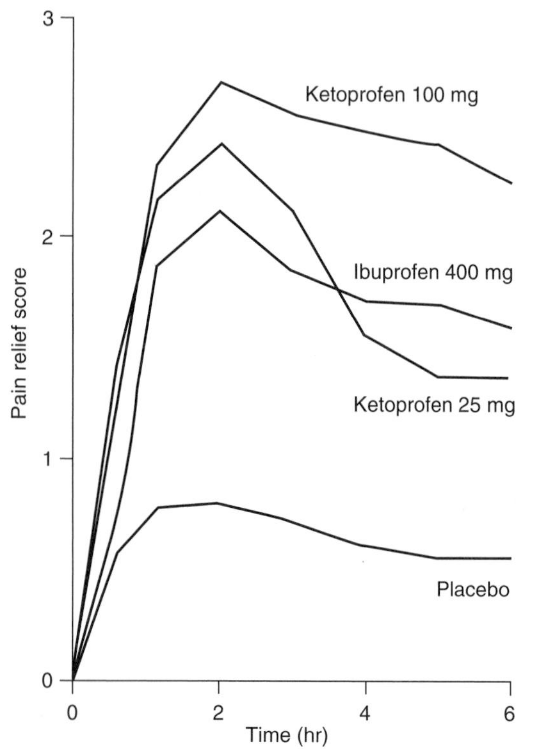

Fig. 21-11 Time-effect curves for placebo, ketoprofen, and ibuprofen. The mean pain relief scores are plotted against time in hours. (Adapted from Cooper SA, Berrie R, Cohn P: Analgesic efficacy of ketoprofen 25 and 100mg compared to ibuprofen 400mg, *Clin Pharmacol Ther* 39:187, 1986.)

Oxaprozin Oxaprozin is currently approved for only rheumatoid arthritis and osteoarthritis. With a half-life of approximately 50 hours, it is typically dosed once a day. Unlike other members of the propionic acid class, oxaprozin produces a significant incidence of photosensitivity, manifested as vesicular eruptions on sun-exposed skin. Like other NSAIDs, oxaprozin is associated with a prolongation of bleeding time, which may persist for more than 8 days after the last dose because of its long half-life.

Adverse effects Although the incidence with some propionic acid derivatives may be less than with aspirin, various gastrointestinal disturbances (epigastric pain, nausea, vomiting, gastric bleeding, and constipation or diarrhea) can occur, and these drugs should be used with caution in patients with a history of peptic ulcer. Long-term high-dose administration for arthritic conditions is far more likely to produce serious adverse events than short-term administration for acute pain. In fact, meta-analyses of OTC doses of ibuprofen (800 to 1200 mg/day) or naproxen sodium (440 to 880 mg/day) taken for 10 or fewer days have revealed a side-effect profile no worse than placebo.[6,73] Propionic acid derivatives can, however, injure the gastric mucosa by suppressing COX-1 activity and therefore decrease the cytoprotection afforded by PGI_2 and PGE_2. CNS effects may include headache, dizziness, drowsiness, vertigo, and visual and auditory disturbances. Skin rashes are relatively common, and immediate allergic reactions have been reported. All the NSAIDs can lead to anaphylactoid reactions in aspirin-intolerant patients (i.e., those susceptible to aspirin-induced asthma). These agents decrease platelet aggregation and adhesiveness and increase bleeding time, although to a lesser degree than aspirin; they should be avoided in patients with bleeding disorders and used with caution in patients receiving anticoagulants. These drugs may promote Na^+ retention, and their use may lead to the formation of edema in susceptible persons. They can interfere with the antihypertensive effects of β-adrenergic blockers, ACE inhibitors, and diuretics if they are administered for more than 1 week.[72] In elderly patients, especially during long-term therapy, the dosage of the propionic acid NSAIDs may have to be reduced by up to 50%.

Indole and indene derivatives

The indole and closely related indene derivatives include several drugs useful in the treatment of acute and chronic inflammatory diseases.

Indomethacin Indomethacin is a methylated indole acetic acid with powerful antiinflammatory properties. Its chemical structure is shown in Figure 21-12. Indomethacin is a potent inhibitor of COX (see Table 21-2) and a more potent antiinflammatory drug in vivo than aspirin. Like the salicylates, it influences numerous biochemical and cellular events that may be involved in the inflammatory process; some of these events may or may not be mediated by PGs.

Clinically, indomethacin produces antipyretic and analgesic effects, the latter being most notable when the pain is associated with an inflammatory condition. Because of its toxic potential, however, indomethacin should not be used as an antipyretic or simple analgesic. An exception to this rule is its use as an antipyretic in Hodgkin's disease. Indomethacin is reserved for those cases of rheumatoid arthritis, ankylosing spondylitis, and osteoarthritis in which less dangerous drugs are ineffective or not tolerated. Indomethacin has also been used as a short-term antiinflammatory agent in the treatment of bursitis, tendonitis, and acute attacks of gouty arthritis. The drug is occasionally administered as a tocolytic and to promote the closure of a patent ductus arteriosus. The mechanism in

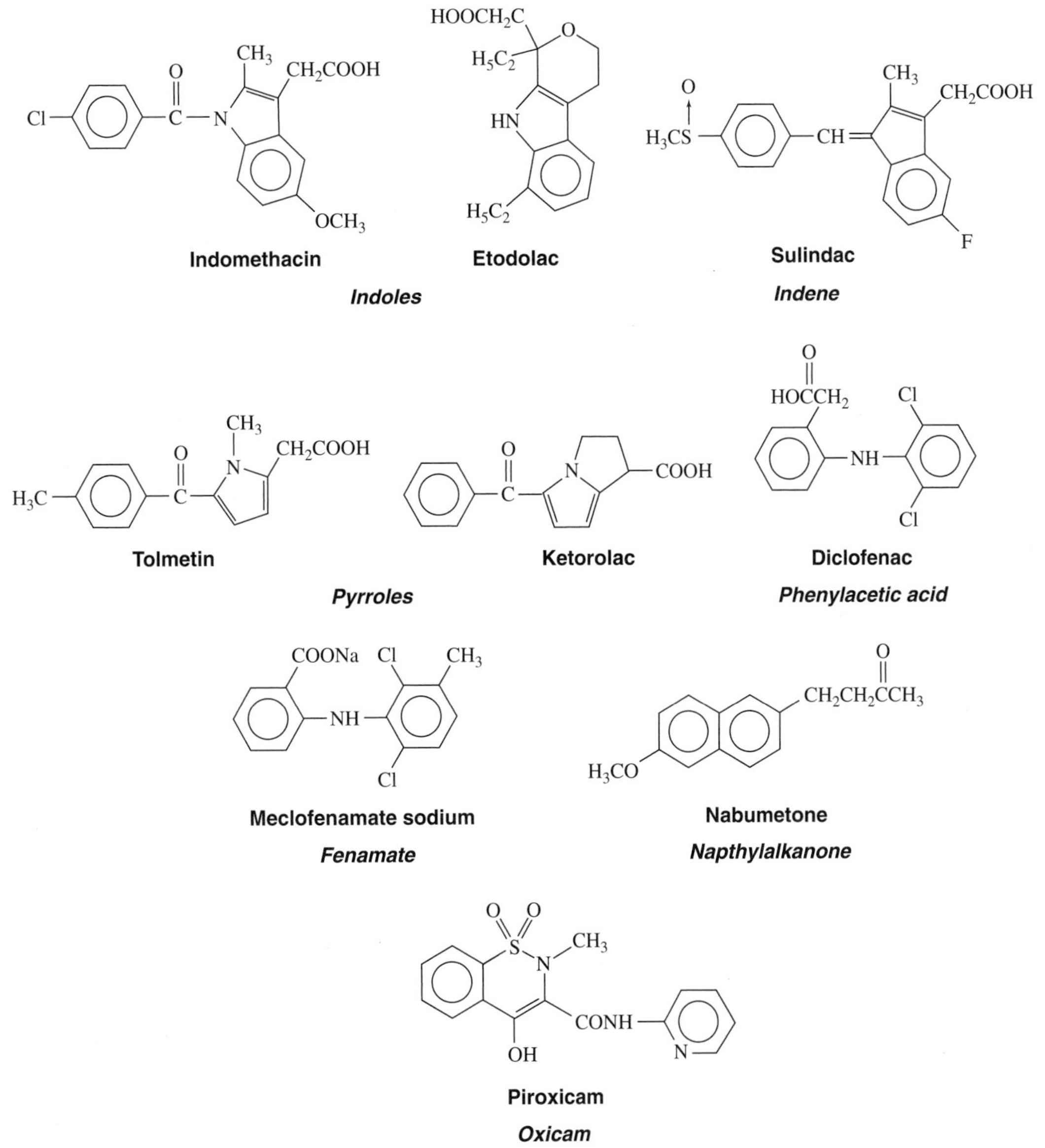

Indomethacin **Etodolac**

Indoles

Sulindac

Indene

Tolmetin **Ketorolac**

Pyrroles

Diclofenac

Phenylacetic acid

Meclofenamate sodium

Fenamate

Nabumetone

Napthylalkanone

Piroxicam

Oxicam

Fig. 21-12 Structural formulas of various aryl- and heteroarylalkanoic acid derivatives. The chemical categories are noted.

both cases is inhibition of PG production. There are no indications for indomethacin in dentistry.

Indomethacin is well absorbed from the gastrointestinal tract, and peak plasma concentrations are reached in 1 to 2 hours. The drug is largely bound to plasma proteins. After a single dose, most of the drug is eliminated in the urine as various metabolites during the next 24 hours. Its plasma half-life is approximately 2.5 hours.

Adverse effects are common with indomethacin therapy. Gastrointestinal disturbances such as epigastric pain, nausea, and diarrhea occur frequently. The drug may also cause perforation of the esophagus, stomach, and duodenum, and the resultant hemorrhage can be fatal. The drug is thus contraindicated in patients with active gastrointestinal lesions or a history of such lesions. CNS effects, including severe headache and confusion, also occur. Psychosis is possible. In addition to dermatologic and allergic reactions, leukopenia, aplastic anemia, thrombocytopenia, and hepatitis have been reported; some of these reactions have also proved fatal. Indomethacin has the potential to interact with many drugs. Simultaneous administration of indomethacin and oral anticoagulants may be hazardous.

Etodolac Etodolac (see Figure 21-12) is an NSAID approved in the United States for the treatment of acute pain and for managing the signs and symptoms of rheumatoid arthritis and osteoarthritis. Although it is classified as a nonselective NSAID, etodolac appears to be approximately threefold more selective for the inducible COX-2 isoenzyme than for the constitutive COX-1 isoenzyme (see Figure 21-6).[55,107,140] This relative activity is thought to explain the lower incidence of gastrointestinal side effects and ulceration seen with long-term dosing compared with other nonselective NSAIDs.[99] Peak plasma concentrations are reached in 1 to 2 hours after oral administration. Etodolac has a plasma half-life of approximately 7 hours, and 200 to 400 mg is taken every 6 to 8 hours for the relief of pain. The daily dose should not exceed 1200 mg. Etodolac has been studied in postsurgical dental pain. Onset of analgesia occurs approximately 30 minutes after oral administration, and its duration is 4 to 6 hours.[52,64] In patients with postimpaction dental pain, etodolac 200 mg provides peak analgesia comparable to aspirin 650 mg but longer in duration. Doses of 400 mg generally provide relief for 5 to 6 hours before half the patients require remedication. An extended-release formulation of etodolac, which can be administered once a day, is available for the treatment of arthritic conditions. Its onset of action, however, is too slow to be used in the treatment of acute postsurgical pain.[64]

Sulindac Sulindac, an indene derivative, is also a sulfoxide (see Figure 21-12). Sulindac is a prodrug that must be reduced to the sulfide before it becomes active as an NSAID. Peak plasma concentrations are reached in approximately 2 hours. Sulindac sulfide has a half-life of approximately 15 hours. Its relatively long half-life probably results from the fact that the drug undergoes enterohepatic circulation. Extensive metabolism yields a sulfone and several conjugates. Sulindac is used to treat rheumatoid arthritis and other inflammatory diseases and is occasionally prescribed as a tocolytic and for treatment of acute gout.

Pyrrole derivatives

The pyrrole acetic acids include tolmetin and ketorolac. Although tolmetin is not used in clinical dentistry, ketorolac enjoys special status because of its parenteral dosage form.

Tolmetin Tolmetin, whose structure is shown in Figure 21-12, has antiinflammatory, antipyretic, and analgesic properties. It is used to treat various inflammatory diseases. Tolmetin has pharmacokinetic properties similar to those of other NSAIDs (well absorbed from the gastrointestinal tract, highly bound to plasma proteins, and highly metabolized). Peak plasma concentrations are reached approximately 20 minutes to 1 hour after oral dosing. It has a half-life of about 5 hours.

Ketorolac Ketorolac (see Figure 21-12) was the first injectable NSAID approved in the United States. It is also available in tablet form for oral use but only after initial intramuscular or intravenous injection. It is recommended that the total course of therapy with ketorolac not exceed 5 days. These limitations follow the drug's relatively high incidence of gastrointestinal ulceration and bleeding complications compared with other NSAIDs. The more than 400-fold selectivity for inhibiting COX-1 over COX-2 (see Figure 21-6) probably accounts for ketorolac's enhanced toxicity. Although ketorolac is marketed as a racemic mixture, only the S-enantiomer is an active analgesic.

Injectable ketorolac has an important application in postoperative pain management in patients who are unable to consume oral analgesics or when the pain is severe and injectable opioids are contraindicated. Clinical trials have shown that, in some circumstances, parenteral ketorolac is as effective as standard doses of intramuscular morphine or meperidine, longer lasting, and with fewer adverse effects.[146] In patients with moderate to severe postoperative pain, 30 mg of intramuscular ketorolac is comparable to 12 mg of morphine and equal or superior to 100 mg of meperidine.[46,51,102,147]

Both the oral and the intramuscular forms are well absorbed. Like other NSAIDs, ketorolac is highly bound (approximately 99%) to plasma proteins. Plasma concentrations of 0.3 μg/ml are estimated to be required for effective analgesia; when plasma concentrations exceed 5.0 μg/ml, side effects are frequent. Onset of analgesia after parenteral ketorolac is similar to that after injectable opioids. The S- and R-isomers have half-lives of about 2.5 and 5 hours, respectively, and are metabolized largely to oxidized and conjugated products.

Initial intramuscular doses of 30 to 60 mg ketorolac are recommended, followed by 15 to 30 mg doses every 6 hours with a maximum daily dose not to exceed 120 mg. The initial intravenous dose is 15 to 30 mg. Oral doses are recommended at 4- to 6-hour intervals. Oral ketorolac (10 mg) has also been evaluated in postoperative dental pain and found to be superior to 650 mg of aspirin, 600 mg of acetaminophen, and combinations of 600 mg acetaminophen/60 mg codeine or 1000 mg acetaminophen/10 mg hydrocodone; it is at least as effective as 400 mg of ibuprofen.[46,49]

Clinical studies have shown that ketorolac does not produce several of the common adverse effects associated with opioid analgesics. It does not depress respiration or cardiovascular function and causes less constipation and drowsiness than equivalent doses of opioids. As with other NSAIDs, physical dependence and tolerance do not develop. The most common adverse effects after ketorolac are drowsiness, dyspepsia, gastrointestinal pain, and nausea. Peptic ulcers and gastrointestinal bleeding have occurred after oral ketorolac. Renal toxicity has also been associated with ketorolac. The drug is contraindicated before surgery because its intense antiplatelet effect is likely to result in increased intraoperative bleeding, which reflects its potent COX-1 blocking activity.

In ophthalmology, ketorolac is instilled as a topical preparation to treat ocular itching associated with seasonal allergic conjunctivitis.

Diclofenac Diclofenac is a phenylacetic acid derivative (see Figure 21-12). It has pharmacokinetic properties and a mechanism of action similar to other NSAIDs. However, it undergoes significant first-pass metabolism in the liver and, in addition to inhibiting COX, may reduce the concentration of arachidonic acid in some inflammatory cells.[13] Diclofenac reaches peak plasma concentrations in 2 to 3 hours after oral use and has a half-life of 1 to 2 hours. The drug is used to treat inflammatory conditions, pain, and dysmenorrhea. Diclofenac is also used topically for ocular inflammation. The adverse effects are similar to other NSAIDs; however, elevation of hepatic enzymes in the plasma is more common and indicates a higher likelihood of producing hepatotoxic effects. In an effort to reduce the ulcerogenic potential of long-term diclofenac therapy, a formulation combining diclofenac with the PG analogue misoprostol has been developed. A 6-month study of long-term NSAID use indicated that misoprostol reduced the incidence of serious drug-induced gastrointestinal complications by 40%.[117] However, misoprostol is an abortifacient and must be used with extreme care in women of child-bearing potential. The reader is referred to Chapter 33 for a more complete discussion of misoprostol and other gastrointestinal drugs.

Fenamates

The fenamates are a group of aspirinlike drugs derived from N-phenylanthranilic acid. The structure of meclofenamate sodium is shown in Figure 21-12. Mefenamic acid is another member of this group approved in the United States. Mefenamic acid is indicated for the relief of moderate pain (therapy not to exceed 1 week) and for relief of primary dysmenorrhea, and meclofenamate is indicated for mild to moderate pain, dysmenorrhea, and arthritis. Their plasma half-lives range from 2 to 4 hours. Meclofenamate has one active metabolite whose elimination half-life is 15 hours.

Mefenamic acid inhibits both the synthesis and activity of PGs. In doses of 250 to 500 mg, its analgesic properties are comparable to those of aspirin. It is superior to aspirin, however, for the treatment of severe dysmenorrhea. The potential for serious blood dyscrasias and gastrointestinal side effects (dyspepsia, diarrhea) limits the use of mefenamic acid to short-term, intermittent administration.

Meclofenamate has been extensively studied as an oral analgesic in the short-term management of acute postsurgical dental pain. In three independent dental studies, 100 mg of meclofenamate appeared to be more effective than 650 mg of aspirin and 600 mg of acetaminophen combined with 60 mg of codeine and as effective as 400 mg of ibuprofen.[23,34,63] However, even the short-term clinical use of meclofenamate and mefenamic acid may be limited by a high (up to 25%) incidence of gastrointestinal disturbances ranging from gastric pain to diarrhea. The ability of these drugs to produce stomach cramping and diarrhea after a week or less of dosing has been demonstrated in two dental pain studies.[24,63] In addition, the fenamates have adverse effects typical of other NSAIDs (tinnitus, gastric bleeding, and impairment of platelet function). More serious toxicities in the form of abnormal renal and hepatic function, hemolytic anemia, and bowel inflammation have been documented.

Oxicams

Piroxicam (see Figure 21-12), the first member of this relatively new class of NSAIDs to be marketed in the United States, is approved for the treatment of rheumatoid arthritis and osteoarthritis. Although it has also been used to treat pain and dysmenorrhea, its onset of analgesic action is too slow to be routinely used for the treatment of dental postoperative pain. Similar to other NSAIDs, piroxicam inhibits platelet aggregation and promotes gastrointestinal bleeding. All these effects are attributed to the inhibition of COX-1.

Piroxicam is at least as effective as aspirin for the treatment of rheumatoid arthritis and appears to be better tolerated. Its major advantage, however, is pharmacokinetic in nature. Piroxicam is well absorbed, with peak plasma concentrations occurring 3 to 5 hours after administration. The drug is highly bound to plasma protein, undergoes considerable enterohepatic recycling, and is eventually eliminated in the urine after being extensively metabolized. The average plasma half-life for piroxicam is 50 hours. This slow elimination rate permits administration of a single daily dose, an advantage for any drug that must be taken on a long-term basis. Of course, it also requires 2 weeks for full therapeutic concentrations to be achieved after the initiation of therapy.

The side effects of piroxicam are similar to those of other NSAIDs. In addition to gastrointestinal upset and the possibility of ulceration and hemorrhage, peripheral edema and renal damage may occur. Like other NSAIDs, this drug should not be administered to a patient susceptible to aspirin-induced bronchospasm.

Meloxicam, a congener of piroxicam, is the newest oxicam derivative to be approved in the United States. Like etodolac, meloxicam is a weakly preferential blocker of COX-2,[41] displaying approximately twofold selectivity over COX-1 in whole blood assay systems (see Figure 21-6).[107] It is currently FDA approved for the treatment of osteoarthritis. In clinical studies of osteoarthritis and rheumatoid arthritis, 7.5 to 15 mg/day of meloxicam has displayed equivalent antiinflammatory efficacy to diclofenac 100 mg/day, naproxen 750 mg/day, or piroxicam 20 mg/day. In addition, meloxicam appears to produce a lower incidence of serious gastrointestinal toxicity than most other NSAIDs, probably as a result of its relative sparing of COX-1 activity.[60] However, gastrointestinal ulceration and bleeding can still occur.

Meloxicam has an elimination half-life of 15 to 20 hours, which supports once-a-day dosing. The major path of metabolism is through hepatic CYP2C9 enzymes; thus there is a theoretical possibility that inhibitors of this enzyme system, such as metronidazole or fluconazole, could cause meloxicam to accumulate in the blood.

Nabumetone

Nabumetone (see Figure 21-12) is a prodrug that is converted to the active naphthylalkanone metabolite 6-methoxy-2-naphthylacetic acid (6MNA) in vivo. The half-life of the active metabolite is approximately 24 hours. Because clinical reports originally suggested that nabumetone produced less gastrointestinal toxicity than antiinflammatory doses of aspirin, naproxen, or indomethacin, it was originally thought to be a selective COX-2 inhibitor. However more recent research has revealed that 6MNA is actually a threefold to fivefold more potent blocker of COX-1 than COX-2.[107,140] Thus at therapeutic doses of nabumetone, COX-1–blocking effects, including gastrointestinal ulceration and platelet inhibition, can occur. The drug is indicated to treat the signs and symptoms of osteoarthritis and rheumatoid arthritis.

Pyrazolones

Phenylbutazone is a congener of the pyrazolones antipyrine, aminopyrine, and dipyrone. The latter agents were used historically as analgesics, antipyretics, and antiinflammatory drugs, but their toxicity and the introduction of phenylbutazone in 1948 led to their abandonment (with the exception of the use of antipyrine as a topical analgesic for earache). Recently, phenylbutazone has also been withdrawn voluntarily by its manufacturer because of its well-documented, serious, and sometimes fatal adverse reactions, as well as the availability of alternative NSAIDs. The most serious of these side effects is bone marrow depression, leading to agranulocytosis, thrombocytopenia, leukopenia, or aplastic anemia. The blood dyscrasias occur most frequently during high-dose therapy and may be manifested initially by fever, stomatitis, and sore throat. Gastrointestinal disturbances associated with COX-1 inhibition are common and range from mucosal irritation to frank ulceration and hemorrhage. Other adverse reactions include skin rashes, hepatitis, jaundice, purpura, and hematuria. Phenylbutazone causes Na^+ retention by the kidney; the resultant edema may be significant in patients with congestive heart failure or hypertension. Phenylbutazone is a good candidate for drug interactions because of its tendency to promote bleeding and gastrointestinal disturbances. Phenylbutazone is also known to inhibit hepatic microsomal enzymes.

Selective Cyclooxygenase-2 Inhibitors

A major advance in NSAID therapy over the last few years has been the introduction of drugs, such as celecoxib and rofecoxib, that selectively inhibit the inducible COX-2 isoform of the COX enzyme system while sparing the constitutive COX-1 isoform. Unlike preferential COX-2 inhibitors such as etodolac and meloxicam, whose COX-2 selectivity does not exceed twofold to threefold, celecoxib and rofecoxib display COX-2 selectivity in the range of eightfold to 35-fold in whole blood assay systems (see Figure 21-6).[107] In fact, the current FDA-approved package inserts for these entities state that, at therapeutic concentrations in human beings, neither drug inhibits COX-1. The selectivity of these so-called "coxibs" has lead to roughly a 50% to 60% reduction in serious gastrointestinal complications—including symptomatic ulcers and gastrointestinal bleeds, perforations, and obstructions—compared with standard NSAIDs (e.g., ibuprofen, naproxen, diclofenac) in long-term safety studies in arthritic patients.[10,116] This reduction represents a major potential health cost savings because clinically important gastroduodenal ulceration occurs in up to 6% of patients on long-term NSAID therapy and results in more than 100,000 hospitalizations and 16,000 deaths annually.[119] Whether selective COX-2 inhibitors offer safety advantages over standard NSAIDs with the typical short-term dosing regimens most commonly used in dental practice is currently unknown.

Celecoxib

Celecoxib (Figure 21-13) is a novel diaryl substituted pyrazole that possesses a sulfonamide group. Its COX-2 selectivity in whole-blood assays approaches eightfold. It is highly protein bound (approximately 97%) and has a plasma elimination half-life of 10 to 12 hours. Its metabolism is mediated primarily by CYP2C9, yielding three inactive metabolites: a primary alcohol, the corresponding carboxylic acid, and its glucuronide metabolite. In randomized trials in patients with rheumatoid arthritis and osteoarthritis, the therapeutic responses seen with celecoxib are equal to that of nonselective NSAIDs, including diclofenac, naproxen, and ibuprofen.[39,112,118] The recommended dose of celecoxib for arthritic conditions is 100 to 200 mg twice per day. Unlike the results of arthritis studies, celecoxib 200 mg was inferior to ibuprofen 400 mg in terms of both analgesic onset and peak effects in patients with acute postsurgical dental pain.[88] Because of this, celecoxib was granted FDA approval for treatment of rheumatoid arthritis and osteoarthritis but not acute pain.

An additional FDA indication for celecoxib is to reduce the number of adenomatous colorectal polyps in patients with familial adenomatous polyposis. This is a genetic condition in which more than 90% of affected individuals develop colorectal cancer. Celecoxib at 400 mg twice per day, which is the recommended dose for this indication, reduced the number of polyps by roughly 25% after 6 months of therapy.[126] COX-2 is known to be overexpressed in human colorectal adenomas and adenocarcinomas,[37] and the ability of celecoxib to inhibit COX-2 probably explains its usefulness in this condition.

As previously stated, the major therapeutic advantage of celecoxib in arthritic pain is one of safety. In a major celecoxib study, 400 mg of celecoxib twice a day, which is two times the maximum antiinflammatory dose, resulted in a reduction of gastrointestinal ulceration, perforations, and bleeds after 6 months by one half compared with large therapeutic doses of ibuprofen or diclofenac.[116] Because celecoxib is a selective COX-2 inhibitor, it has less effect on COX-1 and does not inhibit platelet aggregation or increase bleeding time, which may further enhance its safety with long-term dosing.[79] However, many patients in the arthritic population also require cardioprotective dosages of aspirin. These patients must be reminded that they must take their low-dose aspirin therapy in addition to their antiarthritic dosages of the COX-2 inhibitor.

Despite celecoxib's COX-2 selectivity, patients still must be warned of the potential for the drug, and in fact all specific COX-2 inhibitors, to cause serious gastrointestinal toxicity. Because COX-2 plays a normal constitutive role in the kidney (see Figure 21-3), celecoxib can cause renal toxicity, including Na^+ and water retention, hypertension, and acute renal failure. Like other NSAIDs, celecoxib may interfere with the antihypertensive effects of ACE inhibitors, diuretics, and β-adrenergic blockers. In patients with aspirin intolerance, the use of COX-2 inhibitors may precipitate potentially life-threatening asthmatic or allergic-type reactions. Because celecoxib is a sulfonamide, patients with documented allergies to other sulfonamides (including the thiazide diuretics) should avoid celecoxib. Drug interactions involving celecoxib resemble those of aspirin and other NSAIDs. Recently, reports of significant bleeding episodes have occurred in patients taking warfarin who subsequently received celecoxib. Drugs that are inhibitors of CYP2C9, such as fluconazole and metronidazole, may significantly increase celecoxib blood concentrations.

Rofecoxib

Rofecoxib is a diaryl substituted furanone (see Figure 21-13) with COX-2 selectivity of approximately 35-fold in whole blood assays.[107,140] Its pharmacokinetic properties make it suitable for once-daily administration. The drug is well absorbed orally, with an elimination half-life of 17 hours. Unlike celecoxib, the cytochrome P450 system normally plays only a minor role in the biotransformation of rofecoxib, and inhibitors of this system should not affect the drug's metabolism. Rofecoxib is predominantly reduced in the liver, with the cis-dihydro and trans-dihydro derivatives of rofecoxib accounting for slightly more than half of recovered drug in the urine and a glucuronide of a hydroxy derivative accounting for another 9%. These metabolites are all inactive as COX inhibitors. Although rofecoxib contains a sulfur atom in its structure, it is not a sulfonamide and can be given safely to patients with documented sulfonamide allergies.

Rofecoxib is currently indicated for the treatment of osteoarthritis and for the management of acute pain, including primary dysmenorrhea. The recommended antiinflammatory dose of rofecoxib is 12.5 to 25 mg once a day, whereas

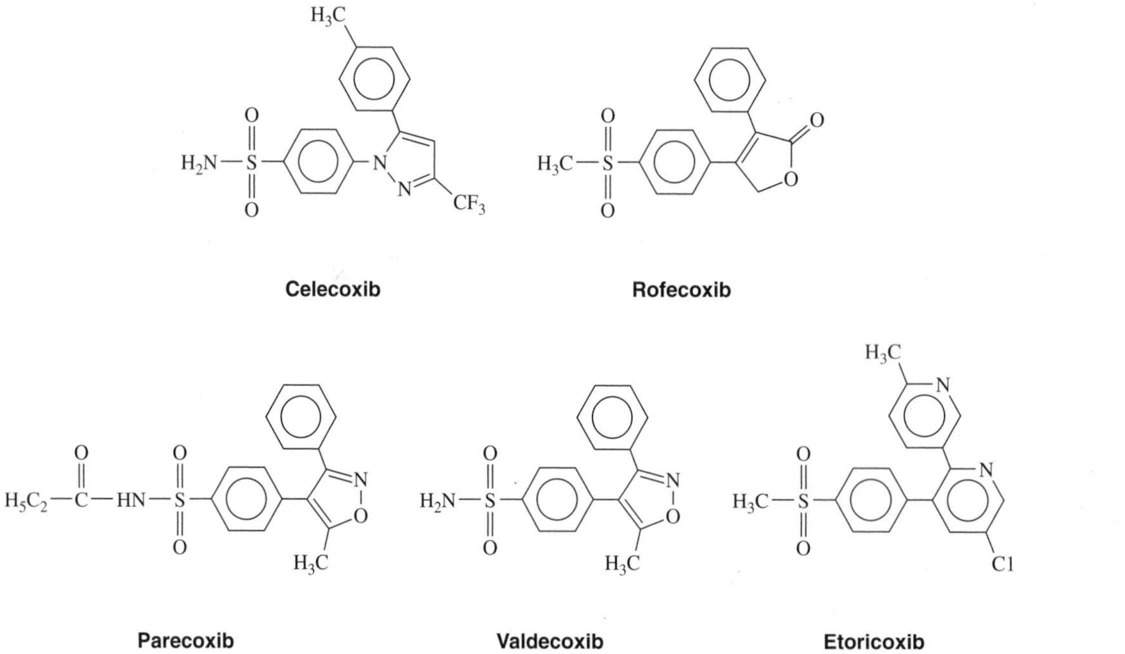

Celecoxib

Rofecoxib

Parecoxib

Valdecoxib

Etoricoxib

Fig. 21-13 Structural formulas of COX-2- selective inhibitors.

the analgesic dose is 50 mg once per day. In large scale studies of osteoarthritis of the hip or knee, rofecoxib has shown therapeutic equivalency to diclofenac and to ibuprofen.[32,112] In acute postsurgical dental pain, 50 mg of rofecoxib was equivalent to 400 mg of ibuprofen in analgesic onset and peak analgesic effect but had a much longer duration of action (24 hours for rofecoxib versus 8 hours for ibuprofen).[38,88,97] Rofecoxib was also more efficacious than 200 mg of celecoxib in analgesic onset, duration, and peak effects (Figure 21-14).[88]

The major safety advantages of rofecoxib are related to its ability to selectively block COX-2. In a major study involving more than 8000 patients, the administration of rofecoxib at twice the maximum antiarthritic dose for up to a year resulted in an approximate 60% reduction in gastrointestinal ulcerations, perforations, obstructions, and bleeds compared with a standard dose of naproxen.[10] Like celecoxib, rofecoxib does not inhibit platelet aggregation or increase bleeding times. In addition, rofecoxib does not alter the antiplatelet effects of low-dose aspirin, which is crucial in patients requiring the cardioprotective effects of aspirin while simultaneously taking a COX-2 inhibitor for acute or chronic inflammatory pain.[56]

Potential adverse reactions with rofecoxib are similar to celecoxib and include serious gastrointestinal toxicity, untoward renal effects (including water and Na^+ retention), hypertension, interference with the blood pressure–lowering effects of certain antihypertensive drugs, and the potential ability to increase blood concentrations and/or toxicity of other drugs with which classic NSAIDs have been shown to interact, including lithium salts and methotrexate. It is again stressed that patients with aspirin salts and NSAID intolerance must avoid COX-2 inhibitors, including rofecoxib.

New COX-2 inhibitors

Three COX-2 inhibitors have recently been developed (see Figure 21-13). Parecoxib is a prodrug that is being proposed as a parenteral analgesic agent. It is converted into the active metabolite valdecoxib by hepatic metabolism. Preliminary research suggests that this drug has analgesic efficacy that approximates that of injectable ketorolac with a longer duration of action.[30] The fact that parecoxib should not inhibit platelet aggregation or increase bleeding times may offer an additional advantage over ketorolac in certain patient populations. Valdecoxib has been approved by the FDA as an oral antiinflammatory and has shown promise as an analgesic agent. It possesses approximately thirtyfold selectivity for the COX-2 isoform.[107] The third member of this group, etoricoxib, is also being developed as an oral antiinflammatory and analgesic. It possesses greater COX-2 selectivity (106-fold) than any of the other COX-2 inhibitors[107] and has demonstrated efficacy in postsurgical dental pain.[89] Whether this additional COX-2 selectivity will enhance the safety profile of this drug is currently unknown.

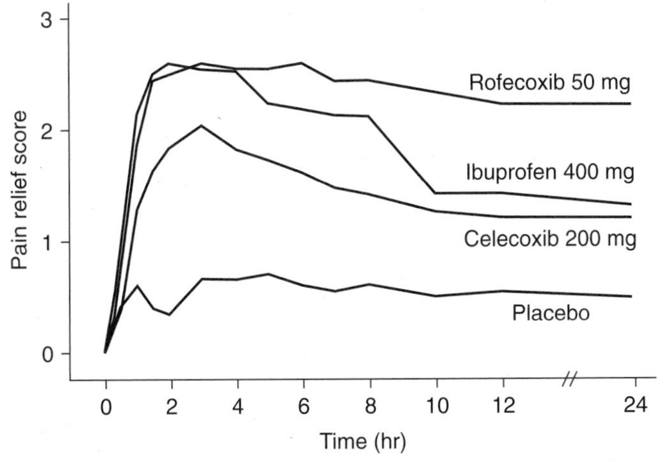

Fig. 21-14 Time-effect curves for placebo, celecoxib, ibuprofen, and rofecoxib. The mean pain relief scores are plotted against time in hours. (Adapted from Malmstrom K, Daniels S, Kotey P, et al: Comparison of rofecoxib and celecoxib, two cyclooxygenase-2 inhibitors, in postoperative dental pain: a randomized, placebo- and active-comparator–controlled clinical trial, *Clin Ther* 21:1653-1663, 1999.)

Implications for Dentistry

The major use of aspirin and other NSAIDs in dentistry is to relieve pain associated with pathologic processes (e.g., pulpitis, dentoalveolar abscesses) or after surgical procedures. In both situations, the antiinflammatory actions of the NSAID may contribute significantly to the therapeutic effect sought. Aspirin at doses between 650 to 1000 mg is an acceptable drug for mild to moderate dental pain. However, for more traumatic surgical procedures such as the removal of impacted third molars, the newer NSAIDs at dosages that approach their analgesic ceiling are more efficacious and sometimes better tolerated than aspirin. In fact, postsurgical dental pain studies that have used ceiling analgesic doses of NSAIDs, such as ibuprofen at 400 mg and naproxen at 500 mg, have displayed efficacy at least equal to that obtained with opioid combination drugs. In addition, the NSAIDs produce far fewer side effects of drowsiness, dizziness, nausea, and vomiting than do opioid-containing analgesics. The recommended dosing schedules of NSAIDs for acute pain of dental origin are shown in Table 21-6.

The role of COX-2 inhibitors in acute postsurgical dental pain still needs to be better defined. Celecoxib is currently not approved and cannot be recommended for acute pain because it is inferior to ibuprofen in postsurgical dental pain models. On the other hand, rofecoxib has analgesic effects that are equal to ibuprofen and with a longer duration of action (see Figure 21-14). One recent oral surgery study also demonstrated that rofecoxib provided greater pain relief than full therapeutic doses of an acetaminophen/codeine combination.[15] Rofecoxib may be ideal when once-a-day dosing is desirable and also as a preemptive analgesic given before the surgical procedure because of its long duration of effect and its lack of antiplatelet action. This enthusiasm must be tempered with the fact that the cost of rofecoxib is extremely high compared with generic or OTC NSAIDs. In addition, when used for a week or less, analgesic dosages of conventional NSAIDs have proved to be extremely safe and efficacious in postsurgical dental pain.

There are few chronic inflammatory diseases solely limited to the oral structures. The temporomandibular joint may be involved in systemic inflammatory diseases that would be treated with NSAIDs. The joint can also be singly affected by an acute or chronic inflammatory process, the cause of which may be known (e.g., trauma, immobilization, malocclusion) or unknown (e.g., nonspecific osteoarthritis). In these cases, an NSAID may be used in conjunction with other therapies such as heat, exercise, bite splints, and joint surgery. It is with the longer-term use of NSAIDs in patients with temporomandibular joint dysfunction or other chronic orofacial pain syndromes that the enhanced gastrointestinal safety of specific COX-2 inhibitors assumes added importance.

Contraindications to the NSAIDs must be heeded. For instance, salicylates must be avoided in children or teenagers with viral or suspected viral infections. The antiplatelet effect of NSAIDs, especially aspirin and ketorolac, must be considered if the patient is at risk from a bleeding abnormality or anticoagulant therapy. Many NSAIDs antagonize the effect of probenecid and sulfinpyrazone. Hypersensitivity to aspirin may indicate a risk to NSAIDs in general, including COX-2 inhibitors. The elimination of methotrexate is reduced with NSAIDs; other drug interactions may occur because of the

Table • 21-6

Some Nonopioid Analgesics Approved for Acute Pain

NONPROPRIETARY (GENERIC) NAME	PROPRIETARY (TRADE) NAME	ANALGESIC DOSAGE*	MAXIMUM DAILY DOSE*
Aspirin	ASA, others	650 to 1000 mg every 4 to 6 hours	4000 mg
Diflunisal	Dolobid	1000 mg to start, then 500 mg every 8 to 12 hours	1500 mg
Acetaminophen	Tylenol, others	650 to 1000 mg every 4 to 6 hours	4000 mg
Ibuprofen	Motrin, Rufen, others	400 mg every 4 to 6 hours	2400 mg
Ibuprofen (OTC)	Advil, Nuprin, others	200 to 400 mg every 4 to 6 hours	1200 mg
Naproxen	Naprosyn	500 mg to start, then 250 mg every 6 to 8 hours	1250 mg
Naproxen sodium	Anaprox	550 mg to start, then 275 mg every 6 to 8 hours	1375 mg
Naproxen sodium (OTC)	Aleve	220 to 440 mg every 8 hours	660 mg
Fenoprofen	Nalfon	200 mg every 4 to 6 hours	1200 mg
Ketoprofen	Orudis	25 to 75 mg every 6 hours	300 mg
Ketoprofen (OTC)	Orudis KT, Actron	12.5 to 25 mg every 4 to 6 hours	75 mg
Diclofenac	Cataflam	50 mg every 8 hours	150 mg
Meclofenamate	Meclomen	50 to 100 mg every 6 hours	400 mg
Mefenamic acid	Ponstel	500 mg to start, then 250 mg every 6 hours	1250 mg
Etodolac	Lodine	200 to 400 mg every 6 to 8 hours	1200 mg
Ketorolac	Toradol	15 to 30 mg IV or 30 to 60 mg IM to start, then 15 to 30 mg IV or IM every 6 hours; 10 to 20 mg orally 6 hours after last parenteral dose, then 10 mg every 4 to 6 hours†	60 to 120 mg IM or IV; 40 mg PO
Rofecoxib	Vioxx	50 mg once a day	50 mg

*Doses are for acute pain only. Higher doses are sometimes used for control of inflammatory disorders.
†Therapy limited to 5 days.
IV, Intravenously; *IM,* intramuscularly; *PO,* orally.

ability of NSAIDs to displace drugs from plasma albumin and otherwise alter their pharmacokinetic properties. The common adverse effects for NSAIDs on the gastrointestinal tract and CNS should be considered, especially when the patient is taking drugs with overlapping toxicity. The NSAIDs can block the therapeutic effects of several antihypertensive drugs. β-Adrenoceptor blockers, ACE inhibitors, and diuretics are among the drugs potentially antagonized by the NSAIDs.

ACETAMINOPHEN

Acetaminophen (N-acetyl-*p*-aminophenol) is the only aniline derivative currently in clinical use. It is widely promoted as the antipyretic analgesic of choice when aspirin cannot be used because of gastric problems or other contraindications. For many years, phenacetin (an acetaminophen analogue) was a common constituent of analgesic preparations, including numerous aspirin-phenacetin-caffeine combinations. Phenacetin has disappeared from use in the United States because of several studies linking long-term administration of such combinations with renal damage. Phenacetin is also capable of producing CNS disturbances (e.g., sedation), hemolytic anemia, and methemoglobinemia.

Chemistry and Classification

The history of acetaminophen dates back to the late 1800s, when the antipyretic activity of aniline derivatives was discovered and several congeners, including acetaminophen, were synthesized. For some reason, two other aniline derivatives, acetanilid and phenacetin, became popular, and acetaminophen was put aside. Chemists eventually realized that acetaminophen was an active metabolite of both of these drugs (Figure 21-15), but it was not until the mid-1900s that acetaminophen became commercially successful.

Mechanism of Action

Acetaminophen has both analgesic and antipyretic activity that is essentially equivalent to that of aspirin. The drug's mechanism of action also appears to stem from an inhibition of PG synthesis, although there may be some differences in the spectrum of COX enzymes that are inhibited.[129] It has been suggested that acetaminophen may be more active than aspirin as an inhibitor of CNS COX (including COX-3, a newly characterized enzyme[141]) and less active in the periphery. This hypothesis is based largely on the differences in the therapeutic and toxic effects of aspirin and acetaminophen rather than on direct experimental evidence. For example, acetaminophen has very weak antiinflammatory effects compared with aspirin. Acetaminophen may be a more selective inhibitor of neuronal PG synthesis than is aspirin. More recent evidence suggests that a peripheral mechanism of acetaminophen may indeed be partially responsible for its analgesic effects.[96] However, the presence of peroxides from leukocytes in inflamed tissues leads to inhibition of acetaminophen caused by the peroxides combining with acetaminophen. This may severely limit any effect of acetaminophen on inflammation. Other proposed mechanisms of action for acetaminophen do not involve PGs and include the activation of spinal serotonergic pathways and the inhibition of nitric oxide synthase.[9,134]

Pharmacologic Effects

Compared with aspirin, acetaminophen exerts relatively few important effects on specific organs or systems. The potency

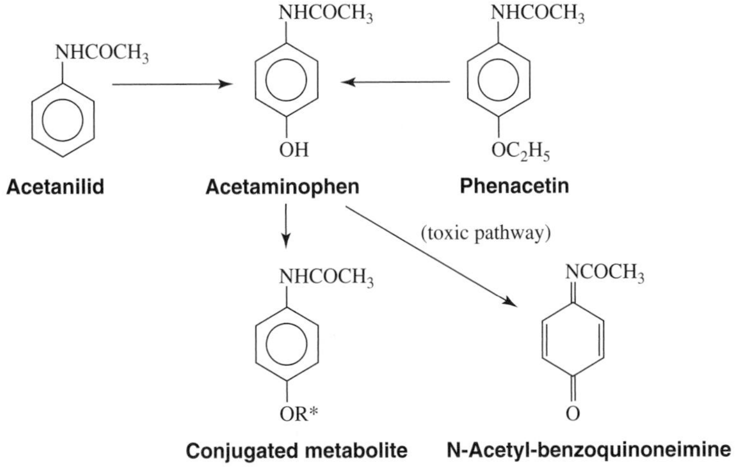

NHCOCH$_3$ NHCOCH$_3$ NHCOCH$_3$

OH OC_2H_5

Acetanilid **Acetaminophen** **Phenacetin**

(toxic pathway)

NHCOCH$_3$ NCOCH$_3$

OR* O

Conjugated metabolite **N-Acetyl-benzoquinoneimine**

Fig. 21-15 Structures and major metabolic pathways of acetaminophen, phenacetin, and acetanilid. **R*, Glucuronate (major), and sulfate (minor) conjugates. N-Acetyl-benzoquinoneimine, produced in high amounts in acetaminophen overdose, forms a conjugate with glutathione that results in depletion of glutathione.

and efficacy of acetaminophen as an antipyretic are similar to those of aspirin. At therapeutic doses, acetaminophen has little if any effect on the cardiovascular or respiratory systems. Acetaminophen does not inhibit platelet aggregation, cause occult bleeding or gastric irritation, affect uric acid excretion, or have as many drug interactions as aspirin. In overdose, the organ most affected is the liver. Acute renal toxicity may also occur. With long-term use, analgesic nephropathy is a possibility, but the risk is low.

Absorption, Fate, and Excretion

Acetaminophen is well absorbed in the small intestine after oral administration. The drug is evenly distributed throughout the body fluids and tissues, and it freely crosses the placenta. The half-life is approximately 2 to 4 hours, and the primary site of biotransformation (by glucuronide conjugation) is the liver (see Figure 21-15). Other minor metabolites include a conjugate with sulfate and various hydroxylated metabolites. A highly reactive and hepatotoxic metabolite, N-acetyl-*p*-benzoquinoneimine (NAPQI), is usually of little significance. However in the case of acetaminophen overdose and in a few individuals who are heavy users of alcohol and then consume acetaminophen, the accumulation of this metabolite can be disastrous. The binding of acetaminophen to plasma proteins is variable but rarely exceeds 40% of the total drug. Elimination is through the kidneys by glomerular filtration and active proximal tubular secretion. There is no competition for secretion with organic acids such as uric acid and aspirin.

General Therapeutic Uses

Although acetaminophen is approximately equipotent to aspirin as both an analgesic and an antipyretic, it is not a true antiinflammatory drug, and thus aspirin and other NSAIDs are far superior for conditions such as rheumatoid arthritis. For patients in whom aspirin and other NSAIDs are contraindicated, acetaminophen is usually the drug of choice. Tables 21-4 and 21-5 list some of the disease states and potentials for drug interactions that make acetaminophen a more acceptable antipyretic analgesic than aspirin or related NSAIDs. Even though acetaminophen is not used to reduce inflammation, it can be effective in treating pain resulting from inflammation. Because of its low toxicity at therapeutic dosages (up to 4 g per day), acetaminophen is still considered first-line therapy for osteoarthritis, despite the fact that NSAIDs are generally more efficacious.[2,112] Acetaminophen remains the antipyretic of choice in children and teenagers because, unlike aspirin, it is not associated with the development of Reye's syndrome.

Therapeutic Uses in Dentistry

The wide publicity given to the adverse effects of aspirin has caused increasing numbers of dentists to substitute acetaminophen for aspirin in the treatment of postoperative dental pain, even though the antiinflammatory effects of acetaminophen are minor. In clinical studies, aspirin and acetaminophen are similar in their effectiveness in relieving pain after the extraction of third molars (Figure 21-16).[20,21]

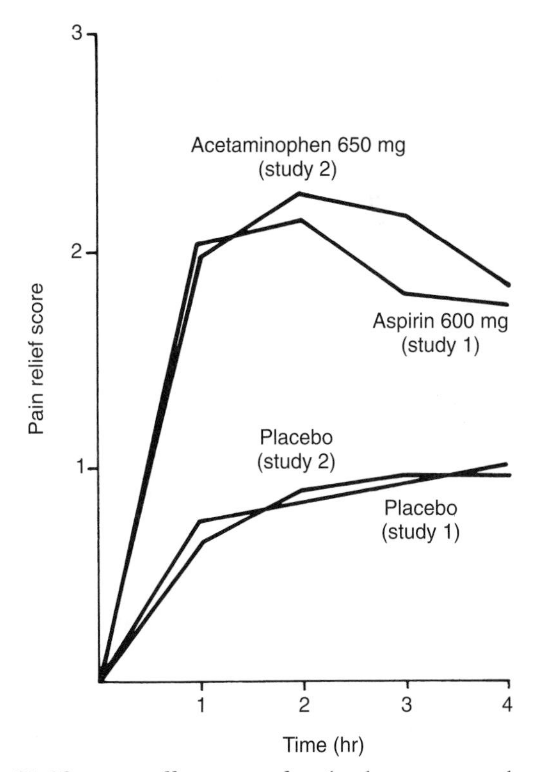

Fig. 21-16 Time-effect curves for placebo, aspirin, and acetaminophen. The mean pain relief scores are plotted against time in hours. (Adapted from Cooper SA, Breen JF, Giuliani RL: Replicate studies comparing the relative efficacies of aspirin and indoprofen in oral surgery outpatients, *J Clin Pharmacol* 19:151-159, 1979; The relative efficacy of indoprofen compared with opioid-analgesic combinations, *J Oral Surg* 39:21-25, 1981.)

Acetaminophen has a positive dose-effect curve for analgesia up to 1000 mg. On the basis of this finding, some clinicians are recommending the use of 1000 mg of acetaminophen rather than the customary 650-mg dose. For postsurgical dental pain, acetaminophen is most often used in combination with an opioid analgesic agent (see below).

Adverse Effects

The potential for adverse effects from acetaminophen seems to be confined to situations in which there is an acute overdose or an interaction with alcohol. At therapeutic doses, acetaminophen does not cause nausea, inhibit platelet aggregation, prolong prothrombin time, or produce the other side affects associated with the use of aspirin or NSAIDs. Allergy to acetaminophen is rare and is generally manifested as skin eruptions. In rare cases, acetaminophen has been associated with neutropenia, thrombocytopenia, and pancytopenia. Unlike phenacetin, acetaminophen rarely produces methemoglobinemia.

Acute overdose from acetaminophen has become a problem because of the extent of its use.[130] In 1992, acetaminophen-containing products accounted for more than 40% of all OTC analgesic drugs sold in the United States, and they remain popular today. Acetaminophen is frequently used in suicide attempts because of its availability in sizable quantities. The therapeutic index for acetaminophen is high; it is estimated that 6 g or more must be ingested within a relatively short time for hepatotoxicity to occur. In children younger than 10 years, a therapeutic overdose, which typically involves multiple dose miscalculations on the part of the parent administering the drug, has also led to severe hepatotoxicity. The degree of liver damage is directly related to the amount of drug ingested, and people with preexisting liver disease are most susceptible.

Hepatotoxicity appears to result from the formation of the highly reactive metabolite NAPQI, which normally reacts rapidly with glutathione and, as a result, is largely neutralized (see Figure 21-15). In acetaminophen overdose, this metabolite depletes glutathione and accumulates, resulting in the alkylation of liver proteins and cellular injury. When enough liver cells are damaged, clinical signs of toxicity, such as nausea and jaundice, appear.[130] In contrast to the rapid onset of toxic signs seen after an overdose with aspirin or related NSAIDs, clinical manifestations of acetaminophen poisoning may not appear until several days after ingestion of the drug, thus making diagnosis and treatment much more difficult than with aspirin overdose. Severe hepatotoxicity after acetaminophen overdose is a life-threatening situation. Fortunately, there is a satisfactory treatment for acetaminophen overdose if initiated in sufficient time. Gastric lavage may be of some benefit if started within a few hours of drug ingestion, even before clinical signs of toxicity appear. N-Acetylcysteine is an effective treatment in many cases of toxicity. It enables the formation of new glutathione and dramatically reduces mortality rates. However, to be effective, N-acetylcysteine must be administered as soon as possible but usually not more than 36 hours after ingestion. A better response is obtained if N-acetylcysteine is given within 10 hours. N-Acetylcysteine is administered orally or intravenously. At present, acetaminophen overdose presents a more dangerous and difficult management problem than does aspirin overdose. The clinician should not be lured into a false sense of security because of acetaminophen's relative freedom from adverse effects at therapeutic doses. To some extent, the dramatic rise in reported cases of acetaminophen toxicity results from a reluctance of the health professions to realize the potential hazards of this drug and to warn their patients of the consequences of misuse.

The potential adverse drug interaction between acetaminophen and alcohol is complex and often difficult to predict.[120] As with acetaminophen overdosage, prolonged alcohol use is associated with hepatotoxicity. In patients who consume alcohol regularly, CYP2E1 is highly induced. CYP2E1 promotes the conversion of acetaminophen to NAPQI. In addition, hepatic glutathione, usually available to bind and inactivate NAPQI, tends to be depleted in chronic alcohol consumers. The dilemma in predicting this drug interaction is that when patients are actively consuming alcohol, CYP2E1 is preferentially occupied by alcohol and not acetaminophen, which may limit the production of NAPQI. This protective effect of alcohol has been demonstrated in suicidal patients showing little hepatotoxicity after ingesting acute overdoses of acetaminophen in combination with large quantities of alcohol. Patients may in fact be at greatest risk of hepatotoxicity when, after prolonged alcohol consumption (which may be as little as a few drinks every day), they stop drinking and begin taking acetaminophen for fever or pain.[58] In this scenario, CYP2E1 is induced, alcohol is no longer present, and the enzyme is free to convert a large portion of the acetaminophen to NAPQI. Our current understanding of this interaction in no way suggests that acetaminophen is a safe drug in alcoholic patients. Other factors that are prevalent in this population, such as reduced glutathione stores, preexisting liver damage, and malnutrition, may further predispose the alcoholic to acetaminophen-induced hepatotoxicity.

COMBINATION ANALGESICS

Nonopioids

Aspirin and acetaminophen are sometimes combined in proprietary compounds (Table 21-7). There is little evidence, however, that either analgesia or antipyresis is enhanced by this combination. A ceiling effect still occurs when the total amount of aspirin and acetaminophen approaches 1 g. The rationale for combining an NSAID with acetaminophen, although still debated, appears to have some justification based on the fact that acetaminophen has some actions that are distinct from those of the NSAIDs. Acetaminophen has been found to inhibit COX-3, a newly characterized cyclooxygenase isozyme.[141]

Many of these combinations also contain caffeine. Caffeine is considered to be an analgesic adjuvant.[77] Caffeine does not appear to have analgesic effects when used alone. However, when 65 to 100 mg of caffeine is combined with traditional analgesics (aspirin, acetaminophen, or ibuprofen), it improves their analgesic efficacy.[44,77] The mechanism for this adjuvant effect is not known but may include the ability of caffeine to block adenosine receptors at free nerve endings or in mast cells, to enhance central catecholamine effects, or to increase the absorption of weak acids such as aspirin.[111] The central vasoconstrictive effects of caffeine probably help alleviate certain types of headache.

Opioid and Nonopioid Analgesics

There is a sound scientific basis for combining NSAIDs or acetaminophen with opioids. The former drugs combat pain principally by interfering with production of biochemical mediators that cause sensitization of nerve endings at the site of injury or spinal cord, whereas the opioids alter CNS perception and reaction to pain. These complementary actions support the use of the drugs in combination.[136] In addition to the fact that these combinations seem reasonable, abundant clinical data exist to support the validity of their combined use.[7,93,94] However, there is a common misconception that such combinations produce a synergistic phenomenon, that is,

Table • 21-7

Some Analgesic Combinations Used in Dentistry

NONPROPRIETARY (GENERIC) NAME	PROPRIETARY (TRADE) NAME	CONTAINS (mg) ASA	APAP	OTHER INGREDIENTS	AVERAGE ADULT DOSE	SCHEDULE
ASA, caffeine	Anacin	400	—	Caffeine, 32	2 q4h	OTC
ASA, APAP, caffeine	Excedrin	250	250	Caffeine, 65	1 to 2 q4h	OTC
ASA, codeine	Empirin with codeine					
	#2	325	—	Codeine, 15	2 q4h	Rx III
	#3	325	—	Codeine, 30	1 to 2 q4h	Rx III
	#4	325	—	Codeine, 60	1 q4h	Rx III
APAP, codeine	Tylenol with codeine					
	#2	—	300	Codeine, 15	2 q4h	Rx III
	#3	—	300	Codeine, 30	1 to 2 q4h	Rx III
	#4	—	300	Codeine, 60	1 q4h	Rx III
APAP, hydrocodone	Lortab 5/500, Vicodin	—	500	Hydrocodone, 5	1 to 2 q4-6h	Rx III
	Lorcet Plus	—	650	Hydrocodone, 7.5	1 q4-6h	Rx III
	Lorcet 10/650	—	650	Hydrocodone, 10	1 q4-6h	Rx III
	Vicodin HS	—	660	Hydrocodone, 10	1 q4-6h	Rx III
	Vicodin ES	—	750	Hydrocodone, 7.5	1 q4-6h	Rx III
	Maxidone	—	750	Hydrocodone, 10	1 q4-6h	Rx III
ASA, oxycodone	Percodan-demi	325	—	Oxycodone, 2.44*	1 to 2 q6h	Rx II
	Percodan	325	—	Oxycodone, 4.88*	1 q6h	Rx II
APAP, oxycodone	Percocet 5/325	—	325	Oxycodone, 5	1 to 2 q4-6h	Rx II
	Tylox	—	500	Oxycodone, 5	1 to 2 q4-6h	Rx II
	Percocet 7.5/500	—	500	Oxycodone, 7.5	1 to 2 q4-6h	Rx II
	Percocet 10/650	—	650	Oxycodone, 10	1 q4-6h	Rx II
ASA, pentazocine	Talwin Compound	325	—	Pentazocine, 12.5	2 q4-6h	Rx IV
APAP, pentazocine	Talacen	—	650	Pentazocine, 25	1 q4-6h	Rx IV
APAP, propoxyphene N	Darvocet N 100	—	650	Propoxyphene N, 100	1 q4h	Rx IV
APAP, tramadol	Ultracet	—	325	Tramadol, 37.5	2 q4-6h	Rx
ASA, caffeine, butalbital	Fiorinal	325	—	Caffeine, 40 Butalbital, 50	1 to 2 q4h	Rx III
APAP, caffeine, butalbital	Fioricet	—	325	Caffeine, 40 Butalbital, 50	1 to 2 q4h	Rx III
ASA, caffeine, butalbital, codeine	Fiorinal with codeine	325	—	Same as Fiorinal, plus codeine, 30	1 to 2 q4h	Rx III
ASA, caffeine, dihydrocodeine	Synalgos-DC	356.4	—	Caffeine, 30 Dihydrocodeine, 16	1 to 2 q4h	Rx III
ASA, caffeine, propoxyphene HCl	Darvon Compound	389	—	Caffeine, 32.4	1 to 2 q4h	Rx IV
ASA, meprobamate	Equagesic	325	—	Meprobamate, 200	1 to 2 q4h	Rx IV
Ibuprofen, hydrocodone	Vicoprofin	—	—	Ibuprofen, 200 Hydrocodone, 7.5	1 q4-6h	Rx III

*Formulation contains a mixture of two different oxycodone salts.

ASA, Aspirin; *APAP,* acetaminophen; *HCl,* hydrochloride; *Rx,* prescription.

NOTE: No attempt has been made to present a complete listing of drug combinations or proprietary preparations (which are available in a dazzling variety of dosage forms). Such listings can be found in a variety of sources, including *Facts and Comparisons* and *Physicians' Desk Reference*. It should be noted that a number of the combinations provide less than optimal amounts of aspirin or acetaminophen. In such cases, taking two tablets instead of one would remedy this problem. However, with some drug preparations such as Empirin or Tylenol with codeine #4, this would result in administration of an excessive amount of the opioid analgesic, and unwanted side effects could occur.

a total effect greater than the sum of individual effects expected from both drugs. No evidence currently supports this belief, and, at best, there is a purely additive effect when drugs from these two classes of analgesics are combined. Indeed, if any synergism does exist, it probably involves toxic effects rather than analgesia.

Another misconception is that the opioid component in an oral analgesic combination is the major contributor to the preparation's overall effectiveness. Clinical studies indicate quite the opposite, showing that the nonopioid component is an equal or, more often, greater contributor to the overall efficacy of the combination for most types of pain. When comparisons are limited to studies evaluating dental pain, there is no question that the aspirinlike drugs provide most of the pain relief.[18,22] The opioids are, however, most often the cause of side effects.[7,26]

The clinical significance of the opioids is that they provide additional analgesia beyond the ceiling effect of the NSAID or acetaminophen alone, and they also contribute a centrally mediated sedative effect. Therefore the most effective combinations are those that use the optimal amount of an aspirinlike drug combined with the appropriate dose of an opioid analgesic.

Analgesic Combinations That Include a Sedative

Some proprietary compounds combine peripherally acting analgesics with either a sedative or both a sedative and an opioid analgesic. The rationale is that patients with pain usually have anxiety, which a sedative drug may help alleviate. Such fixed-dose combined drugs provide a convenient method to administer an analgesic and sedative with one prescription. On the other hand, the use of fixed-dose combinations makes it difficult to adjust the dosage of the various constituents to the individual needs of a patient. Another good argument against the fixed-dose combined drugs is that they increase the potential for adverse drug interactions. This problem is compounded further if the patient receives psychoactive drugs during treatment that could have effects that carry over into the postoperative period.

Examples of sedatives found in the fixed-dose combined drugs are butalbital, meprobamate, and the antihistamines phenyltoloxamine and pyrilamine. There is little published evidence that sedative drugs either adversely affect the pain threshold or in any way contribute to the analgesic efficacy of the combination. However, they are capable of blunting behavioral responses, which sometimes may be mistaken for an increase in the pain threshold.

Oral Analgesic Combinations Used in Dentistry

Although the pharmacologic features of the opioids are discussed thoroughly in Chapter 20, it is appropriate to mention here some of the combinations of opioids and peripherally acting analgesics that are widely used in dentistry. Many opioid analgesics have poor oral/intramuscular (PO/IM) potency ratios because of low oral bioavailability. After oral administration, several opioids are rapidly absorbed into the portal system and mostly transformed to inactive metabolites on their first pass through the liver. For example, to equal the effect of 10 mg of morphine administered intramuscularly, about 60 mg of oral morphine would have to be given, in accord with the drug's PO/IM potency ratio of 0.16. A low PO/IM potency ratio also means that unpredictable and sometimes dangerous effects may occur because individuals show great variability in their metabolic efficiencies. The highest PO/IM potency ratio for any of the commonly used centrally acting analgesics is about 0.5 for drugs such as codeine, hydrocodone, and oxycodone.

Another general problem with the opioid analgesics is their relatively high incidence of undesirable side effects. They all cause nausea and CNS depression, which become more intense as the dosage is increased. Mild CNS depression manifested as sedation may sometimes be useful, but ambulatory dental patients generally want to be able to function normally after they leave the dental office.

Codeine is a commonly used opioid in combination analgesics. Its effective oral dose range is 30 to 90 mg, 30 mg providing only minimal analgesia, 60 mg providing a little more analgesia with considerably more nausea and sedation, and 90 mg approaching the dose at which intolerable side effects appear. Codeine is available in combination with aspirin or acetaminophen. For most patients, 600 to 650 mg of either drug combined with 60 mg of codeine should provide adequate pain relief for most acute dental pain situations.[7,22,23]

Hydrocodone and oxycodone are close analogues of codeine but are approximately 5 and 10 times more potent, respectively.[8] Hydrocodone/acetaminophen combinations (see Table 21-7) are now the most widely prescribed analgesics in the United States. A formulation combining ibuprofen 200 mg with hydrocodone 7.5 mg is also being marketed, but in reality the 200 mg ibuprofen dose is suboptimal. In patients with severe pain, 10 mg of oxycodone combined with either aspirin or acetaminophen is an effective oral analgesic combination, although side effects such as nausea, dizziness, and sedation should be expected.

Propoxyphene (hydrochloride or napsylate) was also very popular in analgesic combinations. However, its therapeutic efficacy is questionable. Some investigators have found that propoxyphene is slightly less potent than codeine, whereas others claim it is no more effective than a placebo. Propoxyphene combinations with aspirin or acetaminophen are listed in Table 21-7. It is usually assumed that 65 mg of propoxyphene hydrochloride is needed to achieve significant analgesia over and above the effect of aspirin or acetaminophen with which it is combined.

Pentazocine, an opioid with mixed agonist-antagonist activity, is available in combination with aspirin and with acetaminophen. It offers no therapeutic advantages over codeine. At the recommended dose of 50 mg, pentazocine is about as effective as 60 mg of codeine. However, most combinations only provide for a maximum of 25 mg of pentazocine per tablet.

Other opioid or opioidlike drugs may be used in combination, but the majority of drug combinations on the market include codeine, hydrocodone, oxycodone, propoxyphene, or pentazocine combined with either aspirin or acetaminophen (see Table 21-7). Opioids such as morphine, meperidine, and oxymorphone have such low PO/IM potency ratios that they are of little use in routine oral analgesic therapy. In general, single-entity opioid analgesics are not the drugs of choice for the management of acute dental pain in ambulatory patients.

Implications for Dentistry

Abundant evidence suggests that dental pain is most amenable to treatment by NSAID analgesics and acetaminophen, and these drugs have become the mainstay for management of acute dental pain. Their use, however, is associated with some risks that are readily reduced by understanding the pharmacologic characteristics of these drugs, including the contraindications and precautions to be followed in selected populations. Opioid combination drugs are most useful in patients with a strong emotional component to their pain, in whom the mood-altering and sedative effects of the opioid are most desirable. Side effects of drowsiness, impaired psychomotor function, and nausea are common with these drugs and should be expected. In addition, the practicing dentist must be aware of the drug-seeking patient who will often request a prescription including a specific opioid, most often oxycodone. Chapter 47 presents a more detailed approach for selecting an appropriate analgesic for particular dental indications.

MISCELLANEOUS AGENTS FOR RHEUMATOID ARTHRITIS

Several groups of compounds unrelated to the NSAIDs and to the adrenal corticosteroids considered in Chapter 35 are useful in suppressing the signs and symptoms of rheumatoid arthritis. These drugs are relatively toxic, and they are for the most part restricted to rapidly progressing or refractory cases of arthritis and patients unable to tolerate standard medications. They are often referred to as *disease-modifying antirheumatic drugs* because they can alter the progression of the disease.[92]

Gold Compounds

Medicinal preparations containing gold historically have been used to treat certain inflammatory conditions. Because of their toxicity, their use is now restricted to rheumatoid arthritis. Gold compounds are generally indicated in active cases where the arthritis steadily progresses despite an adequate regimen of NSAIDs, rest, and exercise therapy. In such cases, chrysotherapy (therapy with aurothioglucose or auranofin) usually induces a partial or complete remission of the disease and not merely a palliation of symptoms. Parenteral gold has been shown to reduce the number of bony erosions in joint tissue.[115] The duration of these remissions is highly variable, however.

The exact mechanism by which gold formulations suppress inflammation is unknown. Gold compounds inhibit PG synthesis, suppress cellular immune reactions, inhibit lysosomal hydrolases, inactivate the classic and alternative complement pathways, and, in particular, diminish the phagocytic activity of mononuclear cells. The relationship of these diverse actions to the observed clinical effects is not clear. Unlike the NSAIDs, gold salts have no antipyretic or analgesic properties in nonrheumatic conditions.

Because conventional gold salts such as aurothioglucose are not well absorbed by the gastrointestinal tract, the dosage is given by intramuscular injection. The distribution of gold is complex and depends on the dose and dosing interval. The plasma half-life increases with each subsequent dose because of tissue binding, and months may be required for mean blood concentrations to reach a plateau. After some period of constant weekly injections, gold accumulates in various tissues to such an extent that it may be continuously excreted for many months after administration has ceased. More than half of an administered dose is eventually eliminated in the urine and the remainder in the feces.

Parenteral chrysotherapy is complicated by a number of occasionally serious adverse reactions. The toxicity of aurothioglucose may initially be manifested by mucocutaneous lesions. These include pruritus, dermatitis (ranging from mild to severe), stomatitis (including glossitis), colitis, and vaginitis. Blood dyscrasias, including leukopenia, agranulocytosis, and aplastic anemia, have been reported. A nitritoid reaction, resembling the orthostatic hypotension, facial flushing, and nausea often seen with nitroglycerin administration, may occur shortly after the injection. Toxic effects involving the liver, kidney, and CNS can also occur. These adverse effects appear to be dose related and may develop at any time during chrysotherapy.

Auranofin is an orally effective form of gold. It appears to be less toxic than parenteral chrysotherapy; the major adverse effect is diarrhea rather than skin rash and bone marrow depression. However, the latter problems can still occur. Auranofin also appears to be less effective than the injectable form of gold. The choice between auranofin and aurothioglucose is based on the seriousness of the illness, responsiveness to previous therapy, and desire to avoid injections.

Antimalarial Agents

Both chloroquine and, more frequently, hydroxychloroquine have antiinflammatory effects that have been used in the treatment of rheumatoid arthritis and lupus erythematosus.[76] The drugs are generally administered in conjunction with other antiinflammatory agents for the relief of mild early rheumatoid arthritis, or they may be used as alternatives to gold compounds or penicillamine (see below) in more severe cases when NSAIDs are no longer effective. Clinical improvement is usually very slow, requiring 3 to 6 months. After this time, if there is no evidence of benefit, the drug is discontinued.

Serious ocular toxicity has been caused by these drugs; the retinopathy is dose related and may progress even after therapy is discontinued. This effect has made the antimalarial drugs controversial as antirheumatic agents and mandates regular ophthalmologic testing during therapy.[4] Other toxic effects include gastrointestinal, dermatologic, and neuropsychiatric disturbances.

Penicillamine

Penicillamine, a degradation product of penicillin used as a chelating agent in the treatment of heavy metal poisoning (see Chapter 52), was first reported in 1970 to be effective in rheumatoid arthritis. Its mode of action is unknown; penicillamine has both immunosuppressive and immunostimulant properties but is devoid of antibacterial activity. Penicillamine, like gold compounds, is indicated in cases of rheumatoid arthritis that are refractory to salicylates or related compounds. As with chrysotherapy, penicillamine must be administered for several months before clinical improvement is noted. Side effects are frequent, usually occurring early in therapy. Skin rash similar to that caused by ampicillin is common, as are gastrointestinal reactions and taste disturbances. To a lesser extent, nephropathy and thrombocytopenia also occur. The drug must be withdrawn from approximately one third of patients because of adverse reactions.[67]

Sulfasalazine

Sulfasalazine is a sulfonamide derivative that has been used for the treatment of ulcerative colitis and, in a delayed release form, for the management of rheumatoid arthritis in patients not adequately responding to NSAIDs. The agent has both antiinflammatory and immunomodulatory effects. After oral administration, sulfasalazine is hydrolyzed by enteric bacteria to yield the sulfonamide sulfapyridine and 5-aminosalicylate. Although 5-aminosalicylate is the active moiety against ulcerative colitis, there is no consensus regarding the drug's mechanism of action in rheumatoid arthritis. Gastrointestinal disturbances are the most frequently observed side effects; blood dyscrasias occurring early in therapy are among the most serious. Patients who have a history of allergy to sulfonamides or salicylates should not receive sulfasalazine.

Immunosuppressants

The immunosuppressants azathioprine and cyclosporine (see Chapter 41) and the antineoplastics cyclophosphamide and methotrexate (see Chapter 42) are effective in relieving symptoms of rheumatoid arthritis.[5] In fact, when NSAID therapy fails to relieve the symptoms, methotrexate has become the initial second-line drug in treating many patients with rheumatoid arthritis. Compared with gold, antimalarials, and penicillamine, methotrexate's onset of action is more rapid and it tends to have better efficacy than do these compounds or the immunosuppressants azathioprine or cyclosporine.[16,71,142] Symptomatic improvement from methotrexate therapy administered once per week can be seen in as little as 3 weeks. Because methotrexate, cyclophosphamide, azathioprine, and cyclosporine are general systemic immunosuppressants and affect a number of components in the inflammatory response, the exact mechanism by which such drugs ameliorate rheumatoid arthritis is unknown. In the treatment of rheumatoid arthritis the dosages of these drugs are less than those used in antineoplastic therapy or organ rejection therapy so the incidence of serious adverse effects is also less. However, these drugs can still cause serious toxicity in this patient population, such as promoting infections, blood dyscrasias, nephrotoxicity, and neoplastic transformation, and they should be used only in patients for whom NSAID therapy has failed. The concomitant use of NSAIDs can displace methotrexate from plasma proteins and thus increase free methotrexate blood concentrations and toxicity. However, this pharmacokinetic interaction appears most important with high-dose methotrexate therapy used in cancer and not low-dose methotrexate therapy used in the treatment of rheumatoid arthritis.[58] In addition, because cyclosporine is metabolized by the CYP3A4 isoenzyme, inhibitors of this enzyme such as erythromycin, clarithromycin, and the azole antifungal drugs can dramatically increase cyclosporine blood concentrations and associated toxicities, including irreversible nephrotoxicity.[62]

Leflunomide is a recently introduced immunomodulatory drug that inhibits dihydroorotate dehydrogenase, an enzyme involved in pyrimidine synthesis. The resulting antiproliferative and antiinflammatory activity is useful in the treatment of active rheumatoid arthritis and produces similar benefits to that of methotrexate. An active metabolite of leflunomide, termed *M1*, is responsible for essentially all of the drug's action. Because M1 has a half-life of approximately 2 weeks, a loading dose schedule must be used to achieve therapeutic concentrations in several days (rather than the 2 months normally required). Adverse effects attributed to leflunomide include alopecia, skin rash, and elevated liver enzymes. The drug should not be taken with other hepatotoxic drugs; coadministration of rifampin can significantly elevate the concentration of M1. A pregnancy category X agent, leflunomide is fetotoxic and contraindicated in pregnant women.

Biologic Agents

Recent advances in biotechnology have lead to the development of biologic agents that selectively target specific pathogenic components of the immune response without causing generalized immunosuppression. Two recently approved intravenously administered agents, infliximab and etanercept, target TNF-α. Infliximab is a chimeric IgG1 monoclonal antibody composed of human constant and murine variable regions,[114] whereas etanercept is a dimeric fusion protein consisting of the extracellular ligand-binding portion of the TNF receptor linked to the Fc portion of human IgG1.[145] Both drugs bind specifically to TNF-α and then inhibit the binding of TNF-α to its receptor located on various inflammatory cell types. Through this action, the biological activity of TNF-α is neutralized, including the ability of TNF-α to induce IL-1 and IL-6, enhance leukocyte migration, and activate neutrophils and eosinophils. These drugs are typically used in patients with the most advanced forms of the disease and in whom methotrexate therapy has failed to alleviate the symptoms. Infliximab is given in combination with low-dose methotrexate therapy, whereas etanercept can be administered alone or in combination with low-dose methotrexate therapy. Infliximab is also approved for the treatment of the signs and symptoms of Crohn's disease. Although these drugs are not generalized immunosuppressants, serious and sometimes fatal infections have been reported in patients receiving either agent. Many of these events have occurred in patients who were receiving concomitant immunosuppressive therapy with drugs such as methotrexate or azathioprine. Infusion reactions such as chills, fever, and urticaria have also been reported and are more likely to occur in patients who have antibodies develop to either infliximab or etanercept.

DRUGS USED TO TREAT GOUT

Gout is an inflammatory disease that stems from elevated concentrations of uric acid in blood and other body fluids. Such elevations may be the result of either increased production (metabolic gout) or decreased excretion (renal gout) of uric acid. Decreased excretion is usually the major contributing factor. Reduced elimination may result from an inability to properly excrete uric acid, from renal disease, or from certain drugs that reduce renal excretion of uric acid. Overproduction may be caused by a primary defect in purine metabolism, such as a deficiency in the enzyme phosphoribosyl transferase, or be caused by certain hematologic disorders, leukemias, cancer chemotherapy, or effects of ethanol.

Essentially all the clinical manifestations of gout derive from the precipitation of sodium urate from extracellular fluids when and where it exceeds the limits of solubility. These manifestations can be divided into four categories: acute gouty arthritis, tophaceous deposits (sodium urate deposits in cartilage, bone, bursae, and subcutaneous tissue in and around joints), uric acid nephrolithiasis, and gouty kidney with various degrees of impairment of renal function. Of all these, gouty arthritis is most frequently the first clinical manifestation of the disease. Intensive study of the mechanism of gouty arthritis has shown it to be an inflammatory reaction to sodium urate microcrystals deposited in synovial fluid. Precisely how these crystals initiate inflammation is not known. The generation of reactive oxygen species has been proposed.[53,133] The crystals can activate Hageman factor and in this way initiate the chain of events leading to bradykinin formation. Large numbers of neutrophils accumulate in the synovium, possibly because of a chemotactic effect of uric acid. These neutrophils actively phagocytize urate crystals, leading to release of lysosomal enzymes and increased lactic acid production. Both these events tend to propagate the inflammatory response, the former by damaging tissue and the latter by lowering the local pH and thus fostering further urate deposition. A glycoprotein released by neutrophils after the ingestion of urate crystals has been shown to replicate the histopathologic characteristics of gout on injection into normal joints.

Although the overall pathogenesis of gouty arthritis is understood, many specific events are still obscure. It is known that acute gouty arthritis often follows a precipitating event. Surgery, injury, alcohol ingestion, dietary excess, emotional crisis, or even the minor stress of walking can elicit an acute attack, but it is not known how these events are related to urate crystal deposition. Another unknown is the reason why less than 10% of gout occurs in women.

Acute gouty arthritis is clinically characterized by severe inflammation of the joint and periarticular tissues. One or several joints may be involved simultaneously, as shown by marked swelling, redness, heat, and intense pain. Lymphadenitis is occasionally present. There may also be systemic signs of inflammation, including fever, leukocytosis, and an increased erythrocyte sedimentation rate. Without treatment, the arthritis gradually subsides over a period of 1 to 2 weeks. The rate of recurrence is variable after an initial attack, but in most patients recurrence is common, usually within a year. With increasing age, the incidence of attacks increases, as does the severity, duration of inflammation, and number of joints affected. The patient may in time rarely be free of gouty arthritis, and the pain, swelling, and stiffness can result in total and permanent disability.

The treatment of gout may involve multiple agents acting at different sites and having distinctly different objectives. Because the pathologic manifestations of the disease result from an elevated extracellular uric acid titer, a rational therapeutic maneuver is to lower urate concentrations. Two approaches toward this end are currently available: the use of uricosuric drugs to increase renal urate clearance and the use of allopurinol to inhibit urate synthesis.

The uricosuric agents most often used are probenecid and sulfinpyrazone (Figure 21-17). Both of these anionic compounds can actually enhance urate retention by blocking its renal tubular secretion or by participating in an anion exchange reaction with urate. At higher doses, however, these agents block the quantitatively more important process of tubular reabsorption of urate, thus increasing the urinary excretion of uric acid and lowering plasma urate concentrations. Uricosuric drugs are used primarily in chronic gout to prevent the formation of new tophi and to slowly mobilize urate deposits in old lesions. They are not useful in treating attacks of gouty arthritis, because mobilization of previously deposited urates may initially increase the severity of the attack. Furthermore, the use of uricosuric drugs may lead to the formation of renal urate stones in the presence of a high plasma uric acid concentration. Maintenance of an alkaline diuresis during therapy with uricosuric agents is important. The pK_a of uric acid is 5.6, and the solubility of the nonionized form is low. Thus an alkaline environment will minimize intrarenal deposition. Both probenecid and sulfinpyrazone are initially given in low doses, which are gradually increased until the desired serum urate concentration is obtained (usually 6 mg/dl); a maintenance dose is then established. Both drugs are generally well tolerated. The most common adverse effects are gastrointestinal disturbances and allergic reactions ranging from dermatitis to anaphylaxis. Although the salicylates are uricosuric at high doses, they are no longer used for this purpose. Because salicylates at ordinary doses may decrease urate excretion (see Table 21-4), they should be used cautiously in patients with gout.

Allopurinol (see Figure 21-17) and its metabolite alloxanthine (oxypurinol) are inhibitors of the enzyme xanthine oxidase. Most of the effect on uric acid appears to be caused by alloxanthine because it has a considerably longer half-life than allopurinol. Also, whereas allopurinol is a competitive inhibitor, alloxanthine is a noncompetitive inhibitor of xanthine oxidase, with a higher potency than allopurinol. Xanthine oxidase catalyzes the oxidation of hypoxanthine to xanthine and then to uric acid. The action of allopurinol is therefore to reduce the biosynthesis of uric acid and lower both blood and urine concentrations. The uric acid precursors do not accumulate in body fluids because they are sufficiently cleared by the kidney. Like the uricosuric agents, allopurinol is indicated for chronic rather than acute gout. It may be preferred in the more severe forms over the uricosuric agents. As with the uricosuric agents, allopurinol may initially increase the number of acute attacks of gouty arthritis unless colchicine prophylaxis, as described below, is used. The toxic effects of allopurinol include allergic reactions involving the skin (e.g., exfoliative, urticarial, and purpuric lesions) and blood (e.g., leukopenia, thrombocytopenia, agranulocytosis). There is a modest incidence of gastric irritation.

In addition to efforts aimed at reducing the extracellular uric acid concentration, another aspect of therapy for gout is management of acute arthritis. This goal entails the short-term use of antiinflammatory agents, some of which (indomethacin, naproxen, and sulindac) have already been described. Although these drugs have no specific actions in gouty arthritis, they can effectively relieve the pain, tenderness, and swelling in affected joints.

The most widely used drug to treat severe gouty arthritis is colchicine, a plant alkaloid with a long history of use in gout (see Figure 21-17). When given at the first indication of an attack, colchicine effects a striking reduction of the emerging signs and symptoms of arthritis. Pain begins to disappear within 4 to 12 hours after oral medication and is completely gone after 24 to 48 hours. Intravenous administration leads to a more rapid onset of action and is preferred for some patients. Colchicine is relatively specific for this condition; the drug has little effect on other inflammatory conditions and it does not have inherent analgesic properties. Colchicine may also be given prophylactically to prevent recurrent attacks.

The antiinflammatory effects of colchicine are believed to derive from its well-known antimitotic activity. It arrests mitosis in metaphase by binding to microtubular protein and preventing spindle formation. By a similar action, colchicine disrupts fibrillar microtubules in neutrophils and other motile cells. The involvement of the microtubular system in cell locomotion could explain colchicine's inhibition of neutrophil migration and phagocytic activity in inflamed joints.[3] This action is thought to inhibit the neutrophil's engulfment of uric acid crystals, preventing the subsequent release of destructive lysosomal enzymes into the extracellular environment.

Colchicine is rapidly absorbed from the gastrointestinal tract. The drug is partially metabolized in the liver, and the metabolites and unchanged drug are excreted in the feces for up to 10 days after a single dose. This finding may explain

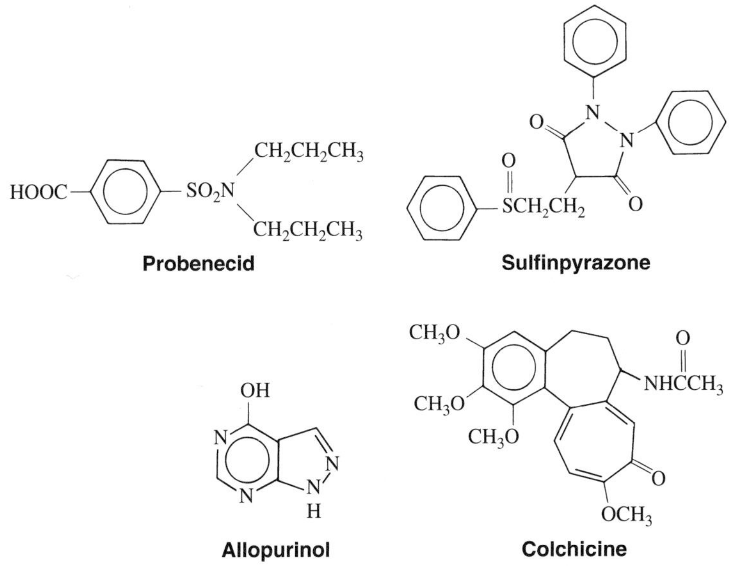

$HOOC-C_6H_4-SO_2N(CH_2CH_2CH_3)_2$

Probenecid

Sulfinpyrazone

Allopurinol

Colchicine

Fig. 21-17 Drugs used in the prevention and treatment of gout.

why the gastrointestinal tract is a frequent site of adverse reactions.

The most common untoward effects of colchicine are nausea, vomiting, and diarrhea. Diarrhea is an important sign because it may signal more serious toxic reactions, such as hemorrhagic gastroenteritis. The gastrointestinal effects of colchicine may result from direct toxicity to intestinal mucosal cells. Long-term use of colchicine may lead to bone marrow depression, myopathy, and alopecia.

NSAIDs, Analgesic Combinations, and Antirheumatic and Antigout Drugs

Nonproprietary (generic) name	*Proprietary (trade) name*
Salicylates*	
Choline magnesium trisalicylate	Trilisate
Choline salicylate	Arthropan
Magnesium salicylate	Magan, Mobidin
Salsalate	Amigesic, Disalcid
Sodium salicylate	—
Sodium thiosalicylate	Asproject, Rexolate
Other NSAIDs*	
Celecoxib	Celebrex
Diclofenac	Voltaren
Flurbiprofen	Ansaid
Indomethacin	Indocin
Meloxicam	Mobic
Nabumetone	Relafen
Oxaprozin	Daypro
Phenylbutazone†	Butazolidin
Piroxicam	Feldene
Sulindac	Clinoril
Tolmetin	Tolectin
Valdecoxib	Bextra
Analgesic combinations‡	
Other Antirheumatic Drugs	
Auranofin	Ridaura
Aurothioglucose	Solganal
Azathioprine	Imuran
Chloroquine	Aralen
Cyclophosphamide	Cytoxan
Etanercept	Enbrel
Gold sodium thiomalate	Aurolate, Myochrysine
Hydroxychloroquine	Plaquenil
Infliximab	Remicade
Leflunomide	Arava
Methotrexate	Rheumatrex
Penicillamine	Cuprimine
Antigout drugs	
Allopurinol	Zyloprim
Colchicine	—
Probenecid	Benemid
Sulfinpyrazone	Anturane

*See also Table 21-6.
†Not currently available in the United States.
‡See also Table 21-7.

Cited References

1. Allison AC: Role of macrophage activation in the pathogenesis of chronic inflammation and its pharmacological control, *Adv Inflamm Res* 7:201-221, 1984.
2. American College of Rheumatology Subcommittee on Osteoarthritis Guidelines: recommendations for the medical management of osteoarthritis of the hip and knee, *Arthritis Rheum* 43:1903-1915, 2000.
3. Asako H, Kubes P, Baethge BA, et al: Colchicine and methotrexate reduce leukocyte adherence and emigration in rat mesenteric venules, *Inflammation* 16:45-56, 1992.
4. Aylward JM: Hydroxychloroquine and chloroquine: assessing the risk of retinal toxicity, *J Am Optom Assoc* 64:787-797, 1993.
5. Bannwarth B, Labat L, Moride Y, et al: Methotrexate in rheumatoid arthritis. An update, *Drugs* 47:25-50, 1994.
6. Bansal V, Dex T, Proskin H, et al: A look at the safety profile of over-the-counter naproxen sodium: a meta-analysis, *J Clin Pharmacol* 41:127-138, 2001.
7. Beaver WT: Mild analgesics: a review of their clinical pharmacology, *Am J Med Sci* 250:577-604, 1965.
8. Beaver WT, Wallenstein SL, Rogers A, et al: Analgesic studies of codeine and oxycodone in patients with cancer, Part I, *J Pharmacol Exp Ther* 207:92-100, 1978.
9. Björkman R, Hallman KM, Hedner T, et al: Acetaminophen blocks spinal hyperalgesia induced by NMDA and substance P, *Pain* 57:259-264, 1994.
10. Bombardier C, Laine L, Reicin A, et al: Comparison of upper gastrointestinal toxicity of rofecoxib and naproxen in patients with rheumatoid arthritis, *N Engl J Med* 343:1520-1528, 2000.
11. Brater DC: Effects of nonsteroidal anti-inflammatory drugs on renal function: focus on cyclooxygenase-2-selective inhibition, *Am J Med* 107:65S-70S, 1999.
12. Brenner BE, Simon RR: Management of salicylate intoxication, *Drugs* 24:335-340, 1982.
13. Brooks PM, Day RO: Nonsteroidal anti-inflammatory drugs—differences and similarities, *N Engl J Med* 324:1716-1725, 1991.
14. Burka JF, Paterson NAM: Evidence for lipoxygenase pathway involvement in allergic tracheal contraction, *Prostaglandins* 19:499-515, 1980.
15. Chang DJ, Christensen KS, Bulloch SE, et al: Rofecoxib was more effective than codeine with acetaminophen for acute postoperative pain, *J Pain* 2(2 suppl 1):45, 2001.
16. Cohen S, Rustein J, Luggen M, et al: Comparison of the safety and efficacy of cyclosporine A and methotrexate in refractory rheumatoid arthritis: a randomized, multicentered, placebo-controlled trial, *Arthritis Rheum* 36:S56, 1993.
17. Cooper SA: The relative efficacy of ibuprofen in dental pain, *Compend Contin Ed Dent* 7:578-588, 1986.
18. Cooper SA, Beaver WT: A model to evaluate mild analgesics in oral surgery outpatients, *Clin Pharmacol Ther* 20:241-250, 1976.
19. Cooper SA, Berrie R, Cohn P: Comparison of ketoprofen, ibuprofen, and placebo in a dental surgery model, *Adv Ther* 5:43-53, 1988.

20. Cooper SA, Breen JF, Giuliani RL: Replicate studies comparing the relative efficacies of aspirin and indoprofen in oral surgery outpatients, *J Clin Pharmacol* 19:151-159, 1979.

21. Cooper SA, Breen JF, Giuliani RL: The relative efficacy of indoprofen compared with opioid-analgesic combinations, *J Oral Surg* 39:21-25, 1981.

22. Cooper SA, Engel J, Ladov M, et al: Analgesic efficacy of an ibuprofen-codeine combination, *Pharmacotherapy* 2:162-167, 1982.

23. Cooper SA, Firestein A, Cohn P: Double-blind comparison of meclofenamate sodium with acetaminophen, acetaminophen with codeine, and placebo for relief of postsurgical dental pain, *J Clin Dent* 1:31-34, 1988.

24. Cooper SA, Hersh EV, Betts NJ, et al: Multidose analgesic study of two mefenamic acid formulations in a postsurgical dental pain model, *Analgesia* 1:65-71, 1994.

25. Cooper SA, Needle SE, Kruger GO: Comparative analgesic potency of aspirin and ibuprofen, *J Oral Surg* 35:898-903, 1977.

26. Cooper SA, Precheur H, Rauch D, et al: Evaluation of oxycodone and acetaminophen in treatment of postoperative dental pain, *Oral Surg Oral Med Oral Pathol* 50:496-501, 1980.

27. Crofford LJ: COX-1 and COX-2 tissue expression: implications and predictions, *J Rheumatol* 24(suppl 49):15-19, 1997.

28. Dahlen SE, Hedqvist P, Hammarström S, et al: Leukotrienes are potent vasoconstrictors of human bronchi, *Nature* 288:484-486, 1980.

29. Dane AK. Treatment of fever in 1982: a review, *Am J Med* 74(suppl):27-35, 1983.

30. Daniels SE, Grossman EH, Kuss ME, et al: A double-blind, randomized comparison of intramuscularly and intravenously administered parecoxib sodium versus ketorolac and placebo in a post-oral surgery pain model, *Clin Ther* 23:1018-1031, 2001.

31. Davies P, Bailey PJ, Goldenberg MM, et al: The role of arachidonic acid oxygenation products in pain and inflammation, *Annu Rev Immunol* 2:335-357, 1984.

32. Day R, Morrison B, Luza A, et al: A randomized trial of the efficacy and tolerability of the COX-2 inhibitor rofecoxib vs. ibuprofen in patients with osteoarthritis. Rofecoxib/Ibuprofen Comparator Study Group, *Arch Intern Med* 160:1781-1787, 2000.

33. Department of Health and Human Services, Food and Drug Administration: Internal analgesic, antipyretic, and antirheumatic drug products for over-the-counter human use; final rule for professional labeling of aspirin, buffered aspirin, and aspirin in combination with antacid drug products, *Fed Regist* 63:56802-56819, 1998.

34. Desjardins PJ, Cooper SA, Mardirossian G: Meclofenamate sodium in dental pain, *Clin Pharmacol Ther* 41:212, 1987.

35. Dionne RA, Cooper SA: Delaying the onset of postoperative dental pain by pretreatment with ibuprofen, *Oral Surg Oral Med Oral Pathol* 45:851-856, 1978.

36. Dubois RN, Abramson SB, Crofford L, et al: Cyclooxygenase in biology and disease, *FASEB J* 12:1063-1073, 1998.

37. Eberhart CE, Coffey RJ, Radhika A, et al: Up-regulation of cyclooxygenase 2 gene expression in human colorectal adenomas and adenocarcinomas, *Gastroenterology* 107:1183-1188, 1994.

38. Ehrich EW, Dallob A, De Lepeleire I, et al: Characterization of rofecoxib as a cyclooxygenase-2 isoform inhibitor and demonstration of analgesia in the dental pain model, *Clin Pharmacol Ther* 65:336-347, 1999.

39. Emery P, Zeidler H, Kvein TK, et al: Celecoxib versus diclofenac in long-term management of rheumatoid arthritis: randomised double-blind comparison, *Lancet* 354:2106-2111, 1999.

40. Endres S, van der Meer JWM, Dinarello CA: Interleukin-1 in the pathogenesis of fever, *Eur J Clin Invest* 17:469-474, 1987.

41. Engelhardt G: Pharmacology of meloxicam, a new non-steroidal anti-inflammatory drug with an improved safety profile through preferential inhibition of COX-2, *Br J Rheumatol* 35(suppl 1):4-12, 1996.

42. Ferriera SH, Vane JR: New aspects of the mode of action of nonsteroid anti-inflammatory drugs, *Annu Rev Pharmacol* 14:57-73, 1974.

43. Flower RJ, Blackwell GJ: The importance of phospholipase-A_2 in prostaglandin biosynthesis, *Biochem Pharmacol* 25:285-291, 1976.

44. Forbes JA, Beaver WT, Jones KF, et al: Effect of caffeine on ibuprofen analgesia in postoperative oral surgery pain, *Clin Pharmacol Ther* 49:674-684, 1991.

45. Forbes JA, Beaver WT, White H, et al: Diflunisal: a new oral analgesic with an unusually long duration of action, *JAMA* 248:2139-2142, 1982.

46. Forbes JA, Butterworth GA, Burchfield WH, et al: Evaluation of ketorolac, aspirin, and an acetaminophen-codeine combination in postoperative oral surgery pain, *Pharmacotherapy* 10(6 pt 2):77S-93S, 1990.

47. Forbes JA, Kolodny AL, Beaver WT, et al: 12-hour evaluation of the analgesic efficacy of diflunisal, acetaminophen, an acetaminophen-codeine combination, and placebo in postoperative pain, *Pharmacotherapy* 3(2 pt 2):47S-54S, 1983.

48. Ford-Hutchinson AW, Bray MA, Doig MV, et al: Leukotriene B, a potent chemokinetic and aggregating substance released from polymorphonuclear leukocytes, *Nature* 286:264-265, 1980.

49. Fricke J, Halladay SC, Bynum L, et al: Pain relief after dental impaction surgery using ketorolac, hydrocodone plus acetaminophen, or placebo, *Clin Ther* 15:500-508, 1993.

50. Fricke JR, Halladay SC, Francisco CA: Efficacy and safety of naproxen sodium and ibuprofen for pain relief after oral surgery, *Curr Ther Res* 54:619-627, 1993.

51. Fricke JR, Jr, Angelocci D, Fox K, et al: Comparison of the efficacy and safety of ketorolac and meperidine in the relief of dental pain, *J Clin Pharmacol* 32:376-384, 1992.

52. Gaston GW, Mallow RD, Frank JE: Comparison of etodolac, aspirin and placebo for pain after oral surgery, *Pharmacotherapy* 6:199-205, 1986.

53. Ghio AJ, Kennedy TP, Rao G, et al: Complexation of iron cation by sodium urate crystals and gouty inflammation, *Arch Biochem Biophys* 313:215-221, 1994.

54. Giugliano D, Ceriello A, Saccomanno F, et al: Effect of salicylate, tolbutamide, and prostaglandin E_2 on insulin responses to glucose in noninsulin-dependent diabetes mellitus, *J Clin Endocrinol Metab* 61:160-166, 1985.

55. Glaser K, Sung ML, O'Neill K, et al: Etodolac selectively inhibits prostaglandin G/H synthetase 2 (PGHS-2) versus human PGHS-1, *Eur J Pharmacol* 281:107-111, 1995.
56. Greenberg HE, Gottesdiener K, Huntington M, et al: A new cyclooxygenase-2 inhibitor, rofecoxib (VIOXX@), did not alter the antiplatelet effects of low-dose aspirin in healthy volunteers, *J Clin Pharmacol* 40:1509-1515, 2000.
57. Gruber CM, Jr: Clinical pharmacology of fenoprofen: a review, *J Rheumatol* 3(suppl 2):8-17, 1976.
58. Haas DA: Adverse drug interactions in dental practice: interactions associated with analgesics. Part I in a series, *J Am Dent Assoc* 130:397-407, 1999.
59. Hamberg M: Inhibition of prostaglandin synthesis in man, *Biochem Biophys Res Commun* 49:720-726, 1972.
60. Hawkey C, Kahan A, Steinbruck K, et al: Gastrointestinal tolerability of meloxicam compared to diclofenac in osteoarthritis patients. International MELISSA Study Group. Meloxicam large-scale international study safety assessment, *Br J Rheumatol* 37:937-945, 1998.
61. Hennekens CH, Buring JE, Sandercock P, et al: Aspirin and other antiplatelet agents in the secondary and primary prevention of cardiovascular disease, *Circulation* 80:749-756, 1989.
62. Hersh EV: Adverse drug interactions in dental practice: interactions involving antibiotics. Part I of a series, *J Am Dent Assoc* 130:236-251, 1999.
63. Hersh EV, Cooper SA, Betts N, et al: Single dose and multidose study of ibuprofen and meclofenamate sodium after third molar surgery, *Oral Surg Oral Med Oral Pathol* 76:680-687, 1993.
64. Hersh EV, Levin LM, Cooper SA, et al: Conventional and extended-release etodolac for postsurgical dental pain, *Clin Ther* 21:1333-1342, 1999.
65. Hersh EV, Levin LM, Cooper SA, et al: Ibuprofen liquigel for oral surgery pain, *Clin Ther* 22:1306-1318, 2000.
66. Hersh EV, Moore PA, Ross GL: Over-the-counter analgesics and antipyretics: a critical assessment, *Clin Ther* 22:500-548, 2000.
67. Hochberg MC: Auranofin or D-penicillamine in the treatment of rheumatoid arthritis, *Ann Intern Med* 105:528-535, 1986.
68. Hurwitz ES: Reyes syndrome, *Epidemiol Rev* 11:249-253, 1989.
69. Hurwitz ES, Barrett MJ, Bregman D, et al: Public Health Service study of Reye's syndrome and medications: report of main study, *JAMA* 257:1905-1911, 1987.
70. Jeffcoat MK, Williams RC, Reddy MS, et al: Flurbiprofen treatment of human periodontitis: effect on alveolar bone height and metabolism, *J Periodontal Res* 23:381-385, 1988.
71. Jeurissen ME, Boerbooms AM, van de Putte LB, et al: Methotrexate versus azathioprine in the treatment of rheumatoid arthritis: a forty-eight week, randomized, double-blind trial, *Arthritis Rheum* 34:961-972, 1991.
72. Johnson AG, Nguyen TV, Day RO: Do nonsteroidal anti-inflammatory drugs affect blood pressure? A meta analysis, *Ann Intern Med* 121:289-300, 1994.
73. Kellstein DE, Waksman JA, Furey SA, et al: The safety profile of nonprescription ibuprofen in multiple-dose use: a meta-analysis, *J Clin Pharmacol* 39:520-532, 1999.
74. Kierch TA, Halladay SC, Hormel PC: A single-dose, double-blind comparison of naproxen sodium, acetaminophen, and placebo in postoperative dental pain, *Clin Ther* 16:394-404, 1994.
75. Kierch TA, Halladay SC, Koschick MS: A double-blind, randomized study of naproxen sodium, ibuprofen, and placebo in postoperative dental pain, *Clin Ther* 15:845-854, 1993.
76. Landewe RB, Miltenberg AM, Verdonk MJ, et al: Chloroquine inhibits T cell proliferation by interfering with IL-2 production and responsiveness, *Clin Exp Immunol* 102:144-151, 1995.
77. Laska EM, Sunshine A, Mueller F, et al: Caffeine as an analgesic adjuvant, *JAMA* 251:1711-1718, 1984.
78. Lecomte M, Laneuville O, Ji C, et al: Acetylation of human prostaglandin endoperoxide synthase-2 (cyclooxygenase-2) by aspirin, *J Biol Chem* 269:13207-13215, 1994.
79. Leese PT, Hubbard RC, Karim A, et al: Effects of celecoxib, a novel cyclooxygenase-2 inhibitor, on platelet function in healthy adults: A randomized, controlled trial, *J Clin Pharmacol* 40:124-132, 2000.
80. Leonards JR: The influence of solubility on the rate of gastrointestinal absorption of aspirin, *Clin Pharmacol Ther* 4:476-479, 1963.
81. Levy DA: Histamine and serotonin. In Weissman G, ed: *Mediators of inflammation*, New York, 1974, Plenum Press.
82. Levy G, Leonards JR: Absorption, metabolism, and excretion of salicylates. In Smith MJH, Smith PK, eds: *The salicylates*, New York, 1966, Interscience.
83. Lewis RA, Austen KF: The biologically active leukotrienes. Biosynthesis, metabolism, receptors, functions, and pharmacology, *J Clin Invest* 73:889-897, 1984.
84. Linnemann CC, Shea L, Partin JC, et al: Epidemiologic and viral studies 1963-1974, *Am J Epidemiol* 101:517-526, 1975.
85. Loll PJ, Picot D, Garavito RM: The structural basis of aspirin activity inferred from the crystal structure of inactivated prostaglandin H_2 synthase, *Nat Structural Biol* 2:637-643, 1995.
86. Malmberg AB, Yaksh TL: Antinociceptive actions of spinal nonsteroidal anti-inflammatory agents on the formalin test in the rat, *J Pharmacol Exp Ther* 263:136-146, 1992.
87. Malmstem CL: Prostaglandins, thromboxanes, and leukotrienes in inflammation, *Semin Arthritis Rheum* 15(2 suppl 1):29-35, 1985.
88. Malmstrom K, Daniels S, Kotey P, et al: Comparison of rofecoxib and celecoxib, two cyclooxygenase-2 inhibitors, in postoperative dental pain: a randomized, placebo- and active-comparator–controlled clinical trial, *Clin Ther* 21:1653-1663, 1999.
89. Malmstrom K, Kotey P, Coughlin H, et al: Efficacy of etoricoxib, naproxen sodium and acetaminophen/codeine in acute dental pain, *Clin Pharmacol Ther* 23:P2, 2001.
90. Mardirossian G, Cooper SA: Comparison of flurbiprofen and aspirin for postsurgical dental pain, *J Oral Maxillofac Surg* 43:106-109, 1985.
91. McCormack K: The spinal actions of nonsteroidal anti-inflammatory drugs and the dissociation between their anti-inflammatory and analgesic effects, *Drugs* 47(suppl 5):28-45, 1994.

92. Menkes CJ: Effects of disease-modifying anti-rheumatic drugs, steroids and non-steroidal anti-inflammatory drugs on acute-phase proteins in rheumatoid arthritis, *Br J Rheumatol* 23 (suppl 3):14-18, 1993.
93. Moertel CG, Ahmann DL, Taylor WF, et al: A comparative evaluation of marketed analgesic drugs, *N Engl J Med* 286:813-815, 1972.
94. Moertel CG, Ahmann DL, Taylor WF, et al: Relief of pain by oral medications. A controlled evaluation of analgesic combinations, *JAMA* 229:55-59, 1974.
95. Moore PA, Hersh EV: Celecoxib and rofecoxib: the role of COX-2 inhibitors in dental practice, *J Am Dent Assoc* 132:451-456, 2001.
96. Moore UJ, Seymour RA, Rawlins MD: The efficacy of locally applied aspirin and acetaminophen in postoperative pain after third molar surgery, *Clin Pharmacol Ther* 52:292-296, 1992.
97. Morrison BW, Christensen S, Yuan W, et al: Analgesic efficacy of the cyclooxygenase-2-specific inhibitor rofecoxib in post-dental surgery pain: A randomized, controlled trial, *Clin Ther* 21:943-953, 1999.
98. Murray MD, Brater DC: Renal toxicity of the nonsteroidal anti-inflammatory drugs, *Annu Rev Pharmacol Toxicol* 33:435-465, 1993.
99. Neustadt DH: Double blind evaluation of the long-term effects of etodolac versus ibuprofen in patients with rheumatoid arthritis, *J Rheumatol* 47(suppl):17-22, 1997.
100. Oates JA, Fitzgerald GA, Branch RA, et al: Clinical implications of prostaglandin and thromboxane A_2 formation, *N Engl J Med* 319:761-767, 1988.
101. O'Brien TP, Roszkowski MT, Wolff LF, et al: Effect of a non-steroidal anti-inflammatory drug on tissue levels of immunoreactive prostaglandin E_2, immunoreactive leukotriene B4, and pain after periodontal surgery, *J Periodontol* 67:1307-1316, 1996.
102. O'Hara DA, Fragen RJ, Kinzer M, et al: Ketorolac tromethamine as compared with morphine sulfate for treatment of postoperative pain, *Clin Pharmacol Ther* 41:556-561, 1987.
103. O'Neill GP, Mancini JA, Kargman S, et al: Overexpression of human prostaglandin G/H synthase-1 and -2 by recombinant vaccinia virus: inhibition by nonsteroidal anti-inflammatory drugs and biosynthesis of 15-hydroxyeicosatetraenoic acid, *Mol Pharmacol* 45:245-254, 1994.
104. Patrono C, Coller B, Dalen JE, et al: Platelet-active drugs: the relationships among dose, effectiveness and side effects, *Chest* 119(1 suppl):39S-63S, 2001.
105. Pedersen AK, Fitzgerald GA: Dose-related kinetics of aspirin, presystemic acetylation of platelet cyclooxygenase, *N Engl J Med* 311:1206-1211, 1984.
106. Reye RDK, Morgan G, Baral J: Encephalopathy and fatty degeneration, *Lancet* 2:749-752, 1963.
107. Riendeau D, Percival MD, Brideau C, et al: Etoricoxib (MK-0663): preclinical profile and comparison with other agents that selectively inhibit cyclooxygenase-2, *J Pharmacol Exp Ther* 296:558-566, 2001.
108. Roszkowski MT, Swift JQ, Hargreaves KM: Effect of NSAID administration on tissue levels of immunoreactive prostaglandin E_2, leukotriene B4, and (S)-flurbiprofen following extraction of impacted third molars, *Pain* 73:339-345, 1997.
109. Roth GJ, Majerus PW: The mechanism of the effect of aspirin on human platelets I. Acetylation of a particulate fraction protein, *J Clin Invest* 56:624-632, 1975.
110. Samuelsson B, Hammarström S: Leukotrienes: a novel group of biologically active compounds, *Vitam Horm* 39:1-30, 1982.
111. Sawynok J, Yaksh TL: Caffeine as an analgesic adjuvant: a review of pharmacology and mechanisms of action, *Pharmacol Rev* 45:43-85, 1993.
112. Schnitzer TJ: Osteoarthritis management: the role of cyclooxygenase-2-selective inhibitors, *Clin Ther* 23:313-326, 2001.
113. Schwartz LB: The mast cell. In Ruddy S, Harris ED, Jr, Sledge CB, et al, eds: *Kelley's Textbook of rheumatology*, ed 5, Philadelphia, 2001, WB Saunders.
114. Siegel SA, Shealy DJ, Nakada MT, et al: The mouse/human chimeric monoclonal antibody cA2 neutralizes TNF in vitro and protects transgenic mice from cachexia and TNF lethality in vivo, *Cytokine* 7:15-25, 1995.
115. Sigler JW, Bluhm GB, Duncan H, et al: Gold salts in the treatment of rheumatoid arthritis. A double-blind study, *Ann Intern Med* 80:21-26, 1974.
116. Silverstein FE, Faich G, Goldstein JL, et al: Gastrointestinal toxicity with celecoxib vs. nonsteroidal anti-inflammatory drugs for osteoarthritis and rheumatoid arthritis: the CLASS study—a randomized controlled trial, *JAMA* 284:1247-1255, 2000.
117. Silverstein FE, Graham DY, Senior JR, et al: Misoprostol reduces serious gastrointestinal complications in patients with rheumatoid arthritis receiving nonsteroidal anti-inflammatory drugs. A randomized, double-blind, placebo-controlled trial, *Ann Intern Med* 123:241-249, 1995.
118. Simon LS, Weaver AL, Graham DY, et al: Anti-inflammatory and upper gastrointestinal effects of celecoxib in rheumatoid arthritis: a randomized controlled trial, *JAMA* 282:1921-1928, 1999.
119. Singh G: Recent considerations in nonsteroidal anti-inflammatory drug gastropathy, *Am J Med* 105(1B):31S-38S, 1998.
120. Slattery JT, Nelson SD, Thummel KE: The complex interaction between ethanol and acetaminophen, *Clin Pharmacol Ther* 60:241-246, 1996.
121. Smith JB, Willis AL: Aspirin selectively inhibits prostaglandin production in human platelets, *Nature* 231:235-237, 1971.
122. Smith WL, DeWitt DL: Biochemistry of prostaglandin endoperoxide H synthetase-1 and synthetase-2 and their differential susceptibility to nonsteroidal anti-inflammatory drugs, *Semin Nephrol* 15:179-194, 1995.
123. Smith WL, Garavito RM, Dewitt DL: Prostaglandin endoperoxide H synthetases (cyclooxygenases)-1 and -2, *J Biol Chem* 271:33157-33160, 1996.
124. Spencer-Green G: Drug treatment of arthritis. Update on conventional and less conventional methods, *Postgrad Med* 93:129-140, 1993.
125. Stechschulte DJ, Orange RP, Austen KF: Detection of slow reacting substance of anaphylaxis (SRS-A) in plasma of guinea pigs during anaphylaxis, *J Immunol* 111:1585-1589, 1973.
126. Steinbach G, Lynch PM, Phillips RK, et al: The effect of celecoxib, a cyclooxygenase-2 inhibitor, in familial adenomatous polyposis, *N Engl J Med* 342:1946-1952, 2000.

127. Stitt JT: Neurophysiology of fever, *Fed Proc* 141:286-292, 1981.
128. Styrt B, Sugarman B: Antipyresis and fever, *Arch Intern Med* 150:1589-1597, 1990.
129. Symposium on analgesics, *Arch Intern Med* 141(special issue):271-406, 1981.
130. Symposium on paracetamol and the liver—overdosage and its management, *J Int Med Res* 4(suppl):149-154, 1976.
131. Swift JQ, Garry MG, Roszkowski MT, et al: Effect of flurbiprofen on tissue levels of immunoreactive bradykinin and acute postoperative pain, *J Oral Maxillofac Surg* 51:112-116, 1993.
132. Szczeklik A, Grylglewski RJ: Prostaglandins and aspirin-sensitive asthma, *Am Rev Respir Dis* 118:799-800, 1978.
133. Thomas MJ: Urate causes the human polymorphonuclear leukocyte to secrete superoxide, *Free Radical Biol Med* 12:89-91, 1992.
134. Tjölsen A, Lund A, Hole K: Antinociceptive actions of spinal nonsteroidal anti-inflammatory agents on the formalin test in the rat, *J Pharmacol Exp Ther* 263:136-146, 1992.
135. Troullos ES, Hargreaves KM, Butler DP, et al: Comparison of the non-steroidal anti-inflammatory drugs, ibuprofen and flurbiprofen, with methylprednisolone and placebo for acute pain, swelling, and trismus, *J Oral Maxillofac Surg* 48:945-952, 1990.
136. Urquhart E: Analgesic agents and strategies in the dental pain model, *J Dent* 22:336-341, 1994.
137. Vane JR, Botting RM: New insights into the mode of action of anti-inflammatory drugs, *Inflammation Res* 44:1-10, 1995.
138. Vogel RI, Desjardins PJ, Major KVO: Comparison of presurgical and immediate postsurgical ibuprofen on postoperative periodontal pain, *J Periodontol* 63:914-918, 1992.
139. Waldman RJ, Hall WN, McGee H, et al: Aspirin as a risk factor in Reye's syndrome, *JAMA* 247:3089-3094, 1982.
140. Warner TD, Guiliano F, Vojnovic I, et al: Nonsteroid drug selectivities for cyclo-oxygenase-1 rather than cyclo-oxygenase-2 are associated with human gastrointestinal toxicity: a full in vitro analysis, *Proc Natl Acad Sci* 96:7563-7568, 1999.
141. Warner TD, Mitchell JA: Cyclooxygenase-3 (COX-3): filling in the gaps toward a COX continuum? *Proc Natl Acad Sci USA* 99:13371-13373, 2002.
142. Weinblatt ME, Kaplan H, Germain BF, et al: Low-dose methotrexate compared with auranofin in adult rheumatoid arthritis: a thirty-six week, double-blind trial, *Arthritis Rheum* 33:330-338, 1990.
143. Williams RC, Jeffcoat MK, Howell TH, et al: Ibuprofen: an inhibitor of alveolar bone resorption in beagles, *J Periodontal Res* 23:225-229, 1988.
144. Williams RC, Jeffcoat MK, Kaplan ML, et al: Flurbiprofen: a potent inhibitor of alveolar bone resorption in beagles, *Science* 227:640-642, 1985.
145. Wooley PH, Dutcher J, Widmer MB, et al: Influence of a recombinant soluble tumor necrosis factor receptor FC fusion protein on type I-I collagen-induced arthritis in mice, *J Immunol* 151:6602-6607, 1993.
146. Wynn RL: Ketorolac (Toradol) for dental pain, *Gen Dent* 40:476-479, 1992.
147. Yee JP, Koshiver JE, Allbon C, et al: Comparison of intramuscular ketorolac tromethamine and morphine sulfate for analgesia of pain after major surgery, *Pharmacotherapy* 6:253-261, 1986.

General References

Dale MM, Foreman JC, Fan T-PD, eds: *Textbook of immunopharmacology*, ed 3, Boston, 1994, Blackwell Scientific.

Famaey JP, Paulus HE, eds: *Therapeutic applications of NSAIDs: subpopulations and new formulations*, New York, 1992, Marcel Dekker.

Glaser KB, Vadas P: Phospholipase A_2 in clinical inflammation. *Molecular approaches to pathophysiology*, Boca Raton, FL, 1995, CRC Press.

Graves DT, Jiang Y: Chemokines, a family of chemotactic cytokines, *Crit Rev Oral Biol Med* 6:109-118, 1995.

Jackson JL, Roszkowski MT, Moore PA: Management of acute postoperative pain. In Fonseca RJ, ed; Frost D, Hersh EV, Levin LM, volume eds: *Oral and maxillofacial surgery, vol 1: anesthesia/dentoalveolar surgery/office management*, Philadelphia, 2000, WB Saunders.

Prescott LF: *Paracetamol (acetaminophen). A critical biographical review*, Bristol, PA, 1996, Taylor & Francis.

Rainsford KD, Powanda MC, eds: *Safety and efficacy of non-prescription (OTC) analgesics and NSAIDs*, Hingham, MA, 1998, Kluwer Academic Publishers.

Ruddy S, Harris ED, Sledge CB, et al, eds: *Kelley's Textbook of rheumatology*, ed 6, Philadelphia, 2001, WB Saunders.

CHAPTER • 22

Histamine and Histamine Antagonists

Clarence L. Trummel

HISTAMINE

Histamine, or β-aminoethylimidazole, is one of a heterogeneous group of biologically active, naturally occurring substances whose physiologic roles are only slowly being defined. In addition to histamine, this group includes another amine (5-hydroxytryptamine), polypeptides (angiotensin, bradykinin, and kallidin), and lipid-derived substances (prostaglandins, leukotrienes, and platelet-activating factor). These compounds have been collectively termed *autacoids.* This designation, derived from the Greek *autos* ("self") and *akos* ("cure"), is sufficiently nonspecific yet still acknowledges the endogenous origin and biologic activities of these substances as well as their certain, although largely uncharacterized, role in the body's economy.

Histamine was the first autacoid to be discovered. After its synthesis in 1907, a series of studies by Dale and Laidlaw of the pharmacologic properties of histamine suggested that this substance might be involved in inflammatory and anaphylactic reactions.[13] These workers observed that the local application of histamine caused redness, swelling, and edema, mimicking a mild inflammatory reaction. They also determined that large doses of histamine given systemically produced profound vascular changes very similar to those seen in shock of traumatic or anaphylactic origin. Although the presence of histamine in animal tissues had been suggested, it was not until 1927 that histamine was conclusively shown to be a natural constituent of mammalian tissues and not the result of bacterial action.[4] This finding provided important support for the work of Lewis and Grant,[26] who had demonstrated earlier that a histaminelike substance ("H substance") was released in the skin after various injuries, including antigen-antibody reactions.

These early studies and those that followed clearly established that histamine is involved in various pathophysiologic phenomena seen after injury to tissue. Since then, a large amount of detailed information regarding the synthesis, storage, release, and actions of histamine has been generated. Despite this, our understanding of the role of histamine in the complex response of cells to injurious stimuli and the relation of this compound to other autacoids is meager. Furthermore, it is increasingly evident that this ubiquitous amine is involved in physiologic processes other than reaction to injury. These processes include gastric secretion,[11] neurotransmission in the central nervous system (CNS),[38,46] and local control of the microcirculation.[59]

Formation, Distribution, and Release

Histamine is widely distributed in nature and is found in plants, bacteria, and animals. Nearly all mammalian tissues contain histamine or have the ability to form it. The histamine content of different tissues varies greatly. In human beings and most other mammals, the highest concentrations are found in lung, skin, and intestinal mucosa; such organs as the pancreas, spleen, liver, and kidney have a low histamine content (Table 22-1). The physiologic significance of this pattern of distribution is not known. Although some tissue histamine may be derived from dietary sources or synthesized by bacteria in the gastrointestinal tract, most of it appears to be formed in situ.

Histamine is synthesized in mammalian tissues by the intracellular decarboxylation of the amino acid histidine (Figure 22-1). This conversion may be catalyzed either by aromatic L-amino acid decarboxylase or by histidine decarboxylase. Histidine decarboxylase is specific for L-histidine, requires pyridoxal phosphate, and appears to be primarily responsible for the synthesis of histamine in human beings.

Histamine is found in most tissues in the mast cell and in blood in a related cell, the basophil.[41,47] These cells synthesize histamine and store it as a proteinaceous complex with heparin or chondroitin sulfate in membrane-bound secretory granules. Histamine in this form is physiologically inactive but can be discharged from the cell by a process called *exocytosis* or *degranulation.* The first step in this process is activation of the cell by an appropriate stimulus. Once the cell is activated, a complex series of events leading to degranulation occurs.[1] These events require an increase in cytosolic Ca^{++} and metabolic energy and involve activation of Ca^{++} dependent protein kinases (protein kinase C and Ca^{++}/ calmodulin-dependent protein kinase), assembly of microtubules, and, finally, fusion of the perigranular membrane with the cell membrane. The granule contents are then released into the extracellular environment and dissociate to yield histamine, heparin, several proteases, and chemoattractants such as tumor necrosis factor α. In addition to release of these preformed mediators, activation of mast cells activates phospholipase A in the cell membrane, with release of arachidonic acid. This is turn is metabolized by the cyclooxygenase pathway to various prostaglandins and thromboxanes and by the lipoxygenase pathway to various leukotrienes.

A small amount of histamine not stored in mast cells or basophils is found in several sites. One of these is certain neurons in the hypothalamus. The function of these histaminergic neurons is not known. Another site of non–mast cell histamine is the enterochromaffinlike cell in the gastric mucosa. These cells synthesize and release histamine, which subsequently stimulates gastric acid secretion by mucosal parietal cells (see Chapter 33). Certain neoplasms collectively known as *carcinoid* can also secrete a variety of bioactive substances, including histamine.[12] These substances likely contribute to the so-called carcinoid syndrome, a prominent feature of which is cutaneous flushing and bronchoconstrictive attacks not unlike that seen with the intravascular administration of histamine.

A variety of conditions (or stimuli) can trigger the release of histamine from mast cells and basophils. These can be grouped into three categories.

1. *Tissue injury.* Any physical or chemical agent that nonspecifically injures tissue, particularly skin or mucosa, causes the immediate release of histamine from mast cells in the affected area. Depending on the severity of injury, histamine continues to be released for several minutes and appears to be largely responsible for the initial sharp increase in vascular permeability that is characteristic of acute inflammation. This histamine-dependent change in permeability is transient (up to 30 minutes) but is followed in 2 to 4 hours by a more prolonged increase in permeability lasting up to 4 hours. Although inhibitors of histamine release or inhibitors of the subsequent action of histamine can block the initial phase of vascular permeability after injury, they have little effect on the secondary or delayed phase, suggesting that autacoids or factors other than histamine mediate the secondary phase.[57] The mechanism by which a nonspecific injury triggers mast cell degranulation is not clear. It could depend on direct physical damage to mast cells or, alternatively, may involve the initial production of factors such as activated complement components or vasoactive polypeptides that then stimulate histamine release.[1,24]
2. *Allergic reactions.* Presentation of a specific antigen to a previously sensitized subject can trigger immediate allergic reactions, ranging in intensity from mild (localized edema, erythema, and itching) to severe (marked fall in blood pressure and bronchospasm). The pathophysiologic manifestations of such reactions are caused in large measure by the release of histamine. This release occurs as a consequence of the binding of specific antigens to allergen-specific reaginic (immunoglobulin E [IgE]) antibodies attached to the plasma membranes of mast cells and basophils by FcεRI receptors (the tetrameric transmembrane high-affinity IgE receptors).[30] Binding of antigen and antibody may cause conformational changes in the membrane, leading to an increase in Ca^{++} permeability. In any case, this antigen-antibody interaction is an appropriate stimulus for the series of events leading to degranulation of these cells.
3. *Drugs and other foreign compounds.* Although drugs that are antigenic (e.g., penicillin) can cause histamine release, a large group of drugs and other chemicals can trigger histamine release directly without a requirement for previous sensitization through an immune response. For convenience, these agents can be classified as *basic histamine releasers, macromolecular compounds,* and *enzymes.*[24] The basic histamine releasers include aliphatic and arylalkyl amines, amides, amidines, diamidines, quaternary ammonium compounds, alkaloids, piperidine derivatives, pyridinium compounds, antimalarial drugs, dyes, and basic polypeptides. The prototypic histamine releaser compound 48/80 and a number of therapeutic agents of interest, such as tubocurarine and morphine, fall into this category. Dextran is an example of a macromolecular compound that causes histamine release. Several enzymes, such as phospholipase A, have been shown to initiate mast cell degranulation, a fact that may explain the release of histamine caused by various insect and snake venoms. The mechanisms by which chemicals trigger histamine release vary. Some agents, typified by compound 48/80, act by stimulating an energy-dependent degranulation process with characteristics similar to anaphylactic histamine release. Other histamine releasers are effective in the absence of energy sources and seem to act by a detergent like effect on cell membranes.

Table • 22-1

Distribution and Content of Histamine in Various Human Tissues and Cells

TISSUE OR CELL	HISTAMINE CONTENT*
Lung	33 ± 10
Mucosa (nasal)	15.6 (range, 5.0 to 38.5)
Stomach	14 ± 4.0
Duodenum	14 ± 0.9
Skin (face)	30.4
Skin (abdomen)	6.6
Pancreas	4.8 ± 1.5
Spleen	3.4 ± 1.0
Bone marrow	3.3 ± 1.5
Kidney	2.5 ± 1.2
Liver	2.2 ± 0.8
Heart	1.6 ± 0.1
Thyroid	1.0 ± 0.1
Skeletal muscle	0.9 ± 0.1
Peripheral nerves	2 to 11
CNS tissue	0 to 0.2
Whole blood	16 to 89 µg/L
Plasma	2.6 µg/L (range, 0 to 15)
Basophils	1080 µg/10^9 cells
Eosinophils	160 µg/10^9 cells
Neutrophils	3.0 µg/10^9 cells
Lymphocytes	0.6 µg/10^9 cells
Platelets	0.009 µg/10^9 platelets

From Van Arsdel PP, Jr, Beall GN: The metabolism and functions of histamine, *Arch Intern Med* 106:714-733, 1960. Copyright 1960, American Medical Association.

*Means or means ± standard error expressed as µg/g unless otherwise indicated.

Metabolism

Histamine of either exogenous or endogenous origin is rapidly inactivated by two routes.[45] The more important of these is methylation of the imidazole ring by the enzyme histamine-N-methyltransferase, which is widely distributed throughout the body. The resultant product is converted to methylimidazole acetic acid by monoamine oxidase. The other route

$$\text{Histidine (HC=C(-CH}_2\text{-CH(COOH)-NH}_2\text{) imidazole ring)} \xrightarrow{\text{Histidine decarboxylase}} \text{Histamine (HC=C-CH}_2\text{-CH}_2\text{-NH}_2\text{)} + CO_2$$

Fig. 22-1 Conversion of histidine to histamine.

involves the oxidative deamination of histamine by diamine oxidase to produce imidazole acetic acid, much of which is subsequently conjugated with ribose. All these metabolites are inactive and, along with a small amount of free histamine, are excreted by the kidney.

Large oral doses of histamine have little effect because histamine is rapidly degraded by intestinal bacteria. Any free histamine that is absorbed is largely inactivated in the intestinal wall and in the liver.

Pharmacologic Effects

Most of the important effects of histamine can be attributed to its actions on smooth muscle and glands. In general, histamine causes relaxation of vascular smooth muscle in smaller blood vessels. It also causes the constriction of some larger blood vessels, the contraction of nonvascular smooth muscle, and the stimulation of secretion of exocrine glands, especially those of the gastric mucosa. These actions are independent of innervation. Different species show considerable variation in the sensitivity of target tissues to histamine. For example, the bronchial smooth muscle of the guinea pig is highly sensitive to histamine, and fatal bronchospasm occurs at concentrations that have minimal effects in other species, including human beings. Within a single species, the actions of histamine are usually reproducible.

The existence of compounds that can selectively block the actions of histamine strongly supports the existence of three specific histamine receptors, H_1, H_2, and H_3.[20] The histamine receptors are G protein–linked receptors. H_1 receptors are associated with $G_{q/11}$, and stimulation of these receptors leads to an increase in intracellular Ca^{++} and Ca^{++}-dependent protein kinase activity. H_2 receptors are linked to G_s, and stimulation of these receptors brings about an increase in intracellular cyclic adenosine 3′,5′-monophosphate. H_3 receptors appear to stimulate G proteins, but less is known about their signaling (see Chapter 1 for more details on the specifics of signal transduction involving G proteins).

H_1 receptors primarily mediate effects on smooth muscle, leading to vasodilation, increased vascular permeability, and contraction of nonvascular smooth muscle. These effects are blocked by the "classic" antihistamines, such as pyrilamine. H_2 receptors mediate the stimulation of gastric acid secretion and may be involved in other effects, such as the direct cardiac stimulation and vasodilation seen after high doses of histamine. A more recently developed group of antihistamines, the H_2-blocking agents, specifically antagonize these effects.[5,6]

During the past decade, H_3 receptors have been identified in a wide variety of tissues, including presynaptic sites on nerve terminals in the CNS and prejunctional sites in gastric mucosa, cardiovascular system, and pulmonary tree.[21] The function of H_3 receptors is not established, but these receptors appear to antagonize stimulatory effects mediated by the activation of H_1 receptors. Their prejunctional location supports their role as autoregulatory receptors in many tissues. H_3 receptors have even been found on adrenergic nerve terminals. Stimulation of these H_3 receptors inhibits the release of norepinephrine.[22] Specific H_3 receptor antagonists have been developed, such as thioperamide; although such compounds have obvious pharmacologic effects, they are not yet beyond the research stage.[54]

Cardiovascular system

The effects of histamine on the circulatory system are complex and vary markedly according to species. In most mammals, histamine causes some constriction of large vessels, both arterial and venous. Histamine also constricts arterioles and increases blood pressure in rats and rabbits. In contrast, the intravenous administration of histamine in human beings and carnivores causes dilation of terminal arterioles, capillaries, and postcapillary venules and leads to a sharp decrease in peripheral resistance and a consequent fall in blood pressure. The dilation of these vessels is caused by histamine stimulation of H_1 receptors on endothelial cells, resulting in the release of nitric oxide, which in turn causes the relaxation of smooth muscle of the arterioles and precapillary sphincters. Stimulation of H_1 receptors also leads to activation of phospholipase A_2 and the generation in endothelial cells of prostacyclin, which contributes to the vasodilation. Histamine also stimulates H_2 receptors on vascular smooth muscle cells, leading to relaxation of small blood vessels. The subsequent increase in arteriolar and capillary blood flow causes, in turn, a passive dilation of postcapillary venules that is accompanied by an increase in their permeability. This increased permeability is initiated by distention or stretching of the venules as well as by a contractile response of the endothelial cells caused directly by histamine; both phenomena contribute to "gaps" between the endothelial cells of the venules and exposure of the basement membrane. These gaps permit the movement of plasma protein and fluid through the basement membrane into the extravascular space, thus causing the formation of edema.[1]

In addition to hypotension, arteriolar dilation induced by histamine leads to cutaneous flushing, especially over the face and upper trunk, and a rise in skin temperature. A short-lived but intense headache caused by dilation of cerebral vessels also occurs. This "histamine headache" is similar in quality and duration to the headache produced by other potent vasodilators, such as amyl nitrite.

The effect of histamine on the terminal vasculature can be illustrated by injection of 10 to 20 μg of the amine into the skin. At the site of the injection, there is first immediate reddening, reflecting vasodilation. This reddening is followed shortly by a zone of erythema, or "flare," extending as an irregular halo for 1 cm or more beyond the original red spot. The flare is presumed to be caused by reflex vasodilation of adjacent small vessels, resulting from the axon reflex, and is abolished by disruption of the peripheral sensory nerves. Finally, the central spot is replaced by a disk of localized edema, or wheal, resulting from increased capillary permeability, and is accompanied by pain and itching. These events constitute the classic triple response first described by Lewis and Grant.[26] It is worthwhile to note that a similar response is elicited by the intradermal injection of antigen in a sensitized person.

Hypotension resulting from moderate doses of histamine is quite transient because reflex circulatory mechanisms come into play and the drug is rapidly inactivated. However, when histamine is given in large doses, there is a progressive fall in blood pressure that resembles that of traumatic or surgical shock. This fall is a consequence of both vasodilation and increased capillary permeability. The increased capillary permeability, in turn, leads to loss of plasma from the vascular compartment and a decrease in the effective blood volume. Venous return to the heart is diminished, so cardiac output declines despite a compensatory tachycardia. There may also be dyspnea caused by bronchoconstriction. In normal human beings, circulatory depression is predominant. Without adequate treatment, death may ensue from histamine shock.

In the intact animal, histamine can cause cardiac stimulation, principally the result of reflex mechanisms triggered by the histamine-induced fall in peripheral vascular resistance. However, histamine also has some direct positive chronotropic and inotropic effects on the heart. The receptors responsible are largely H_2 receptors.[25]

Nonvascular smooth muscle

Histamine generally stimulates contraction of nonvascular smooth muscle to a variable degree depending on the species and tissue. In human beings, the smooth muscle of the bronchioles and gastrointestinal tract is most sensitive to this action; the smooth muscle of other organs, such as the uterus and bladder, is affected to a much lesser extent. People with asthma are highly susceptible to histamine and may have marked bronchial constriction from doses that would cause only minor increases in the airway resistance of normal subjects.

Exocrine glands

Histamine is a potent stimulator of gastric secretion in most species. Low doses of histamine that have minimal effects on blood pressure elicit near-maximal secretion of both acid and pepsin by the gastric glands. On the basis of this sensitivity of the gastric secretory cells to histamine and the presence of histamine in both gastric mucosa and gastric fluid, it is accepted that histamine plays a major physiologic role in gastric secretion. This conclusion is strongly supported by the discovery of H_2 receptor antagonists (see below), which block histamine-stimulated gastric secretion and reduce basal secretion and secretion induced by some other physiologic agents, such as acetylcholine and gastrin.

The relations among potent gastric secretagogues, acetylcholine and the polypeptide hormone gastrin, and histamine are complex (see Figure 33-1). As previously noted, histamine is synthesized by the enterochromaffinlike cells in the gastric mucosa, and its release from these cells is triggered by either gastrin or acetylcholine. The fact that H_2 receptor antagonists inhibit stimulation of gastric secretion by histamine, gastrin, or acetylcholine lends support to the possibility that the latter two agents act by releasing histamine from enterochromaffin-like cells, which then acts directly on the parietal cells through H_2 receptors.[35] However, identification of specific receptors for gastrin and acetylcholine on the parietal cell, plus an ability of gastrin to augment (although moderately) histamine-induced secretion, indicates that gastrin can also cause release of H^+ by acting directly on parietal cells and independently of histamine.

Histamine also stimulates the secretion of catecholamines by the chromaffin cells of the adrenal medulla. This action is of little significance in normal patients, but in patients with pheochromocytoma, release of a large amount of catecholamines occurs. Although histamine can enhance salivary and lacrimal gland secretion, this effect is minimal unless large doses are used.

General Therapeutic Uses

There are currently no valid therapeutic applications for histamine. It is of limited use as a diagnostic tool in the assessment of gastric acid production. In this test, histamine is given subcutaneously in a dose (usually 1 mg) that will stimulate gastric secretion without causing major effects on blood vessels or smooth muscle. The gastric fluid is subsequently sampled and its acid content determined. An isomer of histamine, betazole, can also be used in this test. Betazole has less H_1 receptor activity than histamine and thus offers the advantage of causing a lesser degree of unwanted side effects for a given degree of gastric stimulation. Pentagastrin, a potent synthetic analogue of gastrin, has essentially supplanted both histamine and betazole for the clinical evaluation of gastric secretion. Another use of histamine (in aerosol form) is in testing for nonallergic bronchial hyperreactivity in asthmatics.

Adverse Effects

The toxic effects of histamine are largely predictable on the basis of its pharmacologic actions. In normal persons, these effects are dose dependent. The more prominent manifestations of histamine toxicity are cutaneous flushing, hypotension, headache, visual disturbances, dyspnea, and gastrointestinal disturbances such as nausea, vomiting, and diarrhea. Massive doses may lead to shock and circulatory failure. Histamine, even in low doses, may have serious adverse consequences in elderly persons or those with cardiovascular disease, asthma, or recent gastrointestinal bleeding.

HISTAMINE ANTAGONISTS

Histamine antagonists, or antihistamines, encompass a large group of compounds with the characteristic ability to block the actions of histamine. These compounds do not alter the formation, release, or degradation of histamine but competitively antagonize it at receptor sites. As described above, three groups of antihistamines are now known by their ability to selectively block effects of histamine mediated by H_1, H_2, and H_3 receptors. These three groups of antihistamines are appropriately termed *H_1, H_2, and H_3 receptor antagonists.* However, the generic term *antihistamine* is often used to refer to the "classic" antihistamines, or H_1 antagonists.

The early interest in histamine as a mediator of certain pathologic processes of an allergic nature spurred interest in agents that could block histamine. The first such compound, a derivative of phenoxyethylamine, was reported by Bovet and Staub in 1937.[7] Although this substance could adequately protect guinea pigs against injected histamine or anaphylactic shock, it was too toxic for human use. Other, less toxic compounds with antihistaminic activity were immediately sought. By 1946, numerous compounds with therapeutically useful properties had been found, including phenbenzamine, pyrilamine, diphenhydramine, and tripelennamine. During the following 20 years, hundreds of other compounds with antihistaminic properties were developed.

As the pharmacologic properties of the antihistamines were studied, it became apparent that they had no effect on histamine-induced gastric acid secretion. In 1972, a potent antagonist of histamine-induced gastric secretion was reported.[5] This compound, burimamide, and its subsequently developed congeners offered great potential as therapeutic agents as well as tools for further investigation of the role of histamine in health and disease.

H_1 Receptor Antagonists

Chemistry and classification

Most antihistamines with the ability to block H_1 receptors contain a side chain that resembles the ethylamino group in histamine. These H_1 receptor antagonists, or H_1 antihistamines, can be represented by the following general formula:

$$(\text{Aryl}_1)(\text{Aryl}_2)\text{X}-\overset{|}{\underset{|}{\text{C}}}-\overset{|}{\underset{|}{\text{C}}}-\text{N}(\text{R}_1)(\text{R}_2)$$

In this representation, *aryl* is a heterocyclic aromatic group that may or may not be separated from X by a methylene group. *X* is a carbon, oxygen, or nitrogen atom that connects the side chain to the aryl groups. *R_1* and *R_2* are usually, but not always, methyl groups. The ethylene group in the side chain may also be part of a heterocyclic system containing nitrogen, as in cyclizine. A general conclusion from examination of structure-activity relationships is that a basic nitrogen atom is essential, whether it exists in an aliphatic side chain, as in diphenhydramine, or in a ring structure, as in meclizine (Table 22-2).

By using the general formula just given, most H_1 antihistamines can be grouped according to the substitution made at the X position. Six distinct classes are recognized: (1) alkylamines, in which X is carbon; (2) ethanolamines, in which X is oxygen; (3) ethylenediamines, in which X is nitrogen; (4) piperazines, in which X is carbon linked to a piperazine ring; (5) phenothiazines, in which X is nitrogen as part of a phenothiazine nucleus; and (6) piperidines, in which X is carbon

Table • 22-2

Chemical Classification, Representative Structures, and Dosages of Major H_1 Antihistamines

CLASS	REPRESENTATIVE COMPOUND* (PROPRIETARY NAME)	USUAL ADULT DOSE (ORAL)	DURATION OF ACTION	OTHER COMPOUNDS IN THE SAME CLASS
Alkylamines	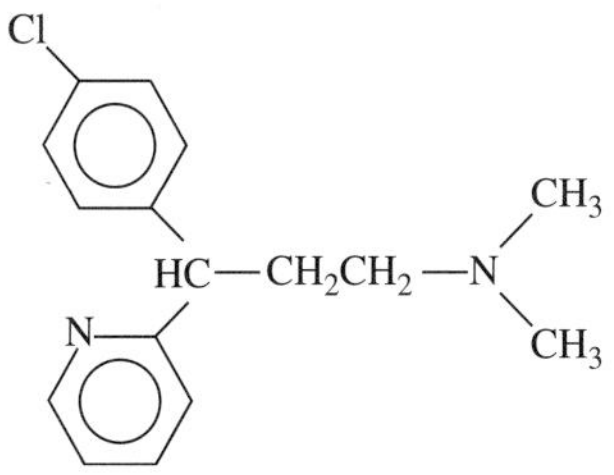 **Chlorpheniramine maleate (Chlor-Trimeton, others)**	4 mg	4-6 hr	Acrivastine (in Semprex-D): 8 mg, 6-8 hr Brompheniramine maleate (Dimetane): 4 mg, 4-6 hr Dexchlorpheniramine maleate (Polaramine): 2 mg, 4-6 hr Tripolidine hydrochloride (Actidil): 2.5 mg, 4-6 hr
Ethanolamines	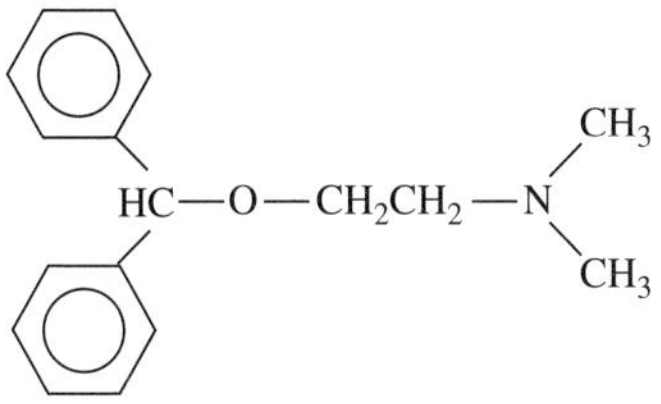 **Diphenhydramine hydrochloride (Benadryl, others)**	25-50 mg	6-8 hr	Carbinoxamine maleate (in Carbiset): 4-8 mg, 6-8 hr Clemastine fumarate (Tavist): 1.34-2.68 mg, 8-12 hr Dimenhydrinate (Dramamine): 50-100 mg, 4-6 hr Doxylamine succinate (Unisom): 12.5-25 mg, 4-6 hr
Ethylenediamines	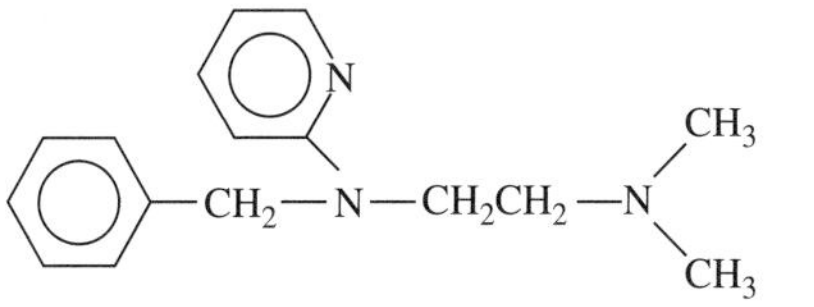 **Tripelennamine citrate (PBZ, others)**	25-50 mg	4-6 hr	Pyrilamine maleate (Nisaval): 25-50 mg, 6-8 hr
Piperazines	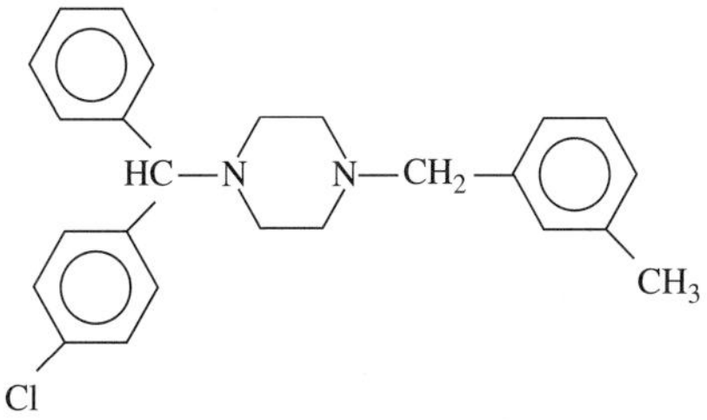 **Meclizine hydrochloride (Bonine, others)**	25-50 mg	24 hr	Cetirizine hydrochloride (Zyrtec): 5-10 mg, 24 hr Cyclizine hydrochloride (Marezine): 50 mg, 4-6 hr Buclizine hydrochloride (Bucladin-S): 50 mg, 4-12 hr Hydroxyzine hydrochloride (Atarax, others): 50-100 mg, 6-24 hr Hydroxyzine pamoate (Vistaril): 50-100 mg, 6-24 hr
Phenothiazines	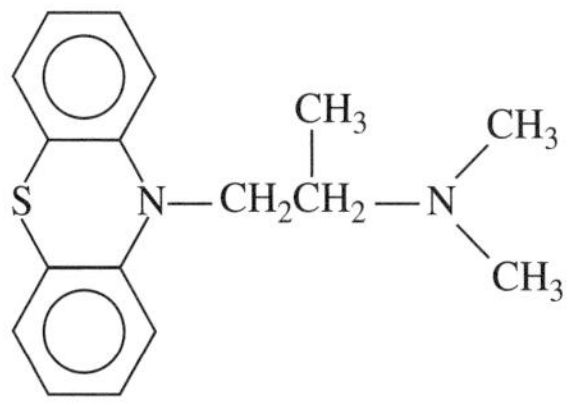 **Promethazine hydrochloride (Phenergan)**	12.5-25.0 mg	4-12 hr	Methdilazine hydrochloride (Tacaryl): 8 mg, 6-12 hr Trimeprazine tartrate (Temaril): 2.5 mg, 6 hr

Continued

Table • 22-2

Chemical Classification, Representative Structures, and Dosages of Major H_1 Antihistamines—cont'd

CLASS	REPRESENTATIVE COMPOUND (PROPRIETARY NAME)	USUAL ADULT DOSE (ORAL)	DURATION OF ACTION	OTHER COMPOUNDS IN THE SAME CLASS
Piperidines	Cl; N–C(=O)–O–CH_2CH_3; N **Loratadine hydrochloride (Claritin)**	10 mg	24 hr	Azatadine maleate (Optimine): 1-2 mg, 8-12 hr Cyproheptadine hydrochloride (Periactin)†: 4 mg, 6-8 hr Fexofenadine hydrochloride (Allegra): 60 mg, 12 hr Levocabastine hydrochloride (Livostin): topical Phenindamine tartrate (Nolahist): 25 mg, 4-6 hr
Phthalazinones	CH_3; N; N-N; O=; CH_2; Cl **Azelastine hydrochloride (Astelin)**	274 μg (topical nasal application; per nostril)	8-12 hr	

*Each structural formula is of the free base form.
†Also a serotonin-receptor antagonist.
The second-generation H_1 antihistamines are acrivastine, azelastine, cetirizine, fexofenadine levocabastine, and loratadine.

linked to a piperidine ring. Levocabastine is a piperidine but does not fit the structural chemistry listed in the six categories above. Azelastine, used only topically on the nasal mucosa, is a phthalazinone and also structurally unrelated to these other categories.

The chemical structures of representative compounds of each of the major classes of H_1 antihistamines are shown in Table 22-2. Despite their structural heterogeneity, the older antihistamines have only minor differences in pharmacologic properties, and these are mainly in potency, duration of action, and intensity of effects on other systems. In the last two decades, several H_1 antihistamines have been developed that differ from older antihistamines in that they are largely devoid of effects on the CNS.[2,52] Because of this difference, this group of agents, which are predominantly piperidine derivatives and include fexofenadine, levocabastine, and loratadine, are often termed *second-generation antihistamines* to distinguish them from the older, or first-generation, antihistamines. Other second-generation H_1 antihistamines include acrivastine (an alkylamine), cetirizine (a piperazine), and azelastine (a phthalazinone).

Pharmacologic effects

The H_1 antihistamines exert a variety of effects. Although the basis of some of these effects is obscure, many clearly result from histamine antagonism. These agents can inhibit the contraction of gastrointestinal and bronchial smooth muscle, the increase in capillary permeability, and the flare and itch components of the "triple response." Although H_1 antihistamines do not block histamine-induced gastric secretion, they do antagonize the increased secretions of the salivary and lacrimal glands and the increased release of epinephrine from the adrenal medulla stimulated by histamine. As with many other pharmacologic inhibitors, the basic mechanism of action can be explained in terms of a competitive blockade of receptors; that is, the antihistamines appear to interact with the H_1 receptors on the target cell, resulting in a decreased availability of these receptors for histamine. This interaction is reversible, or competitive, because the inhibition produced by a given concentration of antihistamine can be overcome by increasing the concentration of histamine (Figure 22-2). No evidence indicates that the antihistamines interfere with the synthesis, release, or biotransformation of histamine. Cetirizine appears to be unique among the antihistamines in that it has been reported to have antieosinophilic activity, so it inhibits the late phase of inflammation in addition to the more immediate histaminic effects.[53,55]

The action of the H_1 antihistamines in antagonizing histamine is specific; that is, the antihistamines "reverse" the effects of histamine by inhibiting its further action, but they have no directly opposing actions of their own. In contrast, epinephrine nonspecifically antagonizes histamine by exerting its own distinct effects, such as vasoconstriction, bronchodilation, and decreased gastrointestinal motility. This type of antagonism is sometimes referred to as *physiologic*. The distinction is important in understanding why a physiologic antagonist such as epinephrine is a more effective agent than an antihistamine in treating systemic histamine toxicity.

As previously indicated, the bronchial smooth muscle of the guinea pig is exquisitely sensitive to histamine, and low doses can trigger lethal bronchospasm. However, the prior administration of an H_1 antihistamine such as pyrilamine can protect the respiratory smooth muscle of these animals from a dose of histamine that is more than 100 times the lethal dose. These agents can similarly protect guinea pigs against the effects of released histamine during experimental anaphylaxis. A quite different situation prevails in human beings. Although H_1 antihistamines can antagonize the histamine-induced contraction

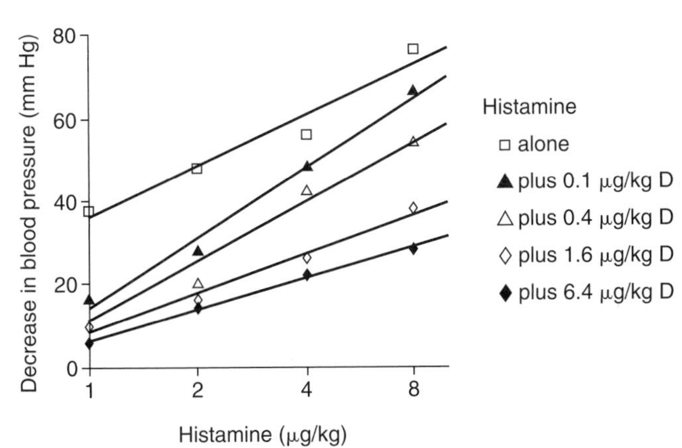

Fig. 22-2 Log dose-response curves illustrating competitive antagonism of histamine by diphenhydramine *(D)*. Decreases in blood pressure *(ordinate)* by graded intravenous doses of histamine *(abscissa)* were determined in anesthetized dogs. The animals then received diphenhydramine (0.1 to 6.4 μg/kg) followed by the same graded doses of histamine. (Data from Chen G, Russell D: A quantitative study of blood pressure response to cardiovascular drugs and their antagonists, *J Pharmacol Exp Ther* 99:401-408, 1950.)

of human respiratory muscle in vitro, these agents are relatively ineffective in relieving bronchospasm associated with asthma, anaphylaxis, and other allergic reactions. This ineffectiveness is caused in part by the involvement of autacoids other than histamine in mediating allergic bronchospasm in human beings. These substances include leukotrienes and kinins, against which the classic antihistamines show little antagonism.

In the human vascular system, H_1 antihistamines are quite effective in antagonizing the increased capillary permeability and consequent edema formation induced by histamine, but their effects on the vasodilation caused by histamine are more complex. H_1 antihistamines can prevent the vasodilation elicited by small doses of histamine; however, a combination of H_1 and H_2 antagonists is required to block large doses. This finding indicates that both receptor subtypes mediate the vascular effects of histamine, with the autacoid having a higher affinity for H_1 receptors.[37,48] The minor direct cardiac stimulation produced by histamine is little affected by H_1 antihistamines because this results largely from H_2 receptor stimulation.

Sedation is a common feature of therapeutic doses of all H_1 antihistamines except second-generation agents. It is usually manifested by drowsiness and may also be accompanied by lassitude, fatigue, dizziness, and incoordination. Sedation appears to be mediated by the inhibition of H_1 receptors in the brain.[40] The ability to cause sedation varies widely among the available first-generation H_1 antihistamines. The most active are the ethanolamines and phenothiazines, whereas the alkylamines have a relatively low incidence of drowsiness.[50] Another clinically useful CNS effect of first-generation H_1 antihistamines is inhibition of nausea and vomiting, especially that associated with motion sickness. These agents also possess mild antiparkinson activity. Large doses of first-generation H_1 antihistamines can cause CNS stimulation that may result in convulsions. Some degree of stimulation—restlessness or insomnia—may occasionally be encountered even at therapeutic doses.

The mechanism of the CNS effects of the H_1 antihistamines is not fully known, although histamine is present in the brain and is thought to play a role as a neurotransmitter. H_1 receptor antagonists have been shown to block histamine-induced depolarizations in human cortical brain slices.[40] This could explain the sedative effects of antihistamines. Although some degree of tolerance to the sedative effects of the H_1 antihistamines usually develops with long-term use, no concomitant decrease in their peripheral antihistaminic effects has been observed. It has been suggested that both the anti–motion sickness and the antiparkinson activities of the H_1 antihistamines are caused by a central cholinergic receptor–blocking action.

Antimuscarinic activity is a feature of most first-generation H_1 antihistamines. The decrease in salivary secretion associated with their use is largely related to this action. Second-generation H_1 antihistamines have little or no antimuscarinic activity. Most antihistamines have some degree of local anesthetic activity. This property is most notable in diphenhydramine, promethazine, pyrilamine, and tripelennamine and has been used clinically in dentistry.[31,56]

Absorption, fate, and excretion

As a group, the older H_1 antihistamines are well absorbed after either oral or parenteral administration. The onset of action varies from 15 to 60 minutes after an oral dose. Effects are typically maximal in 1 to 2 hours, with a duration of 4 to 6 hours, although the duration is longer for some agents (see Table 22-2). In contrast, most second-generation H_1 antihistamines have a considerably longer duration of action. For example, loratadine is transformed to an active metabolite with an average elimination half-time of greater than 24 hours, which allows once-daily dosing.

After absorption, the first-generation H_1 antihistamines are widely distributed in body fluids. However, loratadine and other second-generation agents cross the blood-brain barrier poorly and are barely detectable in brain tissue.[9] This failure to gain access to the CNS largely explains the nearly complete absence of sedation with these drugs. Levocabastine is a second-generation H_1 antihistamine that is only administered topically.

Although the biotransformation of the first-generation H_1 antihistamines has not been studied intensively, the activity of this group appears to be terminated by conversion to inactive metabolites through hydroxylation in the liver.[36] Interestingly, the second-generation antihistamine cetirizine is a metabolite of the first-generation agent hydroxyzine.

The second-generation antihistamines are extensively metabolized in the liver by the CYP3A4 microsomal enzyme (see Chapters 2 and 4). In some cases, such as with loratadine, this results in active metabolites.[50] Concurrent administration of other agents metabolized by this same enzyme can reduce the biotransformation of these particular antihistamines. Other second-generation H_1 antihistamines (e.g., acrivastine and cetirizine) are not metabolized to an active form and are largely excreted unchanged in the urine.

General therapeutic uses

The introduction of the antihistamines into clinical medicine stimulated great interest in these agents and their application in those pathologic states presumed to be caused by histamine release. The early enthusiasm for the antihistamines often led to their irrational use in various clinical situations. Although subsequent experience has brought about a better appreciation of the therapeutic indications and limitations of the antihistamines, they are still often used when their clinical efficacy is doubtful or other agents might be more appropriate.

The most prominent use of the H_1 antihistamines is in countering the manifestations of various allergic conditions, that is, reactions resulting from antigen-antibody combination in the body in which histamine release occurs. The antihistamines have no effect on the interaction of antigens and antibodies or on the release of histamine that may be triggered by this interaction but act by competitively antagonizing the binding of liberated histamine to its receptor. This mechanism of action has several implications for the therapeutic use of the antihistamines. It means that these agents cannot alter the allergic basis of a given disease but can only provide relief from some of the symptoms. It also means the antihistamines are most effective when given before the release of histamine. After histamine release has occurred, an antihistamine can only reduce further undesirable effects, unlike physiologic antagonists that can reverse them. Finally, the competitive nature of antihistamine action means that the effectiveness of these agents in a given situation depends on the relative concentrations of agonist and antagonist. Thus when substantial amounts of histamine are released either locally or systemically, the adverse effects of the antihistamine may preclude attainment of a sufficient concentration of antagonist to be clinically effective.

The clinical applications of the H_1 antihistamines can be summarized as follows:

1. H_1 antihistamines are generally useful in the treatment of nasal allergies of either a seasonal (e.g., hay fever) or perennial (nonseasonal) nature because they relieve rhinorrhea, sneezing, lacrimation, and itching of the eyes and nasal mucosa.[8] Azelastine effective for up to 12 hours when applied topically to the nasal mucosa.[29] This route of administration minimizes unwanted systemic effects such as drowsiness. In chronic or vasomotor (nonallergic) rhinitis, H_1 antihistamines are somewhat less effective.[49] The antihistamines are often combined with decongestants such as pseudoephedrine for the management of allergic symptoms in the upper respiratory tract.
2. A number of allergic dermatoses can be treated with the H_1 antihistamines.[18,50] Both acute and chronic urticaria respond favorably to these agents. Angioedema also responds to antihistamine therapy, although a severe attack involving the larynx almost certainly requires epinephrine for proper management of this serious complication. The H_1 antihistamines may be useful in controlling the itching associated with eczematous pruritus, atopic or contact dermatitis, and insect bites. However, in some situations (e.g., atopic dermatitis), topical corticosteroids are usually more effective. Although the antihistamines are topically effective in treating pruritus and urticaria, it should be noted that topical application can also cause an allergic dermatitis.
3. In systemic anaphylaxis, the H_1 antihistamines have no primary therapeutic role because they cannot control either the marked hypotension or the bronchospasm associated with a severe anaphylactic reaction. Here, the agent of choice is the physiologic antagonist epinephrine. Antihistamines as well as corticosteroids may be given parenterally as an adjunct to the physiologic antagonist, but only after life-threatening problems are controlled. The antihistamines are of some value in treating the itching and urticarial lesions of serum sickness, although other manifestations such as arthralgia are little affected.
4. The H_1 antihistamines have little effect on the acute manifestations of bronchial asthma. The pathogenesis of bronchial asthma is complex, and, as indicated earlier and in Chapter 32, mediators of bronchial muscle constriction other than histamine are involved. The β-adrenergic receptor agonists, and corticosteroids are the primary drugs used to alleviate an acute asthmatic episode. Antihistamines have been used in an attempt to decrease preasthmatic cough in children, although the efficacy of this therapy is not established.
5. H_1 antihistamines, particularly chlorpheniramine, combined with nasal decongestants and analgesics, are widely used for symptomatic relief of the common cold. There are dozens of such preparations on the market, which indicates the popularity of these nostrums. Unless the cold is superimposed on an allergic rhinitis, any relief obtained from this combination stems largely from the drying of the mucosa caused by the anticholinergic action of the antihistamine and the actions of the vasoconstrictor and analgesic. Antihistamines alone are of no proven value in either preventing or shortening the duration of the common cold.
6. A CNS action of the first-generation H_1 antihistamines can be used to prevent or treat nausea and vomiting induced by motion. In general, these agents exert less anti–motion sickness activity than do anticholinergics such as scopolamine. The effectiveness of individual antihistamines varies widely; promethazine, diphenhydramine, dimenhydrinate, and cyclizine are probably the most effective of all. However, the more effective agents also tend to have greater sedative effects, a fact that must be considered in selecting an anti–motion sickness drug. The H_1 antihistamines may also be useful in counteracting nausea and vomiting in vestibular disturbances such as Ménière's disease and other forms of vertigo. They are less effective than prochlorperazine or other phenothiazines for the control of nausea and vomiting after general anesthesia or associated with pregnancy, malignant diseases, radiation sickness, and various drugs.
7. Various over-the-counter (OTC) preparations sold as hypnotics include H_1 antihistamines because of their sedative effect. Because the amounts of antihistamine in such preparations are low, they are of limited value in inducing sleep. However, even in higher doses the antihistamines are less effective sedatives than benzodiazepines and other sedative-hypnotics. Promethazine is widely used as an adjunct to general anesthesia to produce drowsiness as well as to prevent or control nausea and vomiting induced by anesthetic agents and opioid analgesics.
8. Some miscellaneous uses of the H_1 antihistamines include reduction of tremors and muscle rigidity in Parkinson's disease, treatment of headaches of unknown cause, and control of nonhemolytic, nonpyrogenic reactions to blood transfusion. They are also useful in relieving acute dystonias caused by the phenothiazines and other neuroleptics.

Uses in dentistry

The H_1 antihistamines are used in dentistry primarily for their CNS actions rather than for their specific antihistaminic effects. Promethazine, hydroxyzine, and diphenhydraminez-may be used in conscious sedation procedures and as premedication for deep sedation and general anesthesia (see Chapter 18). The sedative effect is increased by the concomitant administration of an opioid analgesic; meperidine and fentanyl are commonly used for this purpose.[27] The preoperative administration of these agents may also cause some inhibition of salivary and bronchial secretions, although more effective anticholinergic drugs should be used if control of secretions is essential. A particular benefit of the antihistamines is their ability to reduce postoperative nausea and vomiting in the outpatient setting.

Although H_1 antihistamines have some local anesthetic activity and their feasibility as local anesthetic agents for dental procedures has been demonstrated,[31,56] they have been little used for this purpose because far more effective agents (e.g., lidocaine) are available. Still, the local anesthetic activity of the antihistamines may be useful when a patient is allergic to conventional local anesthetics.

The H_1 antihistamines can be used as secondary agents in the management of systemic anaphylactic reactions that may occur in the course of dental therapy. They can also be of value in the treatment of allergic lesions of the oral mucosa and as adjuncts in treating angioneurotic edema of the orofacial region.

Adverse effects

At therapeutic doses, the H_1 antihistamines are relatively free of serious adverse reactions. The most common side effects result from CNS depression, which is generally manifested as drowsiness, diminished alertness, lethargy, and decreased motor coordination. The incidence of sedation varies with individual agents, but in general the ethanolamines and the phenothiazines are the most sedating, the ethylenediamines are intermediate, and the alkylamines and piperazines the least. As previously mentioned, loratadine and other second-generation H_1 antihistamines are essentially devoid of sedative or other CNS effects. Sedation caused by antihistamines may be a serious liability in a patient whose daily activities require mental alertness and coordination. In such cases, a reduction of dosage or substitution of agents may be necessary. Gastrointestinal disturbances—nausea, vomiting, and epigastric distress—also occur but are not common. The anticholinergic properties of the antihistamines occasionally cause insomnia, tremors, nervousness and irritability, palpitation, tachycardia, dry mouth, blurred vision, urinary retention, and constipation. The incidence of these effects is dose related.

Serious disturbances of cardiac rhythm have occurred in patients receiving astemizole or terfenadine, second-generation H_1 antihistamines of the piperidine class.[58] These arrhythmias largely involve prolongation of the QT interval, resulting in polymorphic ventricular tachycardia (torsades de pointes) (see Chapter 24), the consequences of which can be fatal.[42] Such cardiotoxic effects usually occur when plasma concentrations of the drugs are increased as a result of either excessive doses or altered hepatic metabolism. The latter can occur as a result of impaired liver function or the concurrent administration of certain drugs, especially the macrolide antibiotics (erythromycin, clarithromycin to a lesser extent) and azole antifungals (ketoconazole, itraconazole) that bind to the CYP3A4 enzyme and interfere with metabolism of the antihistamines. Because of this uncommon but serious problem, terfenadine and astemizole were voluntarily withdrawn from the United States market in 1998 and 1999, respectively. Although loratadine is metabolized by CYP3A4, it does not appear to increase the QT interval even in the presence of drugs that interact with terfenadine and astemizole. Fexofenadine, cetirizine, and acrivastine have not been associated with these arrhythmias or drug interactions.

Large doses of antihistamines can cause marked stimulation of the CNS manifested by hallucinations, excitement, and motor disturbances such as tremors and convulsions. Deaths from overdosage almost invariably occur outside a therapeutic setting (e.g., accidental poisoning in the home).

Allergic reactions to the H_1 antihistamines can occur; they are more frequent after topical application than after oral administration and can complicate the treatment of allergic lesions of the skin or oral mucosa. Allergic reactions can take the form of urticarial, eczematous, bullous, or petechial rashes, fixed drug eruptions, or, more rarely, anaphylaxis.

As with most drugs, various blood dyscrasias (hemolytic anemia, agranulocytosis, pancytopenia, and thrombocytopenia) have been reported after the use of antihistamines. Patients receiving long-term antihistamine therapy should thus be periodically monitored. Although certain piperazine H_1 antihistamines have been shown to be teratogenic in some laboratory animal models, there is no clinical evidence to indicate that antihistamines cause birth defects in human beings. However, the use of these drugs should be avoided during the first trimester of pregnancy. Doxylamine was suspected to cause birth defects when used as an antinausea drug during pregnancy. However, several studies have shown no increase in birth defects with doxylamine, even though it cannot be ruled out that the drug is weakly teratogenic.

Because of their sedative properties, the H_1 antihistamines can potentiate the CNS depressant effects of other agents, such as barbiturates, opioid analgesics, general anesthetics, and alcohol. Although such an interaction may be deliberately sought, as in the preanesthetic use of promethazine, these combinations should otherwise be avoided or monitored closely. Because the antihistamines have antimuscarinic properties, they can produce manifestations of excessive cholinergic blockade if given during therapy with other anticholinergic drugs. Such manifestations (e.g., dry mouth, constipation, blurred vision) are more likely to be troublesome than serious. However, long-term use can have important consequences; for example, if dry mouth persists it can lead to a higher incidence of caries. Second-generation H_1 antihistamines do not have antimuscarinic effects.

Antihistamines are variably excreted in breast milk. Because infants, especially newborns and premature infants, are at higher risk of adverse effects, the use of antihistamines in nursing women should be avoided. Furthermore, antihistamines, like other anticholinergic drugs, may inhibit lactation.

Preparations and doses of drugs used in dentistry

The therapeutic value of the H_1 antihistamines can be encompassed by relatively few agents. Because a large number of preparations are available, the clinician has the task of selecting the most effective drug with the fewest side effects. Because there are few quantitative data on which to base this choice, the clinician should select one or two well-known representatives of each class and become familiar with their therapeutic indications and limitations. These selections can be modified when convincing evidence of an advantage offered by another agent becomes available. Second-generation H_1 antihistamines, because they lack sedative and anticholinergic effects, would appear to meet this criterion. These drugs are expensive, however, and are often best reserved for those persons who are intolerant of established first-generation drugs. In dentistry, the unique pharmacologic profile of the second-generation agents actually precludes them from most applications because sedative and anticholinergic effects are usually desirable outcomes.

Oral doses of established examples of each of the major classes of H_1 antihistamines are given in Table 22-2. For more prescribing information, consult a standard reference for this purpose.[32]

H_2 Receptor Antagonists

Chemistry and classification

The H_2 receptor antagonists, or H_2 antihistamines, are basically structural analogues of histamine (Figure 22-3). Two changes in the histamine molecule are necessary to achieve H_2 receptor–blocking activity.[17] One is modification of the imidazole ring or its substitution by a furan or thiazole ring. A second modification is the presence of a flexible connecting chain linked to a polar substituent capable of hydrogen binding.

The first compound discovered to have the ability to block H_2 receptors was burimamide.[5] Its poor oral absorption and partial-agonist properties led to a search for active congeners. The first of these to be tested was metiamide.[6] Although metiamide is orally effective, it caused a reversible neutropenia during clinical trials. Because the thiourea moiety in the side chain of metiamide was believed to be responsible for this adverse effect, the thiourea group was replaced by a cyanoguanidine group. The resultant compound, cimetidine, became available for clinical use in 1977.[23] Shortly thereafter, ranitidine was approved. It differs from cimetidine and earlier H_2 antagonists in that it is not an imidazole derivative but instead contains a furan ring. Later, two other H_2 receptor antagonists, famotidine and nizatidine, were approved for use. Unlike either cimetidine or ranitidine, famotidine and

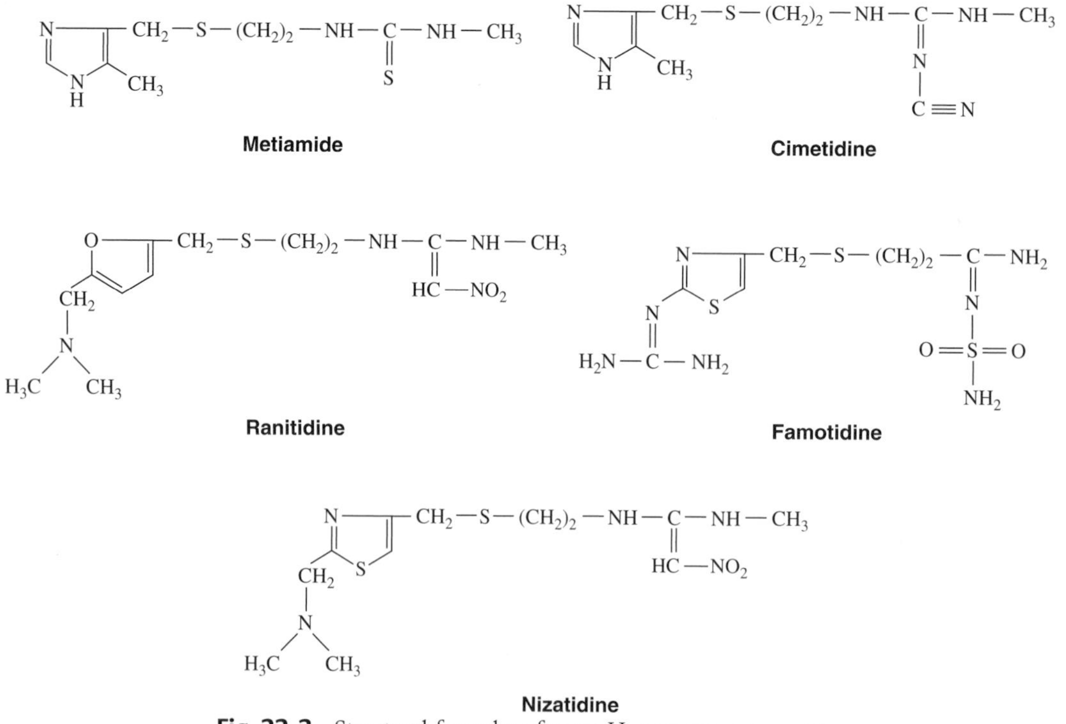

Metiamide

Cimetidine

Ranitidine

Famotidine

Nizatidine

Fig. 22-3 Structural formulas of some H_2 receptor antagonists.

nizatidine are based on a thiazole ring structure (see Figure 22-3).

Several differences between the H_1 and H_2 antihistamines are obvious. The H_1 antihistamines have aryl or heteroaryl rings that are highly lipophilic and bear little resemblance to the imidazole ring of histamine. Their side chains usually have an ammonium group and are mostly positively charged at physiologic pH. In contrast, H_2 antihistamines have a modified imidazole or other heterocyclic ring and a polar but uncharged side chain. The H_2 antihistamines are hydrophilic; this property may account for their rather weak CNS and local anesthetic properties.[17]

Pharmacologic effects

The H_2 antihistamines are potent competitive antagonists of histamine. Because H_2 receptors are strongly implicated in the secretory function of the gastric mucosa, it is not surprising that these compounds cause a marked reduction in H^+ output, pepsin activity, and the total volume of gastric secretion (Figure 22-4). Inhibition of secretion can be attained in the fasting state and after stimulation with food, histamine, betazole, pentagastrin, or caffeine.

Although receptors are found in many tissues, including vascular and bronchial smooth muscle, the H_2 antihistamines have few important effects on physiologic function other than gastric secretion. In certain situations, such as antagonism of a histamine-induced hypotension, a combination of H_1 and H_2 antihistamines is more effective than either alone, which suggests that in such situations both H_1 and H_2 receptors are involved.[37]

Absorption, fate, and excretion

With the exception of famotidine, the H_2 antihistamines are rapidly and completely absorbed after oral administration. All undergo a variable degree of first-pass metabolic degradation in the liver, resulting in an oral bioavailability of approximately 50% for cimetidine, ranitidine, and famotidine and more than 90% for nizatidine. After absorption, the H_2 antihistamines are generally distributed in the total body water. Therapeutic concentrations are reached in approximately 1 to 2 hours. The elimination half-life is 2 to 3.5 hours, except for nizatidine, which has a half-life of 1 to 1.5 hours. Urinary excretion of the parent compound accounts for 60% to 70% of the injected dose of each drug. The remainder is oxidized, the sulfoxide being a major metabolite, and excreted in the urine and feces. Cimetidine (300 mg), the least potent agent, reduces basal gastric acid secretion by at least 80% for 4 to 5 hours, whereas famotidine (20 mg), the most potent, lasts for 10 to 12 hours. Because of the relative safety of these drugs, increased doses can be used to extend the duration of effect.

General therapeutic uses

It has now been demonstrated that *Helicobacter pylori* plays a role in the pathogenesis of most peptic ulcer disease. This organism is a gram-negative rod that can colonize the mucosal surface of the stomach and evoke an inflammatory gastritis. Two lines of evidence implicate *H. pylori* in peptic ulcer disease. First, it is found in most cases (70% to 90%) of active gastric or duodenal ulcers. Second, eradication of the organism by appropriate antimicrobial therapy often leads to remission of symptoms, healing of ulcers, and prevention of recurrence. The fact that *H. pylori* may be found in normal individuals suggests that other risk factors are involved in the genesis of this disease. These observations have altered conventional therapy of peptic ulcer disease; antiinfective measures aimed at *H. pylori* are now frequently combined with control of gastric acid secretion by H_2 antihistamines. The reader is referred to a consensus review for a more detailed discussion of the association between peptic ulcer disease and *H. pylori* infection and the antiinfective strategies for elimination of this putative pathogen.[33] Chapter 33 also discusses antibiotic therapy for *H. pylori*.

The H_2 antihistamines are used clinically for their marked ability to inhibit both basal and stimulated secretion of gastric acid. They are approved for use in a wide variety of gastrointestinal disorders in which reduction of acid secretion may

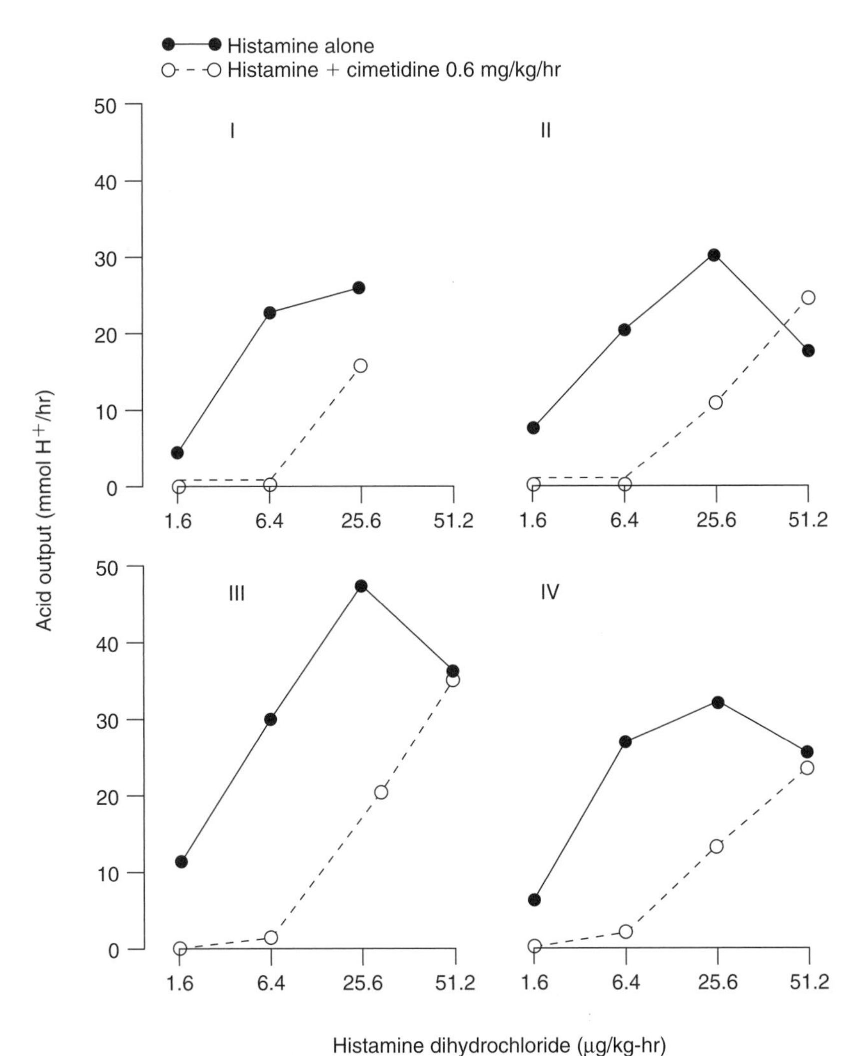

Fig. 22-4 Inhibition of histamine-stimulated gastric acid production by cimetidine in human beings. Histamine dihydrochloride in doses from 1.6 to 51.2 µg/kg per hour was infused intravenously with or without cimetidine at a dose of 0.6 mg/kg per hour for 105 minutes. When cimetidine was given, its administration was begun 15 minutes before the histamine infusion was started. Gastric juice was collected at 15-minute intervals and analyzed for acid concentration; the last four 15-minute intervals were used to establish the dose-response curves. Data shown are individual results from four normal adult subjects (*I* to *IV*). (From Aadland E, Berstad A: Inhibition of histamine- and pentagastrin-stimulated gastric secretion by cimetidine in man. In Creutzfeldt W, ed: *Cimetidine,* Amsterdam, 1978, Excerpta Medica Foundation.)

relieve symptoms, lead to healing, and prevent recurrence of disease once resolved.[16] H_2 antihistamines are generally given orally, but parenteral forms (except for nizatidine) are also available for acute suppression of gastric acid secretion. Oral dosage may be divided into once or twice daily administration; if once daily, the dose is best given at bedtime to block nocturnal gastric acid secretion. A major use of H_2 antihistamines is treatment of active benign gastric ulcers and prophylaxis and treatment of active duodenal ulcers. All the currently available agents (cimetidine, ranitidine, famotidine, and nizatidine) have been shown to be equally effective in appropriate doses in suppressing gastric acid secretion (by up to 90%) and accelerating the healing of duodenal and, to a lesser extent, gastric ulcers.[14] Healing of ulcers generally occurs within 2 to 4 months of therapy; if healing is not achieved in this period, further therapy is unlikely to be successful. Other indications for H_2 antihistamines are the treatment of gastroesophageal reflux (with or without erosive esophagitis) and various pathologic hypersecretory states, such as Zollinger-Ellison syndrome, systemic mastocytosis, and multiple endocrine adenoma.[10,15,39] Although cimetidine and other H_2 antihistamines have been used to treat upper gastrointestinal bleeding caused by liver disease, such as cirrhosis, little evidence supports their effectiveness in these conditions. Finally, H_2 antihistamines may be used before general anesthesia, particularly in patients with gastrointestinal obstruction, to elevate gastric pH and reduce the danger of aseptic pneumonia if gastric contents are aspirated during induction.

H_2 receptor antagonists are among the most widely prescribed drugs in the world. However, data indicate that some uses of H_2 antihistamines might be inappropriate and unwarranted. In a study of 200 patients treated with cimetidine at a university hospital, only 7.5% had an approved indication (e.g., duodenal ulcer disease or pathologic gastric hypersecretion).[44] Because therapy with H_2 antihistamines is not free of adverse effects, there is a clear need to limit these drugs to approved uses until their efficacy in ulcer prophylaxis, nonspecific gastritis, acute gastrointestinal bleeding, and other conditions is better demonstrated.[16]

In addition to cimetidine, the first H_2 receptor antagonist sold over the counter (OTC), the Food and Drug Administration has allowed OTC marketing of the other available H_2 antihistamines for symptomatic relief of occasional heartburn (gastroesophageal reflux), acid indigestion (hyperchlorhydria), or sour stomach. This action reflects the current extensive use of H_2 antihistamines dispensed by prescription for the above conditions and acknowledges their relative safety for unsupervised use. However, their OTC use may delay the diagnosis of more serious disease, such as peptic ulcer or gastric cancer.[34] Given their higher cost and slower onset of action, the H_2 antihistamines will probably not replace the popular and readily available antacids for relief of episodic symptoms caused by hyperacidity.[34]

Adverse effects

The initial impression that cimetidine was generally free of serious adverse effects has been validated by the passage of time and extensive clinical use. The more recently introduced H_2 antihistamines appear to be similarly well tolerated by most people. It has also become apparent that cimetidine and, to a lesser extent, other H_2 antihistamines can cause a variety of toxic reactions and side effects:[28,43] Most untoward responses appear to have no obvious relation to blockade of H_2 receptors. This assumption may simply result from an incomplete understanding of the presence and function of H_2 receptors in tissues other than the gastric mucosa.

The most common adverse effects of cimetidine are manifested in the CNS. These are highly variable and range from minor symptoms (dizziness, lethargy, and fatigue) to more serious disturbances (mental confusion, delirium, focal twitching, hallucinations, and seizures). The CNS effects often appear to be dose related and are most commonly seen in elderly patients or those with impaired liver or kidney function. Cimetidine exerts a number of effects on endocrine function that are generally minor and reversible on cessation of therapy. The most notable of these is gynecomastia; others are elevation of serum prolactin concentrations, galactorrhea, loss of libido, impotence, and reduction in sperm counts. Small but definite increases in serum creatinine concentrations occur in most patients treated with cimetidine. This effect is not associated with other changes in renal function and ceases when the drug is withdrawn. The depression of granulocytes associated with metiamide does not appear to be a problem with cimetidine, but transient leukopenia, granulocytopenia, and thrombocytopenia have been reported. It is difficult to implicate cimetidine as a direct bone marrow suppressant because the cases reported almost always involve the concomitant use of other drugs or the existence of other serious systemic diseases. Although cimetidine enhances cell-mediated immune reactions, no evidence suggests that this phenomenon is related to any of the observed clinical responses. The occurrence of gastric cancer in patients treated with cimetidine has led to the suggestion that the agent may be carcinogenic. This possibility has not been proved, and present information is insufficient to label cimetidine as a carcinogen.

Although cimetidine initially appeared to have no drug interactions of consequence, subsequent clinical reports and laboratory studies indicate that this is not the case. Cimetidine has been shown to increase blood concentrations of numerous drugs, including anticoagulants of the warfarin type, tricyclic antidepressants, various benzodiazepines, phenobarbital, theophylline, propranolol and other β-adrenoceptor blockers, Ca^{++}-channel blockers, lidocaine, estradiol, and phenytoin, thus creating a risk of toxicity. The basis of these interactions appears to be competitive inhibition by cimetidine of the hepatic mixed-function oxidase enzymes responsible for the metabolism of these drugs.[3,19,51] A cimetidine-induced decrease in hepatic blood flow may depress the entry of drugs into the liver and also slow metabolism. Patients receiving cimetidine together with any of the above drugs should be carefully monitored and, if appropriate, reduction of dosages or use of alternative agents should be considered.

Ranitidine, famotidine, and nizatidine appear to have fewer adverse effects than cimetidine. These drugs, for instance, do not exert significant antiandrogenic effects, nor do they influence serum prolactin concentrations. Therefore impotence and gynecomastia do not occur with their use. Mental disturbances are less likely with these drugs, and they have not been reported to elevate serum creatinine activities.[10] Because the binding of these agents to cytochrome P450 enzymes is much less firm than that of cimetidine, they do not significantly inhibit the microsomal metabolism of other drugs. Further investigation and clinical experience are necessary to firmly establish the extent and importance of these differences between cimetidine and the newer H_2 antihistamines.

Antihistamines

Nonproprietary (generic) name	*Proprietary (trade) name*
H_1 receptor antagonists—first generation	
Alkylamines	
Brompheniramine	Bromphen, Dimetane
Chlorpheniramine	Chlor-Trimeton, Teldrin
Dexbrompheniramine	In Bromfed and Drixoral
Dexchlorpheniramine	Polaramine
Triprolidine	Myidil
Ethanolamines	
Clemastine	Tavist
Dimenhydrinate*	Dramamine, Marmine
Diphenhydramine	Benadryl, Sominex
Doxylamine	Unisom
Carbinoxamine	In Rondec
Ethylenediamines	
Pyrilamine	Nisaval
Tripelennamine	PBZ
Piperazines	
Buclizine	Bucladin-S
Cyclizine	Marezine
Hydroxyzine	Atarax, Vistaril
Meclizine	Antivert, Bonine
Phenothiazines	
Methdilazine	Tacaryl
Promethazine	Phenergan, Prothazine
Trimeprazine	Temaril
Piperidines	
Azatadine	Optimine
Cyproheptadine	Periactin
Phenindamine	Nolahist
H_1 receptor antagonists—second-generation (nonsedating)	
Alkylamine	
Acrivastine	In Semprex-D
Piperazine	
Cetirizine	Zyrtec
Piperidines	
Desloratadine	Clarinex
Fexofenadine	Allegra
Levocabastine†	Livostin
Loratadine	Claritin
Phthalazinone	
Azelastine‡	Astelin
H_2-receptor antagonists	
Cimetidine	Tagamet
Famotidine	Pepcid
Nizatidine	Axid
Ranitidine	Zantac

*The chlorotheophylline salt of diphenhydramine.
†For topical ophthalmic use.
‡For topical intranasal use.

CITED REFERENCES

1. Atkinson TP, White MV, Kaliner MA: Histamine and serotonin. In Gallin JI, Goldstein IM, Snyderman R, eds: *Inflammation: basic principles and clinical correlates,* ed 2, New York, 1992, Raven Press.
2. Barnett A, Kreutner W: Pharmacology of non-sedating H_1 antihistamines, *Agents Actions* 33(suppl):181-196, 1991.
3. Bauman JH, Kimelblatt BJ: Cimetidine as an inhibitor of drug metabolism: therapeutic implications and review of the literature, *Drug Intelligence Clin Pharm* 16:380-386, 1982.
4. Best CH, Dale HH, Dudley JW, et al: The nature of the vaso-dilator constituents of certain tissue extracts, *J Physiol* (London) 62:397-417, 1927.
5. Black JW, Duncan WA, Durant CJ, et al: Definition and antagonism of histamine H_2-receptors, *Nature* 236:385-390, 1972.
6. Black JW, Duncan WA, Emmett JC, et al: Metiamide—an orally active histamine H_2-receptor antagonist, *Agents Actions* 3:133-137, 1973.
7. Bovet D, Staub A: Action protectrice des ethers phenoliques au cours de l'intoxication histaminique, *Compt Rend Soc de Biol* 124:547-549, 1937.
8. Busse W: New directions and dimensions in the treatment of allergic rhinitis, *J Allergy Clin Immunol* 82:890-900, 1988.
9. Carter CA, Wajciechowski NJ, Hayes JM, et al: Terfenadine, a nonsedating antihistamine, *Drug Intelligence Clin Pharm* 19:812-817, 1985.
10. Cimetidine and ranitidine [editorial], *Lancet* 1:601-602, 1982.
11. Code CF: Reflections on histamine, gastric secretion, and the H_2 receptor, *N Engl J Med* 296:1459-1462, 1977.
12. Crawford JM: The gastrointestinal tract. In Cotran RS, Kumar V, Collins T, eds: *Robbins' Pathologic basis of disease,* ed 6, Philadelphia, 1999, WB Saunders.
13. Dale HH, Laidlaw PP: Histamine shock, *J Physiol* (London) 52:355-390, 1919.
14. Deakin M, Williams JG: Histamine H_2-receptor antagonists in peptic ulcer disease. Efficacy in healing peptic ulcers, *Drugs* 44:709-719, 1992.
15. Famotidine (Pepcid), *Med Lett Drugs Ther* 29:17-18, 1987.
16. Feldman M, Burton M: Histamine$_2$-receptor antagonists: standard therapy for acid-peptic diseases, *N Engl J Med* 323:1672-1680, 1749-1755, 1990.
17. Ganellin CR, Durant GJ, Emmett JC: Some chemical aspects of histamine H_2-receptor antagonists, *Fed Proc* 35:1924-1930, 1976.
18. Goldsmith P, Dowd PM: The new H_1 antihistamines. Treatment of urticaria and other clinical problems, *Dermatol Clin* 11:87-95, 1993.
19. Hansten PD: Drug interactions of gastrointestinal drugs. In Lewis JH, ed: *A pharmacologic approach to gastrointestinal disorders,* Baltimore, 1994, Williams & Wilkins.
20. Hill SJ: Distribution, properties and functional characteristics of three classes of histamine receptors, *Pharmacol Rev* 42:45-83, 1990.
21. Hollande F, Bali J-P, Magous R: Autoregulation of histamine synthesis through H_3 receptors in isolated fundic mucosal cells, *Am J Physiol* 265:G1039-G1044, 1993.
22. Imamura M, Poli E, Omonivi AT, et al: Unmasking of activated histamine H_3 receptors in myocardial ischemia: their role as regulators of exocytotic norepinephrine release, *J Pharmacol Exp Ther* 271:1259-1266, 1994.
23. Jacobs RS, Catania H: Cimetidine, *Drug Intelligence Clin Pharm* 11:723-726, 1977.
24. Lagunoff D, Martin TW, Read G: Agents that release histamine from mast cells, *Annu Rev Pharmacol Toxicol* 23:331-351, 1983.
25. Levi R, Allan G, Zavecz JH: Cardiac histamine receptors, *Fed Proc* 35:1942-1947, 1976.
26. Lewis T, Grant RT: Vascular reactions of the skin to injury. II. The liberation of a histamine-like substance in injured skin; the underlying causes of factitious urticaria and of wheals produced by burning; and observations upon the nervous control of certain skin reactions, *Heart* 11:209-265, 1924.
27. Malamed SF: *Sedation: a guide to patient management,* ed 4, St Louis, 2003, Mosby.
28. McGuigan JE: A consideration of the adverse effects of cimetidine, *Gastroenterology* 80:181-192, 1981.
29. McTavish D, Sorkin EM: Azelastine: a review of its pharmacodynamic and pharmacokinetic properties and therapeutic potential, *Drugs* 38:778-800, 1989.
30. Metcalfe DD, Costa JJ, Burd PR: Mast cells, and basophils. In Gallin JI, Goldstein IM, Snyderman R, eds: *Inflammation: basic principles and clinical correlates,* ed 2, New York, 1992, Raven Press.
31. Meyer RA, Jakubowski W: Use of tripelennamine and diphenhydramine as local anesthetics, *J Am Dent Assoc* 69:112-117, 1964.
32 *Mosby's drug consult,* St Louis, 2004, Mosby.
33. NIH Consensus Development Panel on *Helicobacter pylori* in peptic ulcer disease. *Helicobacter pylori* in peptic ulcer disease, *JAMA* 272:65-69, 1994.
34. Over-the-counter H_2-receptor antagonists for heartburn, *Med Lett Drugs Ther* 37:95-96, 1995.
35. Parsons ME: The antagonism of histamine H_2-receptors in vitro and in vivo with particular reference to the actions of cimetidine. In Burland WL, Simkins MA, eds: *Cimetidine. Proceedings of the Second International Symposium on Histamine H_2-Receptor Antagonists,* Amsterdam, 1977, Excerpta Medica Foundation.
36. Peets EA, Jackson M, Symchowicz S: Metabolism of chlorpheniramine maleate in man, *J Pharmacol Exp Ther* 180:464-474, 1972.
37. Powell JR, Brody MJ: Identification and blockade of vascular H_2 receptors, *Fed Proc* 35:1935-1941, 1976.
38. Prell GD, Green JP: Histamine as a neuroregulator, *Annu Rev Neurosci* 9:209-254, 1986.
39. Ranitidine (Zantac), *Med Lett Drugs Ther* 24:111-113, 1982.
40. Reiner PB, Kamondi A: Mechanisms of antihistamine-induced sedation in the human brain: H_1 receptor activation reduces a background leakage potassium current, *Neuroscience* 59:579-588, 1994.
41. Riley JF, West GB: The occurrence of histamine in mast cells. In Rocha e Silva M, ed: Histamine and antihistaminics, part 1. *Handbook of experimental pharmacology,* vol 18, Berlin, 1966, Springer-Verlag.
42. Roden DM: Torsades de pointes, *Clin Cardiol* 16:683-686, 1993.

43. Sawyer D, Conner CS, Scalley R: Cimetidine: adverse reactions and acute toxicity, *Am J Hosp Pharm* 38:188-197, 1981.
44. Schade RR, Donaldson RM, Jr: How physicians use cimetidine: a survey of hospitalized patients and published cases, *N Engl J Med* 304:1281-1284, 1981.
45. Schayer RW: Catabolism of histamine in vivo. In Rocha e Silva M, ed: Histamine and antihistaminics, part 1. *Handbook of experimental pharmacology,* vol 18, Berlin, 1966, Springer-Verlag.
46. Schwartz J-C, Barbin G, Duchemin A-M, et al: Histamine receptors in the brain and their possible functions. In Ganellin CR, Parsons ME, eds: *Pharmacology of histamine receptors,* Bristol, 1982, Wright-PSG.
47. Schwartz LB: Mast cells: function and contents, *Curr Opinion Immunol* 6:91-97, 1994.
48. Serafin WE, Babe KS, Jr: Histamine, bradykinin, and their antagonists. In Hardman JG, Limbird LE, Gilman AG, eds: *Goodman & Gilman's The pharmacological basis of therapeutics,* ed 9, New York, 1996, McGraw-Hill.
49. Simons FER, Simons KJ: H1 receptor antagonist treatment of chronic rhinitis, *J Allergy Clin Immunol* 81:975-980, 1988.
50. Simons FER, Simons KJ: The pharmacology and use of H_1-receptor-antagonist drugs, *N Engl J Med* 330:1663-1670, 1994.
51. Somogyi A, Gugler R: Drug interactions with cimetidine, *Clin Pharmacokinet* 7:23-41, 1982.
52. Sorkin EM, Heel RC: Terfenadine. A review of its pharmacologic properties and therapeutic efficacy, *Drugs* 29:34-56, 1985.
53. Spencer CM, Faulds D, Peters DH: Cetirizine. A reappraisal of its pharmacological properties and therapeutic use in selected allergic disorders, *Drugs* 46:1055-1080, 1993.
54. Timmerman H: Histamine H_3 ligands: just pharmacological tools or potential therapeutic agents? *J Med Chem* 33:4-11, 1990.
55. Townley RG: Cetirizine: a new H_1 antagonist with antieosinophilic activity in chronic urticaria, *J Am Acad Dermatol* 25:668-674, 1991.
56. Welborn JF, Kane JP: Conduction anesthesia using diphenhydramine hydrochloride, *J Am Dent Assoc* 69:706-709, 1964.
57. Willoughby DA: Mediation of increased vascular permeability in inflammation. In Zweifach BW, Grant L, McClusky RT, eds: *The inflammatory process,* vol 2, ed 2, New York, 1973, Academic Press.
58. Woolsey RL, Chen Y, Freiman JP, et al: Mechanism of the cardiotoxic actions of terfenadine, *JAMA* 269:1532-1536, 1993.
59. Zweifach BW: Microcirculation, *Annu Rev Physiol* 35:117-150, 1973.

General References

Gallin JI, Snyderman R, eds: *Inflammation: basic principles and clinical correlates,* ed 3, Philadelphia, 1999, Lippincott Williams & Wilkins.

Schwartz JC, Haas HL, eds: *The histamine receptor,* New York, 1992, Wiley-Liss.

Simmons FER, ed: *Histamine and H_1-receptor antagonists in allergic disease,* New York, 1996, Marcel Dekker.

Soll AH: Peptic ulcer and its complications. In Feldman M, Scharschmidt BF, Sleisender MH, eds: *Sleisender & Fordtran's Gastrointestinal disease: pathophysiology, diagnosis, management,* ed 6, Philadelphia, 1998, WB Saunders.

CHAPTER • 23

Drugs Affecting Serotonin, Antimigraine Drugs, and Drugs for Other Pain Syndromes

Robert L. Merrill

PHARMACOLOGY AND CHRONIC PAIN

The management of chronic orofacial pain, as compared with acute pain, requires an in-depth knowledge of pharmacology and pharmacotherapy because chronic pain disorders are a heterogeneous group of conditions with various pathologic mechanisms and characteristics requiring diverse families of medications for treatment. Dentists do not generally use these medications because dentistry has traditionally focused on acute pain problems. The pharmacologic characteristics of opioids are treated in Chapter 20, and those of acetaminophen and nonsteroidal antiinflammatory drugs (NSAIDs) are discussed in Chapter 21. Treatment of acute pain in dentistry is discussed in Chapter 47.

With the recent advances in understanding chronic pain disorders and recognition that these disorders affect the orofacial region, dentists are now being trained to manage chronic pain and use medications normally used only in a medical setting. This chapter will review the medications used for chronic orofacial pain disorders and relate them to known or putative disorders and pain mechanisms.

When a patient is evaluated for chronic orofacial pain, the clinician is faced with the task of determining which of the various potential conditions may be the source of the pain. Generally, after eliminating intracranial and extracranial sources, the clinician has narrowed the differential diagnosis to musculoskeletal, neurovascular, and peripheral or central neuropathic pain, or combinations of these. These categories of pain have different pathophysiologic mechanisms and require different treatment modalities or strategies. Intertwined with the pain issues are psychologic issues that have developed in conjunction with chronic pain. These issues must be dealt with to optimize treatment of pain and obtain a beneficial outcome. Often medications used to treat one condition may be useful for another. This is certainly the case with tricyclic antidepressants, used to treat depression, but which are useful in prophylaxis of migraine and may be the most effective drugs for treating certain neuropathic or musculoskeletal pain disorders. Furthermore, the medications may be used differently in each of the pain categories. To understand chronic orofacial pain, the clinician needs to understand the mechanisms behind the various conditions because this knowledge may be helpful in choosing the medications that would be most beneficial for the patient. This chapter will review the medications used to treat these categories of chronic pain and will also attempt to elaborate on the general and specific mechanisms of action, if known, for each of the medications listed.

This chapter will not discuss the use of opioids for chronic pain other than to indicate that in cases of intractable pain resulting from cancer or other conditions such as chronic neuropathy resulting from failed temporomandibular surgery, long-term use of opioids may be the only option for helping the patient, although this is rare because opioids are generally less effective in treating neuropathic pain than several other drugs.

SEROTONIN (5-HYDROXYTRYPTAMINE, 5-HT)

To understand chronic pain and its pharmacologic management, it is necessary to understand the 5-HT system and its impact on pain modulation. Besides chronic pain, alteration in 5-HT function has been implicated in a number of other clinical conditions, including affective disorders, obsessive-compulsive disorders, schizophrenia, anxiety states, phobic disorders, eating disorders, migraine, and sleep disorders. There is a wide range of drugs that affects 5-HT neurotransmission, including antidepressants (tricyclic antidepressants [TCAS], selective serotonin reuptake inhibitorss [SSRIs], and heterocyclic antidepressants), hallucinogens, anxiolytics, antiemetics, antimigraine agents, atypical antipsychotics, and appetite suppressants. Moreover, a number of other drugs not generally considered to affect the 5-HT system nevertheless have an assumed effect on 5-HT receptors because of the influence they have on conditions that are linked to 5-HT dysregulation, such as migraine.

Historical Aspects

Since 1868, serum *(sero-)* from blood clots was known to possess a substance that caused blood vessels to constrict, increasing their smooth muscle tone (*-tonin*). Subsequent physiologic studies of this vasoconstrictive activity vacillated between some unknown substance and epinephrine as the cause. Eventually, the issue was clarified when it was observed that the serum constricted both frog vascular and rabbit intestinal preparations, whereas epinephrine only caused relaxation of the gut. Because no evidence of epinephrine was found in the blood plasma, it was assumed that vasoconstriction was caused by a substance in the coagulated blood, and by the early 1900s that source was identified with platelets.

Janeway and associates did a thorough investigation of the vasoconstrictive substance and noted that it was not present in uncoagulated or citrated blood, that it was definitely associated with platelets, was soluble in water more than ether or chloroform, and that the factor did not depend on the clot formation but on the disintegration of the platelets in the clot.[28] The substance itself was eventually isolated and named *serotonin* by Rapport et al in 1948.[51] Shortly after this, Rapport identified the agent as 5-HT, and Hamlin and Fischer reported synthesizing it in 1951.[25]

Meanwhile, in Italy, in a separate series of studies, Erspamer and associates isolated a substance from the mucosa of rabbit stomach, and found that it was abundant in the enterochromaffin cells of the gut, could be extracted with alcohol and acetone, was an amine that affected smooth muscle, and was deactivated by deamination. Erspamer named it *enteramine.* By 1952, both serotonin and enteramine had been chemically identified as 5-HT,[13] eventually leading to international wrangling over the naming of 5-HT. It was argued that "enteramine" was inaccurate because the substance was found in places other than the gut and "serotonin" was equally inadequate from the points of origin and pharmacologic action. In 1986 when the International Serotonin Club was organized, American researchers prevailed over the European contingent in naming the substance *serotonin* by arguing that serotonin was the most widely accepted name, 5-hydroxytryptamine was too long, and 5-HT was only an abbreviation (but one used here).[55]

5-HT and pain

Stimulation of the periaqueductal gray (PAG) was shown to modulate nociception on a spinal level.[40] This effect is known as *stimulation-produced analgesia (SPA).* Whereas a number of areas have been studied in animals, human studies of necessity have been limited. In human beings, stimulation of the midbrain region of the PAG and areas slightly more rostral in the periventricular gray matter of the hypothalamus are known to produce SPA. Neurosurgeons were able to demonstrate SPA in human beings by stimulating the equivalent human midbrain sites. Researchers had determined that electrical stimulation of brainstem PAG produced analgesia in animals. Although the exact boundaries of the responsive area were not clearly defined, the sites most responsive to SPA were: ventral to the midbrain cerebral aqueduct; in the PAG; sites lateral to this structure; the rostroventral medulla (RVM), including the midline nucleus raphe magnus (NRM) and reticular formations; the hypothalamus; the frontal lobe; and the spinal cord. Areas outside of the midbrain have not been systematically studied. The majority of the projections from the RVM/PAG are in fact tryptaminergic. Injection of morphine in the PAG has also been shown to have a similar antinociceptive effect, thought to be mediated by activation of a raphe-spinal pathway. Other studies have implicated descending 5-HT fibers as well as other non–5-HT–containing fibers in this process. Increased production of 5-HT in the bulbospinal 5-HT neurons, as shown by Bourgoin in 1980,[4] supports the role of 5-HT in modulation of pain in these pathways. Moreover, studies of the raphe pathways have confirmed that with such stimulation there is a concomitant increase in 5-hydroxyindoleacetic acid (5-HIAA), a major metabolite of 5-HT, in the dorsal horn, implicating activation and degradation of 5-HT in the process.

Anatomical Distribution

5-HT, a biogenic monoamine, is widely distributed throughout the plant and animal kingdom. In mammals, the highest concentrations are found in the enterochromaffin cells of the gastrointestinal mucosa, central nervous system (CNS), and blood platelets. The structure of 5-HT is shown in Figure 23-1. Its most notable features are the hydroxyl group on position 5 of the indole nucleus and the primary amine nitrogen that can accept a proton, making the compound hydrophilic and unable to pass the blood-brain barrier easily. Rapport found the substance in the brain, indicating that it must be synthesized and perform some unidentified function there. It was subsequently assumed that 5-HT was associated with psychiatric disorders such as depression and schizophrenia when it was shown that the psychedelic drug lysergic acid diethylamide (LSD) antagonized 5-HT function. 5-HT is now known to be involved in many of the behavioral and psychiatric disorders such as schizophrenia, obsessive-compulsive disorder, depression, and anxiety, and drugs that have an effect on the 5-HT system have been beneficial in treating these disorders (see Chapter 12).

Despite earlier suggestions that 5-HT was a neurotransmitter synthesized in the brain, the actual localization of

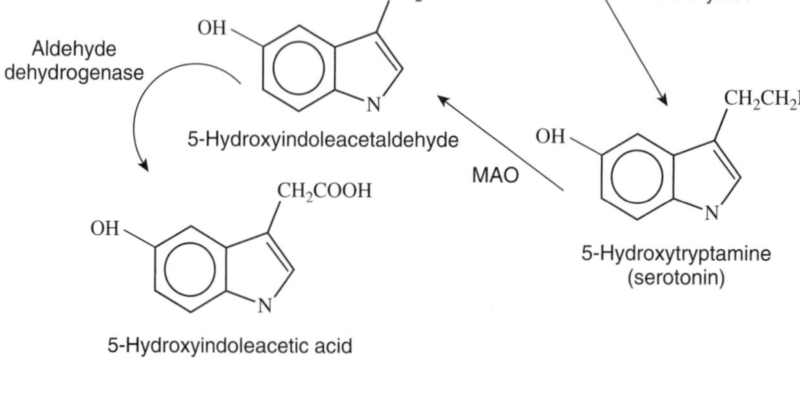

Fig. 23-1 Biosynthesis and metabolism of serotonin. *MAO,* Monoamine oxidase.

5-HT neurons was not determined for at least 10 more years. By using lesioning and fractionation techniques, 5-HT was grossly associated with specific neuronal elements but it was not possible to observe the relationship directly until fluorescence histochemical techniques were developed. This process, however, had inherent problems that made identification a significant challenge. Dahlström and Fuxe, using immunocytochemical techniques, localized 5-HT-associated neurons in nine discrete clusters of cells along the midline of the upper brainstem and pons. These 5-HT–containing cell bodies, designated *B1* to *B9*, corresponded for the most part to the dorsal raphe nuclei. It should be noted, however, that only approximately 40% to 50% of the dorsal raphe nuclei are serotonergic neurons and that some serotonergic nuclei are found outside the midline raphe nuclei area, although the major brain concentration is in the dorsal raphe nuclei.

Additional studies have shown that the lateral and dorsolateral pontine tegmentum, which contain many noradrenergic neurons, are also involved in nociceptive modulation when stimulated, and, furthermore, these sites also send projections to the PAG, the RVM, and the spinal cord. The projections from the lateral and dorsolateral pons are noradrenergic and possess important α_2-adrenergic receptors. In animal studies, norepinephrine applied directly to the spinal cord blocks response to nociception through selective inhibition of the nociceptive dorsal horn neurons (see Chapter 20). Lesioning the white matter of the dorsolateral funiculus of the spinal cord blocks the inhibitory effect of SPA and confirms the existence of a descending modulatory pathway that travels through the dorsolateral funiculus. Further studies of the dorsolateral funiculus projections to the spinal cord have found that the majority of the brainstem projections arise in the RVM and dorsolateral pons, with few projections from the PAG. This would imply that the PAG projections must be relayed through the RVM. This has been confirmed by studies showing that the major neuronal input to the RVM is from the PAG and adjacent structures, and lesioning or blocking RVM cells eliminates the analgesic effect obtained from PAG stimulation.[18]

Anti–5-HT antibody labeling has identified 5-HT in all dorsal horn lamina, but the highest densities are found in lamina I, II, IV, V, and X. The RVM projections terminate mainly in laminae I, II, and V. These areas are important for pain because this is where the central terminals of afferent nociceptors and cell bodies of second-order neurons are found. This dorsal horn area is the major "switchboard" for pain, and stimulation of the PAG and RVM modulate nociceptive activity here (see Chapter 20).

Immunocytochemical studies have also found 5-HT reactive cells in the area postrema, the caudal locus ceruleus, and around the interpeduncular nucleus. Through lesioning studies, it has been observed that the caudal clusters project mainly to the medulla and spinal cord, the rostral clusters project to the telencephalon and diencephalon, and the more centrally located clusters project both rostrally and inferiorly. In general, however, 5-HT cells send axons through virtually every part of the CNS, and recent findings indicate a lack of pattern to this innervation.

Transmission of sensory and particularly nociceptive messages by afferent fibers entering the dorsal horn of the spinal cord is under control of pathways originating in the ventromedial medulla. It had been observed that neurons from the medullary raphe nuclei and particularly the NRM project predominantly to the dorsal horn, including the superficial laminae and the area around the central canal, and are involved in a descending inhibitory pathway for modulation of nociceptive input. As the area was found to have an abundance of 5-HT–containing neurons, researchers postulated that 5-HT was a descending pain modulatory system neurotransmitter. 5-HT–containing neurons are located in the rostroventromedial medulla and caudal pons, and particularly in the NRM, nucleus paragigantocellularis, and the ventral portion of the nucleus gigantocellularis. Recent studies have described other descending projections from the bulbomesencephalon to the spinal cord that do not contain 5-HT and, in fact, are more numerous within the medulla and caudal pons, indicating that descending modulation is not limited to 5-HT fibers.[34]

Immunocytochemical studies of antibodies directed against 5-HT have shown that two distinct types of 5-HT neurons innervate the cerebral cortex of many mammals. The studies have found fine axons with small varicosities originating from the dorsal raphe nuclei and beaded axons with large spherical varicosities originating from the median raphe nuclei. Apparently the two types of axons have different regional and laminar distributions and demonstrate different sensitivities to neurotoxic drugs such as 3,4-methylenedioxymethamphetamine, commonly referred to as "ecstasy." The fine axons appear to be more sensitive to the neurotoxic effects, with loss of functions that may be long term or permanent. Cooper[9] has suggested that lab animal findings may relate to human beings' use of the drug because the doses commonly used by recreational drug users are similar to what are used in animal studies. Ecstasy users have shown a 26% decrease in 5-HIAA, the 5-HT metabolite. The decrease in metabolite may indicate a decrease of 5-HT function in the brain related to loss of some 5-HT neurons. In general, however, the functional distinction between these two types of neurons remains unclear.

Synthesis, Storage, and Fate

5-HT is synthesized from the amino acid L-tryptophan (see Figure 23-1). Although platelets contain relatively large amounts of 5-HT, it only accumulates rather than being synthesized there. Synthesis in the CNS involves active transport of tryptophan through the blood-brain barrier. Tryptophan is derived primarily from the diet, and its elimination from the diet can profoundly lower brain 5-HT. In addition, the active transport of tryptophan is affected by its concentration in the blood and the relative concentration of other amino acids that are transported by the same active transport mechanism. L-Tryptophan is converted in serotonergic neurons containing the enzyme tryptophan hydroxylase (L-tryptophan-5-monooxygenase).

The initial synthesis step is hydroxylation of tryptophan at the 5 position to form 5-hydroxytryptophan (see Figure 23-1). Tryptophan hydroxylase, the enzyme responsible for this reaction, occurs in low concentrations in most tissues, including the brain, and has proved to be difficult to isolate.

Tryptophan hydroxylase has a rate-limiting requirement for oxygen. In addition, mounting evidence suggests that the system adjusts to the amount of tryptophan available. It has been demonstrated that drug treatments affecting the 5-HT system are soon counteracted by a built-in feedback mechanism involving regulation of the synthesis of 5-HT. For example, short-term treatment with lithium salts will initially increase tryptophan uptake, resulting in increased amounts of tryptophan being converted to 5-HT; however, with long-term treatment, increased uptake is still measured, but the synthesis of 5-HT from the increased tryptophan returns to pretreatment levels.

5-Hydroxytryptophan is rapidly decarboxylated to form 5-HT by the aromatic enzyme L-amino acid decarboxylase, which is the same enzyme that catalyzes the decarboxylation of L-dopamine in catecholamine neurons (see Figure 23-1). Because the rate of the reaction is so rapid and requires less substrate than the initial reaction, the action of tryptophan hydroxylase in the first step is regarded as the rate-limiting step in the synthesis of 5-HT, and drugs targeting the action of the decarboxylase have not shown themselves to be effective.

The synthesis of 5-HT is markedly increased with the electrical stimulation of serotonergic soma. This is the result of enhanced conversion of tryptophan to 5-HT and depends on extracellular Ca^{++}. Because, as discussed above, the rate-limiting step is the action of tryptophan hydroxylase on tryptophan, it is likely that Ca^{++} affects the Ca^{++}-dependent phosphorylation of the enzyme, increasing its availability.

Storage and release

Similar to other monoamines, 5-HT is stored in vesicles within the cell. Drugs such as reserpine and tetrabenazine that inhibit the activity of the transporter mechanism within the vesicular membrane deplete the brain content of 5-HT. Furthermore, the storage of 5-HT in vesicles requires an active transport mechanism to transfer the molecule from the cytosol to the storage vesicle.

Metabolism

5-HT is also metabolized in the liver by the enzyme monoamine oxidase (see Figure 23-1). The product of this reaction is 5-hydroxyindoleacetaldehyde, which is further oxidized by aldehyde dehydrogenase to form the final metabolite, 5-HIAA, which is excreted (see Figure 23-1). It had been suggested that increased levels of either of the metabolites of 5-HT or the concentration of 5-HT itself would affect its metabolism, but it has been noted that using monoamine oxidase (MAO) inhibitors to block metabolism does not affect the synthesis of 5-HT, and concentrations will climb to three times greater than controls. Moreover, if the elimination of 5-HIAA is blocked by the drug probenecid, the 5-HIAA levels will continue to rise without apparent feedback inhibition. The implication of these findings is that the synthesis of 5-HT is not affected by changes in concentrations of its metabolites.

Reuptake and transport across body membranes

Presynaptic reuptake of 5-HT from the synaptic cleft is a major mechanism for controlling the synaptic concentration and action of 5-HT. The presynaptic terminals of serotonergic neurons contain high-affinity uptake sites that are involved in this process by using a plasma membrane transporter protein that can transport 5-HT in either direction depending on the concentration gradient. The transporter proteins involved in this process are composed of 12 membrane-spanning proteins that are Cl^- and Na^+ dependent. Although the older TCAs inhibit the reuptake of 5-HT, they also have a variable capacity to inhibit norepinephrine (NE) reuptake as well as affecting other systems and receptors (see Chapter 12). The SSRIs that have shown great utility in moderating depression, anxiety, and obsessive-compulsive disorders also inhibit the 5-HT transporter proteins. These medications are more 5-HT selective with more limited effects on the NE transporter.

5-HT Receptors and Pain

Gaddum and Picarelli in 1957 reported two separate 5-HT receptors in peripheral smooth muscle preparations studied in vitro.[17] Since then, there has been an exponential development of information relating to 5-HT receptor types and functions, and numerous receptor subtypes have recently been identified and cloned. Nevertheless, the complete picture of how 5-HT and its receptors modulate pain remains obscure. There are now seven main family groups of receptors, but current understanding attributes most of the 5-HT actions to the families designated *5-HT*$_1$, *5-HT*$_2$, *5-HT*$_3$, *5-HT*$_4$, and *5-HT*$_7$. Each receptor family is operationally and structurally distinct, having its own separate transducing system. Although other recently identified 5-HT receptors also show characteristics indicative of separate classes or families of 5-HT receptors, not all receptors for 5-HT are fully included in the classification system at this time because of a lack of needed characterization through cDNA cloning and amino acid sequencing of their proteins or data concerning their operational and transductional characteristics. This situation applies to the 5-HT$_{1E}$, 5-HT$_{1F}$, 5-HT$_5$, and 5-HT$_6$ receptors, which have been cloned and their amino acid sequence defined, although their operational and transductional characteristics are unclear and the final nomenclature is unsettled. Fourteen different 5-HT receptor subtypes have been identified.

As indicated above, seven classes or families of 5-HT receptors have been identified and designated *5-HT*$_1$, *5-HT*$_2$, *5-HT*$_3$, *5-HT*$_4$, *5-HT*$_5$, *5-HT*$_6$, and *5-HT*$_7$. Each class has subtypes (with the exception of 5-HT$_3$) and all have been identified in the brain. Localization of the receptors in the CNS and spinal cord is variable and not all 5-HT receptors are found in all locations. Furthermore, within the spinal cord itself there is variability in the location of different receptors. Because 5-HT$_1$, 5-HT$_2$, and 5-HT$_3$ receptors have the highest distribution in the dorsal horn, it is assumed that they are involved in sensory processing. In general, the 5-HT$_1$ family is assumed to be inhibitory and the other classes are thought to be excitatory; however, 5-HT$_2$ and 5 HT$_3$ receptors have been linked to an antinociceptive response as measured by some animal models. This highlights the fact that much work is still to be done before the 5-HT–modulating system is fully understood.

5-HT$_1$ receptors

The 5HT$_1$ family of receptors (Table 23-1) produces its cellular action by inhibiting adenylyl cyclase and opening K^+ channels. Binding studies with autoradiographic ligands have shown binding sites throughout the spinal cord gray matter, raphe nuclei, and substantia gelatinosa, with the higher concentrations in laminae I and II of the dorsal horn and lower in lamina VII in the ventral horn. The hippocampus, the substantia nigra, and dorsal raphe contain the highest concentrations.

5-HT$_{1A}$ receptor Taiwo and Levine[58] have shown that 5HT$_{1A}$ receptors are implicated in peripheral mechanical hyperalgesia. Furthermore, they reported that the hyperalgesia could be blocked by selective. 5-HT$_{1A}$ antagonists injected logically. In various pain models it was also shown that the 5-HT$_{1-3}$ receptors all mediated pain.[12] Powell[50] has suggested that 5HT$_{1A}$ receptor agonists may reduce the effects of morphine in an electric shock model for pain. This same effect was not seen with 5HT$_2$, 5HT$_3$ and α_2–adrenergic receptors.

Autoradiographic studies have demonstrated that half of the spinal cord binding sites involve the 5HT$_{1A}$ receptor, with the greatest concentration in the superficial layers of the dorsal horn in the lumbar cord rather than in the cervico-thoracic segments.[61] The 5-HT$_{1A}$ receptor has been implicated in anxiety but may also be involved in migraine. Antianxiety drugs such as buspirone act as agonists on this receptor.

5-HT$_{1B}$ receptor 5-HT$_{1B}$ is a postsynaptic vascular receptor found primarily on cerebral blood vessels, and to a smaller extent on coronary arteries as well as trigeminal ganglia neurons. Stimulation of the 5-HT$_{1B}$ receptor results in a number of smooth muscle contraction actions such as vasoconstriction, closing of atrioventricular shunts, and bronchoconstriction, as well as platelet aggregation. Since there are a smaller number of receptors on coronary arteries, 5-HT$_{1B}$ agonists cause some degree of coronary artery vasoconstriction.

Table • 23-1

5-HT Receptor Subtypes, Drugs, and Antimigraine Medications

5-HT RECEPTOR	DRUG	AGONIST/ANTAGONIST	ACTION IN MIGRAINE
5-$HT_{1B/1D}$	Triptans, DHE	Agonists	Action on cranial neurovascular receptor to cause vasoconstriction or stimulation of inhibitory receptor to stop release of neuroinflammatory mediators; abort migraine
5-HT_{1F}	Triptans, DHE, ergotamine	Agonists	Blockade of neurogenic dural inflammation
5-HT_2	Methysergide, cyproheptadine, DHE	Antagonists	Suppress action at 5-HT_2 receptor; migraine prophylaxis

DHE, Dihydroergotamine.

5-HT_{1D} receptor The 5-HT_{1D} receptor functions as a presynaptic autoreceptor on trigeminovascular sensory afferent fibers, modulating neurotransmitter release such as 5-HT, substance P (SP), acetylcholine, NE, and calcitonin gene–related peptide (CGRP). 5-HT_{1D} is the most widespread 5-HT receptor in the brain and is thought to be the main 5-HT receptor involved in migraine.

5-HT_2 receptors

5HT_{2A} receptors are found in layers 3 and 5 of the cerebral cortex, the subcortical gray matter, the brainstem, and the spinal cord. These receptors, like the other non–5-HT_1 family of receptors, are excitatory. Activation of 5HT_2 receptors results in closure of K^+ channels and activation of phospholipase C. The 5-HT_{2B} receptor has been associated with cerebrovascular endothelium and it has been suggested that migraine is caused by sensitization of these receptors. Kalkman[30] suggested that as 5-HT bioavailability increased during development of the migraine attack, it was attended by production and release of nitric oxide (NO). Nitroglycerin, a donor of NO, is known to cause headache when used to control angina, and this effect is blocked by indomethacin, which antagonizes the effect of NO. Interestingly, patients suffering from analgesic rebound headache have a greater density of postsynaptic 5-HT_2 receptors on platelet membranes than do migraine patients who do not have analgesic rebound. This implies that chronic ingestion of analgesics causes a depletion of 5-HT and concomitant upregulation of 5-HT_2 receptors.

Even though the exact role of 5-HT neuronal modulation is still not clear in migraine, the medications that seem to give the most benefit have definite 5-HT activity. Furthermore, the role of 5-HT in platelets during the ictal phase of migraine is apparently important but remains to be defined. It seems that all aspects of the 5-HT system come into play during a migraine attack and not only the 5-HT_1 receptors but also 5-HT_2 receptors. It has been observed that some of the most commonly used compounds in migraine prophylaxis, namely propranolol, pizotifen, methysergide, cyproheptadine, amitriptyline, and chlorpromazine, have an antagonistic effect on specific subtypes of the 5-HT_2 receptor family, now known as the 5HT_{2B}/5-HT_{2C} (formerly 5-HT_{1C}) receptors. This hypothesis is supported by previous observations that the 5-HT_2 receptor agonist m-chlorophenylpiperazine (m-CPP) triggers migraine in susceptible individuals when it is administered at doses high enough to activate 5-$HT_{2B/2C}$ receptors.[29]

5-HT_3 receptor

The 5-HT_3 receptor is found mainly in the lower brainstem and on the presynaptic terminals of small-diameter unmyelinated nociceptive afferents in substantia gelatinosa where they may be involved in pain processing. The 5-HT_3 receptor is the only ion-gated cation channel receptor in the 5-HT receptor family. It causes increased conductance for Na^+, K^+ and Ca^{++} and depolarization of the involved cell membrane.[24,46,66] It has been shown that 5HT_3 receptors participate in the nociceptive activity in the dorsal horn and are probably involved in the antinociceptive effect when 5-HT is administered intrathecally.[33] This receptor has also been implicated in emesis associated with migraine. The "triptans" which have been developed for symptomatic treatment of migraine through their agonist action on the 5-$HT_{1D/1B}$ receptors are also antagonist of the 5-HT_3 receptor, relieving nausea.

5-HT_4 receptors

In contrast to the inhibitory effects of the 5-HT_1 receptors, the 5-HT_4 family of receptors is positively coupled to adenylyl cyclase, provoking second messenger activation of cyclic adenosine 3′,5′–monophosphate (cAMP). This receptor has high concentration in the gut and antagonists of the receptor prevent development of increased bowel activity that would be stimulated by 5-HT or 5-HTP sensitization.[52] Ghelardini and colleagues[20] reported that 5-HT_4 agonists had an antinociceptive effect, raising pain thresholds in mice and rats.

5-HT_7 receptors The 5-HT_7 receptor subtype activates adenylyl cyclase with consequent closure of K^+ channels. The 5-HT_7 receptor was recently shown to mediate cerebrovascular smooth-muscle relaxation, independent of any mechanism in the endothelium. Because of its action on the regulation of vascular tone, it has been proposed to have a role in migraine. This has been supported by observations that 5HT_7 receptor–linked relaxation has been observed in dog basilar and middle cerebral arteries, together with other circumstantial evidence such as the high affinity of antimigraine drugs for the 5-HT_7 receptor and the high expression of 5-HT_7 transcripts in both animal and human brain vessels. Furthermore, 5-HT_7 receptor mRNA and second messenger cAMP levels were elevated in cultured smooth-muscle cells from human brain vessels, possibly indicating that this same mechanism is operating in the human brain. This would allow for 5-HT_7 receptor action affecting dilation of meningeal blood vessels without direct interaction with dural blood vessel endothelium.[64,65] These observations may indicate a role for 5-HT_7 receptors in human brain blood vessels during the migraine attack.

Signal transduction pathways

Researchers have identified two major 5-HT receptor–linked signal transduction pathways. One pathway regulates ion channels and the other is a multistep enzyme-mediated pathway. The second pathway requires a G protein to link the receptor to the internal effector molecule. In the case of the 5-HT_1 family of receptors, the link is G_i because the response is inhibition of adenylyl cyclase.

As noted above, the 5-HT_2 G protein–linked family of receptors is coupled to phospholipase C, leading to a variety of intracellular actions. The G protein–type linkage of the 5-HT_2 receptor to its second messenger system is G_q. Activation of adenylyl cyclase was the first signal transduction pathway to be linked to 5-HT receptor activity, but the specific receptor linkages to 5-HT_4, 5-HT_6, and 5-HT_7 were not identified until recently. The 5-HT_4 receptor has been found in the human atrium and guinea pig ileum; the 5-HT_6 found in the cortex has been shown to have a high affinity for TCA drugs, and 5-HT_7 is found in the brain and heart.

The 5-HT_3 receptor, differs from the other 5-HT receptors because it does not have G protein linkage but is associated directly with a ligand-gated ion channel. The receptor has been found on peripheral sensory, autonomic, and enteric neurons and in the cortex, hippocampus, and area postrema, mediating excitation by inducing neurotransmitter release.

Physiologic Function and Drug Intervention

The 5-HT system has been shown to modulate activity in diverse regions of the brain and spinal cord. It is suggested that the system coordinates a variety of sensory and motor patterns associated with behavioral states. 5-HT activity is highest during waking and lowest during sleep. Descending neurons are involved in pain modulation in the dorsal horn and motor activity in the ventral horn. 5-HT activity is absent during rapid eye movement sleep when physical movement is limited, although the animal is in a state of heightened internal arousal. The increased 5-HT activity during waking periods aids in enhancing motor neuron excitability.

Raphe nuclei 5-HT neurons have been shown to display spontaneous discharge activity of one to five spikes per second, releasing 5-HT into the presynaptic cleft. The neurons possess negative feedback autoreceptors that limit the amount of discharge and release of 5-HT. The autoreceptors appear to function only when the discharge and release of 5-HT reaches levels greater than the normal background activity inherent in the neurons. Dysfunction of the autoreceptor regulation has been associated with some forms of neuropathy, and the autoreceptor may provide a therapeutic target for medications. Although in some areas microelectrophoretically administered 5-HT can have an excitatory effect on the discharge rate, the most common response in 5-HT–containing neuron tracts is inhibition of the discharge rate.

It is important to bear in mind that 5-HT released from neurons has both presynaptic and postsynaptic receptor effects. There are many options for affecting the availability of 5-HT directly, either by inhibiting the processes that decreases its availability or enhancing the processes that make it available (Figure 23-2).

Figure 23-2 shows sites of interaction with known drugs that influence the 5-HT system. Of all the options, reuptake blockade of 5-HT by TCAs is the most common mechanism of 5-HT active medications prescribed for the treatment of migraine and chronic pain; however, the issue of availability of 5-HT to help modulate pain has yet to be settled.

DRUGS FOR ACUTE TREATMENT OF MIGRAINE

Sicuteri[56] was the first to note a relationship between 5-HT and migraine in his report on the significant increase in 5-HIAA in the urine of migraine subjects during attacks. Subsequent data, however, did not show a consistent increase in 5-HIAA in all patients with migraine. Nevertheless, the relationship between migraine and 5-HT became solidified at that time and has been further elucidated to the present. Further studies have noted increases in plasma 5-HT, decreases in

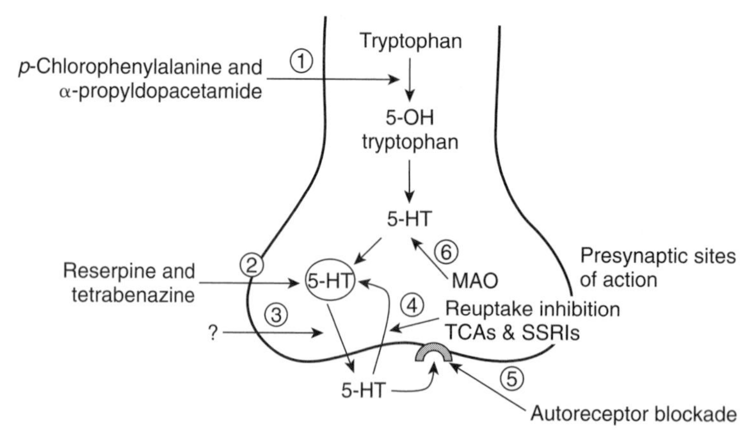

Fig. 23-2 Possible drug sites for intervention. The sites of potential drug action on the 5-HT neuron are enumerated from 1 to 6. *Site 1* represents the modulation of enzymatic action forming the 5-HT precursor and ultimately 5-HT from tryptophan. *Site 2* is a potential target for drugs that affect the storage vesicles of 5-HT. Reserpine and tetrabenazine are known to interrupt the storage and cause release of 5-HT. *Site 3* targets the release mechanism itself; however, there are currently no known agents that act to interrupt or increase the action of the transporter proteins that carry the 5-HT molecule across the membrane. *Site 4* involves the reuptake mechanism that brings 5-HT back into the intracellular environment to be repackaged in the vesicles. A number of drugs inhibit the reuptake of 5-HT (see Chapter 12). *Site 5* refers to the 5-HT autoreceptor. Blockade of this receptor site allows more presynaptic release of 5-HT. *Site 6* focuses on the action of monoamine oxidase that converts the free 5-HT to the metabolic product 5-HIAA. MAO inhibitors such as phenelzine block this action.

5-HT platelet content, and increases in cerebrospinal fluid 5-HIAA content in migraine patients.[15] These observations support the theory that migraine is caused by chronic 5-HT dysregulation. Further support for the role of 5-HT in migraine has come from clinical positron emission tomographic scan studies in patients during migraine attacks showing increased blood flow in the highly serotonergic dorsal raphe nucleus area.

Ergot Derivatives

In the Middle Ages, epidemics of a gangrenous disorder known as "Holy Fire" or "St. Anthony's Fire" were afflicting communities in Europe. The condition was so named because of the attendant burning experienced by the sufferer. The disorder soon became associated with the grain of rye that had been contaminated with the ergot fungus *Claviceps purpurea*. In 1918, the ergot alkaloid ergotamine was isolated from the fungus and was found to have sympatholytic activity (see Chapter 7). Shortly thereafter it was proposed for use as a therapeutic agent for migraine.

Ergotamine has a complex mode of action involving a variety of receptor activities, not only with 5-HT receptors, but with dopamine and NE receptors as well. The vasoconstrictive effect, the most notable characteristic of this medication, can become problematic with overuse, leading to claudication of extremities. The major vasoconstrictive activity is noted in the carotid circulation; the cephalic arteriovenous anastomoses; the pulmonary, cerebral, temporal, and coronary arteries; and the blood pressure. These effects are short lived, although constriction of leg arteries can extend up to 8 hours. Chronic overuse, therefore, becomes a problem, and clinicians need to monitor users carefully.

Ergot derivatives are nonselective partial agonists and antagonists at 5-HT receptors, having high affinity for the 5-HT_{1B}, 5-HT_{1D}, 5-HT_{1F}, and 5-HT_2 receptors and low to moderate affinity for the 5-HT_{1C} and 5-HT_3 receptors. It is currently believed that their primary mode of action in alleviating migraine attacks is through their action on the $5\text{-HT}_{1B/1D}$ receptors, inhibiting neurogenic inflammation and nociceptor activity. Table 23-1 highlights some of the 5-HT receptors as well as related medications and some indications for the drugs.

Ergotamine

Ergotamine is a nonselective 5-HT partial agonist/antagonist and acts at multiple receptors accounting for both therapeutic and adverse effects. For migraine, ergotamine acts primarily as a 5HT_{1D} receptor agonist, inhibiting depolarization of the dural blood vessel–associated nociceptors. Ergotamine's beneficial effect in treating migraine likely occurs by blocking neurogenic inflammation possibly through prejunctional inhibition of neuropeptide release. Ergotamine is commonly available as a tablet or suppository under the name of Cafergot, which is a combination of ergotamine and caffeine. Patients should be instructed regarding the possibility of developing rebound headache if using ergotamine more than two times per week.

Ergotamine is used as an abortive drug at the onset of the migraine attack. Typically, abortive medications have to be taken early in the onset of the migraine because absorption and distribution are impaired as the gastric symptoms of migraine increase. The combination of caffeine with ergotamine speeds gastric absorption, getting the medication into the system more rapidly. In addition to the adverse effects listed in Box 23-1, ergotamine can cause gangrene and damage to blood vessels. Therefore the drug is given for short periods of time at carefully controlled doses.

Box • 23-1

Contraindications and Side Effects of Ergot Alkaloids

Contraindications

Pregnancy
Lactating patients
Renal impairment
Liver impairment
Uncontrolled hypertension
Drug allergy
Peripheral vascular disease

Common Side Effects

Nausea
Vomiting
Restlessness
Irritability
Palpitation
Nervousness
Rebound headache
Claudication
Numbness of fingers and toes
Myalgia
Leg weakness

Other Precautions

Avoid concomitant use of triptans and β blockers

Dihydroergotamine

Dihydroergotamine was introduced in 1945, approximately 10 years after ergotamine. Past and recent studies have determined that the venoconstrictive effect is significantly greater than the arterial effect. It is a nonselective 5-HT receptor partial agonist/antagonist. Additionally, it is a nonselective antagonist at dopaminergic receptors with partial agonist/antagonist activity at α adrenoceptors. The half-life of dihydroergotamine is approximately 10 hours, which is longer than ergotamine and most triptans. This may explain the lower likelihood for rebound adverse effects in headache compared with ergotamine and the shorter-acting triptans (see below). This longer half-life makes dihydroergotamine a useful medication for chronic migraine, which tends to return within hours of treatment with either ergotamine or the shorter–half-life triptans. Dihydroergotamine comes in a parenteral form and as a nasal spray. The parenteral form can be used intravenously, intramuscularly, or subcutaneously. The nasal form has a bioavailability of less than 65%, which may seriously limit its ability to abort a headache in some patients. This medication has definite advantages over the short–half-life triptans and is associated with lower vasoconstrictive potential. Dihydroergotamine is useful in the hospital setting to treat protracted unresponsive migraine. Side effects and contraindications for dihydroergotamine, ergotamine, and the other ergot alkaloids are listed in Box 23-1. Methysergide, a semisynthetic ergot alkaloid, is discussed below.

Triptans

The new family of triptan antimigraine drugs represents the most dramatic advance in the understanding and treatment of migraine. They are classified as $5\text{-HT}_{1B/1D}$ receptor agonists.

Discovery of the first of these drugs, sumatriptan, came after the $5\text{-HT}_{1B/1D}$ receptor was linked with migraine. When it became apparent that the receptor had an inhibitory G protein–linked action on the host vascular and nociceptor neurons, agonist agents were sought that could act with the receptor to stop the attack. Sumatriptan was originally thought to act primarily on nociceptor 5-HT_{1D} receptors, but action was also noted on dilated dural blood vessels. Sumatriptan-sensitive sites of action in the pain transmission pathway have been identified centrally and suggested as additional putative antimigraine targets for brain-penetrant triptan derivatives. Sumatriptan has selective affinity for 5-HT receptor subtypes, 5-HT_{1B}, and 5-HT_{1D}. Recent development of 5-HT receptor subtype–specific compounds and antibodies has allowed a more precise identification of the vascular and neuronal sites of action, thereby providing a basis for a more targeted therapeutic approach.

Moskowitz et al[41,42] developed the concept of neurovascular inflammation in the trigeminovascular system as a migraine mechanism. He observed that sumatriptan's action on peripheral neuronal 5-HT_{1D} receptors blocked subsequent release of neuropeptides such as SP and CGRP that were responsible for the development of neurovascular inflammation with concomitant swelling of the dural blood vessels. He then proposed that the blood vessel dilation and plasma extravasation noted during the migraine attack was an epiphenomenon of the migraine and not the cause of the migraine, as had been proposed by Graham and Wolff.[23]

The 5-HT_{1B} receptor was discovered in human beings after the discovery of the 5-HT_{1D} receptor. It is expressed on human brain blood vessels where it induces contraction of dural blood vessels. An untoward observation of the effect of sumatriptan is the induced contraction of human coronary arteries, which also is most likely mediated by the 5-HT_{1B} receptors. Although the cardiac effect is not severe, it is a concern and has led to some recent efforts to find a compound that would not have an agonistic effect on the coronary 5-HT_{1B} contractile receptors.

Centrally located 5-HT receptor targets in the trigeminal nucleus caudalis have also become the focus of research as potential targets for intervention in acute treatment of migraine. 5-HT_{1B} and 5-HT_{1D} receptors have been identified in the nucleus caudalis. On the basis of protein and mRNA localization studies, presynaptic $5\text{-HT}_{1B/1D}$ and postsynaptic 5-HT_{1F} receptors have been identified. These central 5-HT receptors may be potential sites of action for the new generation of brain-penetrant triptan derivatives (e.g., naratriptan, zolmitriptan, rizatriptan). Identification of the exact nature of these central receptors will be possible when selective receptor subtype compounds become available. Besides the effect on migraine, one of the great benefits for patients with migraine is the relief from nausea that is obtained with the use of the triptans. This may be caused by additional 5-HT receptors in the nucleus tractus solitarius and area postrema, regions of the brain where the blood-brain barrier does not exist. These areas could be accessible even to non–brain-penetrating compounds such as sumatriptan, which could explain some of their antiemetic effects. Additionally, as noted above, the triptans act as 5-HT_3 receptor antagonists, mediating emesis, which gives the drugs an antiemetic effect.

Sumatriptan was the first of the family of triptans to be introduced for the symptomatic treatment of migraine. This agent was designed to act selectively on the $5\text{-HT}_{1D/1B}$ receptor involved in migraine pathophysiology. Seven triptans are currently on the market: sumatriptan, naratriptan, rizatriptan, frovatriptan, almotriptan, eletriptan, and zolmitriptan. There are variable differences between these drugs relating to speed of onset, recurrence rate of headache, side effect profile, and duration of effect, but they all have the same caveats regarding precautions and contraindications. Sumatriptan has the shortest half-life (approximately 2 hours) of all the triptans. This may be a factor in considering recurrence of headache. Within the triptan group, naratriptan and frovatriptan appear to have a recurrence rate comparable to that of dihydroergotamine.

The time to maximal plasma concentration (T_{max}) for a drug can be crucial when used to treat migraine. It is recommended that abortive medications be taken as soon as possible at the onset of the migraine attack to increase the likelihood for successful treatment. If the T_{max} for a drug is too slow, not enough of the drug will get into the system to stop the headache before it is fully developed. Current understanding of migraine pathophysiology has shown that the trigeminal nociceptors become sensitized during the early phase of the migraine attack and the sensitization spreads relatively rapidly to the CNS. After the trigeminal nucleus caudalis has become sensitized, the medications used to abort the headache attacks are less effective. The current recommendation is to take the abortive medication at the onset of the headache and not to wait since efficacy is significantly decreased. The T_{max} and half-lives of the triptans are listed in Table 23-2.

Sumatriptan

One advantage of sumatriptan is the range of delivery options. For some patients, speed is crucial and a delivery system that

Table • 23-2

The Triptans

TRIPTAN AND DOSAGE FORMS	T_{max}	HALF-LIFE
Almotriptan 6.25, 12.5 mg	2.6 hours	3 to 4 hours
Eletriptan 20, 40 mg	2.8 hours	4 hours
Frovatriptan 2.5 mg	2 to 3 hours	26 hours
Naratriptan 1, 2.5 mg	2 to 3 hours	6 hours
Rizatriptan 5, 10 mg	1 hour	2 to 3 hours
Sumatriptan 25, 50, 100 mg	2 hours	2 hours
Sumatriptan 20 mg nasal	1 to 1.5 hours	2 hours
Sumatriptan 6 mg injectable	5 to 20 minutes	2 hours
Zolmitriptan 2.5, 5 mg	1 hour	3 hours

optimizes speed of delivery and bioavailability is a definite advantage. Nausea decreases gastric absorption, slowing the intake of the medication into the system. This problem can be bypassed with the nasal spray or the injection. Both these modalities increase the bioavailability of the medication, enhancing the likelihood of successful intervention. The nasal form of sumatriptan is certainly more effective and more rapid in onset than the nasal form of dihydroergotamine, but the recurrence rate is higher because of the half-life of sumatriptan compared with dihydroergotamine.

Naratriptan

Naratriptan's main advantage is its relatively long half-life of 6 hours. This is less than dihydroergotamine but longer than most, with the exception of frovatriptan. Naratriptan's biggest disadvantage is a delayed onset of action of 2 to 3 hours. For the typical migraine that develops over a half-hour to 1-hour period, this medication may not help because central sensitization may have occurred before the optimal blood concentration of the drug is reached. Studies have looked at using this medication as an add-on, 2 hours after taking a medication with a shorter half-life, such as sumatriptan, to achieve a longer sustained period of relief and diminish the likelihood of recurrence. Additional use is being studied as a prophylactic agent in menstrual migraine during the migraine vulnerability period.

Zolmitriptan

Zolmitriptan has a longer half-life than sumatriptan and a more rapid T_{max}. Although the manufacturers indicated that this drug can be taken further into the attack, nevertheless, the recommendation is to take the drug as early as possible into the attack. Zolmitriptan is also available as a "melt" version that is liquefied in the mouth before it enters the stomach.

Rizatriptan

Rizatriptan has a rapid onset of action similar to zolmitriptan and a T_{max} that is reached in 1 hour. It comes in a tablet form and as a dissolvable wafer that melts on the tongue. The dissolvable version is recommended for patients with nausea.

Frovatriptan

Frovatriptan has a 26-hour half-life, the longest of all of the triptans. This may be a distinct benefit for migraines that last longer than 4 hours, and Géraud[19] reported that frovatriptan had the lowest recurrence rate of all the triptans. The T_{max} of frovatriptan is 2 to 4 hours for a single dose (2.5 mg), which is slower than most of the other triptans. This medication may not be as effective for migraine that develops rapidly because of this pharmacokinetic property.

Eletriptan

Eletriptan is well absorbed after oral administration and has shown a peak plasma concentration occurring approximately 1.5 hours after dosing. In patients with severe migraine the median T_{max} is 2.0 hours. This rapid peak time is definitely an advantage for migraine that develops rapidly. The drug's terminal half-life is approximately 4 hours and Géraud reported that is had a relatively low recurrence rate, compared with rizatriptan, sumatriptan, and zolmitriptan.

Almotriptan

Almotriptan has a half-life of 3 to 4 hours and a relatively low recurrence rate compared with rizatriptan, sumatriptan, and zolmitriptan. Very little has been reported on the 24-hour sustained release preparation of almotriptan.

Box • 23-2

Contraindications, Precautions, and Adverse Reactions to the Triptans

Contraindications and Cautions

Drug allergy
Prinzmetal's (variant) angina
Pregnancy
Breastfeeding
Diabetes
Hepatic disease
Uncontrolled hypertension
Coronary artery disease
Basilar migraine
Use of MAO inhibitor within 14 days
Hemiplegic migraine
Peripheral vascular disease
Cerebrovascular disease
Impaired liver function
Use of ergot derivatives or other anti–5-HT medications

Adverse Reactions

Common
Asthenia
Chest pain
Neck tightness
Jaw tightness
Dizziness
Flushing
Paresthesias

Uncommon
Anaphylaxis
Coronary vasospasm
Acute myocardial infarction
Cardiac arrest
Ventricular tachycardia
Hypertensive crisis
Stroke

Contraindications to ergot derivatives and triptans

Box 23-2 lists the most common contraindications, precautions, and adverse reactions noted with the triptans.

Isometheptene

Isometheptene is a vasoconstrictor similar in action to ergotamine. Midrin is a proprietary combination medication that contains isometheptene plus acetaminophen and dichloralphenazone. This combination is useful in treating mild to moderate migraine headache. The mechanism of action probably relates to a sympathomimetic vasoactivity of isometheptene plus the analgesic effect of acetaminophen. Dichloralphenazone has a mild tranquilizing effect and possibly a central pain inhibitory effect. The medication has to be taken orally at the onset of the headache because delay significantly inhibits the likelihood that it will be effective. It is used for symptomatic treatment of both migraine and tension-type headache and may be combined with an NSAID to increase its effectiveness. This drug should not be used with patients taking MAO inhibitors (see Chapter 12). In addition, it should not be used in patients with partial spinal cord lesions because provocation of hypertensive crises has been reported with sympathomimetic medication use in these patients. It also should not be used concurrently with any of the triptans.

Antiemetics

Phenothiazine derivatives are neuroleptics used to give symptomatic migraine relief. Specifically, they can control the nausea and gastric irritation that accompanies the migraine attack because the medications aid in gastric clearance and gut motility and promote absorption, which is helpful when migraine medications are taken orally. They are available in tablet, suppository, and parenteral forms. The neuroleptics are antagonists at the dopamine D_2 receptor (see Chapter 12). They may cause extrapyramidal reactions such as tardive dyskinesia, although the incidence is low for metoclopramide, promethazine, and prochlorperazine, the most commonly used agents used for nausea. The antiemetic drugs commonly used to particularly reduce the emetic symptoms of migraine are prochlorperazine, metoclopramide, promethazine, and trimethobenzamide.

Clinical Treatment of Migraine

Before deciding on a treatment approach, the frequency of headache must be determined. If a patient is getting a headache less that once per week, then it is appropriate to consider only symptomatic management of the headache unless the infrequent headache is so severe and disabling that it requires more specific interventions. If the headache frequency is more than once per week, preventive medication management needs to be considered. In addition, if the patient has been taking analgesics more than twice per week to treat the headaches, they likely will develop medication-overuse headache, which will require specialized interventions to manage the headache.

The most common approach to treatment of migraine is termed *stepped care.* This treatment strategy starts the patient at the lowest level of therapeutic care, then escalates step by step if the patient does not respond at each given level. The lowest level of therapeutic care usually means simple over-the-counter analgesics. If this fails to help the headache, the patient is then given a prescription for a combination analgesic. If this is not sufficient, then a migraine-specific medication, usually in tablet form, is often given. If this fails, an injectable medication can be used. The problem with this approach is the delay in effective treatment, wasted follow-up visits, failed prescriptions, discouragement, and finally abandonment of care.

Headache specialists now recommend a *stratified care* approach to headache management. This approach immediately takes into account the severity and disability of the migraine attacks and gives the patient the medication appropriate for that situation. This treatment approach limits the long delay in achieving therapeutic benefits.

General guidelines for selecting medications for symptomatic relief of migraine should consider the health status of the patient and the severity and longevity of each attack (Box 23-3). Cost factors also become important, particularly in lower socioeconomic areas where patients may not have adequate health coverage and may not be able to afford some of the expensive medications recently made available.

DRUGS FOR MIGRAINE PROPHYLAXIS AND OTHER CHRONIC PAIN SYNDROMES

The following sections discuss drugs used for prophylayis of migraine and management of other chronic pain conditions, such as cluster headaches, musculoskeletal disorders, and neuropathic pain. Although the use of the medications in each of the conditions may generally be the same, some particular differences are highlighted in the sections under discussion when relevant. Medication selection is still empirical; however, as understanding of the pathophysiologic characteristics of the various disorders and the drug interaction on receptor targets expands, medications will be selected according to what receptors the clinician wants to target.

5-HT Receptor Blockers

Although these drugs act at 5-HT receptors, they may have other actions. They are considered antiserotonin medications because they block the 5-HT_2 receptor. Methysergide, a semisynthetic ergot alkaloid, prevents plasma extravasation in rat dura mater only after long-term administration, an effect that is not noted in short-term use of the drug. Furthermore, Saxena[55] found that methysergide produced only minimal

Box • 23-3

Medications for Aborting Mild, Moderate, and Severe Migraine Headache in a Stratified Treatment Approach

Mild Headache	Moderate Headache	Severe Headache
Acetaminophen	NSAIDs	Ergotamine suppositories plus a prochlorperazine suppository
NSAIDs	Isometheptene	Subcutaneous/nasal sumatriptan
Isometheptene	Ergotamine	Oral naratriptan
Prochlorperazine or metoclopramide for nausea	Nasal DHE	Oral rizatriptan
Caffeine	Prochlorperazine or metoclopramide for nausea	Oral zolmitriptan
	Oral/nasal sumatriptan	DHE intramuscularly
	Oral naratriptan	
	Oral rizatriptan	
	Oral zolmitriptan	

DHE, Dihydroergotamine.

cranial vasoconstriction in vivo during acute migraine attacks. These findings support the observation that methysergide is a better prophylactic agent than an abortive agent. Methylergonovine is an active metabolite of methysergide and is present at a three times greater concentration than methysergide. Its half-life is approximately 220 minutes in contrast to the methysergide half-life of only 60 minutes. Methysergide has an oral bioavailability of 13% because of its extensive first-pass hepatic metabolism to methylergonovine. Methylergonovine maleate is rapidly absorbed orally and has a bioavailability of 60%.

Methylergonovine, the primary metabolite of methysergide, probably accounts for most of methysergide's action in the prophylactic management of chronic migraine as well as cluster headache.[43] These medications are thought to act as agonists on the trigeminovascular afferent 5-HT_{1D} receptors to decrease pain fiber activity and are most useful in resistant migraine and medication-overuse headache. They have peripheral vasoconstrictive activity, although not as great as ergotamine. They also may cause vasoconstriction of the arteries in the carotid bed, where there is a greater concentration of 5-HT_{1B} receptors. The triptans have a greater vasoconstrictive effect on these 5-HT_{1B} receptors, which may explain why they are better abortive medications.

Long-term use of methysergide and methylergonovine has been associated with retroperitoneal, pleuropericardial, and subendocardial fibrosis. Because the majority of patients using the medications do not develop these complications, it is believed that the fibrotic reactions are idiosyncratic. Nevertheless, protocols for medication use have been recommended in the literature and include giving the patient a drug-free holiday every 6 months and obtaining magnetic resonance or computed tomographic imaging with enhancement for retroperitoneal fibrosis and chest radiograph for pleuropulmonary fibrosis. Patients placed on methysergide or methylergonovine should be warned about the possibility of a fibrotic reaction. Because of these potentially extremely serious side effects, methysergide and methylergonovine are reserved for the most recalcitrant chronic headaches. Both drugs are started at the lowest available dose for the formulation and titrated slowly to a maximum daily dose. The patient should be given a drug-free holiday of 30 days after 6 months of use and evaluated as indicated above for fibrotic reactions.

Tricyclic Antidepressants

The opioids and aspirin, acetaminophen, NSAIDs, or combinations have been the most widely prescribed medications for treatment of headache and other pain, but use of TCAs for the treatment of chronic pain, including headaches, is the next most common. Of all the antidepressants, the first-generation TCAs have been shown to be effective in preventive treatment of neuropathic pain, including migraine. The most commonly used drug of this class for neuropathic pain is amitriptyline. The effect of TCAs on pain is distinct from the modulation of depression. It had been thought that 5-HT reuptake inhibition was the primary mode of action until the SSRIs were developed and found to provide little benefit for chronic pain or headache. The mode of action of TCAs may relate to 5-HT receptor activity both presynaptically and postsynaptically, but the exact action is still debated. TCAs may downregulate 5-HT_2 receptors that have been associated with excitatory perivascular inflammation. Additionally, drugs that inhibit the reuptake of both 5-HT and NE seem to have greater benefit than drugs that exclusively inhibit reuptake of either one or the other. Besides migraine, TCAs are useful in treating a number of pain conditions, including tension-type headache, neck pain, and other facial pain syndromes and sleep disturbance. Pain relief for some pain conditions is modest, and the side reactions such as sedation and parasympatholytic effects are particularly bothersome for some patients.

The results of a meta-analysis supported the conclusion that the pain-modulating effect of antidepressants is independent of their antidepressant effect.[47] Furthermore, the benefit for pain occurred within a few days of initiating therapy, whereas the benefit for depression took a much longer time to occur and at a higher dose. It is possible that the 5-HT reuptake blockade alone is not sufficient to relieve pain but enhances the pain-relieving effects of NE reuptake blockade. This would explain why amitriptyline, which inhibits 5-HT reuptake more than NE, is more effective in treating pain than a medication such as desipramine that inhibits reuptake primarily of NE (see Chapter 12). Interestingly, the drugs that inhibit reuptake of 5-HT also ameliorate obsessive-compulsive disorder, but drugs that primarily inhibit NE uptake, such as desipramine, do not.

The choice of a TCA is based on the reported efficacy for migraine and the side effect profile of the medication. The anticholinergic side effects are the most troubling for the patient and are often the major factor that causes the patient to discontinue use of the medication (see Chapter 12). The tertiary amines have stronger anticholinergic effects than the secondary amines but have greater efficacy for pain. The secondary amines are less effective for headache and pain but are better tolerated.

Caution should be exercised when administering TCAs to the elderly and those with a history of cardiac irregularity. It is generally recommended that patients older than 50 years have an electrocardiogram before starting the medication. TCAs should be used with caution in severely depressed and suicidal patients because the margin of safety for overdosing is relatively low as a result of the cardiac conduction–blocking effects (see Chapter 12).

TCAs are typically started at the lowest dose, followed by a slow increase in dose. The patient is advised of the side effects, such as sedation and dry mouth. Weight gain can be a significant problem for most of the TCAs, although protriptyline was associated with modest weight loss in one study that used it for tension-type headache.[8] Many of the side effects decrease as the patient accommodates to the medication. Different dosage forms as well as different drugs can be used to reduce the risk of sedation.

Selective Serotonin Reuptake Inhibitors

Although the analgesic effects of SSRIs have been disappointing, SSRIs may be useful in the overall management of headache and other pain syndromes. For example, if a patient is taking a TCA and getting relief from pain but the consequent sedation is bothersome, addition of fluoxetine, an SSRI, in the morning may help to relieve the sedation, allowing the patient to continue to have the benefit of the TCA. The combination of a TCA with fluoxetine is being used in treating fibromyalgia, probably because of the additional effect of 5-HT reuptake inhibition with drugs that inhibit reuptake of both 5-HT and NE. Addition of another medication that increases 5-HT availability has to be done cautiously, however, because some patients may have 5-HT toxicity or serotonin syndrome develop, a potentially fatal side effect of having too much 5-HT in the system (see Chapter 12).

Another use of the SSRIs relates to their effect with anxiety and obsessive-compulsive behavior. Often patients who have chronic pain syndromes have concomitant anxiety or become fixated on their pain. It has been suggested that the addition of an SSRI with the medication used to ameliorate the pain may actually benefit the patient because it decreases the obsessive component of their pain, allowing them to shift their focus away from the pain issues.

Other Antidepressants

A number of antidepressants are not SSRIs or TCAs but may have utility for chronic pain, although no direct effect on the pain itself. Venlafaxine is more potent as a 5-HT reuptake blocker than as a NE reuptake blocker and has fewer anticholinergic side effects than the TCAs (see Chapter 12). Venlafaxine been noted to be effective in treating chronic pain, neuropathic pain, and migraine.[35] Use of the extended-release form may have fewer side effects.

Although trazodone is more selective as a 5-HT reuptake inhibitor, it has not shown utility for headache or other pain, but it is useful as a sleep medication. Trazodone can cause priapism in men and should be used with caution. It may cause hypotension or syncope, and patients should be closely monitored during the initial phase of treatment. Nefazodone, an analogue of trazodone, is also useful for inducing and maintaining sleep. Additionally, nefazodone is a 5-HT_2 receptor antagonist and has been shown to have a benefit for headache.[53]

β-Adrenergic Receptor Blockers

β Blockers are widely used drugs in the prevention of migraine (Table 23-3). They have not been found useful for preventing tension-type headache and are not as useful as Ca^{++}-channel blockers in prophylaxis of cluster headache. The choice of a β blocker is governed by consideration of potential side effects and the patient's health history. The two β blockers with poor CNS penetration are not lipophilic and are thought to be accompanied by fewer side effects such as depression. Also, these medications are not metabolized in the liver and will not be affected by concomitant use of medications that are affected by the cytochrome P450 enzyme system. The two β blockers with selective β_1 activity are safer to use with patients having a history of asthma; nevertheless, patients should be closely monitored because the selectivity is not exclusive. Because of the risk of stroke, β blockers should not be used with patients who have basilar migraine or other headaches with significant neurologic symptoms. The mechanism of action of the β blockers is undetermined. It was originally assumed that their effect was caused by their vasoactivity, but this is probably only part of the picture. Table 23-3 lists the β blockers with their relative antimigraine efficacy.

Ca^{++}-Channel Blockers

The most widely used Ca^{++}-channel blocker for migraine and cluster headache is verapamil. However, the exact mechanism of action is not known. It is hypothesized that Ca^{++}-channel blockers act on the nociceptive system by interfering with the Ca^{++}-dependent release of SP and possibly other neurotransmitters from sensory nerve terminals. Ca^{++}-channel blockers may also interfere with neurovascular inflammation and the initiation and propagation of Ca^{++}-dependent spreading of cortical depression that is a pathophysiologic feature of migraine. Ca^{++}-channel blockers block the transmembrane influx of Ca^{++} through slow, voltage-dependent ion channels into neurons innervating muscle (see Chapter 26). Fortunately, the inhibitory effect does not affect all Ca^{++}-dependent functions but mainly affects vascular and cardiac functions. Ca^{++} influx can have a cytotoxic effect, a factor that may be involved in migraine during phases of cerebral ischemia, and Ca^{++}-channel blockers are thought to have a protective influence on this process. NO, which is also involved in chronic pain states, is produced through an intracellular mechanism involving Ca^{++} influx after N-methyl-D-aspartate (NMDA) receptor activation, and the Ca^{++}-channel blockers may decrease the production of NO by inhibiting that influx. It has also been noted that 5-$HT_{1D/1B}$ agonists such as sumatriptan abolished NMDA receptor-evoked NO signaling in the brain cortex.[57]

Use of Ca^{++}-channel blockers for the prevention of migraine is not as well founded as β blockers. Verapamil, on the other hand, is one of the most effective medications available for prophylactic management of cluster headache. Generally, the patient is started on a low dose and slowly titrated up to tolerance. The sustained-release versions generally require increased dosing and may not be as effective for headache management as the shorter-acting versions. Problems with bradycardia and hypotension require close monitoring of the patient.

Antihistamines

Antihistamines (see Chapter 22), with the exception of cyproheptadine and hydroxyzine, have not shown particular effectiveness in managing headache. Interestingly, cyproheptadine has a number of nonhistaminic actions that may account for its effectiveness, such as Ca^{++}-channel–blocking activity as well as 5-HT_2 antagonism, making it useful for preventing migraine and managing serotonin syndrome. Cyproheptadine is an important drug for managing childhood migraine. The effect of cyproheptadine in ameliorating headache may be caused by the same mechanism as methylergonovine and methysergide; however, the definitive mechanism is unclear. One study has shown that the combination of propranolol with cyproheptadine had a more beneficial effect on migraine than either drug alone. Sedation, weight gain, and anticholinergic side effects tend to limit the usefulness of the drug.

Hydroxyzine is also used in the management of headache and is commonly given with an opioid in emergency departments to abort acute migraine attacks; however, recent studies have demonstrated that this approach is not as effective as using dihydroergotamine with metoclopramide or an injectable triptan. It is often used as part of the treatment protocol for headache caused by analgesic overuse.

Table • 23-3

β Blockers Useful in Preventing Migraine

NONPROPRIETARY (GENERIC) NAME	ANTIMIGRAINE EFFICACY	RECEPTOR SELECTIVITY	CNS PENETRATION
Propranolol	++++	$\beta_1\beta_2$	Good
Nadolol	++++	$\beta_1\beta_2$	Poor
Timolol	++	$\beta_1\beta_2$	Good
Atenolol	+++	β_1	Poor
Metoprolol	+	β_1	Good

Indomethacin and Indomethacin-Responsive Headaches

A group of uncommon primary headaches demonstrate dramatic remission after the administration of the antiinflammatory drug indomethacin. Because of this unique response, the International Headache Society Classification Committee has included a positive response to indomethacin in the diagnostic criteria for this group of headache disorders. The headaches that are responsive to indomethacin are listed in Box 23-4.

The fact that some of these headache disorders dramatically respond to indomethacin whereas others respond variably and less so has led to speculation regarding the putative pathophysiologic characteristics of these headaches and a mechanism of indomethacin that is unique from other NSAIDs. Indomethacin is a cyclooxygenase-1 and -2 inhibitor similar to the other NSAIDs, but the one outstanding difference is its unique ability to alter cerebral blood flow without inducing vasospasm. It has been observed that indomethacin is able to modulate cerebral blood flow through NO pathways.

Adrenocorticosteroids

Adrenocorticosteroids (see Chapter 35) are useful in the treatment of acute inflammatory pain, headache, and some neuropathic pain. Steroids are used in topical, oral, and injectable forms.

Although corticosteroids are more effective in treatment of cluster headache, they have been found to be useful in treating intractable migraine that has not responded to other forms of therapy. Normally, a high initial dose of steroid is given, then the drug is tapered over a 1- or 2-week period.

This regimen usually terminates the migraine, allowing for the institution of appropriate medications to manage the headache. There has been recent concern regarding avascular necrosis with steroid therapy; although the condition is rare, appropriate consent forms should be obtained when using this group of drugs.

Steroids are thought to act through a number of mechanisms on chronic pain syndromes; for example, steroid modulation of γ-aminobutyric $acid_A$ ($GABA_A$) receptors located outside the blood-brain barrier suppresses neurogenic inflammation and CGRP- and SP-induced plasma extravasation.[45] Drugs that modulate $GABA_A$ receptors may provide a means of targeting the efferent nerves with specific therapies. Steroid hormones modulate neurogenic inflammation related to migraine, cluster headache, and arthritis. Steroids completely block neurogenic extravasation that is mediated by release of neuropeptides such as CGRP and SP.[35] Steroids have also been noted to have an effect on Ca^{++} channels, showing some selectivity in their blocking effects on different high-voltage activated Ca^{++} currents. Some of these effects probably involve directly blocking Ca^{++} channels.[62]

Injectable and oral steroid therapy is effective in management of acute and chronic temporomandibular joint inflammation. Intraarticular corticosteroids reduce pain and swelling associated with inflammatory disease of both muscles and joints. Patients who have inflamed temporomandibular joints are typically started on a protocol including soft diet, moist heat, NSAIDs, and possibly steroids to suppress the joint inflammation.

Cortisone and hydrocortisone injected into the joint are beneficial but they tend to diffuse out of the joint rapidly, thereby not giving a sustained effect. The disodium phosphate ester of betamethasone is used with the insoluble acetate ester form, imparting a rapid effect from the phosphate ester and a sustained effect from the acetate ester. Triamcinolone acetonide and triamcinolone hexacetonide also have very low solubility and a long duration. Up to three injections may be given in a joint, but there should be an interval of 4 weeks between injections.

After nerve injury in which the afferent sensory fibers are crushed or severed, the proximal portion of the nerve is stimulated by nerve growth factor to repair and reestablish a connection with the distal portion. In this process, the proximal terminal forms a mass of neuronal sprouts known as a *neuroma*. The sprouts generate spontaneous ectopic discharges signaling pain centrally. Application of steroids has been shown to reduce the neuronal activity. The reduction in spontaneous discharge is not caused by a reduction in the number of sprouts, but probably arises from a stabilization of the neuronal membrane conductivity.[6] A steroid such as dexamethasone may be injected into the area of the neuroma. Often multiple injections with local anesthetic and steroid are needed to stop the spontaneous discharge.

Corticosteroid therapy is used to control symptoms of acute herpes zoster infection, and experience has shown that the infection is not disseminated with the use of steroids. Esmann,[14] in a double-blind study, showed that steroids were no better than placebo in preventing development of postherpetic neuralgia after zoster infection; however, Keczkes[32] showed that treatment with prednisolone after the development of postherpetic neuralgia reduced the duration of the neuralgia. The Keczkes study also demonstrated that treatment with carbamazepine was no more effective than placebo in modulating the herpetic pain.

Box 23-4

Indomethacin-Responsive Headache Disorders

Exertional or cough headache
Coital headache
Hemicrania continua
Chronic paroxysmal hemicrania
Idiopathic stabbing headache

DRUGS FOR MUSCULOSKELETAL PAIN

Centrally Acting Muscle Relaxants

Centrally acting skeletal muscle relaxants are indicated for relief of acute painful musculoskeletal conditions of local origin but they should be used only as an adjunct to a physical medicine program that includes physical therapy, moist heat and ice, and other nonpharmacologic therapies. There are few studies demonstrating the efficacy of muscle relaxants, and many clinicians are skeptical about their widespread use because of a lack of evidence of benefit apart from the sedative effects of the drugs. There are many causes for muscle spasms, and muscle relaxants are not effective for all causes (see Chapter 13).

The following drugs are generally considered to have muscle-relaxant abilities:

1. *Carisoprodol.* Carisoprodol is metabolized to meprobamate and has habituating potential with development of physical and psychologic dependence. In 1987, the National Institute on Drug Abuse reported that carisoprodol was ranked fifty-fourth of 234 abused drugs. The recommendation is to use it only on a short-term basis.
2. *Cyclobenzaprine.* Cyclobenzaprine is a tricyclic compound similar to TCAs. It has similar side effects

as the TCAs. It is typically chosen for use for patients with myalgia and myofascial pain. It is recommended that this medication be used with caution in older patients and only be used for a short period.[7,39] This drug could be chosen for patients with moderate muscle pain who are not sleeping well. Disturbed sleep is often an accompaniment of musculoskeletal pain, and normalizing the quality and duration of sleep can have a beneficial effect on the pain. The medication is typically taken once a day at bedtime.

3. *Methocarbamol.* Methocarbamol is a skeletal muscle relaxant that is most effective for muscle spasticity. Side effects include seizures, drowsiness, sedation, nausea, and blurred vision.
4. *Metaxalone.* Metaxalone is a skeletal muscle relaxant for acute painful muscle problems. Side effects include leukopenia, hepatotoxicity, rash, dizziness, headache, and nausea.
5. *Baclofen.* Baclofen is primarily a skeletal muscle relaxant, useful in spasticity states. It also has some anticonvulsant activity, making it useful as an alternative drug for trigeminal neuralgia. Side effects include confusion, blurred vision, abdominal pain, and fatigue. Unlike carbamazepine, baclofen is excreted and not metabolized in the liver. Baclofen is a $GABA_B$ receptor agonist. Activation of $GABA_B$ receptors produces analgesia in acute and chronic pain models. Data indicate that a possible mechanism for this effect is a $GABA_B$ receptor–induced blockade of neurokinin-1 receptor gene expression in the spinal cord. GABA is an important neurotransmitter that mediates inhibition in the central nervous system. Approximately 30% to 50% of all synapses are defined as GABAergic. GABA is a neurotransmitter in cortical and hippocampal interneurons. Three pharmacologically different receptor subtypes have been identified: $GABA_A$, $GABA_B$, and $GABA_C$. The $GABA_A$ receptor is postsynaptic and localized in central and peripheral sympathetic neurons. $GABA_B$ is a presynaptic receptor located on central nerve terminals. Its agonist is baclofen. The $GABA_A$ receptor acts directly on a Cl^- ionophore, whereas $GABA_B$ activity is mediated by a G_i protein (see Chapter 13).
6. *Tizanidine.* Tizanidine acts as a central muscle relaxant and has an antinociceptive effect. It is an α_2-adrenergic receptor agonist similar to clonidine that inhibits the release of NE centrally, that is, in the locus ceruleus and spinal cord. Although it is used primarily as a muscle relaxant, one study found it useful for treatment of chronic daily headache.[54] Because of its α_2 agonist activity, it is being used as an intrathecal agent to block sympathetically mediated pain through its effect on the α_2-adrenergic autoreceptors in the sympathetic nervous system.[26] Tizanidine is metabolized in the liver and has been reported to cause elevations in liver enzymes, so the clinician should obtain baseline blood samples to determine alanine aminotransferase and aspartate aminotransferase levels before use and check them during use to make certain the medication is not causing an increase in the enzymes. Common side effects include dry mouth, somnolence, asthenia, and dizziness. The most serious reactions to this medication include hepatotoxicity, bradycardia, and hallucinations. Because of its α_2-receptor agonist activity, it can lower heart rate and blood pressure long term, so these vital signs should be monitored during its use.

Nonsteroidal Antiinflammatory Drugs

NSAIDs are discussed in Chapter 21. Most of the NSAIDs are similar in action; use in orofacial pain is usually limited to acute conditions. However, two NSAIDs, ketorolac and indomethacin, have characteristics that are uniquely useful for headache conditions in addition to their use in musculoskeletal pain.

NSAIDs are often used long term for temporomandibular joint arthritides, but not without adverse effects. (The newer cyclooxygenase-2 inhibitors, thought to be largely free of adverse gastric effects, are also not used long term without problems.) Besides altering platelet function, long-term use of NSAIDs may have a detrimental effect on the endogenous reparative process within the joint. For the most part, NSAIDs are used as temporary measures to stabilize acute flare-ups of pain, and long-term use is not usually recommended.

Injectable ketorolac is a valuable tool for managing acute inflammatory pain conditions and migraine attacks as well as being a preemptive agent after procedures that are likely to cause postprocedure inflammation, such as temporomandibular joint mobilization with lysis, lavage, and manipulation. Ketorolac should not be used in patients whose serum creatinine is greater than 5 mg/dl. The injectable form of ketorolac offers a more rapid and effective medication in acute pain. One study on migraine found that 60 mg of ketorolac intramuscularly was equivalent to 100 mg of meperidine plus 50 mg hydroxyzine. Overuse of the medication can cause acute renal failure and should be limited to 5 days of therapy.

Indomethacin was discussed previously under migraine medications.

Benzodiazepines

The benzodiazepines are not generally used in the management of chronic pain because they are not analgesic. Diazepam is used for short periods as a muscle relaxant and as an antianxiety agent for patients with acute myogenous pain. Clonazepam does not have as great a potential for inducing habituation and is used in chronic neuropathic pain because of its function as an antiseizure medication.

DRUGS FOR NEUROPATHIC PAIN

Trigeminal neuralgia is the most common neuropathy seen in the orofacial environment. Although Jurjani described trigeminal neuralgia in the mid 1100s and postulated that it was caused by vascular compression of the involved nerves, Nicolaus André in 1756 wrote the first comprehensive description of trigeminal neuralgia and coined the term *tic douloureux.* His first patient had had several teeth extracted in an attempt to treat an infection in the maxilla. After the last extraction he wrote

> *What had been regarded as the end of a mild and tolerable ailment, became the source of the sharpest and most uncomfortable pains, I would say the start of a tic douloureux that assailed her night and day, deprived her of sleep, and forbade her some of the bodily functions necessary for life. In fact these periodic agitations became so frequent that they rarely allowed five or six minutes of peace during an entire hour. The patient could not drink, eat, cough, spit or wipe her face without renewing all her pains.*

Trousseau, a French neurologist, proposed that the episodes of tic douloureux were caused by paroxysmal depolarization in the trigeminal pathways similar to the cortical depolarization occurring with epilepsy. He suggested that drugs used to treat epilepsy would be useful for the neuralgic epilepsy. It was not until the early 1940s, however, that another French neurologist, Bourguignon, first tested the drug phenytoin on patients with trigeminal neuralgia. In the early 1960s, Blom, a Swedish neurologist, performed a trial with carbamazepine and found it to be effective for most of his patients. Subsequent studies showed that both these drugs depressed synaptic transmission after maxillary nerve stimulation in the spinal trigeminal nucleus.

The current understanding of neuropathic pain includes a number of disorders that are not discussed in detail here. Trigeminal neuropathy is grossly broken down into disorders involving peripheral and central sensitization mechanisms. The treatment of neuropathy requires an understanding of all these condition and mechanisms. The following sections discuss the medications used to treat neuropathic pain.

Antiseizure Drugs

The mechanisms responsible for the action of antiseizure medications are variable and depend on the type of medication. The medications most effective for trigeminal neuralgia are use-dependent Na^+-channel blockers[59]; however, these medications are not usually the most effective for the other chronic peripheral and central neuropathies.

Carbamazepine

Carbamazepine is considered the gold standard for the management of trigeminal neuralgia, but it is also used to treat other neuropathic pain conditions as well as headache. Although valproic acid is the only anticonvulsant that has been approved for the treatment of migraine and has demonstrated benefit, other anticonvulsants such as carbamazepine have been used successfully in selected cases. For neuropathic pain, the primary mode of action of carbamazepine is thought to be its action as a use-dependent Na^+-channel blocker, inhibiting repetitive neuronal discharge. Structurally, it is similar and related to TCAs.

Before taking carbamazepine, the patient should have baseline laboratory values for liver function and complete blood count, platelet and differential. An extended-release form of carbamazepine is available. This medication only requires a twice-per-day dosing schedule, which is more convenient for the patient and aids in compliance. Initially, liver function tests should be obtained every 30 days to check liver response to the medication (see Chapter 14). Carbamazepine induces CYP3A4 and other subfamilies of the cytochrome P450 system, causing increased metabolism of the drug with lowered serum levels.[60] The result of this effect is noted after 1 to 2 weeks of therapy and requires increasing the dose to obtain better pain control. The inductive effect also reduces the effect of several other drugs.

Gabapentin

Gabapentin has been used for seizures since the mid 1980s but did not become available in the United States until the 1990s. Its use in pain has become a great subject of interest, and numerous papers have described the benefits of gabapentin for treating a variety of chronic pain disorders, including trigeminal neuralgia, diabetic neuropathy, peripheral neuropathy, and migraine.[1,48] Gabapentin is a structural analogue of GABA and was developed as a GABA agonist; however, its mode of action is not through action on GABA receptors. Gabapentin decreases hyperalgesia in the formalin test, a model for centralized neuropathy.[5] It has been hypothesized that the $\alpha_2\delta$ subunit of voltage-dependent Ca^{++} channels maintains mechanical hypersensitivity in neuropathic pain, and recent studies have shown that gabapentin selectively interacts with these units to reduce activity[16]; however, this may not correlate with its therapeutic effects.

Gabapentin crosses membrane barriers using the L-amino acid transporter system. As a substrate of the system gabapentin readily passes the blood-brain barrier; a small amount is also known to cross by passive diffusion. It concentrates in the brain cytosol at a ratio of 10 : 1 compared with the extracellular space. An analgesic effect is attained rapidly but its anticonvulsant effect is delayed, indicating probable different mechanisms for the two effects.

Gabapentin is excreted unchanged in the kidney. It has few interactions with other medications, and the side effect profile is relatively low compared with the other antiseizure drugs. Gabapentin is useful for the management of migraine headache.[11,36,44] The therapeutic range for gabapentin is wide.

Valproic acid

Valproic acid was the first antiepilepsy medication approved by the Food and Drug Administration for migraine. Valproic acid is structurally different from other anticonvulsants, and its mechanism of antiseizure and analgesic action is related to inhibition of Na^+ channels, inhibition of T-type Ca^{++} channels, and facilitation of GABAergic neurotransmission by inhibiting GABA aminotransferase and activating glutamic acid decarboxylase. In seizures, valproic acid may have direct effects on neuronal membranes, inhibiting kindling and reducing excitatory neurotransmission by the amino acids (see Chapter 14). Valproic acid has been shown to block development of neurogenic inflammation in the Moskowitz model of migraine.[36] Valproic acid is also used as a mood stabilizer in manic-depressive disorders (see Chapter 12).

Lamotrigine

Lamotrigine is a novel anticonvulsant drug that is useful for trigeminal neuralgia through its action as a Na^+-channel blocker. The cellular mechanism of Na^+-channel blockade is the same mechanism by which carbamazepine and phenytoin exert their action; however, it is unlikely that Na^+-channel blockade is lamotrigine's only cellular mechanism.

Topiramate

The antiseizure drug topiramate is a monosaccharide derivative that modulates voltage-dependent Na^+ conductance, potentiates GABA-evoked currents, and blocks the kainate and α-amino-3-hydroxy-5-methyl-4-isoxazole propionate (AMPA) subtypes of the glutamate receptor. The Na^+-channel effect and blocking of the metabotropic AMPA and kainate receptor may account for this medication's ability to suppress trigeminal neuralgia and other neuropathic pain states.[31] Topiramate has been shown to have antihyperalgesic and antinociceptive activity in animal models of neuropathic pain.[63]

Oxcarbazepine

Oxcarbazepine is structurally similar to carbamazepine, and its mechanism may involve similar use-dependent inhibition of voltage-dependent Na^+ action potentials. Compared with carbamazepine, oxcarbazepine has an increased tolerability and safety margin. It does not require liver enzymes or complete blood count monitoring, but electrolytes should be checked for Na^+ concentrations, as oxcarbazepine can induce hyponatremia. Oxcarbazepine can be titrated more rapidly than carbamazepine, which is a distinct advantage for patients in an acute phase of trigeminal neuralgia.

Phenytoin

Phenytoin was the first antiseizure medication used to treat neuropathic pain. Its mode of action is similar to carbamazepine. Phenytoin suppresses ectopic discharge of neuromas when applied topically. This effect is probably moderated by a reduction in high-frequency repetitive firing of action potentials by blocking Na^+ channels.[37] Phenytoin is available as an intravenous preparation that has been shown to be beneficial in managing acute flare-ups of neuropathic pain.[38]

Tiagabine

Tiagabine is a potent and selective GABA reuptake inhibitor with antiallodynic effects noted in rodent models of neuropathic pain (see Chapter 14). The antinociceptive effect was related to inhibition of GABA reuptake and resultant increased extracellular GABA levels. Because pretreatment of experimental animals with a $GABA_B$ receptor antagonist eliminated the antinociceptive effect of tiagabine, it is thought that $GABA_B$ receptors are involved in the tiagabine effect.[27] The antiallodynic effects were dose dependent, with significant increases in threshold response to tactile stimulation.

Tiagabine has been compared with valproic acid as having efficacy for prophylactic management of migraine. The mechanism of action probably relates to its GABAergic characteristics.[36] For trigeminal neuralgia, tiagabine is used as an add-on drug in combination with another antiseizure medication when better control of the pain is needed. For migraine, tiagabine is used as a prophylactic agent to decrease the frequency and intensity of migraine attacks.

N-Methyl-D-Aspartate Receptor Antagonists

It has been shown that 90% of C fibers contain glutamate and probably release both glutamate and SP from their peripheral terminals when the stimulus is sufficiently long lasting, at least for several seconds to minutes. Glutamate is an agonist at the NMDA and AMPA receptors but cannot activate the NMDA receptor without the presence of the co-agonist glycine.[8] The NMDA receptor has been considered a potential target for modulating chronic pain; however, the current NMDA receptor antagonists have severe side effects, limiting their usefulness. Blocking the glycine site may provide a target without the profound side effects accompanying the currently available NMDA receptor antagonists. The Ca^{++} channel is normally blocked by Mg^{++}, which is displaced, opening the channel to Ca^{++} influx when the receptor is activated. This event is responsible for the secondary allodynia noted in neuropathic pain. Ketamine is a voltage-dependent blocker of the NMDA receptor channels. The NMDA receptor is an obvious target for pain intervention because it is known to have a role in long-term potentiation and central sensitization. Ketamine and dextromethorphan are both NMDA channel blockers and are effective in reducing NMDA-mediated responses in the dorsal horn nociceptive system. Recent studies have shown that dextromethorphan and ketamine are able to reduce temporal summation hyperalgesia and spontaneous discharge in neuropathic pain.

These agents are used when other medications have failed to provide adequate relief in centralized neuropathies. Ketamine is a strong NMDA receptor antagonist, but its side effects are more disturbing.[10] Dextromethorphan has fewer attendant problems associated with its use but also is only a weak NMDA receptor antagonist with inconsistent benefits. Nevertheless, its antagonistic activity on the NMDA receptor has been reported to be useful for treating chronic pain. Sedation, dizziness, and rash are the most common side effects.

Ketamine may have some use in management of chronic nonresponsive neuropathy; however, as indicated, the side effects become intolerable or difficult to manage. Ketamine is only available for intramuscular or intravenous administration but has been used orally. It is a dissociative anesthetic that is used to provide sedation and anesthesia for short surgical procedures (see Chapter 18). Patients may have adverse psychologic effects, including hallucinations, nightmares, delusions, dissociative reactions, and schizophreniform psychosis. The mechanisms of many relevant drugs used to treat pain are summarized in Box 23-5.

Box • 23-5

Potential Mechanisms of Some Drugs Used to Treat Pain

Mechanism	Drug
5-HT reuptake inhibition	TCAs
NE reuptake inhibition	TCAs
Na^+-channel blockade	Carbamazepine, valproic acid, lamotrigine, phenytoin, topiramate, oxcarbazepine
Ca^{++}-channel blockade	Valproic acid, gabapentin (?)
GABAergic neurotransmission	Gabapentin, valproic acid, baclofen, carbamazepine, topiramate, tiagabine
NMDA receptor antagonism	Ketamine, dextromethorphan
SP depletion	Capsaicin
AMPA receptor antagonism	Topiramate

Drugs That Act at α-Adrenergic Receptors

Atypical odontalgia is a central neuropathic orofacial pain condition that is influenced by the sympathetic nervous system.[22] The use of tizanidine, an α_2-adrenergic receptor agonist, is discussed above as a muscle relaxant. Orofacial pain syndromes mirror pain syndromes in other areas of the body and the underlying mechanisms are similar. In the Graff-Radford and Solberg studies,[22] 60% of the patients diagnosed with atypical odontalgia responded to sympathetic nervous system blockade, relieving their tooth site pain and fulfilling the criteria for a diagnosis of sympathetically maintained pain. Those pain conditions associated with sympathetically maintained pain include reflex sympathetic dystrophy and causalgia. Historically, treatment has involved sympathetic ganglion blockade with local anesthetics or clonidine to stop sympathetic outflow and relieve pain. Phentolamine, an α-adrenergic receptor antagonist, acts on injured nociceptors to reduce sympathetically mediated pain. Continued nociceptor activity is mediated through local sympathetic fiber release of NE, stimulating the α_1-adrenergic receptors and activating the affected nociceptors. α_2-Adrenergic receptors function as autoreceptors on the peripheral terminals of the postganglionic sympathetic nerve. When these receptors are activated, the release of NE from the sympathetic fibers is reduced. Tizanidine, like clonidine, is an α_2-adrenergic receptor agonist that decreases sympathetic release of NE. In sympathetically mediated pain states, it is desirable to either block α_1-adrenergic receptor activity to reduce the postjunctional effect of NE or stimulate α_2-adrenergic receptors to reduce NE release.

Diagnostic Criteria

Box 23-6 lists the diagnostic criteria for the various neuropathic pain conditions found in the orofacial region. It is

Box 23-6

Diagnostic Criteria for Orofacial Neuropathic Pain

C-fiber sensitization	Continuous variable aching pain History of trauma to area No obvious local cause Pain aggravated by local stimuli (hyperalgesia and allodynia) Normal radiograph Positive response to somatic block Response to thermography not defined Sympathetic block does not define this disorder
Traumatic neuralgia	Continuous, variable aching pain May be punctuated by sharp jolts of pain History of trauma to area No obvious local cause Pain aggravated by local stimuli (hyperalgesia and allodynia) Equivocal somatic block (may be varying degree of sympathetic involvement) Normal radiograph Response to thermography depends on sympathetic involvement Response to sympathetic anesthetic block is equivocal
Trigeminal neuralgia	Episodic sharp electriclike pain with periods of remission No obvious local cause Pain is triggered with minor stimulation Normal radiograph Normal thermogram Positive somatic block Sympathetic block does not define this disorder
Sympathetically mediated pain (atypical odontalgia) Complex regional pain syndrome (II or III?)	Continuous, variable, diurnal aching pain History of trauma to area Pain present longer than 4 months Pain aggravated by local stimuli (hyperalgesia and allodynia) No obvious local cause Normal radiograph Equivocal response to somatic block Positive response to sympathetic block (>60%) is not a defining characteristic
Sympathetically independent pain	Continuous, variable, diurnal pain History of trauma to area Pain present longer than 4 months Pain aggravated by local stimuli (hyperalgesia and allodynia) No obvious local cause Normal radiograph Negative response to somatic block Negative response to sympathetic block, although not a defining characteristic

crucial to make an accurate diagnosis before instituting treatment. The selection of medications is a complex issue that involves an understanding of the mechanism of the pain. Trigeminal neuralgia and central neuropathic pain conditions are treated by systemic medications. Surgical interventions are often considered if the disorder does not respond to medication. Peripheral neuropathies are often treated by application of agents to the site of pain. Systemic medications are often added to the regimen for better pain management.

Topical Agents

Topical application of medications to the skin to treat pain has its roots in ancient literature and lore. For example, to treat headache, Aretaeus recommended rubbing the head with rubefacient plants to provoke localized sweating, thought to aid in eliminating humors causing the headache. Compounding pharmacists are able to combine medications in bases such as pleuronic lecithin organogel (PLO) for application to the external skin surface or in bases such as Orabase for intraoral application. Direct application of topical agents to localized areas of inflammation, irritation, and pain offers several advantages: placement of medications directly over the treatment area potentially decreases side effects, and the direct effect of topical agents on the local receptors may have greater effect than systemic medications.

PLO is a gel base that is able to penetrate the epidermal barrier, carrying the agent through the epidermis to the affected locus. Some systemic absorption occurs, but it is significantly less than would be obtained by systemic administration. The combinations of medications are virtually limitless, but the underlying principle for choosing agents to include in the mixture should be based on the assumed pathologic state underlying the painful condition. For example, if the clinician is managing an inflamed temporomandibular joint and the patient is unable or unwilling to take a systemic antiinflammatory drug, an NSAID such as ketoprofen could be included in a PLO base to be applied over the inflamed joint. Presumably the NSAID would decrease pain and inflammation by inhibiting prostaglandin synthesis locally, avoiding significant systemic effects.

In the past, chronic peripheral trigeminal neuropathy has defied treatment, but recent understanding of the pathophysiologic characteristics of the condition has helped to develop treatment approaches with topical agents that inhibit peripheral sensitizing mechanisms such as C-fiber sensitization. When capsaicin-responsive vanilloid receptors were discovered on small-diameter unmyelinated nociceptors (assumed to be C fibers), it was realized that these receptors could be the target for topical intervention. Vanilloid receptor activation causes the affiliated nociceptors to release SP. Long-term application depletes SP stores and temporarily inhibits the neuron's ability to synthesize more. Persistent application of capsaicin desensitizes chronic peripheral neuropathy, rendering relief from pain. Intraoral application is enhanced by fabricating an acrylic stent to cover the affected area when applying a capsaicin mixture. Capsaicin 0.025% is mixed in Orabase-B paste to give a sticky quality to the paste, helping to hold the stent in place and limiting the dispersion of the agent throughout the mouth. Nevertheless, for conditions such as trigeminal neuralgia, systemic drugs or surgical procedures are usually required.

The following are some examples of topical ketoprofen with other agents useful in applications over inflamed muscles and joints. Ketoprofen 10% to 20% can be mixed in a PLO base and applied three to four times per day after wiping the area with a moist washcloth. In this situation, ketoprofen has a local antiinflammatory effect without gastric irritation because of systemic inhibition of cyclooxygenase-1. Patients should be cautioned regarding potential for developing photosensitivity because of the sensitizing properties of the benzophenone moiety of ketoprofen. Ultraviolet light exposure of skin covered with ketoprofen cream promotes the photolysis of erythrocytes. The drug is able to induce photoperoxidation of linoleic acid. Additionally, ketoprofen may induce DNA damage. There is a concern that repeated use of ketoprofen or other topical agents could lead to sensitization, with the possibility of incurring a greater risk of systemic allergic reactions with oral NSAIDs or other drugs.[2]

The most common neuropathies in the orofacial region include trigeminal neuralgia, traumatic trigeminal neuropathy, postherpetic neuralgia, diabetic neuropathy, cancer-induced neuropathy, and AIDS-induced neuropathy. In general, all these neuropathies have common pain mechanisms and similar treatment protocols. Peripheral nerve damage leads to peripheral sensitization and changes in the CNS. Topical medications are useful for neuropathic pain from peripheral sensitization and may be of some use for centralized neuropathy with peripheral pain trigger zones.

To deliver a drug in the orofacial region by topical application, the agent has to penetrate the natural barriers that the facial skin and oral mucosal tissues provide. The pharmaceutical industry has found different ways to improve the absorption of topical medications, increasing the time and contact between the medications and the target tissues and developing different delivery systems such as creams, gels, dissolvable tablets, chewing gum, adhesive patches, polymeric devices, mouth rinses, and medicated lipsticks. The use of topical drug delivery is quite familiar to the dental profession because the application of creams, gels, and rinses to mucosal sites is a daily activity in dental practice.

The medications often used for oral and perioral neuropathies are topical anesthetics and recently, capsaicin. Other compounds such as NSAIDs, sympathomimetic agents, and NMDA antagonists are now being used with variable success. Although it is also possible to have other agents such as carbamazepine, baclofen, or amitriptyline compounded for local delivery, their use in peripheral conditions is controversial because their mechanism of action has been described as central and a peripheral mechanism of action has not been clearly established.

The use of intraoral topical medications is accompanied by some inconveniences. These agents tend to dissolve in saliva and spread throughout the mouth and down the throat. If the topical agent does not have mucosal adhesive properties, it will quickly wash away from the area where it is being applied. Several strategies and delivery systems are being used to counter this problem.

The following medications are delivered through the skin by a transdermal carrier or by placing in a material such as Orabase that adheres to the mucous tissue to enhance and maintain tissue/medication contact for longer periods.

Capsaicin 0.025%

Capsaicin can be applied to the affected area five to six times per day. Capsaicin is known to reduce C-fiber activity where applied. Initial applications cause the typical burning sensation noted when eating spicy food. The burning lasts approximately 10 minutes and then begins to resolve. Repeated application inhibits C-fiber activity, causing immediate release of SP and decreasing further production. The capsaicin should be mixed with Orabase paste in equal parts before application.

Clonidine 0.1% to 0.2%

Clonidine is an α_2-adrenoceptor agonist that is used to reduce sympathetic activity in the target area. This agent should be compounded by a pharmacist to deliver approximately 0.1 mg of clonidine in three applications per day. Clonidine is used for neuropathies that have sympathetic involvement. Thermographic examination of the painful area may show as a cold area, indicating possible sympathetic mediation.

Ketamine 200 mg/ml

Ketamine is applied in a transdermal or mucoadhesive base. Chronic peripheral neuropathic pain may be driven by NMDA receptor activity, hence the rationale for the use of this drug. Although controversial at present, there are reports of NMDA receptor activity in the peripheral area where nerve damage has occurred. Inhibiting NMDA activity may be the reason for these agents providing some benefit.

Eutectic mixture of local anesthetics

The eutectic anesthetic preparation consists of 2.5% prilocaine and 2.5% lidocaine; although effective, it has the inconvenience of a low melting point, rendering it liquid even at room temperature. Covering the application site with an occlusive dressing keeps the anesthetic in the desired area and, if used intraorally, protects the cream from salivary contamination. In the oral mucosa, this mixture is a superior topical anesthetic agent for pain reduction if given sufficient time of contact with the area to be anesthetized.

The rationale for the use of these agents is to decrease self-perpetuating C-fiber activity. It is thought that, if the activity can be reduced for a long enough period, C-fiber function will normalize and not reestablish abnormal activity.

OTHER DRUGS USED FOR OROFACIAL PAIN

Sodium Hyaluronate

Sodium hyaluronate is derived from hyaluronic acid and is available for injection into small joints. Hyaluronic acid is a normal constituent of synovial fluid, responsible for the viscoelastic properties of the fluid. Hyaluronic acid is decreased in osteoarthritis, and use of these products produces viscosupplementation that benefits the joint by augmenting the viscosity of the joint fluid and stimulating endogenous production of hyaluronic acid. The agent also binds to specific hyaluronic acid receptors on the chondrocytes and synoviocytes, acting as a free radical scavenger and reducing the cellular production of prostaglandin E_2 and bradykinin.

Botulinum Toxin Type A

Botulinum toxin type A is used for involuntary movement disorders such as dystonia, blepharospasm, torticollis, and other myotonic and dystonic disorders. Botulinum toxin A causes an irreversible presynaptic blockade of the release of acetylcholine at the motor end plates, inhibiting muscle ability to contract; however, collateral sprouting of motor axons restores function within 3 to 6 months. The effect on muscle pain occurs rapidly, although benefit for the muscle spasms may take 2 to 3 weeks to fully develop; however, it may provide more benefit for the patient than the drug's effect on muscle spasm. Previous treatment for these problems relied on oral medications that were not particularly beneficial. When the toxin was used for muscles involved in the face, it was noted that face wrinkles were eliminated for the 3- to 4-month duration of the muscle endplate block.

Migraine patients who were having these injections for forehead wrinkles began reporting that their migraines had subsided for the duration of the drug's effect. The effectiveness of botulinum toxin for migraine and other headaches is currently being studied.[3] Recent studies have shown benefit for refractory myofascial pain.[49] For a recent review of botulinum toxin A in chronic pain, see Göbel et al.[21]

IMPLICATIONS FOR DENTISTRY

This chapter has reviewed the medications used to treat several pain syndromes, including chronic orofacial pain conditions. The medications traditionally used by dentists to treat their patients are generally limited to antibiotics, antiinflammatory agents, opioids, local or general anesthetics, and benzodiazepines. These medications are used to treat acute pain, inflammation, and infections or to anesthetize patients for surgical procedures. With the development of the field of orofacial pain and the increased understanding of painful non–tooth-related conditions that are seen in the orofacial environment, the dental pharmacopoeia has necessarily expanded to include a vast array of medications that have not generally been considered previously. This array will continue to expand as more pharmaceuticals are developed and the understanding of orofacial pain disorders and their mechanisms broadens.

CITED REFERENCES

1. Backonja MM: Anticonvulsants (antineuropathics) for neuropathic pain syndromes, *Clin J Pain* 16(2 suppl): S67-S72, 2000.

2. Bagheri H, Lhiaubet V, Montastruc J, et al: Photosensitivity to ketoprofen: mechanisms and pharmacoepidemiological data, *Drug Saf* 22:339-349, 2000.

Antimigraine Drugs and Drugs for Neuropathic and other Pain Syndromes

Nonproprietary (generic) name	*Proprietary (trade) name*
Ergots	
Dihydroergotamine	Migranal, DHE 45
Ergotamine	Ergomar, in Cafergot
Triptans	
Almotriptan	Axert
Eletriptan	Relpax
Frovatriptan	Frova
Naratriptan	Amerge
Rizatriptan	Maxalt
Sumatriptan	Imitrex
Zolmitriptan	Zomig
Antiemetics	
Metoclopramide	Reglan
Prochlorperazine	Compazine
Promethazine	Phenergan
Trimethobenzamide	Tigan
TCAs (see Chapter 12)	
β-Adrenergic receptor blockers (see Chapter 7)	
Calcium channel blockers (see Chapter 26)	
Antihistamines (see Chapter 22)	
Centrally acting muscle relaxants	
Baclofen	Lioresal
Benzodiazepines (see Chapter 13)	
Carisoprodol	Soma
Cyclobenzaprine	Cyclobenz
Metaxalone	Skelaxin
Methocarbamol	Robaxin
NSAIDs (see Chapter 21)	
Antiseizure drugs (see Chapter 14)	
NMDA antagonists	
Dextromethorphan	Delsym
Ketamine	Ketalar
α-Adrenergic receptor blocker	
Tizanidine	Zanaflex
Topical drugs*	
Pleuronic lecithin organogel	—
Capsaicin	Theragen
Others	
Botulinum toxin	Botox
Dichloralphenazone	In Midrin
Indomethacin	Indocin
Isometheptene	In Midrin
Sodium hyaluronate	Hyalgan

*See also local anesthetics, Chapter 16.

3. Binder WJ, Brin MF, Blitzer A, et al: Botulinum toxin type A (BOTOX) for treatment of migraine headaches: an open-label study, *Otolaryngol Head Neck Surg* 123:669-676, 2000.
4. Bourgoin S, Oliveras JL, Bruxelle J, et al: Electrical stimulation of the nucleus raphe magnus in the rat: effects on 5-HT metabolism in the spinal cord, *Brain Res* 194:377-389, 1980.
5. Cesena RM, Calcutt NA: Gabapentin prevents hyperalgesia during the formalin test in diabetic rats, *Neurosci Lett* 262:101-104, 1999.
6. Chabal C: Membrane stabilizing agents and experimental neuromas. In Fields HL, Liebeskind JC, eds: *Progress in pain research and management*, Seattle, 1994, IASP Press.
7. Chin MH, Wang LC, Jin L, et al: Appropriateness of medication selection for older persons in an urban academic emergency department, *Acad Emerg Med* 6:1232-1242, 1999.
8. Cohen GL: Protriptyline, chronic tension-type headaches, and weight loss in women, *Headache* 37:433-436, 1997.
9. Cooper JR, Bloom FE, Roth RH: *The biochemical basis of neuropharmacology*, ed 7, New York, 1996, Oxford University Press.
10. Dickenson AH: NMDA receptor antagonists as analgesics. In Fields HL, Liebeskind JC, eds: *Pharmacological approaches to the treatment of chronic pain: new concepts and critical issues*, Seattle, 1994, IASP Press.
11. Di Trapani G, Mei D, Marra C, et al: Gabapentin in the prophylaxis of migraine: a double-blind randomized placebo-controlled study, *Clin Ther* 151:145-148, 2000.
12. Eide PK, Hole K: The role of 5-hydroxytryptamine (5-HT) receptor subtypes and plasticity in the 5-HT systems in the regulation of nociceptive sensitivity, *Cephalalgia* 13:75-85, 1993.
13. Erspamer V, Asero B: Identification of enteramine, the specific hormone of the enterochromaffin cell system, as 5-hydroxytryptamine, *Nature* 169:801-802, 1952.
14. Esmann V, Geil JP, Kroon S, et al: Prednisolone does not prevent post-herpetic neuralgia, *Lancet* 2:126-129, 1987.
15. Ferrari MD, Saxena P: On serotonin and migraine: a clinical and pharmacological review, *Cephalalgia* 13:151-165, 1993.
16. Field M, Hughes J, Singh L: Further evidence for the role of the $\alpha_2\delta$ subunit of voltage dependent calcium channels in models of neuropathic pain, *Br J Pharmacol* 131:282-286, 2000.
17. Gaddum JH, Picarelli ZJ: Two kinds of tryptamine receptor, *Br J Pharmacol* 12:323-328, 1957.
18. Gebhart GF, Sandkuhler JG, Thalhammer J, et al: Inhibition of spinal nociceptive information by stimulation in midbrain of the cat is blocked by lidocaine microinjected in nucleus raphe magnus and medullary reticular formation, *J Neurophysiol* 50:1446-1459, 1983.
19. Géraud G, Keywood C, Senard JM: Migraine headache recurrence: relationship to clinical, pharmacological, and pharmacokinetic properties of triptans, *Headache* 43:376-388, 2003.
20. Ghelardini C, Galeotti N, Casamenti F, et al: Central cholinergic antinociception induced by $5HT_4$ agonists: BIMU 1 and BIMU 8, *Life Sci* 58:2297-2309, 1996.
21. Göbel H, Heinze A, Heinze-Kuhn K, et al: Botulinum toxin A in the treatment of headache syndromes and pericranial pain syndromes, *Pain* 91:195-199, 2001.
22. Graff-Radford SB, Solberg WK: Atypical odontalgia, *J Craniomandib Disord Facial Oral Pain* 6:260-265, 1992.
23. Graham JR, Wolff HG: Mechanism of migraine headache and action of ergotamine tartrate, *Arch Neurol Psychiatry* 39:737-763, 1938.
24. Green GM, Scarth J, Dickenson A: An excitatory role for 5-HT in spinal inflammatory nociceptive transmission: state-dependent actions via dorsal horn $5\text{-}HT_3$ receptors in the anaesthetized rat, *Pain* 89:81-88, 2000.
25. Hamlin K, Fischer F: The synthesis of 5-hydroxytryptamine, *J Am Chem Soc* 73:5007-5008, 1951.
26. Hirata K, Koyama N, Minami T: The effects of clonidine and tizanidine on responses of nociceptive neurons in nucleus ventralis posterolateralis of the cat thalamus, *Anesth Analg* 81:259-264, 1995.
27. Ipponi A, Lamberti C, Medica A, et al: Tiagabine antinociception in rodents depends on $GABA_B$ receptor activation: parallel antinociception testing and medial thalamus GABA microdialysis, *Eur J Pharmacol* 368:205-211, 1999.
28. Janeway T, Richardson H, Park E: Experiments on the vasoconstrictor action of blood serum, *Arch Int Med* 563-603, 1918.
29. Johnson KW, Phebus LA, Cohen ML: Serotonin in migraine: theories, animal models and emerging therapies, *Prog Drug Res* 51:219-244, 1998.
30. Kalkman HO: Is migraine prophylactic activity caused by $5\text{-}HT_{2b}$ or $5\text{-}HT_{2c}$ receptor blockade? *Life Sci* 54:641-644, 1994.
31. Kamiya Y, Andoh T, Furuya R, et al: Comparison of the effects of convulsant and depressant barbiturate stereoisomers on AMPA-type glutamate receptors, *Anesthesiology* 90:1704-1713, 1999.
32. Keczkes K, Basheer AM: Do corticosteroids prevent post-herpetic neuralgia? *Br J Dermatol* 102:551-555, 1980.
33. Kidd EJ, Laporte AM, Langlois X, et al: $5\text{-}HT_3$ receptors in the rat central nervous system are mainly located on nerve fibres and terminals, *Brain Res* 612:289-298, 1993.
34. Kwiat GC, Basbaum AI: The origin of brainstem noradrenergic and serotonergic projections to the spinal cord dorsal horn in the rat, *Somatosens Mot Res* 9:157-173, 1992.
35. Lang E, Hord AH, Denson D: Venlafaxine hydrochloride (Effexor) relieves thermal hyperalgesia in rats with an experimental mononeuropathy, *Pain* 68:151-155, 1996.
36. Leniger T, Wiemann M, Bingmann D, et al: Different effects of GABAergic anticonvulsants on 4-aminopyridine-induced spontaneous GABAergic hyperpolarizations of hippocampal pyramidal cells—implication for their potency in migraine therapy, *Cephalalgia* 20:533-537, 2000.
37. Macdonald RL, Kelly KM: Antiepileptic drug mechanisms of action, *Epilepsia* 36(suppl 2):S2-S12, 1995.
38. McCleane GJ: Intravenous infusion of phenytoin relieves neuropathic pain: a randomized, double-blinded, placebo-controlled, crossover study, *Anesth Analg* 89:985-988, 1999.

39. Merskey H: Pharmacological approaches other than opioids in chronic non-cancer pain management, *Acta Anaesthesiol Scand* 41:187-190, 1997.

40. Morgan MM, Sohn JH, Liebeskind JC: Stimulation of the periaqueductal gray matter inhibits nociception at the supraspinal as well as spinal level, *Brain Res* 502:61-66, 1989.

41. Moskowitz MA: Basic mechanisms in vascular headache, *Neurol Clin* 8:801-815, 1990.

42. Moskowitz MA: The trigeminovascular system, In Olesen J, Tfelt-Hansen P, eds: *The headaches,* New York, 1993, Raven Press.

43. Mueller LGR, Ciervo C: Methylergonovine maleate as a cluster headache prophylactic: a study and review, *Headache* 37:437-442, 1997.

44. Nicolodi M, Sicuteri F: Negative modulators of excitatory amino acids in episodic and chronic migraine: preventing and reverting chronic migraine, *Int J Clin Pharmacol Res* 18:93-100, 1998.

45. Nohr D, Schafer MK-H, Persson S, et al: Calcitonin gene-related peptide gene expression in collagen-induced arthritis is differentially regulated in primary afferents and motoneurons: influence of glucocorticoids, *Neuroscience* 93:759-773, 1999.

46. Obata H, Saito S, Sasaki M, et al: Antiallodynic effect of intrathecally administered 5-HT_2 agonists in rats with nerve ligation, *Pain* 90:173-179, 2001.

47. Onghena P, Van Houdenhove B: Antidepressant-induced analgesia in chronic non-malignant pain: a meta-analysis of 39 placebo-controlled studies, *Pain* 49:201-219, 1992.

48. Otley CC: Gabapentin for the treatment of dysesthetic pain after reconstructive surgery, *Dermatol Surg* 25:487-488, 1999.

49. Porta M: A comparative trial of botulinum toxin type A and methylprednisolone for the treatment of myofascial pain syndrome and pain from chronic muscle spasm, *Pain* 85:101-105, 2000.

50. Powell KR, Dykstra LA: The role of serotonergic receptors in the effects of mu opioids in squirrel monkeys responding under a titration procedure, *Psychopharmacology* 126:42-49, 1996.

51. Rapport M, Green A, Page I: Serum vasoconstrictor (serotonin). IV. Isolation and characterization, *J Biol Chem* 176:1243-1251, 1948.

52. Sanger GJ, Yoshida M, Yahyah M, et al: Increased defecation during stress or after 5-hydroxytryptophan: selective inhibition by the 5-HT_4 receptor antagonist, SB-207266, *Br J Pharmacol* 130:706-712, 2000.

53. Saper JR, Lake AE, Tepper SJ: Nefazodone for chronic daily headache prophylaxis: an open-label study, *Headache* 111:465-474, 2001.

54. Saper JR, Winner PK, Lake AE: An open-label dose-titration study of the efficacy and tolerability of tizanidine hydrochloride tablets in the prophylaxis of chronic daily headache, *Headache* 41:357-368, 2001.

55. Saxena PR: Historical aspects of 5-hydroxytryptamine: discovery and receptor classification. In Olesen J, Saxena PR, eds: *5-Hydroxytryptamine mechanisms in primary headaches,* New York, 1992, Raven Press.

56. Sicuteri F, Testi A, Anselmi B: Biochemical investigations in headache increase in hydroxyindoleacetic acid excretion during migraine attacks, *Arch Allergy Appl Immunol* 19:55-58, 1961.

57. Stepien A, Chalimoniuk M, Strosznajder J: Serotonin $5HT_{1B/1D}$ receptor agonists abolish NMDA receptor-evoked enhancement of nitric oxide synthase activity and cGMP concentration in brain cortex slices, *Cephalalgia* 19:859-865, 1999.

58. Taiwo YO, Levine JD: Serotonin is a directly-acting hyperalgesic agent in the rat, *Neuroscience* 48:485-90, 1992.

59. Tanelian DL, Victory R: Sodium channel-blocking agents: their use in neuropathic pain conditions, *Pain Forum* 4:75-80, 1995.

60. Tateishi T, Asoh M, Nakura H, et al: Carbamazepine induces multiple cytochrome p450 subfamilies in rats, *Chem Biol Interact* 117:257-268, 1999.

61. Thor KB, Nickolaus S, Helke CJ: Autoradiographic localization of 5-hydroxytryptamine$_{1A}$, 5-hydroxytryptamine$_{1B}$ and 5-hydroxytryptamine$_{1C/2}$ binding sites in the rat spinal cord, *Neuroscience* 55:235-252, 1993.

62. Todorovic SM, Prakriya M, Nakashima Y, et al: Enantioselective blockade of T-type Ca^{2+} current in adult rat sensory neurons by a steroid that lacks γ-aminobutyric acid-modulatory activity, *Mol Pharmacol* 54:918-927, 1998.

63. Tremont-Lukats IW, Megeff C, Backonja MM: Anticonvulsants for neuropathic pain syndromes: mechanisms of action and place in therapy, *Drugs* 60:1029-1052, 2000.

64. Villalon CM, Centurion D, Bravo G, et al: Further pharmacological analysis of the orphan 5-HT receptors mediating feline vasodepressor responses: close resemblance to the 5-HT_7, receptor, *Naunyn Schmiedebergs Arch Pharmacol* 361:665-671, 2000.

65. Villalon CM, Terron JA, Ramirez-San JE, et al: 5-hydroxytryptamine: considerations about discovery, receptor classification and relevance to medical research, *Arch Med Res* 26:331-344, 1995.

66. Yakel JL, Shao XM, Jackson MB: The selectivity of the channel coupled to the $5HT_3$ receptor, *Brain Res* 1990; 533:46-52, 1990.

General References

Evans RW, Mathew NT: *Handbook of headache,* Philadelphia, 2000, Lippincott Williams & Wilkins.

Ferrari MD: Systemic biochemistry. In Olesen J, Tfelt-Hansen P, Welch KMA. *The headaches,* New York, 1993, Raven Press.

Frazer A, Hensler JG: Serotonin. In Siegel GJ, Agranoff BW, Albers RW, et al, eds: *Basic neurochemistry: molecular, cellular and medical aspects,* ed 6, Philadelphia, 1999, Lippincott-Raven.

Saper JR, Silberstein SD, Gordon CD, et al: *Handbook of headache management: a practical guide to diagnosis and treatment of head, neck and facial pain,* ed 2, Philadelphia, 1999, Lippincott Williams & Wilkins.

Saper JR, Silberstein SD, Gordon CD, et al: Treatment of intractable, severe migraine: parenteral treatment protocols, hospitalization, and referral guidelines. In Saper JR, Silberstein SD, Gordon CD, et al, eds: *Handbook of headache management: a practical guide to diagnosis and treatment of head, neck and facial pain*, ed 2, Philadelphia, 1999, Lippincott Williams & Wilkins.

Serotonin (5-hydroxytryptamine), histamine and adenosine. In Cooper JR, Bloom FE, Roth RH: *The biochemical basis of neuropharmacology*, ed 8, New York, 2003, Oxford University Press.

CHAPTER • 24

Antiarrhythmic Drugs

Frank J. Dowd

Antiarrhythmic drugs are used to correct or reduce the risk of cardiac arrhythmias (dysrhythmias). They are classified into several categories on the basis of their mechanisms of action and resulting cardiac effects. All antiarrhythmic agents influence impulse generation or impulse conduction in the heart and cause definable electrophysiologic effects.

BASIC CARDIAC ELECTROPHYSIOLOGY

Under normal conditions, the chambers of the heart contract as synchronized rhythmic units driven by electrical impulses generated in and conducted throughout the heart. The normal pacemaker impulse is generated in the sinoatrial (SA) node and travels through the atria to each muscle cell, to the atrioventricular (AV) node, and then through specialized conduction pathways in the common bundle of His, bundle branches, and Purkinje network to reach the ventricular muscle cells. Figure 24-1 illustrates representative action potentials for an SA nodal cell, an atrial muscle cell, an AV nodal cell, a Purkinje fiber, and a ventricular muscle cell.

Three experimental measures are used to characterize the electrophysiologic properties of the heart: automaticity, refractoriness, and conduction velocity. Many of the antiarrhythmic effects of drugs result from changes in these parameters, which in turn are reflected by action potential alterations in various regions of the heart.

Automaticity

Automaticity describes the unique feature of cells of the SA node, AV node, and specialized conducting system to exhibit spontaneous phase 4 depolarization and thus impulse generation. An increase in automaticity refers to an increase in the rate of impulse generation, and, conversely, a decrease in automaticity refers to a decrease in the rate of impulse generation. Under normal conditions, the pacemaker cells of the SA node exhibit the most rapid generation of impulses, making the SA node the controlling pacemaker of the heart. The rate at which pacemaker cells initiate impulses is a function of the rate of phase 4 depolarization, the maximum diastolic potential (MDP), and the magnitude of the threshold potential (Figure 24-2). For example, an increase in the rate of phase 4 depolarization in the SA node raises heart rate, whereas a change in the threshold voltage to a more positive value or an increase in the MDP (hyperpolarization) slows the heart. These functions are under nervous and hormonal control and can be altered by injury or drugs.

Refractoriness

The period after the initiation of an action potential during which another action potential cannot be initiated and propagated regardless of stimulus is known as the *effective refractory period* (ERP; see Figure 24-2). A change in the action potential duration (APD) is accompanied by a similar change in the duration of the ERP, although the ratio of change may not be 1 : 1. If the ERP is lengthened with respect to the APD, the cardiac cells will have repolarized more completely before they respond to a stimulus. Many drugs with antiarrhythmic effects prolong the duration of the ERP and some decrease it.

Conduction Velocity

Conduction velocity in cardiac fibers is altered by several factors, including anatomic characteristics, the electrophysiologic state, pathologic conditions, and many antiarrhythmic drugs. The rate of phase 0 depolarization strongly influences

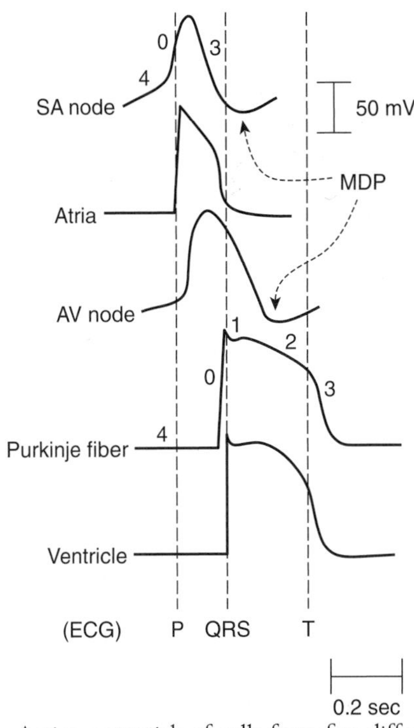

Fig. 24-1 Action potentials of cells from five different regions of the heart. The numbers refer to the phases of the action potential as explained in the text. *Phase 0,* Rapid depolarization; *phase 1,* early repolarization; *phase 2,* plateau phase; *phase 3,* repolarization, which continues until the maximum diastolic potential (MDP) is reached; *phase 4,* steady diastolic potential in the Purkinje fiber, slow spontaneous diastolic depolarization in the SA node and AV node. The action potentials are positioned in temporal relationship to each other as well as to waves of the electrocardiogram (ECG).

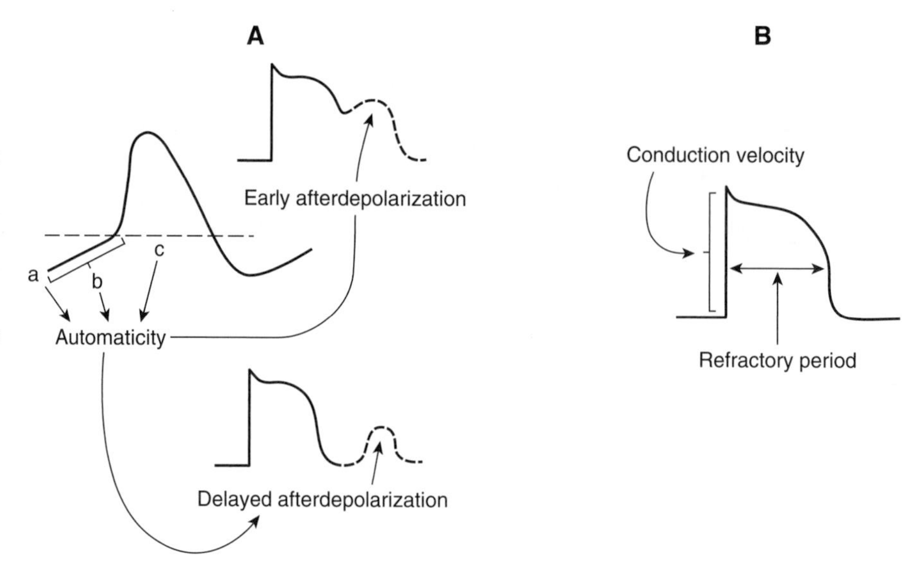

Fig. 24-2 Parameters that are important in arrhythmias and their treatment. **A,** Automaticity is influenced by the level of the MDP *(a)*, the slope of phase 4 *(b)*, the potential at which the threshold *(dashed line)* is reached *(c)*, or by the presence of afterpotentials. **B,** Conduction velocity is directly related to the slope of phase 0. The refractory period is directly related to the duration of the action potential.

the conduction velocity.[4] In turn, the rate (or slope) of phase 0 depolarization (measured as the change in voltage per unit of time [dV/dt]) depends on the membrane potential during phase 4. The more negative the membrane potential at the beginning of phase 0 depolarization, the greater is the maximal dV/dt for phase 0. This relation is illustrated in Figure 24-3. If an antiarrhythmic drug decreases the rate of phase 0 depolarization, it thereby reduces the conduction velocity. In addition to changing the MDP, the drug may also affect conduction velocity by altering the relation between dV/dt during phase 0 and the membrane potential at the beginning of phase 0.

Ion Channels

Ions and the channels that control their movements play major roles in the various phases of cardiac depolarization and repolarization. Figure 24-4 illustrates the membrane action potential in an SA nodal cell and a Purkinje fiber—two characteristically different action potentials—and the flow of ions through specific channels in the Purkinje fiber.

In Purkinje fibers, as well as in atrial and ventricular myocardium, depolarization in phase 0 results from an initial, "fast channel" current of Na^+ in the inward direction. Na^+ channels also contribute to the pacemaker current in phase 4 of pacemaker cells. Another major inward current, carried by Ca^{++} and conducted through "slow channels," contributes to the plateau phase (phase 2) of the action potential. Ca^{++} channels are of two types, T and L. These channels remain open for different periods during the action potential and respond differently to antiarrhythmic drugs.

Outward K^+ currents are responsible for repolarizing the muscle fiber in phase 3 and, by slowly deactivating in phase 4, contribute to spontaneous depolarization in pacemaker cells, notably the SA node, AV node, and (sometimes) His-Purkinje fibers. (Na^+ and Ca^{++} also play roles in depolarization during phase 4.) Thus as K^+ conductance through inwardly rectifying K^+ (Kir) channels falls and Na^+ and Ca^{++} conductance rises, spontaneous depolarization during phase 4 takes place. Another major difference between pacemaker cells (such as those of the SA and AV nodes) and nonpacemaker cells (e.g., cardiac muscle cells) is the slope of phase 0. Phase 0 has a much lower slope in pacemaker cells, where the major membrane event governing depolarization in phase 0 is Ca^{++} influx through slow channels. As indicated, the faster phase 0 depolarization of the myocardium and Purkinje fibers is caused primarily by the Na^+ influx through fast channels. Differential effects on these ion fluxes help explain variations in

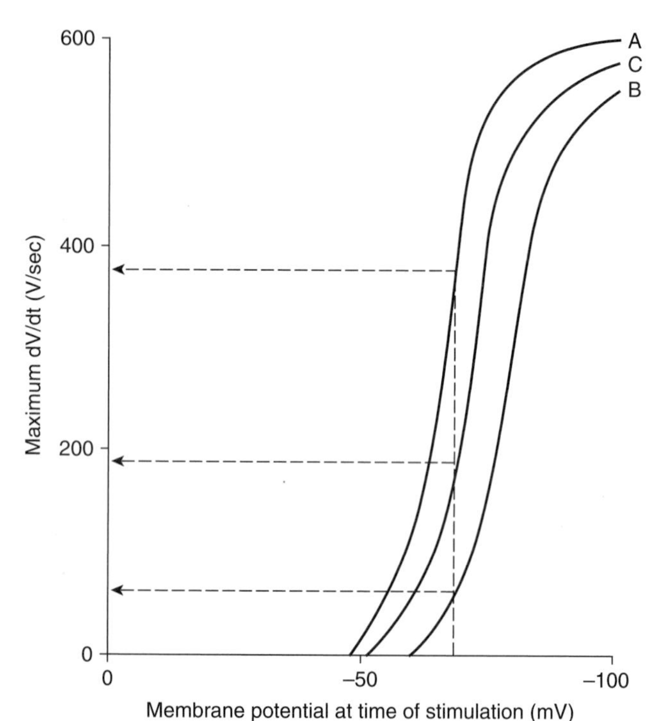

Fig. 24-3 Effect of the membrane potential on the slope of phase 0 depolarization. Small differences in the membrane potential at time of stimulation normally cause large changes in the rate of phase 0 depolarization, as measured by the maximum change in dV/dt *(curve C)*. Drug treatment may alter the membrane potential at the time of stimulation and thus change dV/dt, or it may shift altogether the basic relationship between dV/dt and the membrane potential *(curves A* and *B)*. *Dashed lines* indicate the relation between dV/dt and a given membrane potential (−68 mV) for three different membrane responsiveness curves. (Adapted from Hoffman BF, Bigger JT, Jr: Antiarrhythmic drugs. In DePalma JR, ed: *Drill's Pharmacology in medicine,* ed 4, New York, 1971, McGraw-Hill.)

the therapeutic uses and adverse effects of the antiarrhythmic drugs.

The K^+ current that is responsible for repolarization of the action potential is termed the delayed outwardly rectifying K^+ current (I_K). I_K is made up of several distinct currents

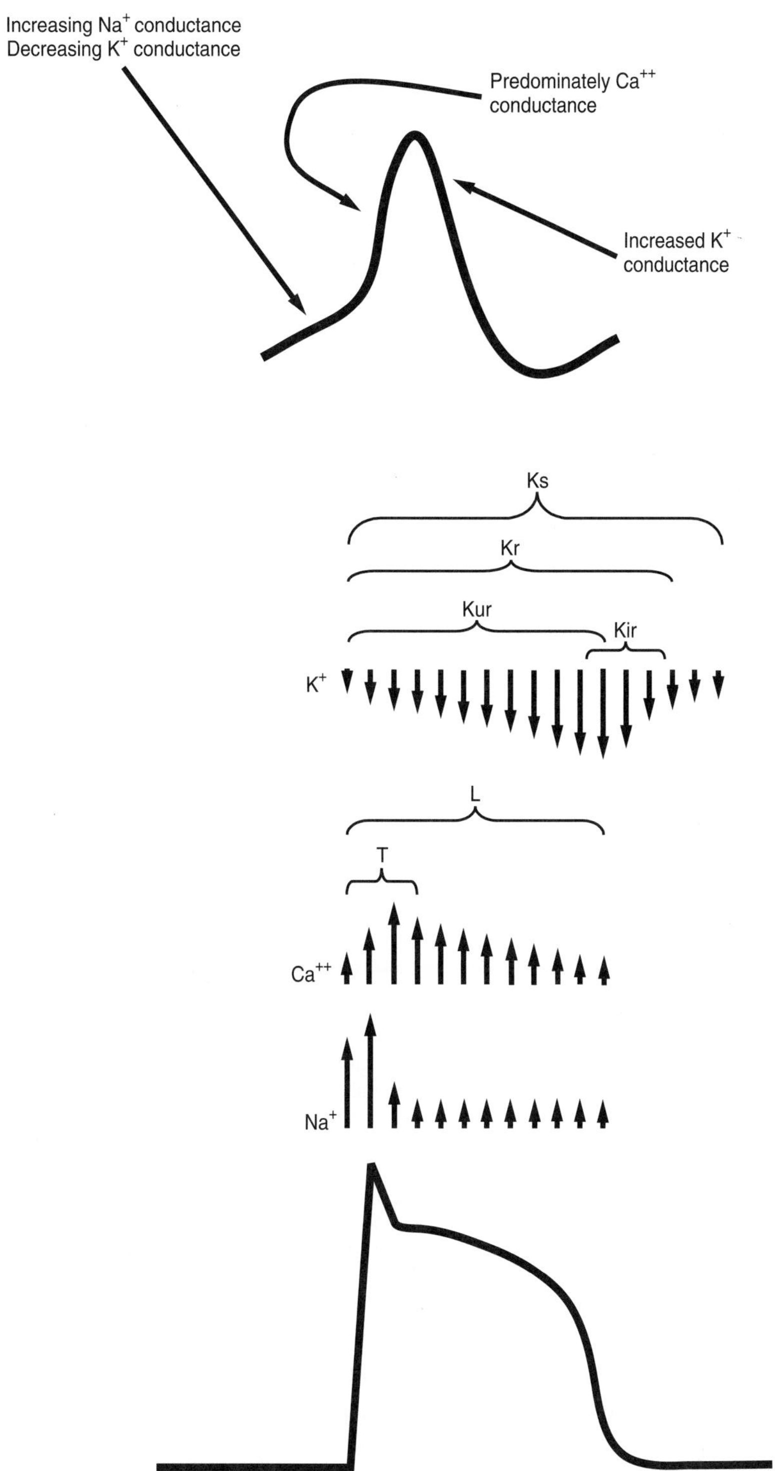

Fig. 24-4 Characteristic membrane action potentials from an SA nodal cell *(top)* and from a Purkinje fiber *(bottom)*. The relative magnitudes of the various ionic fluxes, as they apply to the Purkinje fiber, are shown by the length of the *arrows* above the Purkinje fiber; ↑, a depolarizing current; ↓, a repolarizing current. Differences in ion fluxes for the SA node are described. Predominate channel subtype activities for Ca^{++} and K^+ channels are shown above the respective arrows. In the SA (and AV) node, phase 0 is slower than in the Purkinje fibers and myocardium because phase 0 primarily depends on Ca^{++} influx. There is no discernible phase 2 in the SA node. Phase 3 in the SA node depends on K^+ efflux, as in the other cells of the heart. Phase 4 for SA nodal cells results, in part, from the pacemaker current largely provided by an increase in Na^+ conductance and a gradual decrease in K^+ conductance.

carried through separate channels. Each current and its corresponding channel are defined by the rapidity with which they activate. Thus the K^+ currents I_{Ks}, I_{Kr}, and I_{Kur}, referring to slow-, rapid-, and ultrarapid-activating currents, respectively, are conducted through Ks, Kr, and Kur channels.

The complex interplay of ionic currents that constitute the cardiac action potential is based on the ability of ion channels to sense and respond to variations in the membrane potential. Channels that are in a closed, resting state open when a particular threshold potential is reached. Ions capable of diffusing through these activated channels immediately begin flowing in response to their electrochemical gradients across the cell membrane. Most ion channels then spontaneously close, or become inactivated, over a characteristic time frame, and the ion flux abruptly decreases. Channels in the inactivated state are unresponsive, or refractory, to the original stimulus and will remain so until the membrane potential returns to a value that permits the channels to once again assume the closed, resting conformation. As discussed in subsequent sections of this chapter, many antiarrhythmic drugs bind preferentially to specific conformations of ion channels and therefore exert differing effects on the action potential.

ORIGINS OF ARRHYTHMIAS

Rhythm disturbances, often occurring as a result of myocardial infarction, are the most common cause of death from heart disease. Arrhythmias are thought to originate from abnormal impulse generation, impulse conduction, or both in combination. Some arrhythmias caused by abnormal impulse generation result from increased automaticity. These tachyarrhythmias are usually in response to an increase in the rate of diastolic depolarization (increased slope of phase 4) in pacemaker cells. Phase 4 depolarization can also be altered by autonomic nervous system activity or by drugs. Changes in the MDP and threshold potential voltage can also affect automaticity. Abnormal impulse generation may also be triggered by afterpotentials that occur in cardiac pacemakers affected by drugs, disease, or other disturbances (see Figure 24-2). The induced afterdepolarizations may be early (before repolarization is complete) or delayed (after full repolarization has occurred) and can result in sustained tachyarrhythmias.[25] Excessive intracellular Ca^{++} is a major contributor to delayed afterpotentials, whereas delayed repolarization increases the risk for early afterdepolarizations.

An important example of an alteration in impulse conduction that is easily induced in experimental animals is the phenomenon known as *reentry.* Figure 24-5 shows how a reentrant rhythm may develop. As illustrated, conduction in branch A is normal, whereas impulses in branch B can proceed in only the reverse direction (unidirectional block). A normally conducted impulse through branch A can then be conducted in retrograde fashion through branch B to reexcite an area of tissue (point R) that was previously excited by the normal path of conduction. For this “circus movement” to occur, the tissue at point R must have repolarized to a point at which excitation is possible (which usually means that the retrograde conduction is relatively slow). Thus a wave of reexcitation traveling in a circular path through fiber A, the ventricular muscle, and fiber B can result in a self-sustaining arrhythmia. Reentry is usually a major contributor to atrial fibrillation, an arrhythmia especially common in the elderly.[10]

Another type of conduction abnormality, known as *heart block,* occurs in response to impaired conduction in the AV node or conducting tissues of the ventricular myocardium. In its simplest form (first-degree block), there is excessive delay between atrial and ventricular depolarizations, resulting in a

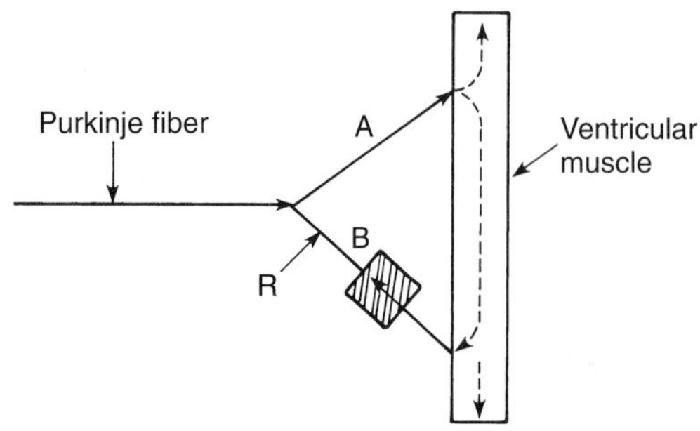

Fig. 24-5 Reentry in the presence of unidirectional block. The *hatched area* in path *B* indicates a unidirectional block of impulse conduction.

prolonged PR interval. In more advanced forms, some (second-degree block) or all (third-degree block) of the impulses from the SA node are prevented from reaching the ventricles, resulting in a ventricular rate that is lower than the atrial rate.

Disturbances in the relationship of the fast and slow electrical responses of certain cardiac cells may play an important role in the genesis of arrhythmias.[23] The *fast response* refers to the rapid phase 0 depolarization caused by rapid Na^+ influx (see Figure 24-4). This kind of activity is seen in atrial and ventricular muscle fibers and specialized conducting fibers. In addition to the rapid inward current carried by Na^+, the fast fibers exhibit a second, slower inward current carried by Ca^{++}. The slower current does not normally constitute a major factor in phase 0 depolarization of the atrial and ventricular myocardium and Purkinje fibers, but it persists after rapid depolarization and is responsible for the prolonged plateau phase characteristic of these fibers. Fibers located in the SA and AV nodes, the AV ring fibers, and the mitral and tricuspid valve leaflets demonstrate the slow response in phase 0, during which the depolarization is carried largely by the inward Ca^{++} current. Although the fast fibers exhibit rapid yet sustained depolarization, and thus remain refractory and conduct impulses safely, the slow fibers exhibit a slow rate of depolarization, low resting potential, and low impulse amplitude, resulting in slow conduction and susceptibility to aberrant stimulation. In some disease states, the fast response may become inactivated, leaving the slow response dominant. These conditions favor the genesis of arrhythmias because of the low safety factor associated with the slow response. It follows from this discussion that there exists in the heart an intricate relationship between conduction velocity, path length, refractory period duration, and impulse generation that, when altered through one or more mechanisms, may result in the development of arrhythmias.[23]

Certain arrhythmias can be traced to defects in one or more ion channels. The long QT syndrome, for instance, results from delayed repolarization in the ventricle. A delayed repolarization can be caused by any depolarizing current, such as a Na^+ current, that lingers into phase 3 of the action potential. It can also result from reduced activity of a repolarizing K^+ current. A defect in the Kr channel is the basis for one type of familial long QT syndrome that can devolve into *torsades de pointes,* a potentially life-threatening ventricular tachyarrhythmia (see below). Torsades may also be elicited by drugs that inhibit Kr channels, including a significant number of antiarrhythmic agents. Whether the delay in repolarization is caused by a hereditary defect or by a drug, it leads to a net enhancement of inward cationic flow, which can trigger early afterdepolarizations (see Figure 24-2). Because the cells in the wall of the ventricle are not equally affected, multiple waves of reentry can occur, initiating torsades. Effort is underway to develop more selective K^+-channel inhibitors as potential antiarrhythmic drugs. Torsades is obviously a major risk of drugs that selectively block Kr channels. The Ks channel is also a possible antiarrhythmic target. In addition to deactivating slowly, it is distinguished from the Kr channel by being inhibited in a use-dependent manner, as occurs with Na^+ channels (see Chapter 16). Therefore drugs acting on the Ks channel would tend to have their greatest effect at high heart rates. For Kr channels, "reverse" use dependence is a characteristic feature. Drugs that block this channel have a greater effect at lower heart rates and tend to promote a long QT interval. Kur channels exist predominately in the atria; inhibiting these channels may contribute to the antiarrhythmic effects of some drugs that are useful in treating atrial arrhythmias.

ELECTROCARDIOGRAPHY AND COMMON ARRHYTHMIAS

Arrhythmias are generally classified as supraventricular (originating in the atria or conducting system not in the ventricle) or ventricular. A few of the most common arrhythmias are described. For comparison, a diagram of the normal electrocardiogram (ECG) is provided in Figure 24-6. In Figure 24-7, representations of ECGs recorded during arrhythmias of ventricular and supraventricular origin are shown.

The first arrhythmia illustrated is a simple sinus tachycardia caused by rapid impulse generation (i.e., increased automaticity) in the SA node. Higher rates of atrial activity often involve reentry, as in atrial flutter (approximately 300 beats/min) or fibrillation (400 to 700 beats/min). Under these conditions, second-degree heart block occurs, as characterized by the failure of some atrial depolarizations to initiate a QRS complex. In a third-degree block (also shown), there is complete dissociation between atrial and ventricular contractions. The ventricular arrhythmias are caused by the development of ectopic foci or reentrant conduction in the ventricles. The first one shown in Figure 24-7 is ventricular tachycardia. In ventricular fibrillation, the most immediately life-threatening arrhythmia, erratic depolarization of different areas of the ventricle totally disorganizes myocardial contraction, renders the heart ineffective, and causes the cardiac output to plummet. Immediate treatment of ventricular fibrillation, usually including defibrillation (precordial direct current shock), must be provided to avert sudden death.

Torsades de pointes (literally meaning twisting of points) is a polymorphic ventricular tachycardia characterized by bizarre shapes in the ventricular depolarization complexes on the ECG (Figure 24-8). As mentioned previously, it often occurs in patients with defective K^+ channel (e.g., Kr) activity and also occurs with certain drugs that delay repolarization of ventricular muscle cells, often by blocking Kr channels. In both cases, QT prolongation precedes and leads to torsades. In Figure 24-8, an excessively long QT interval is followed by

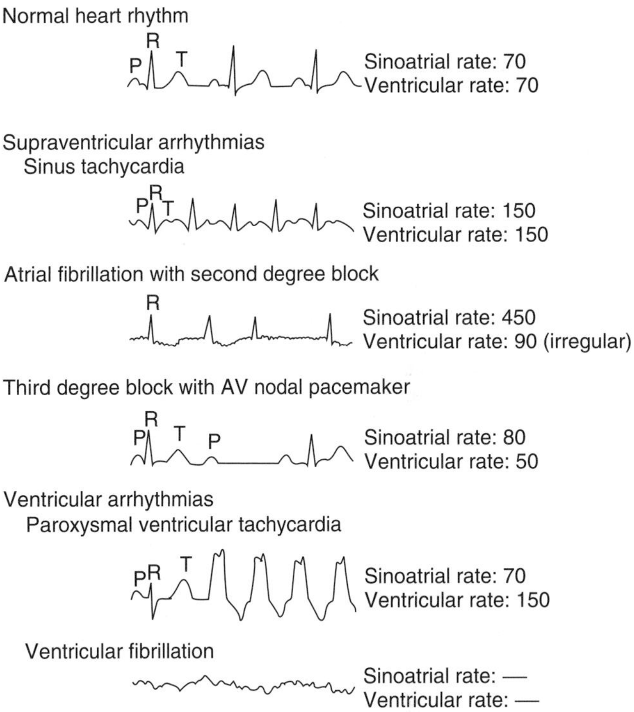

Normal heart rhythm
Sinoatrial rate: 70
Ventricular rate: 70

Supraventricular arrhythmias
Sinus tachycardia
Sinoatrial rate: 150
Ventricular rate: 150

Atrial fibrillation with second degree block
Sinoatrial rate: 450
Ventricular rate: 90 (irregular)

Third degree block with AV nodal pacemaker
Sinoatrial rate: 80
Ventricular rate: 50

Ventricular arrhythmias
Paroxysmal ventricular tachycardia
Sinoatrial rate: 70
Ventricular rate: 150

Ventricular fibrillation
Sinoatrial rate: —
Ventricular rate: —

Fig. 24-7 Various cardiac rhythms as recorded by the ECG. Arrhythmias are classified as supraventricular or ventricular in origin. Rates are given in beats per minute. (Adapted from Shepard RS: *Human physiology*, Philadelphia, 1971, JB Lippincott.)

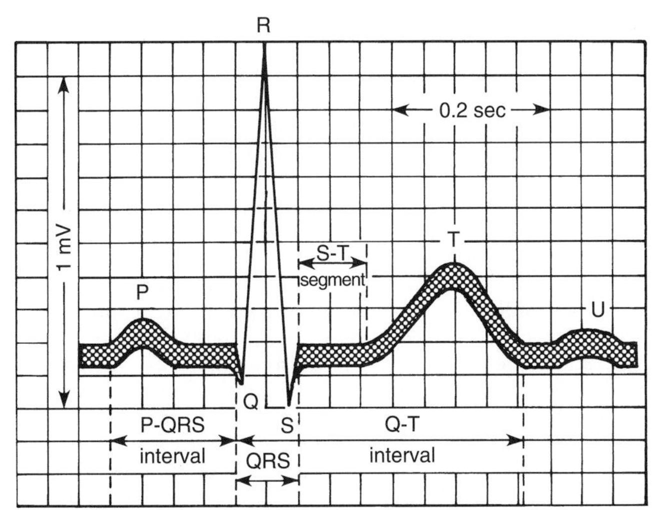

Fig. 24-6 Normal ECG. *P*, Atrial depolarization; *QRS*, ventricular depolarization; *T*, ventricular repolarization. The *U* wave corresponds to interventricular repolarization. (From Milnor WR: The ECG. In Mountcastle VB, ed: *Medical physiology*, ed 14, St Louis, 1980, Mosby.)

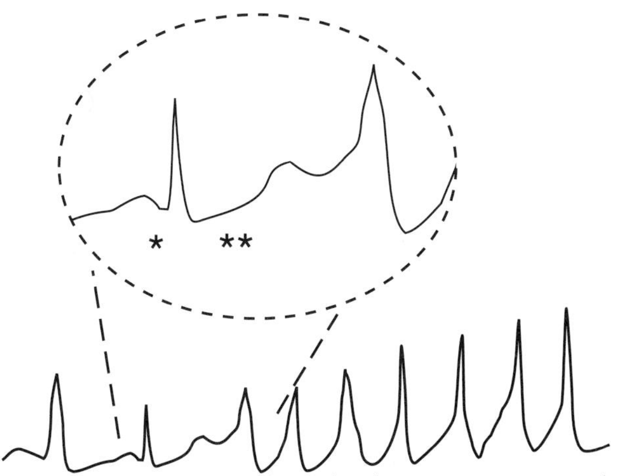

Fig. 24-8 ECG pattern of torsades de pointes. As seen in the enlarged section, the relatively normal P wave and QRS complex (*) are followed by a prolonged QT interval (**) and initiation of polymorphic ventricular tachycardia (non-enlarged section).

a ventricular tachycardia in which each depolarization has a different configuration.

ANTIARRHYTHMIC DRUGS

Antiarrhythmic drugs are used to modify, or restore to normal, aberrant electrophysiologic properties of cardiac muscle. Arrhythmias may result from various disease conditions or drug treatments. However, in all arrhythmias some facet of the normal electrophysiologic system that governs cardiac contraction is behaving abnormally. Several methods of treating arrhythmias are used today. Nonpharmacologic interventions for cardiac arrhythmias include electrical cardioversion, automatic implantable cardioverter devices, ablation therapy, and pacemakers.

The type of arrhythmia is a major factor in the selection of an antiarrhythmic drug. Enhanced impulse generation can be reduced by drugs that slow phase 4 depolarization by reducing the inward Na^+ current or the inward Ca^{++} current. The treatment of reentry includes drugs that reduce Na^+ channel and Ca^{++} channel activity, which then slows conduction velocity. Drugs that block K^+ channels, thereby prolonging repolarization and the refractory period, may also be useful.

The drugs used in the treatment of cardiac arrhythmias are not easily classified because they often have more than one action. Moreover, drugs within each class vary in their magnitudes of action or types of effects produced.[25,26] The most common scheme, originally proposed by Vaughan and Williams,[26] classifies drugs according to certain specific properties. Type I drugs, such as quinidine, lidocaine, and flecainide, depress Na^+ current.[25] The type I agents are further subdivided according to their relative effects on phase 0 depolarization, conduction velocity, and APD. Na^+ channels exist in at least three states: closed, open, and inactivated. At resting membrane potentials the Na^+ channels are closed, except for a Na^+ "leak" associated with phase 4 depolarization for cells that display automaticity. During rapid depolarization (phase 0, especially in Purkinje fibers and ventricular muscle), the Na^+ channels are open. The Na^+ channels then convert to the inactivated state before returning to the resting, closed state. The inactivated state occurs mostly in phase 2 and 3 of the action potential. Class IA and IC drugs bind more selectively to the open state of the channel. Class IB drugs bind more selectively to the inactivated state of the channel. Moreover, since the Purkinje fibers and ventricular myocardial cells have longer plateau phases (phase 2), class IB drugs are able to block Na^+ channels more effectively in these tissues because the Na^+ channels remain in an inactivated state longer during systole. Inasmuch as ischemic ventricular tissue is more depolarized, it, too, is especially sensitive to Na^+ channel blockade by class IB drugs.

Quinidinelike, or type IA, drugs depress phase 0 depolarization at all heart rates. They prolong the APD of the ventricle because they also inhibit K^+ (chiefly Kr) channels (Figure 24-9). Class IB agents, such as lidocaine, block Na^+ channels more selectively, but the rapid onset and recovery of Na^+ channel blockade results in little accumulated lidocaine effect on phase 0 and conduction velocity in healthy tissue at normal heart rates. In damaged or rapidly firing cells, however, lidocaine causes a frequency- or use-dependent block to reduce the slope of phase 0 and lowers phase 4 in ectopic pacemakers and in Purkinje fibers under high sympathetic tone.[25] Thus the faster the heart rate, the greater is the effect of lidocaine. (Use-dependent block is discussed in Chapter 16.) In contrast to other class I agents, lidocaine and related IB antiarrhythmics may actually shorten the APD. Flecainide and other class IC antiarrhythmics are characterized by their profound depression of phase 0 depolarization and slowing of conduction in the atria, AV node, and ventricles at normal heart rates. This pronounced effect results from their slow dissociation from Na^+ channels and accumulation of the channel-blocking effect over several contraction cycles. There is little or no prolongation of the APD.

Propranolol and related β-adrenergic–blocking agents constitute class II drugs and inhibit cardiac stimulation brought on by β-adrenergic agonists. They depress phase 4 depolarization (see Figure 24-9). The class III group, including amiodarone and sotalol, block K^+ channels (chiefly Kr channels) and prolong the APD by delaying phase 3 repolarization.[19] Verapamil and other class IV drugs selectively block Ca^{++} channels (L type) and depress slow fiber conduction (phase 0 of the SA and AV nodes) and phase 4 depolarization (see Figure 24-9). Drugs that cannot be classified by the Vaughan-Williams scheme include digitalis and adenosine.

The various categories of antiarrhythmic agents are outlined in Table 24-1. The action responsible for the classification of each drug, which is usually its major action, is circled. In the discussion of individual agents that follows, reference should also be made to Table 24-2 for the electrophysiologic actions of representative antiarrhythmic drugs. The net effects of the relevant drug classes and various action potentials in the heart are portrayed in Figure 24-9. Pharmacokinetic data for specific drugs are given in Table 24-3. The use of cardiac glycosides for certain kinds of arrhythmias is discussed in Chapter 25.

Quinidine

Quinidine is effective in the treatment of some atrial and (to a lesser extent) ventricular tachyarrhythmias. It was used clinically before its antiarrhythmic properties were discovered. During treatment with quinine and quinidine for patients with malaria, the reversal of atrial fibrillation was noted in some patients. Widespread use of quinidine for supraventricular arrhythmias followed reports from Wenckebach[28] in 1914 and Frey[8] in 1918.

Quinidine, the *d* isomer of quinine, is found in the bark of the cinchona tree, which is indigenous to certain regions of South America. Synthesis of this compound has been accomplished, but the synthesized drug is expensive, and quinidine is still isolated from the natural source. Its structural formula is shown in Figure 24-10.

Pharmacologic effects

Quinidine reduces automaticity and conduction velocity and increases refractoriness. Automaticity is depressed through an increase in the threshold potential and a decrease in the slope of spontaneous diastolic depolarization (phase 4) in pacemaker fibers, particularly at sites other than the SA node. Thus quinidine has the potential to slow or abolish tachyarrhythmias. Quinidine decreases the slope of phase 0 depolarization and thereby decreases conduction velocity in cells such as those of the AV node and ventricular myocardium (see Figure 24-9). By this effect, quinidine may inhibit reentrant pathways. Quinidine influences automaticity and conduction velocity by blocking Na^+ channels, particularly channels in the open state. The rate of recovery from quinidine block is intermediate between class IB and IC antiarrhythmic drugs (see Table 24-1). Therapeutic dosages increase refractoriness by prolonging the duration of the ERP in the ventricle and His-Purkinje system. This effect depends on blockade of K^+ channels, especially Kr channels, and has the potential for preventing or abolishing reentrant rhythms.[27] In the atria, inhibition of Kur channels by quinidine contributes to its antiarrhythmic effect.[11]

In addition to its direct actions on the heart, quinidine exerts a vagolytic action. As a consequence of its antivagal

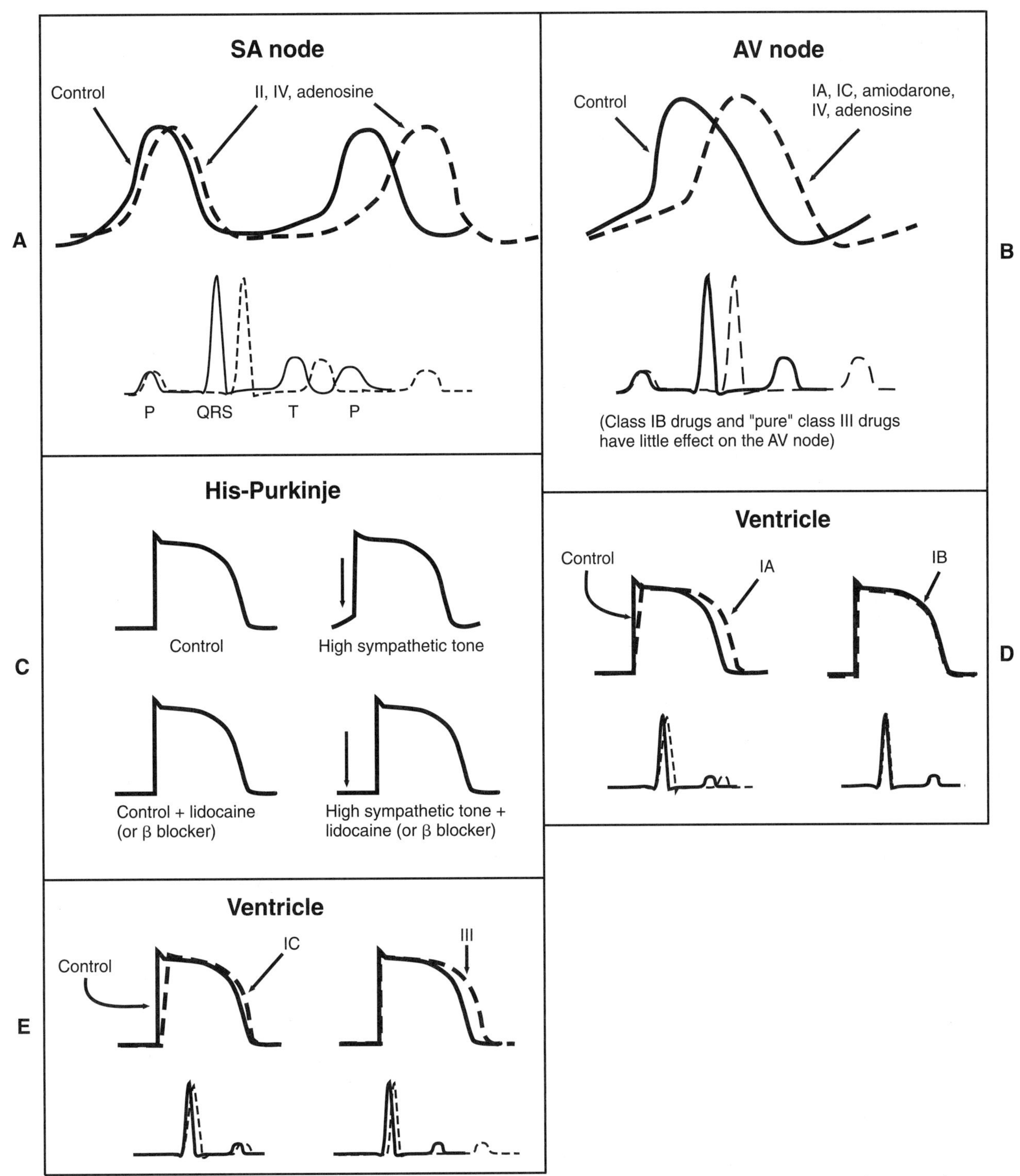

Fig. 24-9 Effect of the various antiarrhythmic drug classes on the action potentials in the SA node (A), the AV node (B), the His-Purkinje system (C), and ventricular muscle (D and E). Where relevant, the corresponding ECG pattern is also shown. Omitted drug classes have little effect on the action potentials depicted. The changes shown do not necessarily imply the same magnitude of change for each drug class. Amiodarone is singled out because although it is classified as a class III drug, it has additional actions. In *(D)*, IB drugs minimally alter the ECG pattern in normal cardiac rhythms.

Table • 24-1

Actions of Antiarrhythmic Drugs

DRUG*	BLOCK Na^+ CHANNELS			BLOCK β RECEPTORS	BLOCK K^+ CHANNELS	BLOCK CA^{++} CHANNELS	OTHER ACTIONS
	SLOW	MEDIUM	FAST				
Class IA							
Quinidine		⊗			x	x	α-Adrenergic blockade, vagolytic action
Procainamide		⊗			x		Ganglionic blockade
Disopyramide		⊗			x		Muscarinic blockade
Class IB							
Lidocaine			⊗				
Tocainide			⊗				
Mexiletine			⊗				
Class IC							
Flecainide	⊗				x		
Propafenone	⊗			x		x	Vagolytic action
Moricizine	⊗						
Class II							
Propranolol			x	⊗			
Esmolol				⊗			
Class III							
Amiodarone			⊗	x	⊗	x	α-Adrenergic blockade, muscarinic blockade
Ibutilide†					⊗		
Dofetilide					⊗		
Bretylium					⊗		Catecholamine release, adrenergic nerve blockade
Sotalol				x	⊗		
Class IV							
Verapamil			x			⊗	α-Adrenergic blockade
Diltiazem						⊗	
Miscellaneous							
Adenosine							A_1-receptor stimulation

*The distinguishing characteristics for the main classes of antiarrhythmic drugs are the following: class I drugs block Na^+ channels. The subclassification is based on the characteristics of the block. The terms *slow, medium,* and *fast* refer to the rates of onset of, and recovery from, Na^+ channel blockade. Class II drugs block β-adrenergic receptors. Class III drugs block K^+ channels. Class IV drugs block Ca^{++} channels. The major action responsible for the classification of each drug is circled.

†Ibutilide is exceptional in that its major action, not shown, is to increase conductance through a slow Na^+ channel.

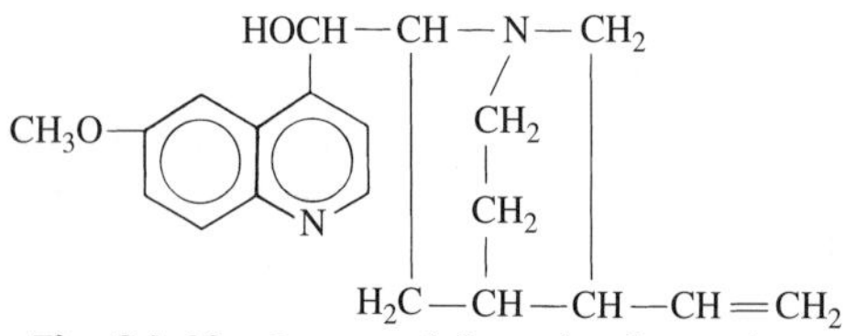

Fig. 24-10 Structural formula of quinidine.

influence on the SA node, quinidine, especially given intravenously, may increase the heart rate. Because the ERP in the atria is decreased by vagal stimulation, quinidine increases the ERP both directly and indirectly. The antivagal action of quinidine on AV nodal conduction is of special importance. By this mechanism, quinidine may increase the conduction velocity and decrease the refractory period of the AV node, which presents a hazard in treating atrial tachyarrhythmias because rapid atrial impulses are more readily conducted to the ventricles. This risk is greatest when the drug is used intravenously.

The ECG changes that result from quinidine administration are predictable from the electrophysiologic effects previously discussed (see Figure 24-9). The antimuscarinic property tends to elicit sinus tachycardia, but with high doses, SA nodal block may result from the drug's direct depressant effects. Increased durations of the QRS complex and the QT interval result, respectively, from decreases in ventricular conduction velocity and lengthening of the ventricular ERP.

In large doses, quinidine causes peripheral vasodilation by blocking α-adrenergic receptor blockade. Hypotension is a possible outcome.[9]

Table • 24-2

Effects of Antiarrhythmic Drug Classes

DRUG CLASS	SA AUTOMATICITY	AV CONDUCTION VELOCITY	ECG CHANGES			AFFINITY FOR Na^+ CHANNELS IN ISCHEMIC TISSUES	ANTIARRHYTHMIC USE	
			PR	QRS	QT		SUPRA	VENT
IA	↓	↑*, ↓	↓*, ↑	↑↑	↑↑	+	Yes	Yes
IB	0	0	0	0	0	+++[†]	No	Yes
IC	0	↓	↑	↑↑↑	0	+	Yes	Yes
II	↓↓	↓↓	↑↑	0	0	+[‡], 0	Yes	Yes
III	↓↓	↓	↑↑	0	↑↑↑	+[§], 0	Yes	Yes
IV	↓↓[‖]	↓↓	↑↑[‖]	0	0	+[¶], 0	Yes	No
Miscellaneous (adenosine)	↓[‖]	↓↓↓	↑↑[‖]	0	0	0	Yes	No

This table does not include unique qualities of individual drugs that may contrast with those of other drugs within the same class. *ECG changes* refer to an increase or decrease in the respective intervals. The number of *plus signs* or *arrows* indicates the relative magnitude of effect or relative affinity for Na^+ channels in ischemic tissue.
*From antimuscarinic and antivagal effects.
†Ischemic tissue is more depolarized and has a higher percentage of inactivated Na^+ channels. Class IB drugs bind most selectively to inactivated Na^+ channels.
‡Propranolol and esmolol can block Na^+ channels in depolarized cells.
§Amiodarone has more blocking effects on Na^+ channels than do other class III drugs.
‖Direct cardiac effect of the drug; does not include reflex effects from vasodilation.
¶Verapamil can block Na^+ channels in the depolarized state, whereas diltiazem has little effect.
Supra, Supraventricular; *Vent*, ventricular; *0*, no or little effect.

Table • 24-3

Pharmacokinetic Properties of Antiarrhythmic Drugs

DRUG CLASS	DRUG	ELIMINATION HALF-LIFE (hr)	PLASMA PROTEIN BINDING (%)	URINARY EXCRETION (%)
IA	Quinidine	4 to 10	85	20
	Procainamide	3 to 4	20	60
	Disopyramide	4 to 10	20 to 60	50
IB	Lidocaine	1.5 to 2	65	<2
	Mexilitine	10 to 12	55	10
	Tocainide	12 to 16	15	40
IC	Flecainide	12 to 27	40	25
	Propafenone	6 to 30	90	<2
	Moricizine	2 to 4	95	<1
II	Esmolol	0.2	55	<2
	Propranolol	4 to 6	90	<2
III	Amiodarone	25 to 100 days	>90	<1
	Bretylium	5 to 10	5	>90
	Sotalol	7 to 15	0	>90
	Ibutilide	2 to 12	40	<5
	Dofetilide	~10	65	80
IV	Verapamil	3 to 7	90	<5
	Diltiazem	4 to 8	75	<5
Miscellaneous	Adenosine	<10 sec	0	0

Absorption, fate, and excretion

Absorption of quinidine after oral administration is fairly rapid and nearly 100%. Depending on the salt formulation, maximum plasma concentrations are reached within 2 hours. Given intramuscularly, peak concentrations occur in 60 minutes. When quinidine is injected intravenously, it should be administered slowly because its therapeutic effects are not instantaneous and overdosage might occur. Moreover, adverse hemodynamic effects are more common with intravenous use. Other pharmacokinetic characteristics are listed in Table 24-3.

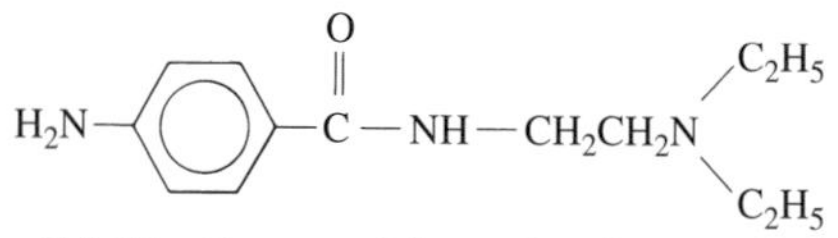

$$H_2N-C_6H_4-C(=O)-NH-CH_2CH_2N(C_2H_5)_2$$

Fig. 24-11 Structural formula of procainamide.

Adverse effects
Quinidine can precipitate a variety of ventricular arrhythmias, including torsades de pointes (see Figure 24-8). As a result of its depressive effects on ion conductance throughout the heart, quinidine modestly reduces myocardial contractility, which might be important in the management of a patient with congestive heart disease. Quinidine can cause a group of symptoms collectively referred to as *cinchonism:* blurred vision, tinnitus, tremor, vertigo, and lightheadedness. Nausea, vomiting, and diarrhea are the most common untoward effects of the drug. The negative inotropic and stronger peripheral vasodilatory effects of quinidine may occasionally lead to hemodynamic deterioration, resulting in hypotension, syncope, and a decrease in coronary blood flow, especially in patients with impaired myocardial function. Intravenous use of the drug presents an added risk of hypotension and syncope.

Immune-mediated reactions may develop with quinidine therapy. Responses include hematologic reactions (thrombocytopenia, hemolytic anemia, agranulocytosis), cutaneous reactions (rash, angioneurotic edema), and very rarely bronchial asthma and anaphylactic shock. Immunologically mediated thrombocytopenia can readily lead to hemorrhagic episodes.

Procainamide
Procaine was shown by Mautz[17] in 1936 to have an action on the heart similar to that of quinidine. Because its duration of action is short, a systematic search was undertaken to find a congener with similar activity but a longer duration. This investigation led to the introduction in 1951 of procainamide as an antiarrhythmic drug. Chemically, procainamide differs from procaine by having an amide linkage instead of an ester linkage (Figure 24-11). Although effective against some ventricular and supraventricular arrhythmias, procainamide is now prescribed less often than many other antiarrhythmic drugs because of its adverse effects. However, it is still used intravenously for acute suppression of ventricular arrhythmias.

Pharmacologic effects
The advantages of procainamide over procaine as an antiarrhythmic are its longer duration of action and its less potent effect on the central nervous system (CNS). The effects of procainamide on the heart are similar to those of quinidine. Both automaticity and conduction velocity are decreased, whereas refractoriness is increased. Like quinidine, procainamide can be described as a cardiac depressant. Procainamide exerts much less of an antivagal effect than does quinidine, but ganglionic blockade has been reported.[30]

The most frequently observed change induced by procainamide in the ECG is an increase in the duration of the QRS complex. Lengthening of the QT and PR intervals is also observed. There are few additional effects on the cardiovascular system when procainamide is administered orally. Intravenous infusion, on the other hand, causes a decrease in blood pressure because of peripheral vasodilation and myocardial depression and occasionally results in centrally mediated mental confusion and hallucination.

Absorption, fate, and excretion
After oral administration, procainamide is rapidly and essentially completely absorbed, with peak plasma concentrations being reached in approximately 90 minutes. Maximum plasma concentrations occur 15 to 60 minutes after intramuscular administration. Because of its short half-life, procainamide is often given in a slow-release preparation.

The major metabolite of procainamide, N-acetylprocainamide (NAPA), also has antiarrhythmic properties. Normally, approximately 25% of an administered dose of procainamide is acetylated in the liver to yield NAPA, but rapid acetylators or patients with renal disease will convert more of the drug to this form. NAPA has a plasma half-life of 6 hours and is eliminated by renal excretion.

Adverse effects
Like quinidine, procainamide can promote ventricular tachycardia when used to treat atrial tachyarrhythmias. It can also elicit other ventricular arrhythmias when given in high doses or to susceptible patients. Hypotension is common with rapid intravenous injection.

The most frequent side effects after oral administration are anorexia, nausea, and vomiting. Other, more rarely seen effects are diarrhea, weakness, flushing, a bitter taste, and CNS manifestations such as hallucinations and depression. Allergic reactions have been reported, and cross-sensitivity to procaine and other derivatives of *p*-aminobenzoic acid should be expected. Allergic reactions associated with procainamide include rashes, fever, chills, neutropenia, and even agranulocytosis. However, the most noteworthy immunologically based reaction is a syndrome similar to systemic lupus erythematosus. Symptoms of lupus occur in up to 30% of patients receiving long-term oral procainamide therapy (more frequently with slow acetylators) and include arthralgia, fever, and occasionally pleuropericarditis, but not renal involvement. The presence of antinuclear antibodies occurs in a high percentage of patients taking procainamide; however, it is widely held that withdrawal of the drug is only required when lupus-like symptoms occur. The syndrome usually disappears after drug withdrawal. NAPA is not associated with a lupuslike reaction.[31]

Disopyramide
Although structurally unrelated to either agent, disopyramide (Figure 24-12) has actions similar to those of quinidine and procainamide. Its effectiveness in the treatment of premature extrasystoles and tachycardias of both supraventricular and ventricular origin has been established. The drug is only occasionally used today.

Pharmacologic effects
Like quinidine, disopyramide decreases the rate of diastolic depolarization (phase 4), particularly in ectopic pacemaker cells; it also decreases the upstroke velocity of the action potential (phase 0) in cardiac fibers and increases the ERP. Disopyramide thus tends to lessen automaticity and conduction velocity. One difference between disopyramide and the other class IA agents is that the PR interval and QRS complex are less affected by disopyramide. Another is that disopyramide is more likely to depress cardiac contractility. Disopyramide also has antimuscarinic effects.

Absorption, fate, and excretion
Disopyramide is almost completely absorbed within several hours after oral administration. Other pharmacokinetic characteristics are listed in Table 24-3.

Adverse effects

The most common side effects of disopyramide are dose dependent and largely result from its antimuscarinic action. These include urinary retention; dryness of the mouth, nose, throat, or eyes; blurred vision; constipation; nausea; and skin rash. Rarely, acute psychosis, cholestatic jaundice, hypoglycemia, and agranulocytosis have occurred, but these disappear on drug withdrawal. As with other class IA antiarrhythmic drugs, various arrhythmias may develop with overdosage. Disopyramide is contraindicated in patients with cardiomyopathy or congestive heart failure because of its relatively pronounced negative inotropic effect.[9]

Lidocaine

Lidocaine has been used as a local anesthetic for more than half a century. Unlike procaine, it has also long been a primary drug for arresting and preventing certain ventricular arrhythmias in emergency situations. For additional discussion of its pharmacologic characteristics, see Chapter 16.

Pharmacologic effects

Lidocaine decreases automaticity but is devoid of antimuscarinic activity. Whereas quinidine affects electrical activity throughout the heart, lidocaine preferentially influences ventricular function. Lidocaine acts by blocking Na^+ channels, particularly inactivated Na^+ channels. This effect on Na^+ channels is rapidly reversed, which restricts its use-dependent blocking effect to patients with rapid heart rates. Because lidocaine has a preferential effect on Na^+ channels in the inactivated state, it preferentially inhibits automaticity in ischemic tissue where membrane depolarization or an enhanced frequency of excitation occurs, such as in the His-Purkinje system (see Table 24-2). Lidocaine also reduces delayed afterdepolarizations seen with digoxin toxicity. Lidocaine does not slow repolarization, but instead may hasten it. Therefore in contrast to the action of quinidine and procainamide, lidocaine tends to shorten the ERP. The drug has little effect on conduction velocity and phase 0.

Lidocaine is usually administered intravenously for the treatment of ventricular ectopic rhythms. Because lidocaine must be administered parenterally, it is largely restricted to emergency situations and hospital settings. Its use is contraindicated in supraventricular arrhythmias because it is largely ineffective against these arrhythmias and excessive ventricular rates may result.

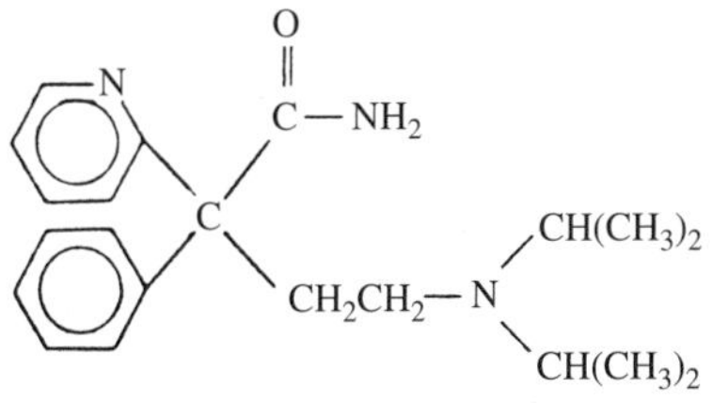

Fig. 24-12 Structural formula of disopyramide.

Absorption, fate, and excretion

As an antiarrhythmic, lidocaine is usually given intravenously by injection or infusion. After intravenous administration, the plasma concentration initially falls rapidly, followed by a slower decrease. For this reason, various loading regimens are used to achieve therapeutic plasma concentrations quickly. Lower constant perfusion rates are then used. Administration is monitored by measurement of plasma concentrations, and the patient is closely observed for neurologic side effects. Both α_1-acid glycoprotein and albumin contribute to plasma protein binding. Lidocaine is broken down in the liver to various metabolites, including N-ethylglycine and 2,6-xylidine. The 2,6-xylidine is further metabolized to 4-hydroxy-2,6-xylidine and largely excreted in the urine. At least two intermediary metabolites, glycinexylidide and monoethylglycinexylidide, have pharmacologic activity.

Adverse effects

Lidocaine exhibits only minor effects on the autonomic nervous system. Arterial pressure is not depressed by lidocaine as much as it is by quinidine. After acutely high dosages or prolonged infusion, lidocaine may cause convulsions and respiratory depression. (These reactions, however, occur only rarely with the dosages and routes of administration used in dentistry.) Cardiac arrest may occur if lidocaine is administered to a patient with preexisting heart block.

Phenytoin

Phenytoin (diphenylhydantoin) has been used since 1938 for the treatment of grand mal epilepsy and other seizure disorders. Although it has been used as an antiarrhythmic drug (class IB), it is now rarely used for this purpose. For a general discussion of its pharmacologic features, see Chapter 14.

Tocainide

Tocainide is a class IB drug along with lidocaine and phenytoin (see Table 24-1). Tocainide closely resembles lidocaine structurally (Figure 24-13) and shares many of that drug's properties. An orally effective drug, tocainide exerts electrophysiologic effects similar to those of lidocaine. A minor difference is that tocainide is more likely to shorten the refractory period in the atria and AV node. It is indicated for life-threatening ventricular arrhythmias that are unresponsive to the more traditional oral drugs.

Tocainide is rapidly and completely absorbed by the oral route. Unlike lidocaine, it does not undergo rapid first-pass metabolism in the liver. Peak plasma concentrations are reached in 1 to 2 hours. The drug is approximately 50% protein bound in the plasma.

The most common adverse reactions are gastrointestinal, including anorexia, nausea, vomiting, and constipation. Neurologic manifestations, including convulsions, are similar to those of lidocaine, as are the cardiac side effects, such as induction of arrhythmias. Agranulocytosis is a rare but potentially fatal reaction that generally occurs with standard doses and early in therapy. Pulmonary fibrosis, interstitial pneumonitis, and bone marrow aplasia are additional toxic effects that limit its use.

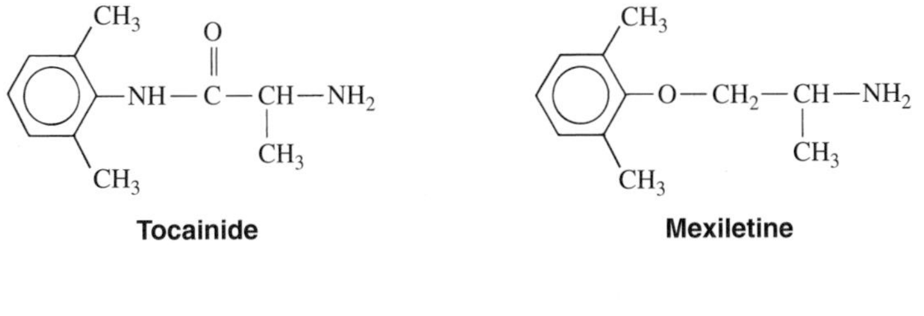

Tocainide

Mexiletine

Fig. 24-13 Structural formulas of tocainide and mexiletine.

Mexiletine

Mexiletine, like tocainide, is a class IB antiarrhythmic drug structurally related to lidocaine (see Figure 24-13). Mexiletine's electrophysiologic properties are similar to those of lidocaine. Conduction velocity in the diseased AV node and ventricular myocardium is more likely to be slowed than with lidocaine. Mexiletine is used primarily to treat life-threatening ventricular arrhythmias.

Mexiletine is well absorbed after oral administration and is useful by both the oral and the intravenous routes. Like tocainide, mexiletine is resistant to first-pass metabolism in the liver, but it does undergo subsequent hepatic metabolism. SA node and AV conduction defects can be worsened by mexiletine, which limits the drug's usefulness in patients with these preexisting problems. Extracardiac adverse reactions include gastrointestinal (nausea, vomiting) and neurologic (tremor, diplopia, dizziness, paresthesias) effects. Hepatitis or agranulocytosis may rarely occur.

Flecainide

A third category of type I antiarrhythmics (class IC) is represented by drugs that are relatively new to clinical use. Flecainide (Figure 24-14) belongs to this class (see Table 24-1). Flecainide is indicated for the treatment of disabling supraventricular arrhythmias and sustained life-threatening ventricular arrhythmias unresponsive to other medications.

Pharmacologic effects

Although possessing some similarity to lidocaine, flecainide and related class IC drugs significantly depress conduction velocity by strongly reducing Na^+ conductance during phase 0 of the action potential.[27] This effect is felt throughout the heart but is especially strong in the atrium and His-Purkinje system. It results from the slow association of drug with, and dissociation from, Na^+ channels, especially channels in the open configuration. Recovery from Na^+-channel blockade is therefore protracted.

Flecainide does not selectively reduce phase 0 in diseased tissues. Rather, it inhibits phase 0 more or less uniformly in diseased and healthy tissues and tends to be effective on reentry mechanisms. Flecainide increases the ERP in atrial and ventricular muscle and widens the QRS complex (as does quinidine). Flecainide also reduces conduction velocity in the AV node but to a lesser degree than in ventricular muscle (see Figure 24-9 and Table 24-2).

Absorption, fate, and excretion

Flecainide is not significantly metabolized on its first pass through the liver and therefore has good bioavailability after oral administration. Approximately 75% of a flecainide dose is eventually metabolized to inactive products. The relatively large range in reported half-lives for the drug stems in part from genetically determined variations in the rate of hepatic metabolism by CYP2D6. As is discussed in Chapter 4, some individuals lack this enzyme. The resulting potential differences in patient response necessitate careful monitoring of drug effects.

Adverse effects

CNS toxicity is the most common adverse effect. Dizziness, blurred vision, tremor, paresthesia, and headache may occur. Nausea and a metallic taste have been reported for flecainide.

The results of the Cardiac Arrhythmia Suppression Trial[2] indicated that flecainide administration to patients with recent myocardial infarction increased the mortality rate in such patients twofold to threefold compared with placebo-treated patients. An arrhythmogenic effect of these drugs is suspected despite the fact that they suppressed premature ventricular depolarizations in these patients.[2] The results of the trial have led to cautions concerning the use of flecainide and its restriction to arrhythmias unresponsive to safer drugs.

Propafenone

Propafenone is classified as a class IC antiarrhythmic because of its strong tendency to depress the maximum rate of depolarization and thereby conduction velocity. The drug is indicated for life-threatening ventricular arrhythmias and is also prescribed for atrial fibrillation and other types of supraventricular arrhythmias. The structure of propafenone is depicted in Figure 24-14.

Pharmacologic effects

Propafenone exerts several actions on the heart. In addition to blocking Na^+ channels, it blocks Ca^{++} channels and exerts β-adrenergic receptor–blocking effects (see Table 24-1). The drug thus reduces the slope of phase 0, prolongs the PR and QRS intervals, and suppresses ectopic pacemakers (see Table 24-2). Negative inotropic effects are possible but usually occur only with high doses.

Absorption, fate, and excretion

Propafenone is well absorbed orally, but approximately 80% of a given dose is destroyed in the first pass through the liver. The same genetic predisposition for efficient or slow metabolism (by CYP2D6) of the drug exists as for flecainide, and the half-life may be prolonged in patients who are slow metabolizers. At least one major metabolite is pharmacologically active.

Adverse effects

Adverse effects include dizziness, blurred vision, dysgeusia, and gastrointestinal symptoms. CNS toxicity appears to be more likely with slow metabolizers. Asthma may be exacerbated in susceptible individuals. Untoward cardiac signs include SA nodal dysfunction, AV nodal block, and worsening of heart failure. The arrhythmogenic potential of the drug must be considered in light of the problems documented for other class IC agents. Competition for metabolism by cytochrome CYP2D6 is the basis for interactions involving propafenone and other drugs. For instance, propafenone may increase the anticoagulant effect of warfarin given concurrently.

Moricizine

Moricizine resembles most closely the class IC antiarrhythmics. However, it is sometimes classified in its own unique category. The structure of moricizine is given in Figure 24-15.

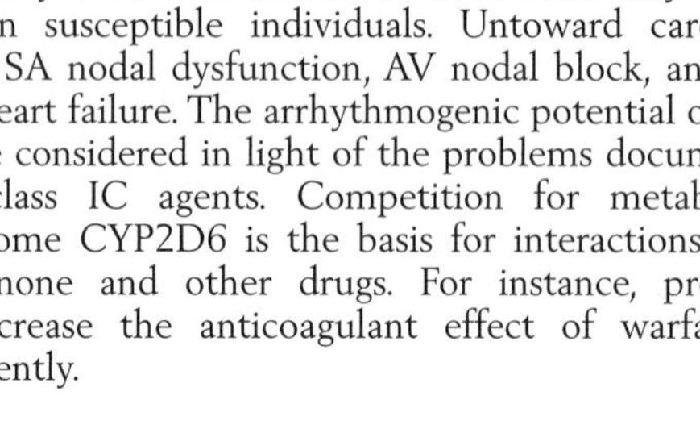

CF_3CH_2O, $C(=O)-NH-CH_2$, HN, OCH_2CF_3

Flecainide

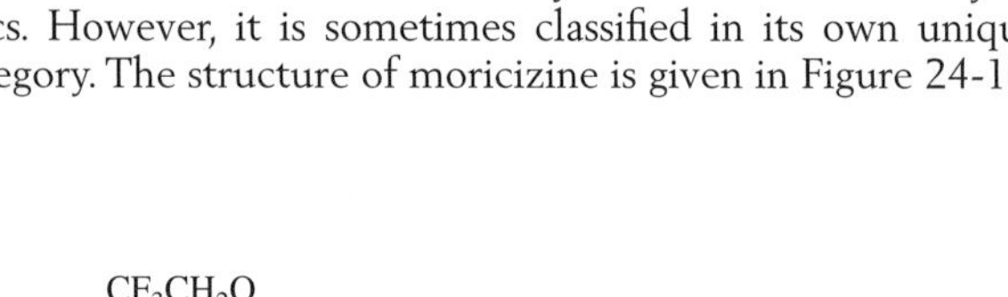

OH, $O-CH_2CHCH_2-NH-C_3H_7$, $CH_2CH_2-C(=O)$

Propafenone

Fig. 24-14 Structural formulas of flecainide and propafenone.

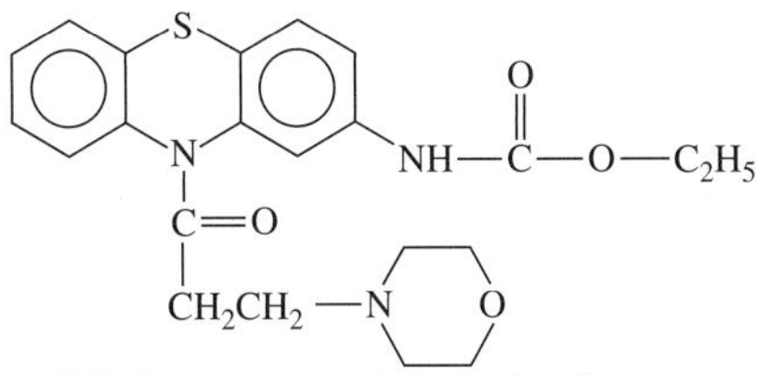

Fig. 24-15 Structural formula of moricizine.

It is used in the treatment of life-threatening ventricular arrhythmias.

Moricizine reduces automaticity by altering the threshold voltage. It is effective against ectopic foci without producing significant negative inotropism. It also is effective in reducing afterdepolarizations. These actions bear resemblance to lidocaine. The slope of phase 0 is reduced, with an increase in the PR and QRS intervals reminiscent of quinidine.[1] AV nodal reentry is inhibited. Despite the fact that moricizine is a phenothiazine, it has little psychotropic effect.

Moricizine is well absorbed orally; however, 60% to 70% of the drug is metabolized in the liver before it reaches the systemic circulation. The drug yields multiple metabolites; one is known to have pharmacologic activity. Dizziness, headache, nausea, and vomiting are common side effects of therapy. SA nodal depression, AV nodal block, and other arrhythmogenic effects occur in approximately 4% of patients being treated for ventricular arrhythmias.

β-Adrenergic Receptor–Blocking Drugs

Since the introduction of propranolol in 1968 for clinical use in the United States, a number of β-adrenergic receptor–blocking agents have been approved. (The β-adrenergic antagonists are discussed in Chapters 7, 26, and 28.) Three β-adrenergic blockers, propranolol, metoprolol, and esmolol, are the primary class II antiarrhythmic drugs (see Table 24-1). Sotalol, a fourth drug with ability to block the β-adrenergic receptor, is discussed under class III drugs. Propranolol is reviewed here as the prototypical agent; special features of the other β blockers are also noted.

Pharmacologic effects

Propranolol, the prototypic type II antiarrhythmic, has two types of effects on the heart: indirect effects as a consequence of blockade of β-adrenergic receptors and "membrane stabilizing" effects similar to those of quinidine. Propranolol decreases automaticity and conduction velocity and increases refractoriness. The drug's greatest effects are on SA nodal automaticity, AV node refractoriness, and (if it exists) His-Purkinje automaticity (see Figure 24-9, Table 24-2).

Activation of the sympathetic nervous system leading to β-receptor stimulation enhances automaticity by increasing the slope of phase 4 depolarization, speeds conduction velocity, and shortens the ERP (especially in the AV node). By blocking β receptors, propranolol can produce opposite effects proportional to the sympathetic input to the heart at the time of administration. In addition to decreasing automaticity in the SA node (and therefore decreasing the heart rate), propranolol variably reduces automaticity and conduction velocity in the atria, AV node, His-Purkinje system, and ventricles. Increased refractoriness in the AV node is an especially important manifestation of blockade. The direct actions of propranolol include decreasing the slope of phase 0 and phase 4 depolarization and prolonging the ERP. The β-adrenergic blockers, with the exception of sotalol, do not appreciably affect repolarization.

The major antiarrhythmic indication for propranolol is in the management of supraventricular tachyarrhythmias in which protection of the ventricles (by interfering with AV transmission) is the major clinical objective. Propranolol is also useful in suppressing paroxysmal supraventricular tachycardia and in treating afterdepolarizations and other ventricular arrhythmias in which catecholamine stimulation is involved. Most ventricular arrhythmias, however, respond only to very large doses. Because propranolol reduces the ratio of oxygen demand to oxygen supply, arrhythmias caused by myocardial ischemia may also be relieved. Although propranolol is effective in treating cardiac glycoside–induced arrhythmias, phenytoin and lidocaine are more useful, especially if AV conduction is impaired, because propranolol tends to exacerbate the AV block induced by digitalis. The β blockers have been shown to reduce the incidence of heart attack and death in patients with previous myocardial infarction. The mechanism is not established but it may relate to an antiarrhythmic mechanism.

Absorption, fate, and excretion

Propranolol is readily absorbed after oral administration, but more than two thirds of the drug is destroyed in its first pass through the liver. Peak plasma concentrations are reached in 1 to 2 hours. The rate of metabolism of propranolol, which involves CYP2D6, varies considerably among individuals, so plasma titers may differ markedly with long-term therapy. Propranolol is metabolized by hydroxylation, deamination, and glucuronide conjugation.

Adverse effects

The important adverse effects of propranolol can be explained by its antagonism of β-adrenergic receptors. Heart rate and myocardial contractility are reduced, at least initially, during therapy. Congestive heart failure and AV block are the major severe cardiac side effects; however, after large doses severe bradycardia or even asystole may occur. Sudden withdrawal of the drug in patients prone to angina pectoris may lead to anginal attacks or even myocardial infarction. Bronchoconstriction is a predictable side effect and may be significant in susceptible persons, such as asthmatics. Propranolol inhibits the glycogenolytic and lipolytic actions of endogenous catecholamines released in response to hypoglycemia and thus complicates therapy of diabetic patients.

β_1-Selective blockers

Metoprolol differs from propranolol in that it is selective for the β_1-adrenergic receptor (cardioselective). Its pharmacologic features are reviewed in Chapter 7. Esmolol is a very short-acting selective β_1-adrenergic receptor blocker that is metabolized by plasma esterases. It is used intravenously for short-term β-adrenergic receptor blockade. The adverse effects of these drugs resemble those of propranolol. Despite their selectivity for β_1-adrenergic receptors, metoprolol and esmolol as well as other β blockers should be avoided, if at all possible, in the asthmatic patient.

Sotalol

Sotalol, a β-adrenergic blocking drug and thus a class II antiarrhythmic, also has properties of the class III drugs. It increases the ERP in addition to its β-adrenergic–blocking activity. The relative importance of its β-blocking properties and its class III antiarrhythmic effects has yet to be determined. Sotalol is well absorbed when taken orally, with a bioavailability of nearly 100%. Sotalol may be useful in supraventricular arrhythmias and in certain cases of ventricular tachycardia. It has been shown to be effective in preventing recurrences of ventricular tachyarrhythmias.[16,24]

Bretylium

Bretylium tosylate is classified as a class III antiarrhythmic because it increases the ERP and delays repolarization without having much effect on conduction velocity. The mechanism involves blockade of K^+ conductance, delaying phase 3 of the action potential. Bretylium was originally developed in the 1950s as an antihypertensive drug but was approved in the United States in 1978 for the treatment of ventricular arrhythmias. The drug has a complex pharmacological profile, some aspects of which are still incompletely understood.

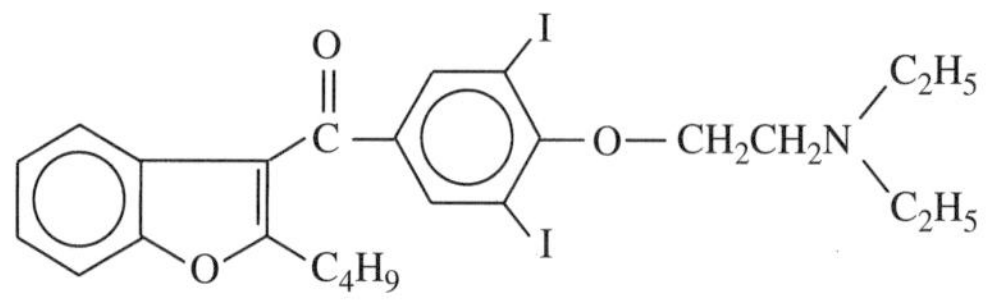

Pharmacologic effects

Bretylium both interferes with sympathetic control of the heart and exerts direct influences on cardiac function. As discussed in Chapter 7, bretylium is classified as an adrenergic neuron blocker because it produces a prolonged inhibition of norepinephrine release from sympathetic nerve endings. Bretylium also initially stimulates norepinephrine efflux and tends to exert an imipraminelike block of the neuronal uptake of catecholamines. Together, these influences on sympathetic function make the drug's effect in any particular patient difficult to predict, especially in the initial phase of therapy.

The effect of bretylium on supraventricular tissues is largely indirect. After an initial catecholamine release, it decreases sympathetic influences, thereby reducing automaticity in the SA node (see Table 24-1). ERP in the AV node is also increased after the initial stimulation. Whereas atrial arrhythmias are often not responsive to the drug, the fact that bretylium significantly increases the ERP in the His-Purkinje system and ventricular myocardium supports the finding that the drug is useful in treating ventricular tachyarrhythmias, including its previous use as an adjunct in treating ventricular fibrillation.[5] A reduction in the differences between refractory periods and APDs in diseased and normal ventricular myocardium by the drug further contributes to a lessened likelihood of reentrant arrhythmias.

Absorption, fate, and excretion

Bretylium can be administered orally, intramuscularly, or intravenously. It is, however, unpredictably absorbed from the gastrointestinal tract, as would be expected from its quaternary ammonium structure.

Adverse effects

The side effects of bretylium can in most cases be explained by its adrenergic-blocking actions. Because of its tendency to produce hypotension (to which tolerance may develop), bretylium is reserved for use in ventricular tachyarrhythmias that are not responsive to other therapeutic measures. Nausea and vomiting may occur even with intravenous use, especially when injected rapidly. Parotid gland pain and swelling may occur in as many as 25% of patients receiving long-term oral therapy, but apparently it does not occur with parenteral use. The initial release of catecholamines induced by bretylium may be associated with hypertension or arrhythmias. Other adverse reactions include diplopia, facial flushing, weakness, and nasal congestion. The actions of bretylium on the adrenergic nerve terminals can be blocked by tricyclic antidepressants, which prevent bretylium from gaining access to the nerve terminal.

Amiodarone

Amiodarone, a benzofuran derivative resembling thyroid hormone (Figure 24-16), was originally introduced in Europe as a coronary vasodilator for the treatment of angina pectoris. It is now widely used for a variety of acute and chronic arrhythmias.

Fig. 24-16 Structural formula of amiodarone.

Pharmacologic effects

Amiodarone's major action is to increase the ERP by slowing the rate of repolarization. Blockade of K^+ channels is involved (see Table 24-1). Repolarization is slowed in the His-Purkinje system as well as in ventricular and atrial myocardium (see Figure 24-9). Although K^+-channel blockade is a major mechanism of action, amiodarone is not as likely to cause torsades as are drugs whose mechanism of action is largely limited to blocking K^+ channels ("pure" Kr-channel blockers). In addition to blocking K^+ channels, amiodarone blocks Na^+ and Ca^{++} channels. Inhibition of these latter channels probably prevents much of the inward depolarizing current that can trigger early afterdepolarizations and torsades. The drug decreases automaticity in the SA node and in ectopic pacemakers but has little effect on automaticity elsewhere in the heart. Conduction velocity is slowed in the AV node by Na^+- and Ca^{++}-channel blockade (see Table 24-1), and the ERP in the AV node is lengthened.[15] Conduction velocity in the His-Purkinje system and ventricular muscle is also slowed. The ventricular fibrillation threshold is increased.

Amiodarone has an active metabolite, desethylamidarone, that contributes to the antiarrhythmic effect. Desethylamidarone binds to thyroid hormone receptors, inhibiting thyroid hormone–induced gene expression.[6] Of the genes normally induced by thyroid hormone, several support the synthesis of certain K^+ channels. This finding is consistent with the fact that amiodarone's effects on K^+ channels are generally delayed compared with those on Na^+ and Ca^{++} channels. Thus long-term therapy with amiodarone is more likely to generate a class III antiarrhythmic effect (K^+-channel block), in large part because of reduction in the number of Kr channels. Short-term therapy, on the other hand, is more likely to limit effects to Na^+ channels, Ca^{++} channels, and β-adrenergic receptors. The resulting cardiac effects appear to be different from those of long-term therapy and avoid many of the adverse effects seen with long-term administration, such as pulmonary fibrosis and hypothyroidism. Amiodarone is a vasodilator, noncompetitively inhibiting the vascular effect of catecholamines.[9] The cardiac effects of catecholamines are likewise inhibited, and coronary arterial resistance is decreased, resulting in increased coronary blood flow.

Amiodarone is used for a variety of arrhythmias, including ventricular extrasystoles, tachycardia, and fibrillation.[14,21] It is also efficacious in some atrial arrhythmias, including atrial fibrillation and flutter as well as supraventricular tachycardia.

Absorption, fate, and excretion

When administered orally, amiodarone's bioavailability is low (20% to 50%). It is also administered intravenously. A highly lipophilic drug, amiodarone is sequestered in tissues, yielding a volume of distribution of approximately 60 L/kg. It is highly bound to protein in plasma. Because the drug would normally take weeks to reach a steady-state concentration after the initiation of therapy, loading doses are routinely used. Amiodarone is extensively metabolized by the liver; a desethyl derivative, which has antiarrhythmic properties as indicated above, has been identified. When the drug is withdrawn, the tissue concentrations drop only gradually as the drug is eliminated. Hence plasma determinations of amiodarone may not reflect tissue concentrations.

Adverse effects

Sinus arrest may occur if amiodarone is given with β-adrenergic blocking drugs or other antiarrhythmics, and AV nodal conduction abnormalities may be exacerbated. Because amiodarone has negative inotropic properties, its use may be associated with a decrease in cardiac function. Some preexisting arrhythmias may be worsened by the drug. Noncardiac adverse reactions are fairly common and occasionally life threatening. The primary concerns are pulmonary fibrosis and pneumonitis, which may become clinically evident in a significant percentage of patients with long-term use and can be lethal. Amiodarone also commonly causes CNS disturbances (ataxia, dizziness), photosensitivity, and hepatic dysfunction as indicated by a rise of liver enzymes in the blood. The skin may take on a blue-gray hue. Corneal microdeposits occur routinely but usually do not interfere with vision and disappear after withdrawal of the drug. Changes in thyroid function (hyperthyroidism and especially hypothyroidism) have been reported, and these may be related to the aforementioned facts that amiodarone resembles thyroid hormone and influences thyroid hormone actions. Furthermore, amiodarone can reduce the action of thyroid hormone by binding to the thyroid hormone receptor and blocking its cellular effects. It has also been shown that amiodarone can inhibit the action of thyroid-stimulating hormone, which could also contribute to a hypothyroid effect by amiodarone.[20] Finally, this drug inhibits the conversion of thyroxine to triiodothyronine in peripheral tissues and causes the buildup of reverse triiodothyronine (see Chapter 34).

Ibutilide and Dofetilide

Ibutilide is classified as a class III drug because it delays repolarization. It blocks Kr channels but more importantly causes the opening of Ca^{++} channels, which then promote Na^{+} influx through slow channels, thereby extending phase 2 of the action potential.[13] The drug is administered intravenously for atrial fibrillation and atrial flutter.[7] It can be used to convert rapidly these arrhythmias to normal sinus rhythm. Torsades de pointes is one of its adverse effects.

Dofetilide is a "pure" class III drug, blocking the Kr channel selectively. It is used for acute conversion of atrial fibrillation and atrial flutter and for short-term maintenance.[18] Dofetilide is available for intravenous and oral use. Predictably, a characteristic adverse effect is torsades in response to the prolonged QT interval that is induced by the drug. The structures for ibutilide and dofetilide are shown in Figure 24-17.

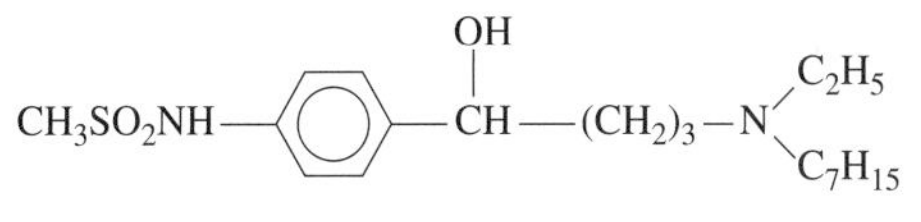

Ibutilide

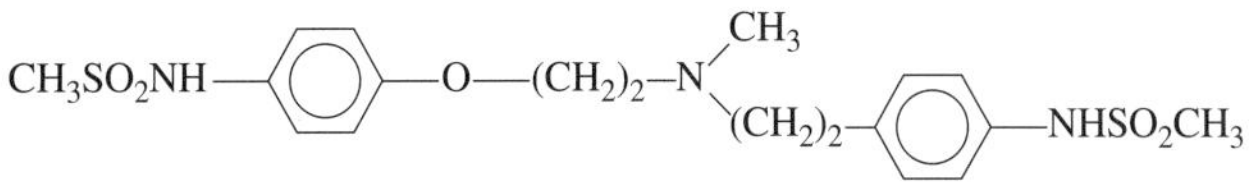

Dofetilide

Fig. 24-17 Structural formulas of ibutilide and dofetilide.

Ca^{++}-Channel Blockers

The Ca^{++}-channel blockers, represented by verapamil, diltiazem, and nifedipine, are used for the treatment of certain cardiovascular diseases. Verapamil and diltiazem are prescribed primarily for their antianginal (see Chapter 26) and antiarrhythmic effects. Nifedipine, which has a relatively greater effect on vascular smooth muscle, is a major antihypertensive drug (see Chapter 28). In each case, the drugs are selective for potential-dependent Ca^{++} channels rather than receptor-operated channels. The potential-dependent Ca^{++} channels are of at least three types: L, N, and T. These channels are distinguished by their electrical properties and anatomic location. The L (long-lasting) channels are selectively inhibited by these drugs. The fact that they are the predominant Ca^{++} channels in the heart and vascular smooth muscle is consistent with the major effects of Ca^{++}-channel blockers on these organs.[3] The N (neuronal) and T (transient) channels are not affected by these channel blockers to a major degree, although the T-type channels play a role in phase 2 of action potentials in the heart (see Figure 24-4).

By interfering with the slow inward current in pacemaker cells, these drugs depress the rate of phase 4 depolarization; thus automaticity in the SA node and the AV node is decreased. The major direct cardiac effect, however, is to reduce conduction velocity and to increase the refractory period of the AV node (see Figure 24-9).[25] Verapamil and diltiazem are useful in treating supraventricular arrhythmias and have been used with success in terminating attacks of paroxysmal atrial tachycardia not responsive to vagal stimulation. Verapamil and diltiazem both have a negative inotropic effect. This effect is less often seen with nifedipine because it is a more potent peripheral vasodilator, and reflex cardiac effects tend to overcome its direct actions. Other aspects of the pharmacologic features of the Ca^{++}-channel blockers are discussed in Chapters 26 and 28.

Adenosine

The endogenous purine nucleoside adenosine is approved for terminating attacks of paroxysmal supraventricular tachycardia. It does not match the profile of any other antiarrhythmic. The structure of adenosine is shown in Figure 24-18.

Pharmacologic effects

Adenosine stimulates the A_1 adenosine receptor in the heart. This receptor is linked to the G protein G_i, which, when activated, increases K^{+} conductance and decreases Ca^{++}-channel activity, leading to hyperpolarization.[25] Adenosine also may reduce the release of norepinephrine from nerve endings. The net effect on the heart is to reduce automaticity in the SA node and Purkinje fibers as well as reduce the AV nodal conduction rate (see Figure 24-9 and Table 24-2). The drug is useful for short-term treatment of supraventricular tachycardia involving reentry with rapid ventricular rate.[29] Adenosine also dilates coronary vessels and reduces contractility.

Adverse effects

Adenosine must be injected intravenously as a bolus because of its extremely short plasma half-life. Adenosine is rapidly transported into tissues, followed by incorporation into purine biosynthetic pathways. A high number of patients have transient flushing and dyspnea with the drug. Arrhythmias, including heart block and even cardiac arrest, may also occur immediately after injection. However, because of the drug's rapid uptake, therapeutic as well as adverse responses are normally short lived.

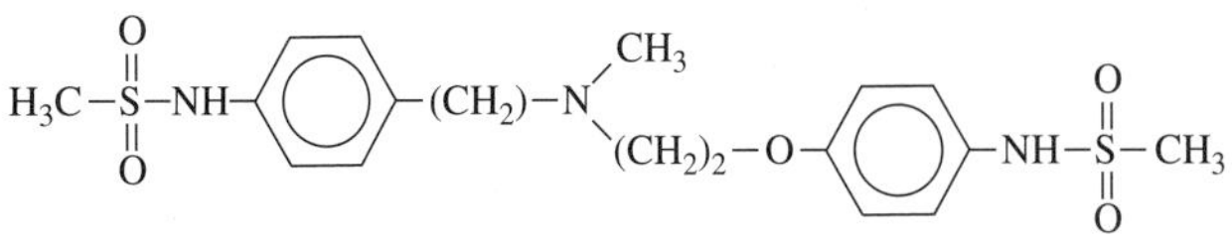

Fig. 24-18 Structural formula of adenosine.

Digitalis

The digitalis glycosides are used in treating certain supraventricular arrhythmias. This use is discussed in Chapter 25.

Indications for Antiarrhythmic Drugs

Table 24-4 reflects the general usefulness of the various agents discussed in this chapter in treating some of the most commonly encountered arrhythmias. It is not intended to be a comprehensive listing of applications of these drugs. Drugs administered orally are largely used to prevent the recurrence of arrhythmias, whereas drugs administered parenterally are usually given to treat acute disorders.[5,12]

Drug Interactions

Antiarrhythmic drugs can participate in a wide variety of drug interactions. Because the margin of safety with these drugs as a group is narrow, clinically significant interactions may develop whenever the activity or plasma concentration of an antiarrhythmic agent is changed. The following discussion is intended to provide an illustrative but not exhaustive list of interactions involving these drugs.

Quinidine may interact with the following drugs to yield the indicated result: with other class I antiarrhythmics and with phenothiazines, additive cardiac effects (quinidine also increases the plasma concentrations of flecainide and propafenone); with digoxin and other digitalis glycosides, increased plasma concentrations of the cardiac glycoside; with rifampin and other hepatic enzyme inducers, decreased plasma quinidine concentrations; with cimetidine and other hepatic enzyme inhibitors, increased quinidine concentrations; with oral anticoagulants, increased likelihood of hemorrhage; with neuromuscular blocking drugs, increased neuromuscular blockade; with systemic antacids that raise urinary pH, reduced urinary excretion of quinidine; and with vasodilators (e.g., nitroglycerin), hypotension. Many of these interactions result from the ability of quinidine to inhibit the activity of CYP2D6.

Quinidine, procainamide, and disopyramide all have antimuscarinic (or antivagal) properties and therefore have additive effects with other antimuscarinic drugs. Drugs that slow AV conduction, such as the β-adrenergic–blocking drugs and amiodarone, can exaggerate the AV conduction effects of drugs with similar actions, possibly leading to bradycardia and heart block. Drugs that have negative inotropic effects (e.g., class IA drugs, the Ca^{++}-channel blockers, and the β blockers) may precipitate heart failure, especially in the presence of other negative inotropic agents. Propranolol and related drugs prevent the tachycardia that normally results from hypoglycemic drugs.

The metabolism of flecainide and propafenone is catalyzed by CYP2D6 in the liver. Drugs that share this same pathway of metabolism will increase each other's elimination half-life.[22] Thus cimetidine and erythromycin can increase the plasma concentrations of flecainide and propafenone. Propranolol and cimetidine reduce lidocaine clearance, whereas induction of hepatic microsomal enzymes by phenobarbital increases it.

Amiodarone increases the effect of warfarin, as well as the concentrations of quinidine, procainamide, and flecainide. There may be more than one mechanism accounting for these interactions. In addition to its effects on metabolism, amiodarone may reduce renal clearance of these drugs by inhibiting the transport function of P-glycoprotein in the kidney.[22] Verapamil, propafenone, amiodarone, and flecainide (as well as quinidine) have been reported to increase plasma digoxin concentrations.[5] These interactions may also involve the P-glycoprotein.

Table • 24-4

Some Indications for Representative Antiarrhythmic Drugs

DRUG	INDICATIONS*
Adenosine	PSVT
Amiodarone	VF, MVT, PVTNQ, AF/F, PAC, PSVT
β-Blockers	PVTNQ, PSVT, AF/F
Bretylium	VF
Dofetilide	AF/F
Flecainide	PAF (prevention), PSVT, VA (prevention of life threatening)
Ibutilide	AF/F
Lidocaine	Acute VA, DVA, PVTNQ
Magnesium salts	PVTLQ
Procainamide	PVTNQ, VA (life threatening)
Propafenone	VT (sustained and life threatening), AF/F
Quinidine	PSVT, AF/F, PAC, PVC
Verapamil	AF/F, PSVT (prevention)

*The suitability of drug versus nondrug therapy for these indications often depends on circumstances. For instance, drug therapy is usually more effective in treating atrial fibrillation of recent origin than if it is long-standing. Moreover, maintenance therapy for atrial fibrillation often differs from strategies for converting atrial fibrillation to normal sinus rhythm.
AF/F, Atrial flutter/fibrillation; *DVA,* digitalis-induced ventricular arrhythmias; *MVT,* monomorphic ventricular tachycardia; *PAC,* premature atrial contractions; *PAF,* paroxysmal atrial fibrillation/flutter; *PVTLQ,* polymorphic ventricular tachycardia with long QT interval; *PSVT,* paroxysmal supraventricular tachycardia; *PVC,* premature ventricular contractions; *PVTNQ,* polymorphic ventricular tachycardia with normal QT interval; *VA,* ventricular arrhythmias; *VF,* ventricular fibrillation; *VT,* ventricular tachycardia.

IMPLICATIONS FOR DENTISTRY

Patients who are being treated on a long-term basis with antiarrhythmic drugs, if under adequate control, are usually not a management problem for the dentist. Because some antiarrhythmic agents may depress cardiovascular function, the potential for an increased incidence of orthostatic hypotension and hypotensive syncope exists. There is also a greater probability that arrhythmias will develop in a patient with a previous history of arrhythmias who is undergoing stressful treatment. The dentist may wish to consult with the patient's cardiologist regarding the use of epinephrine or other adrenergic vasoconstrictors in patients with a significant arrhythmia history.

As described in Chapter 7, the combination of epinephrine and propranolol may lead to hypertensive reactions. Quinidine, disopyramide, and procainamide, because of their antimuscarinic (or antivagal) activity, interact additively with antimuscarinic antisialagogues. This combination can result in enhancement of antimuscarinic side effects. Quinidine blockade of dealkylation reactions by CYP2D6 may limit the effectiveness of certain oral opioid analgesics, especially codeine, that are converted in the liver to highly active metabolites (e.g., codeine metabolized to morphine). The additive effect of lidocaine when used as an antiarrhythmic with all local anesthetics is of special importance to the dentist.

The dentist should be aware of those manifestations of adverse drug reactions that occur in the oral cavity. Quinidine, for instance, has, in a small number of cases, been associated with thrombocytopenia. This reaction may well lead to oral hemorrhaging and petechiae. Blockade of β-adrenergic receptors is associated with a change in the profile of salivary proteins. The implications of this effect on oral health have not been fully determined.

Antiarrhythmic Drugs

Nonproprietary (generic) name	*Proprietary (trade) name*
Adenosine	Adenocard
Amiodarone	Cordarone
Bretylium	Bretylol
Diltiazem	Cardizem
Disopyramide	Norpace
Dofetilide	Tikosyn
Esmolol	Brevibloc
Flecainide	Tambocor
Ibutilide	Corvert
Lidocaine	Xylocaine
Magnesium sulfate	—
Mexiletine	Mexitil
Moricizine	Ethmozine
Procainamide	Pronestyl, Procanbid
Propafenone	Rythmol
Propranolol	Inderal
Quinidine*	Cardioquin, Quinaglute, Quinidex Extentabs
Sotalol	Betapace
Tocainide	Tonocard
Verapamil	Calan, Isoptin

*Several different salts are available for oral and parenteral administration.

CITED REFERENCES

1. Bigger JT, Jr: Cardiac electrophysiologic effects of moricizine hydrochloride, *Am J Cardiol* 65:15D-20D, 1990.
2. CAST investigators: Mortality and morbidity in patients receiving encainide, flecainide, or placebo. The cardiac arrhythmia suppression trial, *N Engl J Med* 324:781-788, 1991.
3. Catterall WA, Striessnig J: Receptor sites for Ca^{2+} channel antagonists, *Trends Pharmacol Sci* 13:256-262, 1992.
4. Dreifus LS, de Azevedo IM, Watanabe Y: Electrolyte and antiarrhythmic drug interaction, *Am Heart J* 88:95-107, 1974.
5. Drugs for cardiac arrhythmias, *Med Lett Drugs Ther* 38:75-82, 1996.
6. Drvota V, Blange I, Häggblad J, et al: Desethylamiodarone prolongation of cardiac repolarization is dependent on gene expression: a novel antiarrhythmic mechanism, *J Cardiovasc Pharmacol* 32:654-661, 1998.
7. Foster RH, Wilde MI, Markham A: Ibutilide: a review of its pharmacological properties and clinical potential in the acute management of atrial flutter and fibrillation, *Drugs* 54:312-330, 1997.
8. Frey W: Weitere Erfahrungen mit Chinidin bei absoluter Herzenregelmassigkeit, *Wein Klin Wochenschr* 55:849-853, 1918.
9. Frumin H, Behrens S, Martyn R, et al: Hemodynamic effects of antiarrhythmic drugs, *J Clin Pharmacol* 31:1070-1080, 1991.
10. Grace AA, Camm AJ: Quinidine, *N Engl J Med* 338:35-45, 1998.
11. Grant AO: Mechanisms of atrial fibrillation and action of drugs used in its management, *Am J Cardiol* 82:43N-49N, 1998.
12. Kowey PR, Marinchak RA, Rials SJ, et al: Intravenous antiarrhythmic therapy in the acute control of in-hospital destabilizing ventricular tachycardia and fibrillation, *Am J Cardiol* 84:46R-51R, 1999.
13. Lee KS, Lee EW: Ionic mechanism of ibutilide in human atrium: evidence for a drug-induced Na^+ current through a nifedipine inhibited inward channel, *J Pharmacol Exp Ther* 286:9-22, 1998.
14. Levine JH, Massumi A, Scheinman MM, et al: Intravenous amiodarone for recurrent sustained hypotensive ventricular tachyarrhythmias. Intravenous Amiodarone Multicenter Trial Group, *J Am Coll Cardiol* 27:67-75, 1996.
15. Lynch JJ, Jr, Sanguinetti MC, Kimura S, et al: Therapeutic potential of modulating potassium currents in the diseased myocardium, *FASEB J* 6:2952-2960, 1992.
16. Mason JW: A comparison of seven antiarrhythmic drugs in patients with ventricular tachyarrhythmias, *N Engl J Med* 329:452-458, 1993.
17. Mautz FR: Reduction of cardiac irritability by the epicardial and systemic administration of drugs as a protection in cardiac surgery, *J Thorac Surg* 5:612-628, 1936.
18. McClellan KJ, Markam A: Dofetilide: a review of its use in atrial fibrillation and atrial flutter, *Drugs* 58:1043-1059, 1999.
19. Nattel S, Singh BN: Evolution, mechanisms and classification of antiarrhythmic drugs: focus on class III actions, *Am J Cardiol* 84:11R-19R, 1999.
20. Pitsiavas V, Smerdely P, Boyages SC: Amiodarone compared with iodine exhibits a potent and persistent inhibitory effect on TSH-stimulated cAMP production in vitro: a possible mechanism to explain amiodarone-induced hypothyroidism, *Eur J Endocrinol* 140:241-249, 1999.
21. Podrid PJ: Amiodarone: reevaluation of an old drug, *Ann Intern Med* 122:689-700, 1995.
22. Roden DM: Mechanisms underlying variability in response to drug therapy: implications for amiodarone use, *Am J Cardiol* 84:29R-36R, 1999.
23. Roden DM, George AL, Jr: The cardiac ion channels: relevance to management of arrhythmias, *Annu Rev Med* 47:135-148, 1996.
24. Singh BN, Kehoe R, Woosley RL, et al: Multicenter trial of sotalol compared with procainamide in the suppression of inducible ventricular tachycardia: a double-blind, randomized parallel evaluation. Sotalol Multicenter Study Group, *Am Heart J* 129:87-97, 1995.
25. Task Force of the Working Group on Arrhythmias of the European Society of Cardiology. The Sicilian gambit. A new approach to the classification of antiarrhythmic drugs based on their actions on arrhythmogenic mechanisms, *Circulation* 84:1831-1851, 1991.

26. Vaughan EM, Williams DM: Classification of antidysrhythmic drugs, *Pharmacol Ther B* 1:115-138, 1975.

27. Wang Z, Fermini B, Nattel S: Effects of flecainide, quinidine, and 4-aminopyridine on transient outward and ultrarapid delayed rectifier currents in human atrial myocytes, *J Pharmacol Exp Ther* 272:184-196, 1995.

28. Wenckebach KF: *Die Unregelmassige Herzt atigkeit und Ihre Klinische Bedeutung,* Leipzig, Germany, 1914, W Engelmann.

29. Wilbur SL, Marchlinski FE: Adenosine as an antiarrhythmic drug, *Am J Cardiol* 79:30-37, 1997.

30. Woosley RL: Antiarrhythmic drugs, *Annu Rev Pharmacol Toxicol* 31:427-455, 1991.

31. Wright JT, Jr: Practical pharmacokinetics of ventricular antiarrhythmic therapy, *Am Heart J* 123:1148-1152, 1992.

General References

Fozzard HA, Arnsdorf MF: Cardiac electrophysiology. In Fozzard HA, Haber E, Jennings RB, eds: *The heart and cardiovascular system: scientific foundations,* ed 2, New York, 1991, Raven Press.

Nattel S: Newer developments in the management of atrial fibrillation, *Am Heart J* 130:1094-1106, 1995.

Singh BN: Current antiarrhythmic drugs: an overview of mechanisms of action and potential clinical utility, *J Cardiovasc Electrophysiol* 10:283-301, 1999.

Spooner PM, Rosen MR, eds: *Foundations of cardiac arrhythmias. Basic concepts and clinical applications in fundamental and clinical cardiology series,* vol 41, New York, 2000, Marcel Dekker.

Woosley RL, Singh SN, eds: *Arrhythmia treatment and therapy. Evaluation of clinical trial evidence,* New York, 2000, Marcel Dekker.

CHAPTER • 25

Cardiac Glycosides and Other Drugs Used in Heart Failure

Frank J. Dowd

Drugs that are currently used in the treatment of heart failure include the diuretics, peripheral vasodilators, angiotensin-converting enzyme (ACE) inhibitors, angiotensin II receptor blockers, and drugs with positive inotropic effects: cardiac glycosides, phosphodiesterase III inhibitors, and catecholamines. Spironolactone is a drug whose mechanism of action includes effects both on cardiac load and cardiac contractility. β-Adrenergic receptor blockers are also used. Drug selection must be made on the basis of many criteria to optimally meet the needs of the patient.

CARDIAC MUSCLE CONTRACTION AND HEART FAILURE

In addition to its role in the action potential, Ca^{++} is intimately involved in the contractile process. Tropomyosin and troponin, which are associated with actin, regulate the interaction between actin and myosin. Troponin consists of three subunits; the binding of Ca^{++} to one of these (troponin C) initiates a series of conformational changes in troponin and tropomyosin that alter the interaction of tropomyosin and troponin I with actin, favoring the coupling of actin with myosin.[34] Adenosine triphosphate (ATP) is hydrolyzed by a myosin-bound adenosine triphosphatase (ATPase) when the actomyosin complex is formed, and chemical energy is then converted into mechanical work.

The contraction of cardiac muscle is initiated by extracellular Ca^{++} entering the cell with the slow inward current. However, the immediate source of contractile Ca^{++} in the heart comes largely from intracellular stores. Ca^{++} entering the cell during an action potential must first traverse the plasma membrane through voltage-sensitive Ca^{++} channels. This influx of Ca^{++} during the slow inward current triggers the release of much larger amounts of intracellular Ca^{++} from the sarcoplasmic reticulum (SR). The sudden rise in cytoplasmic Ca^{++} then stimulates contraction, and the cycle is completed by the active reuptake of Ca^{++} by the SR (and mitochondria) and extrusion from the cell by Na^+-Ca^{++} exchange.

Drugs such as the β-adrenergic receptor agonists increase cardiac contractility by increasing intracellular cyclic 3′,5′-adenosine monophosphate (cAMP), which enhances Ca^{++} influx and accelerates uptake of Ca^{++} by the SR, ultimately making more Ca^{++} available for contraction.[11] The latter effect results from the phosphorylation of phospholamban, a protein associated with the Ca^{++} pump of the SR. The effect of Ca^{++} on troponin may also be enhanced by cAMP.

In heart failure, the heart is unable to maintain the requisite cardiac output. The mechanics underlying this failure are as yet poorly understood. The ability of the SR to participate in the trafficking of Ca^{++} appears to be hindered. Moreover, the Na^+-Ca^{++} exchange sites (Figure 25-1) appear to be increased in heart failure, leading to a decrease in intracellular Ca^{++}.[10] However, there are likely to be multiple biochemical defects in heart failure.

The consequences of heart failure are many. Venous distention occurs because blood is pooled as a result of decreased cardiac output. This is sometimes referred to as *backward failure*. Forward failure entails the decreased perfusion of end organs such as the kidney. Figure 25-2 shows some important adaptive mechanisms that result from heart failure. These changes, including an increase in sympathetic discharge, can compensate for the heart failure. If these and other responses are not sufficient, however, the heart failure becomes uncompensated. Adaptive mechanisms also include an increase in production of angiotensin II, leading to remodeling of the heart over time.[6] Remodeling results in cardiac hypertrophy and several cellular changes, which although they tend to compensate for heart failure, may actually hasten the course of the disease. This cardiac remodeling in heart failure has a parallel in hypertension in which vascular smooth muscle slowly undergoes hypertrophy and hyperplasia.

The pharmacologic features of the ACE inhibitors and other vasodilators, as well as the diuretics, β blockers, and catecholamines, are reviewed elsewhere in this book. They are mentioned in this chapter only in relation to the treatment of heart failure. The cardiac glycosides are not extensively discussed elsewhere in the text. Therefore the cardiac glycosides are discussed more fully than other drugs used for heart failure, although their clinical use has declined because of the increasing reliance on newer drugs.

DRUGS USED IN THE TREATMENT OF HEART FAILURE

Table 25-1 lists the drugs used to treat heart failure and their mechanisms of action. Of the drugs used in long-term therapy, thiazide and loop diuretics, ACE inhibitors, and spironolactone are the most common. The drugs are often used in combination. Heart failure can be classified as *diastolic* or *systolic* failure. In diastolic failure, the heart has inadequate distention and therefore inadequate filling capabilities. Contraction as measured by the ejection function may be normal. This type of heart failure is often seen in patients with hypertension. Systolic heart failure is a deficiency in contractility with a low ejection fraction.[7] Figure 25-3 indicates the drugs used in each type of heart failure.[1]

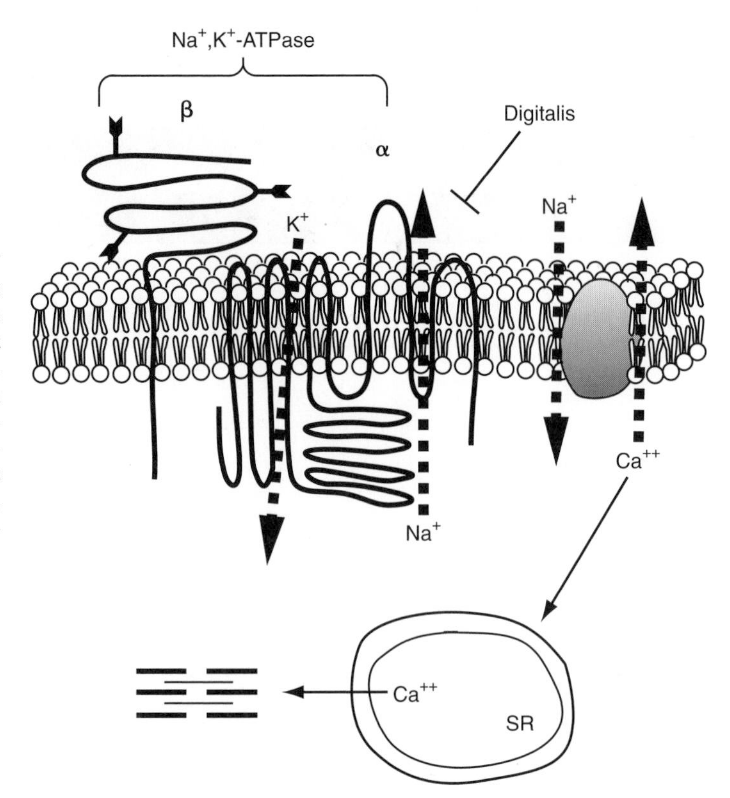

Fig. 25-1 The role of Na^+,K^+-ATPase and the Na^+-Ca^{++} exchange in cardiac contractility and the mechanism of the positive inotropic action of digitalis. Digitalis binds to the extracellular face and transmembrane region of the α subunit of Na^+,K^+-ATPase, thereby inhibiting Na^+ efflux and K^+ influx. The β subunit of Na^+,K^+-ATPase is also shown. The increase in intracellular Na^+ results in reduced binding of Ca^{++} to the Na^+-Ca^{++} exchange system and reduced Ca^{++} efflux. The concentration of intracellular Ca^{++} is increased, hence more Ca^{++} is made available to intracellular storage sites, notably the SR. This leads to enhanced Ca^{++} release to the contractile apparatus and a greater force of contraction.

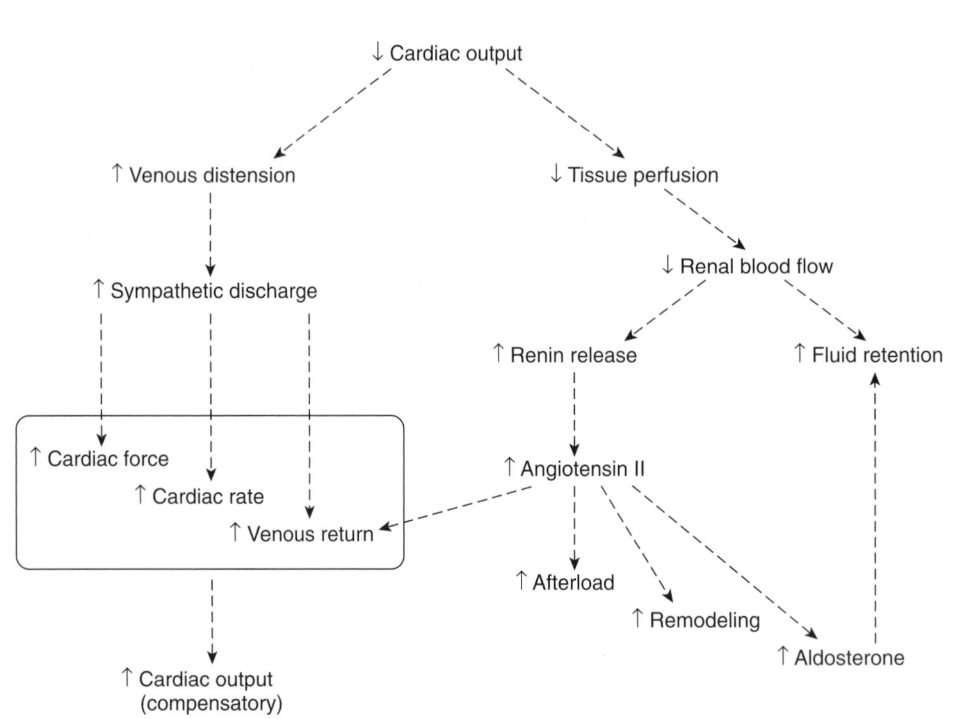

Fig. 25-2 Adaptive mechanisms in heart failure. A decrease in cardiac output leads to a cascade of events that result in a compensatory increase in cardiac output *(box)*. In addition, activation of the renin-angiotensin system leads to changes that put further burden on the failing heart as well as long-term remodeling of the cardiovascular system.

Table • 25-1

Treatment of Heart Failure

DRUG OR DRUG CLASS	MECHANISM(S)
Long-Term Treatment*	
Thiazide and loop diuretics	Reduce fluid volume (reduce preload and afterload)
ACE inhibitors	Reduce effect of angiotensin II, prevent remodeling
Angiotensin II receptor blockers	Reduce effect of angiotensin II, prevent remodeling
Spironolactone	Inhibit effect of aldosterone
Digitalis	Direct cardiotonic effect
β blockers†	Reduce sympathetic effect, prevent remodeling, prevent arrhythmias
Vasodilators‡	Reduce afterload and preload
Short-Term Treatment§	
Dobutamine	Direct cardiotonic effect
Dopamine	Direct cardiotonic effect
Phosphodiesterase III inhibitors	Reduce preload and afterload; direct cardiotonic effect
Nesiritide	Reduce preload and afterload

*Drugs used for long-term therapy are often used together.
†Carvedilol is a β blocker that also blocks α_1 adrenoceptors.
‡*Vasodilators* refer to sodium nitroprusside, hydralazine, Ca^{++}-channel blockers, and α_1-adrenoceptor blockers.
§Usually only for a few days.

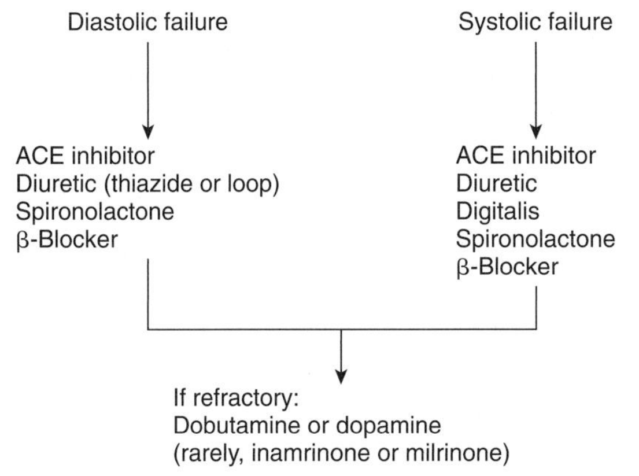

Fig. 25-3 Heart failure and choice of drug. The choice of digitalis depends on the presence of systolic failure, especially if it occurs with atrial fibrillation. Dobutamine, dopamine, inamrinone, and milrinone are reserved for short-term therapy in refractory cases.

CARDIAC GLYCOSIDES

Cardiac glycosides, most notably digitalis, have been used for centuries to treat a number of ailments. The history of their use is marked by an awareness of their therapeutic efficacy as well as their toxic potential. These drugs are currently indicated for the treatment of congestive heart failure and the management of atrial flutter and fibrillation.

Ancient Egyptians first used cardiotonic components from the sea onion, or squill. The Romans subsequently used these drugs as diuretics and heart tonics. Dried toad skin, which contains substances with cardiotonic activity, was used by the Chinese for dropsy and related illnesses. In Africa, the cardiac glycoside ouabain, from *Strophanthus gratus*, was placed on arrows as a poison.

In 1542, Fuchs gave the name *digitalis* to the foxglove plant, which was used for a variety of medicinal purposes. The first detailed scientific study of digitalis on record was made by Sir William Withering[41] of Shropshire, England, in 1785. In his treatise, "An Account of the Foxglove, and Some of Its Medical Uses; With Practical Remarks on Dropsy, and Other Diseases," Withering detailed clinical uses for the leaf of the *Digitalis purpurea* (purple foxglove) plant and described its effects on the heart. His recognition of the potential usefulness of digitalis plant derivatives was occasioned by their extensive use in local folk medicines. Withering ascribed the beneficial effects of digitalis in treating dropsy to a direct diuretic effect, even though he was aware of beneficial effects on the heart as well. He also detailed many toxic effects of the plant.

The history of the use of digitalis since Withering's time has been characterized by a realization of its potential therapeutic benefits on the one hand and its low margin of safety on the other. Advances in digitalis research and clinical use up to the present day have contributed greatly to our knowledge of this drug class.

Chemistry and Classification

The term *digitalis* is often used interchangeably with the term *cardiac glycoside.* Both refer to many compounds, naturally occurring or semisynthetic, that have similar cardiotonic effects. Only one such compound, digoxin, is commonly used clinically in the United States today. Another agent, digitoxin, remains available in Canada and elsewhere and a third compound, of experimental importance, is ouabain. In addition, other plant sources and at least one animal source (certain toads, e.g., *Bufo marinus*) have cardioactive components similar in structure and activity to digitalis. These are mainly of historic and toxicologic interest, although drugs from some of these sources are used in countries other than the United States.

The structure of digoxin is shown in Figure 25-4. The molecule is composed of a steroid ring structure (cyclopentanoperhydrophenanthrene) that in two dimensions resembles the adrenal or nonestrogenic sex steroids. The three-dimensional structure is quite different from these hormones, however, in that the relationship of the C and D rings in cardiac glycosides is in the *cis* rather than the *trans* configuration, as is the case for the steroid hormones. Other distinguishing molecular characteristics include an α,β-unsaturated lactone ring, usually five-membered, at carbon 17 (C_{17}), a hydroxyl group at C_{14}, and a carbohydrate moiety in glycosidic linkage at C_3. The presence of a sugar in glycosidic linkage accounts for the name *glycoside*. These sugars are usually deoxysugars.

Sugar substituents at C_3 can be removed by acid hydrolysis. The products of these reactions are carbohydrates and the appropriate steroids with attached lactone. A steroid plus lactone lacking the sugar group is generically called a *genin* or *aglycone*. Thus the genin of digoxin is digoxigenin.

Mechanism of Action

Digitalis has a direct inotropic effect on the heart; it directly increases the force of contraction. The inotropic action of digitalis does not depend on release of endogenous catecholamines because a reserpinized heart will respond to digitalis. Rather, digitalis has a direct action on heart cells. Cardiac glycosides are known to be specific inhibitors of the Na^+-K^+ pump, specifically Na^+,K^+ activated ATPase (Na^+,K^+-ATPase), which is the enzymatic equivalent of the Na^+-K^+ pump.[32] The active coupled transport of Na^+ and K^+ is the only process of the cell known to be directly affected by low concentrations of cardiac glycosides. The enzyme is located in plasma membranes, and both in vivo and in vitro studies strongly suggest that the site of action of digitalis is the sarcolemmal Na^+,K^+-ATPase.[21,33] It has been estimated that at inotropic concentrations of cardiac glycosides, Na^+,K^+-ATPase is inhibited by 20% to 40%. Na^+,K^+-ATPase is composed of two major subunits. The α subunit has a molecular weight of approximately 100,000 d and contains the digitalis-binding site and the catalytic site for ATP hydrolysis.[24] The β subunit is a glycoprotein and has a molecular weight of approximately 50,000. Its role is less clearly defined; however, it may regulate the assembly and transport of the Na^+-K^+ pump to the plasma membrane. Na^+,K^+-ATPase usually exists in the membrane as a tetramer ($\alpha_2\ \beta_2$). Evidence exists supporting a postulated "γ" subunit, especially in tissues such as the kidney. It is a low molecular weight peptide (approximately 12,000 d) and may play a role in pump regulation.

Inhibition of Na^+,K^+-ATPase leads to a small but significant increase in intracellular Na^+ near the plasma membrane. This increase in Na^+, amounting to approximately 2 mmol/L, reduces the rate of Na^+-Ca^{++} exchange (three Na^+ exchanged into the cell for one Ca^{++} transported out of the cell) because the increase in Na^+ reduces the net binding of Ca^{++} to its binding sites on the exchange system.[14] This alteration results in a reduced efflux of Ca^{++} and an increase in Ca^{++} available to the contractile apparatus.[17,33,42] In addition, the increase in Ca^{++} stimulates the release of additional Ca^{++} from the SR, further stimulating contraction. Digitalis may also increase the influx of Ca^{++} through other channels.[31] The added intracellular Ca^{++} increases the amount of Ca^{++} taken up into the SR during diastole. Therefore after several contractions the amount of Ca^{++} released from the SR is also increased. The positive inotropic effect results from the increased Ca^{++} available for contraction during the systolic phase. The inhibition of Na^+,K^+-ATPase resulting in increased intracellular Na^+ and a reduced diastolic membrane potential has important implications for other ion movements and electrical properties of heart cells. Some of these are indicated below. The relationship between Na^+,K^+-ATPase inhibition by digitalis, and its inotropic effect is shown in Figure 25-1.

The α subunit of Na^+,K^+-ATPase exists in at least four isoforms, whereas three isoforms for the β subunit have been described. Differences in α-subunit isoforms among species and tissues could explain the variable degree of effects of digitalis observed on Na^+,K^+-ATPase in various studies, including the lack of sensitivity of certain rodents to cardiac glycosides.[19] Furthermore, it is possible in human beings that alteration in α isoforms resulting from functional changes in the heart could explain changes in sensitivity to digitalis over time.

Pharmacologic Effects

By far, the most important actions of the digitalis glycosides are those exerted on the cardiovascular system. Resulting changes in hemodynamics may then indirectly influence other systems, yielding beneficial or adverse responses. Some therapeutic effects may be exerted through the nervous system. However, direct actions on the central nervous system (CNS), gastrointestinal tract, and the cardiovascular system also contribute to the toxic profile of digitalis.

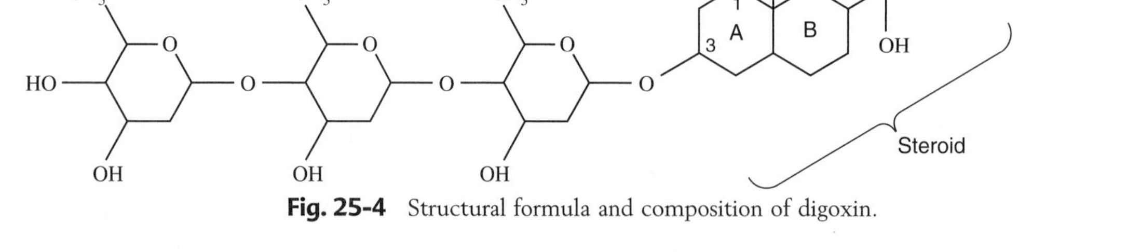

Fig. 25-4 Structural formula and composition of digoxin.

Cardiac effects

Digitalis preparations have two powerful influences on the heart: they increase myocardial contractility and alter electrical activity throughout the heart. A complex interplay of direct actions and autonomically mediated changes contributes to effects clinically observed.

Contractility The experiments of Cattell and Gold[4] clearly showed that cardiac glycosides have direct effects on the isolated heart. In isolated heart preparations, the drugs increase the force of contraction of the myocardium (positive inotropic effect). Maximum tension developed and rate of tension development are both increased, whereas time from onset of contraction to peak contraction is decreased. The duration of the contractile process during systole is abbreviated because of an increase in the rate at which tension is developed. These effects, demonstrated on the cat papillary muscle, are shown in Figure 25-5. The overall cardiodynamic effect of cardiac glycosides on the isolated heart therefore can be summarized as an increased force of contraction caused by an increased rate of force development by the myocardium, resulting in a systolic phase of shorter duration but greater effectiveness.[4,36]

In vivo, many factors complicate the effects of cardiac glycosides on contractility. In the normal intact person, cardiac glycosides directly increase the force of contraction of the heart, but this effect is more than negated by compensatory autonomic reflexes. Cardiac glycosides, in addition to their cardiac effects, constrict peripheral blood vessels by a direct action on vascular smooth muscle. The outcome of such vasoconstriction and the resultant increase in blood pressure is a reduction in myocardial contractile force and cardiac output because of reflex mechanisms.[2] The net effect in normal persons is that reflex mechanisms cancel out the positive effects of digitalis on heart contractility. Furthermore, sarcomere shortening with digitalis in the normal heart somewhat offsets the increased contractility in vivo.

In patients with failing hearts, a different situation prevails. Vasoconstriction, a physiologic sympathetic response to reduced cardiac output, is already significant in peripheral vessels, and digitalis has little additive effect on vascular tone unless administered intravenously. The renin-angiotensin-aldosterone system is also highly activated in heart failure, and antidiuretic hormone is elevated. Therefore in these compromised patients, compensatory mechanisms do not cancel out the cardiac effects of digitalis. Cardiac glycosides increase cardiac output, thus reducing the need for high sympathetic tone in the blood vessels. Sympathetic tone is consequently decreased in the vasculature when these patients receive digitalis, and vasodilation may even result. Furthermore, digitalis enhances baroreceptor sensitivity and thereby corrects an impaired baroreceptor response in patients with heart failure. The net result is to reduce sympathetic activity. The effect of digitalis in vivo therefore depends on the state of the cardiovascular system at the time of administration.

According to Starling's law of the heart, cardiac output, or, more precisely, the ventricular stroke volume, increases as ventricular filling pressure increases. Stated simply, the heart pumps whatever is supplied to it by way of venous return, maintaining a near-optimal heart size. As ventricular end-diastolic pressure increases, ventricular stroke work and stroke volume increase. Normal heart function is within well-defined limits and is described by a single curve (Figure 25-6).

When cardiac contractility is reduced in heart failure, three mechanisms are available by which the heart can compensate for the defect: (1) an increase in ventricular end-diastolic pressure, which enhances cardiac output (Frank-Starling preload mechanism); (2) an increase in number of contractile units (hypertrophy); and (3) use of chronotropic and inotropic reserves of the heart through reflex mechanisms (sympathetic activity). If these mechanisms are sufficient to produce normal cardiac output, the heart failure is said to be *compensated*. In this condition, a new ventricular function curve is generated (see Figure 25-6). For any given ventricular end-diastolic pressure, however, ventricular stroke work, stroke volume, and cardiac output are lower in the failing heart than in the normal heart. Consequently, the heart enlarges to maintain cardiac output, and heart rate increases to help compensate for poor cardiac function.

If the ventricular end-diastolic pressure becomes too elevated (i.e., the heart is working to the far right along the Frank-Starling curve), venous pressures upstream also rise

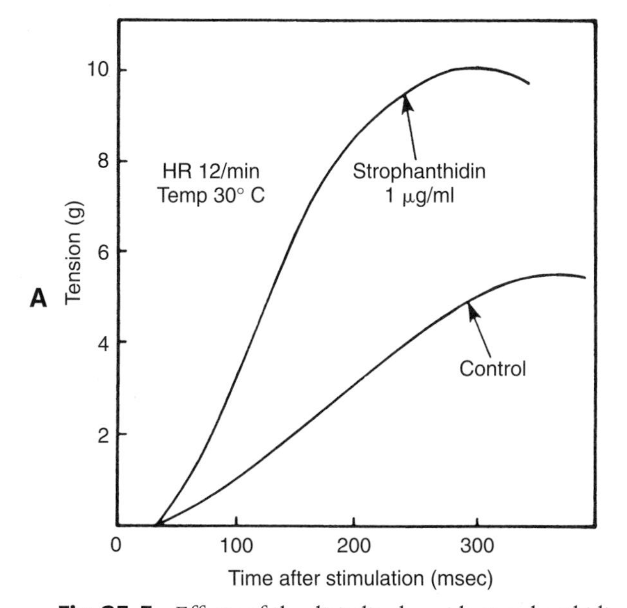

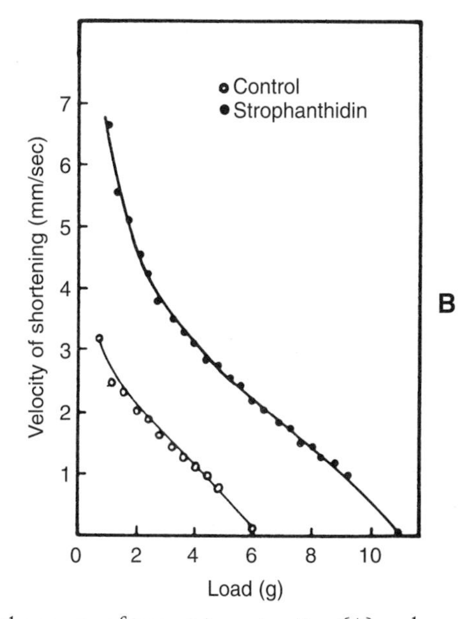

Fig. 25-5 Effects of the digitalis glycoside strophanthidin on the course of isometric contraction **(A)** and the force-velocity relation **(B)** of the cat papillary muscle. (Adapted from Sonnenblick EH, Williams JF, Jr, Glick G, et al: Studies on digitalis. XV. Effects of cardiac glycosides on myocardial force-velocity relations in the nonfailing human heart, *Circulation* 34:532-539, 1966.)

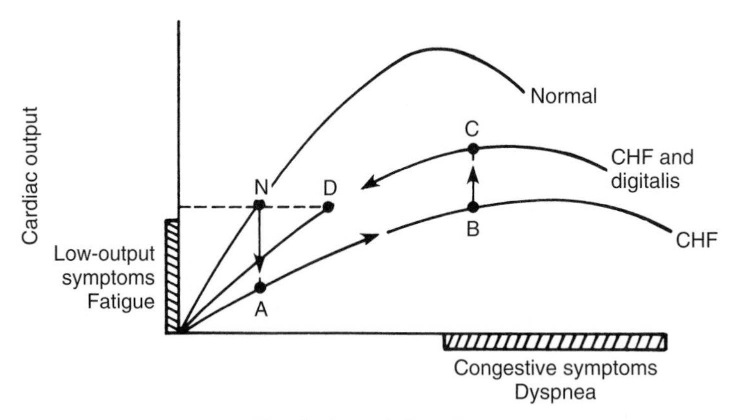

Fig. 25-6 Operation of the Frank-Starling mechanism in the preload compensation for heart failure. The three *curves* represent ventricular function curves in the normal state, in congestive heart failure *(CHF)*, and in heart failure after treatment with digitalis. Points *N* through *D* indicate, in sequence, normal cardiac status *(N)*, depression of contractility with decompensated heart failure *(A)*, Frank-Starling compensation *(B)*, increase in contractility with digitalis *(C)*, and reduction in use of Frank-Starling preload compensation that digitalis allows *(D)*. Points *N, D,* and *B* indicate the same cardiac output on the *vertical axis,* but each point is at a different end-diastolic pressure on the *horizontal axis.* The excessive end-diastolic pressures causing congestive symptoms and the lowered levels of cardiac performance resulting in low-output symptoms are shown by the *hatched areas.* (From Mason DT: Regulation of cardiac performance in clinical heart disease: interactions between contractile state mechanical abnormalities and ventricular compensatory mechanisms, *Am J Cardiol* 32:437-448, 1973.)

excessively, leading to symptoms of "backward" heart failure. Signs and symptoms include pulmonary congestion and dyspnea (left-sided failure) as well as systemic venous distention and edema (right-sided failure). Moreover, if compensatory mechanisms are unable to maintain cardiac output sufficient for the needs of the peripheral tissues, "forward" heart failure ensues. Adverse effects from impaired tissue perfusion include weakness, lassitude, and acute renal failure. In chronic heart failure, aspects of both backward and forward failure interact to produce clinical manifestations. Thus salt and water retention caused by forward failure contributes to the venous hypertension and edema associated with backward failure. Conversely, impaired gas exchange in the congested lungs augments muscle weakness and fatigue associated with reduced cardiac output and delivery of oxygen to skeletal muscle.

In both compensated and decompensated heart failure, digitalis can improve cardiac function so that a greater cardiac output can be achieved without as much reliance on compensatory mechanisms. Figure 25-6 shows that a new ventricular function curve is generated as a result of digitalis. This curve more closely approximates the normal situation.

Heart failure occurs whenever the workload placed on the heart exceeds the ability of the heart to perform. Heart failure often arises from myocardial infarction or hypertension. Myocardial infarction can lead to heart failure as a result of a reduction in the heart's ability to perform work (pump failure).

An increase in total peripheral vascular resistance, as seen in hypertension or as a reflex reaction in congestive heart failure, can contribute to heart failure because of increased outflow resistance on cardiac contraction. The first reaction of the heart to an increase in outflow resistance is often enlargement, resulting in temporary higher efficiency in cardiac function. This is followed, however, by progressive signs of cardiac failure characterized by decreased stroke volume and stroke work, as indicated above. To reduce preload and afterload is an important strategy in treating heart failure associated with increased peripheral vascular resistance.

Cardiac size and rate of contraction Congestive heart failure is accompanied by an increase in heart size. As the heart begins to fail, it is unable to eject as much blood per stroke as the normal heart, and the size of the heart increases, compensating for the loss of contractility. The right or left side of the heart, or both, may be affected.

Digitalis, by increasing the force of contraction, reduces the size of the heart. Digitalis enables the heart to pump with greater force at any given filling pressure. This increased force leads, in turn, to a reduction in both diastolic pressure and cardiac distention.[21]

The reduction in heart size accounts for a greater efficiency of the heart. It can be shown, for instance, that cardiac glycosides can reduce the ratio of oxygen consumption to contractile force in cardiac muscle. The effect is largely caused by a shortened fiber length of cardiac muscle and decreased diastolic wall tension. (Oxygen consumption is highly dependent on wall tension.) The net result of digitalis on the failing heart, therefore, is to increase contractility without a commensurate increase in oxygen consumption—in other words, to improve efficiency.

In the clinical management of congestive heart failure, the administration of digitalis is most often associated with a reduction in heart rate. This reduction results from both a vagal and a direct effect on the heart by digitalis. The cardiac glycosides stimulate the vagus nerve—probably indirectly by an effect on baroreceptors, afferent nerve pathways, and central vagal nuclei—and at therapeutic doses reduce the sympathetic tone of the heart indirectly by improving cardiac function and sensitizing the baroreceptor mechanism.[12] Both effects account for a reduction in heart rate. The effect of digitalis on heart rate during the treatment of certain cardiac arrhythmias is discussed below.

Electrophysiology The effects of digitalis on the electrical properties of the heart can be divided into at least four interrelated categories: automaticity, refractoriness, excitability, and conduction velocity. Because digitalis has both vagal and nonvagal effects on the heart and because the areas of the heart affected by the vagus include the sinoatrial (SA) node, the atrial myocardium, and the upper portions of the atrioventricular (AV) node, a discussion of discrete regions of the heart is necessary.

SINOATRIAL NODE Therapeutic doses of digitalis cause a reduction in SA node automaticity by slowing diastolic depolarization in the cells of the node. This effect is largely vagal because in the presence of atropine, digitalis may actually increase the automaticity of the SA node.

UNSPECIALIZED ATRIAL MYOCARDIUM The vagal effects of digitalis on the atria are more in evidence than the nonvagal, an important distinction because the vagal and nonvagal effects of digitalis are quite different from each other. Digitalis at therapeutic doses, for instance, shortens the atrial refractory period. This effect results from vagal influences of the drug because the drug prolongs the atrial refractory period when the vagus nerve has been blocked by atropine.

The effect on atrial excitability is variable, but at higher therapeutic and toxic doses digitalis decreases excitability. This decrease in excitability is accompanied by a decrease in conduction velocity.

ATRIOVENTRICULAR NODE One of the most important and characteristic effects of digitalis is its effect on the AV node. Under the influence of digitalis, the duration of the effective refractory period (ERP) is increased and conduction velocity decreased. Mechanistically, as the resting membrane potential is reduced in response to inhibition of the Na^+-K^+ pump, the action potential spike is slowed, leading to delayed AV conduction. This inhibition is a direct, or nonvagal, effect of digitalis. However, both vagal and nonvagal effects of digitalis contribute to the slowing of AV conduction. Generally, vagal effects predominate with therapeutic doses of digitalis. Digitalis therapy can lead to various degrees of heart block because of effects on the AV node.

PURKINJE FIBERS The automaticity of the Purkinje fibers is increased by digitalis. Automaticity can be enhanced by an increase in the rate of phase 4 depolarization (see Chapter 24). This effect is heightened if extracellular K^+ is lowered. Digitalis can also cause ectopic beats by inducing oscillatory afterpotentials (see Chapter 24). These afterpotentials are thought to be caused by fluctuations of intracellular Ca^{++} concentrations resulting in increased ionic conductance of the membranes. If the amplitude of these afterpotentials is sufficiently great, they may lead to an action potential. At lower doses of digitalis, excitability is increased; at higher toxic doses, excitability is reduced. Because of the increase in automaticity and development of afterpotentials at these sites, subsidiary pacemaker activity can lead to arrhythmias, especially in the presence of a slow sinus rhythm or heart block.[33] Conduction velocity is reduced and the duration of the ERP is increased in most cases by digitalis, similar to the effects on the AV node. Unlike the situation in the AV node, high or toxic concentrations of digitalis decrease the duration of the ERP of the Purkinje fibers. The duration of the action potential is likewise shortened, and reentrant arrhythmias are more likely to occur, leading to extrasystoles.

UNSPECIALIZED VENTRICULAR MYOCARDIUM In the ventricle, the duration of the ERP is shortened by digitalis. This is caused by activation of a K^+ current resulting from increases in intracellular Na^+ and Ca^{++}. Conduction velocity changes are dose dependent. At lower doses, digitalis increases conduction velocity, whereas at higher and toxic doses, digitalis decreases conduction velocity. Excitability is reduced by digitalis, but only at high concentrations. Lower concentrations may actually increase excitability. The ventricular myocardium is more resistant to reduction in excitability than are the specialized conductive tissues.

SUMMARY The most important direct effects of digitalis on the electrophysiology of the heart can be summarized as follows (Table 25-2): reduced conduction velocity and increased duration of the ERP in the AV node, increased automaticity of subsidiary pacemaker activity in the conductive tissues of the ventricle, and decreased duration of the ERP of the ventricular myocardium. Cardiac vagal effects of digitalis are limited to effects on the atria, the SA node, and the AV node. They consist of a decrease in the duration of the ERP of the atrial myocardium, a decrease in the automaticity of the SA node, and an increase in the duration of the ERP along with a decrease in the conduction velocity of the AV node.

Electrocardiography Therapeutic and toxic effects of digitalis are associated with changes on the electrocardiogram (ECG) that reflect the electrophysiologic effects listed in Table 25-2. They include alterations in the shape of the T wave, the configuration of the ST segment, the lengths of the QT and PR intervals, AV dissociation, and the presence of extrasystoles (Figure 25-7).

Table • 25-2

Electrophysiologic Effects of Digitalis

SITE	AUTOMATICITY	DURATION OF EFFECTIVE REFRACTORY PERIOD	EXCITABILITY	CONDUCTION VELOCITY
SA node	↓,↑A			
Atrial myocardium		↓,↑A	↑*, ↓T	↑*, ↓T
AV node		⇑		⇓
Purkinje fibers	⇑	↑*, ↓ T	↑*, ↓T	↓
Ventricular myocardium		⇓	↑*, ↓T	↑*, ↓T

*Lower therapeutic doses only.
⇑, ⇓, Most important effects; *A*, after atropine; *T*, at toxic doses; ↑, increased; ↓, decreased.

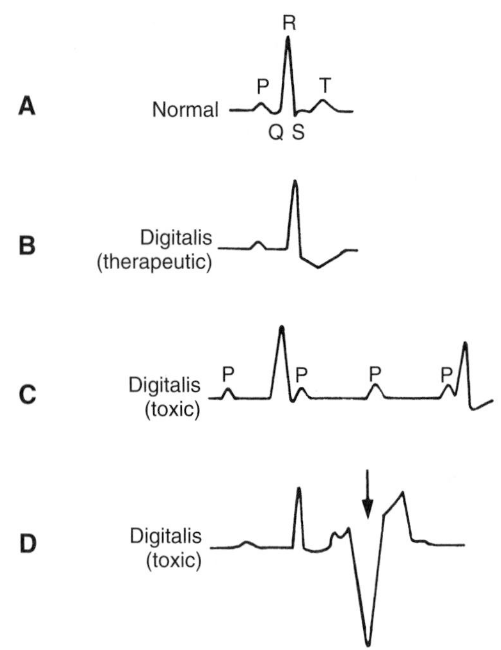

Fig. 25-7 Some effects of digitalis on the ECG (lead II). **A,** Normal ECG. **B,** Typical changes at therapeutic concentrations include depression of the ST segment and lengthening of the PR interval. **C,** Toxic effect of digitalis on AV conduction promotes AV dissociation, such as complete AV block. Notice the lack of relationship between the P waves and QRS complexes. **D,** Toxic effect of digitalis on ventricular impulse generation results in ectopic ventricular beats. An example of an ectopic beat is marked by the *arrow*.

At therapeutic doses, changes often occur in the T wave and the ST segment configuration. The T wave may be inverted or distorted, whereas the ST segment may appear "sunken" (lead II of the ECG). These changes are caused by alterations in the sequence of repolarization of various ventricular myocardial cells. Also at therapeutic doses, the PR interval is lengthened by digitalis as a result of decreased conduction velocity in the AV node. The QT interval, on the other hand, is shortened because of the shortened ventricular action potential.

Although several cardiac effects of digitalis are observed at toxic doses, two effects are typical. The first is heart block caused by excessive reduction in AV nodal conduction; the second is any of several ventricular arrhythmias caused by ectopic pacemaker activity.

Effects on systemic vasculature

Although digitalis is a vasoconstrictor, vasoconstriction by digitalis is usually not observed in patients with congestive heart failure because sympathetic vascular tone is already elevated.[22] In fact, vasodilation often results from digitalis administration because of the improvement in cardiac function.[2] Nevertheless, caution should be used when administering digitalis by the intravenous route because significant vasoconstriction may occur even in the patient with heart failure.

Diuretic effects

Digitalis was at one time thought to act primarily on the kidney because diuresis is such a prominent feature of its use in congestive heart failure. However, the diuretic effect results primarily from improved cardiac function and a direct effect on afferent nerves in the heart that are involved in the central regulation of blood volume. Together, these actions result in reduced peripheral sympathetic tone and increased blood flow to the kidney. Thus glomerular filtration is increased, renin secretion in most cases is lowered, and aldosterone secretion is indirectly inhibited. The retention of Na^+ and water is thereby reduced. Digitalis also promotes fluid mobilization and the lowering of venous pressure, which increases the return of edema fluid to the vascular space and indirectly increases renal excretion.

Some of the diuretic effect of digitalis may result from its direct action on the Na^+-K^+ pump in the kidney, but this is of secondary importance to the diuresis based on improved cardiovascular dynamics and reduced sympathetic activity.

Miscellaneous effects

Cardiac glycosides can cause anorexia, nausea, and vomiting, especially at toxic doses. Excessive salivation often accompanies these effects. Significant neurologic effects of digitalis usually seen in toxic situations are included in the discussion on digitalis toxicity (see below). Although digitalis does contain a steroid ring structure, cardiac glycosides rarely elicit effects associated with steroid hormones. Perhaps the only endocrine influence of any importance is a weak estrogen effect. Digitalis is not an aldosterone receptor antagonist.

Absorption, Fate, and Excretion

Digoxin may be given parenterally in emergencies; the route of choice is intravenous. It should be emphasized that parenteral administration carries with it added risks. By far the most common route is oral. Dose schedules are extremely important for digitalis because attaining a therapeutic effect without toxicity requires precise regulation of the amount of drug administered. Children by and large are less sensitive than adults to digitalis and usually require proportionally larger doses on the basis of weight. Dosages of the cardiac glycosides can be discussed from two aspects: the loading, or digitalizing, dose and the maintenance dose.

The purpose of the loading dose, as in therapy with other drugs, is to build up to a steady-state (plateau) drug concentration faster than would occur with maintenance doses. Maintenance doses, on the other hand, are meant to replace daily losses of a drug during the steady state. Digitalis dosages depend on individual patient variations as well as disease states and concurrent drug therapy. In all cases, patients must be continually monitored, and final judgment on optimal dosages depends on clinical observations.

A comparison of various oral digoxin preparations has shown variability in drug bioavailability, the difference apparently resulting from unequal dissolution rates of the tablets. The highest bioavailability of digoxin has been noted with the use of a solution of digoxin in soft gelatin capsules. Digoxin is excreted by the kidney largely in the active form. The mechanism involves glomerular filtration and tubular secretion and accounts for almost all the elimination of the drug. The pharmacokinetics of digoxin and digitoxin are summarized in Table 25-3.

Adverse Effects

Signs and symptoms

Although allergic reactions to digitalis are rare, toxic reactions are not. Withering himself was well aware of many toxic effects of digitalis when, for instance, he wrote:

> *In the year 1775 my opinion was asked concerning a family recipe for the cure of dropsy. I was told that it had long been kept a secret by an old woman in Shropshire who had sometimes made cures after the more regular practitioners had failed. I was informed also that the effects produced were*

Table • 25-3

Pharmacokinetics of Digoxin

NONPROPRIETARY (GENERIC) NAME	PROPRIETARY (TRADE) NAME	GASTROINTESTINAL ABSORPTION	PEAK DRUG EFFECT*	AVERAGE PLASMA HALF-LIFE	MAIN ROUTE OF ELIMINATION	APPROXIMATE DAILY ADULT ORAL MAINTENANCE DOSE
Digoxin	Lanoxin	60% to 85%†	1 to 5 hours	36 hours	Kidney excretion	0.125 to 0.5 mg
Digitoxin	Digitaline	90% to 100%	4 to 12 hr	7 days	Liver metabolism	0.05 to 0.3 mg

*Intravenous administration.
†Other marketed formulations may yield different absorption percentages.

violent vomiting and purging; for the diuretic effects seemed to have been overlooked. This medicine was composed of twenty or more different herbs; but it was not very difficult for one conversant in these subjects to perceive that the active herb could be no other than foxglove.[41]

Digitalis toxicity represents a significant clinical problem even today. The therapeutic index for clinically useful cardiac glycosides is similar and very low. Toxic signs are often seen at roughly twice the minimum effective dose. In practice, adverse reactions usually result from accumulation of the drug and/or from K^+ depletion caused by diuretic coadministration. Individual differences in patient response do exist and may account for unexpected clinical results; therefore dosages have to be tailored for each patient. The more common toxic effects of digitalis are outlined in Box 25-1.

Extracardiac toxic effects include anorexia, nausea, diarrhea, and vomiting. Gastrointestinal symptoms may also occur at nontoxic concentrations. The mechanism involves stimulation of the chemoreceptor trigger zone of the medulla.[33]

Box • 25-1

Common Signs and Symptoms of Digitalis Toxicity

Gastrointestinal
Salivation
Anorexia
Nausea
Vomiting
Diarrhea

CNS
Headache
Visual disturbances
Fatigue
Drowsiness

Cardiac
AV block
Excessive slowing of the heart
Ventricular extrasystoles
Other arrhythmias

Miscellaneous
Excessive urination

Excessive salivation, headache, fatigue, drowsiness, and abdominal pain often accompany these toxic signs and symptoms. Visual disturbances, such as the appearance of halos and distortions in color perception, can also occur, perhaps because of a direct effect of digitalis on the visual cortex. Objects often appear yellow or green. Giddiness and trigeminal neuralgia are sometimes observed; excessive urination often occurs with digitalis intoxication. Gynecomastia may occasionally develop in men. This side effect is of little value in determining toxicity, however, because it seldom occurs. The drugs may also suppress follicle-stimulating hormone and lead to vaginal cornification. Such effects are probably caused by an interaction with estrogen receptors.

In approximately half the cases of digitalis toxicity, extracardiac signs of toxicity precede the cardiac signs. A typical pattern would be the development of anorexia, followed in 1 or 2 days by nausea and vomiting and other signs. Nevertheless, the absence of extracardiac signs is no guarantee that cardiac toxicity is not occurring.

Cardiac toxicity is the most serious consequence of digitalis therapy. Although it is difficult to characterize specifically cardiac toxicity caused by digitalis, two effects stand out as the most typical—AV nodal block and ventricular tachyarrhythmias.[14] Complete AV dissociation can occur at toxic concentrations of digitalis. This effect is an extension of a therapeutic effect of the drug and is mediated by a reduction in AV nodal conduction. Dropped ventricular beats caused by partial heart block are also a sign of toxicity. The effect on AV conduction accounts in great measure for the excessive slowing of the heart seen in some toxic situations. Thus excessive cardiac slowing may be an important sign of toxicity in many patients.

Digitalis also produces tachyarrhythmias in toxic situations.[33] Increased electrical activity can result in premature beats and extrasystoles of ventricular origin, which may progress to ventricular fibrillation. Tachyarrhythmias may be caused by one of several mechanisms. Some may be caused by increased automaticity of Purkinje fibers, others to a reentry process (see Chapter 24), or finally to delayed afterpotentials whose depolarizations follow quickly on the action potential and in some cases generate a new action potential. Afterdepolarizations are in all likelihood caused by release of intracellular Ca^{++} from overloading of the intracellular Ca^{++} stores. Afterpotentials may also interfere with conduction by reducing the phase 4 resting potential. Other arrhythmias, both of atrial and of ventricular origin, may also occur. Examples of toxic effects on AV conduction and ventricular impulse generation are shown in Figure 25-7.

The arrhythmic effects of digitalis result in large measure from inhibition of cardiac Na^+,K^+-ATPase. Vagal effects of digitalis, however, can contribute to certain cardiac effects, such as heart block. In addition, at toxic concentrations, digitalis may exert significant stimulatory effects on the sympathetic nervous system, and these actions may account for some arrhythmias. Enhanced sympathetic activity is most likely caused by inhibition of Na^+,K^+-ATPase in the CNS and inhibition of active reuptake of norepinephrine at adrenergic nerve endings.

Drug monitoring

Attempts have been made to correlate blood concentrations of cardiac glycosides with signs of toxicity. These attempts offer a technical problem because serum digoxin at therapeutic doses is only 0.7 to 1.2 ng/ml, and toxic effects may start to appear at approximately 2.3 ng/ml.

The plasma concentration of cardiac glycosides can be measured by a specific radioimmunoassay. However, this assay is of limited use in confirming toxic states of patients because of the proximity of toxic and therapeutic plasma titers. Monitoring drug toxicity can best be accomplished by measurement of drug serum concentrations and, more importantly, careful clinical examination. Patient education is a necessary prerequisite for the early detection and prevention of digitalis toxicity.

Treatment of digitalis toxicity

When digitalis toxicity is diagnosed, the drug and any diuretics that may have exacerbated the problem are temporarily discontinued. If digitalis must be readministered before signs of toxicity have abated, small doses are given with constant monitoring. Potassium chloride can be administered intravenously in cases of hypokalemia. Generally, it is not used if AV conduction is significantly impaired because K^+ worsens this condition. Atropine can be helpful in controlling AV block, sinus bradycardia, and SA nodal arrest.

Several antiarrhythmic drugs are useful in treating digitalis toxicity. They are given intravenously in these situations, at least initially. Lidocaine is useful in suppressing ectopic pacemaker activity; however, it has little effect on slowing of AV nodal conduction by digitalis. Propranolol is effective in treating ventricular and supraventricular arrhythmias, but because it retards the AV conduction rate, its usefulness is limited.

Cholestyramine, an anion exchange resin, has been used experimentally to bind digitoxin in the intestine during its enterohepatic circulation. The prevention of reabsorption shortens the half-life of digitoxin but is of little value in hastening the elimination of digoxin.

In severe digitalis toxicity, an antidigoxin drug designated *digoxin immune Fab* may be administered.[14] Digoxin immune Fab consists of antigen-binding fragments derived from sheep antibodies to digoxin. The antidote is given intravenously and inactivates digoxin (or digitoxin) by forming a complex with the drug. The complex is then excreted by the kidney, with an elimination half-life of 15 to 20 hours. Given an adequate dose, the reversal of toxicity is rapid.[16] One potential hazard in its use is the induction of hypokalemia if body stores of K^+ are low. Digoxin immune Fab will also affect radioimmunoassays for digoxin designed to monitor plasma levels of digoxin. Fab fragments, although less likely than the entire antibody to cause an immune response, are associated with some allergic reactions.

General Therapeutic Uses

Congestive heart failure

In the United States, the cardiac glycoside used clinically is digoxin, and the term *digitalis* refers in effect to digoxin. The primary use for digitalis is in the treatment of congestive heart failure. The direct effect of digitalis on the myocardium in most cases enables the heart in congestive failure to increase its contractile force and output.

Digitalis is not very effective when heart failure is caused by infectious or toxic myocarditis or some obstructive cause, such as constrictive pericarditis, and is contraindicated in hypertrophic subaortic stenosis. Digitalis is most effective in those patients with chronic, continuous systolic heart failure in which the ventricle is enlarged at rest, early ventricular filling is rapid, and the compliance of the heart wall has not been reduced because of a condition such as hypertrophy or amyloid infiltration. Furthermore, the best candidates for digitalis have enlarged hearts despite diuretic therapy. It has been shown that patients with a third heart sound, presumably caused by the enlarged heart striking the chest wall, often have improved cardiac function from digitalis, whereas those without this heart sound gain little benefit. Signs such as the third heart sound may help indicate the condition of the heart and predict with greater accuracy the value of using digitalis. At present, however, further work needs to be done to establish the precise predictive criteria for digitalis therapy in various conditions of heart failure.

Although digitalis improves symptoms of heart failure in many patients and reduces hospitalizations of patients receiving other therapy for heart failure,[39] it has not been shown to increase the survival time in these patients.[38,39] Therapy with ACE inhibitors, other vasodilators, spironolactone, other diuretics, and β-adrenergic receptor blockers has been shown to increase the life span in patients with heart failure. Therefore these drugs are replacing digitalis for treating many patients, particularly those with less severe heart failure. This finding illustrates the importance of preload and afterload and other factors in the disease. Digitalis can be used with benefit in combination with other drugs in the treatment of systolic heart failure.[3]

Cardiac arrhythmias

Digitalis is effective in reducing an increased ventricular rate caused by atrial fibrillation. Vagal effects on the AV node account for the majority of the decrease in conduction. This reduction protects the ventricle from atrial electrical impulses arriving in rapid succession. The dosage can be adjusted to titrate the drug to a given ventricular rate. On occasion, atrial fibrillation reverts to normal sinus rhythm during therapy. However, it must be emphasized that this is not the main goal of digitalis therapy, which is to reduce the ventricular rate despite the rapid rate of the atria. The use of digitalis in treating patients with acute atrial fibrillation has declined because of the availability of antiarrhythmics, including the β-adrenergic blockers and Ca^{++}-channel blockers. Digitalis is more appropriately used when systolic heart failure accompanies the atrial fibrillation and where controlling the resting ventricular rate is an added benefit.

CONDITIONS AFFECTING DIGITALIS THERAPY

Disease States

Because of the pharmacokinetic properties of digoxin and digitoxin, patients with kidney or liver hypofunction, respectively, may require downward dosage adjustments of each drug.[33]

Thyroid status has important implications for digitalis therapy. Hypothyroidism increases and hyperthyroidism reduces the sensitivity of the patient to digitalis. The half-life of digoxin is reduced in thyrotoxicosis, in part as a result of increased excretion of the drug. Increased volume of distribution and decreased intestinal absorption of digoxin in hyperthyroid states have also been reported. In addition, sensitivity of the heart itself to cardiac glycosides appears to be a function of thyroid status. This sensitivity may relate to the fact that the number of Na^+,K^+-ATPase active sites appears to vary directly with thyroid function.

Patients with chronic lung disease and cor pulmonale tend to be susceptible to the toxic effects of cardiac glycosides. This enhanced susceptibility is the result of hypoxemia and disturbances in acid-base balance in these patients.

Because the mechanism of action of digitalis in all likelihood involves an increase in a crucial Ca^{++} "pool" in the heart, it is not surprising that high plasma Ca^{++} concentrations can worsen digitalis toxicity. Mg^{++} on the other hand, inhibits many Ca^{++}-induced events; thus Mg^{++} deficiency can increase susceptibility to digitalis toxicity.

Hypokalemia in particular can predispose a patient to digitalis toxicity. Low plasma K^+ concentrations allow greater binding of digitalis to Na^+,K^+-ATPase and independently alter myocardial membrane properties so as to increase cardiac automaticity. Together these factors may account for increased digitalis toxicity at low plasma K^+ concentrations. (For drugs that lower plasma K^+, see the section on drug interactions below.) Loss of intracellular K^+ also plays an important role in digitalis toxicity. When digitalis is administered, intracellular K^+ concentrations gradually decrease, reducing the ratio of intracellular to extracellular K^+. This ratio change and the membrane potential alterations that follow make the heart more sensitive to digitalis toxicity. Reduced intracellular K^+ may be present without a significant reduction in plasma K^+ concentrations. The effects of major electrolyte changes on digitalis toxicity are summarized in Table 25-4.

Pregnancy

Serum concentrations of digoxin are less predictable during pregnancy and usually are higher than in the nonpregnant patient at equal doses.

Drug Interactions

Drugs affect digitalis therapy mainly by reducing its absorption, by altering the rate of its metabolism, by changing plasma and intracellular K^+ concentrations, or by directly influencing the myocardium.

Kaolin-pectin and oral antacids reduce the intestinal absorption of digoxin by forming a complex with the drug. Sulfasalazine, neomycin, and metoclopramide have also been reported to reduce the intestinal absorption of digoxin.

Cholestyramine is used to bind bile acids in the gastrointestinal tract and thereby lower plasma concentrations of cholesterol. It is also able to bind certain drugs in the intestine, including digitalis. Digitalis preparations given concurrently by mouth are therefore prevented from being absorbed. Furthermore, because digitoxin circulates in an enterohepatic cycle, it can be bound by cholestyramine after its initial absorption. The half-life of digitoxin is shortened and the therapeutic effect reduced.

A number of drugs can predispose a patient to digitalis toxicity by lowering plasma K^+ concentrations. These include amphotericin B, corticosteroids, and, most notably, the thiazide and loop diuretics.[33] The clinical problem is a significant one, especially because diuretics are often used with digitalis to treat congestive heart failure or reduce blood pressure. In these situations, supplementation of dietary K^+ or the use of K^+-sparing diuretics is especially important.

Several reports have indicated a substantial interaction between quinidine and digitalis. The most important clinical results of concurrent therapy are enhanced digitalis toxicity and enhanced quinidine toxicity. Adverse reactions can occur at normal therapeutic dosages. Quinidine increases plasma digoxin concentrations by two mechanisms: first, renal clearance of digoxin is decreased; second, digoxin is displaced from tissue stores as a result of quinidine administration. Because of the interaction with digoxin, concurrent therapy usually requires a reduction in the dose of both drugs, although this interaction is highly variable from patient to patient. Quinine, the levo stereoisomer of quinidine, and amiodarone, another antiarrhythmic, also increase plasma digoxin concentrations.

Sympathomimetic amines interact with digitalis because both classes of drugs increase the possibility of ectopic cardiac pacemaker activity. Cardiac arrhythmias are more likely to occur when β-adrenergic receptor agonists are used concurrently with digitalis.

Both cholinergic and anticholinergic drugs alter responses to digitalis. The cholinergic agents enhance and the anticholinergic drugs antagonize the atrial, SA nodal, and AV nodal effects of digitalis. Succinylcholine, by increasing vagal tone and altering the K^+ distribution, may acutely increase digitalis toxicity.

Verapamil, nifedipine, and diltiazem, drugs that block plasma membrane Ca^{++} channels, are used in the treatment of certain cardiac arrhythmias, angina pectoris, hypertension, and other conditions. Because these agents reduce Ca^{++} entry into the cell, it is to be expected that they would have some influence on the effects of digitalis. Verapamil is contraindicated in digitalis toxicity because it may lead to sinus arrest and AV block. Verapamil and diltiazem also increase the plasma concentration of digoxin. On the other hand, the cardiac glycosides tend to reverse the cardiodepressant effect of verapamil, and the dihydropyridine Ca^{++}-channel blockers are useful for heart failure patients with diastolic dysfunction. The interactions and combined uses of the Ca^{++}-channel blockers with digitalis remain subjects of investigation.

Canrenone is a metabolite of spironolactone. Canrenone partially inhibits Na^+,K^+-ATPase and antagonizes the binding of cardiac glycosides to Na^+,K^+-ATPase. These opposing actions account for some complex interactions between digitalis and spironolactone in congestive heart failure. Some evidence supports the possibility that canrenone antagonizes digitalis toxicity. However, spironolactone, especially in the presence of quinidine, reduces digoxin clearance. This may necessitate a reduction in the digoxin dose when used concurrently.[14,18] Spironolactone may also interfere with serum digitalis assays.

In approximately 10% of patients, enteric bacteria, especially *Eubacterium lentum*, metabolize a significant portion of ingested digoxin. In these patients, antibiotics, by inhibiting these bacteria, can increase the amount of digoxin absorbed and thereby increase the potential for digoxin toxicity. This interaction between antibiotics and digoxin has in some cases resulted in a twofold increase in serum digoxin concentrations.

Table • 25-4

Effects of Plasma Electrolyte Concentrations on Digitalis Toxicity

	NORMAL TOTAL PLASMA CONCENTRATION (mmol/L)	DIGITALIS TOXICITY MORE LIKELY IF PLASMA ELECTROLYTE CONCENTRATION IS:
K^+	3.8 to 5.4	Lowered
Ca^{++}	2.2 to 2.8	Raised
Mg^{++}	0.8 to 1.1	Lowered

OTHER DRUG THERAPY FOR CONGESTIVE HEART FAILURE

Diuretics

Therapy of mild congestive heart failure has often involved salt restriction and the use of diuretic drugs to reduce tissue edema and blood volume. The resulting reduction in the preload, or diastolic filling pressure, helps decrease wall tension in the heart and lessen myocardial oxygen demand. The vasodilation caused by the thiazide diuretics also aids in reducing the afterload, or the arterial pressure against which the heart has to pump in moving blood. Diuretics also indirectly reduce sympathetic nervous system activity.

Spironolactone

Spironolactone is a drug commonly used to treat heart failure.[29] Its action as a diuretic is caused by its antagonism of aldosterone at the convoluted tubule of the kidney. However, antagonism of aldosterone leads to several other effects that are beneficial in the patient with heart failure. These are shown in Figure 25-8. K^+-sparing actions help in preventing hypokalemia. Reducing Mg^{++} loss appears to reduce ventricular arrhythmias in patients with heart failure. Because aldosterone can inhibit norepinephrine uptake (uptake 2), spironolactone prevents the enhanced sympathetic activation from aldosterone.[37] Spironolactone also blocks the inhibition of the baroreceptor reflex seen with aldosterone. The consequences of inhibiting the baroreceptor reflex include, among others, the lack of parasympathetic nerve response.[20] The latter response is important in counteracting the adverse effects of sympathetic stimulation such as arrhythmias and cardiac ischemia. Myocardial fibrosis is also inhibited by spironolactone. Thus spironolactone has many salutary effects in heart failure. These beneficial effects also occur when it is used with other drugs such as ACE inhibitors.[40] Because the reduction of aldosterone release by ACE inhibitors is only partial, an added benefit is gained from the use of an aldosterone antagonist.

Angiotensin-Converting Enzyme Inhibitors and Other Vasodilators

The ACE inhibitors are major drugs in the treatment of chronic heart failure.[6] Their primary effect is to reduce afterload and preload. These drugs improve symptoms in patients with heart failure. Enalapril has also been shown to increase survival time in patients with heart failure.[28,35] In addition, there is expectation that the progressive deterioration of the heart may be slowed with the ACE inhibitors. Thus ACE inhibitors appear to control remodeling that occurs with chronic heart failure.[43] Remodeling results from growth of the myocardial cell as well as myocardial fibrosis. This probable cardioprotective effect provides added support for the use of the ACE inhibitors in heart failure. Furthermore, inhibiting the production of angiotensin II or blocking its receptor reduces aldosterone secretion, which in turn reduces the Na^+ and water retention. Reduction of aldosterone release by ACE inhibitors also reduces sympathetic discharge, as described in Chapter 28 (see Figure 25-8). Evidence also suggests that ACE inhibitors stimulate the proliferation of capillaries in the coronary circulation, thereby increasing blood flow.[30] It is not known whether this action of the ACE inhibitors occurs as a result of the decrease in angiotensin II, an increase in bradykinin, or both.[23] In all likelihood, the ability of ACE inhibitors to lower blood pressure in hypertensive patients also contributes to a cardioprotective effect. Early treatment of congestive heart disease with an ACE inhibitor could be a major factor in slowing the progress of the disease as well as in relieving symptoms. These drugs also are useful in combination with digitalis and diuretics in treating heart failure.[25] Angiotensin II antagonists such as losartan and valsartan are additional candidates for treating heart failure.[28] They share the benefits of the ACE inhibitors while avoiding such side effects as angioedema and persistent coughing. The pharmacologic features of angiotensin II antagonists and the ACE inhibitors are discussed in detail in Chapter 28.

Vasodilators such as nitrates and hydralazine also improve tissue perfusion in heart failure and increase survival rates in these patients. The vasodilators are usually administered in combination with other drugs, such as inotropic agents or ACE inhibitors. Disadvantages of the nitrates and hydralazine include the indirect enhancement of sympathetic discharge and activation of the renin-angiotensin pathway. The pharmacologic characteristics of nitrates and hydralazine are discussed in Chapters 26 and 28, respectively.

Inamrinone and Milrinone

Inamrinone and milrinone are bipyridine drugs that have a positive inotropic action on the heart.[18] Their cardiac effects cannot be attributed to an action on Na^+,K^+-ATPase, the β-adrenergic receptor, or adenylyl cyclase. The bipyridines act by inhibiting phosphodiesterase III, also termed *cyclic 3′,5′-guanosine monophosphate–inhibited phosphodiesterase.* As a result of this inhibition, cardiac concentrations of cAMP are elevated and a sympathomimetic effect on the heart is achieved. Inamrinone and milrinone also reduce arterial and venous pressures because of the increase in vascular smooth muscle relaxation, which aids in relieving heart failure. The latter effect is the major mechanism operable in heart failure patients. Both inamrinone and milrinone are available for intravenous use. The half-lives of inamrinone and milrinone are approximately 4 to 6 and 3 hours, respectively. Adverse effects of inamrinone include nausea and vomiting, thrombocytopenia, hepatotoxicity, cardiac arrhythmias, and fever. Milrinone is less likely to cause thrombocytopenia and more likely to cause arrhythmias. The drugs are used clinically for short-term use, especially in cases in which the heart is refractory to other cardiotonic agents and vascular resistance is elevated. Studies have failed to demonstrate long-term benefits,

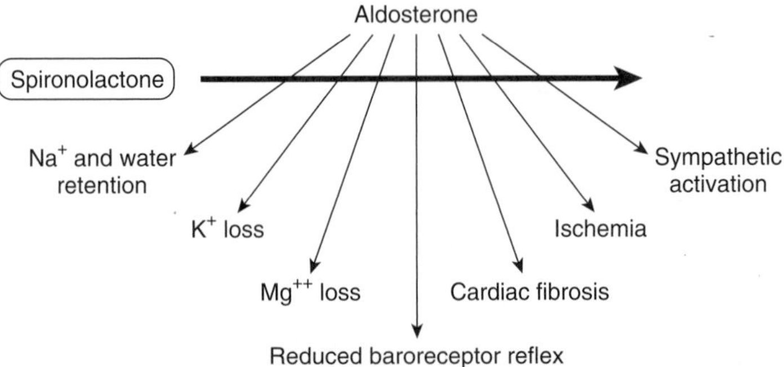

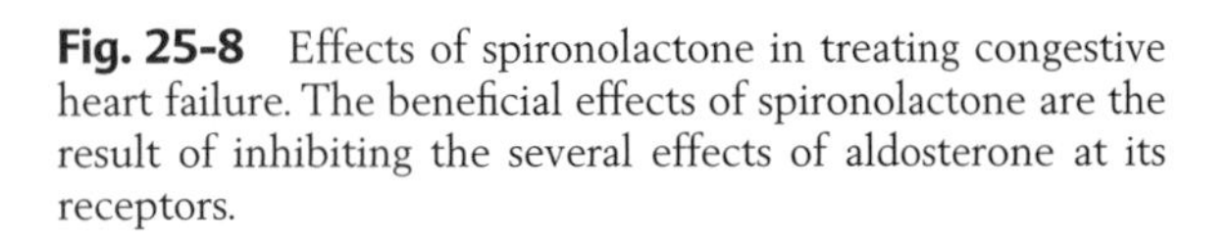
Fig. 25-8 Effects of spironolactone in treating congestive heart failure. The beneficial effects of spironolactone are the result of inhibiting the several effects of aldosterone at its receptors.

however, and evidence indicates that survival is even worsened with long-term administration because of an arrhythmogenic effect of the drugs.[26]

Catecholamines

Drugs that stimulate β_1 adrenoceptors, such as dobutamine and dopamine, are cardiotonic.[18] An undesirable chronotropic response may be obtained; nevertheless, they have use in treating heart failure in the acute setting. Dobutamine is a somewhat selective β_1-adrenergic agonist, which accounts for the positive cardiac inotropic response. A β_2-adrenergic effect appears to account for its effect of reducing vascular resistance. The effect of dobutamine on α-adrenergic receptors is complex. The negative isomer is an α_1-adrenergic agonist, whereas the positive isomer is an α_1-adrenergic antagonist. The combination of both isomers in the clinically available preparation assures primarily a β_1-adrenergic effect of the drug. At low doses, dopamine stimulates D_1-dopaminergic receptors somewhat selectively. This effect accounts for vasodilation of coronary, renal, and mesenteric blood vessels. At somewhat higher doses, dopamine has a greater net effect in stimulating β_1-adrenergic receptors, leading to an inotropic effect. Finally, at still higher doses, dopamine significantly stimulates α_1-adrenergic receptors and increases vascular resistance. Therefore the choice of catecholamine depends largely on the vascular state of the patient. The pharmacologic features of the catecholamines are discussed in Chapter 6.

Adrenergic-Receptor Antagonists

The use of β-adrenoceptor blockers to reduce the adverse cardiac effects of heightened sympathetic discharge that occur as heart failure progresses is a strategy used in the long-term treatment of heart failure. This use is consistent with a neurohumoral component of heart failure.

Carvedilol is a nonselective β- and selective α_1-adrenoceptor blocker used in patients with heart failure. β-Adrenergic blockade may reduce remodeling, whereas α_1-adrenergic blockade reduces preload and afterload. In clinical trials, carvedilol has increased survival times in patients receiving other medications for heart failure.[27] It also has antioxidant properties that result in cell protection against free radicals.[9] The relative importance of each of its three mechanisms in achieving the favorable results is not known.

Nesiritide

Nesiritide is a human B-type natriuretic peptide that is produced using recombinant DNA methods. The drug binds to and stimulates membrane-bound guanylate cyclase, leading to an increase in cyclic GMP in blood vessels. This leads to relaxation of vascular smooth muscle. The half-life of the drug is about 18 minutes; however, the effect of the drug may last several hours. It is used in the acute management of heart failure.

Calcium Sensitizers

Although not yet available in the United States, another strategy in treating heart failure is the use of Ca^{++} sensitizers. These agents increase the sensitivity of the myofilaments to Ca^{++} without overloading the Ca^{++} in the cell or increasing heart rate.[8] It remains to be seen if these drugs will become useful clinical drugs.

Endogenous Digitalislike Compounds

Endogenous digitalislike compounds, sometimes called *endodigins,* have been isolated from various tissues.[15] There is a tendency to draw an analogy between these substances and the enkephalins and endorphins and their action on opioid receptors. It is in this context that investigators are examining chemical substances present in the body that can act like digitalis. Substances that may serve this role include a low molecular weight substance isolated from guinea pig brain and peptides with digitalislike activity in volume-expanded dogs. These substances inhibit Na^+-K^+ pump activity as well as the binding of digitalis to Na^+,K^+-ATPase. Agents exhibiting the latter reaction also bind with antibodies specific for digoxin. Factors that inhibit the Na^+-K^+ pump have been observed in persons with certain types of hypertension.[12] This and other evidence has heightened interest in these factors as potentially important in responding to increased fluid volume. An endogenous digitalislike factor that may arise from the hypothalamus has also been isolated from human cerebrospinal fluid. A steroid with digitalislike activity closely related to ouabain has been detected in human plasma. The physiologic role of these factors is not established.

IMPLICATIONS FOR DENTISTRY

Stress Factors

The practitioner should strive to eliminate needless stress for cardiac patients, especially anxiety or pain associated with dental procedures. It must be emphasized that patients taking digitalis still possess an underlying cardiac defect. Therefore these patients are at special risk in stressful situations because stress puts a greater workload on the heart and stimulates the release of endogenous catecholamines. By increasing the likelihood of ectopic pacemaker activity of the heart, and possibly by temporarily decreasing plasma K^+ concentrations, catecholamines increase the risk of digitalis-induced arrhythmias. Fear and apprehension may also increase the likelihood of adverse CNS reactions to digitalis. One practical conclusion is that antianxiety therapy or analgesics should be used preemptively if emotional stress or pain is likely.

Drug Interactions

The use of catecholamines in local anesthetic injections for patients taking digitalis is not contraindicated but should be approached with special caution. Proper injection technique to avoid intravascular injection should be followed. Many factors influence the decision to use vasoconstrictors in local anesthetic solutions, including the ability to achieve adequate anesthesia without vasoconstrictors and the volume of anesthetic solution required. The chief danger of sympathomimetic vasoconstrictors for patients taking digitalis is that the combination of drugs increases the risk of cardiac arrhythmias if significant amounts of vasoconstrictor enter the vascular space.

The use of gingival retraction cords impregnated with epinephrine is definitely not recommended in digitalized patients. In fact, cardiac disease in general is a contraindication for their use. Considerable amounts of vasoconstrictor may be absorbed systemically from these retraction cords, and the possibility of cardiac arrhythmias developing is significant. If hemostatic retraction cords are to be used in digitalized patients, the cords should be impregnated with an astringent in place of a vasoconstrictor.

The effects of digitalis on the SA node, the atria, and the AV node are mediated primarily by the vagus nerve. Many beneficial effects of digitalis depend on vagal influences. This is especially true in the treatment of atrial fibrillation. Hence, muscarinic and antimuscarinic drugs can influence digitalis therapy. Antisialagogues such as atropine and methantheline should not be used in digitalized patients because they tend to reduce the effects of digitalis. Muscarinic receptor agonists such as pilocarpine enhance the effect of digitalis on the SA node, the atria, and the AV node.

Antibiotic therapy may alter the intestinal flora and, in so doing, increase the absorption of digoxin in those patients whose gastrointestinal flora metabolizes digoxin. Erythromycin has been shown to have this effect. When the need arises, concurrent antibiotic therapy, especially with erythromycin (or other macrolide) or a broad-spectrum antibiotic, should be undertaken with sufficient cognizance given to its possible interaction with digoxin.

Drugs Used in Treating Heart Failure

Nonproprietary (generic) name	*Proprietary (trade) name*
Digoxin	Lanoxin
Dobutamine	Dobutrex
Dopamine	Intropin
Inamrinone	Inocor IV
Milrinone	Primacor
Nesiritide	Natrecor

Other drug classes are covered elsewhere in the text: β-adrenoceptor blockers in Chapter 7 and ACE inhibitors, angiotensin II receptor blockers, diuretics (including spironolactone), and vasodilators in Chapter 28.

CITED REFERENCES

1. ACC/AHA Task Force: Heart failure guidelines, *J Am Coll Cardiol* 26:1376-1398, 1995.
2. Braunwald E, Bloodwell RD, Goldberg LI, et al: Studies on digitalis. IV. Observations in man on the effects of digitalis preparations on the contractility of the non-failing heart and on total vascular resistance, *J Clin Invest* 40:52-59, 1961.
3. Brozena S, Jessup M: Pathophysiologic strategies in the management of congestive heart failure, *Annu Rev Med* 41:65-74, 1990.
4. Cattell M, Gold H: The influence of digitalis glucosides on the force of contraction of mammalian cardiac muscle, *J Pharmacol Exp Ther* 62:116-125, 1938.
5. Cohn JN: Heart failure: future treatment approaches, *J Hypertension* 13:74S-78S, 2000.
6. Cohn JN: Structural basis for heart failure: ventricular remodeling and its pharmacological inhibition, *Circulation* 91:2504-2507, 1995.
7. Coodley E: Newer drug therapy for congestive heart failure, *Arch Intern Med* 159:1177-1183, 1999.
8. Dorigo P, Floreani M, Santostasi G, et al: Pharmacological characterization of a new Ca^{2+} sensitizer, *J Pharmacol Exp Ther* 295:994-1004, 2000.
9. Dunn CJ, Lea AP, Wagstaff AJ: Carvedilol. A reappraisal of its pharmacological properties and therapeutic use in cardiovascular disorders, *Drugs* 54:161-185, 1997.
10. Flesch M, Schwinger RHG, Schiffer F, et al: Evidence for functional relevance of an enhanced expression of the Na^+-Ca^{2+} exchanger in failing human myocardium, *Circulation* 94:992-1002, 1996.
11. Hasenfuss G, Mulieri LA, Allen PD, et al: Influence of isoproterenol and ouabain on excitation-contraction coupling, cross-bridge function, and energetics in failing human myocardium, *Circulation* 94:3155-3160, 1996.
12. Hamlyn JM, Hamilton BP, Manunta P: Endogenous ouabain, sodium balance and blood pressure: a review and a hypothesis, *J Hypertension* 14:151-167, 1996.
13. Hauptman PJ, Garg R, Kelly RA: Cardiac glycosides in the next millennium, *Progr Cardiovasc Dis* 41:247-254, 1999.
14. Hauptman PJ, Kelly RA: Digitalis, *Circulation* 99:1265-1270, 1999.
15. Hollenberg NK, Graves SW: Endogenous sodium pump inhibition: current status and therapeutic opportunities, *Prog Drug Res* 46:9-42, 1996.
16. Kelly RA, Smith TV: Antibody therapies for drug overdose. In Austen KF, Burakoff SJ, Rosen FS, et al, eds: *Therapeutic immunology*, Boston, 2001, Blackwell Scientific.
17. Langer GA: Mechanism of action of the cardiac glycosides on the heart, *Biochem Pharmacol* 30:3261-3264, 1981.
18. Leier CV, Binkley PF: Parenteral inotropic support for advanced congestive heart failure, *Progr Cardiovasc Dis* 41:207-224, 1998.
19. Lingrel JB, Van Huysse J, Obrien W, et al: Structure-function studies of the Na^+,K^+-ATPase, *Kidney Int* 45(suppl 44):S32-S39, 1994.
20. MacFadyen RJ, Barr CS, Struthers AD: Aldosterone blockade reduces vascular collagen turnover, improves heart rate variability and reduces early morning rise in heart rate in heart failure patients, *Cardiovasc Res* 35:30-34, 1997.
21. Mason DT: Regulation of cardiac performance in clinical heart disease: interactions between contractile state mechanical abnormalities and ventricular compensatory mechanisms, *Am J Cardiol* 32:437-448, 1973.
22. Mason DT, Braunwald E: Studies on digitalis. X. Effects of ouabain on forearm vascular resistance and venous tone in normal subjects and in patients in heart failure, *J Clin Invest* 43:532-543, 1964.
23. McDonald KM, Mock J, D'Awia A: Bradykinin antagonism inhibits the antigrowth effect of converting enzyme inhibition in the dog myocardium after discrete transmural myocardial necrosis, *Circulation* 91:2043-2048, 1995.
24. Middleton DA, Rankin S, Esmann M, et al: Structural insights into the binding of cardiac glycosides to the digitalis receptor revealed by solid-state NMR, *Proc Natl Acad Sci* 97:13602-13607, 2000.
25. Opie LH: Fundamental role of angiotensin-converting enzyme inhibitors in the management of congestive heart failure, *Am J Cardiol* 75:3F-6F, 1995.
26. Packer M, Carver JR, Rodeneffer RJ, et al: Effect of oral milrinone on mortality in severe chronic heart failure. The PROMISE Study Research Group, *N Engl J Med* 325:1468-1475, 1991.
27. Packer M, Bristow MR, Cohn JN, et al: The effect of carvedilol on morbidity and mortality in patients with chronic heart failure. The U.S. Carvedilol Heart Failure Study Group, *N Engl J Med* 334:1349-1355, 1996.
28. Pitt B, Poole-Wilson P, Segal R, et al: Effects of losartan versus captopril on mortality in patients with symptomatic heart failure: rationale, design, and baseline characteristics of patients in the losartan Heart Failure Survival Study—ELITE II, *J Card Fail* 5:146-154, 1999.
29. Pitt B, Zannad F, Remme WJ, et al: The effect of spironolactone on morbidity and mortality in patients with severe heart failure. The Randomized Aldactone Evaluation Study Investigators, *N Engl J Med* 341:709-717, 1999.

30. Remme WJ: Bradykinin-mediated cardiovascular protective actions of ACE inhibitors. A new dimension in anti-ischaemic therapy? *Drugs* 54(suppl 5):59-70, 1997.
31. Santana LF, Gomez AM, Lederer WJ: Ca^{++} flux through promiscuous cardiac Na^{+} channels: slip-mode conductance, *Science* 279:1027-1033, 1998.
32. Skou JC: Effect of digitalis glycosides on membrane transport of sodium and potassium. In Marks BH, Weissler AM, eds: *Basic and clinical pharmacology of digitalis,* Springfield, IL, 1972, Charles C Thomas.
33. Smith TW: Digitalis: mechanisms of action and clinical use, *N Engl J Med* 318:358-365, 1988.
34. Solaro RJ, Rarick HM: Troponin and tropomyosin: proteins that switch on and tune in the activity of cardiac myofilaments, *Circ Res* 83:471-480, 1998.
35. SOLVD investigators: Effect of enalapril on survival in patients with reduced left ventricular ejection fractions and congestive heart failure, *N Engl J Med* 325:293-302, 1991.
36. Sonnenblick EH, Williams JF, Jr, Glick G, et al: Studies on digitalis. XV. Effects of cardiac glycosides on myocardial force-velocity relations in the nonfailing human heart, *Circulation* 34:532-539, 1966.
37. Struthers AD: Why does spironolactone improve mortality over and above an ACE inhibitor in chronic heart failure? *Br J Clin Pharmacol* 47:479-482, 1998.
38. The Digitalis Investigation Group: Rationale, design, implementation, and baseline characteristics of patients in the DIG trial: a large, simple, long-term trial to evaluate the effect of digitalis on mortality in heart failure, *Control Clin Trials* 17:77-97, 1996.
39. The Digitalis Investigation Group: The effect of digoxin on mortality and morbidity in patients with heart failure, *N Engl J Med* 336:525-533, 1997.
40. The RALES Investigators: Effectiveness of spironolactone added to an angiotensin-converting enzyme inhibitor and a loop diuretic for severe chronic congestive heart failure (the randomized aldactone evaluation study [RALES]), *Am J Cardiol* 78:902-907, 1996.
41. Withering W: An account of the foxglove, and some of its medical uses; with practical remarks on dropsy, and other diseases, London, 1785, CGJ and J Robinson (reprinted in *Med Classics* 2:305-443, 1937).
42. Yashar, PR, Fransua M, Frishman WH: The sodium-calcium ion membrane exchanger: physiologic significance and pharmacologic implications, *J Clin Pharm* 38:393-401, 1998.
43. Zhu Y-C, Zhu Y-Z, Gchike P, et al: Effects of angiotensin-converting enzyme inhibition and angiotensin II AT1 receptor antagonism on cardiac parameters in left ventricular hypertrophy, *Am J Cardiol* 80(suppl 3A):110A-117A, 1997.

General References

Carson P: Pharmacologic treatment of congestive heart failure, *Clin Cardiol* 19:271-277, 1996.

Cohn JN: The management of chronic heart failure, *N Engl J Med* 335:490-498, 1996.

Hauptman PJ, Kelly RA: Digitalis glycosides. In Hosenpud JD, Greenberg BH, eds: *Congestive heart failure: pathophysiology, diagnosis and comprehensive approach to therapy.* Baltimore, MD, 2000, Williams & Wilkins.

Tauke J, Goldstein S, Gheorghiade M: Digoxin for chronic heart failure: a review of the randomized controlled trials with special attention to the PROVED (Prospective Randomized Study of Ventricular Failure and the Efficacy of Digoxin) and RADIANCE (Randomized Assessment of Digoxin on Inhibitors of the Angiotensin Converting Enzyme) trials, *Prog Cardiovasc Dis* 37:49-58, 1994.

CHAPTER • 26

Antianginal Drugs

Eileen L. Watson and Frank J. Dowd

Angina pectoris (from the Latin, literally meaning "pain in the chest") is usually manifested as severe, transient, retrosternal pain that sometimes radiates to the left arm, back, or jaw. It is frequently accompanied by fear, anxiety, feelings of suffocation, and a sensation of tightening of the chest. There is a wide variation among individuals in the intensity and quality of the pain, and some ischemic episodes may occur without prominent symptoms. The pain and associated changes in the electrocardiogram (e.g., depressed ST segment) result from ischemia (hypoxia) of some area of the myocardium, usually a subendocardial area. The most frequent pathologic cause of angina is epicardial coronary artery atherosclerosis leading to compromised blood flow and reduced oxygen delivery to a region of the myocardium. Angina may also result from vasospasm; even then, the coronary vasoconstriction frequently occurs at an atherosclerotic site on the artery.

As represented in Figure 26-1, the normal response to increased myocardial oxygen demand is satisfied by vasodilation of the small coronary resistance vessels, increased blood flow, and thus increased oxygen supply. In contrast, in the classic anginal patient with exertional (exercise-induced) episodes, significant sclerosis (more than 70% narrowing of the luminal diameter) of the large conductance arteries precludes increased vasodilation in response to increased myocardial work because the poststenotic resistance vessels are already dilated and the resultant demand for oxygen cannot be met. Cardiac determinants of oxygen consumption and factors that can precipitate changes in these determinants are also shown in Figure 26-1.

The intraventricular pressure is important in determining flow in subendocardial regions because of compression of blood vessels in the involved area. Coronary blood flow occurs primarily during diastole, when the intraventricular pressure is least. Increased heart rate decreases the diastolic time more than the systolic and, of course, requires increased oxygen supply in concert with the increased rate of metabolism. Alterations of ventricular size also cause concurrent changes in ventricular work and oxygen demand. Finally, the inotropic state of the myocardium is also a factor in determining oxygen consumption. One of the more important controls of myocardial contractility is exerted by the sympathetic nervous system through catecholamine release.

It is beyond the scope of this chapter to consider in detail the specific changes in the cardiac determinants of myocardial oxygen consumption caused by each of the factors that may precipitate an anginal attack. It is sufficient to say that any factor that compromises the balance between oxygen demand and oxygen supply may cause an attack of angina. Thus anginal pain may follow exercise, emotional upset, or exposure to cold or may occur after meals or smoking. Certain persons have nocturnal attacks of angina, probably because recumbent posture can increase venous return to the heart and therefore cardiac work. Anginal attacks in susceptible patients may also result from self-medication with various drugs, such as cocaine and cold remedies that contain sympathomimetic agents.

There are basically three types of angina pectoris: chronic stable angina (classic exertional angina), variant (Prinzmetal's) angina, and unstable angina (also known as *preinfarction angina, intermediate coronary syndrome, acute coronary insufficiency,* and *accelerated angina*). Chronic stable angina occurs in patients who have fixed atherosclerotic coronary artery disease. Pain in these individuals occurs when the myocardial oxygen requirement reaches a given stable value. Variant angina occurs as a result of coronary artery spasm and a subsequent decrease in coronary blood flow and oxygen supply. These patients usually also exhibit coronary atherosclerosis, although in some it may be minimal. Variant angina is characterized by chest pain occurring at rest and, frequently, during sleep. The third type, unstable angina, refers to a new onset of severe and/or frequent angina, anginal pain at rest, or a sudden worsening of pain in a patient with previously stable exertional angina.[30] The cause of unstable angina is often sudden platelet aggregation or plaque emboli in coronary vessels. The majority of these patients have severe coronary artery disease; coronary spasm may also be involved. Thirty percent of patients with chest pain have unstable angina and up to 20% of these patients will have a myocardial infarct within a year, the majority of these within a month.[18]

Five classes of drugs are used extensively in the treatment of angina pectoris; the sites of action of the β-adrenergic receptor blockers, the Ca^{++} channel blockers (CCBs), and the nitrates/nitrites are shown in Figure 26-2. The first class, the organic nitrites and nitrates, are composed of drugs (e.g., sublingual nitroglycerin) that provide immediate relief from anginal symptoms or provide acute prophylaxis of an attack, as well as nitrate formulations (e.g., topical nitroglycerin, oral isosorbide dinitrate) that are promoted for long-term protection from anginal episodes.

The second class contains the β-adrenergic receptor–blocking agents (β blockers). These are administered on a long-term basis, frequently in conjunction with organic nitrates, to decrease the frequency and severity of anginal attacks.

The third class of drugs useful in the management of angina is composed of CCBs. This class includes verapamil, diltiazem, nifedipine, and others. These agents, like the β blockers, are used prophylactically in angina therapy.[10]

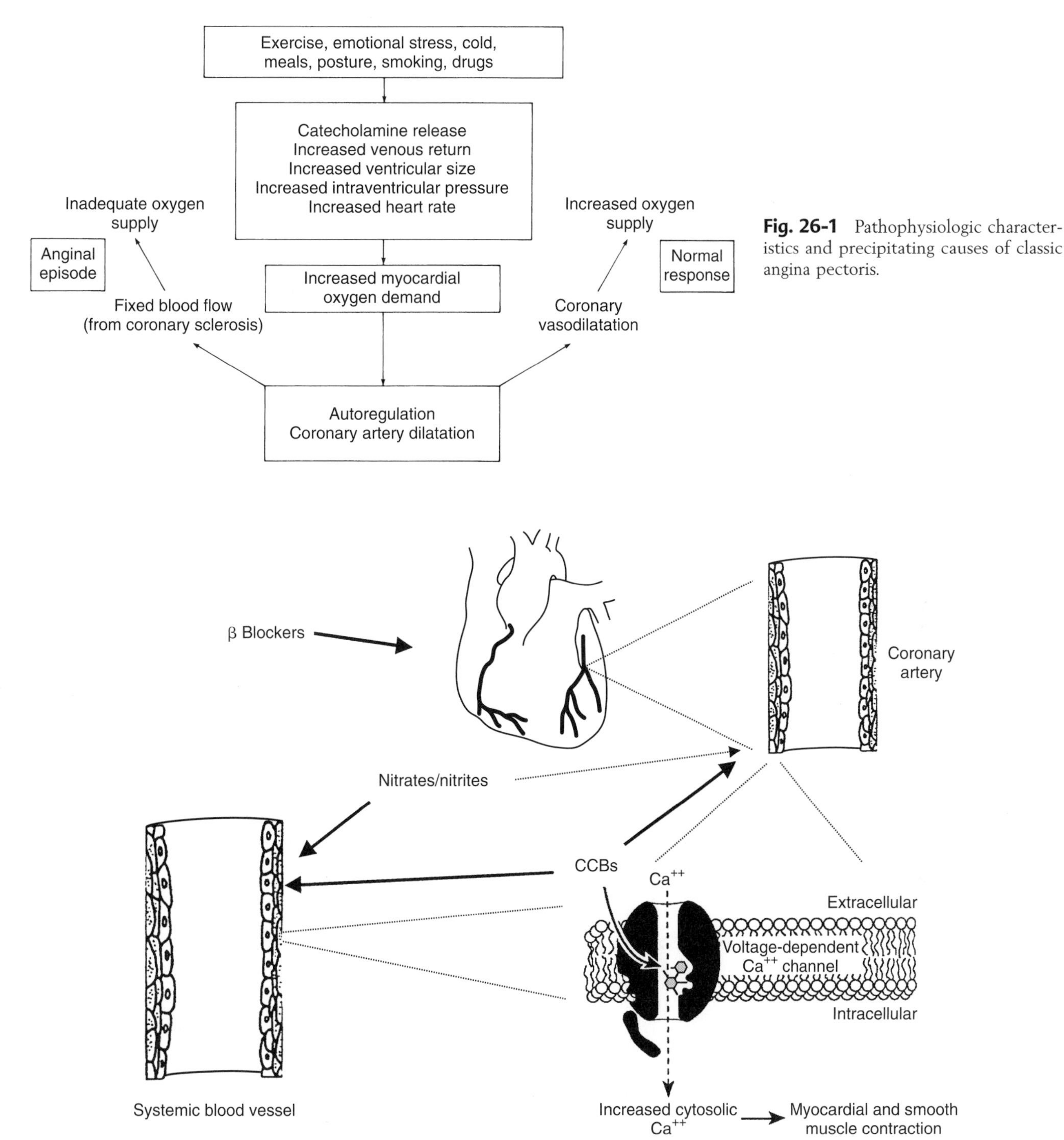

Fig. 26-1 Pathophysiologic characteristics and precipitating causes of classic angina pectoris.

Fig. 26-2 Sites of action of the β-adrenergic receptor blockers, the CCBs, and the nitrates/nitrites. β Blockers reduce the rate and contractility of the heart, thereby reducing energy and oxygen demand of the heart. CCBs reduce vasoconstriction in coronary and noncoronary vessels, increasing coronary blood flow and reducing cardiac load. The nitrates/nitrites act primarily on systemic blood vessels to reduce cardiac load. The effect on coronary arteries is less a factor in alleviating classic angina but plays a major role in variant angina. Three anatomic levels are shown: cardiac anatomy, cell layers of the blood vessel walls, and a blood vessel smooth muscle cell membrane showing a Ca^{++} channel and the effect of CCBs in preventing Ca^{++} entry.

A fourth group of drugs targets blood-clotting mechanisms and is represented by aspirin and the anticoagulants. Aspirin is used in treating stable and unstable angina. The pharmacologic features of aspirin are examined in Chapter 21. It acts by inhibiting platelet aggregation through irreversible inhibition of cyclooxygenase. Anticoagulants are discussed below.

A fifth class is represented by trimetazidine, which acts by other mechanisms. Trimetazidine is a novel antiischemic drug with properties unrelated to changes in myocardial

$H_2C-O-NO_2$
$HC-O-NO_2$
$H_2C-O-NO_2$
Nitroglycerin
(B, C, D, IV, O, S, T)

$H_2C-O-NO$
H_2C
$H_3C-CH-CH_3$
Amyl nitrite
(Inh)

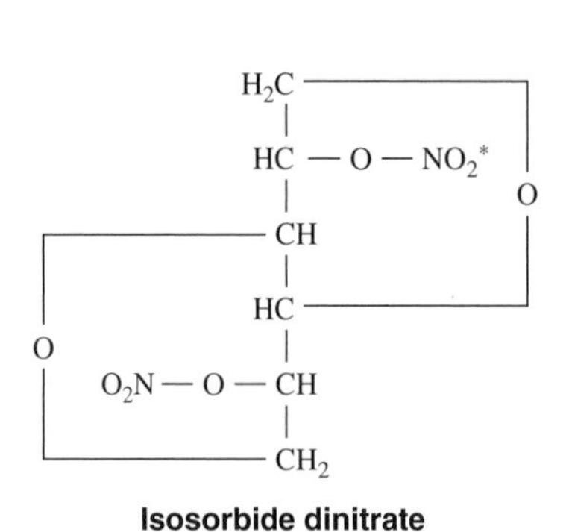

Isosorbide dinitrate
(C, T, TC, TO)

*The nitrate group is replaced by a hydrogen atom in **isosorbide mononitrate** (C, TO).

Fig. 26-3 Structural formulas and methods of administration of selected organic nitrates and amyl nitrite. *B,* Buccal (transmucosal) tablet; *C,* sustained-release capsule or tablet; *D,* transdermal disk; *Inh,* inhalant; *IV,* intravenous injection; *O,* ointment; *S,* lingual spray; *T,* sublingual tablet; *TC,* chewable tablet; *TO,* oral tablet or capsule.

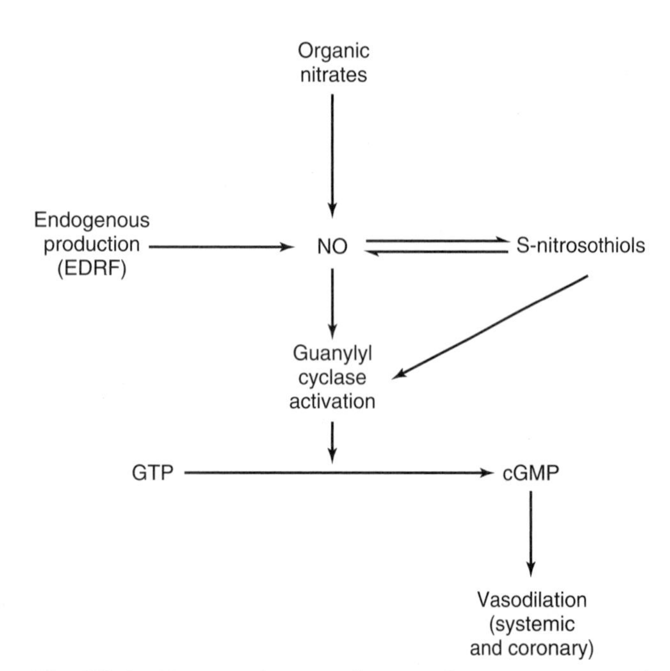

Fig. 26-4 Major mechanism of action of organic nitrates and nitrites. *EDRF,* Endothelium-derived relaxing factor; *GTP,* guanosine triphosphate.

oxygen supply/demand ratio.[4] Although the exact mechanism is unclear, several mechanisms of action are possible: correction of intracellular acidosis, reducing free radical production, and preventing Ca^{++} overload. In addition, it may have anti-inflammatory and antiplatelet effects. These actions cooperate to increase the rate of resynthesis of high energy phosphates within myocardial cells after episodes of ischemia. In several clinical trials, trimetazidine was tested as an antianginal agent; anginal attacks were reduced equally by trimetazidine and the CCB nifedipine, and exercise duration was increased by both treatments.[4] Trimetazidine is generally well tolerated and is associated with minor side effects.

NITRITES AND NITRATES

Amyl nitrite was introduced for use in angina pectoris in 1867, and nitroglycerin (glyceryl trinitrate) was introduced in 1879. Since then, nitroglycerin has remained the drug of choice for the relief of acute symptoms of angina pectoris. Nitroglycerin is administered sublingually as a tablet or aerosol spray and has a quick onset and short duration of action. Various organic nitrates and sustained-release forms of nitroglycerin have been developed in attempts to find a suitable, long-lasting preparation for the control and prevention of anginal pain. Amyl nitrite is used by inhalation for angina pectoris. Its use in the treatment of cyanide poisoning is discussed in Chapter 52.

Chemistry

Nitroglycerin is chemically a simple compound. Figure 26-3 shows its structure and, for comparison, the structures of some of the other organic nitrates marketed for oral, topical, sublingual, buccal, inhalant, or intravenous administration. All the nitrites and nitrates with antianginal activity are esters of nitric or nitrous acid, respectively. The organic nitrites and nitrates are capable of being metabolized to yield the free radical nitric oxide (NO). Research in this area led to the Nobel Prize for physiology/medicine being awarded in 1998 to Robert Furchgott, Louis Ignarro, and Ferid Murad for their discovery of NO as a signaling molecule in the cardiovascular system. NO is thought to be the active intermediate for this broad class of agents, which are appropriately referred to collectively as *nitrovasodilators*.

Pharmacologic Effects

The pharmacologic effects of all the members of this class are similar and are thought to result from actions of NO released by denitration reactions of the parent drugs in the tissues. NO has been shown to stimulate the synthesis of cyclic guanosine 3′,5′monophosphate (cGMP) by a direct action on cytosolic guanylyl cyclase or indirectly by being converted to S-nitrosothiols, which in turn stimulate the enzyme (Figure 26-4). The cGMP then initiates a cascade of reactions involving cGMP-dependent protein kinases leading to the various cellular responses. Previous studies had identified a vasodilator substance released from endothelial cells and referred to as *endothelium-derived relaxing factor.* Experimental evidence from several laboratories clearly indicates that endothelium-derived relaxing factor is either NO or a labile nitroso precursor of it.[16,19]

The most important action of the nitrovasodilators is the direct relaxation of vascular smooth muscle by the metabolite NO, resulting in vasodilation in nearly all vascular beds.[1,15] Nitroglycerin has been shown to cause varying degrees of change in coronary flow in normal and diseased mammalian hearts. Its efficacy in the various types of angina is attributed in part to a preferentially increased oxygen supply to ischemic areas, with variable actions on total coronary blood flow.[17] More importantly, through a reduction in venous tone, there is a reduction in venous pressure, pulmonary arterial pressure, and end-diastolic filling pressure. These actions lead to a decrease in ventricular volume, producing a fall in intramyocardial tension and therefore a drop in myocardial oxygen demand. Arterial smooth muscle is also relaxed by nitroglycerin, although to a lesser degree than is venous smooth muscle. The efficacy of organic nitrates in relieving variant angina probably stems from a direct alleviation of coronary artery spasm.

The nitrates and nitrites relax nonvascular smooth muscle but are largely devoid of actions on tissues other than smooth muscle. Thus bronchial, biliary, and gastrointestinal smooth muscle is relaxed. As is noted in the discussion of toxicity (see below), these actions are of little importance compared with the drugs' cardiovascular actions.

Absorption, Fate, and Excretion

Nitroglycerin is rapidly absorbed after sublingual administration (onset 1 to 3 minutes, duration 30 to 60 minutes). An advantage of the aerosol spray over the sublingual tablet is the better absorption in patients with dry mucous membranes. Nitroglycerin has a much slower onset when applied topically to the skin but has a comparably longer duration of action. Although organic nitrates administered orally are readily absorbed, they are extensively metabolized during the first pass through the liver.

In addition to undergoing denitration reactions in tissues, nitrates are metabolized in the liver by glutathione–organic nitrate reductase. The products of hepatic biotransformation, including the released nitrite ions, are much less effective than the parent compound; they are subsequently excreted in the urine, at least in part, in the form of glucuronide conjugates. Isosorbide dinitrate is exceptional in that its principal metabolite, the mononitrate, is responsible for the majority of its action and is now available separately for clinical use.

Long-Acting Drugs

Although sublingual nitroglycerin is highly effective for the treatment of acute anginal episodes, its short duration of action makes it ill suited for long-term prophylaxis. Several nitrates formulated for oral administration have been marketed for many years for the prevention of anginal attacks. The vasodilatory effects of isosorbide dinitrate were discovered in the 1930s, and the drug was introduced in the 1960s as an oral preparation. When administered sublingually, isosorbide dinitrate, one of the most promising long-lasting agents (see Figure 26-3), was shown to be comparable to nitroglycerin. Unfortunately, when administered orally in recommended dosages, this compound offered no protection against exercise-induced angina. Subsequent investigations showed, however, that large doses of isosorbide dinitrate (and nitroglycerin also) do, in fact, improve exercise tolerance in patients with angina.[22] There is, of course, a concomitantly increased possibility of drug toxicity. Newer long-acting mononitrates, which are major active metabolites of isosorbide dinitrate, offer the advantage of improved bioavailability because they avoid first-pass hepatic elimination. Isosorbide-5-mononitrate, which is at least as effective as isosorbide dinitrate, is available both as immediate-release tablets and as a sustained-release formulation for once-daily administration. The clinical efficacy of a single dose of isosorbide mononitrate formulated as a 30% immediate release/70% sustained release formulation is observed within a few minutes to increase work and exercise capacity.[3] Recent evidence indicates that nitrates reduce platelet aggregation and adhesion in patients with acute myocardial infarction. This suggests a possible added benefit of nitrates.[12]

To avoid the first-pass phenomenon that plagues the orally administered nitrates, nitroglycerin has been prepared in several other forms. The first of these, nitroglycerin ointment, is effective prophylactically but it must be administered every 3 to 4 hours. A further development is the nitroglycerin transdermal system, which comes in the form of an adhesive patch. When applied to the skin, the transdermal patch slowly releases nitroglycerin over a 24-hour period. This system minimizes the potential for toxicity inherent in large-dose oral administration, and it overcomes the inconvenience and frequency of application associated with the ointment. Nitroglycerin is also marketed in a transmucosal preparation. Supplied in a matrix, the drug is made available in a sustained-release fashion when placed between the upper lip and teeth. Swallowing or chewing increases the rate of absorption and could lead to toxicity. The advantages of this preparation are its rapid onset and extended action.

One problem shared by all the long-acting preparations is the development of tolerance. In vitro studies suggest that the cause is a diminished responsiveness of peripheral tissues to the nitrates, caused in turn by cellular thiol group depletion and/or indirect stimulation of salt and water retention.[26] Such tolerance is not observed with the intermittent administration of sublingual nitroglycerin. Intermittent transdermal administration (12 hours on, 12 hours off) has been used to avoid the development of tolerance; however, questions still remain concerning the increased risk of precipitating unstable angina and/or myocardial infarction during the non-treated periods, especially if they occur during the early morning hours.[9] Under certain conditions, N-acetylcysteine, which is a thiol donor, can protect against or reverse nitrate intolerance.[20]

Nitrates have a place in the prophylactic treatment of patients with angina pectoris because their efficacy is not in doubt. However, there are some practical problems associated with their use, such as unreliable absorption, short duration of action, treatment-induced headache, development of nitrate tolerance, and a suggested rebound phenomenon observed during intermittent dosing. Patient convenience regarding the treatment schedule should also be considered. The development of controlled-release formulations that produce sufficiently high nitrate concentrations during part of the day, followed by nitrate-poor rather than nitrate-free intervals, have the potential to prevent both tolerance and rebound phenomena and to produce a sufficiently long duration of action with a convenient once-daily regimen.[20] The combination of both immediate and sustained-release formulations, used once daily, produce a fast onset of action and then a longer period during which nitrate concentrations are sufficient to prevent ischemia during the active part of the day.[3] During the night, nitrate levels fall but offer some protection with low risk of tolerance.

Adverse Effects

Almost all side effects of these drugs are direct results of their effects on the cardiovascular system. Headache is the most common untoward response and can be very severe. Tolerance to this effect may develop in some patients before tolerance to other cardiovascular effects occurs. Orthostatic hypotension resulting in reflex tachycardia, cerebral ischemia, weakness, dizziness, flushing, and syncope may follow drug administration. Syncope is very likely to occur if the patient is standing and immobile while taking medication or has ingested alcoholic beverages. Nitrates should not be administered to a patient taking sildenafil (Viagra) because severe and long-lasting hypotension may occur. Significant hypotension may even cause anginal pain if coronary blood flow is compromised. Because it dramatically reduces placental blood flow, amyl nitrite is contraindicated for use in pregnant women (pregnancy risk category X, see Table 3-7).

Nitrite ions and high doses of nitrates readily oxidize hemoglobin to methemoglobin; large amounts of methemoglobin can seriously impair the oxygen-carrying capacity of the blood, resulting in anemic hypoxia. Infants are especially sensitive to this effect of nitrates because of their relative inability to reduce methemoglobin back to hemoglobin. Drug rash may occasionally occur, most frequently with pentaerythritol tetranitrate and topical nitroglycerin.

β-ADRENERGIC BLOCKING DRUGS

The history and pharmacology of β-blocking agents are reviewed in depth in Chapter 7. In addition, the use of these compounds in the treatment of cardiac arrhythmias and hypertension is discussed in Chapters 24 and 28, respectively. Consideration here is limited to the role that these drugs play in the management of angina pectoris.

An increasing number of β blockers are available for use in the treatment of angina pectoris. All these drugs, whether or not they have partial agonist activity, membrane-stabilizing actions, or general or selective β-blocking properties, can increase the pain-free work capacity of patients with angina pectoris. Some of the most frequently used agents for this purpose include propranolol, metoprolol, atenolol, and nadolol. Selection of β blockers will depend on other clinical factors. Cardioselective agents are of advantage in patients who have pulmonary disease or peripheral vascular disease. However, consideration must be given to the dosage used because all β-blocking drugs have nonselective effects at higher dosages (see Chapter 7).

Pharmacologic Effects

Because exercise and emotional stress are possible precipitating factors in angina (see Figure 26-1), increases in sympathetic nervous system activity can bring on attacks of angina in susceptible persons. Thus the blockade of adrenergic responses can be of benefit in the treatment of this condition.[13] The effects of β blockers that are helpful in treating angina include decreased heart rate and protection from reflex tachycardia, depressed myocardial contractility, decreased cardiac output, and, in some cases, reduced blood pressure. These effects are more prominent when sympathetic activity is elevated, such as during exercise or emotional stress. Total coronary blood flow may actually be reduced after β-receptor blockade, but this reduction in flow seems to be in well-perfused areas and thus is not detrimental in classic angina. Drug-induced vasoconstriction (from unopposed α-receptor activity), however, may be problematic in patients with variant angina.

The beneficial effect of β-receptor–blocking drugs in angina probably results from their common action: blockade of cardiac β-adrenergic receptors. Even though exercise tolerance is improved with β-adrenergic blockade and changes in heart rate and blood pressure with exercise are blunted, the rate-pressure product (heart rate multiplied by the systolic arterial pressure) at which pain occurs is decreased. This finding explains why exercise tolerance is increased less than might be expected on the basis of simple single cardiovascular measurements.

Absorption, Fate, and Excretion

The absorption, fate, and excretion of β-adrenergic antagonists are discussed in Chapter 7.

Use in Treatment of Angina

As mentioned previously, most β blockers are effective in treating the various types of angina pectoris. Their use is, however, questionable in the management of variant angina in the absence of other drugs. Long-term administration of β blockers can make the attacks of angina less frequent and individual attacks less severe. Nonetheless, patients receiving long-term treatment with β-blocking agents usually still require nitroglycerin for the treatment of acute anginal attacks. This combined drug therapy with a β-adrenergic antagonist and nitroglycerin or a related drug works well because the drugs have different mechanisms of action. Additionally, nitrates and β-adrenergic antagonists may work especially well together in angina because β blockers inhibit the reflex tachycardia caused by nitrates and because nitrates (by causing vasodilation) reduce the preload and afterload of the heart and tend to reduce the impact of a negative inotropic effect from β-receptor blockade.[8]

Adverse Effects

As mentioned in Chapter 7, blockade of β receptors may cause bronchoconstriction or prevent the normal response to insulin-produced hypoglycemia in susceptible patients. These problems are less severe with the more selective β_1 blockers, such as metoprolol, which have been used without serious adverse effects in some patients with bronchospastic disease. It should be remembered, however, that drugs such as metoprolol are β_1 selective, not β_1 specific, and therefore are capable of eliciting bronchospasm in susceptible patients. Because of the association between β_2-adrenergic receptors and glycogenolysis and gluconeogenesis in the liver, β_1-selective blockers are associated with less risk of hypoglycemic reactions in diabetics than are the nonselective β-receptor blockers. A problem encountered with both selective and nonselective blockers, since they are related to the inhibition of cardiac β receptors, is that severe myocardial depression and heart failure may occur if initial dosages are too high or if there is concomitant myocardial incompetence (see Chapter 25 for a discussion of the use of β blockers in the treatment of heart failure). For this reason, dosages should be gradually increased until concentrations offering therapeutic effects in the management of angina are reached. The sudden discontinuance of β blockers has been implicated with rebound overstimulation of the heart, worsening of angina, and myocardial infarction.

Ca^{++} CHANNEL BLOCKERS

CCBs are also referred to as *Ca^{++} entry blockers* and, less accurately, as *Ca^{++} antagonists.* These drugs exert their effect on voltage-dependent Ca^{++} channels in vascular smooth muscle and cardiac muscle (see Figure 26-2). This class of drugs (Figure 26-5) includes verapamil, nifedipine, diltiazem, and several other agents. Many of these compounds have been shown to be effective in the prophylactic treatment of chronic stable exertional angina, variant angina, and unstable angina. They have also proved to be useful in the treatment of other cardiovascular disorders such as supraventricular tachyarrhythmias and hypertension (see Chapters 24 and 28). Additional indications for certain CCBs include peripheral

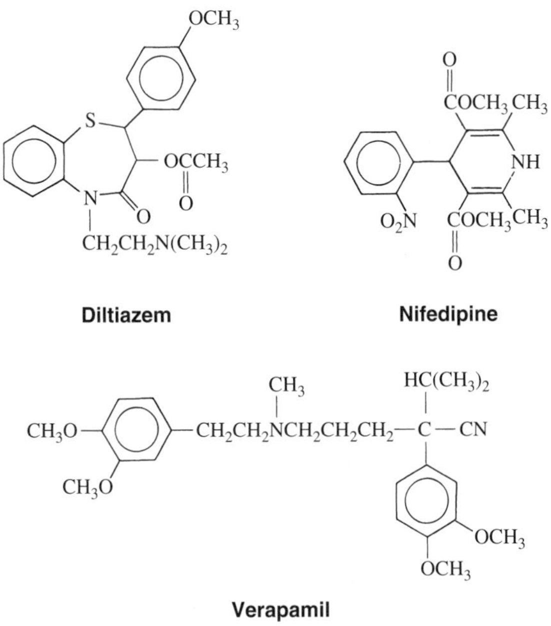

Diltiazem **Nifedipine**

Verapamil

Fig. 26-5 Structural formulas of some CCBs.

Box • 26-1

Cardiovascular Responses to Inhibition of Transmembrane Ca^{++} Influx by CCBs

Myocardium
Excitation-contraction uncoupling
Prevention of Ca^{++} overload

Specialized Pacemaker and Conducting Tissues
Reduction of automaticity
Damping of ectopic pacemakers
Inhibition of reentrant pathways

Vasculature
Vasodilation
Protection against Ca^{++} deposition in vessel walls

vascular disease, hypertrophic cardiomyopathy, and cerebral vasospasm after subarachnoid hemorrhage.[14]

Chemistry and Classification

Verapamil, the first CCB, is a diphenylalkylamine derivative. The only member of its type clinically available, verapamil is closest in pharmacologic profile to diltiazem, a benzothiazepine. The largest category of CCBs consists of the dihydropyridines, of which nifedipine is the prototype. The dihydropyridines are characterized by their prominent arterial vasodilatory properties and relative lack of direct cardiac actions. Bepridil, chemically unrelated to the aforementioned CCBs, like verapamil and diltiazem, is less selective in its action.

Pharmacologic Effects

CCBs exert their primary action on Ca^{++} channels that carry the slow inward Ca^{++} current. The CCBs thus differ from local anesthetics, which are primarily fast-channel blockers inhibiting the rapid inward influx of Na^{+}. Although the primary action of the CCBs is on the slow current, they may also act through other mechanisms. For example, diltiazem, especially at higher doses, has been shown to depress the Na^{+} or fast channels. Bepridil is especially noteworthy in its local anestheticlike inhibition of Na^{+} channels.

Some of the diverse effects of the CCBs can be explained by the roles that Ca^{++} and slow channels have in different cardiovascular cell types (Box 26-1). For instance, in the sinus and atrioventricular (AV) nodes, slow channels are the primary conduit for the generation and propagation of action potentials. They may additionally be involved in regulating sinus node automaticity by altering diastolic depolarization. Ca^{++} channels also govern conduction velocity in the AV node. The actions of CCBs as antiarrhythmics are discussed in Chapter 24.

The CCBs directly and preferentially block voltage-dependent Ca^{++} channels as opposed to receptor-operated channels. By this mechanism, they lower intracellular Ca^{++} activity and interfere with the replenishment of Ca^{++} stores in vascular smooth muscle. Both tonic and phasic muscle contractions are depressed in a dose-dependent manner. The major types of voltage-dependent Ca^{++} channels are designated *L*, *N*, and *T*. Only the L (large, long-lasting current) channel is inhibited by the CCBs. Verapamil, diltiazem, and the nifedipinelike CCBs apparently bind to different receptor sites on the L channel. The degree of binding is influenced by the functional state of the channel (resting, open, or inactivated) in a manner similar to the use dependency described for local anesthetics and Na^{+} channels (see Chapter 16). A CCB of one chemical classification can also affect the binding of another, positively or negatively, through allosteric mechanisms.

CCBs induce both coronary and peripheral arterial dilation. Their action on coronary vessels is especially prominent in those vessels that undergo transient vasospasm in variant angina. The vasodilator action in large measure explains their use as antianginals and antihypertensives.

Although all CCBs directly depress the myocardium and slow conduction velocity in the heart, the overall response in vivo depends on the relative mix of direct and indirect effects of each drug on the cardiovascular system. For verapamil and diltiazem, the direct cardiac effects usually predominate (Table 26-1). Nifedipine, however, typically elicits prominent vasodilation at doses that do not greatly affect Ca^{++} channels in the heart. Reflex sympathetic activity then causes an increase in heart rate and conduction through the AV node and may result in a net positive inotropic effect. Factors that contribute variety to the pharmacologic profile of the different CCBs include the drugs' binding dependence on stimulation frequency, their binding characteristics to L channels in different tissues, and, at least with some agents, their ability to influence other voltage-gated ion channels.

The CCBs are important drugs in the treatment of all forms of angina pectoris. They inhibit Ca^{++} flux in cardiac and smooth muscle[5] and are effective in the treatment of stable angina because of their coronary vasodilator effect, negative inotropic and chronotropic effects, enhancement of diastolic relaxation of the left ventricle, and hypotensive effect mediated through peripheral arterial dilation.[27] These effects lead to an increase in coronary blood flow and myocardial perfusion with a decrease in myocardial oxygen demand.

Absorption, Fate, and Excretion

All the CCBs are rapidly and almost completely absorbed after oral administration. Bioavailability is reduced, however, by extensive first-pass hepatic metabolism. To extend their duration of action, many of the CCBs are marketed in

Table • 26-1

Comparative Pharmacologic Effects of Ca^{++}-Channel Blockers

PARAMETER	VERAPAMIL	DILTIAZEM	NIFEDIPINE	NIMODIPINE	BEPRIDIL
Heart rate	↑, ↓	0, ↓	↑	0	↓
Sinoatrial node automaticity	↓↓	↓↓	0, ↓	0, ↓	↓
AV conduction	↓↓↓	↓↓	0	0	↓
Myocardial contractility	↓↓	↓	↓*	0	↓
Cardiac output	↑, ↓	0, ↑	↑↑	0	0
Peripheral vascular resistance	↓↓	↓	↓↓↓	↓	↓
Coronary vasodilation	↑↑	↑↑	↑↑↑	↑↑	0
Cerebral vasodilation	↑	↑	↑	↑↑↑	—

*The direct myocardial depression of nifedipine is reversed clinically by the hemodynamic effects of vasodilation.
0, No effect; *↑*, slight increase; *↑↑*, moderate increase; *↑↑↑*, strong increase; *↓*, slight decrease; *↓↓*, moderate decrease; *↓↓↓*, strong decrease.

sustained-release formulations. Verapamil and diltiazem are converted in part to active metabolites; biotransformation of nifedipine causes complete inactivation. Most CCBs are highly protein bound, especially to plasma albumin. Excretion of the metabolites is primarily by the kidney.

Use in the Treatment of Angina

The CCBs as a class have been shown to be effective in the treatment of all types of angina regardless of whether coronary spasm is involved.[21] They seem to be especially effective, however, in preventing coronary vasospasm. In chronic stable exertional angina, CCBs may afford relief of pain through one or more mechanisms: coronary and peripheral vasodilation, attenuation of increased heart rate caused by exercise, and/or a negative inotropic effect on the heart.[8]

Adverse Effects

The toxicity of the CCBs varies with the individual agent; however, there are some side effects common to this class of drugs. These side effects include dizziness, headache, and nausea and those related to systemic vasodilation: sensation of heat, facial flushing, hypotension, reflex tachycardia (primarily with nifedipine), and peripheral edema. Verapamil is the most likely, and nifedipinelike drugs the least likely, to reduce myocardial contractility. Both verapamil and diltiazem usually lead to a net decrease in conduction through the AV node. Fortunately, myocardial depression and reduction of AV conduction are rarely a problem clinically with these agents, unless predisposing factors exist.[8] Coadministration with a β-adrenergic antagonist may also lead to a deterioration in cardiac performance,[23] especially when verapamil is used in a patient with abnormal AV conduction. On the other hand, nifedipine and other dihydropyridines, which can reflexly increase AV conduction velocity, are often used to advantage in combination with β-receptor blockers because of their complementary actions. Bepridil is more likely than other CCBs to cause potentially life-threatening arrhythmias such as torsades de pointes. Bepridil also may cause agranulocytosis, and the drug should be used only when safer agents prove ineffective.

The abrupt vasodilation caused by short-acting CCBs may lead to myocardial ischemia. This is especially the case for dihydropyridines such as nifedipine, which have a greater net effect on blood vessels compared with the myocardium. The peripheral vasodilation can significantly reduce coronary blood flow, causing a condition known as *coronary steal.* An increased incidence of a heart attack and sudden death may result, and therefore short-acting dihydropyridines should not be used for angina therapy. Long-acting agents, including slow-release formulations of nifedipine, are now recommended for the treatment of hypertension. It is also for this reason that verapamil and diltiazem are preferred over the dihydropyridines for the treatment of angina.

Drug-induced gingival hyperplasia has been reported during long-term therapy with verapamil, diltiazem, nifedipine, and felodipine. Clinically and histologically, the hyperplasia seen with CCBs resembles that previously described for phenytoin (see Chapter 14) but seems to occur less frequently with the CCBs.[6]

COMBINATION THERAPY

Combination therapy is indicated for the patient who becomes intolerant or continues to have angina with an optimal dosage of a single medication. The rationale for combining a nitrate and a β-adrenergic blocking drug has been previously discussed. Furthermore, if monotherapy fails, nitrates may be used in combination with diltiazem or verapamil, and a β-adrenergic blocking agent may be used with nifedipine. Trimetazidine has also been tested as an antianginal in combination with classic antiischemic compounds. In patients treated with nifedipine, the addition of trimetazidine was able to reduce the number and duration of anginal attacks and also improved exercise capacity.[4] Although combination therapy may be beneficial, consideration must be given to the potential for a higher incidence of untoward effects.

PREVENTION OF MYOCARDIAL INFARCTION

The use of drugs to prevent myocardial infarction (especially reinfarction) has received considerable attention in recent years. In addition to the drugs already discussed, the following classes of drugs are used for this purpose: antiplatelet drugs, cholesterol-lowering drugs, angiotensin-converting enzyme inhibitors, and anticoagulants. Because β blockers have been consistently shown to have a benefit in reducing sudden death in patients with unstable angina, they are now discussed further in this context.

The primary action of β blockers is to inhibit the effects of sympathetic stimulation on the heart. The result is a reduction in heart rate, arterial blood pressure, and the force of myocardial contraction, both at rest and during exercise. These changes reduce the overall myocardial oxygen requirement and in turn limit the intensity, extent, and duration of myocardial ischemia. The combination of the antiarrhythmic and antiischemic actions of β blockers has been shown to have a favorable effect on survival rate after myocardial infarction.

Antiplatelet agents are a much more heterogeneous group than β-adrenergic blockers. These agents have been subclassified as first-generation (aspirin, sulfinpyrazone, and dipyridamole) and second-generation (prostacyclin, prostaglandin E_1, and thromboxane synthase inhibitors) drugs.[28] The first-generation antiplatelet drugs act by the following mechanisms: aspirin, through irreversible inactivation of cyclooxygenase; sulfinpyrazone, through competitive inhibition of cyclooxygenase; and dipyridamole, through phosphodiesterase inhibition or inhibition of adenosine uptake by blockade of adenosine A_2 receptors. These agents have varying effects on platelet aggregation, bleeding time, and platelet survival. The evidence overall indicates a favorable response to the first-generation antiplatelet agents. Aspirin, for example, is effective in reducing the occurrence of myocardial infarction in patients with ischemic heart disease. Furthermore, aspirin can reduce the incidence of transient ischemic attacks in patients with cerebral vascular disease. Dipyridamole is currently used with warfarin in prophylaxis against thromboembolism in patients with prosthetic heart valves. Its mechanism is reduction of platelet aggregation and adhesion by increasing platelet cyclic 3′,5′-adenosine monophosphate and lowering platelet Ca^{++}. Dipyridamole is also a coronary vasodilator that exerts little action on peripheral blood vessels. It seems to act primarily on small cardiac arterioles[24] and is used in certain cardiac imaging procedures. Dipyridamole does not prevent or alleviate anginal attacks, probably because in ischemic areas of the heart near-maximal coronary vasodilation has already occurred. Thus dipyridamole has little additional effect on vasodilation and does not increase collateral blood flow to ischemic areas.

Evidence supporting the efficacy of the second-generation antiplatelet agents is lacking at this time; future studies are needed to determine the worth of these agents or similar drugs in the prevention of myocardial infarction. Ticlopidine, however, a recently marketed thienopyridine antiplatelet drug, has been shown to be at least as effective as aspirin in preventing strokes in a group of patients known to be susceptible to stroke. The drug irreversibly inhibits platelet-fibrinogen binding by inhibiting the effect of adenosine diphosphate on platelets and preventing synthesis of receptors important in aggregation. Unfortunately, ticlopidine may induce life-threatening blood dyscrasias (neutropenia, agranulocytosis). A newer drug of this class, clopidogrel, is less toxic and has use as an aspirin substitute in unstable angina.

Abciximab, a newer antiplatelet agent, is the Fab fragment of a chimeric human-murine monoclonal antibody that binds to glycoprotein (GPIIb/IIIa) receptors on human platelets.[11] This prevents binding of fibrinogen and other aggregating molecules. The drug must be given intravenously. Abciximab reduces the incidence of stroke and death during percutaneous transluminal coronary angioplasty or atherectomy. Bleeding is the most common adverse reaction.[25] Tirofiban and eptifibatide are two other drugs used clinically that are GPIIb/IIIa inhibitors. All three inhibitors are injected. Studies with oral GPIIb/IIIa receptor inhibitors have not been promising.

Epoprostenol is the nonproprietary name assigned to prostacyclin. Given by long-term intravenous infusion, epoprostenol is beneficial for patients with pulmonary hypertension because it causes vasodilation by stimulating prostacyclin (PGI_2) receptors. Epoprostenol inhibits platelet aggregation by stimulating PGI_2 receptors on platelets and activating adenylyl cyclase.

Anticoagulants are discussed in Chapter 31. Heparin, including low molecular weight heparins, is used in unstable angina[2,29]; however, the benefit of warfarin in this setting is not clearly established. Cholesterol-lowering drugs,[31] particularly the statins, are also used to prevent myocardial infarction and coronary artery disease on a long-term basis. This drug class is discussed in Chapter 29. Angiotensin-converting enzyme inhibitors have a beneficial role in that they reduce the risk of myocardial infarction and stroke.[7] They are discussed in Chapters 25 and 28.

IMPLICATIONS FOR DENTISTRY

It has been stated that anginal attacks can be precipitated by physical or emotional stress. Because these situations often arise in the dental operatory, dentists must be aware of the symptoms and treatment of angina. A complete medical history will reveal whether a patient is being treated for angina. If so, the dentist should ensure that the patient has medication (e.g., nitroglycerin) available before a procedure is performed. The patient will know when an attack is imminent; for ready access, the patient's medication may be placed on a nearby tray or counter. Also, nitroglycerin or amyl nitrite should be included on the emergency tray. Although nitroglycerin tablets are now stabilized against breakdown, unused tablets should be discarded 6 months after the original bottle has been opened. The patient should be medicated in a sitting or supine position because standing may lead to hypotension and syncope. In most cases, anginal pain subsides rapidly (2 to 3 minutes), and the patient may have a headache and/or a stinging sensation under the tongue. As a precaution, patients should be treated carefully, be fully informed about the procedure, and, if they feel it necessary, be given prophylactic medication. Preoperative sedation may be helpful and is not contraindicated if significant cardiovascular depression is avoided.

Because the β-adrenergic blocking drugs are cardiac depressants, any drugs that might cause further depression of cardiac function should be used with caution. Conversely, the use of epinephrine in gingival retraction cord is contraindicated because the unopposed vasoconstriction in the presence of nonselective β-adrenergic blockers is more likely to cause hypertension. Similar considerations dictate prudence with, though not necessarily avoidance of, local anesthetics with adrenergic vasoconstrictors. In reference to the CCBs, orthostatic hypotension might be a problem, but cardiac depression is not usually clinically significant. Sensations of heat or facial flushing may be evident in these patients.

As previously mentioned, gingival inflammation and overgrowth occasionally develop in patients as a result of therapy with CCBs, especially when taken concurrently with other agents that promote gingival hyperplasia (phenytoin, cyclosporine). Strict oral hygiene measures, including regular dental prophylaxis, may minimize this problem.

CITED REFERENCES

1. Abrams J: Interactions between organic nitrates and thiol groups, *Am J Med* 91:106s-112s, 1991.
2. Antman EM, McCabe CH, Gurfinkel EP, et al: Enoxaparin prevents death and cardiac ischemic events in unstable angina/non-Q-wave myocardial infarction. Results of the thrombolysis in myocardial infarction (TIMI) 11B trial, *Circulation* 100:1593-1601, 1999.

Drugs Used in the Treatment of Angina Pectoris

Nonproprietary (generic) name	*Proprietary (trade) name*
Nitrates and nitrites	
Amyl nitrite	—
Isosorbide dinitrate	Isordil, Sorbitrate
Isosorbide mononitrate	ISMO, Imdur, Monoket
Nitroglycerin	Nitro-Bid, Nitro disc, Nitro-Dur, Nitrol, Nitrolingual, Nitrostat, Transderm-Nitro
β-Adrenergic blocking drugs	
Atenolol	Tenormin
Carvedilol	Coreg
Metoprolol	Lopressor, Toprol XL
Nadolol	Corgard
Propranolol	Inderal
Timolol	Blocadren
CCBs	
Amlodipine	Norvasc
Bepridil	Vascor
Diltiazem	Cardizem, Dilacor XR
Felodipine	Plendil
Isradipine	DynaCirc
Nicardipine	Cardene
Nifedipine	Adalat, Procardia
Nimodipine	Nimotop
Nisoldipine	Sular
Verapamil	Calan, Isoptin, Verelan
Antiplatelet agents	
Abciximab	ReoPro
Alprostadil (prostaglandin E_1)	Prostin VR Pediatric
Aspirin	—
Clopidogrel	Plavix
Dipyridamole	Persantine
Epoprostenol (prostacyclin)	Flolan
Eptifibatide	Integrilin
Sulfinpyrazone	Anturane
Ticlopidine	Ticlid
Tirofiban	Aggrastat
Cholesterol-lowering drugs	
See Chapter 29	
Other drugs	
Trimetazidine*	Vastarel
Fibrinolytics	
See Chapter 31	

*Not available in the United States.

3. Arthur RM, Mehmel H: A sustained release formulation of isosorbide-5-mononitrate with a rapid onset of action, *Int J Clin Pract* 53:205-212, 1999.
4. Belardinelli R: Trimetazidine and the contractile response of dysfunctional myocardium in ischaemic cardiomyopathy, *Rev Port Cardiol* 5:V35-V39, 2000.
5. Braunwald E: Mechanism of action of calcium-channel-blocking agents, *N Engl J Med* 307:1618-1623, 1982.
6. Butler RT, Kalkwarf KL, Kaldahl WB: Drug-induced gingival hyperplasia: phenytoin, cyclosporine, and nifedipine, *J Am Dent Assoc* 114:56-60, 1987.
7. Farmer JA: Renin angiotensin system and ASCVD, *Curr Opin Cardiol* 15:141-150, 2000.
8. Flaim SF, Zelis R: Clinical use of calcium entry blockers, *Fed Proc* 40:2877-2881, 1981.
9. Fletcher A: Transdermal nitroglycerin. Does it really work in the treatment of angina? *Drugs Aging* 1:6-16, 1991.
10. Fleury J: Long-term management of the patient with stable angina, *Nurs Clin North Am* 27:205-230, 1992.
11. Frishman WH, Burns B, Atac B, et al: Novel antiplatelet therapies for treatment of patients with ischemic heart disease: inhibitors of the platelet glycoprotein IIb/IIIa integrin receptor, *Am Heart J* 130:877-892, 1995.
12. Gebalska J, Wolk R, Ceremuzynski L: Isosorbide dinitrate inhibits platelet adhesion and aggregation in nonthrombolyzed patients with acute myocardial infarction, *Clin Cardiol* 23:837-841, 2000.
13. Heidenreich PA, McDonald KM, Hastie T, et al: Meta-analysis of trials comparing β-blockers, calcium antagonists, and nitrates for stable angina, *JAMA* 281:1927-1936, 1999.
14. Hope RR, Lazzara R: The clinical uses of calcium antagonists, *Adv Intern Med* 27:435-452, 1982.
15. Horowitz JD: Thiol-containing agents in the management of unstable angina pectoris and acute myocardial infarction, *Am J Med* 91:113s-117s, 1991.
16. Ignarro LJ: Biosynthesis and metabolism of endothelium-derived nitric oxide, *Annu Rev Pharmacol Toxicol* 30:535-560, 1990.
17. Kay HB: Angina pectoris: getting the most from drug therapy, *Drugs* 13:276-287, 1977.
18. Mishra B, Jackson G: Unstable angina: a review and practical guide to management, *Int J Clin Pract* 53:530-534, 1999.
19. Moncada S, Radomski MW, Palmer RM: Endothelium-derived relaxing factor. Identification as nitric oxide and role in the control of vascular tone and platelet function, *Biochem Pharmacol* 37:2495-2501, 1988.
20. Olsson G, Allgen J: Prophylactic nitrate therapy in angina pectoris—is there an optimal treatment regimen? *Br J Clin Pharmacol* 34:19s-23s, 1992.
21. Opie LH, Yusuf S, Kubler W: Current status of safety and efficacy of calcium channel blockers in cardiovascular diseases: a critical analysis based on 100 studies, *Prog Cardiovasc Dis* 43:171-196, 2000.
22. Oral isosorbide dinitrate for angina, *Med Lett Drugs Ther* 21:88, 1979.
23. Packer M: Combined beta-adrenergic and calcium-entry blockade in angina pectoris, *N Engl J Med* 320:709-718, 1989.

24. Riley TN: Antianginal agents. In Verderame M, ed: *CRC handbook of cardiovascular and anti-inflammatory agents,* Boca Raton, FL, 1986, CRC Press.

25. Roe MT, Sapp SK, Lincoff AM: Glycoprotein IIb/IIIa inhibitors in acute coronary syndromes, *Cleve Clin J Med* 67:131-140, 2000.

26. Rutherford JD: Nitrate tolerance in angina therapy. How to avoid it, *Drugs* 49:196-199, 1995.

27. Rutherford JD, Braunwald E: Chronic ischemic heart disease. In Braunwald E, ed: *Heart disease: a textbook of cardiovascular medicine,* Philadelphia, 1992, WB Saunders.

28. Sherry S: Platelet inhibitors and myocardial infarction. In Kostis JB, DeFelice EA, eds: *The pharmacological treatment of cardiovascular diseases,* New York, 1986, Elsevier Science.

29. Xiao Z, Theroux P: Platelet activation with unfractionated heparin at therapeutic concentrations and comparisons with a low-molecular-weight heparin and with a direct thrombin inhibitor, *Circulation* 97:251-256, 1998.

30. Yeghiazarians Y, Braunstein JB, Askari A, et al: Unstable angina pectoris, *N Engl J Med* 342:101-114, 2000.

31. Zanger DR, Solomon AJ, Gersh BJ: Contemporary management of angina: part II. Medical managements of chronic stable angina, *Am Fam Physician* 61:129-138, 2000.

General References

Braunwald E, Antman EM, Beasley JW, et al: ACC/AHA guidelines for the management of patients with unstable angina and non-ST-segment elevation myocardial infarction: executive summary and recommendations. A report of the American College of Cardiology/American Heart Association task force on practice guidelines (committee on the management of patients with unstable angina), *Circulation* 102:1193-1209, 2000.

Cohn PF: Concomitant use of nitrates, calcium channel blockers, and β blockers for optimal antianginal therapy, *Clin Cardiol* 17:415-421, 1994.

Denktas AE, Bayes-Genis A, Schwartz RS: New approaches to the pharmacological treatment of angina, *Curr Opin Pharmacol* 1:151-158, 2001.

Weiner DA: Calcium antagonists in the treatment of ischemic heart disease: angina pectoris, *Coronary Artery Dis* 5:14-20, 1994.

Weitz JI, Bates SM: Beyond heparin and aspirin: new treatments for unstable angina and non-Q-wave myocardial infarction, *Arch Intern Med* 160:749-758, 2000.

Yusuf S, Sleight P, Pogue J, et al: Effects of an angiotensin-converting-enzyme inhibitor, ramipril, on cardiovascular events in high-risk patients. The Heart Outcomes Prevention Evaluation Study Investigators, *N Engl J Med* 342:145-153, 2000. [Errata in *N Engl J Med,* 342:748, 1376, 2000.]

CHAPTER • 27

Diuretic Drugs

William B. Jeffries and Dennis W. Wolff

The kidney serves the vital function of maintaining fluid and electrolyte homeostasis. Through the processes of glomerular filtration and selective tubular reabsorption and secretion, the kidney maintains plasma volume and the plasma concentration of electrolytes, glucose, amino acids, and other substances within tight physiologic limits while eliminating metabolic waste products and toxins. The kidneys filter approximately 180 L of plasma each day, one fifth of the cardiac output, producing approximately 1.5 L of urine.

The kidney therefore selectively reabsorbs approximately 99% of the filtered load of water and solute. Many of the filtered solutes are reabsorbed by specific transport proteins located on the luminal membrane of the nephron. Once inside of a nephron cell, solute movement back into the plasma is often directly or indirectly coupled to the actions of Na^+-K^+ activated adenosine triphosphatase (Na^+,K^+-ATPase) located on the basolateral surfaces of the nephron cells. Transepithelial electrochemical potential differences can also drive the reabsorption of various ions by paracellular pathways. The reabsorption of water in the kidney is passive, following osmotic gradients created by the movement of solutes along the nephrons to the extent permitted by the water permeability of the various segments of each nephron.[8] Water readily equilibrates across the nephron as solute is reabsorbed from the tubular fluid or in response to the medullary osmotic gradient as it descends toward the tip of the loop of Henle. However, the ascending portion of the nephron is relatively impermeable to water. The selective reabsorption of solute while trapping water in the lumen in these regions creates the dilute tubular fluid that could ultimately become maximally dilute urine. The solute selectively reabsorbed during the passage of tubular fluid through the ascending loop of Henle creates the medullary osmotic gradient that pulls water from the tubular fluid of the descending loop of Henle and the collecting duct. With the exception of the terminal portions of the collecting duct, where urea is recycled from concentrated urine, relatively little net solute reabsorption occurs in this nephron segment. Instead, this is the portion of the nephron that governs water reabsorption. Antidiuretic hormone (ADH, or vasopressin) determines the extent to which this segment is permeable to water.[18] If ADH is absent, the tubular fluid that reaches the collecting duct will, after some solute exchange, become the maximally dilute excreted urine. If the collecting duct is responding maximally to ADH, the most concentrated urine that the kidney can generate is excreted. This is because ADH makes collecting duct cells permeable to water, which permits passive water extraction from the tubular fluid as it passes through the progressively more concentrated osmotic gradient of the medullary interstitium. Although perhaps not immediately obvious, the more solute that reaches the collecting duct, the greater the volume of urine for any amount of ADH.

In a number of clinical conditions, renal function can become disturbed, producing metabolic abnormalities such as edema. Thus there is a therapeutic need for drugs that modulate renal function.

All the drugs discussed in this chapter affect renal function by inhibiting the reabsorptive capacity of the renal nephrons. This action produces an increase in the rate of urine production. Substances that increase the quantity of urine are called *diuretics.* Many substances produce this effect, including caffeine, alcohol, and even water itself; however, most of the clinically useful diuretics produce their effects by inhibiting Na^+ reabsorption by the nephrons.[8] Such drugs are properly called *natriuretics;* even so, in most circumstances all these drugs are referred to as *diuretics.* All clinically useful diuretics produce their effects by acting at specific segments of the nephron. Common conditions for which diuretics are used include essential hypertension and congestive heart failure.[3,13,15]

CLASSES OF DIURETICS

The discussion of these drugs will proceed up the nephron in a retrograde direction. From Figure 27-1, it is important to note that this takes us from diuretics with a low maximal effect to diuretics with a high maximal effect. Also note that the effects of blockade of Na^+ reabsorption upstream on tubular fluid composition are acted on by downstream mechanisms, mechanisms that act to limit or offset these effects. The discussion begins with the last major region of the nephron that influences net Na^+ excretion. The effects of the various classes of diuretics on urine volume, urine pH, and urine electrolytes are summarized in Table 27-1.

K^+-Sparing Diuretics

The pathway by which Na^+ is reabsorbed in the late distal tubule/cortical collecting duct is shown in Figure 27-2. The apical membrane of these cells contain Na^+ channels. The entry of Na^+ through these channels carries a net positive charge along with it (i.e., Na^+ entry is electrogenic), leaving the lumen with a net negative charge. This lumen-negative charge acts as a driving force for movement in the opposite direction of other cytosolic cations such as K^+ and H^+ by the collecting duct (see Figure 27-2), resulting in Na^+ retention and K^+ excretion. Aldosterone, acting through nuclear receptors in the principal cells of the cortical collecting duct, enhances the conductance of apical Na^+ channels. For a given amount of aldosterone, more Na^+ delivered to this site means

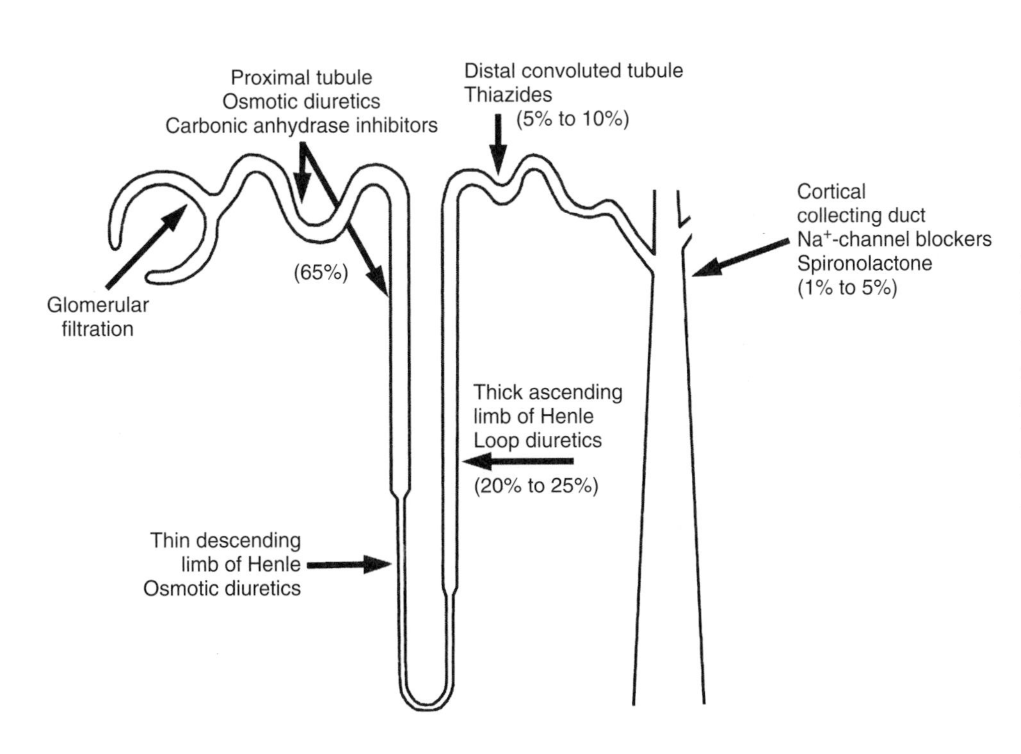

Fig. 27-1 Sites of action of diuretics along the nephron. The percentages shown illustrate the approximate amount of the filtered load of Na^+ that is reabsorbed by each nephron segment. Each diuretic, with the exception of spironolactone, acts on the tubular lumen to produce its effect.

Table • 27-1

Summary of the Urinary Effects and Mechanisms of Action of Diuretic Drugs

	VOLUME (ml/min)	pH	Na^+	K^+	Cl^-	HCO_3^-	MECHANISM OF ACTION
Control	1	6	50	15	60	1	—
Thiazides (e.g., chlorothiazide)	3	7.4	150	25	150	25	Decreases Na^+ and Cl^- cotransport in distal tubule*
Loop diuretics (e.g., furosemide)	8	6	140	10	155	1	Decreases Na^+, K^+, 2 Cl^- cotransport in medullary ascending loop of Henle
Amiloride, triamterene	2	7.2	130	5	120	15	Decreases Na^+ reabsorption in late distal tubule and collecting ducts; less K^+ secretion and Na^+—H^+ exchange
Spironolactone	2	7.2	125	5	120	15	Inhibits aldosterone receptor activation; net effects similar to those of amiloride
Carbonic anhydrase inhibitors (e.g., acetazolamide)	3	8.2	70	60	15	120	Inhibits carbonic anhydrase and H^+ production in proximal tubules; less Na^+ and HCO_3^- reabsorption
Osmotic diuretics (e.g., mannitol)	10	6.5	90	15	110	4	Osmotically retains water in proximal tubule and loop of Henle

Values are average peak diuretic responses in human beings with a normal water and electrolyte balance. Electrolyte concentrations are given in mEq/L.
*Thiazide diuretics also variably inhibit carbonic anhydrase.

more Na^+ reabsorption and more K^+ secretion, a coupled process referred to as *Na^+/K^+ exchange.*[2] It is because of the Na^+/K^+ exchange at this portion of the nephron that any diuretics acting further upstream to block Na^+ reabsorption and therefore increase distal Na^+ delivery result in enhanced urinary excretion of K^+.

Pharmacologic effects

The K^+-sparing diuretics are so named because, by blocking Na^+ reabsorption in the cortical collecting duct region of the nephron, they do not produce the hypokalemic effects of the other natriuretic drugs.[17] The three drugs of this class, spironolactone, triamterene, and amiloride, are structurally dissimilar (Figure 27-3), but each produces similar effects (mild natriuresis with a decrease in K^+ excretion) because of the blockade of Na^+ reabsorption by this pathway.[9] Spironolactone is a 17-spirolactone steroid that is structurally similar to aldosterone and functions as an aldosterone antagonist. Triamterene, a pteridine derivative with structural similarities to folic acid, and amiloride, a pyrazine derivative, exert similar effects by directly blocking the apical membrane Na^+ channels of the principal cells of the collecting duct. By preventing Na^+ entry into these cells, these diuretics reduce the electrogenic driving force for K^+ and/or H^+ secretion in this segment. Thus the net effect is a mild diuresis with a K^+-sparing effect. The amount of additional Na^+ excretion and K^+ retention is small

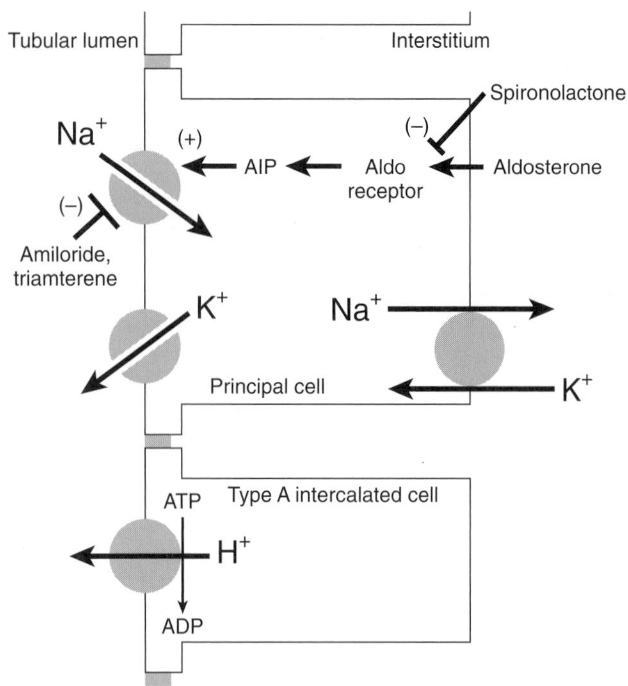

Fig. 27-2 The actions of K$^+$-sparing diuretics in the cortical collecting duct. In this segment, Na$^+$ is transported passively through channels located on the apical membranes of principal cells. The conductance of this channel is enhanced by an aldosterone-induced protein *(AIP)*. The apical entry of Na$^+$ (removal of positive charges) creates a negative electrostatic driving force in the tubule lumen that enhances the secretion of K$^+$ from principal cells and H$^+$ from Type A intercalated cells. Amiloride and triamterene are antagonists of apical membrane Na$^+$ channels, producing a mild natriuresis and preventing K$^+$ excretion in this segment. Spironolactone, by antagonizing the action of aldosterone, prevents AIP activation of Na$^+$ conductance, producing natriuresis with a K$^+$-sparing effect.

when drugs of this class are administered alone. However, when natriuresis from other diuretics is present, the capacity of K$^+$-sparing diuretics to inhibit K$^+$ excretion is significantly increased. This provides the rationale for combining loop and thiazide diuretics with a K$^+$-sparing diuretic to prevent hypokalemia.

Absorption, fate, and excretion

Spironolactone is administered orally and is rapidly absorbed. However, the onset of action takes 2 to 4 days, and full clinical efficacy is not seen for several weeks. Spironolactone is metabolized by the liver and has two active metabolites, canrenone and canrenoate. Canrenone is prescribed as a K$^+$-sparing diuretic in Europe.

Amiloride is given orally, despite its poor gastrointestinal absorption. Diuresis begins within 2 hours, and its duration of action is approximately 24 hours. Amiloride does not undergo metabolism and is excreted unchanged in the urine and feces. Triamterene is better absorbed by the gastrointestinal tract and produces a response within 2 hours of administration. Triamterene has a short plasma half-life and is extensively metabolized to products that are excreted in the urine and feces. However, the duration of diuresis is longer (approximately 14 hours) because the hydroxylated metabolites are also active Na$^+$-channel blockers.

Therapeutic uses

The K$^+$-sparing diuretics are most often used to prevent hypokalemia caused by the thiazide and loop diuretics. Spironolactone, triamterene, and amiloride are each available as combination preparations with thiazide diuretics to facilitate this use. Spironolactone is also sometimes used in the treatment of hyperaldosteronism. More recently, spironolactone has been found to be especially useful in the treatment of congestive heart failure (see Chapter 25). Plasma aldosterone concentration is inappropriately high in patients with congestive heart failure, and it contributes to the development of edema, direct hypertrophic effects on the myocardium, and other adverse effects in heart failure. Spironolactone effectively antagonizes these effects and has been shown to reduce the mortality rate of patients with congestive heart failure.

Adverse effects

The primary toxic effect of the K$^+$-sparing diuretics is hyperkalemia. This effect is most common when these drugs are given alone or concomitantly with other inhibitors of K$^+$ excretion such as angiotensin-converting enzyme inhibitors or angiotensin II receptor antagonists. Dietary K$^+$ supplementation can also precipitate hyperkalemia in patients taking these drugs. Hyperkalemia is infrequent when these drugs are administered in the presence of the loop or thiazide diuretics. Spironolactone, because of its steroid structure, can also produce gynecomastia and/or decreased libido in men. Menstrual irregularities have been reported for women. Triamterene and amiloride infrequently cause other effects such as nausea and vomiting, muscle cramping, and dizziness. Triamterene can sometimes accumulate in the renal pelvis and produce renal stones.

Thiazide Diuretics

The benzothiazide diuretics (commonly referred to as *thiazides*) are derived from 1,2,4-benzothiadiazine-7-sulfonamide 1,1 dioxide. Chlorothiazide (Figure 27-4) was originally synthesized in an attempt to produce more potent carbonic anhydrase inhibitors. Investigators soon observed that although chlorothiazide produced prompt diuresis as predicted, it did not do so by increasing the excretion of $NaHCO_3$. Rather, it produced a large increase in the excretion of NaCl, suggesting a novel natriuretic and diuretic mech-

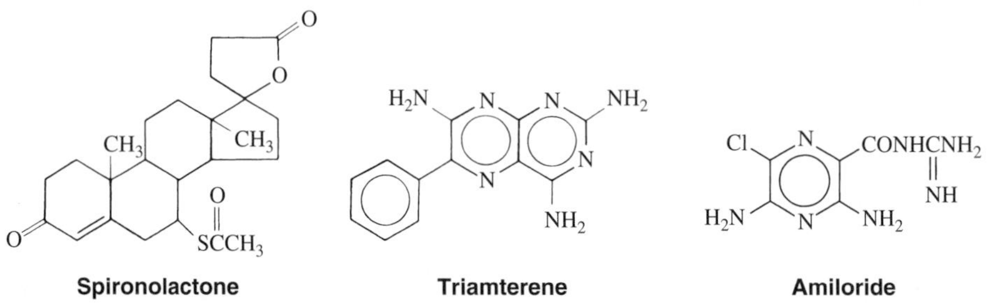

Fig. 27-3 Structural formulas of K$^+$-sparing diuretics.

Spironolactone **Triamterene** **Amiloride**

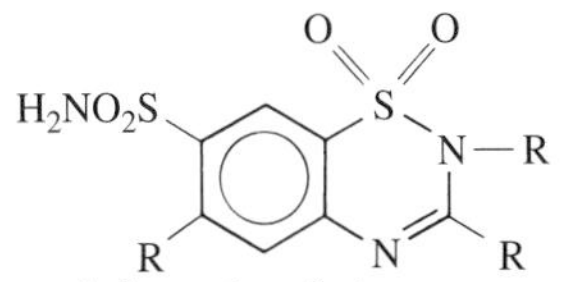

Fig. 27-4 Structural formula of the parent compound of the thiazide diuretics.

anism, inhibition of Na^+-Cl^- cotransport in the distal nephron.[19] Structural congeners of chlorothiazide, including hydrochlorothiazide, hydroflumethiazide, and methyclothiazide, also share this mechanism. Several other compounds (chlorthalidone, indapamide, metolazone, and quinethazone) that are not structurally related to the thiazides also inhibit renal Na^+-Cl^- cotransport and produce natriuresis and diuresis that is indistinguishable from the thiazides. For this reason, it is a common convention to refer to all drugs that inhibit renal Na^+-Cl^- cotransport as "thiazides" regardless of their structure.

Diuretics of the thiazide class available for prescription in the United States are listed in Table 27-2. Hydrochlorothiazide is also available in combination form with the K^+-sparing diuretics (Table 27-3). In addition, there are at least 21 formulations on the market that combine hydrochlorothiazide with an antihypertensive drug.

Pharmacologic effects

The thiazide and thiazide-like diuretics enter the lumen of the nephron by glomerular filtration and through secretion by the organic acid transporters of the proximal tubule. Thus thiazide diuretics can achieve a luminal concentration that is higher than their free plasma concentration. Inhibitors of organic acid transport, such as probenecid, can inhibit the action of the thiazide diuretics by lowering the luminal concentration. When the drug reaches the distal convoluted tubule, it binds to the Na^+-Cl^- cotransporter (most likely at the Cl^- binding site) and inhibits its turnover (Figure 27-5).[14] The result is a reduction in Na^+-Cl^- reabsorption by the distal convoluted tubule and an increase in the amounts of Na^+-Cl^- delivered to the cortical collecting duct.[19] Some of the Na^+ that is delivered to the collecting duct is excreted with an equivalent amount of water, producing natriuresis and diuresis, and some is reabsorbed in the cortical collecting duct as it is exchanged for K^+ or H^+. Thus the thiazides also produce kaliuresis (increased excretion of K^+). In addition to increasing the excretion of Na^+-Cl^- and K^+, thiazide diuretics increase the reabsorption of filtered Ca^{++}. This action distinguishes thiazides from the loop diuretics, which promote Ca^{++} excretion. The mechanism for this action is not completely understood, but Ca^{++} reabsorption appears to be increased at the proximal tubule as a result of decreased glomerular filtration (because of reduced plasma volume) and at the distal convoluted tubule as a direct result of Na^+-Cl^- cotransport inhibition. Ca^{++} influx into the distal

Table • 27-2

Thiazide and Thiazide-Like Drugs Currently Available in the United States

DRUG	PROPRIETARY (TRADE) NAMES	DAILY DOSE (mg)	HALF-LIFE (hr)	DURATION OF DIURETIC ACTION (hr)
Bendroflumethiazide	Naturetin	2.5 to 10	8.5	6 to 12
Chlorothiazide	Diuril	500 to 1000	1 to 2	6 to 12
Chlorthalidone	Hygroton	50 to 100	35 to 50	48 to 72
Hydrochlorothiazide	HydroDIURIL, Microzide, Esidrix, Oretic	12.5 to 100	5.6 to 14.8	6 to 12
Hydroflumethiazide	Saluron	25 to 100	17	18 to 24
Indapamide	Lozol	2.5 to 10	14	12 to 24
Methyclothiazide	Aquatensen, Enduron	2.5 to 10	NA	>24
Metolazone	Diulo, Zaroxolyn	2.5 to 10	14	12 to 24
Polythiazide	Renese	1 to 4	24	24 to 48
Quinethazone	Hydromox	50 to 100	NA	18 to 24
Trichlormethiazide	Metahydrin, Naqua	2 to 8	2.5 to 7.5	<24

NA, Not available.
From *USP dispensing information (USPDI). Drug information for the health care professional,* vol 1, ed 24, Greenwood Village, CO, 2004, Thompson MICROMEDEX.

Table • 27-3

Thiazide and K⁺-Sparing Combination Drugs

PROPRIETARY (TRADE) NAME	THIAZIDE	ADDITIONAL DRUG
Moduretic	Hydrochlorothiazide 50 mg	Amiloride 5 mg
Aldactazide, Spirozide	Hydrochlorothiazide 25 mg	Spironolactone 25 mg
Aldactazide	Hydrochlorothiazide 50 mg	Spironolactone 50 mg
Maxzide	Hydrochlorothiazide 25 mg	Triamterene 37.5 mg
	Hydrochlorothiazide 50 mg	Triamterene 75 mg

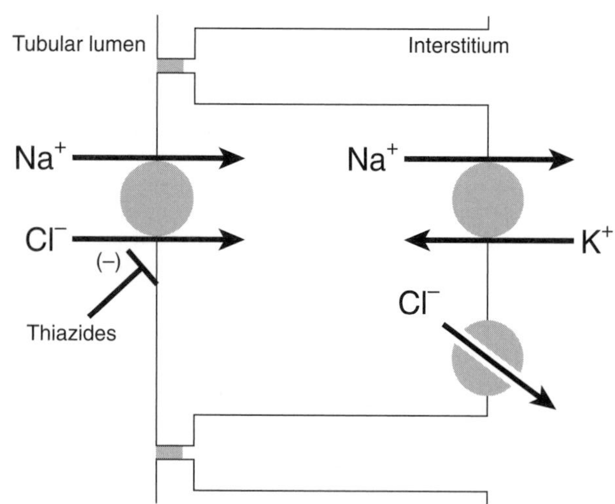

Fig. 27-5 The action of the thiazide diuretics on the distal convoluted tubule. Na^+ and Cl^- enter the cell from the tubular urine by the electroneutral Na^+-Cl cotransporter. Intracellular Na^+ is removed by the action of basolateral Na^+,K^+-ATPase, and Cl^- exits through basolateral Cl^- channels. Thiazides bind to the Cl^--binding site of the Na^+-Cl^- cotransporter, causing an increase in Na^+-Cl^- delivery to more distal tubule segments, increasing Na^+-Cl^- excretion.

convoluted cells is governed in part by hormones such as parathyroid hormone, and its efflux is powered by a basolateral Na^+/Ca^{++} exchanger. Less Na^+ inside the cell from blockade of apical Na^+-Cl^- cotransport creates a larger gradient for the influx of extracellular Na^+ through the basolateral Na^+/Ca^{++} exchanger, resulting in increased Ca^{++} reabsorption. Depending on their structure, some of the thiazides are also weak inhibitors of carbonic anhydrase. This may result in alkalinization of the urine from increased HCO_3^- excretion.

At the level of the whole organism, chronic administration of a thiazide diuretic produces a reduction in the extracellular fluid volume.[1] The fall in blood volume activates the renin-angiotensin system, causing angiotensin II–mediated aldosterone release from the adrenal gland. Aldosterone acts on the cortical collecting duct to increase the conductance of the principal cell Na^+ channels. Thus blood volume reduction leads to aldosterone-induced increases in the recovery of Na^+ in the cortical collecting duct, which in turn further increases the excretion of K^+ in this segment. The thiazides also lead to a long-term decrease in blood pressure. The mechanism for this effect is somewhat controversial. A reduction in blood volume would be expected to lower arterial blood pressure. However, blood volume returns to near normal values after several weeks of thiazide administration. A direct vascular effect, vasodilation caused by reductions in vascular Na^+ content, has therefore been proposed to explain the continued reduction in total peripheral resistance that persists during thiazide administration.[12]

Absorption, fate, and excretion

Absorption of thiazides from the gastrointestinal tract varies with the particular agent. The plasma elimination half-life and duration of diuretic effect for each of the thiazide diuretics are listed in Table 27-2. Plasma protein binding varies considerably among this class of drugs. The parent compounds and/or metabolites are primarily excreted through renal elimination after glomerular filtration and secretion in the proximal tubule.

Therapeutic uses

Thiazide diuretics are primarily used for the treatment of essential hypertension. Both the Joint National Commission VII and the World Health Organization recommend thiazide diuretics as a first-line treatment for essential hypertension because of their demonstrated efficacy and low cost.[3,10,13] (See also Chapter 28.) The antihypertensive dosage of thiazide diuretics should normally not exceed the equivalent of 25 mg/day of hydrochlorothiazide because clinical studies have shown that doses above this produce equivalent antihypertensive effects but greater toxicity. Thiazide diuretics can be given as monotherapy for essential hypertension or as an adjunct agent.[3,6,13] Thiazide diuretics enhance the effectiveness of most other antihypertensive agents, especially vasodilators such as hydralazine and minoxidil, which by themselves promote volume expansion. Thiazide diuretics can also mobilize mild edema and are sometimes used for this purpose, but loop diuretics are generally used to treat edema.

Ca^{++} is absorbed from the diet in response to Ca^{++} loss in the urine, and some people have higher Ca^{++} turnover than others.[5] Excessive Ca^{++} excretion promotes the formation of calcium oxalate kidney stones. Thiazide diuretics can be used to lower the concentration of Ca^{++} in the excreted urine, an effect that can prevent the formation of renal stones.

Thiazide diuretics are also sometimes (paradoxically) useful in the treatment of the polyuria of nephrogenic diabetes insipidus. The plasma volume contraction that occurs from thiazide diuretic use leads to a decreased glomerular filtration rate and other compensatory changes that increase Na^+-Cl^- and water reabsorption in the proximal nephron. Less delivery of water to the collecting duct in nephrogenic diabetes insipidus means less urine volume.[4]

Adverse effects

The thiazide diuretics are generally safe and effective drugs. Toxicity usually is the result of plasma electrolyte disturbances, which can result in extracellular volume depletion, hyponatremia, and hypokalemia. Most prevalent among these is hypokalemia, which results from the combined effects of volume depletion–induced aldosterone release and increased delivery of Na^+ and Cl^- to the collecting duct. Both these effects increase reabsorption of Na^+ through apical channels in the cortical collecting duct, which increases the driving force for the secretion of K^+.

Hypokalemia lowers the resting membrane potential, decreasing the likelihood of action potentials in nerves and muscles. This leads to predictable symptoms such as flaccid muscles, paralytic ileus, confusion and lethargy, and a variety of cardiac arrhythmias such as sinus bradycardia, atrioventricular block, and paroxysmal atrial tachycardia. Hypokalemia also causes hyperglycemia by decreasing insulin production in the pancreatic β cells. Thus hyperglycemia can occur in nondiabetic patients treated with thiazide diuretics, and glucose control can be destabilized in diabetic patients. Because insulin-dependent glucose uptake promotes cellular uptake of K^+, this hyperglycemia blunts the full effects of diuretic-induced hypokalemia. Severe, even fatal, hypokalemia could result if insulin is administered under these circumstances. Hypokalemia can be avoided by eating foods rich in K^+, especially fruits such as bananas, or by taking K^+ supplements. The concomitant use of the K^+-sparing diuretics with thiazide diuretics is an alternative strategy for avoiding hypokalemia, and several combination drugs with hydrochlorothiazide are available for this purpose (see Table 27-3).

Because thiazide diuretics can cause a Na^+ loss in excess of the water loss, they can cause both volume depletion and hyponatremia. Hyponatremia causes systemic cellular edema and brain swelling, leading to symptoms such as irritability, depression, and confusion, whereas plasma volume depletion adds symptoms such as postural hypotension, tachycardia, weak pulse, dry mouth, thirst, and oliguria. Other adverse effects of thiazide diuretics include hypercalcemia and hypophosphatemia, simulating hyperparathyroidism. Thiazide diuretics can also precipitate attacks of gout, a potential consequence of hyperuricemia. Urate is freely filtered by the glomerulus, reabsorbed in the proximal tubule, secreted by more downstream portions of the proximal tubule, and then later largely reabsorbed again. Urate is poorly soluble and its concentration is normally rather close to that at which crystals form. Thiazide diuretics interfere with urate transport in a manner that promotes urate retention.[7] This effect combined with the thiazide diuretic–induced water loss can increase the plasma urate concentration beyond its solubility limits, leading to the formation of urate crystals that can trigger the inflammatory response known as *gout.* Hyperlipidemia was seen in the past when higher doses of thiazide diuretics (e.g., more than 25 mg/day of hydrochlorothiazide) were routinely administered to treat hypertension.[14]

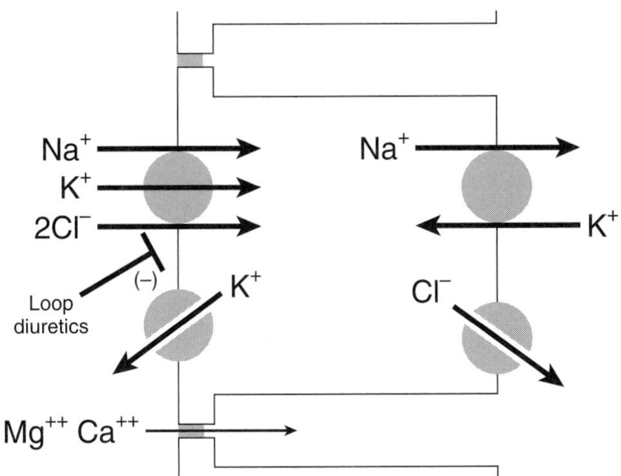

Fig. 27-6 The action of the loop diuretics on the TALH. Na^+, K^+, and Cl^- enter the cell from the tubular urine by the Na^+, K^+, $2Cl^-$ cotransporter. Intracellular Na^+ is removed by the action of basolateral Na^+,K^+-ATPase, and Cl^- exits through basolateral Cl^- channels. K^+ is partially recycled as it exits by an apical channel. This action creates a net positive potential in the tubular lumen, which acts as an electrogenic driving force for the paracellular reabsorption of cations such as Na^+, Mg^{++} and Ca^{++}. Loop diuretics bind to one of the Cl^--binding sites of the Na^+, K^+, $2Cl^-$ cotransporter, causing an increase in Na^+ and Cl^- delivery to more distal tubule segments, increasing Na^+ and Cl^- excretion. K^+ recycling is also disrupted, causing an increase in the excretion of Mg^{++} and Ca^{++}.

Allergic reactions are uncommon with thiazide diuretics but can lead to fever, skin rash, and even interstitial nephritis and renal failure. Patients allergic to sulfonamides should not receive thiazide diuretics.

Loop Diuretics

The loop diuretics are so named for their site of action on the thick ascending limb of the loop of Henle (TALH), where they inhibit Na^+ and Cl^- reabsorption (Figure 27-6). Because 20% to 25% of filtered Na^+ is reabsorbed in this segment, the resulting natriuresis can be of a much larger magnitude compared with other diuretics. Thus these drugs are sometimes referred to as *high ceiling* or *high efficacy* diuretics. Diuretics that act at segments distal to the TALH have a much smaller maximum effect on Na^+ reabsorption. The loop diuretics are structurally dissimilar (Figure 27-7). Furosemide and bumetanide are sulfonamide derivatives of aminobenzoic acid, torsemide is a pyridine sulfonylurea, and ethacrynic acid is an unsaturated ketonic derivative of aryloxyacetic acid.

Pharmacologic effects

Na^+ and Cl^- is reabsorbed in the medullary and cortical TALH by a Na^+, K^+, $2Cl^-$ cotransporter, as described in Figure 27-6.[19] Evidence obtained with radiolabeled bumetanide suggests that loop diuretics bind to one of the Cl^--binding sites on the cotransporter because bumetanide binding is enhanced by Na^+ and K^+ but inhibited by Cl^-. Loop diuretic binding to the Na^+, K^+, $2Cl^-$ cotransporter effectively arrests ion transport, preventing the reabsorption of Na^+ and Cl^-. K^+ reabsorption is also inhibited, which reduces the intraluminal positive electrical potential normally present in the TALH. This in turn reduces the driving force for the paracellular reabsorption of cations in this segment (see Figure 27-6).[19] Additional K^+ excretion occurs in the collecting duct in response to increased Na^+ delivery to the collecting duct and increased aldosterone secretion, as described for the thiazide diuretics. In addition, the amount of titratable acid secreted by the collecting duct is also enhanced by loop diuretics by the same mechanism. Thus loop diuretics increase the excretion of Na^+, K^+, Ca^{++}, Cl^-, H^+, and Mg^{++}. The effect on Ca^{++} is particularly noteworthy because the hypercalciuric effect of the loop diuretics is the opposite of the hypocalciuric effect seen with the thiazides.

At the level of the whole kidney, inhibition of Na^+ and Cl^- reabsorption in the TALH reduces the medullary interstitial osmotic gradient, which is the driving force for water reabsorption by the adjacent descending loops of Henle and collecting ducts. By blocking NaCl reabsorption in the TALH, a more isotonic tubular fluid is delivered to the collecting duct, thereby impairing the ability of the kidney to excrete a dilute urine. The associated reduction in the interstitial

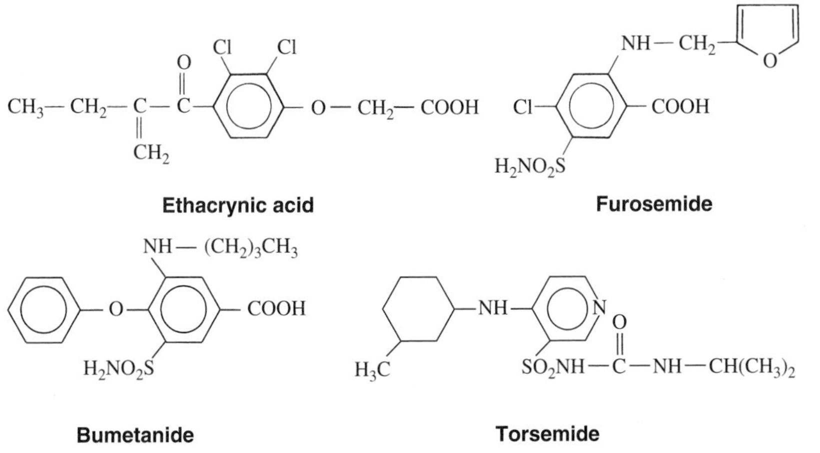

Ethacrynic acid

Furosemide

Bumetanide

Torsemide

Fig. 27-7 Structural formulas of loop diuretics.

medullary gradient means that less water can be extracted from the tubular fluid, impairing the ability of the kidney to excrete a concentrated urine.[16] Thus the urine excreted in the presence of loop diuretics does not differ much from that of plasma, irrespective of ADH levels (i.e., free water clearance is reduced).

At the level of the whole body, loop diuretics reduce the extracellular fluid volume and reduce blood pressure as described for the thiazides, except that these effects are typically of greater magnitude for the loop diuretics. Furosemide also increases venous capacitance, which reduces left ventricular filling pressure. This effect appears to be mediated by prostaglandins and occurs before diuresis. This effect is especially useful with intravenous furosemide to treat acute pulmonary edema.

Absorption, fate, and excretion

Although structurally dissimilar, there is substantial similarity among the loop diuretics regarding absorption, fate, and excretion. Furosemide is available in both oral and injectable forms, with approximately 65% absorption of the oral form. Diuresis begins within 5 minutes of intravenous administration, with a duration of 2 hours, and begins in approximately 30 minutes after oral or intramuscular administration and then lasts 6 to 8 hours. Furosemide is highly protein bound, metabolized by the liver, and excreted in the urine and feces. With normal renal function, it has a half-life of 30 to 70 minutes, but this increases to approximately 9 hours in patients with end-stage renal disease. Torsemide is available in oral and intravenous forms and is rapidly absorbed after oral administration with 80% to 90% bioavailability. Diuresis begins in 30 to 60 minutes and lasts for approximately 6 hours. Torsemide is highly protein bound and is 80% metabolized by the hepatic cytochrome P450 system before excretion in the urine. The half-time for elimination is typically 2 to 4 hours but is increased to 7 to 8 hours by cirrhosis of the liver. Bumetanide is available in both oral and injectable forms. Diuresis begins within 2 to 3 minutes of intravenous administration and 30 to 60 minutes after oral or intramuscular administration and has a duration of approximately 6 hours. Bumetanide is highly protein bound, metabolized by the liver, and excreted in the urine. Ethacrynic acid is available in both oral and intravenous forms. Diuresis begins within 5 minutes of intravenous administration and lasts 2 hours, whereas the onset of the diuretic effect after oral administration requires 30 to 60 minutes and has a duration of approximately 12 hours. Ethacrynic acid is highly protein bound, metabolized by the liver, and excreted in the urine and bile. With normal renal function, ethacrynic acid has a half-life of 2 to 4 hours.

Therapeutic uses

The loop diuretics are predominantly used in the treatment of edema.[10,15] In cardiac failure, low cardiac output results in poor renal perfusion, which causes volume retention.[20] If cardiac dysfunction is severe, this volume retention results in edema and cardiac dilation, which worsen cardiac failure. Fluid retention in the lungs can also produce grave consequences in heart failure. Loop diuretics reduce plasma volume to cause migration of edema fluid from the tissues back into the circulation, from where it can be excreted. Many kidney diseases, both primary and secondary, are characterized by salt and water retention and hyperkalemia. The thiazide diuretics can be used in some of these patients, but they become ineffective when the glomerular filtration rate drops below 30 ml/min. Thus the loop diuretics are the primary drugs of choice for volume management in renal failure. Edema can originate from a primary liver disease. Edema in this setting is the result of low plasma oncotic pressure from hypoalbuminemia, ascites formation, low renal perfusion, and increased aldosterone release. Loop diuretics have a place in the management of this complex syndrome by reducing fluid and electrolyte retention by the kidney. However, some patients with liver disease can be resistant to loop diuretics and these drugs can produce dangerous hypovolemia in others. Therefore great care is needed in the use of loop diuretics in the treatment of edema and ascites in liver disease.

Loop diuretics are also the drugs of choice for the treatment of acute pulmonary edema.[4] In this condition, furosemide is usually administered parenterally, producing a rapid reduction in pulmonary congestion. As stated previously, this response occurs even before the onset of significant natriuresis and appears to be partly caused by a prostaglandin-mediated increase in venous capacitance. This action causes a fall in left ventricular filling pressure, which relieves the pulmonary edema. Longer-term reduction of fluid and electrolyte retention by furosemide maintains the response.

In addition to their use in edema, the loop diuretics are useful in the management of other conditions. In refractory hypertension, loop diuretics are used to combat the fluid and electrolyte retention caused by powerful vasodilators such as minoxidil and hydralazine. In such cases, a K^+-sparing diuretic is also included in the regimen to prevent hypokalemia. Loop diuretics are also used to treat hypercalcemia.[5] As discussed above (see Figure 27-6), loop diuretics decrease Ca^{++} reabsorption in the TALH. In patients with hypercalcemia, furosemide is given intravenously, which produces a prompt reduction in plasma Ca^{++} concentration. To maintain plasma volume and prevent Na^+ and K^+ wasting, normal saline must be infused simultaneously at a rate that matches urine flow.

Adverse effects

Similar to the thiazide diuretics, toxicity from the loop diuretics is usually the result of plasma electrolyte disturbances such as hyponatremia and hypokalemia as well as extracellular volume depletion. The magnitude of these effects can be greater than those produced by the thiazides as a result of the more prominent natriuresis produced by loop diuretics. The hypokalemia produced by loop diuretics occurs by a mechanism similar to that described for the thiazide diuretics (increased exchange of K^+ for Na^+ in the collecting duct) and can be associated with metabolic alkalosis.[7] Again similar to the thiazide diuretics, hypokalemia is the most prevalent among these electrolyte disturbances and exerts a variety of neuromuscular and metabolic effects. Inasmuch as loop diuretics are routinely used to help regulate plasma volume in patients with congestive heart failure, this is the appropriate place to draw attention to an important drug interaction. Digoxin and other digitalislike cardiac glycosides are used to increase myocardial contractility in the failing heart. There are a variety of toxic effects associated with the use of cardiac glycosides (see Chapter 25). Digitalis toxicity increases under conditions of hypokalemia. Therefore thiazide and loop diuretics increase the likelihood and severity of digitalis toxicity.[7]

Hyponatremia causes systemic cellular edema and brain swelling, leading to symptoms such as irritability, depression, and confusion. Plasma volume depletion adds symptoms such as postural hypotension, tachycardia, weak pulse, dry mouth, thirst, and oliguria. Similar to thiazide diuretics, disruption of urate excretion and/or dehydration can lead to hyperuricemia and acute gout. Moreover, some of the loop diuretics can cause potentially severe allergic skin reactions similar to thiazide diuretics.

The adverse effects discussed above are generally shared with thiazide diuretics. In addition, loop diuretics have some adverse effects that are not shared with the thiazide diuretics. Because of their impairment of paracellular reabsorption of Mg^{++} and Ca^{++}, loop diuretics can also cause hypomagnesemia (a risk factor for cardiac arrhythmias and digitalis toxicity) and hypocalcemia (which, in rare instances, can cause tetany). Loop diuretics can cause a variety of gastrointestinal problems, including pancreatitis, jaundice, anorexia, malaise, and abdominal pain. They can elicit thrombocytopenia and, rarely, aplastic anemia or agranulocytosis, and they can cause systemic allergic reactions such as systemic vasculitis. Finally, loop diuretics affect the central nervous system, with the most important adverse effects being tinnitus and hearing loss, vertigo, and paresthesias. Because of the ototoxic effects of loop diuretics, they should not be administered concurrently with other ototoxic drugs such as aminoglycosides.

Carbonic Anhydrase Inhibitors

Acetazolamide is the prototype for this class of drugs, which are nonbacteriostatic sulfonamides, and is among the few members of this class that is still marketed as a diuretic. Carbonic anhydrase inhibitors were among the earliest diuretics available, and the search for new members in this family resulted in the discovery of the thiazide diuretics.

Pharmacologic effects

Acetazolamide is a potent inhibitor of the enzyme carbonic anhydrase, the enzyme that catalyzes the reversible reaction of carbonic acid to form either water and carbon dioxide or HCO_3^- and H^+. By blocking this enzyme, reabsorption of HCO_3^- is impaired in the proximal tubule, which leads to increased delivery of Na^+, K^+, and HCO_3^- to the distal nephron and ultimately an alkaline diuresis.[11]

Absorption, fate, and excretion

Acetazolamide is readily absorbed from the gastrointestinal tract, with peak levels reached in 2 hours. Extended-release capsules are available. Acetazolamide is not metabolized. It is tightly bound to carbonic anhydrase and therefore concentrates in cells with high amounts of this enzyme such as erythrocytes and the renal cortex. It is excreted unchanged in the urine as a result of active secretion and some passive reabsorption and has a half-life ranging from 2.5 to 6 hours.

Therapeutic uses

Carbonic anhydrase inhibitors can be used to treat the edema of congestive failure but are no longer widely used for this purpose. When used to treat edema, best results are obtained when the drug is skipped every other day or every 2 days, giving the kidneys an opportunity to recover lost HCO_3^-. Carbonic anhydrase inhibitors also suppress aqueous humor formation in the eyes and can therefore be used to lower interocular pressure in open-angle glaucoma and before surgery in cases of angle-closure glaucoma. Treatment of glaucoma is the therapeutic indication for most carbonic anhydrase inhibitors that are now on the market. For reasons that are not well established, but perhaps because of the tendency toward acidosis with carbonic anhydrase inhibitors, carbonic anhydrase inhibitors are also useful for treating epilepsy (especially absence seizures in children). A final use for these drugs is the treatment of altitude sickness when taken before the ascent and, if necessary, to suppress symptoms for a few days afterwards.

Adverse effects

Common side effects with carbonic anhydrase inhibitors include a tingling sensation in the extremities, tinnitus, and alterations of taste, loss of appetite, nausea, and vomiting. These side effects are especially common early during therapy. The alkaline diuresis caused by carbonic anhydrase inhibitors can also alter the elimination of other drugs; the excretion of weak acids is increased (an effect sometimes harnessed during treatment for drug toxicities) whereas the excretion of weak bases is decreased. In addition, because these drugs are sulfonamide derivatives, some people do have allergic reactions typical of these kinds of drugs. These usually manifest as rashes but are rarely fatal because of more severe reactions such as anaphylaxis and Stevens-Johnson syndrome.

Osmotic Diuretics

Mannitol is the prototypical osmotic diuretic, a class of drugs that differs from the drugs previously discussed in two important respects: the amounts needed to exert their effects and the site at which they cause diuresis.

Pharmacologic effects

Unlike the other drugs, which are administered in relatively small amounts to block transporters, mannitol is administered intravenously in gram quantities (typically 50 to 200 g over a 24-hour period) and functions as an impermeable solute in the extracellular space. By selectively raising the osmolality of the extracellular space, water is extracted from the intracellular space to equilibrate these osmotic differences. Mannitol is freely filtered at the glomerulus, is poorly reabsorbed (less than 10%), and is not secreted. Mannitol therefore carries water extracted from cells with it into the urine. Thus, in contrast to the other diuretics discussed here, mannitol selectively decreases intracellular volume. (Na^+ and Cl^- excretion is, however, also increased.)

Absorption, fate, and excretion

Mannitol must be administered intravenously to exert its diuretic effects. When administered to treat cerebral edema, decreases in intracerebral volume are seen within 15 minutes and diuresis is evident within 1 to 3 hours. There is little metabolism of mannitol, and it is excreted in the urine with a half-time for elimination of 70 to 100 minutes.

Therapeutic uses

There are three major indications for mannitol administration. The first of these is to increase or maintain urine flow. Maintaining the flow of urine during the oliguric phase of acute renal failure can block the progression of acute renal failure to irreversible chronic renal failure. This effect can also be harnessed to hasten the elimination of toxins from the body that can be trapped in the urine. Second, by extracting intracellular water, mannitol can be administered to decrease brain edema and intracranial pressure. Finally, mannitol is administered preoperatively to lower intraocular pressure before surgery for glaucoma.

Adverse effects

Adverse effects are common both during and after the infusion of mannitol. The redistribution of fluid from the intracellular to the extracellular compartment causes a variety of problems such as pulmonary congestion, electrolyte imbalances, dryness of the mouth, thirst, blurred vision, convulsions, nausea and vomiting, and fever, along with pain, thrombophlebitis, and infection at the injection site. The cardiovascular status of patients must be carefully assessed before administering mannitol because it can cause severe congestive heart failure.

IMPLICATIONS FOR DENTISTRY

The major drug interactions of diuretics are summarized in Table 27-4, and some additional concerns related to herbal remedies are presented at the end of this section. Diuretic therapy does not usually influence dental practice. Nonetheless, epinephrine, sedatives, opioid analgesics, adrenocorticosteroids, and nonsteroidal antiinflammatory drugs used in dentistry can interact with patients on diuretic agents to cause

Table • 27-4

Drug Interactions of Diuretic Agents

DIURETIC	INTERACTING DRUG	EFFECT
Thiazides, loop diuretics, K^+-sparing diuretics	Anticoagulants	Increased concentration of clotting factors from reduction of plasma volume, decreasing anticoagulant effect
	Aspirin, NSAIDs	Natriuresis and hypotensive effect blocked by cyclooxygenase inhibition
	Lithium salts	Decreased Li^+ excretion, leading to increased Li^+ toxicity
	Adrenergic receptor antagonists, α_2-adrenergic receptor agonists, vasodilators, ACE inhibitors, ARBs	Increased antihypertensive response
	Uricosurics	Enhancement of uric acid reabsorption, reducing efficacy of uricosuric agent
Thiazides, loop diuretics	Oral hypoglycemics, insulin	Hypokalemia-induced hyperglycemia
	Nondepolarizing neuromuscular blockers	Hypokalemia-induced potentiation of paralysis
	Adrenergic receptor agonists	Hypokalemia-induced arrhythmias
	Digoxin, digitoxin	Hypokalemia-induced potentiation of digitalis toxicity
	Corticotropin, adrenal steroids	Deceased diuresis, increased hypokalemia
Thiazides	Cholestyramine, colestipol	Decreased thiazide absorption
Loop diuretics	Aminoglycosides, cisplatin	Ototoxicity
	Clofibrate, warfarin	Competition for binding to plasma proteins by furosemide increases their free concentration
	Cephalosporin antibiotics	Increased renal toxicity
K^+-sparing diuretics	ACE inhibitors, K^+ supplements, cyclosporine	Hyperkalemia

ACE, Angiotensin-converting enzyme; *NSAIDs*, nonsteroidal antiinflammatory drugs; *ARBs*, angiotensin II receptor blockers.

adverse effects of clinical importance. Most patients taking diuretics are doing so because of essential hypertension, and the implications of hypertension and its treatment to dental practice are covered in Chapter 28.[13] Extra caution is especially warranted when dental patients have congestive heart failure, cardiac arrhythmias, and any other conditions in which subtle worsening of hypokalemia could have an adverse effect.

As previously discussed, thiazide and loop diuretics are K^+-losing diuretics that can therefore cause hypokalemia. Strategies used to compensate for this K^+ loss include increasing the dietary intake of K^+ or prescribing K^+ supplements or a simultaneous K^+-depleting diuretic. Nonetheless, these patients may still have relatively low plasma K^+ levels. Under these circumstances, the epinephrine present in gingival retraction cords and local anesthetic solutions can produce a transient hypokalemia, which in turn increases the propensity of epinephrine to trigger cardiac arrhythmias.

The use of antiinflammatory dosages of adrenocorticosteroids with even modest mineralocorticoid activity, such as hydrocortisone, can also promote hypokalemia by exaggerating the hypokalemic effect of the thiazide and loop diuretics. Unlike the rapid-onset transient effects of epinephrine on plasma K^+ levels, the hypokalemic effects of adrenocorticosteroids are slow in onset and slow in termination. They therefore may not be of clinical significance until after the patient has left the dental office. Anything that can cause hypokalemia is of greatest concern in patients with congestive heart failure who are receiving digitalis therapy because hypokalemia is a well-known cause of fatal cardiac arrhythmias in this patient population.

Additionally, there is an increased likelihood of syncope in dental patients taking diuretics because of a depletion of intravascular volume. Sedative hypnotics and opioid analgesics are among the drugs that more readily cause orthostatic hypotension in the presence of diuretics.

Nonsteroidal antiinflammatory drugs used for dental pain could antagonize the antihypertensive effect of diuretics. With short-term use, this interaction should not be clinically significant, but it could become relevant if nonsteroidal antiinflammatory drugs were prescribed to treat chronic dental pain.

Most diuretics are in pregnancy class D, meaning that there is a proven risk of fetal harm. Similarly, breastfeeding is generally contraindicated because most of these drugs enter breast milk.

Because various herbal remedies are touted for their diuretic properties, some patients may be taking diuretic therapy without proper medical supervision, and others may choose to combine the use of herbal remedies with contemporary diuretic pharmacotherapy in the potentially erroneous belief that all diuretics work well together. Herbs used as diuretics include dandelion, horsetail, stone root, cleavers, gravel root, hydrangea, pipsissewa, goldenrod, lovage, and parsley. The mechanism of action for these herbs has generally not been established. However, claims that dandelion is a rich source of K^+ while functioning as a K^+-depleting diuretic could be of concern if taken by patients who are also taking a K^+-sparing diuretic. Lastly, the glycyrrhizic acid of "real" (e.g., European) licorice used in candy and for a variety of medicinal purposes has mineralocorticoid properties. Overindulgence in this type of licorice candy has caused hypertension and, if consumed with diuretics, could exacerbate the K^+-depleting effects of thiazide and loop diuretics or inhibit the activities of spironolactone. Thus, the possibility of drug interaction between diuretics and alternative therapies cannot and should not be overlooked.

Diuretic Drugs

Nonproprietary (generic) name	Proprietary (trade) name
Thiazides and related derivatives	
Bendroflumethiazide	Naturetin
Benzthiazide	Exna
Chlorothiazide	Diuril
Chlorthalidone	Hygroton, Thalitone
Hydrochlorothiazide	Esidrix, HydroDIURIL, Hydro-Par
Hydroflumethiazide	Diucardin, Saluron
Indapamide	Lozol
Methyclothiazide	Aquatensen, Enduron
Metolazone	Zaroxolyn, Mykrox
Polythiazide	Minizide, Renese
Quinethazone	Hydromox
Trichlormethiazide	Diurese, Metahydrin, Naqua
Loop diuretics	
Bumetanide	Bumex
Ethacrynic acid	Edecrin
Furosemide	Lasix
Torsemide	Demadex
K^+-sparing agents	
Amiloride	Midamor
Eplerenone	Inspra
Spironolactone	Aldactone
Triamterene	Dyrenium
Osmotic nonelectrolytes	
Glycerin (glycerol)	Osmoglyn
Isosorbide	Ismotic
Mannitol	Osmitrol
Urea	Ureaphil
Carbonic anhydrase inhibitors	
Acetazolamide	Dazamide, Diamox
Dichlorphenamide	Daranide
Methazolamide	Neptazane

Cited References

1. Dustan HR, Tarazi RC, Bravo EL: Diuretic and diet treatment of hypertension, *Arch Intern Med* 133:1007-1013, 1974.
2. Edelman IS: The initiation mechanism in the action of aldosterone on sodium transport, *J Steroid Biochem* 3:167-172, 1972.
3. Ferdinand KC: Update in pharmacological treatment of hypertension, *Cardiol Clin* 19:279-294, 2001.
4. Francisco LL, Ferris TF: The use and abuse of diuretics, *Arch Intern Med* 142:28-32, 1982.
5. Friedman PA: Mechanisms of renal calcium transport, *Exp Nephrol* 8:343-350, 2000.
6. Gifford RW, Jr: Role of diuretics in treatment of essential hypertension, *Am J Cardiol* 58:15A-17A, 1986.
7. Greenberg A: Diuretic complications, *Am J Med Sci* 319:10-24, 2000.
8. Greger R: Physiology of renal sodium transport, *Am J Med Sci* 319:51-62, 2000.
9. Kleyman TR, Sheng S, Kosari F, et al: Mechanism of action of amiloride: a molecular perspective, *Semin Nephrol* 19:524-532, 1999.
10. Lee TH, Goldman L: Which drug for hypertension? *Harvard Heart Lett* 3:1-6, 1992.
11. Maren TH: Carbonic anhydrase: chemistry, physiology, and inhibition, *Physiol Rev* 47:595-781, 1967.
12. Ogilvie RI, Schlieper E: The effect of hydrochlorothiazide on venous reactivity in hypertensive man, *Clin Pharmacol Ther* 11:589-594, 1970.
13. Puschett JB: Diuretics and the therapy of hypertension, *Am J Med Sci* 319:1-9, 2000.
14. Ramsey LE: Thiazide diuretics in hypertension, *Clin Exp Hypertens* 21:805-814, 1999.
15. Reyes AJ: Diuretics in the treatment of patients who present heart failure and hypertension, *Hum Hypertens* 16(suppl 1): S104-S113, 2002.
16. Shankar SS, Brater DC: Loop diuretics: from the Na-K-2Cl transporter to clinical use, *Am J Physiol Renal Physiol* 284:F11-F21, 2003.
17. Stoner LC, Burg MB, Orloff J: Ion transport in cortical collecting tubule: effect of amiloride, *Am J Physiol* 227:453-479, 1974.
18. Strewler GJ, Orloff J: Role of cyclic nucleotides in the transport of water and electrolytes, *Adv Cyclic Nucleotide Res* 8:311-361, 1977.
19. Suki WN, Eknoyan G, Martinex-Maldonado M: Tubular sites and mechanisms of diuretic action, *Annu Rev Pharmacol Toxicol* 13:91-106, 1973.
20. Taylor SH: Diuretic therapy in congestive heart failure, *Cardiol Rev* 8:104-114, 2000.

General References

Acara MA: Renal pharmacology—diuretics. In Smith CM, Reynard AM, eds: *Textbook of pharmacology*, Philadelphia, 1992, WB Saunders.

Better OS, Greger RF, Knauf H, et al: Diuretics. *Handbook of experimental pharmacology*, vol 117, New York, 1995, Springer.

Brater DC: Pharmacology of diuretics, *Am J Med Sci* 319:38-50, 2000.

Francisco LL, Ferris TF: The use and abuse of diuretics, *Arch Intern Med* 142:28-32, 1982.

Hebert SC: Molecular mechanisms, *Semin Nephrol* 19:504-523, 1999.

Puschett JB: Pharmacological classification and renal actions of diuretics, *Cardiology* 84 (suppl 2): 4-13, 1994.

CHAPTER • 28

Antihypertensive Drugs

Frank J. Dowd and William B. Jeffries

Hypertension affects approximately one in four adult Americans.[3] Careful examination of the prevalence of hypertension reveals that it is distributed disproportionately among subgroups in the US population. For example, hypertension increases with advancing age, but its prevalence is much lower in women before menopause than in men of comparable age. There also appears to be a racial component to hypertension[5]: the prevalence is approximately 23% in whites and Mexican Americans but is 32% in African Americans. Because of the asymptomatic nature of this disease, approximately one third of the affected population are unaware of their condition. Isolated systolic hypertension affects more than 15% of all people older than 60 years.[36] Studies suggest that only half the hypertensive population is receiving pharmacologic treatment at all, and, of this fraction, only half has adequate control of blood pressure levels. Because the long-term consequences of hypertension (coronary artery disease, stroke, renal failure, etc.) are so devastating to health, screening programs are essential to detect the disease early so that treatment can be instituted before major complications ensue. Education of the patient is also essential to ensure compliance with recommended therapy because of the insidious nature of the disease and because unpleasant side effects of the drugs used to treat it may actually cause the patient to feel better when not receiving medication. A person is considered hypertensive if his or her systolic and/or diastolic arterial blood pressure is elevated above normal (i.e., systolic arterial pressure more than 140 mm Hg or diastolic arterial pressure more than 90 mm Hg).[13,33]

CLINICAL ASPECTS OF HYPERTENSION

Classification

The severity of hypertension is classified as shown in Table 28-1. Hypertension can arise as a primary disease or as a result of an underlying illness. *Essential hypertension* is a term used to describe the presence of sustained, elevated blood pressure for which no cause is apparent. When this term was coined, it was believed that the elevation of blood pressure was essential to maintain organ perfusion in the afflicted patient. This idea is no longer widely accepted, but the term is still in use. Essential hypertension remains of unknown etiology and represents 80% to 90% of all cases of hypertension. Although much is known about the cardiovascular changes that occur as a consequence of prolonged elevation of blood pressure, no single pathologic change can be cited as the primary cause. Thus many theories abound regarding the causes of essential hypertension, some of which are discussed below.

Secondary hypertension results from a known disorder, such as renal, vascular, or parenchymal disease, or from an endocrine disorder such as pheochromocytoma. Treatment of secondary hypertension usually consists of therapy for the underlying disease process. Hypertension may be either systolic, diastolic, or both. Until recently, less emphasis had been placed on the importance of systolic hypertension. However, recent evidence indicates its close association with untoward outcomes. Treatment of isolated systolic hypertension in the elderly with an antihypertensive drug has been shown to reduce mortality rates, especially from stroke.[27] The results are independent of mean arterial pressure. The risk of heart failure is also decreased with reduction in systolic hypertension.[19] It has been suggested that the incidence of dementia is reduced as systolic pressure is lowered in the elderly.[29]

Regulation of Blood Pressure

Pressure in a hydraulic system is the product of flow through the system and the resistance to such flow. Thus the relationships among mean arterial blood pressure (MAP), cardiac output (CO), and total peripheral resistance (TPR) can be described in the following equation:

$$MAP = CO \times TPR$$

CO is determined by the load presented to the heart (venous return or preload) and the inotropic and chronotropic state of the myocardium. TPR depends on the diameter and compliance (stiffness) of the arterioles. These factors are regulated by the resting vascular smooth muscle tone, intrinsic reactivity of the vasculature, vasoactive substances in the blood, and sympathetic nervous system activity. Another important factor in the governance of blood pressure is the blood volume, which is regulated by the kidneys. The interrelationships among all these factors are illustrated in Figure 28-1.

Blood pressure tends to remain at a constant value, and there are many physiologic control mechanisms to protect the organism from harmful perturbations in blood pressure. Two of the most important regulatory mechanisms are the short-term control afforded by the sympathetic nervous system and long-term control, which is a function of the renal system.[14] Moment-to-moment control of blood pressure largely depends on baroreflexes in which sympathetic nervous system output to the heart, resistance vessels, and capacitance vessels are adjusted in response to feedback from baroreceptors in the carotid sinus and aortic arch. These baroreceptors respond to mechanical stretch (increased pressure) by increasing the firing rate of sensory neurons that innervate blood pressure control areas of the central nervous system (CNS). If blood pressure rises, the resultant increased activity of these sensory neurons inhibits efferent sympathetic nervous system

Table • 28-1

Classification of the Severity of Hypertension by Blood Pressure

STAGE	SYSTOLIC (mm Hg)		DIASTOLIC (mm Hg)
Normal	<120	and	<80
Prehypertension	120 to 139	or	80 to 89
Stage 1	140 to 159	or	90 to 99
Stage 2 to 3	>160	or	>100

Hypertension staging corresponds to the higher of the systolic or diastolic blood pressure values.
From the Seventh Report of the Joint National Committee on the prevention, detection, and treatment of high blood pressure, *JAMA* 289:2534-2573, 2003.

activity, thereby reducing heart rate, vascular tone, and blood pressure. Conversely, if blood pressure suddenly falls, baroreceptor output is reduced, allowing increased peripheral sympathetic discharge. This reflex is responsible for the maintenance of blood pressure during rapid stresses to cardiovascular homeostasis, as induced by a change in posture. Long-term stresses on the maintenance of blood pressure (e.g., alterations in water and salt intake) are handled by the kidneys. A change in blood pressure is sensed by the kidneys as a corresponding change in renal perfusion pressure. This disturbance invokes two compensatory mechanisms. First, the tubular reabsorption of Na^+ and water either decreases (in high perfusion pressure) or increases (in low perfusion pressure). This alteration adjusts blood volume and secondarily changes CO to bring blood pressure back to normal. The kidneys also influence resistance vessel tone more directly by releasing renin (thereby activating the renin-angiotensin system) when renal perfusion is diminished. The resultant increase in vasoactive angiotensin peptides raises peripheral vascular resistance by causing vasoconstriction. Angiotensin peptides also promote volume retention by increasing the release of aldosterone and contribute to muscular hypertrophy and other structural changes in the heart and vasculature (collectively referred to as *remodeling*).

The physiologic mechanisms that control blood pressure are important in the treatment of hypertension in two respects. First, each of these mechanisms represents a potential therapeutic target for lowering blood pressure in the hypertensive patient. Second, because these mechanisms are in place to prevent changes in blood pressure, they become activated in an attempt to restore blood pressure to its former (high) level when steps are taken to reduce the hypertension.

Pathophysiologic Characteristics of Essential Hypertension

The physical findings of a patient with essential hypertension usually reveal that CO is normal and TPR is elevated. In the hypertensive patient, the baroreceptor reflexes function normally but have been "reset" to maintain MAP at a higher than normal value. The reasons for this shift are not yet understood and are the subject of intensive research. It is evident that there is a genetic component to essential hypertension and that certain risk factors lead to a worsening of blood pressure elevation (Box 28-1). In many patients, long-term cardiovas-

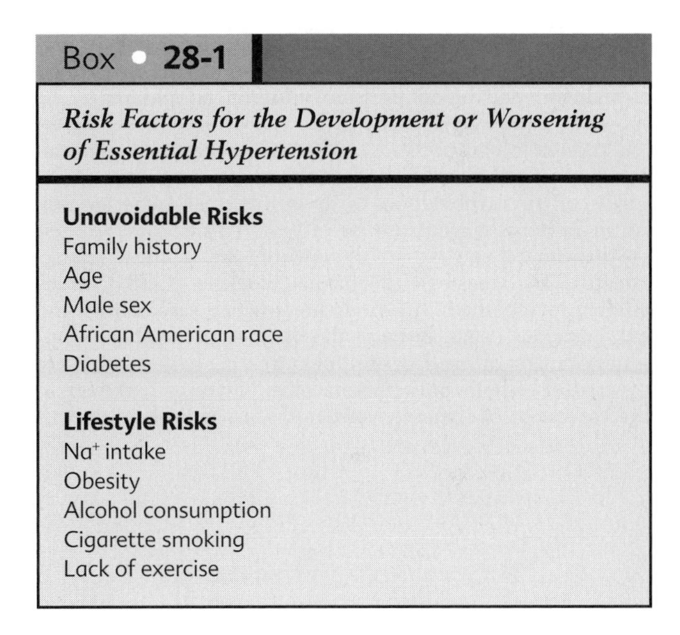
Box • 28-1

Risk Factors for the Development or Worsening of Essential Hypertension

Unavoidable Risks
Family history
Age
Male sex
African American race
Diabetes

Lifestyle Risks
Na^+ intake
Obesity
Alcohol consumption
Cigarette smoking
Lack of exercise

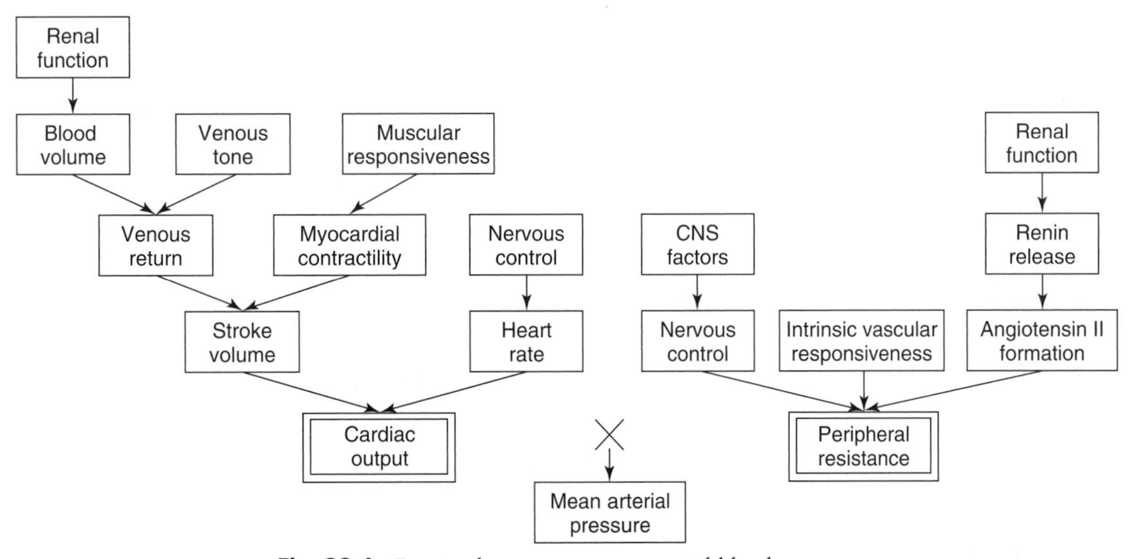

Fig. 28-1 Factors that govern mean arterial blood pressure.

cular complications of hypertension can be controlled solely by making appropriate lifestyle changes.

Although the cause of essential hypertension is unknown, it is well established that high blood pressure leads to cardiovascular and renal disease. In fact, elevated blood pressure is directly correlated with overall mortality (Figure 28-2). The damage caused by decades of elevated arterial pressure can be seen in the form of left ventricular hypertrophy, medial thickening of arteries, and nephropathy.[1,31] These changes contribute to the development of diseases such as congestive heart failure, coronary artery disease, stroke, aneurysm, and renal failure (Box 28-2). Numerous clinical trials have demonstrated a reduction in morbidity and mortality rates after pharmacologic reduction in blood pressure in hypertensive patients. Diabetic patients are particularly vulnerable to targeted organ damage resulting from hypertension. The current standard of care dictates that antihypertensive therapy be prescribed in diabetics whose blood pressure is in the high normal range or above (see Table 28-1). Angiotensin-converting enzyme (ACE) inhibitors are most commonly used for this purpose because of their well-documented protective effects in diabetic patients.[35]

General Aims of Antihypertensive Drug Therapy

Treatment of essential hypertension consists of therapy aimed at reducing the blood pressure into the normal range. As shown in Figure 28-1, many factors play a role in the determination of blood pressure, and, as a consequence, pharmacologic agents with diverse mechanisms of action can be used singly or in combination to treat essential hypertension. Antihypertensive agents can be categorized according to their mechanism of action and therapeutic use: diuretics, drugs affecting angiotensin, Ca^{++}-channel blockers (CCBs), drugs affecting sympathetic function, direct-acting vasodilators, and miscellaneous drugs. Because the basic pharmacologic properties of many of the drugs useful in treating hypertension are covered elsewhere, only pharmacologic features pertinent to the treatment of hypertension are discussed in detail in this chapter. A representation of the major sites of action of antihypertensive agents is shown in Figure 28-3.

DIURETICS

The thiazide diuretics are currently among the initial and most widely used drugs for the management of essential hypertension. The K^+-sparing diuretics are commonly used together with thiazides for their additive effect and to prevent thiazide-induced hypokalemia. The thiazide diuretics may be used alone or in combination with other antihypertensive drugs.

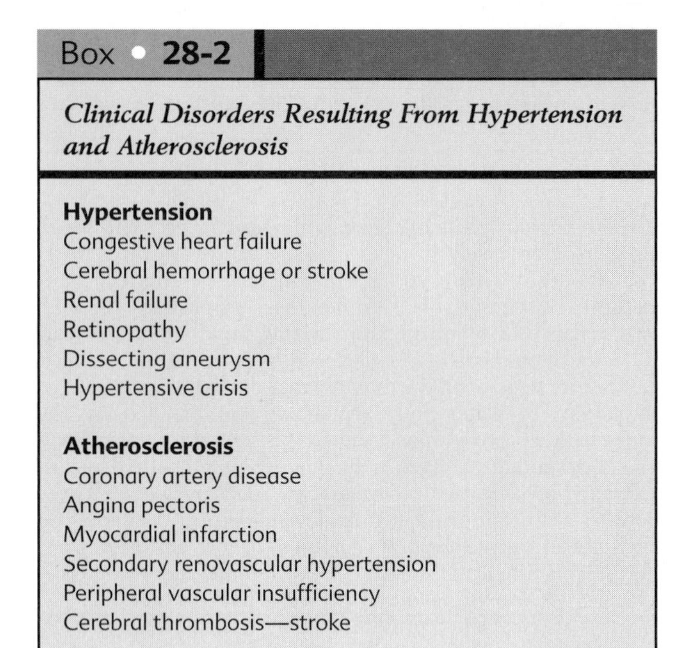

Box • 28-2

Clinical Disorders Resulting From Hypertension and Atherosclerosis

Hypertension
Congestive heart failure
Cerebral hemorrhage or stroke
Renal failure
Retinopathy
Dissecting aneurysm
Hypertensive crisis

Atherosclerosis
Coronary artery disease
Angina pectoris
Myocardial infarction
Secondary renovascular hypertension
Peripheral vascular insufficiency
Cerebral thrombosis—stroke

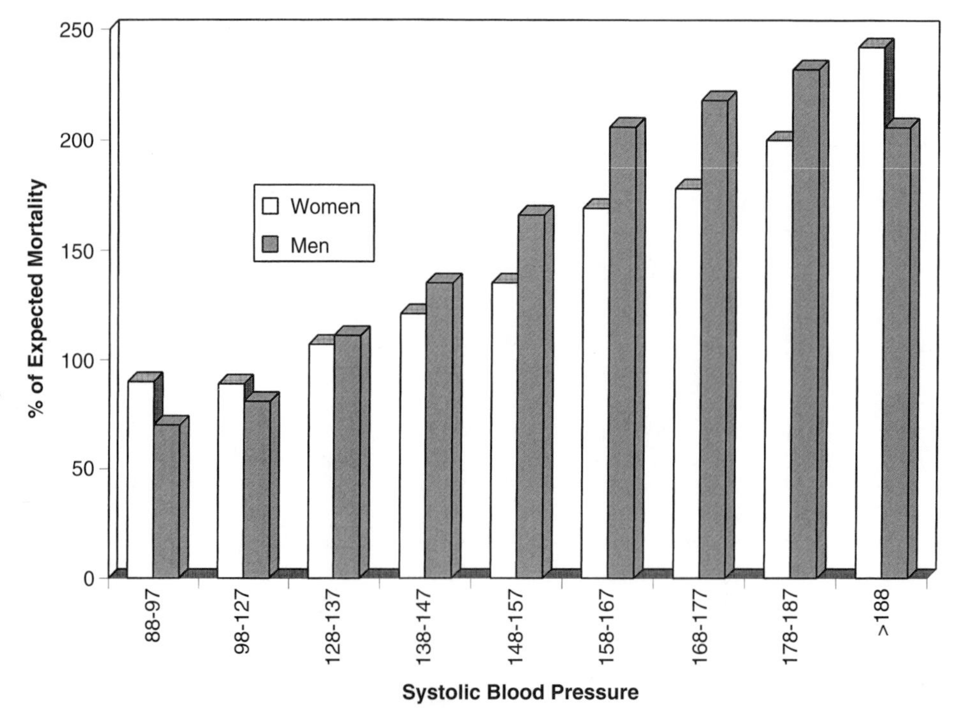

Fig. 28-2 Expected mortality as a function of systolic blood pressure at all ages without regard to treatment. (Adapted from The Society of Actuaries and the Association of Life Insurance Medical Directors of America: *Blood pressure study 1979,* Boston, 1980, The Society.)

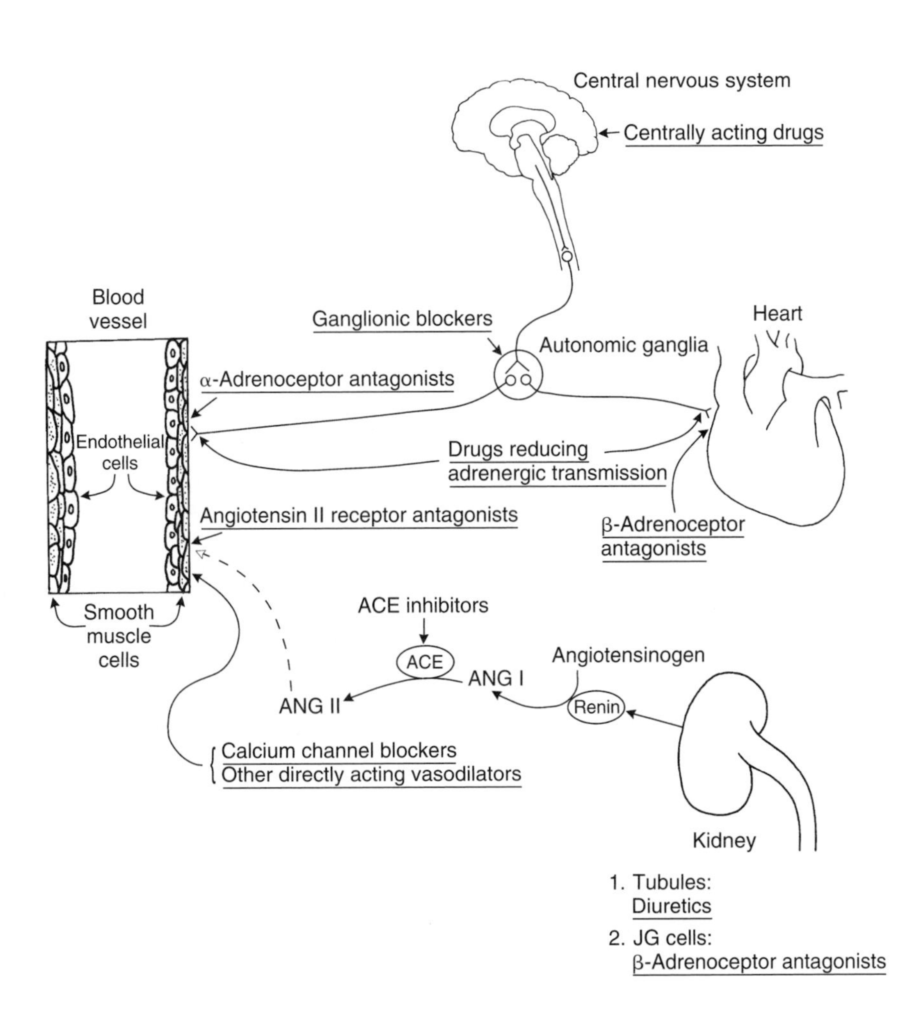

Fig. 28-3 Sites of action of antihypertensive drugs. The diagram indicates by drug class the targets for antihypertensive action. *ANG*, Angiotensin; *JG*, juxtaglomerular.

Loop diuretics such as furosemide are also useful as adjunctive agents in refractory hypertension.

The diuretics reduce plasma volume by increasing Na^+ and water excretion. Initially, this effect lowers blood pressure by decreasing CO. With time, however, CO and extracellular fluid volume return toward normal values, but the hypotensive effect persists because of a reduction in peripheral resistance. It is probable that electrolyte changes in vascular smooth muscle account for the vasodilation. For a complete discussion of diuretics used in the treatment of hypertension, see Chapter 27.

DRUGS AFFECTING ANGIOTENSIN

The role played by the renin-angiotensin system in hypertension has received much attention over the past decade.[8] Renin catalyzes the conversion of angiotensinogen, a glycoprotein found in the blood, to angiotensin I, a decapeptide with little cardiovascular activity (see Figure 28-3). Angiotensin I is activated by conversion to the octapeptide angiotensin II. This reaction is catalyzed by ACE, otherwise known as *dipeptidyl carboxypeptidase* or *peptidyl dipeptidase.* Under its designation as *kininase II*, ACE is also the enzyme that inactivates bradykinin.

Angiotensin II is in turn metabolized by aminopeptidase enzymes to yield the less active and shorter-lived heptapeptide angiotensin III. Increased renin activity thus leads to heightened production of angiotensins II and III, vasoconstriction of peripheral arterioles, and elevation of blood pressure. Moreover, angiotensin peptides stimulate thirst and the secretion of aldosterone and antidiuretic hormone; the resultant increase in extracellular fluid and electrolytes augments the direct pressor effects. Angiotensin II also influences sympathetic nervous system function, both centrally and peripherally, to increase cardiac activity and peripheral vascular resistance.

Patients with essential hypertension can be divided into three groups according to their renin-Na^+ index (i.e., plasma renin activity relative to Na^+ excretion). Approximately 15% of patients have renin concentrations that are higher than normal, 25% have renin concentrations lower than normal, and the remaining 60% exhibit normal renin titers. Renin titers tend to decrease with age. African Americans and the elderly tend to have a higher incidence of low-renin hypertension.

The percentage of hypertensive patients with normal renin activity may be misleading because renin release is ordinarily depressed as the result of increased blood pressure. Thus renin release may still be inappropriately high even in the "normal" group. Although angiotensin II may be the main causative agent in high-renin hypertension and may be a factor in the normal-renin hypertension group, other influences are implicated in low-renin hypertension, and these may contribute to normal-renin hypertension as well.[34]

Pharmacologic intervention to reduce blood pressure can theoretically be made anywhere along the angiotensin system, that is, from the release of renin by the kidney juxtaglomerular cells, to the formation of angiotensin peptides, to the binding of angiotensins II and III to receptors in vascular smooth muscle and other effector sites. In the discussion that follows, attention is limited to those drugs whose primary mechanism of action is interference with the latter two steps in this series of events. It should be recognized, however, that other antihypertensive drugs also affect the renin-angiotensin system. β-Adrenergic receptor antagonists, for instance, inhibit renin release by acting at β_1-adrenergic receptors in the juxtaglomerular apparatus of the kidney. Undesired reflex actions can also occur in which diuretics and direct-acting vasodilators stimulate renin release. Studies indicate that, regardless of the specific drug regimen, treatment of hypertension eventually tends to restore renin to normal levels, whether it was initially high or low.

Angiotensin-Converting Enzyme Inhibitors

The ACE inhibitors are among the most commonly used drugs for the treatment of essential hypertension. Captopril, the first drug of this class to be developed, was specifically designed to disrupt the renin-angiotensin pathway. Its structure is shown in Figure 28-4. Captopril is different from other ACE inhibitors in that it contains a sulfhydryl group. Enalapril, lisinopril, and most of the other ACE inhibitors have an amino acid substitution. Fosinopril, on the other hand, contains a phosphorus linkage.

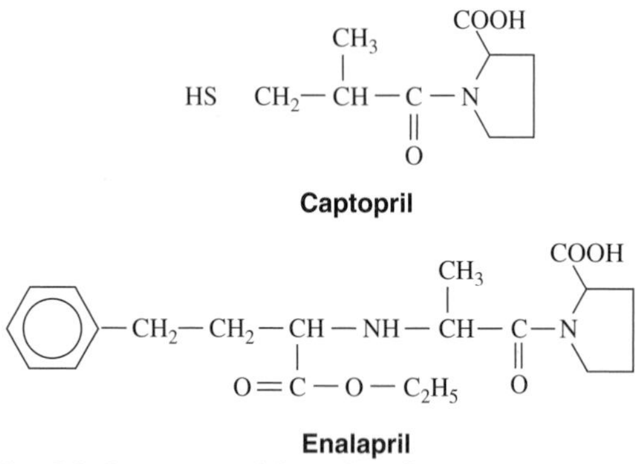

HS CH_2—CH(CH_3)—C(=O)—N (pyrrolidine ring bearing COOH)

Captopril

C_6H_5—CH_2—CH_2—CH($C(=O)—O—C_2H_5$)—NH—CH(CH_3)—C(=O)—N (pyrrolidine ring bearing COOH)

Enalapril

Fig. 28-4 Structural formulas of two ACE inhibitors.

Pharmacologic effects

Drugs that inhibit ACE block the conversion of angiotensin I to angiotensin II (see Figures 28-3 and 28-5).[16] ACE inhibitors markedly decrease blood concentrations of angiotensin II and induce an immediate fall in blood pressure. They may also act to maintain the lowered blood pressure by elevating bradykinin (a potent vasodilator) concentrations in the blood (see Figure 28-5). (As previously mentioned, ACE, as kininase II, is responsible for the breakdown of bradykinin.) Interestingly, ACE inhibitors have an antihypertensive effect even in patients without high renin activities. Over the course of several weeks, blood pressure is progressively reduced, mainly through decreased peripheral resistance, with little effect on CO or renal blood flow. Salt and water retention is not induced, and orthostatic hypotension and tachycardia are not problems. The reduction in angiotensin II concentrations as a result of ACE inhibition leads to a decrease in aldosterone secretion, which in turn results in an increase in Na^+ and water excretion. Correspondingly, there is a net increase in the reabsorption of K^+ in the kidney tubule. Hypokalemia is therefore not an adverse effect of the ACE inhibitors. Indeed, K^+ supplements and K^+-sparing diuretics should not be used concurrently with ACE inhibitors in order to avoid hyperkalemia. With long-term ACE inhibitor therapy, deleterious cardiovascular remodeling may be reduced or even reversed.[7,26] ACE inhibitors are also renal protective and because of this are useful drugs in patients with chronic renal disease and diabetes. In fact, the presence of both high normal (or above) blood pressure and diabetes is a clear indication for the use of an ACE inhibitor.

Absorption, fate, and excretion

The onset of action of captopril is rapid and the duration of effect relatively short, requiring administration two to three times daily. Its elimination half-life is approximately 2 hours. Because food in the gastrointestinal tract significantly reduces the absorption of captopril, the drug should be taken 1 hour before meals. Approximately 40% of captopril is metabolized

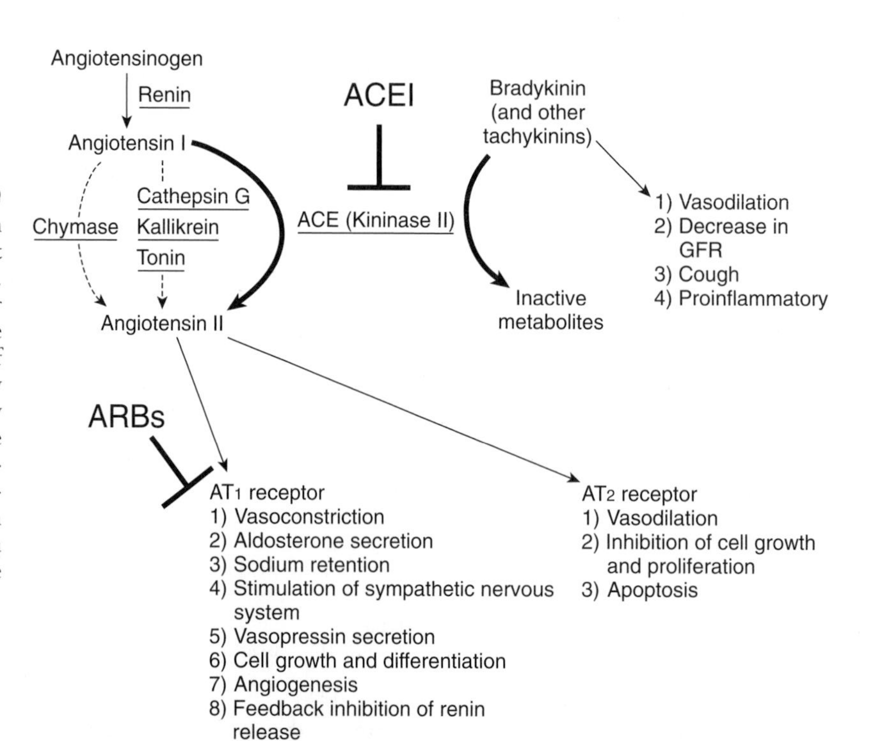

Fig. 28-5 The role of ACE inhibitors *(ACEI)* and angiotensin II receptor blockers (*ARBs*) in treating hypertension. ACEIs block the major but not the only synthetic pathway to angiotensin II. ACEIs also raise the level of bradykinin and other tachykinins, leading to vasodilation as well as some undesirable effects. ARBs block the effect of angiotensin II by whatever synthetic pathway because they block the AT_1 receptor and thereby the response to AT_1-receptor stimulation. The ARBs do not block the AT_2 receptor. This is considered a benefit of ARBs because the AT_2 receptor mediates vasodilation, inhibition of growth and proliferation, and apoptosis. ACE located in tissues is less affected by ACEIs. Enzymes are *underlined*. *GFR*, Glomerular filtration rate.

in the liver, and most of the metabolites as well as the parent drug are excreted by the kidney.

Lisinopril is less well absorbed than captopril, resulting in peak plasma concentrations after approximately 7 hours. The slow elimination half-life of roughly 12 hours permits single daily dosing of the drug. Lisinopril is excreted unchanged in the urine.

Enalapril (see Figure 28-4) is a prodrug that must be hydrolyzed in the liver to become fully active. Its absorption is not influenced by food, however, and it has a longer duration of effect than captopril. The active metabolite enalaprilat, with a plasma half-life of 11 hours, provides for the extended action. Enalaprilat is not absorbed from the gastrointestinal tract but is effective after intravenous administration; it has been marketed for such use in patients unable to take drugs orally. Other ACE inhibitors with an esterified carboxyl side chain are also activated (by hydrolysis) in the liver to "prilat" metabolites that avidly bind to ACE and provide durations of effect sufficient for single daily dosing. The other ACE inhibitors are listed at the end of this chapter. They differ primarily in their pharmacokinetic properties.

Adverse effects

The most frequent side effect of the ACE inhibitors is coughing, which occurs in up to 20% of patients.[9] Altered or reduced taste sensation is also common, especially with captopril. These adverse effects may disappear after continued use. The significance of reported cases of proteinuria is not established at this time. Skin rash; angioedema of the face, mucous membranes of the mouth, or extremities; and flushing, pallor, and hypotension have been documented. Angioedema is a serious condition that demands withdrawal of the drug. Hyperkalemia and neutropenia may rarely occur.

ACE inhibitors may cause renal insufficiency in patients with bilateral renal stenosis. The mechanism is the reduction of renal angiotensin II production, leading to a disproportionate dilation of efferent renal blood vessels compared with afferent vessels. This vascular imbalance results in a significant drop in the glomerular filtration rate. ACE inhibitors, on the other hand, can help preserve renal function in the diabetic patient.[20] Furthermore, ACE inhibitors actually have the beneficial effect of reducing proteinuria in patients with some renal diseases.

Although ACE inhibitors are not known to be teratogenic during the first trimester of pregnancy, they can cause significant developmental defects and fetal death later on. After pregnancy has been established, discontinuance or substitution with another antihypertensive agent is mandatory.

Angiotensin Receptor Antagonists

Losartan (as losartan potassium) was the first orally active angiotensin II receptor antagonist to be introduced (Figure 28-6). Other angiotensin II antagonists include candesartan, eprosartan, irbesartan, telmisartan, and valsartan. These nonpeptide analogues of angiotensin bind to the angiotensin II receptor and competitively inhibit the action of angiotensins II and III.[18] They are selective inhibitors of the AT_1 receptor, the angiotensin receptor subtype that accounts for the major physiologic effects of angiotensin II. The effect is to inhibit the consequences of AT_1 receptor stimulation without affecting potentially beneficial effects mediated by the AT_2 receptor (see Figure 28-5).[24] As is the case with the ACE inhibitors, the AT_1 receptor blockers both reduce the blood pressure and the tissue remodeling seen in hypertension and thereby reduce organ damage resulting from hypertension.[28] Losartan has a half-life of only 1.5 hours, but it is metabolized to an active metabolite with a longer half-life. Valsartan has a plasma half-life of 6 hours; it is excreted in the bile largely in the unchanged form. The half-lives for the other angiotensin II blockers range from 6 hours for eprosartan to 24 hours for telmisartan. The selectivity of angiotensin II antagonists avoids some of the side effects of the ACE inhibitors, namely coughing and angioedema, because the bradykinin pathway is not affected by the angiotensin II antagonists (see Figure 28-5). Orally effective angiotensin II receptor antagonists now constitute a major drug group for treating hypertension.[5]

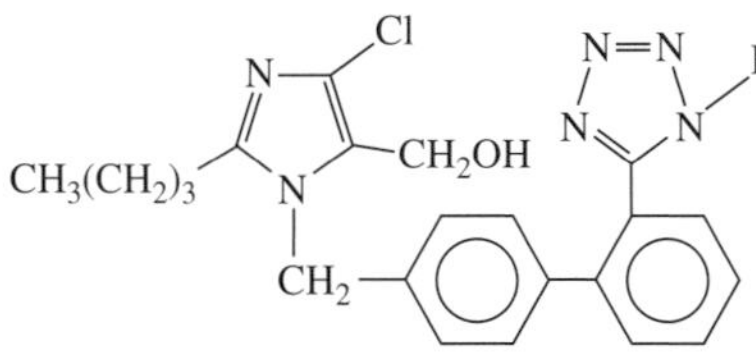

Losartan

Fig. 28-6 Structural formula of losartan.

Ca^{++}-CHANNEL BLOCKERS (CCBs)

Verapamil, diltiazem, and nifedipine were the first CCBs to be marketed. The pharmacologic features of nifedipine and its dihydropyridine congeners, including amlodipine, felodipine, isradipine, nicardipine, nimodipine, nisoldipine, and nitrendipine, are addressed in this chapter. Other CCBs are discussed in Chapters 24 and 26.

Pharmacologic Effects

All CCBs prevent Ca^{++} influx into smooth and cardiac muscle cells. However, the potency of these drugs for each of these actions varies, producing some important clinical distinctions between the dihydropyridines and verapamil and diltiazem. These latter two drugs inhibit Ca^{++} influx into both vascular smooth muscle and the heart with roughly the same potency. Thus the effect of verapamil and diltiazem is to lower blood pressure by vasodilation and reduced CO. On the other hand, dihydropyridines such as nifedipine are much more potent at inhibiting Ca^{++} influx at vascular smooth muscle than in the heart. Therefore, at clinically relevant plasma concentrations, nifedipine produces a pronounced vasodilation with little direct effect on cardiac function. Reflex tachycardia is a common side effect with the dihydropyridines but is almost never seen with verapamil and diltiazem. CCBs are contraindicated in patients with cardiac conduction defects and in heart failure. The CCBs are useful drugs for treating low-renin hypertension.

Dihydropyridines enhance the glomerular filtration rate and renal blood flow. However, some patients taking dihydropyridines develop pedal edema. This condition does not result from fluid retention but rather from precapillary dilation. Renal Na^+ excretion may be enhanced. The antihypertensive effect and an apparent direct renal protective effect of these drugs may make them useful in treating chronic renal failure.

Absorption, Fate, and Excretion

The plasma half-times of most CCBs (diltiazem, isradipine, nicardipine, nifedipine, and verapamil) range from 2 to 8 hours. The half-lives of the others are as follows: amlodipine, 30 to 50 hours; felodipine, 10 to 16 hours; nimodipine, 1 to 2 hours; nisoldipine, 7 to 12 hours; and nitrendipine, 10 to 20 hours. Long-term therapy may be associated with some increase in half-times for some CCBs.

The elimination half-life and duration of action influence the clinical use of these agents. The short time course of nimodipine, along with its relative ability to cross the blood-brain barrier, limits the drug's suitability for the treatment of chronic disease but permits its use to prevent vasospasm subsequent to subarachnoid hemorrhage. Short-acting nifedipine has been associated with an increased cardiovascular mortality rate during long-term use and is no longer used for treating hypertension. The drug's short duration of action causes the blood pressure to wax and wane with each dose. A slow-release version of the drug stabilizes blood concentrations and now is the recommended formulation. In fact, long half-life CCBs or slow-release preparations are recommended for this reason.

Adverse Effects

Toxic reactions and side effects of the CCBs are described in Chapter 26.

DRUGS REDUCING SYMPATHETIC FUNCTION

One of the major homeostatic roles of the autonomic nervous system is control of cardiovascular function. Thus it follows that drugs affecting autonomic activity are useful in controlling blood pressure in essential hypertension. This section describes those drugs that exert their antihypertensive action on the sympathetic division of the autonomic nervous system. These drugs can conveniently be divided into four groups according to their site of action: (1) α-adrenergic receptor–blocking drugs, (2) β-adrenergic receptor–blocking drugs, (3) drugs altering peripheral adrenergic transmission, and (4) drugs acting on the CNS. (It should be pointed out that other drugs that alter adrenergic function, such as monoamine oxidase inhibitors, have been used in treating hypertension, but their use has been in almost all cases superseded by newer agents with fewer adverse effects and greater effectiveness.) Only those actions and side effects pertinent to the antihypertensive use of agents affecting adrenergic function are described here. For discussion of other uses and actions of these drugs, see Chapter 7.

β-Adrenergic Receptor–Blocking Drugs

The structures of several β-adrenergic receptor–blocking drugs are shown in Figure 28-7. Propranolol, the prototype for this class of drugs, and its congeners are not only used as antihypertensives but are used in many other disorders, including cardiac arrhythmias, angina pectoris, and migraine headache. As indicated in Chapter 7, some of these agents, including propranolol, block both β_1 and β_2 receptors, whereas others, such as metoprolol, have a selective effect on β_1 receptors of the heart. Some drugs classified as β-adrenergic blocking drugs are actually partial agonists, and some exert a membrane-stabilizing effect analogous to that of the local anesthetics. Because the local anesthetic action of the β-blocking drugs occurs at doses higher than those used clinically, it may not be clinically relevant.

Pharmacologic effects

The various β-adrenergic receptor–blocking drugs are about equally effective in the management of hypertension, irrespective of subtype selectivity. They can be used alone or in combination with diuretics and other antihypertensive medications. Although much information is available, the exact mechanisms by which these drugs decrease blood pressure remain equivocal. Their effects have been attributed to the following actions: blockade of β_1 receptors resulting in decreased CO, decreased renin secretion, decreased central sympathetic outflow, blockade of prejunctional β receptors on adrenergic nerve endings, and resetting of baroreceptors.[21] Of these mechanisms, the first two are probably the most important for blood pressure control.[21] Some investigators believe that hypertension characterized by high CO or high plasma renin activities represents a specific indication for β receptor antagonist therapy. Partial β receptor agonists produce less bradycardia than β receptor antagonists. Cardioselective β-adrenergic receptor antagonists, having less affinity for bronchial β_2 receptors, are less likely to precipitate asthmatic attacks in susceptible individuals.

Absorption, fate, and excretion

The pharmacokinetics of the β-adrenergic receptor–blocking drugs are strongly influenced by lipid solubility, as illustrated by the highly lipophilic propranolol and the poorly lipid-soluble nadolol and atenolol. Propranolol and most β-adrenergic blocking agents are readily absorbed from the gastrointestinal tract, although bioavailability of an administered dose is often restricted to 50% or less by extensive first-pass metabolism in the liver. The bioavailability of nadolol and atenolol is limited to a similar extent because of incomplete absorption. Plasma protein binding, a factor that also tends to correlate with lipid solubility, ranges from 10% (atenolol) to 90% (propranolol).

Metabolism and excretion also vary with the particular β blocker. Propranolol is almost entirely biotransformed in the liver; nadolol and atenolol are essentially excreted unchanged in the urine; agents of more intermediate lipid solubility show a mixture of elimination pathways. Whereas the plasma half-life of most β-adrenergic receptor antagonists approximates that of propranolol (3 to 5 hours), the slow excretion of nadolol (half-time up to 24 hours) gives the drug an extended duration of action that permits once-daily dosing.

Adverse effects

β-Adrenergic receptor antagonists cause a variety of side effects; tolerance may develop to some but not to others. Those side effects to which early tolerance may develop include nausea, vomiting, anorexia, confusion, dizziness, fatigue, sleep disturbances, and depression.

One of the major toxic effects of the β-adrenergic receptor antagonists is the aggravation of an existing defect in myocardial contractility or atrioventricular conduction. Congestive heart failure and bradyarrhythmias may be exacerbated. (It should be noted, however, that β blockers are used in the treatment of heart failure as discussed in Chapter 25.) Blockade of β receptor–mediated vasodilation may worsen peripheral arterial insufficiency, intermittent claudication, and Raynaud's phenomenon. Bronchospasm may also be induced in asthmatics, particularly with the nonselective β antagonists.

Nonselective β blockers and, to a lesser extent, selective β_1-adrenergic receptor antagonists, inhibit the ability of endogenous catecholamines to elevate plasma glucose concentrations and therefore should be used with caution in patients prone to hypoglycemia or those being treated with insulin or sulfonylureas for diabetes. All blockers can reduce the tachycardia resulting from hypoglycemia. Thus they may mask an important sign used to indicate overdosage of hypoglycemic agents.

Abrupt withdrawal of β-adrenergic receptor antagonists in patients with coronary heart disease increases the likelihood of severe ischemic events and may lead to anginal pain, myocardial infarction, or life-threatening arrhythmia. Abrupt withdrawal in hypertensive patients may result in increased blood pressure and heart rate, palpitation, tremors, and sweating. It is therefore important that dosages be gradually decreased when drug treatment with β blockers is terminated.

Salt and water retention, which is a problem with some antihypertensive medications, has not been reported with the β-adrenergic receptor–blocking drugs. Postural hypotension is also not generally encountered.

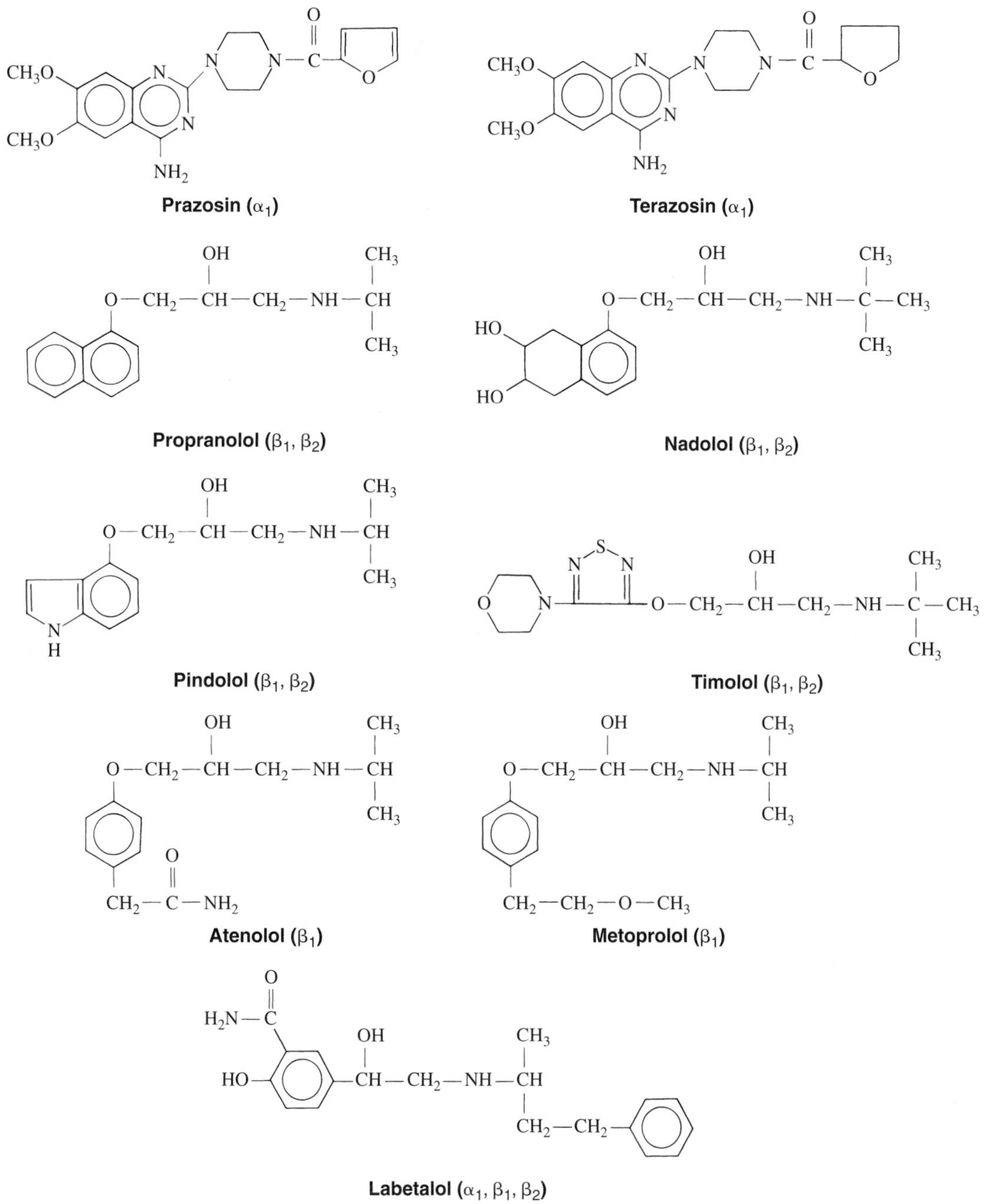

Prazosin (α_1)

Terazosin (α_1)

Propranolol (β_1, β_2)

Nadolol (β_1, β_2)

Pindolol (β_1, β_2)

Timolol (β_1, β_2)

Atenolol (β_1)

Metoprolol (β_1)

Labetalol (α_1, β_1, β_2)

Fig. 28-7 Structures of some α- and β-adrenergic receptor–blocking drugs and their receptor selectivity.

Selective α_1-Adrenergic Receptor—Blocking Drugs

Prazosin is the first of a group of selective α_1-adrenergic receptor–blocking agents used for the treatment of hypertension. Terazosin and doxazosin have a similar action. The chemical structures of these drugs are shown in Figure 28-7, and their general pharmacologic characteristics are discussed in Chapter 7.

Pharmacologic effects

The hypotensive effect of these drugs is ascribed to vasodilation of arterioles and capacitance veins. The action is a result of blockade of α_1 receptors on vascular smooth muscle. Unlike older, nonselective α blockers such as phenoxybenzamine, these drugs have a relatively low affinity for α_2 receptors. They can be used in mild to severe hypertension, either alone, with diuretics, or with other antihypertensive drugs.

Nonselective α-adrenergic receptor blockers are used only occasionally in therapy. Their ability to block both α_1 and α_2 receptors is useful, however, in treating the hypertension resulting from pheochromocytoma. With this disease, both α_1 and α_2 receptors play a major role in the hypertensive response to the elevated circulating catecholamine concentrations. Phentolamine is a competitive antagonist, whereas phenoxybenzamine is a noncompetitive antagonist. Tolazoline is another drug that is a competitive antagonist at both α_1 and

α_2 receptors, with a slight preference for α_2 receptors. It has limited clinical use.

The adverse effects of the nonselective α-adrenergic receptor antagonists are more notable than those of the selective α_1-adrenergic receptor blockers. Inhibition of prejunctional α_2 receptors accounts for the greater reflex tachycardia seen with the nonselective blockers. Furthermore, there is a higher incidence of orthostatic hypotension and fluid retention compared with the selective α_1-adrenergic receptor antagonists.

Absorption, fate, and excretion

Prazosin and terazosin are rapidly absorbed from the gastrointestinal tract and are available only for oral use. Prazosin undergoes more first-pass metabolism than does terazosin or doxazosin. Prazosin is bound significantly to plasma α_1-acid glycoprotein and is excreted principally as glucuronide conjugates, with approximately 90% appearing in the feces and 10% in the urine. The plasma half-life of prazosin (approximately 2 hours) does not correlate with the duration of its hypotensive effect because of tissue binding and the formation of active metabolites, and the drug is administered two to three times daily. Terazosin is eliminated more slowly (half-life of 12 hours), which usually permits dosing once daily. The half-life of doxazosin is approximately 22 hours. Both terazosin and doxazosin are highly bound to plasma proteins and extensively metabolized.

Adverse effects

Prazosin and other α_1-adrenergic receptor blockers produce less reflex tachycardia than do direct vasodilators or nonselective α-adrenergic receptor blockers. Nevertheless, reflex tachycardia may be significant. Syncope from orthostatic hypotension may occur with the initiation of therapy. This heightened response early in therapy has been termed the "first-dose" effect.[22] Postural hypotension usually abates with continued therapy. These drugs share an array of other side effects, including gastrointestinal upset, palpitation, tinnitus, headache, rash, edema, and urinary incontinence. Inhibition of ejaculation may also occur.

α_1-/β-Adrenergic Receptor Blockers

Labetalol is a competitive blocker of α_1, β_1, and β_2 receptors, with a greater affinity for β receptors. It also exerts some β_2-agonistic activity and inhibits norepinephrine uptake by the presynaptic nerve terminal. This extensive pharmacologic profile results from the fact that the drug is actually composed of four different diastereoisomers, each of which has distinct effects. Labetalol has been used singly and in combination with other antihypertensive agents. Used both orally and intravenously, labetalol undergoes significant first-pass metabolism in the liver, accounting for approximately 75% of an oral dose. It has a half-life of approximately 8 hours and is metabolized to the glucuronide conjugate. Labetalol is especially useful in treating pheochromocytoma and hypertensive emergencies. Among its adverse effects are gastrointestinal disturbances, dry mouth, fatigue, nervousness, paresthesias, orthostatic hypotension, and bradycardia. Patients with asthma are at risk of bronchospasm.

Carvedilol is the second drug with mixed α_1- and β-adrenergic receptor–blocking activity to be marketed for the treatment of hypertension. As with labetalol, several stereoisomers contribute to the drug's complex pharmacologic characteristics. The pharmacokinetic profile is similar to that of labetalol; however, one of the isomers of carvedilol, which contributes roughly half of the drug's α-blocking activity, accumulates up to threefold in patients genetically deficient in cytochrome P4502D6 activity. Carvedilol is available only for oral use.

Drugs That Affect Adrenergic Transmission

Guanethidine, guanadrel, and the rauwolfia alkaloid reserpine exert their primary antihypertensive action on peripheral postganglionic adrenergic nerve endings and are thus classified as adrenergic neuron–blocking drugs.

Pharmacologic effects

The ultimate effect of reserpine, guanethidine, and guanadrel is depletion of norepinephrine from adrenergic nerve endings, although the mechanism by which depletion occurs with reserpine differs from that of guanethidine and guanadrel. All three drugs must enter the adrenergic nerve ending to exert an antihypertensive effect. Reserpine inhibits the active uptake of catecholamines into the storage vesicles of the nerve terminal. Inhibition of synaptic transmission occurs in concert with the progressive depletion of neurotransmitter. The mechanisms of action of guanethidine are the same as those of guanadrel. After intravenous injection, guanethidine yields a complex response. Guanethidine may lead to an initial increase in blood pressure caused by the release of catecholamines, which in turn gives way several hours later to extended hypotension associated with inhibition of evoked norepinephrine release. Only the hypotensive effect is usually observed with oral use. The inhibition of norepinephrine release appears to result from a local anesthetic effect on the adrenergic nerve terminal. Competition between norepinephrine and guanethidine for uptake into the nerve terminal and storage in the adrenergic vesicles eventually causes depletion of norepinephrine, but this outcome, while supportive of a decrease in sympathetic activity, is not crucial to the therapeutic effect.

The cardiovascular manifestations that result from these actions and make these agents useful in treating hypertension are decreases in both peripheral resistance and CO.[23] Reserpine enters the CNS, and some of its antihypertensive action may be caused by effects at this site. Guanethidine and guanadrel do not readily cross the blood-brain barrier and thus exert their actions solely on peripheral postganglionic neurons.

Absorption, fate, and excretion

Reserpine is readily absorbed from the gastrointestinal tract but exhibits a slow onset of antihypertensive effect (up to 3 weeks for maximum effect). Its duration of action is long, probably owing to its strong binding to amine transport sites in storage granules. It is excreted as the parent compound and as various metabolites.

Although only available for oral use, guanethidine is poorly absorbed from the gastrointestinal tract, varying from 3% to 30% among different individuals. Guanethidine and its metabolites are slowly excreted in the urine, and small amounts remain in the tissues for prolonged periods (2 weeks). Guanadrel has better absorption, a more rapid onset, and a shorter duration of action than guanethidine.

Adverse effects

The most frequent untoward effects of reserpine are results of actions on either the CNS or the gastrointestinal tract.[22] Sedation is common. Nightmares and emotional depression leading to suicidal tendencies are possible with large doses. Abdominal cramps and diarrhea result because reserpine reduces sympathetic function, resulting in greater parasympathetic effects. Reserpine can also cause nasal congestion. This effect is not serious in adults. However, reserpine passes the placental barrier and can cause nasal congestion, cyanosis, drowsiness, and gastrointestinal disturbances in the newborn when given before term.

The major troublesome adverse effect of guanethidine is orthostatic hypotension. Other side effects include difficulty in ejaculation, nocturia, intestinal cramps, Na^+ and water retention, bradycardia, flushing, weakness, depression, and diarrhea. Guanadrel's pharmacologic properties are essentially the same as those of guanethidine, but its use is associated with a lower frequency of diarrhea.

Centrally Acting Antihypertensive Drugs

Methyldopa, clonidine, guanabenz, and guanfacine are drugs that exert their antihypertensive effect by stimulating α_2 receptors in the brainstem. As a result, these drugs reduce sympathetic outflow from the brain. The structures of methyldopa, clonidine, guanabenz, and guanfacine are shown in Figure 28-8. The structural similarity of methyldopa to the catecholamine transmitter norepinephrine is obvious. Clonidine, guanabenz, and guanfacine are not chemically related to norepinephrine but are very similar in structure to the α-adrenergic receptor–blocking drug tolazoline.

Pharmacologic effects

Methyldopa, a prodrug, is biotransformed in the brain to α-methyldopamine and then to α-methylnorepinephrine. The latter metabolite probably stimulates important α_2-adrenergic receptor sites in the medulla, resulting in inhibition of central sympathetic outflow. In addition, there is evidence that vagal activity to the heart is increased. Clonidine, guanabenz, and guanfacine appear to act directly as central α_2-adrenergic receptor agonists. With all four drugs, the reduction in central sympathetic outflow and increased vagal activity lead to reduced peripheral vascular resistance and CO. It is not certain whether presynaptic or postsynaptic medullary α_2 receptors play the predominant role in mediating the antihypertensive response.

Absorption, fate, and excretion

Methyldopa can be given orally or intravenously (as methyldopate hydrochloride). Approximately 25% to 50% of an orally administered dose of methyldopa is absorbed from the gastrointestinal tract. Although methyldopa and its metabolites appear rapidly in the urine, significant concentrations remain in the body for longer periods. It has a relatively long duration of action (up to 24 hours), probably because α-methylnorepinephrine is not metabolized by monoamine oxidase but is stored in synaptic vesicles in central adrenergic nerve terminals.

Clonidine is available for both oral and parenteral use and is well absorbed after oral administration. Peak plasma concentrations are achieved in 3 to 5 hours; its half-life is approximately 10 hours. Roughly 50% is metabolized in the liver. The remaining clonidine and its metabolites are primarily excreted in the urine.

Approximately 75% of an oral dose of guanabenz is absorbed, but hepatic metabolism decreases bioavailability. Peak plasma concentrations appear between 2 and 5 hours after administration. The plasma half-life is approximately 6 hours. A large percentage of guanabenz is metabolized in the liver and excreted by the kidney. Guanfacine is rapidly and nearly completely absorbed from the gastrointestinal tract. It has a half-life of 14 to 17 hours. The drug is partly hydroxylated, and both parent drug and metabolites are excreted in the urine.

Adverse effects

Untoward effects of methyldopa include drowsiness, depression, nightmares, dry mouth, and nasal stuffiness.[37] The drowsiness caused by this drug, although usually transient, may be particularly bothersome. Orthostatic hypotension may occur but is less frequent than with guanethidine because the baroreceptor reflex is not greatly affected by the centrally acting drugs. Extrapyramidal reactions, prolactin release, and impotence may also occur. Hepatitis, a lupus-like syndrome, drug fever, and blood dyscrasias are rare adverse manifestations.

The most common side effects of clonidine are dry mouth and sedation.[23] The incidence of these effects is high, but some tolerance may develop during long-term therapy. Other side effects include parotid gland pain, nightmares, and insomnia. Constipation and impotence occur in a small percentage of patients treated with clonidine. Other less frequent adverse effects are allergic reactions and orthostatic hypotension. Rebound hypertension has been observed on abrupt withdrawal of clonidine therapy. The sudden withdrawal of clonidine is also associated with tachycardia, anxiety, and insomnia. Thus, when withdrawal is necessary, the dosage should be reduced gradually.

Guanabenz has not been found to cause postural hypotension. Adverse side effects, listed in order of decreasing frequency, are drowsiness, dry mouth, dizziness, weakness, and headache. Guanfacine's side effects are mild and dose related. They include fatigue, dizziness, dry mouth, insomnia, and even impotence, but they tend to be less disturbing than with clonidine or guanabenz. Abrupt withdrawal of both guanabenz and guanfacine has been associated with rebound hypertension.

Direct-Acting Vasodilators

Hydralazine, minoxidil, diazoxide, nitroprusside, nitroglycerin, and epoprostenol are considered together in this section because they exert their primary antihypertensive effect through a direct action on vascular smooth muscle. Figure 28-9 summarizes the functional relationship between vascu-

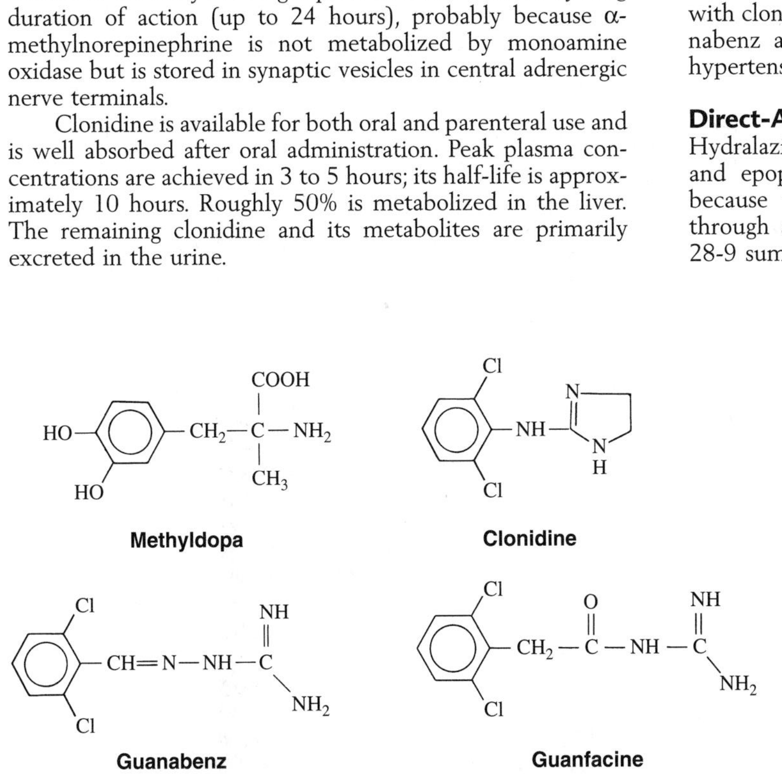

Methyldopa

Clonidine

Guanabenz

Guanfacine

Fig. 28-8 Structural formulas of centrally acting antihypertensive drugs.

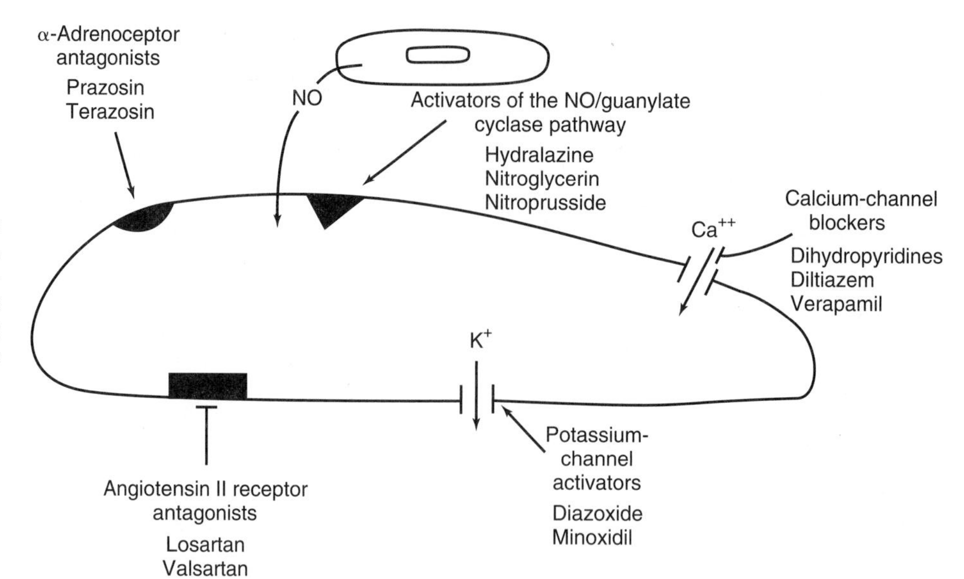

Fig. 28-9 Sites of action of drugs that relax vascular smooth muscle. Five drug types that act on the vascular smooth muscle cell *(bottom)* are depicted. An endothelial cell *(top)* that releases nitric oxide *(NO)* is also shown.

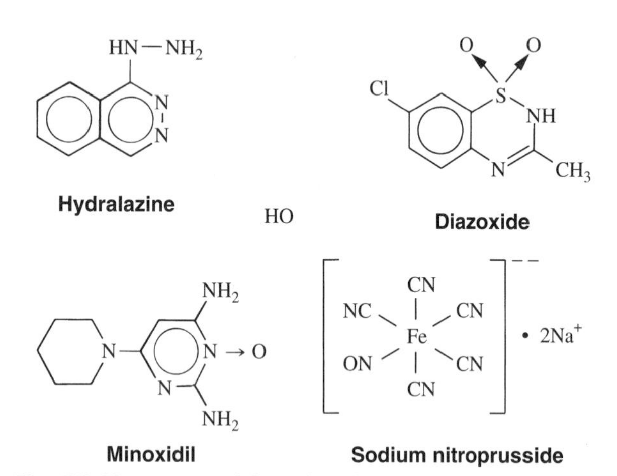

Fig. 28-10 Structural formulas of direct-acting vasodilators.

lar endothelial cells and vascular smooth muscle as well as depicts the site of action of the direct-acting vasodilators and other drugs that relax vascular smooth muscle by inhibiting membrane-bound proteins involved in contractile responses.

Hydralazine

Hydralazine is one of a series of phthalazine derivatives that have been shown to reduce blood pressure and is the only agent of this series available in the United States. The chemical structure of this compound is shown in Figure 28-10.

Pharmacologic effects Hydralazine exerts a preferential effect on arterioles compared with veins. The resulting changes are decreased peripheral resistance, decreased blood pressure, and reflexly increased heart rate, stroke volume, and CO. It stimulates guanylyl cyclase in vascular smooth muscle cells, leading to a decrease in muscle tone. The preferential effect on arterioles reduces the incidence of orthostatic hypotension. Reflex inotropic and chronotropic effects that accompany hydralazine vasodilation may cause exacerbation of existing angina pectoris. Hydralazine has no important therapeutic actions on systems other than the cardiovascular system.

Absorption, fate, and excretion Hydralazine is available for parenteral and oral use. It is readily absorbed from the gastrointestinal tract, and peak blood concentrations are reached in 1 hour. The plasma half-life is also approximately 1 hour; however, hydralazine exhibits a high affinity for vascular muscle and is slowly removed from these sites. Only a small percentage of hydralazine is excreted unchanged, with the major portion undergoing acetylation. A dichotomous distribution exists in the rate of metabolism, with half of the population being characterized as fast acetylators.

Adverse effects A high incidence of side effects is associated with hydralazine therapy. The more common untoward effects are palpitation (and angina in susceptible patients), headache, anorexia, nausea, dizziness, and sweating. Less frequently encountered effects include nasal congestion, flushing, tremors, cramps, postural hypotension, and depression. Tolerance to these effects may develop, especially if the initial dosage is gradually increased. Long-term administration of hydralazine in large doses may cause a syndrome resembling lupus erythematosus, particularly in slow acetylators.

Minoxidil

Minoxidil is another antihypertensive drug that acts chiefly through arteriolar vasodilation. The chemical structure of this piperidinopyrimidine is shown in Figure 28-10. Minoxidil is reserved for use in patients refractory to other therapy.

Pharmacologic effects Minoxidil, like other peripheral vasodilators, reduces blood pressure by decreasing TPR. Minoxidil activates K^+ channels, resulting in hyperpolarization, stabilization of the smooth muscle plasma membrane, and reduced contraction.[25] The drug is a prodrug requiring conversion to minoxidil sulfate (a quantitatively minor metabolite) for its vasodilator effect.

The decrease in blood pressure from minoxidil is accompanied by reflex increases in cardiac function, renin secretion, and fluid retention. These potentially adverse responses may be corrected by coadministration of β-adrenergic receptor–blocking agents and diuretics. Minoxidil has no central depressant effects.

Absorption, fate, and excretion The onset of action of minoxidil after oral administration is rapid, and its hypotensive action is of long duration. This compound is primarily excreted in the urine as the glucuronide conjugate, along with small amounts of the parent compound and hydroxylated derivatives.

Adverse effects The marked fluid retention caused by minoxidil can lead to congestive heart failure. There are reports of pericardial effusion and cardiac tamponade, sometimes with fatal outcomes. As with other vasodilators, the reflex tachycardia may initiate or intensify angina. Dermatologic reactions and breast tenderness may also occur. Finally, abnormal hair growth, or hypertrichosis, is very common and limits the use of this drug. Topical minoxidil is approved, in fact, for the treatment of alopecia and baldness.

Diazoxide

Diazoxide is a nondiuretic thiazide derivative (see Figure 28-10) with direct action as a vasodilator. It reduces blood pressure rapidly, making it useful in hypertensive emergencies and malignant hypertension. Orally, the antihypoglycemic action of diazoxide finds use occasionally in the treatment of hypoglycemia caused by insulin.

Pharmacologic effects Like minoxidil, diazoxide acts by opening K^+ channels. Diazoxide has its major effect on arterioles, with much less effect on capacitance vessels. Intravenous administration of the drug routinely leads to tachycardia and increased CO. Unlike the thiazide diuretics, diazoxide promotes salt and water retention. The opening of K^+ channels accounts for its inhibition of insulin release.

Absorption, fate, and excretion Diazoxide is restricted to the intravenous route for the treatment of hypertension. In plasma it is 90% bound to albumin. Its plasma half-life is 20 to 60 hours. Approximately two thirds of the drug is metabolized in the liver. Excretion of metabolites and the parent drug is by the kidney.

Adverse effects Fluid retention and hyperglycemia can occur, especially if therapy is extended. A diuretic is often required to overcome the fluid retention, and diabetic patients may require added therapy to treat the hyperglycemia. Hyperuricemia, severe hypotension, angina, and cerebral ischemia may occur as well.

Sodium nitroprusside

Sodium nitroprusside (see Figure 28-10) is a direct relaxer of vascular smooth muscle. Its principal uses are to provide controlled hypotension during surgery and to treat hypertensive emergencies, as described later in this chapter.

Pharmacologic effects Nitroprusside is a nitrovasodilator. It generates nitric oxide, which activates guanylyl cyclase in vascular smooth muscle.[17] The resulting relaxation of smooth muscle accounts for its antihypertensive response. The drug affects both veins and arterioles and therefore reduces both preload and afterload. Because both capacitance and resistance vessels are dilated, cardiac ischemia and angina are not as frequently associated with nitroprusside as with arteriolar vasodilators.

Absorption, fate, and excretion Nitroprusside works rapidly after intravenous administration. It is not used orally. In addition to producing nitric oxide, it is converted nonenzymatically to cyanide by red blood cells and then further metabolized to thiocyanate in the liver and kidney. The half-life of nitroprusside is measured in minutes; thiocyanate may persist with a half-life of approximately 3 days. Thiocyanate is excreted by the kidney.

Adverse effects Adverse reactions can be classified as acute or chronic. Acute effects include a precipitous fall in blood pressure, with resultant sweating, vomiting, headache, nervousness, and palpitation. Metabolic acidosis, methemoglobinemia, and cardiac arrhythmias have occurred. Cyanide accumulation may occur in some individuals, leading to toxicity. Thiocyanate may accumulate in patients with renal insufficiency. Thiocyanate may cause psychosis, muscle weakness, and even hypothyroid symptoms.

Nitroglycerin

Nitroglycerin is described in detail in Chapter 26. When given intravenously, nitroglycerin is an effective treatment for perioperative hypertension and to induce controlled hypotension during surgery. Similar in mechanism of action to nitroprusside, nitroglycerin exerts a relatively greater effect on capacitance vessels. Continuous infusion with careful monitoring of blood pressure is required for proper control of blood pressure.

Epoprostenol

Epoprostenol, better known as *prostacyclin*, is a naturally occurring vasodilator (see Chapter 21). Prostacyclin is an autacoid that is released from the endothelium and serves to counterbalance the vasoconstrictor and proclotting influences of thromboxane A_2. As a drug, epoprostenol is an extremely potent and short-acting (half-life of 6 minutes) vasodilator administered by continuous intravenous infusion to patients with primary pulmonary hypertension refractory to other drugs. The annual costs, including the necessary administration pumps, make this therapy prohibitive for many patients.

Fenoldopam

Fenoldopam is a vasodilator that is used in emergency situations.

Pharmacologic effects Fenoldopam (Figure 28-11) is an agonist at D_1 receptors. It stimulates D_1 receptors in blood vessels and results in vasodilation, especially in renal vessels.[15] As such, it increases renal blood flow and lowers blood pressure.

Absorption, fate, and excretion Fenoldopam is given by continuous intravenous administration and has an elimination half-life of approximately 5 minutes. Hepatic metabolism by conjugation accounts for the termination of its pharmacologic effects because the metabolites are inactive. Most of the metabolites are excreted by the kidney.

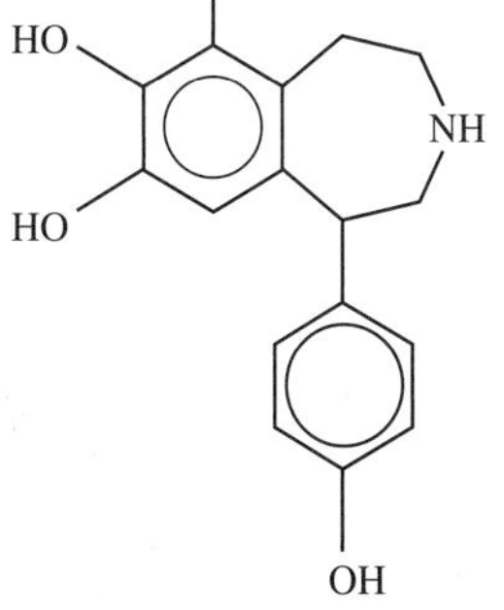

Cl
HO
NH
HO
OH

Fig. 28-11 Structural formula of fenoldopam.

MISCELLANEOUS DRUGS

A number of drugs have limited application in the treatment of hypertension. Some of these agents, such as the monoamine oxidase inhibitors and *Veratrum* alkaloids, were once widely used but have been replaced by more effective or less toxic compounds and will not be considered further. Others are restricted to defined roles exclusive of the routine treatment of essential hypertension and are mentioned briefly.

Ganglionic blocking drugs, discussed in Chapter 10, were once used for the long-term treatment of hypertension. They are rarely prescribed today because of postural hypotension, impotence, and other side effects associated with their use. Trimethaphan infused intravenously is effective in some hypertensive emergencies and to induce a hypotensive state during surgery.

Metyrosine (α-methyltyrosine) is an inhibitor of tyrosine hydroxylase, the rate-limiting enzyme in the formation of norepinephrine and epinephrine. Although not recommended for essential hypertension, metyrosine is useful, often in combination with phentolamine in the pharmacologic amelioration of pheochromocytoma.

Box • 28-3

Drug Treatment for Hypertension

Drugs Used in Monotherapy
Diuretics
ACE inhibitors
Angiotensin II receptor blockers
CCBs
β-Adrenergic receptor blockers
α_1-Adrenergic receptor blockers

Drugs Only Used in Combination
Centrally acting antihypertensive drugs
Hydralazine
Minoxidil
Guanethidine, guanadrel

TREATMENT OF HYPERTENSION

The treatment of hypertension often includes both pharmacologic and nonpharmacologic approaches for optimal control. Although the latter subject is beyond the scope of this discussion, it should be noted that dietary modification to reduce body weight and decrease Na^+ intake causes demonstrable reductions in blood pressure. Na^+ restriction, even within the well-controlled DASH diet, has been shown to reduce blood pressure.[2] The reduction in blood pressure is proportional to the reduction in Na^+ intake.[30] Moreover, restriction of fat intake and alcohol ingestion and cessation of smoking are also important considerations in lessening the dangers of cardiovascular diseases associated with hypertension. Optimal pharmacotherapeutic treatment is based on appropriate diagnosis, proper drug and dose selection, and good patient compliance. Inasmuch as essential hypertension in its early states is asymptomatic, compliance depends strongly on the avoidance of side effects and the simplicity of the therapeutic regimen.

Six drug classes are currently the most commonly used antihypertensive drugs: diuretics, ACE inhibitors, angiotensin II receptor blockers, CCBs, β-adrenergic receptor blockers, and α_1-adrenergic receptor blockers (Box 28-3). Diuretics are considered the most appropriate first choice for most hypertensive patients.[4] A second drug from one of the other categories, such as a β blocker,[33] is often required for blood pressure control.

Therapy needs to be tailored to the patient. For instance, when used alone, ACE inhibitors are usually less effective in African-American patients than in white patients, whereas diuretics may be nearly equally useful in both groups. This selectivity of effect correlates with the typically lower contribution of the renin-angiotensin system to hypertension in African Americans and their greater Na^+ sensitivity. Age may also contribute to the response.[23] In one study, thiazide diuretics were more effective in lowering blood pressure in patients older than 55 years than in those younger than 55 years.[11] Certain disease states can also affect the choice of drug. β-Adrenergic receptor blockers are especially useful in patients with a history of migraine headache, angina pectoris, or myocardial infarction. α-Adrenergic receptor blockers may be particularly useful in certain cases of blood lipid disorders because they can lower low-density lipoprotein and increase the high-density lipoprotein/total cholesterol ratio. Diabetic patients gain added benefit from treatment with an ACE inhibitor because of the renal protective effect of the drugs.

When a single drug is not effective, combination therapy may be required. Drugs such as the β-adrenergic receptor blockers, ACE inhibitors, or angiotensin II receptor blockers, are commonly used with diuretics, sometimes in combination with additional agents. For instance, centrally acting antihypertensives can be combined with CCBs with or without a diuretic. Hydralazine, when used, is combined with a β-adrenergic receptor blocker. The addition of the β blocker prevents the tachycardia resulting from hydralazine and enhances the antihypertensive response. In addition to their hypotensive effect, the diuretics reduce fluid retention caused by some antihypertensive drugs.

Severe hypertension almost always requires use of more than one drug. Furthermore, certain drugs are used only in refractory hypertension. These drugs include guanethidine and minoxidil, each used in combination with a diuretic and other drugs.

Hypertensive Emergencies

In contrast to the gradual increase in blood pressure seen in essential hypertension, a sudden elevation of blood pressure to severely hypertensive levels may sometimes occur. Hypertensive emergencies may arise in the course of any hypertensive disease, including renal hypertension, toxemia of pregnancy,[6] or pheochromocytoma. These situations, regardless of cause, are life threatening and require immediate lowering of blood pressure.[10] Although it is beyond the scope of this discussion to examine in detail the causes of hypertensive emergencies or the pharmacologic management of these conditions, a brief review is provided.

Acute hypertensive episodes can be characterized on the basis of the potential danger to the patient. True emergencies are situations in which greatly elevated blood pressure must be lowered immediately to avoid progression of end-organ damage. Hypertensive urgencies, on the other hand, call for control within several hours to reduce patient risk.[10] Management of a true hypertensive emergency necessitates parenteral therapy and intensive monitoring.[12] Table 28-2 lists the various parenteral drugs indicated for such emergencies and

Table • 28-2

Drugs Used in Acute Hypertension

DRUG	COMMENT
Hypertensive Emergencies (Parenteral)	
Sodium nitroprusside	Often used; requires continuous monitoring
Nitroglycerin	Indicated in patients with ischemic heart disease
Labetalol	Useful in thyrotoxicosis and pheochromocytoma and as a substitute for Na^+ nitroprusside when continuous monitoring is not available; contraindicated in patients with systolic heart failure, airway disease, or heart block
Diazoxide	Occasionally used when continuous monitoring is not available
Fenoldopam	Has rapid onset and short half-life
Hydralazine	Used in hypertensive states associated with pregnancy
Hypertensive Urgencies (Oral Preferred)	
Clonidine	Requires good patient compliance
Captopril	Responses somewhat unpredictable
Labetalol	Refer to labetalol above

salient facts pertaining to their use.[10] Although the rapid control of excessively high blood pressure is sometimes needed to avert necrotizing arteriolitis, hemorrhage, and tissue damage, it is not without risk. A rapid reduction in blood pressure may lead to inadequate tissue perfusion, cerebral ischemia, and angina pectoris. Therefore, when time permits, as in the treatment of hypertensive urgencies, the use of oral medications (see Table 28-2) provides a safer approach that minimizes the possibility of excessive hypotension and lessens the need for constant monitoring.

Antihypertensive Drug Withdrawal Syndrome

Withdrawal of antihypertensive drug therapy has been associated with several signs and symptoms, depending on the abruptness of the withdrawal, the degree of hypertension, and the drugs involved. The classes of drugs involved in withdrawal reactions include the centrally acting agents, β-adrenergic receptor–blocking drugs, neuronal blocking agents, and some vasodilators (e.g., minoxidil, sodium nitroprusside, and nifedipine). Reported responses include rebound hypertension, tachycardia, angina, heart attack, and sudden death.

Recommendations for managing hypertensive patients on drug therapy include encouraging patient compliance and avoiding excessive dosage. To avoid complications, antihypertensive drugs should be withdrawn slowly, and patients should be carefully monitored, especially those with coronary artery or cerebrovascular disease.

IMPLICATIONS FOR DENTISTRY

Drug Interactions

Because there are several categories of antihypertensive drugs (each class having a different mechanism of action), there are numerous possibilities for drug interactions.

Aspirin and other nonsteroidal antiinflammatory drugs (NSAIDs) antagonize a number of antihypertensive drugs (see Chapter 21). For instance, the antihypertensive effect of ACE inhibitors is reduced by aspirin. In addition, the effect of diuretics is inhibited by NSAIDs. This interaction apparently results from the inhibitory effect of the NSAIDs on prostaglandin synthesis. The NSAIDs also reduce the antihypertensive effect of the β blockers. Although the role of prostaglandins in antihypertensive therapy is not known, these autacoids are important in maintaining renal blood flow and urine output. Patients should be advised of this drug interaction; in the event that control of blood pressure is lost, substitution with acetaminophen with or without opioid supplementation is advised.

In general, the use of vasoconstrictors in local anesthesia is not contraindicated in the hypertensive patient, especially in the patient whose blood pressure is well controlled. However, a possible exception to this statement is the patient receiving an adrenergic neuron–blocking or neuron–depleting drug, such as guanethidine or reserpine, or a nonselective β-adrenergic receptor–blocking drug such as propranolol. Use of guanethidine-related drugs on a long-term basis produces supersensitivity to the actions of exogenously administered catecholamines. Injudicious use of sympathomimetic amine vasoconstrictors in local anesthetic solutions could possibly lead to serious disturbances of blood pressure and cardiac rhythm. Nonselective β-adrenergic receptor blockers prevent the fall in peripheral vascular resistance normally caused by doses of epinephrine used in local anesthesia. Unopposed α-agonistic action may then lead to an acute hypertensive episode. To avoid potential complications, the blood pressure of a patient on any of these medications should be taken before and 5 minutes after the injection of a small amount of local anesthetic (e.g., 1 ml of 2% lidocaine with 1:100,000 epinephrine). If no significant reaction is observed, dangerous hypertensive responses to additional local anesthetic are unlikely.

The use of epinephrine-impregnated retraction cord is contraindicated in patients with compromised cardiovascular function, including hypertensive patients. Significant amounts of epinephrine can be absorbed, especially if the gingiva is abraded or multiple teeth are involved.

Although not widely used, the centrally acting sympatholytics, which have a sedative side effect, are important to the dentist. In dealing with patients taking these drugs, the dentist must proceed cautiously when using antianxiety agents or other drugs that depress the CNS. In combination with antihypertensives with sedative side effects, these agents may lead to excessive CNS depression. Use of a smaller dose is advised in the premedication of a patient taking methyldopa, clonidine, guanabenz, guanfacine, or reserpine for hypertension.

Adverse Effects

One adverse effect of significance to the dentist that is associated with antihypertensive medication is orthostatic, or postural, hypotension. After being in a supine position, many patients receiving antihypertensive therapy may be unable to compensate adequately for a sudden change in position. Such patients should be observed carefully at the end of dental appointments. Drugs affecting peripheral adrenergic transmission are most likely to cause orthostatic hypotension, although other drugs may also have this action.

Another adverse effect that has implications in dentistry is inhibition of salivary secretion leading to dry mouth. Xerostomia is especially common in patients medicated with reserpine and the centrally acting antihypertensive agents: methyldopa, clonidine, guanabenz, and guanfacine.

Hypertension Detection

The American Heart Association has stressed the need for more effective hypertension detection, and dentists are encouraged to include blood pressure determinations as a part of routine office visits. Studies indicate that many patients identified by dentists as being hypertensive were unaware of their condition. A majority of those identified sought medical attention to treat the hypertension.

Screening for hypertension in the dental office is a simple procedure that can be carried out effectively by auxiliary personnel. Because hypertension is a dangerous but asymptomatic disease in its early stages, the dentist's efforts to identify and aid these patients by its detection are worthwhile. Furthermore, the dentist can advise against abrupt withdrawal from antihypertensive medication and inform the patient of the possible hazards of such action.

Cited References

1. Alexander RW: Hypertension and the pathogenesis of atherosclerosis. Oxidative stress and the mediation of arterial inflammatory response: a new perspective, *Hypertension* 25:155-161, 1995.
2. Appel LJ, Moore TJ, Obarzanek E, et al: A clinical trial of the effects of dietary patterns on blood pressure, *N Engl J Med* 336:1117-1124, 1997.
3. Burt VL, Whelton P, Rocella EJ, et al: Prevalence of hypertension in the US adult population. Results from the Third National Health and Nutrition Examination Survey, 1988-1991, *Hypertension* 85:305-313, 1995.
4. Chobanian AV, Bakris GL, Black HR, et al: The seventh report on the joint national committee on prevention, detection, and treatment of high blood pressure, *JAMA* 289:2534-2573, 2003.
5. Croog SH, Kong BW, Levine S, et al: Hypertensive black men and women. Quality of life and effects of antihypertensive medications: the Black Hypertension Quality of Life Multicenter Trial Group, *Arch Intern Med* 150:1733-1741, 1990.
6. Cunningham FG, Lindheimer MD: Hypertension in pregnancy, *N Engl J Med* 326:927-932, 1992.
7. Dohi Y, Criscione L, Pfeiffer K, et al: Angiotensin blockade or calcium antagonists improve endothelial dysfunction in hypertension: studies in perfused mesenteric resistance arteries, *J Cardiovasc Pharmacol* 24:372-379, 1994.
8. Dzau VJ: Cell biology and genetics of angiotensin in cardiovascular disease, *J Hypertens* 12:S3-S10, 1994.
9. Fletcher AE, Palmer AJ, Bulpitt CJ: Cough with angiotensin converting enzyme inhibitors: how much of a problem? *J Hypertens* 12:S43-S47, 1994.
10. Franklin SS: Hypertensive emergencies and urgencies. In Glassock RJ, ed: *Current therapy in nephrology and hypertension*, ed 3, St Louis, 1992, Mosby.
11. Freis ED: Veterans Administration Cooperative Study Group on Hypertensive Agents: effects of age on treatment results, *Am J Med* 90:20S-23S, 1991.
12. Gifford RW, Jr: Management of hypertensive crises, *JAMA* 266:829-835, 1992.
13. Guidelines Subcommittee: 1999 World Health Organization—International Society of Hypertension guidelines for the management of hypertension, *J Hypertens* 17:151-183, 1999.
14. Guyton AC: Blood pressure control—special role of the kidneys and body fluids, *Science* 252:1813-1816, 1991.
15. Han G, Kryman JP, McMillin PJ, et al: A novel transduction mechanism mediating dopamine-induced vascular relaxation: opening of BKCa channels by cyclic AMP-induced stimulation of cyclic GMP-dependent protein kinase, *J Cardiovasc Pharmacol* 34:619-627, 1999.
16. Hollenberg NK, Fisher NDL, Price DA: Pathways for angiotensin II generation in intact human tissue. Evidence from comparative pharmacological interruption of the renin system, *Hypertension* 32:387-392, 1998.
17. Ignarro LJ, Lippton H, Edwards JC, et al: Mechanism of vascular smooth muscle relaxation by organic nitrates, nitrites, nitroprusside and nitric oxide: evidence for the involvement of S-nitrosothiols as active intermediates, *J Pharmacol Exp Ther* 218:739-749, 1981.
18. Johnston CI, Risvanis J: Preclinical pharmacology of angiotensin II receptor antagonists. Update and outstanding issues, *Am J Hypertens* 10:306S-310S, 1997.
19. Kostis JB, Laurence-Nelson J, Ranjan R, et al: Association of increased pulse pressure with the development of heart failure in SHEP. Systolic Hypertension in the Elderly (SHEP) Cooperative Research Group, *Am J Hypertens* 14:798-803, 2001.
20. Lewis EJ, Hunsicker LG, Bain RP, et al: The effect of angiotensin-converting-enzyme inhibition on diabetic nephropathy, *N Engl J Med* 329:1456-1462, 1993.
21. Man in't Veld AJ, Van den Meiracker AH, Shalekamp MA: Do beta blockers really increases vascular resistance? Review of the literature and new observations under basal conditions, *Am J Hypertens* 1:91-96, 1988.
22. Materson BJ, Cushman WC, Goldstein G, et al: Treatment of hypertension in the elderly: I. Blood pressure and clinical changes. Results of a Department of Veterans Affairs Cooperative Study, *Hypertension* 15:348-360, 1990.
23. Materson BJ, Reda DJ, Cushman WC, et al: Single-drug therapy for hypertension in men. A comparison of six antihypertensive agents with placebo, *N Engl J Med* 328:914-921, 1993.
24. McConnaughey MM, McConnaughey JS, Ingenito AJ: Practical considerations of the pharmacology of angiotensin receptor blockers, *J Clin Pharmacol* 39:547-559, 1999.
25. Meisheri KD, Cipkus LA, Taylor CJ: Mechanism of action of minoxidil sulfate-induced vasodilation: a role for increased K^+ permeability, *J Pharmacol Exp Ther* 245:751-760, 1988.
26. Parmley WW: Evolution of angiotensin-converting enzyme inhibition in hypertension, heart failure and vascular protection, *Am J Med* 105(1A):27S-31S, 1998.
27. Perry HM, Davis BR, Price TR, et al: Effect of treating isolated systolic hypertension on the risk of developing various types and subtypes of stroke. The Systolic Hypertension in the Elderly Program (SHEP), *JAMA* 284:465-471, 2000.
28. Preston RA: Renoprotective effects of antihypertensive drugs, *Am J Hypertens* 12:19S-32S, 1999.

Antihypertensive Drugs

Nonproprietary (generic) name	*Proprietary (trade) name*
Diuretics	
See Chapter 27	
Agents affecting adrenergic function	
Transmitter synthesis inhibiting	
Metyrosine	Demser
Neuronal blocking or depleting	
Guanadrel	Hylorel
Guanethidine	Ismelin
Reserpine	—
α-Adrenergic receptor blocking	
Doxazosin	Cardura
Phenoxybenzamine	Dibenzyline
Phentolamine	Regitine
Prazosin	Minipress
Terazosin	Hytrin
Tolazoline*	Priscoline
β-Adrenergic receptor blocking	
Acebutolol	Sectral
Atenolol	Tenormin
Betaxolol	Kerlone
Bisoprolol	Zebeta
Carteolol	Cartrol
Metoprolol	Lopressor, Toprol XL
Nadolol	Corgard
Penbutolol	Levatol
Pindolol	Visken
Propranolol	Inderal
Timolol	Blocadren
α- and β-Adrenergic receptor blocking	
Carvedilol	Coreg
Labetalol	Normodyne, Trandate
Ganglionic blocking	
Mecamylamine	Inversine
Trimethaphan*	Arfonad
Centrally acting	
Clonidine	Catapres
Guanabenz	Wytensin
Guanfacine	Tenex
Methyldopa	Aldomet, Amodopa
Direct vasodilators	
Diazoxide	Hyperstat IV
Epoprostenol	Flolan
Fenoldopam	Carlopam
Hydralazine	Apresoline
Minoxidil	Loniten
Nitroglycerin	Nitro-Bid IV, Tridil
Nitroprusside	Nitropress
CCBs	
Amlodipine	Norvasc
Diltiazem	Cardizem, Dilacor XR
Felodipine	Plendil
Isradipine	DynaCirc
Nicardipine	Cardene
Nifedipine	Adalat, Procardia
Nimodipine	Nimotop
Nisoldipine	Sular
Verapamil	Calan, Isoptin
ACE inhibitors	
Benazepril	Lotensin
Captopril	Capoten
Enalapril	Vasotec
Enalaprilat	Vasotec I.V.
Fosinopril	Monopril
Lisinopril	Prinivil, Zestril
Moexipril	Univasc
Perindopril erbumine	Aceon
Quinapril	Accupril
Ramipril	Altace
Trandolapril	Mavik
Angiotensin II receptor blockers	
Candesartan cilexetil	Atacand
Eprosartan	Teveten
Irbesartan	Avapro
Losartan	Cozaar
Olmesartan	Benicar
Telmisartan	Micardis
Valsartan	Diovan
Combination products (examples)	
Amlodipine, benazepril	Lotrel
Bendroflumethiazide, nadolol	Corzide
Captopril, hydrochlorothiazide	Capozide
Chlorthalidone, reserpine	Regroton
Clonidine, chlorthalidone	Combipres
Guanethidine, hydrochlorothiazide	Esimil
Hydralazine, hydrochlorothiazide	Apresazide
Methyldopa, hydrochlorothiazide	Aldoril
Prazosin, polythiazide	Minizide
Propranolol, hydrochlorothiazide	Inderide
Reserpine, hydralazine, hydrochlorothiazide	Ser-Ap-Es
Trandolapril, verapamil	Tarka

*Not currently available in the United States.

29. Rigaud AS, Seux ML, Staessen JA, et al: Cerebral complications of hypertension, *J Hum Hypertens* 14:605-616, 2000.
30. Sacks FM, Svetkey LP, Vollmer WM, et al: Effects on blood pressure of reduced dietary sodium and the dietary approaches to stop hypertension (DASH) diet, *N Engl J Med* 344:3-10, 2001.
31. Schwartz CJ, Valente AJ, Hildebrandt EF: Prevention of atherosclerosis and end-organ damage: a basis for antihypertensive interventional strategies, *J Hypertens* 12:S3-S11, 1994.
32. Siragy H: Angiotensin II receptor blockers: review of the binding characteristics, *Am J Cardiol* 84:3S-8S, 1999.
33. Seventh Report of the Joint National Committee on the prevention, detection, and treatment of high blood pressure, *JAMA* 289:2534-2573, 2003.
34. Taddei S, Virdis A, Mattei P, et al: Vascular renin-angiotensin system and sympathetic nervous system activity in human hypertension, *J Cardiovasc Pharmacol* 23:S9-S14, 1994.
35. The Heart Outcomes Prevention Evaluation Study Investigators: Effects of an angiotensin-converting-enzyme inhibitor, ramipril, on cardiovascular events in high-risk patients, *N Engl J Med* 342:145-153, 2000.
36. Wang JG, Staessen JA: The benefit of treating isolated systolic hypertension, *Curr Hypertens Rep* 3:333-339, 2001.
37. Weber MA: Clinical pharmacology of centrally acting antihypertensive agents, *J Clin Pharmacol* 29:598-602, 1989.

General References

Cruickshank JM, Prichard BNC, eds: *Beta-blockers in clinical practice*, ed 2, New York, 1994, Churchill Livingstone.

Drugs for hypertension, *Med Lett Drugs Ther* 37:45-50, 1995.

Johnston GD: *Fundamentals of cardiovascular pharmacology*, 1999, New York, Chichester.

Oates JA, Brown NJ: Antihypertensive agents and the drug therapy of hypertension. In Hardman JG, Limbard LE, Gilman AG, eds: *Goodman and Gilman's The pharmacological basis of therapeutics*, ed 10, New York, 2001, McGraw-Hill.

Ram CV: Antihypertensive drugs: an overview, *Am J Cardiovasc Drugs* 2:72-89, 2002.

CHAPTER • 29

Lipid-Lowering Drugs

George A. Cook

The transport of lipids in the blood requires their association with proteins. Fatty acids are transported in association with albumin, and triglycerides derived from dietary fat are transported in large macromolecular, cholesterol-containing particles known as *lipoproteins.* Cholesterol plays an essential role in human life as an important component of cell membranes and a precursor of steroid hormones and bile acids in addition to its role in triglyceride transport. Yet it is now beyond doubt that blood cholesterol levels previously thought to be normal are the cause of premature death from coronary artery disease. Atherosclerosis remains the primary cause of premature death in the United States and in other industrialized countries. The major clinical sequelae of elevated lipoprotein levels, known as *hyperlipidemias* or *hyperlipoproteinemias,* are coronary artery disease, cerebral vascular disease, and peripheral vascular disease. The term *hyperlipemia,* which causes acute pancreatitis, is restricted to elevated plasma triglycerides without elevated cholesterol. Because the deposition of cholesterol in arteries is a defining feature of atherosclerosis, strategies for its prevention and treatment include methods to reduce plasma cholesterol. Dentists have an ever-increasing need to understand lipid-lowering drugs as the overall dental patient population of the United States matures and increasing numbers of patients take these drugs for prevention as well as therapy of atherosclerosis. Dentists will also want to follow the development of the cholesterol synthesis inhibitors because of their implication in the stimulation of bone formation.[33,35]

CHOLESTEROL AND ATHEROSCLEROSIS

Atherosclerosis is caused by development of fatty streaks and plaques in large and medium-sized arteries, especially the aorta, coronary arteries, carotids, renal arteries, and the arteries of the legs. Plaques develop in the intimal wall of the vessels after deposition of cholesteryl esters derived from certain lipoproteins. The particular clinical manifestation of atherosclerosis depends on the degree to which the lesions have progressed in a particular part of the vasculature. The presence of atheromatous lesions can have several effects on the circulation to a prescribed area: (1) blood flow may be obstructed by the plaques themselves or by associated thrombi; (2) vascular reactivity, and thus control of blood flow, may be lost; and (3) vessels may become weakened and subject to rupture. Observations of initial lesions in young children have made it obvious that this disease begins at an early age and progresses gradually, with clinical symptoms generally appearing much later in life.[42,51]

Foam cells are a primary characteristic of atheromatous plaques. These cells arise from macrophages that invade the injured arterial endothelium and accumulate large pools of cholesteryl esters from nearby trapped lipoproteins. As with all other cells, macrophages possess a mechanism for converting free cholesterol to cholesteryl esters as a protective mechanism to avoid excessive accumulation of free cholesterol in their membranes. Macrophages also possess scavenger receptors in their plasma membranes that bind chemically modified lipoproteins that arise from free radical–mediated oxidation or glycosylation because of poorly controlled diabetes. The accumulation of foam cells results in a fatty streak visible to the naked eye. Particularly in vascular areas subject to high mechanical shear stresses and turbulent flow, microscopic tearing and disruption of the local endothelium may expose the underlying tissue, resulting in accelerated lipoprotein accumulation, platelet aggregation, and the deposition of fibrin. Eventually, an atherosclerotic plaque forms with a thick fibrous cap covering a necrotic center composed of cellular debris and cholesteryl ester deposits.

Lipoprotein Metabolism

Classification of plasma lipoproteins is based on the density of the complexes, with a lower density indicating higher lipid content (Table 29-1). Chylomicrons are the largest particles and possess the greatest proportion of lipid. The other lipoproteins are very–low-density lipoprotein (VLDL), intermediate-density lipoprotein (IDL), low-density lipoprotein (LDL), high-density lipoprotein (HDL), and lipoprotein(a). Two separate lipoprotein-producing systems or metabolic pathways are responsible for the transport of lipids (Figure 29-1). These are the *exogenous pathway,* producing chylomicrons in the intestinal mucosa primarily from dietary fat, and the *endogenous pathway,* producing VLDL in the liver with triglycerides from hepatic metabolism of dietary carbohydrates.

A crucial factor in the understanding of both physiologic and pathophysiologic aspects of lipoprotein metabolism is the role played by specific *apoproteins,* the proteins associated with lipoprotein particles. Chylomicrons serve to transport dietary lipids to the sites of use and storage. The major protein component of chylomicrons is apoprotein B48, which initially plays an entirely structural role in formation and transport. It forms the amphipathic coating of the particle along with unesterified cholesterol and phospholipid, which surrounds the hydrophobic core containing triglycerides and cholesteryl esters and allows the particle to remain suspended in an aqueous environment. On reaching the capillary endothelium of muscle and adipose tissue, the chylomicron triglycerides are rapidly degraded to fatty acids, glycerol, and monoglycerides by the enzyme lipoprotein lipase. Apoprotein CII serves as a

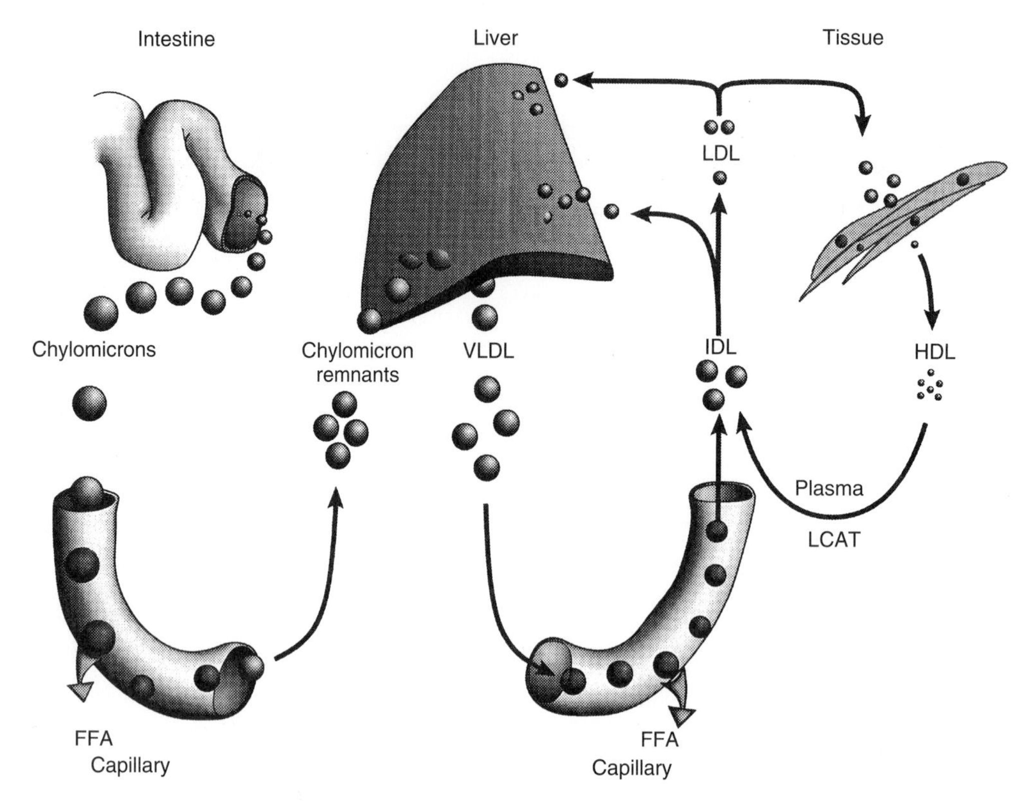

Fig. 29-1 Pathways of lipid transport. *FFA,* Free fatty acid; *LCAT,* lecithin:cholesterol acyltransferase.

Table • 29-1

Classification and Characteristics of Major Plasma Lipoproteins

LIPOPROTEIN	MAJOR LIPIDS	MAJOR APOPROTEINS	DENSITY (g/ml)	DIAMETER (nm)
Chylomicrons	Dietary triglycerides	B48, CI, CII, CIII, E	<0.98	80 to 500
Chylomicron remnants	Dietary cholesteryl esters	B48, E		
VLDLs	Endogenous triglycerides	B100, CII, CIII, E	0.98 to 1.006	30 to 80
IDLs	Cholesteryl esters, triglycerides	B100, CII, CIII, E	1.006 to 1.019	25 to 35
LDLs	Cholesteryl esters	B100	1.019 to 1.063	15 to 25
HDLs	Cholesteryl esters	AI, AII*	1.063 to 1.210	5 to 12
Lp(a)	Cholesteryl esters	B100, (a)	1.055 to 1.085	30

*HDL serves as a reservoir for C and E apoproteins, transferring them to newly synthesized chylomicrons (in exchange for A apoproteins) and VLDL particles and removing them as these particles are depleted of triglyceride.
Lp(a), Lipoprotein(a).

stimulus for endothelial lipase activity. The remaining *chylomicron remnants,* depleted of triglycerides and CII but relatively enriched in cholesterol and apoproteins B48 and E, are then released back into the circulation. The exogenous pathway terminates in the liver, where the chylomicron remnants are actively taken up by hepatocytes. Both apoproteins B48 and E help trigger this receptor-mediated endocytosis. Within the liver, the remnants are digested, releasing the remaining lipids for further metabolism (Figure 29-2).

The hepatic synthesis and release of VLDL particles initiates the endogenous pathway of lipid transport. VLDL is primarily triglyceride and is subject to attack by lipoprotein lipase on activation by apoprotein CII. The resulting IDL particle, greatly reduced in triglyceride content, has two possible fates: (1) a few particles are released and undergo receptor-mediated endocytosis by the liver and lysosomal degradation, or (2) most particles continue further removal of triglyceride and all apoproteins other than B100 to yield LDL. The cholesterol content of LDL is 50% to 60% by weight and normally accounts for 75% of the total plasma cholesterol. Particles of LDL are subject to apoprotein B100–dependent endocytosis by a variety of tissues, most importantly the liver. Excess IDL and LDL, through scavenger uptake by intimal macrophages, account for the cholesterol accumulation in atheromatous lesions. These is no evidence that chylomicrons are involved in this disease process.

The synthesis of cholesterol, regulated by the initial enzyme of the pathway (3-hydroxy-3-methylglutaryl-coenzyme A [HMG-CoA]), is an energetically expensive process because every carbon atom of cholesterol is derived from acetyl-coenzyme A, so the maintenance of total body cholesterol is a priority. This is further exemplified by the fact that there is no mechanism in the human body for removal of cholesterol other than conversion to bile acids. Cholesterol is conserved

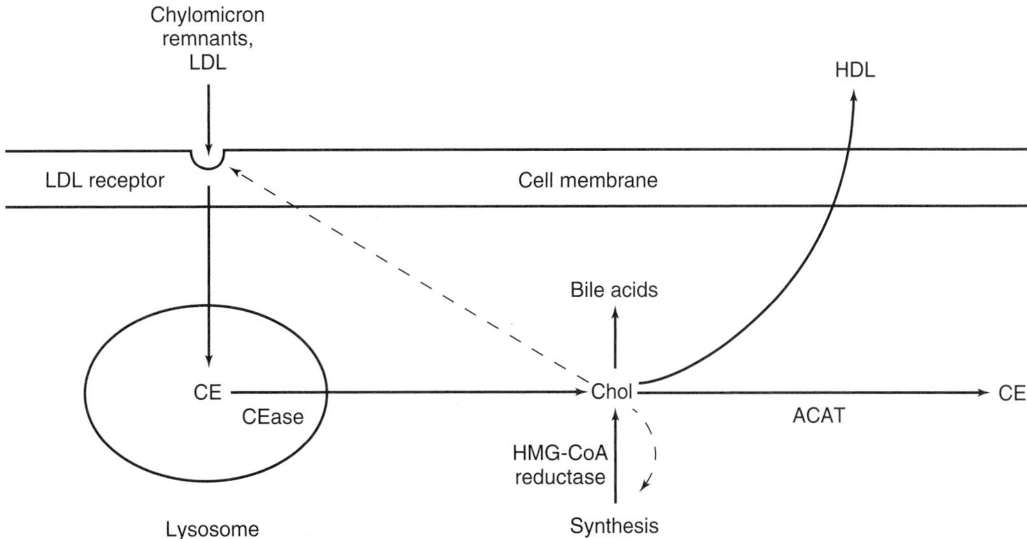

Fig. 29-2 Cholesterol metabolism and transport. Chylomicron remnants and LDL particles are actively taken up by hepatocytes through receptor-assisted endocytosis and are metabolized in lysosomes to yield cholesteryl esters *(CE)*. Cholesterol-rich LDL is similarly transporte and metabolized. In addition, reticuloendothelial cells and phagocytic cells of the vascular wall can ingest LDL by an LDL receptor–independent process. Under the influence of lysosomal acid cholesterol esterase *(CEase)*, cholesterol *(Chol)* is made available to the cell. Cholesterol limits its own intracellular concentration by (1) inhibiting LDL receptor synthesis, (2) stimulating its own reconversion to CE by the enzyme acyl CoA cholesterol acyl transferase *(ACAT)*, and (3) downregulating the production of HMG-CoA reductase, the rate-limiting enzyme of cholesterol synthesis. The inhibitory actions of cholesterol are indicated by *dashed lines*. Cholesterol may also leave the cell to reenter the bloodstream in association with HDL. Cholesterol is converted to bile acids.

through *enterohepatic cycling* and *reverse cholesterol transport*, processes that play important roles in energy conservation as well as sites of action for lipid-lowering drugs. Enterohepatic cycling includes the following processes[43]: (1) synthesis of cholesterol and conversion to bile acids by the liver, (2) secretion of biliary cholesterol and bile acids into the small intestine, (3) absorption of bile acids from the terminal ileum, and (4) transfer through the portal system and reuptake by the liver. Reverse cholesterol transport is the process by which HDL synthesized by the liver and intestine takes up cholesterol from peripheral cells and transports it back to the liver. HDL cholesterol is sometimes referred to as the "good" cholesterol because it represents the amount of cholesterol being removed from most of the body and because higher levels of HDL cholesterol are associated with decreased risk of atherosclerosis. HDL also assists in the removal of triglycerides from the bloodstream by delivering to chylomicrons and VLDL the C and E apoproteins necessary for their processing.

Role of Lipoproteins in Atherosclerosis

The presence of cholesterol as an integral component of arterial plaques has been known for decades, and many studies have been carried out to determine whether abnormal concentrations of cholesterol are involved in the origin or progress of plaque formation. These studies have shown that plasma cholesterol concentrations are higher in patients with coronary artery disease than in normal patients and that the relationship between serum cholesterol concentration and risk of premature death from coronary artery disease is continuous and graded.[46,50] More recent studies of cholesterol reduction therapy in patients with hyperlipidemia have shown that reduction of plasma cholesterol can cause regression of plaque formation as well as decrease the mortality rate from atherosclerosis.[6,53]

An increase in plasma LDL may be caused either by overproduction of its VLDL precursor or, more commonly, by retarded clearance of LDL from the blood. The plasma half-life of LDL is much longer than that of VLDL and IDL. Although LDL receptor–dependent uptake predominates normally, only the alternative phagocytic pathway is available in patients with severe familial hypercholesterolemia, who congenitally lack functional LDL receptors.[7] LDL contains the majority of cholesterol in the plasma, and it is also the lipoprotein group most directly associated with coronary heart disease.[30,49] On the other hand, high plasma concentrations of HDL are inversely related to the risk of coronary heart disease.[11,34,49]

Hyperlipidemia may be primary (i.e., genetic in origin) or result from dietary factors; disease states such as diabetes mellitus, hypothyroidism, or uremia; drugs such as alcohol, oral contraceptives, or glucocorticoids; or a combination of causes. A summary of various types of primary hyperlipidemias is provided in Table 29-2.

Risk Factors in Atherosclerosis

In addition to high plasma cholesterol, several risk factors have been identified with an increased incidence of atherosclerosis. Among these are hypertension, cigarette smoking, sedentary habits, obesity, diabetes mellitus, hypothyroidism, male gender, and a family history of atherosclerosis or diabetes. As shown in Table 29-2, the clinical manifestations of the genetic or familial hyperlipoproteinemias are severe. The lipid-lowering agents to be discussed have proved quite useful in treating many of these disorders and even in reversing the progression of atherosclerosis in patients without specific metabolic defects in lipid metabolism.

THERAPEUTIC AGENTS

Therapy with drugs that lower plasma cholesterol is used to delay or reverse the progression of atherosclerosis and thus

Table • 29-2

Primary Hyperlipoproteinemias: Types and Characteristics

TYPE	LIPOPROTEIN ELEVATED*	BIOCHEMICAL DEFECT (INHERITANCE)†	INCIDENCE	CLINICAL FINDINGS (AGE OF ONSET)	TREATMENT
Monogenic					
Familial lipoprotein lipase deficiency	Chylomicrons (I, V)	Decreased lipoprotein lipase activity (R)	$1:10^6$	Eruptive xanthomas, pancreatitis, abdominal pain, hepatosplenomegaly, lipemia retinalis (childhood)	Fat-free diet
Familial apoprotein CII deficiency	Chylomicrons, VLDL (I, V)	Decreased apoprotein CII activity (R)	$1:10^6$	Pancreatitis, abdominal pain (childhood or adulthood)	Fat-free diet
Familial type 3 hyperlipoproteinemia	Chylomicron remnants, IDL (III)	Dysfunctional apoprotein E plus other defect (R)	$1:10^4$	Palmer lipoproteinemia and tuberous xanthomas, premature atherosclerosis (adulthood)	Correction of other defect (e.g., hypothyroidism), gemfibrozil or clofibrate, nicotinic acid
Familial hypercholesterolemia	LDL (IIa, IIb)	Dysfunctional LDL receptor (D)	1 : 500	Xanthomas, arcus corneae, xanthelasma, early and severe atherosclerosis (childhood or adulthood)	Low cholesterol and saturated fat diet, HMG-CoA reductase inhibitor, bile-acid–binding resin
Familial hypertriglyceridemia	VLDL (rarely chylomicrons) (IV, V)	Unknown; probably multiple subtypes (D)	1 : 500	Obesity, hyperglycemia, hyperinsulinemia, increased incidence of hypertension and atherosclerosis (puberty)	Low saturated fat diet, correct contributing factors, avoidance of alcohol and oral contraceptives, nicotinic acid, gemfibrozil
Multiple lipoprotein-type hyperlipidemia	VLDL, LDL (IIa, IIb, IV)	Unknown; probably multiple subtypes (D)	1 : 250	Premature atherosclerosis (adulthood)	Low saturated fat diet, correction of contributing factors, avoidance of alcohol and oral contraceptives, lipid-lowering drugs
Lp(a) hyperlipoproteinemia	Lipoprotein(a)	Decreased binding to LDL receptor, decreased fibrinolysis	Not determined; wide variance among ethnic groups	Increased incidence of atherosclerosis (adulthood)	Nicotinic acid

Table • 29-2

Primary Hyperlipoproteinemias: Types and Characteristics—cont'd

TYPE	LIPOPROTEIN ELEVATED*	BIOCHEMICAL DEFECT (INHERITANCE)†	INCIDENCE	CLINICAL FINDINGS (AGE OF ONSET)	TREATMENT
Polygenic					
Polygenic hypercholesterolemia	LDL (IIa, IIb)	Unknown but including normal variation in cholesterol metabolism	1 : 24	Increased incidence of atherosclerosis (adulthood)	Low cholesterol and saturated fat diet, HMG-CoA reductase inhibitor, bile-acid–binding resin

*The electrophoretic pattern, or phenotypic expression, of the lipoproteinemia is indicated in parentheses.
†All the monogenic disorders are autosomal.
D, Dominant; *R*, recessive.

decrease the mortality and morbidity rates from the associated clinical manifestations of this disease.[21] Strong evidence supports the idea that correction or lowering of plasma lipid concentrations is beneficial in many instances.[4,26,34,45,49] These drugs are helpful in treating many familial hyperlipidemias, and they are also recommended for use in patients with hyperlipidemias of secondary etiology that cannot be corrected by other means. Lipid-lowering drugs are most frequently administered to patients with a history of ischemic heart disease in an attempt to avoid 3 future fatal episodes of myocardial infarction.

The goal of therapy is to reduce lipid titers as much as possible without producing metabolic derangements or adverse drug effects.[13,46,50] Altering the diet is generally an initial therapeutic measure, along with correcting any disease state or condition contributing to the hyperlipidemia. If nonpharmacologic therapy is insufficient, drug administration should then be considered depending on determinants such as age, gender, presence of ischemic vascular disease, and coexistence of other risk factors. Even when pharmacologic antihyperlipidemic treatment is instituted, however, nonpharmacologic management, including reduction of dietary cholesterol and saturated fatty acids, weight reduction, exercise, and smoking cessation, remains the cornerstone of therapy.

The following hypolipidemic agents are considered in this chapter: (1) derivatives of fibric acid, including clofibrate and gemfibrozil; (2) nicotinic acid; (3) the bile-acid sequestrants cholestyramine and colestipol; (4) probucol; (5) inhibitors of HMG-CoA reductase; (6) cholesterol absorption inhibitors; and (7) other agents. The effects of the major drugs on the various classes of lipoprotein are listed in Table 29-3.

The choice of a drug depends on the lipoprotein profile of the patient, the efficacy of the drug in treating the abnormality, and the ability of the patient to tolerate the agent. Drug therapy to reduce plasma LDL concentrations often begins with an HMG-CoA reductase inhibitor, a bile-acid sequestrant, or a combination of the two in reduced dosages. Multiple drug therapy with agents acting through different mechanisms is common if LDL control is not achieved with a single drug.[27,38] A fibric acid derivative such as gemfibrozil is generally the primary initial agent for the reduction of VLDL concentrations.

Fibric Acid Derivatives

One of the first drugs to be approved for the treatment of hyperlipidemia was clofibrate, a derivative of phenoxyisobutyric acid, which is also known as *fibric acid* (Figure 29-3). Gemfibrozil is safer and more effective than clofibrate, and several second-generation fibrates such as fenofibrate are also more effective. These drugs can influence all the lipoproteins but are most effective in familial type 3 hyperlipoproteinemia and in patients with elevated VLDL concentrations. Fibric acid derivatives act as ligands for the DNA transcription regulator peroxisomal proliferator–activated receptor α (PPARα),[19] thereby modifying rates of synthesis of specific enzymes. They have been shown to increase significantly the activity of extrahepatic lipoprotein lipase, decrease the hepatic synthesis of fatty acids, and increase hepatic fatty acid oxidation. Changes in apoprotein content help increase VLDL catabolism and remnant particle uptake. An inhibition of cholesterol synthesis and an increase in the biliary excretion of cholesterol promote a reduction in LDL in patients without coexisting hypertriglyceridemia. However, the LDL concentration is often increased by the fibrates in patients with elevated amounts of VLDL. Of the more recently developed fibrates, fenofibrate, bezafibrate, and ciprofibrate have been developed in Europe; gemfibrozil and fenofibrate are approved for use in the United States. Recent studies indicate that gemfibrozil is effective in reducing coronary heart disease and stroke by increasing HDL in patients with low HDL and elevated triglycerides.[47,48] The induction of peroxisome proliferation by fibrates has raised the possibility of increased risk of cancer, but recent studies with gemfibrozil have indicated no increased risk of death from noncoronary heart disease–related events.[48] Fibrates also increase blood urea and creatinine, indicating renal dysfunction, but gemfibrozil appears to be devoid of this side effect.[5]

Clofibrate treatment lowers elevated plasma cholesterol and triglyceride concentrations in a majority of patients.[39,40] It also has been shown to lower the plasma free fatty acid concentration.[32] The major effect on lipoprotein is a reduction in plasma VLDL concentrations. The IDL concentration is also reduced, but the effect on LDL depends on the lipid abnormality being treated.[9] Clofibrate was the most commonly prescribed lipid-lowering drug in the early 1970s. A failure to reduce fatal heart attack and cardiovascular complications,

Table • 29-3

Properties of Lipid-Lowering Drugs

	LIPOPROTEIN CONCENTRATIONS	PLASMA CHOLESTEROL	PLASMA TRIGLYCERIDE	TOXICITY	DRUG INTERACTIONS
Clofibrate	↓ VLDL, ↓ IDL	↓	↓	Nausea, diarrhea, myositis, abnormal liver function tests, skin rash, ventricular ectopy, increased incidence of noncardiac death	Enhanced effect of coumarin anticoagulants
Gemfibrozil	↓ VLDL, ↓ IDL, ↑ HDL	↓	↓	Abdominal pain, epigastric pain, diarrhea, nausea, vomiting, flatulence, rash, headache, dizziness, anemia, eosinophilia, leukopenia	Enhanced effect of coumarin anticoagulants; myopathy with HMG-CoA reductase inhibitors
Nicotinic acid	↓ Chylomicrons, ↓ VLDL, ↓ IDL, ↓ LDL, ↑ HDL	↓	↓	Flushing, pruritus, nausea, diarrhea, glucose intolerance, hyperuricemia, hepatotoxicity	Increased hypertensive action of ganglionic-blocking agents
Cholestyramine, colestipol	↑ VLDL (transient), ↓ LDL	↓	May increase modestly in some patients	Constipation, nausea, abdominal pain, flatulence, biliary tract calcification, steatorrhea, hyperchloremic acidosis	Decreased absorption of thiazides, tetracycline, phenobarbital, thyroxine, digitalis, coumarin anticoagulants
Probucol	↓ LDL, ↓ HDL	↓		Diarrhea, flatulence, abdominal pain, nausea, excess perspiration, angioedema, increased QT interval	
HMG-CoA reductase inhibitors	↓ IDL, ↓ LDL, ↑ HDL	↓	↓	Headache, flatulence, abdominal pain, diarrhea, rash, increased creatine kinase and other enzyme activities, myopathy	Enhanced effect of coumarin anticoagulants; myopathy, rhabdomyolysis, renal failure with nicotinic acid, gemfibrozil, erythromycin, cyclosporine
Ezetimibe	↓ LDL, ↓ HDL	↓	↓	Headache, sinusitis, pharyngitis	Cholestyramine binds ezetimibe and lowers its bioavailability. Does not alter bioavailability of digitalis or coumarin anticoagulants

↑, Increase; ↓, decrease.

coupled in some studies with a statistical increase in mortality and morbidity rates from other disorders (e.g., cholelithiasis and gastrointestinal carcinoma),[1] has restricted the use of clofibrate to patients with severe hyperlipoproteinemia intolerant of or unresponsive to gemfibrozil. Infrequent side effects of clofibrate therapy are nausea, diarrhea, muscle cramps, and myalgia. Clofibrate may rarely cause chest pain and cardiac arrhythmias. Clofibrate potentiates the effects of coumarin anticoagulants, in part by displacing them from protein-binding sites, but mostly because fibrates interfere with the synthesis of several clotting factors (fibrinogen and factor VII).

Gemfibrozil is chemically distinct from other fibrates in that it has a propylene connector between the phenoxy and isobutyrate ends of the molecule. The drug has been shown to lower the concentrations of blood triglycerides, cholesterol, VLDL, IDL, and sometimes LDL. It also tends to increase HDL concentrations more reliably than does clofibrate. In contrast to clofibrate, gemfibrozil has been shown to decrease

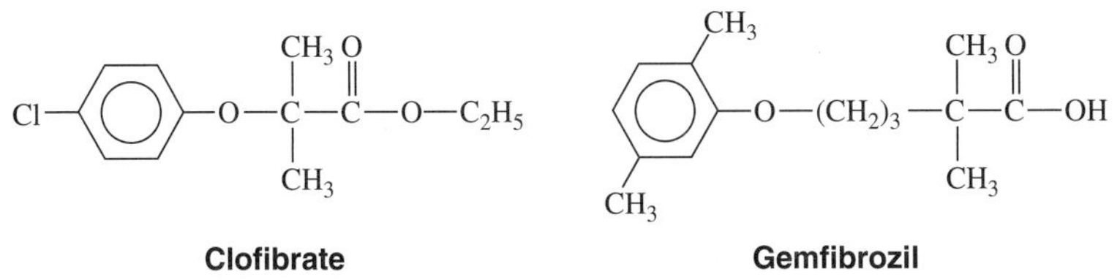

Clofibrate

Gemfibrozil

Fig. 29-3 Structural formula of the fibric acid derivatives clofibrate and gemfibrozil.

the incidence of myocardial infarction by 34% over a period of 5 years.[18] Principal side effects of gemfibrozil include abdominal pain, diarrhea, nausea, and vomiting. Less frequent adverse effects are headache, dizziness, anemia, rash, eosinophilia, and leukopenia. Like clofibrate, gemfibrozil enhances the action of oral anticoagulants and may cause cholelithiasis. When combined with an HMG-CoA reductase inhibitor, muscle damage leading to rhabdomyolysis and myoglobinuria has been reported.

Fenofibrate is the first of the second-generation fibric acid derivatives to be tested in the United States. Although the drug has been available in Europe since the early 1980s, it has not been studied in a large prevention trial, as have clofibrate and gemfibrozil. Nevertheless, the basic pharmacologic features of fenofibrate are similar to that of the previous agents. A potential advantage of the second-generation drugs is their greater ability to reduce LDL concentrations. Side effects include the gastrointestinal disturbances common to all fibrates and the potential for causing cholelithiasis. Bezafibrate and ciprofibrate are not yet approved for use in the United States.

Nicotinic Acid

Nicotinic acid, otherwise known as *niacin*, has been recognized since the late 1930s as a member of the vitamin B complex whose deficiency results in the disease pellagra. In 1955, it was reported that doses of nicotinic acid greater than 1 g (i.e., more than 50 times the recommended daily allowance of niacin as a vitamin) reduce plasma cholesterol concentrations,[2] subsequently lowering triglyceride concentrations.[10] Niacin's function in the body, after conversion to nicotinamide adenine dinucleotide and nicotinamide adenine dinucleotide phosphate, is to act as important enzyme cofactors. Niacin's action as a lipid-lowering drug is not related to its function as a vitamin. Nicotinamide, interchangeable with nicotinic acid as vitamin B_3, has no effect on plasma lipids.

Nicotinic acid is used most often to lower VLDL and LDL while raising HDL levels. It has been used alone or in combination with other lipid-lowering drugs. Its mechanism of action seems to involve inhibition of VLDL synthesis through inhibition of adipose tissue lipolysis and therefore inhibition of subsequent delivery of fatty acids to the liver to produce triglycerides for packaging into VLDL particles.[23] Increased clearance of VLDL may also play a role in the mechanism because of elevated lipoprotein lipase activity. The lipid-lowering effect of nicotinic acid is more dose dependent than is the case with the fibrates, allowing better control of therapy.[9] Nicotinic acid also has the broadest spectrum of activity of the lipid-lowering agents and is potentially useful in most forms of hyperlipidemia.

The major disadvantage of nicotinic acid, which affects 50% or more of the patient population, is its tendency to produce adverse effects sufficient to impair patient compliance or even force cessation of therapy. Common side effects include cutaneous flushing, pruritus, and gastrointestinal distress. If treatment is instituted slowly, with a gradually increasing dosage, tolerance to the cutaneous flushing occurs and therapy can be continued. Aspirin or ibuprofen taken beforehand ameliorates the prostaglandin-dependent flushing. Withdrawal of nicotinic acid is most frequently necessitated by gastric disturbances. Other side effects include hyperuricemia, decreased glucose tolerance, and abnormal liver function tests.

Nicotinic acid is absorbed rapidly, usually reaching a peak plasma concentration in less than an hour. The short half-life is primarily because of rapid excretion of unmetabolized nicotinic acid by the kidneys. This necessitates frequent administration of the drug, usually three times a day with meals. Because of the frequent lack of tolerance, doses are started at 100 mg three times per day and is gradually increased at 100-mg intervals until a dose of 1 to 1.5 g is reached. The usual therapeutic dose is 2 to 6 g/day.

Bile-Acid Sequestrants

Bile-acid sequestrants are nonabsorbable anion exchange resins that bind bile acids in the intestinal lumen, prevent their reabsorption, and promote their excretion in the feces. Enterohepatic cycling of cholesterol is markedly reduced by this mechanism that blocks reabsorption of bile acids from the jejunum and ileum with 95% efficiency and increases excretion rate by tenfold. Bile acids are synthesized in the liver from cholesterol by 7α-hydroxylase, which is regulated through negative feedback by bile acids. Hepatic cholesterol conversion to bile acids is thus accelerated, and plasma cholesterol and LDL concentrations are decreased. LDL concentrations are also reduced by these drugs because of upregulation of LDL receptors and hepatic uptake, whereas the VLDL concentration may be unchanged or even increased.[29] These resins have no effect in patients with homozygous familial hypercholesterolemia who have no functioning LDL receptors.

Cholestyramine and colestipol are the two clinically available drugs in this category (Figure 29-4). They are very large resins that are insoluble in water. The dry resin is mixed with a liquid such as fruit juice and drunk as a slurry. Chloride is released from the resin as bile acids bind to it and the released

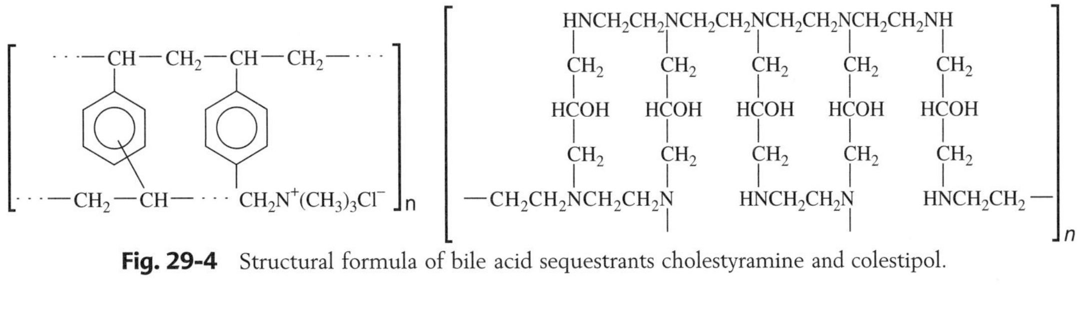

Fig. 29-4 Structural formula of bile acid sequestrants cholestyramine and colestipol.

Cl^- is absorbed, but the resin itself is not absorbed. Because it is not absorbed, it has a high safety factor and absence of serious side effects, but the annoying gastrointestinal side effects (nausea, vomiting, abdominal distention, and constipation) limit the use of these drugs. An unpleasant taste adds to the problem of patient compliance with these agents. Because cholestyramine and the hydrochloride salt of colestipol clinically exchange Cl^- for other anions, hyperchloremic acidosis may develop when large doses are given to small patients. Both resins decrease the absorption, and thus the therapeutic effect, of other drugs such as warfarin, thyroxine, digitalis, propranolol, and thiazides. This interaction can be partially overcome by proper timing of the dosage.

Bile–acid binding resins are used alone or in combination with nicotinic acid and cholesterol synthesis inhibitors. Cholestyramine was used in the Lipid Research Clinics Program Primary Prevention Trial.[30] In this trial of almost 4000 healthy men with hypercholesterolemia, there was a 20% decrease in LDL cholesterol with the resin and a 24% reduction in deaths from myocardial infarction.

The newest bile acid sequestrant to be approved for use in the United States is colesevelam hydrochloride, which is available in tablet form. Colesevelam has been found to lower LDL cholesterol as effectively as cholestyramine[14] but has less danger of interaction with other drugs such as warfarin through adsorption.[15] There are also somewhat fewer gastrointestinal side effects, and, because of the tablet form, compliance is greater.

Probucol

Probucol (Figure 29-5) was originally designed as an antioxidant for the tire manufacturing industry, but it was found to have hypolipidemic effects.[52] Probucol's hypolipidemic mechanism is probably caused by an antioxidant effect on LDL whereby it diminishes scavenger-receptor mediated uptake by macrophages of oxidized LDL.[20] Probucol lowers elevated serum cholesterol and LDL concentrations, but it has no consistent effect on triglycerides.[36] The importance of probucol as a therapeutic agent lies in the fact that it is the only drug that lowers cholesterol and causes regression of xanthomas in patients with homozygous familial hypercholesterolemia.[58] Xanthomas are caused by an accumulation of foam cells in tendons, ligaments, fasciae, and other tissues in a manner similar to the production of atheromatous plaques in arteries. Apparently the regression of xanthomas and decreased plaque formation both result from decreased oxidation of LDL. An early event in atherogenesis is the adhesion of monocytes to the endothelium through adhesion molecules. Probucol has recently been found to inhibit synthesis of one type of adhesion molecule in endothelial cells,[59] thus interfering in the recruitment of monocytes and inhibiting plaque formation. The modest effect of probucol on LDL cholesterol concentrations (10% to 15% reduction) and a greater decline in HDL cholesterol concentrations (20% to 30%) have limited interest in this agent. Decreased HDL may result from interference by probucol with reverse cholesterol transport in peripheral tissues.[56]

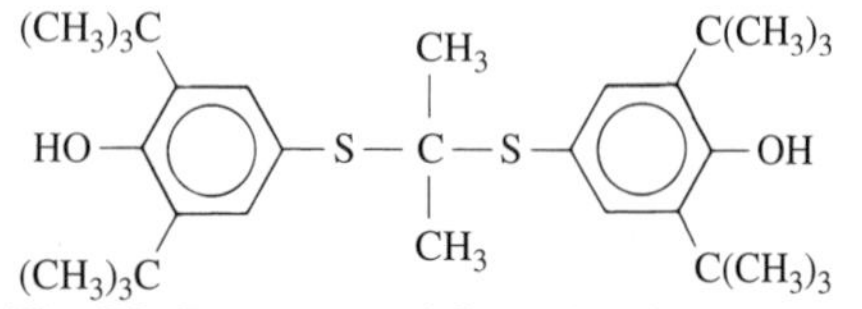

The most frequently encountered side effects of probucol are diarrhea, flatulence, abdominal pain, and nausea. Other, more rarely seen, adverse effects include excessive perspiration and angioedema. Probucol should not be used in patients with significant ventricular conduction defects because it prolongs the QT interval and could predispose the patient to cardiac arrhythmias. In fact, consideration of the risks versus benefits of probucol relative to other lipid-lowering drugs has led to its removal from clinical use in the United States, although it is still available in Canada.

Fig. 29-5 Structural formula of probucol.

HMG CoA Reductase Inhibitors

Several hypolipidemic drugs act by inhibiting HMG-CoA reductase, the enzyme that catalyzes the rate-limiting step in the synthesis of cholesterol.[31] Lovastatin, pravastatin, simvastatin, fluvastatin, cerivastatin, atorvastatin, and rosuvastatin are included in this group.[22,55] These agents structurally resemble an intermediate in the reductase reaction (Figure 29-6) and are potent competitive antagonists of HMG-CoA binding.

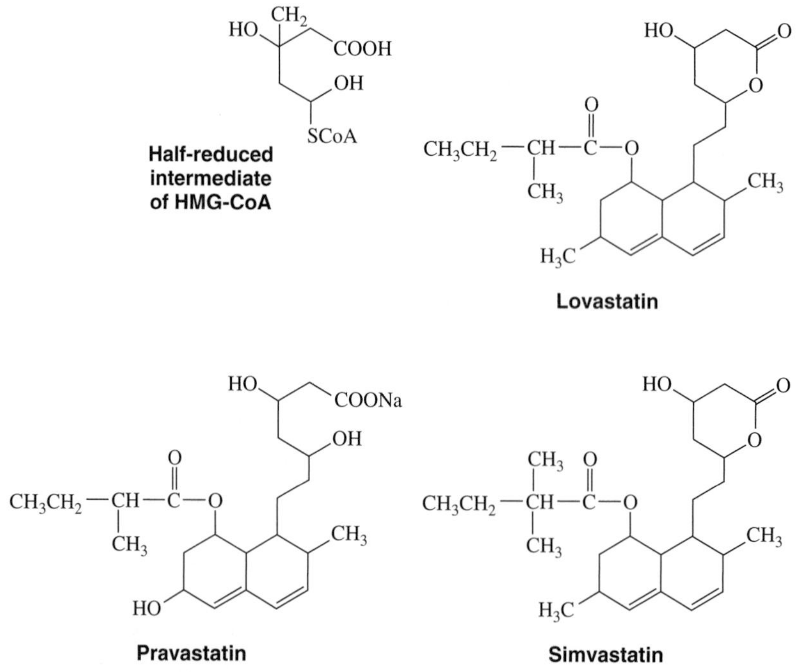

Fig. 29-6 Structural formula of HMG-CoA, half-reduced intermediate, and several HMG-CoA reductase inhibitors.

(Lovastatin and simvastatin are actually prodrugs in that they require cleavage of their lactone ring to become active.)

The antihyperlipidemic effect of this class of drugs depends on inhibition of hepatic HMG-CoA reductase, the rate-controlling enzyme in the pathway of cholesterol synthesis. The subsequent depletion of intracellular cholesterol has two effects: (1) sterol inhibition of the transcription of both HMG-CoA reductase and HMG-CoA synthetase genes is released, resulting in increased synthesis of these two enzymes, but the continuous presence of the drug keeps cholesterol synthesis inhibited in all tissues; and (2) synthesis of hepatic LDL receptors is stimulated, resulting in increased hepatic uptake of LDL and IDL. The net result of these changes is a reduction in LDL and IDL concentrations, a related fall in lipoprotein cholesterol and triglyceride concentrations, and a slight increase in HDL concentrations.[3,27,31,44]

The HMG-CoA reductase inhibitors are the most commonly prescribed lipid-lowering drugs. They are indicated for the treatment of hypercholesterolemia caused by elevated LDL concentrations in patients who have not responded to dietary or other measures.[31,54] Statins may also be useful for the reduction of LDL levels in patients with combined hyperlipidemia (hypercholesterolemia and hypertriglyceridemia).[22] They are ineffective in the rare patient with familial hypercholesterolemia who is homozygous for the defective LDL receptor gene.

Adverse effects of the HMG-CoA reductase inhibitors include myalgia, blurred vision, constipation, diarrhea, gas, heartburn, stomach pain, dizziness, headache, nausea, skin rash, impotence, and insomnia. The incidence varies somewhat among the different agents, with blurred vision more frequent with lovastatin and pravastatin and impotence and insomnia more likely with lovastatin.[22,55] The HMG-CoA reductase inhibitors increase the anticoagulant effect of warfarin. Lovastatin has also been linked with severe myopathy (rhabdomyolysis) when administered in combination with erythromycin, cyclosporine, gemfibrozil, or nicotinic acid. The other HMG-CoA reductase inhibitors have also been found to produce rhabdomyolysis in a small percentage of patients, but there is increased risk with higher doses, in elderly patients, or in combination with other drugs. Cerivastatin was removed from the market by its manufacturer after several deaths attributable to rhabdomyolysis were reported.

Cholesterol Absorption Inhibitors

The most recent class of lipid-lowering drugs to be developed and approved for use are the cholesterol absorption inhibitors.[16] These agents inhibit cholesterol uptake by the intestinal absorptive epithelium. Dietary cholesterol is normally absorbed in the jejunum from bile acid micelles by enterocytes in which the cholesterol is immediately converted to cholesteryl esters for assembly of chylomicrons. The uptake of cholesterol is mediated by specific transporters in the brush border of these cells.[24] The cholesterol absorption inhibitor ezetimibe blocked an elevation in plasma cholesterol in one study in which feeding of high-cholesterol diets increased plasma cholesterol in the control group.[57] This compound also reduced LDL cholesterol in human trials in a concentration-dependent manner at doses as low as 1 mg.[8] In addition to these agents, inhibitors of bile-acid uptake by the intestinal epithelium and inhibitors of acyl CoA cholesterol acyltransferase, the enzyme that produces cholesteryl esters, are also being developed as lipid-lowering drugs.[8] The combination of ezetimibe with an HMG-CoA reductase inhibitors produces even greater control of hyperlipidemia than is possible with either drug used in monotherapy. An advantage of ezetimibe over the bile acid sequestrants is that while inhibiting cholesterol uptake it does not inhibit uptake of triacylglycerols, bile acids, fatty acids, lipid-soluble drugs, or fat-soluble vitamins by the small intestine.

Other Agents

Some agents with moderate antihyperlipidemic activity may be clinically useful for specific patients. These include the very long chain polyunsaturated fatty acids found in fish oil, neomycin, and β-sitosterol. Others, typified by dextrothyroxine, can lower cholesterol concentrations yet provide no therapeutic benefit to the patient.

Fish oils

Evidence exists to support a role for polyunsaturated fish oils in lowering plasma lipid concentrations.[25,45] Specifically, the omega-3 polyunsaturated fatty acids (Ω-3 PUFAs) eicosapentaenoic acid and docosahexaenoic acid have been identified, whether consumed as dietary constituents or as purified supplements. The mechanisms of action of these agents are not clear. Some commercial preparations contain antioxidants, such as vitamin E, in varying concentrations. The actions of the antioxidants and their effect on the action of the fish oils are not defined.

Increasing dietary Ω-3 PUFAs has been shown to increase their concentration in platelet phospholipids. This increase allows them to compete with arachidonic acid for cyclooxygenase in the cascade that normally produces prostaglandins, thromboxanes, and prostacyclins.[25] The prostaglandins derived from the Ω-3 PUFAs have biologic effects different from those derived from arachidonic acid, and this alteration in prostaglandin synthesis is thought to result in a reduction of platelet aggregation and an increase in bleeding time.[17,28] Eicosapentaenoic acid in particular may be converted to prostaglandin I_3, which is an antiaggregatory agent.[28]

Although results vary, some evidence exists to show that fish oils can modestly decrease the levels of plasma cholesterol, triglycerides, and VLDL and modestly increase HDL levels. Patients with severe familial hypertriglyceridemia often have significant improvement on a diet high in fish oil. Before these agents can be recommended for widespread use in hyperlipidemia or to reduce the risk of coronary artery disease, however, long-term studies are needed to establish their safety and efficacy, with special emphasis on contaminants that may be present in some preparations.[25]

Thyroid-active substances

Early animal experiments indicated that the dextroisomers of thyroxine and liothyronine (triiodothyronine) decrease plasma lipid levels with no increase in oxygen consumption, an effect that might be useful in treating hyperlipidemias.[41] However, these compounds have been shown to increase the incidence of angina pectoris and death in patients with coronary artery disease.[11] These findings restrict the use of these drugs as lipid-lowering agents and indicate that they should be used with extreme caution, if at all, in patients with heart disease.

COMBINED-DRUG THERAPY

Lipid-lowering drugs from the different categories are used in combination for three reasons. First, combined-drug therapy may result in a more profound reduction of lipid levels than can be achieved by single-drug therapy. Second, as previously stated, some drugs may actually elevate certain lipid concentrations; thus combined therapy with a drug of another category can be used to overcome this unwanted effect. Third, the use of combined-drug therapy may allow lower doses of the drugs to be used than in single-drug therapy, decreasing potential side effects. Examples of multiple drug therapies having demonstrable value include the combination of a bile-acid sequestrant (cholestyramine or colestipol) with either nicotinic acid[5] or an HMG-CoA reductase inhibitor.[22] Other drug combinations that have been shown to be useful include a bile-acid sequestrant and a fibrate as well as a resin plus nicotinic acid plus an HMG-CoA reductase inhibitor. Colesevelam plus an HMG-CoA reductase inhibitor may also be a useful combination. The newest combined-drug therapy is the use of a cholesterol absorption inhibitor with an HMG-CoA reductase inhibitor. The combination of ezetimibe and atorvastatin achieved a 50% reduction in LDL cholesterol at low doses (10 mg) of each drug. This result was approximately equal to the effect of 80 mg of atorvastatin alone.

RECOMBINANT APOLIPOPROTEIN THERAPY

The use of recombinant proteins to lower total cholesterol in experimental animals has been investigated for several years, and there has been great interest in stimulating reverse cholesterol transport by HDL to remove cholesterol from peripheral tissues and from plaques.[59] Recently, a clinical trial has been completed in which patients had a recombinant mutant, artificial HDL infused into their coronary arteries each week for 5 weeks. The patients showed significant loss of atherosclerotic plaque from the diseased arteries. The artificial HDL was constructed by adding natural phospholipids to a recombinant apolipoprotein called *ApoA I(Milano)*. Normal, nascent HDL contains two molecules of ApoA I plus phospholipids that form a disc-shaped particle that circulates through the bloodstream and accumulates cholesteryl esters before being degraded by the liver. ApoA I(Milano) is a mutant protein discovered in the 1980s in an Italian family with very low HDL but no incidence of heart disease. The mutant protein contains a single substitution of a cysteine residue for a natural arginine. The substitution allows two molecules of ApoA I(Milano) to link together through a disulfide bond and form a mutant HDL particle that remains in circulation for extremely long periods of time compared with natural HDL and greatly enhances its reverse cholesterol transport function. It is possible that clinical use of recombinant apolipoproteins will usher in a new dimension of treatment for coronary artery disease and for hypolipidemic treatment in general.[12,37]

Lipid-Lowering Drugs

Nonproprietary (generic) name	*Proprietary (trade) name*
Atorvastatin	Lipitor
Cerivastatin*	Baycol
Cholestyramine	Questran
Clofibrate	Atromid-S
Colesevelam	WelChol
Colestipol	Colestid
Ezetimibe	Zetia
Fenofibrate	Tricor
Fish oils (n-3 PUFAs)	Max-EPA, Promega, Sea-omega, Super EPA
Fluvastatin	Lescol
Gemfibrozil	Lopid
Lovastatin	Mevacor
Nicotinic acid (niacin)	Niacor, Niaspan, Niacin SR, Slo-Niacin
Pravastatin	Pravachol
Probucol*	Lorelco
Rosuvastatin	Crestor
Simvastatin	Zocor

*Not currently available in the United States.

CITED REFERENCES

1. A co-operative trial in the primary prevention of ischaemic heart disease using clofibrate. Report from the Committee of Principal Investigators, *Br Heart J* 40:1069-1118, 1978.
2. Altschul R, Hoffer A, Stephen JD: Influence of nicotinic acid on serum cholesterol in man, *Arch Biochem Biophys* 54:558-559, 1955.
3. Bilheimer DW, Grundy SM, Brown MS, et al: Mevinolin and colestipol stimulate receptor-mediated clearance of low density lipoprotein from plasma in familial hypercholesterolemia heterozygotes, *Proc Natl Acad Sci USA* 80:4124-4128, 1983.
4. Blankenhorn DH, Nessim SA, Johnson RL, et al: Beneficial effects of combined colestipol-niacin therapy on coronary atherosclerosis and coronary venous bypass grafts, *JAMA* 257:3233-3240, 1987.
5. Broeders N, Knoop C, Antoine M, et al: Fibrate-induced increase in blood urea and creatine: is gemfibrozil the only innocuous agent? *Nephrol Dial Transplant* 15:1993-1999, 2000.
6. Brown BG, Zhao XQ, Sacco DE, et al: Lipid lowering and plaque regression. New insights into prevention of plaque disruption and clinical events in coronary disease, *Circulation* 87:1781-1791, 1993.
7. Brown MS, Goldstein JL: Lipoprotein receptors in the liver. Control signals for plasma cholesterol traffic, *J Clin Invest* 72:743-747, 1983.
8. Brown WV: Novel approaches to lipid lowering: what is on the horizon? *Am J Cardiol* 87(suppl):23B-27B, 2001.
9. Carlson LA, Olsson AG: Hyperlipidaemia and its management. In Oliver MF, ed: *Modern trends in cardiology*, vol 3, London, 1975, Butterworth.
10. Carlson LA, Orö L, Adostman J: Effect of nicotinic acid on plasma lipids in patients with hyperlipoproteinemia during the first week of treatment, *J Atherosclerosis Res* 8:667-677, 1968.
11. Castelli WP, Garrison RJ, Wilson PW, et al: Incidence of coronary heart disease and lipoprotein cholesterol levels. The Framingham study, *JAMA* 256:2835-2838, 1986.
12. Chiesa G, Sirtori C: Recombinant apolipoprotein A-I(Milano): a novel agent for the induction of regression of atherosclerotic plaques, *Ann Med* 35:267-273, 2003.
13. Coronary Drug Project Research Group: The coronary drug project: initial findings leading to modifications of its research protocol, *JAMA* 214:1303-1313, 1970.
14. Davidson MH, Dillon MA, Gordon B, et al: Colesevelam hydrochloride (Cholestagel): a new, potent bile acid sequestrant associated with a low incidence of gastrointestinal side effects, *Arch Intern Med* 159:1893-1900, 1999.
15. Donovan JM, Stypinski D, Stiles MR, et al: Drug interactions with colesevelam hydrochloride, a novel, potent lipid-lowering agent, *Cardiovasc Drugs Ther* 14:681-690, 2000.
16. Dujovne CA, Bays H, Davidson MH, et al: Reduction of LDL cholesterol in patients with primary hypercholesterolemia by SCH 48461: results of a multicenter dose-ranging study, *J Clin Pharmacol* 41:70-78, 2001.
17. Dyerberg J, Bang HO: A hypothesis on the development of acute myocardial infarction in Greenlanders, *Scand J Clin Lab Invest* 42(suppl 161):7-13, 1982.

18. Frick MH, Elo A, Haapa K, et al: Helsinki Heart Study: primary-prevention trial with gemfibrozil in middle-aged men with dyslipidemia: safety of treatment, changes in risk factors, and incidence of coronary heart disease, *N Engl J Med* 317:1237-1245, 1987.

19. Fruchart JC, Staels B, Duriez P: The role of fibric acids in atherosclerosis, *Curr Atheroscler Rep* 3:83-92, 2001.

20. Gillotte KL, Horkko S, Witztum JL, et al: Oxidized phospholipids, linked to apolipoprotein B of oxidized LDL, are ligands for macrophage scavenger receptors, *J Lipid Res* 41:824-833, 2000.

21. Gresham GA: Is atheroma a reversible lesion? *Atherosclerosis* 23:379-391, 1976.

22. Grundy SM: HMG CoA reductase inhibitors for treatment of hypercholesterolemia, *N Engl J Med* 319:24-33, 1988.

23. Grundy SM, Mok HY, Zech L, et al: Influence of nicotinic acid on metabolism of cholesterol and triglycerides in man, *J Lipid Res* 22:24-36, 1981.

24. Hernandez M, Montenegro J, Steiner M, et al: Intestinal absorption of cholesterol is mediated by a saturable, inhibitable transporter, *Biochem Biophys Acta* 1486:232-242, 2000.

25. Herold PM, Kinsella JE: Fish oil consumption and decreased risk of cardiovascular disease: a comparison of findings from animal and human feeding trials, *Am J Clin Nutr* 43:566-598, 1986.

26. Holme I: Effects of lipid-lowering therapy on total and coronary mortality, *Curr Opin Lipidol* 6:374-378, 1995.

27. Illingworth DR: Mevinolin plus colestipol in therapy for severe heterozygous familial hypercholesterolemia, *Ann Intern Med* 101:598-604, 1984.

28. Jorgensen KA, Dyerberg J: Platelets and atherosclerosis, *Adv Nutr Res* 5:57-75, 1983.

29. Levy RI, et al: Dietary and drug treatment of primary hyperlipoproteinemia, *Ann Intern Med* 77:267-294, 1972.

30. Lipid Research Clinics Program: The Lipid Research Clinics Coronary Primary Prevention Trial Results. I. Reduction in incidence of coronary heart disease, *JAMA* 251:351-364, 1984.

31. Mabuchi H, Haba T, Tatami R, et al: Effects of an inhibitor of 3-hydroxy-3-methylglutaryl-coenzyme A reductase on serum lipoproteins and ubiquinone-10 levels in patients with familial hypercholesterolemia, *N Engl J Med* 305: 478-482, 1981.

32. Macmillan DC, Oliver MF, Simpson JD, et al: Effect of ethylchlorophenoxyisobutyrate on weight, plasma volume, total body water, and free fatty acids, *Lancet* 2:924-926, 1965.

33. Maeda T, Matsunuma A, Kawane T, et al: Simvastatin promotes osteoblast differentiation and mineralization in MC3T3-E1 cells, *Biochem Biophys Res Commun* 280:874-877, 2001.

34. Malloy MJ, Kane JP: Agents used in hyperlipidemia. In Katzung BG, ed: *Basic and clinical pharmacology*, ed 6, Norwalk, CT, 1995, Appleton & Lange.

35. Mundy G, Garrett R, Harris S, et al: Stimulation of bone formation in vitro and in rodents by statins, *Science* 286:1946-1949, 1999.

36. Murphy BF: Probucol (Lorelco) in treatment of hyperlipidemia, *JAMA* 238:2537-2538, 1977.

37. Nissen SA, Tsunoda T, Tuzca EM, et al: Effect of recombinant ApoA-I Milano on coronary atherosclerosis in patients with acute coronary syndromes: a randomized controlled trial, *JAMA* 290:2292-2300, 2003.

38. Oberman A, Kreisberg RA, Henkin Y: *Principles and management of lipid disorders: a primary care approach*, Baltimore, 1992, Williams & Wilkins.

39. Oliver MF: Current therapeutics. CXCV. "Atromid-S" and "Atromid," *Practitioner* 192:424-430, 1964.

40. Oliver MF: Further observations on the effects of Atromid and of ethyl chlorophenoxyisobutyrate on serum lipid levels, *J Atherosclerosis Res* 3:427-444, 1963.

41. Oliver MF, Boyd GS: Reduction of serum-cholesterol by dextro-thyroxine in men with coronary heart disease, *Lancet* 1:783-785, 1961.

42. Oster KA: Evaluation of serum cholesterol reduction and xanthine oxidase inhibition in the treatment of atherosclerosis, *Recent Adv Stud Cardiac Structure Metab* 3:73-80, 1973.

43. Packard CJ, Shepherd J: The hepatobiliary axis and lipoprotein metabolism: effects of bile acid sequestrants and ileal bypass surgery, *J Lipid Res* 23:1081-1098, 1982.

44. Perry RS: Contemporary recommendations for evaluating and treating hyperlipidemia, *Clin Pharm* 5:113-127, 1986.

45. Phillipson BE, Rothrock DW, Connor WE, et al: Reduction of plasma lipids, lipoproteins, and apoproteins by dietary fish oils in patients with hypertriglyceridemia, *N Engl J Med* 312:1210-1216, 1985.

46. Report of the National Cholesterol Education Program Expert Panel on Detection, Evaluation, and Treatment of High Blood Cholesterol in Adults. The expert panel, *Arch Intern Med* 148:36-69, 1988.

47. Robins SJ, Collins D, Wittes JT, et al: Relation of gemfibrozil treatment and lipid levels with major coronary events: VA-HIT: a randomized controlled trial, *JAMA* 285:1585-1591, 2001.

48. Rubins HB, Robins SJ, Collins D, et al: Gemfibrozil for the secondary prevention of coronary heart disease in men with low levels of high-density lipoprotein cholesterol. Veterans Affairs High-Density Lipoprotein Cholesterol Intervention Trial Study Group, *N Engl J Med* 341:410-418, 1999.

49. Scandinavian Simvastatin Survival Study Group: Randomised trial of cholesterol lowering in 4444 patients with coronary heart disease: the Scandinavian Simvastatin Survival Study (4S), *Lancet* 344:1383-1389, 1994.

50. Stamler J, Wentworth D, Neaton JD: Is relationship between serum cholesterol and risk of premature death from coronary heart disease continuous and graded? Findings in 356,222 primary screenees of the Multiple Risk Factor Intervention Trial (MRFIT), *JAMA* 256:2823-2828, 1986.

51. Stein EA: Lipids, lipoproteins, and apolipoproteins. In Tietz NW, ed: *Textbook of clinical chemistry*, Philadelphia, 1986, WB Saunders.

52. Steinberg D, Witztum JL: Probucol. In Rifkind BM, ed: *Drug treatment of hyperlipidemia*. New York, 1991, Marcel Dekker.

53. Superko HR, Krauss RM: Coronary artery disease regression. Convincing evidence for the benefit of aggressive lipoprotein management, *Circulation* 90:1056-1069, 1994.

54. The Lovastatin Study Group II: Therapeutic response to lovastatin (mevinolin) in nonfamilial hypercholesterolemia. A multicenter study, *JAMA* 256:2829-2834, 1986.
55. Todd PA, Goa KL: Simvastatin. A review of its pharmacological properties and therapeutic potential in hypercholesterolaemia, *Drugs* 40:583-607, 1990.
56. Tomimoto S, Tsujita M, Okazaki M, et al: Effect of probucol in lecithin-cholesterol acyltransferase-deficient mice: inhibition of 2 independent cellular cholesterol-releasing pathways in vivo, *Arterioscler Thromb Vasc Biol* 21:394-400, 2001.
57. VanHeek M, Compton DS, Davis HR: The cholesterol absorption inhibitor, ezetimibe, decreases diet-induced hypercholesterolemia in monkeys, *Eur J Pharmacol* 415:79-84, 2001.
58. Yamamoto A, Matsuzawa Y, Yokoyama S, et al: Effects of probucol on xanthomata regression in familial hypercholesterolemia, *Am J Cardiol* 57:29H-35H, 1986.
59. Zapolska-Downar D, Zapolski-Downar A, Markiewski M, et al: Selective inhibition by probucol of vascular cell adhesion molecule-1 (VCAM-1) expression in human vascular endothelial cells, *Atherosclerosis* 155:123-130, 2001.

General References

Blankenhorn DH: Hyperlipidemia in patients with vascular disease. In Cooke JP, Frohlich ED, eds: *Current management of hypertensive and vascular diseases,* St Louis, 1992, Mosby.

Blum CB: Comparison of properties of four inhibitors of 3-hydroxy-3-methylglutaryl-coenzyme A reductase, *Am J Cardiol* 73:3D-11D, 1994.

Gold P, Grover S, Roncari DAK, eds: *Cholesterol and coronary heart disease: the great debate,* Park Ridge, NJ, 1992, Parthenon.

Illingworth DR, Tobert JA: A review of clinical trials comparing HMG CoA reductase inhibitors, *Clin Ther* 16:366-385, 1994.

Malloy MJ, Kane JP: Agents used in hyperlipidemia. In Katzung BG, ed: *Basic & clinical pharmacology,* ed 8, New York, 2001, McGraw-Hill.

Milander MM, Kuhn M: Lipid-lowering drugs, *AACN Clin Issues Crit Care Nurs* 3:494-506, 1992.

Schmitz G, Lackner KJ: Lipid-lowering therapy—implications for the prevention of atherosclerosis, *Basic Res Cardiol* 89(suppl 1):185-198, 1994.

USP dispensing information (USPDI). Drug information for the health care professional, vol 1, ed 24, Greenwich Village, CO, 2004, Thomson MICROMEDEX.

Witztum JL: Drugs used in the treatment of hyperlipoproteinemias. In Hardman JG, Limbird LE, eds: *Goodman & Gilman's The pharmacological basis of therapeutics,* ed 10, New York, 2001, McGraw-Hill.

CHAPTER • 30

Antianemic and Hematopoietic Stimulating Drugs

Barton S. Johnson

Hematopoiesis is the intricate system of growth and differentiation of immature pluripotent/multipotent stem cells into all the formed elements of the blood (Figure 30-1). These stem cells, derived embryonically in the liver and later from bone marrow,[55] divide early in development into either myeloid or lymphoid precursors. The myeloid precursors differentiate into the erythrocytes, megakaryocytes (which give rise to thrombocytes [platelets]), neutrophils, and monocytes. The lymphoid precursors give rise to the T-cell and B-cell lymphocytes, natural killer cells, and all their respective subtypes. There is conflicting evidence concerning where the derivation of eosinophils and basophils lies. They may come directly from the pluripotent/multipotent stem cells, or they may be subsets of myeloid precursors. Hematopoietically active bone marrow retains essentially the same mass throughout life, and although bone marrow is found in practically all bones through adolescence, it becomes restricted to the vertebrae, sternum, and ribs after approximately age 20 years.

Hematopoiesis is a dynamic, continuous process because mature cells of the blood have a limited life span in periods of both sickness and health. The hematopoietic system, because of its complexity, ubiquity, and high rate of activity, is often the first organ system to show evidence of underlying systemic disease. The pharmacologic interventions currently available to correct perturbations in marrow function are discussed in this chapter. Conditions such as anemia, thrombocytopenia, neutropenia, and volume depletion are detailed, as well as novel approaches to medical care that involve the hematopoietic system.

ANEMIA

Anemia is composed of a multifactorial group of illnesses with a wide range of underlying causes. As a result, *anemia* is a generic term indicating only that the concentration of hemoglobin in whole blood is below normal. Anemia is not a disease, but a sign of underlying disease. Therefore, when discussing anemia, it is important to diagnose both the nature and the cause of the anemia. There are three general categories of diseases that cause anemia: diseases that cause blood loss, disturb red blood cell production, or increase endogenous destruction of red blood cells. Blood loss can occur either acutely, as in hemorrhage from trauma or surgery, or chronically, as with excessive menstrual bleeding or the occult bleeding of esophageal varices or gastric/duodenal ulcers. Disturbed red blood cell production is associated with nutritional deficiencies, disorders that suppress erythrocyte production (such as in aplastic anemia and with some antiretroviral therapy), and myelophthisic (marrow-displacing) diseases. Finally, anemia can be caused by increased destruction of the red blood cells, such as in sickle cell disease, thalassemia, hemolytic immune reactions, and genetic disorders such as glucose-6-phosphate dehydrogenase deficiency.

When a patient is suspected of having a type of anemia, the first tests to consider are a simple hematocrit and erythrocyte count. These two tests will tell whether the production-to-loss ratio of red blood cells is normal. The *hematocrit* is defined as the ratio of red blood cells to the total blood volume. It is expressed as a percentage and is determined by comparing the packed cell volume (which is made up largely of erythrocytes) to the total volume of centrifuged whole blood. Normal values for women are 36% to 45%, and normal values for men are 38% to 50%. In the anemic patient the hematocrit level is lowered, often into the 20s, and in severe cases into the teens or below. Conversely, the hematocrit rises (referred to as *polycythemia vera* if moderate, *erythroleukemia* if severe) in patients with poor pulmonary function, some chronic cardiac conditions, certain marrow tumors, and in patients living at high altitudes. In acute hemorrhage, because plasma and red cells are lost together, the hematocrit does not initially reflect the loss until the body or exogenous medical intervention has had the opportunity to replenish the lost plasma volume. In these cases, there may be no indication of a problem until several hours later. The erythrocyte (reticulocyte) count is a simple determination of the absolute number of cells (in millions) per microliter. Normal values for women are 3.8 to 5.0 million/μl, and normal values for men are 4.4 to 5.6 million/μl.

After anemia has been detected, it can be characterized by evaluating the hemoglobin in the erythrocytes. Normal amounts of hemoglobin per unit volume of blood (assayed on peripheral blood draw) are 15.2 ± 2.2 g/dl for men and 13.7 ± 2.1 g/dl for women. Hemoglobin is the oxygen-carrying component of red blood cells. It is made up of three components: iron, porphyrin rings, and globin chains. Alterations in any one of these three components can be a cause for a clinical anemia. In normal hemoglobin, iron in the ferrous form (Fe^{++}) is chelated into the middle of the porphyrin chemical ring to yield heme, the nonprotein component of hemoglobin (Figure 30-2). The globin chains comprise the main protein constituents of hemoglobin. There are four forms of globin chains: α (141 amino acids), β (146 amino acids), and two variants of β, namely δ and γ. Approximately 97% of normal hemoglobin (hemoglobin A) consists of two α and two β chains ($\alpha_2\beta_2$); 1% to 2% is made up of the $\alpha_2\delta_2$ combination (hemoglobin A_2). The $\alpha_2\gamma_2$ tetramer forms hemoglobin F, or fetal hemoglobin. Hemoglobin F is the major form during gestation and until approximately 6 months of age. In the adult,

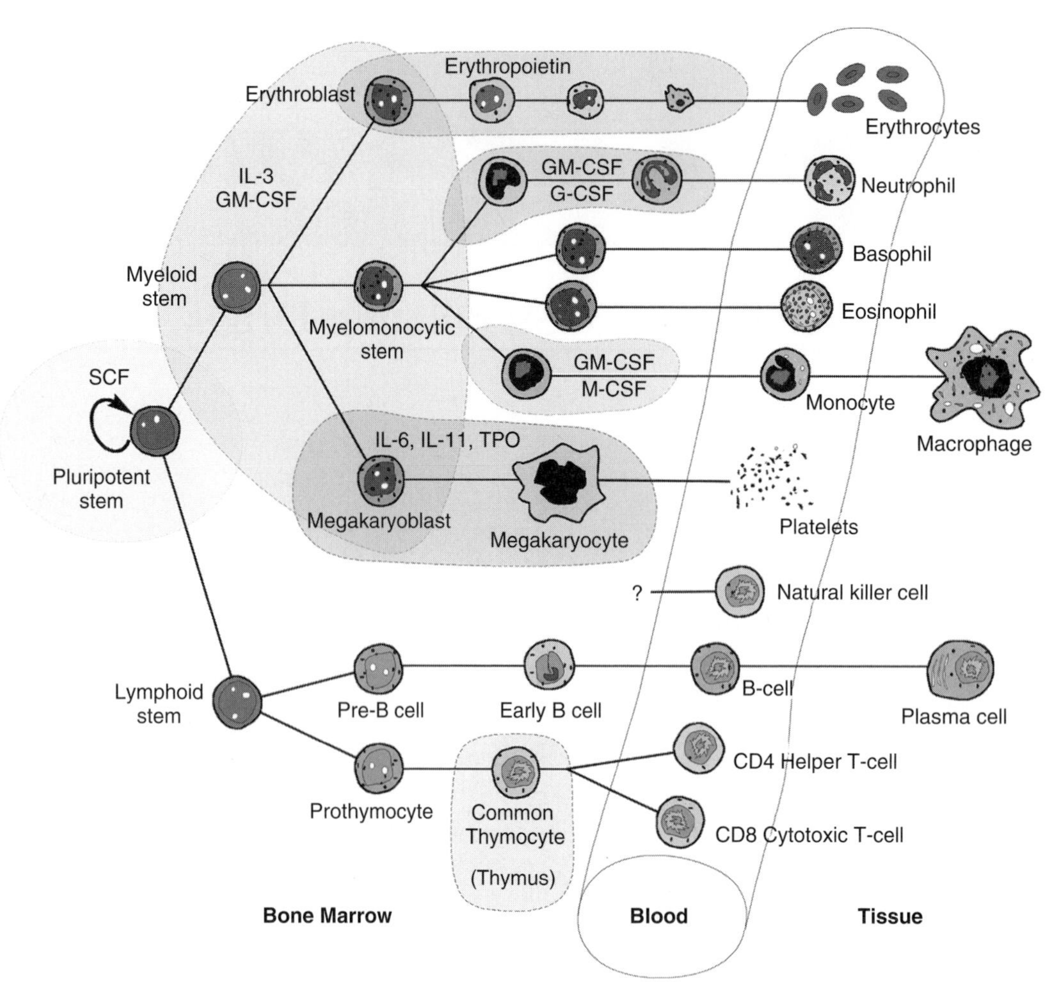

Fig. 30-1 Overview of hematopoiesis. *G-CSF*, Granulocyte colony-stimulating factor; *GM-CSF*, granulocyte/macrophage colony-stimulating factor; *IL-3, IL-6, IL-11*, interleukins-3, -6, and -11, respectively; *M-CSF*, monocyte/macrophage colony-stimulating factor; *SCF*, stem cell factor; *TPO*, thrombopoietin.

it makes up less than 1% of normal hemoglobin. One heme ring is accommodated within each of the four structural folds of the tetramer, allowing each molecule of hemoglobin to bind four oxygen molecules.

Hemoglobin accounts for approximately 95% of the dry weight of mature erythrocytes. Therefore any significant changes in hemoglobin are often directly reflected in the way the erythrocytes look or behave grossly. Classically, laboratory analyses for anemia have reviewed erythrocyte size, shape, and color intensity. The size is determined by the mean corpuscular volume (MCV). The normocytic, or normal size, range is 80 to 100 fl/cell. Cells that are too small are termed *microcytic*, whereas cells that are too large are labeled *macrocytic*. The shape of the red blood cells is also important in diagnosing the cause of anemia. Several terms exist to describe various shapes found on a peripheral blood smear, as reviewed in Box 30-1. The color intensity of the cell is reflected in the mean corpuscular hemoglobin (normally 26 to 34 pg/cell) and the mean corpuscular hemoglobin concentration (normally 31 to 36 g/dl). These two parameters, along with MCV, collectively referred to as the red cell "indices," are extremely helpful in delineating the causes of a particular anemia.

The various kinds of anemia are classified by their typical effect on the erythrocytes (Table 30-1). When anemia results from a loss of blood (intrinsically from hemolysis or extrinsically from hemorrhage) or because of a decrease in production of normal erythrocytes, the cells will still be normal, just fewer in quantity. Therefore these anemias are *normocytic and normochromic*. When anemia is caused by a decrease in the production of properly formed hemoglobin, the cells will tend to be smaller (because hemoglobin composes such a high percentage of erythrocyte content) and paler in color. These forms of anemia are known as *microcytic and hypochromic* and are usually the result of defective or inadequate iron absorption. Forms of anemia that cause the red blood cells to mature incompletely, and therefore be larger cells, are known as *macrocytic* or *megaloblastic* anemia. They generally occur as a result of a deficiency in vitamin B_{12}, folic acid, or both nutrients. In these forms of anemia, the cells may also have a darker or *hyperchromic* color.

Iron and Iron Deficiency Anemia: Nutrition and Physiologic Characteristics

Iron deficiency anemia is the most common cause of anemia worldwide and may occur for many reasons: inadequate nutrition in relation to rate of growth (qualitative or quantitative); defective absorption, transport, or storage (e.g., congenital atransferrinemia or inability to release iron from transferrin to the red blood cells and their precursors); or blood loss from hemorrhage (most commonly gastrointestinal), menstruation,

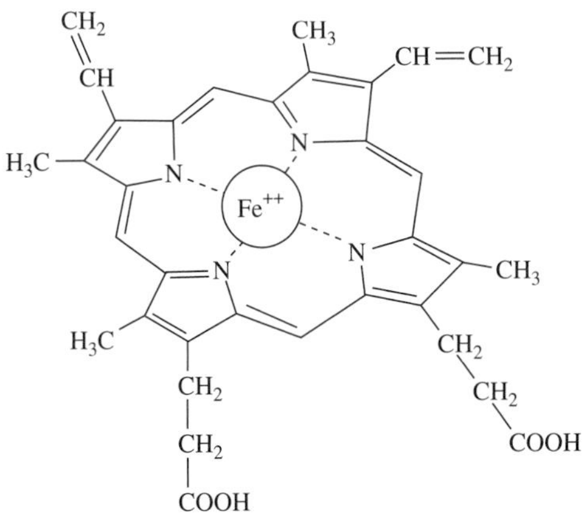

Heme

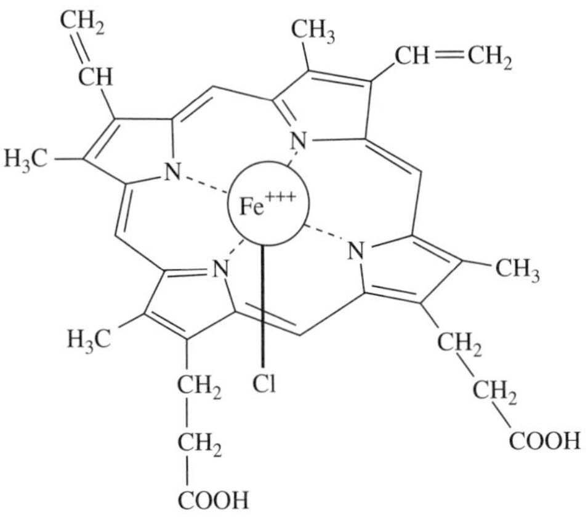

Hemin

Fig. 30-2 Structural formulas of heme and hemin.

or blood donation. In the United States, iron deficiency anemia is found in up to 25% of infants, 6% of children, 3% of menstruating women, and 10% of pregnant women.[42] Only 0.2% of adult men have iron deficiency anemia, however, and women taking oral contraceptives tend to have lower rates because progestins reduce menstrual blood loss. Children between 6 months and 2 years of age are particularly vulnerable because of their high growth rate coupled with weaning off breast milk and onto bovine milk. Cow's milk is low in absorbable iron and may irritate the intestines. Pregnancy may precipitate iron deficiency anemia by rapidly increasing the blood volume, sometimes requiring two to five times the normal intake of iron. According to a World Health Organization technical report,[16] women who have sufficient iron reserves to support the increase in hemoglobin production during pregnancy and who breast feed their infants are generally capable of meeting their iron needs by diet alone, although supplementation is still recommended. In a nonpregnant, normal, healthy person, the iron reserves and recycling are so effective that even extreme reduction of iron intake may be insufficient to cause severe anemia.[11]

Men average 3.8 g total iron (50 mg/kg) and women average 2.3 g (35 to 42 mg/kg). Most (approximately 60% to 80%) of the iron in the body is incorporated into hemoglobin (Figure 30-3). Therefore anemia is the primary presenting sign of iron deficiency. Approximately 10% to 25% is sequestered in reticuloendothelial cells in the storage forms ferritin and hemosiderin (described below) and another 10% to 15% is associated in parenchymal cells with myoglobin. Less than 1% is used in various enzymes, most notably the cytochromes, and trace amounts are linked to the plasma transport protein transferrin. The amount of stored iron varies with intake and demand, averaging 400 mg in women and 1000 mg in men.

The average American ingests 10 to 20 mg of iron per day. Iron is obtained through the diet, most commonly by heme or iron complexed to various organic compounds. Foods considered high in iron (more than 0.5% by weight) are liver, heart, oysters, egg yolks, and yeast. Other meats and green vegetables have somewhat less iron. Absorption of iron from dietary sources is ordinarily 10% efficient or less, but it increases when iron stores are depleted. Therapeutic iron, generally in the form of inorganic salts or complexes, has an even poorer absorption profile than dietary iron because the Fe^{++} must be liberated from the salt before it can be absorbed across the intestinal mucosa.

Iron absorption occurs along the entire length of the intestine, but maximum absorption occurs in the duodenum and proximal jejunum. This is not surprising because iron is

Table • 30-1

Classification of Anemia by Cause and Presentation

MICROCYTIC	MACROCYTIC	NORMOCYTIC
Decreased Production		
Iron deficiency Thalassemia Anemia of chronic disease	Megaloblastic: vitamin B_{12} deficiency, folate deficiency Nonmegaloblastic: myelodysplasia, chemotherapy, hepatitis	Aplastic anemia Bone marrow infiltration Carcinoma Lymphoma
Increased Destruction		
		Intrinsic hemolysis Extrinsic hemolysis
Blood Loss		
		Acute hemorrhage Chronic hemorrhage

Box 30-1

Descriptive Terms of Red Cell Morphologic Characteristics

Term	Description
Poikilocytosis	Irregular erythrocyte shape
Anisocytosis	Irregular erythrocyte size
Polychromasia	Change in the amount of hemoglobin
Sickling	Sickle cell disease and trait
Targeting	"Bull's-eye" look to the erythrocytes caused by hemoglobin C and liver disease
Leptocytes	Hemoglobin in the border with pigmentation in the center; found in thalassemia, obstructive jaundice, any hypochromic anemia, hemoglobinopathy, and after splenectomy
Spherocytes	Round erythrocytes (not biconcave), caused by hereditary spherocytosis, or by immune or microangiopathic hemolysis
Schistocytes	Fragments of erythrocytes; found in hemolytic transfusion reactions, microangiopathic hemolysis, other severe anemias
Acanthocytes	Distorted ("thorny") erythrocytes with protoplasmic projections; seen in severe liver disease and with high titers of bile, fats, or toxins
Howell-Jolly bodies	Smooth, round remnants of nuclear chromatin; seen in megaloblastic and hemolytic anemias and after splenectomy
Nucleated erythrocytes	Found in severe bone marrow stress (e.g., hemorrhage, hemolysis), marrow replacement by tumor, extramedullary hematopoiesis

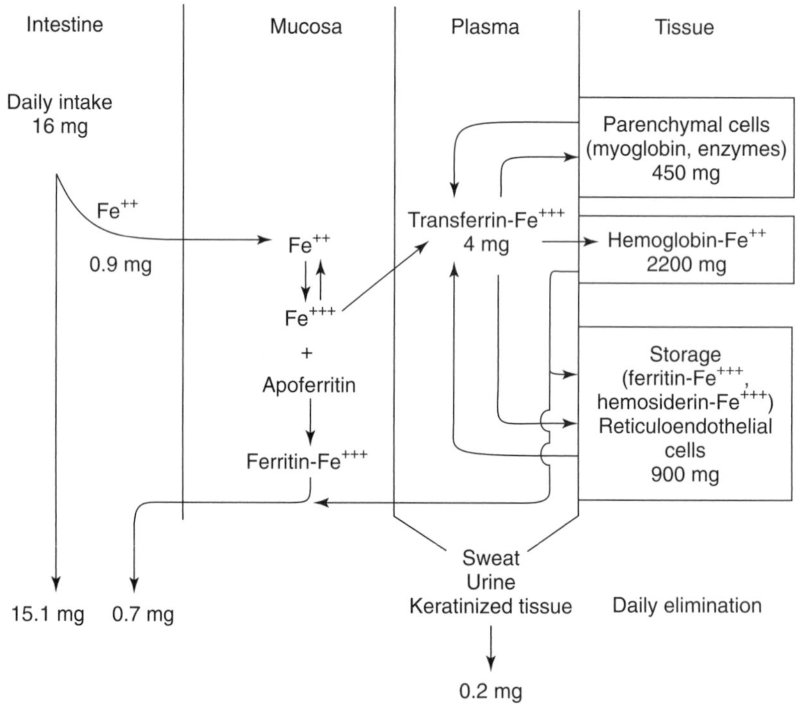

Fig. 30-3 Absorption, excretion, and storage of iron within the body of a 70-kg man. The amounts of iron absorbed, excreted, and stored in the three major compartments are expressed in milligrams. Note the balance between daily absorption and excretion.

absorbed primarily as Fe^{++}, and an acid medium favors the breakdown of salts to the ionic form. In the lower portions of the gastrointestinal tract there is a trend toward increasing alkalinity, which favors the formation of less soluble iron salts and complexes. Iron ingested as heme iron is absorbed five to seven times more efficiently than Fe^{++} salts.[20] Iron absorption is hindered by coffee, tea, phosphates, and antacids, particularly calcium carbonate and aluminum or magnesium hydroxide. Absorption of nonheme iron is facilitated by vitamin C. There is conflicting evidence regarding whether ethanol ingestion retards iron absorption,[15] but it is known that approximately 50% of alcoholics exhibit some iron depletion or anemia.[42]

Iron is absorbed by active transport across the intestinal mucosa, where it is converted intracellularly to ferric iron (Fe^{+++}). Depending on the body's acute need for iron, the Fe^{+++} is either bound to transferrin or converted to ferritin or hemosiderin for storage in the intestinal mucosa. Transferrin is a transport glycoprotein electrophoretically migrating with the β globulins; it specifically binds two molecules of Fe^{+++}. It enters the plasma and carries the Fe^{+++} to the bone marrow and developing erythroblasts. The erythroblasts present membrane transferrin receptors that bind diferric transferrin and then internalize the complex by endocytosis. Inside the cell, the transferrin receptor, transferrin, and Fe^{+++} are broken apart, with the iron being used in hemoglobin synthesis and the transferrin and transferrin receptor being carried back intact to the surface for recycling. The typical developing erythroblast can process 25,000 to 50,000 transferrin molecules per minute.

A test for transferrin is the total iron-binding capacity (TIBC). In the normal adult, approximately 20% to 50% of the transferrin is replete with Fe^{+++}. In an iron-deficient person, the transferrin saturation may drop to 15% or less. Therefore the capacity to bind iron is considerably greater, and the TIBC value rises. Normal values are 250 to 450 µg/dl.

If the body is not in acute need of iron, most of the ingested iron is stored as ferritin. Twenty-four apoferritin monomers bind together to form a hollow spherical shell 130 Å in diameter and fenestrated with small pores through which up to 4000 Fe^{++} atoms can enter. Once inside, the Fe^{++} is oxidized to Fe^{+++} and stored in the form of hydrous ferric oxide phosphate. Ferritin, the resulting apoferritin-iron complex, is a very effective storage mechanism, allowing the binding and release of iron to occur rapidly and efficiently. Mature ferritin is found in virtually all cells of the body and in plasma. Although the amount in plasma is small, it does reflect the total ferritin stores in the body and is measured to diagnose iron deficiency anemia. Normal values for serum ferritin are 16 to 300 mg/ml in men and 4 to 160 mg/ml in women.

The other, minor storage component of iron is hemosiderin. It is found in the monocyte/macrophage system of the marrow and in the Kupffer cells of the liver. Hemosiderin is an insoluble compound that appears to be aggregated ferritin cores partially or completely stripped of the apoferritin protein shell. In pathology (hemosiderosis), it can be found in large quantities in most tissues of the body.

The concentration of iron in the plasma at any one time represents a balance between the absorption rate, storage capacity, rate of hemoglobin formation, and rate of iron excretion. Iron is remarkably well conserved in the body; less than 0.1% is excreted on a daily basis, or approximately 0.5 to 1.0 mg/day. The major pathway of iron excretion is through the feces by exfoliation of gastrointestinal cells and their intracellular stores of ferritin when the mucosal cells are replaced by new epithelium. Iron is also lost in considerably smaller amounts by excretion through urine, exfoliation of dermal cells, and perspiration. Menstruation causes the amount of lost iron to roughly double to 2 mg/day. Uncommon sources of iron loss include excessive blood loss or excessive destruction of erythrocytes. Hemorrhage depletes heme iron, whereas excessive turnover of erythrocytes releases it back into the circulation, where it can be recycled. The normal person can lose as much as a quarter to a third of the erythrocyte mass through hemorrhage without need for iron therapy. Because iron is so well conserved in the body and most people have large reserves, chronically insufficient intake of iron is almost always the cause of iron deficiency anemia.

Pathophysiologic Characteristics

Iron deficiency is manifested as signs and symptoms of anemia (pale color, fatigue, tachycardia, tachypnea on exertion). Severe cases, which are rare in first-world nations, may show progressive skin and mucosal changes, such as angular cheilosis and brittle fingernails and toenails. Splenomegaly may be present if hemolysis is occurring. The classic intraoral finding is a red-appearing, sore, smooth tongue caused by atrophy of the dorsal filiform papillae. In very severe cases, Plummer-Vinson syndrome may occur, which is iron deficiency anemia coupled with the formation of esophageal webs and resultant dysphagia. This syndrome is also associated with pharyngeal or esophageal squamous cell carcinoma. Many iron-deficient patients have pica, an unusual craving for specific foods or unnatural food items (e.g., ice cubes, soil, paint chips) that may or may not contain iron.

The laboratory findings of iron deficiency anemia reflect the severity of the loss. In the first stage, there is a normocytic anemia without changes in erythropoiesis. The ferritin stores are depleting, so the serum ferritin values fall while the TIBC rises. As anemia progresses and the stores are depleted, the erythrocytes become affected, resulting in a decrease in the MCV, mean corpuscular hemoglobin, erythrocyte count, hemoglobin, and hematocrit.

Therapeutic Use

Because the intuitive treatment of any disease state that is accompanied by extreme fatigue, weakness, and loss of color includes increased dietary intake, it is not surprising that the ancient Greeks, Hindus, and other early peoples turned to iron in many forms simply because it represented "strength." Although Sydenham is generally credited with the first rational use of iron (iron filings in wine) for treating anemia in 1681, it was not known that iron was actually present in blood until 30 years later, when Lemery and Geoffry demonstrated its presence. Shortly thereafter it was shown by an Italian physician, Menghini, that foods with iron actually increase blood iron, but it was not until approximately 1830 that a pill containing iron (ferrous sulfate and potassium carbonate, 1:1) was introduced into medicine by Pierre Blaud,[6] an event that marked the beginning of modern treatment of iron deficiency anemia. An excellent history is presented by Fairbanks and Beutler.[15]

Iron therapy is indicated in iron deficiency anemia; it is contraindicated in anemia of any other cause. Iron is available in the form of Fe^{++} salts (sulfate, gluconate, and fumarate), which are reasonably well absorbed, and a Fe^{+++}-containing compound (iron polysaccharide), which is not as well absorbed. The most commonly used Fe^{++} preparation, and the agent of choice for uncomplicated iron deficiency anemia, is ferrous sulfate. It is normally given in doses (325 mg three times a day) much larger than should theoretically be needed because of its limited absorption (no more than 15%). The response to oral iron preparations is usually evident in 5 to 10 days and is first manifested by an increase in reticulocytes. Adverse effects associated with orally administered iron are gastrointestinal symptoms, chiefly nausea and vomiting, because of direct irritation of the stomach. The patient will have black stools as a result of therapy, which may obscure the diagnosis of melena. The drug is unquestionably best absorbed when taken between meals, but gastrointestinal distress is lessened if the medication is taken with meals and if the dose is started at a lower level and slowly increased with time. Generally, the hematocrit returns halfway to normal in approximately 3 weeks and is fully corrected in roughly 8 weeks. To replenish iron stores, a course of therapy of 3 to 6 months is generally required.

Although parenteral iron preparations are available, they are not generally used because of the simplicity of oral medication and the much greater risk of serious side effects and higher expense. Iron should be administered parenterally only if the oral preparations are inadequately absorbed or poorly tolerated, such as in patients with enteritis or colitis, or if it is absolutely necessary to replace a serious iron deficit quickly. The classic parenteral form is iron dextran, a sterile colloidal solution of ferric hydroxide and low–molecular-weight dextran, which is administered by intramuscular or intravenous injection. Adverse reactions include pain and staining at the site of injection (intramuscular), urticaria, fever, arthralgia, lymphadenopathy, nausea, and vomiting. Rarely, severe, even fatal, anaphylactic reactions have occurred after the use of this preparation. Another parenteral form, iron sucrose, is a polynuclear ferric hydroxide sucrose complex. It is believed that the antigenic potential of iron dextran lies in the Fe^{++} and dextran polysaccharides and therefore that this preparation is less allergenic. Iron sucrose is commonly used in patients undergoing renal dialysis who are receiving erythropoietin (EPO) therapy.

Acute iron poisoning is not uncommon, particularly because many of the iron formulations are brightly colored and attractive to children. Ingestion of large doses of iron causes the transferrin to become saturated, and free iron enters the blood in excess. Unbound iron is toxic and has caused severe gastrointestinal disturbances and circulatory collapse. Chelating agents have been used in the treatment of acute iron toxicity; deferoxamine, a potent and specific iron-chelating compound, is capable of removing iron from both ferritin and transferrin but not from hemoglobin. It is, however, no substitute for more immediate measures, such as inducing vomiting, gastric lavage, and fluid administration, that should be carried out in the event of iron poisoning.

Perhaps the most important consideration for the dental professional is the finding that people who are taking oral iron supplements may have altered absorption profiles of other drugs. The quinolone class of antibiotics, tetracyclines, and thyroid replacement hormones all form complexes with iron and result in significantly poorer (up to 36% less) absorption profiles. Simply having the patient stagger the iron and the other medication by 2 or more hours is usually sufficient to avoid this difficulty.

OTHER MINERALS AND HEMATOPOIESIS

Copper deficiency, although extremely rare in human beings, has been reported as the cause of anemia in intestinal bypass surgery patients.[20] Copper is required for the operation of several copper-containing enzymes (e.g., cytochrome oxidase and monoamine oxidase) and may be essential for iron absorption. Interestingly, too much zinc in the diet can result in copper deficiency.[21]

Cobalt is not essential for hematopoiesis except in the form of vitamin B_{12}, as described later in this chapter. It is therefore surprising that elemental cobalt can stimulate red cell formation to the point of polycythemia in human beings. This effect is thought to be derived from the release of erythropoietin (EPO) by the kidneys. Unfortunately, the metal's toxic effects limit its clinical application.

Lithium salts used in the treatment of manic-depressive illness, frequently induce a selective leukocytosis involving neutrophils, eosinophils, and monocytes and may even increase platelet formation.[7] This effect is a true increase in blood cell proliferation, and lithium has been used in aplastic anemia, specific leukemias, and thrombocytopenia, albeit with limited success.

PORPHYRIA

Although iron deficiency anemia is by far the most commonly encountered form of anemia, it is not the only disorder in which insufficient functional heme is produced. The porphyrias, a cluster of disorders that involve decreased or disordered production of the porphyrin ring, can be associated with anemia depending on the variety and severity of the diseases' presentation. Heme, of course, is a major component of hemoglobin, but it is also crucial to several enzyme systems, most notably the large family of cytochrome P450 enzymes involved in steroid synthesis and drug metabolism.

Porphyrin is produced in an eight-step process that takes place both in the mitochondria and in the cytosol. The two principal cell types involved are the developing erythroblasts and reticulocytes of the bone marrow (mature erythrocytes lack mitochondria and are therefore unable to synthesize porphyrin) and the liver hepatocytes. As a result, two general classifications of porphyria exist—erythropoietic and hepatic—that are further divided into nine varieties (Table 30-2), each corresponding to a particular enzyme deficiency in the synthetic pathway of porphyrin. These deficiencies may be genetic in nature or caused by medications.

The acute exacerbations usually occur when there is a significant demand for heme synthesis that cannot be met by the limited enzyme function. This deficiency in heme inhibits the negative feedback cycle on δ-aminolevulinic acid synthase, causing induction of this rate-limiting enzyme. However, because the heme synthesis pathway is damaged, induction instead leads to the excessive production in the liver of the porphyrin precursors δ-aminolevulinic acid and

Table • 30-2

Classification of the Porphyrias

PORPHYRIA	SITE OF EXPRESSION	PRINCIPAL CLINICAL FEATURE
Acute intermittent porphyria	Liver	Neurologic
δ-Aminolevulinic acid dehydratase deficiency porphyria (rare)	Liver	Neurologic
Hereditary coproporphyria	Liver	Neurologic, photosensitivity
Porphyria cutanea tarda	Liver	Photosensitivity
Variegate porphyria	Liver	Neurologic, photosensitivity
Hepatoerythropoietic porphyria	Liver, bone marrow	Photosensitivity
Congenital erythropoietic porphyria	Bone marrow	Photosensitivity
Erythropoietic protoporphyria	Bone marrow	Photosensitivity
X-linked sideroblastic anemia	Bone marrow	Hemolytic anemia

porphobilinogen, which build up and cause the acute symptoms. This accumulation of protoporphyrin precursors results in neurologic disorders, photocutaneous disturbances, or both.

Probably the most common genetic form of porphyria is acute intermittent porphyria. Its mode of transmission is autosomally dominant and results from a partial enzymatic deficiency (less than 50% of normal) in the third step of porphyrin synthesis. Because synthetic activity is diminished but not lost, most patients remain asymptomatic throughout normal life. Acute exacerbations, which give rise to the name, have highly variable symptoms that last between days and months. The most common presentation is one of a neurologic nature, including mental changes, seizures, and acute sensory neuropathies such as abdominal pain, chest and back pain, and limb pain. The severity of the pain can be great enough to mimic other acute disorders and result in unnecessary surgical intervention such as laparotomy. Motor neuropathies, especially in the cranial nerves, are often seen. Occasionally, motor paralysis of the respiratory diaphragm has resulted in death. Gastrointestinal disturbances, primarily nausea, vomiting, and diarrhea, are common.

Several events can precipitate an attack. Physiologic stressors, such as surgery, excessive alcohol intake, illnesses, and infections, may induce hepatic heme oxygenase, which breaks down heme. Endocrine changes, such as may occur around a woman's menses, or synthetic estrogens and progestins, may also induce an attack. Many medications commonly used in dentistry and medicine (Box 30-2) are metabolized by, and induce the synthesis of, the cytochrome P450 enzyme system, leading to increased accumulation of porphyrin precursors.[32] The unsafe medications should be avoided in susceptible porphyric patients, which also includes individuals with hereditary coproporphyria and variegate porphyria. Poor nutritional intake has also been associated with acute attacks.

Porphyria cutanea tarda is the most common porphyria and is representative of the erythropoetic porphyrias. Symptomatology commonly includes photosensitivity, which results from sequestration of protoporphyrins in the skin and subsequent deposition of iron in the integument. Porphyrin and its precursors undergo photoactivation at 400 nm in the presence of oxygen, causing cellular destruction by release of oxygen free radicals. Therefore, in skin exposed to light, the porphyrins become photoexcited, and clinically evident cellular damage occurs. Porphyrin-laden erythrocytes also undergo phototoxicity when circulating through light-penetrated tissues. The damage may be sufficient to result in hemolytic anemia.

Management of acute intermittent porphyria has been primarily aimed at avoiding exacerbating conditions. Adequate caloric intake, prompt diagnosis and treatment of infections (including odontogenic and other orofacial infections), and care in not taking medications known to trigger attacks are strategies the patient can use to minimize the risk of developing a crisis. In those patients who have photoreactive porphyria, avoidance of sunlight, wearing clothing to cover the skin, and generous use of sunscreen lotion are helpful. If an acute attack occurs that is not amenable to glucose infusion, a medication of choice is lyophilized hemin with sodium carbonate. Hemin is ferric heme that has a Cl^- on one of the two available coordination sites for the Fe^{+++} (see Figure 30-2). On mixing with sterile water, the hemin is converted in the resulting alkaline solution to hematin by replacement of the Cl^- with an OH^- group. Hematin serves as an enzymatic inhibitor of porphyrin synthesis by decreasing the concentration of the precursors porphobilinogen and δ-aminolevulinic acid. The reconstituted drug is unstable, however, and has been frequently associated with thrombophlebitis and increased coagulopathy. The palliative use of opioid analgesics is also often indicated during porphyric exacerbations.

Box 30-2

Drugs Considered Safe or Unsafe for Use in Patients with Acute Intermittent Porphyria, Variegate Porphyria, and Hereditary Coproporphyria

Safe	Unsafe
Acetaminophen	Alcohol
Amitriptyline	Alkylating agents
Aspirin	Barbiturates
Atropine	Carbamazepine
Chloral hydrate	Chlordiazepoxide
Clorazepate	Chlorpropamide
Diazepam	Chloroquine
Digoxin	Clonidine
Diphenhydramine	Dapsone
Glucocorticoids	Ergots
Guanethidine	Erythromycin
Hyoscine	Estrogens, synthetic
Ibuprofen	Food additives
Imipramine	Glutethimide
Insulin	Griseofulvin
Labetalol	Hydralazine
Lithium	Ketamine
Naproxen	Meprobamate
Nitrofurantoin	Methyldopa
Opioid analgesics	Metoclopramide
Penicillamine	Nortriptyline
Penicillin and derivatives	Pentazocine
Phenothiazines	Phenytoin
Procaine	Progestins
Propranolol	Pyrazinamide
Streptomycin	Rifampin
Succinylcholine	Spironolactone
Tetracycline	Succinimides
Thiouracil	Sulfonamides
Vitamins B and C	Theophylline
	Tolazamide
	Tolbutamide
	Valproic acid

THALASSEMIA

In addition to problems affecting iron and porphyrin, several disorders of the third component of hemoglobin—the globin chains—can also lead to clinical anemia. Grouped together, these disorders are called the *thalassemias*.

As discussed previously, normal hemoglobin A is composed of two α- and two β-globin chains. When there is a genetic defect in the production of the α chains, the patient has α-thalassemia. Similarly, a defect in the β chains results in β-thalassemia. Sickle cell anemia, although normally addressed as a separate entity, is a variant of β-thalassemia. The thalassemias generally result in a decreased production of their respective protein chains. As a result, hemoglobin synthesis is impaired, and a non–iron-deficient, hypochromic, microcytic anemia ensues.

There are two pairs of genes encoding the α-globin chains, both located on chromosome 16. When all four α-globin genes are defective, the fetus will develop hydrops fetalis, a condition incompatible with life. If there is a defective mutation in one of the four genes, the individual will be clinically normal but called a *silent carrier.* If two genes are affected, the patient is labeled as having *α-thalassemia minor.* The hematocrit is mildly depressed (32% to 40%), and there is a marked decrease in erythrocyte size (MCV of 60 to 75 fl). All the iron parameters are normal. If three genes are affected, the patient is diagnosed with *α-thalassemia intermedia,* also known as *hemoglobin H disease.* Hemoglobin H is composed of tetramers of β-globin (β_4), resulting from a relative excess of β-globin chains compared with the α chains. Hemoglobin H has a high affinity for oxygen and therefore binds it too tightly for efficient tissue delivery. It is rather unstable, being prone to denaturation by oxidative medications (such as the sulfonamides) and infectious conditions. The hematocrit in hemoglobin H disease is markedly depressed (22% to 32%), and the anemia is hypochromic and microcytic in nature (MCV, 60 to 70 fl). Clinical signs of the disease include pallor and splenomegaly.

The β-thalassemias exhibit a similar variability in severity based on which mutations in the genome are present. Most of the β-thalassemias result from point mutations in the gene, which create premature stop codons or cause difficulties with RNA transcription. As a result, the afflicted β chain may be either reduced (β^+) or absent (β^0). Because the δ or γ forms of hemoglobin can substitute for the β form, the β-thalassemias typically have decreased ratios of hemoglobin A ($\alpha_2\beta_2$) and increased ratios of hemoglobin A_2 ($\alpha_2\delta_2$) and hemoglobin F ($\alpha_2\gamma_2$). The total amount of useful hemoglobin, however, is usually severely depressed, decreasing oxygen transport capability. Further clinical disease occurs because of a relative excess of α-globin chains, which precipitate and cause damage to both the developing erythrocytes and the circulating peripheral erythrocytes. The intramedullary destruction of reticulocytes triggers a hyperplastic response by the bone marrow, resulting in increased marrow spaces and subsequent pathologic fractures and osteopenia. Peripherally, the destruction of the red blood cells may lead to a potentially life-threatening hemolytic anemia, splenomegaly, hepatomegaly, and hyperbilirubinemia.

The correct diagnosis of a thalassemia condition is crucial to proper treatment. Mild forms of the disease need no treatment. More severe forms typically require transfusion support and folate supplementation. Iron therapy should be avoided because there is often hemosiderosis/iron overload because of insufficient complete hemoglobin production. Patients requiring chronic transfusions are particularly susceptible to iron overload. In these cases, deferoxamine can be used to chelate iron and suppress the progression of hemosiderosis. Splenectomy may be required if severe hemolysis is occurring. Finally, allogenic bone marrow transplantation may be required to correct the defect in severe cases.

Sickle Cell Anemia

Sickle cell anemia is technically a variant of β-thalassemia. A point mutation in the number 6 position of the β-globin chain causes a valine to be substituted for glutamic acid. As an autosomal recessive disorder, sickle cell *anemia* occurs when both alleles are positive for the sickle variant. Sickle cell *trait* occurs in the heterozygous state, where partial penetrance ($\alpha_2\beta^s\beta$) can occur. The abnormal β chain is designated β^s, and the resulting tetramer of $\alpha_2\beta^s_2$ is known as *hemoglobin S.* The significance of hemoglobin S is that in the severely deoxygenated state the globin tetramers are capable of coalescing into long, straight, spiral polymers that act as deforming filaments within the red blood cell. The cell loses its typical biconcave disk shape and its inherent pliability that is so important for moving through the microvasculature. These deformed and hardened erythrocytes are much more prone to automembrane damage and hemolysis even as the sickled shape makes them likely to cause microvascular occlusion and endothelial vascular damage.

Sickle cell anemia generally first presents in the homozygous patient by the age of 6 months, when hemoglobin F is downregulated and hemoglobin S becomes the dominant form of hemoglobin in the erythrocyte. Many patients with homozygous disease can have relatively normal lives as long as they avoid situations in which moderate to severe hypoxic stress can develop.[29] Acute crises of sickling occur when the globin tetramers are deoxygenated for a sufficient time to allow polymerization into the deforming filamentous form. Small infections, such as odontogenic infections, may or may not cause an acute crisis. Even though acidosis can develop, unless the red blood cells are severely hypoxic, they will reoxygenate at the lungs before developing significant polymers and distorted cells. However, if the hypoxic stress is great, such as with more severe infection, acute sickling will occur. The episodes are extremely painful, often lasting several hours to days. Treatment for the acute crisis is aimed at hydration, oxygenation, and resolution of the underlying precipitating factor. Many patients require opioid analgesics to help them through a crisis.

The patient with sickle cell anemia who is prone to repeated acute crises will have a variety of chronic complications from the disease. The erythrocytes containing hemoglobin S have a shortened life span compared with those containing hemoglobin A, and episodes of sickling accelerate their demise, resulting in a chronic hemolytic-type anemia. The anemia predisposes the patient to diminished oxygen transport capability (furthering the likelihood of a sickling crisis), and the breakdown by-products of the erythrocytes can produce clinical jaundice, hepatomegaly, and splenomegaly. At the same time, chronic and repeated microvascular occlusive episodes can cause renal infarction, stroke, retinopathy, cardiomyopathy, and hepatic damage from occlusive ischemic necrosis. Many patients develop significant microvascular damage in the spleen because of its slow, tortuous microcirculation. In some cases, the spleen ultimately undergoes reactive fibrosis and becomes a small, scarred, essentially nonfunctional organ (autosplenectomy). In severe cases of sickle cell anemia, death can occur from multisystem organ failure.

Two strategies have been used in the long-term management of sickle cell anemia: bone marrow transplantation and pharmacotherapy. In one controlled study, definitive cure was demonstrated in 36 (86%) of 42 cases by bone marrow transplantation from an antigen-matched sibling, with five of the six failures cured by subsequent engraftment.[23] Bone marrow transplantation replaces the pluripotent stem cells of the marrow with those of a person without the genotype, thereby erasing the genetic defect. Although bone marrow transplantation is significantly more predictable than in years past, there is still a significant (more than 10%) mortality rate associated with the procedure, and the implications of chronic graft-versus-host disease must be weighed. This approach is generally reserved for severe cases that exhibit recurrent sickle crises.

Although still experimental, pharmacologic therapy has shown at least partial success in both β-thalassemia and sickle cell anemia. This approach is based on the premise that any measure that increases the quantity of β-like globin molecules in erythrocytes is beneficial.[31] Several antineoplastic agents—cytarabine, hydroxyurea, 5-azacytidine, as well as interferon γ, butyrates, and EPO with or without hydroxyurea—have been used to stimulate the formation of hemoglobin F. Hemoglobin F transports oxygen as effectively as does hemoglobin A, and it circumvents the genetic abnormalities associated with defective β-globin synthesis. In addition, hemoglobin F suppresses the polymerization of hemoglobin S, further helping reduce the effects of the disease. Although not a cure, this therapy has been recommended by the National Institutes of Health for adult patients, as long as they are closely monitored hematologically, to reduce the pain and organ damage of sickle cell anemia.[3]

VITAMIN B_{12}, FOLIC ACID, AND MEGALOBLASTIC ANEMIA

Deficiency Syndromes

Vitamin B_{12} and folic acid are two nutritional supplements that are crucial to normal DNA synthesis. When one or both of these are deficient, all rapidly dividing cells throughout the body, but especially those of the bone marrow and gastrointestinal epithelium, begin to have difficulties with proliferation and differentiation caused by inhibition of mitosis and cytokinesis. Primarily, DNA synthesis is impaired; the resulting cells therefore have large RNA/DNA ratios, increased cytoplasmic compartments, and unusual, immature nuclear forms. In hematopoiesis, the deficiency causes the cells to assume a characteristic macrocytic and often oval or irregular shape that resembles the less mature blast forms, hence the term *megaloblastic anemia*.[2] Protein synthesis is also adversely affected, resulting in substandard cell membranes and shortened life spans, causing the anemia to have a hemolytic component as well.

Although the diagnosis of megaloblastic anemia is most commonly made because of the characteristic changes in erythrocytes, all hematopoietic cell types are affected, which in rare cases can result in pancytopenia. The myeloid-derived cells released into the bloodstream may include macroovalocytes, hypersegmented polymorphonuclear leukocytes, and oversized platelets. Depending on which cell types are adversely affected, there may be not only clinical fatigue caused by erythropoietic depression, but also leukopenia and thrombocytopenia, with an increased potential of infection (particularly in the urinary tract) and hemorrhage.[2]

It must be emphasized that even though both folic acid and vitamin B_{12} have similar effects on the developing erythrocytes, the overall clinical presentations of their respective deficiency states differ greatly. The similarity comes from the sharing of a common biochemical pathway. The major difference is that neurologic manifestations often occur with vitamin B_{12} deficiency but not with folic acid deficiency. Folate deficiency alone is characterized by pallor, anemia, fatigue, and glossitis. Vitamin B_{12} deficiency results in the same signs and symptoms as folate deficiency but also causes inadequate myelin synthesis and epithelial replacement in the gastrointestinal tract. Symptoms of vitamin B_{12} deficiency therefore include gastrointestinal disturbances, weight loss, hepatomegaly, splenomegaly, and prominent neurologic disturbances related to inadequate myelin formation and maintenance. Paresthesias involving the peripheral nerves are the most common presenting symptoms. There is also decreased vibration and positional sense. Reflexes may be altered, and motor disturbances, including weakness and loss of sphincter tone, may occur. As the disease progresses, the posterior columns are affected, resulting in difficulty with balance. In advanced cases, cerebral dysfunction may lead to the loss of memory, confusion, or dementia and other neuropsychiatric changes. It is very important to diagnose correctly and treat a vitamin B_{12} deficiency early because most of these neurologic findings can be reversed in the early stages. Patients with more advanced cases have permanent neurologic damage. On occasion, neurologic changes occur without hematopoietic alterations.

Although any interruption in DNA synthesis, maturation, or division of marrow stem cells can give rise to a megaloblastic anemia, virtually all cases seen clinically result from vitamin B_{12} or folic acid deficiency. The cause may be insufficient dietary intake, decreased absorption, decreased utilization, or increased destruction of either or both of these two essential nutrients. Other, rarer causes include chemical agents that interfere with purine metabolism (such as chemotherapeutic drugs) and an intestinal parasite, the fish tapeworm (*Diphyllobothrium latum*), which competes rather successfully with the host for available vitamin B_{12}.

One particular variety of vitamin B_{12} deficiency is *pernicious anemia*. Historically, some anemic patients did not respond to iron supplementation, and their disease was characterized as pernicious, meaning fatal. Although pernicious anemia was described by Addison[1] and others in the early 1800s, it remained for Minot and Murphy[35] in 1926 to demonstrate the value of raw liver in treating the disease. Castle[8] showed in 1927 that a carrier glycoprotein secreted into the intestinal lumen by the gastroparietal cells plays a crucial role in reversing the lethal course of pernicious anemia. This finding led to the isolation of vitamin B_{12} two decades later.[46,51]

Vitamin B_{12}

Nutrition and physiologic characteristics

Vitamin B_{12} is a generic term for cyanocobalamin and hydroxocobalamin, two stable forms of cobalamin. Cobalamins are unique in that they are the only cobalt-containing organic compounds known to occur in nature, and they represent the only known biologic example of a metal-carbon bond.[41] The cobalamins are composed of a nearly planar macrocyclic corrin ring (similar to porphyrin) covalently linked to a trivalent cobalt atom by four coordination bonds in a manner similar to iron binding in heme (Figure 30-4).[34] The nucleotide 5,6-dimethylbenzimidazole is bound perpendicularly below this ring structure to both the corrin ring and the cobalt atom, whereas various R groups above the ring are bound solely to the cobalt atom. Four forms of the cobalamins have significant biochemical activity in vivo. Cyanocobalamin has a cyanide moiety as its R group; hydroxocobalamin has a hydroxyl. Hydroxocobalamin is converted endogenously to either deoxyadenosylcobalamin (5'-deoxyadenosyl R group) or methylcobalamin (methyl R group), the major form of cobalamin in plasma.

The cobalamins are essential cofactors in three human enzymatic processes. Deoxyadenosylcobalamin activates methylmalonyl coenzyme A (CoA) mutase, a mitochondrial enzyme that converts potentially toxic methylmalonyl CoA to the easily metabolized succinyl CoA. Methylmalonyl CoA is produced in the catabolism of propionate, which is formed during the breakdown of valine and isoleucine. In vitamin B_{12} deficiency, it is believed that accumulation of methylmalonyl CoA results in aberrant fatty acid synthesis and metabolism, causing nonphysiologic fatty acids to be incorporated into cell membranes of the central nervous system, leading to the neurologic symptoms already described.[4]

In a separate enzymatic pathway, methylcobalamin serves as a cofactor for methionine synthase, a cytoplasmic methyltransferase that converts homocysteine and 5-methyltetrahydrofolate to methionine and tetrahydrofolate. As will be discussed later, tetrahydrofolate is the precursor to many folate cofactors, several of which are crucial to DNA synthesis. When vitamin B_{12} is deficient, 5-methyltetrahydrofolate (derived from dietary folate) accumulates and tetrahydrofolate (the metabolically useful product) declines, leading to megaloblastic anemia. Because of the common factor of folic acid, pharmacologic vitamin B_{12} can sometimes ameliorate a folic acid deficiency and vice versa. As stated previously, however, folic acid alone cannot correct the induced

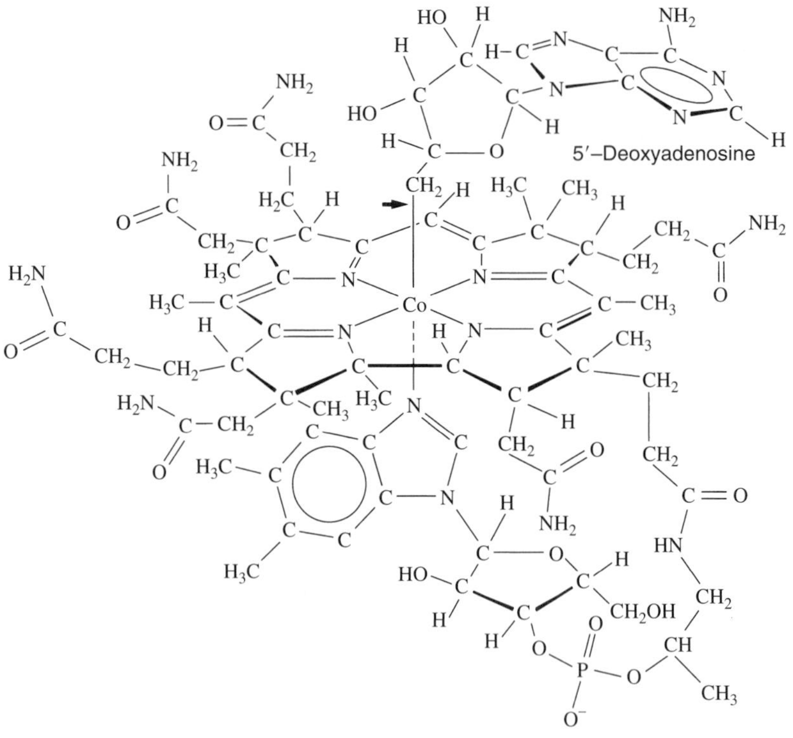

Fig. 30-4 Hemelike corrin ring structure of deoxyadenosylcobalamin, one of the active coenzyme forms of vitamin B_{12}. Current therapeutic agents cyanocobalamin and hydroxocobalamin, respectively, have CN or OH substituted for the 5′-deoxyadenosyl moiety at the bond indicated by the *arrow*. Methylcobalamin (CH_3 substituted) as well as deoxyadenosylcobalamin are active coenzyme forms. (Adapted from McGilvery RW, Goldstein GW: *Biochemistry: a functional approach*, ed 3, Philadelphia, 1983, WB Saunders.)

neurologic changes associated with decreased vitamin B_{12} activity. A deficiency of methionine, an essential amino acid whose daily utilization is approximately twice the normal dietary intake, may contribute to the degenerative nervous system changes that can occur in pernicious anemia.

The third vitamin B_{12}–dependent enzyme is leucine 2,3-aminomutase, which permits the interconversion of leucine and β-leucine. It is not known at this time how interruption of this pathway may contribute to human disease.

The sole natural and commercial source of cobalamin is synthesis by microorganisms. Many animals can use vitamin B_{12} produced by their own enteric bacteria, but because microbial synthesis in human beings is limited to the large intestine, a site too distal for effective absorption, human beings must derive their vitamin B_{12} exogenously. Foods rich in vitamin B_{12} include shellfish, such as oysters and clams (greater than 10 μg/100 g tissue), and mammalian organ meats (liver, kidney, and heart). The average daily diet contains 5 to 30 μg of vitamin B_{12}, of which 20% to 30% is absorbed. Daily intake of 1 to 3 μg does little more than compensate for daily loss, but normally more than 1000 times this amount (up to 4 mg) is stored in the liver.

Vitamin B_{12} is quite lipophobic and depends heavily on transfer mechanisms to be absorbed from the gastrointestinal tract. Cobalamin transport is mediated by several different proteins.[20,27] When first ingested, the cobalamin liberated from food interacts with *R proteins* in the stomach. These proteins bind tightly to cobalamin and protect it from acidic degradation, but they do not have any ability to transport the cobalamin across the enteric mucosa. As the R protein–cobalamin complex moves into the duodenum and the pH rises, pancreatic proteases degrade the R protein from around the cobalamin. The cobalamin is next adsorbed onto *intrinsic factor*, a glycoprotein secreted by the stomach parietal cells that has very specific cobalamin-binding properties. The intrinsic factor–cobalamin complex is carried to the ileum, where highly specific receptors on cells of the ileal microvilli transport it across the cell membrane. In the enterocytes, the intrinsic factor is broken down, liberating the cobalamin. A plasma polypeptide, *transcobalamin II*, then binds the cobalamin to carry the vitamin into the portal bloodstream. Receptors for this protein-cobalamin complex are ubiquitous but are especially rich in the liver. If the vitamin is needed in the tissues, it is taken up by the respective cells by endocytosis. If there is surplus, the cobalamin is moved to the hepatocytes for storage. Inside the cell, the cobalamin is freed by lysosomal enzymes, and the transcobalamin II is recycled back for reuse.

Transcobalamin II is the active transport protein, yet most of the circulating cobalamin is bound to two other transcobalamins—I and III—with transcobalamin I being the principal binding protein. Both proteins are also known to exist in saliva, bile, milk, and other fluids. It is not known if transcobalamin I functions as a storage reserve of vitamin B_{12} or if it is involved in the excretion of nonuseful corrinoid moieties.[27] Dietary foodstuffs do have other corrin-containing compounds, and it has been theorized that transcobalamin I binds all corrin compounds, not just vitamin B_{12}. The bound complexes are excreted into the intestine by the bile. In the intestine, vitamin B_{12} is reabsorbed with the assistance of intrinsic factor, whereas the other corrin compounds are excreted in the feces.

The enterohepatic cycling of cobalamin emphasizes the striking ability of the body to retain cobalamin. Normal hepatocyte turnover releases 3 to 4 μg of cobalamin into the bile each day, but the vitamin is essentially quickly rebound by intrinsic factor in the small intestine and reabsorbed. Thus very little new vitamin B_{12} is required in the diet each day. In fact, as long as the ability of the body to transport cobalamin across the intestinal wall and reabsorb the bile-secreted cobalamin is intact, a diet completely devoid of vitamin B_{12} may not produce clinical symptoms for as long as 20 years.[27]

Pathophysiologic characteristics

Vitamin B_{12} deficiency can be difficult to diagnose. Typically, the MCV of the erythrocytes will be markedly increased, usually to between 110 and 140 fl. However, if there is a concurrent iron deficiency anemia, the combination of microcytic and macrocytic anemias may result in relatively normal-sized cells. Other times, the cells are normocytic for obscure reasons. The peripheral blood smear is abnormal, showing anisocytosis and poikilocytosis, along with the characteristic macroovalocytes. Multilobulated neutrophils are typical. Hemolytic changes, resulting in increased plasma bilirubin and lactic dehydrogenase, as well as increased iron and saturated transferrin, may also be found. Serum vitamin B_{12} concentrations, normally 150 to 350 pg/ml, are less than 100 pg/ml. Currently, interest has been placed in measuring homocysteine and methylmalonic acid concentrations as good indicators of vitamin B_{12} deficiency, especially because a rise in homocysteine has been shown to be a significant risk factor for cardiovascular disease.[28]

It is rare to see a person with dietary vitamin B_{12} insufficiency, especially in first-world nations. Only vegans, the strictest of vegetarians who eat no animal products whatsoever (including dairy products), may show dietary insufficiency. Even then, small amounts of vitamin B_{12} may be available in the diet from microorganisms of legumes or exogenous application of cobalamins to grain and cereal products. As previously mentioned, dietary deficiency may take up to two decades to become clinically evident.

A more common difficulty is with malabsorption of dietary cobalamin. In these patients, the transport proteins are defective for one reason or another, so not only is the primary absorptive capacity decreased or lost, but the ability of the body to recycle enterohepatic cobalamin is also impaired. These patients have a much more rapid onset of symptoms, usually 3 to 6 years. Three basic causes exist: inadequate production of intrinsic factor in the stomach, altered ileal ability to absorb the intrinsic factor–cobalamin complex, and pancreatic disease, in which transfer of the cobalamin from the R proteins to intrinsic factor is interrupted.

Pernicious anemia is a hereditary autoimmune disease in which antibodies develop against intrinsic factor.[5,27] Even though the disorder is hereditary, the patient is usually middle-aged or older with age-related chronic atrophic gastritis. The antibodies (immunoglobulin [Ig] G or IgM) may either bind to intrinsic factor and prevent cobalamin binding, or they may bind to the intrinsic factor–cobalamin complex to prevent the complex from binding to the ileal receptors. In the classic form, other problems such as IgA deficiency, polyglandular endocrine insufficiency, and predisposition to gastric carcinoma are also found. Additional causes of decreased gastric secretion resulting in a condition similar to pernicious anemia include severe nonautoimmune gastritis, atrophic gastritis, and surgical resection. Surgical gastrectomy results in loss of intrinsic factor, usually in proportion to the amount of stomach removed. Total or near-total gastrectomy will cause vitamin B_{12} deficiency and require supplemental therapy.

Ileal problems may also lead to vitamin B_{12} deficiency. Luminal stasis may allow significant enteric bacterial overgrowth, leading to "blind loop syndrome." Here, the vitamin is "stolen" by the bacteria and therefore is unavailable to the host. Other conditions, such as carcinoma, Crohn's disease and other inflammatory bowel disorders, or surgical resection, may similarly induce a vitamin B_{12} deficiency. Not surprisingly, because vitamin B_{12} deficiency results in decreased DNA synthesis of rapidly dividing cells, the enterocytes themselves begin to suffer inhibition of mitosis and cytokinesis as the availability of cobalamin drops. Thus as the disease progresses it becomes increasingly self-perpetuating in that the enterocytes become defective and further lose their ability to absorb cobalamin. Pancreatic disease decreases the absorption of vitamin B_{12} by impairing the secretion of bicarbonate and pancreatic proteases necessary to degrade the R protein–cobalamin complex in the small intestine.

Finally, certain drugs such as *p*-aminosalicylic acid can reduce cobalamin absorption. Megadoses of vitamin C may cause vitamin B_{12} to be converted to nonuseful analogues, some of which may actually harbor antivitamin B_{12} activity.[19] Long-term exposure to nitrous oxide has been shown in pigs and human beings to result in megaloblastic anemia by inhibiting methionine synthase activity. The nitrous oxide irreversibly oxidizes the exposed cobalt atom after the methylcobalamin cofactor of methionine synthase has transferred its methyl group to homocysteine. In so doing, nitrous oxide permanently inactivates the enzyme.

Therapeutic use

Various preparations are used for vitamin B_{12} therapy, most commonly cyanocobalamin and hydroxocobalamin. Both are given by intramuscular or deep subcutaneous injection. Hydroxocobalamin is more highly protein bound and remains in circulation longer, but the more popular form is cyanocobalamin because hydroxocobalamin has been associated with the development of antibodies to the transcobalamin II–vitamin B_{12} complex. Neither form of cobalamin should be given intravenously.

Oral cobalamin is a relatively ineffective and expensive therapy because it relies on the same protein transport systems that have usually gone awry. However, in very high doses, sufficient vitamin B_{12} can be passively absorbed across the intestinal wall to correct some deficiencies. Although oral vitamin B_{12} is often formulated with intrinsic factor concentrate or liver extract to aid in the absorption process, these are not recommended over preparations of cobalamin only. The oral route is generally reserved for patients who cannot tolerate intramuscular injections.

Initial treatment of pernicious anemia involves twice-weekly intramuscular injections of vitamin B_{12} for several months. Such treatment brings about a rapid change in the bone marrow from megaloblastic to normoblastic erythropoiesis (usually in 2 to 3 days), with improving relief of the glossitis, neuritis, and spinal cord degeneration in several months. As the blood picture improves, the interval between doses can be increased to 2 or 3 weeks. Because the hepatic stores are so great after they are replenished, the patient can eventually be put on maintenance therapy involving an injection every 1 or 2 months, but it must be continued for life. Neurologic damage that is not reversed after 12 to 18 months of therapy must be considered permanent.

Large doses of cobalamin are promptly excreted in the urine and to a lesser extent in the feces. There have been no reports of toxic effects from cyanocobalamin or hydroxocobalamin other than occasional allergic responses to impurities in the preparations. There is no evidence that large doses of cyanocobalamin result in cyanide poisoning.

Folic Acid

Nutrition and physiologic characteristics

In the course of an attempt to isolate vitamin B_{12} to treat another form of macrocytic anemia peculiar to Hindu women, a different hematopoietic factor, folic acid (folacin or pteroylglutamic acid), was recognized and isolated.[36,60] Because the hematologic picture produced by vitamin B_{12} deficiency is almost indistinguishable from that of folic acid deficiency, it is not surprising that the paths of discovery of these two essential antianemic factors were so entwined.

Although not usually referred to as such, folic acid fits the definition of a vitamin. It occurs widely in nature as polyglutamate conjugates, but is an essential nutrient in microgram quantities for human beings. Folic acid itself is formed from glutamic acid, *p*-aminobenzoic acid, and pterin, as is shown in Figure 30-5. Fresh green vegetables (e.g., asparagus, broccoli,

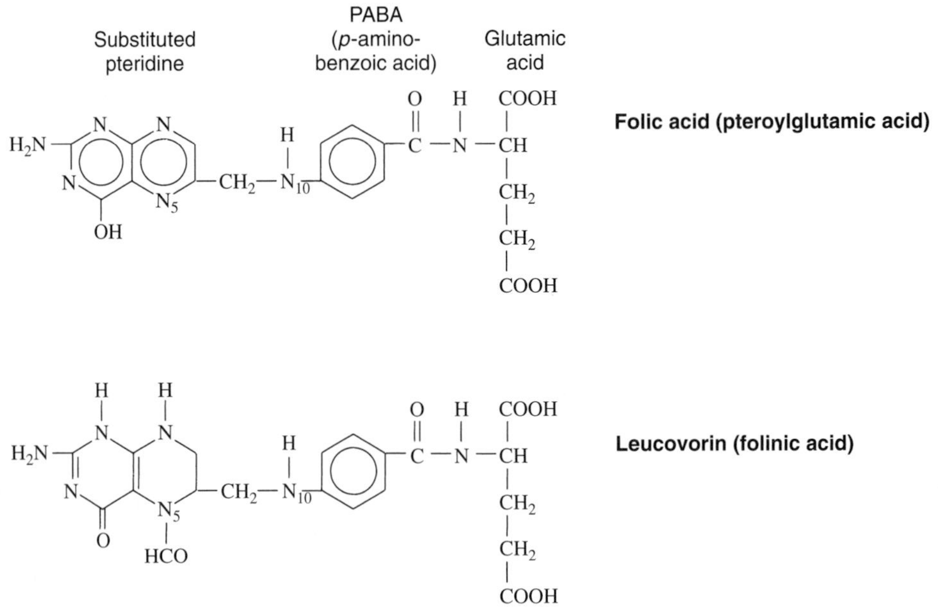

Substituted pteridine | PABA (p-aminobenzoic acid) | Glutamic acid

Folic acid (pteroylglutamic acid)

Leucovorin (folinic acid)

Fig. 30-5 Structural formulas of folic acid and leucovorin.

spinach, lettuce) are an excellent source of folic acid. Fruits such as bananas, lemons, and melons have high amounts, and liver, kidney, yeast, and mushrooms are also abundant in folate conjugates. Prolonged cooking destroys folic acid, especially when the conjugates are in dilute aqueous solution.

Absorption occurs primarily in the proximal jejunum, and it depends on specific mucosal membrane carboxypeptidases (conjugases) that hydrolyze the dietary polyglutamates to yield folic acid. In the mucosa, folic acid is reduced by dihydrofolate reductase and methylated to 5-methyltetrahydrofolate before entering the bloodstream.[20] Once in tissues, the compound is demethylated by vitamin B_{12}–dependent methionine synthase. The product, tetrahydrofolate, is then conjugated with 1-carbon moieties to yield several active coenzyme forms that are essential for purine and thymidylate synthesis. Tetrahydrofolate is also involved in the conversion reactions of several amino acids. Figure 30-6 illustrates the major metabolic pathways and interactions of folate and vitamin B_{12}.

The minimum daily folate requirement for human beings is approximately 50 μg, but because of less than complete absorption and special requirements for lactating women and certain other persons, a daily intake of 400 μg of free folate is recommended. Folate is stored to some extent in cells as polyglutamates, primarily as the pentaglutamate, and is recycled through the enterohepatic pathway similarly to cobalamin. However, the resorptive process is far less efficient than with B_{12}, and deficient intake may appear as megaloblastic anemia within a month.

Pathophysiologic characteristics

Folic acid deficiency has the same hematologic profile as cobalamin deficiency. As previously mentioned, folic acid deficiency causes a megaloblastic anemia essentially without neurologic manifestations. In patients who are folate deficient, serum folate concentrations are less than 3 ng/ml and erythrocyte folate is less than 150 ng/ml.

Despite the fact that folates are abundant in many foods, deficiency still occurs from many different causes. Various malabsorption syndromes disturb the absorption of folic acid by the intestines. Phenytoin and other antiepileptic drugs, oral contraceptives, and antimalarial drugs cause folate deficiency by inhibiting folate conjugases in the intestinal wall. The antimetabolites methotrexate and trimethoprim inhibit dihydrofolate reductase and lead to a megaloblastic anemia with prolonged use.

Elderly patients and persons of low economic status may have an inadequate intake of folate simply from poor nutrition. Overcooking of folate-containing foods, if consistently performed, can lead to folate deficiency. Pregnancy greatly increases the maternal requirement for folate, and a marginal diet can become inadequate to meet the growing demands of the fetus. Interestingly, there is strong evidence that maternal folate deficiency, especially before conception, is implicated in fetal neural tube defects such as spina bifida.[37] Chronic debilitating disease, such as cancer and myeloproliferative disorders, may predispose a patient to folic acid deficiency. Alcoholism and other hepatic diseases are definitely correlated with folate deficiency caused by generally poor nutritional status, malabsorption difficulties across the intestinal wall, and depleted liver stores.

Therapeutic use

Folate deficiency can often be treated with simple dietary supplements, such as an additional piece of fresh fruit daily. The vitamin is available in oral tablet form, is included in most multivitamin preparations, and is also supplied for injection in the form of sodium folate or the calcium salt of folinic acid (citrovorum factor) under the nonproprietary name of *leucovorin* (see Figure 30-5). Leucovorin has been used to counteract the effects of folic acid antagonists (e.g., the dihydrofolate reductase inhibitors methotrexate and trimethoprim) used in cancer or malaria chemotherapy. A recent study demonstrated that even simple use of folic acid or folinic acid greatly improved the side effects of methotrexate therapy in patients with rheumatoid arthritis, allowing better tolerance of the chemotherapeutic agent.[58] The response to oral folic acid therapy is rapid, and an improvement in the hematologic picture is seen 5 to 10 days after beginning daily administration of folic acid. Adverse effects directly attributable to folic acid have not been reported.

HEMATOPOIETIC GROWTH FACTORS

Perhaps the most exciting advance in the pharmacologic management of anemia and related disorders has been the

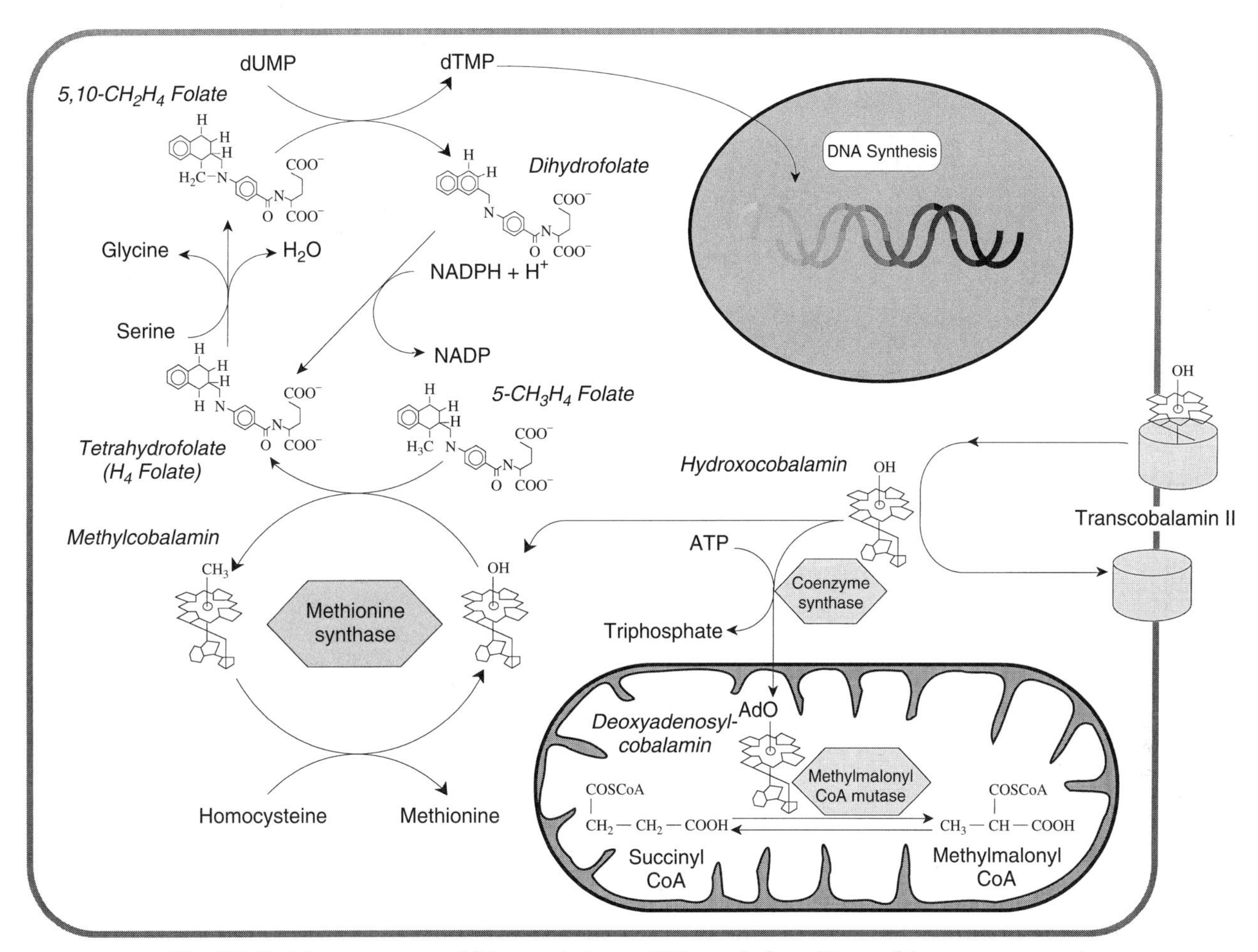

Fig. 30-6 Major pathways of folate and vitamin B12 metabolism. Dietary folates are converted to 5-methyltetrahydrofolate (5-CH3H4 folate). Demethylation by the enzyme methionine synthase yields tetrahydrofolate, an acceptor of single-carbon units in the metabolism of histidine (not shown) and serine. The folate products of these reactions provide carbon units for the synthesis of purines and, as shown for 5,10-methylenetetrahydrofolate (5,10-CH2H4 folate), the conversion of deoxyuridylate (dUMP) to thymidylate (dTMP). Vitamin B12, carried to the cell by transcobalamin II in the form of hydroxocobalamin, is converted to methylcobalamin and deoxyadenosylcobalamin, necessary cofactors for methionine synthase and methylmalonyl CoA mutase, respectively. NADP, Nicotinamide adenine dinucleotide phosphate; NADPH, reduced nicotinamide adenine dinucleotide phosphate.

introduction of hematopoietic growth factors to the therapeutic armamentarium. Numerous diseases and iatrogenic disorders can cause all or part of a patient's hematopoietic system to produce insufficient cells; the result is usually a pancytopenia with different degrees of individual cell line depression. Examples of causative maladies include the many varieties of leukemia, myeloproliferative disorders, lymphomas, aplastic anemia, and end-stage renal disease, as well as therapies such as cytotoxic chemotherapy, ionizing radiation, stem cell transplants, and bone marrow transplantation. Other causes include side effects of medications such as the sulfonamides, phenytoin, zidovudine, and carbamazepine. In the past, the only recourse was to transfuse the patient with whole blood or appropriate replacement components of blood. In severe instances, a bone marrow transplant may have been necessary. Although not a panacea, the introduction of several hematopoietic growth factors has greatly reduced the need for transfusion therapy in many patients with various forms of hematopoietic depression. All these products are derived from their respective human genes that have been subcloned into mammalian, bacterial, or yeast expression systems so that large quantities can be obtained.

Erythropoietin (EPO)/Darbepoetin

Background and physiologic characteristics

EPO was the first growth factor to be identified and successfully cloned into a recombinant vector. The gene is located on chromosome 7q11-22, and the final endogenous protein is a 165-amino-acid glycoprotein with a molecular weight of 30,400. Native EPO is formed primarily in the kidneys and, to a smaller degree, in the liver.[13] It is the major humoral regulator of red blood cell production and does not appear to have any effect on other cell lineages.

EPO expression is regulated in the kidney in response to the local oxygen tension by signaling mechanisms that are not well understood but are suspected to involve a membrane-bound, oxygen-sensitive heme protein.[18] The newly formed EPO moves to the bone marrow, where it attaches to EPO receptors on the cell membranes of myeloid stem cells, causing the cells in the presence of other regulatory factors to differentiate into erythroblasts and ultimately into erythrocytes. Once committed to the erythrocytic line, these cells become dependent on continued EPO for their survival. If EPO is removed, the cells die within one or two cell cycles. As a result, it has been postulated that EPO may be an apoptosis inhibitor rather than a differentiation stimulator. Bone marrow sensitivity to EPO is somewhat dependent on the availability of iron; various inflammatory mediators suppress EPO secretion and stem cell stimulation.

Pathophysiologic characteristics

In disease states, EPO synthesis may be disrupted (as in end-stage renal disease), the protein may be prematurely cleared (as in the anemia associated with rheumatoid arthritis), or the target stem cells may not be responsive to it (as in some myeloproliferative disorders). In all cases of depressed synthesis or accelerated catabolism, the plasma EPO will be low. If the problem is decreased tissue responsiveness, plasma EPO levels may be increased 100 times above normal.

Therapeutic use

Two forms of pharmacologic EPO are currently available. The recombinant form of the endogenous glycoprotein known as *epoetin alfa* has been available for several years and has been well tolerated. It generally requires intravenous or subcutaneous dosing three times a week. A newer form, darbepoetin alfa, has been approved for use and only requires dosing once a week. Darbepoetin differs from epoetin in that it contains five N-linked oligosaccharide chains instead of only three such chains in epoetin. Its pharmacologic profile is believed to be similar to that of epoetin alfa.

Both forms of EPO are currently approved for use in the anemia of chronic renal failure and cancer chemotherapy. Epoetin alfa has also been extensively studied for use in a host of other conditions that result in anemia or pancytopenia for which there is insufficient production of EPO in relation to the metabolic needs of the patient. One study demonstrated that the use of EPO with supplemental iron significantly improved the health status of patients with congestive heart failure and anemia.[50] Treated patients experienced relative improvements in serum creatinine and left ventricular ejection fraction, resulting in better renal function and a reduced need for diuretics. The authors concluded that correction of anemia markedly enhanced cardiac function in these patients.[50]

Epoetin alfa has the most consistent effect when plasma EPO is low, but exogenous EPO has also been successful in treating some conditions in which endogenous titers are already high and the target stem cells appear to be resistant to the effects of the protein. Epoetin alfa is also used in the treatment of chronic anemia associated with acquired immune deficiency syndrome, but results have been inconsistent. On the positive side, epoetin alfa can often stabilize a patient's hematopoietic profile enough to resume zidovudine therapy. Zidovudine has the unfortunate side effect of depressing the bone marrow, thus complicating the anemia to the point at which it may be necessary to discontinue the medication.

Epoetin alfa is sometimes used to prepare patients for autologous blood donation before nonemergency surgery. In these instances, the patient is phlebotomized normally and then put on a course of epoetin alfa for a few weeks before surgery. Just before the surgery, they can be phlebotomized again to maximize the available yield of autologous blood. Epoetin alfa has also been used in persons who require blood products but will not allow transfusions for religious reasons. It must be noted that epoetin alfa solutions contain human albumin, a blood product. For this reason, the patients may still refuse the therapy unless the diluent can be changed.[47]

Epoetin alfa can be given intravenously and is well absorbed, but the subcutaneous route is preferred because of a greater persistence of each dose in the plasma. (Epoetin alfa has a half-life of 6 to 9 hours after intravenous injection but 24 to 30 hours after subcutaneous administration.) Less medication needs to be given, resulting in lower cost and fewer adverse effects. Contraindications for its use include uncontrolled hypertension and allergy to albumin or mammalian cell–derived products. Adverse reactions include aggravation of existing hypertension, seizures, headache, and nausea. Patients receiving epoetin alfa therapy may need increased heparin doses during hemodialysis.[43] Failure of epoetin alfa most commonly results from the development of a significant iron deficiency caused by the increased production of hemoglobin. For this reason, close monitoring of the iron stores (TIBC, iron, ferritin) should be performed routinely, with iron supplementation given as necessary. The rate of hematocrit increase should not exceed 4% per week to avoid depleting the iron stores. Clinically significant results are usually seen in 2 to 6 weeks.

Myeloid Growth Factors

Background and physiologic characteristics

Several additional growth factors are currently approved for use by the Food and Drug Administration, and others are undergoing clinical trials. Two currently available myeloid growth factors, granulocyte colony-stimulating factor (G-CSF) and granulocyte/macrophage colony-stimulating factor (GM-CSF), are crucial to the early and intermediate development of the myeloid line of hematopoiesis. G-CSF is a lineage-specific growth factor for the neutrophil line, whereas GM-CSF is a stimulator for granulocytes and monocytes (with some erythrocyte and megakaryocyte effect as well; see Figure 30-1). In addition to increasing the numbers of neutrophils, both also activate the neutrophils and monocytes/macrophages in the tissues. Their names are derived from their ability to stimulate colony formation of hematopoietic stem cells when grown in semisolid media.

Recombinant human G-CSF, assigned the nonproprietary name of *filgrastim*, is synthesized in an *Escherichia coli* bacterial expression system. It is a 175-amino-acid polypeptide. A pegylated derivative known as *pegfilgrastim* is produced by covalently linking a large polyethylene glycol moiety to the active polypeptide.

G-CSF binds to cell surface receptors present on the progranulocytes and stimulates them to proliferate and mature. The more differentiated cells are known to have two to three times more G-CSF receptors on their surface, which appears to correlate with increased functional activity in the presence of the drug. Exactly how the G-CSF upregulates transcription in the nucleus is not currently known, but part of the therapeutic benefit of this medication is from enhanced neutrophilic activity as well as increased numbers.

GM-CSF has been produced in mammalian cells, yeast, and *E. coli*.[48] The commercially available form, from yeast, is a 127-amino-acid glycopeptide with a leucine substitution at position 23. Sargramostim is the nonproprietary designation. (Two other forms are in clinical trials; molgramostim is bacterially derived and nonglycosylated and regramostim is mammalian derived and glycosylated.) Like G-CSF, GM-CSF both stimulates terminal proliferation and differentiation of the granulocyte lineage. Unlike G-CSF, it also stimulates the monocytic lineage. As with G-CSF, the mechanism by which the intracellular changes occur is not known. It does appear, however, to require interleukin-3 (IL-3) stimulation to get a maximal differentiative response.[25]

Four additional growth factors have been cloned, purified, and made available for investigational laboratory and clinical studies. They are stem cell factor (SCF), monocyte/macrophage-CSF (M-CSF), thrombopoietin (TPO), and IL-3. These four, coupled with G-CSF and GM-CSF, round out the six "classic" known hematopoietic stimulating agents.

SCF has been assigned the nonproprietary name of *ancestim*. SCF, as the name implies, is crucial for the survival and proliferation of the early pluripotent/multipotent and myeloid/lymphoid stem cells. The immature stem cells produce and "autostimulate" themselves with their own SCF production to maintain a sufficient population of pluripotent/multipotent cells to keep the marrow supplied with adequate precursors for the various differentiation pathways. Interestingly, SCF alone does not push the stem cells toward maturation but maintains their immaturity. However, when coupled with other growth factors, SCF acts synergistically to "bump" the cells into a committed pathway, where most of these early intermediates begin to lose their need for this particular factor. As the cells continue to move toward maturation, SCF is no longer necessary.

M-CSF, as the name implies, promotes the growth and differentiation of monocyte progenitor cells, but only at high concentrations. More important, however, may be its ability to activate monocyte-macrophage cytotoxicity, as demonstrated by its ability to increase the survival of patients with invasive fungal infections.[39] It remains to be seen how M-CSF may be significantly different in function from GM-CSF.

TPO has been tested in two forms. The first is a full-length, 332-amino-acid recombinant human glycoprotein molecule known as *rhTPO*. The other is a pegylated truncated 163-amino-acid form of the protein in which the receptor-binding N-terminal domain is intact. It is known as *pegylated megakaryocyte growth and development factor* (PEG-MGDF). As the TPO name suggests, it stimulates the megakaryocytic lineage, which results in increased platelet production by as much as tenfold. Thus far, the medication has been used in cancer chemotherapy patients to hasten platelet recovery after thrombocytopenic nadirs are reached. Both the full-length and truncated versions appear to work equally well, but PEG-MGDF has caused neutralizing antibodies to develop in some patients.

IL-3 is encoded by a gene located near the gene for GM-CSF. Endogenous supply is essentially from activated T cells, mast cells, and natural killer cells.[17] IL-3 is a multilineage, broader-acting hematopoietic growth factor important in initiating early and intermediate stages of hematopoietic differentiation. It appears to be a crucial early trigger for the shift from pluripotent/multipotent stem cells down any of the myeloid differentiation pathways. IL-3 mediates its effects by the retinoic acid (vitamin A) receptors.[25] Once "nudged" this way, the cells show irreversible commitment and go on to become one of the myeloid stems that will later differentiate into the granulocytic, erythroid, monocytic, or megakaryocytic lineages. Note that IL-3 by itself has little differentiative activity, but it does appear to be involved in the crucial first step to bring stem cells out of the pluripotent/multipotent stage. As the cells mature, they become less dependent on its actions.

Interleukin-11 (IL-11), in the recombinant form of oprelvekin, is the first growth factor to gain approval for the management of thrombocytopenia. IL-11 is produced by fibroblasts and stromal cells in bone marrow. It binds to a spelcific receptor but acts with other growth factors to simulate the growth of both myeloid and lymphoid cell lines. The primary therapeutic benefit is a significant decrease in the need for platelet transfusions in patients receiving chemotherapy for nonmyeloid cancers.

Pathophysiologic characteristics

Any of the diseases or therapeutic interventions that adversely affect the hematopoietic system may cause leukopenia, thrombocytopenia, or pancytopenia. Congenital or acquired bone marrow failure states, hematopoietic neoplasms, cancer chemotherapy, and total body ionizing radiation therapy are the most common causes for hematopoietic disruption.

Therapeutic use

Stimulating and/or accelerating the recovery of the bone marrow (especially the neutrophils) after disease or medical therapy is the primary indication for the myeloid growth factors G-CSF and GM-CSF. Similarly, in clinical trials TPO is being used to hasten the recovery of platelet counts in patients with thrombocytopenia. When so used, the window of immunosuppression and hemorrhagic vulnerability of leukopenic and thrombocytopenic patients has been significantly shortened, greatly improving chances for survival while decreasing morbidity.

Filgrastim administered intravenously or subcutaneously is generally well tolerated, with the most common side effect being bone pain that clears on discontinuance of the medication. Rare serious reactions include anaphylaxis and splenic rupture. Pegfilgrastim is administered subcutaneously as a single dose after chemotherapy.

Sargramostim is administered intravenously. At normal doses, it does not significantly alter the megakaryocyte (and therefore thrombocyte) or erythrocyte lineages. It does have, however, significantly more severe side effects, especially at higher doses. The most common are fever, malaise, arthralgia, myalgia, and increased vascular permeability, which can lead to pleural and pericardial effusions.

SCF is given generally in conjunction with filgrastim and sargramostim. Its use is still investigational, and possible side effects associated with its administration include fever, chills, rash, myalgia, injection site irritation, and edema. In high doses, it can produce mast cell activation with associated symptoms.[59] IL-3 is usually given subcutaneously in daily doses in conjunction with GM-CSF and has been well tolerated.

Oprelvekin is injected daily for up to 3 weeks after a course of chemotherapy is completed. The therapeutic goal is to reach a platelet count of 50,000/μL. Impaired renal excretion of Na^+ may lead to fluid retention, hypokalemia, pulmonary edema, and atrial arrhythmias.

RED BLOOD CELL SUBSTITUTES AND PLASMA EXTENDERS

In recent years, considerable research has been focused on developing products that could substitute for blood on a temporary basis.[14] As the population ages and grows and as surgeries become more sophisticated and therapies (such as for cancer) affect marrow function, more blood products are required for these procedures. Some patients have rare blood types that are simply unavailable at their hospital in significant quantities. In major trauma, large amounts of blood (up to 20 units or more) might be required emergently, and careful screening, typing, and crossing is time consuming. In times of war or natural disaster, urgent blood requirements can easily outstrip supplies. Testing blood for disease transmission risk is becoming increasingly complex (and costly) and remains problematic with some viruses; as a result, it is often not done in third world nations. Finally, adherents of some religious groups will not accept blood product transfusions from another person.

As a result of these issues, several different products have been developed to serve as artificial blood capable of binding oxygen and supporting gaseous exchange in the lungs and peripheral tissues. Although *artificial blood* is technically a misnomer because these compounds do not have any of the cellular, immunologic, hemostatic, or hormonal constituents of whole blood, they do have the potential advantage that they could be manufactured in great quantities without the worry of viral contamination. Many of them can be stored for long periods, administered in the field, and therefore serve as an emergency bridge to keep the patient alive until better solutions can be found. A less ambitious goal is to use artificial colloids to help maintain the normal volume and oncotic pressure of blood after acute hemorrhage.

These products can be divided into the following major groups: hemoglobin preparations, perfluorocarbon oxygen transport fluids, and plasma extenders.

Hemoglobin

The first approach to oxygen-transport compounds was to prepare solutions of hemoglobin tetramers ($\alpha_2\beta_2$). The rationale was to purify hemoglobin molecules to avoid the antigenic determinants (ABO) found in the erythrocyte membrane while inactivating any viruses that may be present. It rapidly became clear, however, that after hemoglobin is removed from the erythrocyte, its properties change significantly.[40] Free tetrameric hemoglobin has a significantly higher affinity for oxygen (i.e., a leftward shift in the oxyhemoglobin desaturation curve) because of the lack of 2,3-diphosphoglycerate found in the erythrocyte, which allosterically reduces the affinity of hemoglobin for oxygen. In addition, the injected free hemoglobin rapidly dissociates into a dimeric or monomeric form that is cleared from the plasma by the kidneys, often with renal damage if sufficient dimers exist. Finally, the oncotic effect of the free hemoglobin molecules in the plasma greatly limits the amount that can be given safely. As a result, several modified hemoglobin products have been investigated in an attempt to circumvent these problems.[40]

The first modification was to polymerize the hemoglobin by cross-linking the α or β chains into polyhemoglobin. In this form, the normal hemoglobin tetramers are intramolecularly stabilized, preventing breakdown into dimers, while at the same time they are intermolecularly linked to other tetramers to form polymers, usually with three to six tetramers each. These approaches resulted in significantly larger molecules that were much more difficult to clear, giving significantly higher half-lives, as much as 30 hours. The hemoglobin was also modified to have a lower oxygen affinity by pyridoxylation of the β-globin chain. These modified hemoglobin solutions were shown to support life after near-complete transfusion in baboons and sheep.[44] However, in human clinical trials, the results were not as promising. Severe side effects such as renal failure and dyspnea caused some trials to be discontinued. In the acidic ascending loop of Henle, the hemoglobin molecules precipitated, causing renal damage.

Further research indicated that most of the problems with polyhemoglobin preparations were caused by a significant percentage of intramolecularly cross-linked single tetramers existing among the polytetramers.[9] Removal of these single units gave much better results. Two formulations have been developed that essentially eliminate the single tetramers: glutaraldehyde cross-linked human pyridoxylated polyhemoglobin and *o*-raffinose cross-linked human polyhemoglobin. (Concern exists over the possible transmission of bovine spongiform encephalitis, or "mad cow" disease; however, the manufacturer obtains its hemoglobin from a single controlled herd, which is carefully screened for prions.)[9,33] These later-generation polyhemoglobin products are showing good promise in phase III trials. They are well tolerated, provide better plasma oxygenation in the microvasculature than erythrocytes, and are able to be stored for more than a year with good results.[54]

In a completely different approach, recombinant human hemoglobin ($\alpha_2\alpha_2$) tetramers have been synthesized in *E. coli*.[22] These tetramers effectively prevent breakdown to the dimer form and have a modified 2,3-diphosphoglycerate pocket yielding a more favorable oxygen dissociation curve. Unfortunately, in clinical trials this product has shown significant vasoactivity because it scavenges free nitric oxide, a potent vasodilator. Normal ($\alpha_2\beta_2$) hemoglobin releases nitric oxide from its cysteine residues whenever it gives off oxygen, which causes capillary vasodilation and facilitates oxygenation. These recombinant tetramers apparently have nitric oxide–binding sites and end up causing the opposite effect. A second-generation recombinant human hemoglobin is being developed in an attempt to modify the nitric oxide–binding site on the molecule to reduce the hypertensive effect.[9]

Yet another approach has been to conjugate the individual hemoglobin tetramers to macromolecules such as polyethylene glycol, dextran, or polyoxyethylene derivatives.[26,40] Some products have been well tolerated in early clinical trials, but it remains to be seen how they will fare when more data are gathered. These formulations have also been tested in patients undergoing radiotherapy for cancer as a means to oxygenate hypoxic tumor tissue and increase its radiosensitivity.

Finally, much research is aimed at encapsulation methods to create an artificial red blood cell.[45] Free hemoglobin has a short half-life of about 24 hours and has to be ultrapure to avoid adverse reactions, problems that could be minimized by encapsulation. One way to encapsulate hemoglobin is with the use of liposomes, but to date many of the liposomal products have been phagocytized by the reticuloendothelial system. Polyactide membrane nanocapsules (about 150 nm in diameter) may be a potential solution to this problem. Polyactide is broken down into carbon and water, circumventing the need for lipid structures. Consideration is even being given to include superoxide dismutase, catalase, carbonic anhydrase, and other enzymes with the nanocapsules to prevent the accumulation of methemoglobin.[9,49]

Perfluorochemicals

In a remarkable experiment that caught the attention of the lay press in 1966, a fluid containing oxygenated fluorocarbon was demonstrated to be able to support respiration of mice immersed in it.[10] Goldfish were kept alive for weeks under an oil monolayer with only the fluorocarbon and bubbles of oxygen. Even cats were able to support respiration in these compounds, although they all quickly succumbed on return to room air respiration from massive pulmonary edema.[52] These compounds, referred to as *perfluorocarbons* (PFCs), are large organic compounds in which all the hydrogen atoms are replaced with fluorine and act as a solvent for oxygen (Figure 30-7).[26,56] It is important to note that, unlike the chemical binding of oxygen to the porphyrin-iron binding sites of hemoglobin, the oxygen dissolution in PFCs is a passive process in which the gas simply occupies spaces within the PFC liquid.[33] As a result, the oxygen dissociation curves are not sigmoid as with hemoglobin, but linear, and the amount of oxygen dissolved in the PFCs is proportional to the partial pressure of the gas in solution. A disadvantage is that to reach a high solubility of the oxygen in the PFCs (approximately 25% in current formulations), up to 95% oxygen must be administered. On the other hand, hyperbaric oxygen therapy causes the PFCs to carry even more oxygen because of its increased pressure.

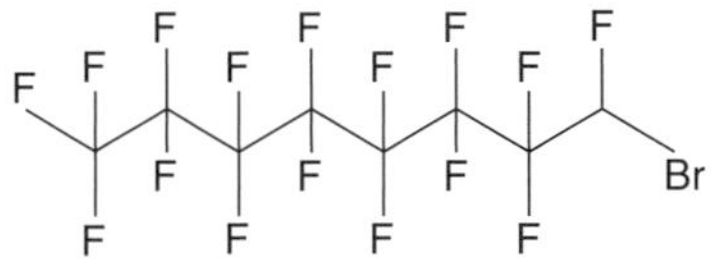

Perflubron

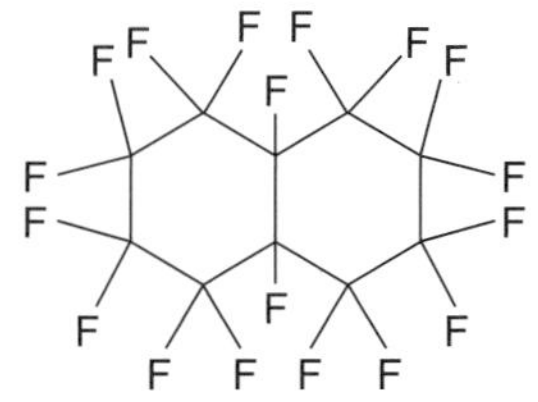

Perfluorodecalin

Fig. 30-7 The perfluorochemicals perflubron (linear) and perfluorodecalin (cyclic).

The PFCs, being large hydrocarbons, are not soluble in plasma. As a result, the primary difficulty in developing this technology has been to find an appropriate way to emulsify the compounds for injection that ensures both effectiveness and biocompatibility. Currently, egg yolk phospholipids or safflower oil is the emulsifier most commonly used. After emulsification, the particles are approximately 0.1 μm in diameter (considerably smaller than erythrocytes), which allows a significantly higher amount of surface area to be available for gas exchange. It is believed that in high-flow arterioles the PFC emulsion occupies the external luminal area next to the endothelium because of erythrocyte streaming. In the slower microvasculature, the PFCs occupy the plasma space surrounding erythrocytes and enter partially occluded vessels that exclude erythrocytes. Thus the oxygenation of microvascular tissue is believed to be significantly better.[33]

The first-generation PFC emulsions had only an approximately 10% concentration of PFCs; newer products have up to 83%. A first-generation product, Fluosol-DA 20, was approved for use in the United States for perfusion of coronary arteries after percutaneous transluminal angioplasty but was later withdrawn from the market.[57] The two most studied products currently available are perflubron and perfluorodecalin.

PFCs have numerous potential uses. The first is as an oxygen carrier in instances of significant blood loss.[53] It has been shown that the reinfusion of stored autologous blood can be significantly delayed or reduced with the concomitant use of these products. Although only researched in the animal model, in instances of severe blood loss these chemicals may be able to carry the patient until surgery can correct the source of blood loss and blood transfusions can be provided. Another interesting investigational use of these chemicals is in cases of acute respiratory distress syndrome. In a technique known as *partial liquid ventilation,* the lung is filled with PFCs to a volume approximately equal to the residual volume. Because of an extremely low surface tension, the liquid spreads rapidly and uniformly across the respiratory network, opening up collapsed alveoli and facilitating gas exchange. Third, because of its bromine substitution, perflubron makes an excellent contrast dye. Uses so far have included gastrointestinal endoscopy and bronchography. The material also has good acoustic impedance, making it an echogenic compound useful in ultrasound applications. Finally, these chemicals are being investigated for use in oxygenating hypoxic tumors before administering ionizing radiation and/or chemotherapy.[33]

PFCs are not metabolized but are primarily transported to the lung on plasma phospholipids and excreted unchanged by exhalation. A lesser percentage undergoes phagocytosis by reticuloendothelial cells of the liver (Kupffer's cells) and spleen macrophages. Transient alterations in the hepatic metabolism of drugs such as lidocaine have been noted in animals when the reticuloendothelial system has become saturated with PFCs. No cytotoxic or antigenic effects have been reported.

Synthetic Plasma Extenders

In applications where support of oxygenation is not as crucial but blood volume needs supplementation to avoid hypotension, artificial colloids have been developed to serve as plasma extenders. These preparations help maintain the normal oncotic pressure of blood and can reduce, but not eliminate, the need for blood transfusion. There is no true substitute for lost whole blood except whole blood, but within fairly wide limits of total hemoglobin various colloidal solutions can be substituted to sustain an acceptable blood pressure. Whole plasma is obviously the most effective replacement; however, individual units of plasma pose a risk of viral infection equal to that of individual units of whole blood. Five percent plasma protein solution (pooled plasma heated to 60° C for 10 hours to minimize the risk of cross-infection) or 5% human albumin is a suitable alternative. Unfortunately, the former preparation may cause hypotension, and both are expensive and unacceptable to certain religious groups because of their human origins.

In theory, the development of a synthetic substitute to fulfill the oncotic functions of plasma proteins would be an ideal approach. To be of more value than isotonic saline solution as an oncotic substitute, a substance must be relatively inert, nontoxic, and nonallergenic and have a molecular size and weight in excess of those that can be easily filtered across the glomerulus. Of the many materials that have been tested, the most suitable have proved to be polysaccharide derivatives, namely dextran and hetastarch.[38]

Dextran

A branched polysaccharide, dextran is produced by certain bacteria and consists of as many as 200,000 glucose molecules interconnected by glucosidic linkages to produce a molecular weight of approximately 4×10^7 d. Controlled hydrolysis of this material can yield a wide range of molecules that are then fractionated according to size. Available dextrans for injection include two forms: high–molecular-weight dextran, a 6% solution of dextran with a mean molecular weight of approximately 70,000 or 75,000 d depending on manufacturer, and low–molecular-weight dextran, having a weight of approximately 40,000 d. The main advantage of the smaller material, which of course can escape more readily across the glomerular membranes, is the fact that it seems to improve microcirculation by reducing the rouleaux formation and red cell sludging that usually accompanies hemorrhagic and other forms of shock. Dextran can interfere with blood typing, which therefore must precede dextran injection, and it impairs platelet function, resulting in an iatrogenic form of von Willebrand's disease. Fibrin formation is also impaired. The major disadvantage of the dextrans is their antigenic potential. Enteric bacteria produce dextran, and a small percentage of the population has antibodies for dextran in the blood. Fortunately, when dextran is used as a plasma extender, a massive dose is usually given that overwhelms the immune response (immunologic paralysis), and anaphylactic risk is as low as, or lower than, that of blood transfusion. This risk can be further reduced by prophylactic administration of dextran 1, a monovalent hapten that binds to immunoglobulins without triggering an allergic response.

Hetastarch

Hetastarch is a hydroxyethylated derivative of amylopectin, with a mean molecular weight of 450,000 d and a range of 10,000 to 1 million d. The lower-weight molecules (less than 50,000 d) are excreted by glomerular filtration (33% within 24 hours); remaining molecules are metabolized slowly over a 2- to 3-week period to smaller products by plasma α-amylase activity.[24] The volume expansion produced by this agent lasts approximately 24 to 36 hours. Hematologically, there appears to be no obvious advantage of hetastarch over dextran; however, hetastarch is said to have a low incidence of anaphylaxis and may have less of an effect on blood clotting. Besides being effective as a volume expander, hetastarch has been found useful in leukapheresis (the harvesting of granulocytes for patient use) and as a priming fluid for extracorporeal pumps used in coronary surgery.

IMPLICATIONS FOR DENTISTRY

The dentist is often in a unique position as the first health professional to observe manifestations of anemia in a patient. In fact, because the oral signs frequently precede a drop in hemoglobin below the normal range, the dentist may be able to diagnose the disease before it has caused symptoms warranting medical attention. Because anemia is simply a sign of an underlying hematopoietic disorder, the blood cells are frequently the earliest biologic indicators of diseases such as cancer, malnutrition, or conditions of drug toxicity. The response may take the form of granulocytopenia, hemolytic or aplastic anemia, or thrombocytopenia with associated immunosuppression and defective hemostasis leading to spontaneous hemorrhage, internal bleeding, and purpura. Patients with these difficulties may have oral mucositis, intraoral or circumoral viral outbreaks, fungal infections, and serious bacterial infections of odontogenic origin. The dentist should recognize these signs, understand the gravity of the situation, and attempt to ensure that the patient receives proper medical evaluation. Anemic conditions can run the gamut from easily corrected nutritional deficiency states to life-threatening disorders, and the sooner the patient is diagnosed the better the chances are for correcting the underlying problem.

Patients who are undergoing therapy for these same diseases and taking many of the medications described in this chapter are increasingly encountered in dental practice. The dentist who has knowledge of the way these medications function and why they are being given will be better able to identify the presence or history of a particular disease and to make appropriate decisions about how to manage the patient's overall care.

As a final concern, dental professionals should know about the relationship between chronic nitrous oxide inhalation and pernicious anemia. Megaloblastic responses to nitrous oxide were first recognized in 1956 when the gas was used for sedation of patients with tetanus.[30] More recently, persons habituated to inhaling nitrous oxide have been found to develop neuropathies similar to those seen with vitamin B_{12} deficiency.[12] It is now recognized that nitrous oxide readily interacts with the cobalt atom in cobalamin, which in turn is oxidized and rendered inactive as a cofactor for methionine synthtase. The potential implications for health care workers chronically exposed to nitrous oxide and for patients receiving nitrous oxide therapeutically are covered, respectively, in Chapters 17 and 18.

Antianemic Drugs

Nonproprietary (generic) name	*Proprietary (trade) name*
Iron preparations	
Ferrous fumarate	Feostat, Ircon, Hemocyte, Nephro-Fer
Ferrous gluconate	Fergon
Ferrous sulfate	Feosol, Fer-In-Sol, Fer-Gen-Sol, Mol-Iron, Feratab, Fero-Gradumet
Iron dextran	INFeD, DexFerrum
Iron sucrose	Venofer
Iron polysaccharide	Hytinic, Niferex, Nu-Iron, Fe-Tinic, Ferrex
Iron-chelating agent	
Deferoxamine	Desferal Mesylate
Hematopoietic factors	
Darbepoetin alfa	Aranesp
Epoetin alfa	Epogen, Procrit
Filgrastim (G-CSF)	Neupogen
Oprelvekin	Neumega
Pegfilgrastim	Neulasta
Sargramostim (GM-CSF)	Leukine
Vitamin B_{12} preparations	
Cyanocobalamin	—
Hydroxocobalamin	—
Folic acid preparations	
Folate sodium	Folvite
Folic acid	—
Leucovorin (folinic acid)	—
Heme derivative	
Hemin	Panhematin
Oxygen carrier fluid	
Perflubron	Adato-Deca, Imagent GI, Fluosol DA, Oxygent
Plasma volume extenders	
Dextran, high molecular weight	Dextran 70, Gentran 70, Macrodex
Dextran, low molecular weight	Dextran 40, Rheomacrodex, 10% LMD, Gentran 40
Hetastarch	Hespan
Human albumin	Albumarc, Albuminar, Albutein, Buminate, Plasbumin
Plasma protein fraction	Plasmanate, Plasmatein, Protenate

G-CSF, Granulocyte colony-stimulating factor; *GM-CSF*, granulocyte/macrophage colony-stimulating factor.

Cited References

1. Addison T: Anemia—disease of the supra-renal capsules, *London Med Gazette* 43:517, 1849. Cited by Kass L: *Pernicious anemia*, Philadelphia, 1976, WB Saunders.
2. Allen RH: Megaloblastic anemias. In Bennett JC, Plum F, eds: *Cecil Textbook of medicine*, ed 20, Philadelphia, 1996, WB Saunders.
3. Atweh G, Loukopoulos D: Pharmacologic induction of fetal hemoglobin in sickle cell disease and β-thalassemia, *Semin Hematol* 38:367-373, 2001.
4. Babior BM: The megaloblastic anemias. In Beutler E, Lichtman MA, Coller BS, et al, eds: *Williams Hematology*, ed 6, New York, 2001, McGraw-Hill.
5. Besa EC: Megaloblastic anemia. In Rose LF, Kaye D, eds: *Internal medicine for dentistry*, ed 2, St Louis, 1990, Mosby.
6. Blaud P: Sur les maladies chlorotiques, et sur un mộde de traitement spécifiques dans ces affections, *Rev Med Française Etrangère* 45:341-367, 1832.
7. Boggs DR, Joyce RA: The hematopoietic effects of lithium, *Semin Hematol* 20:129-138, 1983.
8. Castle WB: Observations on the etiologic relationship of achylia gastrica to pernicious anemia. I. Effect of administration to patients with pernicious anemia of contents of normal human stomach recovered after ingestion of beef muscle, *Am J Med Sci* 178:748-764, 1929.
9. Chang T: Red blood cell substitutes, *Baillieres Clin Haematol* 13:651-667, 2000.
10. Clark LC, Jr, Gollan F: Survival of mammals breathing organic liquids equilibrated with oxygen at atmospheric pressure, *Science* 152:1755-1756, 1966.
11. *Control of nutritional anaemia with special reference to iron deficiency: report of an IAEA/USAID/WHO joint meeting*, World Health Organization technical report, series no 580, Geneva, 1975, World Health Organization.
12. Deacon R, Lumb MJ, Perry J: Vitamin B_{12}, folate and nitrous oxide, *Med Lab Sci* 39:171-178, 1982.
13. Dessypris EN, Krantz SB: Erythropoietin: regulation of erythropoiesis and clinical use, *Adv Pharmacol* 21:127-147, 1990.
14. Dietz NM, Joyner MJ, Warner MA: Blood substitutes: fluids, drugs, or miracle solutions? *Anesth Analg* 82:390-405, 1996.
15. Fairbanks VF, Beutler E: Iron deficiency. In Beutler E, Lichtman MA, Coller BS, et al, eds: *Williams Hematology*, ed 6, New York, 2001, McGraw-Hill.
16. FAO-WHO Expert Group: *Requirements of ascorbic acid, vitamin D, vitamin B_{12}, folate, and iron*, World Health Organization technical report, series no 452, Geneva, 1970, World Health Organization.
17. Ganser A: Clinical results with recombinant human interleukin-3, *Cancer Invest* 11:212-218, 1993.
18. Goldberg MA, Dunning SP, Bunn HF: Regulation of the erythropoietic gene: evidence that the oxygen sensor is a heme protein, *Science* 242:1412-1415, 1988.
19. Herbert V, Drivas G, Foscaldi R, et al: Multivitamin/mineral food supplements containing vitamin B_{12} may also contain analogues of vitamin B_{12}, *N Engl J Med* 307:255-256, 1982.
20. Hillman RS: Hematopoietic agents: growth factors, minerals, and vitamins. In Hardman JG, Limbird LE, Gilman AG, eds: *Goodman & Gilman's The pharmacological basis of therapeutics*, ed 10, New York, 2001, McGraw-Hill.
21. Hoffman HN II, Phyliky RL, Fleming CR: Zinc-induced copper deficiency, *Gastroenterology* 94:508-512, 1988.
22. Hoffman SJ, Looker DL, Roehrich JM, et al: Expression of fully functional tetrameric human hemoglobin in *Escherichia coli*, *Proc Natl Acad Sci USA* 87:8521-8525, 1990.
23. Hoppe C, Walters M: Bone marrow transplantation in sickle cell anemia, *Curr Opin Oncol* 13:85-90, 2001.
24. Hulse JD, Yacobi A: Hetastarch: an overview of the colloid and its metabolism, *Drug Intell Clin Pharm* 17:334-341, 1983.
25. Johnson B, Mueller L, Si J, et al: The cytokines IL-3 and GM-CSF regulate the transcriptional activity of retinoic acid receptors in different in vitro models of myeloid differentiation, *Blood* 99:746-753, 2002.
26. Kahn RA, Allen RW, Baldassare J: Alternate sources and substitutes for therapeutic blood components, *Blood* 66:1-12, 1985.
27. Kapadia CR, Donaldson RM, Jr: Disorders of cobalamin (vitamin B_{12}) absorption and transport, *Annu Rev Med* 36:93-110, 1985.
28. Klee G: Cobalamin and folate evaluation: measurement of methylmalonic acid and homocysteine vs vitamin B_{12} and folate, *Clin Chem* 46:1277-1283, 2000.
29. Lane PA: Sickle cell disease, *Pediatr Clin North Am* 43:639-664, 1996.
30. Lassen HCA, Henricksen E, Neukirch F, Kristensen HS: Treatment of tetanus: severe bone-marrow depression after prolonged nitrous-oxide anaesthesia, *Lancet* 1:527-530, 1956.
31. Ley TJ, Nienhuis AW: Induction of hemoglobin F synthesis in patients with thalassemia, *Annu Rev Med* 36:485-498, 1985.
32. Linker CA: Blood. In Tierney LM, Jr, McPhee SJ, Papadakis MA, eds: *Current medical diagnosis & treatment*, ed 42, New York, 2003, McGraw-Hill.
33. Lowe KC: Perfluorinated blood substitutes and artificial oxygen carriers, *Blood Rev* 13:171-184, 1999.
34. McGilvey RW, Goldstein GW: *Biochemistry, a functional approach*, ed 3, Philadelphia, 1983, WB Saunders.
35. Minot GR, Murphy WP: Treatment of pernicious anemia by a special diet, *JAMA* 87:470-476, 1926.
36. Mitchell HK, Snell EE, Williams RJ: The concentration of "folic acid," *J Am Chem Soc* 63:2284, 1941.
37. MRC Vitamin Study Research Group: Prevention of neural tube defects: results of the Medical Research Council Vitamin Study, *Lancet* 338:131-137, 1991.
38. Mudge GH, Weiner IM: Agents affecting volume and composition of body fluids. In Hardman JG, Limbird LE, Gilman AG, eds: *Goodman & Gilman's The pharmacological basis of therapeutics*, ed 10, New York, 2001, McGraw-Hill.
39. Nemunaitis J, Shannon-Dorcy K, Appelbaum FR, et al: Long-term follow-up of patients with invasive fungal disease who received adjunctive therapy with recombinant human macrophage colony-stimulating factor, *Blood* 82:1422-1427, 1993.
40. Ogden JE, Parry ES: The development of hemoglobin solutions as red cell substitutes, *Int Anesthesiol Clin* 33:115-129, 1995.
41. Orten JM, Neuhaus OW: *Human biochemistry*, ed 10, St Louis, 1982, Mosby.

42. Paige DM: *Clinical nutrition*, ed 2, St Louis, 1988, Mosby.
43. *Physicians' desk reference*, ed 58, Montvale, NJ, 2004, Medical Economics.
44. Rabinovici R, Neville LF, Rudolph AS, Feuerstein G: Hemoglobin-based oxygen-carrying resuscitation fluids, *Crit Care Med* 23:801-804, 1995.
45. Rabinovici R, Rudolph AS, Ligler FS, et al: Biological responses to exchange transfusion with liposome-encapsulated hemoglobin, *Circ Shock* 37:124-133, 1992.
46. Rickes EL, Brink NG, Koniuszy FR, et al: Crystalline vitamin B_{12}, *Science* 107:396-397, 1948.
47. Ridley DM, Dawkins F, Perlin E: Erythropoietin: a review, *J Nat Med Assoc* 86:129-135, 1994.
48. Ries CA, Santi DV: Agents used in anemias: hematopoietic growth factors. In Katzung BG, ed: *Basic & clinical pharmacology*, ed 8, Norwalk, CT, 1998, Appleton & Lange.
49. Shibuya-Fujiwara N, Hirayama F, Ogata Y, et al: Phagocytosis in vitro of polyethylene glycol-modified liposome-encapsulated hemoglobin by human peripheral blood monocytes plus macrophages through scavenger receptors, *Life Sci* 70:291-300, 2001.
50. Silverberg DS, Wexler D, Sheps D, et al: The effect of correction of mild anemia in severe, resistant congestive heart failure using subcutaneous erythropoietin and intravenous iron: a randomized controlled study, *J Am Coll Cardiol* 37:1775-1780, 2001.
51. Smith EL: Purification of anti-pernicious anemia factors from liver, *Nature* 161:638-639, 1948.
52. Spiess BD: Perfluorocarbon emulsions: one approach to intravenous artificial respiratory gas transport, *Int Anesthesiol Clin* 33:103-113, 1995.
53. Spiess BD, Cochran RP: Perfluorocarbon emulsions and cardiopulmonary bypass: a technique for the future, *J Cardiothorac Vasc Anesth* 10:83-90, 1996.
54. Sprung J, Kindscher JD, Wahr JA, et al: The use of bovine hemoglobin glutamer-250 (Hemopure) in surgical patients: results of a multicenter, randomized single-blinded trial, *Anesth Analg* 94:799-808, 2002.
55. Till JE, McCulloch EA: Hemopoietic stem cell differentiation, *Biochim Biophys Acta* 605:431-459, 1980.
56. Tremper KK, Anderson ST: Perfluorochemical emulsion oxygen transport fluids: a clinical review, *Annu Rev Med* 36:309-313, 1985.
57. Tremper KK, Friedman AE, Levine EM, et al: The preoperative treatment of severely anemic patients with a perfluorochemical oxygen-transport fluid, Fluosol-DA, *N Engl J Med* 307:277-283, 1982.
58. van Ede AE, Laan RF, Rood MJ, et al: Effect of folic or folinic acid supplementation on the toxicity and efficacy of methotrexate in rheumatoid arthritis: a forty-eight week, multicenter, randomized, double-blind, placebo-controlled study, *Arthritis Rheum* 44:1515-1524, 2001.
59. Vose JM, Armitage JO: Clinical applications of hematopoietic growth factors, *J Clin Oncol* 13:1023-1035, 1995.
60. Wills L, Clutterbuck PW, Evans BDF: A new factor in the production and cure of macrocytic anaemias and its relation to other haemopoietic principles curative in pernicious anaemia, *Biochem J* 31:2136-2147, 1937.

General References

Babior BM: The megaloblastic anemias. In Beutler E, Lichtman MA, Coller BS, et al, eds: *Williams Hematology*, ed 6, New York, 2001, McGraw-Hill.

Cooper BA, Rosenblatt DS: Disorders of cobalamin and folic acid metabolism. In Handin RI, Lux SE, Stossel TP, eds: *Blood: principles and practice of hematology*, Philadelphia, 1995, JB Lippincott.

Fairbanks VF, Beutler E: Iron deficiency. In Beutler E, Lichtman MA, Coller BS, et al., eds: *Williams Hematology*, ed 6, New York, 2001, McGraw-Hill.

Hillman RS, Ault KA: *Hematology in clinical practice*, ed 3, New York, 2002, McGraw-Hill.

Sassa S, Kappas A: Disorders of heme production and catabolism. In Handin RI, Lux SE, Stossel TP, eds: *Blood: practice and principles of hematology*, Philadelphia, 1995, JB Lippincott.

Tierney LM, Jr, McPhee SJ, Papadakis MA, eds: *Current medical diagnosis & treatment*, ed 42, New York, 2003, McGraw-Hill.

CHAPTER • 31

Procoagulant, Anticoagulant, and Thrombolytic Drugs

Barton S. Johnson

Because the practice of dentistry frequently involves procedures that cause bleeding, the dentist is often confronted with the need to maintain hemostasis. The practitioner must therefore be familiar with the physiologic processes of hemostasis and the myriad conditions that cause abnormalities of these processes. Complicating matters, modern medicine has developed several therapies for systemic disease that purposefully use medications that alter normal hemostasis. When appropriate, the dentist will need to eliminate or make alterations in the dosage of these compounds before surgery. Only with a clear understanding of the complex process of hemostasis and the various drugs that can affect it will the clinician be able to manage safely patients with inherited or acquired bleeding disabilities.

HEMOSTASIS

Large or intermediate arteries and veins are generally not severed intentionally without prior ligation, but it is common during the extraction of teeth and other oral surgical procedures to cut small arteriolar, venous, and capillary vessels. Extensive blood loss may occur if hemostasis is delayed. The formation of a patent clot requires four distinct yet interdependent steps: vessel constriction; platelet adhesion, activation, and aggregation; cross-linking of fibrin by the coagulation cascade; and limitation of the blood clot to the area of damage only. Later, a fifth step will become necessary: the breakdown of the clot so that repair and remodeling can occur. Each of these five distinct processes will be discussed in turn.

VASCULAR CONSTRICTION

In the laboratory animal, transection of small arteries and arterioles that contain smooth muscle has revealed several patterns of hemorrhagic flow. Generally, after a sudden surge of blood there is a moderate to severe reduction in flow, apparently caused by contraction of vascular smooth muscle initiated directly by the trauma. This initial hemostasis is independent of blood coagulation and platelet agglutination because it occurs in heparinized animals. Furthermore, it is maintained only for a short period (5 to 20 minutes). The vessel wall is lined with endothelial cells that constitutively secrete nitric oxide and prostacyclin, both of which are potent smooth muscle relaxing agents.[29] Nitric oxide and prostacyclin diffuse down to the vascular smooth muscle beneath the endothelial cells, effect relaxation, and therefore maintain luminal patency. On injury, this effect is disrupted and the now unopposed muscle layer reflexly and rapidly constricts, greatly narrowing the lumen. The effect is short lived; after a few minutes the constrictive effect wanes and the muscle layers begin to relax again. However, this brief period of constriction does provide the healthy individual sufficient time for the platelets and coagulation cascade to seal the injured site.

PLATELET ADHESION, ACTIVATION, AND AGGREGATION

Adhesion

The next major event is the adhesion of platelets at the severed edges of the vessel. In normal untraumatized blood vessels, platelets show little tendency to adhere to the endothelium, in part because prostacyclin, again elaborated by the endothelial cells, induces cyclic adenosine 3′,5′-monophosphate synthesis in platelets and thus inhibits platelet adhesion. Endothelium-derived relaxing factor (e.g., nitric oxide), also normally secreted by the endothelial cells, is another natural inhibitor of platelet adhesion. However, injury to the intima, even if the vessel wall remains intact, leads to exposure of subendothelial extracellular matrix proteins such as collagen, fibronectin, von Willebrand factor (vWF), thrombospondin, and laminin.[37] Platelets have a high density of surface receptors that respond to these proteins, and they undergo an extremely rapid localization to the site of injury and begin the formation of a platelet plug or thrombus. Two main receptors are involved in adhesion: the glycoprotein (GP) Ia/IIa heterodimer, which binds to collagen directly but weakly; and the GP Ib/IX/V heterotrimer, which binds with high shear strength to connective tissue vWF associated with the collagen surface.[21,29,37,58] Note that the Ib-vWF linkage is more of a "tethering" of the platelet to the substrate; later the adhesion is firmed up by GP IIb/IIIa activation. If vessels without a muscular sheath are severed, the immediate hemostatic action of the platelet plug is especially important. Indeed, the true significance of the platelet in hemostasis is most evident in the management of the patient with thrombocytopenia.

Activation

Activation of the platelets is a crucial step in forming a proper thrombus. Activation can occur from a variety of agonists, some of which are strong, some of which are weak, and some of which are dose dependent. Examples include thrombin, adenosine diphosphate (ADP, from red blood cells or other platelets), thromboxane A_2 (TXA_2), 5-hydroxytryptamine (5-HT, serotonin), epinephrine, vasopressin, fibrinogen, immune complexes, plasmin, and platelet-activating factor. Most of the plasma-derived agonists exert their effect by a number of G protein–linked membrane receptors. However, the strongest agonist for platelet activation is binding of vWF to the GP Ib/IX/V heterotrimeric receptors.[13,20,29,37] When one of these receptors is bound by its specific agonist, an intraplatelet protein cascade begins that ultimately causes activation of Ca^{++} pumps and movement of Ca^{++} from stores in the platelet's dense tubular system to the general intracellular matrix.[45] This intracellular rise in Ca^{++}, in turn, causes several other changes.

In the resting state, the platelets have internal cytoskeletal actin; as the Ca^{++} level increases, the actin is initially fragmented into smaller subunits, causing a change from the normal discoid shape of the platelet to a spherical conformation. These smaller actin subunits are then rapidly reassembled into very-long actin monomers, which cause the platelet to change shape and sprout filopods. As will be discussed later, these filopods are important in ultimate clot retraction.[45] Meanwhile, as the filopods are developing, the rising intracellular Ca^{++} levels act on cytoplasmic vesicles known as α and *dense (δ) granules* (Figure 31-1) and cause them to rise to the surface and degranulate their contents. The dense granules harbor ADP, adenosine triphosphate, the vasoconstrictor 5-HT, as well as Ca^{++} and inorganic pyrophosphate.[26] The α granules contain numerous proteins involved in coagulation, adhesion, cellular mitogenicity, protease inhibition, and other functions (Box 31-1). Most notably, fibrinogen, coagulation factors, vWF, fibronectin, high–molecular-weight kininogen, plasminogen, plasminogen activator inhibitor-1 (PAI-1), platelet-derived growth factor, GP IIb/IIIa, and thrombospondin are all found within these vesicles.[26]

Release of the dense granule ADP into the extracellular milieu has an autocatalytic effect on the platelet from which it came and also stimulates nearby platelets. The ADP will bind to its own purinergic receptors, most notably $P2Y_1$ and $P2Y_{12}$. Activation of both of these proteins is required for maximal aggregation of the platelets to one another. $P2Y_1$ stimulation acts to mobilize Ca^{++} (autocatalytic effect), which leads to further shape change and transient aggregation. $P2Y_{12}$ activation causes inhibition of adenylyl cyclase (blocking conversion of adenosine triphosphate to cyclic adenosine 3′,5′-monophosphate), potentiation of secretion of the α and dense granules, and sustained aggregation. ADP also binds the transmembrane protein $P2X_1$, an ion channel receptor linked to influx of Ca^{++} into the platelet.

Box • 31-1

Contents of Platelet α Granules

α_2-AP	Interleukin-1B
α_2-Macroglobulin	Multimerin
Albumin	P-Selectin
β-Thromboglobulin	PAI-1
CD63	Platelet factor 4
C1-inhibitor	Platelet-derived growth factor
Endothelial cell growth factor	Protein S
Epidermal growth factor	Thrombospondin
Factors V, XI, XIII	TFPI
Fibrinogen	Transforming growth factor-β
Fibronectin	Vascular endothelial growth factor
GMP 33	Vitronectin
High—molecular-weight kininogen	vWF
IgA, IgG, IgM	

AP, Antiplasmin; *Ig,* immunoglobulin; *TFPI,* tissue factor pathway inhibitor.

Fig. 31-1 **A,** Platelet adhesion and aggregation. Exposed collagen at the site of injury stimulates initial weak platelet adhesion by the GP Ia/IIa receptors. Stronger adhesion follows by the GP Ib/IX/V/vWF complex. This triggers platelet activation that leads to initial aggregation by the GP IIb/IIIa receptors binding the GP Ib/IX/V complex. This low-shear bond is later supplanted by a pair of GP IIb/IIIa receptors interacting with fibrinogen to create high-strength mature fibrin "ropes" interconnecting the two, then cross-linking to others. **B,** Platelet activation. *Lower left, moving clockwise:* Contact with the compromised vessel wall by platelet membrane GPs Ia/IIa and Ib/XI/V, stabilized by vWF, causes the platelets to become activated and begin moving Ca^{++} out of their tubular stores. The increased intracellular Ca^{++}, in turn, causes actin to break down and reassemble in long chains, resulting in filopod formation. The rise in Ca^{++} causes conversion of the GP IIb/IIIa from its inactive form to the active form. The dense granules move to the surface and release many activating substances, one of which is ADP. ADP stimulates $P2Y_1$ and $P2Y_{12}$ receptors, both of which accelerate the activation process. Note that the thienopyridine medications block the $P2Y_{12}$ receptors. The rise in Ca^{++} also causes α degranulation, resulting in the release of many substances important for further aggregation. Finally, platelet membrane phospholipids yield arachidonic acid *(AA)*, which is then converted by cyclooxygenase (COX) to prostaglandins G_2 *(PGG_2)* and H_2 *(PGH_2)*. Thromboxane synthase *(TS)* converts these to TXA_2, which, acting on a G protein–linked receptor, is a potent catalyst of platelet aggregation by accelerating further release of stored platelet Ca^{++}. Irreversible acetylation of COX by aspirin blocks TXA_2 synthesis and impairs platelet aggregation. *HMWK,* High–molecular-weight kininogen; *PDGF,* platelet-derived growth factor; *PPi,* pyrophosphate.

Aggregation

As the activated platelets interact with one another, they begin to aggregate. Aggregation is initiated by the Ca^{++}-mediated conformational activation of GP IIb/IIIa, a heterodimeric transmembrane protein. GP IIb/IIIa is a protein receptor complex unique to platelets and is expressed at extraordinarily high density on the surface of the platelets—some 80,000 to 100,000 per platelet, at an average of distance of only 20 nm from one another. Another 20,000 to 40,000 units are stored in the α granules and are released on the surface or in the local plasma milieu during degranulation. In the circulating, unactivated platelet, the GP IIb/IIIa receptor has little affinity for its ligands (primarily fibrinogen), so intravascular thrombus formation is minimized. However, on activation the GP undergoes a conformational change, which imparts high affinity for its ligands. Several proteins have the specific amino acid sequence necessary for binding to the GP IIb/IIIa receptor; the known ones are fibrinogen, fibronectin, vitronectin, and vWF.

As the α and dense granule contents are released extracellularly, nearby platelets are activated so their GP IIb/IIIa receptors are modified to the active form. The ligand proteins bind to the surface-associated GP IIb/IIIa of adjacent platelets, forming bridges. At low shear rates, fibronectin and fibrinogen (stabilized by thrombospondin, another GP from the α granules[6]) suffice as the main adhesive proteins, whereas vWF is necessary for proper adhesion in areas of high shear.[5] Interestingly, microvascular video imaging studies show that initially the thrombus formation is rather inefficient. Platelets bind quickly, but a significant percentage of them break free and float away. As a result, thrombus formation is much slower

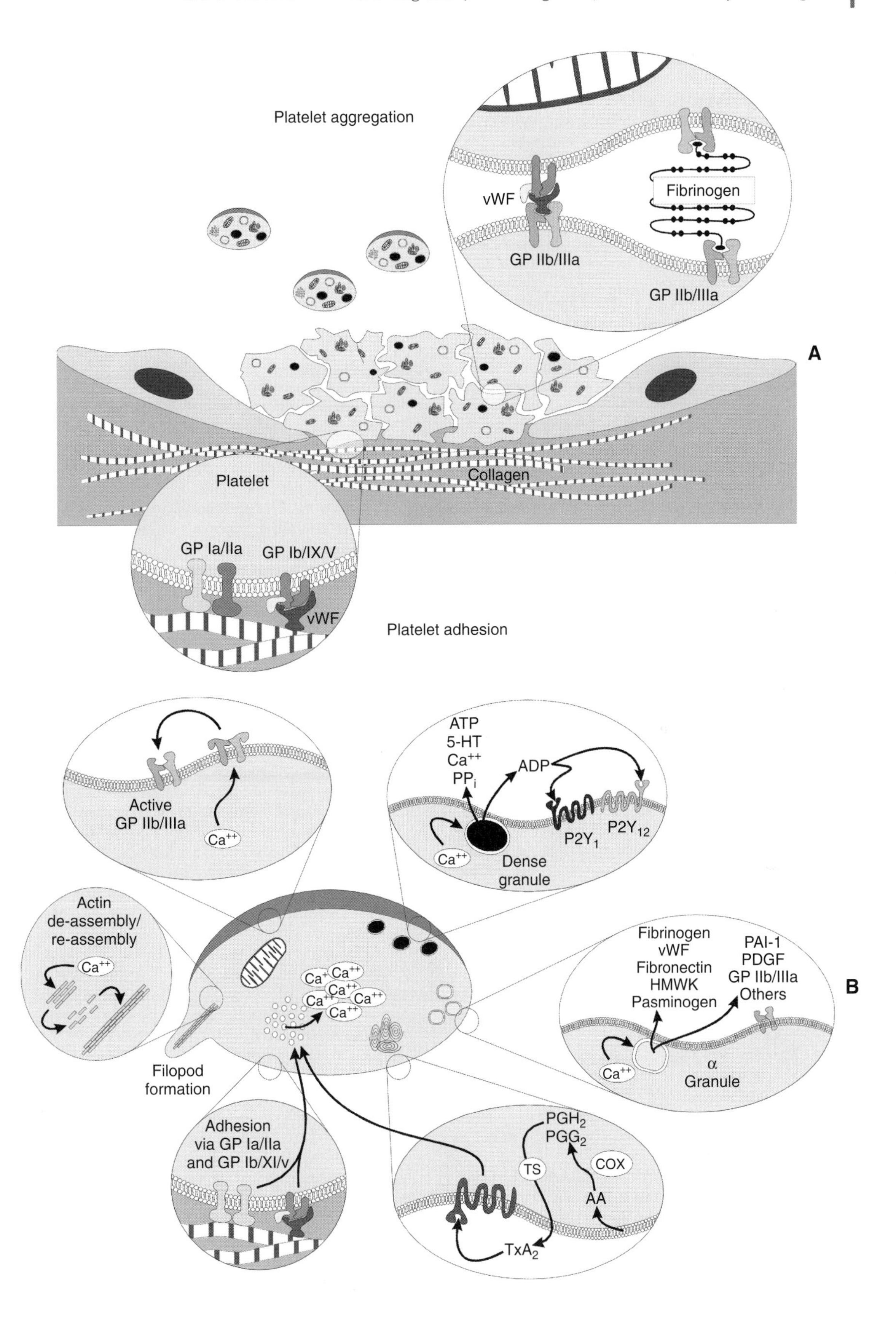
Platelet aggregation
vWF
Fibrinogen
GP IIb/IIIa
GP IIb/IIIa
A
Platelet
Collagen
GP Ia/IIa
GP Ib/IX/V
vWF
Platelet adhesion
Active
GP IIb/IIIa
Ca++
ATP
5-HT
Ca++
PPi
ADP
P2Y1
P2Y12
Ca++
Dense
granule
Actin
de-assembly/
re-assembly
Ca++
Fibrinogen
vWF
Fibronectin
HMWK
Pasminogen
PAI-1
PDGF
GP IIb/IIIa
Others
B
Ca++
α
Granule
Filopod
formation
Adhesion
via GP Ia/IIa
and GP Ib/XI/v
PGH2
PGG2
TS
COX
AA
TxA2

than if all the platelets that physically aggregate remained bound.

Several other events occur simultaneously with activation and aggregation, but the two most important are generation of TXA_2 and platelet-assisted generation of thrombin. Both these proteins serve to accelerate the platelet-activation response and therefore accelerate thrombus formation. TXA_2 is generated when platelet phospholipases are activated during platelet aggregation, which in turn release arachidonic acid from glycerophospholipids of the platelet membrane. Arachidonic acid serves as the substrate for cyclooxygenase (COX) to yield the prostaglandin endoperoxides PGH_2 and PGG_2, evanescent but potent inducers of further aggregation and secretion. The prostaglandins are also modified by thromboxane synthase to produce TXA_2, a short-acting, extremely potent inducer of platelet aggregation, granule secretion, and vasoconstriction. TXA_2 acts at its own protein-linked receptor.

Perhaps the most interesting effect of platelet activation is the procoagulant activity the platelets impart. In the normally resting platelet, the outer membrane has negatively charged phospholipids (including phosphatidylserine) sequestered almost exclusively on the inner side or leaflet by processes that are not fully understood. When an activating ligand binds, the resultant increase in intracellular Ca^{++} causes a membrane enzyme ("scrambalase") to evert the phosphatidylserine to the outer leaflet while simultaneously causing the membrane to form small evaginated microvesicles. Factor Va and VIIIa (discussed below) bind to these phosphatidylserine moieties and recruit factors Xa and IXa, respectively. The interaction of these complexes en toto accelerates the conversion of prothrombin to thrombin by a factor of 2.4×10^6. Additionally, the binding of activated coagulation factors to the platelets appears to protect the factors from plasma inhibitors while directing the bulk of the coagulation cascade to the site of injury. Note that the α granules have factor V and IX in them; the former appears to be complexed with multimerin protein (see Box 31-1).

As the thrombin is generated, it acts to activate other platelets by its G protein–linked receptors. The thrombin receptors are interesting in that they appear to be unique "suicide" receptors, requiring proteolytic cleavage to transmit an activating signal. Thrombin is a serine protease, and it acts on the receptors by cleaving the protein at the serine-42 residue, near the amino terminus. The new amino terminus acts as a "tethered ligand" to double back and stimulate the transmembrane protein to activate. Hence this receptor has been named the *protease-activated receptor (PAR)*. There are four such thrombin receptors, PAR-1 through PAR-4, with only PAR-1 and PAR-4 expressed by human platelets.[38] Thrombin-induced activation appears to upregulate GP IIb/IIIa activation while downregulating GP Ib/IX/V activity. Therefore the platelets appear to be converted from a mainly adhesive role to an aggregate role when thrombin is present.

Two other important activities of platelets warrant mention. The first is that the α granules contain P-selectin, a membrane protein that helps recruit and tether neutrophils and monocytes into the local area. It is believed that this activity is crucial for generating a local inflammatory response at the site of injury. Second, platelets are also essential in clot retraction, an event that facilitates wound healing by bringing the severed ends of small blood vessels into closer apposition. Clot retraction, or syneresis, occurs when the filopodia expressed by platelets during activation attach to fibrin strands and contract. A number of actin-binding proteins are present in platelets.[5] On activation, phosphorylated myosin monomers polymerize into filaments next to the long-chain actin filaments, which then slide past one another to generate a contractile force in the presence of adenosine triphosphate.

COAGULATION CASCADE

Although it is possible to separate the numerous events of hemostasis (e.g., platelet aggregation, formation of fibrin, retraction of the blood clot), the whole process occurs synergistically.[12] The fundamental clotting interactions were known by the early 20th century, primarily through the discovery of thrombin by Schmidt[50] in 1872 and formulation of the basic clotting scheme by Morawitz[43] in 1905. This simple scheme, in which thromboplastin, in the presence of Ca^{++}, promotes the conversion of prothrombin to thrombin, which in turn produces fibrin from fibrinogen, remains the backbone of the clotting mechanism. However, in recent years the classic coagulation cascade has undergone significant revision to recognize that many of the factors involved are actually enzymatic cofactors and that the majority of the reaction occurs on cell and platelet membranes (Figure 31-2). Many refinements in the understanding of blood coagulation have come about through study of "experiments of nature" in which discrete defects of the clotting process have been identified in patients with bleeding diatheses, as illustrated by the factors and deficiency states listed in Table 31-1.

Initiation of coagulation after injury is a complex process involving an initial pathway of thrombin generation, which then autocatalyzes a secondary burst of additional thrombin generation sufficient to convert fibrinogen to fibrin (see Figure 31-2). Before the process is described, a brief review of the critical factors and cofactors and how they function is warranted.

Vitamin K–Dependent Clotting Factors

In the liver, the vitamin K–dependent clotting factors are factors II (prothrombin), VII, IX, and X, along with protein C. They all share remarkable homologic characteristics, and molecular genetic evidence suggests they are all derived from a common ancestral precursor gene. The five proteins have similar structural elements. They all have a prepro leader that is cleaved away posttranslationally, followed by an amino-terminal γ-carboxyglutamic acid (Gla) domain with 9-12 Gla residues. This is followed by a hydrophobic domain and finally a serine protease domain in which the carboxy-terminal region becomes activated by cleavage of key arginine residues.

The amino terminus Gla domain is crucial for the lipid binding of these proteases to their substrate membranes. In the presence of seven Ca^{++} ions intercalated within the three-dimensional structure of the Gla domain, the proteins undergo a conformational change that places their hydrophilic domain at one end of the three-dimensional protein structure, with the hydrophobic moieties facing outward. This is crucial because it allows the protein to settle into the lipid membrane and exert its effects locally rather than systemically in the vasculature. Before the Gla domain can bind Ca^{++}, each of the Gla residues must be posttranslationally carboxylated by a specific γ-glutamyl carboxylase that requires the prepro leader sequence of amino acids to bind to the protein. This carboxylase enzyme requires oxygen, carbon dioxide, and vitamin K to function (see Figure 31-7). For every Gla residue carboxylated, one molecule of reduced vitamin K is converted to its epoxide form. A separate enzyme, vitamin K epoxide reductase, converts the vitamin K back to the reduced form. This latter enzyme is the target of the warfarin anticoagulants and is discussed in greater detail later.

Each of the clotting factors mentioned is a protease with activity directed at substrate arginyl residues. Activated factors VII, IX, and X each have a cofactor associated with them. VIIa (a for activated) binds to tissue factor (TF), IXa binds to VIIIa, and Xa binds to Va. The cofactors all serve to bind to both the substrate and the enzyme and approximate each to the

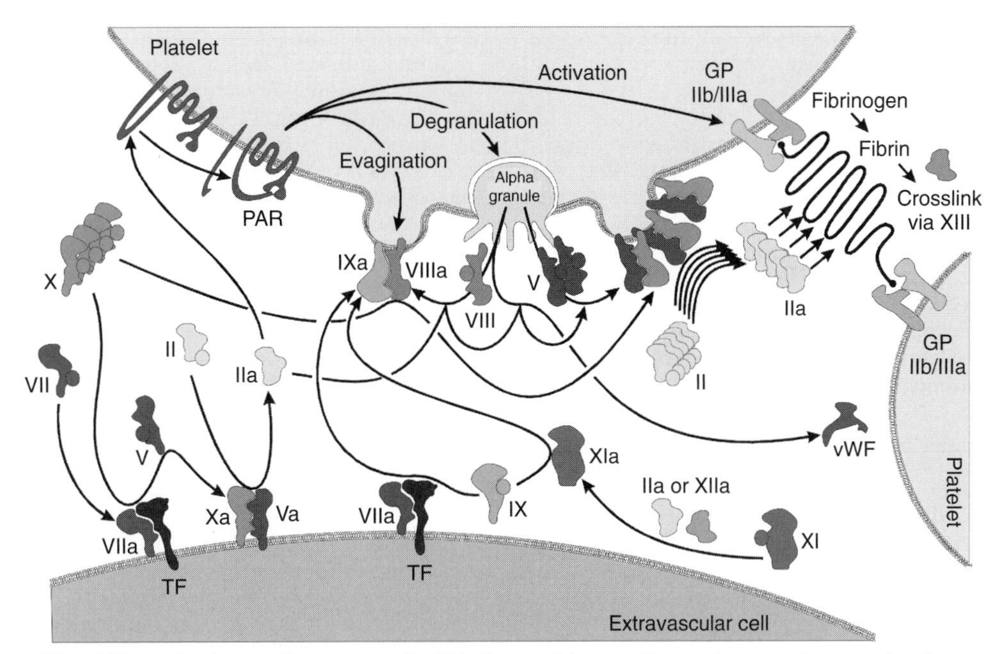

Fig. 31-2 Blood coagulation cascade. TF (factor III) on cell membranes of exposed subendothelial matrix cells combines with circulating factor VIIa (activated by Ca^{++}) to form an activating complex for factor X and factor IX. Factor Xa, locally bound to the membrane by factor Va, converts prothrombin (factor II) to thrombin (factor IIa). Meanwhile, converted factor IXa diffuses to adjacent platelets where it is bound to the platelet membrane by factor VIIIa. The complex acts to accelerate factor Xa conversion, leading to additional factor Va binding and ultimately vastly increased thrombin formation. Fibrin, after it is formed from fibrinogen by the proteolytic action of thrombin, is cross-linked and stabilized by factor XIIIa. Thrombin, a serine protease, accelerates the entire cascade by catalyzing cleavage of XI to XIa, stimulating platelets to activate by the transmembrane PAR, and stimulates conversion of XIII to XIIIa (not shown).

Table • 31-1

Blood Clotting Factors

INTERNATIONAL NUMBER OR TERM*	PLASMA FACTOR AND ALTERNATIVE NAMES†	CAUSE OR DESCRIPTION OF DEFICIENCY
I	Fibrinogen	Liver disease
II	Prothrombin	Liver disease or vitamin K deficiency
III	TF, thromboplastin	Deficiency of TF probably does not occur
IV	Ca^{++}	Never deficient without tetany
V	Proaccelerin	Parahemophilia, rare
VII	Proconvertin	Liver disease or vitamin K deficiency
VIII	Antihemophilic globulin, AHF A	Hemophilia A, 80% of hemophilics
IX	Christmas factor, AHF B	Hemophilia B (Christmas disease), depressed with vitamin K deficiency
X	Stuart-Prower factor	Liver disease or vitamin K deficiency
XI	Plasma thromboplastin antecedent, AHF C	Factor XI hemophilia (hemophilia C)
XII	Hageman factor	Generally no clinical symptoms but may have thromboses, rare
XIII	Fibrin-stabilizing factor, Laki-Lorand factor, fibrinase	Delayed bleeding, defective healing, rare
PF3	Platelet factor 3	Thrombocytopenia
—	Protein C	Liver disease or vitamin K deficiency
—	Protein S	Liver disease or vitamin K deficiency
—	Protein M	Liver disease or vitamin K deficiency
vWF	von Willebrand factor	vWD types I, IIa, IIb, IIc, III
Pre-K	Prekallikrein, Fletcher factor	
HMWK	High–molecular-weight kininogen	

*Roman numerals were assigned in 1958 by the International Committee on Blood Clotting Factors. Factor VI, originally assigned to prothrombin converting principle (prothrombinase), has since been abandoned.
†Most sources currently use factor numbers.
AHF, Antihemophilic factor; *TF,* tissue factor.

other, as well as to conformationally modify the enzyme to have greater activity in the presence of substrate.

Enzymatic Cofactors

TF is a unique protein normally constitutively found expressed on the cell surfaces of many extravascular cell types. Unlike the other coagulation cofactors, it is a transmembrane protein homologous to the receptors for interleukin-10 and interferon-α, -β, and -γ. It therefore appears to have both procoagulant and signal transduction functions. Interestingly, it can be induced to become expressed on the cell surfaces of intravascular monocytes and endothelial cells in response to some bacterial products and inflammatory cytokines, perhaps as part of the body's immunologic defense system. P-selectin, secreted by platelet α granules, can also induce TF expression in monocytes when binding to the activated platelets.

When injury occurs and the vasculature gains exposure to cells with TF on their surface, circulating factor VII rapidly binds to TF and undergoes proteolytic cleavage to VIIa by mechanisms that are not well understood. The TF/VIIa complex serves two crucial functions: it cleaves factor X to Xa and factor IX to IXa, both of which have distinct and separate functions. Newly formed factor Xa rapidly binds to circulating factor V and activates it to Va. The factor Xa/Va complex settles into the adjacent cellular membrane (by the hydrophobic Gla domain), where it acts on circulating prothrombin to generate a very small amount of thrombin. This tiny amount of thrombin is insufficient to significantly cleave fibrinogen but instead serves four crucial functions that set up the area for a much larger burst of thrombin formation: (1) nearby platelets are activated by their PAR receptors, which causes degranulation; (2) additional factor V liberated from the platelet α granules is activated (note that thrombin activates V much more efficiently than Xa does); (3) factor VIII is both activated and dissociated from vWF; and (4) factor XI is activated. Factor Xa exerts its effect locally; any factor Xa that escapes the TF/VIIa complex area is rapidly destroyed by TF pathway inhibitor (TFPI) or antithrombin III (ATIII), both of which are discussed later.

Unlike the factor Xa/Va complex, activation of factor IXa by TF/VIIa results in an enzyme that is not restricted to the nearby cell surface because it is not inhibited by TFPI, and ATIII is much more sluggish against it. As a result, factor IXa diffuses through the plasma over to nearby activated platelets. As previously discussed, activated platelets rapidly place factors Va and VIIIa on their cell surfaces. The diffusing factor IXa binds tightly to the VIIIa cofactor, and this IXa/VIIIa complex efficiently activates factor X to Xa. As before, the Xa then binds to adjacent Va and this time a much larger burst of prothrombin conversion to thrombin occurs. This much larger amount of thrombin formation is sufficient to begin cleaving fibrinogen and start clot formation as well as continue to perform the activating functions listed previously.

Fibrinogen and Factor XIII

The final phase of blood clotting consists of the thrombin-mediated proteolytic cleavage of fibrinogen to fibrin. Fibrinogen consists of a mirror-image dimer in which each monomer is composed of three intertwined and disulfide bond–linked polypeptide chains. In the dimer, the amino terminus of all six polypeptides meet in the middle of the linear molecule to form the N-terminal disulfide knot, or *E domain*. The carboxy termini of the three polypeptides at each opposite end form a globular protein cluster known as the *D domain*. Between the E and D domains, the polypeptide chains form a helical coil-coil structure.

Thrombin binds to the central E domain and cleaves off peptides from the knot to expose binding sites in the E domain that match the corresponding D domains of two neighboring fibrinogen molecules. The monomers thus begin to form a staggered "ladder" protofibril. As the monomers continue to associate, branch points occur that allow the fibrin meshwork to become more like a net and thicken. The initial clot is not stable, being held together primarily by hydrogen bonds. With time, however, the fibrin strands become cross-linked with covalent bonds by the action of a transglutaminase, fibrin-stabilizing factor XIII. This factor cross-links proteins between the γ-carbon of glutamine in one protein and the ε-amino group of lysine in the other.

Entrapped in this coagulum are white blood cells and intact platelets that then promote clot retraction, as previously described. These events are followed by the inflammatory processes of organization and wound healing, which require, among other things, an effective proteolytic (fibrinolytic) mechanism described later in this chapter.

Other Coagulation Cascade Proteins

It has long been known that patients with factor XI deficiency do not demonstrate severe bleeding profiles. Activated by thrombin, factor XIa cleaves factor IX to IXa. It is thought that this factor boosts the levels of IXa, but as only an enhancer. Lack of the protein causes mild to moderate clinical bleeding. Factor XII, prekallikrein, and high–molecular-weight kininogen have all been implicated in the activation of platelets when exposed to a negatively charged surface such as glass or kaolin. It is believed that these proteins act on factor XII to activate it to XIIa, which then activates factor XI to XIa, and ultimately IX to IXa. This method of "surface activation" is used to initiate the activated partial thromboplastin time (aPTT) test to determine how well the factor IXa system is functioning.

REGULATION OF COAGULATION

In this discussion of hemostatic mechanisms, consideration should be given to the natural inhibitors of blood clotting. As important as the procoagulant process is, it is equally important to ensure that inappropriate clotting does not occur. The intent of the clotting system is to seal a site of vascular compromise; powerful antithrombotic mechanisms must come to play to ensure that clotting remains limited to the injured area. Several mechanisms of antithrombosis have been elucidated; they are detailed below and summarized in Figure 31-3. At the heart of the matter is how to control the extremely efficient clotting cascade after it is initiated.

Strict control of the coagulation cascade is mediated by several proteins that act as natural anticoagulants, all of which rely on the first traces of thrombin from the nearby wound site to activate them. In general, the theory is simple: bind or degrade any activated procoagulant proteins if they escape the site of injury. At the same time, the site of injury must be protected from invasion/inclusion of these same inhibitory proteins.

Because thrombin is the major procoagulant protein, it makes sense that inactivation of it is a high priority. An elegant mechanism exists that, instead of destroying thrombin, uses thrombin to catalyze an important set of anticoagulant proteins, the protein C/protein S system. In the microcirculation, where there is a high cell surface/volume ratio, the protein C/protein S system predominates. Vascular endothelial cells normally constitutively express thrombomodulin on their membranes. Thrombomodulin is a transmembrane cofactor protein with no known enzymatic activity. It serves to bind the thrombin that escapes from the surface of nearby platelets but is not carried off in the vascular flow. Thrombomodulin, as the name implies, alters the conformation of the thrombin and effectively removes its ability to cleave fibrinogen,

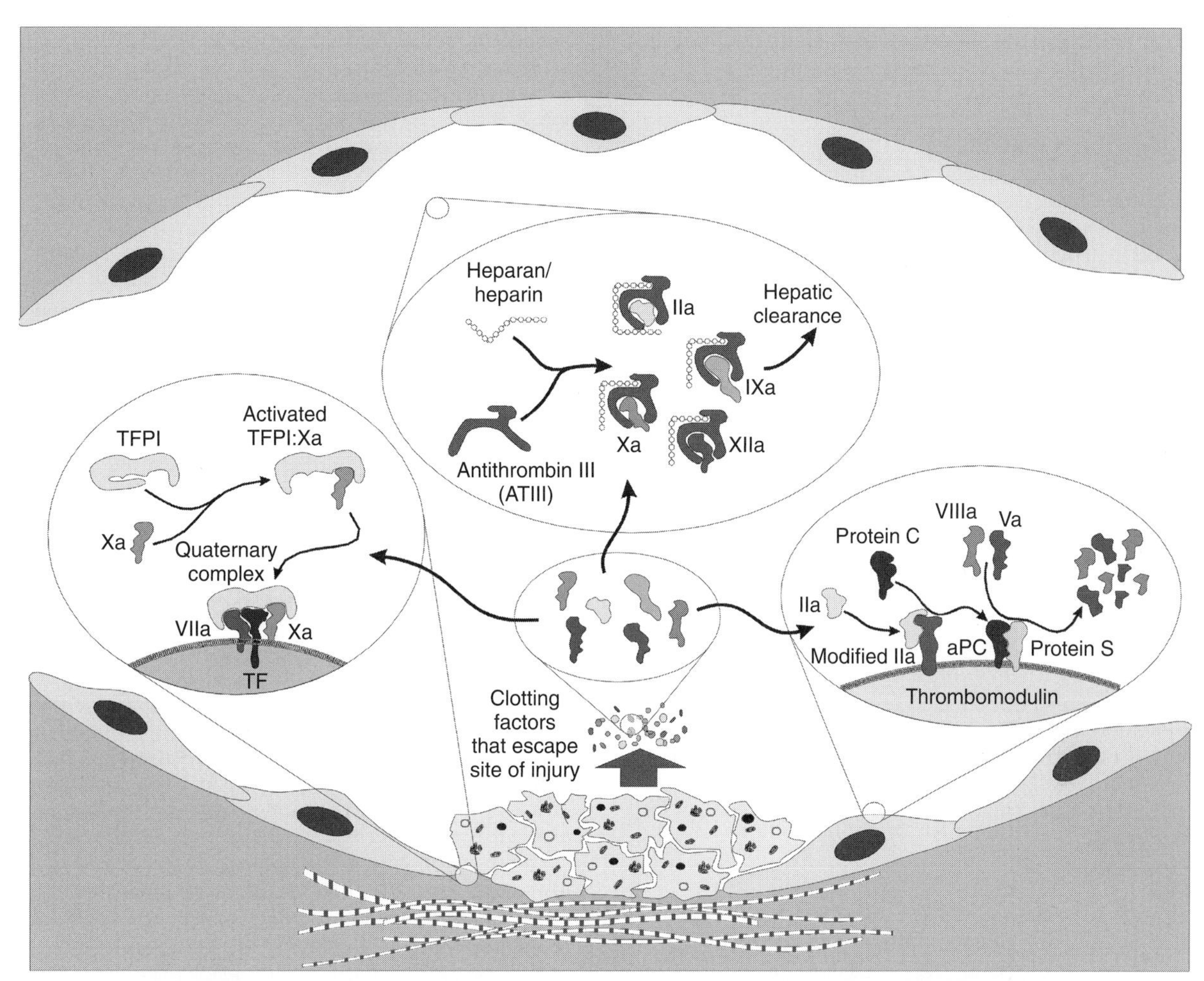

Fig. 31-3 The clotting inhibition system: examples of proteins that help limit fibrin formation to the site of the vascular injury by inactivating clotting factors. ATIII undergoes conformational change in the presence of heparin/heparan, which then allows it to bind and sequester factors IIa (thrombin), IXa, Xa, and XIIa. It is later cleared in the liver. When trace amounts of thrombin bind to thrombomodulin on intact endothelial cell membranes, the thrombin-thrombomodulin dimer undergoes a conformational change that allows it to activate protein C, which then is bound down to the membrane by protein S to form a protease complex specific for factors Va and VIIIa. Loss of these two factors disrupts the coagulation cascade sufficiently to prevent disseminated intravascular coagulation. A final inhibitor, TFPI, is first activated by factor Xa and then binds to the TF/VIIa complex to interrupt conversion of additional factor X.

activate platelets, and activate factors V and VIII. Instead, the new conformation of thrombin imparts a 2000 times greater affinity for activation of the vitamin K–dependent protein C.[16] Activated protein C (aPC) has considerable homologic characteristics with the other vitamin K–dependent factors, complete with a Gla domain, hydrophobic domain, and active serine protease domain. aPC's cofactor is protein S, a membrane-bound moiety that has no inherent activity. However, when aPC is bound, the complex efficiently cleaves and destroys any factors Va and VIIIa that might have been liberated from the platelet surfaces, thus slowing coagulation and protecting the normal person against random intravascular coagulation.[40]

Another protein, ATIII, is a serine protease inhibitor ("serpin") found in the plasma. It inhibits clotting by covalently binding 1 : 1 to the active sites of thrombin and the other serine proteases (factors IXa, Xa, and XIIa). This reaction is normally relatively slow but is accelerated 1000-fold in the presence of heparan sulfate, a proteoglycan synthesized on the surfaces by endothelial cells. (A similar effect is achieved therapeutically by administration of the closely related agent heparin sulfate, as described later.) Note that ATIII only binds to these factors without destroying them; reactivation by unbinding probably does not occur physiologically. The ATIII-protease complexes are cleared in the liver. It is believed that ATIII is responsible for complexing to proteases that escape into the circulation.

Finally, as briefly mentioned earlier, TFPI is a protease inhibitor found in low concentrations in the plasma, mostly bound to circulating lipoproteins or to endothelial cell membrane heparans. It is capable of inactivating both factor Xa and the TF/VIIa complex; it must first bind Xa before it can bind to the TF/VIIa complex. TFPI appears to be the major inhibitor of free-floating factor Xa, and it may be responsible for shifting the activation of factor IX from the TF/VIIa complex to thrombin-activated factor XI. The inhibitor is found in high concentrations in patients with hemophilia A and B, presumably because factors VIII and IX normally keep these conditions in check. This finding offers one explanation for why hemophilics bleed despite normal concentrations of

TF, factor VIIa, and factor Xa at the site of injury. TFPI is synthesized in both liver and endothelial cells.[62]

PROCOAGULANT AGENTS

In medical and dental practice it is essential to take maximum precautions to avoid serious hemorrhage. This admonition is particularly true for hemophilic patients, patients with hematopoietic disease, and patients receiving therapies known to affect hemostasis. Conservative precautions, which may include the administration of clotting factors and/or hospitalization, are prudent in these cases. In contrast, normal patients usually require no more than temporary hemostatic assistance (e.g., pressure packs, hemostatic forceps, ligation, or other locally active measures) to facilitate normal hemostasis and allow clotting to take place. Table 31-2 outlines various methods of controlling bleeding.

Local Measures

A perplexing hemostatic problem may arise from continued, slow oozing of blood from small arterioles, veins, and capillaries. These vessels cannot be ligated, and measures such as pressure packs and dressings, vasoconstrictor agents, and procoagulants must be used. Styptics or astringents, once extensively used, are no longer viewed as rational procedures for routine hemostasis in most applications; however, some astringents are commonly used for gingival retraction. Tranexamic acid mouthwash has been shown to have hemostatic properties,[52] but it has been removed from the US market for an indeterminate time.

Dressings

Bleeding caused by dentoalveolar surgery can most often be controlled by applying pressure with sterile cotton gauze. If this treatment is inadequate, the clinician must localize the source of bleeding as originating either within the soft tissues or within the bony structures. Soft tissue bleeding may be controlled by hemostats, ligation, electrocautery, or application of microfibrillar collagen or collagen sheets (on broad bleeding surfaces). Microfibrillar collagen, made from purified bovine skin collagen, is used topically to arrest certain hemorrhagic conditions that do not respond to conventional methods of hemostasis. Collagen accelerates the aggregation of platelets and therefore may have limited effectiveness in patients with platelet disorders or hemophilia.

Bleeding from bony structures, especially from extraction sockets, can be controlled by a variety of means. If initial attempts to achieve hemostasis with sterile cotton gauze and pressure do not succeed, a collagen plug or gelatin sponge may be inserted within the bony crypt. The collagen plug, like microfibrillar collagen, serves to accelerate the aggregation of platelets as well as form a physical barrier. The gelatin sponge facilitates platelet disruption and can absorb 40 to 50 times its own weight in blood, both of which aid in blood coagulation. It is resorbed in 4 to 6 weeks. Because it is gelatin, it must be applied dry; once moistened, it becomes difficult to handle. For this reason, many practitioners prefer the use of either denatured cellulose preparations or collagen sponge.

Denatured cellulose sponge or gauze serves as both a physical plug and a chemical hemostatic. The apparent coagulation-promoting action stems from the release of cellulosic acid, which denatures hemoglobin. Cellulosic acid, like tannic acid, inactivates thrombin; thus the use of cellulose sponge in conjunction with this procoagulant is ineffective. Two forms of cellulose sponge, oxidized cellulose and oxidized regenerated cellulose, are available. Both these materials cause delayed healing, particularly the oxidized cellulose, which notably interferes with bone regeneration and epithelialization. Although regenerated cellulose is said to have less inhibitory action, neither dressing should be left permanently in the wound if it can be removed.

Topically Applied Clotting Factors

The most physiologic hemostatic aids are the blood clotting factors themselves. Assuming an otherwise normal clotting system, topical thrombin is often used clinically. If given intravenously, thrombin causes extensive thrombosis and death. Topically applied thrombin (particularly in conjunction with a compatible matrix such as gelatin sponge) operates as a hemostatic, particularly if the patient has a coagulation deficiency or is receiving oral anticoagulants, because all that is required for clotting is a normal supply of platelets, fibrinogen, and factor XIII in the plasma. In the event that blood flows too freely, temporary physical hemostasis must be attained before topical thrombin can be of practical value. The use of thrombin is not without problems. Currently available thrombin, especially the bovine products, may be relatively crude preparations that still contain plasmin, a fibrinolytic agent (discussed below). Antibodies may also be generated to the bovine thrombin or bovine factor V; the latter can cross-react with human factor V and lead to an acquired inhibition and bleeding.

One of the more promising hemostatic aids to appear in recent years is fibrin sealant, also sometimes referred to as *fibrin glue.*[7] With this agent, the concept of the application of topical thrombin is taken one step further. Bovine or human thrombin and calcium chloride are mixed in one of two syringes; purified human fibrinogen with factor XIII, aprotinin, and other plasma proteins (fibronectin and plasminogen) are in the second syringe. The two solutions are mixed in a single delivery barrel, where the thrombin cleaves the fibrinogen to fibrin monomers. Initially, they are gelled by hydrogen bond formation, but in 3 to 5 minutes factor XIII in the

Table • 31-2

Methods of Controlling Bleeding

DESIRED RESULT	PHYSIOLOGIC METHODS	PHYSICAL METHODS	CHEMICAL AGENTS
Hemostasis	Vasoconstriction, platelet plugs, clot retraction	Pressure, electrocautery, cooling, sutures	Epinephrine, astringents-styptics*
Clotting	Procoagulants: thrombin, platelets, other clotting factors	Physical matrixes: gelatin, cellulose, collagen	Topical thrombin, fibrin sealant, antifibrinolytics

*Chemicals that denature protein include aluminum, zinc, iron, and silver salts; alcohol; tannic acid; and cellulosic acid.

presence of the Ca^{++} initiates cross-linking and increases the tensile strength of the clot.[7] As the clot solidifies, the sealant becomes milky white. The rate of fibrin clot formation depends on the concentration of the thrombin; 4 IU/ml produces a clot in approximately 1 minute, whereas 500 IU/ml requires only a few seconds. The strength of the clot, on the other hand, depends on the concentration of the fibrinogen. If used in an area where the clot is likely to break down too soon, or in patients with compromised hemostasis, a protease inhibitor such as aprotinin can be added to delay fibrinolysis. Aprotinin functions by inhibiting plasmin, which is generally carried along with the thrombin. The term *glue* arises from the fact that in many medical applications this material has been literally used to adhere tissues together naturally.

Fibrin sealant is now commercially available in the United States. The protein fractions are lyophilized and require careful reconstitution at 37° C under sterile conditions; proper mixing of the materials requires approximately 30 minutes to perform. As a result, the emergent use of this material is difficult; typically it is finding more use in planned surgeries in patients with known bleeding disorders. It is also an expensive medication; 1 ml of the material currently costs approximately $300. However, it does work well to stop the microbleeding and oozing that often accompany dental procedures.

If commercially manufactured fibrin sealant is unavailable, a crude but effective preparation can be made by mixing cryoprecipitate (discussed below), which will have approximately 20 mg/ml fibrinogen within it and the requisite factor XIII, with bovine thrombin and calcium chloride. Of course, because the fibrinogen is derived from human donors, care must be taken to ensure that any potential for viral transmission is kept to a minimum; for elective surgeries, autologous cryoprecipitate can be prepared.

Astringents and Styptics

The terms *astringents* and *styptics* are interchangeable, referring to different concentrations of the same drugs. Many chemicals have vasoconstrictive or protein-denaturing ability, but relatively few are appropriate for dentistry. The suitable preparations are primarily salts of several metals, particularly zinc, silver, iron, and aluminum. Aluminum and iron salts are quite acidic (pH 1.3 to 3.1) and therefore irritating.[61] Furthermore, iron causes annoying, though temporary, surface staining of the enamel, whereas silver stains may be quite permanent.

Currently, astringents are generally only used in dentistry to aid hemostasis while retracting gingival tissue. Other applications, such as controlling bleeding after surgery, are not looked on as favorably as in the past, when 20% ferric subsulfate (Monsel's solution) and 8% zinc chloride were among the most popular agents used. Aluminum and iron salts function by denaturing blood and tissue proteins, which then agglutinate and form plugs that occlude the capillary orifices. In a rabbit mandible model, when ferric sulfate salts were left in an osseous wound, there was an intense foreign body reaction and delayed healing in many of the experimental sites compared with the control sites.[39] When the salts were irrigated and the coagulum curetted away, this response was markedly diminished with no persistent inflammation or delay of osseous repair.[30] It is therefore imperative that if these compounds are to be used in the practice of dentistry, they be used briefly and with copious irrigation and debridement to remove the breakdown products. They should not be applied to areas of exposed osseous material in order to avoid inflammation or complications of retarded healing such as the distressful dry socket. Tannic acid (0.5% to 1.0%) is an effective astringent; it also precipitates proteins, including thrombin, but is often incompatible with other drugs and metal salts used therapeutically. Finally, the use of an astringent in a patient with even a mild bleeding tendency may provide temporary hemostasis but then lead to a larger area of delayed oozing after the chemically affected tissue sloughs.

Vasoconstrictors

Temporary hemostasis may be obtained with adrenergic vasoconstrictor agents, generally epinephrine. Obviously, such vasoconstrictors should be applied topically or just under the mucosa only for restricted local effects and for very short periods to avoid prolonged ischemia and tissue necrosis. Because some of the drug is absorbed systemically, particularly in inflamed and abraded tissue, cardiovascular responses may occur. Epinephrine solutions and dry cotton pellets impregnated with racemic epinephrine are available for topical application, but other methods to control bleeding are generally preferred. Other vasoconstrictive agents, such as 0.5% tetrahydrozoline or 0.5% oxymetazoline, have been suggested for use as better hemostatic agents for gingival cord retraction because of their much more neutral pH than epinephrine or the astringent salts.[61]

Systemic Measures

Patients with acquired or genetic bleeding disorders usually have deficiencies in platelet number, platelet function, or faulty or missing clotting factors. Bleeding may develop several hours after trauma or surgery. Uncontrolled bleeding does not generally appear with superficial abrasions, but hemarthrosis and hemorrhage are common with deeper injuries. Thrombocytopenia is frequently drug induced or associated with other myelogenous diseases; hemophilia disorders are generally inherited. In either case, with proper evaluation and supportive therapy (Table 31-3), extensive surgery can usually be accomplished without serious incident.

Platelet disorders

Patients with a platelet count of less than 50,000/mm^3 are at risk for surgical or other trauma but generally do not demonstrate spontaneous hemorrhage until the count drops below 5000 to 10,000/mm^3. Platelet transfusion should be reserved for acute situations because alloimmunization to injected platelets readily occurs. One unit of platelet concentrate (equal to the platelets derived from one unit of whole blood) elevates the platelet count in adults from 4000 to 10,000/mm^3. Platelet recovery is low in patients with hypersplenism and may be undetectable in patients with immune thrombocytopenia. Drug-induced disease generally is alleviated by withdrawal of the offending drug. Idiopathic forms may benefit from corticosteroid administration, splenectomy, injections of vincristine (an immunosuppressive agent also used in cancer chemotherapy), or, acutely, after high doses of intravenous immunoglobulin. Finally, patients receiving aspirin therapy should consider reducing or discontinuing their aspirin intake for 4 to 7 days before anticipated surgery, if feasible, depending on the nature and extent of the planned procedure.

Hemophilia

All forms of hemophilia are genetically based disorders of coagulation. They may range in severity from mild to moderate to severe; this designation greatly affects what dental interventions can occur. The most common forms of hemophilia are the result of a deficiency in factor VIII or IX (hemophilia A and B, respectively). Although the transmission of hemophilia A or B is hereditary and X-linked, nearly half of all cases arise spontaneously as new mutations.[55] Any child or adult with newly discovered hemophilia should have counseling with the family as provided by hemophilia treatment centers. Bleeding disorders (especially of the mild variety) are often

Table • 31-3

Procoagulant Preparations Used in the Management of Bleeding Disorders

NONPROPRIETARY (GENERIC) NAME	PROPRIETARY (TRADE) NAMES	CONTENT	THERAPEUTIC USE
Factor VIII Products			
Antihemophilic factor, porcine	Hyate-C	400 to 700 porcine units/vial; contains platelet aggregation factor	Hemophilia A; patients with inhibitor antibodies to human factor VIII
Antihemophilic factor, plasma derived	Humate-P, Profilate SD, Koate HP	250, 500, and 1000 IU/vial; contains albumin and small amounts of other proteins	Hemophilia A
Antihemophilic factor, plasma derived, purified by heparin ligand or immunoaffinity column	Alphanate, Hemofil M, Monoclate-P, Monarc-M	250, 500, 1000, and 1500 IU/vial; contains albumin	Hemophilia A
Antihemophilic factor, recombinant	Bioclate, Helixate, Kogenate, Recombinate	250, 500, and 1000 IU/vial; contains albumin and trace amounts of animal protein	Hemophilia A; patients without HIV or viral hepatitis
Factor IX Products			
Factor IX complex	Bebulin VH Konyne 80, Profilnine SD, Proplex T	500, 1000, and 1500 IU/vial; also contains significant amounts of factors II, VII, and X	Hemophilia B
Factor IX human complex, purified	Alphanine, SD Mononine	500, 1000, and 1500 IU/vial; contains small amounts of factors II, VII, and X	Hemophilia B
Factor IX, recombinant	BeneFIX	250, 500, and 1000 IU/vial	Hemophilia B; patients without HIV or viral hepatitis
Factor VIIa Product			
Factor VIIa, recombinant	NovoSeven	60, 120, and 240 KIU/visit	Hemophilia A or B; patients with inhibitors for factors VIII or IX
Mixed Factor Products			
Anti-inhibitor coagulant complex (factor VIII inhibitor bypassing activity)	Autoplex T, FEIBA VH	≥80 IU/bag; contains other clotting factors; prepared from single donors	Hemophilia A, vWD, hypofibrinogenemia, DIC, Kasabach-Marrot syndrome
Antihemophilic factor, cryoprecipitated	—	≥80 IU/bag; contains other clotting factors; prepared from single donors	Hemophilia A, vWD, hypofibrinogenemia, DIC, Kasabach-Marrot syndrome

Unless otherwise noted, all products are derived from human plasma or, in the case of recombinant products, based on human genes.
DIC, Disseminated intravascular coagulopathy; *IU*, international units; *vWD*, von Willebrand's disease.

first discovered after dental procedures, such as extractions or periodontal surgery.

Hemophilia A occurs when there is a deficiency in circulating factor VIII activity. Factor VIII accelerates blood coagulation by serving as a cofactor in the platelet membrane in the enzymatic activation of factor X by the factor IXa/VIIIa complex (see Figure 31-2). In the inactive state, factor VIII is an asymmetric protein molecule. The normal amount of factor VIII antigen[27] averages 100 U/dl, with a range of 50 to 180 U/dl. Mild hemophilia occurs when the patient's blood has 5% to 30% of normal factor VIII activity. Moderate disease is defined as 1% to 4% factor VIII, and severe hemophilia shows less than 1% factor VIII. People with more than 40% normal factor VIII antigen clot normally.

The gene for factor VIII resides on the long arm of the X chromosome (Xq28),[55] resulting in an X-linked pattern of inheritance. In severe factor VIII hemophilia, gene inversions account for 45% of mutations, whereas other patients have point mutations that often cause a premature stop codon to be inserted, resulting in incomplete mRNA transcription. Generally, only males with a faulty factor VIII gene on their only X chromosome show phenotypic expression of severe disease, at a rate of 1 in 10,000. Females who carry an affected X chromosome typically do not show phenotypic disease because the normal factor VIII gene on the other X chromosome provides sufficient protein to allow normal clotting. However, expression of the normal gene may become depressed during development if key progenitor cells favor the chromosome with the defective gene. The result is that some carrier females are phenotypically mild (or rarely, moderate) hemophilics, with factor VIII concentrations between 15% and 25% of normal. Referred to as "symptomatic carriers," their bleeding tendency is often not uncovered until they encounter a significant insult, such as extraction of teeth, orthognathic surgery, or extensive periodontal surgery. For this reason, all female relatives of hemophilics should have interviews, and possibly blood tests, to determine both their carrier status and their factor VIII activity.

Hemophilia B was discovered when it was noted that combining plasma from different hemophilics sometimes allowed normal clotting; it was deduced that the second sample corrected the defect in the first. It was later determined that deficiencies in factor IX were responsible for approximately one fifth of the forms of hemophilia. Older literature refers to factor IX deficiency as "Christmas disease," named after the surname of the first family studied with this variant of hemophilia.

Like hemophilia A, the gene for factor IX is on the X chromosome (Xq27.3)[55] and therefore shows the same familial pattern of expression: affected males and carrier females. Because this gene is considerably smaller than the factor VIII gene (34 kd versus 186 kd), most of the genetic variations have been identified in kindreds. Like factor VIII deficiency, partial or whole gene deletions or insertions lead to severe hemophilia B, as do nonsense point and some missense mutations. Also like hemophilia A, there are mild, moderate, and severe forms of the disease, and female symptomatic carriers do occur. Hemophilias A and B are clinically indistinguishable.

von Willebrand's disease

Originally described by Erik von Willebrand in 1926, von Willebrand's disease (vWD) is an autosomal dominant hemorrhagic disorder resulting from a quantitative or qualitative deficiency of the vWF GP. Both males and females are affected equally; the defect is in an autosomal dominant gene located on chromosome 12.[23] vWD may be the most common inherited bleeding disorder, with many cases remaining undiagnosed.

The vWF GP is produced in vascular endothelial cells and megakaryocytes and is stored both intracellularly in the α granules of platelets and circulated in the plasma as multimeric polymers. The high–molecular-weight multimers are necessary for normal biologic activity, presumably from more ligand-binding domains. vWF has three important functions. The first is to form a tight but noncovalent complex with factor VIII protein (in a ratio of approximately 1 factor VIII to 100 vWF), thereby stabilizing factor VIII and slowing its clearance from the circulation. Second, vWF promotes normal, high-shear platelet adhesion to the subendothelium on injury and exposure of subendothelial matrix proteins. The latter function is mediated by the GP Ib/IX/V tetramer found on the platelets, and the vWF involved is bound to the subendothelial matrix proteins. Third, vWF is one of the proteins that binds to the multiple platelet membrane GP IIb/IIIa receptors, along with fibrinogen, to help stabilize the aggregating platelets.

As an aside, one of the first antistaphylococcic antibiotics, ristocetin, was found to cause thrombocytopenia in many patients because of spurious binding to the platelet membrane (mechanism undetermined) that mediated enhancement of the binding of vWF, resulting in aggregation and resultant thrombosis and depletion thrombocytopenia. Although the antibiotic was removed from the therapeutic market as a result, it is now used in an assay for vWD. By using washed platelets, ristocetin, and plasma from the affected patient, a positive correlation occurs between the amount of *functional* vWF present and the amount of ristocetin necessary to induce platelet aggregation. When the ristocetin cofactor assay (as it is known) is compared with tests that show the amount of vWF protein present in the plasma, diagnosis of the type of vWD can be made.

The hematologic disorder in vWD can present as either structural or quantitative changes in vWF. Three types of disease exist. Type 1 vWD is associated with a mild quantitative defect in the amount of vWF produced. Titers of vWF antigen and ristocetin cofactor activity are comparable. This is the most common type (80%) and is most often manifested by mucocutaneous bleeding. Type 2 vWD is a defect in the production of the high–molecular-weight multimers, causing a significant decrease in platelet adhesion and normal or mildly decreased vWF antigen. Type 3 vWD is characterized by severe bleeding disorders from an essential lack of any vWF, with concomitantly low concentrations of factor VIII and decreased platelet adhesion. This third type, fortunately, is rare, usually occurring only in homozygous or compound heterozygous offspring of parents with mild or asymptomatic variants of vWD.

Treatment

Treatment of either variety of hemophilia or vWD requires the restoration of the appropriate factor so that factor complex IXa/VIIIa activity is sufficient.[19] For the treatment of hemophilia A, there are a variety of factor VIII replacement products (see Table 31-4).[22,55] Because the half-life of factor VIII is 8 to 12 hours, the patient must be reinfused with at least half the original dose at approximately 12-hour intervals to prevent rebleeding from surgical wounds.

Until recently, the only way to obtain factor VIII was by pooled human blood products. Initially, the most common method was to use cryoprecipitate. Cryoprecipitate is the cold-insoluble (precipitated) protein fraction derived when fresh frozen plasma is thawed at 4° C.[51] It is primarily composed of factor VIII, fibrinogen, and vWF. Classically, it has been one of the mainstays of factor VIII hemophilia treatment but has declined in use with development of methods to purify factor VIII from whole blood, reduce the infectious risk with virucidal treatments, and manufacture recombinant factor VIII. Like plasma, cryoprecipitate is not virally inactivated. The most common use of cryoprecipitate currently is as a source of fibrinogen for the treatment of disseminated intravascular coagulopathy.[4] For congenital bleeding disorders, cryoprecipitate is used for the treatment of vWD. Single-donor cryoprecipitate (after desmopressin stimulation of the donor) is still the preferred method of treating vWD for some families.

Modern plasma-derived factor VIII products have greatly reduced the risk of viral transmission by donor screening and viral inactivation protocols. Two methods are currently being used to inactivate viruses—heat and solvent detergent. All viruses that have lipid envelopes are readily destroyed, including the human immunodeficiency (HIV), hepatitis B, and hepatitis C viruses. Viruses that do not have lipid envelopes, such as the B-19 parvovirus and hepatitis A virus, can still be transmitted in the solvent detergent or heat-inactivated products. A vaccination for hepatitis A is now available, and patients with hemophilia or vWD are clearly encouraged to receive it early in life.

Some manufacturers additionally purify their factor VIII protein products from the pooled factor VIII proteins on affinity columns, both increasing the specific activity of the preparation and further decreasing the risk of viral transmission. Those products are, of course, more expensive. The porcine factor VIII product does not transfer HIV or hepatitis, although some allergic reactions may occur. It is particularly useful for inhibitor patients (discussed below) because, on average, the cross-reactivity between species is approximately 25% that of human products.

Two recombinant factor VIII products are currently being marketed in the United States. They are derived from stable transfection of the human factor VIII cDNA into Chinese hamster ovary or baby hamster kidney cells, with resultant transcription and protein production. The protein derived is virus free, has a high specific activity, and, because of cost considerations, has been primarily used in individuals who are HIV and hepatitis virus negative. Of concern is the fairly high (38%) incidence of inhibitor formation, but the inhibitors are usually low titer and controllable with low-dose daily infusions of factor VIII protein to build immune tolerance over time. Current products contain pasteurized albumin for stabilization, so there remains some risk of nonlipid-envelope viral transmission.

Another approach to the treatment of mild hemophilia A or type 1 vWD was introduced in 1977 when it was discovered that desmopressin, the synthetic 1-desamino-8-D-arginine analogue of vasopressin (antidiuretic hormone), could prevent bleeding in many of these patients. This medication causes factor VIII, vWF, and plasminogen activator to be released from storage sites on the vascular endothelium. In many patients with mild hemophilia or type 1 vWD, the protein structures are normal but concentrations are low. With desmopressin, transient increases of two to three times the patient's baseline concentrations can be achieved, which may be sufficient to allow adequate hemostasis during minor surgery. For those hemophilics who use single donors (usually a parent or sibling) as their sole source of factor product to decrease the risk of viral transmission, desmopressin can be given to the donor before donation to double or triple the amount of factor VIII recovered.

Desmopressin is subject to peptic hydrolysis and is therefore injected or insufflated intranasally. Mild facial flushing is normal during the infusion, with headache, nausea, and lightheadedness as common side effects. Because of its antidiuretic properties, water intake must be restricted for 12 hours to avoid volume overload (note that the drug is also used as an aid for children with bed-wetting difficulties). The medication is contraindicated in type 2B vWD because sudden release of large multimers of vWF may cause intravascular platelet aggregation and resultant thrombocytopenia. Types 2 and 3 vWD usually require replacement therapy for both factor VIII and vWF instead.[51]

The advantage of desmopressin over vasopressin is that this derivative retains the factor VIII–releasing activity but lacks the vasoconstrictor action of vasopressin. Most importantly, desmopressin is devoid of the risk of viral transmission inherent in the blood-derived products. Desmopressin also has the capacity to stimulate an increase in tissue-type plasminogen activator (t-PA), an action useful in the treatment of thromboses.

Historically, factor IX concentrates have been difficult to purify. The most common factor IX preparations are known as "factor IX complex" because, although they have high amounts of factor IX protein, they also contain factors II, X, and some factor VII as well (see Table 31-4).[54,55] Disseminated intravascular coagulopathy, because of the presence of the excessive extra clotting factors (some partially activated), is occasionally a problem, so in some preparations heparin has been added to reduce thrombin generation during storage. These concentrates are still in use simply because of cost considerations. Like factor VIII concentrates, they are subjected to various forms of viral inactivation to reduce the transmission of HIV, hepatitis B, and hepatitis C.

In 1990, two high-purity factor IX concentrates were marketed. They contain essentially no factor II or factor VII and only small amounts of factor X. Purified factor IX concentrates have markedly reduced the risk of thrombosis. Although these preparations are treated with solvent detergent or ultrafiltration, there remains some uncertainty about viral transmission with their use.

A recombinant factor IX preparation was licensed in 1997. Like all recombinant products, it is essentially virus free; it is produced in Chinese hamster ovary cells. A major difficulty in developing this product is the extensive posttranslational modifications the protein undergoes: 11 disulfide bonds, one β-hydroxylation, one sulfation, one phosphorylation, and 12 γ-carboxylations must all occur to activate the protein. The recombinant product has several differences from the native protein: only approximately 60% is fully carboxylated, 15% gets sulfated, and only 1% is phosphorylated. As a result, the protein is not quite as efficacious as it could be, so the patients typically require an average of 1.5 times more protein than highly purified plasma-derived protein to get sufficient increases in plasma factor IX. The cost is also substantially higher on a per-unit basis.[41,56]

One aspect of blood product replacement therapy that is often overlooked is the cost. On average, a patient with severe hemophilia A uses between 50,000 and 100,000 units of factor VIII per year, at a 2002 wholesale cost range from $0.30 to $1.00 per unit. Therefore, in an average year, the nonretail cost ranges from $10,000 to $90,000 depending on the type of product used and the extent of use required. Younger hemophilics, to avoid potential viral exposure, generally use the more expensive recombinant products.

As a hope for the future, correction of hemophilia by viral vector– or nonviral-mediated gene transfer is actively being pursued. In one study,[33] the cDNA for canine factor IX was inserted in a retroviral vector and infused into the portal vein of four dogs with severe hemophilia B that had undergone partial hepatectomy. As their livers regenerated, the virus was integrated into hepatocyte DNA, causing a very low (0.1% of normal) level of factor IX to be produced. The protein was still being produced more than 2 years later in one of the animals. Although the concentrations are not high enough to be of clinical relevance, the model does show that the gene can be stably transferred. In a more recent study, dermal fibroblasts obtained from six patients by skin biopsy were grown in culture and transfected with the factor VIII gene. Cells that produced the protein were selected, cloned, and propagated in vitro, and later administered into the patient's peritoneal cavity. In four of the six patients, detectable levels of factor VIII were found, with two of them surpassing the 1% threshold considered to be therapeutic. Unfortunately, by 10 months after administration, all four had reverted to undetectable levels.[49]

Clearly, gene therapy is in its infancy, but great strides have been made. In the clotting cascade, posttranslational modifications (numerous with factor IX) often present great challenges beyond simply expressing the gene itself. However, if the right expression system can ultimately be found, correction of these genetic defects may someday be achieved.

Inhibitors

A confounding problem in treating hemophilics is the development of antibody inhibitors against the deficient factor.[42] Approximately 10% of patients with severe hemophilia A express a high titer of inhibitor, usually within the first few years of being treated with factor VIII concentrates. Multiple approaches must be used to protect these patients against bleeding crises. The most crucial task is to determine whether the patient carries low-titer or high-titer antibodies. Patients with low-titer antibodies can often be given excessive amounts of factor replacement, thereby depleting the inhibitor antibody sufficiently to allow the remaining factor to promote hemostasis. Although low-titer inhibitors may persist for years, they do not show the typical alloantibody boost response after exposure to human factor VIII concentrates. Care must be exercised in using this method for elective procedures because there is the risk that in some patients the additional factor challenge will boost the titer from a low- to a high-titer inhibitor, making future crisis intervention more difficult.

In patients who have high-titer inhibitors, preventing or reducing hemorrhage risk is of utmost importance. Daily infusion of high-, medium-, or low-dose factor replacement, with the hope of developing immune tolerance, has often been successful. Concomitant administration of immunosuppressant medications such as cyclophosphamide and prednisone may further depress antibody formation. This approach is much more effective with autoantibody inhibitors than with alloimmune responses. A short course of daily intravenous infusion of immunoglobulin G has sometimes reduced titers as well. After immune tolerance is achieved, most patients require continued low-dose prophylactic factor infusions at least weekly.[42]

In an acute hemorrhagic situation, or in the emergent dental crisis, porcine factor VIII is sometimes useful. The protein is fully functional in human beings, but inhibitor antibodies directed against the human form tend not to be strongly cross-reactive. Side effects include fever, chills, headache, vomiting, and rarely anaphylaxis. Continued use can result in development of species-specific antibody or, occasionally, immune tolerance to the human antigen.

Finally, factor VIIa is now available for use in hemophilics with high-titer inhibitors to factor replacement therapy. It is a recombinant protein derived in baby hamster kidney cells transfected with the factor VII cDNA and therefore has no risk of transmission of human pathogenic viruses. During processing it spontaneously activates to VIIa. The protein as a therapeutic agent functions like its endogenous counterpart: by combining with TF present at all sites of injury to stimulate conversion of factors IX and X to their respective activated analogues. Because TF is only found at the site of injury, disseminated coagulation has not been a difficulty. Also, factor VIIa is not rapidly inactivated by ATIII, giving it a sufficient half-life to allow hemostasis. It does have a much shorter half-life (only 2 to 3 hours) than either factors VIII or IX, however, and requires high doses every 2 hours in the dental setting. The drug has the limitation that its mechanism is to achieve sufficient thrombin formation via that part of the coagulation cascade that is intended for only small amounts of thrombin generation. It does seem to work well for initial hemostasis, but there have been difficulties with breakthrough bleeding 48 hours or so after surgery (unpublished data). The use of topical fibrin sealant in conjunction with this product seems to be a wise choice. It should also be noted that the current cost of this medication is expensive—several thousand dollars per dose.

AGENTS THAT PROMOTE OR INHIBIT FIBRINOLYSIS

Fibrinolytics

Achieving hemostasis is a crucial aspect of the coagulation system; limiting its spread is another, and remodeling or breaking down clots when they are no longer necessary is a third aspect of the process of vascular repair. As healing occurs, it is necessary to remove all or part of the fibrin that has been deposited to restore blood flow to the affected tissue; this is mediated by the protease plasmin (Figure 31-4). When fibrin is initially deposited, thrombin stimulates adjacent endothelial cells to release t-PA and urokinase (u-PA). A serine protease with a fibrin-binding domain, t-PA must adhere to the fibrin molecules to function. This binding occurs on lysine residues of the fibrin. Once adhered, t-PA binds plasminogen (also by a lysine residue) and cleaves the plasminogen to liberate plasmin, also a serine protease. Note that plasmin also has the ability to bind directly to fibrin. u-PA acts independently of fibrin, and instead activates plasminogen to plasmin in the circulation. Plasmin associated with t-PA on the fibrinogen both lyses the fibrin, releasing fibrin degradation products, and degrades factors V and VIII, inhibiting further clotting. t-PA can associate with circulating plasminogen but does not effectively activate it unless both are bound to the fibrin, which is an important consideration in the therapeutic use of this compound.[11]

As expected, strict control mechanisms for plasmin activity exist. Without such control, circulating plasmin would cause systemic fibrinolysis and oozing of previously clotted sites. Three proteins are intimately involved. The first, α_2-antiplasmin (α_2-AP), is a serpin (serine protease inhibitor) that is synthesized in the liver and is efficient at neutralizing any free plasmin circulating in the blood. Conversely, binding of the plasmin to fibrin (independently or by t-PA) protects it from attack by α_2-AP, which appropriately restricts plasmin's activity to the wound site. The second control protein, PAI-1, is a serpin synthesized by the endothelial cells in response to thrombin stimulation, with specificity for t-PA as its substrate. PAI-1 is in molar excess in the plasma compared with t-PA, effectively inhibiting t-PA's systemic conversion of plasminogen to plasmin unless (as with α_2-AP and plasmin) the t-PA can "hide" and be protected from it by binding to fibrin.[62] The third control protein is PAI-2, which functions like PAI-1, only with specificity for u-PA. The liver also functions to clear the bloodstream of any free active plasmin, further helping to prevent systemic fibrinolysis.

Therapeutic measures designed to induce or facilitate fibrinolysis are available for use in relieving certain types of thromboses, most notably in the event of acute myocardial infarction. These agents may also be of value in patients with life-threatening pulmonary emboli, infarctive stroke, or deep venous thrombosis. All these agents function by activating the conversion of plasminogen to plasmin with subsequent natural fibrinolysis. One of the medications now used is the natural activator, u-PA. The parent compound is cleaved twice, first to high–molecular-weight u-PA, then to low–molecular-weight u-PA. As with the endogenous form, the low–molecular-weight u-PA loses its fibrin-binding domain, causing it to be effective at activating circulating plasminogen to plasmin. In pharmacologic doses, this results in systemic fibrinolysis.

t-PA is now produced by recombinant DNA techniques. It is marketed under the nonproprietary name of *alteplase.* Because t-PA is naturally more fibrin specific than are preparations containing streptokinase or u-PA, it is the first thrombolytic agent recommended by the American Heart Association in the management of myocardial thrombosis.[28] Note, however, that at pharmacologic doses it imparts some circulating plasminogen conversion. A deletion mutation variant of t-PA is available by the nonproprietary name of *reteplase.* It is similar in activity and side effects to t-PA.

Streptokinase, an exotoxin from certain β-hemolytic streptococci, also serves as an activator of plasminogen.[28] It is different from t-PA and the u-PA family in that it is not an enzyme and does not proteolytically cleave plasminogen to plasmin. Instead, it binds noncovalently to plasminogen and confers plasminlike proteolytic activity on the plasminogen-streptokinase complex.[40] The complex then cleaves other molecules of plasminogen, liberating active plasmin. Because streptokinase is an exogenous protein originating in bacteria, there is a higher incidence of adverse and allergic reactions with this medication. Like the u-PA family, streptokinase is

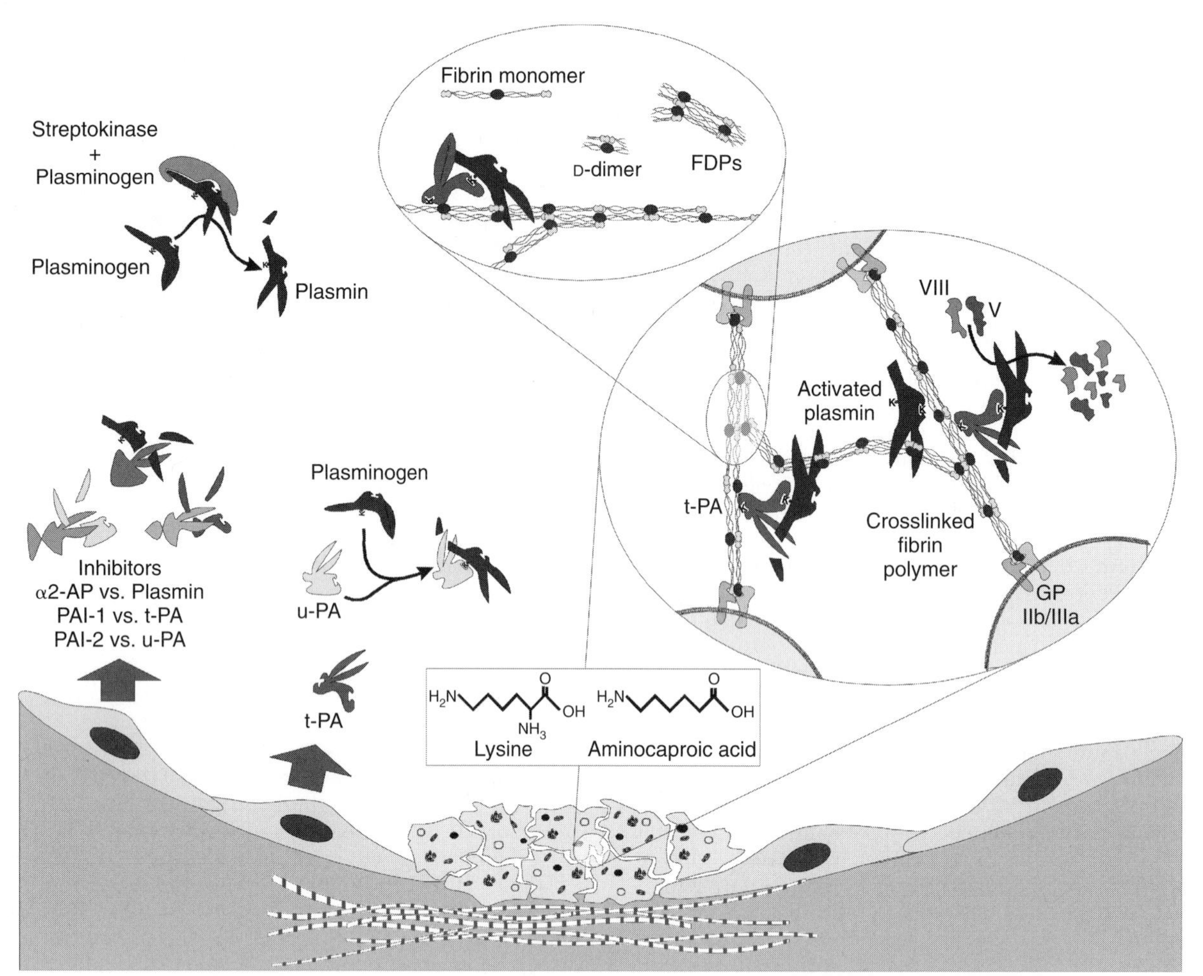

Fig. 31-4 Fibrinolysis. Thrombin formation causes adjacent endothelial cells to release t-PA and u-PA. t-PA adheres to lysine residues on the fibrin molecules and adsorbs plasminogen onto it, also by lysine binding. t-PA's proteolytic action converts the plasminogen to plasmin at the wound site, whereas u-PA converts it in the free circulation. Plasmin acts to degrade factors V and VIII and proteolytically cleave the fibrin. Various fibrin degradation products *(FDPs)* are liberated, including the D-dimer formed from two fibrin molecule "ends" linked to one fibrin molecule "middle." Aminocaproic acid interferes with plasminogen conversion by occupying lysine sites in both t-PA and plasminogen. The endothelial cells also release several inhibitors: PAI-1 destroys any free circulating t-PA, while PAI-2 inhibits u-PA. Both serve to limit the plasminogen activation primarily to the clot site. Another protein, circulating α_2-AP, neutralizes any free plasmin in the bloodstream, also restricting plasmin's activity to the wound site. Shown also are the pharmacologic fibrinolytic agents. Exogenous t-PA functions similarly to endogenous t-PA. Interestingly, streptokinase combines with plasminogen to create a complex that cleaves other plasminogen molecules to free circulating plasmin. As a result, systemic fibrinolysis is more common with this medication. Not shown is streptokinase formulated with exogenous acylated plasminogen, which spontaneously deacylates on mixing with the plasma to form the same streptokinase-plasminogen complex.

quite efficient at converting circulating plasminogen to plasmin, causing systemic fibrinolysis. It has been shown, however, that there is no greater mortality rate with this product than with t-PA when used for the treatment of acute myocardial infarction.[28]

A similar medication, anistreplase (anisoylated streptokinase plasminogen activator complex), is a combination of streptokinase with an acylated plasminogen, forming an inactive complex that spontaneously deacylates in plasma. The deacylated form is the same as the streptokinase-plasminogen complex previously discussed. Anistreplase has the advantage that it does not seem to be inhibited by endogenous serpins because of the acylated plasminogen protein, but it has the disadvantage that it still causes systemic fibrinolysis.[40]

The many available plasminogen activators have made possible effective treatment reducing ischemic myocardial necrosis if given within 30 to 60 minutes after the onset of chest pain.[28] There is a 47% success rate in thrombolysis if the products are given 1 hour from onset of symptoms. Results are poor if given after a 3- to 6-hour delay. Because intracoronary infusions require cardiac catheterization, intravenous administration of these agents has been investigated.[35] The disadvantage of their intravenous injection is that the fibrinolytic effect occurs throughout the body, thus placing the patient at risk for intracranial bleeding and other hemorrhagic sequelae. The use of fibrin-specific antibodies that can be conjugated to plasminogen activators may promote more specific thrombolysis at the site of thrombosis.

Antifibrinolytics

In some circumstances it is advantageous to limit fibrinolytic activity (e.g., after surgery in a hemophilic patient who may be prone to breakthrough bleeding as the wound heals). The drug used for this purpose is aminocaproic acid (sometimes referred to as *ε-aminocaproic acid*), which competitively inhibits plasminogen and plasminogen activators from binding to fibrin. Aminocaproic acid is a lysine analogue that binds to the plasminogen and plasmin, masking their ability to bind to fibrin. The usual dose of aminocaproic acid is 50 to 100 mg/kg every 6 hours for 10 days. In the tablet form (500 mg) this requires the average adult patient to take six or seven tablets every 6 hours. As a result, compliance can be difficult. A concentrated syrup form exists for pediatric use (250 mg/ ml), and experience indicates that adult patients generally are more compliant about taking the liquid form of the medication, especially after oral surgical procedures.

A related product, tranexamic acid, was available in the United States but has been removed indefinitely from the market. The drug has the advantages that it is more potent and less rapidly cleared by the kidneys, and so could be given in doses of 25 mg/kg every 8 hours for 10 days, thus improving compliance. The cost for a 10-day course is comparable to that of aminocaproic acid.

Side effects of these medications include unwanted thrombosis in patients who are prone to deep venous thrombosis and cardiovascular disease. Careful consideration and consultation with the physician is important before using these medications in such patients.

ANTICOAGULANTS

Although dentists are unlikely to ever prescribe an anticoagulant agent, it is essential that they be aware of any hemostatic deficiency in the patient, whether pathologic or therapeutic in origin. Anticoagulants are being used with ever-increasing frequency by the medical profession, and it is becoming common for dentists to encounter patients who are taking these medications. There are now three classes of anticoagulants in clinical use: direct-acting agents, which are capable of acting in vitro as well as in vivo; indirect-acting agents, which interfere with the synthesis of coagulation system proteins; and the platelet inhibitors, of which three subclasses exist: COX inhibitors, GP IIb/IIIa antagonists, and ADP receptor antagonists. Dentists should be familiar with the pharmacologic features of each class and understand if, how, and, more importantly, when their effects should be modified.

Direct-Acting Anticoagulants: Heparins

First extracted by McLean in 1916, heparin is at present the only systemically effective direct-acting anticoagulant. Although salts of ethylenediaminetetraacetic acid, citrate, and oxalate are useful Ca^{++} chelators and are routinely used in vitro to prevent clotting of blood samples taken for clinical testing, they cannot serve as systemic anticoagulants. They would indiscriminately bind free Ca^{++} necessary for muscle and nerve activity, causing tetany to occur before any anticoagulant action could be realized. Certainly, the development of a nontoxic synthetic alternative capable of heparinlike activity would be of tremendous value, but to date those drugs (heparinoids) that have been tested have invariably produced unacceptable side effects. Continuing advances in the understanding of heparin, however, suggest that the future of synthetic direct-acting anticoagulants is bright.

Heparin is a linear mucopolysaccharide primarily composed of repeating units of D-glucosamine in 1,4 glucosidic linkage with D-glucuronic and L-iduronic acid. These disaccharide residues, which are partially esterified (up to 40%) with sulfuric acid, make heparin the strongest organic acid normally occurring in the body. Ten to 15 of these chains, each with 200 to 300 monosaccharide units, are attached to a core protein to give the final proteoglycan as the storage form of heparin in mast cells. Because the polysaccharide chains are variable in length, and the sulfation reactions are variable, endogenous heparin is a heterogeneous mixture of molecules, with molecular weights varying from 4000 to 40,000, none of which has been completely characterized. At present, commercial preparations are made primarily from porcine intestinal mucosa and bovine lung, but recombinant DNA techniques will probably make this source obsolete. Figure 31-5 depicts one of 40 to 50 repetitive sequences found in commercial preparations, a pentasaccharide segment of heparin that is believed to include an essential binding site for anticoagulant activity.

Heparin is produced endogenously in mast cells, where it is stored in a large macromolecular form complexed with histamine. Both heparin and histamine are released together, providing a physiologic example of a fixed-drug combination, the significance of which is not yet fully understood. Many investigators have attempted to explain the in vivo maintenance of blood fluidity by the presence of heparin in plasma. Historically, such attempts have been frustrated by methodologic limitations and by the strong tendency of heparin to bind with various proteins. An important feature of heparin's activities, and one that is obscured by a narrow focus on plasma heparin concentrations, is the fact that the vascular epithelium can concentrate heparin against a gradient of 100 : 1. It has been proposed that adsorbed heparinlike mucopolysaccharides (termed the *heparans*) are major contributors to the normally strong electronegative charge maintained by the vascular epithelium. This property is made use of in the manufacture of such prosthetic devices as heart valves, in which ionizable heparin is incorporated into the surface plastic to inhibit thrombus generation.

Mechanism of action

Heparin appears to interfere with blood coagulation in several ways. Heparin functions by binding tightly to the plasma protease inhibitor ATIII, causing a conformational change in the

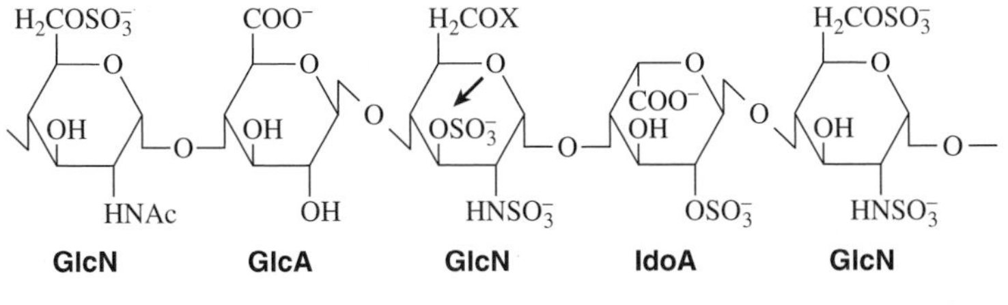

Fig. 31-5 Pentasaccharide sequence of heparin. This sequence, unique in its high affinity for ATIII (binding site indicated by *arrow*), also reflects the general structure of heparin: repeating units of sulfate-substituted glucosamine *(GlcN)*, glucuronic acid *(GlcA)*, and iduronic acid *(IdoA)* residues. *Ac*, Acetyl group; *X*, H or SO_3^-.

inhibitor that exposes its active site and accelerates its activity 1000-fold. ATIII is a "suicide" serine protease inhibitor that covalently binds the serine proteases (factors IXa, Xa, and XIIa), resulting in the permanent inactivation of both the protease and the ATIII protein. As a result, factor Xa–mediated conversion of prothrombin to thrombin does not occur, and, because thrombin is not available, factors V, VIII, and XIII are also not activated. In the form of a true catalyst, heparin is not destroyed in this process. The heparin-ATIII complex dissociates on binding of a protease to ATIII, releasing intact heparin for renewed binding to another ATIII molecule.

At higher concentrations, the heparin-ATIII complex binds to and inactivates thrombin itself (also a serine protease), inhibiting its proteolytic action on fibrinogen. Thrombin must form a ternary complex with the heparin-ATIII for this to occur, and only higher–molecular-weight moieties of heparin are capable of producing the effect; molecules of less than 18 monosaccharides are incapable of inhibiting thrombin. The effects of heparin on platelets are likewise complex. In part, because thrombin is not formed or is rendered inactive, platelet activation is usually reduced. More troubling, heparin may also sometimes induce a transient, anomalous platelet aggregation and significant thrombocytopenia in 1% to 5% of patients, independent of other aggregating agents. Two varieties of heparin-induced thrombocytopenia (HIT) exist: a relatively benign nonimmune process and an immune-mediated process. The latter, known as type II, can have as much as a 20% to 30% mortality rate. It is believed that complexing of the heparin to platelet factor 4 results in antibody formation and subsequent activation of the platelets. In this syndrome, the difficulty is not with bleeding but with runaway thrombosis. As the platelets activate, they form thrombi, which account for much of the clinical presentation. Of course, as the platelets are used up, thrombocytopenia occurs. Patients with a history of HIT are far more likely to have a repeat problem, as would be expected with immunologic phenomena.[24,59]

Heparin also exhibits the ability to promote lipid clearance from the bloodstream. In this capacity it releases and stabilizes lipoprotein lipase, which hydrolyzes the triglycerides of chylomicrons and very–low-density lipoproteins to free fatty acids, which can then be rapidly absorbed by tissue cells. This effect occurs at low physiologic blood concentrations, and it has been shown that all heparin molecules are capable of activating lipoprotein lipase, whereas only approximately 30% of heparin molecules in commercial fractions have anticoagulant properties. Because the anticoagulant property of heparin, as well as its antilipemic action, depends on the presence of ATIII in the plasma, heparin cannot act as an anticoagulant in a system composed of isolated clotting factors alone, and it cannot function as a lipemia-clearing agent in the absence of cofactor.

Low–molecular-weight heparins

Much research activity has focused upon the use of low–molecular-weight heparin (LMWH) fractions for the prevention of thrombosis.[3,18] Unfractionated heparin consists of heterogeneous combinations of various-sized sulfated mucopolysaccharides. Because only high–molecular-weight heparins (those with 18 or more specific saccharide sequences) can bind thrombin and inactivate it, attention has turned to the LMWHs. They are poor inhibitors of thrombin, but they do retain the ability to catalyze ATIII to inhibit the other serine proteases, most notably factor Xa. As a result, they have at least some advantage in that they have antithrombotic activity without completely destroying the coagulant activity thrombin imparts on factors V, VIII, XII, and XIII.[3,18] A problem with the LMWHs is that they are all prepared by fractionating heparin, and different methods impart different ratios of anticoagulant and antithrombotic activity.[17] Enoxaparin and dalteparin currently are the most commonly used medications in this class; the one selected by the physician will depend on the degree of anticoagulation desired for the patient.

Similar to the LMWHs, a new synthetic pentasaccharide, fondaparinux, has recently been marketed. This medication is a selective factor Xa inhibitor, and three studies have shown that it is more effective than enoxaparin in the prevention of deep venous thrombosis (with concurrent risk of pulmonary embolism) after hip and knee surgery.[1,15,36] Clearly, more specific products will likely be developed that mimic the basic actions of heparin.

Absorption, fate, and excretion

All available forms of heparin must be administered parenterally because they are highly charged and rapidly hydrolyzed in the gastrointestinal tract. Unfractionated heparin is usually infused intravenously but may be given by deep subcutaneous or fat depot injection. It should not be injected intramuscularly because of the risk of deep muscle hematoma. Heparin has a dose-dependent biologic half-life of 1 to 5 hours when given intravenously, and it is removed primarily by the liver. Two distinct advantages of the LMWHs are that they are generally administered subcutaneously, and their effects are prolonged compared with unfractionated heparin because they are less readily neutralized by platelet factor 4 (platelet antiheparin), which permits single- or twice-daily dosing. Moreover, LMWHs cause more release of t-PA and have less lipoprotein lipase–activating capacity than does the unfractionated drug.[3,58]

Heparin activity is best monitored by the partial thromboplastin (PTT) or the activated PTT (aPTT), both of which measure drug effects on the intrinsic pathway and are sensitive to low doses of heparin. The PTT is much less sensitive (or may be completely normal) to LMWHs, but fortunately there is less individual variability to the LMWHs, with body weight being highly correlated to amount of anticoagulation for a given dose. This allows standardized doses to achieve a more consistent anticoagulant effect, lessening the need for monitoring. The prothrombin time, routinely used to monitor oral (indirect-acting) anticoagulants, is of little value because it does not respond to inhibition of the thrombin-catalyzed part of the coagulation cascade, and heparin is diluted out in the procedure.

Antidotes

The action of heparin can be readily terminated by intravenous injection of one of several highly positively charged compounds, including protamine sulfate, toluidine blue dye, or hexadimethrine bromide. Only protamine, however, is currently recommended for this purpose. Protamine is a highly basic compound that combines with heparin as an ion pair to form a stable complex that can no longer bind to ATIII.[35] Because protamine may itself have anticoagulant (antithromboplastic) effects, only enough drug should be given to neutralize the heparin (approximately 1 mg protamine/100 units unfractionated heparin). The drug should be given intravenously but very slowly (5 mg/min) to avoid depression of the myocardium and vascular smooth muscle. Anticoagulant rebound is often seen after protamine administration because of more rapid clearance of protamine compared with heparin.

Other Direct-Acting Anticoagulants

Direct thrombin inhibitors

It has long been known that leeches secrete a potent anticoagulant in their saliva. In many centers, medicinal leeches (*Hirudo medicinalis*) are still used to help patients combat venous thromboembolic events. The active component has been isolated and identified as hirudin, a 65–amino-acid polypeptide chain that is a specific thrombin inhibitor. It works by stoichiometrically binding to thrombin at two sites, the fibrinogen-binding site and the active protease site. As such, it is the most powerful naturally occurring anticoagulant known.

Hirudin has many advantages over heparin. As a direct thrombin inhibitor, it is able to inhibit clot-bound thrombin that the heparin-ATIII complex cannot reach. As would be expected with a direct inhibitor, it also has caused more severe bleeds. A recombinant analogue, lepirudin, has been approved for the treatment of thrombosis associated with heparin-induced thrombocytopenia (HIT) syndrome. Unfortunately, up to 50% of the patients develop immunoglobulin G antibodies against the hirudins, so the aPTT must be monitored closely. Bivalirudin is a semisynthetic analogue consisting of 20 amino acids. It differs from hirudin in that it produces only transient inactivation of the thrombin protease site. Bivalirudin was recently shown to prevent blood clots better than did heparin in patients undergoing angioplasty.[9,48]

Several low–molecular-weight thrombin inhibitors have been developed. They bind to the active protease site of thrombin and inhibit its action. Argatroban is the only currently approved medication in this class, and it has been associated with an increased mortality rate when treating patients with HIT type II. Further clinical trials are underway.

Miscellaneous agents

Danaparoid functions similarly to heparin, but it is composed of a mixture of glycosaminoglycans, including heparan sulfate, dermatan sulfate, and chondroitin sulfate. It works primarily by binding with ATIII to diminish factor Xa activity and has been used for HIT type 2 treatment.

Lastly, aprotinin is a broad-spectrum protease inhibitor. It selectively blocks the activation of the major thrombin receptor PAR-1. As discussed earlier, this receptor is activated by thrombin cleaving a portion away, allowing the "new" N-terminus to autostimulate signal transduction. Aprotinin blocks this proteolytic cleavage, thus inhibiting the receptor from thrombin activation. It does not stop the platelet from ADP-, collagen-, or epinephrine-induced activation because those receptors do not require proteolytic cleavage, and thus does not fully inhibit clot formation. The medication is often used during cardiopulmonary bypass surgery because it helps protect the platelets from forming thrombi under the influence of thrombin liberated from platelets while in the bypass circuit.[38]

Indirect-Acting Anticoagulants: Coumarin-Indandiones

Discovery of the prothrombin-depressant action of spoiled sweet clover by Roderick in 1929 led to the isolation and synthesis of dicumarol (bishydroxycoumarin) by Campbell and Link in the 1940s. These advances introduced a new era of relatively inexpensive, self-administered oral anticoagulant therapy. Since then, several other coumarin compounds have been introduced, as have drugs of a related group, the indandiones. Because there is little qualitative difference in the action of any of these agents, they are referred to here as a single group, the coumarin-indandiones. The indandiones, however, are generally more toxic.

Mechanism of action

The indirect anticoagulants act by competitively inhibiting vitamin K epoxide reductase, an enzyme essential for the synthesis of many coagulation factors by the liver. (The structural similarity between these drugs and vitamin K is shown in Figure 31-6.) Vitamin K serves as a cofactor with oxygen and carbon dioxide in the γ-carboxylation of glutamic acid residues of several proteins, including the clotting factors II, VII, IX, and X, as well as proteins C and S. The carboxyglutamic acid moieties formed are able to chelate Ca^{++}, which promotes conformational change and eversion of hydrophobic domains, allowing the factors to settle into the platelet or endothelial cell membrane and bind cofactors. Vitamin K is oxidized in the carboxylation process, and must be reduced enzymatically to regain cofactor activity. The coumarin-indandiones inhibit this reduction (Figure 31-7).

The most sensitive indicator of vitamin K deficiency, or of dicumarol anticoagulation, is the depression of factor VII. Prothrombin (factor II) is the most resistant of the factors affected. This apparent ordering of sensitivity is a reflection of the plasma half-lives of the clotting factors. Factor VII is initially depressed because its half-life is only 4 to 8 hours. Prothrombin, with a half-life of 2 to 3 days, is the last to be diminished.

Because of the close relationship between hypovitaminosis K and spontaneous hemorrhaging in patients and animals receiving coumarin-indandione drugs, it is generally assumed that there is a direct causal relation between coagulation impairment and hemorrhage. This has never been proved, however, and there is reason to doubt that the incoagulability of blood per se is sufficient to cause spontaneously leaky vessels. It appears, in fact, that vitamin K may have physiologic functions not yet fully realized, including an important

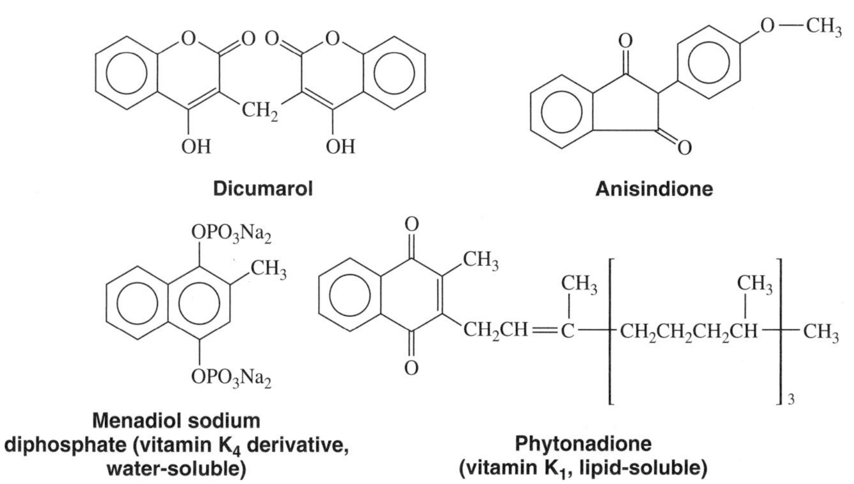

Dicumarol

Anisindione

Menadiol sodium diphosphate (vitamin K_4 derivative, water-soluble)

Phytonadione (vitamin K_1, lipid-soluble)

Fig. 31-6 Structural formulas of several indirect-acting anticoagulants and analogues of vitamin K.

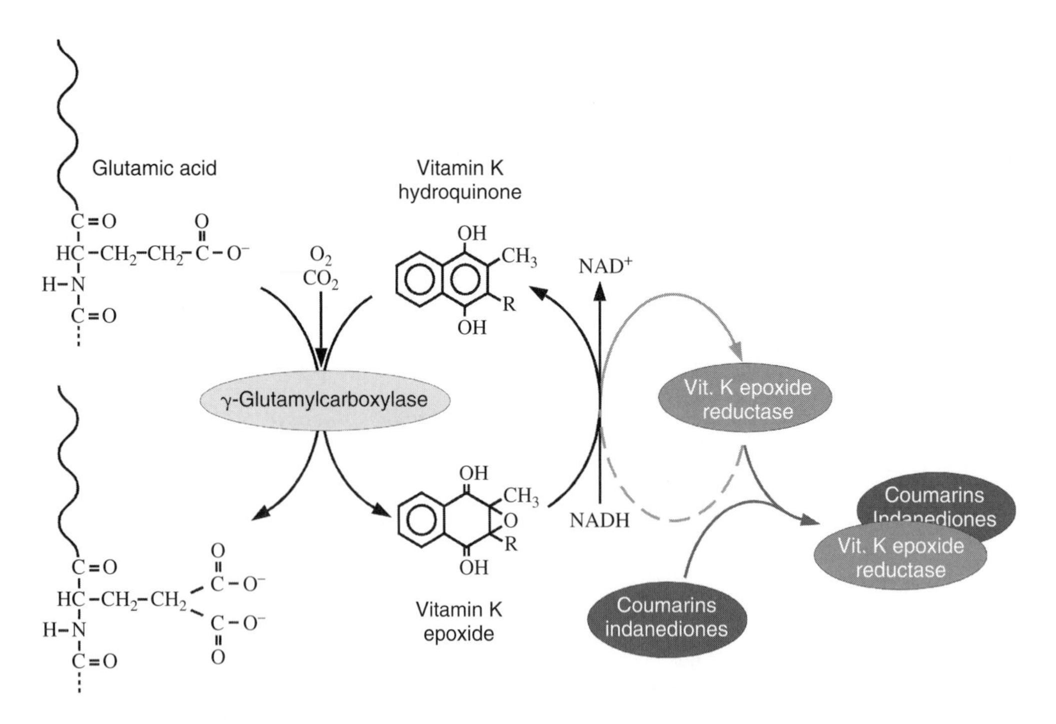

Fig. 31-7 Inhibition of synthesis of vitamin K–dependent clotting factors by coumarin-indandione anticoagulants. In the final posttranslational modification of prothrombin (factor II), factor VII, factor IX, factor X, protein C, and protein S, vitamin K is oxidized to the epoxide in the process of carboxylating glutamic acid residues on the amino end of each protein. The resultant γ-carboxyglutamic acid groups serve to chelate Ca^{++} ions and conformationally change to expose a hydrophobic domain that will settle into phospholipid membranes, anchoring the factors for normal hemostasis. The indirect-acting anticoagulants prevent the restoration of vitamin K by competitively inhibiting vitamin K epoxide reductase, the enzyme responsible for reducing vitamin K epoxide by nicotinamide adenine dinucleotide *(NADH)*. *R*, Hydrocarbon side chain of vitamin K.

role in carboxylation of bone proteins necessary for Ca^{++} binding.

Adverse effects

The indirect anticoagulants notably produce adverse reactions in the presence of certain drugs and medical conditions. These effects most often arise from interference with vitamin K absorption or metabolism, competition for the drug-binding sites of proteins, or competition for or activation of the hepatic microsomal enzymes responsible for biotransformation. By far the most important toxic effect of the coumarin-indandiones is hemorrhage.

Any change in the absorption or availability of vitamin K from the intestine obviously affects the balance between the anticoagulant and vitamin K in the liver and is reflected in the prothrombin time. A fall in vitamin K uptake may result from a disease such as sprue (biliary stasis with concomitant loss of fat-emulsifying bile salts) or from the use of mineral oil for laxation. In patients with marginal amounts of vitamin K in the diet, it can reflect the depressed bacterial synthesis of vitamin K in the intestine resulting from administration of a wide range of antimicrobial agents. Thus sensitivity to the coumarin-indandione drugs may be increased by sulfisoxazole, chloramphenicol, tetracycline, neomycin, and other bacteriostatic or bactericidal drugs, among others. A great deal of attention has been directed in recent years toward the effects of oral contraceptive agents on the blood coagulation mechanism. In this regard, it is interesting to note that oral estrogen, such as that used in contraceptive preparations, greatly increases vitamin K_1 absorption in experimental animals.[31] Estrogen also promotes procoagulant synthesis in animals with experimentally induced hypovitaminosis K; however, this finding does not appear to be very relevant clinically.[32]

The coumarin compounds are highly protein bound in the plasma (warfarin approximately 99%). This association creates a tremendous reserve of drug in the bloodstream, a very small displacement of which could easily double the concentration of active free drug. Many unrelated compounds that are highly protein-bound theoretically may complete for this protein binding by the coumarins and potentiate their action. Some antiinflammatory agents, the antiepileptic agent phenytoin, and clofibrate, a drug capable of lowering blood cholesterol, are examples of drugs reported to compete successfully with indirect anticoagulants for albumin binding sites. It has been suggested that part of the salicylate potentiation of dicumarol may also result from this kind of mechanism.

Only trace amounts (approximately 1%) of the coumarin-type anticoagulants are excreted unchanged; thus hepatic biotransformation serves as the principal route of elimination. Warfarin is a racemic mixture of both an R- and S-enantiomer. The R-enantiomer, a weak anticoagulant, is metabolized primarily by CYP1A2, with 2C19 and 3A4 providing minor pathways. The S-enantiomer, a potent anticoagulant, is metabolized by CYP 2C9.[25] Medications that either inhibit or induce these various hepatic microsomal enzymes affect the patient's response to warfarin. For example, certain agents, particularly rifampin, phenytoin, and the barbiturates (including phenobarbital, which is only partially metabolized), are capable of hepatic microsomal enzyme induction, which in turn tends to desensitize the patient to the coumarin compounds. Microsomal enzyme induction may also occur with chloral hydrate, ethanol, and other drugs. In some instances, a reverse sensitization may be demonstrated in which the coumarin compounds potentiate these and other drugs by inhibiting their metabolism through competition for microsomal enzymes or, more importantly, are potentiated, leading to overaccumulation of anticoagulant and generalized hemorrhaging. Various drug-warfarin interactions are listed in Box 31-2.

A number of other drug interactions involving oral anticoagulant agents do not involve vitamin K absorption, carrier protein displacement, or biotransformation. Anabolic steroids such as norethandrolone are thought to diminish

Box 31-2

Drug-Drug Interactions Involving Coumarin-Indandione Derivations

Drugs That May Increase Response of the Coumarin-Indandione Derivatives

Acetaminophen	Diflunisal	Ketoprofen	Sertraline
Alcohol (acute intoxication)	Disulfiram*	Lovastatin	Streptokinase
Allopurinol	Erythromycin	Meclofenamate	Sulfinpyrazone
Aminosalicylic acid	Ethacrynic acid	Mefenamic acid	Sulfonamides
Amiodarone*	Fenofibrate	Methylthiouracil	Sulindac
Anabolic steroids	Fenoprofen	Metronidazole*	Tamoxifen
Azithromycin	Fluoroquinolones	Miconazole	Tetracyclines
Capecitabine	Fluoxetine	Nalidixic acid	Thiazides
Cefixime	Flutamide	Neomycin (oral)	Thyroid drugs
Celecoxib	Fluvastatin	Pentoxifylline	Tramadol
Chloral hydrate	Fluvoxamine	Phenylbutazone*	Tricyclic antidepressants
Chloramphenicol	Gemfibrozil	Propafenone	Urokinase (u-PA)*
Cimetidine	Glucagon	Propoxyphene	Vitamin E
Clofibrate	Ibuprofen	Propylthiouracil	Zafirlukast
Cotrimoxazole	Indomethacin	Quinidine	Zileuton
Danazol	Influenza virus vaccine	Rofecoxib	
Diazoxide	Isoniazid	Salicylates*	

Dietary or Herbal Supplements That May Increase Response to Coumarin-Indandione Derivatives

Agrimony	Bromelains	Ginkgo biloba	Poplar
Alfalfa	Buchu	Ginseng (Panax)	Prickly ash (northern)
Aloe gel	Capsicum	Horse chestnut	Quassia
Angelica (dong quai)	Cassia	Horseradish	Red clover
Aniseed	Celery	Inositol nicotinate	Senega
Arnica	Chamomile (German/Roman)	Licorice	Sweet clover
Asafetida	Clove	Meadowsweet	Sweet woodruff
Aspen	Dandelion	Nettle	Tamarind
Black cohosh	Fenugreek	Onion	Tonka beans
Black haw	Feverfew	Parsley	Wild carrot
Bladder wrack (Fucus)	Garlic	Passion flower	Wild lettuce
Bogbean	German sarsaparilla	Pau d'arco	Willow
Boldo	Ginger	Policosanol	Wintergreen

Drugs That May Decrease Response to Coumarin-Indandione Derivatives

Alcohol (chronic alcoholism)*	Corticosteroids	Methaqualone	Spironolactone
Aminoglutethimide	Corticotropin	Nafcillin	Trazodone
Atorvastatin	Ethchlorvynol	Oral contraceptives containing estrogens*	Sucralfate
Barbiturates*	Glutethimide		Vitamin K
Carbamazepine	Griseofulvin	Raloxifene	
Clozapine	Mercaptopurine	Rifampin	

Dietary or Herbal Supplements That May Decrease Response to Coumarin-Indandione Derivatives

Agrimony	Goldenseal	Mistletoe	St. John's wort
Coenzyme q10 (ubidecarenone)		Yarrow	

*Concurrent use should be avoided if possible.
From *American Hospital Formulary Service Drug Information*, Bethesda, MD, 2002, American Society of Health-System Pharmacists.

procoagulant synthesis and increase the affinity of receptors for the oral anticoagulants. Aspirin is representative of drugs that inhibit platelet function. In addition to their potentiation of the anticoagulants, platelet inhibitors have potentially important antithrombotic effects of their own (discussed later). Finally, there are many still unexplained interactions, such as the lethal hemorrhagic effects of adrenocorticotropin, reserpine, and various stress situations.

Antidotes

Except where an emergency demands the replacement of whole blood or plasma, the usual antidote for coumarin-indandione toxicity is vitamin K administered parenterally in fairly high concentrations. Because the coumarin-indandiones inhibit recycling of vitamin K, simple administration of more "fresh" vitamin K obviates the need for recycling the epoxide form immediately. Unfortunately, this therapy depends on the temporal synthesis of clotting factors, and significant shortening of the prothrombin time cannot be expected to occur for several hours. Of the two major congeners, vitamin K_1 (naturally occurring, lipid-soluble phytonadione) and vitamin K_4 (as water-soluble menadiol salts), the more efficient drug is vitamin K_1. Natural vitamin K_1 is not water soluble, but it is now available in solubilized form (with a polyoxyethylated fatty acid derivative), thus reducing both the hazard of injecting an emulsion intravenously and the added delay of oral administration. Subcutaneous or intramuscular administration provides obvious improvement in coagulation in as little as 1 to 3 hours, but normal hemostasis may not be achieved for up to 24 hours.

Anticoagulants: General Pharmacologic Characteristics and Therapeutic Uses

The principal pharmacologic action of both the direct- and indirect-acting anticoagulants is interference with some step in the blood coagulation process. Beyond this, neither type has outstanding effects on the cardiovascular, respiratory, or other systems except in the case of the coumarin-type agents through competition with other drugs for protein binding sites and drug-metabolizing enzymes.

There are many indications in medicine for the use of anticoagulants, including myocardial infarction, cerebrovascular thrombosis, pulmonary embolism, venous thrombosis, rheumatic heart disease, mechanical cardiac valves, and renal dialysis. Cardiovascular compromise, such as that seen in atrial fibrillation or congestive heart failure, causes decreased flow of blood and therefore presents a greater risk for thrombosis in areas of stasis.[36] Atherosclerotic plaques, especially in hypertensive patients, are risks for intimal tears, with resultant thrombus formation. Both heparin and oral anticoagulants are useful in the treatment and prevention of these disorders. Heparin, although it is costly and requires parenteral administration, acts immediately and is more effective than coumarin-indandiones in arterial thrombosis. The oral anticoagulants, most commonly warfarin, provide a less expensive, more easily administered, and more readily controlled form of sustained therapy. It has become quite commonplace to see patients treated with anticoagulants for long periods of time for these various reasons, and anticoagulation clinics are a staple in most medical centers. The dentist must be able to manage such patients appropriately without causing undue harm either from excessive bleeding or increasing thrombosis risk.

PLATELET INHIBITORS

As is discussed in Chapter 21, drugs that interfere with platelet function are increasingly being recommended for prophylaxis of arterial and venous thrombosis. In recent years, many different agents have been developed and marketed with considerable success. These agents can be divided into three essential groups: the COX inhibitors, the ADP receptor inhibitors, and the GP IIb/IIIa inhibitors. Each has unique characteristics in managing thrombosis, and the dentist will undoubtedly find patients with one or more of these medications in their drug profiles.

Cyclooxygenase Inhibitors

Aspirin (acetylsalicylic acid) is the prototypic and most commonly recognized COX inhibitor. Inexpensive and readily available, it is prescribed in doses between 81 and 325 mg/day to reduce the risk of myocardial infarction, particularly in men with a history of unstable angina, or in any patient at risk for ischemic stroke. The antihemostatic effect of aspirin is ascribed to irreversible acetylation of COX isozyme 1 (COX-1). (Isozyme 2 is also inhibited but is involved in inflammatory and pain pathways. Note that aspirin is a more potent inhibitor of COX-1 than COX-2, which explains its ability to impart antithrombotic activity at much lower doses than pain control requires.) COX-1 is required to synthesize platelet TXA_2 from arachidonic acid. Disruption of this pathway results in decreased platelet ADP release and aggregation. Because platelets are incapable of synthesizing new COX, the inhibition by aspirin lasts for the life of the platelet. The seemingly fortuitous effect on TXA_2 may be offset theoretically by a similar inhibition of prostacyclin synthesis in the vascular endothelium, which could theoretically facilitate thrombotic activity. However, the nonreversible nature of this inhibition and the relative insensitivity of COX-2–dependent prostacyclin synthesis to aspirin removes this concern.

When aspirin therapy is used in combination with thrombolytic therapy after acute myocardial infarction, there are significant reductions in mortality rate and in the incidence of major complications.[47] Interestingly, ibuprofen has been shown to prevent the platelet inhibition of aspirin. In one study, aspirin was given either 2 hours before or 2 hours after acetaminophen, ibuprofen, or diclofenac. When ibuprofen was given before the aspirin, a 54% decrease in the TXB_2 (a stable metabolite of TXA_2) effect was seen. In all other arms of the study, no change was noted.[10]

ADP Receptor Inhibitors

As detailed earlier, ADP will bind to its own receptor proteins $P2Y_1$ and $P2Y_{12}$, which results in maximal aggregation of the platelets to one another. Two medications are currently available that irreversibly inhibit the $P2Y_{12}$ receptor by what is believed to be a covalent bond to the receptor. They are the thienopyridine compounds ticlopidine and clopidogrel. Both are inactive until metabolized in the liver to their active forms, and both have similar pharmacologic profiles. Because they only bind to the $P2Y_{12}$ receptor, the $P2Y_1$-mediated ADP effects still occur. This results in the platelets still undergoing shape change and transient aggregation, but sustained aggregation and potentiation of granule secretion is inhibited. Clinically, the patients are likely to have sustained bleeding as a result of the action of these drugs. No reversal agents are available. Because the inhibition lasts the lifetime of the platelet,[44] stopping antiplatelet therapy for 3 to 7 days before surgery should be considered. This will give the platelets time to turn over sufficient unaffected platelets.[20]

Glycoprotein IIb/IIIa Receptor Inhibitors

Activation of the GP IIb/IIIa receptors is a crucial near-final step in platelet aggregation, and platelets genetically deficient in these receptors (i.e., Glanzmann thrombasthenia) display a much more profound inhibition to aggregation than those altered by the relatively limited effects of aspirin or the thienopyridines. As a result, attention has been focused on developing agents that can antagonize the GP IIb/IIIa receptors. The first agent, a monoclonal antibody named *abciximab*, is a mouse-human chimeric protein. The highly variable region of the antibody is from the mouse and is directed against the human GP IIb/IIIa protein complex. However, the Fc region is human so as to not engender an immunogenic response. The medication has also been shown to bind to the vitronectin receptor on the endothelial cells, contributing further to its antithrombotic activity. No allergic or anaphylactic reactions have been reported, but the medication can result in severe thrombocytopenia.

Molecular analysis of the GP IIb/IIIa receptors indicates that they recognize a specific arginine-glycine-aspartic acid (RGD) sequence found in many of the adhesive molecules to which they bind (such as vWF). As a result, peptide analogues have been developed to bind at this RGD sequence and compete for the active sites. (The venom of several species of viper all contain peptides with similar RGD homologic features; these peptides are referred to as *disintegrins* and are known to bind to the GP IIb/IIIa receptors as well in an antagonistic fashion.)[53] Cyclic peptides bind better than linear ones, and one that is currently available is the peptide eptifibatide. Rather than an RGD sequence, it has a lysine-glycine-aspartic acid (KGD) sequence that imparts improved specificity for the GP IIb/IIIa receptor.

Finally, a variety of nonpeptide agents that can compete for binding with the GP IIb/IIIa receptor have been developed. Like eptifibatide, they have structure and charge characteristics that mimic the RGD sequence and therefore compete for the receptor's docking. Not being peptides, they have the advantage that they might be engineered to be orally acting. Currently, tirofiban (a tyrosine derivative) and lamifiban have been approved, with xemilofiban and sibrafiban in clinical trials.

Herbal and Dietary Supplements

There is great academic interest in the surging herbal and dietary supplement use in current society and whether these agents may have pharmacologic action. Many of these agents have been implicated in directly modifying the coagulation status of patients or indirectly interacting with Western medications to increase or decrease their pharmacokinetic profiles (see Box 31-2). Chapter 56 details the current knowledge about many of these compounds. As more data become available, it will be necessary for the dentist to be knowledgeable about what these medications might do in the patient who requires dentoalveolar or other oral surgery.

IMPLICATIONS FOR DENTISTRY

Anticoagulants

There are no accepted indications for the use of anticoagulants in the practice of dentistry. However, many patients requiring dental treatment receive some form of medical anticoagulation therapy for the reasons previously cited. Such patients present three kinds of problems to the dentist: their therapeutic regimen may result in excessive bleeding after oral and periodontal surgery unless there is appropriate prior modification; modification of their therapeutic regimen in preparation for surgery may predispose them to thromboembolic events; and they may present a real danger of drug interaction between their anticoagulants and agents commonly used in dental practice, such as some antibiotics, sedatives, and analgesics. It is essential for the dentist to have a complete and thorough knowledge of the patient's drug history and what options are available when treating patients in whom anticoagulant therapy is involved.

Any intended oral surgical therapy in anticoagulated patients requires preliminary planning and consultation with the patient's physician. The coumarin-indandione anticoagulants are monitored by the prothrombin time, which is now expressed in international normalized ratio (INR) units. The prothrombin test is performed by adding a source of TF and Ca^{++} to a patient's citrated blood sample and measuring the amount of time necessary to coagulate the sample. Previously, this value has been expressed in seconds or as a ratio of the patient's value to a laboratory-specific control. Because various laboratories use TF from different sources (human, rabbit, recombinant), there have been wide variations in the reported values and the resulting amount of anticoagulation. In an effort to normalize the activity of the various forms of TF, a formula has been developed that accounts for the various inherent sensitivities of TF as well as individual laboratory methods. The resultant ratio, the INR, can be compared with any other INR value with high accuracy.[2] The test should not be called "the INR" because the assay is a measurement of prothrombin time, with the results reported as an INR. Other tests, such as the aPTT, will likely have INR units attached to them soon.

Because the prothrombin time INR is derived from an exponential formula, small changes in anticoagulation result in large changes in the INR value as the anticoagulation progresses. It is generally agreed that for the coumarin-indandiones a prothrombin time INR value of 2.5 to 3.0 is considered ideal. Prosthetic heart valves and other instances in which more anticoagulation is required may have a target value of 3.5 to 4.0, with higher values being acceptable.[60] Although there are no official recommendations from the American Dental Association on the topic of prothrombin time INR and dental treatment, one report[8] recommends that an INR of 4.0 be used as the upper limit for simple oral surgical procedures and that a maximum of 3.0 be targeted for procedures likely to result in significant blood loss, such as multiple extractions with alveoloplasty. The authors state, and several others have agreed,[8,14,34,60] that it is unusual to have significant clinical bleeding when the INR is less than 3.0 (Figure 31-8).

If a patient is anticoagulated to a high prothrombin time INR value, the dentist may wish to consult with the physician about the possibility of reducing the anticoagulation to an INR of 3.0 or less. A unilateral request by a dentist for a patient to discontinue or decrease coumarin without consulting the physician is at best poor medical practice because, even if the coumarin is ultimately to be decreased, the physician is the appropriate person to alter and follow the dosages perioperatively. This adjustment may take several days to a week to accomplish. Current medical practice often places the responsibility of the anticoagulation management with an anticoagulation clinic that tracks the prothrombin time INR on a consistent basis, and as such is a reliable resource to help guide the dentist and patient in making therapeutic decisions. Some patients have erratic responses to the coumarin class of anticoagulants, with unpredictable highs and lows in their INR despite the best efforts of the medical team to stabilize it. In these patients, the prudent dentist will obtain a prothrombin time INR on the day of surgery and be prepared to reschedule the appointment if the value is too high to be safe. In the emergent patient, reversal with vitamin K and use of local hemostatic measures (collagen plugs, suturing, topical thrombin, fibrin sealant) may be indicated; in severe cases the administration of fresh frozen plasma may be necessary.

If the anticoagulant is heparin, the drug may be totally withheld for a period of 1 to 6 hours (this is dose dependent; consult with the medical doctor), or a coumarin agent may be gradually substituted before surgery. If the heparin is to be restarted after surgery, typically waiting at least 1 hour is advisable to allow the clot time to fully form. The use of local hemo-

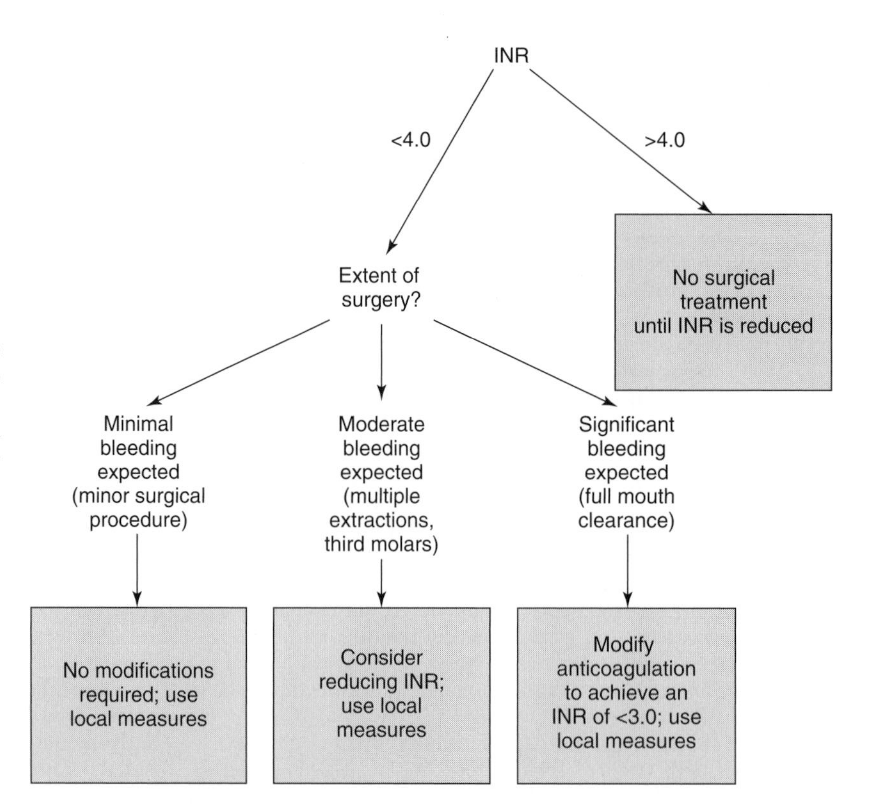

Fig. 31-8 Flow chart for determining the appropriateness of dental therapy based on the INR of the prothrombin time. (From Beirne OR, Koehler JR: Surgical management of patients on warfarin sodium, *J Oral Maxillofac Surg* 54:1115-1118, 1996.)

static agents may be considered for further hemorrhage control and, in rare cases, protamine infusion may be necessary.

Patients who are taking an LMWH such as enoxaparin have an interesting dilemma. Because LMWHs stimulate ATIII to be active against factor Xa but have relatively little stimulation of the enzyme against thrombin (factor IIa), the prothrombin time and aPTT in these patients are both usually normal. In fact, a special factor Xa assay (costly and not always available in every medical center) is used to monitor these medications when needed. The question arises, then: What should a dentist do when patients are using these agents on a daily basis? Data are limited; one author suggests that the LMWH should be discontinued for 12 hours before the surgical event.[57] However, it could be argued that for simple surgical procedures (dentoalveolar surgery, periodontal surgery), if there is sufficient thrombin generation to maintain the aPTT at a normal value, then perhaps no adjustment to the regimen needs to be made. Until further data become available, it is advisable to discuss each situation with the physician and arrive at a consensus decision.

Similar lack of clinical data exists for dentoalveolar surgery when patients are taking antiplatelet medications such as the thienopyridines and the various GP IIb/IIIa inhibitors. Because platelet inhibition can result in profound clinical bleeding, it is advisable to contact the physician and discuss strategies for limiting the risk to the patient. As previously discussed, many of these agents irreversibly alter the platelets, so between 3 and 7 days off these medications may be necessary to ensure a good response. Local measures coupled with platelet transfusion as required may be necessary if the clinical situation is emergent or too risky to have the patients off these medications for several days.

Hemophilics

Managing the patient with hemophilia and other coagulopathies has become significantly easier in recent years, but many issues require careful consideration before proceeding. Patients who were once believed to be inoperable are now being routinely treated in many hospitals and dental offices. The most difficult problem a hemophilic faces is not the threat of exsanguination from a small laceration, but rather the problems encountered from a massive muscle bleed or chronic joint disease resulting from hemarthroses. In the dental arena, there are many procedures that potentially can cause significant bleeding in a hemophilic. Surgical procedures, of course, must be planned so that replacement factor can be given preoperatively and postoperatively. It is recommended that tight primary closure not be used so that any accumulation of blood will preferentially drain into the oral cavity and be identified rather than fill critical spaces in the head and neck region. Similarly, the dentist must take care that simple nerve block injections of local anesthetic are adequately covered by factor replacement to reduce the risk of hemorrhage into one of the parapharyngeal areas. The use of a commercial intraosseous anesthetic delivery system is a rational consideration for patients in whom block anesthesia is contraindicated. Profound anesthesia can usually be easily obtained with minimal hemorrhage risk when these systems are used in hemophilic patients.

Associated disorders that commonly occur with hemophilics may affect the delivery of dental care as well. Hemophilics often have associated joint disorders from hemarthrosis. Any spontaneous or trauma-induced bleeding into the synovial space of a joint may cause permanent damage if inflammatory by-products, produced as the blood breaks down, damage the surrounding cartilaginous and bony structures. Knees, ankles, and elbows are the most commonly affected, and many hemophilics have permanent limitation of motion in their joints by the time they reach adulthood. Joint replacement surgery is common in the older population of severe hemophilic patients. As a result, mobility in and out of the operatory, and positioning in the chair itself, may be compromised.

Because of the historic necessity of transfusing hemophilics with pooled human blood products before recombinant factor replacements were available or the products were treated with heat or solvent detergent to inactivate viruses, many hemophilic patients were infected with HIV, hepatitis

B, and hepatitis C viruses. Seroconversion to HIV began around 1979 and accelerated rapidly until the mid-1980s. Many of these patients have since died. Screening donors for hepatitis B began in the 1970s, in 1985 for HIV, and in 1990 for hepatitis C. This has significantly reduced the viral risk but it has not eliminated it. Noninfected hemophilics (primarily children and teens) are now being given the more expensive recombinant factor replacements, whereas infected hemophilics more often select the pooled human-derived, virally inactivated products. In uninfected patients in whom no recombinant factor replacement is available, and especially in families with vWD that is not responsive to desmopressin, the use of single-donor cryoprecipitate (usually a family member) for all necessary transfusions has proved effective in reducing the risk for viral transmission.

When surgical procedures are required in hemophilic patients, it is imperative that the dentist work closely with a hematologist well versed in the care of these patients. The dentist should describe the nature of the proposed surgery, the expected amount of bleeding, and the normal postoperative course after the procedure. In this way, a hemophilia treatment center can best plan how much and which kinds of factor replacement (or other pharmacologic intervention, such as desmopressin) are most appropriate. Depending on the training, location (office versus hospital), and experience of the treating dentist, the blood product or factor replacement may be given in the dental office, the medical office, or perhaps at home by the patient. Most of the products have an in vivo half-life of several hours, allowing the patient to receive the product at another site and then go to the dental office for treatment with no reduction in hemostatic ability.

The normal healing mechanism of a wound site involves breakdown and reestablishment of newer fibrin matrixes as

Agents That Affect Coagulation and Hemostasis

Nonproprietary (generic) name	*Proprietary (trade) name*
Astringents-styptics	
Aluminum chloride	Hemodent
Negatol	Negatan
Tannic acid compound	Amertan
Vasoconstrictor	
Epinephrine	Adrenalin
Topical procoagulants	
Absorbable gelatin film	Gelfilm
Absorbable gelatin powder	Gelfoam
Absorbable gelatin sponge	Gelfoam, SURGIFOAM
Carboxymethylcellulose	In Orabase
Microfibrillar collagen	Avitene
Oxidized cellulose	Oxycel
Oxidized regenerated cellulose	Surgicel
Thrombin	Thrombin-JMI, Thrombogen
Systemic procoagulants	See Table 31-4
Fibrinolytics	
Alteplase (t-PA)	Activase
Anistreplase	Eminase
Fibrinolysin, human	in Elase
Reteplase	Retavase
Streptokinase	Streptase
Tenecteplase	TNKase
Urokinase (u-PA)	Abbokinase
Fibrinolysis inhibitors	
Aminocaproic acid	Amicar
Aprotinin	Trasylol
Tranexamic acid*	Cyklokapron
Direct-acting anticoagulants	
Unfractionated heparin, heparinoids	
Danaparoid	Organ
Heparin†	—
LMWHs	
Ardeparin	Normiflo
Dalteparin	Fragmin
Enoxaparin	Lovenox
Fondaparinux	Arixtra
Tinzaparin	Innohep
Direct thrombin inhibitors	
Argatroban	Novastan
Bivalirudin	Angiomax
Hirudin	*Hirudo medicinalis*‡
Lepirudin	Refludan
Indirect-acting anticoagulants	
Anisindione	Miradon
Dicumarol (bishydroxycoumarin)	—
Phenindione*	Hedulin
Warfarin	Coumadin
Antidotes for anticoagulants	
Menadiol* (vitamin K_4)	Synkayvite
Phytonadione (vitamin K_1)	AquaMEPHYTON, Konakion
Protamine sulfate	—
Platelet inhibitors	
Abciximab	ReoPro
Aspirin	—
Clopidogrel	Plavix
Dipyridamole	Persantine
Eptifibatide	Integrilin
Lamifiban*	—
Sibrafiban*	—
Ticlopidine	Ticlid
Tirofiban	Aggrastat
Xemilofiban*	—

*Not currently available in the United States.
†Available in calcium and sodium salts.
‡Organism of origin.

the tissue heals. In a patient with a coagulopathy, the normal breakdown of fibrin can result in a rebleeding episode a few days later. Stabilization of the clot with an antifibrinolytic medication such as aminocaproic acid helps reduce the incidence of bleeding episodes several days postoperatively. In many cases, the use of aminocaproic acid can greatly reduce or eliminate the need for additional blood or factor replacement. The recommended dose is 100 mg/kg in children and 6 g every 6 hours for adults, but lower doses (e.g., 50% of the recommended dose) may be sufficient. Adjunctive measures, such as the use of local hemostatic agents (microfibrillar collagen, suturing, or fibrin sealant[46]), may be helpful as well.

Cited References

1. Bauer K, Eriksson BI, Lassen MR, et al: Fondaparinux compared with enoxaparin for the prevention of venous thromboembolism after elective major knee surgery, *N Engl J Med* 345:1305-1310, 2001.
2. Beirne OR, Koehler JR: Surgical management of patients on warfarin sodium, *J Oral Maxillofac Surg* 54:1115-1118, 1996.
3. Bergqvist D: Low molecular weight heparins, *J Intern Med* 240:63-72, 1996.
4. Bick RL: Disseminated intravascular coagulation and related syndromes: a clinical review, *Semin Thromb Hemost* 14:299-338, 1988.
5. Blockmans D, Deckmyn H, Vermylen J: Platelet activation, *Blood Rev* 9:143-156, 1995.
6. Bornstein P: Thrombospondins: structure and regulation of expression, *FASEB J* 6:3290-3299, 1992.
7. Brennan M: Fibrin glue, *Blood Rev* 5:240-244, 1991.
8. Campbell J, Alvarado F, Murray RA: Anticoagulation and minor oral surgery: should the anticoagulation regimen be altered? *J Oral Maxillofac Surg* 58:131-135, 2000.
9. Carswell C, Plosker GL: Bivalirudin: a review of its potential place in the management of acute coronary syndromes, *Drugs* 62:841-870, 2002.
10. Catella-Lawson F, Reilly MD, Kapoor SC, et al: Cyclooxygenase inhibitors and the antiplatelet effects of aspirin, *N Engl J Med* 345:1809-1817, 2001.
11. Collen D, Topol EJ, Tiefenbrunn AJ, et al: Coronary thrombolysis with recombinant human tissue-type plasminogen activator: a prospective, randomized, placebo-controlled trial, *Circulation* 70:1012-1017, 1984.
12. Davie EW, Fujikawa K, Kisiel W: The coagulation cascade: initiation, maintenance, and regulation, *Biochemistry* 30:10363-10370, 1991.
13. DeGroot PG, Sixma JJ: Platelet adhesion, *Br J Haematol* 75:308-312, 1990.
14. Devani P, Lavery KM, Howell CJ: Dental extractions in patients on warfarin: is alteration of anticoagulant regime necessary? *Br J Oral Maxillofac Surg* 36:107-111, 1998.
15. Eriksson B, Bauer KA, Lassen MR, et al: Fondaparinux compared with enoxaparin for the prevention of venous thromboembolism after hip-fracture surgery, *N Engl J Med* 345:1298-1304, 2001.
16. Esmon CT: The regulation of natural anticoagulant pathways, *Science* 235:1348-1352, 1987.
17. Fareed J, Hoppensteadt DA: Are the available low-molecular-weight heparin preparations the same? *Semin Thromb Hemost* 22(suppl 1):77-91, 1996.
18. Frydman A: Low-molecular-weight heparins: an overview of their pharmacodynamics, pharmacokinetics, and metabolism in humans, *Haemostasis* 26(suppl 2):24-38, 1996.
19. Furie B, Limentani SA, Rosenfeld CG: A practical guide to the evaluation and treatment of hemophilia, *Blood* 84:3-9, 1994.
20. Gachet C: ADP receptors of platelets and their inhibition, *Thromb Haemost* 86:222-232, 2001.
21. George JN, Nurden AT, Phillips DR: Molecular defects in interactions of platelets with the vessel wall, *N Engl J Med* 311:1084-1098, 1984.
22. Gill JC: Therapy of factor VIII deficiency, *Semin Thromb Hemost* 19:1-12, 1993.
23. Ginsburg D, Bowie EJW: Molecular genetics of von Willebrand disease, *Blood* 79:2507-2519, 1992.
24. Hammeke M: Heparin-induced thrombocytopenia type II: criteria for diagnosis and options for treatment, *University of Washington Drug Therapy Topics* 31:11-16, 2002.
25. Hansen P, Horn J: Drug interaction tables, *University of Washington Academic Medical Center drug formulary,* ed 18, Seattle, WA, 2001, University of Washington, p 49-55.
26. Harrison P, Cramer EM: Platelet α-granules, *Blood Rev* 7:52-62, 1993.
27. Hathaway WE, Goodnight SH, Jr: *Disorders of hemostasis and thrombosis: a clinical guide,* New York, 1993, McGraw-Hill.
28. Hazinski MF, Cummins RO, Field JM, eds: *2000 Handbook of emergency cardiac care for healthcare providers,* Dallas, 2000, American Heart Association.
29. Hillman R, Ault K: *Hematology in clinical practice,* ed 3, New York, 2002, McGraw Hill.
30. Jeansonne BG, Boggs WS, Lemon RR: Ferric sulfate hemostasis: effect on osseous wound healing. II. With curettage and irrigation, *J Endod* 19:174-176, 1993.
31. Jolly DW, Craig C, Nelson TE, Jr: Estrogen and prothrombin synthesis: effect of estrogen on absorption of vitamin K_1, *Am J Physiol* 232:H12-H17, 1977.
32. Jolly DW, Kadis BM, Nelson TE, Jr: Estrogen and prothrombin synthesis. The prothrombinogenic action of estrogen, *Biochem Biophys Res Commun* 74:41-49, 1977.
33. Kay MA, Rothenberg S, Landen CN, et al: In vivo gene therapy of hemophilia B: sustained partial correction in factor IX-deficient dogs, *Science* 262:117-119, 1993.
34. Kearon C, Hirsch J: Management of anticoagulation before and after elective surgery, *N Engl J Med* 336:1506-1511, 1997.
35. Kennedy JW, Gensini GG, Timmis GC, et al: Acute myocardial infarction treated with intracoronary streptokinase: a report of the Society for Cardiac Angiography, *Am J Cardiol* 55:871-877, 1985.
36. Klein A, Grimm RA, Murray RD, et al: Use of transesophageal echocardiography to guide cardioversion in patients with atrial fibrillation, *N Engl J Med* 344:1411-1420, 2001.
37. Kottke-Marchant K, Corcoran G: The laboratory diagnosis of platelet disorders, *Arch Pathol Lab Med* 126:133-146, 2002.
38. Landis RC, Haskard DO, Taylor KM: New anti-inflammatory and platelet–preserving effects of aprotinin, *Ann Thorac Surg* 72:S1808-1813, 2001.
39. Lemon RR, Steele PJ, Jeansonne BG: Ferric sulfate hemostasis: effect on osseous wound healing. I. Left in situ for maximum exposure, *J Endod* 19:170-173, 1993.

40. Loscalzo J: An overview of thrombolytic agents, *Chest* 97(suppl):117S-123S, 1990.
41. Lynch TJ: Biotechnology: alternatives to human plasma-derived therapeutic proteins, *Baillieres Best Pract Res Clin Haematol* 13:669-688, 2000.
42. Macik BG: Treatment of factor VIII inhibitors: products and strategies, *Semin Thromb Hemost* 19:13-24, 1993.
43. Morawitz P: *Die Chemie der Blutgerinnung, Ergebnisse der Physiologie, Biologischen Chemie, und Experimentellen Pharmakologie* 4:307-422, 1905.
44. O'Reilly RA: Drugs used in disorders of coagulation. In Katzung BG, ed: *Basic and clinical pharmacology,* ed 6, Norwalk, CT, 1995, Appleton & Lange.
45. Parise L, Smyth SS, Coller BS: Platelet morphology, biochemistry and function, In Beutler E, Lichtman MA, Coller BS, et al, eds: *Williams Hematology,* ed 6, New York, 2001, McGraw-Hill.
46. Rakocz M, Mazar A, Varon D, et al: Dental extractions in patients with bleeding disorders. The use of fibrin glue, *Oral Surg Oral Med Oral Pathol* 75:280-282, 1993.
47. Ranjadayalan K, Umachandran V, Timmis AD: Clinical impact of introducing thrombolytic and aspirin therapy into the management policy of a coronary care unit, *Am J Med* 92:233-238, 1992.
48. Raskob G, Hull RD, Pineo GF: Heparin, hirudin, and related agents. In Beutler E, Lichtman MA, Coller BS, et al, eds: *Williams Hematology,* ed 6, New York, 2001, McGraw-Hill.
49. Roth D, Tawa NE, Jr, O'Brien JM, et al: Nonviral transfer of the gene encoding coagulation factor VIII in patients with severe hemophilia A, *N Engl J Med* 344:1735-1742, 2001.
50. Schmidt A: Neue Untersuchung über die Faserstoffgerinnung, *Pfluegers Archiv fur die Gesamte Physiologie des Menschen und der Tiere* 6:413-420, 1872.
51. Scott JP, Montgomery RR: Therapy of von Willebrand disease, *Semin Thromb Hemost* 19:37-47, 1993.
52. Sindet-Pedersen S, Ramstrom G, Bernvil S, et al: Hemostatic effect of tranexamic acid mouthwash in anticoagulant-treated patients undergoing oral surgery, *N Engl J Med* 320:840-843, 1989.
53. Smith JB, Theakston RD, Coelho AL, et al: Characterization of a monomeric disintegrin, ocellatusin, present in the venom of the Nigerian carpet viper, *Echis ocellatus, FEBS Lett* 512:111-115, 2002.
54. Thompson AR: Factor IX concentrates for clinical use, *Semin Thromb Hemost* 19:25-36, 1993.
55. Thompson AR: Molecular biology of the hemophilias, *Prog Hemost Thromb* 10:175-214, 1991.
56. Thompson AR: Recombinant factor IX for the treatment of hemophilia B, *Semin Hematol* 35:(suppl 2):1-3, 1998.
57. Todd D, Roman A: Outpatient use of low-molecular weight heparin in an anticoagulated patient requiring oral surgery: case report, *J Oral Maxillofac Surg* 59:1090-1092, 2001.
58. Walsh PN: Platelet-mediated coagulant protein interactions in hemostasis, *Semin Hematol* 22:178-186, 1985.
59. Warkentin T, Kelton JG: Temporal aspects of heparin-induced thrombocytopenia, *N Engl J Med* 344:1286-1292, 2001.
60. Webster K, Wilde J: Management of anticoagulation in patients with prosthetic heart valves undergoing oral and maxillofacial operations, *Br J Oral Maxillofac Surg* 38:124-126, 2000.
61. Woody RD, Miller A, Staffanou RS: Review of the pH of hemostatic agents used in tissue displacement, *J Prosthet Dent* 70:191-192, 1993.
62. Wu KK, Thiagarajan P: Role of endothelium in thrombosis and hemostasis, *Annu Rev Med* 47:315-331, 1996.

General References

Beutler E, Lichtman MA, Coller BS, et al, eds: *Williams Hematology,* ed 6, New York, 2001, McGraw-Hill.

Hillman RS, Ault KA: *Hematology in clinical practice,* ed 3, New York, 2002, McGraw-Hill.

Majerus PW, Tollefesen, DM: Anticoagulant, thrombolytic, and antiplatelet drugs. In Hardman JG, Limbird LE, Gilman AG, eds: *Goodman and Gillman's The pharmacological basis of therapeutics,* ed 10, New York, 2001, McGraw-Hill.

McEvoy G, Miller J: *American Hospital Formulary Service Drug Information 2002,* Bethesda, MD, 2002, American Society of Health-System Pharmacists.

Ravel R: *Clinical laboratory medicine: clinical application of laboratory data,* ed 6, St Louis, 1995, Mosby.

Tierney LM, Jr, McPhee SJ, Papadakis MA, eds: *Current medical diagnosis & treatment,* ed 41, Stamford, CT, 2002, Lange Medical Books/McGraw-Hill.

CHAPTER • 32

Drugs Acting on the Respiratory System*

Bruno Kreiner and Jeffrey D. Bennett

A variety of drugs exert direct or indirect effects on the respiratory system. This chapter focuses on agents used to support or stimulate respiration, medications for the asthmatic patient, and drugs that improve ventilation or provide symptomatic relief from respiratory infection or obstruction. The basic pharmacologic features of some drugs discussed here are presented in other chapters.

AGENTS USED TO SUPPORT OR STIMULATE RESPIRATION

Oxygen

Oxygen is a colorless, odorless, and tasteless gas. Although it is not flammable, it vigorously supports combustion. Oxygen is an essential emergency drug in the dental office and is indicated in all emergencies other than hyperventilation syndrome. The deprivation of oxygen by any mechanism is termed *hypoxia*.

A reduction of both arterial blood oxygen tension (PaO_2) and total oxygen content (hypoxic hypoxia) can develop by several mechanisms. Inadequate oxygenation of normal lung tissue can occur as a result of (1) airway obstruction by a foreign body, edema, or bronchial constriction; (2) insufficient pulmonary ventilation as a complication of disease or depression of respiration by morphine or similar drugs; (3) deficiency of oxygen in the inspired air, such as at high altitudes; or (4) inadequate oxygenation caused by abnormal pulmonary function (e.g., in pulmonary edema, pulmonary fibrosis, or emphysema) or anatomic arteriovenous shunts (e.g., in congenital heart disease).

Administration of oxygen is most effective when hypoxia is a result of insufficient pulmonary ventilation. It is of benefit as an adjunctive agent in supporting the cardiovascular system when hypoxia is a result of impaired circulation.

The central nervous system (CNS) is particularly vulnerable to the effects of hypoxia. As the PaO_2 decreases, mental aberrations, impaired judgment, disorientation, loss of visual acuity and sense of time, and impaired coordination occur. Loss of consciousness ensues when the oxygen saturation of hemoglobin decreases acutely to approximately 65%. (The rapidity of the fall in PaO_2, as well its absolute value, is important because the CNS may adapt to chronic oxygen deprivation.) Cyanosis may or may not be evident. Approximately 5 g of unoxygenated hemoglobin are usually required in adults to show signs of cyanosis. This amount typically requires a total hemoglobin concentration of approximately 14 g/dl, with a hemoglobin oxygen saturation of 65%.

Cerebral hypoxia, produced in animals by the arrest of cerebral circulation, causes unconsciousness within seconds. Arrest for even 2 minutes has been shown experimentally to produce histologic changes in the cerebral cortex and blood vessels. Some return of function occurred in animals surviving 6 minutes of cephalic stasis, but in those surviving 8 minutes, irreversible damage resulted, and consciousness was never restored.[21]

Adverse effects

There are situations, more likely to be encountered in the hospital than in the dental office, when the administration of oxygen can produce untoward effects. Although every cell is a potential target for oxygen toxicity, cells of the respiratory tract are uniquely susceptible to oxygen's cytotoxic effects because they are exposed to the greatest concentration of the gas. The cytotoxicity of oxygen is believed to result from partially reduced oxygen products (free radicals) generated during normal cellular metabolism. The partially reduced oxygen products, including the superoxide anion, hydrogen peroxide, and the hydroxyl radical, interact with tissue components to damage cellular integrity and function. Oxygen toxicity develops as a function of the concentration and duration of administration.

One manifestation of oxygen toxicity is respiratory tract irritation, which can occur after inhalation of 80% to 100% oxygen at atmospheric pressure for 12 to 24 hours. A progressive decrease in vital capacity is accompanied by a sore throat, coughing, nasal congestion, and substernal pain. Continued administration of oxygen at high concentrations is likely to produce even more severe complications. On the other hand, long-term administration of oxygen at a concentration of 50% or less does not produce these severe effects (although ciliary dysfunction probably occurs at oxygen concentrations of 30% or more).

In some clinical situations the response of the medullary respiratory centers to carbon dioxide is so depressed that respiration is maintained by the reflex hypoxic stimulus mediated by the carotid body and aortic arch chemoreceptors. Chronic pulmonary disease or severe barbiturate overdosage may present such a situation. The administration of oxygen here may eliminate the hypoxic drive to respiration and produce apnea and respiratory acidosis. These problems can be circumvented by provision of artificial ventilation along with oxygen therapy.

Premature infants who require oxygen supplementation for any substantial length of time are usually not exposed to oxygen concentrations greater than 40%. Oxygen is administered only to those infants who need it and for the shortest time possible because a high concentration of oxygen is considered to be a factor in the development of retrolental fibroplasia and, ultimately, blindness.[53] Retinal damage can

*The authors wish to recognize Dr. Glenn Housholder for her past contributions to this chapter. See the Acknowledgments.

also occur in adults if 100% oxygen is inhaled at hyperbaric conditions (pressures of 2 to 3 atm). The patient with compromised retinal circulation is particularly susceptible.

Long-term low-flow oxygen therapy

Long-term low-flow oxygen therapy (LTOT) has emerged as a useful tool in the care of selected patients with chronic obstructive lung disease.[59,60] Technologic improvements in oxygen delivery systems have led to extensive use of LTOT. There are three major sources of supplemental oxygen for home or institutional use: oxygen cylinders, liquid oxygen, and oxygen concentrators. Oxygen is usually administered by nasal cannula; however, at times a jet-mixing mask or other device may be prescribed.

The results of two controlled studies[29,32] clearly demonstrated that the long-term administration of oxygen for at least 15 hours/day in severely hypoxic patients with chronic obstructive pulmonary disease significantly improved life expectancy. Additionally, improvement has been documented in neuropsychologic function, exercise tolerance, and dyspnea, as well as quality of life (although quality of life has also been shown to decrease with LTOT).

Patients selected for LTOT require oxygen in the range of 1 to 3 L/min, a flow rate adequate to provide the benefits of oxygen therapy without significant risk of respiratory depression from abolition of the hypoxic stimulus to breathe. Although patients receiving this therapy must remain under close medical supervision, complications appear to be negligible.

Preparation

Oxygen is available as a compressed gas at approximately 2000 psi. As with other therapeutic gases, oxygen is marketed in steel cylinders that, for safety's sake, have a unique color code (green) and a pin-indexed or otherwise noninterchangeable connector system. A two-stage, grease-free regulator is typically used to provide oxygen at flow rates and pressures commensurate with therapeutic needs.

Doxapram

Doxapram is one of a class of general CNS stimulants known as *analeptics*, which collectively have had only marginal success in the treatment of ventilatory insufficiency. The difference between the analeptic and convulsant doses of these drugs is small, and their use is generally discouraged in clinical situations such as drug-induced coma, overdose of inhalation anesthetics, shock, hypoxemia, increased intracranial pressure, and acute or chronic lung disease. In the rare cases in which analeptic therapy is elected, doxapram is the safest drug in this category. Even so, large doses of doxapram produce tonic-clonic convulsions, and repeated administration of the drug is contraindicated.

Doxapram stimulates ventilation by increasing tidal volume and ventilatory rate. Respiratory stimulant effects appear to be exerted by a direct excitatory action on medullary respiratory centers and carotid chemoreceptors. There is some evidence that doxapram may prevent or reverse opioid- and anesthetic-induced ventilatory depression. Doxapram hastens arousal when administered immediately after general anesthesia, but the clinical usefulness of the drug is limited. Doxapram may also be administered to treat acute hypercapnia in patients with chronic obstructive pulmonary disease.

DRUGS USED TO TREAT ASTHMA

Bronchial asthma is a disease distinguished by excessive irritability of the respiratory tree. Whether induced by an allergen or chemical irritant (extrinsic asthma) or by an intrinsic factor such as infection or emotional distress (intrinsic asthma), an asthma attack is characterized by a diffuse airway obstruction related to bronchial and bronchiolar constriction coupled with hypersecretion of viscous mucus. This reversible condition is marked by hypertrophy of the bronchial smooth muscle and by the presence of intraluminal mucous plugs and submucosal edema. Asthma is now viewed to be a clinical syndrome characterized by signs and symptoms of intermittent, and potentially reversible, airflow limitation superimposed on a background of inflammation.[26] The airway obstruction follows an acute bronchoconstrictor response to the spasmogenic stimulus, peaking within 10 to 20 minutes.[8] This early response is probably caused by mast cell mediators, such as histamine and several proteases, platelet-activating factor, and certain prostaglandins and leukotrienes.

A late asthmatic phase begins 3 to 4 hours after exposure, peaks within 4 to 8 hours, and may last for as long as 12 hours. The initial activation of mast cells releases chemotactic factors that recruit inflammatory cells, such as eosinophils and neutrophils. During the next several hours, the mast cells also synthesize and release a variety of cytokines that promote, among other things, leukocyte chemotaxis. The late-phase response is characterized by the resulting influx of inflammatory cells. Activation of recruited inflammatory cells causes concentrations of chemical mediators (e.g., histamine, leukotrienes, bradykinin, prostaglandins) again to increase, thus contributing to the bronchoconstrictive reaction and to the development of bronchial hyperreactivity (BHR). *BHR* refers to an increased contractile response of airway smooth muscle, and the degree of BHR correlates with the clinical severity of the disease.[36] As a result of the existent hyperresponsiveness, symptoms may then develop in response to nonallergenic as well as to allergenic stimuli. Many asthmatic patients thus become trapped in a vicious circle of repeated exacerbations of their disease.

Recognition of the role of inflammation in the pathophysiologic features of asthma has led to a change in the therapeutic approach to treatment.[35] Traditionally, enhanced contraction of bronchial smooth muscle was considered to be the major pathologic event; hence, bronchodilators were the drugs of choice. It is now recommended that asthma be treated as a persistent inflammatory disease rather than as an episodic bronchospastic disorder.[8,40] The regular use of antiinflammatory drugs, preferably inhaled corticosteroids, is now viewed as first-choice therapy for anything more than occasional mild asthma. Regular or frequent therapy with inhaled β_2-adrenergic bronchodilators alone is not recommended. Instead, they should be reserved for pretreatment of exercise-induced asthma or for relief of acute exacerbations when steroid therapy is inadequate. In recent years, leukotriene modifiers have been added to the antiinflammatory armamentarium for the treatment of asthma. Various other therapeutic measures may also be used. The prompt administration of antibiotics is indicated for respiratory infections of nonviral origin. Sedatives may be used to minimize emotional stress; expectorants may aid in the removal of secretions. Finally, avoiding tobacco and environmental irritants or allergens may help prevent episodes of asthma.

Drugs commonly used for the treatment of acute and chronic asthma are identified in Table 32-1 along with some salient features of their pharmacologic characteristics.

Antiinflammatory Drugs

Corticosteroids

Corticosteroids have been of major importance for decades in the clinical management of patients with bronchial asthma. The mechanisms by which their beneficial effects are achieved in this disease are still not fully understood, although they are

Table • 32-1

Drugs Commonly Used in the Treatment of Asthma

DRUG CLASS	NONPROPRIETARY (GENERIC) NAME (PROPRIETARY [TRADE] NAME)	MECHANISM OF ACTION IN ASTHMA	BENEFITS	ADVERSE EFFECTS	TYPICAL DOSE
Selective β_2-adrenergic agonists	Albuterol (Proventil, Ventolin), metaproterenol (Alupent), pirbuterol (Maxair), salmeterol (Serevent)	Stimulation of β_2 receptors in lung	Rapid bronchodilation and minimal systemic effects with inhalation (except with salmeterol, which produces slow, sustained bronchodilation)	Tachycardia, tremor, potential for overuse	2 Puffs every 4 to 6 hours, up to every 2 hours if needed for short periods (salmeterol: 2 puffs every 12 hours)
Nonselective adrenergic agonists	Epinephrine (Adrenalin)	Stimulation of β_2 and α receptors in lung	Rapid bronchodilation and relief of mucosal congestion	Arrhythmia, tachycardia, hypertension, tremor	0.01 ml/kg up to 0.5 ml subcutaneously of 1:1000 solution
Antimuscarinic agents	Ipratropium (Atrovent)	Blockade of M_3 muscarinic receptors	Bronchodilation and decreased secretions; especially effective in patients with COPD	Tachycardia, xerostomia	2 to 3 puffs every 6 to 8 hours
Methylxanthines	Theophylline (Theo-24, Theo-Dur)	Phosphodiesterase inhibition, adenosine receptor blockade	Bronchodilation and antiinflammatory effects	Anorexia, nausea and vomiting, arrhythmias, tachycardia; highly variable dose response	100 to 300 mg every 6 to 12 hours
Inhaled glucocorticoids	Beclomethasone (Beclovent), budesonide (Pulmicort), flunisolide (AeroBid), fluticasone (Flovent), triamcinolone (Azmacort)	Stimulation of steroid receptors; modulation of gene expression	Reduced airway inflammation and hyperreactivity with good prophylactic control and reduced systemic drug effects	Hoarseness, oropharyngeal candidiasis; growth suppression in children with high doses of potent drugs	2 to 12 puffs twice daily depending on potency of agent
Oral (systemic) glucocorticoids	Prednisone (Deltasone, Sterapred), methylprednisolone (Medrol)	Stimulation of steroid receptors; modulation of gene expression	Reduced airway inflammation and hyperreactivity; best used for acute exacerbations of asthma	Na^+ retention, hyperglycemia, increased appetite, increased susceptibility to infections, mood disturbances, osteoporosis	Tapering doses from 40 to 60 mg daily to 5 to 10 mg every other day
Leukotriene synthesis inhibitors	Zileuton (Zyflo)	Inhibition of 5-lipoxygenase	Decreased inflammation; may reduce need for steroid use	Hepatotoxicity (mild), inhibition of drug metabolism	600 mg every 6 hours
Leukotriene antagonists	Montelukast (Singulair), zafirlukast (Accolate)	Blockade of cys-LT1 receptors	Decreased inflammation; may reduce need for steroid use	Inhibition of warfarin metabolism (zafirlukast only)	Montelukast, once daily; zafirlukast, twice daily
Khellin derivatives	Cromolyn (Intal), nedocromil (Tilade)	Unknown	Inhibition of mast cell degranulation and leukocyte activation and chemotaxis	None significant	2 Puffs every 6 hours

From McNally D: Wheezing. In Bennett JD, Rosenberg MB, eds: *Medical emergencies in dentistry,* Philadelphia, WB Saunders, 2002.
COPD, Chronic obstructive pulmonary disease; *cys-LT1,* cysteinyl leukotriene 1.

believed to be a consequence of the common pattern of corticosteroid action, as described in Chapter 35. The ultimate expression of the corticosteroid effect occurs as a result of new protein synthesis within the target cell, and several hours are required for DNA transcription and RNA translation to occur. Consequently, an immediate therapeutic response cannot be expected to follow the administration of a corticosteroid, and these agents cannot be used as a substitute for adrenergic or xanthine bronchodilators in acute asthma. In this situation, however, clinical studies have shown a more rapid therapeutic response when sympathomimetics are used in combination with systemic steroids.[48]

Corticosteroids act on many sites to help reverse the pathologic process of bronchial asthma.[48] They enhance the β_2-adrenergic response by increasing the number of β_2 receptors in human lung cells and leukocytes, thus lowering the response threshold of β_2-receptor activation to catecholamines and potentiating the stimulation of adenylyl cyclase. The corticosteroids decrease the release of prostaglandins and leukotrienes and other arachidonic acid metabolites. By inhibiting the synthesis of leukotrienes C_4, D_4, and E_4, these drugs suppress smooth muscle contraction, vascular permeability, and airway mucous secretion. The inhibition of leukotriene B_4 production influences the migration and function of leukocytes. Corticosteroids produce eosinopenia, which may help to prevent the cytotoxic effects of proteins and other inflammatory mediators released from eosinophils.

Corticosteroids influence the establishment of inflammatory processes by inhibiting the formation of cytokines and other mediators that induce the recruitment, proliferation, and activation of leukocytes and by direct inhibition of the activation of cells already at the site. As a result, corticosteroids are effective in preventing the late asthmatic responses and in decreasing BHR.[5,8] They are not prophylactic against acute bronchospasm because they do not inhibit the early asthmatic response.[10]

Topical steroid aerosols Aerosol corticosteroids have been intensively investigated in an attempt to minimize potential adverse effects of these drugs, as described in Chapter 35. Aerosolization allows the drug to be deposited directly into the lung, where it might be expected to exert a local action at much lower doses than are needed orally. Cortisone, hydrocortisone, prednisone, prednisolone, and dexamethasone in aerosol form have been evaluated, but they are all absorbed into the circulation and consequently can produce systemic side effects.

Beclomethasone dipropionate (BDP), triamcinolone acetonide, flunisolide, fluticasone, and budesonide are currently available for administration by metered-dose inhalers. These drugs provide potent topical antiinflammatory activity safely with few systemic side effects. Since their introduction in the 1970s, inhaled corticosteroids have been effective and safe for the long-term treatment of asthma. Their regular use has allowed many patients to discontinue systemic steroids or to significantly reduce the doses required. BDP has been in clinical use longer than the other inhaled corticosteroids and consequently has been the most extensively studied. After inhalation, approximately 10% of the drug reaches the lung; the remainder is swallowed or adheres to the upper airways. In the lung, BDP is partially metabolized to the monopropionate (BMP) and, more slowly, to free beclomethasone. Both BDP and BMP are believed to cause the therapeutic effect.[55] When the swallowed drug is absorbed from the gastrointestinal tract, it is rapidly inactivated during its first pass through the liver. The drug and its metabolites are excreted principally in the feces, with less than 10% appearing in the urine. Only when large doses are inhaled is first-pass metabolism inadequate and systemically active concentrations of drug attained.

At recommended doses, BDP achieves reasonable control in adult and child asthmatic patients without apparent adrenal suppression. Impaired adrenal function has been reported in patients maintained on five times the recommended daily dose. The major side effects associated with BDP are dryness of the mouth and an increased incidence of oral candidiasis, the latter often preventable with oral rinsing. Side effects may also include voice changes.

Inhaled steroids are formulated for twice-daily administration, but in many instances the dosing schedule is increased up to four times per day. This more frequent regimen may lead to lack of compliance and compromise therapy. In an attempt to improve inhaled steroid therapy, the newest agents fluticasone and budesonide were developed with higher affinity for the glucocorticoid receptor and with prolonged binding times, allowing for less frequent administration. However, no inhaled steroid has proved superior to any other in equivalent dose, and the newer agents have an increased incidence of systemic effects, including growth retardation and a decrease in bone density.

Oral corticosteroids Oral steroids are the most effective drugs for acute exacerbations of asthma unresponsive to bronchodilators. Even when the acute attack responds to bronchodilators, many patients are treated with oral corticosteroids for a period of up to 10 days to decrease symptoms and prevent early relapse.

Commonly used oral corticosteroids for the treatment of asthma include prednisolone, prednisone, and methylprednisolone.[5] Currently, prednisone is the most frequently prescribed oral agent. It has a plasma half-life of approximately 3 hours and a clinically active half-life of 18 to 36 hours. Prednisolone has a slightly shorter plasma half-life. If taken once a day in the morning, either drug allows the adrenal glands several hours to recover between doses. The effects on ventilatory capacity can be seen within 1 hour, although the maximum effect occurs at 9 to 10 hours. Prednisone is biologically inactive until it is converted to prednisolone in the liver.[55] Liver dysfunction can impair this conversion. Methylprednisolone is a good alternative to prednisone or prednisolone, especially if large doses are required, because of its lower mineralocorticoid properties.

The continued use of oral corticosteroids in pharmacologic doses can cause adrenal suppression and hyperadrenocorticism. The risk of adrenal suppression depends on the dosage, as well as on the duration of action of the specific drug and the length of treatment. Prednisone and prednisolone produce fewer complications than do longer-acting preparations such as betamethasone and dexamethasone. In fact, the administration of a short-acting drug for a brief time (7 to 10 days) is generally not associated with significant toxicity.

An alternate-day regimen for oral corticosteroids has been developed. This strategy was much more important before the introduction of inhaled steroids. Patients have fewer adverse reactions on this regimen, with the short-acting compounds causing the least adrenal suppression. Nevertheless, all patients receiving long-term corticosteroid therapy should be continually monitored by the physician, and dose-dependent side effects such as osteoporosis, diabetes, cataracts, and poor wound healing should be expected.

Parenteral corticosteroids Parenteral corticosteroids may be indicated in severe acute asthma. Hydrocortisone sodium succinate and methylprednisolone sodium succinate are commonly administered by intravenous injection or infusion. The intravenous route allows the dose to be rapidly adjusted to clinical need.

The necessity for systemic corticosteroid treatment in acute severe asthma has been controversial for more than a decade. Clinical trials have shown that steroids hasten improvement in arterial hypoxemia and reduce the incidence of subsequent asthma relapses compared with bronchodilator treatment alone.

Nonsteroidal prophylactic drugs

Cromolyn Cromolyn is a nonbronchodilating, nonsteroidal drug used for prophylactic treatment of asthma. It is a synthetic derivative of khellin, the agent in extracts of the *Ammi visnoga* plant that produces smooth muscle relaxation. It is administered by inhalation. Although the mechanism of action is not fully understood, it is known that cromolyn inhibits the release of mediators from mast cells, as well as other inflammatory cells, probably by inhibiting the inflow of Ca^{++} into the mast cells.[8,58] The drug inhibits both early and late asthmatic responses and is effective in the long-term treatment of chronic asthma. Other biologic effects, including inhibition of afferent pulmonary nerve fiber receptors that contribute to reflex bronchoconstriction, may also be relevant to its therapeutic action.

Clinically, cromolyn is ineffective in the treatment of acute attacks of asthma, including status asthmaticus. It functions exclusively as a prophylactic agent in the management of chronic symptoms. Maximum benefit is obtained only after 4 weeks of treatment. Cromolyn has also been shown to be useful as a premedication before a challengelike exercise, where the drug, similarly to steroids and leukotriene inhibitors, reduces airway hyperactivity. Both long-term and short-term studies have documented clinical improvement in patients taking cromolyn, with a low incidence of adverse effects. Indeed, cromolyn is one of the least toxic medications used for asthma. Most adverse reactions have been mild and have consisted mainly of wheezing, coughing, and dryness of the throat. There have been rare reports, however, of eosinophilia with pulmonary infiltration, pulmonary granulomatosis, and the development of subacute and acute allergic reactions. Generally, any patient who demonstrates a reaction other than a transitory irritative response is removed from cromolyn therapy.

During cromolyn treatment, patients are maintained on regular medication, such as oral bronchodilators. In cromolyn-treated patients receiving corticosteroids, there have been reports of a decreased corticosteroid requirement, which permits many patients to convert from a daily steroid schedule to an alternate-day program or to discontinue steroids completely.[41] A decreased requirement for sympathomimetic and xanthine bronchodilators has also been noted. This medication-sparing effect is one of the major advantages of cromolyn therapy. Cromolyn is generally available in a metered-dose aerosol unit and in a nebulizer solution. The availability of liquid cromolyn has been a major benefit to many asthmatics, especially young children.

Nedocromil Nedocromil is a novel and potent antiinflammatory drug with many properties and effects in common with cromolyn.[9] It inhibits the immediate bronchoconstrictor response to allergen challenge, probably as a result of preventing the release of mast cell mediators. It also inhibits the late-phase asthmatic response and aids in reducing BHR by blocking the effect of peptide-activating factors on inflammatory cells. Nedocromil, like cromolyn, is essentially free from systemic toxicity. Both drugs are highly ionized (more than 99%) at physiologic pH, and their inability to penetrate cells, coupled with the lack of an extracellular route of metabolism, results in their being excreted unchanged in the urine (approximately 80%) and feces (approximately 20%). Clinical experience has shown that nedocromil is well tolerated by the majority of patients, but a bitter taste and, less frequently, headache and nausea have been reported.

Ketotifen Ketotifen, an oral agent with cromolynlike activity, has been tested in the management of mild to moderate bronchial asthma and allergic disorders. It has strong antihistaminic (H_1) actions and powerful antianaphylactic properties.[20] Inhibition of the release or activity of proinflammatory mediators may contribute to the prophylactic effect of ketotifen. Some evidence suggests that ketotifen also interferes with Ca^{++} flux. It does not appear to affect smooth muscle contraction.

In asthmatic patients, the clinical benefit of ketotifen is usually detectable only after 6 to 12 weeks of treatment. The delayed onset has not been satisfactorily explained. Comparative clinical trials have shown that the oral administration of ketotifen and the inhalation of cromolyn have a similar prophylactic efficacy.[1] As with cromolyn, an important benefit of ketotifen treatment is that dosages of bronchodilators and corticosteroids can be reduced during therapy.

The major side effect of ketotifen is sedation, which is experienced by 10% to 15% of patients during the first week of treatment. Drowsiness diminishes with time. The drug is well tolerated and the oral route of administration promotes patient compliance. Currently, ketotifen is approved for topical use in the treatment of allergic conjunctivitis.

Leukotriene modifiers The newest approach to the treatment of asthma is to prevent or inhibit the effect of leukotrienes on the airway. This approach results from the concept that chronic asthma is, to a large extent, an inflammatory disease. Leukotrienes, being mediators of inflammation, cause leukocyte recruitment, stimulate bronchoconstriction, and increase capillary permeability, resulting in edema. At the same time, they stimulate mucus secretion and impair mucociliary clearance.

Leukotrienes are derived from arachidonic acid, which is released from cellular membrane phospholipids by the enzyme phospholipase A_2. Arachidonic acid is metabolized by one of two pathways: the cyclooxygenase pathway, producing prostaglandins, thromboxanes, and prostacyclin, or the 5-lipoxygenase pathway, yielding the cysteinyl leukotrienes C_4, D_4, and E_4.[47] To enter this latter pathway, arachidonic acid is presented to 5-lipoxygenase by a nuclear membrane protein, 5-lipoxygenase–activating protein.[27] Leukotriene A_4 and, subsequently, leukotriene B_4 are synthesized, neither of which has any bronchoconstrictor activity. In certain inflammatory cells, leukotriene A_4 is converted into leukotriene C_4. Leukotriene C_4 is secreted extracellularly and metabolized into leukotrienes D_4 and E_4 (see Figure 21-2). Inhaled leukotrienes C_4 and D_4 are more potent than histamine in inducing airflow obstruction in normal individuals.[16,23] All cysteinyl leukotrienes (C_4, D_4, and E_4) occupy the same receptors, are potent bronchoconstrictors, and have been implicated in the pathogenesis of asthma and allergy.

Antileukotriene therapy involves two mechanisms.[7] 5-Lipoxygenase inhibitors impede leukotriene synthesis, and leukotriene receptor antagonists block the cysteinyl leukotriene receptors.[15] Leukotriene modifiers are highly effective in preventing aspirin-induced asthma, but inhaled corticosteroids are more effective in improving airflow obstruction in other forms of asthma. Antileukotriene therapy is maintenance therapy recommended for persistent asthma that requires daily bronchodilator treatment. These drugs are frequently used as adjuvants to inhaled corticosteroids in poorly controlled patients treated by a combination of other drugs.[34] Several randomized, double-blind, placebo-controlled studies have shown that patients treated with leukotriene modifiers have fewer asthma attacks over time, decrease the amount of β_2-adrenergic agonists inhaled daily for acute exacerbations, and require diminished dosages of inhaled corticosteroids for maintenance.[34]

5-Lipoxygenase Inhibitors Zileuton, an inhibitor of 5-lipoxygenase, is used in maintenance therapy for chronic asthma. This drug reduces cysteinyl leukotriene production by approximately 70%. Because of its rapid hepatic metabolism (half-life of 2 to 3 hours), zileuton is administered four times a day. The drug is given orally and is well absorbed from the gastrointestinal tract. Headache and irritation of the gastric mucosa are typical adverse effects. The most notable and serious side effect is liver toxicity. The drug is contraindicated in patients with active liver disease, and all patients require periodic liver function tests while taking it. Zileuton inhibits the CYP2C9 enzyme and decreases the clearance of theophylline by as much as 50%. On initiation of combined therapy with theophylline, the dosage of theophylline should be reduced by half and serum concentrations closely monitored.[19] Clearance of warfarin is also reduced, causing a concomitant increase in prothrombin time that must be monitored.[3] The metabolism of some other drugs (e.g., propranolol) may be affected as well.

Leukotriene Receptor Antagonists Several leukotriene receptor antagonists have been developed, including zafirlukast, montelukast, and pranlukast. Zafirlukast was the first leukotriene antagonist to be approved in the United States for the management of chronic asthma. The drug is rapidly absorbed after oral administration. It is approved for use in children 12 years of age and older. Unlike zileuton, its bioavailability is significantly decreased in the presence of food. For this reason, zafirlukast is administered 2 hours before meals. Zafirlukast has a half-life of approximately 10 hours and is given two times a day. It is metabolized in the liver and can inhibit the metabolism of warfarin and possibly phenytoin and carbamazepine, all of which are metabolized by the CYP2C9 enzyme. Periodic monitoring for increased prothrombin times is necessary in patients receiving warfarin therapy. Rarely, elevation of liver enzymes has been observed, which returned to normal when the drug was discontinued. Severe hepatitis has been reported after administration of zafirlukast.[44] Zafirlukast is also associated with gastrointestinal disturbances and headache.

Montelukast has the advantage of being administered only once daily, usually in the evening. It is approved for use in children as young as 6 years of age. Montelukast is not believed to cause significant hepatotoxicity, and periodic liver testing is not a requirement for this drug.

Pranlukast is used mostly in Japan. The therapeutic effect is noted after approximately 2 weeks of treatment. In a 4-year follow-up study, no significant side effects were reported with the drug.[33]

Methotrexate Methotrexate is a well-known immunosuppressive chemotherapeutic drug used for the treatment of various diseases. Methotrexate inhibits the enzyme dihydrofolate reductase, preventing folate-dependent nucleic acid synthesis. The drug has been used during the last decade as an adjuvant for the treatment of severe glucocorticoid-dependent asthma. The low doses used do not significantly inhibit nucleic acid synthesis but have an antiinflammatory action. There is often a decrease in white blood cell count, and the patient should be monitored to detect this change. The rationale for methotrexate in the treatment of asthma came from the observation that corticosteroid doses can be reduced when combination therapy with methotrexate is prescribed. Some studies have found a reduction of steroid dosages by up to 25%, but others have been unable to show this effect.[28] Because methotrexate produces no direct effect on pulmonary function, it is added to the treatment of asthma patients only for its steroid-sparing effect in patients unresponsive to steroids or taking high doses with severe side effects. The objective is to reach the lowest possible oral steroid dose. Low doses of methotrexate are not free of side effects. Liver toxicity, pneumonitis, and *Pneumocystis carinii* pneumonia have been observed.[62] There is also a small possibility for delayed malignancy.

BRONCHODILATORS

β_2-Selective Adrenergic Agonists

The pharmacologic characteristics and structure-activity relationships of adrenergic drugs with bronchodilating properties are discussed in Chapter 6. These agents have long provided effective means of obtaining symptomatic relief in the treatment of asthma. The early asthmatic response can be completely reversed by bronchodilators such as epinephrine and the β_2-selective adrenergic agonists.

The rationale for their use can be explained in part by advances in understanding of the cyclic adenosine 3′,5′-monophosphate (cAMP) second messenger system. The release of spasmogens and inflammagens—primarily histamine, leukotrienes, prostaglandins, and thromboxane A_2—from mast cells and basophils is regulated by the autonomic nervous system. The mast cell has, among others, β_2-adrenergic receptors that respond to agonists by stimulating adenylyl cyclase and increasing the concentration of cAMP, as discussed in detail in Chapters 1, 5, and 6. The accumulation of cAMP leads to the activation of protein kinases, which bring about the characteristic responses of the cell. In bronchial smooth muscle, cAMP-dependent protein kinase inhibits the contractile mechanism by affecting myosin light-chain kinase and by lowering the myoplasmic Ca^{++} concentration through sequestration of Ca^{++} in intracellular stores and extrusion of Ca^{++} out of the cell.[56] The ultimate expression of these actions is bronchial dilation.

Inhaled short-acting β_2-selective adrenergic agonists are normally the drugs of choice for managing acute bronchospasm because they are less likely to activate other adrenergic receptors and to stimulate the heart. Salmeterol, a long-acting partial agonist at β_2 receptors, plays a unique role in the long-term management of asthma.

Metaproterenol

Metaproterenol is a derivative of the nonselective β-adrenergic blocker isoproterenol in which the hydroxyl group is moved from C_4 to C_5 of the benzene nucleus in the molecule (see Table 6-1). This structural change produces a predominantly β_2-stimulant action. It also protects metaproterenol from enzymatic degradation by catechol-O-methyltransferase (COMT), thus prolonging the drug's duration of action.

An effective clinical response is obtained after inhalation or oral administration of metaproterenol. However, as with all the β_2-selective sympathomimetic drugs, selectivity of action is less apparent when the drug is given orally. Inhalation produces a peak effect in 30 to 60 minutes, and there is sustained improvement in pulmonary function tests for up to 5 hours. Tachycardia and tremor are two common side effects, but the incidence and severity of cardiac reactions are less than with isoproterenol.

Terbutaline

Terbutaline, a congener of metaproterenol, is of clinical interest because of its long duration of action (3 to 6 hours), its availability in an injectable form, and a side effect profile equivalent to metaproterenol. For patients with spontaneous asthma, terbutaline is reported to provide greater protection against bronchoconstriction than an equivalent dose of metaproterenol.[2] Terbutaline from the aerosol-metered dose inhaler stimulates bronchial β_2 receptors more selectively than do oral or parenteral forms of the drug. Tolerance to the aerosol does not appear to develop with continued use over several months. The most common side effect of therapeutic doses is a slight tremor, which may be particularly noticeable in the elderly. Other side effects, typically seen with nonselective β blockers, are infrequent. Terbutaline is the only drug used as a bronchodilator that has good safety data supporting its use during pregnancy.

Albuterol

Albuterol, the most commonly prescribed β_2-adrenergic bronchodilator, is similar in pharmacologic profile (and in resistance to COMT) to terbutaline. It is available in tablet form, as a sustained-release tablet, and as a metered-dose pressurized aerosol. As with terbutaline, pulmonary β_2 specificity is greater with aerosol delivery than it is with an oral dose.[35] When administered by a metered-dose inhaler, albuterol is more effective and longer lasting than metaproterenol. Adverse reactions to albuterol are similar to those of other β_2-adrenergic receptor agonists.

Pirbuterol

Pirbuterol is a relatively selective β_2-adrenergic agonist that is structurally related to albuterol. When administered by inhalation, its onset and duration of action are comparable to those of albuterol. It is less potent on a weight basis.

Isoetharine

Isoetharine, an agent with modest selectivity for β_2 receptors, is available only for inhalation. The duration of action is 1 to 3 hours.

Bitolterol

Bitolterol is a predominantly β_2-specific sympathomimetic that functions as a prodrug, remaining inactive until it is metabolized by ester hydrolysis to release the active moiety colterol. Bitolterol is unique in that the 3- and 4-hydroxy groups are esterified. Available in a metered-dose inhaler for oral inhalation, bitolterol has a rapid onset (3 to 4 minutes) of bronchodilator activity, which persists for at least 5 hours in most patients and up to 8 hours in some. The major side effects include tremor, nervousness, headache, and palpitation.

Salmeterol

Salmeterol is a long-acting, highly selective β_2-adrenergic agent structurally related to albuterol. Synthesis of salmeterol combined the active head group of albuterol to take advantage of its bronchodilatory effects with an extended lipophilic tail to prolong its duration of action. The lipophilic tail allows the drug to remain in the tissue for longer periods of time, diminishing its systemic uptake.[25] The drug provides bronchodilation usually lasting at least 12 hours, presumably by forming a stable complex with the hydrophobic environment around the β_2 receptor.

Compared with albuterol, salmeterol has greater β_2 receptor selectivity but decreased intrinsic efficacy. The receptor selectivity and the intrinsic efficacy differences of the drug minimize cardiac side effects. However, cardiac effects are not completely absent because human cardiac tissue contains β_2 adrenoceptors. The low intrinsic efficacy also contributes to a decreased incidence of receptor desensitization, a significant problem with more powerful β adrenergic receptor agonists.[30]

Incorporating a long-acting β_2 agonist into the therapeutic regimen has several advantages. Clinical trials have shown salmeterol to be more efficacious than albuterol in (1) reducing variation in diurnal peak expiratory flow rates; (2) decreasing nocturnal symptoms, asthma exacerbations, and the need for rescue medication; and (3) increasing overall lung function.[13,37] Some antiinflammatory effects have also been noted in animal studies. However, most clinical studies do not demonstrate that salmeterol inhibits the accumulation or activity of airway inflammatory cells.[18,39] Of equal importance is the subjective assessment of improved quality of life associated with the use of salmeterol compared with albuterol or placebo.[24,46] The combination of salmeterol with an inhaled corticosteroid has been shown to be beneficial. Several studies have demonstrated that the administration of salmeterol with a lower dose of corticosteroid results in improved pulmonary function compared with a larger dose of corticosteroid administered alone.[17,63] In addition to the improved physiologic response, the administration of salmeterol decreases the potential of systemic effects of corticosteroids.

Salmeterol is relatively slow in onset (approximately 10 minutes), and maximal bronchodilation takes hours. Therefore it is not indicated for the symptomatic relief of acute asthma. Side effects, such as tachycardia, tremor, hypokalemia, and hyperglycemia, are minimal at standard doses.

Other Adrenergic Agonists

Epinephrine

Epinephrine may be administered by oral inhalation from a nebulizer or metered-dose inhaler. The inhaler is generally favored because it is effective, less expensive, and more portable. The therapeutic effect is weak and transient compared with the longer-acting β_2 agonists immune to metabolism by COMT. Signs of overdose include nervousness, restlessness, sleeplessness, bronchial irritation, and tachycardia. Inhalation of recommended dosages may minimize reactions other than bronchodilation. However, patients will frequently have palpitation and tremors that increase with increased use. The occurrence of these signs and symptoms usually limits the use of this drug because patients tend not to tolerate these effects.

Parenteral epinephrine is reserved for acute episodes of asthma requiring immediate relief when inhaled β_2-selective agonists have proved ineffective or could not be effectively administered. In such cases, 0.2 to 0.5 mg may be injected subcutaneously or intramuscularly to produce bronchodilation. Because epinephrine produces α- as well as β-adrenergic receptor stimulation, it can also improve respiration by relieving congestion of the bronchial mucosa.

Ephedrine

Ephedrine stimulates α and β receptors by both a direct action and through the release of endogenous catecholamines. Its pharmacologic effects are similar to those of epinephrine. Ephedrine was once widely used in treating mild to moderate asthma because of its oral efficacy and longer duration of action. It is not as effective as epinephrine in severe attacks because its bronchodilator action is weaker. Ephedrine may be administered at bedtime to prevent nocturnal wheezing. The tendency of ephedrine to produce tachyphylaxis when taken for long periods has limited its use in chronic asthma.

Ephedrine is marketed as a single-entity drug and as a component in fixed-dose combination products. It was often combined with theophylline, sedatives, or expectorants. Until the U.S. Food and Drug Administration banned its sale, ephedrine was widely used in the form of ephedra and related herb products.

The adverse reactions are similar to those of epinephrine. In addition, there may be CNS stimulation, the most common signs of which are nervousness, excitability, and insomnia. There is little reason to recommend ephedrine over the more recently developed β_2-specific bronchodilators.

Isoproterenol

Isoproterenol is the prototypic nonselective β-receptor agonist. It acts on β_1 receptors to increase the rate and force of cardiac contractions and on β_2 receptors located in the smooth muscle of the bronchi, blood vessels, and other locations. Oral inhalation is still used for the treatment of asthmatic attacks but has been largely superseded by the more selective β_2 agonists. Isoproterenol has a rapid onset but a short duration of action. Excessive administration of the drug can produce adverse effects, such as nervousness, headaches, and severe arrhythmias (including ventricular fibrillation), as well as tolerance and refractoriness.

Other Bronchodilators

Theophylline

Theophylline (1,3-dimethylxanthine) is a naturally occurring plant alkaloid closely related to caffeine and theobromine. The drug has been used for the treatment of asthma for more than a half century. Its clinical efficacy has traditionally been attributed to its bronchodilatory effect. This effect was believed to be mediated through inhibition of phosphodiesterase enzymes that catalyze the breakdown of cAMP and cyclic guanosine 3′,5′-monophosphate. Experimental studies subsequently determined that significant inhibition of phosphodiesterase activity required concentrations several times higher than those usually achieved clinically. In recent years, however, it has been discovered that a family of phosphodiesterases exist and that bronchodilation may be mediated by inhibition of two specific isoenzymes, phosphodiesterases III and IV. Other mechanisms of action that may contribute to the bronchodilatory effect of theophylline include blockade of adenosine receptors, stimulation of catecholamine release, alteration of prostaglandin synthesis or function, and inhibition of Ca^{++} flux.[6] Theophylline has also been shown to have antiinflammatory (Table 32-2), bronchoprotective, and immunomodulatory effects. Additional effects that may contribute to the efficacy of theophylline include stimulation of respiration, increased diaphragmatic contractility, and increased mucociliary clearance.[31] Clearly, there is no consensus on how theophylline acts to relieve asthma.[35]

Theophylline is insoluble in aqueous solutions and is often prepared in salt form to increase aqueous solubility and hasten systemic absorption. Some of the theophylline salts are also combined with other agents such as adrenergic drugs, expectorants, or sedatives.

The availability of theophylline in various forms allows for several modes of administration. The salt aminophylline (theophylline ethylenediamine), which contains approximately 85% theophylline by weight, is the only preparation used for intravenous injection. It is one of several salts available for oral use. The rectal administration of theophylline, in the form of a retention enema, is an effective way to achieve rapid action in acute asthma. Rectal suppositories, however, are unreliably and sometimes lethally absorbed and frequently irritating. Extended-release formulations of theophylline purportedly permit therapeutic plasma concentrations with minimal peak-trough fluctuations at dosage intervals of 8 to 12 hours for some drugs and 24 hours for others. These preparations differ substantially in the rate and sometimes the extent of absorption and therefore are not interchangeable. The absorption of several theophylline preparations is affected by food, and unacceptable fluctuations in plasma concentrations occur in some patients.

At therapeutic doses, approximately 60% of theophylline is bound to plasma proteins. It undergoes extensive hepatic biotransformation, yielding several metabolites.[57] Less than 10% is excreted unchanged in the urine. The half-life of theophylline averages 3.5 hours in children and 8 hours in adults.

Many drug interactions involving theophylline are attributed to changes in the rate of theophylline metabolism. Phenytoin, phenobarbital, carbamazepine, and rifampin increase microsomal enzyme activity, thus increasing theophylline clearance and reducing serum concentrations by up to 40%. On the other hand, increased serum concentrations (typically by 20% to 100%) and prolonged half-lives are seen with alcohol, cimetidine, propranolol, zileuton, and certain antibiotics (e.g., erythromycin and ciprofloxacin). A single large dose of alcohol decreases theophylline clearance for approximately 24 hours.

Theophylline exerts numerous pharmacologic effects. These include stimulation of respiration, augmentation of cardiac rate and force of contraction, diuresis, and relaxation of smooth muscle, particularly in the bronchi and in blood vessels other than cerebral vessels.

Table • 32-2

Antiinflammatory Effects of Theophylline

TARGET	EFFECT
In Vitro	
Mast cells	Decreased mediator release
Macrophages	Decreased release of reactive oxygen species
Monocytes	Decreased cytokine release
Eosinophils	Decreased basic protein release, increased/decreased release of reactive oxygen species
T-lymphocytes	Decreased proliferation, decreased cytokine release
Neutrophils	Decreased release of reactive oxygen species
In Vivo	
Experimental animals	Decreased late response to allergen (guinea pigs), decreased airway responsiveness to allergen and platelet-activating factor (guinea pigs, sheep), decreased airway inflammation after endotoxin and allergen (guinea pigs, rats), decreased plasma exudation (guinea pigs)
Asthmatic patients	Inhibition of late response to allergen, increased CD8+ cells in peripheral blood, decreased T lymphocytes in airways

From Barnes PJ, Pauwels RA: Theophylline in the management of asthma: time for reappraisal? *Eur Respir J* 7:583, 1994.

Although some therapeutic effect against asthma may accrue in concentrations as small as 5 μg/ml, and bronchodilation continues to increase linearly with concentrations greater than 20 μg/ml, the typical goal is to maintain serum concentrations between 10 and 15 μg/ml for the entire dosing interval to optimize the potential benefit against the risk of adverse effects. Because the dose required to achieve a target theophylline concentration varies up to fourfold among otherwise similar patients even in the absence of factors known to alter theophylline clearance, it must be individualized on the basis of peak serum concentration measurements.

Theophylline toxicity is largely dose dependent.[43] Mild adverse effects may be observed with serum concentrations less than 20 μg/ml. Transient caffeinelike effects such as nausea, vomiting, abdominal discomfort, headache, and insomnia are more common when theophylline therapy is initiated. Metabolic changes, including hypokalemia, hyperglycemia, and acid-base disturbances, may be noted at higher concentrations.[49,50] Serious toxicity involving seizures, cardiac arrhythmias, and even death may occur when serum concentrations exceed 30 μg/ml. Seizures are often resistant to anticonvulsant therapy.[51] Activated charcoal is administered orally to prevent the absorption of theophylline ingested accidentally or purposefully in overdose. Extracorporeal removal of the drug may be indicated when serum measurements indicate potentially life-threatening concentrations.[52]

Theophylline salts, including aminophylline, have no role in the emergency management of acute asthmatic attacks because they provide no benefit over inhaled bronchodilators and may promote toxic effects such as CNS stimulation and cardiac arrhythmias. The oral use of theophylline in the long-term management of chronic asthma is well recognized, even though some authors claim that this drug is rarely indicated. Although the drug is inexpensive and still widely prescribed throughout the world, the availability of newer, better tolerated agents has limited its use in the United States. When theophylline is prescribed, the regimen that is chosen depends on the frequency of asthma attacks. For example, the patient who has only an occasional attack may require treatment for the episode and for a week or so thereafter. Some asthmatic patients have marked airway obstruction between attacks, even while they are apparently asymptomatic; for these cases, the long-term use of theophylline at 6-hour intervals has proved advantageous in diminishing the need for oral or inhaled steroids.[38]

Anticholinergics

Alkaloid anticholinergic agents were used for asthma therapy during the 1800s. It was later shown that cholinergic mechanisms are responsible for resting airway tone and that reflex bronchoconstriction is mediated by vagal pathways. In modern medicine, three anticholinergic drugs have been used for the treatment of asthma: atropine, glycopyrrolate, and, most importantly, ipratropium.

Ipratropium, an atropine derivative, was the first anticholinergic drug specifically approved for use as a bronchodilator. The drug probably produces bronchodilation by antagonizing the action of acetylcholine at its muscarinic receptors on bronchial smooth muscle and limiting the release of mediators from mast cells. It demonstrates a high degree of bronchoselectivity when delivered in small doses by inhalation.[11] The bronchodilation achieved in some patients is nearly equivalent to that produced by β agonists, but the onset of action is slower (20 minutes, maximum effect at 1 to 2 hours). The addition of ipratropium to a β_2 agonist may elicit a response in severe asthma of greater magnitude[42] and longer duration[22] than produced by either drug by itself. Available in a metered-dose inhaler alone or combined with albuterol, ipratropium is used in the treatment of chronic obstructive pulmonary disease, including chronic bronchitis and emphysema.

At therapeutic doses, ipratropium does not inhibit salivary secretion, induce significant cardiovascular effects, or affect urinary flow or intraocular pressure. The only side effects reported with any regularity have been a bad taste and dry mouth after inhalation.

Implications for Dentistry

To provide the most effective and the safest dental care for the asthmatic patient, it is important for the dentist to know the patient's history of asthma and how this medical problem is being managed. Important questions the dentist should ask are whether the patient is being maintained on corticosteroids, by what route, and whether the patient has received this therapy in the last 6 to 12 months. Patients often do not realize that one of their inhalers is a steroid. The answers to these questions help determine, at least to some extent, the likelihood of the patient requiring asthma medication during dental treatment and whether the patient might manifest signs of adrenal hypofunction under the stress of dental procedures.

A major consideration is how the patient reacts to dental appointments. Many persons become apprehensive and anxious about impending visits to the dental office, and it is known that emotional factors play an active role in precipitating or exacerbating asthmatic symptoms. For this reason, the asthmatic patient should be questioned about the medication the physician has prescribed for acute attacks and should be requested to bring antiasthma medication to the dental office in case it is needed during the appointment.

If the patient is a candidate for preoperative or postoperative sedation, hydroxyzine is a good choice; diazepam or another suitable benzodiazepine is a reasonable alternative. Unusually large doses of sedative drugs may be required if the patient is receiving continuous treatment with a CNS stimulant such as theophylline or ephedrine. A better solution is for the patient's physician to update the therapeutic regimen with nonstimulating antiasthmatic drugs.

The concomitant use of theophylline and erythromycin, an antibiotic commonly prescribed in dentistry, can lead to increased serum concentrations of the bronchodilator and toxic reactions, particularly if relatively high dosages are used. Erythromycin forms a stable complex with certain hepatic cytochrome P450 enzymes, thus inhibiting their ability to metabolize other drugs.[14] Erythromycin may reduce the clearance of theophylline by 20% to 50% in some patients.[12] Asthma patients stabilized on theophylline who receive erythromycin should be monitored for increased serum theophylline concentrations, which can occur quickly and necessitate an immediate reduction in dosage.

Another consideration is the choice of an analgesic for the asthmatic patient. Aspirin and aspirin-containing compounds should be avoided if there is a question of patient intolerance or nasal polyps because asthmatic episodes can be precipitated in some patients in minutes to hours after ingestion of these drugs.[54] Asthmatic patients unable to tolerate aspirin may also react adversely to indomethacin, mefenamic acid, propionic acid derivatives (e.g., ibuprofen), and the fenamate analgesics. Large doses of morphine and especially meperidine can produce bronchial constriction by releasing histamine from mast cells. Inasmuch as these drugs have been reported to precipitate asthmatic attacks in anesthetized patients, they should certainly be avoided during an asthmatic attack. Their action to decrease the respiratory drive, which is shared by other opioid analgesics, is a dangerous liability to the patient whose airway resistance may be many times greater than normal.

If an asthmatic attack does occur in the dental office, drug therapy may be indicated. The inhalation of a β_2-selective adrenergic bronchodilator is generally safe and effective; however, subcutaneous injection of 0.2 to 0.5 ml of 1:1000 epinephrine (equivalent to 0.2 to 0.5 mg) may be needed for severe episodes.

DRUGS USED TO IMPROVE VENTILATION

Numerous drugs are used to improve ventilation or to provide symptomatic relief of some uncomfortable symptoms of respiratory infection. These include bronchodilators (discussed in previous sections), antitussives, nasal decongestants, intranasal steroids, expectorants, and mucolytic agents.

Antitussives

Coughing is a protective reflex that clears the respiratory tract of accumulated secretions or noxious substances. A productive cough, with the elimination of excessive secretions, is beneficial, but a nonproductive cough may impair rest and increase discomfort. An ideal antitussive agent should decrease the frequency and intensity of coughing but still allow adequate elimination of excessive secretions from the respiratory tract.

Opioid analgesics

The ability of opioid analgesics to suppress coughing parallels their analgesic effect and their abuse potential. Because of their side effects and addiction liability, the more potent drugs, such as morphine and hydromorphone, are not commonly used as antitussives.

Codeine is the most useful opioid for cough suppression. At therapeutic doses and for short-term use, its addiction potential is minimal and depressed ventilation is infrequent. Overdosage can result in respiratory depression, convulsions, hypotension, and tachycardia.

Hydrocodone, like codeine, acts centrally on the medullary cough center. Hydrocodone appears to be three times more potent in antitussive activity than codeine. It also has a somewhat greater abuse potential. At therapeutic doses, the most common side effects include nausea, constipation, and dizziness. Long-term use should be accompanied by a plan for supporting bowel function. Lactulose, for example, may be prescribed to minimize constipation.

Other drugs

Other drugs that act centrally on the medullary cough center include benzonatate, dextromethorphan, and noscapine. These agents generally produce fewer adverse reactions than the traditional opioid drugs.

Benzonatate is an antitussive structurally related to tetracaine. Although the primary action of benzonatate is apparently depression of the central cough mechanism, it may also act by inhibiting the stretch receptors of the respiratory mucosa. The most common adverse reactions include nausea, constipation, headache, drowsiness, and vertigo. Nasal congestion, as well as numbness of the tongue, mouth, and pharynx, have been noted if the capsules are chewed before swallowing.

Dextromethorphan, the methyl ester of the dextroisomer of the opioid levorphanol, appears to be the most popular cough suppressant. In one clinical study, the antitussive effects of 60 mg of dextromethorphan did not differ significantly from those of 30 mg of codeine phosphate.[4] In over-the-counter (OTC) mixtures, it is often used in combination with other agents such as bronchodilators, antihistamines, and expectorants. It has no addiction liability or analgesic properties. Side effects are minimal at recommended doses.

Noscapine is one of the isoquinoline series of opium alkaloids. It has no analgesic activity or abuse potential but expresses effective antitussive activity with few adverse reactions. At high doses, nausea, headache, and drowsiness have been reported. Noscapine is occasionally included in multientity OTC preparations.

Nasal Decongestants

The most commonly used nasal decongestants are adrenergic agents. These drugs act by stimulating excitatory α-adrenergic receptors of vascular smooth muscle, thereby constricting the dilated arterioles within the nasal mucosa. This constriction reduces blood flow in the edematous area and opens obstructed nasal passages.

Most of these drugs are used topically. Topical application may cause temporary stinging, burning, or drying of the mucosa. Rebound congestion occurs after the use of many of these agents, often causing misuse of the drugs. Prolonged topical use may be irritating enough to induce a chronic swelling of the nasal mucosa; discontinuing the drug remedies this situation.

Phenylephrine, an α_1-adrenergic receptor agonist, is a widely used decongestant. It is less potent than the catecholamines but its duration of action is longer. Pseudoephedrine is a closely related drug.

Both ephedrine and epinephrine are effective decongestants, but they are seldom used in this capacity. Ephedrine can produce swelling of the nasal mucosa and tachyphylaxis, as well as CNS stimulation, palpitation, and transient hypertension. Epinephrine frequently produces rebound nasal congestion as well as the typical symptoms of CNS and cardiovascular stimulation, such as anxiety, palpitation, restlessness, dizziness, and headache. The adverse reactions produced by either drug disappear rapidly after the medication is discontinued.

Propylhexedrine is administered by nasal inhalation. It has essentially no toxic effects when used clinically, and it can even be used for those patients in whom the pressor effect of ephedrine is to be avoided.

Oxymetazoline is an effective decongestant with a long duration of action. It is available as a solution and as a spray. The adverse reactions associated with its use are mild and include stinging or drying of the nasal mucosa, headache, palpitation, and insomnia. Similar drugs include naphazoline, tetrahydrozoline, and xylometazoline.

Intranasal Steroids

Adrenal corticosteroids administered by nasal spray are effective for the relief of seasonal and perennial rhinitis. In this use, these drugs share many of the characteristics of steroids given by inhalation for the management of asthma. Drugs that are used for both purposes include beclomethasone, flunisolide, triamcinolone, budesonide, and fluticasone. Therapeutic benefits normally begin after several days of continuous use (one to three times per day, depending on the drug) but may be delayed for up to 3 weeks.

When used appropriately, systemic effects are minimal. Local candidiasis of the mouth and pharynx has been reported on occasion. Rinsing the mouth after use helps prevent such occurrences. Overdosing can produce adrenal suppression and the side effects reported in Chapter 35 for corticosteroids given orally.

Expectorants and Mucolytics

Agents administered to stimulate the flow of respiratory tract secretions are termed *expectorants*. Mucolytic agents are used to reduce the viscosity of respiratory tract secretions. Both drug groups enhance the movement of secretions upward and outward by ciliary movement and coughing.

Expectorants are believed to act by stimulating receptors in the gastric mucosa, thus initiating the reflex secretion of respiratory tract fluid. This action is assumed to increase the volume and decrease the viscosity of the secretions. There is little clinical evidence of the efficacy of these agents.

Potassium iodide is an example of a drug used traditionally as an expectorant and for which there is little proof of effectiveness. It is readily absorbed and produces untoward reactions on prolonged use. Iodism, characterized by skin rash, fever, parotitis, and lacrimal gland enlargement, can be produced. Thyroid enlargement or decreased thyroid function can also occur. Sensitivity reactions can develop, and anaphylaxis has occasionally been reported.

Ammonium chloride is another example of a drug used traditionally to stimulate the flow of respiratory secretions. It is used most frequently in multientity mixtures. It is readily absorbed and can produce metabolic acidosis if large doses are administered.

Guaifenesin (glyceryl guaiacolate) is available as an ingredient in various tablets and syrups. In clinical evaluations[45] it reportedly increased sputum volume; facilitated removal of sputum; and reduced cough frequency, cough intensity, and chest discomfort when compared with a matching vehicle. Nausea and gastrointestinal upset may occasionally occur, but no serious adverse reactions have been reported.

Drugs Acting on the Respiratory System

Nonproprietary (generic) name	*Proprietary (trade) name*
Emergency drugs	
Aromatic ammonia spirit	Aromatic Ammonia Aspirols
Doxapram	Dopram
Oxygen	—
Corticosteroids (inhalation and/or intranasal)	
Beclomethasone	Beclovent, Beconase AQ, QVAR, Vancenase AQ
Budesonide	Pulmicort, Rhinocort
Dexamethasone	Decadron
Flunisolide	AeroBid, Nasalide
Fluticasone	Flonase, Flovent, in Advair
Mometasone	Nasonex
Triamcinolone	Azmacort, Nasacort
Adrenergic bronchodilators	
Albuterol	Proventil, Ventolin
Bitolterol	Tornalate
Ephedrine	—
Epinephrine	Nephron, Primatene Mist
Ethylnorepinephrine	Bronkephrine
Formoterol	Foradil
Isoetharine	—
Isoproterenol	Isuprel
Levalbuterol	Xopenex
Metaproterenol	Alupent
Pirbuterol	Maxair
Procaterol*	Pro-Air
Salmeterol	Serevent, in Advair
Terbutaline	Brethine
Xanthines	
Aminophylline (theophylline ethylenediamine)	Phyllocontin, Truphylline
Oxtriphylline	Brondecon, Choledyl
Theophylline	Elixophyllin, Slo-Phyllin
Theophylline, extended-release	Slo-Phyllin Gyrocaps, Theo-Dur
Agents limited to prophylaxis or chronic treatment of asthma	
Cromolyn	Intal, Nasalcrom
Ketotifen*	Zaditen
Montelukast	Singulair
Nedocromil	Tilade
Zafirlukast	Accolate
Zileuton	Zyflo
Anticholinergic bronchodilators	
Atropine	Day-Dose Atropine Sulfate
Ipratropium	Atrovent
Antitussives	
Benzonatate	Tessalon Perles
Caramiphen edisylate	In Rescaps-D S.R.
Codeine	—
Dextromethorphan	Pertussin, Vicks Formula 44
Diphenhydramine	Bydramine, Diphen Cough
Hydrocodone	In Hycodan
Hydromorphone	In Dilaudid Cough Syrup
Noscapine	—
Nasal decongestants	
Ephedrine	Pretz-D, Vicks Vatronol
Epinephrine	Adrenalin Chloride
Naphazoline	Privine
Oxymetazoline	Afrin, Dristan Long Acting
Phenylephrine	Alconefrin, Neo-Synephrine
Phenylpropanolamine*	Propagest
Propylhexedrine	Benzedrex
Pseudoephedrine	Novafed, Sudafed
Tetrahydrozoline	Tyzine
Xylometazoline	Otrivin
Expectorants and mucolytics	
Acetylcysteine	Mucomyst, Mucosil
Ammonium chloride	In Efricon Expectorant Liquid
Guaifenesin	Halotussin, Robitussin
Iodinated glycerol	Iophen, Organidin
Potassium iodide	Pima
Syrup of ipecac	—
Terpin hydrate	—

*Not currently available in the United States.

Syrup of ipecac is a traditional expectorant and has been used widely in combination with other drugs in OTC mixtures. At higher doses it is an effective emetic, but it is no longer recommended for emergency home use to cause vomiting.

Acetylcysteine (N-acetyl-L-cysteine) is used in the hospital setting to reduce the viscosity of respiratory tract secretions.[61] The mucolytic action of acetylcysteine, when applied directly to the airways either by nebulization or instillation, is believed to result from the free sulfhydryl group cleaving certain disulfide bonds in glycoprotein macromolecules through a sulfhydryl-disulfide interchange reaction, thereby forming smaller mixed disulfides of acetylcysteine and glycoprotein subunits, with a resultant decrease in viscosity. The drug may cause mild gastrointestinal disturbances, including nausea, vomiting, and stomatitis. It can produce varying degrees of airway obstruction in hyperreactive asthmatics. Acetylcysteine should be used only where a suction apparatus is available and when patient strength and cooperation can help clear secretions because it produces large amounts of secretions that must be removed.

Cited References

1. Adachi M, Kobayashi H, Aoki N, et al: A comparison of the inhibitory effects of ketotifen and disodium cromoglycate on bronchial responses to house dust, with special reference to the late asthmatic response, *Pharmatherapeutica* 4:36-42, 1984.
2. Arner B: A comparative clinical trial of different subcutaneous doses of terbutaline and orciprenaline in bronchial asthma, *Acta Med Scand Suppl* 512:45-48, 1970.
3. Awni WM, Hussein Z, Granneman GR, et al: Pharmacodynamic and stereoselective pharmacokinetic interactions between zileuton and warfarin in humans, *Clin Pharmacokinet* 29(suppl 2):67-76, 1995.
4. Aylward M, Maddock J, Davies DE, et al: Dextromethorphan and codeine: comparison of plasma kinetics and antitussive effects, *Eur J Respir Dis* 65:283-291, 1984.
5. Barnes PJ: Corticosteroids: mode of action and place in management. In Clark TJH, Godfrey S, Lee TH, et al, eds: *Asthma*, ed 4, London, 2000, Arnold.
6. Barnes PJ, Pauwels RA: Theophylline in the management of asthma: time for reappraisal? *Eur Respir J* 7:579-591, 1994.
7. Bisgaard H: Leukotriene modifiers in pediatric asthma management, *Pediatrics* 107:381-390, 2001.
8. Chesnutt MS, Lazarus SC: Asthma therapy in the nineties: focus on inflammation, *Hosp Formul* 27:466-487, 1992.
9. Church MK, Polosa R, Rimmer SJ: Cromolyn sodium and nedocromil sodium: mast cell stabilizers, neuromodulators, or anti-inflammatory drugs? In Kaliner MA, Barnes PJ, Persson CGA, eds: *Asthma: its pathology and treatment. Lung biology in health and disease*, vol 49, New York, 1991, Marcel Dekker.
10. Cockcroft DW: Airway hyperresponsiveness in asthma, *Hosp Pract* 25:111-129, 1990.
11. Cugell DW: Clinical pharmacology and toxicology of ipratropium bromide, *Am J Med* 81(suppl 5A):18-22, 1986.
12. Cummins LH, Kozak PP, Gillman SH: Erythromycin's effect on theophylline blood levels, *Pediatrics* 59:144-145, 1977.
13. D'Alonzo GE, Nathan RA, Henochowicz S, et al: Salmeterol xinafoate as maintenance therapy compared with albuterol in patients with asthma, *JAMA* 271:1412-1416, 1994.
14. Descotes J, André P, Evreux JC: Pharmacokinetic drug interactions with macrolide antibiotics, *J Antimicrob Chemother* 15:659-664, 1985.
15. Drazen J: Clinical pharmacology of leukotriene receptor antagonists and 5-lipoxygenase inhibitors, *Am J Respir Crit Care Med* 157:S233-S237, 1998.
16. Drazen JM: Comparative contractile responses to sulfidopeptide leukotriene in normal and asthmatic human subjects, *Ann NY Acad Sci* 524:289-295, 1998.
17. Faurschou P, Steffensen I, Jacques L: Effect of addition of inhaled salmeterol to the treatment of moderate-to-severe asthmatics uncontrolled on high-dose inhaled steroids. European Respiratory Study Group, *Eur Respir J* 9:1885-1890, 1996.
18. Gardiner PV, Ward C, Booth H, et al: Effect of eight weeks of treatment with salmeterol on bronchoalveolar lavage inflammatory indices in asthmatic, *Am J Respir Crit Care Med* 150:1006-1011, 1994.
19. Granneman GR, Braeckman RA, Locke CS, et al: Effect of zileuton on theophylline pharmacokinetics, *Clin Pharmacokinet* 29(suppl 2):77-83, 1995.
20. Grant SM, Goa KL, Fitton A, et al: Ketotifen. A review of its pharmacodynamic and pharmacokinetic properties, and therapeutic use in asthma and allergic disorders, *Drugs* 40:412-448, 1990.
21. Grenell RG: Central nervous system resistance. I. The effects of temporary arrest of cerebral circulation for periods of two to ten minutes, *J Neuropathol Exp Neurol* 5:131-154, 1946.
22. Higgins RM, Stradling JR, Lane DJ: Should ipratropium bromide be added to beta-agonists in treatment of acute severe asthma? *Chest* 94:718-722, 1988.
23. Horwitz RJ, McGill KA, Busse WW: The role of leukotriene modifiers in the treatment of asthma, *Am J Respir Crit Care Med* 157:1363-1371, 1998.
24. Hyland ME, Kenyon CA, Jacobs PA: Sensitivity of quality of life domains and constructs to longitudinal change in a clinical trial comparing salmeterol with placebo in asthmatics, *Qual Life Res* 3:121-126, 1994.
25. Johnson M, Butchers PR, Coleman RA, et al: The pharmacology of salmeterol, *Life Sci* 52:2131-2143, 1993.
26. Lee TH, Hawrylowicz CM: Inflammatory mediators and cytokines in asthma. In Clark TJH, Godfrey S, Lee TH, et al, eds: *Asthma*, ed 4, London, 2000, Arnold.
27. Lewis RA, Austen KF, Soberman RJ: Leukotrienes and other products of the 5-lipoxygenase pathway. Biochemistry and relation to pathobiology in human diseases, *N Engl J Med* 323:645-655, 1990.
28. Marin MG: Low-dose methotrexate spares steroid usage in steroid-dependent asthmatic patients: a meta-analysis, *Chest* 112:29-33, 1997.
29. Medical Research Council Working Party: Long term domiciliary oxygen therapy in chronic hypoxic cor pulmonale complicating chronic bronchitis and emphysema, *Lancet* 1:681-686, 1981.
30. Moore RH, Khan A, Dickey BF, et al: Long-acting inhaled β_2-agonists in asthma therapy, *Chest* 113:1095-1108, 1998.
31. Murciano D, Aubier M, Lecocguic Y, et al: Effects of theophylline on diaphragmatic strength and fatigue in patients with chronic obstructive pulmonary disease, *N Engl J Med* 311:349-353, 1984.

32. Nocturnal Oxygen Therapy Trial Group: Continuous or nocturnal oxygen therapy in hypoxemic chronic obstructive lung disease: a clinical trial, *Ann Intern Med* 93:391-398, 1980.
33. Obase Y, Shimoda T, Tomari S, et al: Efficacy and safety of long-term treatment of asthmatic patients with pranlukast, a cysteinyl-leukotriene-receptor antagonist: four-year followup study, *Ann Allergy Asthma Immunol* 87:43-47, 2001.
34. O'Byrne PM, Israel E, Drazen J: Antileukotrienes in the treatment of asthma, *Ann Intern Med* 127:472-480, 1997.
35. Parson GH: Treatment of asthma in adults. In Gershwin ME, Albertson TE, eds: *Bronchial asthma: principles of diagnosis and treatment*, ed 4, Totowa, NJ, 2001, Humana.
36. Pauwels R, Persson CGA: Xanthines. In Kaliner NA, Barnes PJ, Persson CGA, eds: *Asthma: its pathology and treatment. Lung biology in health and disease*, vol 49, New York, 1991, Marcel Dekker.
37. Pearlman DS, Chervinsky P, LaForce C, et al: A comparison of salmeterol with albuterol in the treatment of mild-to-moderate asthma, *N Engl J Med* 327:1420-1425, 1992.
38. Piafsky KM, Ogilvie RI: Dosage of theophylline in bronchial asthma, *N Engl J Med* 292:1218-1222, 1975.
39. Ramage L, Cree IA, Dhillon DP: Comparison of salmeterol with placebo in mild asthma: effect on peripheral blood phagocyte function and cytokine levels, *Int Arch Allergy Immunol* 105:181-184, 1994.
40. Randall T: International consensus report urges sweeping reform in asthma treatment, *JAMA* 267:2153-2154, 1992.
41. Read J, Rebuck AS: Steroid-sparing effect of disodium cromoglycate ("Intal") in chronic asthma, *Med J Aust* 1:566-569, 1969.
42. Rebuck AS, Chapman KR, Abboud R, et al: Nebulized anticholinergic and sympathomimetic treatment of asthma and chronic obstructive airway disease in the emergency room, *Am J Med* 82:59-64, 1987.
43. Reilly KM, Salluzzo R: Theophylline toxicity, *Resid Staff Physician* 37:55-57, 1991.
44. Reinus JF, Persky S, Burkiewicz JS, et al: Severe liver injury after treatment with the leukotriene receptor antagonist zafirlukast, *Ann Intern Med* 133:964-968, 2000.
45. Robinson RE, Cummings WB, Deffenbaugh ER: Effectiveness of guaifenesin as an expectorant: a cooperative double-blind study, *Curr Ther Res* 22:284-296, 1977.
46. Rutten-van Molken MP, Custers F, van Doorslaer EK, et al: Comparison of performance of four instruments in evaluating the effects of salmeterol on asthma quality of life, *Eur Respir J* 8:888-898, 1995.
47. Samuelsson B, Dahlen SE, Lindgren JA, et al: Leukotrienes and lipoxins: structures, biosynthesis, and biological effects, *Science* 237:1171-1176, 1987.
48. Schleimer RP: Effects of glucocorticosteroids on inflammatory cells relevant to their therapeutic applications in asthma, *Am Rev Respir Dis* 141:S59-S69, 1990.
49. Sessler CN, Theophylline toxicity: clinical features of 116 consecutive cases, *Am J Med* 88:567-576, 1990.
50. Shannon M: Hypokalemia, hyperglycemia and plasma catecholamine activity after severe theophylline intoxication, *J Toxicol Clin Toxicol* 32:41-47, 1994.
51. Shannon M: Life-threatening events after theophylline overdose: a 10-year prospective analysis, *Arch Intern Med* 159:989-994, 1999.
52. Shannon MW: Comparative efficacy of hemodialysis and hemoperfusion in severe theophylline intoxication, *Acad Emerg Med* 4:674-678, 1997.
53. Southorn PA, Powis G: Free radicals in medicine. II. Involvement in human disease, *Mayo Clin Proc* 63:390-408, 1988.
54. Szczeklik A: The cyclooxygenase theory of aspirin-induced asthma, *Eur Respir J* 3:588-593, 1990.
55. Szefler SJ: Glucocorticoid therapy for asthma: clinical pharmacology, *J Allergy Clin Immunol* 88:147-165, 1991.
56. Tattersfield AE: β-agonists: mode of action and place in management. In Clark TJH, Godfrey S, Lee TH, et al, eds: *Asthma*, ed 4, London, 2000, Arnold.
57. Thompson RD, Nagasawa HT, Jenne JW: Determination of theophylline and its metabolites in human urine and serum by high-pressure liquid chromatography, *J Lab Clin Med* 84:584-593, 1974.
58. Thomson NC: Non-steroidal prophylactic agents: mode of action and place in management. In Clark TJH, Godfrey S, Lee TH, et al, eds: *Asthma*, ed 4, London, 2000, Arnold.
59. Tiep BL: Long term oxygen therapy. In Hodgkin JE, ed: Chronic obstructive pulmonary disease, *Clin Chest Med* 11:505-521, 1990.
60. Tiep BL: *Portable oxygen therapy: including oxygen conserving methodology*, Mount Kisco, NY, 1991, Futura.
61. Ventresca GP, Cicchetti V, Ferrari V: Acetylcysteine. In Braga PC, Allegra I, eds: *Drugs in bronchial mucology*, New York, 1989, Raven Press.
62. Wenzel SE, New approaches to anti-inflammatory therapy for asthma, *Am J Med* 104:287-300, 1998.
63. Woolcock A, Lundback B, Ringdal N, et al: Comparison of addition of salmeterol to inhaled steroids with doubling of the dose of inhaled steroids, *Am J Respir Crit Care Med* 153:1481-1488, 1996.

General References

Clark TJH, Godfrey S, Lee TH, et al, eds: *Asthma*, ed 4, London, 2000, Arnold.

Emond SD, Camargo CA, Jr, Nowak RM: 1997 National Asthma Education and Prevention Program guidelines: a practical summary for emergency physicians, *Ann Emerg Med* 31:579-589, 1998.

Page CP, Barnes PJ, eds: *Pharmacology of asthma. Handbook of experimental pharmacology*, vol 98, New York, 1991, Springer-Verlag.

Undem BJ, Lichtenstein LM: Drugs used in the treatment of asthma. In Hardman JG, Limberd LE, Gilman AG, eds: *Goodman & Gilman's The pharmacological basis of therapeutics*, ed 10, New York, 2001, McGraw-Hill.

CHAPTER • 33

Drugs Acting on the Gastrointestinal Tract*

David H. Shaw

Some of the most frequently used drugs are those that exert an effect on the gastrointestinal tract. Digestive diseases are reported to afflict 12% of all American adults and account for 16% of all absences from work.[21] The likelihood that a patient coming into the dental office may be on a regimen of one or more of these agents is high. Included in this group of drugs are various anticholinergics and antihistamines, antacids, proton pump inhibitors, antiemetics, laxatives, antidiarrheal or antispasmodic drugs, stimulants, and miscellaneous agents. Some of these are sold over the counter (OTC) without prescription and may be used at the discretion of the patient. Knowing that these drugs are being used may influence the choice of a dental therapeutic agent. Furthermore, a gastrointestinal disturbance arising during the course of dental treatment may be attributable to one of these agents.

Many of the drugs discussed here are described in detail in other parts of the book. This chapter focuses on those drugs that are used exclusively for their effect on the gastrointestinal tract, as well as those with a wider spectrum of activity that have application to gastrointestinal disorders. Some drugs that act on the gastrointestinal tract and are likely to be used in dentistry are listed in Table 33-1.

DRUGS USED IN PEPTIC ULCER THERAPY

Peptic ulcer disease (PUD) is a common malady afflicting 10% to 15% of the population at some time in life. It has been estimated that in the American population, approximately 2% of men and 1.5% of women have peptic ulcers.[10] Although PUD is a painful condition that can seriously affect the quality of life, it is rarely fatal. Economically it is a major illness, with billions of dollars spent in treatment and lost in decreased wages and work productivity. Peptic ulcers are characterized by spontaneous healing and recurrence. The primary complication is spontaneous hemorrhage, which may be life threatening. However, the greater portion of the 3000 deaths from this disease per year in the United States is caused by perforation of the gastrointestinal wall, which occurs much less frequently.[10]

Throughout most of the twentieth century, therapy for PUD was directed at suppression of acid secretion or neutralization of secreted acid. This approach was based on the long-held assumption that ulcers develop only because of increased gastric acid secretion. The cause of PUD is now thought to be related to mucosal exposure to gastric acid and pepsin with a very strong association with *Helicobacter pylori* infection, or the breakdown of normal mucosal defenses from the use of nonsteroidal antiinflammatory drugs (NSAIDs).[10] *H. pylori* infects more than half of the US population older than 60 years and accounts for 80% of all stomach ulcers and more than 90% of all duodenal ulcers.[2] Because only 15% to 20% of *H. pylori*–infected patients are estimated to have PUD develop in their lifetime, other factors must play a role in the development of this disease. Several studies have demonstrated the presence of *H. pylori* in saliva,[19] but the relation between its presence in the mouth and infection in the stomach is not known. The oral cavity may be a permanent reservoir for *H. pylori*, and a person-to-person route is the most probable mode of transmission.[54] The current cornerstone of therapy for peptic ulcers involves a triple combination regimen of a proton pump inhibitor (e.g., lansoprazole) or an H_2-receptor antihistamine (e.g., ranitidine) with two antibiotics (e.g., clarithromycin and amoxicillin). Other therapeutic approaches include antacids, topical cytoprotectants, antimuscarinic agents, and exogenous prostaglandin.

Proton Pump Inhibitors

Proton pump inhibitors (PPIs) are drugs that irreversibly inhibit H^+, K^+-activated adenosine triphosphatase (H^+, K^+-ATPase, commony called the *proton pump*), in the gastric parietal cell (Figure 33-1), the final common pathway for acid secretion.[56] The PPIs have become the drug class of choice for treating acid-related gastrointestinal diseases such as PUD and gastroesophageal reflux disease (GERD). Currently there are five members of the PPI class available by prescription in the United States: esomeprazole, lansoprazole, omeprazole, pantoprazole, and rabeprazole (Table 33-2). Omeprazole is also available OTC. When taken orally, all five effectively reduce basal and stimulated acid secretion by up to 100%. They are longer lasting and substantially more potent than H_2-receptor antagonists in the short-term treatment of PUD and GERD and relief of heartburn.[45]

PPIs are prodrugs that accumulate selectively in the acid environment of the secretory canaliculus of the gastric parietal cell. The PPI is protonated in this acid environment to the active form of the drug.[30] Because the PPIs bind covalently to the proton pump (rabeprazole may be the exception), synthesis of new pumps or activation of resting pumps is required to restore pump activity.[56] This irreversible inhibition of the pump explains why the duration of action of this class extends beyond the elimination half-life of 0.5 to 2 hours (see Table 33-2).[30]

The most common adverse effects reported with PPIs are headache, diarrhea, and nausea, but the frequency is only slightly above that seen with a placebo.[22] Safety concerns with long-term use of PPIs have been caused by the slight increase in serum gastrin accompanying their use, because gastrin-induced neoplasms have been reported in animal

*The author wish to recognize Dr. Glenn Housholder for her past contributions to this chapter. See the Acknowledgmets.

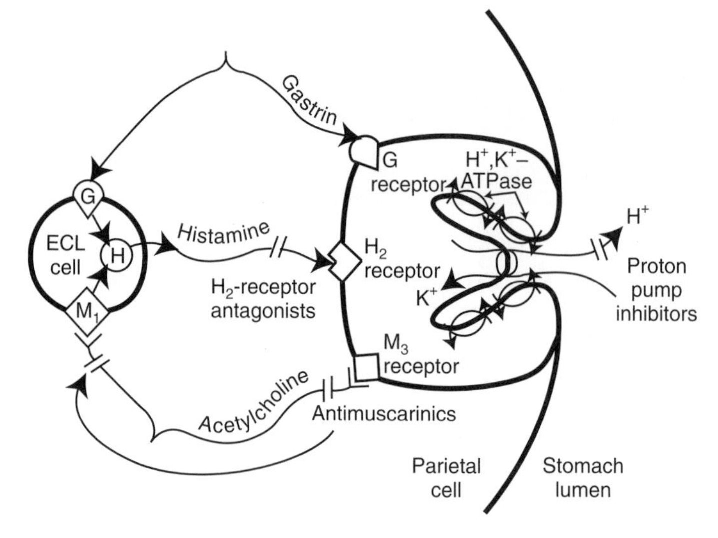

Fig. 33-1 The physiologic control of H^+ secretion by the gastric parietal cell, with the site of action of the major antisecretory drugs. Included is an endocrine cell that secretes histamine (enterochromaffinlike [*ECL*] cell) and an acid-secreting parietal cell.

Table • 33-1

Drugs Useful in Dentistry That Affect the Gastrointestinal Tract

THERAPEUTIC USE	DRUG	DOSE*
Antisialagogue	Atropine sulfate (Sal-Tropine)	0.3 to 1.2 mg
	Scopolamine hydrobromide (Scopace)	0.4 to 0.8 mg
	Glycopyrrolate (Robinul)	1 to 2 mg
	Propantheline bromide (Pro-Banthine)	7.5 to 30 mg
Antiemetic	Dimenhydrinate (Dramamine)	50 to 100 mg
	Meclizine (Antivert)	25 to 50 mg
	Promethazine hydrochloride (Phenergan)	25 mg
	Trimethobenzamide hydrochloride (Tigan)	250 mg

*Adult, oral route.

Table • 33-2

Comparison of the Proton Pump Inhibitors (PPIs)

DRUG	BIOAVAILABILITY (%)	PEAK PLASMA TIME (hr)	ELIMINATION HALF-LIFE (hr)	ORAL DOSE INTERVAL (hr)
Esomeprazole (Nexium)	>50	1.5	1.7	24
Lansoprazole (Prevacid)	>80	1.7	1.5	24
Omeprazole (Prilosec)	35	0.5 to 3.5	0.5 to 1.0	24
Pantoprazole (Protonix)	>77	2.4	1	24
Rabeprazole (Aciphex)	52	2 to 5	1 to 2	24

models.[22] To date, none of the PPIs has been associated with an increased risk of gastric cancers in patients receiving long-term therapy.

All PPIs increase gastric pH and may alter the absorption of drugs that are weak bases or acids or formulated as pH-dependent controlled-release products. Absorption of aspirin, digoxin, and midazolam has been reported to increase, and ketoconazole absorption is decreased when administered with a PPI,[22] but the clinical significance is not clear. PPIs can also alter the hepatic metabolism of other medications. All PPIs are metabolized to varying degrees by specific hepatic cytochrome P450 (CYP) isoenzymes and may interfere with the medications metabolized by these same enzymes. Specifically omeprazole, but not the other PPIs, has been shown to inhibit the metabolism of diazepam, causing a 15% to 25% increase in diazepam concentrations.[22] However, few clinically important drug interactions have been reported despite the enormous popularity of the PPIs.

H_2-Receptor Antihistamines

Histamine is one of the primary mediators of gastric acid secretion, along with acetylcholine and gastrin. The final common

Table • 33-3

Comparison of H_2 Antihistamines

DRUG	BIOAVAILABILITY (%)	PEAK PLASMA TIME (hr)	ELIMINATION HALF-LIFE (hr)	ORAL DOSE INTERVAL (hr)*
Cimetidine (Tagamet)	60 to 70	0.75 to 1.5	2	6 to 24
Famotidine (Pepcid)	40 to 45	1 to 3	3	12 to 24
Nizatidine (Axid)	>90	0.5 to 3	1.5	12 to 24
Ranitidine (Zantac)	50 to 60	1 to 3	2.5	12 to 24

*For treatment of duodenal or gastric ulcer.

pathway is through the proton pump (see Figure 33-1). As discussed in Chapter 22, H_2 receptors are located on the acid-secreting parietal cells of the stomach. These cells release acid when stimulated by histamine and so contribute to ulcer formation. The H_2-receptor antihistamines are reversible, competitive antagonists of histamine at the H_2 receptors and thus block acid secretion. Both the duration and degree of acid suppression are dose dependent. These are highly selective agents in that they do not affect the H_1 receptors and are not anticholinergic. Cimetidine, the first of these drugs to enjoy widespread use, revolutionized the treatment of duodenal ulcers.

A single dose of cimetidine or any of the other H_2-receptor antagonists currently available for prescription or nonprescription use in the United States (famotidine, nizatidine, and ranitidine) (Table 33-3), reduces the volume of basal and food-stimulated gastric acid secretion by more than 90%. The drugs are somewhat less effective, however, in reducing nocturnal secretion of gastric acid. Nevertheless, numerous clinical studies have confirmed their effectiveness in promoting healing of gastric and duodenal ulcers as well as preventing their recurrence.

H_2-receptor blockers, in addition to their antisecretory actions, also accelerate ulcer healing by the induction of endogenous prostanoid synthesis. Endogenous gastric prostanoid synthesis in patients with untreated duodenal ulcer is significantly lower than in normal subjects. This fact, coupled with the almost complete inhibition of prostanoid synthesis by gastric mucosa in patients receiving long-term NSAID therapy, suggests that decreased endogenous prostanoid synthesis may contribute to the pathogenesis of mucosal damage.

The H_2 blockers are commonly administered orally, and the antisecretory activity usually begins within 1 hour of administration and persists for 6 to 12 hours.[39] They have an oral bioavailability of 40% to more than 90%, achieve peak plasma concentrations in 0.5 to 3 hours, and are eliminated with a terminal half-life of 1.5 to 3 hours (see Table 33-3). The drugs undergo some metabolism in the liver; the remainder of the parent drug is eliminated unchanged by the kidney. The duration of effectiveness varies with the drug, dose, and medical condition being treated, ranging from 4 hours for a low dose of cimetidine for hypersecretory disorders up to 24 hours for all these agents when used to treat duodenal and gastric ulcers.

Comparative studies of the H_2 blockers demonstrate that the four drugs in this class are essentially equal in clinical effectiveness regarding ulcer treatment even though they express varying potencies in their ability to block pentagastrin-stimulated gastric acid secretion in the research laboratory.

Cimetidine appears unique among H_2 blockers in exerting biologic effects that are unrelated to gastric H_2-receptor occupancy. For example, cimetidine therapy, particularly when prolonged and at high doses, can cause antiandrogenic effects. These reversible effects result from the ability of cimetidine to compete for dihydrotestosterone binding at androgen-binding sites and to inhibit the CYP metabolism of estradiol.[13] As many as 50% of patients with Zollinger-Ellison syndrome who are treated with high doses of cimetidine for long periods of time experience impotence and development of gynecomastia. Substitution of ranitidine for cimetidine reverses these effects, and no antiandrogenic effects have been reported after therapeutic doses of famotidine or nizatidine.

Of importance to the dentist is the ability of cimetidine to decrease the hepatic oxidative biotransformation of a number of other drugs, including lidocaine and diazepam. Both cimetidine and ranitidine are ligands for multiple CYP enzymes (see Table 2-3), with cimetidine exhibiting a much higher affinity and thus inhibiting hepatic microsomal enzyme activity to a much greater extent. The clinical use of ranitidine does not appear to have a significant effect on the metabolism and elimination of other drugs, and this statement also applies to famotidine and nizatidine, which have shown no effect on hepatic CYP enzymes.

The widespread use of cimetidine has revealed a variety of central nervous system (CNS) manifestations (e.g., headache, lethargy, confusion, forgetfulness), especially in the elderly. Impaired renal function in the older patient may contribute to these reactions. Similar effects have been reported for ranitidine and famotidine but appear to be less common.

Antibiotics

The evidence that PUD (as well as gastritis and possibly gastric adenocarcinoma) is directly linked to infection by the gram-negative organism *H. pylori* is now well established.[23] Cultures taken from biopsy material are positive for *H. pylori* in approximately 95% of specimens collected from duodenal ulcers and 75% of biopsies taken from gastric ulcers, compared with a roughly 25% incidence in asymptomatic control subjects.[5] Experimentally, gastric inoculation of *H. pylori* in experimental animals results in ulceration.[32]

These findings have led to the routine use of antibiotic therapy for the eradication of ulcers. Significant reduction in both clinical symptoms and histologic evidence of ulcers has been achieved. In an early study of patients with confirmed duodenal ulcers, antibiotic plus H_2-blocker treatment reduced the incidence of ulcer relapse by tenfold compared with placebo plus H_2-blocker treatment.[27] More recently, the use of a PPI with two antibiotics has assumed a major role in therapy because the PPIs not only add antisecretory properties but have been shown to demonstrate anti–*H. pylori* properties in vitro.[49] This multiple drug therapy is recommended because bacterial resistance is a problem. The combined use of bismuth subsalicylate, tetracycline, and metronidazole (along with an H_2 blocker) is highly effective, but the use of amoxicillin and clarithromycin with lansoprazole is better tolerated. A clinical study of this latter regimen resulted in an eradication rate of 86%.[44] Although future studies are required to determine the exact interaction between bacterial infection and other prognostic factors (e.g., smoking, alcohol, NSAIDs) important in ulcer formation, it is now recommended that all patients with ulcers infected with *H. pylori* be treated with therapy that combines an antisecretory drug with two or more antimicrobial agents.[46]

Gastric Antacids

Gastric antacids are weak bases that buffer or neutralize gastric hydrochloric acid and thereby increase gastric pH. This reduction in gastric acidity makes them useful in the treatment of PUD as well as heartburn and upset stomach caused by overeating or eating certain foods. Through acid neutralization, antacids reduce the proteolytic activity of pepsin, which is completely inactivated above a pH of 4. Overuse of antacids is discouraged because excessive neutralization may stimulate acid rebound; however, this response may be of little clinical significance because the added acid load may be compensated for by the buffers in the antacid. Antacids may also enhance ulcer healing beyond and independent of their acid-neutralizing property by enhancing the gastric mucosal defense mechanism through the stimulation of prostaglandin production or in the binding of unidentified substances that may be injurious to the mucosa. A comparison of selected tablet antacid formulations is shown in Table 33-4.

Prostaglandins are known to inhibit gastric acid secretion and exert cytoprotective properties. The actions of antacids on the gastric mucosa illustrate that the overall effect of antacid therapy is far more complex than simple acid neutralization.

Antacids have a rapid onset of action that depends on how fast the product dissolves in gastric acid. Generally, antacid suspensions dissolve more easily than tablets or powders for a faster response. The duration of action of an antacid in the stomach is influenced by the gastric emptying time, which is slowed by food in the stomach and patient variability in gastric secretory capacity. Generally, antacids taken on an empty stomach have a duration of action of approximately 30 minutes, whereas antacids taken after a full meal may neutralize acid for up to 3 hours.

Four primary compounds are currently used, alone or in combination, in antacid products: sodium bicarbonate, magnesium salts, aluminum salts, and calcium carbonate. The following is a discussion of these commonly used antacid preparations.

Sodium bicarbonate

Sodium bicarbonate is widely available in the form of baking soda and in combination products. It reacts almost instantaneously to neutralize gastric acid. Sodium bicarbonate is referred to as a "systemic" antacid because it has the capability of being absorbed into general circulation and altering systemic pH. The potential for Na^+ overload and systemic alkalosis limits its use to short-term relief of indigestion. Na^+ overload resulting from repeated use of large doses may contribute to fluid retention, edema, congestive heart failure, and renal failure. Sodium bicarbonate is contraindicated in patients on a low-salt diet.

Magnesium salts

Several magnesium salts (carbonate, hydroxide, oxide, trisilicate) have antacid properties. Magnesium hydroxide (milk of magnesia) is used most often and has a rapid onset of action and high neutralizing capacity. The risk of Mg^{++} overload is low and significant only in patients with impaired renal function. A disadvantage is its laxative effect, and few ulcer patients can tolerate it as the sole antacid for any length of time.

Magnesium trisilicate is much weaker than magnesium hydroxide, and therefore substantially more of the drug is required for the same degree of neutralization. Its onset of action is slow, and it reacts with gastric acid to form silicon dioxide in the stomach. Silicate kidney stones have been reported after its prolonged use. It is generally used in combination with other antacids such as aluminum hydroxide and calcium and magnesium carbonates.

Aluminum salts

Aluminum may be administered in several salt forms (aminoacetate, carbonate, hydroxide, phosphate) but aluminum hydroxide gel is the most potent buffer and is used the most frequently. Aluminum hydroxide dissolves slowly and is poorly absorbed. Liquid formulations provide a more rapid response than solid forms. Toxicity, other than occasional nausea and vomiting, is rare. The formation of insoluble salts limits its absorption. However, patients with impaired renal function who take aluminum antacids long term may not clear the Al^{+++}, resulting in hyperaluminemia and accumulation of Al^{+++} in other tissues. Its most common side effect is constipation, which may lead to intestinal obstruction. The constipating effect of aluminum-containing antacids is dose related and can be managed with stool softeners or laxatives or minimized when the drug is taken with magnesium hydroxide. Because the Al^{+++} can combine with phosphate in the gut to form insoluble aluminum phosphate, which is then excreted in the feces, prolonged use of large doses of aluminum hydroxide may result in phosphate depletion, particularly when phosphate intake is low. Anorexia, malaise, and muscle weakness are characteristic of phosphate depletion. The tendency of Al^{+++} to combine with phosphate has been used by nephrologists to prevent the formation of renal phosphatic calculi.

Calcium carbonate

Calcium carbonate produces a potent and prolonged neutralization of gastric acid. Approximately 90% of the ingested calcium forms insoluble salts in the gut and is excreted in the

Table • 33-4

Comparison of Selected Tablet Antacid Formulations

PROPRIETARY (TRADE) NAME	mEq ACID-NEUTRALIZING CAPACITY PER TABLET	DOSE EQUIVALENTS (TABLETS)
Maalox TC	28	3
Riopan Plus 2	30	3
Mylanta II	23	4
Tums E-X	15	6
Mylanta	11.5	7
Tums	10	8
Gelusil	11	8
Rolaids, Sodium-Free	8.5	10
Gaviscon	0.5	160

Adapted from Berardi RR, ed: *Handbook of nonprescription drugs*, ed 13, Washington, DC, 2002, American Pharmaceutical Association, p 275.

feces. The remaining Ca^{++} is absorbed into the systemic circulation. Extensive use of calcium-containing antacids may cause or exacerbate hypercalcemia, which is characterized by neurologic symptoms and reduced renal function. This effect is rare in healthy patients with normal renal function. Calcium-containing antacids are associated with acid rebound and increased serum gastrin concentrations. These effects have not been shown to delay ulcer healing and may be caused by a direct effect of Ca^{++} on the gastric mucosa.[25] Calcium carbonate has a chalky taste and may produce constipation, which reduces its desirability as an antacid. Because some Ca^{++} is absorbed, calcium-containing antacids are marketed as a source of dietary Ca^{++}.

Alginic Acid

Alginic acid is not an antacid, but because of its unique mechanism of action it is added to various antacid formulations to increase their effectiveness in the treatment of heartburn and relieve the symptoms of GERD. In the presence of saliva, alginic acid reacts with sodium bicarbonate to form sodium alginate. Gastric acid causes the alginate to precipitate, forming a foaming, viscous gel that floats on the surface of the gastric contents.[37] This provides a relatively pH-neutral barrier during episodes of acid reflux and enhances the efficacy of drugs used to treat GERD, although the FDA considers alginic acid to be of questionable value. Alginic acid products are not indicated for the treatment of PUD.

Sucralfate

Sucralfate, a complex of aluminum hydroxide and sulfated sucrose, is used in clinical practice to prevent and treat several gastrointestinal diseases, including PUD, GERD, and dyspepsia. After oral administration the drug disperses in the stomach and, in the presence of acid, forms a viscous suspension that binds with high affinity at the ulcer site. This produces an adherent, physical cytoprotective barrier that covers the ulcer and protects it from further attack by damaging agents (e.g., acid, pepsin, bile salts).

Although sucralfate has multiple actions,[8,47] it possesses no meaningful antacid properties. A key element in the acute gastroprotective actions of sucralfate is its ability to maintain mucosal vascular integrity and blood flow. It enhances bicarbonate and mucus secretion, increases mucosal hydrophobicity, and induces a rise in mucosal concentration of prostaglandin—all factors considered important in tissue healing.[8] An increase in local fibroblast growth factors, and possibly other growth factors, has also been proposed to explain the powerful ulcer-healing actions of sucralfate, which occur independently of a decreased gastric acid concentration in the stomach and duodenum.[8] Because it is minimally absorbed from the gastrointestinal tract, sucralfate is considered a remarkably safe agent. For this reason, sucralfate is a therapy of choice in the management of acid-related diseases during pregnancy.[9] It does require an acid pH to be activated and so should not be administered concomitantly with antacids, H_2 receptor antagonists, or PPIs. The most common side effect is constipation (up to 15%). Other reactions include dry mouth, nausea, vomiting, headache, and rashes.

For short-term treatment of an acute duodenal ulcer, the efficacy of sucralfate therapy is comparable to that of cimetidine. The use of a topical sucralfate suspension has been advocated in the prevention or treatment of stomatitis caused by chemotherapy or radiation,[4,20] despite studies that showed no substantial benefits from sucralfate in inhibiting radiation-induced esophagitis.[40]

Antimuscarinic Drugs

The use of antimuscarinic drugs (muscarinic receptor antagonists) for the treatment of PUD declined dramatically after the introduction of the H_2-blocker cimetidine. As is discussed in Chapter 9, antimuscarinic agents (e.g., atropine) are not selective inhibitors of gastric acid secretion, and therapeutic benefits for the treatment of gastrointestinal disease accrue only at doses that cause sufficient side effects to impair patient compliance. However, antimuscarinic drugs with activity relatively selective for gastric M_1 muscarinic receptors have been developed. Pirenzepine and telenzepine, selective M_1-receptor antagonists, are currently available in other countries for the treatment of PUD, but they have not yet been approved for use in the United States. Pirenzepine and telenzepine block gastric acid secretion to a greater extent than they inhibit smooth and cardiac muscle and salivary gland function. The reason is that the M_1 receptor is not the major muscarinic receptor in most smooth muscle, cardiac muscle, or salivary glands. In clinical studies both pirenzepine and telenzepine are as effective as cimetidine in the treatment of PUD, although the ulcer healing rates are somewhat lower. Pirenzepine and telenzepine have a low incidence of side effects because of their selective inhibition of gastric acid secretion; this will likely make them a valuable addition to current agents used in the treatment of PUD.

Prostaglandins

Misoprostol, a synthetic prostaglandin E_1 analogue, is the best studied of the prostaglandin derivatives. Although the prostaglandins have direct cytoprotective effects on the gastroduodenal mucosa, as noted above, the ulcer-healing effect of misoprostol and other prostaglandin analogues appears to be caused by the inhibition of acid secretion.[13] These agents interact with a basolateral receptor of the parietal cell that causes the inhibition of adenylyl cyclase. This results in reduced production of cyclic 3′,5′-adenosine monophosphate, the major second messenger for histamine-induced acid secretion. Doses of misoprostol (200 mg four times a day) produce duodenal and gastric ulcer healing rates that are comparable to those with cimetidine (300 mg four times a day). The drug is useful in preventing gastric (but not duodenal) ulceration associated with the use of NSAIDs.[50] The most common side effects are abdominal pain (7% to 20%) and diarrhea (13% to 40%) and are dose related. Misoprostol stimulates contraction of the uterus, which contraindicates its use in women of childbearing age. This property, however, makes it useful in women undergoing elective termination of pregnancy by facilitating expulsion of the uterine contents.

Clinical experience with other prostaglandin E analogues (e.g., enprostil) is too limited to predict their place in ulcer therapy.

Implications for Dentistry

Whether a patient is taking a regimen of a PPI, H_2 blocker, or antacids or has a history of a gastric or duodenal ulcer is important information for the dentist because this can influence the choice of a therapeutic agent or time of drug administration. The use of aspirin as an analgesic is contraindicated because of its irritating effect on gastric mucosa. This is particularly true for the elderly patient.[24] All NSAIDs share the ulcerogenic property of the salicylates. In fact, NSAIDs are estimated to cause 30% of ulcers.[26] Acetaminophen may be used as an alternative analgesic because it produces minimal damage to gastric mucosa compared with aspirin. For acute dental pain, a cyclooxygenase-2–selective inhibitor, such as rofecoxib, may also be used if the patient is currently ulcer free because it is at least as efficacious and significantly less ulcerogenic than either aspirin or ibuprofen.

As previously mentioned, PPIs may cause a profound inhibition of gastric acid secretion that may influence the absorption of drugs in which gastric pH influences bioavailability (e.g., ketoconazole, ampicillin), although the clinical significance of this interaction has yet to be determined. Likewise, the theoretical risk of increasing the response to diazepam when coadministered with PPIs, especially omeprazole, has to date little clinical significance.

Systemic corticosteroids, as used after oral surgical procedures, are potentially ulcerogenic. Even topical steroids used in the management of oral lesions should be avoided in the patient with an ulcer because of the possibility that absorption through the mucosa will occur.

The choice of a preoperative or postoperative sedative is particularly important for the ulcer patient. For instance, chloral hydrate is quite irritating, and gastrointestinal side effects such as nausea and vomiting can occur. Diazepam is appropriate for selected patients because, in addition to producing sedation, it can suppress the nocturnal secretion of gastric acid. Furthermore, absorption of orally administered diazepam is increased by the use of aluminum hydroxide, whereas magnesium salts retard its absorption. For the patient being treated with cimetidine or omeprazole, however, a prudent choice might be lorazepam or oxazepam, antianxiety drugs not dependent on hepatic oxidative biotransformation. They are eliminated in the urine as glucuronide conjugates, the formation of which is not impaired by either cimetidine or omeprazole.

Pretreatment with cimetidine for a day or more may cause much higher plasma concentrations of diazepam taken on a regular basis, a more pronounced sedative effect, and slowed elimination of the drug. However, the significance of such cimetidine-induced drug interactions is likely to be patient or population specific. The manifestations of the diazepam-cimetidine interaction may be clinically insignificant in young adults, but the interaction could be important in the elderly or in patients on multiple medications. If a course of diazepam therapy is prescribed for a dental patient on cimetidine, its dosage should be reduced.

As previously mentioned, cimetidine inhibits the hepatic metabolism of lidocaine and presumably other amide local anesthetics. Fortunately, this interaction is of little practical concern in view of the low dosages of lidocaine typically required for intraoral anesthesia.

Aluminum hydroxide gels, antacids containing calcium and magnesium salts and sodium bicarbonate impair the absorption of the tetracyclines. This action is shared by milk and milk products and appears to result from chelation and an increased gastric pH. Sucralfate can also reduce the absorption of several drugs, including tetracycline, when administered concomitantly. A reasonable general approach for prescribing tetracycline or other drugs to the dental patient receiving sucralfate therapy would be to separate the administration of each drug by several hours. This approach resulted in a negligible effect on tetracycline absorption when tested in animals.[38]

ANTISIALAGOGUES

The short-term control of salivary flow is often helpful in dental procedures (e.g., occlusal adjustment and impression taking) but is not an officially accepted indication for these drugs. Blockade of acetylcholine at muscarinic receptor sites can have dramatic effects on the secretory function of the salivary glands. The recommended oral doses for blocking excessive salivation are relatively free of side effects (see Table 33-1).[57]

The pharmacologic characteristics of the antimuscarinic drugs are presented in Chapter 9. These drugs block the action of acetylcholine on the muscarinic receptor sites of effector cells innervated by postganglionic parasympathetic cholinergic nerves. They are used in dentistry to control excessive salivation and as a preanesthetic medication. In medicine, they are used as antispasmodics.

Salivary secretion is readily inhibited by antimuscarinic drugs. The prototypes for this class are the belladonna alkaloids atropine and scopolamine. These drugs, some of which are listed in Table 33-1, can be used to control salivation, but many patients have unpleasant side effects such as difficulty in swallowing because of excessive dryness in the mouth and throat, as well as inhibition of sweating. Scopolamine in particular may impair psychomotor activity and is not often used to reduce salivary secretion in the typical dental setting. A complete discussion of these effects is found in Chapter 9. The decision to use an antisialagogue depends in part on the patient's medical history. Atropine is contraindicated in patients with prostatic hypertrophy or narrow-angle glaucoma, and the topical use of atropine is absolutely contraindicated in all forms of glaucoma. Atropine should be administered with caution in patients with cardiovascular disease because it can increase the pulse rate and cardiac workload. It may also antagonize the vagal effects of digitalis. Toxic effects are not uncommon, particularly in children, who have increased susceptibility to heat prostration from inhibition of sweating.

The synthetic anticholinergic drugs propantheline and glycopyrrolate have also been used in dental procedures to control excessive salivation. Because they are quaternary amines, they are ionized at body pH and are unable to cross the blood-brain barrier. The resultant freedom from CNS effects constitutes a distinct advantage over atropine and scopolamine. However, both drugs are also less well absorbed, and propantheline is less selective in controlling salivation. Precautions for their use in dentistry are similar to those for atropine and scopolamine.

EMETICS

Emergencies may arise that might be handled by an agent that induces a forceful emptying of the stomach. However, many authorities now question the efficacy of emesis in the management of acute poisoning episodes, especially when treatment is initiated more than 1 hour after ingestion of the toxic substance. Instead, the favored treatment is the administration of activated charcoal as an adsorbent for most drugs and chemicals. The use of activated charcoal in poison management has dramatically increased over the past 15 years, whereas the use of ipecac syrup has significantly decreased.[35]

If an emetic is desired, syrup of ipecac, available OTC, remains a popular choice, despite a recommendation by the American Academy of Pediatrics that it no longer be used routinely to treat accidental poisonings in the home. Syrup of ipecac is a mixture of plant alkaloids (principally emetine) that acts centrally on the medullary chemoreceptor trigger zone (CTZ) and locally by irritation of the stomach and duodenum. Vomiting occurs 15 to 30 minutes after oral administration. Because emesis may not occur if the stomach is empty, the drug should be followed by a drink of water. Adverse reactions to ipecac syrup include diarrhea, lethargy, and prolonged vomiting[34]; however, such responses are rare if the recommended dose is not exceeded. The oral dose is 15 ml in children from 6 months to 12 years and 30 ml in older children and adults. It should be noted that a poison control center should be contacted in all cases in which poisoning is suspected for information needed to determine the appropriate treatment approach.

Apomorphine, a dopamine receptor agonist derived chemically from morphine, has been used as an emetic in a supervised medical setting. Because excessive dosages may cause significant respiratory depression, apomorphine is now considered too dangerous for this use and is infrequently used as an emetic.

ANTIEMETICS

There are numerous drugs available that have demonstrated antiemetic actions (see Table 33-1). Nausea and vomiting are complex processes that are not fully understood. The vomiting center in the medulla appears to coordinate the associated motor activities after input from the CTZ, cerebral cortex, and vestibular apparatus. The identification of the neurotransmitters and their receptors within these sites has provided a likely target for the disruption of the emetic process. Cancer chemotherapeutic agents and other chemical stimuli activate the CTZ by dopamine or 5-hydroxytryptamine (5-HT, or serotonin) receptor activation. Motion sickness, on the other hand, results from an acetylcholine-mediated response from vestibular disturbances. Drugs or drug classes useful as antiemetics include the phenothiazines, metoclopramide, droperidol, H_1 antihistamines, anticholinergics, 5-HT_3 antagonists, cannabinoids, and corticosteroids.

The pharmacologic features of phenothiazines are discussed in Chapter 12. The phenothiazines are dopamine antagonists and inhibit stimulation of the CTZ. Most of the phenothiazines are not effective for motion sickness, but they are often used successfully for the nausea of pregnancy, postoperative emesis, or vomiting induced by radiation or cancer chemotherapy. Among the most commonly used agents are chlorpromazine and prochlorperazine. Trimethobenzamide, a nonphenothiazine antiemetic, also inhibits the CTZ and has the same range of action as the phenothiazines.

Nausea and vomiting, sometimes very marked, are almost universal sequelae of cancer chemotherapy. The protracted bouts of severe drug-induced vomiting, which may be only slightly relieved by standard antiemetic therapy, have led to the inability of some patients to complete courses of potentially curative treatment.[3] Chemotherapy-induced nausea and vomiting were found to respond to high doses of the dopaminergic D_2 receptor antagonist metoclopramide. Approximately 40% to 60% of cancer patients treated with cisplatin (a highly emetogenic drug) responded to the antiemetic effect of metoclopramide in well-controlled clinical trials. Metoclopramide acts both peripherally and centrally. Peripherally, it stimulates the release of acetylcholine and sensitizes smooth muscle to acetylcholine. Centrally, it blocks D_2 receptors in the CTZ. Additionally, high-dose metoclopramide was shown to inhibit 5-HT_3 receptors,[43] which may be more responsible for its antiemetic effect.[3] High-dose metoclopramide, like other dopamine antagonists, may cause extrapyramidal symptoms and sedation, particularly in young and elderly patients. Prolonged use has been associated with tardive dyskinesia.[42] Droperidol, an anti-D_2 dopamine receptor neuroleptic, is an antiemetic used in anesthesia for the prophylactic management of postoperative nausea and vomiting.

As pointed out in Chapter 22, certain H_1-receptor histamine antagonists are effective antiemetics. All possess significant anticholinergic actions that contribute to their antiemetic efficacy. Diphenhydramine, dimenhydrinate, meclizine, and cyclizine are especially useful in treating the nausea and vomiting associated with motion sickness, pregnancy, and the postoperative state. It should be emphasized, however, that these drugs should not be used during pregnancy unless absolutely necessary. The antihistamines are not of significant value in relieving nausea associated with the administration of cytotoxic drugs. Promethazine, a phenothiazine antihistamine without significant dopamine-blocking activity, is effective in vertigo and motion sickness. Its sedative action is advantageous in the treatment of postoperative nausea and vomiting. The nonsedating H_1 antihistamines such as loratadine are ineffective against motion sickness because they penetrate poorly into the CNS.

The anticholinergic scopolamine is effective in the prevention and treatment of motion sickness, but its oral use is limited by its sedative and antimuscarinic actions. A transdermal sustained-release preparation of scopolamine when applied to the postauricular area effectively prevents motion sickness for up to 72 hours with minimal side effects.

The recognition that 5-HT_3 receptor blockade by high-dose metoclopramide contributes to its antiemetic activity led to the development of ondansetron, a potent, highly selective competitive 5-HT_3-receptor antagonist.[3,42] The 5-HT_3 receptor is found in both the gastrointestinal tract and the CNS. Ondansetron is more effective than high-dose metoclopramide in the 24 hours after chemotherapy, and there is some evidence that it is equally effective in the following 4 days. It is generally well tolerated, although during clinical trials, constipation, abdominal discomfort, headache, sedation, dry mouth, blurred vision, and anxiety were noted in some patients. Importantly, extrapyramidal effects have not been reported. At this time, the relative efficacy and safety of ondansetron and its congeners granisetron and dolasetron have made them drugs of first choice for the management of chemically induced nausea.

The cannabinoids are indicated when conventional antiemetics fail to relieve the nausea and vomiting associated with cancer chemotherapy. Dronabinol, or Δ-9-tetrahydrocannabinol, is the main psychoactive constituent in marijuana (see Chapter 51). Investigation of its use as an antiemetic was undertaken after anecdotal reports that marijuana smokers had less nausea and vomiting in association with cytotoxic agents than did other patients. Dronabinol given orally has been shown to be significantly better than placebo and comparable to metoclopramide in reducing chemotherapy-induced vomiting in selected patients. The use of dronabinol is limited by its tendency to produce acute, and often intolerable, mental disturbances, particularly in older patients who are unaccustomed to marijuana-like side effects.

Corticosteroids such as dexamethasone and methylprednisolone have been reported to be effective for cancer chemotherapy–induced nausea and vomiting. The mechanism of this effect is not known, but it may be related to a reduced synthesis of prostaglandins. Prostaglandin E has been shown to induce nausea and vomiting (see Chapter 21). Sedative-hypnotics such as the benzodiazepines may help prevent anticipated nausea and vomiting associated with chemotherapy; lorazepam is most commonly used.

Just as combinations of antineoplastic drugs with different modes of action are used in cancer chemotherapy (see Chapter 42), combinations of different antiemetic drugs are being used to treat the nausea and vomiting associated with the use of antineoplastics.[41] Combinations of anti-emetics are often more effective than single-agent therapy because of multiple sites of emetic action by antineoplastic agents, as well as the potential for additive or even synergistic effects of several antiemetics with different mechanisms of action.

Droperidol, metoclopramide, dexamethasone, and the 5-HT_3 blockers are useful as antiemetics when used prophylactically to reduce the incidence of postoperative nausea and vomiting. In a recent comparison of the first three antiemetics, the choice was not a significant predictor of postoperative nausea and vomiting. In fact, the choice of antiemetic drug given for prophylaxis had little effect on clinical outcome or patient satisfaction.[12] Ondansetron and granisetron are now widely used when there is expectation of postoperative nausea and vomiting.

LAXATIVES

Laxatives are used to relieve acute and chronic constipation, treat anorectal disorders (hemorrhoids), and prepare the bowel for examination (colonoscopy). Constipation occurs in all age groups but is especially common during pregnancy[11] and in the elderly.[31] Most cases are self-limiting or are self-treated with diet or a laxative (cathartic). Laxatives are well known, highly advertised, and the most overused OTC drugs having a therapeutic effect on the gastrointestinal tract. Well over $675 million are spent each year in the United States for laxative preparations.[53] Traditionally, these drugs have been generally classified as stimulants (or irritants), wetting agents, saline cathartics, bulk-forming agents, and lubricants (Figure 33-2). Although that taxonomy is used in this chapter, it must be recognized that these categories are somewhat arbitrary and not necessarily reflective of the pathophysiologic principles of altered intestinal fluid and electrolyte transport and of the multiplicity of effects generated by laxatives.

Stimulants

A large number of laxatives belong to the stimulant category. As a group, these drugs are thought to act as a local irritant of the intestinal mucosa that increases propulsive activity, or they may increase motility by a selective action on the intramural nerve plexus of intestinal smooth muscle. The exact mechanism is not completely understood. All the stimulant laxatives increase mucosal permeability, resulting in movement of fluid and electrolytes into the intestinal lumen.[6]

Castor oil is obtained from the seeds of *Ricinus communis* and is hydrolyzed in the small intestine by pancreatic lipase to glycerol and ricinoleic acid, an unsaturated hydroxy fatty acid that is the active moiety. Castor oil evokes the secretion of water and electrolytes in the colon and small intestine and increases small bowel peristaltic activity to produce a very prompt cathartic effect in 2 to 6 hours.

Phenolphthalein was a widely used stimulant laxative found as an ingredient in numerous OTC preparations; however, the FDA banned its use in laxatives in 1997 because of reports of its association with carcinogenic tumors in laboratory rats. Products previously containing phenolphthalein have been reformulated.

Bisacodyl is structurally related to phenolphthalein and has similar pharmacologic actions. After oral administration, approximately 5% of a therapeutic dose is absorbed from the digestive tract with no apparent systemic effects. The laxative effect is obtained in 6 to 8 hours but can be accelerated by administration in suppository form. The major toxicity is diarrhea with overdosage.

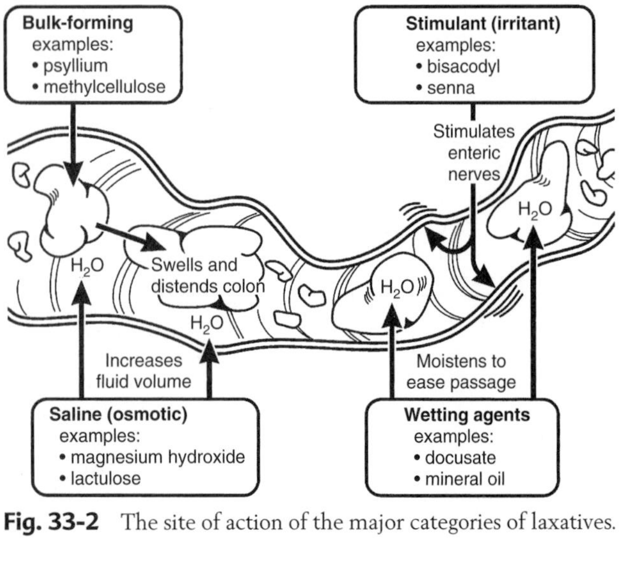

Some of the most extensively used stimulant laxatives are in the anthraquinone group, which includes senna and cascara sagrada. These preparations contain emodin (or anthracene) alkaloids in an inactive glycoside form. The glycosides are hydrolyzed within the colon by the action of bacteria to liberate the active principle.[33] A small percentage of the active form may be absorbed and excreted in the bile and other body fluids. The laxative action is limited primarily to the colon and is produced in 6 to 8 hours. Cascara sagrada is considered to be milder than senna. In general, adverse reactions to these agents relate to excessive catharsis and may include severe abdominal pain.

Wetting Agents and Lubricants

Docusate sodium (dioctyl sodium sulfosuccinate) and docusate calcium (dioctyl calcium sulfosuccinate) act like detergents and are used to soften the stool when it is desirable to lessen the discomfort or the strain of defecation. These drugs are anionic surfactants that produce their effect by lowering the surface tension and allowing intestinal fluids and fatty substances to penetrate the fecal mass. They usually require 1 to 3 days to exert their full effect if used alone, but they may be combined with other laxatives in OTC preparations. These agents are not thought to interfere with the absorption of nutrients from the intestinal tract, and they are not appreciably absorbed. Docusate is frequently recommended for elderly patients because it is associated with so few side effects.[15] Diarrhea and mild abdominal cramps are the only adverse effects reported.

Mineral oil (liquid petrolatum) may be considered together with the surface-active agents because it also softens the stool. Mineral oil acts as a lubricant and coats the intestinal contents, preventing the absorption of fecal water. It produces a cathartic action in 6 to 8 hours after oral administration and 5 to 15 minutes if given rectally. Its use is attended by several potential hazards not associated with the other agents. Prolonged oral use or administration with meals can reduce the absorption of the fat-soluble vitamins (A, D, E, and K). Lipid pneumonia can result from the accidental aspiration of the oil. Mineral oil is absorbed to a limited extent from the intestinal tract; therefore its use with a wetting agent (docusate), which could increase its absorption, is contraindicated. Significant absorption of mineral oil may occur if used repeatedly. The seepage of oil through the anal sphincter may occur and produce pruritus ani or other perianal conditions.

Saline Cathartics

The saline cathartics are salt solutions containing one or more ions that are poorly absorbed from the gastrointestinal tract.[55] Available preparations include magnesium salts (hydroxide, sulfate, or citrate), sodium phosphate (monobasic or dibasic), and sodium biphosphate. The salt solutions osmotically increase the water content of feces and fluid volume in the intestinal lumen. This increases the intraluminal pressure, which exerts a mechanical force to stimulate peristalsis. It has also been postulated that magnesium salts increase colonic motility by causing the release of cholecystokinin. Oral administration of these agents generally results in the production of a fluid to semifluid stool within 30 minutes to 3 hours. If given rectally, laxation occurs in 2 to 5 minutes. Some absorption of the saline cathartics does occur, and consequently systemic effects may be noted. For this reason, the sodium salts are contraindicated in patients on a low-salt diet and in patients with edema or congestive heart failure.

Fig. 33-2 The site of action of the major categories of laxatives.

Magnesium and potassium salts are contraindicated in patients with impaired renal function. Magnesium sulfate (Epsom salt), which is an effective and frequently used cathartic, may cause serious loss of body water with repeated use. Milk of magnesia, a suspension of magnesium hydroxide, is a widely used OTC preparation. Abdominal cramps and dehydration are reported adverse reactions from saline laxatives.

Bulk-Forming Agents

This group of agents includes polycarbophil and other natural and semisynthetic cellulose derivatives such as psyllium and methylcellulose. They possess the property of absorbing water and expanding, thereby increasing the bulk of the intestinal contents.[15] The elevated luminal pressure stimulates reflex peristalsis, and the increased water content serves to soften the stool. These agents are not absorbed and do not interfere with the absorption of nutrients from the gastrointestinal tract. Several days of medication may be required to achieve the full therapeutic benefit of these agents, although the usual onset of action is 12 to 24 hours. Some patients prefer to add foods such as bran or dried fruit (e.g., prunes and figs) to their diet that exert the same effect rather than use a bulk-forming laxative. These laxatives have the advantage of having few systemic effects and are least likely to produce laxative abuse. Cellulose agents may physically bind with other drugs if administered concurrently (e.g., salicylates, warfarin, digitalis glycosides) and hinder their absorption and thus reduce their desired effect. Patients should also not take a calcium polycarbophil laxative within 2 hours of taking tetracycline for the same reason.

Laxatives with psyllium come in a powdered mixture containing approximately 50% powdered psyllium seeds and 50% dextrose or sucrose. Sugar-free products containing aspartame are also available. Psyllium seeds are rich in a hemicellulose that forms a gelatinous mass with water. The refined hydrophilic colloid from the seeds is the most widely used form of this agent. Methylcellulose is indigestible and not absorbed systemically.

Miscellaneous Agents

Several preparations, notably glycerin, lactulose, and polyethylene glycol, do not readily fit into the categories of laxatives described above.[14,15,55] Glycerin is used in suppository form to promote defecation. It osmotically dehydrates exposed rectal tissue; the resultant irritation promotes evacuation of the lower bowel within 30 minutes. Lactulose is a semisynthetic disaccharide. In the large intestine, lactulose is metabolized by enteric bacteria to various acids and carbon dioxide. The acidification and increased osmolarity of the bowel contents cause fecal softening and a more normal bowel movement. Up to 2 days may be required for a therapeutic effect to occur. A polyethylene glycol prescription formulation is available that acts osmotically to retain water in the gut to produce laxation. It is not metabolized by bowel flora and is not significantly absorbed.[14] These osmotic agents are often the mainstay of therapy for chronically constipated persons.

ANTIDIARRHEAL AGENTS

One out of every six illnesses of adults and children involves the digestive system, and one of the more common complaints is diarrhea. The antidiarrheal agents generally available in the past lacked gastrointestinal specificity or demonstrated efficacy, often produced undesirable side effects, and even possessed abuse potential.

Attapulgite

Attapulgite is a hydrated magnesium aluminum silicate with a crystalline structure that allows for a large surface area that adsorbs up to eight times its weight in water. It is 33 times more adsorbent than kaolin[17] and has replaced kaolin-pectin in Kaopectate. Its use in the treatment of diarrhea is based on its purported ability to adsorb bacteria, toxins, and various noxious materials in the gastrointestinal tract. In the colon, it may act as an adsorbent or protectant, but the adsorption is not selective. It also may adsorb several drugs, including the tetracyclines and anticholinergics, and reduce their systemic absorption. It is generally used to treat mild nonspecific acute diarrhea. However, it is much less effective than the opioid derivatives. Controlled clinical studies demonstrating the efficacy of attapulgite are lacking.

Opioid Preparations

The opioids are effective and prompt-acting antidiarrheal agents. As is discussed in Chapter 20, they enhance tone in the anal sphincter and in segments of the longitudinal muscle of the gastrointestinal tract while inhibiting propulsive contraction of circular and longitudinal muscle. Codeine has been shown to cause a marked slowing of fluid movement through the jejunum but to have no effect on the movement of fluid through the ileum or colon.[51] By increasing the contact time of luminal fluid with mucosal cells, therapeutic doses of codeine increase net intestinal absorption and thereby reduce stool volume.

Diphenoxylate

Diphenoxylate, a Drug Enforcement Administration (DEA) Schedule V (C-V) prescription drug, is a congener of meperidine and was synthesized in the search for compounds similar to the opioid analgesics in actions on the gastrointestinal tract but devoid of their CNS effects. The efficacy of diphenoxylate was found to be approximately equal to that of camphorated tincture of opium in patients with diarrhea of various causes. Inasmuch as diphenoxylate is structurally related to meperidine, there was concern about its abuse potential, but in the several decades of experience with it, diphenoxylate has emerged as having an addiction liability comparable to that of codeine, which is further diminished by the incorporation of atropine (as in Lomotil) and by the low water solubility of diphenoxylate salts, which prevents parenteral administration.

Various minor side effects have been reported. These include abdominal cramps, nausea, weakness, drowsiness, xerostomia, gingival swelling, partial intestinal obstruction, and urinary retention. In patients with inflammatory bowel disease, diphenoxylate has caused toxic megacolon and, in patients with severe liver disease, hepatic coma. Toxic doses have produced respiratory depression and unconsciousness, which can be effectively reversed by the opioid antagonists. Although clinical studies have indicated only minimal, if any, drug interactions during diphenoxylate therapy, the drug may potentially augment the actions of barbiturates, alcohol, opioids, and antianxiety and antipsychotic drugs.

Difenoxin, the principal active metabolite of diphenoxylate, is a DEA Schedule IV (C-IV) prescription antidiarrheal drug that is effective at one fifth the dosage of diphenoxylate. Atropine is added to the formulation to discourage deliberate overdose.

Loperamide

Loperamide, a long-acting derivative of both haloperidol and diphenoxylate, is the most selective antidiarrheal opioid currently available for clinical use because it has a distribution within the body different from other opioids. Although drugs such as meperidine penetrate the blood-brain barrier and interact with CNS opioid receptors to modify intestinal motor function, only small concentrations of loperamide reach the brain. Therefore its effects are thought to result mainly from interactions with peripheral opioid receptors. When loperamide is administered orally at therapeutic doses, the effect on the gastrointestinal tract is not accompanied by any significant CNS opioid effect. Large amounts of the drug become concentrated in target tissues along the gastrointestinal tract. One hour after oral administration, most of the drug (85%) is distributed to the gastrointestinal tract, 5% to the liver, and less than 0.04% to the brain.

Loperamide exerts its antidiarrheal effect by altering motor function in the intestine, which results in increased capacitance of the intestine and a delay in the passage of fluid through it.[52] This action is analogous to that of codeine. In spite of differences in distribution and other pharmacologic properties, the action of both the traditional opioid antidiarrheal drugs and loperamide appear to be the same, an inhibition of propulsion through the intestine.

Adverse effects of loperamide include abdominal pain and distention, constipation, nausea and vomiting, dry mouth, and drowsiness or dizziness. Allergic reactions, including skin rash, have been reported. Unlike diphenoxylate and difenoxin, loperamide is available OTC. After years of extensive use, there has been no evidence of drug abuse or physical dependence. It is a safe and effective antidiarrheal agent.

Agents Used for the Prevention of Traveler's Diarrhea

The risk of travelers from the United States acquiring a diarrheal illness while visiting developing countries is reported to be 40% to 46%.[16,28] The most common infecting organism is enterotoxigenic *Escherichia coli*, which is primarily acquired through contaminated food (e.g., raw vegetables) and water, including ice.[1] The ingested bacteria produce enterotoxins that cause the sudden onset of loose stools, commonly referred to as *traveler's diarrhea*. This is usually a self-limiting illness lasting only several days. Less common pathogens that may cause this disorder include *Salmonella*, *Shigella*, *Campylobacter*, and *Giardia*.

Several approaches to the prevention of traveler's diarrhea have been evaluated. However, because of the potential for drug resistance and adverse reactions, many physicians do not prescribe drugs prophylactically, instructing the traveler instead to begin treatment promptly when symptoms occur. When prophylaxis is used, once daily dosing with a quinolone antibiotic is the recommended treatment of choice.[1] Antibiotics recommended from this group include ciprofloxacin (500 mg), levofloxacin (500 mg), ofloxacin (300 mg), or norfloxacin (400 mg). Bismuth subsalicylate (Pepto-Bismol) has also been shown to be particularly active against mild to moderate traveler's diarrhea, although it is considered less effective than antibiotics. A regimen of 520 mg (30 ml of the liquid suspension or two tablets) taken four times a day is effective for the prevention of traveler's diarrhea[18] but, when taken after the onset of diarrhea, will also diminish the number of loose bowel movements and relieve abdominal cramps. The preparation is well tolerated, and constipation is not a problem. The mechanisms of action of bismuth subsalicylate are complex and incompletely understood. It does possess an antibacterial effect, but this may not be its major action. Salicylate is absorbed, but its exact role is undetermined. Approximately 99% of the orally administered bismuth is not absorbed but is excreted as insoluble salts in the feces. The small amount that is absorbed may, although rare, reach toxic levels after ingestion of high doses. Symptoms of bismuth toxicity include ataxia and encephalopathy. Bismuth may react with bacterial H_2S, causing a grayish-black discoloration of the tongue and feces.

An effective treatment for traveler's diarrhea uses loperamide (4 mg loading dose, then 2 mg orally after each loose stool, to a maximum of 16 mg/day) plus a single dose of ciprofloxacin (750 mg), levofloxacin (500 mg), or ofloxacin (400 mg). This regimen usually relieves symptoms within 24 hours.[1] The antimicrobial combination product trimethoprim-sulfamethoxazole has been used with success in the past, but resistance to it has become common in many areas. It may still be an effective treatment option, especially for children. Fluids and oral rehydration salt packets are helpful in maintaining fluid balance.

In countries where traveler's diarrhea is prevalent, what one ingests or avoids ingesting may be as important as chemoprophylaxis in reducing the risk. Common sense is an important preventive measure.

GASTROINTESTINAL STIMULANTS

Drugs that stimulate smooth muscle of the gastrointestinal and urinary tracts are used in the treatment of nonobstructive urinary retention, paralytic ileus, gastrointestinal atony, and postoperative abdominal distention. Cholinomimetic agents such as bethanechol are effective in these situations by promoting gastrointestinal motility (see Chapter 8). Bethanechol is a useful agent because it is resistant to metabolism by cholinesterase enzymes, its actions are essentially muscarinic, and its effects on the gastrointestinal tract are much more pronounced than those on the cardiovascular system. The side effects of bethanechol are those typical of other cholinergic drugs, but serious adverse reactions are rare with therapeutic doses. This drug is contraindicated in patients with obstructive ileus, obstructive urinary retention, peptic ulcer, bronchial asthma, hyperthyroidism, or serious cardiac disease.

Gastroparesis (gastric stasis) is a clinical syndrome characterized by delayed gastric emptying that leads to debilitation. It is most commonly seen in patients with diabetes mellitus and is characterized by intractable nausea, vomiting, early satiety, abdominal pain, and bloating.[29] Therapeutic success often remains elusive. The use of prokinetic agents is the best option for acute exacerbations and long-term maintenance therapy. Metoclopramide, cited earlier for its antiemetic action, and the macrolide antibiotic erythromycin have prokinetic actions that are commonly used in the management of gastroparesis. Erythromycin acts as a motilin receptor agonist to stimulate gastrointestinal activity (see Chapter 39). Metoclopramide, possessing both cholinomimetic and dopamine antagonist properties, is also useful in this syndrome because the drug stimulates the motility of the upper gastrointestinal tract.[48] Metoclopramide augments esophageal peristalsis, gastric antral contractions, and the rate of intestinal transit. Additionally, metoclopramide increases the resting pressure of the lower esophageal sphincter but reduces that of the pyloric sphincter. It does not stimulate gastric, biliary, or pancreatic secretions and has little effect on colonic motor activity. Oral administration of metoclopramide is indicated for relief of symptoms associated with diabetic gastroparesis. The usual duration of therapy is 2 to 8 weeks, depending on the response. An injectable form of metoclopramide is also approved for use in facilitating intubation of the small intestine and the passage of barium into the intestine for radiographic procedures. Of particular concern to the dentist is that the use of opioids or anticholinergic drugs will antagonize the gastrointestinal effects of metoclopramide.

Cisapride, a prokinetic agent structurally related to metoclopramide, facilitates gastrointestinal motility presumably by increasing the peripheral release of acetylcholine. Unlike metoclopramide, it does not bind to dopamine receptors and is devoid of extrapyramidal side effects. It has demonstrated efficacy for treating constipation, gastroparesis, and GERD.[36] However, cisapride was associated with serious cardiac arrhythmias and was removed from the United States market in 2000. A derivative of cisapride, norcisapride, is under development and may have a better safety profile.

ANTISPASMODICS

Irritable bowel syndrome (IBS) is the most common disorder diagnosed by gastroenterologists and one of the most common gastrointestinal conditions encountered by family practice physicians.[7] Symptomatic treatment includes loperamide combined with increased dietary fiber.

Naturally occurring belladonna alkaloids and their derivatives, including propantheline, possess antispasmodic activity and may also be useful as adjuncts in the management of IBS and in selected patients with other spastic disorders of the gastrointestinal tract (e.g., diverticulitis, neurogenic colon). Their anticholinergic effects on smooth muscle and secretory glands, as discussed above and in Chapter 9, reduce spastic contractions and hypermotility.

ADVERSE REACTIONS OF THE GASTROINTESTINAL SYSTEM TO DRUGS

The gastrointestinal tract must be considered a target for the adverse side effects of many drug groups, some important to dentistry. For example, the opioid analgesics may produce constipation, nausea, and vomiting. Aspirin-containing analgesic compounds are associated with gastric distress, fecal blood loss, and ulceration. All antiinflammatory agents, in fact, share the ulcerogenic action of aspirin. The sedative-hypnotic chloral hydrate may be prescribed by the dentist for the child or elderly patient. A major complaint against its use is the gastric irritation it produces.

Antibiotic agents are often associated with gastrointestinal distress. Erythromycin preparations commonly cause nausea. Diarrhea, enterocolitis, and pseudomembranous colitis are possible outcomes from the administration of tetracyclines, clindamycin, and extended-spectrum penicillins.

Many drugs not directly related to dentistry cause a wide spectrum of gastrointestinal effects. Important examples include the antineoplastic drugs, digitalis glycosides, and oral contraceptives.

Drugs Acting on the Gastrointestinal Tract

Nonproprietary (generic) name	*Proprietary (trade) name (selected)*
Antacids	
Algenic acid, sodium bicarbonate, magnesium carbonate	Gaviscon
Aluminum carbonate gel	Basaljel
Aluminum hydroxide gel	Amphojel
Calcium carbonate	Tums, Alka-Mints
Magaldrate (aluminum magnesium hydroxide sulfate)	Riopan
Magnesium hydroxide	Milk of Magnesia
Magnesium hydroxide/ aluminum hydroxide	Maalox, Gelusil, Mylanta
Magnesium oxide	Mag-Ox 400, Uro-Mag
Sodium bicarbonate	Bell/ans
Sodium bicarbonate/aspirin	Alka-Seltzer
Sodium citrate	Citra pH
H_2-receptor antagonists	
Cimetidine	Tagamet, Tagamet HB
Famotidine	Pepcid, Pepcid AC
Nizatidine	Axid, Axid AR
Ranitidine	Zantac, Zantac 75
***H. pylori* agents (combination packages)**	
Bismuth subsalicylate, metronidazole, tetracycline	Helidac
Lansoprazole, amoxicillin, clarithromycin	Prevpac
Prostaglandin analogue	
Misoprostol	Cytotec
PPIs	
Esomeprazole	Nexium
Lansoprazole	Prevacid
Omeprazole	Prilosec, Prilosec OTC
Pantoprazole	Protonix
Rabeprazole	Aciphex
Ulcer-adherent complex	
Sucralfate	Carafate
Antisialagogue*	
See Tables 9-5 and 33-1	
Emetic	
Ipecac syrup	Ipecac
Antiemetics†	
Alosetron	Lotronex
Buclizine	Bucladin-S Softabs
Chlorpromazine	Thorazine
Cyclizine	Marezine
Dimenhydrinate	Dramamine
Diphenhydramine	Benadryl
Dolasetron	Anzemet
Dronabinol	Marinol
Granisetron	Kytril
Meclizine	Bonine, Antivent
Metoclopramide	Reglan

Continued

Drugs Acting on the Gastrointestinal Tract—cont'd

Nonproprietary (generic) name	*Proprietary (trade) name (selected)*
Antiemetics[†]—cont'd	
Ondansetron	Zofran
Perphenazine	Trilafon
Phosphorated carbohydrate solution	Emetrol
Prochlorperazine	Compazine
Promethazine	Phenergan
Scopolamine, oral	Scopace
Scopolamine, transdermal	Transderm-Scop
Thiethylperazine	Torecan
Triflupromazine	Vesprin
Trimethobenzamide	Tigan
Laxatives	
Bisacodyl	Dulcolax
Cascara sagrada	Cascara Sagrada
Castor oil	Purge
Docusate calcium	Surfak Liquigels
Docusate sodium	Colace
Docusate/casanthranol	Peri-Colace
Glycerin, liquid	Fleet Babylax
Glycerin, suppositories	Sani-Supp
Lactulose	Chronulac
Magnesium hydroxide	Milk of Magnesia
Magnesium sulfate	Epsom Salt
Methylcellulose	Citrucel
Mineral oil	Milkinol
Polycarbophil	FiberCon
Polyethylene glycol–electrolyte solution	CoLyte
Polyethylene glycol	MiraLax
Psyllium	Metamucil, Fiberall
Sennosides	ex-lax, Senokot
Antidiarrheal agents	
Antibiotics	See Chapter 39
Attapulgite	Diasorb
Bismuth subsalicylate	Pepto-Bismol
Difenoxin with atropine	Motofen
Diphenoxylate with atropine	Lomotil
Loperamide	Imodium
Opium tincture, camphorated	Paregoric
Gastrointestinal stimulants	
Erythromycin	See Chapter 39
Dexpanthenol	Ilopan
Metoclopramide	Reglan
Antispasmodics	
Loperamide	Imodium
Anticholinergics	See Chapter 9

*See Table 33-1 and Chapter 9.
[†]See also Table 33-1.

Cited References

1. Abramowicz M: Advice for travelers, *Med Lett Drugs Ther* 41:39-42, 1999.
2. Anderson J, Gonzalez J: *H. pylori* infection: review of the guideline for diagnosis and treatment, *Geriatrics* 55:44-49, 2000.
3. Andrews PLR, Rapeport WG, Sanger GJ: Neuropharmacology of emesis induced by anti-cancer therapy, *Trends Pharmacol Sci* 9:334-341, 1988.
4. Barker G, Loftus L, Cuddy P, et al: The effects of sucralfate suspension and diphenhydramine syrup plus kaolin-pectin on radiotherapy-induced mucositis, *Oral Surg Oral Med Oral Pathol* 71:288-293, 1991.
5. Befrits R, Granstrom M, Rylander M, et al: *Helicobacter pylori* in 205 consecutive endoscopy patients, *Scand J Infect Dis* 25:185-191, 1993.
6. Beubler E: Laxatives: how they work. In Barbara L, Miglioli M, Phillips SF, eds: *New trends in pathophysiology and therapy of the large bowel,* New York, 1983, Elsevier Science.
7. Camilleri M: Management of the irritable bowel syndrome, *Gastroenterology* 120:652-668, 2001.
8. Candelli M, Carloni E, Armuzzi A, et al: Role of sucralfate in gastrointestinal diseases, *Panminerva Med* 42:55-59, 2000.
9. Charan M, Katz PO: Gastroesophageal reflux disease in pregnancy, *Curr Treat Options Gastroenterol* 4:73-81, 2001.
10. Crawford J: The oral cavity and gastrointestinal tract. In Kumar V, Cotran R, Robbins S, eds: *Basic pathology,* ed 6, Philadelphia, 1997, WB Saunders.
11. Cummings JH: Constipation. In Misiewicz JJ, Pounder RE, Venables CW, eds: *Diseases of the gut and pancreas,* ed 2, Oxford, 1994, Blackwell Scientific Publications.
12. Darkow T, Gora-Harper M, Goulson DT, et al: Impact of antiemetic selection on postoperative nausea and vomiting and patient satisfaction, *Pharmacotherapy* 21:540-548, 2001.
13. Del Valle J, Cohen H, Laine L, et al: Acid-peptic disorders. In Yamada T, Alpers DH, Owyang C, eds: *Textbook of gastroenterology,* ed 3, Philadelphia, 1999, JB Lippincott.
14. DiPalma JA, DeRidder PH, Orlando RC, et al: A randomized, placebo-controlled, multicenter study of the safety and efficacy of a new polyethylene glycol laxative, *Am J Gastroenterol* 95:446-450, 2000.
15. Donatelle EP: Constipation: pathophysiology and treatment, *Am Fam Physician* 42:1335-1342, 1990.
16. Duchini A, Rodgers VD: Diarrhea in the international traveler, *Curr Treat Options Gastroenterol* 2:251-257, 1999.
17. Dukes GE: Over-the-counter antidiarrheal medications used for the self-treatment of acute nonspecific diarrhea, *Am J Med* 88(suppl 6A):24S-26S, 1990.
18. DuPont HL, Ericsson CD, Johnson PC, et al: Prevention of travelers' diarrhea by the tablet formulation of bismuth subsalicylate, *JAMA* 257:1347-1350, 1987.
19. Ferguson DA, Li C, Patel NR, et al: Isolation of *Helicobacter pylori* from saliva, *J Clin Microbiol* 31(10):2802-2804, 1993.

20. Ferraro JM: Sucralfate suspension for mouth ulcers, *Drug Intel Clin Pharm* 19:480, 1985.
21. Garcia G: Gastrointestinal disorders. In Carruthers S, Hoffman B, Melmon K, et al, eds: *Clinical pharmacology*, ed 4, St Louis, 2000, McGraw-Hill.
22. Garnett WR: Considerations for long-term use of proton-pump inhibitors, *Am J Health Syst Pharm* 55:2268-2279, 1998.
23. Goodwin CS, Mendall MM, Northfield TC: *Helicobacter pylori* infection, *Lancet* 349:265-269, 1997.
24. Griffin MR, Piper JM, Daugherty JR, et al: Nonsteroidal anti-inflammatory drug use and increased risk for peptic ulcer disease in elderly persons, *Ann Intern Med* 114:257-263, 1991.
25. Hade JE, Spiro HM: Calcium and acid rebound: a reappraisal, *J Clin Gastroenterol* 15:37-44, 1992.
26. Hawkey CJ: Non-steroidal anti-inflammatory drugs and peptic ulcers, *BMJ* 300:278-284, 1990.
27. Hentschel E, Brandstatter G, Dragosics B, et al: Effect of ranitidine and amoxicillin plus metronidazole on the eradication of *Helicobacter pylori* and the recurrence of duodenal ulcer, *N Engl J Med* 328:308-312, 1993.
28. Hill DR: Occurrence and self-treatment of diarrhea in a large cohort of Americans traveling to developing countries, *Am J Trop Med Hyg* 62:585-589, 2000.
29. Hoogerwerf WA, Pashricha PJ, Kalloo AN, et al: Pain: the overlooked symptom in gastroparesis, *Am J Gastroenterol* 94:1029-1033, 1999.
30. Horn J: The proton-pump inhibitors: similarities and differences, *Clin Ther* 22:266-280, 2000.
31. Koch T, Hudson S: Older people and laxative use: literature review and pilot study report, *J Clin Nurs* 9:516-525, 2000.
32. Krakowka S, Morgan DR, Kraft WG, et al: Establishment of gastric *Campylobacter pylori* infection in the neonatal gnotobiotic piglet, *Infect Immun* 55:2789-2796, 1987.
33. Leng-Peschlow E: Senna and its rational use, *Pharmacology* 44(suppl 1):1-52, 1992.
34. Lipscomb JW, Burda AM, Holbrook MG: Response in children to 15 ml or 30 ml doses of ipecac syrup, *Clin Pharm* 5:234-235, 1986.
35. Litovitz TL, Klein-Schwartz W, Dyer KS, et al: 1997 annual report of the American Association of Poison Control Centers Toxic Exposure Surveillance System, *Am J Emerg Med* 16:443-497, 1998.
36. Longo WE, Vernava AM III: Prokinetic agents for lower gastrointestinal motility disorders, *Dis Colon Rectum* 36:696-708, 1993.
37. Mandel KG, Daggy BP, Brodie DA, et al: Alginate-raft formulations in the treatment of heartburn and acid reflux, *Aliment Pharmacol Ther* 14:669-690, 2000.
38. Marks IN: Sucralfate—safety and side effects, *Scand J Gastroenterol* 26(suppl 185):36-42, 1991.
39. Marsh TD: Nonprescription H2-receptor antagonists, *J Am Pharm Assoc* 37:552-556, 1997.
40. McGinnis WL, Loprinzi CL, Buskirk SJ, et al: Placebo-controlled trial of sucralfate for inhibiting radiation-induced esophagitis, *J Clin Oncol* 15:1239-1243, 1997.
41. Merrifield KR, Chaffee BJ: Recent advances in the management of nausea and vomiting caused by antineoplastic agents, *Clin Pharm* 8:187-199, 1989.
42. Milne RJ, Heel RC: Ondansetron. Therapeutic use as an antiemetic, *Drugs* 41:574-595, 1991.
43. Miner WD, Sanger GJ: Inhibition of cisplatin-induced vomiting by selective 5-hydroxytryptamine M-receptor antagonism, *Br J Pharmacol* 88:497-499, 1986.
44. Misiewicz JJ, Harris AW, Bardhan KD, et al: One week triple therapy for *H. pylori:* a multicentre comparative study, *Gut* 41:735-739, 1997.
45. Naunton M, Peterson GM, Bleasel MD: Overuse of proton pump inhibitors, *J Clin Pharm Ther* 25:333-340, 2000.
46. NIH Consensus Development Panel on *Helicobacter pylori* in Peptic Ulcer Disease: *Helicobacter pylori* in peptic ulcer disease, *JAMA* 272:65-69, 1994.
47. Rees WDW: Mechanisms of gastroduodenal protection by sucralfate, *Am J Med* 91(suppl 2A):58S-62S, 1991.
48. Ricci DA, Saltzman MB, Meyer C, et al: Effect of metoclopramide in diabetic gastroparesis, *J Clin Gastroenterol* 7:25-32, 1985.
49. Richardson P, Hawkey CJ, Stack WA: Proton pump inhibitors: pharmacology and rationale for use in gastrointestinal disorders, *Drugs* 56:307-335, 1998.
50. Roth SH: Misoprostol in the prevention of NSAID-induced gastric ulcer: a multicenter, double-blind, placebo-controlled trial, *J Rheumatol* 17(suppl 20):20-24, 1990.
51. Schiller LR, Davis GR, Santa Ana CA, et al: Studies on the mechanism of the antidiarrheal effect of codeine, *J Clin Invest* 70:999-1008, 1982.
52. Schiller LR, Santa Ana CA, Morawski SG, et al: Mechanism of the antidiarrheal effect of loperamide, *Gastroenterology* 86:1475-1480, 1984.
53. Snyder K: The state of the o-t-c marketplace, *Drug Topics* 141:82-90, 1997.
54. Song Q, Spahr A, Schmid RM, et al: *Helicobacter pylori* in the oral cavity: high prevalence and great DNA diversity, *Dig Dis Sci* 45:2162-2167, 2000.
55. Tedesco FJ, DiPiro JT: Laxative use in constipation, *Am J Gastroenterol* 80:303-309, 1985.
56. Welage LS, Berardi RR: Evaluation of omeprazole, lansoprazole, pantoprazole, and rabeprazole in the treatment of acid-related diseases, *J Am Pharm Assoc* 40:52-62, 2000.
57. Yagiela JA: Agents affecting salivation. In Ciancio SG, ed: *ADA Guide to dental therapeutics*, ed 3, Chicago, 2003, American Dental Association.

General References

Allan SG: Antiemetics, *Gastroenterol Clin North Am* 21:597-611, 1992.

Graham DY: Therapy of *Helicobacter pylori:* current status and issues, *Gastroenterology* 118 (2 suppl 1):S2-S8, 2000.

Pandolfino JE, Howden CW, Kahrilas PJ: Motility-modifying agents and management of disorders of gastrointestinal motility, *Gastroenterology* 118(2 suppl 1):S32-S47, 2000.

Rabine JC, Barnett JL: Management of the patient with gastroparesis, *J Clin Gastroenterol* 32:11-18, 2001.

Watcha MF, White PF: Postoperative nausea and vomiting. Its etiology, treatment, and prevention, *Anesthesiology* 77:162-184, 1992.

Wolfe MM, Sachs G: Acid suppression: optimizing therapy for gastroduodenal ulcer healing, gastroesophageal reflux disease, and stress-related erosive syndrome, *Gastroenterology* 118:S9-S31, 2000.

CHAPTER • 34

Pituitary, Thyroid, and Parathyroid Pharmacology

Gail T. Galasko

HYPOTHALAMIC AND PITUITARY HORMONES

The pituitary gland consists of an anterior lobe (adenohypophysis) and a posterior lobe (neurohypophysis). It is connected to the hypothalamus, which lies above it, by the stalk that contains neurosecretory fibers and capillaries. The hypophyseal portal system drains the hypothalamus and perfuses the anterior pituitary. A number of releasing factors or regulating hormones that are produced by the hypothalamus are carried to the anterior pituitary by this portal system. These hypothalamic releasing factors stimulate the anterior pituitary to produce and secrete a number of tropic hormones, which in turn stimulate target glands to produce hormones. The hypothalamic releasing factors, anterior pituitary hormones produced, target glands, and target gland hormones are shown in Table 34-1.

Pituitary hormone secretion is regulated by negative feedback. For anterior pituitary hormones, secretion of releasing factors from the hypothalamus is decreased when the concentration of target gland hormones is high and increased when it is low.

POSTERIOR PITUITARY HORMONES

The posterior lobe of the pituitary secretes two homologous peptide hormones, vasopressin and oxytocin. Both these hormones are synthesized in the hypothalamus and transported via the neurosecretory fibers of the stalk to the posterior pituitary, where they are stored and released. Both are nonapeptides and their structures are similar.

Vasopressin

Vasopressin (antidiuretic hormone) acts on the kidney to increase water reabsorption. It increases total peripheral resistance and has an important role in the long-term control of blood pressure. Vasopressin also has a vasoconstrictor action that plays a role in the short-term regulation of arterial pressure. There are two subtypes of vasopressin receptors. V_1 receptors, which are $G_{q/11}$ protein–linked, produce their action by stimulation of phospholipase C and formation of inositol triphosphate. This is the pathway responsible for the vasoconstrictor action of vasopressin. V_2 receptors, which are G_s protein–linked, are linked to stimulation of adenylyl cyclase and stimulation of cyclic 3′,5′-adenosine monophosphate production. Stimulation of V_2 receptors by vasopressin leads to its antidiuretic effect. Lack of antidiuretic hormone leads to diabetes insipidus, resulting in polyuria and polydipsia.

Pharmacokinetics

Vasopressin may be given intravenously, intramuscularly, or intranasally. Because the drug is rapidly metabolized in the liver and kidney, the half-life is approximately 20 minutes.

Therapeutic uses

Vasopressin and desmopressin acetate, a long-acting synthetic analogue that acts predominantly at V_2 receptors, are used in the treatment of diabetes insipidus. The receptors mediating this effect are located on the cells of the collecting duct in the kidney. Vasopressin is also used to control bleeding in certain conditions (such as colonic diverticular bleeding). Vasopressin stimulates the release of von Willebrand factor and clotting factor VII and is used to treat deficiencies of these factors in certain types of hemophilia. Desmopressin is also used to decrease nocturnal enuresis.

Oxytocin

Oxytocin receptors are $G_{q/11}$ protein–linked receptors that, when stimulated, lead to an increase in intracellular Ca^{++} and muscle contraction. Oxytocin causes contraction of uterine smooth muscle and may play a role in the initiation of labor. Oxytocin also stimulates milk ejection in lactating mothers by stimulating myoepithelial cells around the alveoli of the mammary glands.

Pharmacokinetics

Oxytocin has a circulating half-life of 5 minutes. It is not bound to plasma protein and is metabolized in the liver and kidneys.

Therapeutic uses

Oxytocin is used intravenously for stimulation of labor and to induce postpartum lactation in cases of breast engorgement.

ANTERIOR PITUITARY HORMONES

Growth Hormone

Growth hormone (GH, or somatotropin) is the most abundant of the anterior pituitary hormones. The principal form of GH is a 191-amino-acid single-peptide chain with two sulfhydryl bridges. GH for pharmacologic use is produced by recombinant DNA techniques and contains either the 191-amino-acid sequence of somatotropin, recombinant human GH, or 192 amino acids consisting of somatotropin plus an extra methionine at the amino terminal end. These preparations are equipotent.

Table • 34-1

Hypothalamic Stimulatory Releasing Factors, Corresponding Anterior Pituitary Tropic Hormones, Target Glands, and Target Gland Hormones

HYPOTHALAMIC HORMONE	PITUITARY HORMONE	TARGET ORGAN	HORMONE PRODUCED
Corticotropin-releasing hormone	Adrenocorticotropin	Adrenal cortex	Glucocorticosteroids, mineralocorticosteroids, androgens
GH-releasing hormone	GH (somatropin)	Liver, bone, other tissues	IGFs
Gonadotropin-releasing hormone	Follicle-stimulating hormone, luteinizing hormone	Gonads	Estrogen, progesterone, testosterone
Thyrotropin-releasing hormone	Thyroid-stimulating hormone	Thyroid	T_4, T_3

GH, Growth hormone; *IGF*, insulinlike growth factor; *T_3*, triodothyronine; *T_4*, thyroxine.

Actions
GH has both direct and indirect effects. Its action is through cell surface receptors. The direct actions of GH include lipolysis in fat cells and stimulation of hepatic glucose output. These effects are opposite to those of insulin. The anabolic and growth-promoting effects of GH are indirect and are mediated by insulinlike growth factor type 1 (IGF-1). IGF-1 stimulates chondrogenesis as well as skeletal and soft tissue growth. IGF-1 increases mitogenesis, increasing cell number rather than cell size. GH-releasing hormone from the hypothalamus stimulates GH release. Somatostatin from the hypothalamus inhibits GH release as well as release of gastrointestinal secretions.

In contrast to the direct effects of GH, those mediated by IGF-1 are insulinlike. IGF-1 acts through cell membrane receptors that resemble those of insulin. In fact, insulin at high doses may act at IGF-1 receptors and vice versa (see Chapter 36). In pharmacologic doses, GH causes an initial insulin-like effect followed by an effect antagonistic to that of insulin.

Pharmacokinetics
Circulating endogenous GH has a half-life of 20 to 25 minutes, although slow-release forms are available allowing injections once or twice a month. Human GH can be given subcutaneously, with peak plasma levels reached at 2 to 4 hours. Metabolism takes place in the liver and the kidney.

Therapeutic uses
GH (somatrem, somatropin) is used in the treatment of growth failure in children (pituitary dwarfism), wasting in AIDS, and somatotropin-deficiency syndrome. Short-term treatment of GH-deficient adults results in increased lean body mass, decreased fat mass, increased exercise tolerance, and improved psychologic well-being. It is sometimes abused by athletes[6] or used for its antiaging effect. It is a potent anabolic agent and may have a role in clinical management of burn injuries.[17] The GH-releasing hormone analogue sermorelin is used to treat GH deficiency in children who have growth retardation and diagnostically to determine the GH-releasing capacity of the pituitary. Octreotide, a somatostatin analogue, is used to inhibit irritable bowel syndrome, pain from pancreatitis, and variceal bleeding.

Adverse effects
GH may induce relative insulin resistance. It has been documented to cause diabetes in AIDS patients[19] and decreased insulin sensitivity that is dose dependent, with a possible increase in type 2 diabetes in children.[5] Arthralgia, especially in the hands and wrist, may occur. Patients may have headaches, especially in the first few months of therapy, and should be carefully observed (monitored) because of the possibility of intracranial hypertension.

Table • 34-2

Hypothalamic Inhibitory Releasing Factors, Anterior Pituitary Hormones Inhibited, and Target Glands

HYPOTHALAMIC HORMONE	PITUITARY HORMONE INHIBITED	TARGET ORGAN
Dopamine	Prolactin	Breast
Somatostatin	GH	Liver, bone, other

Prolactin
Prolactin is an anterior pituitary hormone that is similar in structure to GH. Prolactin increases the growth of the secretory epithelium in the breast and stimulates the production of milk. Although prolactin is not used clinically, the secretion of prolactin can be altered by certain drugs. Because dopamine inhibits prolactin release (Table 34-2), drugs that affect dopamine levels or dopamine receptors in the pituitary affect prolactin release. Bromocriptine, cabergoline, and pergolide are dopamine-receptor agonists that are used to inhibit prolactin release and reduce the size of pituitary prolactin-releasing tumors.

Thyroid-Stimulating Hormone (Thyrotropin)
Thyrotropin (TSH) is a glycoprotein hormone consisting of two subunits (α and β). Secretion is pulsatile and follows a circadian rhythm, with levels of TSH being highest during sleep at night. TSH secretion is controlled by thyrotropin-releasing hormone (TRH), which in turn is inhibited by thyroid hormone negative feedback. Because TRH is stimulated by cold and decreased by severe stress, TSH is also affected by these conditions. TSH stimulates the thyroid to synthesize thyroglobulin and the thyroid hormones thyroxine and triiodothyronine. An increase in the amount of free thyroid hormone in the circulation results in decreased TSH gene transcription and decreased TSH secretion.

The TSH receptor is G protein–coupled. The effects of TSH are mediated by stimulation of adenylyl cyclase and increased cyclic 3′,5′-adenosine monophosphate formation in the thyroid cell. TSH also causes activation of phospholipase C. TSH is used for diagnostic purposes and to stimulate iodine (^{131}I) uptake in some patients with thyroid cancer (see below).

THYROID HORMONES

The active principles of the thyroid gland are iodine-containing amino acid derivatives of thyronine. They are formed from iodinated tyrosine residues. The structures are shown in Figure 34-1.

Synthesis of Thyroid Hormones

The synthesis of thyroid hormones is shown schematically in Figure 34-2. The first step is uptake of iodide by the thyroid gland. This step may be inhibited by ions of similar size and charge such as perchlorate. Iodide uptake is followed by oxidation of iodide to hypoiodate and then iodination of tyrosyl groups of thyroglobulin to form iodotyrosyl groups. Tyrosine residues within the thyroglobulin molecule may be monoiodinated to monoiodotyrosine (MIT) or diiodinated to form diiodotyrosine (DIT). This step is catalyzed by thyroperoxidase and is rapid. Iodotyrosyl residues are then coupled to form iodothyronyl residues within thyroglobulin. This may be either MIT plus DIT to form T_3 or DIT plus DIT to form T_4. The ratio of $T_4 : T_3$ formed is approximately 4 : 1. The coupling of iodotyrosyl groups is also catalyzed by peroxidase enzyme. Thyroid hormones are then released by proteolysis of thyroglobulin. Most of the hormone released is T_4, which is converted to T_3 in peripheral tissues. Triiodothyronine is about four times more potent than thyroxine.

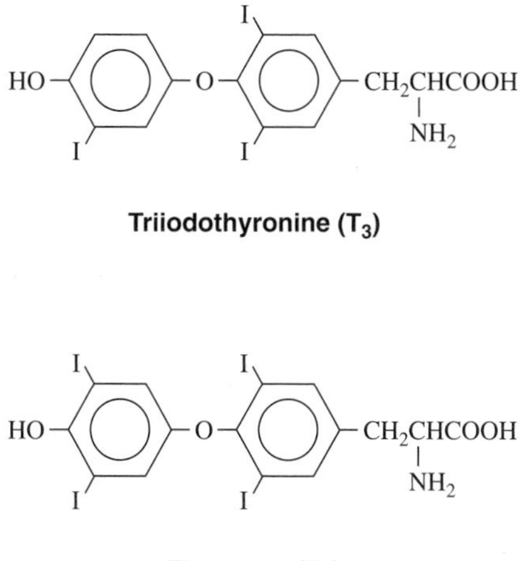

Triiodothyronine (T_3)

Thyroxine (T_4)

Fig. 34-1 Structure of thyroid hormones.

Control of Thyroid Hormone Secretion

The effect of TSH on the thyroid gland is to stimulate the synthesis and secretion of thyroid hormones T_4 and T_3 (see previous discussion). In addition to TSH, the iodine concentration in the blood plays an important role in regulating the uptake of iodide and formation of thyroid hormones in the thyroid gland. Iodination and thyroid hormone release can both be inhibited by larger doses of iodides.

The hypothalamic-pituitary-thyroid axis is stimulated by cold and decreased in severe stress. It is under negative feedback control of the thyroid hormones, which act both on the hypothalamus to decrease TRH synthesis and secretion and on the pituitary to block the action of TRH.

Actions of Thyroid Hormones

Thyroid hormones act by diffusing across the cell membrane and binding to intracellular receptors in target tissues. T_4 is converted to T_3 inside the cell. T_3 has greater affinity than T_4 for the receptors. The action of thyroid hormones leads to an increase in transcription, resulting in synthesis of proteins that

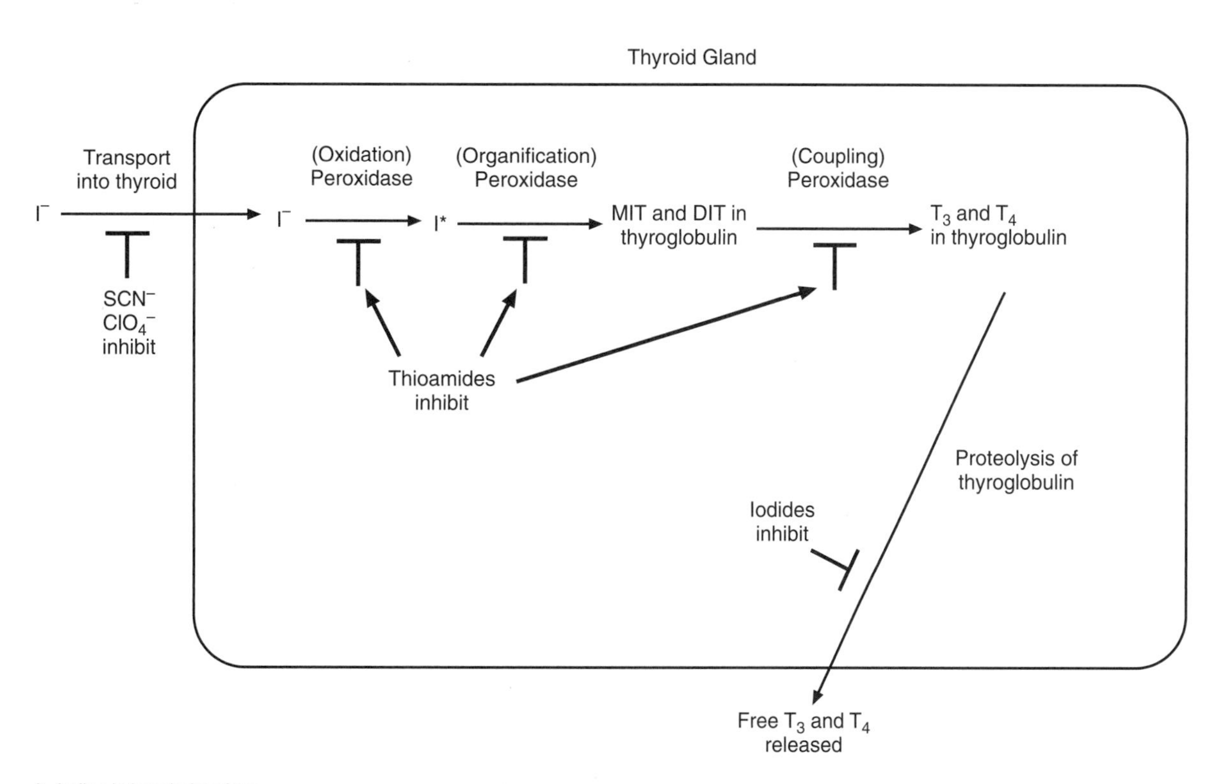

Fig. 34-2 Synthesis of thyroid hormones and sites of action of various antithyroid drugs. *DIT*, Diiodotyrosine; *MIT*, monoiodotyrosine.

produce many of the actions of thyroid hormones. Thyroid hormones are extremely important in normal development and metabolism. They have a critical effect on growth, partly by direct action and partly by potentiating GH. Thyroid hormones are important for a normal response to parathyroid hormone and calcitonin. They are crucial for nervous and skeletal tissues. Thyroid deficiency during development causes cretinism, characterized by mental retardation and dwarfism.

In addition, thyroid hormones are regulators of metabolism in most tissues. They increase basal metabolic rate and resting respiratory rate. Thyroid hormones stimulate the heart, resulting in the heart beating more rapidly and with greater force, and an increase in cardiac output. Energy utilization in skeletal muscle, liver, and kidney is also markedly stimulated. T_3 sensitizes the heart to the effects of circulating endogenous catecholamines by a direct effect on Ca^{++} channels,[9] and, in addition, thyroid hormones cause an increase in myocardial β-adrenergic receptors.[20]

Pharmacokinetics

The thyroid hormones are highly protein bound, the major plasma-binding protein being thyroxine-binding globulin. They are also bound by thyroxine-binding prealbumin and albumin. The half-life of T_4 is normally 6 to 7 days, shortened to 3 to 4 days in hyperthyroidism. T_3 binds more loosely to plasma proteins and has a half-life of approximately 2 days.

THYROID DISORDERS

Worldwide, the most common cause of thyroid disorders is iodine deficiency. In the United States, the leading cause of hypothyroidism is Hashimoto's thyroiditis, an autoimmune disease. Graves' disease (diffuse toxic goiter), also an autoimmune disorder, is the most common cause of hyperthyroidism in the United States.

Hypothyroidism

Thyroid deficiency during development causes cretinism, which is characterized by gross retardation of growth and mental deficiency. In the adult, thyroid deficiency results in hypothyroidism and, in more severe cases, myxedema. Hypothyroidism is a common endocrine disorder affecting 1.4% to 2.0% of women and 0.1% to 0.2% of men.[7] The prevalence of both overt and subclinical hypothyroidism is significantly greater in women than in men and increases dramatically in women after age 40 years, affecting 5% to 10% of women older than 50 years.[2] Subclinical hypothyroidism is common, especially among older women.[18] It has been suggested that this may be associated with an increased mortality rate, particularly from cardiovascular disease and a subtle decrease in myocardial contractility.[11] Subclinical hypothyroidism is associated with a small increase in low-density lipoprotein cholesterol and a decrease in high-density lipoprotein cholesterol, changes that increase risk of atherosclerosis and coronary artery disease.[11] Cognitive impairment occurs in hypothyroidism, and attention, motor speed, memory, and visual spatial organization are all significantly impaired.[4] In addition, hypothyroidism is an important risk factor for carpal tunnel syndrome.[15]

Signs and Symptoms of Hypothyroidism

Typical symptoms include lethargy, fatigue, loss of energy/ambition, slowing of intellectual and motor activity, decreased appetite, increased weight, and skin that is dry, cold, and coarse. Hair loss, including loss of the outer third of eyebrows, occurs. Hypothyroid patients display cold intolerance, bradycardia, hypotension, and increased capillary fragility, as well as show an exaggerated response to central nervous system depressants such as sedatives and narcotic analgesics.

Replacement Therapy

Animal products include desiccated thyroid, which is composed of animal thyroid glands. Numerous preparations of T_4, levothyroxine sodium, are available and are the most commonly used thyroid replacement medication. Liothyronine sodium (T_3) and liotrix, a mixture of T_4 and T_3 in a 4 : 1 ratio, are also available. Evidence is now accumulating that the combination of T_3 and T_4 is better than T_4 alone in a substantial minority of patients.[3]

Pharmacokinetics

The thyroid hormones are well absorbed after oral administration. However, absorption of T_4 may be decreased by food, Ca^{++} preparations, and aluminum-containing antacids. Absorption of T_4 is best if it is taken on empty stomach in the morning. Absorption of T_3, which is almost completely absorbed, is not affected by food.

Levothyroxine has a half-life of approximately 7 days. It therefore takes about a month to reach steady state. The half-life of liothyronine is shorter (less than 2 days), as is its duration of action.

Hyperthyroidism

Hyperthyroidism may be caused by Graves' disease (diffuse toxic goiter), an autoimmune disorder, or toxic nodular goiter. Graves' disease is the most common cause of hyperthyroidism in the United States. In hyperthyroidism (thyrotoxicosis), there is an excess of thyroid hormones, resulting in a high metabolic rate, increased heart rate and contractility, and increased sensitivity to catecholamines. Other signs and symptoms include increased appetite but decreased weight, weakened skeletal muscles or muscle wasting, increased body temperature, sensitivity to heat, nervousness, and tremor. Exophthalmus may be present in Graves' disease.

Treatment

Hyperthyroidism may be treated surgically or pharmacologically. The most common treatments are described below.

DRUGS USED IN THE TREATMENT OF HYPERTHYROIDISM

The major drugs used to inhibit production of thyroid hormones are radioactive iodine (^{131}I), the thiourylenes, and iodide.

Radioactive Iodine

The ^{131}I isotope has a half-life of 8 days and emits both γ radiation and β particles. Given orally, it is concentrated in the thyroid, where the β particles destroy the gland. Symptoms of hyperthyroidism begin to improve in a few days to a few weeks, but 2 to 3 months are often required for a complete effect.

^{131}I is selective for the thyroid gland. Advantages of the use of ^{131}I include the comparative low cost because surgery is not required, and the fact that no deaths have been reported resulting from this treatment. The disadvantage of this treatment is that hypothyroidism frequently occurs as a delayed effect. However, it is now believed that hypothyroidism may represent the end stage of hyperthyroidism rather than overtreatment with ^{131}I. ^{131}I should be avoided in children and pregnant patients. Uptake of low-dose ^{131}I may be used as a test of thyroid function.

Thiourylenes

Within this group of drugs, propylthiouracil and methimazole are the most important antithyroid drugs used in the United

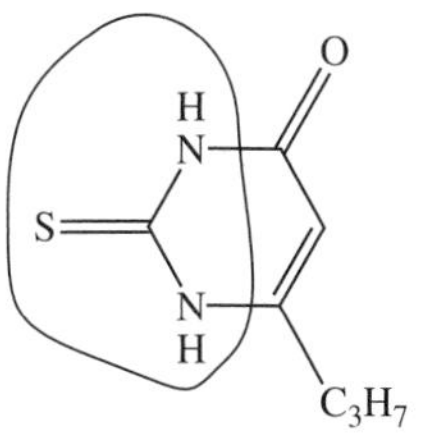

Propylthiouracil

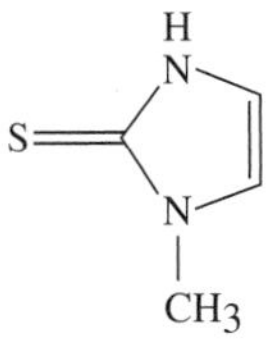

Methimazole

Fig. 34-3 Chemicaml structures of propylthiouracil and methimazole. The thiocarbamide group is *circled* in propylthiouracil.

States (Figure 34-3). These drugs are related to thiourea and contain a thiocarbamide group that is essential for their antithyroid activity.

Mechanism of action

The thiourylenes inhibit thyroid peroxidase, thereby decreasing iodide oxidation, iodination of tyrosines, and coupling of iodotyrosyl and iodothyronyl residues (see Figure 34-2). As a result, less thyroid hormone is synthesized. Propylthiouracil also inhibits the peripheral conversion of T_4 to T_3.

Pharmacokinetics

The thiourylenes are given orally. Methimazole is distributed throughout body water and has a plasma half-life of 6 to 15 hours. An average dose produces more than 90% inhibition of thyroid incorporation of iodide within 12 hours, but the clinical response takes weeks to manifest itself because of the long half-life of T_4 and because there may be stores of hormone in the thyroid that need to be depleted. The actions of propylthiouracil may be seen more quickly because of the inhibition of peripheral conversion of T_4 to T_3.

Adverse effects

Side effects include occasional, reversible, yet rapidly developing agranulocytosis as well as rashes, pain, stiffness in joints, paresthesias, and loss or depigmentation of hair.

Therapeutic uses

The thiourylenes are used to control hyperthyroidism in anticipation of spontaneous remission, before surgery, or together with ^{131}I to hasten recovery from hyperthyroidism.

Ionic Inhibitors

The ionic inhibitors interfere with the concentration of iodide by the thyroid gland. They are monovalent anions that resemble iodide. Examples include thiocyanate and perchlorate. Thiocyanate, which is not used therapeutically, may be formed during the digestion of certain foods such as cabbage and has an antithyroid effect.

Iodide

Iodide is the oldest remedy for thyroid disorders. Iodine/odides are required for thyroid hormone synthesis (see Figure 34-2); however, high concentrations of iodide limit its own transport. In addition, high concentrations of iodide inhibit synthesis of iodotyrosines and iodothyronines (organification) and inhibit thyroid hormone release. These effects, which depend on intracellular concentrations of iodide, are transient. High plasma iodide concentrations also inhibit release of thyroid hormones. Iodide has been used preoperatively in preparation for thyroidectomy because it makes the gland less vascular. Iodide is also used together with antithyroid drugs and propranolol to treat thyrotoxic crisis.

Adverse effects

Hypersensitivity to iodides is the major adverse effect. Iodism, which is chronic iodine toxicity, has a number of adverse effects, including unpleasant taste, burning in the mouth and throat, soreness of teeth and gingiva, and increased salivation. Symptoms similar to those of a head cold commonly occur, as do skin eruptions, gastric irritation, and diarrhea. Inflammation of the larynx, tonsils, and lungs and enlargement of the parotid and submandibular glands may occur. Iodide concentrates in salivary glands.

IMPLICATIONS FOR DENTISTRY

Subclinical hypothyroidism and hyperthyroidism are common, well-defined conditions that often progress to overt disease. The clinical presentation of thyroid disorders is often subtle in older adults and may be confused with normal aging.

Hypothyroidism

Hypothyroidism is 5 to 6 times more common than hyperthyroidism. Hypothyroidism affects 7 to 10 times as many women as men and the incidence of the disease increases sharply with age in women after age 40 years, affecting 5% to 10% of women older than 50 years.[2,18] Subclinical states may contribute to hyperlipidemia, cardiac dysfunction, and osteoporosis.[18]

The dentist may be in a position to detect signs and symptoms of subclinical thyroid disease and refer the patient for medical evaluation and treatment. This is very important in hypothyroidism, in which signs and symptoms are subtle and similar to those of depression (Box 34-1). As a result, the disease may not be diagnosed.

Subclinical hypothyroidism in younger individuals may show as delayed eruption of teeth, malocclusion, and skeletal retardation. Other oral manifestations of hypothyroidism include tongue enlargement and scalloping. Hypothyroid patients have increased capillary fragility and show an exaggerated response to CNS depressants such as sedatives and opioids.

Box 34-1

Common Signs of Hypothyroidism and Depression

- Depressed mood
- Decreased interests
- Weight gain
- Disturbed sleep
- Muscle weakness/slow speech
- Disturbed concentration and cognition
- Feelings or guilt or inadequacy/inability to cope

Clinical hypothyroidism or myxedema may be recognized by a patient's dull expression; puffy eyelids; alopecia of the outer third of the eyebrows; dry, rough skin; dry, brittle, coarse hair; increased size of tongue; slowing of physical and mental activity; anemia; constipation; and increased sensitivity to cold.

In patients with myxedema, stressful situations such as surgery, trauma, or infections may precipitate myxedematous coma. This occurs predominantly in elderly women and has a greater than 50% mortality rate.[1]

Hyperthyroidism

Thyrotoxicosis is characterized by warm, moist skin; a rosy complexion; weight loss; fine, friable hair; and nail softening. Profuse sweating is common in these patients. Achlorhydria may occur, and approximately 3% of those affected develop pernicious anemia. Hyperthyroid individuals cannot sit still, are nervous, emotionally labile, and always moving. They display tremor of the hands and tongue and muscle weakness. In thyrotoxicosis there is increased bone loss. In these patients there is also increased stroke volume and heart rate as well as palpitations. Supraventricular arrhythmias may occur. Graves' ophthalmopathy may be recognized by eyelid retraction, proptosis, and a bright-eyed stare. Patients who are hyperthyroid are highly sensitive to epinephrine. Propranolol alleviates adrenergic symptoms such as sweating, tremor, and tachycardia.

Oral complications of thyrotoxicosis include osteoporosis of the alveolar bone. Dental caries and periodontal disease appear more frequently. In children, teeth and jaws develop more rapidly, and there is early loss of deciduous teeth and early eruption of permanent teeth. Changes in the gingiva resulting from hyperthyroidism may lead to ill-fitting dentures.

HORMONES OF CALCIUM HOMEOSTASIS

Parathyroid Hormone

The parathyroid glands (there are usually four) are embedded within the posterior surface of the thyroid. The principal cells secrete parathyroid hormone (PTH), which is formed by proteolysis of a larger precursor. PTH is a single-chain polypeptide containing 84 amino acids and has a molecular weight of approximately 9500. Loss of the first 2 amino acids eliminates most biologic activity.

Regulation of secretion

The principal factor in control of PTH secretion is plasma Ca^{++} concentration. High plasma Ca^{++} concentration decreases PTH secretion; low Ca^{++} concentration stimulates it. Ca^{++} regulates PTH secretion by a G protein–coupled, cell surface Ca^{++}-sensing receptor. Phosphate regulates PTH secretion indirectly by forming complexes with Ca^{++}. Increases in phosphate concentration reduce Ca^{++} levels and hence increase PTH secretion.

Pharmacologic effects

PTH regulates Ca^{++} and phosphate, causing an increase in plasma Ca^{++} and a decrease in plasma phosphate concentrations. The primary function of PTH is to maintain a constant extracellular Ca^{++} concentration.

The most important target tissues for PTH are bone and kidney. In bone, PTH increases Ca^{++} and phosphate release by increasing bone resorption. It acts on the osteoblast to induce osteoclast differentiation factor (also called *receptor for activating nuclear factor kappa B ligand* and the earlier term *tumor necrosis factor-related activation-induced cytokine*), which in turn stimulates osteoclast activity, resulting in increased bone turnover. Both bone formation and bone resorption are enhanced by PTH. With constant dosing, PTH increases bone resorption. However, when PTH is given intermittently at low doses, it stimulates both cortical and trabecular bone growth.[13] The use of low-dose PTH pulsing as a treatment for osteoporosis is currently under study.

In the kidney, PTH increases reabsorption of Ca^{++} and Mg^{++} and decreases reabsorption of phosphate. PTH also increases conversion of vitamin D to its active form, 1,25-dihydroxyvitamin D (calcitriol), which is then secreted into the circulation and acts in the gastrointestinal tract to increase the absorption of Ca^{++}.

Pharmacokinetics

PTH has a half-life of minutes, with clearance occurring mostly in the liver and kidney.

Calcitonin

Calcitonin is secreted by the parafollicular cells of the thyroid gland. Calcitonin is synthesized as a prohormone and processed to the hormone. There is considerable species variation in calcitonin. Human calcitonin is a single-chain peptide composed of 32 amino acids and has a molecular weight of 3600. A disulfide bridge between positions 1 and 7 is essential for biologic activity.

Control of secretion

Elevated extracellular Ca^{++} concentration is the most important stimulator of calcitonin secretion. Calcitonin release is also stimulated by gastrointestinal tract hormones, including cholecystokinin and gastrin.

Actions

Calcitonin acts on G protein–linked cell surface receptors located on target tissues. It lowers plasma Ca^{++} and phosphate concentrations mainly by acting on bone to inhibit osteoclast activity and bone resorption. Calcitonin also acts on the kidney to increase urinary excretion of Ca^{++} and phosphate.

Therapeutic uses

Calcitonin is used in the treatment of Paget's disease, in which there is excessive, disorganized bone remodeling, and in some patients with osteoporosis. Salmon calcitonin, which is more potent and has a longer half-life than mammalian calcitonin, is typically used in therapy. It is given by injection or nasal spray.

Adverse effects

Nausea and gastrointestinal tract effects are the most common adverse effects. Rash with itching and swelling may also occur.

Vitamin D

Vitamin D is the name given to two related substances, cholecalciferol (vitamin D_3) and ergocalciferol (vitamin D_2). Both are active in human beings and are able to prevent or cure rickets. Cholecalciferol is formed in the skin from 7-dehydrocholesterol by the action of ultraviolet irradiation; ergocalciferol comes from plants. Vitamin D is also found in dietary products.

The major action of vitamin D is control of Ca^{++} homeostasis. Vitamin D acts to facilitate absorption of Ca^{++} and phosphate from the small intestine, interacts with PTH to enhance mobilization of Ca^{++} and phosphate from bone, and decreases excretion of Ca^{++} and phosphate by the kidney. In addition, vitamin D has effects on bone remodeling.

The net effect of vitamin D is to increase both serum Ca^{++} and serum phosphate. This is different from the net effect

Table • 34-3

Effects of PTH and Vitamin D on Bone, Gastrointestinal Tract, and Kidney

ORGAN	PTH	VITAMIN D
Bone	Low doses increase bone formation; high doses increase bone resorption	Secalcifediol may increase bone formation; calcitriol increases bone resorption
Gastrointestinal tract	Increases Ca^{++} and phosphate absorption (by increased calcitriol production)	Calcitriol increases Ca^{++} and phosphate absorption
Kidney	Decreases Ca^{++}, increases phosphate excretion	Decreases Ca^{++} and phosphate excretion
Overall effect	Increases serum Ca^{++}, decreases serum phosphate	Increases serum Ca^{++} and serum phosphate

of PTH, which is to increase serum Ca^{++} and reduce serum phosphate. The effects of PTH and vitamin D are shown in Table 34-3.

Vitamin D is a prohormone that is a precursor to a number of biologically active metabolites. Cholecalciferol is biotransformed to 25-hydroxycholecalciferol (25[OH]D, calcifediol) in the liver and further converted to 1,25-dihydroxy vitamin D (1,25$[OH]_2$D, calcitriol) and 24,25-dihydroxy vitamin D (24,25$[OH]_2$D, secalcifediol) in the kidney.

Calcitriol is biologically the most active metabolite of Vitamin D (Figure 34-4).[25] It stimulates Ca^{++} and phosphate absorption from the gastrointestinal tract. Calcitriol is required for bone mineralization, although it directly stimulates bone resorption.[8] In the kidney it slightly increases Ca^{++} and phosphate reabsorption. Receptors for calcitriol are found in a variety of tissues, including bone, gut, and kidney. These are intracellular receptors, as are typical of other steroid hormone receptors. Calcitriol binding to its receptors leads to a selective increase in transcription and production of proteins such as Ca^{++}-binding proteins in the gastrointestinal tract. Calcitriol may also act directly on the membrane to alter Ca^{++} flux. In addition to its classic effects (discussed above), calcitriol has a number of other actions, including regulation of PTH secretion, cytokine production, and proliferation and differentiation of a number of cells. Secalcifediol stimulates bone formation and is essential for fracture healing.[22]

Calcifediol (25[OH]D) is more potent than calcitriol in stimulating renal reabsorption of Ca^{++} and phosphate and may be the major metabolite involved in the regulation of Ca^{++} flux and contractility in muscle.

High levels of Ca^{++} and phosphate reduce the amount of 1,25-dihydroxyvitamin D produced by the kidney and also decrease the amount of 24,25-dihydroxyvitamin D. Calcitriol directly inhibits PTH secretion by a direct action on PTH gene transcription.

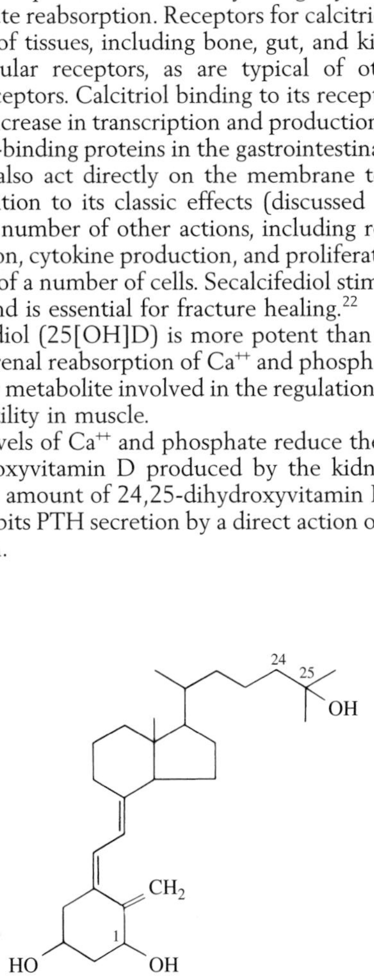

Fig. 34-4 Structural formula of the primary active form of vitamin D: 1,25-dihydroxycholecalciferol (calcitriol).

Pharmacokinetics

Vitamin D is usually given orally. After absorption, vitamin D and its metabolites circulate in plasma bound to vitamin D–binding protein, which is an α globulin. Vitamin D (cholecalciferol) has a plasma half-life of 19 to 25 hours but is stored in fat for prolonged periods. The major circulating form is calcifediol, which has a half-life of 19 days. The half-life of calcitriol is 3 to 5 days.

Calcifediol and calcitriol are available for clinical use as vitamin D. In addition, doxercalciferol and paricalcitol have been approved for treatment of secondary hyperparathyroidism in patients with renal failure.

Bisphosphonates

Members of this group of drugs include etidronate, tiludronate, pamidronate, risedronate, and alendronate and are modeled after pyrophosphate (Figure 34-5).

The major action of the bisphosphonates is inhibition of bone resorption. Because bone formation is coupled to

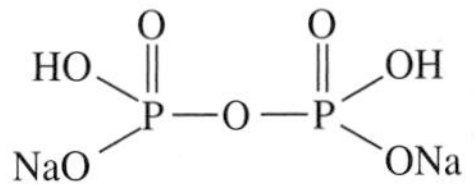

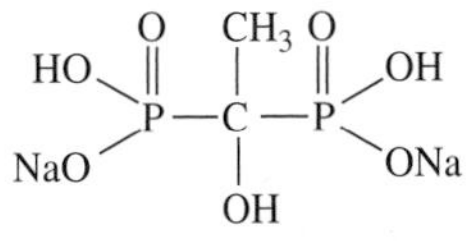

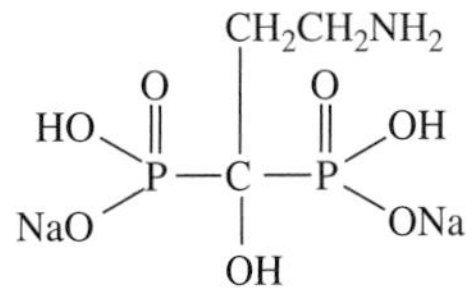

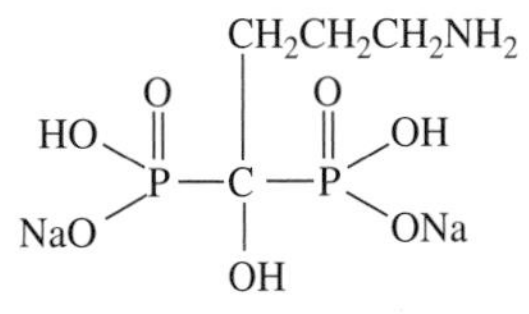

Fig. 34-5 Chemical structures of pyrophosphate and some bisphosphonates.

resorption, a secondary, indirect decrease in bone formation may also occur. This is seen with etidronate.

The mechanism of action of the bisphosphonates is not completely understood. It is believed that they are incorporated into bone matrix and taken into the osteoclast during resorption, incapacitating it. There is evidence that alendronate and tiludronate inhibit protein tyrosine phosphatases, leading to detachment of osteoclasts from bone surface and inhibition of the osteoclast proton pump.[14,21]

Pharmacokinetics

The bisphosphonates are poorly absorbed after oral administration. Food significantly decreases the absorption. It is suggested that these drugs should be taken only with water, after an overnight fast, and 2 hours before breakfast. Bioavailability is reduced if coffee or orange juice is taken concurrently with these drugs.

The bisphosphonates, unlike pyrophosphate, are not metabolized and are excreted unchanged in the urine. Plasma levels decrease by more than 95% within 6 hours, but the terminal half-life may exceed 10 years because they are slowly released from the skeleton, to which they bind.

Therapeutic uses

Bisphosphonates are used in the treatment of diseases in which there is rapid bone turnover or excessive osteolytic activity.[23] They are used in the treatment of osteoporosis, Paget's disease, and malignant bone disease. In the treatment of osteoporosis, both alendronate and risedronate have been shown to decrease the incidence of fractures significantly and improve bone mineral density.[10,26] These two drugs do not have the effect of decreasing bone formation that is seen with etidronate.

In cancer, inhibition of osteolysis has proved effective therapy for malignancy-associated hypercalcemia and for adjunctive therapy in delaying or preventing cancer-related skeletal pain. Therapy reduces the incidence of fractures and may reduce the need for radiation therapy. In Paget's disease, bisphosphonates reduce the rapid bone turnover rate and slow the disease progression.[12]

Hypothalamic, Pituitary, Thyroid, and Parathyroid Drugs

Nonproprietary (generic) name	*Proprietary (trade) name*
Hypothalamic and pituitary drugs*	
Desmopressin	DDAVP, Stimate
Octreotide	Sandostatin
Oxytocin	Pitocin, Syntocinon
Sermorelin	Geref
Somatrem	Protropin
Somatropin	Genotropin, Humatrope, Nutropin, Nutropin AQ, Norditropin, Serostim, Saizen
Vasopressin	Pitressin Synthetic
Drugs used to inhibit prolactin release	
Bromocriptine	Parlodel
Cabergoline	Dostinex
Pergolide	Permax
Thyroid hormone and TSH preparations	
Levothyroxine	Eltroxin, Levothroid, Levoxyl, Synthroid
Liothyronine	Cytomel, Triostat
Liotrix	Thyrolar
Thyroid desiccated	Armour Thyroid, Thyroid, Strong, Thyroid USP, Thyrar, S-P-T
Thyrotropin (recombinant human TSH)	Thyrogen
Antithyroid agents	
Iodide (^{131}I) sodium	Iodotope, Sodium iodide ^{131}I Therapeutic
Methimazole	Tapazole
Potassium iodide	Lugol's solution, Pima, SSKI
Propylthiouracil	PTU
Drugs affecting Ca^{++} metabolism	
Bisphosphonates	
Alendronate	Fosamax
Etidronate	Didronel
Pamidronate	Aredia
Risedronate	Actonel
Tiludronate	Skelid
Calcium salts	
Calcium acetate	Phos-Ex, PhosLo
Calcium carbonate	Cal-Sup, Os-Cal, Tums
Calcium chloride	—
Calcium citrate	Citracal
Calcium glubionate	Neo-Calglucon
Calcium gluceptate	—
Calcium gluconate	—
Calcium lactate	—
Tricalcium phosphate	Posture
Vitamin D	
Calcifediol	Calderol
Calcitriol	Calcijex, Rocaltrol
Cholecalciferol	Delta-D
Dihydrotachysterol	DHT, Hytakerol
Doxercalciferol	Hectorol
Ergocalciferol	Calciferol, Drisdol
Paricalcitol	Zemplar
Other drugs	
Calcitonin (salmon)	Calcimar, Miacalcin, Salmonine

*Gonadotropins are covered in Chapter 37.

Adverse effects

The most common adverse effects of bisphosphonates are gastrointestinal tract disturbances.[16] Esophagitis can occur with oral preparations. To prevent this, oral preparations are given with liberal amounts of water and with the patient in an upright position. Proton pump inhibitors (see Chapter 33) can also be used with benefit. The use of an intravenous form of bisphosphonate such as pamidronate is another alternative.

Cited References

1. Bailes BK: Hypothyroidism in elderly patients, *AORN J* 69:1026-1030, 1999.
2. Bonar BD, McColgan B, Smith DF, et al: Hypothyroidism and aging: the Rosses' survey, *Thyroid* 10:821-827, 2000.
3. Bunevicius R, Kazanavicius G, Zalinkevicius R, et al: Effects of thyroxine as compared with thyroxine plus triiodothyronine in patients with hypothyroidism, *N Engl J Med* 340:424-429, 1999.
4. Capet C, Jego A, Denis P, et al: Is cognitive change related to hypothyroidism reversible with replacement therapy? *Rev Med Intern* 21:672-678, 2000.
5. Clayton PE, Cowell CT: Safety issues in children and adolescents during growth hormone therapy—a review, *Growth Horm IGF Res* 10:306-317, 2000.
6. De Palo EF, Gatti R, Lancerin F, et al: Correlations of growth hormone (GH) and insulin-like growth factor I (IGF-I): effects of exercise and abuse by athletes, *Clin Chim Acta* 305:1-17, 2001.
7. Elliott B: Diagnosing and treating hypothyroidism, *Nurse Pract* 25:92-94, 99-105, 2000.
8. Gardiner EM, Baldock PA, Thomas GP, et al: Increased formation and decreased resorption of bone in mice with elevated vitamin D receptor in mature cells of the osteoblastic lineage, *FASEB J* 14:1908-1916, 2000.
9. Gotzsche LB: L-Triiodothyronine acutely increases Ca^{2+} uptake in the isolated, perfused rat heart. Changes in L-type Ca^{2+} channels and β-receptors during short- and long-term hyper- and hypothyroidism, *Eur J Endocrinol* 130:171-179, 1994.
10. Harris ST, Watts NB, Genant HK, et al: Effects of risedronate treatment on vertebral and nonvertebral fractures in women with postmenopausal osteoporosis: a randomized controlled trial. Vertebral Efficacy with Risedronate Therapy (VERT) Study Group, *JAMA* 282:1344-1352, 1999.
11. Kahaly GJ: Cardiovascular and atherogenic aspects of subclinical hypothyroidism, *Thyroid* 10:665-679, 2000.
12. Lourwood DL: The pharmacology and therapeutic utility of bisphosphonates, *Pharmacotherapy* 18:779-789, 1998.
13. Morley P, Whitfield JF, Willick GE: Parathyroid hormone: an anabolic treatment for osteoporosis, *Curr Pharm Des* 7:671-687, 2001.
14. Murakami H, Takahashi N, Tanaka S, et al: Tiludronate inhibits protein tyrosine phosphate activity in osteoclasts, *Bone* 20:399-404, 1997.
15. Palumbo CF, Szabo RM, Olmsted SL: The effects of hypothyroidism and thyroid replacement on the development of carpal tunnel syndrome, *J Hand Surg* [Am] 25:734-739, 2000.
16. Peter CP, Kindt MV, Majaka JA: Comparative study of potential for bisphosphonates to damage gastric mucosa of rats, *Dig Dis Sci* 43:1009-1015, 1998.
17. Ramirez RJ, Wolf SE, Herndon DN: Is there a role for growth hormone in the clinical management of burn injuries? *Growth Horm IGF Res* 8(suppl B):99-105, 1998.
18. Samuels MH: Subclinical thyroid disease in the elderly, *Thyroid* 8:803-813, 1998.
19. Schauster AC, Geletko SM, Mikolich DJ: Diabetes mellitus associated with recombinant human growth hormone for HIV wasting syndrome, *Pharmacotherapy* 20:1129-1134, 2000.
20. Seppet EK, Kaasik A, Minajeva A, et al: Mechanisms of thyroid hormone control over sensitivity and maximal contractile responsiveness to β-adrenergic agonists in atria, *Mol Cell Biochem* 184:419-426, 1998.
21. Skorey K, Ly HD, Kelly J, et al: How does alendronate inhibit protein-tyrosine phosphatases? *J Biol Chem* 272: 22472-22480, 1997.
22. St-Arnaud R: Novel findings about 24,25-dihydroxyvitamin D: an active metabolite? *Curr Opin Nephrol Hypertens* 8:435-441, 1999.
23. Theriault RL, Hortobagyi GN: The evolving role of bisphosphonates, *Semin Oncol* 28:284-290, 2001.
24. Van den Brande JL: A personal view on the early history of the insulin-like growth factors, *Horm Res* 51:149-175, 1999.
25. van Leeuwen JP, van den Bemd GJ, van Driel M, et al: 24,25-Dihydroxyvitamin D_3 and bone metabolism, *Steroids* 66:375-380, 2001.
26. Watts NB: Treatment of osteoporosis with bisphosphonates, *Rheum Dis Clin North Am* 27:197-214, 2001.

General References

Angusti T, Codegone A, Pellerito R, et al: Thyroid cancer prevalence after radioiodine treatment of hyperthyroidism, *J Nucl Med* 41:1006-1009, 2000.

Bilezikian JP, Meng X, Shi Y, et al: Primary hyperparathyroidism in women: a tale of two cities—New York and Beijing, *Int J Fertil Womens Med* 45:158-165, 2000.

Bindels AJ, Westendorp RG, Frolich, M, et al: The prevalence of subclinical hypothyroidism at different total plasma cholesterol levels in middle aged men and women: a need for case-finding? *Clin Endocrinol* 50:217-220, 1999.

Bjoro T, Holmen J, Kruger O, et al: Prevalence of thyroid disease, thyroid dysfunction and thyroid peroxidase antibodies in a large, unselected population. The Health Study of Nord-Trondelag, *Eur J Endocrinol* 143:639-647, 2000.

Brownlie BE, Rae AM, Walshe JW, et al: Psychoses associated with thyrotoxicosis—"thyrotoxic psychosis." A report of 18 cases, with statistical analysis of incidence, *Eur J Endocrinol* 142:438-444, 2000.

Carter-Su C, King AP, Argetsinger LS, et al: Signaling pathway of GH, *Endocr J* 43(suppl):S65-S70, 1996.

Cohen MM: Merging the old skeletal biology with the new. II. Molecular aspects of bone formation and bone growth, *J Craniofac Genet Dev Biol* 20:94-106, 2000.

Franklyn JA: Thyroid disease and its treatment: short- and long-term consequences, *J R Coll Physicians Lond* 33:564-567,1999.

Gerland K, Bataille-Simoneau N, Basle M, et al: Activation of the Jak/Stat signal transduction pathway in GH-treated rat osteoblast-like cells in culture, *Mol Cell Endocrinol* 168:1-9, 2000.

Hellgren G, Albertsson-Wikland K, Billig H, et al: Growth hormone receptor interaction with Jak proteins differs between tissues, *J Interferon Cytokine Res* 21:75-83, 2001.

Hunter I, Greene SA, MacDonald TM, et al: Prevalence and aetiology of hypothyroidism in the young, *Arch Dis Child* 83:207-210, 2000.

Kroll MH: Parathyroid hormone temporal effects on bone formation and resorption, *Bull Math Biol* 62:163-188, 2000.

Lal SO, Wolf SE, Herndon DN: Growth hormone, burns and tissue healing, *Growth Horm IGF Res* 10(suppl B):S39-S43, 2000.

McCarthy TL, Ji C, Centrella M: Links among growth factors, hormones, and nuclear factors with essential roles in bone formation, *Crit Rev Oral Biol Med* 11:409-422, 2000.

Murray RD, Shalet SM: Growth hormone: current and future therapeutic applications, *Expert Opin Pharmacother* 1:975-990, 2000.

Pirich C, Mullner M, Sinzinger H: Prevalence and relevance of thyroid dysfunction in 1922 cholesterol screening participants, *J Clin Epidemiol* 53:623-629, 2000.

Rack SK, Makela EH: Hypothyroidism and depression: a therapeutic challenge, *Ann Pharmacother* 34:1142-1145, 2000.

Rosen CJ: Growth hormone and aging, *Endocrine* 12:197-201, 2000.

Rosen CJ, Rackoff PJ: Emerging anabolic treatments for osteoporosis, *Rheum Dis Clin North Am* 27:215-233, 2001.

Skripitz R, Andreassen TT, Aspenberg P: Strong effect of PTH (1-34) on regenerating bone: a time sequence study in rats, *Acta Orthop Scand* 71:619-624, 2000.

Vallejo-Bolanos E, Espana-Lopez AJ, Munoz-Hoys A, et al: The relationship between bone age, chronological age and dental age in children with isolated growth hormone deficiency, *Int J Paediatr Dent* 9:201-206, 1999.

Weigel RJ: Nonoperative management of hyperparathyroidism: present and future, *Curr Opin Oncol* 13:33-38, 2001.

Wimalawansa SJ: Prevention and treatment of osteoporosis: efficacy of combination of hormone replacement therapy with other antiresorptive agents, *J Clin Densitom* 3:187-201, 2000.

Yonemura K, Suzuki H, Fujigaki Y, et al: New insights on the pathogenesis of hypercalcemia in primary hyperparathyroidism, *Am J Med Sci* 320:334-336, 2000.

CHAPTER • 35

Adrenal Corticosteroids

Clarence L. Trummel

The adrenal gland is the source of a diverse group of hormones essential to metabolic control, regulation of water and electrolyte balance, and regulation of the body's response to stress. The medullary portion of the gland secretes epinephrine and norepinephrine on sympathetic stimulation. These hormones and their physiologic effects and pharmacologic actions have been previously discussed (see Chapters 5 and 6). Using cholesterol as a substrate, the adrenal cortex produces a large number of substances collectively known as *corticosteroids*. Certain corticosteroids and their synthetic analogues are used in medicine for replacement in adrenal insufficiency. They are used even more widely for an array of nonadrenal diseases, primarily for their notable ability to suppress the acute or chronic inflammation that accompanies injury and many diseases. Unfortunately, when corticosteroids are administered in hyperphysiologic doses over long periods, as they often are in chronic inflammatory disorders, severe and even lethal toxicity can result. To properly understand the therapeutic applications and limitations of this group of drugs, the physiologic role of the corticosteroids must be reviewed.

GENERAL PHYSIOLOGIC AND PHARMACOLOGIC ACTIONS

By using cholesterol as a substrate, the adrenal cortex synthesizes and secretes two types of steroid hormones—the 19-carbon androgens and the 21-carbon corticosteroids. The latter group can be considered derivatives of pregnane (Figure 35-1). The corticosteroids can be further classified on the basis of their major actions. Some compounds, such as hydrocortisone (the nonproprietary name for the natural hormone cortisol), have relatively greater effects on carbohydrate metabolism, as measured by liver glycogen deposition, and are thus termed *glucocorticoids*. They also possess potent antiinflammatory actions and are used therapeutically for that purpose. Others, represented by aldosterone, are most active in enhancing sodium retention and are referred to as *mineralocorticoids*. These corticosteroids do not have antiinflammatory effects (Table 35-1). The structures of hydrocortisone and aldosterone are shown in Figure 35-1.

The corticosteroids are not stored to any extent in the adrenal gland but are continuously synthesized and secreted. There is a strong diurnal variation in this process; plasma concentrations of cortisol are several-fold higher at 8 AM than at 4 PM. Production of all corticosteroids except aldosterone is directly regulated by the blood concentration of adrenocorticotropic hormone (ACTH) secreted by the anterior pituitary (adenohypophysis). In turn, circulating corticosteroids act on both the hypothalamus and adenohypophysis to suppress the release of ACTH, completing the control loop linking the pituitary and the adrenal cortex (Figure 35-2). By this negative feedback mechanism, the administration of large doses of corticosteroids can prevent the tropic influence of this hormone on the adrenal cortex, thus completely suppressing the adrenal production of corticosteroids. Aldosterone secretion is controlled primarily by a direct effect of angiotensin II on the adrenal cortex. Hyponatremia and hyperkalemia also favor the release of aldosterone. ACTH has only a minor stimulatory effect on the release of aldosterone.

The corticosteroids play diverse and complex roles in the body economy of mammalian organisms. They are involved in carbohydrate, protein, lipid, and purine metabolism; electrolyte and water balance; and the functions of the cardiovascular, nervous, and immune-inflammatory systems, as well as the kidney, skeletal muscle, bone, and most other organs and tissues. It is not surprising, then, that the hormones of the adrenal cortex play a major role in the ability of animals to withstand stressful events. Without the adrenal cortex, life is possible only when food and large amounts of salt and water are regularly ingested, a constant ambient temperature prevails, and infection and other perturbing events are absent.

Most of the diverse actions of corticosteroids appear to be achieved by regulating gene expression. The glucocorticoids enter target cells and bind to cytosolic receptors. These receptors exist in a complex with several proteins, including heat shock protein and an immunophilin. Binding by the hormone or a synthetic analogue alters the conformation of the receptor, freeing it from the associated proteins. The hormone-receptor complex migrates to the nucleus and binds to the glucocorticoid-responsive elements on DNA of affected genes. The DNA-binding domain on the receptor is distinct from the drug-binding domain. Gene expression is then regulated either negatively or positively to render the characteristic and complex glucocorticoid signature for modification of protein synthesis.[11] The mechanism of action of mineralocorticoids has been less well studied but appears to be similarly based on regulation of transcription in renal and other target cells.

Consistent with the mechanism described, the major effects of corticosteroids are not manifested for several hours. However, other less apparent effects are more immediate. These likely occur through other receptor mechanisms involving the plasma membrane of target cells.[12]

The pharmacologic effects of the glucocorticoids are largely exaggerations of the physiologic functions of the endogenous corticosteroids. These effects thus simulate the pathologic features of Cushing's syndrome, a metabolic disorder resulting from an excess of corticosteroids, primarily

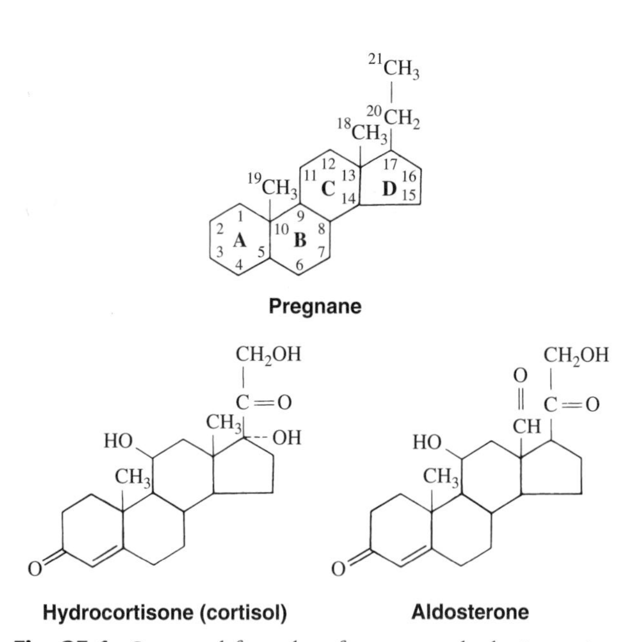

Fig. 35-1 Structural formulas of pregnane, the basic corticosteroid nucleus, and hydrocortisone (cortisol) and aldosterone, the prototypic glucocorticoid and mineralocorticoid, respectively.

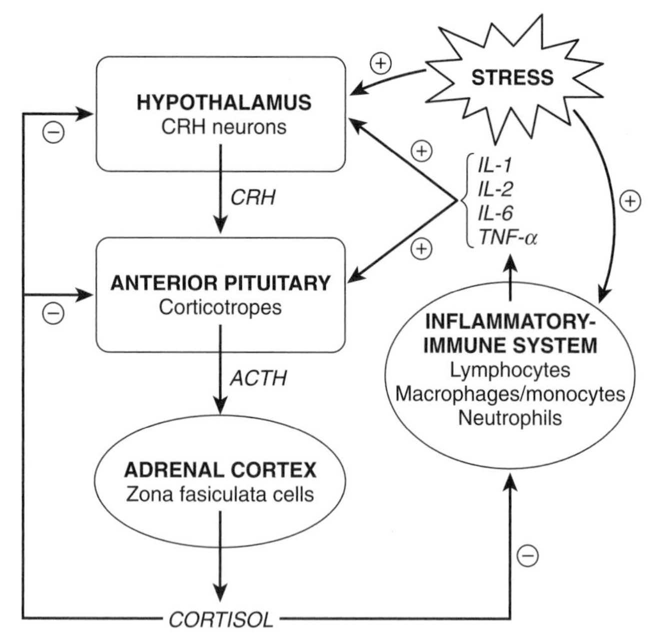

Fig. 35-2 The hypothalamic-pituitary-adrenal axis and its relationship to stress and the inflammatory-immune system. Cortisol exerts a negative feedback control on the secretion of corticotropin-releasing hormone (*CRH*) and ACTH. Physiologic or psychologic stress increases cortisol secretion directly through neural mechanism or by activation of the inflammatory-immune system and production of cytokines, interleukin-1 *(IL-1)*, interleukin-2 *(IL-2)*, interleukin-6 *(IL-6)*, and tumor necrosis factor–α *(TNF-α)*.

Table • 35-1

Potencies of Some Commonly Used Corticosteroids (Relative to Hydrocortisone)

	LIVER GLYCOGEN DEPOSITION*	SODIUM RETENTION
11-Desoxycorticosterone	0	100
Aldosterone	0.1	3000
Cortisone	0.8	0.8
Hydrocortisone	1	1
Prednisolone	4	0.8
Triamcinolone	5	0
Fludrocortisone	10	3000
Dexamethasone	25	0
Betamethasone	25	0

*Generally paralleled by antiinflammatory activity.

cortisol. A review of these features and their pathophysiologic basis is helpful in understanding the pharmacologic and toxic actions of the glucocorticoids.[13]

Carbohydrate and Protein Metabolism

Through several actions, glucocorticoids exert prominent anti-insulin effects. Glucocorticoids decrease the peripheral use of glucose by decreasing the cellular uptake of glucose. In the liver, glucocorticoids specifically stimulate glucose synthesis from amino acids (gluconeogenesis)[6]; concurrently, they mobilize amino acids by inhibiting protein synthesis in muscle, connective tissues, and skin (antianabolic effect). These actions are reflected in the parallel increases in blood glucose, liver glycogen, and urinary nitrogen excretion seen after the administration of glucocorticoids. As a consequence of these actions, prolonged high titers of glucocorticoids cause clinical manifestations of protein wasting: retardation of linear growth in children, wasting of the skin and increased capillary fragility resulting in ecchymoses, loss of muscle tissue leading to weakness (which may be extreme), and osteoporosis associated with enhanced bone resorption.

Lipid Metabolism

The effects of glucocorticoids on lipid metabolism further antagonize the actions of insulin. Glucocorticoids inhibit fatty acid synthesis and exert a permissive action on fatty acid mobilization from adipose tissue by lipolytic hormones. Long-term administration of large doses of glucocorticoids causes redistribution of fat from peripheral stores to more central locations on the back, shoulders, abdomen, and face; the result is termed *centripetal obesity*. Cutaneous striae form on areas of the trunk where the skin is stretched by the accumulation of fat.

Electrolyte and Water Balance

Excesses or deficiencies of corticosteroid hormones are associated with severe disturbances in electrolyte and fluid balance. These disturbances result from three actions of corticosteroids on the kidney: stimulation of reabsorption of Na^+ from the tubular fluid and increased urinary excretion of K^+ and H^+ ions. Thus excessive concentrations of corticosteroids lead to Na^+ retention, hypokalemia, alkalosis, and expanded extracellular fluid volume. These changes are manifested clinically by edema and hypertension; they may lead to left ventricular hypertrophy and predispose the patient to congestive heart failure and stroke. In corticosteroid deficiency (Addison's disease), essentially the opposite occurs (loss of Na^+, hyperkalemia, reduced extracellular fluid volume, and generalized cellular hydration) and, if severe, may quickly lead to death.

Antiinflammatory Properties

The glucocorticoids are potent inhibitors of the inflammatory response. This antiinflammatory activity is independent of the initiating stimulus and occurs at multiple points throughout the course of the process (see Figure 35-2). Several contributory actions are especially prominent. Glucocorticoids, by their action on gene expression, induce the production of lipocortin, a protein inhibitor of phospholipase A_2. The resulting decrease in the production of arachidonic acid leads to a reduction in the synthesis of prostaglandins (PGs) and leukotrienes, important mediators of inflammation. This effect is particularly important in macrophages, monocytes, endothelial cells, and fibroblasts. Glucocorticoids also suppress the synthesis of cyclooxygenase. The net result of these two actions is an inhibition of neutrophil, eosinophil, and monocyte chemotaxis (from inhibition of leukotriene B_4 synthesis), inhibition of capillary permeability and bronchoconstriction (from decreased leukotrienes C_4 and D_4, as well as $PGF_{2\alpha}$), and inhibition of the vascular and inflammatory responses to PGI_2 and PGE_2. In addition, glucocorticoids inhibit the production of eosinophils, basophils, monocytes, and lymphocytes; the synthesis of various cytokines (interleukins and tumor necrosis factor–α) in macrophages, lymphocytes, monocytes, and endothelial cells; and the release of histamine. Furthermore, glucocorticoids inhibit the synthesis of adhesion molecules in endothelial cells; this impairs the attachment of inflammatory cells and hinders their recruitment to sites of inflammation.

Immune Responses

The glucocorticoids are widely used to suppress undesirable immune reactions such as graft rejection. The mechanism involved is complex but involves glucocorticoid inhibition of T-lymphocyte activation and proliferation. Production of plasma cells is also inhibited. These effects on both T and B lymphocytes appear to be largely caused by the reduced production of cytokines, as described previously. Glucocorticoids impair the ability of inflammatory cells to migrate into sites of immunologic or inflammatory reactions. Phagocytosis and subsequent digestion (processing) of antigen by macrophages, events necessary for the development of some immune responses, are inhibited. Finally, glucocorticoids suppress antibody production.

ABSORPTION, FATE, AND EXCRETION

All the natural and synthetic corticosteroids except desoxycorticosterone are well absorbed from the gastrointestinal tract. Significant amounts of these drugs may also be absorbed from sites of local application, such as the skin, mucous membranes, and eye. In normal circumstances, more than 90% of circulating corticosteroids are bound to plasma proteins, principally α-globulin (corticosteroid-binding globulin, also known as *transcortin*), which has a high affinity but low capacity for these compounds, and albumin, which has the opposite characteristics.

Hydrocortisone is rapidly degraded in the liver by reduction, conjugated with glucuronic acid, and excreted in the urine. Most other corticosteroids are similarly metabolized, although at different rates. The plasma half-life of hydrocortisone is approximately 1.5 hours. Synthetic analogues of hydrocortisone generally have longer half-lives; for example, the potent long-acting compound dexamethasone has a plasma half-life of roughly 4 hours and a tissue half-life of approximately 2 days. Because the corticosteroids act by modifying gene expression, the time course of effect bears little correspondence to the plasma concentration.

The major metabolic products of corticosteroid metabolism found in the urine, the 17-hydroxycorticosteroids and 17-ketosteroids, were formerly measured by clinical laboratories to assess adrenal-pituitary function. This method has been largely supplanted by direct measurement of plasma cortisol concentrations by radioimmunoassay.

GENERAL THERAPEUTIC USES

The glucocorticoids are used clinically in two ways. The first and most intuitive is replacement therapy. Insufficient production of corticosteroids can result from a defect in the adrenal cortex, anterior pituitary, or hypothalamus; these defects may be congenital or acquired. Depending on the degree of insufficiency, the outcome may be either acute or chronic. Acute adrenal insufficiency (adrenal crisis) is a life-threatening emergency characterized by extreme weakness, gastrointestinal symptoms, dehydration, and hypotension. It frequently follows abrupt cessation of long-term high-dose therapy with glucocorticoids and stems from a drug-induced suppression of adrenal-pituitary function (which may require as long as 2 years for full recovery). The features of chronic adrenal insufficiency (Addison's disease) are similar to but milder than those of the acute state. Treatment of adrenal insufficiency, regardless of the cause, requires replacement with appropriate corticosteroids.

In addition to replacement therapy, the glucocorticoids are used on a purely empirical basis in a large number of conditions (Box 35-1). These conditions, though varied, are generally characterized by chronic inflammatory and immune phenomena and are associated with tissue destruction and functional impairment. For this reason it is widely assumed that the salutary effects of glucocorticoid therapy in these diseases are related to suppression of inflammation and immune reactions. In none of these conditions do the corticosteroids have specific actions on the basic disease process, despite their ability in some cases to produce dramatic improvement and even remission of signs and symptoms. The destructive aspects of the primary disease may continue unchecked; in rheumatoid arthritis, for example, glucocorticoids can effectively relieve the distressing inflammation and pain, but deterioration of affected joints progresses.[8] The use of corticosteroids in other than replacement therapy must therefore be considered palliative. Because of their lack of specificity and their considerable potential for causing harm, the long-term use of corticosteroids to treat inflammatory disorders should be viewed with caution. Before corticosteroids are considered, less toxic agents and nonpharmaceutical measures should be used to the maximum extent possible. This approach is well illustrated in rheumatoid arthritis. Systemic corticosteroids should seldom be necessary in this disease and, in any case, should not be used as the initial agent. Most patients improve considerably with large, regular doses of a nonsteroidal anti-inflammatory analgesic drug (NSAID) combined with application of heat and appropriate physical therapy. This program may be supplemented by other drugs, such as gold salts. Patients in whom these drugs are ineffective or intolerable are candidates for corticosteroid therapy, but corticosteroids should be used in the smallest possible dosage for the shortest period of time as adjuncts to other measures.

The use of glucocorticoids in the treatment of asthma involves several strategies to minimize systemic toxicity. Depending on the severity of an acute asthmatic attack, intravenous or oral administration can be used, with doses tapering off as the condition subsides.[4] Inhaled steroids are preferred for long-term therapy because they minimize systemic uptake.[2]

When corticosteroids are used on a long-term basis, they are often administered on alternate days to minimize suppression of the pituitary-adrenal axis. Giving a glucocorticoid every other day between 6 and 9 AM mimics the normal diurnal pattern of corticosteroid secretion. Such a regimen appears to lessen suppression of the adrenal cortex and permits increased endogenous corticosteroid production in response to stress. Unfortunately, alternate-day therapy may not adequately control symptoms in some cases, especially in patients with rheumatoid arthritis and ulcerative colitis. Glucocorticoid therapy for periods up to 1 week usually does not cause significant suppression of pituitary or adrenal function.

Box • 35-1

Some Conditions Treated with Corticosteroids

- Adrenal insufficiency (acute or chronic, primary or caused by anterior pituitary insufficiency)
- Cerebral edema and increased intracranial pressure (brain tumors, meningitis, trauma, cerebrovascular accidents)
- Collagen vascular diseases
  - Lupus erythematosus
  - Polymyositis
  - Polyarteritis nodosa
  - Chronic granulomatous disorders (sarcoidosis and others)
  - Temporal (giant cell) arteritis
  - Mixed connective tissue disease syndrome*
- Dermatologic disturbances
  - Psoriasis
  - Dermatitis (atopic, allergic, irritant)
  - Pemphigus
  - Lichen planus
- Gastrointestinal diseases
  - Ulcerative colitis
  - Crohn's disease
  - Celiac disease
- Hematologic diseases
  - Malignancies (acute and chronic lymphocytic leukemia, lymphoma, multiple myeloma)
  - Hemolytic anemia (autoimmune or drug-induced)
  - Idiopathic thrombocytopenic purpura
- Hepatic diseases
  - Chronic active hepatitis
  - Alcoholic hepatitis (severe forms with hepatic encephalopathy)
- Hypercalcemia (sarcoid, malignancies, vitamin D intoxication)
- Multiple sclerosis (acute episodes)
- Nephrotic syndrome
- Ocular diseases with inflammatory or allergic components
- Pulmonary disorders
  - Asthma
  - Chronic bronchitis (acute episodes)
  - Aspiration pneumonia
- Rheumatic diseases and joint ailments
  - Rheumatic arthritis
  - Rheumatic carditis
  - Osteoarthritis (intraarticular administration)
  - Bursitis (intracapsular administration)
- Shock
- Solid tumors (breast)
- Tissue grafts and organ transplants

*Must be differentiated from scleroderma, which is usually not altered by corticosteroids.

THERAPEUTIC USES IN DENTISTRY

The glucocorticoids have rather limited applications in dentistry. As in medicine, they are used largely to reduce the signs and symptoms of unwanted inflammatory reactions. These potential uses fall into the following general categories: oral ulcerations, pulpal hypersensitivity, temporomandibular joint pain, postoperative sequelae, and anaphylaxis and other allergic reactions.

Oral Ulcerations

Various ulcerative lesions of the oral mucosa may be treated by the application of glucocorticoids. Relief of symptoms and abbreviation of the clinical course are usually obtained, regardless of the cause of the ulceration. Applicable conditions are denture-induced and other traumatic ulcers, recurrent ulcerative (aphthous) stomatitis, erosive lichen planus, erythema multiforme, pemphigus, desquamative gingivitis and stomatitis, geographic tongue, and angular stomatitis (cheilitis). Although diseases such as pemphigus are usually treated with systemic glucocorticoids, further improvement of associated oral ulceration may be obtained by topical application of glucocorticoids. Despite the fact that herpetic ulcers may respond favorably, the use of glucocorticoids to treat this condition is contraindicated because suppression of the host response may allow dissemination of the herpes virus. It is thus important for the therapist to make a careful diagnosis of oral ulcers before instituting glucocorticoid therapy.

The benefit of glucocorticoids applied topically is greatest when the period of contact with the tissue is maximal. Retention at the site of application, of course, is difficult in the oral cavity. A partial solution is to apply the drug in a paste that adheres to the mucosa and resists dissolution and displacement. One such vehicle is carboxymethylcellulose in a base of polyethylene resin and mineral oil (Orabase); it is available with or without a glucocorticoid. Symptomatic relief of many oral ulcers, particularly those likely to be limited in duration, may be obtained with the adhesive paste alone.

Pulpal Hypersensitivity

Hypersensitivity of the dental pulp can result from various conditions that induce an inflammatory response in the pulp; these include operative trauma, invasion of the pulp by bacteria or their products, and exposure of dentin to the oral environment. Glucocorticoids have been variously applied directly or indirectly to the pulp to reduce pain.[5,10] Although success has been claimed, the efficacy of this therapy is not established and therefore cannot be recommended.

Temporomandibular Joint Disorders

Pain originating in the temporomandibular joint may have many possible causes, including trauma, bruxism, anatomic anomalies, rheumatoid arthritis, and psychophysiologic disorders. Treatment of such conditions should be conservative and based on careful diagnosis. NSAIDs, antianxiety muscle relaxant drugs, carbamazepine, and tricyclic antidepressants have proved useful for short-term pharmacotherapy. Nondrug approaches include rest, heat, gentle stretching, bite-plane appliances, and occlusal adjustments. In relatively refractory cases of temporomandibular joint pain or when acute pain is initially so severe that it precludes a course of conservative therapy, intraarticular injection of a glucocorticoid such as prednisolone or dexamethasone may be beneficial. Relief of symptoms may be full or partial, permanent or temporary (especially if the underlying cause of the disorder is not corrected). Although deterioration of the articular surfaces of the joint has been claimed to result from intraarticular injection of corticosteroid, the weight of available evidence does not support such an association. Nevertheless, the best responses to intraarticular injection seem to occur in persons free of radiographic changes in the joint.

Postoperative Sequelae

Glucocorticoids are often used to lessen postoperative complications, mainly edema and trismus, after dental surgical procedures. Although the risk of adverse effects from a short, intensive course of glucocorticoids is slight, whether the benefits obtained justify such "prophylactic" use is controversial at this time. What is certain, however, is that careful surgical technique is of primary importance in the reduction of uncomfortable postoperative sequelae.

Anaphylaxis and Other Allergic Reactions

The immunosuppressant and antiinflammatory effects of the glucocorticoids may be used to treat the manifestations of various allergic reactions, such as urticaria, contact dermatitis, angioneurotic edema, allergic rhinitis and conjunctivitis, insect bites, drug reactions, and serum sickness. Because histamine is an important mediator in most of these conditions, H_1 antihistamines are major drugs in the treatment of milder reactions involving histamine release (e.g., urticaria). Systemic glucocorticoids are useful in more severe responses. In anaphylaxis, even though epinephrine is the drug of choice, large doses of glucocorticoids may be beneficial in reducing bronchospasm and laryngeal edema. In this situation, the glucocorticoids also act to increase the cardiac and vascular effects of catecholamines. In addition, because the maximal effects of glucocorticoids are delayed for several hours after administration, the prolonged duration of action of glucocorticoids can afford added benefit. The glucocorticoids are thus not the primary drugs in treating the life-threatening cardiovascular failure of anaphylaxis; they add a supplemental benefit after the administration of epinephrine.

ADVERSE EFFECTS

Although glucocorticoids are valuable agents in some situations, they have considerable potential to cause greater harm than good. Actualization of this potential depends on, among other factors, the intensity and duration of therapy. A single large dose or a short course of moderate doses of hydrocortisone causes few adverse effects. If, however, more than 20 to 30 mg of hydrocortisone (or its equivalent) is given daily for more than a week, some manifestations of glucocorticoid toxicity are likely to appear. In general, these manifestations are predictable from a knowledge of the pathologic features of endogenous Cushing's disease.

The major adverse effects of glucocorticoid therapy are listed in Box 35-2 and are summarized below. The frequency and severity of adverse effects correlate with the dose and duration of therapy, the age and condition of the patient, and the disease being treated.

Hyperglycemia and Glycosuria

A diabetic-like state stems from the antiinsulin action of the glucocorticoids. It is usually mild and controllable with diet, insulin, or both. In diabetics, the requirement for insulin or oral hypoglycemic agents is increased.

Myopathy

Large doses of glucocorticoids, especially the more potent fluorinated synthetic compounds, cause muscle wasting, manifested chiefly as weakness of the musculature of the limbs. Significant reduction of muscle mass in the extremities can occur. Recovery may be incomplete after cessation of therapy.

Osteoporosis and Osteonecrosis

Osteoporosis is a common sequel of long-term glucocorticoid therapy and can lead to compression fractures of the vertebrae and to an increased susceptibility to traumatic fractures.[1] In postmenopausal women and others prone to develop osteoporosis, this complication may be especially serious. Several mechanisms are responsible. Glucocorticoids reduce Ca^{++} absorption from the intestine and increase renal excretion of Ca^{++}. Resorption of bone occurs through an increase in parathyroid hormone release and a direct inhibitory effect of

Box • 35-2

Major Adverse Effects of Glucocorticoid Therapy

Neurologic	Insomnia, agitation, mania, withdrawal syndrome
Infectious	Increased infections, opportunistic infections
Vascular	Hypertension, increased atherosclerotic disease risk
Skin and mucosa	Atrophy
Skeletal	Reduced Ca^{++} absorption, osteoporosis, avascular osteonecrosis, impaired growth
Muscular	Myopathy, wasting
Metabolic	Glucose intolerance, obesity, hyperlipidemia
Reproductive	Hypogonadism
Gastrointestinal	Peptic ulcer
Ocular	Cataracts

glucocorticoids on osteoblasts. Aseptic osteonecrosis may involve the large joints, especially the head of the femur. The condition is often progressive, necessitating joint replacement.

Studies indicate that concurrent treatment with bisphosphonates such as alendronate can reduce bone wasting in patients receiving long-term glucocorticoid therapy.[9]

Suppression of growth

In growing persons, glucocorticoids can inhibit skeletal growth and maturation.

Negative Nitrogen Balance

A net nitrogen loss results from the imbalance between protein synthesis and degradation. It reflects the antianabolic effects of the glucocorticoids in cutaneous and musculoskeletal tissues.

Peptic Ulcer

There is an increased incidence of gastric ulcers in patients treated with glucocorticoids, especially those with rheumatoid arthritis. Because such patients are often concurrently receiving aspirin or other NSAIDs, it is difficult to implicate only the glucocorticoids in the pathogenesis of these ulcers.[7] Nonetheless, when they occur, ulcers associated with glucocorticoid therapy have a high incidence of complications, such as hemorrhage and perforation. The mechanism is likely related to the decreased synthesis of PGI_2 and PGE_2, which provide protection for the gastric mucosa.[1]

Ocular Effects

Increased intraocular pressure, which may produce irreversible damage, and posterior subcapsular cataracts can result from either topical or systemic administration of glucocorticoids. Children and diabetic persons are particularly susceptible to untoward ocular effects.

Central Nervous System Effects

Psychologic disturbances can occur during glucocorticoid therapy. These reactions are reversible and range in severity from mild (euphoria, insomnia, or nervousness) to pronounced (manic-depressive or schizophrenic psychosis).

Edema and Hypokalemia

Although water retention with hypokalemia is a potentially serious complication of glucocorticoid therapy, the incidence and severity can be greatly minimized by dietary sodium restriction and by the use of a synthetic glucocorticoid essentially devoid of mineralocorticoid activity.

Altered Distribution of Body Fat

Long-term treatment with glucocorticoids often causes changes in the distribution of body fat deposits, leading to the classic "cushingoid" appearance. The most characteristic of these changes are a round ("moon") face, accumulation of fat in the back of the neck ("buffalo hump") and supraclavicular region, and increased abdominal fat. The obese trunk may markedly contrast with the thin, wasted extremities. The enhanced lipolysis seen with glucocorticoids leads to these changes; however, the reason for the redistribution is not known.

Increased Susceptibility to Infection

Because of the effect on inflammation and the immune system, the body's reaction to infectious agents is depressed by glucocorticoids. Fungal, bacterial, and viral pathogens that would otherwise cause localized or no infection may become widely disseminated with serious or fatal consequences. Latent tuberculosis may be reactivated after the initiation of glucocorticoid therapy.

Suppression of Pituitary-Adrenal Function

Prolonged administration of glucocorticoids (greater than physiologic amounts for more than 1 week) results in suppression of ACTH and, consequently, suppression of adrenal corticosteroid production; the degree of suppression is dose related. Abrupt withdrawal or significant reduction of glucocorticoid dosage can thus precipitate acute adrenal insufficiency. Moreover, acute exacerbation of the disease being treated may occur during withdrawal. Cessation or reduction of glucocorticoid therapy must therefore be done slowly and with great caution to permit the recovery of normal pituitary and adrenal function.

Miscellaneous Effects

Acne, thinning of the skin, hirsutism, weight gain, intestinal perforation, pancreatitis, hyperlipidemia, hypertension, hepatomegaly, and poor wound healing may occur during long-term glucocorticoid therapy.

IMPLICATIONS FOR DENTISTRY

Patients treated with large doses of glucocorticoids for long periods present special problems in dentistry. As noted previously, such patients are likely to have a decreased resistance to infection and a poor wound healing response. Actual or potential sources of infection in the oral cavity, such as carious teeth and inflamed tissues, should be promptly treated. If surgical procedures are necessary, they should be as conservative, atraumatic, and aseptic as possible. Preoperative antimicrobial prophylaxis may be indicated in some cases.

A second consideration in patients treated with glucocorticoids is suppression of pituitary-adrenal function. The degree of adrenal suppression depends on the length of treatment, the frequency and manner of administration, and the glucocorticoid preparation used (glucocorticoid potency of individual agents may vary more than 25-fold; see Table 35-1). A person with intact adrenal function responds to a stressful situation such as anxiety, an acute infection, or a surgical procedure with an increased release of ACTH and production of cortisol. Patients with suppressed adrenal function, however, are unable to increase cortisol production. In assessing the degree of suppression, a good guideline is to assume that any patient who has received 30 mg of hydrocortisone or its equivalent for 4 or more weeks or 80 mg of hydrocortisone for more than 2 weeks has some degree of adrenal suppression.[3] It is a time-honored but unproven notion that these patients may develop signs and symptoms of adrenal insufficiency. Therefore, during stressful dental situations (surgery or acute infection), it is often recommended that the dose of glucocorticoids be increased in such patients to compensate for the lack of endogenous hormone. The dose is usually at least double or triple the patient's maintenance dose, depending on the degree of suppression of adrenal function and the severity of the stressful event. When the period of stress is over, the dose is gradually reduced over several days to the maintenance level.

A major surgical procedure performed under general anesthesia constitutes a maximally stressful episode and may require essentially complete corticosteroid replacement in a patient with adrenal suppression. One commonly accepted approach is to give 100 mg of cortisone acetate intramuscularly approximately 8 hours before the procedure. Sufficient hydrocortisone or its equivalent is then given intravenously during the procedure so that the total dose on the day of the operation is 300 mg of hydrocortisone or its equivalent. If the postoperative course is uneventful, corticosteroid dosage is tapered off over a 2- to 3-day period (e.g., 300 mg of hydrocortisone on the day of the procedure, 150 mg the following day, 75 mg on the next day, and the usual maintenance dose

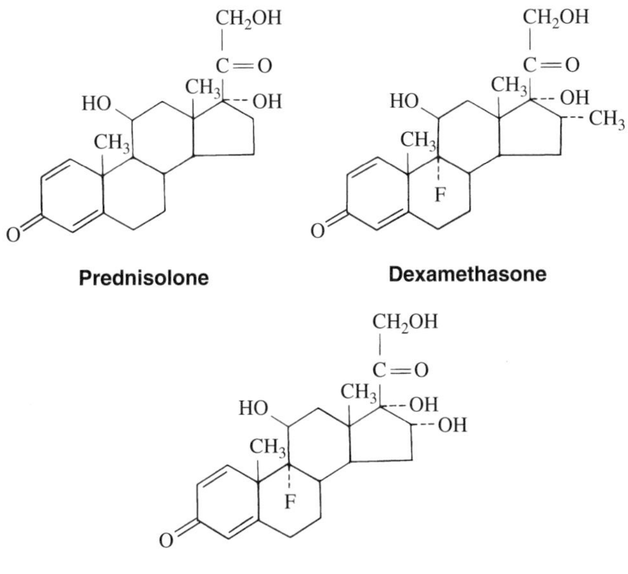

Prednisolone

Dexamethasone

Triamcinolone

Fig. 35-3 Structural formulas of three synthetic glucocorticoids: prednisolone, dexamethasone, and triamcinolone.

Box 35-3

Biologic Half-Lives* of Commonly Used Corticosteroids

8 to 12 hr (Short-Acting)
Cortisone
Hydrocortisone

18 to 36 hr (Intermediate-Acting)
Methylprednisolone
Prednisolone
Prednisone
Triamcinolone

36 to 72 hr (Long-Acting)
Betamethasone
Dexamethasone
Paramethasone

*Biologic half-life of corticosteroid is defined as the period of suppression of the hypothalamus-pituitary-adrenal axis.

on the third postoperative day).[3] A low-dose alternative is to infuse 25 mg of hydrocortisone during the induction of anesthesia, followed by a continuous infusion of 100 mg during the next 24 hours. Because recovery of glucocorticoid-induced adrenal suppression may be slow, dental patients formerly treated for prolonged periods with glucocorticoids and assumed to have adrenal suppression by the above criteria may need to receive glucocorticoids during stressful situations for 1 year after cessation of glucocorticoid therapy. It is obvious that consultation with the patient's physician is essential for the optimal management of a person who is receiving or has received long-term glucocorticoid therapy.

PREPARATIONS

A large number of glucocorticoids are available in various forms for local, oral, and parenteral administration. These include the natural hormone hydrocortisone and synthetic compounds prepared by modifying the chemical structures of hydrocortisone and other natural hormones. Three of these are shown in Figure 35-3. Relative to hydrocortisone, the synthetic compounds are, in varying degrees, longer acting and more potent. These differences are the basis for classifying the glucocorticoids as short-acting (less than 12 hours), intermediate-acting (12 to 36 hours), and long-acting (more than 36 hours) (Box 35-3). Representatives of these three categories are hydrocortisone, prednisolone, and dexamethasone, respectively. The intermediate and long-acting compounds also have a greater ratio of glucocorticoid to mineralocorticoid activity. Consequently, these agents are preferred for long-term use in the treatment of chronic inflammatory disorders because they cause less disturbance of electrolyte and fluid balance than does hydrocortisone.

In the clinical management of inflammatory or allergic disorders, the dosage of glucocorticoids varies widely according to such factors as the nature, severity, and probable duration of the condition being treated and the patient's response. In acute or life-threatening situations, a glucocorticoid should be given in sufficient doses to control the disorder quickly; treatment should then be discontinued as soon as possible. In the long-term management of chronic diseases such as rheumatoid arthritis, alternate-day therapy with the minimum dosage that achieves an acceptable reduction of symptoms is the regimen of choice.

Table 35-2 lists a few of the many different preparations currently available, some of the dosage forms, and a range of doses for a given route of administration.

Glucocorticoids

Nonproprietary (generic) name	*Proprietary (trade) name*
Beclomethasone	Beclovent, Vanceril
Betamethasone	Celestone
Cortisone	Cortone
Dexamethasone	Decadron, Dexone, Hexadrol
Fludrocortisone	Florinef
Flunisolide	AeroBid
Hydrocortisone (cortisol)	Cortef, Hydrocortone, Solu-Cortef
Methylprednisolone	Depo-Medrol, Medrol, Solu-Medrol
Prednisolone	Delta-Cortef, Predalone, Pediapred
Prednisone	Deltasone, Orasone
Triamcinolone	Aristocort, Kenacort, Kenalog

CITED REFERENCES

1. Adachi JD, Bensen WG, Hodsman AB: Corticosteroid-induced osteoporosis, *Semin Arthritis Rheum* 22:375-384, 1993.
2. Barnes PJ: Inhaled glucocorticoids for asthma, *N Engl J Med* 332:868-875, 1995.

Table • 35-2

Some Commonly Used Corticosteroid Preparations

NONPROPRIETARY (GENERIC) NAME	PROPRIETARY (TRADE) NAME	RELATIVE POTENCY	USUAL ADULT DOSE	ROUTE OF ADMINISTRATION	PREPARATIONS
Hydrocortisone	Hydrocortone	1	20 to 240 mg/day	Oral	Tablets: 5, 10, and 20 mg
Hydrocortisone acetate	Orabase HCA	1	2 to 3 times daily	Topical	Paste: 0.5%, containing gelatin, pectin, and sodium carboxymethylcellulose in a polyethylene and mineral oil base
	Hydrocortone acetate	1	5 to 50 mg	Intraarticular	Suspension: 25 and 50 mg/ml
Hydrocortisone sodium succinate	Solu-Cortef	1	100 to 500 mg/day	Intravenous or intramuscular	Powder: 100, 250, 500, and 1000 mg
Prednisone	Deltasone, Orasone	4	5 to 60 mg/day	Oral	Tablets: 1, 2.5, 5, 10, 20, 25, and 50 mg
Prednisolone	Delta-Cortef	4	5 to 60 mg/day	Oral	Tablets: 5 mg
Prednisolone acetate	Econopred	4	1 to 2 drops	Ophthalmic	Suspension: 0.12% and 1%
Triamcinolone acetonide	Kenalog in Orabase	5	2 to 3 times daily	Topical	Paste: 0.1%, with gelatin, pectin, and sodium carboxymethylcellulose in a polyethylene and mineral oil base
Triamcinolone diacetate	Aristocort	5	5 to 40 mg every 1 to 8 weeks	Intraarticular	Suspension: 25 and 40 mg/ml
Dexamethasone	Decadron	25	0.75 to 9.0 mg/day	Oral	Tablets: 0.25, 0.5, 0.75, 1, 1.5, 2, 4, and 6 mg
Dexamethasone acetate	Decadron-LA	25	1 to 5 mg*	Intraarticular	Suspension: 8 and 16 mg/ml
Betamethasone	Celestone	25	0.6 to 7.2 mg/day	Oral	Tablets: 0.6 mg

*Dose recommended for the temporomandibular joint.

3. Blonde LRR, Tullman MJ, Redding SW: Endocrinologic disease. In Tullman MJ, Redding SW, eds: *Systemic disease in dental treatment*, New York, 1982, Appleton-Century-Crofts.
4. Goldstein RA, Paul WE, Metcalfe DD, et al: Asthma, *Ann Intern Med* 121:698-708, 1994.
5. Mosteller JH: The ability of a prednisolone solution to eliminate pulpal inflammation, *J Prosthet Dent* 13:754-760, 1963.
6. Pilkis SJ, Granner DK: Molecular physiology of the regulation of hepatic gluconeogenesis and glycolysis, *Annu Rev Physiol* 54:885-902, 1992.
7. Piper JM, Ray WA, Daugherty JR, et al: Corticosteroid use and peptic ulcer disease: role of nonsteroidal anti-inflammatory drugs, *Ann Intern Med* 114:735-740, 1991.
8. Ramos-Remus C, Sibley J, Russell AS: Steroids in rheumatoid arthritis: the honeymoon revisited, *J Rhematol* 19: 667-670, 1992.
9. Saag KG, Emkey R, Schnitzer TJ, et al: Alendronate for the prevention and treatment of glucocorticoid-induced osteoporosis. Glucocorticoid-Induced Osteoporosis Intervention Study Group, *N Engl J Med* 339:292-299, 1998.
10. Swerdlow H, Stanley HR, Sayegh FS: Minimizing pulpal reactions with prednisolone therapy, *J Oral Ther Pharmacol* 1:593-601, 1965.
11. Webster JC, Cidlowski JA: Mechanism of glucocorticoid-receptor mediated repression of gene expression, *Trends Endocrinol Metab* 10:396-402, 1999.
12. Wehling M: Novel aldosterone receptors: specificity-conferring mechanism at the level of the cell membrane, *Steroids* 59:160-163, 1994.
13. Williams GH, Dluhy RG: Disorders of the adrenal cortex. In Braunwald E, Fauci AS, Isselbacher KJ, et al, eds: *Harrison's Principles of internal medicine*, ed 15, New York, 2001, McGraw-Hill.

General Reference

Schimmer BP, Parker KL: Adrenocorticotropic hormone; adrenocortical steroids and their synthetic analogs; inhibitors of the synthesis and actions of adrenocortical hormones. In Hardman JG, Limbird LE, Gilman AG, eds: *Goodman & Gilman's The pharmacological basis of therapeutics*, ed 10, New York, 2001, McGraw-Hill.

CHAPTER • 36

Insulin, Oral Hypoglycemics, and Glucagon*

Gail T. Galasko

THE ENDOCRINE PANCREAS

The pancreas has both exocrine and endocrine functions. The acinar cells, which secrete digestive enzymes, comprise the exocrine system. The islets of Langerhans, which represent the endocrine system, contain four types of cells, each of which synthesizes and secretes different polypeptide hormones, as shown in Table 36-1. Insulin is produced by the β cells, which comprise most (60% to 80%) of the islet and form its central core. The β cell is the primary glucose sensor for the islet.

Insulin

Insulin is a polypeptide containing 51 amino acids. It has a molecular weight of approximately 5800. It is composed of two chains (called the *A* and *B chains*) that are joined by two disulfide bridges. Insulin is formed by proteolysis of a large, single-chain precursor, proinsulin. In proinsulin, shown in Figure 36-1, the A and B chains are connected by C peptide. Proinsulin is converted to insulin when the C peptide is removed. This occurs within the secretory granules of the pancreatic β cell. Approximately equimolar amounts of insulin and C peptide are stored in the granules and released by exocytosis when the β cell is stimulated. C peptide has no known biologic function, but it can serve as an index of insulin secretion. Units of insulin, originally defined by activity, are now defined on the basis of weight. There are approximately 28 U/mg of insulin.

Insulin is a member of a family of related peptides known as *insulin-like growth factors (IGFs)*. IGF-I and IGF-II have molecular weights of approximately 7500 and structures that are homologous to proinsulin.[5] The receptors for insulin and IGF-I are closely related.[8] Insulin can bind to the receptor for IGF-I with low affinity and vice versa. The growth promoting actions of insulin appear to be mediated, at least in part, through the IGF-I receptor. In contrast to insulin, the IGFs are produced in many tissues, where they are more important in regulating growth than in regulating metabolism. IGFs mediate the anabolic and growth-promoting effects of growth hormone. IGF-I and IGF-II were originally known to have *nonsuppressible insulin-like activity* because of their ability to produce insulin-like effects in adipocytes that were not suppressed by the addition of antiinsulin antibodies.

Regulation of Insulin Secretion

The pancreas secretes insulin into the portal vein. Insulin secretion is a tightly regulated process designed to provide stable concentrations of glucose in the blood during both fasting and feeding. Regulation of plasma glucose is achieved by the coordinated interplay of various nutrients, gastrointestinal hormones, pancreatic hormones, and autonomic neurotransmitters. A basal secretion of insulin is present during fasting periods.[20] This is followed by a rapid rise in insulin secretion after ingestion of a meal. Glucose is the principal stimulus to insulin secretion in human beings. It is more effective in provoking insulin secretion when taken orally than when administered intravenously.[9]

Actions of Insulin

The classic action of insulin is to lower the blood glucose concentration. Insulin does this by affecting both glucose utilization and production. Although liver, muscle, and fat are the important target tissues for regulation of glucose homeostasis by insulin, insulin exerts potent regulatory effects on other cell types as well. Insulin stimulates glucose transport into muscle and fat by promoting translocation of the intracellular transporter, glucose transporter 4 (Glut 4), to the cell surface (Figure 36-2).[19] Insulin does not stimulate glucose uptake into the liver, but it inhibits hepatic glucose production. Insulin inhibits catabolic processes such as breakdown of glycogen, fat, and protein. Both glycogenolysis and gluconeogenesis are inhibited. Insulin affects the activities of a variety of enzymes involved in intracellular utilization and storage of glucose, amino acids, and fatty acids. Thus both glycolysis (utilization) and glycogen synthesis (storage) are promoted. These enzymes catalyze phosphorylation or dephosphorylation reactions. The effects of insulin are summarized in Table 36-2.

In addition to the short-term metabolic effects, insulin has other, longer-term actions. It affects synthesis of key enzymes and is believed to have important growth-regulating effects in vivo. Insulin regulates gene transcription,[18] affecting protein synthesis, and increases cell proliferation and differentiation.

Pharmacokinetics

Insulin is biotransformed in a variety of tissues, including the liver, kidney, and skeletal muscle. Almost half the insulin secreted by the pancreas is destroyed by the liver before it reaches the general circulation. Metabolism of insulin results in the production of inactive peptides. The half-life of exogenous insulin in plasma is approximately 8 minutes in nondiabetic and uncomplicated diabetic subjects.

Insulin Receptor Interactions

The insulin receptor in mammalian cells is a large transmembrane glycoprotein. It is composed of two α subunits and two β subunits linked by disulfide bonds to form a β-α-α-β heterotetramer. Binding of hormone to the α subunits of the insulin receptor leads to the rapid intramolecular autophosphorylation of tyrosine residues in the β subunits. This initiates a series of events that culminate in a cascade

*The authors wish to recognize Dr. William Warner for his past contributions to this chapter. See the Acknowledgments.

of phosphorylation or dephosphorylation reactions. This is shown schematically in Figure 36-2.

PUTATIVE MEDIATORS OF INSULIN ACTION

There is evidence that insulin acts by synthesis of second messengers that enter the cell to mediate some of the hormone's actions on intracellular enzymes (e.g., phosphorylation, dephosphorylation). These mediators are of the inositolphosphoglycan (IPG) class.[12] The IPGs represent a new family of second messengers or mediators that are increasingly being implicated as having an important role in signal transduction, not only for insulin but also for other hormones and growth factors. They are discussed later in this chapter.

Table • 36-1

Pancreatic Islet Secretions

CELL TYPE	HORMONE SECRETED
α (A) Cell	Glucagon
β (B) Cell	Insulin, amylin (islet amyloid polypeptide)
δ (D) Cell	Somatostatin
F (PP) Cell	Pancreatic polypeptide

Diabetes Mellitus

Diabetes mellitus is a group of syndromes characterized by hyperglycemia. Virtually all forms of diabetes mellitus are due to either a decrease in the circulating concentration of insulin (insulin deficiency) or a decrease in the response of peripheral tissues to insulin (insulin resistance).

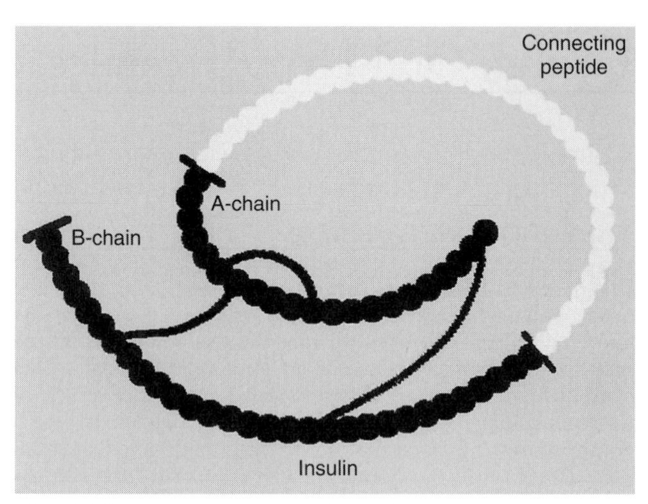

Fig. 36-1 Structure of proinsulin. When connecting peptide is removed, insulin is formed. The A and B chains of insulin are shown in *black;* C peptide is *white.*

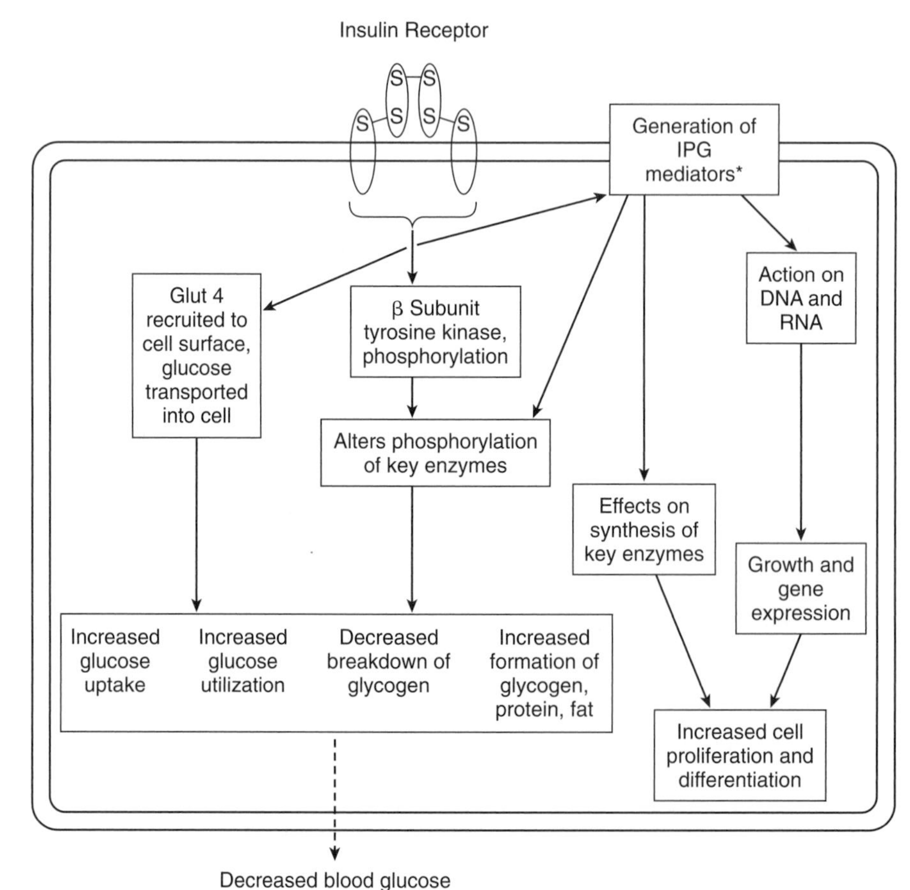

Fig. 36-2 Insulin signaling pathways. *Glut 4,* Glucose transporter 4.

Table • 36-2

Metabolic Actions of Insulin

TYPE OF METABOLISM	ACTION OF INSULIN	MAJOR TARGET TISSUE*
Carbohydrate	Increases glucose transport	Muscle, fat
	Increases glycogen synthesis	Liver, muscle
	Decreases gluconeogenesis	Liver
	Increases glycolysis	Liver, muscle
	Increases glucose oxidation	Fat
Fat	Increases lipogenesis	Liver, fat
	Decreases lipolysis	Liver, fat
	Increases synthesis of triglycerides	Fat
Protein	Decreases protein breakdown	Liver
	Increases protein synthesis	Muscle, various
	Increases amino acid uptake	Muscle, various

*Insulin exerts potent regulatory effects on other cell types in addition to liver, muscle, and fat, the classically important target tissues for glucose regulation.

The disease has two major forms. Currently, the preferred nomenclature is *type 1* and *type 2* diabetes mellitus. Older names include *juvenile onset* or *insulin-dependent* diabetes mellitus for type 1 and *maturity onset* or *non–insulin-dependent* diabetes mellitus for type 2.

Evidence indicates that the incidence of both type 1 and type 2 diabetes mellitus is increasing worldwide. It is predicted that the prevalence will double by 2010.[11] Type 2 diabetes is becoming increasingly common and is an emerging problem in children and adolescents, particularly minorities.[6] Major risk factors for type 2 diabetes are obesity and physical inactivity. It is reported that the incidence of type 1 diabetes is increasing by approximately 3.0% per year.[21]

Type 1 diabetes mellitus

There is considerable evidence that type 1 diabetes is an autoimmune disease of the pancreatic β cell, resulting in degeneration. In type 1 diabetes there is an absolute lack of insulin. Both genetic predisposition and environmental components are involved, with the incidence in homozygous twins being approximately 50%.[25] Approximately 5% to 10% of diabetics have type 1 diabetes.

Type 2 diabetes mellitus

Approximately 90% to 95% of diabetics have type 2 diabetes mellitus. There is no significant loss of β cells from the islets in type 2 diabetes. In contrast to type 1 diabetics, in type 2 diabetics the mean plasma concentration of insulin over a 24-hour period is essentially normal or even elevated. Rather, in type 2 diabetes, target cells are relatively insensitive to insulin.[10] This is known as *peripheral resistance to insulin.* Impaired glucose metabolism in muscle is a key feature of type 2 diabetes. Genetic predisposition is important in type 2 diabetes; there is greater than 95% concordance in identical twins.[25] In addition, most type 2 diabetics are obese. Type 2 diabetics have impaired glucose taste detection,[15] which may reflect a generalized defect in glucose sensitivity, including the glucose-sensing pancreatic β cells.

Glycosylation of hemoglobin

Nonenzymatic glycosylation of proteins can occur as a result of elevated blood glucose concentrations. Hemoglobin is glycosylated on its amino terminal valine residue to form the glycosyl valine adduct, termed *hemoglobin* $A1_C$ *(*$HbA1_C$*)*.[28] Because the half-life of $HbA1_C$ is the same as that of the red blood cell, the concentration of $HbA1_C$ in the circulation can be used to assess the severity of the glycemic state over an extended period (4 to 12 weeks) prior to sampling.

Insulin Therapy

Insulin is the mainstay for treatment of virtually all type 1 and many type 2 diabetic patients. When necessary it may be administered intravenously or intramuscularly. However, long-term treatment relies on subcutaneous injection of the hormone.

Subcutaneous administration of insulin differs from physiologic secretion of insulin in two major ways. First, the kinetics of absorption are relatively slow and thus do not mimic the normal rapid rise and decline of insulin secretion in response to ingestion of nutrients. Second, the injected insulin diffuses into the peripheral circulation instead of being released into the portal circulation. Any preferential effect of secreted insulin on hepatic metabolic processes is thus eliminated.

Insulin preparations

Insulin occurs in the pancreas complexed with zinc and is extracted in the form of zinc insulin, which is not water soluble at neutral pH. This can be converted to the sodium salt, which is water soluble at neutral pH. Although pork insulin is derived directly from pigs, human insulin is made by genetic engineering with *Escherichia coli* (Lilly) or yeast (Novo Nordisk). It is called *human insulin* because its structure is the same as that of normal human insulin, but it is not obtained from human tissues.

Insulin preparations are classified according to their duration of action into ultrashort-, short-, intermediate-, and long-acting preparations. Insulin products available in the United States are listed in Table 36-3.

Ultrashort- and short-acting insulin preparations Ultrashort- and short-acting insulin preparations are soluble. They have a rapid onset and ultrashort or short durations of action. They are dispensed as clear solutions at neutral pH. Soluble insulin preparations are the only insulin preparations that may be given intravenously.

Table • 36-3

Insulin Preparations

PREPARATION	ONSET	PEAK	DURATION
Ultrashort-Acting			
Insulin lispro (Lilly)*	~5 minutes	1 hour	3 to 4 hours
Short-Acting			
Iletin II Regular (Lilly)	30 to 120 minutes	4 to 6 hours	6 to 8 hours
Humulin R (Lilly)	30 to 60 minutes	2 to 4 hours	≤16 hours
Novolin R (Novo Nordisk)	30 minutes	2.5 to 5 hours	8 hours
Velosulin BR (Novo Nordisk)†	0.5 hours	1 to 3 hours	8 hours
Intermediate-Acting			
Humulin N (Lilly)	1 to 2 hours	4 to 12 hours	≤24 hours
Humulin L (Lilly)	1 to 3 hours	6 to 15 hours	24 hours
Lente Iletin II (Lilly)‡	4 to 6 hours	8 to 14 hours	24 hours
Novolin L (Novo Nordisk)	2.5 hours	7 to 15 hours	22 hours
Novolin N (Novo Nordisk)	1.5 hours	4 to 12 hours	24 hours
NPH Iletin II (Lilly)	4 to 6 hours	8 to 14 hours	24 hours
Premixed (% NPH/ % Regular)§			
Humulin 70/30 (Lilly)	30 to 60 minutes	2 to 4 hours	≤24 hours
Humulin 50/50 (Lilly)	30 to 60 minutes	2 to 4 hours	≤24 hours
Novolin 70/30 (Novo Nordisk)	30 minutes	2.5 to 5 hours	24 hours
Long-Acting			
Glargine (Aventis)	2 to 5 hours	5 to 24 hours	18 to 24 hours
Humulin U (Lilly)	4 to 8 hours	16 to 18 hours	36 hours

*Insulin lispro is an insulin preparation in which two amino acids near the carboxyl terminal of the B chain are reversed, namely proline at B28 and lysine at B29. As a result, there is a lowered tendency for this insulin to form hexamers, resulting in very rapid absorption.
†A phosphate-buffered preparation for use with a pump.
‡Insulin Iletin II is a pure pork insulin preparation.
§The premixed insulin preparation has the shorter onset of action of the regular insulin and the longer duration of action of the NPH insulin.
L, Lente; *R*, regular; *N*, NPH; *U*, ultralente; *BR*, buffered regular.

Intermediate- and long-acting insulin preparations Intermediate- and long-acting preparations contain particles and are cloudy suspensions at neutral pH. They contain either protamine in phosphate buffer (neutral protamine Hagedorn [NPH] insulin) or varying concentrations of zinc in acetate buffer (lente, ultralente preparations). The duration of action depends on the size of the particles present. The larger the particles, the more slowly they dissolve and hence the longer the duration of action of the preparation.

NPH insulin is a protamine zinc suspension of insulin, at neutral pH, developed in Hagedorn's laboratory. Isophane insulin is NPH insulin in which there is no excess of either protamine or insulin. For therapeutic purposes, dosages and concentrations of insulin are expressed in units. All commercial preparations of insulin are supplied in solution at a concentration of 100 U/ml (approximately 3.7 mg/ml).

Insulin analogues These include insulin lispro and insulin glargine. Insulin lispro is an insulin preparation in which two amino acids near the carboxyl terminal of the B chain are reversed, namely proline at B28 and lysine at B29. As a result, there is a lowered tendency for this insulin to form hexamers, resulting in very rapid absorption. Insulin glargine is also an insulin analogue. It has two extra amino acids added on and one that is different from human insulin. As a result of these changes, it precipitates in subcutaneous tissue from which it is slowly absorbed. Its duration of action is longer and its time-action profile is flatter than NPH. Thus it causes less hypoglycemia at night.

Pharmacokinetics

Insulin is given by injection, usually subcutaneously. Absorption of insulin after subcutaneous administration is affected by the site of injection, the subcutaneous blood flow, the volume and concentration of the injected insulin, and the presence of circulating insulin antibodies. Insulin absorption is usually most rapid from the abdominal wall, followed by the arm, buttock, and thigh. Increased subcutaneous blood flow (brought about by massage, hot baths, and exercise) increases the rate of absorption. Soluble insulins may also be given intravenously. The onset of action of insulin after intravenous injection is very fast, but the duration of action is short.

Adverse effects

Hypoglycemia is the most common adverse reaction to insulin. This may result from an inappropriately large dose, a mismatch between the time of peak delivery of insulin and food intake, increased sensitivity to insulin (e.g., adrenal insufficiency), or increased insulin-independent glucose uptake (exercise). The more vigorous the attempt to achieve euglycemia, the more frequent the episodes of hypoglycemia.

The most frequent symptoms of hypoglycemia include sweating, tremor, blurred vision, weakness, hunger, confusion, and altered behavior. This may be followed by loss of consciousness. Hypoglycemia may be confused with inebriation by onlookers.

With long-standing type 1 diabetes, the mechanisms for counteracting hypoglycemia can be blunted or absent in a significant number of patients, thus putting them at higher risk of developing hypoglycemia. Mild to moderate hypoglycemia may be treated by ingestion of glucose. When hypoglycemia is severe, it should be treated with intravenous glucose or an injection of glucagon.

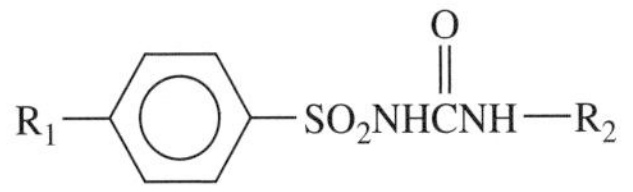

ORAL HYPOGLYCEMIC AGENTS

Sulfonylureas

The sulfonylureas are sulfonamide derivatives (Figure 36-3). They are traditionally divided into two groups or generations of agents. Second-generation sulfonylureas are considerably more potent than the earlier drugs. The sulfonylureas available in the United States are shown in Table 36-4.

Mechanism of action

The sulfonylureas are only effective in patients with functioning pancreatic β cells. These drugs stimulate release of insulin by blocking adenosine triphosphate (ATP)-dependent K^+ current in pancreatic β cells. The effects of the sulfonylureas are initiated by their binding to and blocking an ATP-sensitive K^+ channel.[1,22,23] Glimepiride has been shown to have an additional effect, that is, it increases the sensitivity of peripheral tissues to insulin.[13] This may be true for the other sulfonylureas (especially second-generation drugs) as well.[4] The predominant effect is on insulin secretion.

Pharmacokinetics

The sulfonylureas are well absorbed after oral administration. Glipizide absorption is delayed by food. All sulfonylureas are highly bound to plasma protein (90% to 99%). Plasma protein binding is least for chlorpropamide and greatest for glyburide. Sulfonylureas are metabolized in the liver and excreted in the urine.

R_1—(benzene ring)—$SO_2NHC(=O)NH—R_2$

General structure of sulfonylureas

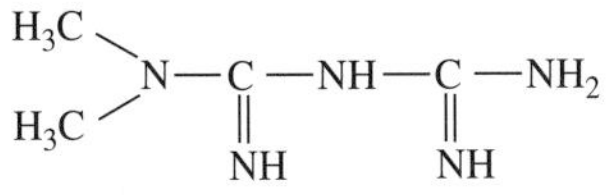

$(H_3C)_2N—C(=NH)—NH—C(=NH)—NH_2$

Metformin

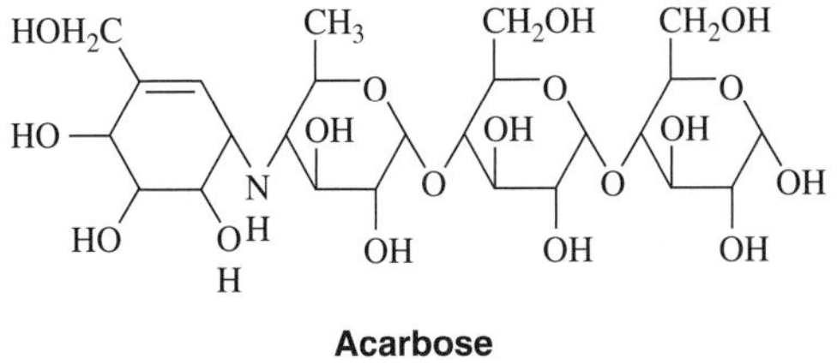

Acarbose

Fig. 36-3 Chemical structures of the sulfonylureas, metformin and acarbose.

The half-life and extent of metabolism varies considerably among the first-generation sulfonylureas. Metabolism of chlorpropamide is incomplete, and approximately 20% of the drug is excreted unchanged, which can be a problem for patients with impaired renal function.

Therapeutic uses

Sulfonylureas are used to control hyperglycemia in type 2 diabetics who cannot achieve appropriate control with changes in diet and exercise alone.

Adverse effects

Adverse effects are infrequent, occurring in approximately 4% of patients taking first-generation drugs and perhaps slightly less often in patients receiving second-generation agents. The most important adverse effect is hypoglycemia, which, if severe, can lead to coma. Hypoglycemia is a particular problem in elderly patients with impaired hepatic or renal function who are taking longer-acting sulfonylureas.

Table • 36-4

Sulfonylureas Available in the United States

NONPROPRIETARY (GENERIC) NAME	PROPRIETARY (TRADE) NAME	ONSET (hr)	SERUM HALF-LIFE (hr)	DURATION OF ACTION (hr)
First Generation				
Acetohexamide	Dymelor	1	6 to 8	12 to 24
Chlorpropamide	Diabinese	1	36	24 to 60
Tolazamide	Tolinase	4 to 6	7	12 to 24
Tolbutamide	Orinase	1	4.5 to 6.5	6 to 12
Second Generation				
Glimepiride	Amaryl	2 to 3	9	10 to 24
Glipizide (glydiazinamide)	Glucotrol, Glucotrol XL	1 to 3	2 to 4	12 to 24
Glyburide (glibenclamide)	Diaβeta, Micronase, Glynase Pres Tab	1 to 4*	4 to 10	10 to 24

*Micronized forms have a faster onset of action.

The sulfonylureas have a sulfonamide structure, which is the basis for cross-sensitivity with antibacterial sulfonamide drugs. Hypersensitivity reactions occur with some regularity. Other adverse effects of sulfonylureas include nausea and vomiting, hematologic reactions (especially agranulocytosis and aplastic and hemolytic anemias), cholestatic jaundice, and dermatological effects. Sulfonylureas are teratogenic in animals (large doses). Patients taking sulfonylureas tend to gain weight, which is a problem in type 2 diabetics who tend to be obese.

Sulfonylureas have a disulfiram-like effect. In patients who take alcohol concurrently, sulfonylureas may decrease aldehyde dehydrogenase, causing acetaldehyde accumulation (see Chapter 43). As a result, the patient may have flushing, headache, nausea, vomiting, sweating, and hypotension shortly after alcohol ingestion. This reaction is not as likely to occur with a single occasional drink.

Drug interactions

As can be seen in Box 36-1, a number of drugs interact with the sulfonylureas by enhancing or decreasing their effect on blood glucose concentration.

Contraindications

Contraindications to the use of sulfonylureas include hypersensitivity to sulfonylureas and drugs that have similar structures (see above) and pregnancy. Caution should be exercised in cases of reduced renal or hepatic function. Patients with ketoacidosis should receive insulin, not an oral hypoglycemic.

Meglitinides

Members of this group approved for use in the United States are repaglinide and nateglinide. The structure of repaglinide is shown in Figure 36-4. These drugs are only effective in patients with functioning pancreatic β cells. Like the sulfonylureas, they stimulate release of insulin by blocking ATP-dependent K^+ channels in pancreatic β cells.[22] They may be used alone or in combination with metformin (see below) and may be given to patients who are allergic to sulfonamides.[24]

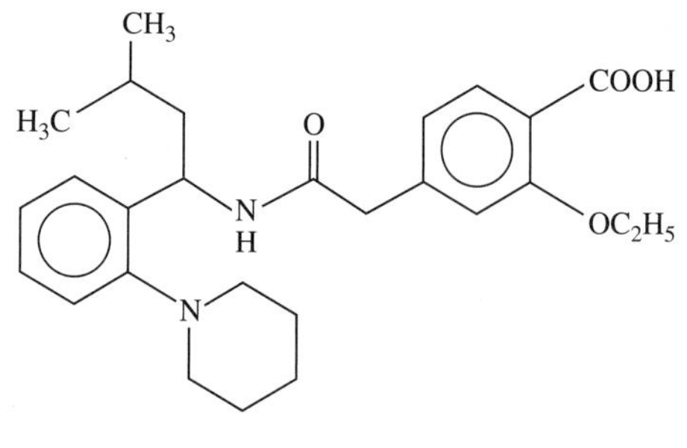

Repagliuide

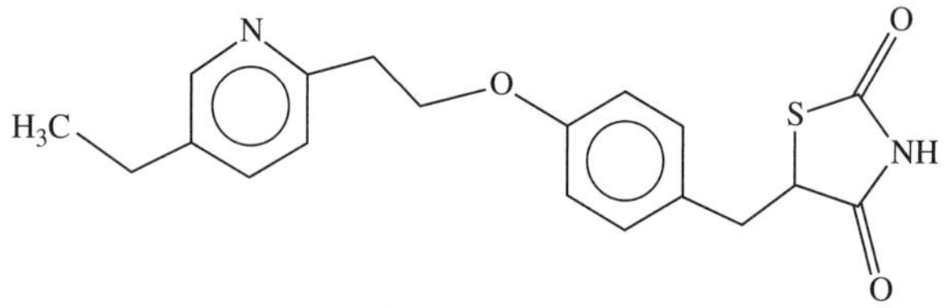

Pioglitazone

Fig. 36-4 Chemical structures of repaglinide and pioglitazone.

Pharmacokinetics

Repaglinide and nateglinide are rapidly absorbed after oral administration. They are metabolized primarily by the liver. Repaglinide peak plasma levels occur within 1 hour and the plasma half-life is 1 hour. It is recommended that this drug be taken just before each meal. Nateglinide is most effective if taken 1 to 10 minutes before a meal. These drugs offer the advantage of rapid and short-term control over blood glucose.

Adverse effects

Hypoglycemia is the major adverse effect of repaglinide and is most likely to occur if a meal is delayed or skipped or in patients with hepatic insufficiency.

Drug interactions

Ketoconazole, miconazole, and erythromycin decrease biotransformation and potentiate the effect of repaglinide. Nonsteroidal antiinflammatory drugs, salicylates, sulfonamides, and other highly protein-bound drugs may potentiate the hypoglycemic effects of repaglinide.

Biguanides

Metformin is currently the only biguanide approved for use in the United States (see Figure 36-3). Phenformin and buformin, two other biguanides, are widely used in Europe and elsewhere.[7] Phenformin was withdrawn from the United States in 1977 because of its ability to cause lactic acidosis.

Mechanism of action

The mechanism of action of the biguanides is different from that of the sulfonylureas or meglitinides. Biguanides lower blood glucose concentrations by several different actions. They decrease hepatic gluconeogenesis, improve tissue sensitivity to insulin, increase peripheral glucose uptake and utilization, and decrease intestinal absorption of glucose.[27] Biguanides do not

Box 36-1

Sulfonylurea Drug Interactions

Drugs that Increase the Effect of the Sulfonylureas

Antihistamines (H_2 antagonists)
Azole antifungals
Clofibrate
Magnesium salts
Methyldopa
Monoamine oxidase inhibitors
Oral anticoagulants
Salicylates
Sulfonamides
Tricyclic antidepressants
β-Adrenergic receptor blockers

Drugs that Decrease the Effect of the Sulfonylureas

Calcium salts
Corticosteroids
Diazoxide
Estrogens
Phenothiazines
Sympathomimetics
Thiazide diuretics
Thyroid hormones

cause hypoglycemia. In addition, patients do not gain weight, in contrast to the sulfonylureas. The action of the biguanides does not depend on functioning pancreatic β cells, and they are often used in combination with sulfonylureas.[3]

Pharmacokinetics

Approximately 50% to 60% of an oral dose of metformin is absorbed after oral administration. Food decreases the extent of absorption and delays it slightly. Protein binding is minimal, and metformin is excreted unchanged in the urine by tubular secretion. Approximately 90% is excreted within 24 hours. It has a plasma half-life of approximately 6 hours.

Adverse effects

Gastrointestinal tract symptoms such as nausea, anorexia, vomiting, diarrhea, flatulence, and cramps are common adverse effects of metformin (biguanides) but are generally transient. Metformin may cause a decrease in vitamin B_{12} levels, possibly by decreasing absorption from the B_{12} intrinsic factor complex. Lactic acidosis is a rare but serious complication of the biguanides. When it occurs, it is fatal in roughly 50% of patients.

Contraindications

Biguanides are contraindicated in patients with renal disease, hepatic disease, or conditions predisposing to tissue anoxia (including cardiopulmonary dysfunction) because of concern regarding lactic acidosis.

Thiazolidinediones

Thiazolidinediones currently available are pioglitazone and rosiglitazone. The structure of pioglitazone is shown in Figure 36-4.

The thiazolidinediones are a relatively new class of oral antidiabetic drugs that act by increasing insulin sensitivity in tissues. They depend on the presence of insulin for their activity. Thiazolidinediones enhance the effect of circulating insulin by improving target cell response. They have post-receptor insulin-mimetic activity, affecting insulin receptor kinase activity and insulin receptor phosphorylation. They decrease hepatic gluconeogenesis and increase insulin-dependent glucose uptake in muscle and fat.[14] Thiazolidinediones act synergistically with sulfonylureas and metformin.

The first thiazolidinedione to be introduced, in January 1997, was troglitazone but it has been removed from the market because of hepatotoxicity.

Pharmacokinetics

Thiazolidinediones are taken with or without food. They are metabolized by the cytochrome P450 oxidative enzyme system.

Drug interactions

Concurrent administration of pioglitazone with oral contraceptives containing ethinyl estradiol and norethindrone results in decreased plasma concentrations of the contraceptive and can result in loss of contraceptive effect. Ketoconazole has been shown to inhibit pioglitazone metabolism in vitro.

MISCELLANEOUS DRUGS USED IN THE TREATMENT OF DIABETIC PATIENTS

α-Glucosidase Inhibitors

Acarbose and miglitol are the α glucosidase inhibitors approved for use in the United States. The structure of acarbose is shown in Figure 36-3. The α-glucosidases facilitate digestion of complex starches, oligosaccharides, and disaccharides into monosaccharides, allowing them to be absorbed from the small intestine. The α-glucosidase inhibitors are competitive, reversible inhibitors of intestinal α-glucosidases.[17,26] In addition, acarbose also inhibits α-amylase. The α-glucosidase inhibitors delay absorption of most carbohydrates. This limits the postprandial rise in glucose. They do not directly affect insulin secretion.

Pharmacokinetics

The α-glucosidase inhibitors are taken at the beginning of meals. Absorption of acarbose is poor. It is metabolized in the gastrointestinal tract, principally by intestinal bacteria. Miglitol is absorbed after oral administration.

Adverse effects

Adverse effects include flatulence, diarrhea, and abdominal pain from the presence of undigested carbohydrates in the lower gastrointestinal tract. These effects tend to decrease with continued use. α-Glucosidase inhibitors do not cause hypoglycemia when given alone. However, hypoglycemia may occur with concurrent sulfonylurea therapy. Hypoglycemia should be treated with glucose, not sucrose, because breakdown of sucrose may be inhibited. Miglitol has minor lactase inhibitory activity but should not induce lactose intolerance.

Drug interactions

Miglitol decreases plasma concentrations of several drugs, including glyburide and metformin.

Contraindications

Contraindications include hypersensitivity to the drug, inflammatory bowel disease, and intestinal obstruction.

Inositolphosphoglycans

A considerable amount of evidence suggests that interaction of insulin with its receptor leads to the release of low–molecular-weight inositolphosphoglycans (IPGs), which enter the cell and act as mediators of insulin action. IPG mediators have been shown to reproduce a variety of short-term effects of insulin (see Figure 36-2). Two families of IPG insulin mediators have been isolated. Myoinositol is a major component of one; chiroinositol is a major component of the other. Studies have shown the presence of hypochiroinositoluria in type 2 diabetics. In addition, there is both decreased chiroinositol content and decreased chiroinositol mediator activity in type 2 diabetics.[2] There is evidence that chiroinositol, on its own, decreases elevated blood glucose concentrations in diabetic monkeys and rats.

Angiotensin-Converting Enzyme Inhibitors

Captopril and other angiotensin-converting enzyme inhibitors have been shown to delay the onset and significantly reduce the progression of diabetic nephropathy and retinopathy. They are routinely given to type 1 diabetics to decrease the incidence of these complications of the disease.[16]

GLUCAGON

Glucagon is synthesized in the α cells of the pancreatic islets. It is a 29-amino-acid peptide with a molecular weight of approximately 3500. Like insulin, it is formed from a larger precursor molecule by proteolytic cleavage. Glucagon binds to specific G_s protein–linked receptors in the liver, causing an increase in adenylyl cyclase activity and production of cyclic 3′,5′-adenosine monophosphate. This ultimately results in an increase in glycogen phosphorylase activity as well as a decrease in glycogen synthase. Thus, glucagon increases blood glucose concentration by decreasing glycogen synthesis, stimulating breakdown of stored glycogen, and increasing gluconeogenesis in the liver. It does not affect skeletal muscle glycogen, presumably because of a lack of receptors in skeletal muscle. Glucagon has potent inotropic and chronotropic effects on the heart. These are similar to effects resulting from β-adrenergic receptor stimulation.

Pharmacokinetics

Glucagon is rapidly degraded in the plasma, liver, and kidney. Its half-life is 3 to 6 minutes.

Therapeutic uses

Glucagon may be used in the emergency treatment of severe hypoglycemic reactions (sufficient to cause unconsciousness). It is given parenterally. Glucagon is also used to reverse the cardiac effects of toxic amounts of β-adrenergic receptor blockers.

Adverse effects

Adverse effects include nausea (usually transient) and vomiting.

IMPLICATIONS FOR DENTISTRY

In the United States there are approximately 16 million diabetics (approximately 6% of the population), about a third of whom are not aware that they have the disease. The incidence of diabetes is rapidly increasing. Between 1990 and 1998 the number of diagnosed diabetics increased 30%, and it is predicted that the prevalence will double by 2010. Type 2 diabetes is becoming increasingly common and is an emerging problem in children and adolescents, particularly minorities. Dentists can expect to have an increasing number of diabetic patients, many of whom are unaware of their condition.

Diabetes mellitus is a complex, chronic disease that is characterized by hyperglycemia. It is not a curable disease, and the need for lifelong compliance is a problem for many patients. Complications of the disease include neuropathy, microangiopathy, and macrovascular disease. Diabetic neuropathy may cause numbness, tingling, or a deep burning pain. This may present as oral paresthesias and burning mouth. Diabetics are more susceptible to infection and have an impaired ability to deal with infection. They also have delayed wound healing. In addition, infection, stress (emotional or physical), or surgical procedures commonly disturb control of diabetes.

A number of oral complications may occur in diabetes. These include xerostomia; infection; poor healing of wounds or lesions; and an increased incidence and severity of caries, candidiasis, gingivitis, periodontal disease, and periapical abscesses. Diabetics often have progressive periodontal disease and may have multiple periodontal abscesses. Diabetics may have burning mouth syndrome or loss of sensation. Type 2 diabetics have impaired sweet taste detection (glucose and sucrose).

In addition, patients may become hypoglycemic. Signs and symptoms of mild hypoglycemia include hunger, weakness, tachycardia, pallor, and sweating. Tachycardia may be masked by β-adrenergic receptor blockers. β-Blockers, especially the nonselective ones, also tend to worsen the hypoglycemia.

Signs of moderate hypoglycemia include incoherence, uncooperativeness, belligerence, lack of judgment, and poor orientation. If hypoglycemia is severe, the patient may become unconscious.

Diabetics are more susceptible to infection and may need antimicrobial therapy more often. Morning appointments are usually best for diabetic patients because that minimizes the chance of stress-induced hypoglycemia. A source of sugar should be readily available. Patients taking α-glucosidase inhibitors need glucose, not sucrose, because breakdown of sucrose may be inhibited by these drugs.

Hypoglycemic and Hyperglycemic Agents

Nonproprietary (generic) name	*Proprietary (trade) name*
Hypoglycemic agents	
Acarbose	Precose
Acetohexamide	Dymelor
Chlorpropamide	Diabinese
Glimepiride	Amaryl
Glipizide	Glydiazinamide, Glucotrol, Glucotrol XL
Glyburide	Glibenclamide, Micronase, Diaβeta, Glynase Pres Tab
Insulin	See Table 36-3
Metformin	Glucophage, Riomet
Miglitol	Glyset
Nateglinide	Starlix
Pioglitazone	Actos
Repaglinide	Prandin
Rosiglitazone	Avandia
Tolazamide	Tolinase
Tolbutamide	Orinase
Hyperglycemic agents	
Glucagon	—
Glucose	Insta-Glucose

CITED REFERENCES

1. Aguilar-Bryan L, Nichols CG, Wechsler SW, et al: Cloning of the beta cell high-affinity sulfonylurea receptor: a regulator of insulin secretion, *Science* 268:423-426, 1995.
2. Asplin I, Galasko G, Larner J: Chiro-inositol deficiency and insulin resistance: a comparison of the chiro-inositol- and the myo-inositol-containing insulin mediators isolated from urine, hemodialysate, and muscle of control and type II diabetic subjects, *Proc Natl Acad Sci USA* 90:5924-5928, 1993.
3. Bailey CJ: Biguanides and NIDDM, *Diabetes Care* 15:755-772, 1992.
4. Beck-Nielsen H, Hother-Nielsen O, Pedersen O: Mechanism of action of sulfonylureas with special reference to the extrapancreatic effect: an overview, *Diabetic Med* 5:613-620, 1988.
5. Cohick WS, Clemmons DR: The insulin-like growth factors, *Ann Rev Physiol* 55:131-153, 1993.
6. Dabelea D, Pettitt DJ, Jones KL, et al: Type 2 diabetes mellitus in minority children and adolescents. An emerging problem, *Endocrinol Metab Clin North Am* 28:709-729, 1999.
7. DeFronzo RA, Goodman AM: Efficacy of metformin in patients with non-insulin-dependent diabetes mellitus. The Multicenter Metformin Study Group, *N Engl J Med* 333:541-549, 1995.

8. Duronio V, Jacobs S: Comparison of insulin and IGF-I receptors. In Kahn CR, Harrison LC, eds: *Insulin receptors, part B. Clinical assessment, biological responses and comparison to the IGF-I receptor,* New York, 1988, Alan R Liss.
9. Ganda OP, Soeldner JS, Gleason RE, et al: Metabolic effects of glucose, mannose, galactose, and fructose in man, *J Clin Endocrinol Metab* 49:616-622, 1979.
10. Groop LC: Insulin resistance: the fundamental trigger of type 2 diabetes, *Diabetes Obes Metab* 1(suppl 1):S1-S7, 1999.
11. Heine RJ: Diabetes in the next century: challenges and opportunities, *Neth J Med* 55:265-270, 1999.
12. Huang LC, Fonteles MC, Houston DB, et al: Chiroinositol deficiency and insulin resistance. III. Acute glycogenic and hypoglycemic effects of two inositol phosphoglycan insulin mediators in normal and streptozotocin-diabetic rats in vivo, *Endocrinology* 132:652-657, 1993.
13. Kawamori R, Morishima T, Kubota M, et al: Influence of oral sulfonylurea agents on hepatic glucose uptake, *Diabetes Res Clin Pract* 28:S109-S113, 1995.
14. Lawrence JM, Reckless JP: Pioglitazone, *Int J Clin Pract* 54:614-618, 2000.
15. Lawson WB, Zeidler A, Rubenstein A: Taste detection and preferences in diabetics and their relatives, *Psychosom Med* 41:219-227, 1979.
16. Lewis EJ, Hunsicker LG, Bain RP, et al: The effect of angiotensin-converting-enzyme inhibition on diabetic nephropathy. The Collaborative Study Group, *N Engl J Med* 329:1456-1462, 1993.
17. Mertes G: Safety and efficacy of acarbose in the treatment of type 2 diabetes: data from a 5-year surveillance study, *Diabetes Res Clin Pract* 52:193-204, 2001.
18. O'Brien RM, Granner DK: Regulation of gene expression by insulin, *Physiol Rev* 76:1109-1161, 1996.
19. Olson AL, Pessin JE: Structure, function, and regulation of the mammalian facilitative glucose transporter gene family, *Annu Rev Nutr* 16:235-256, 1996.
20. O'Meara NM, Sturis J, Blackman JD, et al: Analytical problems in detecting rapid insulin secretory pulses in normal humans, *Am J Physiol* 264:E231-E238, 1993.
21. Onkamo P, Vaananen S, Karvonen M, et al: Worldwide increase in incidence of type I diabetes—the analysis of the data in published incidence trends, *Diabetologia* 42:1395-1403, 1999.
22. Panten U, Burgfeld J, Goerke F, et al: Control of insulin secretion by sulfonylureas, meglitinide and diazoxide in relation to their binding to the sulfonylurea receptor in pancreatic islets, *Biochem Pharmacol* 38:1217-1229, 1989.
23. Philipson LH, Steiner DF: Pas de deux or more: the sulfonylurea receptor and K^+ channels, *Science* 268:372-373, 1995.
24. Pratley RE, Foley JE, Dunning BE: Rapid acting insulinotropic agents: restoration of early insulin secretion as a physiologic approach to improve glucose control, *Curr Pharm Des* 7:1375-1397, 2001.
25. Pyke DA: Diabetes: the genetic connections, *Diabetologia* 17:333-343, 1979.
26. Sels JP, Huijberts MS, Wolffenbuttel BH: Miglitol, a new alpha-glucosidase inhibitor, *Expert Opin Pharmacother* 1:149-156, 1999.
27. Stumvoll M, Nurjan N, Perriello G, et al: Metabolic effects of metformin in non-insulin-dependent diabetes mellitus, *N Engl J Med* 333:550-554, 1995.
28. Tchobroutsky G, Charitanski D, Blouquit Y, et al: Diabetic control in 102 insulin-treated out-patients, *Diabetologia* 18:447-452, 1980.

General References

Banting FG, Best CH, Collip JB, et al: Pancreatic extracts in the treatment of diabetes mellitus, *Can Med Assoc J* 12:141-146, 1922.

Bevan P: Insulin signaling, *J Cell Sci* 114:1429-1430, 2001.

Cheatham B, Kahn CR: Insulin action and the insulin signaling network, *Endocrine Rev* 16:117-142, 1995.

Cianciola LJ, Park BH, Bruck E, et al: Prevalence of periodontal disease in insulin-dependent diabetes mellitus (juvenile diabetes), *J Am Dent Assoc* 104:653-660, 1982.

Fujimoto WY, Bergstrom RW, Boyko EJ, et al: Preventing diabetes—applying pathophysiological and epidemiological evidence, *Br J Nutr* 84:173-176, 2000.

Granner DK, O'Brien RM: Molecular physiology and genetics of NIDDM, *Diabetes Care* 15:369-395, 1992.

Hermann LS, Schersten B, Bitzen PO, et al: Therapeutic comparison of metformin and sulfonylurea, alone and in various combinations, *Diabetes Care* 17:1100-1109, 1994.

Jacobs DB, Hayes GR, Lockwood DH: In vitro effects of sulfonylureas on glucose transport and translocation of glucose transporters in adipocytes from streptozocin-induced diabetic rats, *Diabetes* 38:205-211, 1989.

Kahn CR: Banting Lecture, Insulin action, diabetogenes, and the cause of type II diabetes, *Diabetes* 43:1066-1084, 1994.

Kilgour E, Larner J, Romero G: The generation of inositolglycan mediators from rat liver plasma membranes: the role of guanine nucleotide binding proteins, *Biochem Biophys Res Comm* 186:1151-1157, 1992.

Koffler M, Ramirez LC, Raskin P: The effect of many commonly used drugs on diabetic control, *Diabetes Nutr Metab* 2:75-93, 1989.

Larner J: Four questions times two: a dialogue on the mechanism of insulin action dedicated to Earl W. Sutherland, *Metabolism* 24:249-255, 1975.

Lilley K, Zhang C, Villar-Palasi C, et al: Insulin mediator stimulation of pyruvate dehydrogenase phosphatases, *Arch Biochem Biophys* 296:170-174, 1992.

Martikkala V, Sundvall J: Prevention of type 2 diabetes mellitus by changes in lifestyle among subjects with impaired glucose tolerance, *N Engl J Med* 344:1343-1350, 2001.

Meglasson MD, Matschinsky FM: Pancreatic islet glucose metabolism and regulation of insulin secretion, *Diabetes Metab Rev* 2:163-214, 1986.

Nathan DM: Long-term complications of diabetes mellitus, *N Engl J Med* 328:1676-1685, 1993.

Nathan DM: Prevention of long-term complications of non-insulin-dependent diabetes mellitus, *Clin Invest Med* 18:332-339, 1995.

Partanen J, Niskanen L, Lehtinen J, et al: Natural history of peripheral neuropathy in patients with non-insulin-dependent diabetes mellitus, *N Engl J Med* 333:89-94, 1995.

Saltiel AR, Osterman DG, Darnell JC: Role of glycosyl phosphoinositides in insulin action, *Cold Spring Harb Symp Quant Biol* 53 Pt. 2:955-963, 1988.

Saltiel AR, Siegel MI, Jacobs S, et al: Putative mediators of insulin action: regulation of pyruvate dehydrogenase and adenylate cyclase activities, *Proc Natl Acad Sci USA* 79:3513-3517, 1982.

Scheen AJ: Non-insulin-dependent diabetes mellitus in the elderly, *Bailliers Clin Endocrinol Metab* 11:389-406, 1997.

Seltzer HS: Drug-induced hypoglycemia, *Endocrinol Metab Clin North Am* 18:163-183, 1989.

Sweet LJ, Dudley DT, Pessin JE, et al: Phospholipid activation of the insulin receptor kinase: regulation by phosphatidylinositol, *FASEB J* 1:55-59, 1987.

Van den Brande JL: A personal view on the early history of the insulin-like growth factors, *Horm Res* 51:149-175, 1999.

Visscher TL, Seidell JC: The public health impact of obesity, *Annu Rev Public Health* 22:355-375, 2001.

White MF, Kahn CR: The insulin signaling system, *J Biol Chem* 269:1-4, 1994.

Yalow RS, Berson SA: Immunoassay of endogenous plasma insulin in man, *J Clin Invest* 39:1157-1175, 1960.

Yarden Y, Ullrich A: Growth factor receptor tyrosine kinases, *Annu Rev Biochem* 57:443-478, 1988.

CHAPTER • 37

Steroid Hormones of Reproduction and Sexual Development*

Angelo J. Mariotti

The central focus of endocrinology is on specific regulatory molecules (i.e., hormones) that govern reproduction, growth and development, and maintenance of the internal environment, as well as energy production, utilization, and storage. As a result of these global demands within the organism, it is not surprising that the actions of hormones are complex and diverse in nature. A single hormone may elicit a different outcome in a variety of tissues or a variety of hormones may be required to produce a single, particular effect in a group of tissues. For example, estrogens can function independently to stimulate growth of the breast (promotion of fat accumulation, connective tissue development, and ductal growth), yet must work in concert with other hormones (prolactin, progesterone, placental lactogen, glucocorticoids, thyroxine, and oxytocin) to regulate lactation. In spite of the complex and diverse nature of hormones, it is possible to categorize these compounds into two classes depending on their chemical structure: the peptide/amino acid derivative hormones and the steroid hormones.

Steroid hormones are derivatives of cholesterol and consist of a combination of three rings of six carbon atoms each (phenanthrene) and one ring of five carbon atoms (cyclopentane) to form a complex hydrogenated cyclopentanoperhydrophenanthrene ring system (Figure 37-1). Steroid hormones can be further divided into three principal sets: corticosteroid hormones (glucocorticoids and mineralocorticoids), calcium-regulating steroid hormones (vitamin D and its metabolites), and gonadal or sex steroid hormones (estrogens, androgens, and progestins).

The past 50 years have dramatically improved our perceptions concerning the actions of sex steroid hormones in health and disease. Although there is no doubt of the importance of sex steroid hormones in reproductive endocrinology, evidence has accrued that gonadal hormones have a much broader role in human tissues. Androgens, estrogens, and progestins are now believed to be directly or indirectly involved in the regulation of various diverse tissues such as the brain, heart, kidney, skin, liver, and tissues of the oral cavity. Reports of the effects of sex steroid hormones in the periodontium, a unique structure composed of two fibrous (gingiva and periodontal ligament) and two mineralized (cementum and alveolar bone) tissues, have been noted for more than a century. The effect of sex steroid hormones on each periodontal tissue has heightened interest in defining the specific relationships among androgens, estrogens, and progestins and their role in normal function and disease in the periodontium.

Since the identification of gonadal hormones in the early twentieth century, the use of these agents has exploded. Today both steroidal and nonsteroidal compounds with properties of sex steroid hormones are extensively used in the prophylaxis or treatment of disease as well as for population control. Although dentists do not typically prescribe these agents, their ubiquitous presence in the population requires a careful understanding of the actions and interactions of sex steroids with other pharmacologic agents as well as how they affect structures in the oral cavity.

STRUCTURE AND FUNCTION

Androgens

Androgens (Figure 37-2) are derived from a 19-carbon tetracyclic hydrocarbon nucleus known as *androstane.* One of the most potent androgenic hormones, testosterone, is synthesized by the Leydig cells of the testes, the thecal cells of the ovary, and the adrenal cortex. In men, testosterone is the principal plasma androgen and is reduced to dihydrotestosterone, the mediator of most actions of the hormone.[33] The irreversible metabolic conversion of testosterone to dihydrotestosterone occurs only in tissues that contain the enzyme 5α-reductase.[50] Testosterone (but not dihydrotestosterone) can also be aromatized to estradiol by a number of extragonadal tissues (primarily adipose tissue and skeletal muscle), a common route of estrogen production in men. In women, the major plasma androgen is androstenedione (androst-4-ene-3,17-dione), which can be secreted into the bloodstream or converted into either testosterone or estradiol by the ovary. Once secreted into the bloodstream, the majority of androgens are transported to their sites of action by a hepatic-secreted carrier protein designated as *sex hormone–binding globulin* (44% bound) as well as serum albumins and other proteins (54% bound).[7] Secreted plasma androgens are also metabolized to physiologically weak or inactive molecules consisting of either 17-ketosteroids or polar compounds (diols, triols, and conjugates) for excretion by the kidney or liver.[20]

Androgens may be administered orally, topically, or through intramuscular injections (Table 37-1). Testosterone is generally not administered enterally because extensive first-pass hepatic metabolism rapidly reduces plasma concentrations. An increase in the bioavailability of androgens can be accomplished by intramuscular injections in an oil vehicle, by transdermal application, or by alkylation at C17, which significantly decreases hepatic metabolism and makes oral administration therapeutically possible.

The biologic activities of androgens are manifested in virtually every tissue of the body. The more important functions of androgens include (1) male sexual differentiation of wolffian ducts, external genitalia, and brain in utero; (2) development of adult male phenotype, including growth and

*The authors wish to recognize Dr. William Warner for his past contributions to this chapter. See the Acknowledgments.

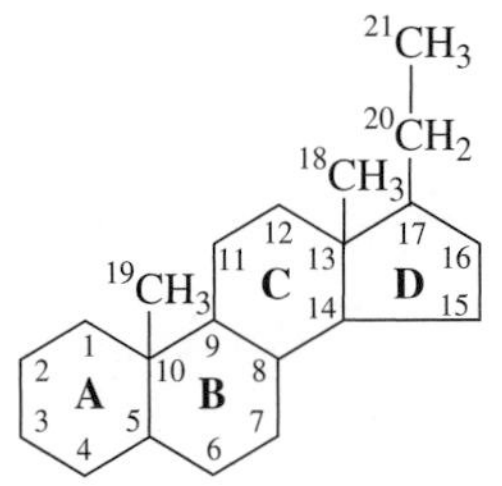

Fig. 37-1 Ring structure for pregnane and numbering system for steroids. Progesterone contains 21 carbons. Androgens, estrogens, and some progestins lack carbons 20 and 21. Estradiol and synthetic estrogenic steroids have an aromatic ring A and therefore lack carbon 19.

maintenance of male sex accessory organs as well as anabolic actions on skeletal muscle, bone, and hair; 3) facilitation of human sexual behavior; and (4) regulation of specific metabolic processes in the liver, kidney, and salivary glands.[33]

Estrogens

The estrogens (Figure 37-3)—estrone, estradiol, and estriol—are characterized by an aromatic A ring, a hydroxyl group at C3, and either hydroxyl groups (C16 and C17) or a ketone group (C17) on the D ring. Estradiol is the most potent estrogen and is secreted by the ovary, testes, placenta, and peripheral tissues. Estrone is also secreted by the ovary; however, the principal source in both women and men is through extragonadal conversion of androstenedione in peripheral tissues.[43] In premenopausal women, the most abundant physiologic estrogen is estradiol and in men and postmenopausal women the most abundant estrogen in the plasma is estrone.[53] Like other lipid-soluble hormones, estrogens are transported in the blood principally bound to carrier proteins; for example, estradiol in the plasma is bound by either albumin (60%) or sex hormone–binding globulin (38%), leaving only 2% of the hormone free.[52] Both estradiol and estrone are metabolized principally to estriol, which is the major estrogen detected in the urine.

Estrogens may be administered orally, topically, or through intramuscular injections (Table 37-2). Although estradiol is available for enteral administration, it is generally not used in this manner because concentrations in the bloodstream remain low due to extensive hepatic metabolism.[10] An increase in the half-life of estrogenic compounds can be accomplished by synthetic substitutions on the C or D ring (see Figure 37-3). For example, the half-life of estradiol is a few minutes, whereas the half-life of ethinyl estradiol (ethinyl substitution at the C17 position) may be greater than 13 hours. Nonsteroidal compounds may also have estrogenic activity, and examples of such compounds include diethylstilbestrol, flavones, isoflavones, as well as certain pesticides (e.g., p,p′-DDT) and plasticizers (e.g., bisphenol A).

The biologic activities of estrogens in women include (1) development, growth, and maintenance of secondary sex characteristics; (2) uterine growth; (3) pulsatile release of luteinizing hormone from the pituitary; (4) thickening of the vaginal mucosa; and (5) ductal development in the breast. In the male, the physiologic significance of estrogens is largely unknown but may be involved in the regulation of plasma androgen and estrogen levels as well as sexual behavior.

Progestins

Progestins (Figure 37-4), or steroids that have progestational activity, are derived from a 21-carbon saturated steroid hydrocarbon known as *pregnane.* The principal progestational hormone secreted into the bloodstream is progesterone, which is synthesized and secreted by the corpus luteum, placenta, and adrenal cortex. As with the androgens, most of the progesterone is transported in the bloodstream by plasma

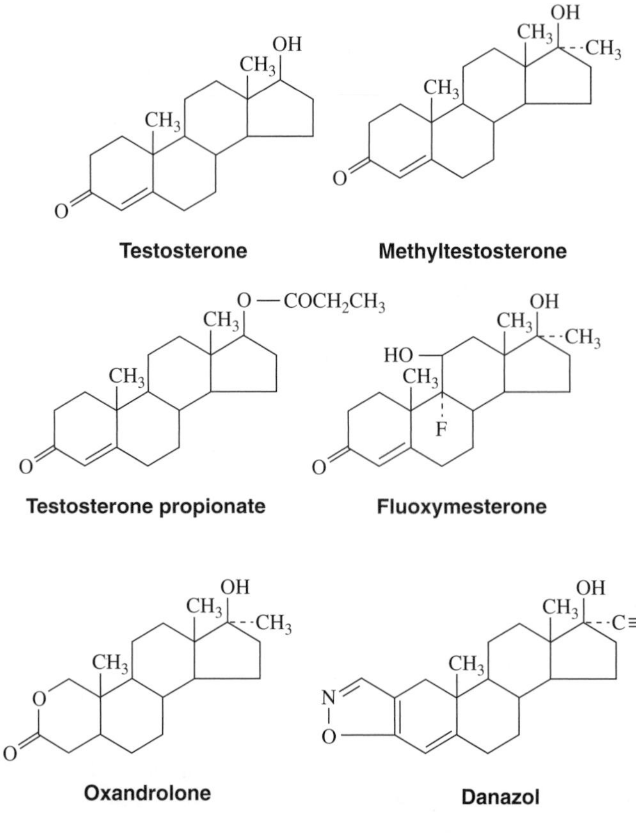

Fig. 37-2 Structural formulas of testosterone and some other androgens.

Table • 37-1

Examples of Anabolic-Androgenic Drugs

NONPROPRIETARY (GENERIC) NAME	PROPRIETARY (TRADE) NAME	INDICATIONS	DOSE	MISCELLANEOUS
Danazol	Danocrine	Endometriosis, fibrocystic breast disease, hereditary angioedema	Oral, 800 mg/day	Suppresses pituitary-ovarian axis; weak androgen
Fluoxymesterone	Halotestin	Delayed puberty in males, hypogonadism, breast cancer	Oral, 10 to 40 mg/day depending on indication	Methylated androgens are more likely to cause jaundice
Methyltestosterone	Android, Testred, Virilon	Delayed puberty in males, hypogonadism, breast cancer	Oral, 5 to 200 mg/day depending on indication	Methylated androgens are more likely to cause jaundice
Oxandrolone	Oxandrin	Catabolic or tissue-depleting processes	Oral, 2.5 to 20 mg/day depending on indication	Methylated androgens are more likely to cause jaundice
Testosterone propionate	Testex	Lichen sclerosus, microphallus	Injected or topical (ointment)	The ester forms of testosterone increase its duration of action

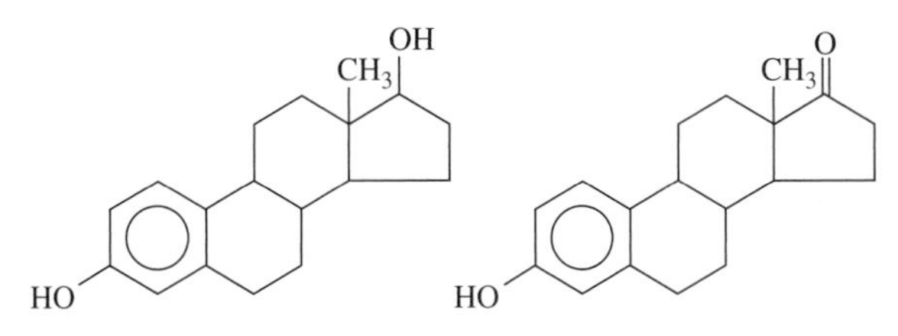

OH
CH3
C≡CH
HO
Ethinyl estradiol

OH
CH3
C≡CH
H3C—O
Mestranol

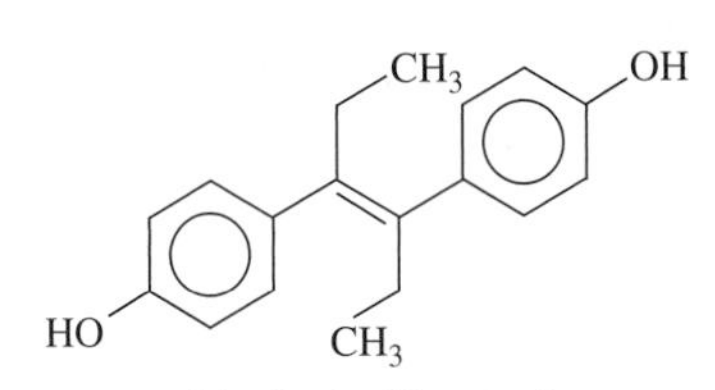

Fig. 37-3 Structural formulas of estradiol and some other estrogens.

Table • 37-2

Examples of Estrogenic Drugs

NONPROPRIETARY (GENERIC) NAME	PROPRIETARY (TRADE) NAME	INDICATIONS	DOSE	MISCELLANEOUS
Diethylstilbesterol	Stilphostrol	Prostatic carcinoma	Oral, 1 mg/day	Not available in United States, Canada only
Ethinyl estradiol	Estinyl	Breast carcinoma, prostatic carcinoma, menopausal vasomotor symptoms, estrogen deficiency from surgery, ovarian failure or hypogonadism, contraception	Oral, 0.02 to 0.15 mg/day depending on indication	Used in combination with progestins in oral contraceptives
Conjugated estrogens	Premarin	Menopausal symptoms, prevention of postmenopausal bone loss, atrophic vaginitis, hypoestrogenism	Oral, 0.3 to 1.25 mg/day (more in certain circumstances); IV or IM (for hormone imbalance), up to 50 mg/day; vaginal cream, 0.5 to 2 g/day	

IV, Intravenous; *IM,* intramuscular.

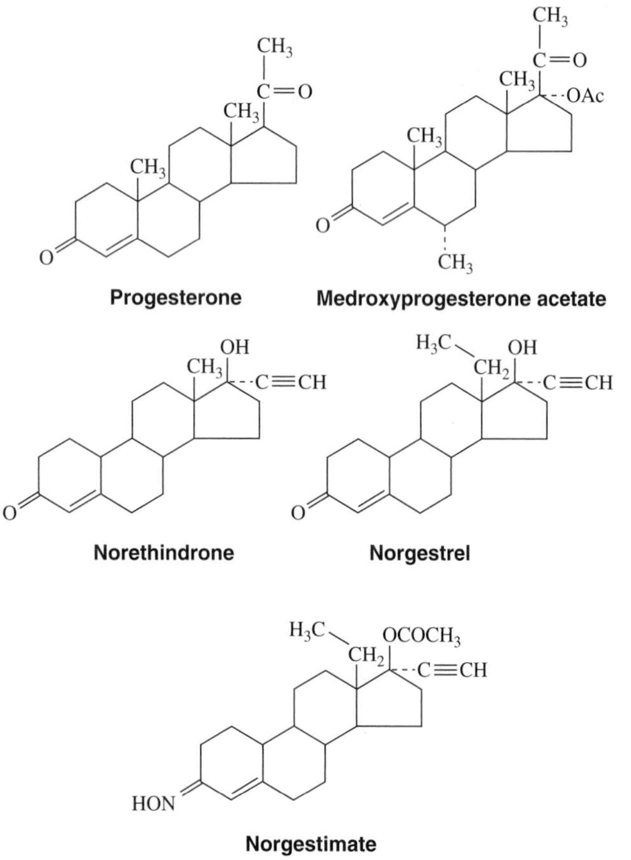

Progesterone

Medroxyprogesterone acetate

Norethindrone

Norgestrel

Norgestimate

Fig. 37-4 Structural formulas of progesterone and some progestins.

proteins; however, progesterone in human beings is primarily nonspecifically bound to globulin and albumin proteins. The fate of plasma progesterone depends on hepatic, extrahepatic, and extra-adrenal metabolism. Both 5-α-dihydroprogesterone and deoxycorticosterone are the most probable active progesterone metabolites. Metabolic inactivation of progesterone to pregnanediol is accomplished by the liver.

Progestins may be administered orally, topically, or through intramuscular injections (Table 37-3). Progesterone is available for enteral administration; however, it is generally not administered in this manner because concentrations in the bloodstream remain low because of extensive first-pass hepatic metabolism. An increase in the bioavailability of progestins can be accomplished by intramuscular injections in oil, by vaginal suppositories, or by ethinyl substitution at C17, which significantly decreases hepatic metabolism.

The biologic activities of progestins are principally observed during the luteal phase of the menstrual cycle and pregnancy. Progesterone is necessary for glandular endometrial development prior to nidation, development of mammary lobules and alveoli, as well as the maintenance of pregnancy (i.e., endometrial gland function, decreased excitability of myometrium, and possible effects on the immune system to decrease rejection of the developing fetus). Progesterone also decreases hepatic secretion of very–low-density lipoprotein and high-density lipoprotein, diminishes insulin action, stimulates the hypothalamic respiratory center, elevates basal core body temperature at ovulation, and enhances sodium excretion by the kidneys.

MECHANISM OF ACTION

In the bloodstream, sex steroid hormones exist in extremely low concentrations (in the femtomolar to nanomolar range) yet are capable of regulating differentiation and growth in selected tissues distant from the site of secretion. The actions of sex steroid hormones become even more intriguing when one considers that the distinct biologic effects of these hormones depend on nominal differences between relatively small (molecular weight approximately 300) molecules. For example, testosterone, which is capable of powerful virilizing effects, differs from estradiol only by one carbon atom and four hydrogen atoms. (Estradiol is aromatic, as are the other estrogens.) These differences in molecular structure of steroid

Table • 37-3

Examples of Progestins

NONPROPRIETARY (GENERIC) NAME	PROPRIETARY (TRADE) NAME	INDICATIONS	DOSE	MISCELLANEOUS
Medroxyprogesterone acetate	Provera, Depo-Provera	Dysfunctional uterine bleeding, endometrial carcinoma, contraception	Oral and injectable (IM), 5 to 20 mg/day orally or 150 mg IM for 3 months to 400 mg IM per month depending on indication	
Norethindrone	Aygestin, Micronor, Nor-QD	Dysfunctional uterine bleeding, endometriosis, contraception	Oral, variable depending on indication	For contraception, 0.35 mg/day
Norgestrel	Ovrette	Contraception	Oral, 0.075 mg/day	

hormones change biologic activity. Specificity of hormone response also depends on the presence of intracellular proteins or receptors, which specifically recognize and selectively bind the hormone and act in concert with the hormone ligand to regulate gene expression.

The current hypothesis of sex steroid hormone action[2] begins with the absorption of the hormones into the bloodstream, where they circulate, principally bound (approximately 98%) to plasma proteins. In the circulation, the unbound or free hormone can enter the cell by diffusion and bind to receptors. These large intracellular protein receptors are located in the nucleus of the cell. When the steroid hormone is bound to the receptor, it transforms the receptor to an active configuration and the activated receptor-steroid hormone complex binds with high affinity to specific nuclear sites (e.g., discrete DNA sequences, the nuclear matrix, nonhistone proteins, the nuclear membrane). Once the receptor-hormone complex is bound to nuclear regulatory elements, a coactivator is usually recruited to the promoter region to allow gene activation and transcription of messenger RNA. After the nuclear interaction, the receptor-hormone complex dissociates, leaving an unoccupied receptor and the steroid hormone. The dissociated receptor is thought to be in an inactive configuration that requires conversion to a form that can bind the steroid again, and the steroid hormone is metabolized and eliminated from the cell.

Although the regulation of gene transcription by hormone-receptor complexes in the nucleus appears to be the major biologic action of sex steroid hormones, these molecules also have other behaviors that are distinct from actions at nuclear receptors. Androgens, estrogens, and progestins have membrane effects and can influence the production of second messenger systems, which can in turn affect neural transmission, the transport of Ca^{++} ions into cells, and the intracellular concentration of polyamines.[29]

Steroid Hormone Receptor Structure

The receptors for steroid hormones are able to initiate a wide assortment of responses yet are very similar to one another, not only in their mechanism of action but also in their structure.[9,23] Generally, steroid hormone receptors consist of asymmetric protein subunits with long (10 : 1) axial ratios. These subunits, which form either dimers or tetramers at low ionic strengths, range in weight from 80 to 100 kd. As a class of regulatory proteins, the different steroid hormone receptors have a high degree of homology. Each protein can be divided into six sections, designated as regions *A* through *F*.[33] The A/B regions located at the N-terminal are exceedingly variable in size (50 to more than 500 amino acids) and have negligible amino acid similarities between different receptors. The C region, located between the N- and C-terminus, is a remarkably conserved area that contains the DNA-binding domain. The hydrophilic D region is not conserved in length or sequence but may serve as a hinge between the hormone-binding and DNA-binding domains. The E/F regions located at the C-terminal are similar in size (250 to 300 amino acids), have moderate amino acid homology among the different steroid receptor proteins, and contain the hormone-binding domain. Areas in both the N-terminal and C-terminal are responsible for the transcriptional activation of the DNA.[13,24]

From these six regions, two important binding domains are present for sex steroid hormone receptors. In one binding domain, the functional activation of the receptor depends on a distinct, high-affinity binding site for a specific hormone. This steroid hormone binding domain is a large hydrophobic region located near the C-terminal. The other receptor binding domain recognizes specific sites on DNA. This DNA-binding domain of the steroid receptor is a highly conserved area that contains a tetrahedral arrangement of four cysteine residues around a zinc ion to form a zinc fingerlike structure.[31] On activation of the receptor, the receptor-steroid complex binds to a specific site on the DNA that is referred to as a *steroid responsive element.* Steroid responsive elements are unique for each receptor but have common nucleotide characteristics.

THERAPEUTIC USES

Androgens

The least controversial and principal indication for androgen therapy is for the treatment of testosterone deficiency in adolescent boys or adult men. Transdermal testosterone preparations have been used to mimic normal serum levels for testosterone-deficient boys to develop normal genitalia and secondary sex characteristics and for the normal virilization of hypogonadal men. Other less common and more controversial applications for androgens include uses for male senescence, female hypogonadism, enhancement of athletic performance, male contraception, catabolic and wasting states, angioneurotic edema, and blood dyscrasias.

Estrogens

The two principal reasons for the prescription of estrogens are for the prevention of conception and to reduce the sequelae associated with declining hormone levels after menopause.

Oral contraceptives are among the most widely used medications in the world and most often are a combination of estrogens and progestins (Table 37-4). Combination oral contraceptives principally affect conception by suppressing the surge of luteinizing hormone, which consequently prevents ovulation (Figure 37-5).[25] The estrogen component of combination oral contraceptives usually contains either ethinyl estradiol or mestranol. In these preparations, the estrogen content ranges from 20 to 50 μg, and pills containing less than 35 μg are usually considered low-dose contraceptives. The combination oral contraceptives are available as either monophasic, biphasic, or triphasic preparations. Monophasic preparations maintain a fixed dose of estrogen and progesterone over a 21-day period; the biphasic contraceptives maintain a fixed dose of estrogen but increase the progestin dose over a 21-day period, and the triphasic preparation may have varying amounts of estrogen and progestin for 21 days. Both biphasic and triphasic oral contraceptives were designed to more closely approximate the ratios of estrogen and progesterone during the menstrual cycle. The progestin in the oral contraceptive also protects the endometrium of the uterus against the proliferative action of the estrogen. Thus the inclusion of a progestin reduces the risk of endometrial cancer.

Another major use of estrogen has been in postmenopausal women for the prevention of osteoporosis-related fractures to vertebral or long bones. Osteoporosis is characterized by reduced bone mass as well as microarchitectural deterioration of both cortical and trabecular bone and presents as a major public health problem among the elderly. In the United States, one in three postmenopausal women are affected by osteoporosis[21]; by the age of 90 years, one in two women and one in six men are likely to sustain an osteoporosis-related fracture. Of the affected elderly, between 12% and 20% will die of fracture-related complications,[21] making osteoporosis the twelfth leading cause of death in the United States.[34] Furthermore, it is estimated that more than $15 billion will be required to treat the 1.3 million Americans who annually have an osteoporosis-related fracture and its sequelae.[21] As the elderly population continues to increase, so will the incidence of osteoporosis and its complications.[14,17,34] To reduce the incidence of osteoporosis, treatment with estrogen, in combination with exercise and an appropriate diet, should begin before there is significant bone loss. It should be noted that estrogens can prevent further bone loss but cannot restore lost bone; therefore the benefits of estrogen replacement therapy require continuous use of the drug. Estrogen replacement therapy has also been shown to be effective in the treatment of vasomotor symptoms associated with menopause (e.g., hot flashes, paresthesia, hyperhidrosis) as well as postmenopausal urogenital atrophy. Orally or locally administered

Table • 37-4

Examples of Contraceptive Agents

PROPRIETARY (TRADE) NAME	ESTROGEN	PROGESTIN
Ovcon-35 (monophasic), Jenset (biphasic), Tri-Norinyl (triphasic)	Ethinyl estradiol	Norethindrone
Genora 1/50 (monophasic), Intercon 1/50 (monophasic), Ortho-Novum 1/50 (monophasic)	Mestranol	Norethindrone
Ortho-Cyclen (monophasic), Ortho Tri-Cyclen (triphasic)	Ethinyl estradiol	Norgestimate
Lo/Ovral (monophasic), Ovral (monophasic)	Ethinyl estradiol	Norgestrel
Depo-Provera	—	Medroxyprogesterone acetate
Norplant System	—	Norgestrel

Most combinations are marked in a variety of strengths and estrogen/progestin ratios.

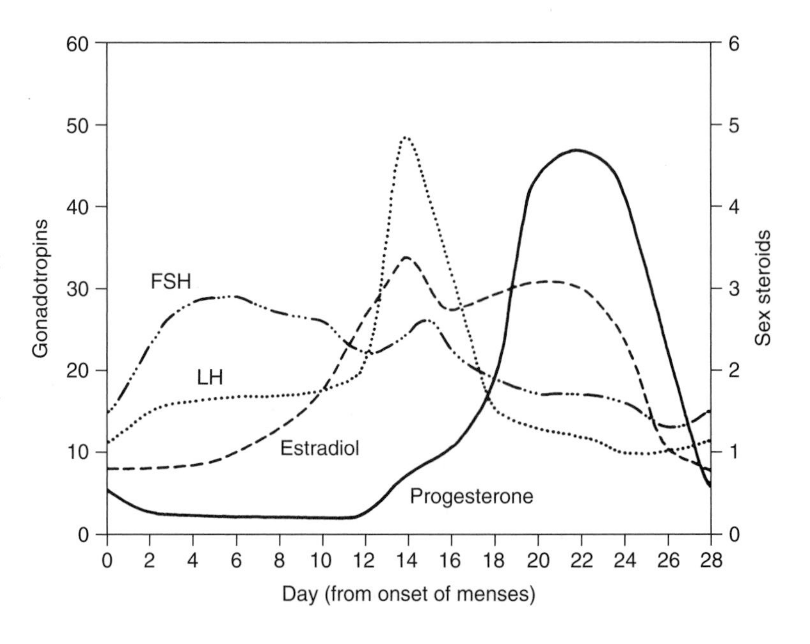

Fig. 37-5 Hormonal changes during the normal menstrual cycle. The gonadotropins, follicle-stimulating hormone *(FSH)*, and luteinizing hormone *(LH)* are measured in mU/ml; the sex steroids estradiol and progesterone are plotted in units (1 unit = 100 pg/ml estradiol and 2 ng/ml progesterone). Combination oral contraceptives prevent ovulation by inhibiting LH (and FSH) secretion, resulting in no LH peak at mid-cycle.

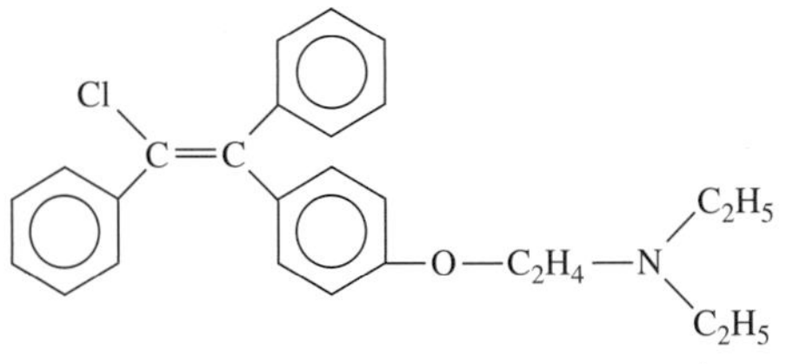

Clomiphene

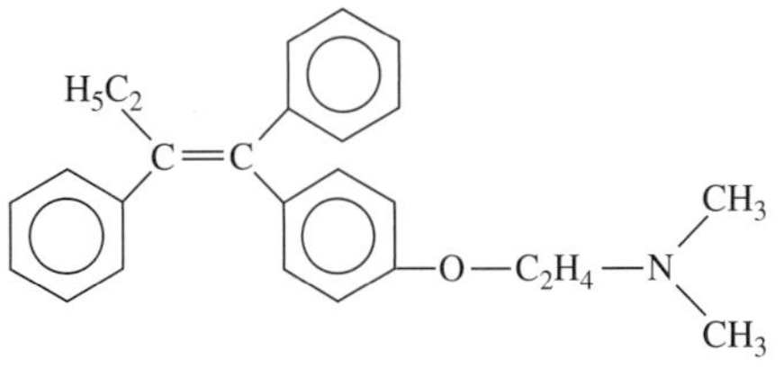

Tamoxifen

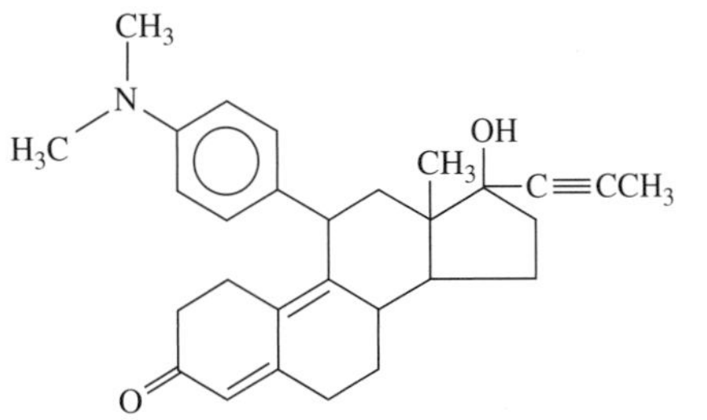

Mifepristone

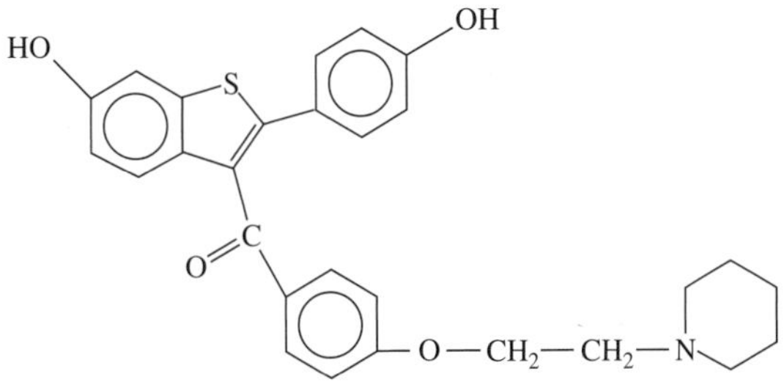

Raloxifene

Fig. 37-7 Chemical structures of antiestrogens (including partial agonists) and the antiprogestin mifepristone.

Tamoxifen and toremifene are examples of drugs that are often referred to as antiestrogens even though they are partial agonists. They also display tissue selectivity, as does raloxifene. Tamoxifen has been approved for the adjunctive treatment of breast neoplasms and as a prophylactic agent for women who are at high risk for breast cancer. Toremifene is used for the treatment of metastatic, estrogen receptor–positive breast cancer in postmenopausal women. Unlike raloxifene, tamoxifen, and toremifene, clomiphene shows little if any tissue selectivity. It is a drug that has been shown to act as an estrogen antagonist (actually a partial agonist) in all tissues studied. Clomiphene has been approved to promote ovulation in women. Therapeutic estrogen synthesis inhibitors involve blocking the activity of aromatase, the enzyme responsible for the conversion of testosterone to estradiol. Aromatase inhibitors (e.g., exemestane, anastrozole) have been used for the adjunctive treatment of breast cancer patients who have been unresponsive to tamoxifen.

Progestins

Agents that block the effect of progesterone (see Figure 37-7) are primarily potent, competitive antagonists of the progesterone receptor (see Table 37-5). Progesterone receptor antagonists such as mifepristone can be used as contraceptives and abortifacients as well as for the treatment of endometriosis, leiomyomas, breast cancer, and meningiomas.[4] In the United States, mifepristone is primarily used for the termination of early pregnancy (defined as 49 days or less).

IMPLICATIONS FOR DENTISTRY

The homeostasis of the periodontium is a complex, multifactorial relationship that involves, at least in part, the endocrine system. The assertion that hormone-sensitive periodontal tissues exist relies on several salient observations, including the retention and metabolic conversion of sex steroid hormones in the periodontium as well as the presence of steroid hormone receptors in periodontal tissues.[29] These biologic findings correlated with clinical observations confirm an increased prevalence of gingival diseases with fluctuating sex steroid hormone levels, even when oral hygiene remained unchanged. For example, the dramatic rise in steroid hormone levels during puberty has been accompanied by an increase in gingival inflammation in circumpubertal individuals of both sexes. Further evidence of the relationship between sex steroid hormones and the periodontium occurs during pregnancy, when the prevalence and severity of gingival disease has been reported to be elevated until parturition.[3,26] A cross-sectional study examined 121 pregnant and 61 postpartum women for changes in gingival inflammation and found the prevalence and severity of the gingival inflammation were significantly higher in the pregnant versus the postpartum patients, even though plaque scores remained the same between the two groups.[44] Furthermore, gingival probing depths are larger,[26,32] bleeding on probing or toothbrushing is increased,[3,32] and gingival crevicular fluid is elevated in pregnant women. Finally, women who are pregnant also exhibit a significant prevalence (0.5% to 0.8%) of localized gingival enlargements.[26,32] These pregnancy-induced gingival overgrowths are reversed after parturition.

In contrast to pregnancy, when hormone levels are significantly elevated, during menopause ovarian function is declining and there is a reduction in the production and secretion of sex steroid hormones. During this period, the question has arisen whether osteoporosis can affect the periodontal attachment apparatus. Although theories for the pathogenesis of osteoporosis are diverse, it is known that estrogen deficiency is an important factor in bone loss.[46] In addition, positive correlations between estrogens and bone density have been demonstrated.[46] Considering these findings, it is not surprising that bone mass from edentulous mandibles has been shown to differ by age and sex. Several cross-sectional studies have demonstrated decreased bone mass and density[22] as well as reduced bone mineral content[48] in edentulous mandibles of postmenopausal women. A variety of studies have attempted to provide insight into the relationship of osteoporosis to periodontitis but the results of these studies have been equivocal.[11,12,28,36,41,47,49]

In addition to the intentional prescription of estrogens, new compounds that have estrogenic activity are being released into the environment. Many environmental estrogens do not bind tightly to estrogen receptors and are poorly absorbed from the gastrointestinal tract, yet the constant exposure, bioaccumulation in adipose tissue, and persistence in the environment have heightened consideration of these chemicals as possible toxic agents in human beings. Currently, the prescribed use of Bis-GMA–based resins for restoration of the dentition has increased the concern of dentists about the safety of what were was once considered inert materials.[45] On the basis of existing research, we must accept that certain impurities may be present in some Bis-GMA–based resins and release of impurities from such restorations is potentially estrogenic.[45] Under extreme conditions, these impurities are capable of inducing weak estrogenic effects on target tissues. Moreover, the amounts of bisphenol A that may be present as an impurity or produced as a degradation product from dental restorations, including sealants, are quite small and far below the doses needed to affect the reproductive tract.[30]

Hormones of Reproduction and Related Drugs

Nonproprietary (generic) name	*Proprietary (trade) name*
Estrogens	
Chlorotrianisene	Tace
Conjugated estrogens	Premarin
Diethylstilbestrol*	Stilphostrol
Dienestrol	Ortho Dienestrol
Esterified estrogens	Menest
Estradiol	Estrace, Estraderm
Estrogenic substance	Gravigen Aqueous
Estropipate	Ogen
Ethinyl estradiol	Estinyl
Quinestrol	Estrovis
Selective estrogen receptor modifier	
Raloxifene	Evista
Tamoxifen	Nolvadex
Toremifene	Fareston
Progestins	
Hydroxyprogesterone	Hylutin
Levonorgestrel	Norplant
Medroxyprogesterone	Provera
Megestrol	Megace
Norethindrone	Aygestin
Norgestrel	Ovrette
Progesterone	—
Oral contraceptives	
See Table 37-4	
Anabolic-androgenic drugs	
Danazol	Danocrine
Ethylestrenol	Maxibolin
Fluoxymesterone	Halotestin
Methandrostenolone	—
Methyltestosterone	Oreton Methyl, Android
Nandrolone	Durabolin
Oxandrolone	Oxandrin
Oxymetholone	Anadrol-50
Stanozolol	Winstrol
Testosterone	Testex
Testolactone	Teslac
Gonadotropins	
Choriogonadotropin alpha	Ovidrel
Chorionic gonadotropin	Pregnyl
Follitropin alpha	Gonal-F
Follitropin beta	Follistim
Menotropins	Pergonal
Urofollitropin	Fertinex
Gonadotropin-releasing hormone analogues	
Gonadorelin	Factrel
Goserelin	Zoladex
Histrelin	Supprelin
Leuprolide	Lupron
Nafarelin	Synarel
Antiestrogens	
Clomiphene	Clomid
Antiprogestin	
Mifepristone (RU-486)	Mifeprex
Antiandrogens	
Bicalutamide	Casodex
Cyproterone	Androcur
Flutamide	Eulexin
5α-Reductase inhibitor	
Finasteride	Proscar
Aromatase inhibitors	
Anastrozole	Arimidex
Exemestane	Aromasin
Letrozole	Femara

*Not currently available in the United States.

The specific relationship of sex steroid hormones to periodontal endocrinopathies remains an enigma; however, the most reasonable explanations of hormone action in the periodontium have focused on hormone effects on microbial organisms, the vasculature, the immune system, and specific cells in the periodontium.[29]

When one considers the primary functions of sex steroid hormones, the periodontium would appear to be an odd target; however, given the influence of sex steroid hormones on periodontium, the health and lifestyles of women may be significantly affected.

PEPTIDE HORMONES

Human menopausal gonadotropins (menotropins) that contain both follicle-stimulating hormone and luteinizing hormone, urofollitropin, and chorionic gonadotropin are used as fertility drugs in women and in men with hypogonadism and cryptorchidism. These drugs, derived from the urine of postmenopausal (menotropins, urofollitropin) and pregnant (chorionic gonadotropin) women, are injected intramuscularly. Short-acting gonadotropin-releasing hormone analogues such as gonadorelin, given in a pulsatile manner, are used to increase fertility in women and to treat cryptorchidism in men. Long-acting gonadotropin-releasing hormone analogues such as leuprolide are used to treat precocious puberty, prostate cancer, and estrogen-dependent tumors in women. (The long-acting nonpulsatile administration of the drugs inhibits release of the gonadotropins.) The gonadotropin-releasing hormone analogues are given intravenously, subcutaneously, and by nasal spray.

CITED REFERENCES

1. Alonso LC, Rosenfield RL: Oestrogens and puberty, *Best Pract Res Clin Endocrinol Metab* 16:13-30, 2002.
2. Amanatullah DF, Zafonte BT, Pestell RG: The cell cycle in steroid hormone regulated proliferation and differentiation, *Minerva Endocrinol* 27:7-20, 2002.
3. Arafat AH: Periodontal status during pregnancy, *J Periodontol* 45:641-643, 1974.
4. Cadepond F, Ulmann A, Baulieu EE: RU486 (mifepristone): mechanisms of action and clinical uses, *Annu Rev Med* 48:129-156, 1997.
5. Cobasso A: Peliosis hepatis in a young adult bodybuilder, *Med Sci Sports Exerc* 26:2-4, 1994.
6. Dickinson BD, Altman RD, Nielsen NH, et al: Drug interactions between oral contraceptives and antibiotics, *Obstet Gynecol* 98:853-860, 2001.
7. Dunn JF, Nisula BC, Rodbard D: Transport of steroid hormones: binding of 21 endogenous steroids to both testosterone-binding globulin and corticosteroid-binding globulin in human plasma, *J Clin Endocrinol Metab* 53:58-68, 1981.
8. El-Ashiry GM, EL-Kafrawy AH, Nasr MF, et al: Comparative study of the influence of pregnancy and oral contraceptives on the gingivae, *Oral Surg Oral Med Oral Pathol* 30:472-475, 1970.
9. Evans RM: The steroid and thyroid hormone receptor superfamily, *Science* 24:889-895, 1988.
10. Fotherby K: Bioavailability of orally administered sex steroids used in oral contraception and hormone replacement therapy, *Contraception* 54:59-69, 1996.
11. Grodstein F, Colditz GA, Stampfer MJ: Hormone use and tooth loss: a prospective study, *J Am Dent Assoc* 127:370-377, 1996.
12. Groen J, Menczel J, Shapero S: Chronic destructive periodontal disease in patients with presenile osteoporosis, *J Periodontol* 33:1-23, 1968.
13. Gronemeyer H, Turcotte B, Quirin-Stricker C, et al: The chicken progesterone receptor: sequence, expression and functional analysis, *EMBO J* 6:3985-3994, 1987.
14. Hildebolt CF: Osteoporosis and oral bone loss, *Dentomaxillofac Rad* 26:3-15, 1997.
15. Jick H, Derby LE, Myers MW, et al: Risk of hospital admission for idiopathic venous thromboembolism among users of postmenopausal oestrogens, *Lancet* 348:981-983, 1996.
16. Kaufman AV: An oral contraceptive as an etiologic factor in producing hyperplastic gingivitis and a neoplasm of the pregnancy tumor type, *Oral Surg Oral Med Oral Pathol* 28:666-670, 1969.
17. Kelsey JL: *Osteoporosis: prevalence and incidence*, Consensus development conference summary, Bethesda, MD, 1984, National Institutes of Health.
18. Key TJ, Verkasalo PK, Banks E: Epidemiology of breast cancer, *Lancet Oncol* 2:133-140, 2001.
19. Knight GM, Wade B: The effects of hormonal contraceptives on the human periodontium, *J Periodont Res* 9:18-22, 1974.
20. Kochakian CD, Arimasa N: The metabolism in vitro of anabolic-androgenic steroids in mammalian tissues. In Kochakian CD, ed: *Anabolic-androgenic steroids*, New York, 1976, Springer-Verlag.
21. Krejci CB: Osteoporosis and periodontal disease: is there a relationship? *J West Soc Periodontol Abstract* 44:37-42, 1996.
22. Kribbs PJ: Comparison of mandibular bone in normal and osteoporotic women, *J Prosthet Dent* 63:218-222, 1990.
23. Krust A, Green S, Argos P, et al: The chicken oestrogen receptor sequence: homology with v-erbA and the human oestrogen and glucocorticoid receptors, *EMBO J* 5:891-897, 1986.
24. Kumar V, Green S, Stack G, et al: Functional domains of the human estrogen receptor, *Cell* 51:941-951, 1987.
25. Lobo RA, Stanczyk FZ: New knowledge in the physiology of hormonal contraceptives, *Am J Obstet Gynecol* 170:1499-1507, 1994.
26. Löe H, Silness J: Periodontal disease in pregnancy. I. Prevalence and severity, *Acta Odontol Scand* 21:533-551, 1963.
27. Lynn BD: "The pill" as an etiologic agent in hypertropic gingivitis, *Oral Surg Oral Med Oral Pathol* 24:333-334, 1967.
28. Manson J: Bone morphology and bone loss in periodontal disease, *J Clin Periodontol* 3:14-22, 1976.
29. Mariotti A: Sex steroid hormones and cell dynamics in the periodontium, *Crit Rev Oral Biol Med* 5:27-53, 1994.
30. Mariotti A, Söderholm KJ, Johnson S: The in vivo effects of Bis-GMA on murine uterine weight, nucleic acids and collagen, *Eur J Oral Sci* 106:1022-1027, 1998.
31. Miller J, McLachlan AD, Klug A: Repetitive zinc-binding domains in the protein transcription factor IIIA from *Xenopus* oocytes, *EMBO J* 4:1609-1614, 1985.
32. Miyazaki H, Yamashita Y, Shirahama R, et al: Periodontal condition of pregnant women assessed by CPITN, *J Clin Periodontol* 18:751-754, 1991.

33. Mooradian AD, Morley JE, Korenman SG: Biological actions of androgens, *Endocr Rev* 8:1-28, 1987.
34. Owen RA, Melton LF, Gallagher FC, et al: The national cost of acute care of hip fractures associated with osteoporosis, *Clin Orthop* 150:172-176, 1980.
35. Pankhurst CL, Waite IW, Hichs KA, et al: The influence of oral contraceptive therapy on the periodontium—duration of drug therapy, *J Periodontol* 52:617-620, 1981.
36. Payne JB, Reinhardt RA, Nummikoski PV, et al: Longitudinal alveolar bone loss in postmenopausal osteoporotic/osteopenic women, *Osteoporos Int* 10:34-40, 1999.
37. Pettersson K, Gustafsson J-A: Role of estrogen receptor beta in estrogen action, *Annu Rev Physiol* 63:165-192, 2001.
38. Pike MC, Peters RK, Cozen W, et al: Estrogen-progestin replacement therapy and endometrial cancer, *J Natl Cancer Inst* 89:1110-1116, 1997.
39. Preshaw PM, Knutsen M, Mariotti A: Experimental gingivitis in women using oral contraceptives, *J Dent Res* 80:2011-2015, 2001.
40. Rasmussen JE: The effect of antibiotics on the efficacy of oral contraceptives, *Arch Dermatol* 125:1562-1564, 1989.
41. Ronderos M, Jacobs DR, Himes FH, et al: Associations of periodontal disease with femoral bone mineral density and estrogen replacement therapy: cross-sectional evaluation of US adults from NHANES III, *J Clin Periodontol* 27:778-786, 2000.
42. Shapiro S, Kelly FP, Rosenberg L, et al: Risk of localized and widespread endometrial cancer in relation to recent and discontinued use of conjugated estrogens, *N Engl J Med* 313:969-972, 1985.
43. Siiteri PK, MacDonald PC: Role of extraglandular estrogen in human endocrinology. In Greep RO, Astwood EB, Geiger SR, eds: *Endocrinology, vol II. Female reproductive system. Handbook of physiology.* Washington, DC, 1973, American Physiology Society.
44. Silness J, Loe H: Periodontal disease in pregnancy. II. Correlation between oral hygiene and periodontal condition, *Acta Odontol Scand* 22:121-135, 1963.
45. Söderholm KJ, Mariotti A: BIS-GMA–based resins in dentistry: are they safe? *J Am Dent Assoc* 130:201-209, 1999.
46. Steinberg KK, Freni-Titulaer LW, Depuey EG, et al: Sex steroids and bone density in premenopausal and perimenopausal women, *J Clin Endocrinol Metab* 69:533-539, 1989.
47. Tezal M, Wactawski-Wende F, Grossi SG, et al: The relationship between bone mineral density and periodontitis in postmenopausal women, *J Periodontol* 71:1492-1498, 2000.
48. Von Wowern N: Bone mineral content of mandibles: normal reference values—rate of age-related bone loss, *Calcif Tissue Int* 43:193-198, 1988.
49. Weyant RJ, Perlstein ME, Churak AP, et al: The association between osteopenia and periodontal attachment loss in older women, *J Periodontol* 70:982-991, 1999.
50. Wilson JD: Metabolism of testicular androgens. In Greep RO, Astwood EB, Geiger SR, eds: *Endocrinology, vol V. Male reproductive system. Handbook of physiology.* Washington, DC, 1975, American Physiology Society.
51. Writing Group for the Women's Health Initiative Investigators: Risks and benefits of estrogen plus progesterone in healthy postmenopausal women: principal results from the Women's Health Initiative randomized controlled trial, *JAMA* 288:321-333, 2002.
52. Wu CH, Motohashi T, Abdel-Rahman, et al: Free and protein-bound plasma estradiol-17 during the menstrual cycle, *J Clin Endocrinol Metab* 43:436-445, 1976.
53. Yen SS: The biology of menopause, *J Reprod Med* 18:287-296, 1977.

General References

Mariotti A: Sex steroid hormones and cell dynamics in the periodontium, *Crit Rev Oral Biol Med* 5:27-53, 1994.

Williams RH: *Textbook of endocrinology,* ed 9, Philadelphia, 1998, WB Saunders.

CHAPTER • 38

Principles of Antibiotic Therapy*

Thomas J. Pallasch

INFECTIOUS DISEASE PAST AND PRESENT

In 1967 the United States Surgeon General declared that "The time has come to close the book on infectious diseases." In 1993, 17 million people died of infectious diseases throughout the world, with 11.4 million deaths (mostly of children) caused by bacterial diarrhea and pneumonia. In the same year, 15.6 million died of cardiovascular disease and cancer combined.[64] The four primary disease killers caused by infection are the same as in 1900: diarrhea, pneumonia, tuberculosis, and malaria.[18] Up to one third of the world population has tuberculosis, and Africa accounts for 90% of the 300 to 500 million new cases of malaria annually, with 1.5 to 2.7 million deaths per year. In World War II, 55 million people were killed; by 2010, 65 million will have died of AIDS.

To be fair, the Surgeon General was only echoing the prevailing wisdom of the 1960s era of optimism regarding antibiotics. In the late 1950s the medical community became alarmed at the extent and rapidity of *Staphylococcus aureus* resistance to the penicillins, erythromycin, and tetracyclines and the discovery that bacteria could transfer the genes for antibiotic resistance among themselves. In the early 1960s, however, came a plethora of new antibiotics: cephalosporins, the β-lactamase–resistant penicillins, lincosamides, and new aminoglycosides. The belief that humankind would always stay several steps ahead of the microbes because they could not possibly match our intelligence was widely accepted. Assumptions are the genesis of most disasters, and, as one of "Murphy's laws" states, "Optimism indicates that the situation is not clearly understood."

The Centers for Disease Control and Prevention (CDC) estimates that 65,000 to 90,000 deaths annually in US hospitals are from nosocomial (hospital-acquired) infections. This figure may be a significant underestimate and may in fact be closer to 200,000 to 300,000 because infectious disease deaths may be misclassified as cardiac arrest or respiratory or renal failure instead of their underlying microbial causes. In 1977, 100,000 gram-negative nosocomial bacteremic deaths were estimated annually in the United States[54]; bloodstream infections (septicemia and bacteremia) alone, among all nosocomial infections, may now be the eighth leading cause of death in the United States.[110,111] Hospitals are currently plagued by vancomycin-resistant enterococci, vancomycin- or glycopeptide-intermediate–resistant *S. aureus*, and coagulase-negative staphylococci (CoNS) and other multiply antibiotic-resistant microorganisms, particularly *Streptococcus pneumoniae* and extended β-lactamase–producing enteric bacilli. The community is now beset by methicillin-resistant *S. aureus*, which was once thought only the problem of the hospital, penicillin- and macrolide-resistant *S. pneumoniae* and viridans group streptococci (VGS), β-lactamase–producing *Haemophilus influenzae* and *Moraxella catarrhalis*, and widespread fluoroquinolone resistance. The oral cavity is home to β-lactam–resistant VGS and β-lactamase–producing *Prevotella* and *Porphyromonas*.

Mechanisms for resistance to antibiotics have likely always existed in some form to allow microbes to ensure their survival against competing microorganisms and find a niche in their environment to survive and thrive. However, our current problems are of human origin—we disturbed this delicate microbial ecology for our own benefit, never realizing how formidable microbial retaliation would be. We are approaching the loss of one of our greatest gifts.

The importance of two medical discoveries that have essentially doubled the human lifespan in first-world countries since the 1850s—anesthesia and the control of infectious diseases—cannot be overestimated. Without the ability to operate internally within the human body free of excruciating pain, the gains of medical and dental surgery would be void. In the United States in 1776, the average lifespan was less than 40 years of age. In England in 1853, infectious disease was responsible for 37% of all deaths. At the beginning of the twentieth century in the United States, the infant mortality rate was 100 per 1000; now it is less that 10 per 1000.[64] A child in 1900 had a 10% chance of death between ages 1 and 4 years from pneumonia or diarrhea.[64] Typhus, typhoid, diphtheria, whooping cough, yellow fever, malaria, influenza, measles, smallpox, and streptococcal and staphylococcal infections all laid to rest many adults, infants, and children.

Even before the advent of the modern germ theory of disease in the 1870s, many surmised that filth had a substantial bearing on disease. The "sanitary movement" began in Great Britain in the 1850s and the United States in the 1870s with improvement in wages, housing, education, and personal hygiene. Civil engineers cleaned the streets, water, and air, and cities removed refuse and their attendant rodent vectors of disease. Waste disposal, clean water, and hand hygiene by public health engineering have reduced the transmission of 35 to 40 infectious diseases.[30]

The modern era of infectious disease began with the first visualization of microbes by Anton van Leeuwenhoek in 1683, the "animicules" of dental plaque scraped from his upper gingiva and killed with salt (the first periodontal chemotherapy).[44] In 1776, Edward Jenner administered the first smallpox vaccination, in 1848, Ignaz Semmelweiss introduced clean surgical operating technique ("gentlemen, wash your

*The authors wish to recognize Dr. Edward Montgomery for his past contributions to this chapter. See the Acknowledgments.

hands"), and in 1854, John Snow demonstrated the link between cholera and drinking water.[44]

In the 1860s, Louis Pasteur first used the word *germ* for living entities that produced disease, and Joseph Lister used carbolic acid to disinfect wounds. In the 1870s, Robert Koch proved the bacterial causation of anthrax and tuberculosis, and in the 1880s, Pasteur developed anthrax and rabies vaccines. In 1891, Paul Ehrlich demonstrated that antibodies were responsible for immunity, and in 1897, Ivanowski and Beiternick discovered viruses. The mosquito vector for yellow fever was demonstrated in 1900, *Treponema pallidum* was found to be the cause of syphilis in 1905, HIV was identified in 1983, *Helicobacter pylori* was discovered as a cause of peptic ulcer in 1984, and the West Nile virus was identified in 1999.[44]

In the early 1900s, Paul Ehrlich used the term *magic bullet* for his predicted chemical that would affect only microbial cells and have no effect on mammalian cells. He later used fuchsin and mercury (Salvarsan) to treat syphilis. In 1928, Alexander Fleming, through serendipity, discovered that a mold, *Penicillium chrysogenum*, lysed staphylococci, which was later developed to its full potential by the isolation of penicillin from *Penicillium notatum* by Florey et al at Oxford in the late 1930s and early 1940s. The first use of penicillin was in 1941 on an English police constable with streptococcal and staphylococcal skin abscesses and in the United States in 1942 on Anne Miller, who had streptococcal toxemia of pregnancy. All this has possibly overshadowed arguably the greatest of all medical advances: the demonstration in 1935 by Gerhard Domagk that sulfanilamide could be safely used systemically to treat infectious disease. The "dreaded disease of summer" (poliomyelitis) declined from 57,879 cases in the United States in 1953 to 72 cases in 1965 with the advent of the polio vaccine.[66] By 1977 smallpox was eradicated from the world as a contagious disease. Between 1900 and 1997, the American lifespan increased by 60% to a median age of 76.[18]

The developing world, unfortunately, has been quite a different story. In 1998 the World Health Organization determined that infectious disease caused 25% (13 million) of the 54 million deaths in the world that year, with pneumonia (3.5 million), AIDS (2.3 million), diarrhea (2.2 million), tuberculosis (1.5 million), malaria (1.1 million), and measles (1 million) the top killers.[18] The incidence of emerging infections (defined by the Institute of Medicine as new, reemerging, or drug-resistant infections whose incidence has increased in the last 2 decades or whose incidence threatens to increase) has increased.[18] Now included in this category are Legionnaire's disease, toxic shock syndrome, respiratory syncytial virus, Lyme disease, Nipah virus, hantavirus, the hemorrhagic viral diseases (Dengue, Ebola, Marburg), *Escherichia coli* O157:H7, malaria, yellow fever, cholera, and multidrug-resistant tuberculosis. All these and more are potentially transmitted by 500,000 world refugees and 1.6 billion annual airline passengers, 500 million of which cross borders each year.[64]

All of the media attention to these potential pathogens has led to a second "germ panic" with the revival of the focal infection theory of disease,[68] which alleges that many or most current diseases are caused by various microbes: cardiovascular disease, various forms of emotional disorders such as obsessive compulsive disorder and Tourette's syndrome, autism and schizophrenia, preterm births, chronic fatigue syndrome, and multiple sclerosis. The first germ panic of 1900 to 1940 was fostered by the focal infection theory as espoused by Hunter et al, in which a localized infection in one area of the body could move and then occur elsewhere in the body and cause various pathologic conditions such as arthritis, neuritis, myalgia, osteomyelitis, endocarditis, brain abscess, skin abscess, pneumonia, anemia, indigestion, gastritis, pancreatitis, colitis, diabetes, emphysema, goiter, thyroiditis, Hodgkin's disease, "obscure fever," nervous diseases, headache, mental apathy, and mental incompetence.[68] Interestingly, all these were disorders for which medicine at the time (and many currently) had no explanations and no answers.

These foci of infection were conveniently located in areas of the body readily accessible to surgery (particularly in the wealthy): teeth, tonsils, and the facial sinuses, leading to an excessive number of dental extractions, tonsillectomies, and other surgeries in the first half of the twentieth century.[40,68,114,115] The resurrection of the foci of infection concept today is based on limited scientific evidence and questionable studies that lack attention to sound epidemiologic methods.

On very rare occasions, microbes leave the oral cavity and metastasize to other areas of the body to initiate a nonspecific inflammatory infectious process manifested as liver, splenic, or brain abscesses or bacterial endocarditis. These microorganisms are almost always VGS and almost never pathogens associated with periodontal disease. That these metastatic infections are so rare is truly remarkable and speaks well for our immune defense mechanisms, particularly in the oral cavity and blood, and the reticence of microorganisms to leave their ecologic niches for foreign environments. Currently little evidence suggests that the oral cavity is the source of significant systemic disease.[67,68]

PATTERNS OF ANTIBIOTIC USE AND MISUSE

Antibiotics are the most widely abused prescribed drugs on the basis of inappropriate indications, dosages, and duration of use. Approximately half of all antibiotics used in hospitals are given to patients without signs or symptoms of infection, in many cases to "prevent" infections and to ensure that "everything was done" to avoid later criticism. Antibiotics are often used as "drugs of fear"[42] to cover for potential errors of omission or commission and thereby prevent a claim of negligence. The abuse of negligence (tort) law has been a major contributing factor to the massive overuse of antibiotics and the attendant mortality rate associated with highly antibiotic-resistant microorganisms.

In hospitals, one third of antibiotics are used empirically, one third for prophylaxis, and one third with appropriate culture and sensitivity tests.[64] Because hospitals save money by not using culture and sensitivity tests, the demand has been for broader-spectrum antibiotics, which has created a vicious cycle by further disturbing the hospital microbial ecology and fostering even greater microbial resistance.[92]

Outpatient antibiotic use is characterized by the "80 : 80 rule": 80% of all antibiotics are used in the community and 80% are used for respiratory infections, the vast majority of which are viral in cause and not amenable to antibiotic therapy.[64] Of the 50% of people with acute respiratory illness who seek medical treatment, 50% to 80% may receive an antibiotic, but pneumonia (the only respiratory tract disorder requiring an antibiotic) may account for only 2% of these cases.

The prescribing of antibiotics can vary 15-fold among physicians; those who tend to prescribe many drugs also prescribe many antibiotics. Antibiotic prescriptions are a quick way to end an office visit and reduce return visits.[85]

Dentists prescribe between 7% and 11% of all common antibiotics (β-lactams, macrolides, tetracycline, metronidazole, clindamycin), and abuse of such antibiotics can be substantial.[17] In England, between 33% and 87% of various antibiotics were judged to be inappropriately prescribed by dentists according to the Dental Practitioners Formulary.[69] Experts in England are in agreement that antibiotics are used too long for the management of orofacial infections and that shorter durations are more appropriate and reduce the selection of drug-resistant microbes.[53]

In a survey of 505 Canadian dentists, the average length of antibiotic therapy was 6.92 days (range, 1 to 21 days), and

17.5% did not use the 1997 American Heart Association (AHA) guidelines for endocarditis prophylaxis.[26] Two thirds of the dentists used antibiotic prophylaxis for patients with rheumatic fever without rheumatic heart disease, 25% for patients with HIV/AIDS, 70% for prosthetic joints, and two thirds for restorative dentistry not associated with significant bleeding even though not advocated by the AHA.

Twenty percent of dental specialists did not use AHA prophylaxis for patients with cardiac valve prostheses. The study concluded that antibiotics are underused for symptomatic infections, overused for surgical prophylaxis, and commonly used at suboptimal dosing with prolonged dosing schedules and often not according to antibiotic prophylaxis guidelines.[26]

In a survey of antibiotic use by 1606 members of the American Association of Endodontists, 12.5% used antibiotics as an analgesic for posttreatment pain, 37.3% as antibiotic prophylaxis after surgery, 44.8% after incision and drainage without systemic involvement or patient immunosuppression, and between 12% and 54% for situations in which they are not effective: (1) irreversible pulpitis with moderate to severe symptoms with or without apical periodontitis; (2) asymptomatic necrotic pulps with chronic apical periodontitis but no swelling; (3) necrotic pulps with acute apical periodontitis, no swelling, and moderate to severe symptoms; and (4) asymptomatic necrotic pulps with chronic periapical periodontitis with or without a sinus tract.[116] The authors concluded that not much had changed in the past 25 years.

Inappropriate antibiotic use in dentistry includes (1) antibiotic therapy initiated after surgery to prevent an infection unlikely to occur and not documented effective for this purpose by clinical trials, (2) failure to use prophylactic antibiotics according to the principles established for such use, (3) as analgesics in endodontics, (4) overuse in situations in which patients are not at risk for metastatic infections, (5) treatment of chronic adult periodontitis almost totally amenable to mechanical therapy, (6) administration instead of mechanical therapy for periodontitis, (7) long-term administration in the management of periodontal disease, (8) antibiotic therapy instead of incision and drainage, (9) administration to avoid claims of negligence, and (10) administration in improper situations, dosage, and duration of therapy.[64]

ANTIBIOTIC MECHANISMS OF ACTION

To appreciate how microbes defend themselves against chemicals in their environment, one must first determine how antimicrobial agents kill microbes or prevent their replication.

Antibiotics are chemicals most often, but not always, derived from microorganisms (commonly yeasts and fungi) that are intended in nature to perform as part of the system that maintains the ecologic balance in the microbial world. This system is composed of various entities such as bacteriophages (bacterial viruses), cationic peptides, antibiotics, and the quorum-sensing system that conveys chemical messages to microbes regarding metabolic activities, surface adhesion, colony formation, virulence, and the presence of chemicals intended to do harm. Virtually all clinically useful antibiotics are derived from naturally occurring entities, with only three synthetically produced: sulfonamides, fluoroquinolones, and oxazolidinones.

Antimicrobials affect the viability of microorganisms by five known processes: (1) inhibition of cell wall synthesis, (2) alteration of cell membrane integrity, (3) inhibition of ribosomal protein synthesis, (4) suppression of deoxyribonucleic acid (DNA) synthesis, and (5) inhibition of folic acid synthesis (Table 38-1, Figure 38-1). Microbial cell wall synthesis inhibition and membrane effects are extracytoplasmic, and inhibition of nucleic acid, protein, and folic acid synthesis is intracytoplasmic. Drugs that affect bacterial cell wall or membrane integrity and DNA synthesis are usually but not always bactericidal (inducing cell death), and protein and folic acid synthesis inhibitors are usually bacteriostatic (preventing cell growth or replication).

Whether an antimicrobial agent is bactericidal (cidal) or bacteriostatic (static) can also depend on its concentration at the infected site and the particular offending organism because some static drugs become cidal at high concentrations. The previous preference for cidal drugs over static antibiotics (cidal drugs allegedly do not rely on host defenses) has become less distinct recently because of the appreciation of the long postantibiotic effects (continued antibiotic activity when the drug blood levels have declined) of bacteriostatic drugs.

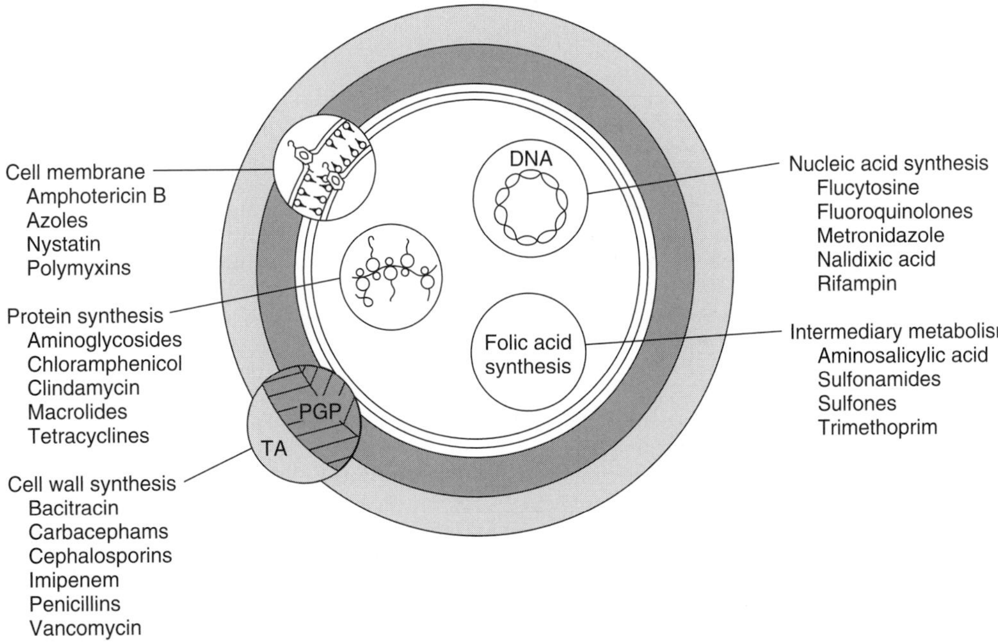

Fig. 38-1 Site and mechanism of action of antimicrobial agents. *TA*, Teichoic acid; *PGP*, peptidoglycan.

Table • 38-1

Mechanisms of Action of Common Antibiotics

ANTIMICROBIALS	MECHANISMS
Inhibition of Cell Wall Synthesis	
β-Lactams	Inhibit PBPs responsible for the final three-dimensional structure of the rigid bacterial cell wall; initiate autolysin activity
Glycopeptides	Complex with muramyl peptide precursors to block the effect of transglycosylase and transpeptidase enzymes at a stage just before the β-lactams
Alteration in Cell Membrane Integrity	
Polymyxins	Disrupt cell membrane osmotic integrity by displacing divalent metals from membrane lipid phosphates
Cationic antimicrobial peptides	Disrupt cell membrane integrity by causing voids to form in the membrane
Inhibition of Ribosomal Protein Synthesis	
Macrolides	Inhibit peptidyl transferase; increase dissociation of peptidyl tRNA from ribosome
Lincosamides	Attach to same ribosomal P site of the 50S ribosome as the macrolides
Tetracyclines	Inhibit binding of tRNA to mRNA at 30S ribosomal subunit
Aminoglycosides	Attach to 30S ribosomal subunit; induce formation of lethal proteins
Streptogramins	Bind to 50S ribosomal subunit to prevent peptide extrusion from the ribosome
Oxazolidinones	Prevent initiation complex necessary for bacterial translation
Inhibition of Nucleic Acid Synthesis	
Metronidazole	Intracellular reduction to form DNA-damaging nitro, nitroso, and hydroxylamine compounds
Fluoroquinolones	Inhibit topoisomerase IV and DNA gyrase to prevent DNA supercoiling and replication; affect SOS DNA repair system resulting in unbalanced growth, vacuole formation, filamentation, and lysis
Inhibition of Folic Acid Synthesis	
Sulfonamides	Inhibit folic acid synthesis by blocking conversion of PABA to dihydrofolic acid; inhibit dihydropteroate synthase
Trimethoprim	Block next step in folic acid synthesis by inhibiting conversion of dihydrofolic acid to tetrahydrofolic acid; inhibit dihydrofolate reductase

PABA, *p*-Aminobenzoic acid; *PBPs*, penicillin-binding proteins.
From Pallasch TJ: Global antibiotic resistance and its impact on the dental community, *J Calif Dent Assoc* 28:215-233, 2000; Salyers AA, Whitt DD: *Bacterial pathogenesis: a molecular approach*, ed 2, Washington DC, 2002, ASM Press.

Cell Wall Synthesis Inhibitors

The principal cell wall inhibitors are the β-lactam antibiotics and glycopeptides. Bacterial cell walls are rigid and composed of alternating peptidoglycan (murein) units of N-acetyl-D-glucosamine and N-acetylmuramic acid (NAM). These are cross-linked via short peptides by amide linkages to a D-alanyl group on NAM. Various bacterial enzymes (transglycosylases, transpeptidases, carboxypeptidases, endopeptidases), termed *penicillin-sensitive enzymes* or *penicillin-binding proteins* (PBPs), catalyze the formation of the rigid cell wall by incorporating new peptidoglycan into existing peptidoglycan by attaching a free amino group on the NAM-pentapeptide to a terminus opened by displacement of D-alanine. β-Lactam antibiotics competitively inhibit this final transpeptidation reaction to prevent three-dimensional rigid cell wall formation. The internal osmotic pressure of the bacterium causes lysis of the bacterial cell because the wall is no longer an effective barrier.

Additionally, in some organisms the β-lactams inhibit the inhibitor (derepression) of an endogenous bacterial autolysin (N-acetyl-muramyl-L-alanine amidase) that, once activated, will cause the lysis of the bacterial cell wall, initiating bacterial suicide. Microbes that lose this autolysin system can become tolerant to antibiotics, with the antibiotic becoming bacteriostatic instead of bactericidal.

The glycopeptides inhibit gram-positive bacterial cell wall synthesis by complexing with the D-alanyl–D alanine portion of the muramyl peptide precursors to inhibit the action of transglycosylase and transpeptidase at a stage just before that of the β-lactams.

Alteration in Cell Membrane Integrity

Polymyxin B disrupts the integrity of the cell membrane by displacing calcium and magnesium from membrane lipid phosphate groups. Cationic antimicrobial peptides are part of our natural skin and mucosal defense system and act by disrupting cell wall or membrane integrity by an effect on the gram-negative lipopolysaccharide component that literally puts holes in the wall or membrane.

Inhibition of Ribosomal Protein Synthesis

The macrolides bind to the P site of the 50S ribosomal subunit to inhibit RNA-dependent protein synthesis by inhibiting peptidyl transferase or by increasing the dissociation of peptidyl tRNA from the ribosome. Clindamycin similarly attaches to the same 50S subunit and can compete with the macrolides for this site. Cross-resistance between these two disparate antibiotics is common. Tetracyclines attach to the 30S ribosomal subunit to block ribosomal protein synthesis by inhibiting the binding of tRNA to mRNA on the ribosome. The aminoglycosides attach to the 30S subunit to inhibit ribosomal protein synthesis but may also induce the formation of abnormal bactericidal proteins. The streptogramins (quinupristin-dalfopristin) each bind to two different sites on the 50S subunit of the 70S ribosome to prevent newly synthesized peptide chains from extruding from the ribosome. The oxazolidinone, linezolid, attaches to the 50S ribosome near the interface with the 30S subunit to prevent the initiation complex required for bacterial translation.

Inhibition of Nucleic Acid Synthesis

The 5′ nitro group of metronidazole is reduced in sensitive obligate anaerobes by nitro reductase to cell toxic nitro, nitroso, and hydroxylamine compounds that damage DNA or inhibit its synthesis. The fluoroquinolones inhibit both topoisomerase IV and DNA gyrase that control the supercoiling of DNA and DNA replication, recombination, and repair. The fluoroquinolones may also induce the SOS response, which constitutes a repair system of DNA (the bacterial response to DNA damage) that normally functions to inhibit cell division to prevent the replication of damaged DNA. When the SOS repair system is affected by the fluoroquinolones, unbalanced growth, vacuoles, filamentation, and cell lysis occur.

Inhibition of Folic Acid Synthesis

The sulfonamides and trimethoprim are antimetabolites that inhibit sequential steps in the bacterial synthesis of folic acid essential for one-carbon transfers in nucleic acid synthesis. Mammalian cells do not synthesize folic acid but acquire it from the environment. The sulfonamides are structural analogues of *p*-aminobenzoic acid (PABA) and block the conversion of PABA to dihydrofolic acid by inhibiting tetrahydropteroic acid synthetase, which has greater affinity for the sulfonamides than PABA. Trimethoprim blocks the next step in folic acid synthesis by inhibiting dihydrofolate reductase that catalyzes the conversion of dihydrofolic acid to tetrahydrofolic acid.

MICROBIAL RESISTANCE TO ANTIBIOTICS

Microbial resistance to antibiotics has become a major factor in determining when and which antibiotic is used, as well as dosages and length of administration. It also has spurred renewed interest in antibiotic pharmacokinetics and pharmacodynamics.

Procedures designed to reduce antibiotic-resistant pathogenic microorganisms have been developed: education of health care providers and the general public, improved hand-washing techniques, better hospital infection control, isolation of patients with highly resistant bacteria, control of antibiotic use in hospitals through formularies and pharmacist oversight, and the removal of antibiotics for growth promotion in agricultural animals. Unfortunately, many of these programs have had little effect to date.

All microbial resistance is local; the patterns and extent of this resistance are determined by the use of antibiotics in a particular community. What is true in Florida may not be true in Los Angeles or in Paris, London, Rome, or New Delhi. If tetracyclines are used widely in the community for acne or Lyme disease, a high resistance level to the drug is likely to be present in that locale. If not, the microbial resistance level is likely to be low. If an antibiotic or its analogue has been used widely in agriculture, this may strongly influence resistance patterns—even to the point of rendering a new antibiotic far less useful. In Taiwan, virginiamycin (a streptogramin) has been used for more than 2 decades as a growth promoter in food animals. When quinupristin-dalfopristin, a new streptogramin, was tested on human bacterial isolates before its clinical introduction, more than 50% of some pathogens were already resistant to the drug. Antibiotics are truly societal drugs that cumulatively affect the individual receiving the drug and many others as well.[47]

Microorganisms have developed seven known mechanisms to evade the bactericidal or bacteriostatic actions of antimicrobials: (1) enzymatic inactivation, (2) modification/protection of the target site, (3) limited access of antibiotic (altered cell membrane permeability), (4) active drug efflux, (5) failure to activate the antibiotic, (6) use of alternate growth requirements, and (7) overproduction of target sites (Table 38-2).[64,83]

Enzymatic inactivation is one of the more common methods and is typified by the β-lactamase hydrolysis of penicillins and cephalosporins and acetyltransferases that inactive chloramphenicol, aminoglycosides, and tetracyclines. Altered target sites include ribosomal point mutations for the tetracyclines, macrolides, and clindamycin; altered DNA gyrase and topoisomerase for the fluoroquinolones; and modified PBPs for VGS and pneumococci. Most microorganisms have developed ways to alter their cell wall or membrane permeability to limit access of the antibiotic to its receptor by deleting outer membrane proteins or closing membrane pore channels. Altering antibiotic access to the cell interior usually does not confer a high level of resistance on the organism and must be combined with another mechanism for significant resistance potential. Several hundred efflux proteins are available that extrude waste products from the microbial cell but that now have been adapted over time to eliminate antibiotics specifically from the cell interior virtually as fast as they can enter. Enterococci can evade destruction by developing alternate metabolic growth requirements (auxotrophs). Sulfonamide resistance may occur from the overproduction of PABA, and some enteric organisms evade β-lactam antibiotics by overproducing β-lactamase (hyper–β-lactamase producers).

Antibiotic tolerance occurs when the antibiotic no longer kills the microorganism but merely inhibits its growth or multiplication. Tolerant microorganisms start to grow after the antibiotic is removed, whereas resistant microorganisms multiply in the presence of the antibiotic. Tolerance is usually caused by the loss of autolysin activity through a failure to create or mobilize the autolytic enzymes. Vancomycin tolerance in *Streptococcus pneumoniae* is unique; a mutation in the sensor-response system controls the bactericidal autolysin activity.

Most agree that the major factor in the development and maintenance of antibiotic resistance in microbes is their ability to eliminate sensitive microorganisms and allow resistant ones to multiply and dominate. Although this selection process is no doubt crucial, other factors also contribute. Lengthy antibiotic regimens are commonly advocated to kill all the resistant strains or prevent stepped resistance (the development of resistance by a sequence of mutations occurring over several generations of microbial multiplication). Theoretically, if the antibiotic is given long enough, all these mutants are exposed to the antibiotic and killed at cell division. This is the rationale for taking the entire prescribed antibiotic rather than

Table • 38-2

Antibiotic Resistance Mechanisms

MECHANISMS	ANTIMICROBIAL DRUGS AND EXAMPLES OF MECHANISMS
Enzymatic antibiotic inactivation	• β-Lactams by β-lactamases • Aminoglycosides by aminoglycoside-modifying enzymes • Chloramphenicol by acetyltransferases • Streptogramins by acetyltransferases • Tetracyclines by enzymatic oxidation
Modification/protection of target site	• β-Lactams: altered PBPs • Fluoroquinolones: altered DNA gyrase or topoisomerases • Rifampin: altered RNA polymerase • Sulfonamides: altered dihydropteroate synthase • Trimethoprim: altered dihydrofolate reductase • Macrolide-lincosamide-streptogramin B aggregate gene (MLS_b): methylation of adenine on 23S rRNA • Glycopeptides: change of D-Ala-D-Ala to D-Ala-D-lactate in cell wall • Tetracyclines: ribosomal protection
Limiting access of antibiotic	• β-Lactams, fluoroquinolones, most antibiotics: altered outer membrane porins • Most antibiotics: reduced membrane transport
Active antibiotic efflux	• Tetracyclines: *tet* genes • Fluoroquinolones: *Nor A* genes
Failure to activate antibiotic	• Metronidazole: decreased flavodoxin production
Use of alternate growth requirements	• Enterococcal auxotrophs
Overproduction of target sites	• Sulfonamides: overproduction of PABA • Enteric bacilli: overproduction of β-lactamase

From Polk R: Optimal use of modern antibiotics: emerging trends, *Clin Infect Dis* 29:264-274, 1999; Smith H: Host factors that influence the behavior of bacteria pathogens in vivo, *Int J Med Microbiol* 290:207-213, 2000.

stopping the antibiotic when the patient is well. This concept is false for three reasons: (1) microbial mutations rarely occur during antibiotic treatment, (2) stepped resistance occurs even with prolonged antibiotic use,[5] and (3) most antibiotic resistance is gained by the transfer of genetic material between microbes, which is greatly enhanced by low-dose, prolonged antibiotic therapy.[47] Combination antibiotic therapy against the stepped resistance seen with *Mycobacterium tuberculosis* is unique for this organism but should not be extrapolated to all microbes. Also, a directive to "take all the antibiotic" assumes that the prescriber knows exactly how long the duration of the infection will be, which is not possible.

Microbial resistance is most likely to occur when subtherapeutic antibiotic doses are used—those that do not kill or inhibit the microorganism but rather allow it to perceive the chemical as a threat to its survival and to react by mutation to resistance, acquisition, or transfer of resistance genes/virulence factors or induction (expression) of latent resistance genes.[31,47] The gastrointestinal tract is a massive reservoir for resistance genes readily transferred within and between enteric microbial species,[88] a process greatly enhanced by antibiotics that readily induce the expression or transfer of resistance genes: tetracyclines, imipenem, cefoxitin, and clavulanic acid.[77]

Bacteria-carrying resistance genes may have a reduction in "fitness" (a biologic cost) that results in slower growth rates, loss of virulence, and an increased biologic burden (synthesis of nucleic acids). However, studies indicate that many bacteria can adapt to this new genetic burden or even require resistance genes for survival. If this becomes common then removal of the antibiotic from the environment will have little effect on lowering resistance in the hospital or community, a point that may already have been reached with some microbes.

SPECIFIC RESISTANCE MECHANISMS

β-Lactamases

The most important acquired mechanism for β-lactam resistance, particularly in gram-negative microorganisms, is the production of various β-lactamases that hydrolyze the β-lactam ring to form a linear metabolite incapable of binding to PBPs. In 1984, 19 plasmid-mediated β-lactamases were known, with the number now having risen to more than 340 chromosomally and plasmid-mediated β-lactamases—70 of the TEM-1 and TEM-2 and 20 of the SHV-1 types alone.[11]

β-lactamases have been variously classified by Richmond-Sykes (I to V), Ambler (A to D), and Bush (1 to 4).[11] β-Lactamase enzymes can be chromosomally mediated or easily transferred by transposable elements. Many are of the TEM type (from a patient named Temoniera in Greece, in whom a β-lactamase was isolated in the early 1960s) or the SHV type (sulfhydryl variable).[11] The most pressing difficulties with the β-lactamases are their widespread dissemination throughout the microbial environment, ability to move between widely disparate organisms, tendency to rapidly inhibit new antibiotic agents, and increasing resistance to β-lactamase inhibitors (clavulanic acid, sulbactam, and tazobactam). β-Lactamases have been observed in numerous gram-positive and gram-negative pathogens. The cohabitation of staphylococci and enterococci on human skin in hospitals has likely led to the incorporation of β-lactamase genes into enterococci after the latter organisms had successfully avoided this transfer for billions of years.

Point mutations have recently appeared in TEM and SHV β-lactamases, resulting in extended-spectrum β-lactamases in *Klebsiella pneumoniae* that hydrolyze the latest cephalosporins (cefotaxime, ceftazidime, cefepime) and aztreonam. Certain enteric microorganisms *(Escherichia coli, Citrobacter freundii, K. pneumoniae, Proteus mirabilis)* can produce massive amounts of TEM-1 β-lactamase (hyper–β-lactamase producers) that can overwhelm β-lactamase inhibitors. Metallo–β-lactamases possess the broadest spectrum of inhibitory activity and hydrolyze all β-lactam antibiotics except monobactams (aztreonam) and are not inhibited by any of the β-lactamase inhibitors currently available.

Multidrug Antibiotic Efflux Pumps

A mechanism by which bacteria move an antibiotic out of the cell as soon as it enters was first detected in *E. coli* by Levy in 1978; the first gene (*qac*A) encoding a multidrug efflux protein was subsequently detected in an isolate of *S. aureus*.[64] Currently more than 50 such systems have been described, and these cytoplasmic membrane transport proteins (multidrug efflux pumps) have likely evolved to protect the cell from foreign chemical invasion and allow its secretion of cell metabolic products.[106] Efflux pumps operate in *E. coli, Pseudomonas aeruginosa*, staphylococci, *Streptococcus pyogenes* and *pneumoniae*, *Bacillus subtilis, Pasturella multocida, Neisseria gonorrhoeae*, mycobacteria, and enterococci.[106] For the tetracyclines these efflux pumps are the major mechanism for resistance and are becoming increasingly so for the fluoroquinolones.[106] Efflux pumps are classified into five main groups: the major facilitator family; the small/staphylococcal multidrug resistance family; the resistance, nodulation, and cell division family; the adenosine triphosphate binding cassette superfamily; and the multidrug and toxic compound extrusion family.[106]

These chromosomal and plasmid-mediated efflux transporter proteins may be quite specific for antibiotics and metabolic product substrates and are regulated by a number of genes and gene products. Repressors are also present and are highly regulated to prevent the accidental overproduction of efflux pumps. The tetracyclines derepress this system, leading to an overproduction of efflux proteins and increasing resistance to themselves and any other antibiotics carried by these proteins.[75]

Transposable Elements

Microorganisms possess three mechanisms for genetic variation: (1) local nucleotide changes in the genome, (2) rearrangement of genomic sequences, and (3) horizontal acquisition of DNA from other microorganisms. Such genetic alterations have allowed for their evolution and survival for 3.5 billion years. The rearrangement of genes and particularly the acquisition of new genetic information are commonplace and are now the major mechanism controlling microbial resistance to antibiotics.

In the 1950s, McClintock described genetic controlling elements that did not follow the Mendelian laws of genetics and acquired an independent existence (selfish genes, jumping genes). In the early 1970s, Hedges and Jacob first used the term *transposon* for a mobile genetic element conveying resistance to ampicillin. Microbes acquire new genetic information by three mechanisms—transformation, transduction, and conjugation—and use a number of transposable elements such as bacteriophages, transposons, integrons, and plasmids.

During transformation bacteria acquire "naked" DNA from their environment to incorporate into their genome. Such genetic transformations are uncommon and require unique circumstances involving genes, binding, uptake, and integration. On the other hand, at least 50 bacteria are sufficiently competent to acquire environmental genes from their fellow microbes, plants, yeasts, and animals. Both VGS and *S. pneumoniae* have the DNA recognition sites and a quorum-sensing peptide (competence-stimulating peptide) that allows for the acquisition of each other's genes when released into the environment on their death. Because they coinhabit the oropharynx and penicillin resistance occurs in a stepwise manner with gradual amino acid mutations in at least four PBPs for high penicillin resistance, this resistance likely evolved over a period of many years and indicates that transformation is a slow but ultimately efficient mechanism for genetic change.

Transduction is the movement of DNA from one bacterium to another by a bacteriophage (bacterial virus) intermediary. Conjugation is the self-transfer of genetic information by plasmids or transposons to other microorganisms, generally by physical contact with a sex pilus in gram-negative organisms and stimulated by various pheromones (small peptides). Mobile elements commonly require site-specific combination sites but not DNA segment identity, allowing for broad DNA movement. Mobile elements of various types include bacteriophages, transposons, plasmids, integrons, and shufflons.

Transposons are DNA segments that cannot self-replicate but can self-transfer between plasmids, bacteriophages, and chromosomes. Transposons can recruit as many genes as required for their purpose, and the mechanisms that control this process are essentially unknown. That we know so little about a system with so much potential for genetic change is worrisome. Between 30% and 40% of the human genome is composed of transposable element sequences or gene sequences directly derived from them.[22]

Plasmids may be conjugative (self-transmissible) or non-conjugative (unable to effect their own transfer) and may be narrow range (replication in only one or a few hosts) or broad range (replication in many hosts). Too great a concentration of plasmids in one microorganism is usually intolerable because of the high energy costs to maintain it; therefore plasmids have an autoregulatory system (iterons) that allows them to determine their own rate of replication.

Plasmids may also be constitutive (ongoing formation) or inductive (formed only when stimulated or induced by a foreign chemical). Plasmids carry resistance genes and virulence genes or pathogenicity islands that carry all the components necessary to damage the host directly or initiate host responses, such as inflammation, that harm the host. Plasmids are common in oral and gastrointestinal *Bacteroides, Porphyromonas*, and *Prevotella* isolates.

Researchers once hoped that resistance genes and their transporters would pose such a fitness problem for bacteria (requiring so much energy) that bacteria no longer exposed to the antibiotic would lose their resistance genes. However, such genes may become so important for bacterial functions that they become permanent. The tetracycline efflux pumps can become necessary for bacterial survival by functioning in Na^+-K^+ exchange across the bacterial membrane.[7] The problem is compounded when the resistance gene for a particular antibiotic becomes part of an integron-containing multiple antibiotic resistance gene array. Eliminating the one antibiotic does nothing; all the antibiotics must be eliminated from the environment for the integron to be lost.

Integrons

Antibiotic resistance has been further enhanced by the discovery of the integron, a genetic element that captures and disseminates genes by site-specific integration of DNA (gene cassettes) that can mediate resistance, virulence, and biochemical functions.[73] Integrons have three distinct genes encoding for an integrase enzyme, a recombination site, and a promoter element.[73] Integrons resemble bundled products with a computer operating system; they package resistance determinants to allow for widespread gene dissemination.

Each gene is a cassette, and up to five genes may commonly be present in one integron.[73] Recently, superintegrons have been isolated in *Vibrio cholerae* that contain hundreds of gene cassettes that encode many bacterial functions beyond those of resistance and virulence. Gene cassettes have been identified for all antibiotics except fluoroquinolones, and they also exist for quaternary ammonium compounds. Integrons cannot promote self-transfer because they lack transporter genes but they are commonly associated with transposons and conjugative plasmids.

MICROBIAL RESISTANCE: DISEASE AND ORGANISM INSTITUTIONAL RESISTANCE

Nosocomial Infections

A nosocomial infection (NI) is an infection neither present nor incubating at hospital admission that develops at least 48 hours after admission without proven prior incubation. The CDC has variously estimated that of the 40 million people hospitalized in the United States annually, 2 to 4 million have an NI, resulting in 90,000 deaths.[64] The CDC estimates 500,000 surgical site infections annually with 20,000 annual deaths. This has been estimated to result in one death every 6 minutes from an NI with the likelihood of an NI increasing by 6% per hospital day. In other parts of the world morbidity and mortality rates for NIs may reach 25%. The mortality rate for methicillin-resistant *S. aureus* (MRSA) and nosocomial pneumonia is 50% even with vancomycin therapy, and the mortality rate from bloodstream intensive care unit NIs is also 50%, which may alone account for 150,000 deaths.[64] In the preantibiotic era, the mortality rate from gram-negative bacteremia was 30% to 40%; in the antibiotic era it may approach 25% to 40%.

As astounding as these CDC numbers are, they may be a significant underestimate of the true devastation of NIs[111] because pathologists commonly list the cause of death by general pathologic diagnosis rather than the causative microorganisms; multiple cause-of-death data do not allow for extraction of microbial causation information. If the microbial cause of death were listed rather than the terminal result, such as congestive heart failure, renal failure, or respiratory failure/cardiac arrest (the eventual cause of death for everyone), the reported NI mortality rate would likely make the list of the 10 leading causes of death in the United States,[93,111] with fatal bloodstream NIs alone ranking from fourth to eighth on this list.[64,110]

The major offending nosocomial pathogens are currently MRSA, methicillin-resistant coagulase-negative staphylococci (MRCoNS; vancomycin-resistant enterococci (VRE); multiple-antibiotic-resistant *S. pneumoniae*; *Candida*; and extended-spectrum or ampicillin C (ampC) β-lactamase–producing *K. pneumoniae*, *P. aeruginosa*, *P. mirabilis*, *Citrobacter*, and *Enterobacter*, with a rising incidence of vancomycin– or glycopeptide–intermediate-resistant *S. aureus* strains (vancomycin–intermediate-resistant *S. aureus* and glycopeptide–intermediate-resistant *S. aureus*, *VISA*, *GISA*). Approximately 50% to 60% of all nosocomial pathogens are resistant to multiple antibiotics, and in some intensive care units there is a 27% to 70% chance of acquiring an infection from one of these organisms.[64]

Long-Term Care Facilities

Currently 2.5 million people reside in long-term care facilities (LTCFs) in the United States; approximately 43% of the US population that turned 65 years in 1990 will spend time in a LTCF.[64] Pneumonia caused by *S. pneumoniae*, *S. aureus*, and *P. aeruginosa* is a major cause of death, with LTCF infection rates of 5 to 15 of 100 residents a month or 5 to 6 per 100 resident days. Antibiotics account for 40% of all drugs used in LTCFs, with 50% to 70% of residents receiving at least one antibiotic per year. Some or much of this antibiotic use is considered inappropriate.[64]

LTCFs have become septic reservoirs for highly and multiply antibiotic-resistant microorganisms: MRSA, MRCoNS, VRE, *E. coli*, *Enterobacter*, and *Citrobacter*. The oropharynx, external nares, and skin are often colonized with these microorganisms. Of particular concern is *K. pneumoniae* expressing extended spectrum and ampC β-lactamases conferring resistance to the carbapenems and third-generation cephalosporins, which are then transferred to acute care hospitals on admission of LTCF residents, with the return transfer of multiply antibiotic-resistant organisms from the acute care facility to the LTCF.

Day Care Centers

Microorganism transmission at day care centers (DCCs) is endemic through contaminated body fluids (saliva, urine, feces) and fomites (toys, other surfaces).[64] The most commonly transmitted diseases are respiratory (rhinitis, sinusitis, pharyngitis, bronchitis, and pneumonia). Causative organisms include adenovirus types II and V, respiratory syncytial virus, parainfluenza virus B, influenza type B, *Neisseria meningitidis*, and *Mycobacterium* tuberculosis. Diarrhea caused by rotavirus, adenovirus, *Shigella*, *Salmonella*, *E. coli*, *Yersinia enterocolitica*, *Giardia lamblia*, and *Entamoeba histolytica* is the second most common affliction.

Other DCC-transmitted diseases include otitis media, herpesviruses, hepatitis A and B, and whooping cough.[65] Critical factors for disease transmission are the age of the child (toilet training, immune system maturity) and the size of the facility (the larger the size, the greater the number of infections). Of greater significance is the finding that 20% to 60% of children attending DCCs are carriers of antibiotic-resistant *S. pneumoniae*. Antimicrobial use both individually and in the general community is strongly associated with nasopharyngeal carriage of penicillin-resistant *S. pneumoniae* in children.[65] In an 8-month study of child care centers, the prevalence of antibiotic use was 36% versus 7% in child care homes and 8% in the child's own home.[76] The annual rate of antibiotic use is 3.6 times greater in child care centers than in the home and five times longer in duration.[64]

Tradition holds that MRSA is found only in institutions (hospitals, LTCFs); however, MRSA is now a community pathogen and is increasingly detected in children and adults with no known risk factors such as recent hospitalizations, prolonged antibiotic therapy, or contact with hospital personnel. In a study of two DCCs, 3% of children at one and 24% of children at another were carriers of MRSA; a third DCC exhibited a 24.4% carriage rate.[64] Fortunately, some MRSA may be susceptible to tetracycline, clindamycin, trimethoprim/sulfamethoxazole, rifampin, gentamicin, and vancomycin.

AGRICULTURAL MICROBIAL RESISTANCE

Antibiotic use in agricultural animals (beef and veal cattle, broiler chickens, and hogs) began after World War II to treat bovine mastitis and to act as a growth promoter, resulting in a 4% to 6% increase in animal body weight. As early as 1972 the US Food and Drug Administration (FDA) found widespread antibiotic resistance in *Salmonella* isolates.

Currently 25 million pounds of antibiotics (primarily tetracyclines, streptomycin and penicillin, and fluoroquinolones) are used annually in animal husbandry in the United States, and 50,000 pounds are sprayed on fruit trees.[64] This results in significant concentrations of free antibiotics or their microbial resistance genes in the possibly 1.4 billion tons of manure placed on the soil of the United States annually.

The Environmental Protection Agency has found antibiotics in wells and groundwater not removed by filtration plants in several states, presumably leached from lagoons of manure.

In Denmark, 24 kg of vancomycin were used in human beings and 24,000 kg of avoparcin (a vancomycin analogue) were used in animal feed in 1994, and from 1992 to 1996 Australia imported 582 kg per year of vancomycin for human use and 62,642 kg of avoparcin for animal husbandry.[65] Avoparcin use was never approved in the United States but has been responsible for a high carriage rate of VRE in the European population. In Dutch fecal pig samples, *E. coli* has demonstrated a resistance rate of 70% to 94% to amoxicillin, 78% to 98% to oxytetracycline, 62% to 96% to tetracycline, 24% to 46% to vancomycin, and 6% to 8% to quinupristin-dalfopristin. The issue is an important one because the CDC estimates more than 6 million cases of food poisoning annually in the United States with 325,000 hospitalizations and 5000 deaths.[64]

The evidence is unequivocal that agricultural antibiotic use has contributed to multiply antibiotic resistant microorganisms resistant to ampicillin, amoxicillin, tetracycline, erythromycin, aminoglycosides, chloramphenicol, sulfonamides, methicillin/oxacillin, vancomycin, everinomycin, and streptogramins.[64] These resistance genes are carried by staphylococci, *Salmonella, Campylobacter, Enterococcus, E. coli,* and *Y. enterocolitica,* with the same molecular gene patterns in both animals and human beings indicating gene transfer between species. Antibiotic-resistant *Enterobacter, E. coli,* and *Salmonella* have been found on vegetables and meat, posing a risk of transfer to the home environment.[29,101]

The use of antibiotics as growth promoters has been banned in Sweden since 1986, and in the past few years Denmark, Finland, Norway, and Germany have done the same with no detrimental effects on competition in the European Union food market and at no increase in costs. The prevalence of VRE has declined in some areas, but not always if the genes are linked in transposable elements with other resistance or virulence genes.[2] In Denmark the VRE resistance gene was not reduced in the population until tylosin (an erythromycin analogue) was also banned because both genes were found on the same plasmid.[2]

In 1969 the Swan Committee in the United Kingdom recommended that no antibiotic be used in farm animals if the same drug is used in human beings and selects for antibiotic resistance. More than 30 years have passed with little attention to these recommendations, with the exception of the aforementioned European countries.

RESISTANCE IN MAJOR MICROBIAL PATHOGENS

Streptococcus pneumoniae

Microbial resistance to antibiotics in *S. pneumoniae* is most serious because the organism is responsible for 3000 cases of meningitis, 50,000 cases of bacteremia, 500,000 cases of pneumonia, and 2 million cases of otitis media in the United States annually and 3 to 5 million deaths annually worldwide.[64] Resistance to the sulfonamides was first detected in 1943 and to penicillin in the late 1960s in Australia and New Guinea. The mechanism of penicillin resistance is a single point mutation in PBP2x or PBP2b, with an altered PBP2a requiring mutation also in pBP2x (the organism has six PBPs).

High penicillin resistance (usually a plasma concentration of 2 μg/ml or greater) is seen in 14% of US, 6.8% in Canadian, 10.4% in European, and 17.8% in Asian-Pacific isolates.[37] Resistance of the pneumococcus to penicillin can vary significantly with geographic area, for example, 38.8% in Tennessee, 15.3% in Maryland, 65.3% in Japan, 60.8% in Vietnam, 15.6% to 48.2% in Latin America, and 79.7% in Korea.[64]

Tolerance to vancomycin has been detected in an isolate responsible for meningitis as well as high-level resistance to quinupristin-dalfopristin and cefotaxime. Tetracycline resistance in *S. pneumoniae* is currently low but is increasing, which may pose a significant problem because doxycycline has become an important drug for community and nosocomial-acquired pneumonia caused by *S. pneumoniae, Mycoplasma pneumoniae, Legionella pneumophila,* and *Chlamydia pneumoniae.*

Methicillin-Resistant Staphylococci

In a 1999 review of more than 10,000 bloodstream infections at 49 US hospitals, *S. aureus* accounted for 16% and CoNS for 32% of all isolates, with most of the CoNS being methicillin resistant.[64] Some isolates are only susceptible to vancomycin, others are susceptible to linezolid and quinupristin-dalfopristin, and still others are susceptible to older agents such as macrolides, tetracyclines, aminoglycosides, rifampin, clindamycin, sulfonamides, and fluoroquinolones. The mechanism of methicillin resistance is an altered PBP2 (PBP2a or PBP2′) conferred through a *mec*A gene that results in a much lower binding affinity of methicillin for the PBP2a. This mode of resistance requires the cooperation of both PBP2 and PBP2a sites and two enzymes, one natural and one environmentally acquired.

The first MRSA isolate was detected in the United Kingdom in 1961 and was rare in the United States until 1976. MRSA then spread throughout the hospital by nasal secretions, hands, clothing, bedding, air currents, fomites, and skin boils (furuncles). The anterior nares is the prime carrier site of *S. aureus* in human beings, with 80% of people either persistent or intermittent carriers and possibly up to 25% of healthy persons colonized with CoNS. High concentrations of staphylococci are also found in the throat, axilla, and perineum (groin and upper thighs).

Enterococci

Of the 17 species of enterococci found in the human oral cavity and gastrointestinal and genitourinary tracts, *Enterococcus faecalis* accounts for 90% of human infections and *E. faecium* for approximately 10%.[64] Enterococcal infections are classic examples of a relatively harmless commensal organism becoming a serious pathogen by the acquisition of multiple resistance genes.

Enterococci are intrinsically resistant to the cephalosporins and have varying degrees of resistance to aminoglycosides, macrolides, tetracyclines, and clindamycin. Vancomycin resistance, particularly in *E. faecium*, has been of major concern since the late 1980s. Enterococci cause 800,000 NIs annually in the United States, with more than 50% caused by vancomycin-resistant *E. faecium;* resistance is more than 90% in *E. faecium* bacteremias. Currently 17% of enterococcal strains in the United States are resistant to vancomycin.[49] VRE infections, particularly of the bloodstream type, are becoming extremely difficult to treat. Doxycycline has recently been enlisted in the treatment of VRE.[49] Enterococcal resistance is further complicated by the observations that (1) streptococci, staphylococci, and enterococci often share the same resistance genes; (2) the β-lactamase in enterococci is identical to that in staphylococci, indicating sharing of genetic information; (3) enterococci can transfer resistance genes, particularly for vancomycin to staphylococci and other organisms, in vitro and animal models; (4) staphylococci and enterococci coinhabit the skin; and (5) the possibility exists that vancomycin resistance may one day appear in many VGS.[64]

Helicobacter Pylori

Chronic gastritis, peptic ulcer, and gastric cancer have been linked to *H. pylori.* Depending on the geographic area and the prevalence of antibiotic use, alarming reports have appeared of resistance to all antibiotic agents used in its management: metronidazole, clarithromycin, tetracycline, and amoxicillin. Resistance to metronidazole acquired by a decreased ability to reduce its nitro group ranges from 10% to 50% in developed countries and up to 100% in developing countries, where it is widely used to treat parasitic diseases. Resistance to amoxicillin ranges from 0% in The Netherlands to 18% in Mexico to 72% in Shanghai, China. Resistance to clarithromycin ranges from 1.7% in The Netherlands to 10% to 12% in the United States to 24% in Mexico.

Tetracycline has recently been added to antibiotic regimens, and resistance rates are 0% in The Netherlands, 5.3% in Korea, and 58.8% in Shanghai, China, with the disturbing possibility that tetracycline-resistant *H. pylori* may exhibit cross-resistance with metronidazole. Metronidazole resistance in *H. pylori* may decrease the effectiveness of *its* therapy by 37.7% and clarithromycin resistance by 55%.[24] The widespread use of systemic metronidazole and tetracycline is difficult to justify in the management of a relatively trivial, mechanically responsive disease such as periodontitis when such a practice may promote resistance in a microbial pathogen responsible for very serious diseases such as peptic ulcer and gastric cancer.

Human Immunodeficiency Virus

The current therapy for HIV infection entails highly active antiretroviral therapy (HAART; see Chapter 40) with a combination of drugs that interfere with several steps in viral replication: reverse transcriptase inhibitors, protease inhibitors, and the new integrase inhibitors that prevent HIV from integrating into the genome of the host cell. Difficulties have arisen with this therapeutic approach because the virus provides for reservoirs of replication-competent HIV in resting CD4 T lymphocytes throughout many years of intensive HAART. It is estimated that more than 60 years of HAART may be necessary to eradicate the virus from these reservoirs.[64] More than 50% of HIV-infected persons in the United States receiving HAART are resistant to one or more of the drugs, and 78% of those with measurable viral loads are resistant to at least one drug, encompassing about 100,000 people in the United States.[94] From 1994 to 2000, 14% of new HIV cases had one or more HIV mutations associated with antiretroviral drug resistance; in 2000 it was 27%. Approximately 25% of newly infected, therapy-naïve people carry at least one key HIV drug-resistant mutant.[72]

ANTIBIOTIC RESISTANT DISEASES

Otitis Media

Antibiotic therapy of middle ear infections is second only to upper respiratory tract infections as a cause of microbial resistance in the community. The microorganisms are *S. pneumoniae* (20% to 50%), *H. influenzae* (10% to 30%), and *M. catarrhalis* (5% to 20%), with penicillin resistance rates of 31% for *S. pneumoniae,* 31% to 57% for *H. influenzae,* and more than 90% for *M. catarrhalis.*[64] The longer the antibiotic treatment for otitis media, the greater the pressure for selection of drug-resistant *S. pneumoniae.* Consequently the therapy of otitis media may now require very high doses of amoxicillin or second- and third-generation cephalosporins.

Malaria

Malaria accounts for 500,000 to 2 million deaths annually worldwide. Resistance to sulfadoxime and pyrimethamine is widespread in South America and East Asia and chloroquine resistance is high in Africa, but resistance to amodiaquine, quinine, and quinidine is only moderate.[112] Resistance to the antimalarials is a classic example of the deleterious effects of suboptimal doses of antimicrobials because resistance rises most rapidly in *Plasmodia* when exposed to subtherapeutic concentrations with long half-life drugs and for long periods of time.[112]

Tuberculosis

Multidrug-resistant *Mycobacterium tuberculosis* has emerged as a major health problem, with a 9% to 12% prevalence rate of resistance to one and 2.2% to two first-line drugs (isoniazid and rifampin) in 35 countries. Directly observed treatment to ensure patient compliance has reduced single-drug resistance but is less successful for multidrug-resistant strains and does not prevent their transmission. The use of second-line drugs results in a 4 to 10 times greater failure rate and 100 times greater cost.

The antimicrobial chemotherapy of tuberculosis is different from other microbial infections because the causative organism has a long generation time, dormancy, and low metabolic activity and is commonly located in areas where antibiotic penetration is poor, such as empyema purulence, pulmonary cavities, and solid caseous material. Resistance to the drugs used against tuberculosis (isoniazid, rifampin, pyrazinamide, ethambutol, aminoglycosides, fluoroquinolones, ethionamide, clarithromycin, and cycloserine) is almost exclusively gained by chromosomal mutations with only rare transposable elements.

SPECIFIC ANTIMICROBIAL AGENT RESISTANCE

Vancomycin

The long-feared arrival of vancomycin resistance in MRSA was realized in El Salvador, Japan, France, and the United States between 1996 and 1999.[64] Because the glycopeptides (vancomycin, teicoplanin) are the only consistently effective agents against MRSA, the appearance of such resistance has the potential for microbiologic disaster because 50% of nosocomial *S. aureus* and 80% of CoNS are methicillin resistant. Fortunately, some of these strains are at least for now susceptible to streptogramins, tetracyclines, trimethoprim/sulfamethoxazole, chloramphenicol, and fluoroquinolones. Recently streptogramin resistance has been reported in GISA. Vancomycin tolerance is now found in *S. pneumoniae,* group G streptococci, *Streptococcus bovis, Streptococcus mitis,* and *Staphylococcus epidermidis* and *haemolyticus.* Possibly 2% to 3% of all *S. pneumoniae* strains are tolerant to vancomycin.[60] In 1994, 61% of all surveyed hospitals reported VRE versus 23% in 1992.[64] The mortality rates for bloodstream infections with VRE is 36% versus 16% for vancomycin-sensitive enterococci. Five genes (*van*A, *van*B, *van*C, *van*D, *van*E) modulate vancomycin resistance with spread by all transposable elements.

One mechanism of vancomycin resistance is caused by an altered peptidoglycan terminus of D-ala-D-lac rather than the usual D-ala-D-ala, which results in reduced vancomycin binding and failure to prevent rigid cell wall synthesis.[13] Resistance in VISA may be caused by the production of abnormal mucopeptides (false binding sites) in the cell wall that bind vancomycin and prevent its access to the peptidoglycan receptor or increase peptidoglycan within the cell wall to produce thickened cell walls.[14] The mechanism for vancomycin tolerance in *S. pneumoniae* is unique: a mutation in the sensor-response system controlling autolysin activity necessary to kill bacteria.[64] This sensor system is also required for the bactericidal activity of the β-lactams, fluoroquinolones, and aminoglycosides.

Macrolides

Within 1 year of its introduction in 1952, erythromycin resistance was detected in the United States, Japan, and Europe; after 6 months of use at the Boston City Hospital virtually all staphylococci were resistant to the drug. The current global resistance rate for erythromycin is approaching epidemic proportions. In the United States, resistance in *S. pneumoniae* and *S. pyogenes* has reached 40% to 60% in some areas. In Taiwan, where the macrolides are over-the-counter drugs, resistance rates are among the highest in the world: 80% for MRSA, 30% for methicillin-sensitive *S. aureus,* 58% for *S. pneumoniae,* and 42% for *S. pyogenes.* In a 1995 to 1999 CDC study of 15,481 invasive isolates of *S. pneumoniae,* macrolide use increased 13% in adults and 320% in children younger than 5 years, and macrolide resistance increased from 10.6% of isolates in 1995 to 20.4% in 1999.[64]

In 66 VGS isolates from the blood of neutropenic cancer patients, 68.8% of those highly resistant to penicillin were also resistant to erythromycin, as were 43.6% of the *S. mitis* isolates.[64] Of much concern is the ability of VGS to confer the *mef*A resistance gene (M phenotype) to *S. pneumoniae* and *S. pyogenes* because 50% to 60% of the VGS in the pharynx possess the M phenotype. VGS may provide a reservoir for erythromycin resistance genes available for transfer to various other streptococci.

The principal mechanism for resistance to the macrolides is by an *erm* (*e*rythromycin *r*esistant *m*ethylase) gene encoding an enzyme that catalyzes the demethylation of the 2058 residue of bacterial 23S ribosomal RNA, resulting in decreased macrolide binding to its ribosomal receptor site (a ribosomal protection mechanism).[64] The *erm* genes are both constitutive and inducible with induction on exposure to the 14- and 15-membered but not the 16-membered macrolides. Approximately 21 *erm* genes have been identified.[79] *Erm* genes are often associated with other antibiotic resistance genes, particularly those for tetracycline (*tet*Q, *tet*M), making it possible to select for resistance to both drugs while using only one. Macrolide resistance genes are also commonly combined with resistance genes for the lincosamides (clindamycin) and streptogramins (quinupristin-dalfopristin) in the MLS_B aggregate. Because resistance has now been detected in the new ketolide analogues of the macrolides, a new designation has arisen of MLKS resistance (*m*acrolide, *l*incosamide, *k*etolide, *s*treptogramin).

Other macrolide resistance mechanisms include active efflux encoded by *mef*A and *mef*E genes for 14- and 15-membered macrolides and esterification by phosphorylation or glycosylation to inactivate the macrolides.[79]

Fluoroquinolones

Resistance to the fluoroquinolones was detected early after their introduction and was easily predictable because it required only a single point mutation and its precursor, nalidixic acid, demonstrated rapid resistance development. Unfortunately, little attention was paid to this potential for serious difficulties with this group of antibiotics.

Resistance to the fluoroquinolones is chromosomally mediated by three mechanisms: (1) target alteration by point mutations for DNA gyrase (serine 83 and aspartate 87 of *gyr*A) and topoisomerase IV (serine 79 and aspartate 83 of *par*C), (2) active efflux pumps, and (3) reduction in permeability from loss of outer membrane protein F (OmpF). No bacterial enzyme capable of metabolizing the fluoroquinolones has yet been detected, and the significance of a transferable resistance plasmid in *K. pneumoniae* is unknown. Microorganisms displaying efflux mechanisms include VGS, staphylococci, enterococci, *S. pneumoniae, Enterobacteriaceae, P. aeruginosa, Campylobacter jejunum, Bacteroides fragilis,* and *N. gonorrhoeae.*

Clinical microbial resistance to the fluoroquinolones has become widespread, necessitating the development of newer agents that are only marginally better than the older agents and still susceptible to the same resistance mechanisms. Resistance in *N. gonorrhoeae* rose in Japan from 6.6% in 1993 to 1994 to 24.4% in 1997 to 1998.[64] A single 500-mg antibiotic prophylaxis dose of ciprofloxacin increased the percentage of resistant *E. coli* in the colon from 3% to 12%.[108]

Tetracyclines

Microbial resistance to the tetracyclines is widespread, inducible, transposable, and sometimes permanent because the genes for tetracycline resistance are commonly associated with other antibiotic resistance genes on transposons, bacteriophages, and plasmids. None of these resistance genes may be lost until all antibiotics whose resistance genes are carried on the transposable element are eliminated from the environment or, conversely, tetracycline may select for all antibiotic resistance genes carried on the element. Because tetracyclines have been rediscovered as effective therapy for nosocomial VRE and MRSA and community-acquired *S. pneumoniae* and *H. pylori,* the unwarranted use of tetracycline poses potentially serious clinical difficulties.

Three mechanisms exist for tetracycline resistance: drug efflux pumps, ribosomal protection, and enzymatic inactivation.[16] At least 29 different tetracycline resistance genes *(tet)* have been characterized, with at least 19 for specific and nonspecific efflux pumps, eight for ribosomal protection, and the *tet*X gene for enzymatic activation.[16] Resistance determinants encoding at least one of these mechanisms is likely in most genera of bacteria.

The major mechanism for tetracycline resistance is drug efflux and *tet* efflux genes that encode at least 300 different active efflux proteins[16] and in gram-negative bacteria are widely distributed and associated with large conjugative plasmids that carry resistance genes for other antibiotics, heavy metals, bacterial toxins, and virulence factors. Any chemical that selects for one of these genes can select for them all. Nine genes encode for cytoplasmic ribosomal proteins that bind to the ribosome to alter its configuration and prevent tetracycline from attaching to its receptor.[16] Enzymatic inactivation is encoded by a *tet*X gene currently present only in *Bacteroides.* Mutation in the *tet*A and *tet*B genes promotes efflux resistance in the new glycylcyclines.

Since the 1970s, resistance to the tetracyclines has become common in *Enterobacteriaceae,* staphylococci, streptococci, *Bacteroides, H. influenzae,* and *P. aeruginosa,* ranging from 25% to 97% of all isolates.[16] Considering the close association of tetracycline resistance genes with transposable elements, this is not surprising. Thirty-nine genera of gram-negative bacteria and 23 of gram-positive organisms have acquired tetracycline resistance with an ongoing process of new gene discovery. Oral VGS have acquired *tet*M, *tet*O, *tet*L, and *tet*K genes, as have *S. pneumoniae* and *S. pyogenes.*

Not only is tetracycline almost exclusively associated with multiple drug resistance, it may also induce bacterial expression of resistance genes. The drug also downregulates a repressor gene that controls efflux mechanisms. Only nanomolar amounts of tetracycline are necessary to derepress this efflux control system. After that, regardless of the concentration, tetracycline can stimulate its own microbial cell efflux and that of other intracellular chemicals.

Subinhibitory levels of tetracycline that are allegedly insufficient to prevent microbial growth or stimulate resistance as used in agriculture and some therapeutic regimens increase antibiotic resistance in streptococci and staphylcococci.[64] Tetracycline promotes gene transfer by stimulating the frequency of bacterial conjugation, and colonic *E. coli* may only express tetracycline and other resistance genes when the drug is present. Resistance gene (*tet*Q) transfer in the colon is widespread and occurs readily by conjugative transfer with more than 95% of DNA sequence homology with *erm*F and *erm*G genes for erythromycin.[88]

With standard tetracycline doses, within 24 hours more than 95% of coliform bacteria in the gastrointestinal tract show resistance to tetracycline that lasts as long as the drug is present and for at least 4 to 6 months or longer in some cases after tetracycline is discontinued.[71] Family members of people taking the tetracyclines for acne may have a 1000 times greater chance of multidrug-resistant bacteria than those whose members do not take tetracycline.[55]

For a long time it was assumed that the massive resistance to tetracyclines observed from the 1960s to the 1980s would always remain and that the drugs were essentially useless against most major pathogens, particularly those of a nosocomial nature. To the contrary, recent clinical studies document a very low level of tetracycline resistance (in some studies 1.3%) in common outpatient pathogens: *S. pneumoniae, H. influenzae,* C. *pneumoniae* and *trachomatis, M. pneumoniae* and *hominis,* and *Ureaplasma urealyticum.* Tetracyclines have now become accepted, if not primary, antibiotics against community-acquired *S. pneumoniae* and many are life saving against VRE and MRSA.[64]

The advocates of long-term low doses of doxycycline for periodontitis maintain that such doses produce a maximum blood level of 0.79 ± 0.285 μg/ml and that such blood/tissue levels do not adversely affect oral bacteria or increase levels of resistance.[102] Limited data are presented regarding resistance in other body areas (colon, skin). Ample evidence suggests that such blood levels of tetracyclines, particularly doxycycline, are therapeutic and even life saving at 0.06 to 0.25 μg/ml or lower, many times below the 0.79 ± 0.285 μg/ml or less seen with 20 mg twice/day.[64] A choice must be made between long-term therapy with tetracycline for whatever benefit, if any, it may have in periodontitis and the possibility of losing these drugs again by resistance development for serious and sometimes life-threatening diseases.

Triclosan and Other Biocides

Approximately 75% of liquid soaps and 30% of bar soaps (average, 45%) in the United States contain triclosan or triclocarban, and both chemicals are widely found in toothpastes, plastics, towels, carpets, woods, food preparation surfaces, paints, and other personal use products (more than 700 to date). Triclosan is a broad-spectrum antimicrobial agent touted to have a nonspecific mechanism of action that does not foster microbial resistance. This concept may no longer be tenable because triclosan specifically inhibits an enoyl-aryl protein reductase enzyme to alter microbial cell membrane fatty acid synthesis. Resistance to triclosan in *E. coli* is by mutation in the *fabl* gene for this carrier protein, resulting in increased triclosan minimal inhibitory concentrations (MICs).[70] If a specific enzyme is involved in triclosan activity then resistance is feasible and awaits further delineation. Similar reductase resistance targets have been detected in *S. aureus* and *P. aeruginosa,* and an efflux pump mechanism has been observed in *E. coli* and *P. aeruginosa* that is intrinsically resistant to triclosan.

Microbial resistance to other biocides, disinfectants, and antiseptics is increasingly documented with a multidrug resistance plasmid (pSAJ1) carrying resistance genes to aminoglycosides, chlorhexidine, benzalkonium chloride, and ethidium bromide and transferable to *E. coli.* Microbes that express the *mar* regulon (Mar protein) are resistant to tetracyclines, chloramphenicol, triclosan, and pine oil. Quaternary ammonium resistance is mediated by *qac* A-E genes for efflux mechanisms in staphylococci, pseudomonads, and *Enterobacteriaceae* with sequence homology to tetracycline efflux genes. A significant risk exists that widespread biocide use will result in increased resistance to these topical products in clinical pathogens and also to systemic antibiotics, particularly if biocide resistance genes are carried on the same transposable elements as antibiotic resistance genes.

Heavy Metal Resistance

Microbial resistance to the heavy metals (e.g., silver, mercury, lead) is widespread in nature among varied microorganisms. The most widely studied has been mercury resistance both systemically and in the oral cavity. Not only do microorganisms develop genetic resistance mechanisms to the toxic effects of heavy metals (mercury damages thiol-containing enzymes), but these genes are also associated with antibiotic-resistance genes (penicillin, aminoglycosides, tetracyclines, chloramphenicol) in transposable elements and induce the transfer of resistance genes among microorganisms.[114]

Six heavy metal resistance mechanisms have been detected: (1) reduced membrane permeability, (2) active efflux, (3) intracellular sequestration by proteins, (4) extracellular sequestration, (5) enzymatic intracellular detoxification, and (6) target modification.[10] Reduced membrane permeability is relatively simple, but the major resistance mechanism is active efflux with the adenosine triphosphatase energy-driven system. Metallothioneins sequester metals intracellularly to prevent access to vital cellular constituents, whereas yeast and fungi secrete glutathione that binds heavy metals extracellularly to prevent access to the outer membrane. Mercury resistance genes of the *mer* operon code for two enzymes: organomercurial lyase, which hydrolyzes the mercury-carbon bond in organomercurial compounds, and mercuric ion reductase, which reduces mercury to its metal ion form for ready efflux.[10] Narrow-spectrum, mercury-resistant organisms have only the *mer*A gene for mercuric ion reductase, and broad-spectrum–resistant organisms possess both the *mer*A and *mer*B genes for both enzymes, making the broad-spectrum organisms resistant to mercury in all its organic and inorganic forms.[10]

Controversy has arisen regarding the potential effect of dental amalgam mercury on the resistance patterns of oral and fecal bacteria (interestingly, silver has not been studied). Monkeys given 12 to 16 occlusal amalgams at one time demonstrated that shortly after placement, mercury-resistant bacteria increased in the oral cavity and feces and were associated with resistance to several antibiotics (ampicillin, tetracycline, aminoglycosides).[114] Clinical studies in three separate populations (persons in whom all amalgams had been removed, those never having had an amalgam, and persons with a varying number of amalgams) demonstrated no differences in the MICs of oral and fecal microorganisms in their resistance patterns to tetracycline, chlorhexidine, cefuroxime, penicillin, and mercury chloride.[45,61]

The animal studies placed a very high number of amalgams at one time with no data on their mercury content or the occlusal volume of the restoration and studied the resistance patterns for a maximum of 12 weeks, at which time the fecal mercury level had fallen so low as to not present any selective advantage to resistance.[98] If the mercury resistance genes are only transient and are later lost, then the effect of mercury on the oral and fecal bacteria would likely be insignificant. Conversely, if the metal resistance genes become permanent residents of the oral or fecal flora, associate as part of a multidrug-resistant transposable element, or significantly induce resistance gene transfer among bacteria, then a significant problem could exist. At least one study documents such gene transfer[114]; further study is warranted. Currently no compelling evidence indicates that dental amalgam possesses any significant long-term adverse effect on microbial resistance patterns in the oral or fecal flora.

New vaccines are on the horizon against staphylococci, enterococci, and VGS. New antibiotics will be developed but progress in developing new classes of drugs is limited. Meanwhile, the public, agribusiness, and health practitioners must use antimicrobial agents with much wisdom and circumspection. In the words of Norman Simmons: "We screwed up, and we ought to say so and apologize. Doctors were handed the wonderful gift of antibiotics but are destroying them through indiscriminate use. We know what to do, we should use them less."[91]

FACTORS INFLUENCING ANTIMICROBIAL THERAPY

The goal of microbial culture and sensitivity testing is to predict the outcome of treatment for an infection managed with an antibiotic agent. Identification of the microorganism(s) allows for the ideal choice of antimicrobial agent. Empirical antibiotic therapy remains satisfactory for infections in which the microbial cause is likely to be either routinely predictable or unlikely to be associated with drug-resistant strains but may not be satisfactory for nonpredictable infections.[39]

The mere recovery of an organism from an infection does not necessarily indicate that it is involved in disease causation.[58] Orofacial infections are characterized by a rapid onset, prompt resolution with the elimination of the source, and a multiplicity of potential pathogens. Orofacial infections differ substantially from infections elsewhere in the body, where the onset is typically slow with protracted resolution and commonly monomicrobial in causation with rarely an opportunity to perform incision and drainage. Orofacial infections, if treated properly and caused by antibiotic-sensitive organisms, are commonly in remission before the culture tests are available. Because of their polymicrobial cause, determining the etiologic pathogens is difficult to impossible.

The issue of whether microbial culture and sensitivity tests are required or even desirable for the management of orofacial infections has been debated.[32,109] Because of the clinical features of orofacial infections (rapid onset and resolution, polymicrobial nature, well-established pathogens), routine culture and sensitivity tests are unlikely to be necessary, much less useful, unless the infection is very serious or fails to respond to diligent intervention. Polymicrobial infections defy the detection of the precise offending pathogens. In the future, real-time polymerase chain reaction may be readily and cheaply available.

The breakpoints for MIC determinations are established in the United States by the National Committee for Clinical Laboratory Standards (NCCLS) but can vary widely throughout the United States and the rest of the world. One locale may use 0.1 μg/ml for penicillin resistance, whereas another may use 1.0 μg/ml. These breakpoints should reflect the reasonable blood level of the antibiotic that can be achieved by conventional and practical doses. Sometimes breakpoints are used that, although approved by the NCCLS, cannot be attained in the body except by unusual dosing. The use of such breakpoints can imply lack of resistance when for all clinical purposes the organism is indeed resistant. The NCCLS recommendations are currently under criticism for just such difficulties. As stated by Jacobs et al[38]: "Many of the NCCLS breakpoints are actually higher than the peak concentrations of the agent in serum and tissue, so that clinically achievable concentrations can never reach, let alone exceed, the concentrations needed to inhibit organisms for which the MICs are at or close to the susceptibility breakpoint value."

ANTIBIOTIC PHARMACOKINETICS AND PHARMACODYNAMICS

Despite being used clinically for more than 60 years, antibiotic unit doses, dosing intervals, and duration of therapy are not generally established for the majority of infections.[41,74] Because antibiotics produced such remarkable cures not previously encountered and were essentially nontoxic drugs, clinicians would often forgo clinical trials and merely administer the drug until the patient got well or died. Very few clinical studies were ever performed on dosage, with one of the only being the 10-day therapy for the treatment of streptococcal sore throat, which was then extrapolated to most infections—10 days for all infections regardless of cause and locale. This was another case of an assumption determining therapy without any scientific basis.

Many dosing guidelines are empirical and should not be relied on blindly[6,104]; substantial resistance is encountered to changing package insert dosages even in the light of new data and understanding of antibiotic pharmacokinetics and pharmacodynamics.[34] The formula approach does not take into account mechanism of actions or postantibiotic effects, host-microbe interactions, or whether the antibiotic effect is concentration or time dependent. It does not incorporate clinical data on microorganism virulence, anatomic location of the infection, whether incision and drainage can be established, microbial resistance, the physical signs and symptoms of the patient, and the status of the host defense mechanisms.

Formulas are a poor way to treat multifactorial infections unique to each patient as antibiotic therapy is not an exact science. Suspicion lingers that because of the common practice of inadequate antibiotic dosing, many patients get well by themselves with the antibiotic contributing little to their recovery. A clear understanding of current concepts of antibiotic pharmacokinetics (dose, absorption, distribution, metabolism, excretion) and pharmacodynamics (serum concentrations, dosing, host-microbe interaction, postantibiotic effects) are essential to achieving optimal efficacy and reducing microbial resistance.

PRINCIPLES OF ANTIBIOTIC DOSING

The goal of antibiotic therapy is to aid the body's defenses to clear the tissues of the microbial pathogens by achieving antibiotic levels in the infected area equal to or greater than the MIC.[46] To accomplish this, the organism must be susceptible and the drug concentration must be sufficient at the infected site until the next dose. Local factors that interfere with antibiotic activity must be minimized, with all efforts being made to eliminate the organism(s) physically (incision and drainage). Host defenses need to be adequate to eventually eradicate the pathogen and associated metabolic products (toxins).[46]

Minimal Inhibitory Concentration

The MIC is the lowest antibiotic concentration that prevents growth of microorganisms after an 18- to 24-hour incubation period with a standard organism inoculation of 10^4 to 10^5 cfu/ml. The minimal bactericidal concentration, which is rarely used as a clinical measure, is the lowest concentration of the antibiotic that causes the complete destruction of the organism or permits survival of less than 0.1% of the inoculum. Because the concentration of the antibiotic cannot be measured at the site of the infection, the serum antibiotic concentration and the MIC serve as surrogate markers attempting to quantify antibiotic activity.

Although useful, the MIC has certain inherent difficulties. The MIC is only a point in time and tells nothing about the true antibiotic activity at the locus of the infection (antibiotic pharmacodynamics). The concentration of organisms (inoculum size) at the site of the infection is commonly 10^8 to 10^{10} cfu/ml, many times greater than that used to determine the MIC in the laboratory. The growth of microorganisms in vitro is exponential, whereas growth in vivo can be very slow to none.[46] The laboratory MIC determination is also subject to considerable variables, including temperature, inoculum size, pH, and growth medium, that may substantially differ from those occurring in the patient. However, the MIC can be useful in determining certain guides to antibiotic dosing: (1) the ratio of the peak drug concentration in the serum to the MIC (peak/MIC ratio), (2) the duration of time the serum drug concentration exceeds the MIC (time above the MIC), and (3) the ratio of the 24-hour area under the curve to the MIC (AUC_{24}/MIC ratio).[46] The AUC is the measure of the drug exposure to the bacteria over time. The time above the MIC is very important in the efficacy of the time-dependent β-lactam antibiotics, linezolid, and, to some extent, the macrolides and clindamycin. The ratio of the 24-hour AUC to the MIC is important for the concentration-dependent aminoglycosides and fluoroquinolones. A general rule of thumb is that the concentration of the antibiotic in the blood should exceed the MIC by a factor of two to eight times to offset the tissue barriers that restrict access to the infected site.[58]

All this applies only if the offending microorganism can be cultured and the MICs determined. Such determinations are not commonly performed in outpatient medicine, not as often as they should in hospitals, and virtually never in dentistry. Yet these principles are useful and have led to the concepts of concentration-dependent versus time-dependent antibiotics.

Concentration-Dependent Versus Time-Dependent Antibiotics

Depending on their mechanism of action, some antibiotics are much more effective if very high blood (and presumably tissue) concentrations are reached periodically (peak and trough effects, concentration-dependent) and others are more effective if the blood levels are maintained above the MIC for as long a time as possible (time-dependent). The antibacterial activity of the aminoglycosides, metronidazole, and fluoroquinolones is critically dependent on high drug concentrations at the infected site because the killing rate is proportional to the drug concentration.[46] Conversely, some antibiotics such as the β-lactams and vancomycin are less dependent for their activity on tissue concentrations and are much more effective with a long time of exposure of the microorganism to the antibiotic (time-dependent killing).

Because these agents require organisms in the process of cell division for their activity, antibiotics with slow time-dependent killing should ideally be continually present in the infected area because bacteria divide at different times and at different rates. Bacterial cell walls can only be inhibited while being formed; β-lactams have no effect on cells with fully formed cell walls. The goal of dosing with the cell wall inhibitors is to maximize the time of exposure to active drug levels and maintain their blood and tissue concentrations above the organism's MIC for as long as possible.[46] For pragmatic purposes, the blood/tissue concentrations of the β-lactams should exceed the organism MIC for at least 60% to 70% of the dosing interval for pathogens with a short or no postantibiotic effect and 40% to 50% for those with long postantibiotic effects.[19]

Increasing the dosage of β-lactams to gain tissue concentrations more than four to five times the MIC does not result in increased killing and may even end in a paradoxic or "Eagle effect" in which very high β-lactam concentrations produce reduced rates of microbial killing.[62,65] It may then be theoretically possible to have too high a dose of an antibiotic, but little or no evidence suggests that this paradoxic effect contributes to antibiotic failures.

Time-dependent killing with current package insert dose regimens is relatively easy to achieve with long half-life β-lactams such as amoxicillin but difficult with short half-life penicillin V, cephalexin, or cephradine, which have about 45-minute half-lives or less. If the peak blood level of these agents is achieved 1 hour after oral administration and the standard formulas for half-lives and blood levels are at work (50% of the drug left at one half-life, 25% at two half-lives, 12.5% at three half-lives), at 4 hours from the original dosing, less than 12.5% of the peak blood level of the short-half life β-lactam remains. Unless the organism is very sensitive to the β-lactam (something not known without culture and sensitivity tests), this concentration is unlikely to be above the MIC, leading to at least a 2-hour time period below the MIC because the package insert dosing interval for these agents is typically 6 hours. This considerable time period below the MIC allows for more rapid regrowth of the organism and increased risk of the emergence of resistant strains, both of which are associated with therapeutic failure. Therefore these dosing intervals merit serious reassessment.

Postantibiotic Effects

The concepts of time-dependent or concentration-dependent killing primarily involve bactericidal antibiotics that either inhibit nucleic acid or cell wall synthesis. For bacteriostatic antibiotics (macrolides, clindamycin, tetracyclines) that act by ribosomal protein synthesis inhibition and possess long postantibiotic effects (PAEs), such critical blood and tissue concentrations are considerably less imperative. A PAE is the persistent suppression of microbial growth after short-term exposure to an antimicrobial agent.

The concept of the PAE is gaining increasing interest as an important corollary to concentration-dependent versus time-dependent dosing. The antibiotic concentration may be well below the MIC or the drug may even no longer be present, yet suppression of bacterial replication persists and the organism may be more susceptible to phagocytosis and the postantibiotic leukocyte effect (PALC, the greater susceptibility of microorganisms to white cells after exposure to antibiotics). Humoral and cellular immune processes undergo altered morphologic characteristics and lose their adhesive properties, which may be important in the antibiotic prevention of bacterial endocarditis. The PAE may also render bacteria less susceptible to cell wall inhibitors but allow for longer dosing intervals for bacteriostatic agents.

Virtually all antibiotics have demonstrable PAEs but the duration is most significant with intracellular bacteriostatic agents and least with the β-lactams. Various factors influence the PAE: the particular organism, inoculum size, growth medium, organism growth phase, antibiotic mechanism of action, antibiotic concentration, and exposure time to the antibiotic. β-Lactam antibiotics have a short PAE (1 to 3 hours) in gram-positive organisms and no PAE in gram-negative species. Under ideal circumstances antibiotics that suppress ribosomal protein synthesis may have 5- to 10-hour PAEs, whereas the fluoroquinolones and aminoglycosides possess intermediate PAEs of 2 to 4 hours.[28]

The exact mechanism for PAEs is unknown but is related to the time necessary to recover from sublethal structural and metabolic alterations that prevent resumption of bacterial regrowth (replication).[28] The precise clinical benefits of PAEs are difficult to determine but likely allow for less concern about rigid dosing intervals for bacteriostatic agents and undermine the old clinical adage that bactericidal antibiotics are always superior to bacteriostatic agents.

Microbial Persistence and Regrowth

The next antibiotic dose must be given before significant microbial regrowth can recur.[46] Microbial regrowth is not related to resistance but rather to the subpopulation of organisms that is not inhibited or killed during a given dosing interval (the residual bacteria at the end of each dosing cycle), which can then reestablish themselves and continue growth. The size of the residual population is related to the initial population size (inoculum size), bactericidal activity, organism MIC, any postantibiotic effects, antibiotic pharmacokinetics, and the doubling time of the organism.[46] The doubling time of VGS in bacterial endocarditis and *S. pneumoniae* in pneumonia can be every 20 minutes, whereas the doubling time for *Treponema pallidum* in syphilis may be up to 36 hours. Any rapidly expanding or spreading infection implies a very rapid microbial doubling time and a necessity to reduce the residual population available for regrowth to as low a number as possible.

Dosing and Resistance

The antibiotic concentration in the tissues should ideally exceed the MIC by a factor of eight to 10 times to reduce or prevent the emergence of a resistant subpopulation.[46] The likelihood for the emergence of resistant strains during antibiotic therapy increases with greater spontaneous mutations, reduced host ability to eliminate the mutants, and, most importantly, the concentration of the antibiotic at the site of infection (the greater the concentration the less likely the emergence of resistance; the lower the concentration the greater the risk of resistance emergence).[46]

The less time the pathogen is exposed to sub-MIC doses, the less the chance of resistance mutations.[84] The ability of the resistant subpopulation to develop and overgrow decreases exponentially with greater antibiotic concentrations.[103]

Antibiotic Loading Doses

Because most acute orofacial infections begin and peak rapidly, high antibiotic blood levels must be achieved quickly. This is best and often only achieved with oral loading doses (two to four times the maintenance dose).[62,65,113] An antibiotic loading dose should be used whenever the half-life of the antibiotic is longer than 3 hours or a delay of 12 hours or longer to achieve therapeutic blood levels is unacceptable. If an antibiotic loading dose is not used, approximately four maintenance doses spaced at the recommended intervals are required to achieve a steady-state blood level of the antibiotic. Most antibiotics useful in orofacial infections have half-lives of less than 3 hours, but the acute nature of orofacial infections necessitates therapeutic blood levels earlier than 12 hours. With antibiotics having exceptional bioavailability, such as amoxicillin, a loading dose is not as crucial as with penicillin V or cephalexin, which are not as rapidly or as well absorbed.

Duration of Antibiotic Dosing

There is a natural but irrational tendency to treat infections for longer than necessary when shorter durations would be just as effective and decrease the overall selection pressure or microbial resistance.[21,53] On the other hand, determining the optimal duration of antibiotic treatment is usually difficult because bacterial kinetics and effects of drugs are not precisely known. Although some bacteria may occasionally mutate to resistance in a stepwise fashion and the presence of the antibiotic and high or prolonged doses might stop these mutants from attaining complete resistance, the reality of today is that virtually all resistance occurs by transposable element gene transfer promoted by the use of antibiotics, particularly at low doses and for long durations.[47,64]

Antibiotics should be used aggressively and for as short a time as is compatible with patient remission of disease.[62,65] With infectious diseases that do not rebound (return at cessation of the antibiotic), the proper duration of the antibiotic is determined by the time required for the patient's host defenses to gain control of the infection. The ideal antibiotic duration is the shortest time that will prevent both clinical and microbiologic relapse. The only practical guide to effectiveness of antibiotic therapy and hence the duration of therapy is clinical improvement of the patient as judged by remission of the infection. Antibiotic success is best determined by clinical improvement.

Four misconceptions are the major reasons for the unnecessary prolonged use of antibiotics: (1) prolonged antibiotic therapy destroys resistant bacteria, (2) prolonged antibiotic therapy is necessary to prevent oral rebound infections, (3) antibiotic dosages and duration of therapy can be extrapolated from one infection to another, and (4) the antibiotic prescriber knows how long the infection will last.

Certain infections (fungal, urinary tract, respiratory) tend to recur once the antibiotic is terminated because the organisms may not be eliminated but only suppressed. Orofacial infections rarely if ever rebound, particularly if the source of the infection is eradicated. All too often in medicine the temptation has been to extrapolate from one infection to another regarding dosage and duration of therapy. Many regimens have been based on the 10-day therapy against Group A beta-hemolytic streptococcal sore throat with little thought that such therapy might not apply to infections in the rest of the body.

Even experts get caught up in the adage to finish the course of the antibiotic and "make sure you take it all." Again, in many cases this is based on a fallacious assumption—that the prescriber knows beforehand just how long the particular infection will last. This is unlikely considering the number of variables involved in any given infectious process. The dentist should prescribe a reasonable amount of antibiotic (commonly for 3 to 5 days) with an initial loading dose (probably unnecessary with amoxicillin) and then reevaluate the patient shortly into the infection (in 1 or 2 days) and monitor the patient's progress until he/she is well. Prescription refills are designed for additional antibiotic administration if necessary. The antibiotic is terminated when, in the dentist's best clinical judgment, the patient's host defenses have gained control of the infection and it is well on its way to or at termination.

Incision and Drainage

The reduction in the inoculum size of the infecting organism is paramount in the management of infections. As stated by Cunha and Ortega,[20] "Most patients who develop abscesses and are being treated with antibiotics cannot hope to be cured by antibiotics alone," and "Surgical drainage remains the cornerstone of the therapeutic approach in the patient with abscesses."

With some clinical infections (pericoronitis, indurated cellulitis) the infection is too diffuse or has no nidus that would respond to incision and drainage. With the vast majority of orofacial infections, incision and drainage is imperative because (1) antibiotics do not diffuse well into infected areas; (2) some antibiotics are inactive at abscesses because of acidic pH and other reasons; (3) abscess microorganisms may not be dividing or may be at a very low metabolic state, negating the effects of antibiotics, particularly the β-lactam cell wall inhibitors; and (4) high levels of antibiotic inhibitors (β-lactamases or other enzymes) may be present to inactivate the antibiotic.[62,65]

Antibiotic Dosing Variables

Additional pharmacokinetic factors determining antibiotic efficacy include diffusion to the site of the infection, lipid solubility, plasma protein binding, inoculum effect, surface area to volume ratio, pregnancy, age, and renal and hepatic function.

The ease with which antibiotics penetrate to the site of infection follows the same path as other drugs and is guided by their pK_a, tissue pH, and lipid and water solubility. Lipophilic antibiotics such as the tetracyclines, macrolides, and fluoroquinolones pass through tissue barriers better than hydrophilic β-lactams. The tetracyclines and macrolides are highly concentrated within cells, making them effective against intracellular pathogens and also providing for a drug depot within macrophages. The β-lactams, vancomycin, and aminoglycosides are principally confined to the extracellular fluid. Diffusion through the capillary endothelium is relatively easy for rifampin, metronidazole, and chloramphenicol, difficult for the β-lactams and aminoglycosides, and intermediate for the tetracyclines, fluoroquinolones, and trimethoprim.

Only the antibiotic not bound to plasma protein is free to diffuse through capillary walls and other barriers to its site of action. The degree of plasma protein binding can vary from 80% to 96% for oral antistaphylococcal penicillins, clindamycin, and doxycycline; down to 50% to 80% for penicillin V and G, erythromycin, and tetracycline; to less than 25% for amoxicillin, ciprofloxacin, cephalexin, metronidazole, and aminoglycosides. Protein binding may increase with infection, inflammation, malignancy, and diabetes and decrease with cirrhosis, burns, and malnutrition. The clinical significance of antibiotic protein binding is currently debated but, all things being equal, drugs with lower protein binding may be preferable.

The inoculum effect (loss of antibiotic efficacy against dense microbial populations) may significantly affect antibiotic activity and the ability of the drug to penetrate to the core of the infection. A large mass of bacteria results in a decreased growth rate, less phagocytic activity, increased β-lactamase activity, more glycocalyx production, and reduced pH. The deleterious effect of inoculum size can be eliminated by early and vigorous antibiotic therapy combined with mechanical removal of the microorganisms (incision and drainage, scaling, and root planing). Antibiotics penetrate poorly into dense biomasses.

The antibiotic concentration at the site of the infection also depends on the ratio of the surface area of the vascular bed to the volume of the tissue compartment to be supplied.[80] With a high vascular bed-to-volume ratio (high vascularity and low infection volume), as is found in areas of inflammation and minimal purulence, the antibiotic concentration (except for β-lactams) may be similar to that of blood; in areas of low vascular bed-to-volume ratio (low vascularity and high infection volume), the antibiotic concentration may be much lower than serum. Incision and drainage can create a high vascularity, low infection volume situation that promotes better antibiotic penetration.

In pregnancy, all tetracyclines are contraindicated because of their tooth-staining effects and hepatotoxicity. The estolate form of erythromycin is contraindicated because it has a greater tendency to induce cholestatic hepatitis, including during pregnancy. Metronidazole and fluoroquinolones affect DNA synthesis and have been studied for any teratogenic, mutagenic, or carcinogenic effects. None appears to exist, but metronidazole carries a warning that its use should be avoided if possible in the first trimester of pregnancy. Similar caution should be exercised for the fluoroquinolones.

Very little data exist on the effect of hepatic disease on antibiotic pharmacokinetics, but impaired renal function or renal failure can have significant effects on antibiotic blood levels. As a rule in renal dysfunction, the dosage interval is increased for concentration-dependent antibiotics and the dose is decreased for time-dependent antibiotics.[27,34] In renal dysfunction, dosage modification is required for many antibiotics. Clindamycin, dicloxacillin, azithromycin, and doxycycline do not require dosage adjustment in renal dysfunction.[34,48] The central nervous system effects of the fluoroquinolones, the toxic effects of aminoglycosides, the platelet aggregation from some penicillins, and the deafness associated with the macrolides may be seriously increased with renal insufficiency.[48]

The following modifications should be used for antibiotics used in dentistry in patients with renal failure: amoxicillin (increase dose interval to 8 to 12 hours with moderate failure and to 24 hours with severe failure); ciprofloxacin (reduce dosage by 25% to 50%); cephalexin (increase dosage interval to 8 to 12 hours); cefaclor (decrease dose by 50%); cephradine (decrease dose by 50% with moderate and 75% with severe renal failure); metronidazole (decrease dosage by 25% with severe renal failure); clarithromycin (decrease dose by 25% to 50%); and erythromycin (decrease dose by 25% to 50%).[48]

Drug pharmacokinetics in neonates (first month of life) and infants (1 month to 2 years) may differ substantially from children (2 to 13 years) and adults.[62,65] Infants and neonates have a significantly greater percentage of body weight compared with body water, leading to a greater volume of distribution and increased serum half-lives. Other factors in neonates and infants versus children and adults are reduced gastric emptying and acidity, plasma protein binding, and reduced glomerular filtration rate. Renal function may be assumed to be totally functional by age 1 year.[12]

The elderly must also be considered substantially different from younger adults because of normal aging processes, underlying illness, and reduced host defenses predisposing to more serious infections[62,65] as well as altered pharmacokinetics: reduced total body water and lean body mass (more body fat) and reduced cardiac output, gastric acid, gastric emptying time, and renal function. Age may have little effect on most antibiotic pharmacokinetics, but renal insufficiency must always be a concern. The elderly also tend to be noncompliant about taking medication because of impaired memory, hearing, and vision; fear of drug interactions; perceived ineffectiveness of antibiotics; or the desire to save the medication for "the next time" because of the high cost of drugs.

COMBINATION ANTIBIOTIC THERAPY

Some established but limited situations may require combining antibiotics. The use of more than one antibiotic agent to treat an infection is often controversial because the efficacy of such therapy is likely to be microorganism specific and may promote the emergence of resistant organisms since many antibiotic resistance genes are now carried on multiple gene transposable elements. A common empirical reason for combined antibiotic therapy is to broaden the antibacterial spectrum when confronted with a probable polymicrobial infection of unknown origin.[8] Other proposed benefits include a reduction of dose for each agent (rarely done clinically), antibiotic synergism, and a decrease in adverse drug reactions. In most cases, unless documented by certain laboratory tests (fractional inhibitory concentration, checkerboard or time-killing curve methods) or proven empirical data, the disadvantages of combination antibiotic therapy commonly outweigh its advantages; the more drugs are present, the greater the likelihood of adverse reactions, antibiotic antagonism, increased financial costs, greater microbial resistance, greater environmental spread of resistance genes, and increased risk of superinfections (appearance of a new infection when treating a primary one).[62,65]

Antibiotic synergism is the combined effect of two or more antibiotics that is greater than the sum of the antibiotics individually. Antibiotic combinations that have been documented to be synergistic are (1) cell wall inhibitors and aminoglycosides, (2) β-lactams with β-lactamase inhibitors, (3) β-lactams that act on different PBPs, (4) streptogramin combinations, and (5) sulfonamides and trimethoprim.[4,62,65] Other combinations that may be synergistic include doxycycline and aminoglycosides for brucellosis; amoxicillin, tetracycline, macrolides, and metronidazole for *H. pylori;* vancomycin, rifampin, and aminoglycosides for MRSA; penicillin and clindamycin for group A streptococci; and fluoroquinolones and macrolides for *L. pneumophila*. A special case exists in the treatment of active tuberculosis in which the use of combination antibiotic therapy is required, not because of a synergistic effect of antibiotics, but because of the necessity of reducing the growth of strains of *M. tuberculosis* resistant to a single or multiple drugs.

Antibiotic antagonism (a decrease in the efficacy of two or more antibiotic agents in combination) is not well documented clinically. Some examples of antagonism include penicillin and macrolides in the treatment of *S. pneumoniae*, β-lactam induction of β-lactamase production in enteric bacilli and the macrolide and lincosamide combination against *S. aureus* leading to induction of MLS_b resistance.[4]

ANTIBIOTIC FAILURES

The inability of antibiotic therapy to control and eliminate an infection can be the result of a number of factors (Box 38-1) that primarily involve microbial resistance, poor antibiotic pharmacokinetics, faulty dosing, and inadequate host response to the infection.[62,65] Antibiotic failures are marked by persistent fever, lack of clinical improvement, and clinical deterioration of the patient.[20]

Box 38-1

Common Reasons* for Antibiotic Failure

- Failure to surgically eradicate the source of the infection
- Too low a blood antibiotic concentration
- Inability of the antibiotic to penetrate to the site of infection
- Impaired/inadequate host defenses
- Patient failure to take the antibiotic
- Inappropriate choice of antibiotic
- Limited vascularity or blood flow
- Decreased tissue pH or oxygen tension
- Slow microbial growth
- Emergence of antibiotic resistance
- Delay in diagnosis
- Incorrect diagnosis
- Antibiotic antagonism

*Listed in decreasing order of probable importance.
From Cunha BA, Ortega AM: Antibiotic failures, *Med Clin North Am* 79:663-672, 1995; Pallasch TJ: How to use antibiotics effectively, *J Calif Dent Assoc* 21:46-50, 1993; Pallasch TJ: Pharmacokinetic principles of antimicrobial therapy, *Perio 2000* 10:5-11, 1996.

A common factor in antibiotic failures is patient noncompliance with the prescribed antibiotic regimen. The most common reason for antibiotic failure in orofacial infections is a lack of or inadequate incision and drainage. A typical initial reaction to an apparent antibiotic failure is to add an additional antibiotic in the assumption that the current antibiotic has an inadequate spectrum of activity against the pathogen when the most likely reason is poor antibiotic penetration to the infected site.[20] The specter of increased microbial resistance in the oral cavity will play a greater role in antibiotic failures with an anticipated increased spread of oral infections to the orbit and submandibular regions.

HOST-MICROBE-ANTIBIOTIC INTERACTIONS

Host Defenses

Except in immunocompromised patients, antibiotics do not cure patients; patients cure patients. The innate immune system of the human being provides a wide variety of defense mechanisms to recognize the microbial pathogen, activate effector mechanisms to isolate and destroy the invader, and eventually eliminate its waste products. Antibiotics gain time for this system, initially overwhelmed by the invasion and rapid multiplication of the organism, to reestablish its control of our defense against microbial pathogens.

Microorganisms attempting to gain access to the interior of their host first encounter the physical barriers of the skin and mucosa along with skin-associated lymphoid tissue, dendritic (antigen-processing) cells, defensins, cathelicidins and associated cationic antimicrobial peptides, and secreted immunoglobulin A that increases mucosal stickiness.[83] If these barriers are then breached, both specific and nonspecific defenses assert their protective effects.

Antibiotics and Immune Function

The assumption that antibiotics act synergistically with the immune system against microbial pathogens seems reasonable, but this is not always the case. Antibiotics may assist by the PAE and PALC activities and by altering microbial adherence and virulence. Conversely, antibiotics, most notably the tetracyclines, may reduce macrophage and polymorphonuclear cell (PMN) chemotaxis, decrease phagocytic activity, and reduce the oxidative burst. Some antimicrobials may reduce inflammation (macrolides), whereas most are capable of releasing microbial toxins (endotoxins) on microbial cell death. Generally most cell wall inhibitors have no effect on the immune system, whereas the fluoroquinolones, imipenem, and some cephalosporins may enhance the immune response.[43] The data on the macrolides are presently equivocal and the tetracyclines, rifampin, sulfamethoxazole/trimethoprim, aminoglycosides, and chloramphenicol may impair immune function. The clinical significance of these interactions is currently unknown but does imply that host-microbe-antibiotic interactions are complex.

Microbial Virulence

The virulence (pathogenicity) of a microorganism depends on five necessary traits: the ability to colonize, penetrate, grow, inhibit, or avoid host defenses, as well as induce host damage.[90] Microbial virulence is highly regulated by population density, growth phases, osmolality, pH, iron/ion concentrations, temperature, adhesin expression,[23] and "quorum sensing": the ability of microbes to convey the information for all these factors to each other to maintain optimum existence and occasionally attack their hosts.

The genes for virulence are contained in pathogenicity "islands" that are distinct genetic elements encoding virulence factors for pathogenic bacteria acquired by horizontal gene transfer and fully capable of enclosure in integrons for transfer to other bacteria. These pathogenicity islands contain the genes for adherence factors (adhesins, fimbriae), toxins (hemolysins, enterotoxins), iron uptake systems, apoptosis, and mobile elements (transposons, integrons, insertion sequence elements).[35]

ANTIBIOTIC ADVERSE REACTIONS

The following section contains a discussion of adverse drug reactions, some of which are unique to antibiotics; others are not exclusive to antimicrobials but are clinically more significant than the common adverse reactions seen with most drugs.

Antibiotic Teratology

Few studies have been published regarding the ability of antibiotics to cause birth defects. Most antibiotics are in the FDA class B or C categories (see Table 3-7), indicating little if any risk. Several studies have followed the long-term use of metronidazole; its use in pregnancy does not appear to be associated with any increased rate of birth defects, preterm delivery, or low birth weight. Studies on aminoglycosides, cephalosporins, and oxacillin have likewise shown no teratogenic effects.

Antibiotic-Induced Mania

Acute mania has been described in association with clinical antibiotic therapy. A total of 103 cases have been reported worldwide, making such reactions rare but disconcerting. The prime causative agents are clarithromycin followed by the fluoroquinolones and isoniazid.[3] Other antibiotics less commonly implicated are metronidazole, erythromycin, sulfamethoxazole/trimethoprim, and amoxicillin.[3] All but two of these reactions were reversible with antibiotic discontinuance and are likely to be due to the antibiotic, although some occurred in patients taking other medications that could cause mania. The mechanism may be related to altered γ-aminobutyric acid (GABA) activity in the brain because fluoroquinolones and isoniazid are GABA antagonists.[3]

Long QT Interval

The long QT interval syndrome is a cardiac disorder caused by ion channel abnormalities that prolong the time interval between the beginning of the QRS complex and the end of the T wave on the electrocardiogram (see Chapter 24). The long QT syndrome may be either congenital or acquired, with the congenital mutations in the genes controlling the cardiac K^+ channels. The acquired form is caused either by metabolic disorders or certain drugs. Metabolic disorders include reduced blood K^+, Ca^{++}, and Mg^{++}, and diseases include heart failure, myocardial ischemia, mitral valve prolapse, and liver and renal disorders. Antibiotics that have been implicated in the cause of torsades de pointes include fluoroquinolones (gatifloxacin, levofloxacin, moxifloxacin, sparfloxacin), macrolides (erythromycin, clarithromycin), and clindamycin.[100]

The FDA Adverse Event Reporting System has analyzed 202 cases of macrolide- or fluoroquinolone-induced torsades de pointes: 77% were caused by macrolides and 23% by fluoroquinolones; 89% to 95% were in older patients; 9% to 13% were fatal; the mean time to the adverse event was 4 to 5 days; and 42% to 62% had cardiac disease, 7% to 11% had renal disease, and 17% had low blood K^+ or Mg^{++} levels.[87] The risk rate has been estimated to be 1 per 1 million exposures to ciprofloxacin, 3 per 1 million exposures to clarithromycin, and 14.5 per 1 million exposures to sparfloxacin.

Antibiotics and Oral Contraceptives

In response to a few case reports, the FDA in the 1980s issued a warning that antibiotics may interfere with the action of oral contraceptives, potentially resulting in unwanted pregnancies. The proposed mechanisms of reduced contraceptive blood levels leading to decreased efficacy include (1) increased urinary/fecal excretion from antibiotic-induced diarrhea, (2) increased microsomal liver metabolism, (3) receptor displacement, (4) reduced gastrointestinal absorption, and (5) reduced enterohepatic circulation. The antibiotic rifampin stimulates the liver metabolism of the oral contraceptives, reducing blood levels. No other experimental data or controlled clinical studies have documented the interference of any other antibiotics with the activity of oral contraceptives.

The most likely theoretical mechanisms are the gastrointestinal reduction in free estrogen or a reduction in enterohepatic circulation. Several studies document no effect of antibiotics on the blood levels of ethinyl estradiol, norethindrone, and progesterone in patients taking doxycycline (100 mg/day for 7 days),[57] tetracycline (500 mg every 6 hours for 10 days),[56] and ciprofloxacin (500 mg three times per day for 7 days).[51] No effort has been made to determine whether the failure rate of the oral contraceptives in women taking antibiotics is greater than the normal failure rate of oral contraceptives in women not taking antibiotics. No official authoritative body has ever examined this alleged drug interaction to investigate the evidence and make a recommendation. The initial FDA response has never been updated.

From a purely scientific point of view, no reason exists to believe that any antibiotics except rifampin interfere with the action of oral contraceptives. However, from a medicolegal point of view the dentist may wish to advise the patient taking oral contraceptives and receiving antibiotics to use an additional contraceptive method or perform abstinence during the time the antibiotic is present and for several days after its termination to allow for complete antibiotic excretion (usually 5 times the half-life of the drug). The oral contraceptive should never be stopped during antibiotic therapy as it is the single most effective means of contraception with the exception of sexual activity abstinence.

Antibiotic-Induced Agranulocytosis

Various antibiotics have been implicated as rare causative agents in reduced blood neutrophil counts with accompanying signs and symptoms of fever and septicemia or septic shock. The median onset of the agranulocytosis is 12 to 14 days after beginning antibiotic therapy. The mortality rate in the literature from all drug-induced agranulocytosis is 6% to 20%, with antibiotics possibly causing 20% of the cases. The most commonly involved antibiotics are sulfonamides and β-lactams, followed by aminoglycosides and macrolides.

Antibiotic-Induced Photosensitivity, Photoallergy, and Phototoxicity

Antibiotics (along with the phenothiazine antipsychotics) are among the most common drugs inducing skin reactions on exposure to sunlight. Photosensitivity may occur in one of two forms: (1) phototoxicity, in which chemicals (drugs) are deposited in the skin, absorb ultraviolet light, and then transfer the energy to local tissue, resulting in inflammatory responses; or (2) photoallergy, in which sunlight causes a hapten to become a complete antigen in the skin, eliciting an immediate or a delayed allergic reaction. The signs and symptoms (erythema, urticaria, eczema, lichenoid dermatitis, bullous lesions) may be the same but the mechanisms are different (photoallergy may need a sensitizing dose unless the drug is continually taken for 5 to 10 days or longer). The most common antibiotics that induce photosensitivity are sulfonamides, tetracyclines, and fluoroquinolones. Photosensitivity is managed by discontinuing the drug, avoiding sunlight, and wearing protective clothing.

Antibiotic Effects on Body Flora and Superinfection

The question of whether human exposure to antibiotic doses at the low concentrations seen in agriculture and aquaculture, as therapy for inflammatory or other diseases, or in the food and water supply alters body flora or promotes emergence of resistant microbes or the transfer of resistance genes is of crucial importance to public health.

Some data from veterinary studies indicate that daily doses of tetracycline at 15 mg per 60 kg/day of animal body weight or 2 mg/day of oxytetracycline may have no effect on gastrointestinal carbohydrate or fat metabolism and do not cause any increase in antibiotic-resistant enteric bacilli. However, 20 mg of oxytetracycline twice a day can promote such resistance.[99] Several studies have been unable to document the transfer of resistance genes from animals to farmers or shared resistance plasmids between farm animals and farmers. At times when resistance is not detected, the chosen breakpoint for such a determination was extremely high (e.g., 32 μg/ml for vancomycin), which is not comparable to concentrations achieved with human doses.

On balance, the evidence is substantial that antimicrobial agents at any dose or concentration for virtually any length of time do select for resistance and promote the acquisition and transfer of drug-resistant genes.[64] Many of these species exhibit extraordinary resistance patterns: 50% to 100% of *Salmonella*, staphylococci, and enteric bacilli are resistant to tetracycline and 32% to 47% are resistant to β-lactams, with 49.7% exhibiting polyantibiotic resistance; 30% of *S. aureus* is resistant to ciprofloxacin and 47% to tetracycline; 72% of *Campylobacter* in human beings and 99% in chickens and pigs are resistant to ciprofloxacin; and *E. coli* exhibits 70% to 94% resistance to amoxicillin, and 62% to 98% resistance to tetracycline.[1,29,52,81,107] If the very low (nanogram/nanomolar) concentrations of antibiotics found in the food chain and used in nature to control bacterial ecologic niches induce such resistance patterns, then the assumption (until proven otherwise) must be that subtherapeutic dosages in human beings will do the same. *Subtherapeutic* is not synonymous with biologically or pharmacologically inactive. If microbes employ nanogram amounts of antibiotics to control their own microbial ecology (kill fellow microorganisms, promote resistance gene expression and transfer), it is difficult to believe that micrograms would not do the same in humans.

Of possibly greater importance is the ability of antibiotics to induce microbial resistance or promote the transfer of resistance genes from one species to another. The mere presence of a β-lactam antibiotic produces a 100- to 1000-fold increase in induction of β-lactamase in microorganisms producing extended-spectrum β-lactamases.[50] *E. coli* carries resistance genes that are not expressed until tetracycline is present.[59] Concentrations of tetracyclines at 0.1 to 1 μg/ml per gram in meat cause the dissemination of resistance genes in the human gastrointestinal tract,[33] and 1 μg/ml of tetracycline in drinking water results in a tenfold increase in the transfer of conjugative plasmids from *E. faecalis* to *Listeria monocytogenes*.[25]

In oral plaque biofilm, tetracycline resistance genes can be transferred from *B. subtilis* to streptococci, illustrating that nonoral bacteria have the potential to transfer genes to opportunistic oral microorganisms.[78] The presence of tetracycline increases the conjugative transfer of Tn916 by a factor of 19 to 119 times in matings between *B. subtilis* and *B. thuringiensis* and 15 times between *E. faecalis* and *B. thuringeinsis*[89] and *subtilis*.[105] The self-transfer of *Bacteroides* conjugative transposons can be increased 100- to 1000-fold by the presence of low levels of tetracycline (1 μg/ml)[96,97] because of the transcription of a three-gene operon near the middle of a transfer element.[82]

Oral streptococci can harbor tetracycline resistance genes in dental plaque and disseminate such genes by mobile elements to other microflora: *E. faecalis*, *Veillonella*, and other streptococci.[78] Salyers et al[82] state that "the fact that tetracycline acts as an inducer of transfer gene expression illustrates how the use of an antibiotic could accelerate the spread of antibiotic resistance genes not only by selecting for their acquisition but also by stimulating their transfer."

A significant and unappreciated adverse effect of antibiotics is the potential to decrease colonization resistance of indigenous anaerobic flora in the digestive tract and other anatomic areas (skin, oral mucosa). The role of colonization resistance is to limit the concentration of potentially pathogenic flora of either an exogenous or endogenous nature in a given body part. Removal of indigenous flora by antibiotics can promote growth of microorganisms not sensitive to the drug (a superinfection). Many superinfections result from a reduction in the endogenous microorganisms important for colonization resistance, with the most notable example being antibiotic-induced diarrhea and colitis.

Antibiotic-Induced Diarrhea and Pseudomembranous Colitis

Adverse colonic effects of antibiotics range from simple diarrhea (antibiotic-associated diarrhea) to mucosal inflammatory diarrhea/colitis (antibiotic-associated colitis), with or without associated *Clostridium difficile* (*C. difficile*–associated colitis), to potentially fatal pseudomembranous colitis. Of the 25 million people affected by serious diarrhea annually in the United States, approximately 10% of these cases are the result of antibiotics, particularly broad-spectrum agents.[63] The vast majority of these antibiotic-associated diarrhea cases are not clinically significant and respond to drug discontinuance and rehydration if necessary.

Nevertheless, a significant portion of these are a manifestation of "benign" colitis or the far more menacing pseudomembranous colitis caused by toxins from *C. difficile*. Approximately 3 million cases of *C. difficile*–associated diarrhea (CDAD) or colitis (CDAC) may occur annually in the United States, primarily in hospitalized patients.[63] The outpatient toll of CDAD or CDAC is approximately 20,000 cases per year, with a range of 7.7 to 20 cases per 100,000 patient-years worldwide.

Pseudomembranous colitis was first described in 1893 as "diphtheric colitis" and before the introduction of antibiotics was ascribed to staphylococci, heavy metal intoxication, sepsis, surgical shock, and uremia. Antibiotic-associated pseudomembranous colitis (PMC) was described in the 1950s with the advent of penicillins, tetracyclines, and chloramphenicol. In 1977 the association of PMC with a toxin from *C. difficile* was discovered and the relationship between the organism and antibiotic-associated diarrhea and PMC was established in 1978.[63]

Virtually all cases of CDAD, CDAC, and PMC are associated with antibiotics, with 92% of patients exposed to the antibiotic within 2 weeks of onset of the diarrhea and 100% within 8 weeks, of which 87% were nosocomially acquired.[63] Any antibiotic is capable of inducing diarrhea, colitis, or PMC but the most common agent involved is amoxicillin, followed by third-generation cephalosporins and clindamycin. When the colonic flora are disturbed by antibiotics or disease, the colonization resistance of the gastrointestinal tract is reduced by the suppression of natural antagonists of *C. difficile* such as *Bacteroides*, *Lactobacillus*, pseudomonads, staphylococci, streptococci, peptostreptococci, enterococci, and *E. coli*. It is no accident that these antibiotics are involved because their antibacterial spectrum includes these microbial antagonists of *C.*

difficile. Antibiotic-associated colitis and CDAC are classic superinfections.

C. difficile is a spore-forming, gram-positive obligate anaerobic bacillus commonly acquired by cross-infection by oral ingestion and also widely found in rivers, seas, lakes, swimming pool water, soil, domestic animals, and raw vegetables. *C. difficile* is cultured in up to 19% of patients with antibiotic-associated diarrhea without colitis, 60% of those with antibiotic-associated colitis without PMC, and 95% with PMC.[63]

CDAC is caused by cytotoxins (A and B) that gain access to the intestinal mucosa to alter Rho proteins (guanosine triphosphate–binding proteins) to disrupt the F-actin structures and cause cell rounding and eventual intestinal cell death.[63] The initial diarrhea may appear as early as 1 to 10 days or as late as 6 to 10 weeks after initiating the antibiotic therapy. The incubation period after exposure to or acquisition of *C. difficile* may be less than 1 week, with a median time of diarrhea onset of 2 days.

As the disease progresses the signs and symptoms include fever; diarrhea with abdominal tenderness; profuse green, watery, foul-smelling, bloody diarrhea with abdominal distention; and fecal and blood leukocytosis. The onset of PMC is heralded by high fever, marked abdominal tenderness, dehydration, and the initiation of 2 to 20 mm in diameter raised adherent yellow plaques interspersed between relatively normal colonic mucosa. From patchy epithelial necrosis these plaques may proceed to ulcerations overlaid by a pseudomembrane consisting of fibrin, mucus, leukocytes, and cellular debris. In fulminant colitis, the colonic muscle tone may be lost, resulting in toxic colonic dilation (toxic megacolon), paralytic ileus, or colonic perforation with peritonitis. CDAD is diagnosed by the presence of diarrhea and one of the following: (1) a pseudomembrane on colonoscopy, (2) positive cytotoxin stool assay for toxin B, (3) a stool assay for toxins A and B, or (4) a positive stool culture for *C. difficile*.[63]

In 15% to 25% of CDAD cases the diarrhea resolves with only antibiotic discontinuance. The antibiotic of choice for unresolved CDAC or PMC is metronidazole (250 mg orally four times per day or 500 mg three times per day) for 10 days.[63] Vancomycin (125 mg orally four times per day for 10 days) is now reserved only for those cases that do not respond to metronidazole or in severely ill patients because of concerns about selection of vancomycin-resistant organisms in the hospital. Other therapies that have been attempted are bacitracin, fusidic acid, teicoplanin, vancomycin plus rifampin, vancomycin in tapering doses, and the re-establishment of the colonic flora with probiotics: lactobacilli, nonenterotoxigenic *C. difficile*, and *Saccharomyces boulardii*.

Resolution of CDAD occurs in an average of 2 to 4 days with metronidazole and 2.6 to 4.2 days with vancomycin.[63] The hospital stay for patients acquiring antibiotic-associated diarrhea may be extended to 18 to 21 days. Studies on the mortality rates associated with nosocomial CDAD are virtually nonexistent but several have reported a 3% to 17% death rate. The mortality rate associated with community-acquired CDAC or PMC is very low.[36,95]

The range for relapse and recurrence rates of CDAD is 4.8% to 66%, with an average of 20% appearing reasonable.[63] Relapse may be caused by the incomplete eradication of *C. difficile* and recurrence to the acquisition of a new organism. Most individuals with recurrence or relapse respond to the same initial metronidazole or vancomycin regimen, but refractory CDAD can occasionally become persistent and elude long-term cure for years. Risk factors for recurrence include acquisition during the spring, female sex, diarrhea that resolves but then recurs within 2 weeks after the antibiotic treatment is terminated, and, most importantly, those receiving antibiotics again within 2 months of the initial recurrent CDAD.

The fear of inducing a potentially fatal case of PMC has led to a reluctance to use clindamycin because early and faulty preliminary data reported a 10% association of PMC with the drug.[63] More recent data indicate that antibiotic-associated diarrhea and CDAC associated with clindamycin in community use of the drug is very low. The overall risk rate for community-acquired *C. difficile*–associated PMC from retrospective data may be as low as 1 per 10,000 antibiotic prescriptions and the risk of hospitalization 0.5 to 1.0 per 100,000 patient-years.[36] In a study of 376,590 antibiotic prescriptions given to more than 280,000 patients over a 4-year period, four cases of acute antibiotic-associated colitis were detected.[95] The incidence rate was calculated to be 1.6 per 100,000 persons exposed to ampicillin, 2.9 per 100,000 to dicloxacillin, and 2.6 per 100,000 to tetracycline with no antibiotic-associated diarrhea seen in the 1509 patients receiving oral or topical clindamycin.

In another retrospective study, 51 cases of CDAD were detected in 662,500 person-years (7.7 per 100,000 person-years).[36] All patients recovered and only six were hospitalized. The overall risk rate for community-acquired CDAD in this study was less than 1 per 10,000 antibiotic prescriptions, and the risk of hospitalization was 0.5 to 1.0 per 100,000 patient-years.[36] Therefore the risk for hospitalization from community-acquired, antibiotic-induced diarrhea or colitis seems to be very low.[36,95]

On the basis of the above epidemiologic data it appears that the fears of significant PMC associated with the outpatient use of clindamycin are unfounded. Statistically, PMC is more likely to occur with amoxicillin than clindamycin. Clinicians should refrain from unnecessary antibiotic therapy in patients within the first 2 months after the elimination of CDAD. Any elective dental procedure requiring antibiotic treatment or prophylaxis would best be postponed for this 2-month period. If antibiotic therapy is required, the use of antibiotics far less commonly associated with CDAD (penicillin V, macrolides) is appropriate.

NEW ANTIMICROBIAL APPROACHES

The current pattern of formulating "new" antibiotics that are merely derivatives of existing antibiotics will not solve the problems of microbial resistance. Entirely new approaches to unique mechanisms of antibiotic action attacking heretofore unknown microbial metabolic processes will require a much better basic understanding of microbial life and considerable risk-taking on the part of the pharmaceutical industry.

Some of these approaches are currently under study: (1) inhibiting species-specific enzymes, (2) employing bacteriophages, (3) using our natural cationic peptide antibiotics, (4) inhibiting glycosyltransferases that control bacterial membrane lipopolysaccharide synthesis, (5) using antisense RNA inhibitors, (6) sequestering the iron necessary for microbial survival, (7) sequencing the bacterial genome to identify unique antibiotic targets, (8) improving the immune system's ability to recognize and destroy microbial pathogens, (9) developing highly specific narrow-spectrum antibiotics to target specific microbes identified by real-time polymerase chain reaction, (10) developing chemicals that inhibit microbial surface adhesion, and (11) interfering with microbial quorum sensing so that bacteria misread signals for virulence, adherence, and growth.

Peptide antibiotics and cationic antimicrobial peptides are natural antibiotics that function as a component of all immune systems of living species. Some 500 cationic antimicrobial peptides have been isolated, with some living species possessing 30 or more entities. Nonribosomally synthesized peptides include the gramicidins, polymyxins, bacitracins, and glycopeptides; the ribosomally synthesized peptides include defensins, cathelicidins, cecropins, and magainins.

The peptide antibiotics function to kill all invading microorganisms (bacteria, viruses, parasites, fungi), elicit the inflammatory response and immunoglobulin G production, recruit neutrophil and T cells, increase phagocytosis and chemotaxis, and participate in apoptosis.[86] The cationic antimicrobial peptides are located in epithelial cells, neutrophils, and macrophages and on the epithelial surfaces of the skin, mucosa (including the oral cavity), lungs, kidneys, and gastrointestinal tract. The cationic antimicrobial peptides may act on the microbial membrane to disrupt its permeability.

The use of cationic antimicrobial peptides as antibiotic agents is hampered by their destruction in gastric acid; however, they may function as topical agents because they appear to be essentially nontoxic and nonallergenic. The cationic antimicrobial peptides have been used experimentally in the management of oral mucositis and to sterilize catheter sites.

An intriguing approach to the control of pathogenic bacteria is the possibility of interfering with their ability to communicate with each other. Quorum sensing is the process by which microbes exchange signaling chemicals (autoinducers) that allow the bacterial population to coordinate gene expression for virulence, symbiosis, conjugation, sporulation, mobility, apoptosis, antibiotic production, and biofilm development.[15] Quorum sensing is related to the size of the colony; a single autoinducer from a single microbe is incapable of inducing change, but when the colony reaches a critical density (quorum), a threshold of autoinduction is reached and gene expression begins.

The autoinducers can be specific to each bacterial species and usually consist of acetylated homoserine lactones in gram-negative and oligopeptides in gram-positive bacteria. A boron-containing sensor, AI-Z, has been identified as a possible universal signal for interspecies communication.[15] Quorum sensing may explain how microorganisms can build geometrically perfect colonies without ever seeing them. Interference with these signals for virulence or adhesiveness may prove to be of significant benefit to human beings.

Some of these new approaches pose difficulties. Bacteriophages are bacterial viruses that are specific for a single bacterium and require precise identification of the pathogen to be effective. Cationic peptides are a vital part of our natural defense to microbial pathogens and have protected us for millions of years but are not stable in the gastrointestinal tract and may only be effective topically. If resistance were to occur to these peptides when used as therapeutic agents then a "Satan bug" might be created that is unaffected by our most basic defense mechanism.[9] Just such resistance has been detected in *P. gingivalis*, which secretes a peptide that destroys cationic peptides.[117] Widespread resistance of this type would be catastrophic. Soil microorganisms serve as potential reservoirs for new antibiotic agents, but to date only 1% have been identified and these organisms appear very difficult to grow in the laboratory.

Cited References

1. Aarestrup FM, Agerso LY, Ahrens P, et al: Antimicrobial susceptibility and presence of resistance genes in staphylococci from poultry, *Vet Microbiol* 74:353-364, 2000.
2. Aarestrup FM, Seyfarth AM, Emborg H-D, et al: Effect of abolishment of the use of antimicrobial agents for growth promotion and occurrence of antimicrobial resistance in fecal enterococci from food animals in Denmark, *Antimicrob Agents Chemother* 45:2054-2059, 2001.
3. Abouesh A, Stone C, Hobbs WR: Antimicrobial-induced mania (antibiomania): a review of spontaneous reports, *J Clin Psychopharmacol* 22:71-81, 2002.
4. Acar JF: Antibiotic synergy and antagonism, *Med Clin North Am* 84:1391-1406, 2000.
5. Ahmad M, Urban C, Mariano N, et al: Clinical characteristics and molecular epidemiology associated with imipenem-resistant *Klebsiella pneumoniae, Clin Infect Dis* 29:352-355, 1999.
6. Ambrose PG, Jr, Owens RC, Grasela D: Antimicrobial pharmacodynamics, *Med Clin North Am* 84:1431-1446, 2000.
7. Barbosa TM, Levy SB: The impact of antibiotic use on resistance development and persistence, *Drug Resist Update* 3:303-311, 2000.
8. Bouza E, Munoz P: Monotherapy versus combination therapy for bacterial infections, *Med Clin North Am* 84:1357-1389, 2000.
9. Breithaupt H: The new antibiotics: can novel antibacterial treatments combat the rising tide of drug resistant infections? *Nature Biotechnol* 17:1165-1169, 1999.
10. Bruins MR, Kapil S, Oehme FW: Microbial resistance to metals in the environment, *Ecotoxicol Environ Safety* 45:198-207, 2000.
11. Bush K: New β-lactamases in gram-negative bacteria: diversity and impact on the selection of antimicrobial therapy, *Clin Infect Dis* 32:1085-1089, 2001.
12. Butler DR, Kuhn RJ, Chandler MH: Pharmacokinetics of anti-infective agents in paediatric patients, *Clin Pharmacokinet* 26:374-395, 1994.
13. Cetinkaya Y, Falk P, Mayhall CG: Vancomycin-resistant enterococci, *Clin Microbiol Rev* 13:686-707, 2000.
14. Chadwick PR, Wooster SL: Glycopeptide resistance in *Staphylococcus aureus, J Infect* 40:211-217, 2000.
15. Chen X, Schauder S, Potier N, et al: Structural identification of a quorum-sensing signal containing boron, *Nature* 415:545-549, 2002.
16. Chopra I, Roberts M: Tetracycline antibiotics: mode of action, applications, molecular biology, and epidemiology of bacterial resistance, *Microbiol Mol Biol Rev* 65:232-260, 2001.
17. Cleveland JL, Kohn WC: Antimicrobial resistance and dental care: a CDC perspective, *Dent Abstr* 43:108-110, 1998.
18. Cohen ML: Changing patterns of infectious disease, *Nature* 406:762-767, 2000.
19. Craig WA: Pharmacokinetic/pharmacodynamic parameters: rationale for antimicrobial dosing in mice and men, *Clin Infect Dis* 26:1-10, 1998.
20. Cunha BA, Ortega AM: Antibiotic failures, *Med Clin North Am* 79:663-672, 1995.
21. Cunney RJ, Smith EG: The impact of laboratory reporting practice on antibiotic utilization, *J Int Antimicrob Agents* 14:13-19, 2000.
22. Deragon JM, Capy P: Impact of transposable elements on the human genome, *Ann Med* 32:264-273, 2000.
23. Donnenberg MS: Pathogenic strategies of enteric bacteria, *Nature* 406:768-774, 2000.
24. Dore MP, Leandro G, Realdi G, et al: Effect of pretreatment antibiotic resistance to metronidazole and clarithromycin on outcome of *Helicobacter pylori* therapy: a meta-analytical approach, *Dig Dis Sci* 45:68-76, 2000.

25. Doucet-Populaire F, Trieu-Cuot P, Dosbaa I, et al: Inducible transfer of conjugative transposons Tn/1545 from *Enterococcus faecalis* to *Listeria monocytogenes* in the digestive tracts of gnotobiotic mice, *Antimicrob Agents Chemother* 35:185-187, 1991.
26. Epstein JB, Chong S, Le ND: A survey of antibiotic use in dentistry, *J Am Dent Assoc* 131:1600-1609, 2000.
27. Estes L: Review of pharmacokinetics and pharmacodynamics of antimicrobial agents, *Mayo Clin Proc* 73:1114-1122, 1998.
28. Fuursted K: Postantibiotic effects in vitro, *APMIS Suppl* 90:1-23, 1999.
29. Gebreyes WA, Davies PR, Morrow WEM, et al: Antimicrobial resistance of *Salmonella* isolates from swine, *J Clin Microbiol* 38:4633-4636, 2000.
30. Greene VW: Personal hygiene and life expectancy improvements since 1850: historic and epidemiologic associations, *Am J Infect Control* 29:203-206, 2001.
31. Guillemot D, Carbon C, Balkau B, et al: Low dosage and long treatment duration of β-lactam: risk factors for carriage of penicillin-resistant *Streptococcus pneumoniae*, *JAMA* 279:365-370, 1998.
32. Heimdahl A: Culturing the exudate of an odontogenic infection: a useful procedure [letter]? *Oral Surg Oral Med Oral Pathol Oral Radiol Endod* 90:2-4, 2000.
33. Heimdahl A, Nord CE: Influence of doxycycline on the normal human flora and colonization of the oral cavity and colon, *Scand J Infect Dis* 15:293-302, 1983.
34. Henry NK, Hoecker JL, Rhodes KH: Antimicrobial therapy for infants and children: guidelines for the inpatient and outpatient practice of pediatric infectious diseases, *Mayo Clin Proc* 75:86-97, 2000.
35. Hentschel U, Hacker J: Pathogenicity islands: the tip of the iceberg, *Microbes Infect* 3:545-548, 2001.
36. Hirschhorn LR, Trnka Y, Onderdonk A, et al: Epidemiology of community-acquired *Clostridium difficile*–associated diarrhea, *J Clin Infect Dis* 169:127-133, 1994.
37. Hoban DJ, Doern GV, Fluit AC, et al: Worldwide prevalence of antimicrobial resistance in *Streptococcus pneumoniae, Haemophilus influenzae*, and *Moraxella catarrhalis* in the SENTRY Antimicrobial Surveillance Program, 1997-1999, *Clin Infect Dis* 32(Suppl 2):S81-S93, 2001.
38. Jacobs MR, Applebaum PC, Zhanel GG, et al: Authors reply: assumed versus approved breakpoints, *Antimicrob Agents Chemother* 44:3243-3245, 2000.
39. Jorgensen JH, Ferraro ML: Antimicrobial susceptibility testing: general principles and contemporary practices, *Clin Infect Dis* 26:973-980, 1998.
40. Kopeloff N: *Why infections?* London, 1926, Alfred A Knopf.
41. Kunin CM: Dosage schedules of antimicrobial agents: a historical review, *Rev Infect Dis* 3:4-11, 1981.
42. Kunin CM: Editorial response: antibiotic Armageddon, *Clin Infect Dis* 25:240-241, 1997.
43. Labro M-T: Interference of antibacterial agents with phagocyte functions: immunomodulation or "immuno-fairy tales"? *Clin Microbiol Rev* 13:615-650, 2000.
44. Lederberg J: Infectious history, *Science* 288:287-293, 2000.
45. Leistevuo J, Järvinen H, Österblad M, et al: Resistance to mercury and antimicrobial agents in *Streptococcus mutans* isolates from human subjects in relation to exposure to dental amalgam fillings, *Antimicrob Agents Chemother* 44:456-457, 2000.
46. Levison ME: Pharmacodynamics of antibacterial drugs, *Infect Dis Clin North Am* 14:281-291, 2000.
47. Levy SB: *The antibiotic paradox*, New York, 1992, Plenum Press.
48. Livornese LL, Jr, Slavin D, Benz RL, et al: Use of antibacterial agents in renal failure, *Infect Dis Clin North Am* 14:371-390, 2000.
49. Low DE, Keller N, Barth A, et al: Clinical prevalence, antimicrobial susceptibility, and geographic resistance patterns to enterococci: results from the SENTRY Antimicrobial Surveillance Program, 1997-1999, *Clin Infect Dis* 32(Suppl 2):S133-S145, 2001.
50. Low DE, Kellner JD, Wright GD: Superbugs: how they evolve and minimize the cost of resistance, *Infect Dis Reports* 1:464-469, 1999.
51. Maggiolo F, Puricelli G, Dottorini M, et al: The effect of ciprofloxacin on oral contraceptive steroid treatments, *Drug Exp Clin Res* 17:451-454, 1991.
52. Manie T, Khan S, Brozel VS, et al: Antimicrobial resistance of bacteria isolated from slaughtered and retail chickens in South Africa, *Lett Appl Microbiol* 26:253-258, 1998.
53. Martin MV, Longman LP, Hill JB, et al: Acute dentoalveolar infections: an investigation of the duration of antibiotic therapy, *Br Dent J* 183:135-137, 1997.
54. McCabe RM, Kreger DE, Johns M: Type-specific and cross-reactive antibodies in gram-negative bacteremia, *Engl J Med* 287:261-267, 1977.
55. Miller YW, Eady EA, Lacey RW, et al: Sequential antibiotic therapy for acne promotes the carriage of resistant staphylococci on the skin of contacts, *J Antimicrob Chemother* 38:829-837, 1996.
56. Murphy AA, Zachur HA, Charache P, et al: The effect of tetracycline on levels of oral contraceptives, *Am J Obstet Gynecol* 164:28-33, 1991.
57. Neely JL, Abate M, Swinker M, et al: The effect of doxycycline on serum levels of ethinyl estradiol, norethindrone, and endogenous progesterone, *Obstet Gynecol* 77:416-420, 1991.
58. Neu HC: Current practices in antimicrobial dosing, *Rev Infect Dis* 3:12-18, 1981.
59. Nguyen TN, Phan QG, Duong LP, et al: Effects of carriage and expression of the Tn10 tetracycline resistance operon on the fitness of *Escherichia coli* K12, *Molec Biol Evol* 6:213-225, 1989.
60. Novak R, Henriques B, Charpentier E, et al: Emergence of vancomycin tolerance in *Streptococcus pneumoniae*, *Nature* 399:590-593, 1999.
61. Osterblad M, Leistevuo J, Leistevuo T, et al: Antimicrobial and mercury resistance in aerobic gram-negative bacilli in fecal flora among persons with and without dental amalgam fillings, *Antimicrob Agents Chemother* 39:2499-2502, 1995.
62. Pallasch TJ: How to use antibiotics effectively, *J Calif Dent Assoc* 21:46-50, 1993.
63. Pallasch TJ: *Clostridium-difficile*–associated diarrhea and colitis, *J Calif Dent Assoc* 27:405-413, 1999.
64. Pallasch TJ: Global antibiotic resistance and its impact on the dental community, *J Calif Dent Assoc* 28:215-233, 2000.
65. Pallasch TJ: Pharmacokinetic principles of antimicrobial therapy, *Perio 2000* 10:5-11, 1996.

66. Pallasch TJ, Gill CJ: Microbial resistance to antibiotics, *J Calif Dent Assoc* 14:25-27, 1986.
67. Pallasch TJ, Slots J: Oral microorganisms and cardiovascular disease, *J Calif Dent Assoc* 28:204-214, 2000.
68. Pallasch TJ, Wahl MJ: Focal infection: new age or ancient history? *Endod Topics* 4:32-45, 2003.
69. Palmer NO, Martin MV, Pealing R, et al: An analysis of antibiotic prescriptions from general dentist practitioners in England, *J Antimicrob Chemother* 46:1033-1035, 2000.
70. Perencevich EN, Wong MT, Harris AD: National and regional assessment of the antibacterial soap market: a step toward determining the impact of prevalent antibacterial soaps, *Am J Infect Control* 29:281-283, 2001.
71. Petrocheilou V, Richmond MH, Bennett PM: The persistence of R-plasmid–carrying *E. coli* in a married couple, one of whom was receiving antibiotics, *Contrib Microbiol Immunol* 6:178-188, 1979.
72. Phillips A: Will the drugs still work? Transmission of resistant HIV, *Nat Med* 7:993-994, 2001.
73. Ploy MC, Lambert T, Couty J-P, et al: Integrons: an antibiotic resistance gene capture and expression system, *Clin Chem Lab Med* 38:483-487, 2000.
74. Polk R: Optimal use of modern antibiotics: emerging trends, *Clin Infect Dis* 29:264-274, 1999.
75. Putman M, vanVeen HW, Konings WN: Molecular properties of bacterial multidrug transporters, *Microbiol Mol Biol Rev* 64:672-693, 2000.
76. Reves RR, Murray BE, Pickering LK, et al: Children with trimethoprim- and ampicillin-resistant fecal *Escherichia coli* in day care centers, *J Infect Dis* 156:758-762, 1987.
77. Rice LB, Bonomo RA: The red menace: emerging issues in antimicrobial resistance in gram-negative bacilli, *Curr Infect Dis Reports* 1:338-346, 1999.
78. Roberts AP, Pratten J, Wilson M, et al: Transfer of a conjugative transposon, Tn 5397 in a model oral biofilm, *FEMS Microbiol Lett* 177:63-66, 1999.
79. Roberts MC, Sutcliffe J, Courvalin P, et al: Nomenclature for macrolide and macrolide-lincosamide-streptogramin B resistance determinants, *Antimicrob Agents Chemother* 43:2823-2830, 1999.
80. Ryan DM, Cars O, Hoffstedt B: The use of antibiotic serum levels to predict concentrations in tissues, *Scand J Infect Dis* 18:381-388, 1986.
81. Saenz Y, Zarazaga M, Lantero M, et al: Antibiotic resistance in *Campylobacter* strains isolated from animals, foods, and humans in Spain in 1997-1998, *Antimicrob Agents Chemother* 44:267-271, 2000.
82. Salyers AA, Shoemaker NB, Li LY: In the driver's seat: the *Bacteroides* conjugative transposons and the elements they mobilize, *J Bacteriol* 177:5727-5731, 1995.
83. Salyers AA, Whitt DD: *Bacterial pathogenesis: a molecular approach*, ed 2, Washington DC, 2002, ASM Press.
84. Schrag SJ, Beall B, Dowell SF: Limiting the spread of resistant pneumococci: biological and epidemiologic evidence for the effectiveness of alternative interventions, *Clin Microbiol Rev* 13:588-601, 2000.
85. Scott G: Prevention and control of infections in intensive care, *Intensive Care Med* 26(Suppl 1):S22-S25, 2000.
86. Scott MG, Hancock RE: Cationic antimicrobial peptides and their multifunctional role in the immune system, *Crit Rev Immunol* 20:407-431, 2000.
87. Shaffer D, Singer S, Korvick J: *Macrolide and fluoroquinolone associated torsades de pointes: review of the FDA Adverse Event Reporting System*, 41st Annual ICAAC Meeting, A-635, Chicago, December 2000.
88. Shoemaker NB, Vlamakis H, Hayes K, et al: Evidence for extensive resistance gene transfer among *Bacteroides* spp. and among *Bacteroides* and other genera in the human colon, *Appl Environ Microbiol* 67:561-568, 2001.
89. Showsh SA, Andrews RE, Jr: Tetracycline enhances Tn916-mediated conjugal transfer, *Plasmid* 28:213-214, 1992.
90. Smith H: Host factors that influence the behavior of bacteria pathogens in vivo, *Int J Med Microbiol* 290:207-213, 2000.
91. Smith R: Action on antimicrobial resistance. Not easy but Europe can do it, *Br Med J* 317:764, 1998.
92. Spratt BG: Antibiotic resistance: counting the cost, *Current Biol* 6:1219-1221, 1996.
93. Stein F, Trevino R: Nosocomial infections in the pediatric intensive care unit, *Pediat Clin North Am* 41:1245-1257, 1994.
94. Stephenson J: "Sobering" levels of drug-resistant HIV found, *JAMA* 287:704-705, 2002.
95. Stergachis A, Perera DR, Schnell MM, et al: Antibiotic-associated colitis, *West J Med* 140:217-219, 1984.
96. Stevens AM, Sanders JM, Shoemaker NB, et al: Genes involved in production of plasmidlike forms by a *Bacteroides* conjugal chromosomal element share amino acid homology with two-component regulatory systems, *J Bacteriol* 174:2935-2942, 1992.
97. Stevens AM, Shoemaker NB, Li LY, et al: Tetracycline regulation of genes on *Bacteroides* conjugative transposons, *J Bacteriol* 175:6134-6141, 1993.
98. Summers AO, Wireman J, Vimy MJ, et al: Mercury released from dental "silver" fillings provokes an increase in mercury- and antibiotic-resistant bacteria in oral and intestinal floras of primates, *Antimicrob Agents Chemother* 37:825-834, 1993.
99. Tancrede C, Barakat R: Ecological impact of low doses of oxytetracycline on human intestinal microflora, *J Vet Med* 42:35-39, 1989.
100. Tatro DS: Drug-induced prolongation of the QT interval and torsades de pointes, *Drug facts and comparison news* Sept:67-70, 2001.
101. Teuber M: Spread of antibiotic resistance with food-borne pathogens, *Cell Mol Life Sci* 56:755-763, 1999.
102. Thomas J, Walker C, Bradshaw M: Long-term use of sub-antimicrobial dose doxycycline does not lead to changes in antimicrobial susceptibility, *J Periodontol* 71:1472-1483, 2000.
103. Thomas JK, Forrest A, Bhavnani SM, et al: Pharmacodynamic evaluation of factors associated with the development of bacterial resistance in acutely ill patients during therapy, *Antimicrob Agents Chemother* 42:521-527, 1998.
104. Thompson RL, Wright AJ: General principles of antimicrobial therapy, *Mayo Clin Proc* 73:995-1006, 1998.
105. Torres OR, Korman RZ, Zahler SA, et al: The conjugative transposon Tn925: enhancement of conjugal transfer by tetracycline in *Enterococcus faecalis* and mobilization of chromosomal genes in *Bacillus subtilis* and *E. faecalis*, *Mol Gen Genet* 225:395-400, 1991.
106. Van Bambeke F, Balzi E, Tulkens PM: Antibiotic efflux pumps, *Biochem Pharmacol* 60:457-470, 2000.

107. van den Bogaard AE, London N, Stobberingh EE: Antimicrobial resistance in pig faecal samples from The Netherlands (five abattoirs) and Sweden, *J Antimicrob Chemother* 45:663-671, 2000.

108. Wagenlehner F, Stower-Hoffman J, Schneider-Brachert W, et al: Influence of a prophylactic single dose of ciprofloxacin on the level of resistance of *Escherichia coli* to fluoroquinolones in urology, *Int J Amtimicrob Agents* 15:207-211, 2000.

109. Walton RE: Culturing the exudate of an odontogenic infection: a useful procedure [editorial]? *Oral Surg Oral Med Oral Pathol Oral Radiol Endod* 88:525, 1999.

110. Wenzel RP, Edmond MB. The impact of hospital-acquired bloodstream infections, *Emerg Infect Dis* 7:174-177, 2001.

111. White MC: Mortality associated with nosocomial infections: analysis of multiple cause-of-death data, *J Clin Epidemiol* 46:95-100, 1993.

112. White NJ: Drug resistance in malaria, *Br Med Bull* 54:703-715, 1998.

113. Wilkowske CJ: General principles of antimicrobial therapy, *Mayo Clin Proc* 66:931-941, 1991.

114. Wireman J, Liebert CA, Smith T, et al: Association of mercury resistance with antibiotic resistance in gram-negative fecal bacteria of primates, *Appl Environ Microbiol* 63:4494-4503, 1997.

115. Woods AC: Focal infection, *Am J Ophthalmol* 25:1423-1444, 1942.

116. Yingling NM, Byrne BE, Hartwell GR: Antibiotic use by members of the American Association of Endodontists in the year 2000: report of a national survey, *J Endod* 28:396-404, 2002.

117. Zasloff M: Antimicrobial peptides of multicellular organisms, *Nature* 415:389-395, 2002.

CHAPTER • 39

Antibacterial and Antibiotic Drugs*

Thomas J. Pallasch

OROFACIAL INFECTIONS

Infectious diseases are commonly and mistakenly managed as if they all were essentially the same, when in fact the opposite is true since few diseases are associated with more variables than are infectious disease. Each infectious disease process is uniquely dependent on its anatomic location, etiologic microorganism(s) and virulence patterns, accessibility to surgical drainage, signs and symptoms, and, most importantly, the host response to the process. Pneumonia is quite different from otitis media, which differs from a urinary tract infection, which in turn does not resemble infective endocarditis.

Orofacial infections are unique and do not mimic infections in other anatomic locations. They can be chronic (e.g., periodontitis), chronic-subacute with acute exacerbations (e.g., pericoronitis, periodontal abscesses), or intensely acute (e.g., necrotizing gingivitis, periapical abscesses, or cellulitis with or without extension into the orbital or submandibular spaces). Acute orofacial infections commonly arise very rapidly and may easily spread into fascial planes because of their streptococcal component; they are often rapidly terminated by incision and drainage along with antibiotic therapy if appropriate and necessary. The accessibility of orofacial infections to mechanical incision and drainage procedures is often not shared with other bodily infections except those of surgical sites and prosthetic devices.

As with other infectious diseases, various orofacial infections share a commonality among their etiologic microbial pathogens. Otitis media and sinusitis are almost always associated with *Streptococcus pneumoniae, Moraxella catarrhalis,* or *Haemophilus influenzae,* whereas orofacial infections commonly yield viridans group streptococci (VGS), *Prevotella, Porphyromonas, Fusobacteria, Peptostreptococcus, Eubacterium, Veillonella,* and *Actinomyces*. Otitis media or sinusitis is usually associated with only one of its three pathogens, whereas orofacial infections are polymicrobial in nature with two to eight or more microbial species involved. This makes determining the precise etiologic microbe virtually impossible—if indeed only one is the cause. In orofacial infections it is essentially impossible to determine which are the principal pathogens and which are only commensals.

Many infections are monomicrobial in etiology and are caused by microorganisms that, by their nature, are primary pathogens capable of producing disease in the absence of other factors. Orofacial pathogens are rarely if ever primary pathogens but rather are usually opportunists that cause disease when local or systemic variables change—such as trauma, necrosis, tissue oxidation, microbial acquisition of virulence or resistance genes, loss of microbial antagonist(s) from antibiotic therapy, and probably most often a reduction or loss of host immune defense mechanisms. A thorough knowledge of the commonalties and vagaries of oral microbial pathogens is as important as the effective use of antibiotic agents in the successful management of orofacial infections.

Oral Microbial Pathogens and Associated Oral Infections

Acute orofacial infections

The quantifiable data from 12 clinical studies from 1976 to 1996 on the microbiology of acute orofacial infections is presented in Table 39-1. The average number of isolates per case was 3.6, with a maximum of 12. The information in Table 39-1 indicates that acute orofacial infections are polymicrobial, dominated by anaerobes, and often contaminated by a variety of microorganisms, particularly from the pharynx, sinuses, and gastrointestinal tract.

Substantial commonality exists in the microbial cause of acute orofacial cellulitis, pulpal infections, periodontal abscesses, periimplantitis, pericoronitis, acute necrotizing gingivitis, osteomyelitis, and their serious extensions (Ludwig's angina, mediastinal infections). These entities differ primarily in quantitative rather than qualitative microbiologic characteristics. Rapidly spreading infections often have a VGS component because streptococci possess various "spreading factors" (hyaluronidase, streptokinase, streptodornase) that promote rapid movement by fascial planes. Staphylococci rarely move except in blood, whereas gram-negative oral anaerobes may move in tissue but rarely in blood to cause metastatic infections elsewhere; streptococci move easily in both blood and tissue.

Metastatic infections from *Porphyromonas gingivalis, Prevotella intermedia,* and *Prevotella nigrescens* and other anaerobic periodontal pathogens appear to be very rare,[58,72] whereas respiratory tract infections may commonly precede pericoronitis. Staphylococci isolated from facial cellulitis are most likely contaminants because these organisms are not a normal component of the subgingival flora residing primarily on oral mucosal surfaces. They can be a major factor in the cause of oral mucositis. Anterior nares carriage of *Staphylococcus aureus* occurs permanently in 20% and intermittently in 60% of the population.[45] Subgingival staphylococci may appear because of selection by local or systemic antibiotic therapy.[19] Retropharyngeal abscesses appear to have the same microbial cause as facial cellulitis.

*The authors wish to recognize Dr. Edward Montgomery for his past contributions to this chapter. See the Acknowledgments.

Table • 39-1

Microorganisms Associated with Acute Orofacial Abscesses Based on 2339 Isolates in 12 Studies from 1976 to 1996

MICROORGANISM	NUMBER OF ISOLATES	PERCENT OF TOTAL (%)
Aerobes/Facultative		
VGS	470	20.1
Staphylococcus aureus/epidermidis	136	5.8
β-Hemolytic streptococci	68	2.9
TOTAL	674	28.8
Anaerobes		
*Prevotella/Porphyromonas**	641	27.4
Peptostreptococcus	388	16.6
Fusobacteria	181	7.7
Eubacterium	87	3.7
Veillonella	58	2.5
Actinomyces	47	2.0
TOTAL	1402	59.8

Each of the following species is less than 1% of total but together constitute 11.3% of all isolates: *Acinetobacter, Actinobacillus actinomycetemcomitans, Arachnia, Citrobacter, Corynebacterium, Eikenella corrodens, Clostridia, Enterobacter, Escherichia coli,* group A, B, C, D, and G streptococci, *Haemophilus influenzae, Klebsiella pneumoniae, Lactobacillus, Neisseria, Propionibacterium acnes, Serratia,* and spirochetes (most likely contaminants).
*Most studies list as *Bacteroides.*

Box • 39-1

Microorganisms Isolated from Pulpal/Periapical Infections

Aerobic/Facultative

Gram-Positive Cocci
Staphylococci
VGS*

Gram-Positive Bacilli
Lactobacillus
Corynebacterium
*Eikenella corrodens**

Anaerobic

Gram-Positive Cocci
*Peptostreptococcus micros**

Gram-Negative Cocci
*Veillonella**

Gram-Positive Bacilli
*Actinomyces**
Bifidobacterium
Eubacterium
Clostridia
Propionibacterium

Gram-Negative Bacilli
Bacteroides
*Fusobacteria**
*Porphyromonas**
*Prevotella**

Treponemes*
Treponema denticola
Treponema macrodentium
Treponema oralis
Treponema pectinovorum
Treponema socranskii
Treponema vincentii

*Major oral pathogens.
VGS, Viridans group streptococci.

Pulpal and periapical pathogens

It may be somewhat artificial to separate acute orofacial infections from the microbiologic features of pulpal and periapical lesions as acute facial cellulitis is most often a sequela to dentition-derived infections. Yet this is often done in the literature, and at times it is difficult to determine precisely what type of infection is being studied, making a review of both of these entities necessary.

A number of studies have attempted to determine the significance and quantity of microbial pathogens responsible for pulpal and periapical infections. Some maintain that certain microorganisms work synergistically to initiate orofacial infections, whereas others have concluded that each pulpal infection has its own distinct flora. More recent studies have isolated a high prevalence of black-pigmented anaerobes (*Prevotella nigrescens* and *intermedia, Porphyromonas gingivalis* and *endodontalis*); however, this may reflect better anaerobic isolation technique rather than a shift in pathogenic flora. The percent of obligate anaerobes isolated varies with the particular study from 21% to 80%, again possibly reflecting the skill in taking the culture. These infections are polymicrobial, with the number of species isolated varying from one to 33, with five to seven species commonly reported as an average. Achieving a general consensus of the major pathogenic microorganisms responsible for pulpal/periapical infections is hampered by methodologic difficulties: small sample sizes, lack of randomization or use of consecutive case series, varying expertise in culturing, presence or absence of dental caries or periodontal disease, and bacterial contamination of cultures. The major exception is VGS, which is prominent in both periodontal health and acute orofacial infections.

The commonly isolated microorganisms associated with pulpal/periapical lesions appear to be VGS, other streptococci (β-hemolytic, β-hemolytic, group D), *Fusobacteria, Peptostreptococcus micros, Lactobacilli, Actinomyces, Porphyromonas, Prevotella, Veillonella, Eubacteria,* and *Bacteroides forsythus.* Other microorganisms found less commonly or rarely include *Propionibacterium acnes, Candida albicans, Enterococcus,* staphylococci, *Pseudomonas aeruginosa, Enterobacter aerogenes, Serratia marcescens, Eikenella corrodens, Streptococcus pneumoniae, Corynebacterium, Capnocytophaga, Selenomonas,* and *Wolinella* (Box 39-1). A significant portion of these may be contaminants.

Periodontal abscesses

The acute periodontal abscess is characterized as a lesion of periodontal breakdown located within the gingival wall of the periodontal pocket and manifested as a localized accumulation of purulence.[34] The acute periodontal abscess may result from an exacerbation of local periodontitis pathology, after periodontal debridement procedures, or from the lodgment of a foreign object in the periodontal pocket (popcorn husks, dental floss, calculus).[34] The microbial cause of the periodontal abscess is similar to that of adult periodontitis and the flora is commonly indistinguishable from the microflora of the subgingival plaque in adult periodontitis.[34] The predominant microflora are *Porphyromonas gingivalis* (55% to 100% of isolates), *Prevotella intermedia* (25% to 100%), *Fusobacterium nucleatum* (44% to 65%), *Actinobacillus actinomycetemcomitans* (25%), *Campylobacter rectum* (80%), *Prevotella melaninogenicus* (22%), and *Treponema denticola* (71%)[34]; other organisms include *Peptostreptococcus micros* and *Bacteroides forsythus*.[34] It has been estimated that 74% may be anaerobes and 67% gram-negative rods, with streptococci significant only at the base of the abscess.[63]

The principal and sometimes only therapy of the periodontal abscess is incision and drainage through the external tissue and compression of the soft tissue wall.[34] Curettage or root planing is not usually required unless a reasonable chance exists to eliminate the periodontal pocket.[34] The abscess tends to readily fistulate and rarely results in metastasis or acute orofacial cellulitis, possibly because VGS have been replaced by periodontal pathogens that do not spread by fascial planes as do streptococci. On fistulization the lesion is self-limiting, as opposed to dentoalveolar abscesses of pulpal origin, which may readily end in cellulitis.

Often the periodontal abscess can be treated simply with incision and drainage without antibiotics because it is rarely associated with fever, malaise, lymphadenopathy, and other signs of systemic involvement; the periodontal abscess may necessitate antibiotic therapy only if the signs and symptoms of systemic involvement or cellulitis are present or incision and drainage cannot be performed.[34,51,69] This is in contrast to the antibiotic therapy of the pulpal/periapical infection, which should be more aggressive because there is a much greater tendency to spread into the fascial planes. If antibiotic therapy of a periodontal abscess is indicated, the situation is classic for short-term, high-dose therapy as opposed to commonly longer therapy for the dentoalveolar abscess.[51,70] Periodontal pathogens rarely if ever metastasize to the heart or other organs and tissues.[71,72]

Acute necrotizing ulcerative gingivitis

The microbiology of acute necrotizing ulcerative gingivitis (trench mouth, Vincent's infection) is characterized primarily by *Treponema, Fusobacteria, Selenomonas,* and *Prevotella intermedia* and secondarily by *Veillonella, Neisseria, Capnocytophaga, Eikenella corrodens, Bacteroides, Actinomyces,* and gram-positive cocci.[56]

Pericoronitis

The microbial flora of pericoronitis are a complex mixture of organisms resembling that of both periodontitis or gingivitis,[50] often with a high concentration of VGS. Common microorganisms found in 40% or more of samples include *Stomatococcus, Rothia dentocariosa, Actinomyces naeslundii* and *israelii, Prevotella, Neisseria, Haemophilus, Peptostreptococcus micros, Capnocytophaga, Corynebacterium, Bifidobacteria,* and treponemes.[50] Other less common isolates include coagulase-negative staphylococci (CoNS), *Lactobacilli, Veillonella, Fusobacteria,* and *Porphyromonas*.[50]

Periimplantitis

The microbial causes of chronic adult periodontitis, refractory periodontitis, and periimplantitis (an inflammatory process of the tissues surrounding an osseointegrated implant resulting in loss of supporting bone) are remarkably similar, differing primarily in the quantitative and not qualitative isolation of the predominant species: *Bacteroides forsythus, Fusobacterium nucleatum, Porphyromonas gingivalis, Prevotella intermedia* and *nigrescens, Campylobacter rectum,* and treponemes (spirochetes).[53] The healthy dentulous or implant periodontium usually exhibits fewer of the above organisms and is dominated by VGS, *Actinomyces, Veillonella, Eikenella corrodens,* and *Capnocytophaga*.[49]

Periimplantitis results from a shift in periodontal flora with facultative anaerobic streptococci (VGS) and nonmotile rods replaced by gram-negative anaerobic bacilli and spirochetes, much the same as occurs in periodontitis.[49,53] The issue of whether implant success is compromised in patients with periodontitis (treated or untreated) is controversial but it appears reasonable to postulate that the gingival sulcus in patients with periodontitis is a reservoir for periodontal microbial pathogens.[73] Host resistance and factors that reduce immunity (stress) are as likely a complicating factor in periimplantitis as they are in refractory or rapidly progressive periodontitis.

Osteomyelitis

The microbial cause of oral osteomyelitis varies to some extent with the anatomic site and very much with the era in which the cultures were taken. Before the advent of sophisticated anaerobic culturing techniques, the majority of isolates were *Staphylococcus aureus*.[39] It now appears that staphylococci are more likely a contaminant and that oral osteomyelitis is associated with the usual microbial suspects: VGS, *Actinomyces, Fusobacterium nucleatum, Veillonella parvula, Eubacterium, Eikenella corrodens, Prevotella,* and *Porphyromonas*.[39]

Ludwig's angina

As first described by Wilhelm Fredric von Ludwig in 1836, Ludwig's angina is characterized by a massive bilateral edema of the mouth floor with pathognomonic elevation of the tongue against the palate and posterior pharyngeal wall along with glottic edema, resulting in potentially life-threatening airway obstruction. Hence the vernacular terms of "morbus strangulatoris," "angina maligne," and "garotillo" (hangman's noose).

Ludwig's angina involves the connective tissues, fascia, and muscle and spreads by fascial planes through the submandibular, sublingual, and submental spaces and potentially on to the pharynx, retropharyngeal region, and mediastinum.[67] Approximately 70% to 80% of cases are of odontogenic origin, with 99% exhibiting bilateral swelling in the neck, 95% an elevated tongue, 89% fever, and 51% trismus.[67] In 71 cultured patients, 35% of species were VGS, 28% were "other" streptococci, 14% were staphylococci, and 27% were *Porphyromonas* and *Prevotella* and other anaerobes, with a few isolates of *Pseudomonas aeruginosa, Klebsiella pneumoniae, Haemophilus influenzae, Streptococcus pneumoniae,* and *Escherichia coli*.[60] The heavy preponderance of streptococci again emphasizes the ability of these organisms to move through tissue rapidly.

Mediastinal infections

Rarely oral microorganisms may traverse anatomic pathways to locate in the mediastinum. The microbial flora is typically diverse, with the single predominant organisms again being VGS, followed by *Porphyromonas, Prevotella, Fusobacteria,* and staphylococci. Rare isolates included *Escherichia coli, Pseudomonas aeruginosa, Clostridium perfringens, Enterobacter, Enterococcus, Haemophilus influenzae, Klebsiella pneumoniae,* and *Proteus vulgaris*.

Microbial Resistance in Orofacial Pathogens

The data on the antibiotic sensitivity of these orofacial pathogens suffer from major difficulties in that they are very limited, depend on the local antibiotic use in the community, are commonly time dated (what may have been true 5 years ago may not be true today), and crucially dependent on what mean inhibitory concentration (MIC) is chosen as the breakpoint for resistance (the higher the breakpoint, the lower the number of organisms labeled "resistant"). The breakpoint is the MIC for the organism, above which it is considered to be resistant (blood or tissue levels of the antibiotic above this MIC will likely not kill or inhibit its growth).

Even though information on microbial resistance patterns in orofacial pathogens is limited, it is adequate to determine that difficulties exist. Until lately it was and may still be the impression in dentistry that the oral cavity somehow has remained relatively unscathed by the antibiotic resistance epidemic that has plagued other human microbial ecological systems. It is now apparent that no such immunity exists and that oral pathogenic microbes may demonstrate substantial antibiotic resistance that can compromise treatment.

In the 1950s and 1960s it was apparent that oral streptococci and *Streptococcus pneumoniae* (pneumococcus) coinhabit the oropharynx (but not the oral cavity) and had the potential for gene transfer between species. Later it became apparent that both VGS and pneumococci possessed identical β-lactam resistance mechanisms: an altered penicillin binding protein–2b that greatly decreased the affinity of penicillin for its receptor. The genes for this resistance spread from oral streptococci to oropharyngeal *Streptococcus pneumoniae* with devastating effects on the management of one of the world's worst microbial killers.

In the 1970s, viridans and anaerobic streptococci were universally sensitive to the β-lactams, with 90% to 99% also sensitive to erythromycin and clindamycin. In 1983 a high rate of penicillin resistance in VGS was detected in South Africa in the oral flora of children with a similar high penicillin resistance in pneumococci.[31] Currently β-lactamase enzymes are common in oral microorganisms, and VGS (*S. milleri, S. mutans, S. salivarius, S. sanguis, S. mitis* groups) with altered penicillin binding proteins (PBPs) are increasingly resistant to the β-lactams and macrolides.

In children treated for otitis media and exposed to repeated antibiotics who had samples taken of their supragingival plaque, 60% of *Streptococcus sanguis* isolates were resistant to at least one antibiotic, 26% to at least two antibiotics, 32% resistant to amoxicillin, 24% to penicillin V, and 20% to both amoxicillin and penicillin V.[27] In 139 cultures of VGS isolated from mixed orofacial infections, 23% were resistant to penicillin G, 45% to erythromycin, 46% to clindamycin, and 44% to levofloxacin; 100% were sensitive to minocycline.[47] Reports of 23% to 81% resistance rates of VGS to ampicillin and amoxicillin in both hospitalized patients and those in the community are not uncommon, again depending on the breakpoint chosen for resistance.

In a cohort of Japanese children at high risk for bacterial endocarditis, 31.7% of VGS exhibited resistance at MICs of 4 to 16 µg/ml.[64] Children treated with long-term penicillin for the prevention of rheumatic fever were found to have resistance rates of 78% to 81%. The problem is further compounded because many oral streptococci are multiply antibiotic resistant with reduced sensitivities to cephalosporins, macrolides, and clindamycin,[47] as demonstrated by a Taiwan study showing a 20% to 50% resistance rate to clindamycin and 30% to 70% resistance to tetracycline in penicillin-resistant *Streptococcus oralis*.[86]

In the United States, 40% to 50% of sampled VGS are resistant at MICs equal to or greater than 0.25 µg/ml,[41] whereas in a study of 43 US medical centers from 1993 to 1994, 352 VGS blood cultures exhibited a resistance rate of 13.4% at MICs greater or equal to 4 µg/ml (high resistance) and 42.9% at MICs of 0.25 to 2.0 µg/ml (intermediate resistance).[24] Intermediate resistance commonly escalates to high resistance over time.

Of considerable concern is the high β-lactam resistance rate in VGS in patients with neutropenia associated with hematologic malignancies and those at risk for infective endocarditis. Approximately 18% to 21% of bacteremias experienced by immunocompromised patients may be caused by VGS, particularly *Streptococcus mitis* with a 3.2% to 40% resistance rate to penicillin G and cephradine,[75] with some at MICs of 0.25 to 4 µg/ml for penicillin and 2 to 32 µg/ml for cephradine.

Approximately 25 studies have detected β-lactamase production in *Prevotella* and *Porphyromonas* species associated with periodontitis or acute orofacial infections. The prevalence of β-lactamase in these clinical isolates ranges from 11% to 100% depending on study year and type of organisms, but most studies document a 30% to 50% median/mean prevalence of β-lactamase in pigmented and nonpigmented gram-negative anaerobes in the oral cavity. Commonly these organisms presently remain susceptible to β-lactam/β-lactamase inhibitor combinations, metronidazole, and azithromycin.

β-Lactamase production is also present in oral *Veillonella, Fusobacterium, Capnocytophaga, Pseudomonas aeruginosa*, and *Bacteroides forsythus*. Lengthy or repeated antibiotic exposure increases the presence of β-lactamase in oral *Prevotella, Porphyromonas*, and *Fusobacteria*.[35,66] Resistance genes may be shared between family members.[46]

Resistance to the fluoroquinolones in VGS is increasing and the resistance factors can be transferred between VGS, *Streptococcus constellatus*, and *Streptococcus pneumoniae*, providing for efflux mechanisms or point mutations in topoisomerase IV or DNA gyrase. Methicillin-resistant *Staphylococcus aureus* (MRSA) may be present in the oral cavity of children for 5 or more years.[84]

In a study of gingival crevicular fluid microorganisms found in periodontitis patients and their sensitivities to seven antibiotics at two different time periods (1980-1985 and 1991-1995), the resistance rates increased by 172% to tetracycline, 193% to doxycycline, 133% to penicillin G, 238% to amoxicillin, 116% to erythromycin, and 108% to clindamycin.[93] VGS demonstrated variable sensitivities: 85% to 100% to penicillin G, 75% to 100% to amoxicillin, 46% to 100% to clindamycin, and 34% to 74% to tetracyclines.

Veillonella were 83% to 100% sensitive to tetracyclines, 89% to penicillin G, 67% to amoxicillin, 86% to erythromycin, and 94% to clindamycin. *Peptostreptococcus micros* was 67% to 82% susceptible to both tetracycline and amoxicillin, 82% to erythromycin, 95% to penicillin G, and 91% to clindamycin. The breakpoint MICs used for resistance determination in this study were high in some cases: 4 µg/ml for various tetracyclines and 2 µg/ml for penicillins, erythromycin, and clindamycin. Many studies use lower breakpoints that would likely have demonstrated an even higher percentage of resistance strains.

The resistance patterns for orofacial pathogens depends on a number of variables: frequency and duration of exposure to antibiotics both from health care providers and the environment, age, family member exposure to antimicrobials, patterns of antibiotic use in geographical locales, and the particular MICs chosen as breakpoints for resistance. Breakpoints too high will underestimate levels of microbial resistance and those too low will overestimate it. The proper breakpoint is the MIC commonly attained in human beings by reasonable doses.

The oral cavity is as much a part of the microbial world of antibiotic resistance as any other portion of the body and is subject to the same forces that ensure microbial survival elsewhere. The more we look for microbial resistance in the oral environment the more we are likely to find. It is probable that antibiotic failures in the management of orofacial infections will continue to rise, resulting in more severe orofacial infections and a greater dependence on vigorous incision and drainage and sophisticated antibiotic therapy unless wise and judicious use of antimicrobials becomes the universal rule.

ANTIBACTERIAL ANTIMICROBIAL DRUGS

Antibacterial drugs are primarily classified according to their chemical class and mechanism of action.[4] They also can be distinguished based on spectrum and adverse effects. In addition to these aspects of antimicrobial drugs, the therapeutic uses, including dental applications, of each class of drugs are discussed.

β-Lactam Antibiotics

Penicillin has been said to have "brought more curative power to a barefoot, itinerant care provider in the deepest reaches of Africa than the collective powers of all the physicians in New York City."[59] Yet with the seemingly infinite ability of human beings to push a system until it breaks, we now have a multiplicity of microorganisms that were initially exquisitely sensitive to the antimicrobial effects of the penicillins but that are now highly resistant to their killing power. Still, the β-lactam antibiotics remain the most widely used antibiotics in the world because of their broad spectrum of activity and relative lack of toxicity despite a relatively high incidence of allergy.

The β-lactams are composed of five different groups of antibiotics, with the β-lactam nucleus as the common feature: the penicillins, cephalosporins, carbapenems, monobactams, and carbacephems. The penicillins and cephalosporins are the most important with the carbapenems (imipenem, meropenem, ertapenem), monobactams (aztreonam), and carbacephems (loracarbef) reserved for serious infections such as nosocomial (hospital-acquired) infections. The β-lactams as a group have the widest spectrum of antimicrobial activity but range from an extremely narrow spectrum (β-lactamase–resistant penicillins) to a very wide spectrum (imipenem and some cephalosporins).

Penicillins

Penicillin is a generic term for a group of antibiotics that share the β-lactam ring nucleus, similar adverse drug reactions, and mechanism of action, but differ in their antibacterial spectrum, pharmacokinetics, and resistance to β-lactamase enzymes.

Chemistry and classification Penicillin is a cyclic dipeptide consisting of two amino acids (D-valine, L-lysine), a particular molecular configuration unknown in higher life forms (Figure 39-1). The synthesis in 1958 of the basic structure of the penicillins (6-aminopenicillanic acid) allowed for its manipulation by the addition of various side chains to the β-lactam and thiazolidine rings. Different salts (sodium, potassium, procaine, benzathine) were also created for pharmacokinetic purposes. On the basis of these modifications, the penicillins can be divided into four groups: penicillin G and its congeners, β-lactamase–resistant (stable) penicillins, extended-spectrum penicillins, and extended-spectrum penicillins with β-lactamase inhibitors (Table 39-2).

Acid-stable penicillins are those resistant to breakdown in stomach acid, indicating their usefulness as oral drugs. Penicillin V, amoxicillin, and cloxacillin are examples. Other examples are listed in Table 39-2 as orally useful drugs.

Penicillinase-resistant penicillins are those resistant to some β-lactamases (see below). Bacteria, particularly staphylococci, develop resistance to the penicillins chiefly through the elaboration of β-lactamase enzymes (penicillinases) that inactivate the penicillins by cleavage of the 6-aminopenicillanic acid nucleus to yield penicilloic acid derivatives. The production of staphylococcal penicillinase is encoded in a plasmid and may be transferred to other bacteria. Methicillin was the first semisynthetic derivative to be introduced that was stable in the presence of β-lactamase. Subsequently, nafcillin and three isoxazolyl derivatives (oxacillin, cloxacillin, and dicloxacillin) were marketed. The structural formulas for these semisynthetic derivatives are shown in Table 39-2.

Extended-spectrum penicillins are represented by two groups of penicillin derivatives. One group includes ampicillin, the first extended-spectrum penicillin to be introduced; amoxicillin, a close congener of ampicillin; and bacampicillin, a drug that is rapidly hydrolyzed in vivo to yield ampicillin (which then accounts for its pharmacologic and toxicologic effects).

The second group contains carbenicillin, the first penicillin to demonstrate activity against *Pseudomonas* and indole-positive *Proteus* species, and ticarcillin, mezlocillin, and piperacillin, drugs with improved activity against *Pseudomonas aeruginosa*.[65] The molecular structures of these agents are depicted in Table 39-2. Carbenicillin for injection is no longer available in the United States, but carbenicillin indanyl, the oral form, remains in use.

Mechanism of action and antibacterial spectrum Early in the discovery of penicillin, it was noted that the drug acted only on rapidly dividing organisms, and it was later determined that bacterial cell wall precursors (the Park nucleotides) accumulated in sensitive bacteria exposed to the penicillins. Penicillin was determined to be a structural analogue of D-alanine; the final step in the formation of the bacterial rigid cell wall was a transpeptidation reaction involving the enzymatic removal of a terminal D-alanine to allow for the formation of the completed peptidoglycan cell wall. The β-lactams are then competitive inhibitors of various enzymes (transpeptidases, carboxypeptidases), collectively termed the *penicillin-sensitive enzymes*, or more commonly the *PBPs*. The β-lactams promote the formation of cell wall–deficient microorganisms of different shapes (oval, oblong, spherical) depending on the particular PBP affected, which then cannot maintain their internal osmotic pressure and eventually burst. The mechanism of action of the β-lactams is a classic example of Paul Ehrlich's goal of the "magic bullet": a chemical that inhibits a cellular activity present only in bacteria (a rigid cell wall) and not found in mammalian cells.

In some bacterial species the β-lactams have an additional mechanism of action as they activate an enzyme, muramyl synthetase, responsible for the separation of daughter cells after cell division. Activation of this enzyme in the absence of cell division produces lysis of the cell wall (autolysis) and literally bacterial suicide.

Considering these mechanisms it is then apparent why consistently high blood levels of the β-lactams are required for optimum success (not all bacteria divide at the same time) and why the penicillins do not kill rapidly (it takes time for enzyme inhibition and eventual microorganism rupture). This realization that the β-lactams kill slowly has raised questions about the mechanism of action in endocarditis prophylaxis: whether they act only (or at all) by microbial killing or rather by cell wall alteration to retard attachment of the bacteria to damaged cardiac valves.

Penicillin G and penicillin V are narrow-spectrum antibiotics, demonstrating activity against mostly gram-positive

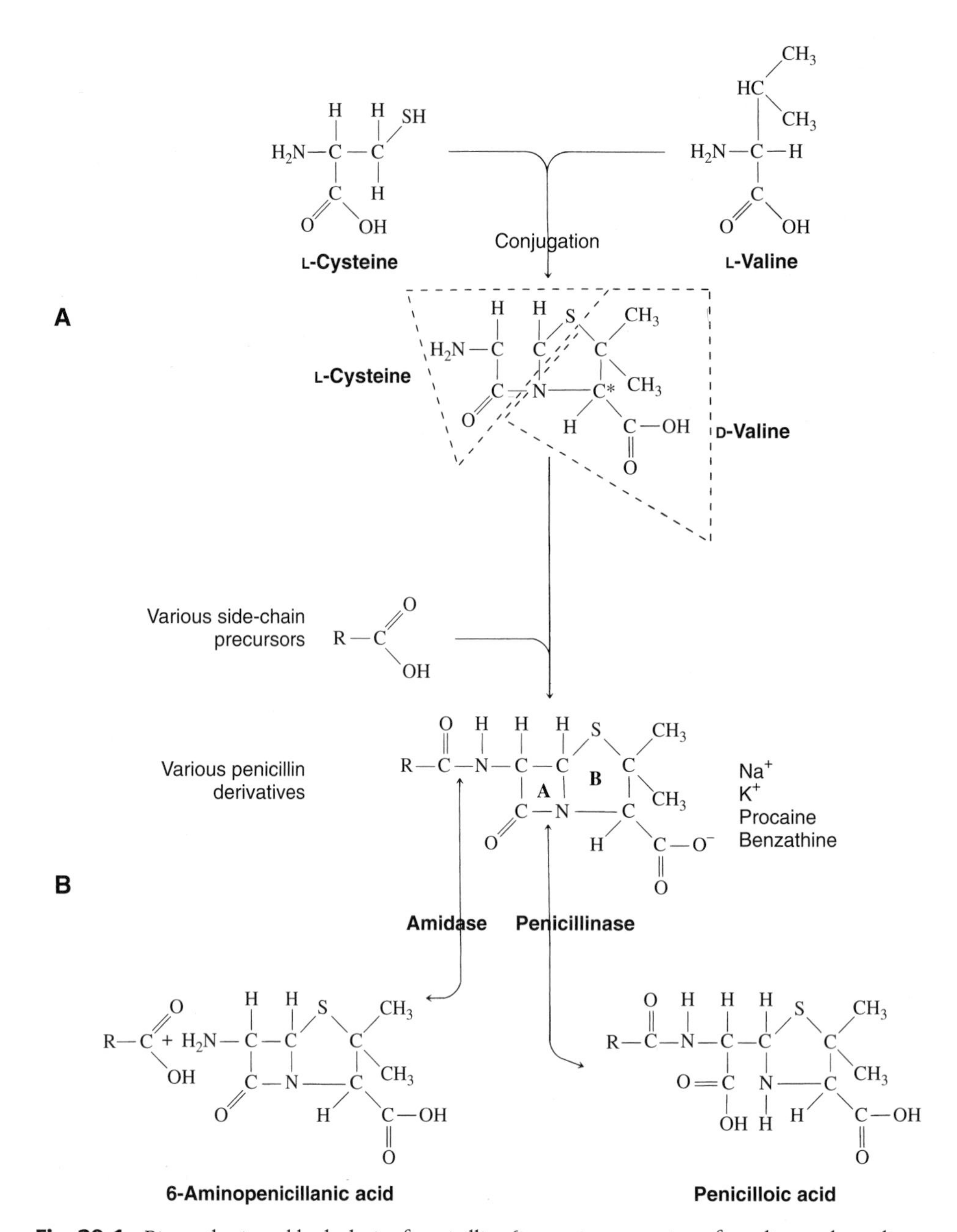

Fig. 39-1 Biosynthesis and hydrolysis of penicillins (isomeric conversion of L-valine and D-valine during conjugation). **A,** β-Lactam ring; **B,** thiazolidine ring.

Table • 39-2

Structures and Characteristics of the Penicillin Derivatives

R—C(=O)—NH—[β-lactam ring (C=O, N) fused to thiazolidine ring (S, CH_3, CH_3, COOH)]

NONPROPRIETARY NAME	R SIDE CHAIN	PROPRIETARY NAME(S)	ROUTE OF ADMINISTRATION
Penicillin G and Congeners			
Penicillin G	C_6H_5—CH_2—	Pfizerpen	IM, IV, Oral*
Penicillin V	C_6H_5—O—CH_2—	PenVee-k, Veetids	Oral
Benzathine penicillin G	Same as penicillin G	Bicillin L-A, Permapen	IM
Procaine penicillin G	Same as penicillin G	Wycillin	IM
Procaine + benzathine penicillin G	Same as penicillin G	Bicillin C-R	IM
β-Lactamase-Resistant Penicillins			
Methicillin[†]	2,6-(OCH_3)$_2$-phenyl—	Staphcillin	IM, IV
Nafcillin	2-OCH_3-naphthyl—	Unipen, Nafcil	Oral, IM, IV
Oxacillin	phenyl-isoxazolyl (N, O, CH_3)—	Bactocill	Oral, IM, IV
Cloxacillin	Cl-phenyl-isoxazolyl (N, O, CH_3)—	Cloxapen	Oral
Dicloxacillin	Cl,Cl-phenyl-isoxazolyl (N, O, CH_3)—	Dynapen, Dycill	Oral
Extended-Spectrum Penicillins			
Aminopenicillins			
Ampicillin	C_6H_5—CH(NH_2)—	Omnipen, Principen	Oral, IM, IV
Bacampicillin	1-Ethoxycarbonyl-oxyethyl ester of ampicillin	Sectrobid	Oral
Amoxicillin	HO—C_6H_4—CH(NH_2)—	Amoxil, Trimox	Oral

Continued

Table • 39-2

Structures and Characteristics of the Penicillin Derivatives—cont'd

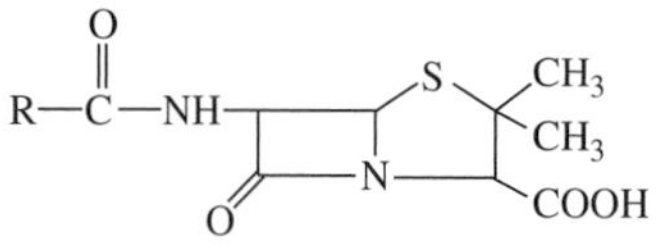

NONPROPRIETARY NAME	R SIDE CHAIN	PROPRIETARY NAME(S)	ROUTE OF ADMINISTRATION
Extended-Spectrum Penicillins—cont'd			
Carboxypenicillins			
Carbenicillin indanyl	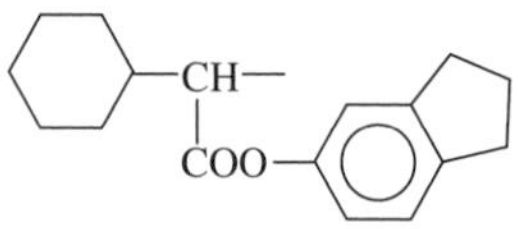	Geocillin	Oral
Ticarcillin	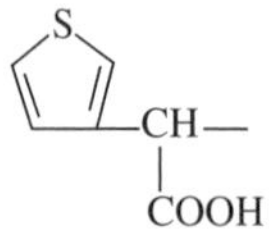	Ticar	IM, IV
Ureidopenicillins			
Mezlocillin	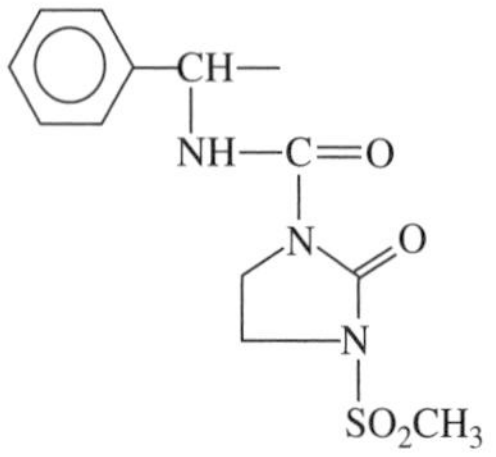	Mezlin	IM, IV
Piperacillin	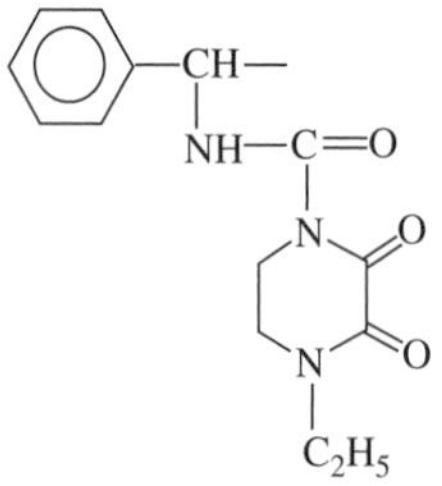	Pipracil	IM, IV
Extended-Spectrum Penicillins Plus β-Lactamase Inhibitors			
Amoxicillin plus clavulanate		Augmentin	Oral
Ampicillin plus sulbactam		Unasyn	IM, IV
Piperacillin plus tazobactam		Zosyn	IV
Ticarcillin plus clavulanate		Timentin	IV

*Poorly absorbed by the oral route.
†Discontinued in the United States.
IM, Intramuscular; *IV*, intravenous.

cocci and gram-positive bacilli as well as gram-negative cocci. Other penicillins have an extended spectrum and greater activity against some gram-negative bacilli.

The penicillins as agents of choice in treating specific organisms are listed in Box 39-2 (primarily according to the *Medical Letter of Drugs and Therapeutics*).[15,29,96] Amoxicillin or penicillin V are drugs of choice against VGS, peptostreptococci, *Eikenella corrodens, Fusobacterium nucleatum, Actinomyces israelii, Clostridium tetani* and *perfringens, Leptotrichia buccalis, Neisseria,* and non–β-lactamase–producing *Prevotella* and *Porphyromonas*.[15,29,96] Amoxicillin plus clavulanate is additionally effective against *Klebsiella pneumoniae, Enterobacter, Moraxella catarrhalis, Bacteroides fragilis,* non–methicillin-resistant and β-lactamase–producing staphylococci, and β-lactamase–producing *Prevotella* and *Porphyromonas*.[29]

Amoxicillin and penicillin V are the initial drugs of choice in orofacial infections in nonallergic patients but are ineffective against streptococci (VGS) with altered PBPs. The clinical impact of antibiotic failures against these resistant streptococci and gram-negative β-lactamase–producing oral anaerobes is likely to be significant but has yet to be determined by clinical studies. On the basis of the antimicrobial spectrum of penicillin G and V, as well as other clinical characteristics, the drugs are useful in the treatment of a large number of diseases (Box 39-3).

Bacterial resistance Bacteria evade the killing effects of the β-lactams by three mechanisms: reduced drug binding to PBPs (altered target sites), hydrolysis by β-lactamase enzymes (enzymatic inactivation), or development of tolerance by the

Box • 39-2

The Penicillins as Drugs of Choice or Alternative Agents (Penicillin G, Penicillin V, Ampicillin, or Amoxicillin Unless Otherwise Indicated)

*Acinetobacter**
Actinomyces israelii
Bacillus anthracis
*Campylobacter fetus**
Capnocytophaga canimorsus
*Citrobacter freundii**
Clostridium perfringens
Clostridium tetani
Eikenella corrodens
*Enterobacter**
Erysipelothrix rhusiopathiae
Fusobacterium nucleatum
Group A, B, C, and G streptococci
Listeria monocytogenes
Neisseria meningitidis
Pasturella multocida
Peptostreptococcus micros
*Serratia marcescens**
Proteus mirabilis
Spirillum minus
Streptobacillus moniliformis
Staphylococcus aureus/epidermidis†
Streptococcus bovis
Treponema pallidum
VGS

From Choice of antibacterial drugs, *Med Lett Drugs Ther* 43:69-78, 2001; *Facts and comparisons,* St Louis, 2002, Facts and Comparisons; Wright AJ: The penicillins, *Mayo Clin Proc* 74:290-307, 1999.
*Imipenem/meropenem.
†β-Lactamase–resistant penicillins.

loss of the autolysis mechanism (penicillin becomes bacteriostatic instead of bactericidal). In most species the principal mechanism is β-lactamase production.

Absorption, fate, and excretion The important pharmacokinetic properties of the oral penicillins are listed in Table 39-3.[10,62] Penicillin G (benzylpenicillin) it rarely used orally because of its poor gastric absorption rate. If it is prescribed orally it should be given at doses four to five times greater than those used parenterally. Both penicillin V and amoxicillin are well absorbed orally, with amoxicillin considerably superior in its half-life and peak serum concentrations. Better oral absorption argues for the use of amoxicillin over penicillin V, but both drugs are effective in microorganism-sensitive orofacial infections and are equally inactive against VGS with altered PBPs.

Box • 39-3

Disease Entities for Which Penicillin G or V or Amoxicillin are of Major Use

Abscesses, including orodental
Bacteremia (gram-positive)
Endocarditis
Gas gangrene
Mastoiditis
Meningitis
Orodental infections
Osteomyelitis
Pericarditis
Periodontal infections
Pharyngitis
Pneumonia
Rat-bite fever
Scarlet fever
Suppurative arthritis
Syphilis
Vincent's stomatitis
Weil's disease
Wound infections

These diseases are caused by a variety of gram-positive cocci and bacilli and some gram-negative organisms, spirochetes, and anaerobic microorganisms. Susceptibility testing may be essential for some to determine therapeutic MICs.

Procaine penicillin G and benzathine penicillin G are repository forms prepared for intramuscular injection with slow release from the injection site (Figure 39-2). The free non–protein-bound serum concentration of the penicillins is penicillin G (0.9 μg/ml), penicillin V (0.8 μg/ml), dicloxacillin (0.45 μg/ml), and amoxicillin (6.2 μg/ml).[10] The route of excretion is primarily by the kidneys, with limited liver

Table • 39-3

Pharmacokinetics of Various Oral Penicillins

PENICILLIN	ORAL ABSORPTION (%)	HALF-LIFE (hr)	PEAK SERUM LEVELS (μg/ml)	PROTEIN BINDING (%)	FOOD AFFECTS ABSORPTION (ACID LABILE)
Penicillin G	20	0.5	2	45 to 68	Yes
Penicillin V	60 to 73	0.5	4	75 to 89	No
Amoxicillin	75 to 90	0.7 to 1.4	7.5	17 to 20	No
Dicloxacillin	35 to 76	0.3 to 0.9	15	95 to 97	Yes
Amoxicillin-clavulanate	75 to 90	0.7 to 1.4	7.5	17 to 20	No

From Cars O: Efficacy of beta-lactam antibiotics: integration of pharmacokinetics and pharmacodynamics, *Diag Microbiol Infect Dis* 27:29-33, 1997; Neu HC: Penicillins. In Mandell GL, Douglas RG, Jr, Bennett JE, eds: *Principles and practice of infectious diseases,* ed 5, New York, 1990, Churchill Livingstone.

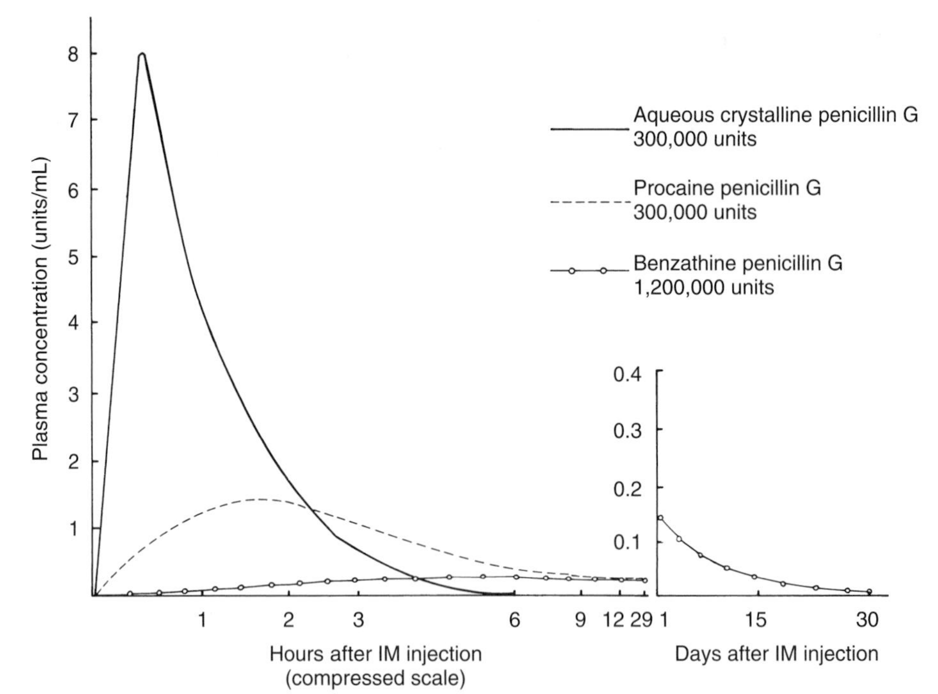

Fig. 39-2 Comparative plasma concentrations of penicillin G obtained from soluble versus repository intramuscular (IM) dosage forms.

metabolism: penicillin G (20% metabolized), penicillin V (50%), dicloxacillin (10%), and amoxicillin (10%).[10]

The β-lactam antibiotics produce time-dependent killing of bacteria, therefore frequent dosing is required to maintain relatively constant blood levels with as little fluctuation as possible.[88] The killing power of the β-lactams is maximum at three to four times the MIC of susceptible microorganisms.[88] The prime determinant of the efficacy of β-lactams is the length of time the concentration of the drug in the infected area is above the MIC of the infecting organism.[88]

The serum and tissue concentrations of the β-lactams should be above the MIC for 50% to 70% of the dosing interval to be maximally effective.[18] The current package insert recommends dosing intervals of 6 hours for penicillin V and first-generation oral cephalosporins. Some drugs have very short half-lives (30 to 45 minutes),[29] and consequently 6-hour dosing intervals may result in very low serum levels in the last 2 or 3 hours. Continuous intravenous penicillin is receiving greater attention as a way to circumvent this problem.

β-Lactamase inhibitors Currently three agents are available to bind irreversibly to the catalytic site of susceptible β-lactamases to prevent hydrolysis of β-lactam antibiotics: clavulanic acid, sulbactam, and tazobactam. Clavulanic acid is derived from *Streptomyces clavligerus*, sulbactam is a semisynthetic penicilloic acid sulfone, and tazobactam is chemically related to sulbactam.[8] All β-lactamase inhibitors have the same mechanism of action: to bind to the active site of β-lactamases where they are then converted to an inactive product by β-lactamase ("suicide inhibition").[8] Only clavulanic acid is orally absorbed. Clavulanic acid is combined with amoxicillin, sulbactam with ampicillin, and tazobactam with piperacillin.

The β-lactamase inhibitors are generally effective against plasmid-mediated β-lactamases found in methicillin-sensitive *Staphylococcus aureus (MSSA)*, *Haemophilus influenzae* and *ducreyi*, *Escherichia coli*, *Klebsiella pneumoniae*, *Proteus mirabilis*, *Listeria*, *Neisseria gonorrhoeae*, all anaerobes, and some *Enterobacteriaceae*. They are generally ineffective against chromosomally mediated β-lactamases found in *Enterobacter*, *Pseudomonas aeruginosa*, *Morganella morganii*, *Serratia marcescens*, and organisms producing inducible extended-spectrum β-lactamases.

The sole therapeutic use of the β-lactamase inhibitors is to prevent the hydrolysis of penicillins in the management of β-lactamase–producing microorganisms responsible for otitis media and sinusitis *(Streptococcus pneumoniae, Haemophilus influenzae, Moraxella catarrhalis)*, nosocomial pneumonia (MSSA or *Klebsiella pneumoniae*), intraabdominal abscesses from β-lactamase–producing anaerobes and other microorganisms, and some upper respiratory tract infections. β-lactam/β-lactamase inhibitor combinations offer no advantage against non–β-lactamase–producing microorganisms and are ineffective against MRSA, many CoNS and enterococci, and the inducible β-lactamases produced by *Pseudomonas aeruginosa*, *Serratia marcescens*, *Enterobacter cloacae*, *Citrobacter freundii*, and *Morganella morganii*.[8] These β-lactam/β-lactamase inhibitor combinations can often be useful as alternate antibiotics against *Bacteroides*, *Moraxella catarrhalis*, *Escherichia coli*, *Klebsiella pneumoniae*, indole-positive *Proteus*, *Providencia rettgeri* and *stuartii*, *Eikenella corrodens*, *Pasturella multocida*, and *Pseudomonas pseudomallei* (see Box 39-2).[15]

Therapeutic uses in dentistry Because the oral route is the safest, most convenient, and least expensive mode of drug administration, it is favored in the treatment of dental patients. Currently penicillin V is the most frequently prescribed antibiotic for chemotherapy of infections of dental origin, but amoxicillin has significantly superior pharmacokinetics. Parenteral penicillin G is largely reserved for severe infections in patients or situations in which the oral route is compromised (as in malabsorption syndrome and vomiting).

In some instances, penicillins G and V and amoxicillin are unsuitable for treating oral infections. Some dental infections are caused by β-lactamase (penicillinase)–producing organisms and in such cases the appropriate antibiotic is a penicillinase-resistant penicillin derivative, erythromycin, or clindamycin. Patients who have been receiving extended prophylactic therapy with penicillin for the prevention of rheumatic fever generally require another antibiotic if they acquire an infection or require endocarditis prophylaxis. Certain periodontal infections are associated with both gram-positive and gram-negative aerobic and anaerobic microorganisms for which an antimicrobial agent with a more extended antibacterial spectrum such as amoxicillin or more commonly a β-lactam/β-lactamase agent combined with metronidazole may be the agents of choice. Table 39-4 summarizes antimicrobial therapy based on pathogens. It emphasizes the importance of penicillin V and amoxicillin.

Adverse effects The adverse effects of the penicillins are both allergic and nonallergic in nature.

Penicillin allergy Allergic reactions to the penicillins are common; allergic fatalities are far less common. Allergy to the penicillins ranges from 0.7% to 8% in various studies, with a 0.7% to 4% chance of an allergic reaction (average of 2%) during any given course of penicillin therapy.[41,42] Most allergic manifestations are maculopapular or urticarial skin reactions.

Penicillin may be the most common cause of anaphylactic death in the United States, accounting for 75% of all cases and 400 to 800 annual deaths. However, these numbers may be low estimates. Penicillin-induced anaphylaxis is most common in adults between the ages of 20 and 49 years.[41,42] Estimates of severe penicillin anaphylaxis range from 0.004% to 0.015% of persons exposed and, from the point of view of number of exposures, possibly 1 in 1200 to 1 in 2500 penicillin exposures. The fatality rate from penicillin anaphylaxis by all routes of administration may be 1 in 60,000 patient courses (16 per 1 million),[68,70] but data regarding penicillin allergy are limited.

Eventually 1% to 10% of the general population exposed to therapeutic penicillin will have an allergic reaction, with a higher positive history with increased age. Retrospective studies suggest that the incidence of allergy varies with the route of administration: oral (0.3%), intravenous (2.5%), and intramuscular (5%), but this lower incidence by the oral route has been questioned because of limited data.[68,69] With higher oral doses (3.5 g of amoxicillin), the allergy rate may approach that of intramuscular penicillin, indicating that the dose as well as the route may be a determining factor in penicillin allergy. Fatal anaphylactic reactions after oral penicillin are well documented.[68,70]

It is probable that an acute penicillin allergic reaction is less common in children and the elderly, but fatal reactions may be more likely in the elderly because of their compromised cardiopulmonary function. Whether certain individuals are predisposed to penicillin allergy remains unsettled. Risk factors for penicillin allergies include multiple allergies to other drugs, particularly other antibiotics (the "multiple allergy syndrome'), or those with atopic disease (asthma, allergic rhinitis, nasal polyps). Several studies indicate a higher rate of penicillin allergy in persons with a history of other drug allergies while others indicate no such increased risk.[68,70] It is possible that those with multiple drug allergies or atopy may have more severe penicillin allergic reactions. Allergy to the procaine component of procaine penicillin G has been detected.

In persons with a positive history of penicillin allergy, 15% to 40% will demonstrate allergy on reexposure to penicillin, and those with a positive history of penicillin allergy have a four to six times greater likelihood of a subsequent reaction than those with a negative history.[68,70] Some patients may retain their penicillin-specific immunoglobulin (IgE) antibodies indefinitely, while most will lose them over time. The serum half-life of penicillin IgE antibodies ranges from 10 to more than 1000 days; therefore the risk of recurrent penicillin allergy is higher in persons with long half-life antibodies or repeated penicillin exposures. Little data are available regarding whether the 60% to 85% not exhibiting allergy on reexposure will reacquire the IgE antibodies to penicillin and then have an allergic reaction to the drug on the next (third) exposure by resensitization. In a study of patients with a positive history of penicillin allergy (25 with urticaria/angioedema, 19 with anaphylaxis, 19 with pruritic skin rash) and a negative skin test for penicillin allergy, none had an allergic reaction to three successive 10-day courses of penicillin.[78] The average length of time from the penicillin allergic reaction to rechallenge was 25 years (range, 5 to 50 years), indicating that patients commonly lose their antibodies to penicillin. This study, however, provides no information on patients with a more recent history of penicillin allergy.

Because variable IgE antibody levels to penicillin are commonplace, skin testing for penicillin allergy becomes problematic. The incidence of positive skin tests in persons with a history of penicillin allergy range from 4% to 91% depending on the accuracy of the patient history, the haptens in the test solution, and the time elapsed between the allergic reaction and the skin test.[68,70] It is possible that penicillin skin tests may only be reliable for 72 hours after the test is performed.[68,70]

Penicillin skin testing can be of considerable value in determining who might have a severe anaphylactic reaction. Approximately 95% of penicillin-allergic individuals form the penicilloyl-protein conjugate (the major antigenic determinant) and approximately 5% form the 6-aminopenicillanic acid and benzylpenamaldic acid minor antigenic determinants (Figure 39-3).[68,70] Penicillin skin tests with both the major and minor antigenic determinants eliciting a negative skin test virtually eliminate the risk for a serious IgE-mediated reaction. A positive skin reaction to the minor determinant mixture indicates a high risk for anaphylaxis.

The penicillins are primarily associated with IgE-mediated (Gell and Coombs type I) allergic reactions but may also induce types II (cytotoxic) or III (immune complex). Type I signs and symptoms include skin erythema, itch, angioedema, urticaria, wheezing, hypotension, and bronchospasm resulting from mast cell/basophil release of histamine along with other tissue allergic mediators. Type II reactions are caused by circulating IgM or IgG antibodies that attach to blood cells and induce blood dyscrasias: hemolytic anemia, leukopenia, thrombocytopenia, and aplastic anemia. Type III reactions result from the deposition of soluble immune complexes on blood vessels, basement membranes resulting in serum sickness, vasculitis, and glomerulonephritis.

Allergic reactions to the penicillins can also be classified according to their time of onset. Immediate IgE reactions begin within seconds to 1 hour after drug exposure and are the most life threatening (it is an allergy truism that the more rapid the onset of the allergic reaction, the more serious the consequences). Accelerated reactions begin from 1 to 72 hours after antigen exposure and are usually manifested as urticaria or angioedema. Late reactions occur after 72 hours and are characterized by type II and type IV (eczema-like) Gell and Coombs reactions. Ninety-six percent of all fatal anaphylactic reactions occur within the first 60 minutes after penicillin exposure.[68,70]

Some other adverse reactions to the penicillins are likely to be autoimmune in origin and have an obscure etiology: maculopapular rashes, eosinophilia, Stevens-Johnson syndrome, and exfoliative dermatitis. A maculopapular rash is seen in 2% to 3% of persons late in penicillin therapy.

Nonallergic adverse effects Ticarcillin, mezlocillin, and piperacillin may cause abnormal coagulation times; abnormal liver function tests may occur with the β-lactamase–

Table • 39-4

Drugs Used To Treat Infections Caused by Specific Microorganisms

MICROORGANISM	DRUG OF FIRST CHOICE	ALTERNATIVE DRUGS*
Gram-Positive Cocci		
Staphylococcus species		
Methicillin-sensitive	A penicillinase-resistant penicillin (e.g., cloxacillin)	First generation cephalosporin, vancomycin, clindamycin, amoxicillin-clavulanate, ampicillin-sulbactam, piperacillin-tazobactam, imipenem, meropenem, a fluoroquinolone
Methicillin-resistant	Vancomycin with or without gentamicin or rifampin	Quinupristin-dalfopristin, linezolid, a fluoroquinolone, a tetracycline, trimethoprim-sulfamethoxazole
Intermediate sensitivity to vancomycin	Quinopristin-dalfopristin, linezolid	Vancomycin with nafcillin or oxacillin
Streptococcus pyogenes	Penicillin G or V	A cephalosporin, erythromycin, vancomycin, clindamycin, clarithromycin, azithromycin
Streptococcus viridans group		
Oral infections	Penicillin G or V	Erythromycin, clindamycin, a cephalosporin
Bacteremia or endocarditis	Penicillin G with or without gentamicin	Ceftriaxone, vancomycin
Streptococcus, anaerobic *(Peptostreptococcus)*	Penicillin G or V	A cephalosporin, clindamycin, vancomycin
Streptococcus pneumoniae	Penicillin G or V, amoxicillin	A cephalosporin, trimethoprim-sulfamethoxazole, erythromycin, clindamycin, clarithromycin, azithromycin, levofloxacin, gatifloxacin, moxifloxacin, meropenem, imipenem
Enterococcus species	Ampicillin, amoxicillin, or penicillin G with gentamicin	Vancomycin with gentamicin, linezolid, quinupristin-dalfopristin
Gram-Negative Cocci		
Neisseria gonorrhoeae	Ceftriaxone, cefixime, ciprofloxacin, gatifloxacin	Cefotaxime, spectinomycin, penicillin G
Neisseria meningitidis	Penicillin G	Cefotaxime, ceftriaxone, chloramphenicol, a fluoroquinolone
Moxarella (Branhamella) catarrhalis	A fluoroquinolone, cefuroxime	Trimethoprim-sulfamethoxazole, amoxicillin-clavulanate, erythromycin, clarithromycin, azithromycin, a tetracycline, cefotaxime, ceftizoxime, ceftriaxone, cefixime
Gram-Positive Bacilli		
Bacillus anthracis	Ciprofloxacin, a tetracycline	Penicillin G, erythromycin
Clostridium difficile	Metronidazole	Vancomycin
Clostridium perfringens	Penicillin G, clindamycin,	Imipenem, meropenem, ertapenem, metronidazole, chloramphenicol
Clostridium tetani	Metronidazole	Penicillin G, doxycycline
Corynebacterium diphtheriae	A macrolide	Penicillin G
Corynebacterium species (diphtheroids)	Vancomycin or penicillin G with gentamicin	Erythromycin
Gram-Negative Bacilli		
Bacteroides, oropharyngeal strains	Penicillin G	Cefotetan, cefoxitin, clindamycin, metronidazole, ampicillin-sulbactam
Capnocytophaga canimorsus	Penicillin G or V	Cefotaxime, ceftriaxone, clindamycin, ciprofloxacin, imipenem, meroperem
Eikenella corrodens	Ampicillin, amoxicillin-clavulanate	Erythromycin, tetracycline, ceftriaxone
Escherichia coli	Cefotaxime, ceftizoxime, ceftriaxone, ceftazidime	Ciprofloxacin, ampicillin with or without gentamicin, tobramycin or amikacin, aztreonam, an extended-spectrum penicillin with a penicillinase inhibitor, trimethoprim-sulfamethoxazole, imipenem, meropenem, ertapenem

Table • 39-4

Drugs Used To Treat Infections Caused by Specific Microorganisms—cont'd

MICROORGANISM	DRUG OF FIRST CHOICE	ALTERNATIVE DRUGS*
Gram-Negative Bacilli—cont'd		
Fusobacterium species	Penicillin G, penicillin V	Clindamycin, metronidazole, cefoxitin, erythromycin
Haemophilus influenzae	Cefotaxime, ceftriaxone, trimethoprim-sulfamethoxazole	Ampicillin or amoxicillin with or without a penicillinase inhibitor, cefaclor, cefuroxime, ciprofloxacin, clarithromycin
Klebsiella pneumoniae	Cefotaxime, ceftizoxime, ceftriaxone, ceftazidime, cefepime	An aminoglycoside, aztreonam, ciprofloxacin, ofloxacin, imipenem, meropenem, ertapenem, mezlocillin, a penicillin with a penicillinase inhibitor, piperacillin
Legionella pneumophila	Azithromycin or ciprofloxacin or other fluoroquinolone with or without rifampin	Trimethoprim-sulfamethoxazole, erythromycin, doxycycline, with or without rifampin
Leptotrichia buccalis	Penicillin G, penicillin V	Clindamycin, a tetracycline, erythromycin
Proteus mirabilis	Ampicillin or amoxicillin	An aminoglycoside, a cephalosporin, ciprofloxacin, aztreonam, imipenem, meropenem, ertapenem
Pseudomonas aeruginosa	Ticarcillin, piperacillin, or mezlocillin, with an aminoglycoside	Aztreonam, ceftazidime, cefepime or imipenem with an aminoglycoside, ciprofloxacin
Salmonella typhi	Ceftriaxone, ciprofloxacin, or levofloxacin	Amoxicillin, ampicillin, trimethoprim-sulfamethoxazole, azithromycin, chloramphenicol
Shigella	A fluoroquinolone	Trimethoprim-sulfamethoxazole, ampicillin, azithromycin, ceftriaxone
Other Microorganisms		
Mycobacterium tuberculosis	Isoniazid with rifampin and pyrazinamide with or without ethambutol or streptomycin	Ethambutol, cycloserine, amikacin, ciprofloxacin, ofloxacin, capreomycin, kanamycin, ethionamide, clofazimine, aminosalicylic acid, (in combinations)
Actinomyces israelii	Penicillin G	Doxycycline, erythromycin, clindamycin
Nocardia asteroids	Trimethoprim-sulfamethoxazole	Minocycline, sulfisoxazole, amikacin, imipenem, meropenem, amoxicillin-clavulanate, ceftriaxone, linezolid
Treponema pallidum	Penicillin G	Ceftriaxone, doxycycline
Chlamydia psittaci	Doxycycline	Chloramphenicol
Rickettsia	Doxycycline, tetracycline	Chloramphenicol, rifampin, a fluoroquinolone
Candida albicans		
Oral lesions	Nystatin, clotrimazole, fluconazole, or ketoconazole	Itraconazole
Systemic infections	Amphotericin B with or without flucytosine	Fluconazole, itraconazole, ketoconazole
Viruses†		
Herpes simplex		
Orolabial	Penciclovir	
Keratitis	Acyclovir	Trifluridine, foscarnet
Genital infection	Acyclovir	Valacyclovir, famciclovir
Encephalitis	Acyclovir	
Human immunodeficiency virus	Zidovudine with another nucleoside analogue, plus a protease inhibitor†	Zidovudine with another nucleoside analogue, plus nevirapine
Influenza A	Rimantadine	Amantadine, zanamivir, oseltamivir

*Listing does not include all alternative drugs.
†See Chapter 40.

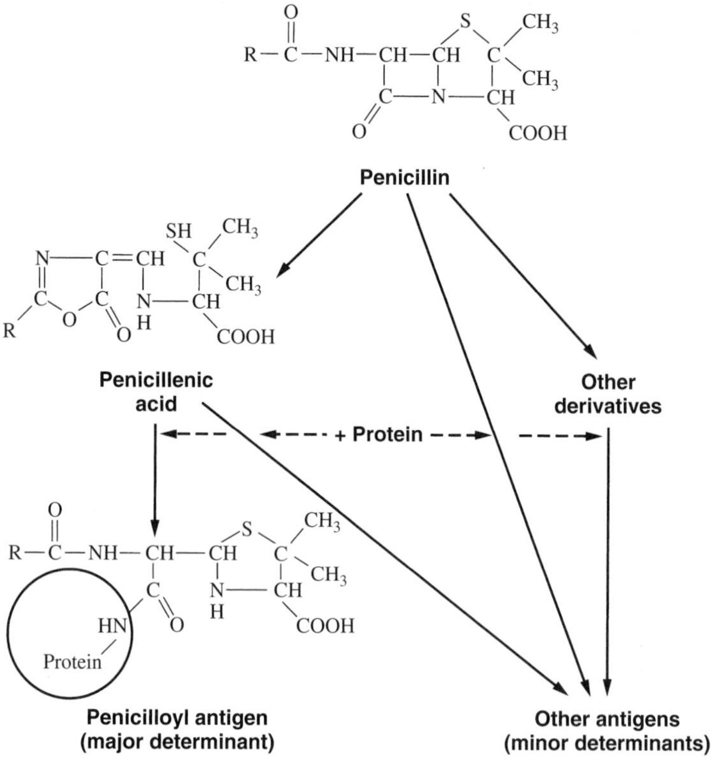

Fig. 39-3 Antigenic determinants of penicillin allergy.

resistant penicillins and Na^+ overload may be seen with the antipseudomonal penicillins. Large intravenous doses of penicillins may induce hyperexcitability, seizures, and hallucinations. Amoxicillin is the most common cause of antibiotic-induced diarrhea/colitis because of its spectrum and widespread use. The penicillins are Food and Drug Administration (FDA) pregnancy B drugs.

Approximately 5% to 10% of persons receiving ampicillin or amoxicillin may have a mild pruritic rash, usually beginning on the body trunk and then extending to the face, extremities, and extensor portions of the knees and elbows. This nonallergic "ampicillin/amoxicillin rash" is not associated with antibody formation and is of unknown cause. It does not appear to increase the risk of true penicillin allergy. The rash may begin 24 hours to 28 days after the drug is begun and may last for 90 minutes to 7 days. The incidence of ampicillin/amoxicillin rash is 95% to 100% in persons with cytomegalovirus infection/mononucleosis and 22% in persons given both ampicillin and allopurinol.

Rare and reversible disorders reportedly associated with the penicillins include acute pancreatitis, neutropenia, aseptic meningitis, and hepatotoxicity and increased prothrombin time/international normalized ratio (INR) in patients taking the oral anticoagulants either through impaired platelet function or altered gastrointestinal microbial flora. Untoward bleeding may occur also in patients not taking the coumarin anticoagulants and is dose dependent, with a maximum effect 3 to 7 days after the penicillin is begun, with a return to a normal bleeding time in up to 72 to 96 hours; this bleeding has been reported after a dental extraction.[7] The mechanism is likely from an altered adenosine diphosphate–mediated platelet aggregation response and is seen most commonly in patients with underlying chronic illnesses associated with hypoalbuminemia and uremia.

Drug interactions The oral penicillins (penicillin G, penicillin V, amoxicillin) may be antagonized by bacteriostatic antibiotics (tetracycline, erythromycin, clindamycin). Nonsteroidal antiinflammatory drugs and probenecid may increase the serum half-lives of the penicillins by decreasing their renal excretion. Persons taking β-adrenergic blocking drugs may have a diminished or nonexistent response to a β-adrenergic receptor agonist given for the treatment of penicillin-induced anaphylactic bronchospasm.

Contraindications The penicillins are generally contraindicated in persons allergic to the drugs but it is well documented that some persons with a previous allergic history may subsequently tolerate the drugs without allergic manifestations. The best policy is to refrain if possible from penicillin administration to anyone with a positive history. The penicillins may be contraindicated in some persons taking the coumarin anticoagulants because untoward bleeding may occur, but this appears to be highly unpredictable and rare in occurrence.

Dosage The standard package insert doses for amoxicillin are given in Table 39-5. Amoxicillin has excellent and rapid oral absorption, yields high blood levels, and has a longer half-life than penicillin V. Based on pharmacokinetic studies, the package insert intervals of 6 hours for short half-life β-lactams (penicillin V, cephalexin, cephradine) appear inappropriate and 4-hour dosing intervals will provide more constant blood and tissue levels for these time-dependent antibiotics. As with all acute infections, a loading dose of two to four times the maintenance dose is appropriate, with the possible exception of amoxicillin due to its superior pharmacokinetics.

Cephalosporins

The isolation of the fungus *Cephalosporinium acremonium* (now *Acremonium chrysogenum*) in 1948 by Brotzu from the harbor sewage of Sardinia and the subsequent isolation of the active nucleus of cephalosporin C (7-amino-cephalosporinic

Table • 39-5

Recommended Doses of Some Antibiotics

ANTIBIOTIC	DOSE
β-Lactams	
Penicillin V	Adult: 250 to 500 mg every 6 hours; child (<12 years): 250 to 500 mg every 6 hours
Amoxicillin	Adult: 250 to 500 mg every 8 hours; child (<20 kg): 20 to 40 mg/kg in 8-hour divided doses or 6.7 to 13.3 mg/kg every 8 hours
Amoxicillin/clavulanate	Adult: 250 to 500 mg every 8 hours; child: 25 to 40 mg/kg per day in 8-hour divided doses or 6.6 to 13.3 mg/kg every 8 hours
Dicloxacillin	Adult: 125 to 500 mg every 6 hours; child (<20 kg): 50 to 100 mg/kg per day in 6-hour divided doses or 3.125 to 6.25 every 6 hours
Cephalexin	Adult: 125 to 1000 mg every 6 hours; child: 25 to 100 mg/kg per day in 4 divided doses
Cephradine	Adult: 250 to 1000 mg every 6 hours; child: 25 to 100 mg/kg per day in 2 or 4 divided daily doses
Cefaclor	Adult: 250 to 500 mg every 8 hours; child: 20 to 40 mg/kg per day in divided doses every 8 hours
Macrolides	
Erythromycin	Adult: 250 to 500 mg (stearate, base, or estolate salts) or 400 mg ethylsuccinate salt every 6 hours; child: 30 to 50 mg/kg per day in divided doses every 6 hours
Azithromycin	Adult: 500 mg every 12 hours; child: 5 to 12 mg/kg per day
Clarithromycin	Adult: 250 to 500 mg every 12 hours; child: 7.5 mg/kg twice daily up to 500 mg twice daily
Miscellaneous Antibiotics	
Clindamycin	Adult: 150 to 450 mg every 6 hours; child: 8 to 20 mg/kg per day in 3 or 4 equal doses
Metronidazole	Adult: 250 to 750 mg every 8 hours, not to exceed 4 g in 24 hours
Ciprofloxacin	Adult: 250 to 500 mg every 12 hours; child: 25 mg/kg per day divided every 12 hours
Doxycycline	Adult: 200 mg on day 1 (100 mg every 12 hours) then 100 mg daily; child (age 8 or older): 4.4 mg/kg in two divided doses on day 1 then 2.2 mg/kg daily
Linezolid	Adult: 375 to 625 mg every 12 hours

From Amsden GW: Tables of antimicrobial agent pharmacology. In Mandell GL, Bennett JE, Dolin R, eds: *Mandell, Douglas and Bennett's Principles and practice of infectious diseases,* Philadelphia, 2000, Churchill Livingstone; *Facts and comparisons,* St Louis, 2002, Facts and Comparisons; Neu HC: Penicillins. In Mandell GL, Douglas RG, Jr, Bennett JE, eds: *Principles and practice of infectious diseases,* ed 5, New York, 1990, Churchill Livingstone; Pallasch TJ: Antibiotics for acute orofacial infections, *J Calif Dent Assoc* 21:34-44, 1993; Wright AJ: The penicillins, *Mayo Clin Proc* 74:290-307, 1999.

acid) by Florey and Abraham at Oxford University contributed in large measure to a golden age in antimicrobial chemotherapy. Unfortunately the massive use and misuse of the cephalosporins because of their broad antibacterial spectrums combined with low toxicity and allergenicity has resulted in widespread microbial resistance to these agents.

Chemistry and classification The cephalosporins are closely related to the penicillins, with a 6-membered dihydrothiazine ring replacing the 5-membered thiazolidine ring of penicillin (Figure 39-4). Both contain the β-lactam ring, as do the monobactams and carbapenems discussed below. Side chain modification of the 7-APA nucleus has led to differences in antibacterial spectrum, pharmacokinetics, susceptibility to various β-lactamases, affinity for different PBPs, and occasionally adverse reactions.

The cephalosporins are most commonly classified according to their "generations": first generation (introduced in the 1960s), second generation (1970s), third generation (1980s), and fourth generation (cefepime in 1997) (Box 39-4).[6,29,42,57] Ceftidoren is a third-generation agent introduced in 2001. It is useful to examine the cephalosporins according to their antibacterial spectrum and therapeutic uses (Table 39-6).[29]

The cephalosporins evolved from early agents primarily active against gram-positive microorganisms (first generation) to those with a greater gram-negative spectrum (second generation) to those with greater activity against various nosocomial pathogens: *Pseudomonas aeruginosa, Bacteroides fragilis,* and organisms producing extended spectrum and ampicillin C (ampC) β-lactamases. The demand for wider spectrum cephalosporins to avoid having to isolate the organism via culture and sensitivity tests (and thereby save money) has been a major factor in microbial resistance to these agents. Technically the second-generation agents include both true cephalosporins and the cephamycins (cefoxitin, cefotetan, cefmetazole), which are derived from *Streptomyces* rather than *Cephalosporinium.*

Mechanism of action and antibacterial spectrum The cephalosporins possess a mechanism of action identical to the penicillins: inhibition of bacterial cell wall peptidoglycan synthesis by inhibition of penicillin-sensitive enzymes (transpeptidases, carboxypeptidases) that are responsible for the final three-dimensional structure of the rigid bacterial cell wall. Each bacterial species may have different PBPs, and the affinity of the cephalosporins for these PBPs can vary greatly.[42] Most cephalosporins bind to PBP1 and PBP3 of gram-negative organisms[6] and, depending on which PBPs are inhibited, the resulting bacterial cells may take different shapes: oval, round, or filamentous.[6] The antibacterial spectrum, susceptible microorganisms, and drugs of choice or alternate indications are listed in Table 39-6.[6,15,42,57]

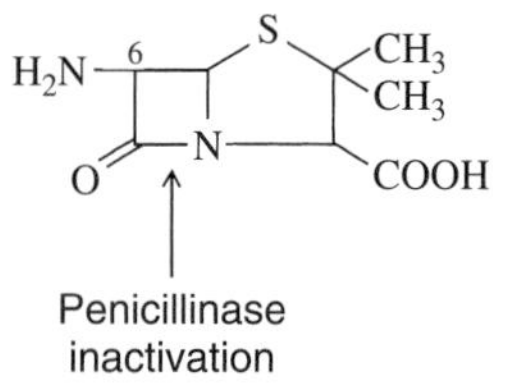

Penicillinase inactivation

6-Aminopenicillanic acid

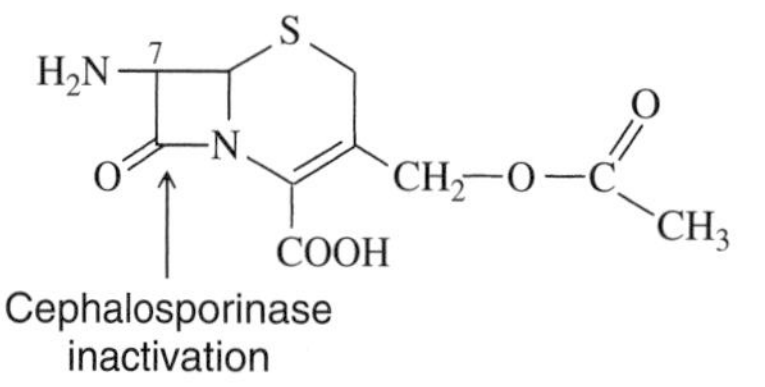

Cephalosporinase inactivation

7-Aminocephalosporanic acid

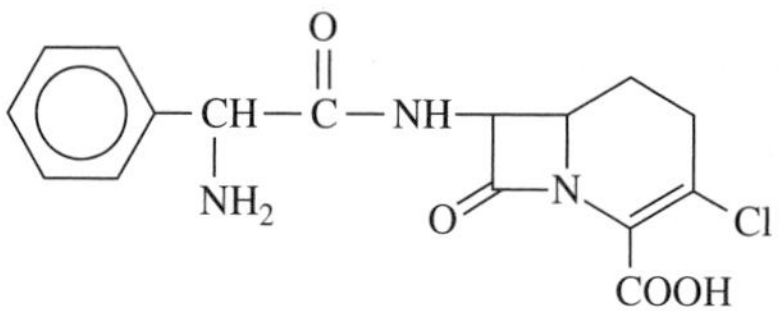

Loracarbef

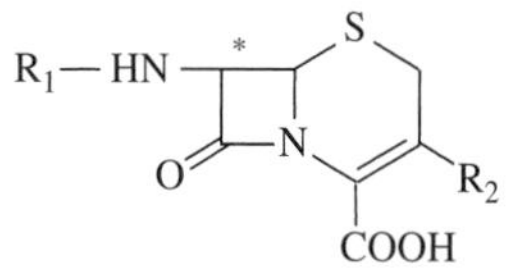

General structure of cephalosporin derivatives

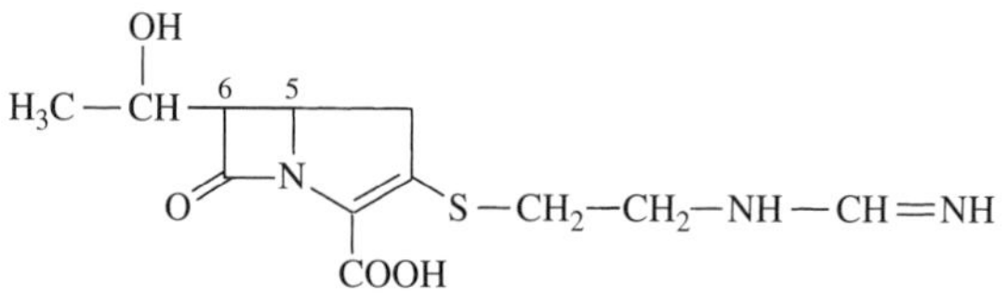

Imipenem

Fig. 39-4 Comparison of basic nuclei of penicillins and cephalosporins. *A methoxy group is added to the 7 carbon in cephamycins. Included for comparison are the structures of imipenem, a carbapenem antibiotic, and loracarbef, a carbacephem.

Box 39-4

Classification of the Cephalosporins by Generations and Classification of Other β-Lactam Antibiotics

Cephalosporins

First Generation

Cefadroxil (Duricef)*
Cefazolin (Ancef, Kefzol, Zolicef)†
Cephalexin (Biocef, Keflex, Keftab)*
Cephalothin (Keflin)†
Cephapirin (Cefadyl)†
Cephradine (Velosef)‡

Second Generation

Cefaclor (Ceclor)*
Cefamandole (Mandol)†
Cefonicid (Monocid)†
Cefotetan (Cefotan)†
Cefoxitin (Mefoxin)†
Cefmetazole (Zefazone)†
Cefprozil (Cefzil)*
Cefuroxime (Ceftin, Kefurox, Zinacef)‡
Loracarbef (Lorabid)*

Third Generation

Cefdinir (Omnicef)*
Cefixime (Suprax)*
Cefoperazone (Cefobid)†
Cefotaxime (Claforan)†
Cefpodoxime (Vantin)*
Ceftazidime (Ceptaz, Fortaz, Tazicef, Tazidime)†
Ceftibuten (Cedax)*
Cefditoren (Spectracef)*
Ceftizoxime (Cefizox)†
Ceftriaxone (Rocephin)†

Fourth Generation

Cefepime (Maxipime)†

Other β-Lactam Antibiotics

Carbapenems

Imipenem (with cilastatin in Primaxin)†
Meropenem (Meronem)†
Ertapenem (Invanz)†

Monobactams

Aztreonam (Azactam)†

From Asbel LE, Levison ME: Cephalosporins, carbapenems, and monobactams, *Infect Dis Clin N Am* 14:435-447, 2000; *Facts and comparisons*, St Louis, 2002, Facts and Comparisons; Karchmer AW: Cephalosporins. In Mandell GL, Bennett JF, Dolin R, eds: *Principles and practice of infectious diseases*, ed 5, New York, 2000, Churchill Livingstone; Marshall WF, Blair JE: The cephalosporins, *Mayo Clin Proc* 74:187-195, 1999.

*Oral.
†Parenteral.
‡Oral and parenteral.

Table • 39-6

Classification of Cephalosporins According to Disease and Antibacterial Spectrum

	ANTIBACTERIAL SPECTRUM	THERAPEUTIC USES	AGENTS
Group 1	*Staphylococcus aureus* *Streptococcus pneumoniae* and *pyogenes* *Haemophilus influenzae* *Escherichia coli* *Klebsiella pneumoniae* *Proteus mirabilis* *Moraxella catarrhalis* *Neisseria gonorrhoeae* VGS	Skin and skin structures Urinary tract infections Respiratory tract infections Bone *(Staphylococcus aureus)* Septicemia Tonsillitis Pharyngitis	Cefazolin Cephapirin Cefdinir Ceftibuten Cefprozil Loracarbef Cephradine Cefadroxil Cephalexin Cefpodoxime
Group 2	*Staphylococcus aureus* *Streptococcus pneumoniae* and *pyogenes* *Escherichia coli* *Haemophilus influenzae* *Proteus mirabilis and vulgaris* *Enterobacteriaceae* *Klebsiella pneumoniae* *Bacteroides fragilis* *Clostridium perfringens* *Moraxella catarrhalis* *Streptococcus agalactiae* (group B streptococcus) *Neisseria meningitides* *Peptostreptococcus*	Skin and skin structures Urinary tract infections Lower respiratory tract infections Acute otitis media Sexually transmitted diseases Sinusitis Chronic bronchitis Community-acquired pneumonia Mild to moderate abdominal infections	Cefmetazole Cefoxitin Cefuroxime Cefonicid Ceftriaxone Cefixime Cefdinir
Group 3	*Streptococcus pneumoniae* *Haemophilus influenzae* *Staphylococcus aureus* *Klebsiella pneumoniae* *Escherichia coli* *Proteus mirabilis* *Enterobacteriaceae* *Bacteroides fragilis* *Streptococcus agalactiae* *Clostridia* *Neisseria gonorrhoeae* CoNS *Fusobacterium nucleatum* *Peptostreptococcus* *Pseudomonas aeruginosa*	Meningitis Lower respiratory tract infections Skin infections Urinary tract infections Sexually transmitted diseases Septicemia Bone and joint infections Pelvic inflammatory disease Intraabdominal infections Peritonitis	Cefoperazone Cefotaxime Ceftriaxone Cefotetan Ceftazidime Cefamandole Cefditoren Cefoperazone, Ceftazidime or Cefoperazone (For *Pseudomonas aeruginosa,* Cefoperazone or Ceftazidime
Group 4	*Streptococcus pyogenes* *Staphylococcus aureus* *Klebsiella pneumoniae* *Pseudomonas aeruginosa* *Enterobacteriaceae* *Bacteroides fragilis*	Pneumonia Moderate to severe skin and abdominal infections Prophylaxis for febrile neutropenia	Cefepime

From Asbel LE, Levison ME: Cephalosporins, carbapenems, and monobactams, *Infect Dis Clin North Am* 14:435-447, 2000; Choice of antibacterial drugs, *Med Lett Drugs Ther* 43:69-78, 2001; *Facts and comparisons,* St Louis, 2002, Facts and Comparisons; Karchmer AW: Cephalosporins. In Mandell GL, Bennett JF, Dolin R, eds: *Principles and practice of infectious diseases,* ed 5, New York, 2000, Churchill Livingstone; Marshall WF, Blair JE: The cephalosporins, *Mayo Clin Proc* 74:187-195, 1999.

The first-generation agents are intended for gram-positive aerobes, facultative cocci, and MSSA. Cefazolin is commonly used as single-dose antibiotic prophylaxis for clean-clean hospital surgery. The second-generation drugs have variable antistaphylococcal activity, a greater gram-negative spectrum, and some activity against anaerobes (cefotetan, cefoxitin). The third-generation agents are most active against gram-negative organisms and penicillin-resistant *Streptococcus pneumoniae*, with a subset effective against *Pseudomonas aeruginosa*. Cefoperazone, ceftazidime, and cefsulodin have good antipseudomonal activity. Fourth-generation drugs have a wider antibacterial spectrum and good activity against *Pseudomonas*, penicillin-resistant *Streptococcus pneumoniae*, VGS, multiple–drug-resistant *Streptococcus pneumoniae* and *Enterococcus*, MRSA, and hyper–β-lactamase–producing organisms. New potential fourth-generation agents include cefilidin, cefpirone, cefclidin, cefoselis, cefpirime, and cefluprenan.[6]

Bacterial resistance The major mechanism of resistance to the cephalosporins is the microbial elaboration of various β-lactamases (cephalosporinases). The first-generation agents are very sensitive to β-lactamase hydrolysis, with the second to fourth generations more resistant to β-lactamases. Moderate stability is demonstrated by cefonicid, loracarbef, cefdinir, and cefixime; moderate to high stability by cefoxitin, cefuroxime, ceftriaxone, cefotaxime, ceftizoxime, cefmetazole, and cefotetan; and high stability by cefoperazone, cefpodoxime, and ceftazidime.[6,29,42,57] The current concern is the microbial production of extended-spectrum β-lactamases derived from point mutations on TEM-1, TEM-2, and SHV-1 β-lactamases (see Chapter 38) that result in high-level resistance to ceftazidime, aztreonam (a monobactam), and third-generation cephalosporins in highly pathogenic nosocomial *Escherichia coli, Klebsiella pneumoniae,* and *Enterobacter cloacae.*[42]

Absorption, fate, and excretion The oral cephalosporins are generally well absorbed, with all except cefadroxil and cefprozil having their absorption delayed but not reduced by food.[29] Cephalosporins are hydrophilic and widely distributed in extracellular fluid but do not enter the cells of the immune system (macrophages, polymorphonuclear leukocytes) as do the lipophilic macrolides, tetracyclines, and lincosamides. Only cefuroxime of the first- and second-generation agents penetrates into the cerebrospinal fluid. Plasma protein binding ranges from 10% for ceftibuten to 80% to 90% for cefazolin, cefoxitin, and cefoperazone. The plasma protein binding is 10% for cephalexin, 25% for cefaclor, and 8% to 17% for cephradine. The serum half-lives of some oral cephalosporins are cephalexin (50 to 80 minutes), cephradine (48 to 80 minutes), and cefaclor (35 to 54 minutes).[29] In patients with end-stage renal disease, these half-lives may rise to 19 to 22 hours for cephalexin, 8 to 15 hours for cephradine, and 2 to 3 hours for cefaclor.

General therapeutic uses The cephalosporins have wide applications in the treatment of infections. Tables 39-4 and 39-6 indicate their clinical importance as antimicrobial drugs. The utility of these drugs depends on the generation.

First-generation drugs are used to treat infections caused by staphylococci and streptococci. They also are useful in surgical and endocarditis prophylaxis. Some gram-negative bacilli such as *Proteus mirabilis* and *Klebsiella pneumoniae* may be sensitive.

Second-generation drugs have limited use, although a subset of this group represented by cefoxitin has good activity against many gram-negative anaerobes.

The third-generation drugs have become prominent in the treatment of serious gram-negative infections, both coccal and bacillary. They are very useful in treating meningitis, pneumonia, gonorrhea, and sepsis from sensitive organisms. Cephalosporins are often given with aminoglycosides for gram-negative bacilli infections. It is important to note that there are significant individual differences between members of the third-generation drugs, and not all indications apply to each member.

Fourth-generation cephalosporins are resistant to many β-lactamases and are effective in treating some gram-negative bacilli that produce β-lactamases.

Therapeutic uses in dentistry The cephalosporins have good activity against many orofacial pathogens but limited activity against oral anaerobes. These β-lactam antibiotics are also time-dependent agents without significant postantibiotic effects, and the serum and tissue concentrations of the cephalosporins should remain above the organism's MIC for at least 60% of the dosing interval to retard organism regrowth as much as possible.[18] At the current package dosing intervals of 6 hours for the short half-life oral cephalosporins (cephalexin, cephradine, cefaclor), it is unlikely that these serum levels will be attained. At three half-lives after ingestion (approximately 4 hours), only 12.5% of the β-lactam remains in the blood or tissue and may well be below the organism's MIC. Brief peak blood concentrations followed by a significant period below the organism's MIC are not ideal for time-dependent antibiotics and allow for recovery of the pathogen(s) from β-lactam cell wall formation inhibition.[17] Shortening the dosing interval to 4 hours for these agents may resolve this pharmacokinetic difficulty.

Adverse effects Serious adverse reactions associated with the cephalosporins are rare, with the major concern being the potential for cross-allergy with the penicillins. Unusual adverse reactions include transient increases in liver enzymes, nephrotoxicity, reversible neutropenia, eosinophilia and thrombocytopenia, aseptic meningitis, and disulfiram-like reactions associated with cephalosporins with the methylthiotetrazole side chain (cefotetan, cefoperazone, cefamandole). Pseudomembranous colitis is rare with the first- and second-generation agents but is more common with the third-generation cephalosporins, possibly because of their anti-*Bacteroides* activity (*Bacteroides* and antagonistic *Clostridium difficile* in the colon). Some cephalosporins (cefoperazone, cefotetan, cefmetazole, cefmenoxime) may induce hypoprothrombinemia by reduced synthesis of vitamin K–dependent clotting factors.

The inherent allergic potential of the cephalosporins along with their cross-allergenicity with the penicillins is of major concern. Cutaneous allergic reactions to the cephalosporins (rash, pruritus, urticaria) are commonly reported to occur in 1% to 3% of patients. Serum sickness or a morbilliform rash may be seen in children receiving cefaclor. Stevens-Johnson syndrome and toxic dermal necrolysis have been reported.[29] In 6573 patients receiving the cephalosporins, 73 (1.1%) exhibited an allergic reaction.[20]

Anaphylactic reactions to the cephalosporins appear to be rare, with an incidence ranging from 0.0001% to 0.1% of those exposed.[43] In 9388 patients without a history of penicillin allergy given the cephalosporins, two anaphylactic reactions were reported (0.2%).[43] In a retrospective study of 350,000 adverse drug reactions, six fatal cases of cephalosporin-induced anaphylaxis were reported, with three of the six cases in patients with a history of penicillin allergy.[74]

The issue of cross-sensitivity between the cephalosporins and penicillins has never been satisfactorily resolved. Estimates range from 1.1% (the same as the allergy incidence to the cephalosporins in the general population) to 18% in the earliest studies.[68,70] Penicillin-allergic individuals may have a fourfold greater risk of allergy to the cephalosporins than persons not allergic to the penicillins, but penicillin-allergic individuals have a three to four times greater risk of allergy to any drug. No skin test is available to detect cephalosporin allergy, and experience with desensitization is limited and not standardized.

It is generally agreed that the cephalosporins can be given in reasonable safety to patients with a history of a mild skin reaction to the penicillins or a positive penicilloyl-polylysine (major determinant mixture) skin test.[68,70] Cephalosporins are generally contraindicated in patients with a positive penicillin skin test to the minor determinant mixture or a history of local or systemic penicillin anaphylaxis (severe urticaria, bronchospasm, hypotension, exfoliative dermatitis) unless the cephalosporins are mandated in the management of a life-threatening infection and anaphylaxis antidotal therapy is readily available.

Drug interactions Antacids decrease the plasma concentrations of cefaclor, cefdinir, and cefpodoxime; H_2 histamine receptor antagonists reduce the plasma concentrations of cefpodoxime and cefuroxime, and iron supplements reduce the gastric absorption of cefdinir.[29] Food decreases the oral absorption of cefuroxime and cefpodoxime. Cefmetazole, cefoperazone, and cefotetan may induce a disulfiram reaction with ethanol and also hypoprothrombinemia. Nephrotoxicity may be seen with the combination of cephalosporins with aminoglycosides or loop diuretics. Cephalosporins may produce a false-positive reaction for urine glucose with Benedict's solution and cephradine a false-positive for urinary proteins with tests using sulfosalicylic acid.[29]

Contraindications The cephalosporins are contraindicated in patients allergic to the drugs and in persons with a history of severe penicillin reactions or a positive skin test reaction to the penicillin minor determinant mixture.

Other β-lactam antibiotics

Carbapenems Carbapenems are derivatives of thienamycin (from *Streptomyces cattleya*) and differ from the penicillins by the replacement of the sulfur by a methylene group in the 5-membered ring of the β-lactams (see Figure 39-4). Currently three carbapenems are available for parenteral use in the United States: imipenem, meropenem, and ertapenem. Imipenem is combined with cilastatin to reduce the hydrolysis of imipenem by a renal peptidase.

The carbapenems have a very wide antibacterial spectrum, a high specificity for PBP2 of both gram-positive and gram-negative microorganisms (resulting in ovoid organisms), and are not hydrolyzed by most β-lactamases.[33] The carbapenems are drugs of choice for the management of infections caused by *Campylobacter fetus, Citrobacter freundii, Enterobacter, Acinetobacter, Serratia marcescens,* and *Rhodococcus equi* and alternate drugs against MSSA, penicillin- or non–penicillin-resistant *Streptococcus pneumoniae, Bacillus subtilis* and *cereus, Clostridium perfringens, Bacteroides, Escherichia coli, Klebsiella pneumoniae, Proteus mirabilis,* indole-positive *Proteus, Providencia stuartii, Capnocytophaga canimorsus, Haemophilus influenzae,* and *Pseudomonas aeruginosa.*[15]

Microorganisms that are generally resistant to the carbapenems include *Enterococcus faecium, Pseudomonas cepacia, Stenotrophomonas maltophilia, Flavobacteria, JK Corynebacterium,* MRSA and methicillin-resistant CoNS. Organisms with varying resistance include *Pseudomonas aeruginosa, Serratia marcescens,* penicillin-resistant *Streptococcus pneumoniae, Klebsiella pneumoniae,* and vancomycin-resistant *Enterococci.* Metallo–β-lactamases derived from *Klebsiella pneumoniae, Pseudomonas cepacia,* and *Stenotrophomonas maltophilia* readily metabolize the carbapenems and also induce the production of cephalosporinases that significantly increase microbial resistance to the third-generation cephalosporins.[6] Microbial resistance to the carbapenems is via the loss of an outer membrane protein thereby retarding cell wall penetration of the drugs, altered PBPs in *Enterococcus faecium* and MRSA, and hydrolysis by metallo– and other β-lactamases.[33]

The carbapenems are classified as FDA pregnancy B or C drugs, are cross-allergenic with other β-lactams, may raise the level of serum liver transaminases, may induce pseudomembranous colitis, and are associated with a 3% to 4% incidence of skin rash. Combined with cyclosporin they may increase central nervous system (CNS) toxicity and seizures when combined with ganciclovir.

Monobactams Aztreonam is a monocyclic β-lactam (monobactam) lacking the thiazolidine ring of penicillin (Figure 39-5).[6,33] It is only available parenterally. It does not bind to the PBPs of gram-positive or anaerobic microorganisms; therefore its spectrum is limited to aerobic gram-negative species (binding to PBP3 to produce filamentous organisms), primarily *Enterobacteriaceae, Klebsiella pneumoniae, Proteus mirabilis, Citrobacter freundii, Yersinia enterocolitica, Pasturella multocida, Salmonella, Shigella, Providencia Neisseria, Haemophilus,* and *Pseudomonas aeruginosa.* Aztreonam can be combined with clindamycin, metronidazole, and vancomycin and can be used with the aminoglycosides (which have a similar antibacterial spectrum) in the management of infections caused by *Escherichia coli, Klebsiella pneumoniae, Proteus mirabilis, Providencia stuartii, Serratia marcescens,* and *Pseudomonas aeruginosa.* Aztreonam is metabolized by β-lactamases elaborated by *Klebsiella pneumoniae* and *Pseudomonas aeruginosa.* Aztreonam is not the initial drug of choice for any infection.[15]

Aztreonam is an FDA pregnancy B drug and lacks cross-allergenicity with the β-lactams. Aztreonam induces β-lactamase production and may be synergistic with the renal and ototoxicity of the aminoglycosides.

Macrolide and Ketolide Antibiotics

Chemistry and classification

The macrolide antibiotics are characterized by large 14-, 15-, or 16-membered lactone rings. Box 39-5 details the macrolides available in the United States. Erythromycin, as derived from *Streptomyces erythreus,* was introduced in 1952 and azithromycin and clarithromycin in 1991 and 1992, respectively. Azithromycin is a 15-membered macrolide with an added nitrogen and N-methylation (making it technically an azalide), whereas clarithromycin is formed by the alkylation of a hydroxyl group of erythromycin (a 14-membered ring) (Figure 39-6). Troleandomycin is a synthetic derivative of oleandomycin, dirithromycin is a prodrug yielding erythromycylamine in the intestine, and telithromycin is a derivative of erythromycin A and a 14-membered macrolide with a 3-keto group substitution.[29]

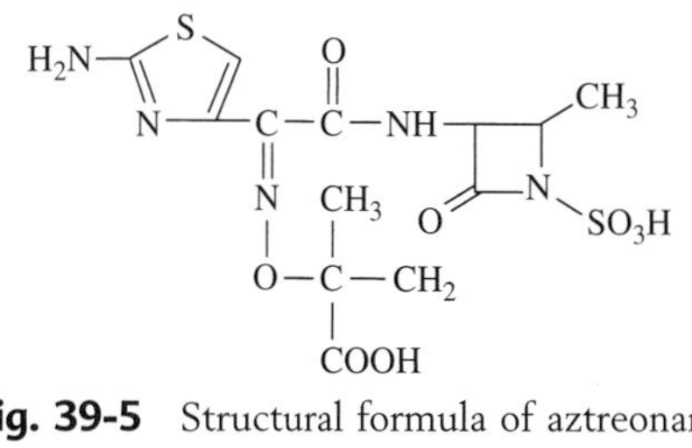

Fig. 39-5 Structural formula of aztreonam.

Box • 39-5

Macrolide Preparations Available in the United States

Nonproprietary (Generic) Name	Proprietary (Trade) Name
Erythromycin base (film-coated)	Erythromycin Filmtabs
Erythromycin (enteric-coated)	E-Base, E-Mycin, Ery-Tab, Eryc
Erythromycin stearate	Erythrocin Stearate
Erythromycin ethylsuccinate	E.E.S., EryPed
Erythromycin estolate	Ilosone
Erythromycin lactobionate	—
Erythromycin gluceptate	Ilotycin Gluceptate
Clarithromycin	Biaxin
Azithromycin	Zithromax
Dirithromycin	Dynabac
Troleandomycin	TAO

From *Facts and comparisons*, St Louis, 2002, Facts and Comparisons.

Box • 39-6

Macrolides as Agents of Choice or Alternate Drugs

Drugs of Choice	Alternate Agents
Bartonella henselae	*Actinomyces israelii*
Bartonella quintana	*Bacillus anthracis*
Bordetella pertussis	*Borrelia burgdorferi*
Campylobacter jejuni	*Capnocytophaga canimorsus*
Chlamydia trachomatis	*Chlamydia pneumoniae*
Clostridium diphtheriae	*Corynebacterium JK group*
Haemophilus drucreyi	*Eikenella corrodens*
Legionella pneumophila	*Erysipelothrix rhusiopathiae*
Mycobacterium avium	*Helicobacter pylori*
Mycoplasma pneumoniae	*Leptotrichia buccalis*
Ureaplasma urealyticum	*Mycobacterium kansasii*
	Mycobacterium leprae
	Mycobacterium marinum
	Streptococcus pneumoniae
	Streptococcus pyogenes

From Choice of antibacterial drugs, *Med Lett Drugs Ther* 43:69-78, 2001; *Facts and comparisons*, St Louis, 2002, Facts and Comparisons.

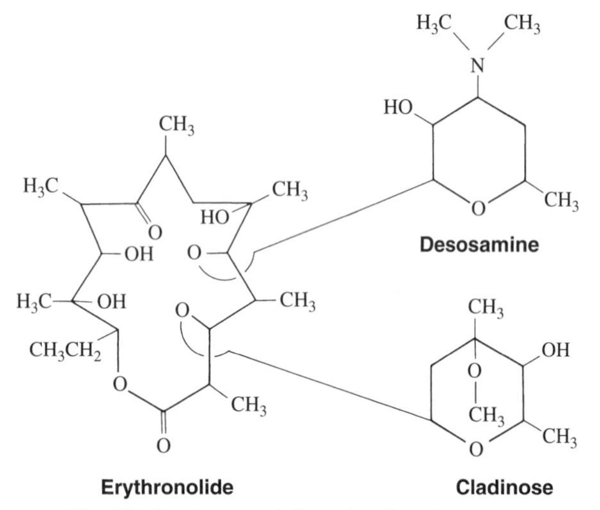

Fig. 39-6 Structural formula of erythromycin.

Mechanism of action and antibacterial spectrum

The mechanism of action of the macrolides is to reversibly bind to the P site of the 50S ribosomal subunit and inhibit RNA-dependent protein synthesis by stimulating the dissociation of peptidyl t-RNA from the ribosome.[17,29]

Box 39-6 lists the infections for which the macrolides are drugs of choice or alternate agents.[29,76] Generally the macrolides have similar activity against gram-positive aerobic/facultative staphylococci and streptococci, gram-negative anaerobes *(Moraxella catarrhalis, Bordetella pertussis, Legionella pneumophila)*, and *Mycoplasma pneumoniae,* but differing activity against other microorganisms. *The Medical Letter*[15] lists erythromycin as a drug of choice against *Corynebacterium diphtheriae, Bartonella henselae* and *quintana, Bordetella pertussis,* and *Ureaplasma urealyticum;* azithromycin against *Haemophilus ducreyi, Legionella pneumophila,* and *Chlamydia trachomatis;* clarithromycin against *Mycobacterium fortuitum/chelonae* complex; erythromycin or azithromycin against *Campylobacter jejunum;* azithromycin or clarithromycin against *Mycobacterium avium;* and erythromycin, azithromycin, and clarithromycin are recommended as equally effective against *Chlamydia pneumoniae.*

Erythromycin is an alternative drug against *Bacillus anthracis, Corynebacterium JK* group, *Erysipelothrix rhusiopathiae, Eikenella corrodens, Haemophilus ducreyi, Leptotrichia buccalis, Actinomyces israelii,* and *Rhodococcus equi;* azithromycin is recommended against *Shigella* and *Bartonella henselae* and *quintana;* clarithromycin against *Mycobacterium kansasii, marinum,* and *leprae;* clarithromycin or azithromycin against *Bordetella* pertussis and upper respiratory infections, *Ureaplasma urealyticum,* and *Borrelia burgdorferi;* and erythromycin, azithromycin, and clarithromycin are recommended as equally effective against *Streptococcus pyogenes, Streptococcus pneumoniae,* and *Moraxella catarrhalis.*

Microorganisms generally resistant to the macrolides include *Haemophilus influenzae, Peptostreptococcus, Actinobacillus actinomycetemcomitans, Pasturella, Fusobacterium, Mycobacterium* tuberculosis, MRSA, and *Enterobacteriaceae.* Marginally affected organisms include *Prevotella* and *Porphyromonas.*[3]

Bacterial resistance

The major mechanism for microbial resistance is demethylation of the 2058 residue of the gene coding for the 23S ribosomal RNA peptidyl transferase region, resulting in reduced macrolide binding (ribosomal protection).[17] The *erm* (*e*rythromycin-*r*esistant *m*ethylase) gene responsible for the ribosomal protection is often associated with tetracycline resistance genes and is frequently combined with the resistance genes for lincosamides (clindamycin) and the streptogramins (quinupristin/dalfoprinstin) to form the macrolide-lincosamide-streptogramin B (MLS_B) aggregate, which confers resistance to all three antibiotic groups simultaneously. Other macrolide resistance mechanisms include active efflux genes encoding for transport efflux proteins and an esterification gene that codes for inactivation of the macrolides by phosphorylation and glycosylation.[17]

Absorption, fate, and excretion

Despite relatively minor structural modifications, the macrolides have somewhat distinct pharmacokinetic properties.[29] Erythromycin and azithromycin are available for oral and intravenous use, whereas the remaining agents are only used orally. Bioavailability ranges from 10% for dirithromycin to 40% to 50% for azithromycin, clarithromycin, and erythromycin. Food in the stomach may increase or have no effect on the absorption of azithromycin, but the remaining macrolides should be taken 1 hour before or 2 hours after a meal, except for the estolate and ethylsuccinate salts of erythromycin, which may be taken without regard to meals.

Erythromycin base is poorly resistant to gastric acid and is prepared with enteric coating or as various salts (stearate), esters (ethylsuccinate), or salts of esters (estolate), which protect against gastric acid degradation. The macrolides are best absorbed in the small intestine and when given orally in standard doses generally produce adequate tissue MIC concentrations of 0.5 μg/ml for azithromycin, 1 to 3 μg/ml for clarithromycin, and 0.3 to 2 μg/ml for erythromycin.[29] Erythromycin may have a variable absorption rate resulting in tissue concentrations ranging from 0.3 to 2 μg/ml. The time to maximum blood concentrations of a single dose is 2.2 hours for azithromycin, 2 to 3 hours for clarithromycin, and 1.6 hours for erythromycin. Impaired renal function may reduce the excretion of the macrolides, with the elimination half-life of erythromycin rising from 1.6 hours to 5 to 6 hours in anuric patients. Clarithromycin and erythromycin are primarily eliminated in the urine and azithromycin in the bile, although erythromycin may also undergo significant biliary excretion. The average serum half-lives are 68 hours for azithromycin, 3 to 7 hours for clarithromycin, and 1.6 hours for erythromycin.

A remarkable property of the macrolides as well as the highly fat soluble tetracyclines and clindamycin is their selective uptake by phagocytic cells and fibroblasts that then function both as repository drug depots and as a drug delivery system to areas of inflammation and infection. These cells concentrate the macrolides and then transport them to areas of tissue pathology where they are then released for their anti-infective and antiinflammatory properties. The tissue concentrations of azithromycin may reach 100 to 1000 times that of blood and persist long after blood levels have declined because of their significant postantibiotic effects.[54] The tissue concentration of azithromycin may exceed the microorganism MIC for 2 to 10 days, and the elimination half-life in abscesses may be up to 4 days.

General therapeutic uses

Macrolides are often indicated for treating community-acquired bacterial pneumonia because of their action against a number of causative organisms. However, microbial resistance is becoming increasingly common. They are useful against various chlamydial infections and a number of gram-positive coccal infections. They are also active against *Corynebacterium*. The 14-membered macrolides possess antiinflammatory effects distinct from their antimicrobial actions by decreasing proinflammatory cytokine release from phagocytes, which may prove useful in the management of rheumatoid arthritis, cystic fibrosis, asthma, and chronic sinusitis. General therapeutic uses are listed in Table 39-4 and Box 39-6.

Therapeutic uses in dentistry

Erythromycin has a long and successful history of use against acute orofacial infections, particularly in β-lactam–allergic patients. Its spectrum of activity is good to excellent against gram-positive aerobic/facultative cocci (streptococci, some staphylococci). Its spectrum is not generally favorable against the gram-negative anaerobes associated with orofacial infections: *Prevotella*, *Porphyromonas*, *Fusobacterium*, and *Veillonella*. However, azithromycin has been observed to be effective against oral spirochetes and pigmented anaerobes.[77] Azithromycin at 500 mg/day for 3 days has demonstrated comparable efficacy to amoxicillin/clavulanic acid at 625 mg three times daily for 5 to 10 days in the management of acute periapical abscesses.[1] The macrolides are also useful for endocarditis prophylaxis.

Clarithromycin is most active against gram-positive anaerobes (*Actinomyces*, *Propionibacterium*, *Lactobacillus*), whereas erythromycin is more active than azithromycin for these organisms. Azithromycin has the best activity against gram-negative anaerobes (*Fusobacteria*, *Prevotella*, *Porphyromonas*, *Wolinella*, *Selenomonas*, and *Actinobacillus actinomycetemcomitans*). Azithromycin may be more active against streptococci and staphylococci than erythromycin and clarithromycin and has much less propensity for drug interactions. Prolonged use of erythromycin and possibly other macrolides may lead to a superinfection with gram-negative enteric bacilli.

Adverse effects

Serious toxicity with the macrolides is rare but occasionally significant. The most important adverse effects include epigastric pain, ototoxicity (deafness), ventricular arrhythmias (torsades de pointes), acute pancreatitis, mania, cholestatic hepatitis, the hypersensitivity syndrome, and certain drug interactions.

Cholestatic hepatitis is much more common with the estolate form of erythromycin than with other forms of erythromycin or the other macrolides. This reaction can be misdiagnosed as viral hepatitis. Symptoms usually appear after approximately 10 days of erythromycin use, disappear 2 to 4 weeks after drug discontinuance with no residual effects, and readily reappear with drug readministration. This reaction is less common in children.

The most common serious adverse reaction associated with the macrolides, particularly erythromycin, is potentially severe epigastric pain resulting from stimulation of the gastric smooth muscle motilin receptor.[11] Motilin is a regulatory peptide of the gastrointestinal tract that stimulates enzyme secretions by the stomach and pancreas and induces strong phasic contractions of the stomach. The most significant agonists of the motilin receptor are the 14-membered macrolides (erythromycin), whereas azithromycin and clarithromycin are lesser stimulants.

Approximately 30 cases have been reported of macrolide-induced hearing loss, with at least two cases judged to be irreversible. The majority appear associated with erythromycin doses exceeding 4 g/day or from accumulation of lesser doses in patients with impaired renal or hepatic function. In patients with renal impairment, the dose of erythromycin should be no greater than 1.5 g/day. Ototoxicity is particularly common in patients with HIV/AIDS, given the use of macrolides as prophylaxis for *Mycobacterium avium* infections. All the macrolides induce ototoxicity, possibly by an effect on the auditory nerve pathways, and tinnitus has been observed even with therapeutic doses of azithromycin.

The long QT interval syndrome is characterized by delayed ventricular repolarization that triggers ventricular tachyarrhythmias, most notably torsades de pointes, resulting in syncope, seizures, or sudden death. The long QT interval syndrome may be either congenital or acquired, and the list of drugs, diseases, and metabolic disorders inducing torsades de pointes is long and impressive (see Chapter 24).

At least four cases of acute pancreatitis associated with erythromycin have been reported and several cases of mania have been associated with clarithromycin in patients with and without HIV/AIDS. Stevens-Johnson syndrome (erythema multiforme) may occur with erythromycin along with a hypersensitivity syndrome associated with azithromycin and clarithromycin consisting of fever, rash, hepatitis, interstitial nephritis, oliguria, and xerostomia. Azithromycin and erythromycin are classified as FDA pregnancy B drugs and clarithromycin, dirithromycin, and troleandomycin as pregnancy C drugs.[29]

Drug interactions

The macrolides are associated with many drug interactions (Table 39-7).[85] Erythromycin and clarithromycin, either through their inhibition of the liver microsomal enzyme drug metabolizing system or their effect on gastrointestinal microbial flora, increase the serum levels of fluconazole, ranitidine, alfentanil, benzodiazepines, tacrolimus, theophylline, vinblastine, bromocriptine, buspirone, carbamazepine, cyclosporine, digoxin, disopyramide, ergot alkaloids, felodipine, oral anticoagulants, methylprednisolone, and omeprazole.[29] Azithromycin and dirithromycin do not affect the liver microsomes. Macrolide blood levels may be increased by fluconazole, H_2-receptor antagonists, and omeprazole and decreased by theophylline. Antacids reduce the rate but not the total amount of macrolide absorption, and the combination of the macrolides and oral contraceptives may result in cholestasis. Bacteriostatic macrolides may interfere with the bactericidal effect of cell wall inhibitors. Concomitant administration with fluoroquinolones, pimozide, or cisapride may lead to torsades de pointes.

After only 3 days of administration, the macrolides may seriously reduce cardiac glycoside metabolism in the gastrointestinal tract by *Eubacterium lentum*, resulting in digitalis toxicity because the microorganism may metabolize up to 30% to 40% of the drug.[87] The macrolides may potentiate the anticoagulant effect of oral anticoagulants. Concomitant use of the macrolides may increase the myopathy and rhabdomyolysis seen with the "-statin" anticholesterol agents.[29]

Contraindications

The macrolides are contraindicated in patients with allergy to the drugs and those with a history of previous allergic cholestatic hepatitis and in combination with other drugs that may induce torsades de pointes. The maximum daily dose should be 4 g in adults with normal renal function and 1.5 g per day with impaired renal function.

Ketolides

The ketolides (e.g., telithromycin) are derivatives of erythromycin A specifically designed for activity against bacteria responsible for community-acquired respiratory tract infections. Telithromycin is a 14-membered macrolide with a 3-keto group substitution.[98] The oral bioavailability of telithromycin is approximately 55%, with maximum serum concentrations of 1.9 μg/ml at 1 to 3 hours. Its elimination half-life is 13.4 hours; the drug has a long postantibiotic effect and is highly concentrated in white blood cells and pulmonary tissue. It is primarily metabolized in the liver. Telithromycin inhibits bacterial protein synthesis by binding to the 50S ribosomal subunit to inhibit translation at the peptidyl transferase site. The drug also inhibits formation of the bacterial 50S and 30S ribosomal subunits.

Telithromycin is active against a wide spectrum of respiratory pathogens: *Streptococcus pneumoniae, Haemophilus*

Table • 39-7

Drug Interactions Associated with the Macrolides

MACROLIDE	INTERACTING DRUG(S)	ADVERSE REACTION
E	Grepafloxacin, sparfloxacin	Torsades de pointes
All	Warfarin	Bleeding
All	Cyclosporins	Nephrotoxicity and neurotoxicity
All	Theophylline	Decreased macrolide blood levels, increased theophylline toxicity
All	Benzodiazepines	Increased CNS depression
C, E	Carbamazepine	Carbamazepine toxicity
C, E	Digitalis	Digitalis toxicity
E, T	Methylprednisolone	Increased steroid effects
C, E, T	Buspirone	Increased CNS depression
C, E, T	Tacrolimus	Renal toxicity
C, E, T	Rifampin	Reduced macrolide activity
C, E, T	Ergot alkaloids	Peripheral ischemia
C, E, T	Pimozide	Torsades de pointes
C, E, T	Cisapride	Cardiotoxicity

From *Facts and comparisons,* St Louis, 2002, Facts and Comparisons; Tatro DS: *Drug interaction facts,* St Louis, 2001, Facts and Comparisons Wolters Kluwer.

Drug interaction is potentially severe or life-threatening and its occurrence has been suspected, established or probable in well-controlled studies. "All" includes E, C, and T, as well as azithromycin and dirithromycin.

E, Erythromycin; C, clarithromycin; *T,* troleandomycin.

influenzae, Moraxella catarrhalis, Chlamydia pneumoniae, Mycoplasma pneumoniae, and *Legionella pneumophila* as well as group A and B streptococci *(Streptococcus pyogenes* and *agalactiae), Enterococcus, Clostridia, Neisseria, Helicobacter pylori,* and both MRSA and MSSA.[98] It is also active against some anaerobes: *Porphyromonas, Prevotella, Eikenella corrodens,* and some *Bacteroides.* Telithromycin may be effective against *Streptococcus pneumoniae* with *mef*E and *erm*B resistance genes and gram-positive cocci with MLS_B resistance.

Staphylococcus epidermidis is intrinsically resistant to telithromycin, and *Streptococcus pneumoniae* and *pyogenes* isolates have appeared in Germany, Mexico, and Canada with very high telithromycin resistance (more than 100 μg/ml) because of the *erm*B and L4 mutations. In Central and Eastern Europe, *Streptococcus pyogenes* presently has a 1.5% resistance rate to telithromycin and 12.3% to erythromycin. Telithromycin may select for staphylococci and *Bacteroides fragilis* in the gastrointestinal tract.

The most frequent adverse reactions associated with telithromycin are diarrhea (12% to 20%), nausea (2% to 12%), dizziness (2% to 5%), and headache (2.5% to 5%). Telithromycin is an inhibitor of the liver microsomal enzyme cytochrome P450 system and will be expected to increase blood levels of a number of drugs.[98] Like the macrolides, telithromycin may prolong the QT interval. It is classified as an FDA pregnancy B drug.

Telithromycin has no place in the management of acute or chronic orofacial infections unless dictated by sensitivity testing. It should be reserved for highly and multiply resistant microbial pathogens, particularly of the respiratory tract.

Lincosamides

Clindamycin and lincomycin are the only lincosamide antibiotics (Figure 39-7). Lincomycin was isolated from *Streptomyces lincolnensis* in 1962, and clindamycin (7-chloro-7-deoxy-lincomycin) was introduced in 1966. Clindamycin is used almost exclusively because of its greater efficacy and superior pharmacokinetics.

Mechanism of action and antibacterial spectrum

The receptor site for the lincosamides is identical to that of the macrolides, chloramphenicol, and streptogramins: the 23S subunit of the 50S bacterial ribosome resulting in bacteriostatic inhibition of microbial protein synthesis.

Clindamycin has significant activity against many gram-positive and gram-negative anaerobic and facultative/aerobic microorganisms: *Bacteroides, Prevotella, Porphyromonas, Veillonella, Peptostreptococcus,* microaerophilic streptococci, *Actinomyces, Eubacteria, Clostridium* (except *Clostridium difficile*), and *Propionibacteria;* gram-positive organisms generally susceptible to clindamycin include *Streptococcus pneumoniae;* VGS; *Corynebacterium,* Group A, B, C, and G streptococci, and *Streptococcus bovis,* with variable susceptibility in staphylococci.[29,30] Also susceptible are *Leptotrichia buccalis, Bacillus cereus* and *subtilis, Capnocytophaga canimorsus,* and some β-lactamase—producing staphylococci.

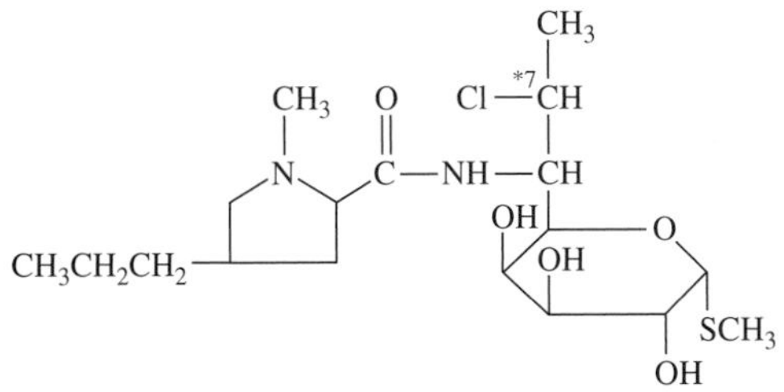

Microorganisms with intrinsic resistance to the lincosamides include *Enterococcus, Enterobacteriaceae, Haemophilus influenzae, Neisseria meningitidis, Mycoplasma pneumoniae,* and most MRSA, with increasing resistance in *Streptococcus pneumoniae* and *Streptococcus pyogenes* and 12% to 20% resistance rates in *Prevotella, Porphyromonas, Fusobacteria,* and *Peptostreptococcus* in the hospital setting.

Fig. 39-7 Structural formula of clindamycin. Substitution of the chlorine atom on the 7 carbon with a hydroxyl group yields lincomycin.

Bacterial resistance

Resistance to clindamycin occurs by three mechanisms: (1) alteration of 23S ribosomal RNA of the 50S ribosomal subunit by adenine methylation (ribosomal protection), (2) an altered single 50S ribosomal protein at the receptor site (receptor alteration), or (3) inactivation in some staphylococcal strains by a nucleotidyl transferase (drug inactivation).

Adenine methylation is plasmid mediated and confers MLS_B resistance. The M phenotype macrolide resistance in *Streptococcus pneumoniae* does not confer resistance to clindamycin. If erythromycin resistance in staphylococci is inducible and not constitutive, the microorganisms are resistant only to the 14- and 15-membered macrolides and remain sensitive to the lincosamides, streptogramins, and 16-membered macrolides. Constitutive resistance in staphylococci of the MLS_B type confers resistance to all these antibiotics simultaneously.

Absorption, fate, and excretion

Clindamycin is well absorbed orally with a 90% bioavailability not appreciably reduced by food. The time to oral peak serum levels is 45 to 60 minutes, with mean peak serum levels of 2.5 μg/ml and an elimination half-life of 2.4 to 3.0 hours.[29] With renal failure the elimination half-life increases to 6 hours, with a doubling of the serum level. The drug penetrates well into bone, but not cerebrospinal fluid, is metabolized primarily in the liver (greater than 90%), and is highly concentrated in the bile, where it may alter colonic flora for up to 2 weeks after it is discontinued. Clindamycin in a manner similar to the macrolides is concentrated preferentially in polymorphonuclear cells, alveolar macrophages, and abscess tissue.

General therapeutic uses

Clindamycin is used in the treatment of certain infections caused by susceptible strains of streptococci, staphylococci, pneumococci, or anaerobes such as *Bacteroides.* Clindamycin may be indicated in the treatment of refractory bone infections. Clindamycin is also useful in treating certain conditions involving anaerobes, such as infections of the female genital tract, pelvic infections, and abdominal penetrating wounds. It can also be used in combination for *Pneumocystis carinii* and for toxoplasmosis.

Therapeutic uses in dentistry

Although amoxicillin or penicillin V remain drugs of choice for acute orofacial infections, a resurgence in clindamycin use may be appropriate as the oral microbial resistance to the β-lactams continues to rise. It is anticipated that oral microbial resistance to clindamycin will also increase proportionately along with the specter of MLS_B resistance shared with macrolides and streptogramins.

Adverse effects

Minor adverse reactions associated with clindamycin include nausea and vomiting, abdominal pain, esophagitis, glossitis, stomatitis, allergy, reversible increase in serum transaminase levels, reversible myelosuppression, metallic taste, maculopapular rash (3% to 10%), and diarrhea (2% to 20%, average of 8%).[29] High intravenous doses of clindamycin may result in a neuromuscular blockade similar to that of the aminoglycosides, tetracyclines, and polymyxin B.

The major concern with clindamycin has been its purported propensity to induce antibiotic-induced diarrhea and colitis, most notably pseudomembranous colitis, based on early reports of an incidence as high as 10%. It is now apparent that the association of clindamycin with these colonic disorders in outpatient use is much less than previously reported, although nonetheless real (see Chapter 38).

In a large retrospective study, the overall risk rate for community-acquired *Clostridium difficile*–associated pseudomembranous colitis was determined to be as low as 1 per 10,000 antibiotic prescriptions, with a risk rate for hospitalization of 0.5 to 1.0 per 100,000 patient years.[36] In a study of 376,590 antibiotic prescriptions given to more than 280,000 patients over a 4-year period, four cases of acute antibiotic-induced colitis were detected.[81] The incidence rate was calculated to be 1.6 in 100,000 persons exposed to ampicillin, 2.9 in 100,000 to dicloxacillin, and 2.6 in 100,000 to tetracycline, with no cases in patients receiving clindamycin.[81]

Although antibiotic-associated diarrhea is common in the outpatient environment and readily managed by drug discontinuance, it appears that serious antibiotic-induced colitis and potentially lethal pseudomembranous colitis are rare. Such forms of colitis are more likely to occur with amoxicillin than clindamycin simply based on the much greater use of the former antibiotic, but this might change if clindamycin is used more often clinically.

Care should be taken with patients who have recently recovered from *Clostridium difficile*–associated diarrhea or colitis for 2 months after the cessation of the disease. Any elective dental procedure requiring antibiotic therapy or prophylaxis is best postponed for this 2-month period. If antibiotic therapy is required, antibiotics far less associated with antibiotic-induced diarrhea (penicillin V, macrolides) are appropriate.

Drug interactions

Clindamycin acts synergistically with nondepolarizing (curarelike) neuromuscular blocking drugs in blocking neurotransmission at skeletal muscle. Clindamycin oral absorption is slowed by kaolin-pectin antidiarrheal drugs.[29]

Contraindications

Clindamycin is contraindicated in patients allergic to the drug and in combination with curare-like neuromuscular blocking drugs. All antibiotics should be avoided if possible for 2 months following antibiotic-induced colitis.

Metronidazole

Metronidazole (Figure 39-8) is a synthetic nitroimidazole patterned after a naturally occurring antiparasitic substance that was isolated from a *Streptomyces* species in 1955. The drug was

CH_2CH_2OH
O_2N N CH_3
N

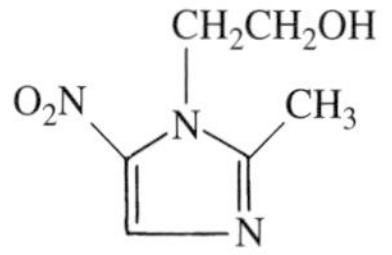

Fig. 39-8 Structural formula of metronidazole.

introduced into medicine in 1959 and was quickly found to possess strong trichomonacidal activity. Since then, metronidazole has become the drug of choice for a variety of protozoal infections. A chance observation that the symptoms of acute necrotizing ulcerative gingivitis were relieved in a woman receiving metronidazole for the treatment of vaginal trichomoniasis stimulated research on the drug's antibacterial effects, culminating in its approval in 1981 for the treatment of anaerobic bacterial infections. Its extensive use in treating parasitic diseases worldwide has led to significant resistance to the drug where parasites are a major problem. It was soon discovered that the drug possessed exceptional activity against obligate anaerobic and microaerophilic microorganisms, including those involved in acute orofacial infections, periodontitis, and acute necrotizing ulcerative gingivitis.

Mechanism of action and antibacterial spectrum

The antimicrobial activity of metronidazole requires entry into the cell and then reduction of its nitro group to produce metabolites that damage DNA, eventually inducing cell death. Metronidazole is active only against bacteria that are obligate anaerobes. It is a concentration-dependent rather than time-dependent antibiotic. Because metronidazole metabolites interfere with nucleic acid synthesis, concerns have been raised regarding its potential for mutagenicity, carcinogenicity, and teratogenicity.

Metronidazole penetrates all bacterial cells equally well. In sensitive anaerobes, however, the nitro moiety of the drug is enzymatically reduced, and it is this metabolite that is the active form of the drug. Metronidazole is almost always bactericidal. The drug reacts with bacterial DNA, causing inhibition of DNA replication, fragmentation of existing DNA, and, in low doses, mutation of the bacterial genome.

Bacterial resistance

Microbial resistance to metronidazole is relatively limited probably because of its limited clinical use except in developing countries, where it is widely used to manage parasitic diseases. A notable exception to this generalization is the high level of resistance in *Helicobacter pylori* in developed countries. Resistance to metronidazole is both chromosomally and plasmid-mediated by a reduction in activity or expression of several genes (*rdx*A, *nim*A, *nim*B) that control nitroreductase activity, which in turn reduces the concentration of active metronidazole metabolites within the microbial cell.

Limited resistance is seen in *Trichomonas vaginalis, Bacteroides, Gardnerella vaginalis, Campylobacter fetus, Leptotrichia buccalis,* and *Treponema pallidum.* High level metronidazole resistance in *Trichomonas vaginalis* has been detected in 1 of 2000 to 1 of 3000 cases. Between 1994 and 1997 in five US medical centers the sensitivity rate to metronidazole was 85% to 100% in *Prevotella*, 80.9% to 96.7% in *Peptostreptococcus,* and 93.3% to 100% in *Fusobacterium*, with a decline in sensitivity in *Fusobacterium* and *Peptostreptococcus* from 100% to 93.3% and 100% to 95%, respectively.[28] Subinhibitory concentrations of metronidazole may increase resistance rates in various periodontal pathogens: *Fusobacteria, Prevotella, Porphyromonas,* and *Peptostreptococcus.*[48] *Bacteroides* strains resistant to metronidazole also acquire enhanced virulence properties.[23]

The most striking resistance to metronidazole has occurred in *Helicobacter pylori*, the etiologic agent in some cases of peptic ulcer and gastric cancer. The resistance rates range from 10% to 50% in developed countries and 100% in developing countries, where the drug is used for parasitic diseases. *Helicobacter pylori* resistance may significantly reduce the efficacy of other agents used along with metronidazole (omeprazole, bismuth, tetracycline, clarithromycin) and also increase macrolide resistance in *Helicobacter pylori*.

Absorption, fate, and excretion

Metronidazole is almost completely absorbed from the gastrointestinal tract (oral bioavailability approaches 100%) so that serum levels are essentially the same whether the drug is administered orally or intravenously.[29] Food may delay peak serum levels of metronidazole but not the total amount absorbed. Metronidazole attains a peak blood level orally in 1 to 2 hours, has a wide volume of distribution, excellent CNS penetration, an elimination half-life of 8 hours, and is biotransformed into five metabolic products, all of which have anti-anaerobic activity. The pharmacokinetics of metronidazole are the same in pregnant and nonpregnant women, its metabolism is reduced in the presence of severe hepatic dysfunction, and its pharmacokinetics are not significantly altered with renal impairment.[29]

General therapeutic uses

The principal medical indications for metronidazole are anaerobic abdominal and CNS infections, bacterial vaginosis, protozoan and *Helicobacter pylori* infections, and the management of *Clostridium difficile*—associated diarrhea and colitis.[15] Metronidazole is very active against obligate anaerobes (*Bacteroides, Porphyromonas, Prevotella, Fusobacterium, Peptostreptococcus, Clostridium*), many of which are associated with periodontitis as well as various human parasites (*Trichomonas vaginalis, Gardnerella vaginalis, Entamoeba histolytica, Balantidium coli*). Metronidazole has variable activity against *Mycobacterium hominis, Campylobacter fetus, Treponema pallidum, Helicobacter pylori,* and *Capnocytophaga canimorsus. Actinobacillus actinomycetemcomitans, Eikenella corrodens, Actinomyces,* and *Propionibacterium* are commonly resistant to metronidazole. The combination of metronidazole with amoxicillin may significantly enhance its activity against *Actinobacillus actinomycetemcomitans,* apparently by increasing cellular uptake of metronidazole.[91]

Three studies have used antibiotics (metronidazole, clindamycin) during pregnancy in an attempt to prevent preterm delivery in women with bacterial vaginosis, and all have been unsuccessful.[9,44,92] These results may weaken the potential association between periodontal disease and preterm birth, since metronidazole is active against both periodontal pathogens and those associated with bacterial vaginosis.

Therapeutic uses in dentistry

Metronidazole is highly effective against gram-negative anaerobic pathogens responsible for both acute orofacial infections and chronic periodontitis. Its combination with a β-lactam antibiotic for oral infections may be indicated for serious acute orofacial infections and in the management of refractory/rapidly progressive periodontitis.

Metronidazole is a concentration-dependent and not time-dependent antibiotic, a fact that is not reflected in the current package insert dosing regimen for the drug. The promiscuous use of metronidazole for classic chronic adult periodontitis is a misuse of the drug and may contribute to the increasing resistance of metronidazole seen with parasites, *Helicobacter pylori*, and other microorganisms.

Adverse effects

Minor adverse reactions associated with metronidazole include reversible neutropenia, metallic taste, dark or red-brown urine, skin rash, urethral or vaginal burning sensation, gynecomastia, and nausea and vomiting. Rare major adverse reactions include pancreatitis, pseudomembranous colitis, peripheral neuropathy, disulfiram reaction when combined with ethanol, and CNS toxicity consisting of seizures, encephalopathy, cerebellar dysfunction, paresthesias, mental confusion, and depression. These neurologic reactions generally only occur with high prolonged cumulative doses.

Because metronidazole affects DNA synthesis, a number of studies have addressed its potential to cause birth defects. Its use in pregnancy does not appear to be associated with any congenital abnormalities, preterm delivery, or low birth weight in newborns and the drug has an FDA pregnancy B classification. There also is no increase in cancer in women who take metronidazole during pregnancy, making in it very unlikely that the drug is carcinogenic.[79]

Drug interactions

Barbiturates may reduce the efficacy of metronidazole and cimetidine may reduce its liver metabolism. The concurrent use of metronidazole and ethanol may result in acute psychosis and the disulfiram reaction (flushing, tachycardia, nausea and vomiting), although for most individuals the risk is minor.[29] Metronidazole may increase lithium blood levels, decrease the body clearance of phenytoin,[29] and significantly increase blood warfarin levels by decreasing its liver metabolism.

Tetracyclines and Glycylcyclines

The tetracyclines are a group of broad-spectrum, bacteriostatic antibiotics that have been extensively used in the treatment of numerous and varied infections. Their widespread use, and often misuse, has resulted in the appearance of many bacterial strains that are resistant to these drugs, which has curtailed their clinical usefulness. Paradoxically, the clinical use of the tetracyclines has had a recent resurgence of interest with the growing realization that the drugs may be lifesaving in the treatment of serious nosocomial infections from highly and multiply antibiotic-resistant methicillin-resistant staphylococci and vancomycin-resistant enterococci. This may be related to the almost complete lack of use of the tetracyclines in hospitals for several decades, possibly leading to the loss of tetracycline resistance genes in this environment. Because of the advent of widespread resistance of *Helicobacter pylori* to metronidazole and the macrolides, the tetracyclines have gained importance in the treatment and prevention of peptic ulcers and gastric cancer and have also emerged as a prophylactic agent in the prevention of multi–drug-resistant malaria and the management of community-acquired pneumonia, particularly in penicillin and macrolide-resistant strains.

The tetracyclines are a group of antibiotics with a similar antibacterial spectrum but differing pharmacokinetic properties created by various chemical substitutions on the hydronaphthacene four-ringed nucleus. The first tetracycline was marketed in 1948 as chlortetracycline isolated from *Streptomyces aureofaciens.* Along with oxytetracycline, tetracycline, and demeclocycline, these four drugs constitute the first-generation tetracyclines. The second generation agents introduced from 1965 to 1972 include minocycline, methacycline, and doxycycline.[16] The glycylcyclines are third-generation agents. The first microorganism clinically detected resistant to the tetracyclines was a *Shigella dysenteriae* strain in 1953.

Chemistry

The structure of tetracycline is shown in Figure 39-9. As is implied by the name ("tetra," four; "cycline," ring), all the tetracyclines are derivatives of a four-ringed nucleus and differ structurally only with regard to the chemical moieties attached at the 2, 5, 6, and 7 positions of the nucleus. Various derivatives exhibit somewhat different pharmacologic properties, such as differences in absorption, protein binding,

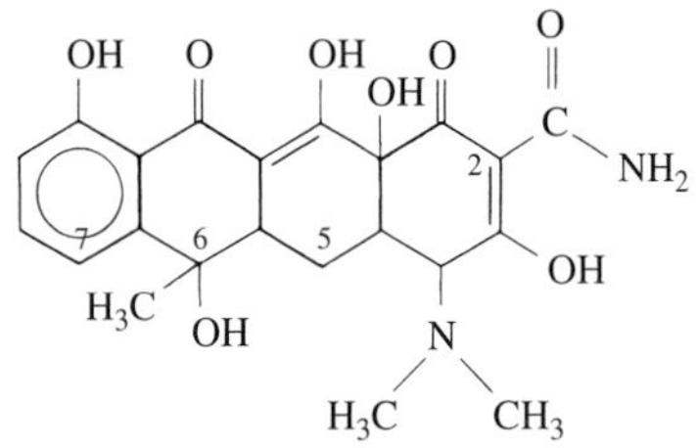

Fig. 39-9 Structural formula of tetracycline.

Box • 39-7

Tetracyclines as Drugs of Choice

Brucella
*Borrelia burgdorferi**
Borrelia recurrentis
Chlamydia pneumoniae
Chlamydia psittaci
Chlamydia trachomatis
*Ehrlichia chaffeensis**
*Ehrlichia ewingii**
Helicobacter pylori
Mycobacterium marinum†
Mycoplasma pneumoniae
Pseudomonas mallei
*Rickettsiae**
Vibrio cholerae
Vibrio vulnificus
Yersinia pestis

From Choice of antibacterial drugs, *Med Lett Drugs Ther* 43:69-78, 2001; Chopra I, Roberts M: Tetracycline antibiotics: mode of action, applications, molecular biology, and epidemiology of bacterial resistance, *Microbiol Molec Biol Rev* 65:232-260, 2001; Standiford HC: Tetracyclines and chloramphenicol. In Mandell GL, Bennett JE, Dolin R, eds: *Mandell, Douglas and Bennett's Principles and practice of infectious diseases,* ed 5, Philadelphia, 2000, Churchill Livingstone.
*Specifically doxycycline.
†Specifically minocycline.

metabolism, excretion, and degree of activity against susceptible microorganisms.

Mechanism of action and antibacterial spectrum

The tetracyclines inhibit bacterial protein synthesis by preventing the association of aminoacyl-tRNA with the bacterial ribosome.[16] The drugs must transverse the gram-negative microbial outer membrane via OmpF and OmpC porin channels or through the gram-positive cell wall in its electronegative hydrophobic form and attach to a single high-affinity binding site on the ribosomal 30S subunit and protein 7 on the 16S rRNA base.[16]

Some important therapeutic uses of the tetracyclines are listed in Box 39-7. The tetracyclines are drugs of choice against *Helicobacter pylori,* various *Chlamydiae,* rickettsiae and *Ehrlichia, Bacillus anthracis,* and *Vibrio cholerae.* The list of indications for which the tetracyclines serve as alternate drugs is impressive,[15,29] including nosocomial infections from life-threatening staphylococci and enterococci, community-acquired pneumonia due to highly antibiotic-resistant pathogens, and the chemoprevention of chloroquine/mefloquine-resistant malaria.[2]

It is imperative with the tetracyclines, as with all antibiotics, that a determination be made of the risk-benefit ratio associated with their use. The severity of the disease and likely response to the drugs are key considerations.

Bacterial resistance

Microbial resistance to the tetracyclines is widespread, transposable, inducible, and commonly permanent because their resistance genes are almost always combined in transposable elements with the genes for resistance to other antibiotics (multidrug resistance gene cassettes). Of the three mechanisms for tetracycline resistance (drug efflux, ribosomal protection, and enzymatic inactivation), drug efflux is the most important, with at least 300 different active efflux proteins capable of extruding tetracycline from the bacterial cell.[16,80]

The tetracyclines are one of the most active chemical inducers of microbial resistance gene expression and also downregulate a repressor gene that controls efflux activity for not only tetracyclines but possibly other antibiotics as well. Only nanomolar amounts of tetracycline are necessary to derepress this system and greatly increase antibiotic efflux from bacterial cells.[16] Tetracycline also promotes the mobility of resistance determinants (transfer of resistance genes between bacteria) by stimulating the frequency of bacterial conjugation.[82] Considering these extraordinary properties of the tetracyclines to induce and promote microbial resistance not only to themselves but also other antibiotics, it would appear prudent to restrict their use to serious medical infections and restrict their use for most cases of periodontitis, where they may have limited or even undocumented value.

Absorption, fate, and excretion

The tetracyclines are adequately but variably absorbed from the gastrointestinal tract with significant differences in bioavailability: chlortetracycline, 30%; demeclocycline, tetracycline, and oxytetracycline, 60% to 80%; and minocycline or doxycycline, 95% to 100%.[29] Dairy products, Ca^{++}, Mg^{++} and aluminum compounds, and Na^{+} bicarbonate significantly impair tetracycline absorption either by chelation or altered gastric pH.[29] Their serum protein binding ranges from 20% to 40% for oxytetracycline to 80% to 95% for doxycycline, and the percent excreted unchanged in the urine ranges from 70% for oxytetracycline to 30% to 42% for doxycycline and 12% to 16% for minocycline.[29] With renal impairment only doxycycline and minocycline do not have increased half-lives and can then be administered with reasonable safety. Other tetracyclines may accumulate in conditions of renal impairment, resulting in high blood levels and possible liver necrosis and death.

The tetracyclines are metabolized in the liver to a varying degree depending on the individual drug and are highly concentrated in the bile at levels three to five times higher than serum.[97] The more recent tetracyclines are more lipid soluble with greater tissue distribution than the earlier tetracyclines. Enterohepatic circulation and incomplete absorption may lead to high drug concentrations in the feces, particularly with the older agents.[29] Doxycycline may to some degree be found in the feces as an inactive form, and it is as yet unknown if this metabolic product is as capable of inducing resistance gene expression or transfer as the parent compound. The serum half-lives of the various agents are oxytetracycline, tetracycline, and demeclocycline, 12 to 16 hours; methacycline, 14 to 16 hours; minocycline, 11 to 18 hours; and doxycycline, 15 to 25 hours.[29] Peak serum concentrations of 3 to 5 μg/ml are reached in 2 hours after the usual therapeutic doses.[97] Box 39-8 lists the tetracycline preparations that are available in the United States.

Box 39-8

Commercially Available Tetracycline Preparations

Nonproprietary (Generic) Name	Proprietary (Trade) Name
Tetracycline hydrochloride	Tetralen, Panmycin, Sumycin, Tetracyn, Tetracap
Oxytetracycline hydrochloride	Terramycin
Demeclocycline hydrochloride	Declomycin
Doxycycline hyclate	Vibramycin, Doxy Caps
Minocycline hydrochloride	Minocin, Vectrin, Dynacin

General therapeutic uses

Some important indications for the tetracyclines are listed in Table 39-4 and Box 39-7. These lists of pathogenic microorganisms and associated diseases make it difficult to rationalize the widespread use of the tetracyclines in the management of periodontitis when it is amenable to mechanical therapy. The degree of benefit of the use of tetracyclines in periodontal disease has to be weighed against the risk of developing resistant strains of microorganisms, resistance gene transfer, and induction of latent resistance genes. A careful consideration of risk-benefit is appropriate when tetracyclines are employed systemically for the management of periodontitis, particularly if the benefit is marginal at best. Acne can be a serious psychological disease in adolescents sensitive to the scorn of their peers and long-term tetracycline use is reasonable based on risk-benefit analysis, but this does not apply to periodontitis.

Tetracyclines are major drugs in treating rickettsial diseases, *Mycoplasma*, *Chlamydia*, *Helicobacter pylori*, and *Borrelia*. (*Borrelia burgdorferi* is the causative agent of Lyme disease.) Many other bacteria nominally within their range of activity should not be treated, at least initially, with a tetracycline because of the large number of resistant strains.

The tetracyclines have been used in the treatment of acne using both oral and topical preparations. Tetracyclines are concentrated in the skin and are effective against *Propionibacterium acnes* and may also have an antiseborrheic action to reduce skin lipids. Because tetracyclines are deposited in bone, they can be used to measure the rate of bone growth. Other indications include the plague, tularemia, cholera, brucellosis, and certain protozoal infections.

Therapeutic uses in dentistry

The use of tetracyclines in the management of acute orofacial infections is widely considered inappropriate because of their bacteriostatic activity and extensive microbial resistance, but with the advent of oral microbial pathogens increasingly resistant to the β-lactams, macrolides, and clindamycin this concept may have to be reconsidered. Systemic tetracyclines in the management of chronic adult periodontitis must be carefully evaluated for risk-benefit ratio considering their limited efficacy (questionable clinical efficacy and limited data on long-term efficacy) and their propensity to induce microbial resistance gene expression, stimulation of drug efflux mechanisms, and common association with multiple resistance genes to other antibiotics in transposable elements. Tetracyclines are effective in the management of localized juvenile periodontitis (LJP) and its associated organism, *Actinobacillus actinomycetemcomitans*. Tetracyclines also appear to inhibit inflammatory matrix metalloproteinase activity. Tetracyclines may also be used subgingivally.

Adverse effects

Tetracyclines have a long list of adverse drug reactions. The tetracyclines may induce photosensitivity, nephrogenic diabetes insipidus (demeclocycline), blood dyscrasias, liver dysfunction (high doses and especially during pregnancy), pseudotumor cerebri and bulging fontanelles (adults and infants, respectively), *Candida albicans* overgrowth, gastrointestinal difficulties (nausea, vomiting, diarrhea, pancreatitis), and various allergic manifestations, including urticaria, serum sickness, angioneurotic edema, and anaphylaxis.[29]

Minocycline in conventional doses is associated with skin, nail, and hair pigmentation and a systemic lupus erythematosus–like syndrome, mainly in adolescents taking the drug for acne. This syndrome is usually reversible but may require corticosteroid therapy and the absolute risk appears to be low (52.8/100,000 uses). Sixteen cases of autoimmune hepatitis have been described.

Minocycline is the only tetracycline that induces vestibular toxicity (ataxia, loss of balance), possibly because of its high concentration in the lipid-rich cells of the inner ear. The tetracyclines in general are one of the few groups of drugs that are toxic if ingested beyond their expiration date, inducing a Fanconi-like syndrome (azotemia, kidney damage). Tetracycline-induced acute interstitial nephritis may result in acute renal failure. The hepatotoxicity is relatively rare except at high doses and is most likely to occur during pregnancy, leading to an absolute contraindication to the drugs in pregnancy.

The chelation properties of the tetracyclines are responsible for their deposition in calcifying teeth, bone, and cartilage and these drugs have been used as vital stains to determine bone growth. Tetracycline staining is not permanent in tissues that are remodeled (bone, cartilage) but is permanent in those that are not remodeled (teeth). Tetracyclines then should not be used in children younger than 8 years unless other antibiotics are unlikely to be effective or are contraindicated.[29] The tetracyclines most likely to stain the dentition severely are tetracycline and demeclocycline with oxytetracycline, chlortetracycline, and doxycycline the least likely, but the magnitude of the staining may depend more on dose and duration than the drug itself. Deposition of tetracyclines in bone and teeth eliminates their antimicrobial activity. Because of the deleterious staining effects on the teeth, the tetracyclines are classified by the FDA as pregnancy D drugs. Tetracyclines should not be used in pregnancy both because of staining of teeth and potential hepatotoxicity.

Drug interactions

The tetracyclines and all other antimicrobial ribosomal protein synthesis inhibitors may reduce the efficacy of antibiotic cell wall inhibitors, which rely on cell wall division for their action. Polyvalent cations (aluminum, Ca^+, zinc, iron, magnesium, bismuth) may decrease gastric tetracycline absorption by chelation. Na^+ bicarbonate alters the gastric pH and reduces absorption of tetracyclines.

Tetracyclines may reduce insulin requirements and may alter lithium blood levels.[29] Serum blood levels of digoxin may be increased in 10% of patients and serum levels of the tetracyclines may be reduced from increased hepatic metabolism induced by barbiturates, carbamazepine, and the hydantoins.[29] The addition of tetracyclines to the coumarin anticoagulants (warfarin) may greatly increase the latter's effect on the INR

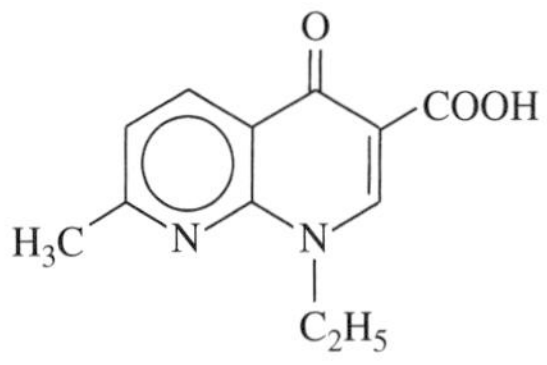

Nalidixic acid

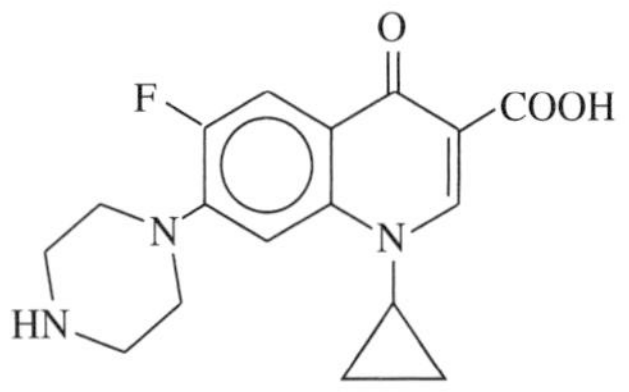

Ciprofloxacin

Fig. 39-10 Structural formulas of nalidixic acid, a quinolone antibiotic, and ciprofloxacin, a fluoroquinolone derivative.

and lead to serious bleeding episodes. The effect is due in part on the inhibitory effect of tetracyclines on the intestinal flora that produce vitamin K (see Chapter 31).

Contraindications

The tetracyclines are contraindicated in children up to the age of 8 years, in cases of allergy, during pregnancy, during lactation, and in those with sulfite sensitivity.

Glycylcyclines

The glycylcyclines are synthetic derivatives of minocycline that may be effective against some tetracycline-resistant bacteria as well as *Streptococcus pneumoniae* resistant to the macrolides and penicillin where the *Streptococcus pneumoniae* possess a lower MIC for the macrolides and penicillins than for tetracycline, minocycline, and doxycycline.[37] Unfortunately, the resistance gene for the glycylcyclines is carried on the same transposon as the resistance genes for the macrolides and tetracycline, making the use of the glycylcyclines potentially limited. Tigilcycline is a glycylcycline presently undergoing clinical trials.

Fluoroquinolones

The fluoroquinolones were introduced in the 1980s and are C6 fluorine derivatives of nalidixic acid, which is a byproduct of chloroquine (Figure 39-10). Nalidixic acid (a quinolone) was discovered in the 1960s and is still available but has the undesirable properties of CNS stimulation, rapid development of microbial resistance, poor pharmacokinetics, and chondrotoxicity (damage to cartilage). The terms *fluoroquinolone* and *quinolone* are often used interchangeably; however, this is technically incorrect as nalidixic acid, oxolinic acid, and cinoxacin are the only true quinolones (devoid of the fluorine substitution).

The fluoroquinolones/quinolones are currently classified much as the cephalosporins into first, second, third, and fourth generations depending on the time of their introduction into medicine and to a lesser extent their antibacterial spectrum (Boxes 39-9 and 39-10).[5,61,94] The first fluoroquinolone (norfloxacin) was synthesized in 1978 as a 6-fluorinated derivative of nalidixic acid with a piperazine ring at position 7. Ciprofloxacin was synthesized in 1981 and marketed in 1986. The newer fluoroquinolones have improved activity against *Streptococcus pneumoniae, Staphylococcus aureus,* gram-positive cocci, anaerobes, *Pseudomonas aeruginosa,* and various other organisms (see Table 39-4).[5,15,94] Potential new agents include the 2-pyridones and the desfluoroquinolones.

Box 39-9

Generational Classification of the Fluoroquinolones/Quinolones

First Generation*
Cinoxacin (Cinobac)
Nalidixic acid (NegGram)
Oxolinic acid

Second Generation
Ciprofloxacin (Cipro)
Enoxacin (Penetrex)
Fleroxacin
Lomefloxacin (Maxaquin)
Levofloxacin (Levaquin)
Norfloxacin (Noroxin)
Ofloxacin (Floxin)
Rulfloxacin

Third Generation
Gatifloxacin (Tequin)
Grepafloxacin
Pazufloxacin
Sparfloxacin (Zagam)
Tosulfloxacin

Fourth Generation
Clinafloxacin
Gemfloxacin
Moxifloxacin (Avelox)
Trovafloxacin (Trovan)

From Andriole VT: The future of the quinolones, *Drugs* 58(suppl 2):1-5, 1999; Naber KG, Adam D: Classification of fluoroquinolones, *Int J Antimicrob Agents* 10:255-257, 1998; Walker RC: The fluoroquinolones, *Mayo Clin Proc* 74:1030-1037, 1999.
*Quinolones.

Mechanism of action and antibacterial spectrum

DNA gyrase and topoisomerases are enzymes involved in the crucial processes of DNA replication, transcription, and recombination. DNA gyrase has two subunits (A and B) regulated by two genes (*gyr*A and *gyr*B), with topoisomerase IV encoded by *par*C and *par*E genes. Both enzymes are responsible for supercoiling DNA, forming double-stranded DNA, and maintaining DNA in its physiologically stable and biologically active state. Topoisomerase IV nicks double-stranded DNA and seals the nicked DNA while DNA gyrase guides the passage of the DNA through the interior of the enzyme complex. Both enzymes are then responsible for supercoiling DNA, allowing for its fit into the bacterial cell. The fluoroquinolones stabilize the enzyme complex after strand breakage and before resealing, thereby preventing DNA supercoiling.

The fluoroquinolones are broad-spectrum antibiotics that were initially greeted with great enthusiasm because they

Box 39-10

Classification of the Fluoroquinolones Based on Antibacterial Spectrum

Group I (Urinary Tract Infections)
Norfloxacin (Noroxin)

Group II (Broad Spectrum)
Ciprofloxacin (Cipro)

Enoxacin (Penetrex)
Ofloxacin (Floxin)

Group III (Greater Gram-Positive Activity)
Levofloxacin (Levaquin)
Sparfloxacin (Zagam)

Group IV (Greater Gram-Positive/Antianaerobic Activity)
Gatifloxacin (Tequin)
Moxifloxacin (Avelox)
Trovafloxacin (Trovan)

From Naber KG, Adam D: Classification of fluoroquinolones, *Int J Antimicrob Agents* 10:255-257, 1998.

were orally effective against some of the most pathogenic nosocomial microorganisms: *Staphylococcus aureus, Pseudomonas aeruginosa*, and *Streptococcus pneumoniae*. Then, as with all orally effective antibiotics, the fluoroquinolones were used widely throughout the community, often in infections for which older agents were still effective. This has led to widespread resistance to these agents and ultimately a race to produce new fluoroquinolones, which unfortunately are only marginally better in many cases.

The fluoroquinolones are most active against aerobic bacilli and cocci: *Enterobacteriaceae, Haemophilus influenzae, Neisseria gonorrhoeae* and *meningitidis, Moraxella catarrhalis,* and *Pseudomonas aeruginosa*. The fluoroquinolones can be classified according to their antibacterial spectrum (see Box 39-10) with considerable overlap: group I (mainly for urinary tract infections), group II (broad spectrum), group III (greater activity against streptococci, enterococci, staphylococci) and group IV (greater activity against anaerobes).[61] *The Medical Letter* lists the fluoroquinolones as drugs of choice in the management of infections caused by penicillin-resistant *Streptococcus pneumoniae, Neisseria gonorrhoeae, Bacillus anthracis, Salmonella typhi* and other *Salmonella, Shigella, Bartonella henselae, Legionella pneumophila, Pseudomonas aeruginosa* (urinary tract infection), and *Rhodococcus equi*, and as an alternate drug for a myriad of infections (see Table 39-4 and Box 39-11).[15]

The in vitro MICs for sensitive microorganisms range from 0.008 to 1.0 µg/ml, whereas the maximum serum concentrations range from 1.1 to 5.7 µg/ml.[29] MSSA may have MICs of 0.06 to 0.25 µg/ml but MRSA and ciprofloxacin-resistant *Staphylococcus aureus* have MICs of 1 to 4 to 8 to 18 µg/ml for some fluoroquinolones, respectively.

The MICs for the fluoroquinolones against VGS range from 0.12 to 8 µg/ml, with various fluoroquinolones and their MICs against oral anaerobic pathogens are 0.25 to 128 µg/ml.

Box 39-11

Fluoroquinolones as Drugs of Choice or Alternate Agents for Various Infections

Drugs of Choice	Alternate Agents
Bartonella henselae	*Acinetobacter*
Campylobacter jejuni	*Aeromonas*
Legionella pneumophila	*Bacillus anthracis*
Neisseria gonorrhoeae	*Calymmatobacterium granulomatis*
Penicillin-resistant *Streptococcus pneumoniae*	*Capnocytophaga canimorsus*
Pseudomonas aeruginosa (urinary tract)	*Chlamydia pneumoniae*
Salmonella typhi and other *Salmonella*	*Chlamydia trachomatis*
Shigella	*Citrobacter freundii*
	Enterobacter
	Enterococcus (urinary tract)
	Erysipelothrix rhusiopathiae
	Escherichia coli
	Haemophilus drucreyi
	Haemophilus influenzae (respiratory tract)
	Klebsiella pneumoniae
	MRSA
	Moraxella catarrhalis
	Mycobacterium pneumoniae
	Mycobacterium tuberculosis
	Neisseria meningitidis
	Proteus (indole-positive)
	Proteus mirabilis
	Pseudomonas aeruginosa (non—urinary tract)
	Rickettsiae
	Serratia marcescens
	Stenotrophomonas maltophilia
	Vibrio cholerae

From Choice of antibacterial drugs, *Med Lett Drugs Ther* 43:69-78, 2001.

Moxifloxacin, gatifloxacin, and trovafloxacin have the best activity against anaerobes but the effect is highly variable depending on the species.

Bacterial resistance

Three mechanisms account for microbial resistance to the fluoroquinolones: mutations in DNA gyrase and topoisomerase IV, drug efflux pumps, and reduction in microbial outer membrane permeability.[5,94] The target alterations are accomplished by simple point mutations in DNA gyrase (*gyr*A) and topoisomerase IV (*par*C). Significant and sometimes extensive resistance has been detected in *Neisseria gonorrhoeae, Salmonella* and *Shigella, Escherichia coli, Campylobacter jejuni,* and many gram-negative anaerobes. Microorganisms displaying efflux mechanisms include VGS, *Enterococcus, Streptococcus pneumoniae, Enterobacteriaceae, Pseudomonas aeruginosa,* and *Bacteroides fragilis.*

Absorption, fate, and excretion

The fluoroquinolones are well absorbed orally with a 70% and 90% bioavailability for ciprofloxacin and levofloxacin, respectively.[29] Food generally delays the peak concentration of ciprofloxacin and levofloxacin but has no effect on gatifloxacin and moxifloxacin. The percent excreted by the kidneys ranges from 27% to 73% and protein binding from 15% to 35%.[29] Fluoroquinolone half-lives vary from approximately 4 hours for ciprofloxacin and norfloxacin to 7 to 8 hours for gatifloxacin, lomefloxacin, and sparfloxacin, to 9 to 12 hours for moxifloxacin and trovafloxacin.[29] Pharmacokinetic improvements have included longer half-lives to allow for once-daily dosing and greater volumes of distribution for better tissue penetration. The postantibiotic effects of the fluoroquinolones vary from 1 to 4 hours.

General therapeutic uses

Fluoroquinolones are used to treat urinary tract infections and bacterial diarrhea (e.g., traveler's diarrhea[2]) because of their activity against many of the causative organisms (see Table 39-4). Because the fluoroquinolones vary in their pharmacokinetics and in their spectra, some, but not all, fluoroquinolones are employed for upper and lower respiratory tract infections, *Pseudomonas aeruginosa* infections, genital diseases caused by gonococci and *Chlamydia,* as well as Legionnaires disease and tuberculosis.

Therapeutic uses in dentistry

The fluoroquinolones are not indicated for any acute orofacial infections unless dictated by culture and sensitivity tests. Drugs with better antimicrobial spectrums are readily available. The drugs possess concentration-dependent killing not reflected in their package insert doses and they are not predictably synergistic with the β-lactams and aminoglycosides (may be additive or indifferent). Ciprofloxacin may be useful for the management of rapidly progressive or refractory periodontitis associated with *Enterobacteriaceae* as dictated by culture and sensitivity tests.

Adverse effects

The major adverse effects associated with the fluoroquinolones include the gastrointestinal tract, the CNS, skin, and cartilage.[29] Less common systems involved are the cardiovascular, hepatic, and renal systems. The incidence of each adverse effect may vary between the different drugs because of chemical substitutions on the quinolone nucleus.

Gastrointestinal adverse reactions include nausea and vomiting, dyspepsia and heartburn, and abdominal pain.[29] CNS effects include mild neuropathy (headache, dizziness, malaise, restlessness, bad dreams) possibly caused by central γ-aminobutyric acid inhibition or activity at the N-methyl-D-aspartate receptor. Dermatologic toxicity includes rash, pruritus, exfoliative dermatitis, Stevens-Johnson syndrome, and phototoxicity likely caused by dose-related ultraviolet light activation of reactive oxygen from the fluoroquinolones in the skin. Anaphylactic and anaphylactoid reactions occur at a rate of 0.46 to 1.23 per 100,000 drug exposures, with an onset of 3 to 30 minutes after drug administration.

Chondrotoxicity includes arthralgia, joint swelling, tendinitis, and tendon rupture (primarily the Achilles tendon). In a recent study of 42 cases of tendinitis and tendon rupture, the majority of individuals took normal doses with a median 6 days (range, 1 to 510 days) until the onset of signs and symptoms (pain, edema, dysfunction, erythema, warmth), with 93% occurring within 30 days of the onset of drug intake.[90] These disorders were more likely to occur in men, patients with a median age of 68 years and with concomitant corticosteroid therapy, diabetes mellitus, renal failure, other musculoskeletal disorders, or involvement in sports activity.[90] The tendinitis usually resolved with drug discontinuance. In animals given the fluoroquinolones, changes have occurred in all immature joint cartilage (epiphyseal growth plate), possibly by chelation of the Mg^{++} ion.[29] These agents are not approved for children younger than 18 years, with the exception of ciprofloxacin.[90]

Other possible adverse effects include induction of a prolonged QT interval (torsades de pointes), transient increase in liver enzymes, neutropenia, serum sickness, allergic vasculitis, and renal crystalluria. Because these antibiotics affect DNA, they have been investigated as possible teratogens. At extremely high in vitro doses of 100 to 750 μg/ml for 24 hours, the fluoroquinolones have induced genotoxicity in the chromosomal aberration test; however, a clinical study of 200 women exposed to ciprofloxacin and norfloxacin during gestation demonstrated no increase in fetal malformations or musculoskeletal defects.[55]

Anecdotal reports in Europe have claimed an association between fluoroquinolones and suicidal behavior, but a study of individuals receiving the drugs for 31 to 180 days could detect no increase in suicidal behavior.[40] Two cases of possible exacerbation of myasthenia gravis have been reported.

Drug interactions

An important drug interaction with the fluoroquinolones is the potential increase in CNS toxicity with the concomitant use of nonsteroidal antiinflammatory drugs and methylxanthines.[29] The combination of sparfloxacin, gatifloxacin, and moxifloxacin with the tricyclic antidepressants, erythromycin, phenothiazines, and antiarrhythmic agents (quinidine, procainamide, disopyramide) may increase the risk of torsades de pointes.[29] Fluoroquinolones may reduce the liver clearance of warfarin and procainamide and increase the toxicity of cyclosporin.[29] Cimetidine may increase fluoroquinolone blood levels and antacids and sucralfate may reduce their gastric absorption. The fluoroquinolones may induce urine false-positives for opioid drugs by immunoassay techniques.

Contraindications

Ciprofloxacin should be used with caution during pregnancy and with children. For children younger than 18 years other fluoroquinolones are contraindicated.[29] Phototoxicity may occur on skin areas exposed to sunlight, and sunscreens are not always effective.[29]

Aminoglycosides

The era of the aminoglycosides began in 1943 with the isolation of streptomycin by Waksman and the further development of kanamycin (1957), gentamicin (1963), tobramycin (1968), amikacin (1972), and netilmicin (1975). The aminoglycosides are amino sugars bound by glycosidic bridges to a hexose nucleus.

Chemistry

Streptomycin is produced by *Streptomyces griseus.* The other aminoglycosides are elaborated by various species of *Streptomyces* and *Micromonospora* or, in the case of amikacin and netilmicin, are semisynthetic derivatives of naturally occurring aminoglycosides. As the name implies, these agents consist of a highly polar amino base attached by glycosidic linkage to one or more sugars. Streptomycin, for example, is composed of three elements: streptidine (the amino base) and the two sugar moieties streptose and N-methyl-glucosamine (Figure 39-11).

Mechanism of action and antibacterial spectrum

The aminoglycosides bind irreversibly to the 30S ribosome to interfere with the reading of the microbial genetic code and to inhibit protein synthesis. The aminoglycosides are generally bactericidal and their efficacy in several cases can be greatly enhanced by the concomitant use of cell wall inhibiting β-lactams and glycopeptides.

The activity of the aminoglycosides is primarily directed toward gram-negative bacilli and mycobacteria. The spectrum includes *Enterobacteriaceae* as well as *Pseudomonas aeruginosa*. There are some differences between the aminoglycosides regarding their efficacy toward specific microorganisms: amikacin for gentamicin-resistant gram-negative bacilli, gentamicin and doxycycline for brucellosis, gentamicin and penicillins for *Campylobacter* infective endocarditis, tobramycin against *Acinetobacter* and *Pseudomonas aeruginosa*, and streptomycin for tularemia and plague. Most *Enterobacteriaceae* remain sensitive to the aminoglycosides. Significant resistance has occurred in enterococci.[25] Gentamicin is the most commonly used aminoglycoside, often acting synergistically with ampicillin, penicillin G, ceftriaxone, vancomycin, and rifampin.[25] Some of the original indications for the aminoglycosides have been supplanted by the safer extended-spectrum β-lactams and the fluoroquinolones.[25]

Bacterial resistance

Three resistance mechanisms exist presently for the aminoglycosides: ribosomal mutations (less affinity for the 30S ribosome), reduced intracellular transport (primarily in staphylococci and pseudomonads), and, most commonly, plasmid-mediated aminoglycoside-modifying enzymes: acetyltransferases, adenyltransferases, and phosphotransferases.

Absorption, fate, and excretion

The aminoglycosides are poorly absorbed orally and do not penetrate well into the CNS, bronchial secretions, or certain microbial cells *(Rickettsia, Chlamydia)* but are effective intracellularly in the treatment of tuberculosis, plague, brucellosis, and tularemia. The aminoglycosides are classic concentration-dependent antibiotics commonly administered in high parenteral doses repeated after the blood levels have fallen to a low concentration (peak and trough dosing). Single daily dosing is becoming more common, taking advantage of the long postantibiotic effect of the aminoglycosides, a reduction in cost, and lessening of renal toxicity. The normal elimination half-lives of the aminoglycosides are 2 to 3 hours, which can be extended to 24 to 100 hours in end-stage renal disease.[29] The aminoglycosides are excreted primarily by glomerular filtration.

General therapeutic uses

The parenteral aminoglycosides currently available include amikacin, gentamicin, kanamycin, netilmicin, streptomycin, and tobramycin. Kanamycin and neomycin are available for oral use for gastrointestinal infections. The aminoglycosides are primarily indicated for infections caused by gram-negative aerobic bacteria. These include *Pseudomonas aeruginosa*, *Serratia*, *Klebsiella*, *Enterobacter*, and *Proteus*. The aminoglycosides are often combined with a penicillin or cephalosporin for various infections (see Table 39-4). Their use in tuberculosis is described below.

Therapeutic uses in dentistry

The aminoglycosides have no uses in orofacial infections unless dictated by culture and sensitivity tests.

Adverse effects

The major adverse effects of the aminoglycosides are renal toxicity and both auditory and vestibular ototoxicity.[25] Nephrotoxicity is caused by inhibition of an intracellular lysosomal phospholipase in the renal proximal tubules, resulting in aminoglycoside accumulation and subsequent reduced glomerular filtration, reduced water and Na^+ transport, reduced mitochondrial respiration, and reduced renal protein synthesis resulting in renal necrosis.[25] The incidence of some degree of nephrotoxicity can be as high as 10% to 20%.

A primary target for toxicity of the aminoglycosides is the hair cells of the inner ear; the initial loss of the outer hair cells

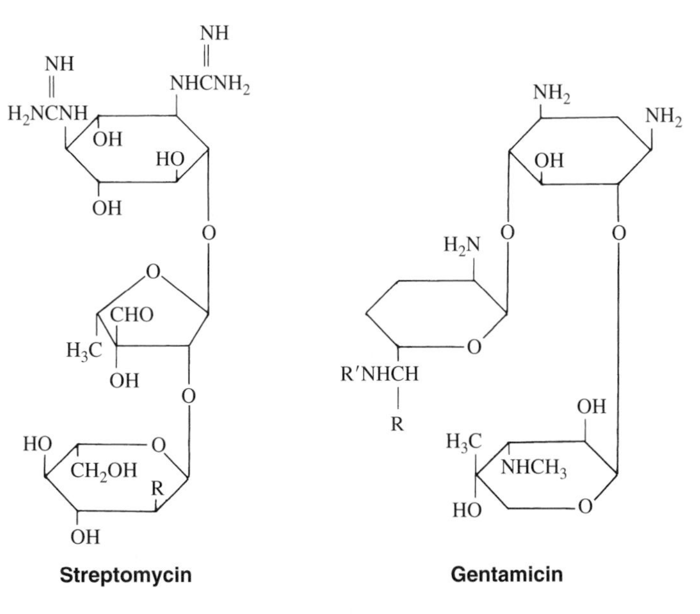

Streptomycin **Gentamicin**

Fig. 39-11 Structural formulas of streptomycin and gentamicin. R for streptomycin is CH_3NH. Commercial preparations of gentamicin contain three closely related gentamicins: C_1 ($R = CH_3$, $R' = CH_3$), C_{1a} ($R = H$, $R' = H$), and C_2 ($R = CH_3$, $R' = H$).

eventually damages the inner ear cochlear hair cells (type II).[25] Further damage may occur to the cochlear sensory epithelium and the spiral ganglion cells required for cochlear implants. Vestibular (type I) hair cell damage occurs at the apex of the macula and often earlier than the cochlear hair cell damage.[32] Initial signs and symptoms are hearing loss at the higher frequencies, which increases with dose, duration, and noise exposure.[32] The incidence of cochlear damage may be as high as 15%. Other adverse reactions associated with the aminoglycosides include neuromuscular blockade of the curare type, rare blood dyscrasias, headache, dizziness, and urticarial and peripheral neuropathy.

Drug interactions

The nephrotoxicity of aminoglycosides is increased by vancomycin, cephalosporins, and methoxyflurane. Loop diuretics increase auditory toxicity.

Vancomycin

Vancomycin is the most important glycopeptide antibiotic, originally isolated from *Streptomyces orientalis* in Borneo in 1956 and introduced into medicine in 1958. Other glycopeptides include teicoplanin and daptomycin. The glycopeptides are seven-membered peptide chains with two sugars: vacosamine and glucose. Vancomycin is poorly absorbed from the gastrointestinal tract and causes severe pain when given intramuscularly. It is administered intravenously for systemic infections or orally in the treatment of pseudomembranous colitis. Its elimination half-life is 6 hours and it has a postantibiotic effect of 1.5 to 3 hours.

Mechanism of action and antibacterial spectrum

Vancomycin inhibits gram-positive bacterial cell wall synthesis by complexing with the D-alanyl-D-alanine portion of the peptide precursor units to inhibit the transglycosylase reaction in peptidoglycan synthesis.[95] This inhibition is at the second stage of bacterial cell wall synthesis before the action of the penicillins at the third stage. Vancomycin may also affect cytoplasmic membrane permeability and RNA synthesis and, as with the β-lactams, requires active cell replication. Because of its large molecular size, vancomycin cannot traverse the outer cell membrane of gram-negative bacteria.

The activity of vancomycin is almost exclusively against aerobic and anaerobic gram-positive species: staphylococci, streptococci (*Streptococcus pneumoniae*, VGS, β-hemolytic streptococci), *Corynebacterium*, peptostreptococci, enterococci, nutritionally variant streptococci *(Abiotrophia)*, Bacillus, *Listeria*, and *Clostridia*.[95] Occasionally *Neisseria gonorrhoeae* is susceptible. Vancomycin is a drug of choice against MRSA, methicillin-resistant CoNS, *Corynebacterium jeikeium*, and multiple–antibiotic-resistant *Streptococcus pneumoniae*. It may also be indicated for serious enterococcal infections and in patients who cannot tolerate the β-lactams. *The Medical Letter* lists vancomycin as a drug of choice for MRSA, penicillin-resistant *Streptococcus pneumoniae*, MSSA or *Staphylococcus epidermidis*, *Bacillus cereus* and *subtilis*, *Corynebacterium JK* group, *Rhodococcus equi*, and as an alternate drug for enterococcal endocarditis, VGS, group A and B streptococci, *Streptococcus bovis*, *Peptostreptococcus*, and *Clostridium difficile*.[15]

Bacterial resistance

Vancomycin resistance is caused by an altered peptidoglycan terminus (D-ala-D-lac instead of the usual D-ala-D-ala), resulting in reduced vancomycin binding and failure to prevent cell wall synthesis.[12] Resistance in vancomycin-intermediate *Staphylococcus aureus* (VISA) and glycopeptide-intermediate *Staphylococcus aureus* (GISA) may be due to the production of abnormal peptides ("false binding sites") in the cell wall that bind vancomycin and prevent its attachment to its receptor or possibly to an increase of peptidoglycan resulting in thickened cell walls.[13] A form of resistance is seen in *Streptococcus pneumoniae* by a unique mutation in the sensor-response system that controls autolysin activity necessary to kill certain bacteria.[65]

General therapeutic uses

Vancomycin is used for serious gram-positive infections caused by such organisms as methicillin-resistant staphylococci and *Streptococcus pneumoniae*. It is also useful for non–vancomycin resistant enterococcal infections. It is effective in treating enterocolitis caused by *Clostridium difficile;* however, metronidazole should be used for this situation if at all possible because of the significant risk of promoting vancomycin enterococcal resistance. Vancomycin may also be useful in treating multiple antibiotic-resistant VGS infections.

Therapeutic uses in dentistry

The glycopeptides have no uses in the management of acute or chronic orofacial infections unless dictated by laboratory culture and sensitivity tests.

Adverse effects

The major adverse drug reactions associated with vancomycin include transient or permanent ototoxicity, hypotension, reversible neutropenia, renal toxicity, skin rash, and the "red man" (red neck) syndrome. The auditory toxicity of vancomycin is rare if the peak blood levels are kept below 40 to 50 μg/ml but can be exacerbated by the combination with the aminoglycosides. The red man syndrome results from the direct histamine release from mast cells manifesting as pruritus, erythematous rash of the head, neck, face, and upper torso along with hypotension mimicking anaphylactic shock.[95] This glycopeptide-induced anaphylactoid reaction may occur with the first drug exposure, is tachyphylactic in nature, and can be reduced significantly by the slow infusion of vancomycin over a 1-hour period and premedication with antihistamine drugs.[95] To reduce the development of resistant bacteria, vancomycin use is contraindicated or discouraged for routine surgical prophylaxis.

Drug interactions

Vancomycin-induced nephrotoxicity or ototoxicity is increased with the concomitant use of aminoglycosides and neuromuscular blockade with curare-like agents.

Streptogramins

Quinupristin/dalfopristin is a 30/70 mixture of streptogramins A and B recently approved for intravenous use in the United States.

Mechanism of action and antibacterial spectrum

Quinupristin and dalfopristin bind sequentially to different sites of the 50S subunit of the 70S ribosome to prevent newly synthesized peptide chains from extruding from the ribosome, resulting in cell death.

Quinupristin/dalfopristin is used to treat life-threatening vancomycin-resistant *Enterococcus faecium* (*Enterococcus faecalis* is resistant) and skin or skin-structure infections from *Staphylococcus aureus* and *Streptococcus pyogenes*. The drug is additionally approved in the United Kingdom for nosocomial pneumonia. In vitro the drug combination is active against *Enterococcus faecium*, MRSA, MSSA, methicillin-resistant CoNS, methicillin-sensitive CoNS, penicillin-sensitive and penicillin-resistant *Streptococcus pneumoniae, Neisseria meningitidis, Moraxella catarrhalis, Legionella pneumophila, Mycoplasma pneumoniae,* and *Clostridium perfringens.* Its spectrum closely resembles that of vancomycin and linezolid.

Bacterial resistance

Microbial resistance occurs by three mechanisms: decreased ribosomal binding by methylation of an adenine residue, drug efflux, and enzymatic inactivation. This resistance belongs to the MLS_B type, potentially conferring cross-resistance to all these antibiotics. The streptogramin group also contains virginiamycin and pristinamycin, which have been used for years in some countries as animal growth promoters, resulting in microbial resistance in human beings even before the drugs were clinically employed. Currently, intermediate resistance has been detected in *Staphylococcus aureus* and *Enterococcus faecium,* with vancomycin and streptogramin resistance genes detected on the same plasmid. *Enterococcus faecium* resistance may occur during drug use and quinupristin/dalfopristin selects for superinfection with *Enterococcus faecalis.*

General therapeutic uses

Quinupristin/dalfoprinstin should be reserved for life-threatening and multiply antibiotic resistant infections from *Enterococcus faecium,* staphylococci, and some streptococci encountered primarily in the hospital.

Adverse effects

Adverse effects associated with the streptogramins include possible severe arthralgias and myalgias, elevation in conjugated serum bilirubin, and significant inhibition of the liver microsomal CYP3A4 drug metabolizing system.

Drug interactions

The streptogramins decrease the liver metabolism of Ca^{++} channel blockers, immunosuppressant drugs, corticosteroids, several anticancer agents, 3-hydroxy-3-methylglutaryl coenzyme A reductase inhibitors (statins), HIV protease inhibitors, quinidine, nonsedating antihistamines, sildenafil, opioids, and benzodiazepines.

Oxazolidinones

The oxazolidinones (eperezolid, linezolid) were synthesized in 1987, and linezolid was approved for use in the United States in 2000. Linezolid is the first totally synthetic new antibiotic released in approximately 40 years.

Mechanism of action and antibacterial spectrum

Linezolid has a unique mechanism of action by binding to the 50S ribosome subunit near the interface with the 30S subunit to prevent the initiation complex required for bacterial translation.[14,21,22] This unique mechanism may possibly limit cross-resistance with other antibiotics.[22]

Linezolid is approved in the United States for the management of vancomycin-resistant *Enterococcus faecium,* nosocomial and community-acquired pneumonia from *Staphylococcus aureus* and penicillin-sensitive *Streptococcus pneumoniae,* and complicated skin and skin structure infections from MRSA, MSSA, methicillin-resistant CoNS, *Streptococcus pyogenes,* and *Streptococcus agalactiae.*[29]

Linezolid has demonstrated in vivo and in vitro bacteriostatic activity against penicillin-resistant VGS, beta-hemolytic streptococci, *Bacillus, Listeria, Corynebacterium, Moraxella catarrhalis, Pasturella multocida, Bacteroides fragilis,* and antibiotic-resistant mycobacteria.[21] Linezolid has little useful clinical activity against *Enterobacteriaceae, Acinetobacter, Pseudomonas aeruginosa,* and most gram-negative species, with some activity against mycobacteria and chlamydiae. Very high MICs are seen with *Fusobacterium, Porphyromonas, Prevotella,* and *Veillonella.*

Bacterial resistance

Microbial resistance to linezolid has been detected in isolated cultures of vancomycin-resistant enterococci, *Escherichia coli,* and laboratory strains of *Staphylococcus aureus.* The recent reports of clinical isolates of *Enterococcus faecium* and *Staphylococcus aureus* resistant to linezolid is disconcerting because the drug has been available only for a short period of time. The mechanism of resistance appears to be a 62,576 T mutation in the gene encoding the central loop domain of 23S rRNA.[22]

Absorption, fate, and excretion

Linezolid, with a near 100% oral bioavailability, produces peak blood levels at 1 to 2 hours, and can also be administered parenterally. It has an elimination half-life of 4.4 to 5.5 hours and a postantibiotic effect of 0.6 to 1.4 hours.[29]

General therapeutic uses

Linezolid is at this time highly effective against three of the five most important nosocomial pathogens: *Staphylococcus aureus, Streptococcus pneumoniae,* and enterococci and should be reserved for highly and multiply antibiotic-resistant microorganisms. The ability of *Staphylococcus aureus* to mutate to resistance after only a few months of exposure to the drug is disconcerting. Linezolid has no use in orofacial infections.

Adverse effects

Approximately 2% to 3% of patients receiving linezolid experience nausea and vomiting, diarrhea, headache, tongue discoloration, taste alteration, or fungal superinfections and very rarely pseudomembranous colitis.[29] The most serious adverse reaction is myelosuppression (anemia, leukopenia, pancytopenia, thrombocytopenia), which may occur in an average of 2.4% of patients. Linezolid requires weekly blood monitoring tests. The safety of the drug has not been established beyond 28 days of use. It is classified as an FDA pregnancy C drug.

Drug interactions

Linezolid is a weak monoamine oxidase inhibitor and should be used with caution with drugs that release catecholamines and foods containing tyramine. Linezolid may precipitate the serotonin syndrome (confusion, agitation, seizures, hypertension, tachycardia, sweating, myoclonus, muscle rigidity, trismus, death)[29] but the clinical significance of this drug effect is as yet unknown.

Sulfonamides

The era of effective and safe systemic antibiotic therapy began in 1932 with the discovery by Gerhard Domagk that a dye (prontosil) protected laboratory animals from streptococcal infections. Domagk determined that the active antibacterial portion of prontosil was sulfanilamide, which was subsequently first used in the United States in 1935. Trimethoprim was introduced in 1968 as a synergistic agent with the sulfonamides and the combination of sulfamethoxazole and trimethoprim is the most commonly used sulfonamide preparation today. Arguably the discovery of prontosil by Domagk ranks with the discovery of the anesthetic properties of nitrous oxide by Horace Wells, the work on penicillin by the Oxford group, and the discovery by Jenner of vaccinations as among the greatest of all medical discoveries.

Chemistry

All the sulfonamides are derivatives of *p*-aminobenzenesulfonamide (Figure 39-12). For antibacterial activity, the sulfur must be attached directly to the benzene ring, and the *p*-amino group (N_4) must be a primary amine in vivo. Substitutions on the amino group (N_1) of the sulfonamide moiety confer differences in rates of absorption and excretion of these drugs and, to some degree, in variations of antibacterial activity. The sulfonamides are weak acids with limited water solubility, particularly in solutions of low pH. This property may present problems for the excretion of these drugs in an acidic urine.

Mechanism of action and antibacterial spectrum

Both the sulfonamides and trimethoprim interfere with the microbial synthesis of folic acid necessary for life in some microorganisms. Mammals acquire folic acid from their diet. The sulfonamides competitively inhibit the incorporation of para-aminobenzoic acid into tetrahydropteroic acid as the sulfas have a greater affinity for tetrahydropteroate synthetase than para-aminobenzoic acid (Figure 39-13). Trimethoprim inhibits bacterial dihydrofolate reductase with 50,000 to 100,000 times greater affinity for the bacterial than the human enzyme. This, in turn, blocks the conversion of dihydrofolic acid to tetrahydrofolic acid, resulting in the reduced synthesis of folinic acid, purines, and DNA. The sulfonamides and trimethoprim inhibit successive steps in the synthesis of folic acid and eventually bacterial nucleotides and DNA.

The sulfonamides and trimethoprim are intended primarily for respiratory, urinary, and gastrointestinal infections.[15] *The Medical Letter* lists this combination as drugs of choice for *Yersinia enterocolitica, Aeromonas, Burkholderia cepacia, Stenotrophomonas maltophilia, Nocardia,* and generally for bronchitis and upper respiratory tract infections as well as alternate drugs for some *Enterobacteriaceae, Moraxella catarrhalis,* MRSA, *Streptococcus pneumoniae, Listeria monocytogenes, Bartonella henselae, Brucella, Legionella pneumophila, Vibrio cholerae, Yersinia pestis, Mycobacterium marinum,* and *Pseudomonas pseudomallei.*[15] Species that have intrinsic resistance or that can become highly resistant include enterococci, *Bacillus anthracis,* various *Enterobacteriaceae, Pseudomonas aeruginosa, Streptococcus pneumoniae,* and *Corynebacterium diphtheriae.*

Pteridine moiety — *p*-Aminobenzoic acid moiety — Glutamic acid moiety

Folic acid

***p*-Aminobenzoic acid** **Typical sulfonamide**

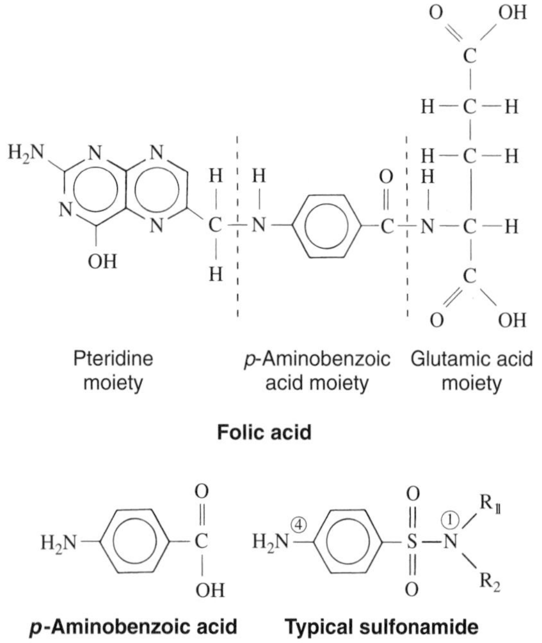

Fig. 39-12 Structural formulas of folic acid, a sulfonamide, and *p*-aminobenzoic acid.

Bacterial resistance

Transferable microbial resistance to the sulfonamides and trimethoprim occurs by three principal mechanisms: increased cell permeability barriers and efflux proteins, decreased sensitivity or alterations in target enzymes (dihydropteroate synthase and dihydrofolate reductase), and the acquisition of new target enzymes. Trimethoprim-sulfamethoxazole resistance in *Streptococcus pneumoniae* occurs via a single amino acid substitution in dihydrofolate reductase. Chromosomal resistance by mutations in the dihydropteroate synthetase gene occurs in *Escherichia coli,* staphylococci, *Pneumocystis carinii, Campylobacter, Streptococcus pneumoniae, Streptococcus pyogenes,* and *Neisseria meningitidis.*

It is discouraging to note that despite a determined effort to drastically reduce sulfonamide use in the United Kingdom, the resistance rate in *Escherichia coli* not only did not decline but actually increased.[26] As is now common, the resistance genes for trimethoprim-sulfamethoxazole are carried on transposable elements along with the resistance genes for other antibiotics, possibly necessitating the removal of all from the environment before resistance declines.

Absorption, fate, and excretion

The sulfonamides are classified as short-, medium-, or long-acting and topical agents (solely for gastrointestinal tract use) according to their absorption properties, solubility, and gastrointestinal tolerance. The short- to medium-acting agents include sulfisoxazole, sulfamethoxazole, sulfamethizole, and sulfadiazine. Sulfadoxine is a long-acting agent with a 100- to 230-hour elimination half-life. Various other sulfonamide preparations include those used topically for burns (silver sulfadiazine, mafenide), vaginal and ophthalmic preparations,

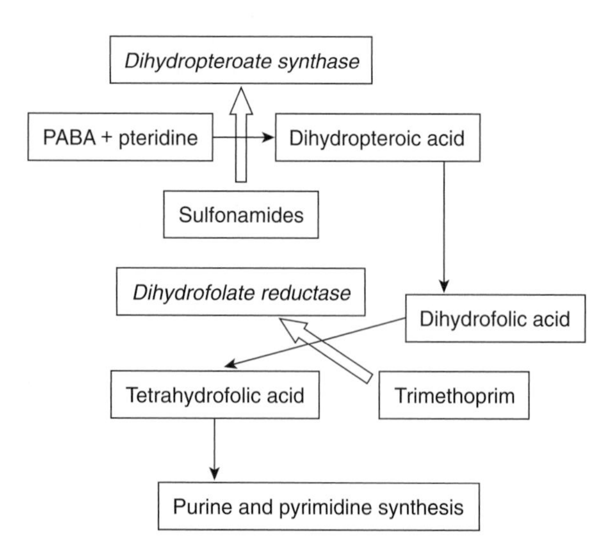

Fig. 39-13 Sites of inhibition of folic acid synthesis by sulfonamides and trimethoprim. Note the effect of the two drugs on this common pathway and the effect on purine and pyrimidine synthesis. *PABA, p*-aminobenzoic acid.

and drugs for the management of ulcerative colitis (salicylazosulfapyridine). The oral sulfonamides are 70% to 100% bioavailable with a large volume of distribution and ready penetration into the CNS. The drugs are metabolized by acetylation and conjugation in the liver and excreted by glomerular filtration.

General therapeutic uses

The primary clinical uses of a sulfonamide alone or trimethoprim/sulfamethoxazole are acute bronchitis, community-acquired pneumonia, *Legionella pneumophila* and *Pneumocystis carinii* pneumonia, uncomplicated urinary tract infections, male genitourinary tract infections, traveler's diarrhea from enterotoxigenic *Escherichia coli, Shigella, Nocardia asteroides,* toxoplasmosis, malaria (sulfadoxine in combination with pyrimethamine), *Neisseria meningitidis* prophylaxis, trachoma, chancroid, rheumatic fever, and Wegener's granulomatosis. Some sulfonamides are also used in special cases such as in burns, and in certain cases of ophthalmic, gastrointestinal, and skin disorders (Table 39-8). There are no indications for the sulfonamides/trimethoprim in the management of orofacial infections.

Adverse effects

Approximately 8% of those receiving sulfonamides and trimethoprim have some form of adverse reaction: nausea and vomiting, blood dyscrasias, and crystalluria (less soluble preparations, such as sulfadiazine, precipitate in the urine), with 3% to 5% experiencing allergy in any of its forms from skin rash and pruritus to major skin eruptions (Stevens-Johnson syndrome, epidermal necrolysis, exfoliative dermatitis, photosensitivity) to anaphylaxis.[29] Stevens-Johnson syndrome is much more likely to occur with long-acting sulfonamides. Up to 70% of patients with AIDS have some form of skin rash and fever from the sulfonamides/trimethoprim.

Drug interactions

Trimethoprim/sulfamethoxazole increases the clinical activity of the oral anticoagulants, thiopental, methotrexate, hydantoins, sulfonylureas, and tolbutamide and decreases the activity of cyclosporine.[29] The sulfonamides are displaced from plasma protein by aspirin, other nonsteroidal antiinflammatory drugs, and probenecid. Para-aminobenzoic acid (present in some health foods) will compete against the effect of the sulfonamides.

Contraindications

Contraindications for the use of sulfonamides include allergy to sulfonamides and other related drugs: sulfonylureas, thiazide, loop and carbonic anhydrase inhibitor diuretics. Health foods and possibly sunscreens containing para-aminobenzoic acid (PABA) are contraindicated because PABA competes against the sulfonamide.

Chloramphenicol

Chloramphenicol (Chloromycetin) is a broad-spectrum antibiotic isolated in 1949 from *Streptomyces venezuelae.* It is bacteriostatic because of its inhibition of bacterial protein synthesis by reversible binding to the peptidyl transferase component of the 50S ribosomal subunit. Chloramphenicol is unique among naturally occurring antibiotics in that it contains a nitrobenzene group, which is attached to a propanediol moiety linked to a dichloroacetamide side chain. Its structure is illustrated in Figure 39-14. Resistance occurs by both plasmid and chromosomal-mediated chloramphenicol acetyltransferase, which metabolizes chloramphenicol to an inactive form.

Chloramphenicol may be active against a wide range of microorganisms: gram-positive and gram-negative bacteria, spirochetes, rickettsiae, *Mycoplasma,* and *Chlamydia.* Common pathogens sensitive to chloramphenicol include

$$O_2N{-}C_6H_4{-}\underset{\text{OH}}{\mathrm{CH}}{-}\underset{\mathrm{CH_2OH}}{\mathrm{CH}}{-}\mathrm{NH}{-}\underset{\mathrm{O}}{\mathrm{C}}{-}\mathrm{CH(Cl)_2}$$

Fig. 39-14 Structural formula of chloramphenicol.

Table 39-8

Classification, by Use, of Selected Sulfonamide and Trimethoprim Preparations

USE	NONPROPRIETARY (GENERIC) NAME	PROPRIETARY (TRADE) NAME
Systemic infections	Sulfadiazine	—
	Sulfamethoxazole*	Gantanol
	Sulfisoxazole*	Gantrisin
	Erythromycin-sulfisoxazole	Eryzole, Pediazole
	Trimethoprim*	Proloprim, Trimpex
	Trimethoprim-sulfamethoxazole*†	Bactrim, Cotrim, Septra, Sulfatrim
Urinary tract infections	Sulfacytine	Renoquid
	Sulfamethizole	Thiosulfil Forte
Dermatitis herpetiformis	Sulfapyridine	—
Local use in gastrointestinal tract	Sulfasalazine	Azulfidine
Ophthalmic use	Sulfacetamide sodium	Blef-10, Sodium Sulamyd
Topical use, burns	Mafenide	Sulfamylon
	Silver sulfadiazine	Silvadene, Thermazene

*These drugs are also used in the treatment of urinary tract infections.
†Also used in the treatment of *Pneumocystis carinii* pneumonia in AIDS patients.

Salmonella typhi, other *Salmonella, Streptococcus pneumoniae, Haemophilus influenzae,* and *Neisseria meningitidis.* Enterococci are variably resistant and MRSA, methicillin-resistant CoNS, and *Pseudomonas aeruginosa* are completely resistant. Because of its propensity to induce bone marrow depression and aplasia, chloramphenicol is not the current drug of choice for any infection but is an alternate drug for gastrointestinal *Bacteroides,* as well as *Clostridium perfringens, Proteus mirabilis, Brucella, Salmonella typhi* and other *Salmonella, Francisella tularemia, Fusobacteria, Haemophilus influenzae, Pseudomonas mallei* and *pseudomallei, Yersinia pestis, Chlamydia psittaci,* various *Ehrlichia, Vibrio vulnificus,* and rickettsial diseases (Rocky Mountain spotted fever, tick-bite fever, Q fever, and typhus).[29]

The most significant adverse reactions associated with chloramphenicol are reversible and irreversible bone marrow depression seen with topical, oral, and parenteral use.[80] The reversible type is dose related (greater than 4 g/day) and possibly caused by inhibition of mitochondrial protein synthesis resulting in anemia, leukopenia, or thrombocytopenia. "Idiosyncratic" bone marrow aplasia is not dose related, may begin weeks or months after the drug is terminated, and is manifested by an often fatal aplastic anemia, the incidence of which appears to be 1 in 24,500 to 1 in 40,800 patients receiving chloramphenicol by any route of administration. This is 13 times greater than the spontaneous random occurrence of aplastic anemia in the general population. Topical use is associated with a risk of three cases in 440,000 uses. The cause of this idiosyncratic aplastic anemia is unknown but may be due to a genetically determined liver metabolite.

The "gray baby syndrome" associated with chloramphenicol is caused by toxicity resulting from the inability of the immature liver of neonates to detoxify the drug by conjugation.[80] The signs and symptoms include abdominal distress, cyanosis, vomiting, circulatory collapse, and possibly death. There are no indications for chloramphenicol in the management of orofacial infections. The drug is rarely used because of its major adverse effects.

Bacteriophages

Bacteriophages are bacterial viruses that invade bacterial cells and can induce cell lysis by disrupting microbial metabolism.[83] Bacteriophages literally punch holes in microbial cell membranes and are one of the most ubiquitous entities on earth, found in or on salt and fresh water, soil, plants, animals, and human beings. Bacteriophages are composed of either RNA or DNA with a protein coat, have either a spherical or rod shape, and contain less than 10 to several hundred genes.[52] Bacteriophages thrive when horizontal transfer of genetic material between microorganisms is common.[52] Bacteriophages came into clinical use in World Wars I and II almost exclusively in Germany, Russia (Georgia), and Eastern Europe (Poland), with claims of 75% to 100% cures of various infections from staphylococci, pseudomonads, *Shigella, Salmonella, Escherichia coli,* and *Klebsiella pneumoniae.*[83]

The difficulties with bacteriophage therapy are lack of clinical proof of efficacy with controlled clinical studies, the potential for autoantibodies developed against the bacteriophages that may decrease their efficacy, microbial resistance development, and unknown activity against intracellular pathogens. The merits of bacteriophage therapy include high, but not absolute, specificity for a single pathogenic organism, thereby greatly reducing the risk for superinfections and resistance development; apparent safety, although this has not been studied in clinical trials; and ease of chemical manipulation to affect newly emerging pathogens.[83]

Microbial cells can mutate to resist bacteriophages or not even recognize these entities.[52] As with cationic peptides, if microorganisms develop resistance mechanisms to the bacteriophages then human beings will have lost another essential host defense mechanism. Proper use of bacteriophages requires very specific identification of the microbial pathogen since they are specific for each individual microbial species, making them of limited or no value in the treatment of polymicrobial disease such as pneumonia and orofacial infections.

Topical Antibiotics

Bacitracin

Bacitracin is a polypeptide antibiotic derived from *Bacillus subtilis* that functions to block cell wall formation by interfering with the dephosphorylation of the lipid compound that carries peptidoglycans to the growing microbial cell wall.[89] The antibacterial spectrum of bacitracin is gram positive: staphylococci, streptococci, *Corynebacterium,* and *Clostridium,* with rare resistance seen in staphylococci. Bacitracin is too toxic to be used parenterally; allergic contact dermatitis has been reported on occasion. Bacitracin is commonly combined with neomycin and polymyxin B in over-the-counter topical antibiotic preparations, but evidence for efficacy is limited.[89]

Neomycin

Neomycin is an aminoglycoside derived from *Streptomyces fradiae* and binds to the 30S ribosomal subunit to inactivate bacterial DNA polymerase and cause misreading of the genetic code to produce lethal proteins. Neomycin has a wide antibacterial spectrum against both gram-positive and gram-negative bacteria but is poorly effective against streptococci and *Pseudomonas aeruginosa.*[89] It is useful as a topical antibiotic and in the management of hepatic coma by reducing nitrogen-producing bacteria in the gastrointestinal tract.[89]

Polymyxin B

Polymyxin B was isolated from *Bacillus polymyxa* and functions as a cationic detergent to disrupt the microbial cell membrane, causing a leak in cell constituents. Its spectrum is gram negative and it is particularly useful against *Pseudomonas aeruginosa.* The drug is not used parenterally because it commonly will induce paresthesias, ataxia, and slurred speech.

Mupirocin

Mupirocin has a unique chemical structure composed of a short fatty acid chain linked to monic acid; it inhibits bacterial RNA and protein synthesis by binding to isoleucyl-tRNA synthetase to prevent incorporation of isoleucine into the cell wall protein chain.[89] The antimicrobial spectrum for mupirocin includes staphylococci (MRSA, MSSA, methicillin-resistant CoNS), *Pseudomonas aeruginosa,* streptococci, fungi, anaerobes, and *Enterobacteriaceae.*[89] Irreversible resistance has been detected in *Staphylococcus aureus* and CoNS either by altering the binding sites on isoleucyl-tRNA transferase or by a plasmid resistance gene, *mvp*A, that creates a modified isoleucyl tRNA synthetase.[89] Organisms inherently resistant include enterococci, *Corynebacterium,* and *Propionibacterium acnes.* The primary use of mupirocin is as a topical application for skin infections: impetigo, folliculitis, burns, and leg ulcers.[89] Mupirocin is also used to reduce or eliminate the nasal carriage of staphylococci, particularly MRSA.[89] Unfortunately its widespread use is associated with an 11% to 63% reinfection rate from resistance development or reinfection from other body areas.[89]

Fusidic acid

Fusidic acid is a highly lipid soluble agent that readily penetrates skin and is useful in deeper skin infections such as boils, pyoderma, and impetigo.[89] Its action is to inhibit bacterial protein synthesis by interfering with elongation factor G. Particularly sensitive organisms include *Staphylococcus aureus, Corynebacterium,* and *Clostridium.*[89]

Urinary Antiseptics

Nitrofurantoin

Nitrofurantoin is prepared in various suspension forms and, as with all urinary antiseptics, has limited bioavailability, low volumes of distribution, and high urinary excretion rates. Its mechanism of action is unknown but may involve inhibition of cell wall formation or DNA synthesis after its enzymatic activation in the bacterial cell.[38] Its antibacterial spectrum includes *Escherichia coli, Citrobacter, Staphylococcus saprophyticus, Enterococcus faecalis,* group B streptococci, *Klebsiella pneumoniae,* and *Enterobacter,* with inherent resistance in *Proteus, Providencia, Morganella, Serratia, Acinetobacter,* and *Pseudomonas aeruginosa.*[29,38] Adverse drug reactions include severe gastrointestinal upset (nausea and vomiting, anorexia, cramping), hepatitis, pneumonitis, peripheral neuropathy, and bone marrow depression.[29,97] Pulmonary pneumonitis may be acute, subacute, or chronic with an incidence for the acute form of 1 in 100,000 users.[38] Hemolytic anemia may occur in persons deficient in glucose-6-phosphate dehydrogenase. Nitrofurantoin and the other agents listed below are indicated for uncomplicated urinary tract infections and cystitis.

Fosfomycin

Fosfomycin is a broad-spectrum bactericidal antiseptic converted in the blood to free acid fosfomycin. Its mechanism of action is to inactivate enolpyruvyl transferase responsible for the condensation of uridine diphosphate-N-acetylglucosamine with *p*-enolpyruvate, one of the initial steps in microbial cell wall synthesis.[29] The antimicrobial spectrum for fosfomycin includes *Escherichia coli, Enterococcus faecalis, Citrobacter, Enterobacter, Klebsiella pneumoniae, Proteus mirabilis,* and *Serratia marcescens.* Adverse reactions are mild and include diarrhea, vaginitis, rash, and headache. Fosfomycin use is commonly restricted to only a single dose because of rapid microbial resistance.[29]

Methenamine

The hydrolysis of methenamine results in the liberation of ammonia and formaldehyde as its active ingredient. The mechanism of action of methenamine is to denature proteins and amino acids.[38] Methenamine has a broad spectrum of activity against *Escherichia coli,* staphylococci, and enterococci, with significant resistance in *Enterobacter aerogenes, Proteus vulgaris,* and *Pseudomonas aeruginosa.*[29] Adverse reactions include pruritus, urticaria, nausea and vomiting, cramping, headache, dizziness, proteinuria, hematuria, and precipitation of urate crystals in the urine.[29]

Nalidixic acid

Because of its high microbial resistance rates and CNS toxicity, the quinolone nalidixic acid is presently relegated to the management of urinary tract infections from gram-negative microorganisms: *Klebsiella pneumoniae, Escherichia coli, Proteus mirabilis* and *vulgaris,* and *Providencia. Pseudomonas aeruginosa* is resistant to nalidixic acid. Its mechanism of action is the same as the fluoroquinolones: inhibition of DNA gyrase and topoisomerase IV. The major adverse effects are CNS toxicity (dizziness, weakness, headache, papilledema, and rare seizures and psychosis) along with blood dyscrasias, photosensitivity, and hemolytic anemia in glucose-6-phosphate dehydrogenase–deficient individuals.

Drugs Used to Treat Tuberculosis

Successful treatment of tuberculosis caused by *Mycobacterium tuberculosis* became possible only with the advent of chemotherapeutic agents. Multiple drug-resistant strains of *M. tuberculosis* have arisen, especially among patients with HIV/AIDS. Because of the rapid development of antimicrobial resistance in strains of *M. tuberculosis,* a combination of agents is always employed for treatment. The primary antituberculosis drugs are isoniazid, rifampin, pyrazinamide, ethambutol, and streptomycin. For recurrent infections, or cases that exhibit microbial resistance, a group of secondary drugs are available, including ethionamide, cycloserine, amikacin, kanamycin, capreomycin, ciprofloxacin, ofloxacin, and aminosalicylic acid. These agents are generally less active and often more toxic than the primary drugs.

Typical therapy consists of isoniazid, rifampin, and pyrazinamide for 2 months followed by isoniazid and rifampin for 4 months or, alternatively, isoniazid and rifampin for 9 months.[15] However, until the results of sensitivity tests dictate the regimen, tuberculosis therapy should begin with four drugs: isoniazid, rifampin, pyrazinamide, and ethambutol or streptomycin for 2 months, followed by 4 months of isoniazid and rifampin.[15] Other options are available in multiple–drug-resistant tuberculosis. The pharmacologic features of isoniazid, rifampin, pyrazinamide, and ethambutol are described here. Streptomycin, an aminoglycoside antibiotic, has been previously discussed.

Isoniazid

Isoniazid, the name of which derives from its chemical designation of isonicotinic acid hydrazide, is the most important drug for the treatment and prophylaxis of tuberculosis. Its spectrum of activity, however, is limited to *M. tuberculosis* and one species of atypical mycobacteria, *Mycobacterium kansasii.*

Isoniazid inhibits the synthesis of mycolic acids, unique and necessary components of the cell wall of mycobacteria. The drug is bactericidal to actively growing tubercle bacilli but not to dormant organisms. Resistance to isoniazid occurs by spontaneous mutation of the bacterial chromosome (at a rate of 1 in 106 divisions), resulting in the failure of the bacterium to take up the drug, possibly as a result of an alteration in mycolic acid synthesis. Most established infections can be expected to harbor at least several resistant bacteria. There is no cross-resistance between isoniazid and other antituberculosis drugs except ethionamide.

Isoniazid is well absorbed after either oral or parenteral administration, but the oral route is preferred for reasons of convenience and maximum therapeutic effect. The drug is well distributed into all body fluids, including the caseous material of the tubercle-infected foci. Isoniazid is mainly metabolized in the liver and excreted in the urine as metabolites. Genetic differences in the rate of biotransformation are seen, but these appear to have little effect on therapeutic efficacy. The plasma half-life is prolonged in patients with hepatic dysfunction.

One important adverse reaction with isoniazid is peripheral neuritis caused by an isoniazid-induced increase in the excretion of pyridoxine. This adverse effect is more common in slow acetylators. This reaction and other symptoms of pyridoxine deficiency can be prevented by prophylactic administration of vitamin B_6 (15 to 50 mg daily). Other adverse effects include allergic reactions (fever, rashes, hepatitis), fatal hepatic necrosis (rarely), xerostomia, epigastric distress, hematologic reactions, and convulsions in seizure-prone patients (although administration of isoniazid to patients taking phenytoin has been without problems except for the potential of pharmacokinetic effects on phenytoin metabolism). A nonallergic hepatitis of some severity has also been reported, and subsequent studies have shown that the incidence of hepatic damage increases with age and in those who regularly drink alcohol.

Isoniazid is effective prophylaxis against tuberculosis and approved for single-drug therapy for prophylaxis. It is also the most important drug used in tuberculosis therapy for reasons of effectiveness, expense, convenience of administration, and relative safety.

Rifampin

Rifampin is a semisynthetic derivative of one of the rifamycins, a group of macrocyclic antibiotics produced by *Streptomyces mediterranei*. Rifampin is effective against a number of gram-positive and gram-negative bacteria in addition to *M. tuberculosis* and most other species of *Mycobacterium*. Its mechanism of action involves inhibition of DNA-dependent RNA polymerase. Mammalian RNA polymerase does not bind the drug, and RNA synthesis in host cells is therefore unaffected. Resistance can develop rapidly to rifampin, frequently in a single step, by alteration of the target enzyme.

Rifampin is generally well absorbed from the gastrointestinal tract after oral administration. The drug is distributed throughout the body and imparts an orange-red color to the urine, saliva, sweat, tears, sputum, and feces. It is secreted in the bile and undergoes enterohepatic recirculation prolonging its half-life. Elimination occurs by hepatic deacetylation and excretion in the urine and feces.

Rifampin may be of use in prophylaxis of tuberculosis in contacts of patients infected with isoniazid-resistant organisms. The drug has proven effective in certain diseases refractory to conventional therapy, for example, rifampin in combination as an option in treating resistant *Streptococcus pneumoniae* and methicillin-resistant staphylococci.

The incidence of adverse reactions to rifampin is relatively low (4%), and the most common is liver toxicity. Gastrointestinal disturbances, suppression of T-lymphocyte function, neurologic disorders, and a variety of allergic reactions, including soreness of the mouth and tongue, have been reported. Decreased effectiveness of oral anticoagulants, oral contraceptives, estrogens, and glucocorticoids has occurred with concomitant administration of rifampin as rifampin induces liver microsomal enzymes. If the drug is used sporadically, a flulike syndrome (possibly immune related) may develop, sometimes leading to renal failure, hepatorenal syndrome, hemolysis, and thrombocytopenia. The drug should be taken according to a prescribed regimen. Because rifampin can cause a reddish-orange color in body fluids, staining of soft contact lenses may occur.

Pyrazinamide

Pyrazinamide is the pyrazine analogue of nicotinamide. It had widespread use in the 1960s but proved to be hepatotoxic in the doses used and was relegated to secondary status after the development of isoniazid and rifampin. More recently, pyrazinamide in reduced dosage has reemerged as the third most important antituberculosis agent.

Pyrazinamide is active against a variety of mycobacteria, including *M. tuberculosis*. It appears to function as a prodrug, relying on amidase enzymes in the mycobacteria to convert it to the active pyrazinoic acid form. Resistance to the drug in *M. tuberculosis* infection is associated with the loss of pyrazinamidase activity. The mechanism of action of pyrazinamide is inhibition of mycolic acid synthesis, most likely by inhibiting fatty acid synthase I.

Pyrazinamide is well absorbed after oral administration and is distributed throughout the body. It is metabolized primarily in the liver and excreted largely in the urine. Although pyrazinoic acid is an intermediate metabolite, it may be inactive against intracellular mycobacteria because it is not taken up intracellularly.

Pyrazinamide is administered with other antituberculosis drugs to decrease the duration of therapy required to effect a cure of uncomplicated tuberculosis. Hepatotoxicity is the most common adverse effect, but this has been less evident with the lower dosages currently used. Other toxic effects associated with current regimens are relatively benign or infrequent. Gastrointestinal disturbances, arthralgias, fever, and rash have been noted. Pyrazinamide may cause hyperuricemia and therefore the drug represents a risk in patients with gout.

Ethambutol

Ethambutol is a synthetic agent that inhibits arabinosyl transferases, which are important in cell wall synthesis of sensitive mycobacteria. It is active against almost all strains of *M. tuberculosis* and *M. kansasii*. Other *Mycobacterium* species show variable sensitivity, and other bacteria are not affected by the drug. Ethambutol is tuberculostatic, and resistance develops, although slowly, if it is used alone.

Ethambutol is given orally because of good absorption from the gastrointestinal tract. Distribution into various body compartments is adequate. The major route of excretion of ethambutol is by renal tubular secretion and glomerular filtration, with the drug appearing in the urine mostly as unchanged drug and as two metabolites. Dosage adjustment is required in the presence of renal impairment.

Adverse reactions to ethambutol are infrequent, the most notable being optic neuritis, with symptoms of decreased visual acuity and loss of the ability to perceive the color green. Other adverse effects include gastrointestinal upset, peripheral neuritis, allergic reactions, usually appearing as skin rashes or drug fever, and increased retention of uric acid.

Streptomycin

Streptomycin is the only first-line antituberculosis drug that has to be given parenterally. Its pharmacologic features are discussed above with the other aminoglycosides.

Second-line drugs

A number of second-line drugs are used to treat tuberculosis. These are useful in cases of resistance to first-line drugs. They include ethionamide, capreomycin, aminosalicylic acid, cycloserine, and select members of the aminoglycoside and fluoroquinolone group of drugs.

Drugs Used to Treat Leprosy

Although leprosy is rarely seen in the United States, the World Health Organization estimates that 12 million cases exist throughout the world. Leprosy is a bacterial disease caused by the tubercle bacillus *Mycobacterium leprae*. Five clinical types of leprosy are recognized, ranging from the skin lesion of tuberculoid leprosy to the neuropathies and spontaneous amputations occurring in disseminated lepromatous disease. Patients may be infectious or noninfectious, depending on the type, duration, and effectiveness of therapy. Generally, this disease can be treated successfully with drugs. Treatment may be as short as 2 to 4 years or extend throughout life, depending on the severity and type of disease.

The sulfones, dapsone in particular, are the major drugs used in the treatment of leprosy. These chemical relatives to the sulfonamides are bacteriostatic against *M. leprae*, with a mechanism of action similar to that of the sulfonamides. These sulfones are used orally. Other drugs, normally used in combination with the sulfones, are rifampin and clofazimine. Clarithromycin and amoxicillin-clavulanate may also be beneficial.

Antibacterial Antibiotics*

Nonproprietary (generic) name	*Proprietary (trade) name*
Aminoglycosides	
Amikacin	Amikin
Gentamicin	Garamycin, Jenamicin
Kanamycin	Kantrex
Neomycin	Mycifradin
Netilmicin	Netromycin
Paromomycin	Humatin
Streptomycin	—
Tobramycin	Nebcin
Antituberculosis drugs (not included elsewhere in this list)	
Aminosalicylate sodium	Tubasal
Capreomycin	Capastat Sulfate
Cycloserine	Seromycin
Ethambutol	Myambutol
Ethionamide	Trecator-SC
Isoniazid	Nydrazid
Pyrazinamide	—
Rifabutin	Mycobutin
Rifampin	Rifadin, Rimactane
Topical antibiotics	
Bacitracin	Baciguent
Mupirocin	Bactroban
Neomycin	Myciguent
Polymyxin B	Aerosporin
Bacitracin with neomycin and polymyxin B	Neosporin
Miscellaneous agents	
Chloramphenicol	Chloromycetin
Clofazimine	Lamprene
Colistimethate	Coly-Mycin M
Colistin	In Coly-Mycin S
Dapsone	—
Fosfomycin	Monurol
Lincomycin	Lincocin
Linezolid	Zyvox
Methenamine	Hiprex, Mandelamine, Urex
Metronidazole	Flagyl
Nitrofurantoin	Furadantin, Macrodantin
Quinupristin-dalfopristin	Synercid
Spectinomycin	Trobicin
Telithromycin	Ketek
Troleandomycin	TAO
Vancomycin	Vancocin

*Agents not shown here are listed in various tables throughout this chapter.

Cited References

1. Adriaenssen CF: Comparison of the efficacy, safety and tolerability of azithromycin and co-amoxiclav in the treatment of acute periapical abscesses, *J Int Med Res* 26:257-265, 1998.
2. Advice for travelers, *Med Lett Drugs Ther* 44:33-38, 2002.
3. Alvarez-Elcoro S, Enzler MJ: The macrolides: erythromycin, clarithromycin, and azithromycin, *Mayo Clin Proc* 74:613-634, 1999.
4. Amsden GW: Tables of antimicrobial agent pharmacology. In Mandell GL, Bennett JE, Dolin R, eds: *Mandell, Douglas and Bennett's Principles and practice of infectious diseases,* Philadelphia, 2000, Churchill Livingstone.
5. Andriole VT: The future of the quinolones, *Drugs* 58(suppl 2):1-5, 1999.
6. Asbel LE, Levison ME: Cephalosporins, carbapenems, and monobactams, *Infect Dis Clin N Am* 14:435-447, 2000.
7. Bandrowsky T, Vorono AA, Borris TJ, et al: Amoxicillin-related postextraction bleeding in an anticoagulated patient with tranexamic acid rinses, *Oral Surg Oral Med Oral Pathol Oral Radiol Endod* 82:610-612, 1996.
8. Bush LM, Johnson CC: Ureidopenicillins and beta-lactam/beta-lactamase inhibitor combinations, *Infect Dis Clin North Am* 14:409-433, 2000.
9. Carey JC, Klebanoff MA, Hauth JC, et al: Metronidazole to prevent preterm delivery in pregnant women with asymptomatic bacterial vaginosis, *N Engl J Med* 342:534-540, 2000.
10. Cars O: Efficacy of beta-lactam antibiotics: integration of pharmacokinetics and pharmacodynamics, *Diagn Microbiol Infect Dis* 27:29-33, 1997.
11. Catnach SM, Fairclough PD: Erythromycin and the gut, *Gut* 33:397-401, 1992.
12. Cetinkaya Y, Falk P, Mayhall CG: Vancomycin-resistant enterococci, *Clin Microbiol Rev* 13:686-707, 2000.
13. Chadwick PR, Wooster SL: Glycopeptide resistance in *Staphylococcus aureus, J Infect* 40:211-217, 2000.
14. Champney WS, Miller M: Linezolid is a specific inhibitor of 50S ribosomal subunit formation in *Staphylococcus aureus* cells, *Curr Microbiol* 44:350-356, 2002.
15. Choice of antibacterial drugs, *Med Lett Drugs Ther* 43:69-78, 2001.
16. Chopra I, Roberts M: Tetracycline antibiotics: mode of action, applications, molecular biology, and epidemiology of bacterial resistance, *Microbiol Molec Biol Rev* 65:232-260, 2001.
17. Chu DTW: Recent developments in macrolides and ketolides, *Curr Opinion Microbiol* 2:467-474, 1999.
18. Craig WA, Ebert SC: Killing and regrowth of bacteria in vitro: a review, *Scand J Infect Dis* 22(suppl 1):63-70, 1990.
19. Dahlen G, Wikstrom M: Occurrence of enteric rods, staphylococci and *Candida* in subgingival samples, *Oral Microbiol Immunol* 10:42-46, 1995.
20. Dash CH: Penicillin allergy and the cephalosporins, *J Antimicrob Chemother* 1(Suppl 3):107-118, 1975.
21. Diekema DI, Jones RN: Oxazolidinones: a review, *Drugs* 59:7-16, 2000.
22. Diekema DI, Jones RN: Oxazolidinone antibiotics, *Lancet* 358:1975-1982, 2001.

23. Diniz CG, Cara DC, Nicoli JR, et al: Effect of metronidazole on the pathogenicity of resistant *Bacteroides* strains in gnotobiotic mice, *Antimicrob Agents Chemother* 44:2419-2423, 2000.

24. Doern GV, Ferraro MJ, Brueggeman AB, et al: Emergence of high rate of antimicrobial resistance among viridans group streptococci in the United States, *Antimicrob Agents Chemother* 40:891-894, 1996.

25. Edson RS, Terrell CL: The aminoglycosides, *Mayo Clin Proc* 74:519-528, 1999.

26. Enne VI, Livermore DM, Stephens P, et al: Persistence of sulphonamide resistance in *Escherichia coli* in the UK despite national prescribing restriction, *Lancet* 357:1325-1328, 2001.

27. Erickson PR, Herzberg MC: Emergence of antibiotic resistant *Streptococcus sanguis* in dental plaque of children after frequent antibiotic therapy, *Pediat Dent* 21:181-185, 1999.

28. Erwin ME, Fix AM, Jones RN: Three independent yearly analyses of the spectrum and potency of metronidazole: a multicenter study of 1,108 contemporary anaerobic clinical isolates, *Diag Microbiol Infect Dis* 39:129-132, 2001.

29. *Facts and comparisons,* St Louis, 2002, Facts and Comparisons.

30. Falagas ME, Gorbach SL: Clindamycin and metronidazole, *Med Clin North Am* 79:845-867, 1995.

31. Farber BF, Eliopoulos GM, Ward JI, et al: Multiply resistant viridans streptococci: susceptibility to β-lactam antibiotics and comparison of penicillin-binding protein patterns, *Antimicrob Agents Chemother* 24:702-705, 1983.

32. Forge A, Schacht J: Aminoglycoside antibiotics, *Audiol Neurootol* 5:3-22, 2000.

33. Hellinger WC, Brewer NS: Carbapenems and monobactams: imipenem, meropenem, and aztreonam, *Mayo Clin Proc* 74:420-434, 1999.

34. Herrera D, Roldan S, Sanz M: The periodontal abscess: a review, *J Clin Periodontol* 27:377-386, 2000.

35. Herrera D, van Winkelhoff AJ, Dellemijn-Kippuw N, et al: β-Lactamase producing bacteria in the subgingival microflora of adult patients with periodontitis: a comparison between Spain and The Netherlands, *J Clin Periodontol* 27:520-525, 2000.

36. Hirschhorn LR, Trnka Y, Onderdonk A, et al: Epidemiology of community-acquired *Clostridium difficile*–associated diarrhea, *J Infect Dis* 169:127-133, 1994.

37. Hoellman DB, Pankuch GA, Jacobs MR, et al: Antipneumococcal activities of GAR-936 (a new glycylcycline) compared to those of nine other agents against penicillin-susceptible and -resistant pneumococci, *Antimicrob Agents Chemother* 44:1085-1088, 2000.

38. Hooper DC: Urinary tract agents: nitrofurantoin and methenamine. In Mandell GL, Bennett JF, Dolin R, eds: *Mandell, Douglas and Bennett's Principles and practice of infectious diseases,* ed 5, Philadelphia, 2000, Churchill Livingstone.

39. Hudson JW: Osteomyelitis of the jaws: a 50-year perspective, *J Oral Maxillofac Surg* 51:1294-1301, 1993.

40. Jick SS, Vasilakis C, Martinez C, et al: A study of the relation of exposure to quinolones and suicidal behavior, *Br J Clin Pharmacol* 45:77-81, 1998.

41. Jones RN, Wilson WR: Epidemiology, laboratory detection, and therapy of penicillin-resistant streptococcal infections, *Diag Microbiol Infect Dis* 31:453-459, 1998.

42. Karchmer AW: Cephalosporins. In Mandell GL, Bennett JF, Dolin R, eds: *Principles and practice of infectious diseases,* ed 5, New York, 2000, Churchill Livingstone.

43. Kelkar PS, Li JT: Cephalosporin allergy, *N Engl J Med* 345:804-809, 2001.

44. Klebanoff MA, Carey JC, Hauth JC, et al: Failure of metronidazole to prevent preterm delivery among pregnant women with asymptomatic *Trichomonas vaginalis* infection, *N Engl J Med* 345:487-493, 2001.

45. Kluytmans J, van Belkum A, Verbrugh H: Nasal carriage of *Staphylococcus aureus:* epidemiology, underlying mechanisms, and associated risks, *Clin Microbiol Rev* 10:505-520, 1997.

46. Kononen F, Saarela M, Kanervo A, et al: β-Lactamase production and penicillin susceptibility among different ribotypes of *Prevotella melaninogenica* simultaneously colonizing the oral cavity, *Clin Infect Dis* 20(suppl 2):S364-S366, 1995.

47. Kuriyama T, Karasawa T, Nakagawa K, et al: Bacteriologic features and antimicrobial susceptibility in isolates from orofacial odontogenic infections, *Oral Surg Oral Med Oral Path Oral Radiol Endod* 90:600-608, 2000.

48. Larsen T, Fiehn N-E: Development of resistance to metronidazole and minocycline in vitro, *J Clin Periodontol* 24:254-259, 1997.

49. Lee KH, Maiden MF, Tanner AC, et al: Microbiota of successful osseointegrated dental implants, *J Periodontol* 70:131-138, 1999.

50. Leung WK, Theilade E, Comfort MB, et al: Microbiology of the pericoronal pouch in mandibular third molar pericoronitis, *Oral Microbiol Immunol* 8:306-312, 1993.

51. Lewis MA, MacFarlane TW: Short-course high dosage amoxycillin in the treatment of acute dentoalveolar abscess, *Br Dent J* 162:175, 1987.

52. Lindqvist BH: Bacteriophage and gene transfer, *APMIS* 106(suppl 84):15-18, 1998.

53. Listgarten MA, Lai C-H: Comparative microbiological characteristics of failing implants and periodontally diseased teeth, *J Periodontol* 70:431-437, 1999.

54. Lode H, Borner K, Koeppe P, et al: Azithromycin—a review of key chemical, pharmacokinetic and microbiological features, *J Antimicrob Chemother* 37:1-8, 1996.

55. Loebstein R, Addis A, Ho E, et al: Pregnancy outcome following gestational exposure to fluoroquinolones: a multicenter prospective controlled study, *Antimicrob Agents Chemother* 42:1336-1339, 1998.

56. Loesche WJ, Syed SA, Laughon BE, et al: The bacteriology of acute necrotizing ulcerative gingivitis, *J Periodontol* 53:223-230, 1982.

57. Marshall WF, Blair JE: The cephalosporins, *Mayo Clin Proc* 74:187-195, 1999.

58. Matto J, Asikainen S, Vaisanen M-L, et al: Role of *Porphyromonas gingivalis*, *Prevotella intermedia*, and *Prevotella nigrescens* in extraoral and some odontogenic infections, *Clin Infect Dis* 25(suppl 2):S194-S198, 1997.

59. McDermott W, Rogers DE: Social ramifications of control of microbial diseases, *Johns Hopkins Med J* 151:302-312, 1982.

60. Moreland LW, Corey J, McKenzie R: Ludwig's angina: report of a case and review of the literature, *Arch Intern Med* 148:461-466, 1988.

61. Naber KG, Adam D: Classification of fluoroquinolones, *Int J Antimicrob Agents* 10:255-257, 1998.

62. Neu HC: Penicillins. In Mandell GL, Douglas RG, Jr, Bennett JE, eds: *Principles and practice of infectious diseases,* ed 5, New York, 1990, Churchill Livingstone.

63. Newman MG, Sims TN: The predominant cultivable microbiota of the periodontal abscess, *J Periodontol* 50:350-354, 1979.

64. Nishi J, Yoshinaga M, Nomura Y: Prevalence of penicillin-resistant viridans streptococci in the oral flora of Japanese children at risk for endocarditis, *Circulation* 99:1274-1275, 1999.

65. Novak R, Henriques B, Charpentier E, et al: Emergence of vancomycin tolerance in *Streptococcus pneumoniae, Nature* 399:590-593, 1999.

66. Nyfors S, Kononen T, Takal A, et al: β-Lactamase production by oral anaerobic gram-negative species in infants in relation to previous antimicrobial therapy, *Antimicrob Agents Chemother* 43:1591-1594, 1999.

67. Owens BM, Schuman NJ: Ludwig's angina, *Gen Dent* 42:84-87, 1994.

68. Pallasch TJ: Antibiotics for acute orofacial infections, *J Calif Dent Assoc* 21:34-44, 1993.

69. Pallasch TJ: Pharmacokinetic principles of antimicrobial therapy, *Periodontol* 2000 10:5-11, 1996.

70. Pallasch TJ: Principles of pharmacotherapy: III. Drug allergy, *Anesth Prog* 35:178-189, 1988.

71. Pallasch TJ, Slots J: Antibiotic prophylaxis and the medically compromised patient, *Periodontol 2000* 10:107-138, 1996.

72. Pallasch TJ, Wahl MJ: Focal infection: new age of ancient history? *Endod Topics* 4:32-45, 2003.

73. Papaioannou W, Quirynen M, Nys M, et al: The effect of periodontal parameters on the subgingival microbiota around implants, *Clin Oral Implant Res* 6:197-204, 1995.

74. Pumphrey RS, Davis S: Under-reporting of antibiotic anaphylaxis may put patients at risk [letter], *Lancet* 353:1157-1158, 1999.

75. Reinert RR, von Eiff C, Kresken M, et al: Nationwide German multicenter study on the prevalence of antibiotic resistance in streptococcal blood isolates from neutropenic patients and comparative in vitro activities of quinupristin/dalfopristin and eight other antimicrobials, *J Clin Microbiol* 39:1928-1931, 2001.

76. Schlossberg D: Azithromycin and clarithromycin, *Med Clin N Am* 79:803-815, 1995.

77. Sefton AM, Maskell JP, Beighton D, et al: Azithromycin in the treatment of periodontal disease: effect on microbial flora, *J Clin Periodontol* 23:998-1003, 1996.

78. Solensky R, Earl HS, Gruchalla RS: Lack of penicillin resensitization in patients with a history of penicillin allergy after receiving repeated penicillin courses, *Arch Intern Med* 162:822-826, 2002.

79. Sorensen HT, Larsen H, Jensen ES, et al: Safety of metronidazole during pregnancy: a cohort study of risk of congenital abnormalities, preterm delivery, and low birth weight in 124 women, *J Antimicrob Chemother* 44:854-856, 1999.

80. Standiford HC: Tetracyclines and chloramphenicol. In Mandell GL, Bennett JE, Dolin R, eds: *Mandell, Douglas and Bennett's Principles and practice of infectious diseases,* ed 5, Philadelphia, 2000, Churchill Livingstone.

81. Stergachis A, Perera DR, Schnell MM, et al: Antibiotic-associated colitis, *West J Med* 140:217-219, 1984.

82. Stevens AM, Shoemaker NB, Li Ly, et al: Tetracycline regulation of genes on *Bacteroides* conjugative transposons, *J Bacteriol* 175:6134-6141, 1993.

83. Sulakvelidze A, Alavidze Z, Morris JG, Jr: Bacteriophage therapy, *Antimicrob Agents Chemother* 45:649-659, 2001.

84. Suzuki J, Komatsuzawa H, Sugai M, et al: A long-term survey of methicillin-resistant *Staphylococcus aureus* in the oral cavity of children, *Microbiol Immunol* 41:681-686, 1997.

85. Tatro DS: *Drug interaction facts,* St Louis, 2001, Facts and Comparisons, Wolters Kluwer.

86. Teng L-J, Hsueh P-R, Chen Y-C, et al: Antimicrobial susceptibility of viridans group streptococci in Taiwan with an emphasis on the high rates of resistance to penicillin and macrolides in *Streptococcus oralis, J Antimicrob Chemother* 41:621-627, 1998.

87. Thalhammer F, Hollenstein UM, Locker GJ, et al: Azithromycin-related toxic effects of digitoxin, *Br J Clin Pharmacol* 45:91-92, 1998.

88. Trunidge JD: The pharmacodynamics of β-lactams, *Clin Infect Dis* 27:10-22, 1998.

89. Tunkel AR: Topical antibiotics. In Mandell GL, Bennett JF, Dolin R, eds: *Mandell, Douglas and Bennett's Principles and practice of infectious diseases,* ed 5, Philadelphia, 2000, Churchill Livingstone.

90. van der Linden PD, van Puijenbroek EP, Feenstra J, et al: Tendon disorders attributed to fluoroquinolones: a study of 42 spontaneous reports in the period 1988 to 1998, *Arthitis Rheum Care Res* 45:235-239, 2001.

91. Van Winkelhoff AJ, Tijhof CJ, De Graaff J: Microbiological and clinical results of metronidazole plus amoxycillin therapy in *Actinobacillus actinomycetemcomitans*-associated periodontitis, *J Periodontol* 63:52-57, 1992.

92. Vermeulen GM, Bruinse HW: Prophylactic administration of clindamycin 2% vaginal cream to reduce the incidence of spontaneous preterm birth in women with an increased recurrence risk: a randomised placebo-controlled double-blind trial, *Br J Obstet Gynaecol* 106:652-657, 1999.

93. Walker CB: The acquisition of antibiotic resistance in the periodontal microflora, *Periodontol 2000* 10:79-88, 1996.

94. Walker RC: The fluoroquinolones, *Mayo Clin Proc* 74:1030-1037, 1999.

95. Wilhelm MP, Estes L: Symposium on antimicrobial agents—part XII. Vancomycin, *Mayo Clin Proc* 74:928-935, 1999.

96. Wright AJ: The penicillins, *Mayo Clin Proc* 74:290-307, 1999.

97. Yao JDC, Moellering RC, Jr: Antibacterial agents. In Murray PR, Baron EJ, Pfaller MA, et al, eds: *Manual of clinical microbiology,* ed 7, Washington, DC, 1999, American Society for Microbiology Press.

98. Yassin HM, Dever LL: Telithromycin: a new ketolide antimicrobial for treatment of respiratory tract infections, *Expert Opin Investig Drugs* 10:353-367, 2001.

CHAPTER • 40

Antifungal and Antiviral Agents

No-Hee Park and Mo K. Kang

Although the management of systemic fungal and viral diseases lies within the realm of medicine, the dentist is called on to treat localized and superficial lesions in and around the oral cavity. This chapter discusses drugs that are of use in the management of such localized lesions and drugs whose use may indicate that a patient has a potentially communicable disease, a defective immune response, or both.

ANTIFUNGAL AGENTS

Fungal diseases may take the form of superficial infestations involving the skin or mucous membranes or systemic (deep) infections involving various internal organs. The superficial mycoses are generally managed with topical drugs. Topical agents considered in this chapter are those with activity against mucocutaneous infections caused by *Candida albicans*, the fungus most commonly observed in oral lesions. Often these infections are rather benign, as in denture stomatitis, but they may indicate a serious medical condition such as immunodeficiency. The systemic fungal infections are subdivided into two groups according to the status of the patient and the type of infecting organism. *Opportunistic mycoses* occur in debilitated and immunocompromised patients, such as those with AIDS, leukemia, or lymphoma, and in patients who are receiving immunosuppressive agents or broad-spectrum antibiotics. The fungi involved include *Candida*, *Aspergillus*, and *Cryptococcus* species and various phycomycetes. They are particularly dangerous and carry a high mortality rate.[40] *Endemic mycoses* are caused by various pathogens distributed unevenly throughout the world and have a relatively low incidence in temperate climates. Examples of endemic mycoses that occur in the United States include blastomycosis, histoplasmosis, coccidioidomycosis, and sporotrichosis.

A number of antifungal agents have been developed (Table 40-1). Two polyene antibiotics are of special interest: amphotericin B, the drug of choice for most deep mycoses,[1] and nystatin, an agent useful in the treatment of oral candidiasis. A third polyene, natamycin, is limited to ophthalmologic use. Flucytosine is a pyrimidine analogue used infrequently as a single agent but commonly used with amphotericin B in severe fungal infections. Miconazole, ketoconazole, and clotrimazole are representative imidazole antifungals. Ketoconazole was a major advance in systemic antifungal therapy; clotrimazole has become a widely used topical agent. Itraconazole, fluconazole, and saperconazole are triazole derivatives. These newer drugs are welcome therapeutic alternatives at a time when the incidence of systemic fungal infections is rising. Several other antifungal agents (e.g., voriconazole, caspofungin) with different mechanisms of action are also being developed to help control the pathogens with resistance to currently available drugs.[27] Additional antifungal preparations are available for the treatment of superficial fungal infections of the skin (e.g., tolnaftate, ciclopirox, undecylenic acid) or for systemic treatment of dermatophytosis (e.g., griseofulvin). With the exception of griseofulvin, these drugs are not included in this chapter. The interested reader is referred to the general references on antifungal agents for their description.

Amphotericin B

Amphotericin B is an antifungal agent obtained from *Streptomyces nodosus*, an actinomycetes found in the soil. It is a member of the polyene family of antibiotics, so called because their structure contains a large lactone (macrolide) ring with numerous conjugated double bonds (Figure 40-1). The polar hydroxylated portion and the nonpolar hydrocarbon sequence lend an amphophilic character to the molecule. The polyenes are unstable in solution because of the unsaturated chromophore region, which is easily photo-oxidized. Amphotericin B exerts either fungistatic or fungicidal activity depending on the concentration of the drug, the pH, and the fungus involved. Peak activity occurs at a pH between 6.0 and 7.5. Amphotericin B has a broad spectrum of antifungal activity and is effective against *Candida* species, *Histoplasma capsulatum*, *Cryptococcus neoformans*, and *Coccidioides immitis*. The primary mechanism of antifungal action of amphotericin B results from its binding to ergosterol, a component of the cell membrane of sensitive fungi.[33] This binding forms channels in the membrane, altering its permeability and causing leakage of Na^+, K^+, and H^+ ions. Amphotericin B also binds to a lesser extent to cholesterol of the mammalian plasma membrane, which accounts for most of the toxicity associated with its use. In addition, amphotericin B may stimulate the function of host macrophages, and this immunomodulation is mediated by the oxidized form of amphotericin B.[9] Finally, amphotericin B increases the ability of *C. albicans* to induce the synthesis of tumor necrosis factor-α.[58]

Resistance to amphotericin B is associated with a replacement of ergosterol with other sterols in the fungal plasma membrane. A parallel fall in virulence generally occurs, however, and resistance has not been a problem clinically except for rare instances involving *Candida* other than *C. albicans*.

Amphotericin B is not absorbed from the skin or mucous membranes and is poorly and inconsistently absorbed from the gastrointestinal tract. Because of its insolubility in an aqueous media, the drug is reconstituted in a solution of the bile salt deoxycholate immediately before use. For systemic infections, amphotericin B is administered by slow intravenous

Table • 40-1

Mechanisms of Action and Clinical Uses of Antifungal Agents

ANTIFUNGAL AGENT	MECHANISM OF ACTION	CLINICAL USES
Amphotericin B	Binding to ergosterol of fungal membrane	Topical: superficial candidiasis; intravenous: severe, progressive systemic fungal infection*
Nystatin	Binding to ergosterol of fungal membrane	Topical: oral candidiasis
Clotrimazole	Inhibition of ergosterol synthesis	Topical: oral candidiasis, superficial fungal infections†
Fluconazole	Inhibition of ergosterol synthesis	Oral: systemic and localized candidiasis, cryptococcal meningitis, systemic blastomycosis, and coccidioidomycosis
Itraconazole	Inhibition of ergosterol synthesis	Oral: systemic fungal infections,* dermatophyte infections
Ketoconazole	Inhibition of ergosterol synthesis	Topical: superficial fungal infections†; oral: systemic fungal infections,* mucocutaneous candidiasis, severe, unresponsive cutaneous dermatophyte infections
Miconazole	Inhibition of ergosterol synthesis	Topical: cutaneous candidiasis and vulvovaginitis, superficial fungal infections†
Flucytosine	Inhibition of nucleic acid synthesis	Oral: systemic candidiasis and cryptococcosis
Griseofulvin	Disruption of mitotic spindle	Oral: fungal infections of skin, hair, and nails
Caspofungin	Inhibition of fungal cell wall synthesis	Intravenous: severe, invasive aspergillosis

*Systemic fungal infections include aspergillosis, blastomycosis, candidiasis, chromomycosis, cryptococcosis, coccidioidomycosis, histoplasmosis, paracoccidioidomycosis, phycomycosis, and sporotrichosis. Indications for specific drugs vary.
†Superficial fungal infections caused by pathogenic dermatophytes, yeasts, and *Malassezia furfur.*

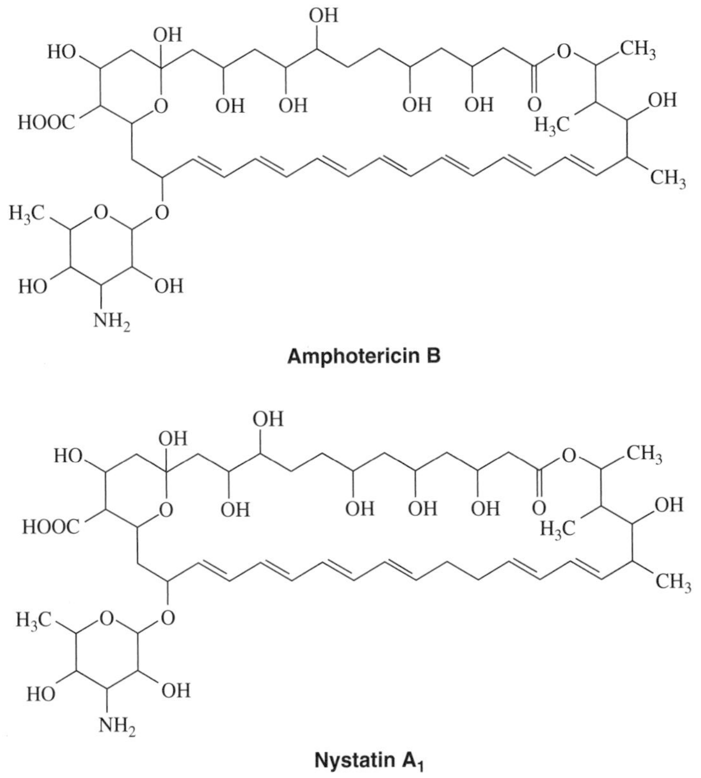

Amphotericin B

Nystatin A_1

Fig. 40-1 Structural formulas of polyene antifungal agents. Nystatin A_1 is one of three compounds found in the commercial nystatin preparation.

infusion (over a period of 2 to 6 hours each day). The drug is bound in plasma to various lipoproteins and in tissues to cholesterol-containing membranes. Recent studies showed that amphotericin B lipid complex or liposomal amphotericin B preparations could be used for systemic infections, particularly in premature infants and other immune-compromised patients.[34] Amphotericin B can also be prepared in colloidal dispersion with sodium cholesteryl sulfate in a 1 : 1 discoidal complex. The colloidal amphotericin B demonstrated reduced peak plasma levels, prolonged residence time, and reduced renal and hepatic toxicity compared with the conventional amphotericin B preparations.[28] The exact metabolic pathway of amphotericin B is not known, but most of the drug is biotransformed and then slowly excreted by the kidney over the next 2 months. The plasma concentration of amphotericin B is unaffected by renal disease; thus no dosage adjustment needs to be made in patients with compromised renal function. Amphotericin B applied topically as a 3% cream, ointment, or lotion is useful in the treatment of superficial *Candida* infections. Because C. *albicans* infection can readily occur in patients receiving broad-spectrum antibiotics, these agents are sometimes administered with amphotericin B or nystatin. However, the efficacy of fixed-ratio combinations has not been proved and does not reflect sound therapy.

The only adverse effects accompanying the topical application or oral administration of amphotericin B are local irritation and mild gastrointestinal disturbances. As an intravenous agent, however, amphotericin B is the most toxic antibiotic in current use. Intravenous amphotericin B causes many side effects such as hypotension and delirium along with fever, nausea, vomiting, abdominal pain, anorexia, headache, and thrombophlebitis. Hypochromic, normocytic anemia is induced by amphotericin B, and leukopenia and thrombocytopenia occur rarely. Allergic reactions of all types have been reported, including anaphylaxis. All patients receiving intravenous amphotericin B show some degree of nephrotoxicity. Permanent damage of the kidneys, however, does not occur in patients receiving a cumulative dosage of less than 4 g during a normal therapeutic interval of several weeks. Great caution should be exercised when amphotericin B is used with other nephrotoxic drugs. Because amphotericin B can cause hypokalemia, it can increase digitalis toxicity. The toxic effects of cyclosporine may also be increased.

Nystatin

Nystatin is a polyene antibiotic obtained from *Streptomyces noursei*. Its structure is similar to that of amphotericin B (see Figure 40-1). Nystatin is relatively insoluble in water and unstable except as a dry powder.

Nystatin has a spectrum of activity slightly narrower than that of amphotericin B but is nevertheless active against a number of species of *Candida*, *Histoplasma*, *Cryptococcus*, *Blastomyces*, and the dermatophytes *Epidermophyton*, *Trichophyton*, and *Microsporum*. As with amphotericin B, nystatin is either fungistatic or fungicidal depending on the concentration of the drug present, the pH of the surrounding medium, and the nature of the infecting organism. The mechanism of action of nystatin is also similar to that of amphotericin B. In vitro, some species of *Candida*, such as C. *tropicalis*, can develop resistance to nystatin, but resistance is rarely observed clinically.

Nystatin is not appreciably absorbed from the skin, mucous membranes, or gastrointestinal tract. After oral administration, the bulk of the administered dose appears unchanged in the feces. Because of unacceptable systemic toxicity, nystatin is never given parenterally. However, a newer form of nystatin encapsulated in liposomes showed reduced systemic cytotoxicity, making it an active systemic antifungal agent.[27] Also, the liposomal nystatin has been suggested to target *Candida* species that are resistant to amphotericin B.[6]

Nystatin is used primarily to treat candidal infections of the mucosa, skin, intestinal tract, and vagina. Although the efficacy of oral nystatin for enteric candidiasis has been questioned, topical nystatin remains a drug of choice for the treatment of candidal infections of the oral cavity (oral moniliasis, thrush, denture stomatitis). It has also been used prophylactically in immunocompromised patients.[43] For the treatment of oral candidiasis, 2 to 3 ml of a suspension containing 100,000 units/ml of nystatin are placed in each side of the mouth, swished, and held for at least 5 minutes before swallowing. This regimen is repeated every 6 hours for at least 10 days or for 48 hours after remission of symptoms. Alternatively, one to two lozenges (200,000 units per each) may be used four to five times per day. For denture stomatitis, nystatin ointment (100,000 units/g) can be applied topically every 6 hours to the tissue surface of the denture.

Nystatin is well tolerated, and only mild and transient gastrointestinal disturbances such as nausea, vomiting, and diarrhea have occurred after oral ingestion. The major complaint associated with nystatin is its bitter, foul taste.

Griseofulvin

Griseofulvin was first isolated from *Penicillium griseofulvum dierckx* in 1939, but its antifungal activity was not known until 1946. It exerts a fungistatic effect against *Microsporum*, *Epidermophyton*, and *Trichophyton* species that infect skin, hair, and nails. Griseofulvin interacts with polymerized microtubules, causing the disruption of the mitotic spindle and eventually fungal mitosis.

Griseofulvin is variably absorbed from the gastrointestinal tract; micronization of the primary drug particles (see Chapter 2) and ingestion with a fatty meal improve bioavailability. Although most of the absorbed drug is inactivated in the liver by dealkylation, the plasma half-life is fairly long (approximately 20 hours), and griseofulvin readily reaches the skin, hair, and nails, where it binds avidly to newly synthesized keratin and inhibits fungal invasion through surface keratin. Serious side effects are uncommon, but griseofulvin may induce nausea, vomiting, diarrhea, fatigue, headache, and mental confusion. The drug may also cause hematologic and dermatologic reactions. As an inducer of cytochrome P450 enzymes, griseofulvin is contraindicated in patients with acute intermittent porphyria and may participate in a number of drug interactions, potentially decreasing the effectiveness of drugs such as warfarin and oral contraceptives.

Flucytosine

Flucytosine, a fluorinated analogue of cytosine (5-fluorocytosine, Figure 40-2), is a synthetic antimycotic agent orally effective in the treatment of systemic fungal infections, in particular those caused by yeasts. Flucytosine has a limited antifungal spectrum compared with amphotericin B and is mainly effective against *Candida* and *Cryptococcus*. It is also active against some species of *Cladosporium* and *Phialophora*, the latter being etiologic agents for chromoblastomycosis.

Flucytosine is taken up within sensitive fungal cells by cytosine permease, where it is converted to 5-fluorouracil by the enzyme cytosine deaminase. The 5-fluorouracil is then further metabolized to yield 5-fluorodeoxyuridine monophosphate, a competitive inhibitor of thymidylate synthetase. The formation of thymidine monophosphate from deoxyuridine monophosphate is thus blocked and the synthesis of DNA impaired. 5-Fluorouridine triphosphate is also formed in fungal cells, leading to the synthesis of defective RNA. Selective toxicity is achieved with flucytosine because mammalian

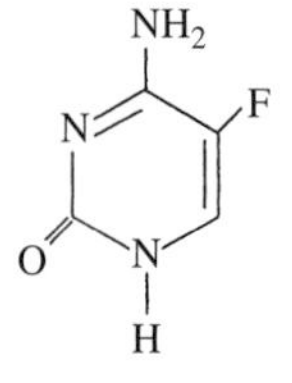

Flucytosine

Fig. 40-2 Structural formula of flucytosine.

cells do not readily take up the drug or convert it to 5-fluorouracil.

Flucytosine is indicated for the treatment of systemic candidiasis and cryptococcosis; however, resistance to flucytosine frequently develops during therapy of these infections. Mechanisms of resistance include decreased flucytosine uptake by fungal cells (altered permease) and decreased synthesis of the active nucleotide metabolites (decreased deaminase and other enzyme activities). Flucytosine is therefore normally used in combination with amphotericin B, which appears to increase fungal uptake of flucytosine and to result in synergistic effects against certain fungal diseases. Perhaps more importantly, coadministration permits a reduction in the dose of amphotericin B.

Flucytosine is well absorbed from the gastrointestinal tract, and the peak plasma concentration is attained within 1 to 2 hours after oral administration. The drug is widely distributed throughout the body; it attains a concentration in cerebrospinal fluid approximately 65% to 90% that of the plasma. Flucytosine has a half-life of 3 to 6 hours and is excreted unchanged in the urine.

The major toxicity of flucytosine is depression of the bone marrow, resulting in anemia, leukopenia, and thrombocytopenia. This effect is dose related and is reversible. Because flucytosine is excreted mainly through the kidneys, it is advisable to measure the plasma concentration of the drug periodically, especially because it is normally given with the highly nephrotoxic amphotericin B. An elevation of hepatic enzymes in plasma and hepatomegaly occurs in approximately 5% of patients receiving flucytosine. Lastly, flucytosine may cause nausea, vomiting, diarrhea, and (rarely) severe enterocolitis. These toxic effects may result from the formation and release of 5-fluorouracil by fungi and intestinal microbes.

Ketoconazole

Ketoconazole (Figure 40-3) is the only imidazole antifungal compound routinely used systemically. It was also the first oral antifungal agent to be approved for the treatment of deep systemic mycoses. The imidazoles and the triazoles (discussed below) are members of the azole class of antifungal drugs. They are synthetic compounds.

The antifungal spectrum of ketoconazole and the other imidazole antifungal drugs is broad, including yeasts, dermatophytes, and various species of *Histoplasma, Coccidioides, Paracoccidioides, Cladosporium, Phialophora, Blastomyces,* and *Aspergillus.* The mode of action is not fully established. Imidazoles (e.g., ketoconazole, miconazole, clotrimazole) and triazoles (e.g., itraconazole and fluconazole) inhibit an enzyme involved in the synthesis of ergosterol. More specifically, one of the nitrogen atoms of the azole ring binds to the heme moiety of the fungal cytochrome P450 enzyme lanosterol 14-α-demethylase, thereby inhibiting the conversion of lanosterol to ergosterol.[17] However, the addition of ergosterol fails to reverse the antifungal effect in vitro, and other mechanisms must be invoked to explain the activity of these compounds against several protozoa and bacteria in which ergosterol is not an important membrane constituent. The addition of 14-α-methyl sterols such as lanosterol, whose concentrations increase as a result of azole therapy, may disrupt cell membranes even in the presence of ergosterol. Other antifungal actions ascribed to ketoconazole and similar drugs, perhaps related to the changes caused by lanosterol, include inhibition of purine transport, interference with mitochondrial respiration, and alteration of the composition of nonsterol membrane lipids. Acquired resistance to the imidazoles has not been a significant problem clinically; however, it can develop in *C. albicans.*[53] Refractory mucosal candidiasis in immunocompromised patients has been ascribed to the *Candida* species with cross-resistance to clotrimazole and other azole compounds.[44]

Ketoconazole is well absorbed from the gastrointestinal tract, provided that the stomach contents are acidic. Therefore drugs that increase gastric pH, such as antacids and H_2 antihistamines, markedly reduce its absorption. The bioavailability of ketoconazole is likewise reduced in achlorhydric patients.[36] Such patients should be given acidifying agents (e.g., orange juice) before ketoconazole administration. The peak plasma concentration after oral administration is reached in 1 to 2 hours. Ketoconazole is readily distributed to most body compartments, but penetration into the central nervous system (CNS) is poor. After extensive metabolism in the liver, the drug is excreted mainly through the bile. The terminal

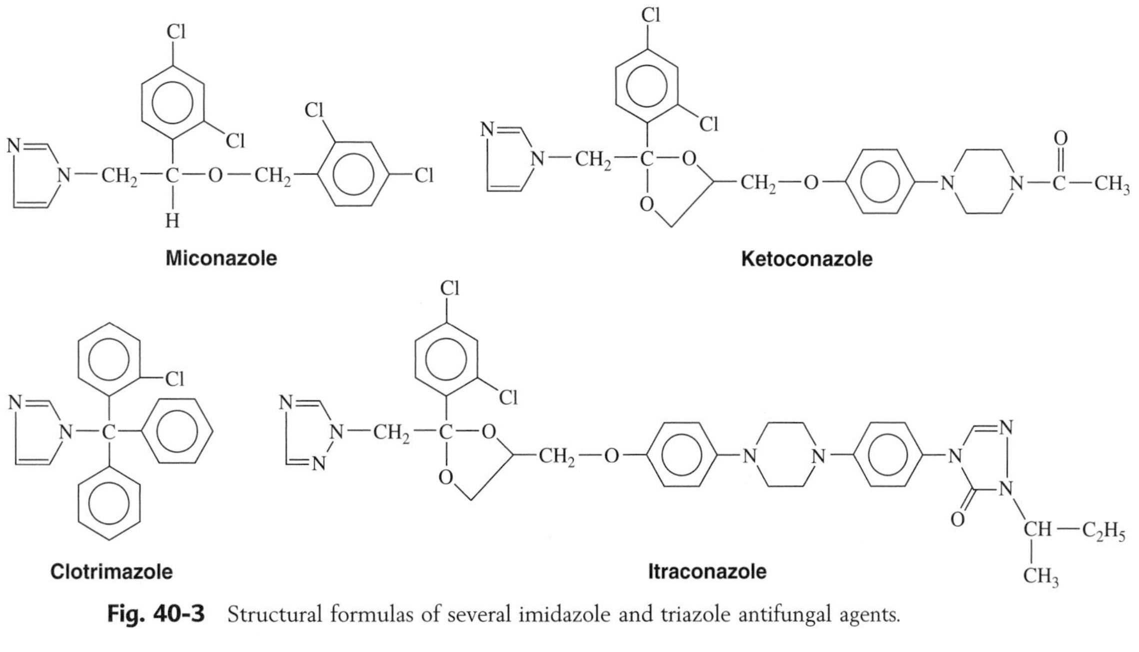

Miconazole

Ketoconazole

Clotrimazole

Itraconazole

Fig. 40-3 Structural formulas of several imidazole and triazole antifungal agents.

half-life is 7 to 10 hours, but saturation of metabolism occurs with long-term therapy, resulting in a longer half-life and permitting once-a-day dosing. Ketoconazole is useful in the treatment of blastomycosis, histoplasmosis, coccidioidomycosis, and paracoccidioidomycosis. Ketoconazole is also effective against chronic mucocutaneous candidiasis, but relapses may occur on discontinuation of the drug. Effective treatment of deep-seated candidiasis often requires many months for complete cure. Although reports indicate the successful treatment of oral candidiasis with systemic ketoconazole, it should be reserved for cases refractory to more conventional therapy with topically applied agents.[45] Ketoconazole is effective against oral and pharyngeal candidiasis in patients with advanced AIDS.[7,52]

Nausea and vomiting are the most common untoward effects of ketoconazole, but the incidence can be reduced by administering the drug with food. Other side effects include anorexia, headache, epigastric pain, gingival bleeding, paresthesia, rash, and thrombocytopenia. Severe hepatic toxicity occurs in approximately 0.01% of persons; thus the drug should be used cautiously. Ketoconazole markedly inhibits the synthesis of testosterone and estradiol, which may lead to gynecomastia and menstrual irregularities, respectively. Alterations of adrenal steroid synthesis may also occur. Ketoconazole inhibits the metabolism of cyclosporine, phenytoin, the sulfonylureas, and warfarin. Isoniazid increases the metabolism of ketoconazole.

Miconazole

Miconazole (see Figure 40-3) was the first imidazole antifungal drug to be approved for both topical and parenteral use. Its systemic use is now severely limited because of its toxicity and the availability of less dangerous alternatives.

Cutaneous candidiasis and vulvovaginitis caused by *C. albicans* respond rapidly and reliably to a 2% miconazole nitrate cream. Oral candidiasis is also effectively treated; however, a specific formulation for intraoral use is not available. Other topical uses of miconazole are for the treatment of cutaneous infections caused by *Epidermophyton*, *Microsporum*, and *Trichophyton*. Parenteral administration of miconazole can be useful for the treatment of coccidioidomycosis, paracoccidioidomycosis, cryptococcosis, systemic candidiasis, and mucocutaneous candidiasis, but it is considered only a second-line drug. On rare occasions miconazole may be administered intrathecally for fungal meningitis.

Untoward effects after the topical administration of miconazole are rare, but burning, skin maceration, itching, and redness can develop. The most common side effect after intravenous injection of the drug is thrombophlebitis at the injection site. Nausea and vomiting may occur in concert with drug administration and last for a few hours afterward. Less common toxicities from systemic use include allergic reactions, fever, hyperlipidemia, anemia, thrombocytosis, hyponatremia, and seizures. Some of these effects, as well as a potentiation of oral anticoagulant action, have been attributed to the emulsifying agent used in the intravenous formulation.

Clotrimazole

Clotrimazole is an imidazole antifungal drug used for various mucosal and cutaneous infections. The antifungal spectrum and mechanism of action are similar to ketoconazole and the other imidazole derivatives. Although clotrimazole is restricted to topical use, a preparation specifically suited for intraoral application is marketed.

For the treatment of oral candidiasis, clotrimazole is available as a 10-mg troche. Slow dissolution in the mouth results in the binding of clotrimazole to the oral mucosa, from which it is gradually released to maintain at least fungistatic concentrations for several hours. The swallowed drug is variably but poorly absorbed. It is metabolized in the liver and eliminated in the feces along with the unabsorbed drug.

One troche dissolved in the mouth five times a day for 2 weeks is the standard regimen for oropharyngeal candidiasis. Patient compliance is believed to be enhanced by the more pleasant taste of clotrimazole compared with nystatin. Clotrimazole also appears to be highly effective and is the drug of choice for the treatment of oral candidiasis in patients with AIDS.[52,58,59] For cutaneous candidiasis and dermatophytoses, a 1% cream or lotion is equivalent to topical miconazole.

Irritation associated with topical clotrimazole, though unlikely, is qualitatively similar to that described for miconazole. Occasionally, minor gastrointestinal upset may follow oral ingestion of the drug.

Itraconazole

Itraconazole is a water-insoluble triazole compound that shows a broader spectrum of antifungal activity and a faster clinical effect compared with ketoconazole. Like ketoconazole, itraconazole is well absorbed from the gastrointestinal tract when it is given with meals. It is highly bound to plasma proteins (more than 99%), and has a long half-life (approximately 20 hours after a single dose, up to 60 hours at steady state). Although the concentrations of itraconazole in saliva and cerebrospinal fluid are negligible, tissue concentrations are two to five times higher than that of plasma. The drug is mostly metabolized in the liver and partially eliminated in the bile.

When given in therapeutic doses, itraconazole exerts effective antifungal activity against paracoccidioidomycosis, blastomycosis, aspergillosis, histoplasmosis, sporotrichosis, candidiasis, and various dermatophytoses. Previous studies show that itraconazole is effective for suppressive therapy and primary treatment of histoplasmosis in patients seropositive for HIV.[37,54] Adverse effects and drug interactions are qualitatively similar to those noted for ketoconazole. However, itraconazole and related triazoles are more specific for fungal 14-α-demethylase and do not affect mammalian steroid metabolism as greatly.[16]

Fluconazole

Fluconazole is a water-insoluble fluorine-substituted bistriazole with effective antifungal activity in immunocompetent and immunocompromised patients. The antifungal activity of fluconazole is similar to that of ketoconazole. However, fluconazole is significantly less potent as an inhibitor of mammalian steroid synthesis, indicating more specific antifungal actions than ketoconazole. It is well absorbed from the gastrointestinal tract (the drug is also available for intravenous injection), weakly bound to plasma proteins (12%), and well distributed throughout the body. Peak plasma concentrations are reached within 2 hours after oral administration; concentrations in the cerebrospinal fluid are generally more than 50% of the corresponding plasma values. Fluconazole has a long plasma half-life of 20 to 50 hours in adults and approximately 17 hours in children. Fluconazole is excreted largely unchanged in the kidney.

Fluconazole is active in suppressive therapy and primary treatment of cryptococcal meningitis, which may occur in patients with AIDS.[32] It is effective in the treatment of mucosal candidiasis, including oropharyngeal and esophageal candidiasis.[7] Weekly use of fluconazole was suggested to have prophylactic value against mucosal candidiasis in HIV seropositive patients.[47] It is also used in the primary treatment of coccidioidal meningitis as well as for blastomycosis and histoplasmosis. In one study, it was found to be more effective against oral candidiasis than nystatin in immunocompromised children.[26] It may also be effective in candidiasis resistant to the polyenes and the imidazoles.[38]

Nausea, vomiting, gastric pain, headache, and rashes are the most common adverse effects. Increases in serum transaminases have been reported in less than 5% of individuals receiving fluconazole. Seizures, anaphylaxis, and exfoliative dermatitis are rare occurrences. The drug interactions generally resemble those of itraconazole. However, gastric pH has little effect on the oral absorption of fluconazole (antacids and H_2 antihistamines do not interact), and fluconazole has less effect on drug metabolism than ketoconazole.

Other Imidazoles and Triazoles

Terconazole, a triazole, is supplied in a vaginal suppository for vaginal candidiasis. Butoconazole and tioconazole are imidazoles that are also used topically for vulvovaginitis. Oxiconazole and sulconazole are used topically for infections caused by dermatophytes. Saperconazole is an investigational water-insoluble, lipophilic fluorinated triazole with a broad spectrum of antifungal activity including the dimorphic fungi, phaeohyphomycetes, and species of *Cryptococcus* and *Aspergillus*.[42] The plasma half-life of saperconazole is approximately 20 hours after a single oral dose. Other pharmacologic effects of saperconazole are similar to those of itraconazole.

Caspofungin

Caspofungin, the first of a new class of antifungal agents was recently approved by the Food and Drug Administration (FDA) for invasive aspergillosis (Figure 40-4). It is an echinocandin with antifungal activity against a wide variety of fungal pathogens, including *Candida*,[5] *Pneumocystis*, *Aspergillus*, and *Histoplasma* species. Caspofungin disrupts the formation of the fungal cell wall by inhibiting the enzyme 1,3-β-D-glucan synthase, which is necessary for β(1,3)-D-glucan polymerization in filamentous fungi. This mechanism of action is different from those of amphotericin B and the azole compounds. For this reason, combination therapy of caspofungin and other antifungal agents has been suggested and yielded synergistic effects against cryptococcal species.[19] Caspofungin showed higher therapeutic efficacy against candidal infections compared with amphotericin B in immunocompromised patients.[9,30] Caspofungin is of particular importance in patients with life-threatening systemic fungal infection who cannot tolerate amphotericin B or azole therapy; it is generally well tolerated when administered parenterally. The manufacturer recommends daily intravenous infusion of 70 mg caspofungin acetate for the first day, followed by 50 mg/day thereafter. The common adverse effects resemble histamine-mediated symptoms, such as rash, facial swelling, pruritus, or sensation of warmth. One case of anaphylaxis was also reported with the initial administration of the drug. Table 40-1 contains a summary of the mechanisms of action and clinical uses of antifungal drugs.

Treatment of Oral Candidiasis

Candidiasis is by far the most common type of oral fungal infection. Regardless of which drug is used, therapy for 2 weeks is required. Even more extended treatment may be necessary. Clotrimazole, in the form of oral troches, is highly effective in most cases. On swallowing, however, clotrimazole can cause an increase in plasma concentrations of hepatic enzymes and may rarely lead to hepatitis. If patients have liver disease or are at greater risk of liver toxicity (e.g., alcoholics), nystatin oral pastilles or rinses are preferred. For more extensive disease or difficult cases, such as patients with AIDS, systemic antifungal therapy may be indicated.[43,59] Oral ketoconazole (200 mg/day) can be used; however, it is also potentially hepatotoxic. Ketoconazole can be combined with topical nystatin if necessary. Oral fluconazole (100 to 200 mg/day) is another systemic drug useful for oral candidiasis. The risk of causing liver abnormalities is less with fluconazole than with ketoconazole.[16] If the infection is resistant to these drugs, oral itraconazole (200 mg/day) is another alternative.[20] In extreme cases, intravenous amphotericin B with or without flucytosine may be considered.[20] The toxicity of this drug must be carefully weighed, and consultation with a specialist in infectious disease is essential. Surgery may be helpful to remove a condensed lesion after medical therapy. The occurrence of oral candidiasis with lichen planus is common. In these cases a topical antifungal drug may be applied with a topical

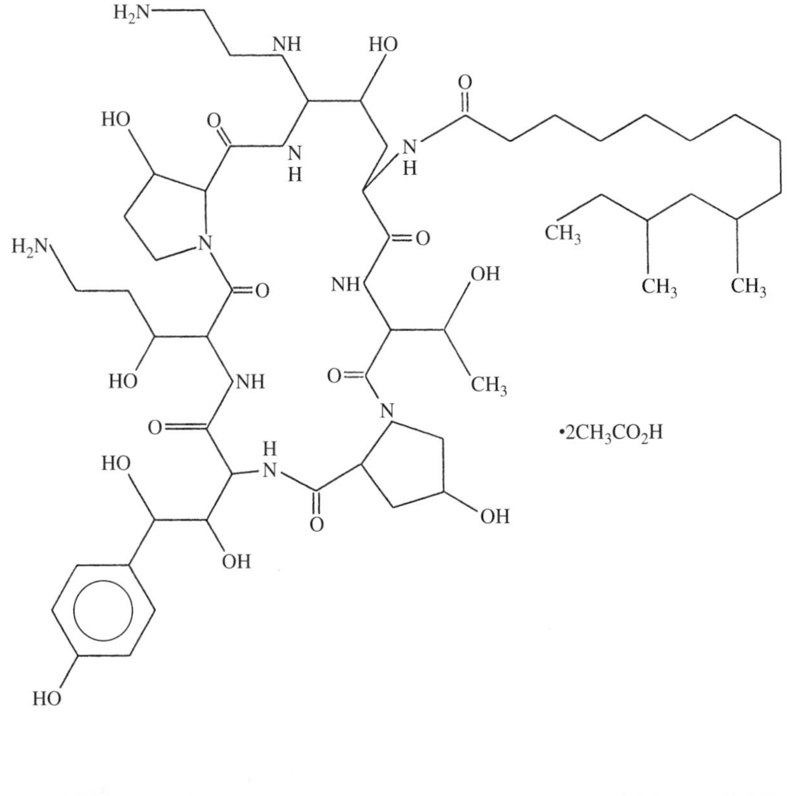

Fig. 40-4 Structural formula of caspofungin.

corticosteroid. It has been suggested that clotrimazole be given with a topical steroid in patients with oral lichen planus for prophylaxis against candidiasis.[59] Chlorhexidine oral rinses may also be of some use in treating oral candidiasis.

ANTIVIRAL AGENTS

Advances in the pharmacologic control of viral infections have lagged behind achievements in the chemotherapy of other microbial diseases. The reason for this delay, which applies as well to the therapeutic management of neoplastic disorders (see Chapter 42), has been the difficulty in attaining an adequate degree of selective toxicity. Indeed, when the First Conference on Antiviral Agents, sponsored by the New York Academy of Sciences, was held in 1965, there were no more than a half-dozen scientists in the United States who believed that safe and effective antiviral agents could be identified. Because the replication of viruses was known to use metabolic machinery essential for the function of normal cells, it seemed to be nearly impossible to find agents that would inhibit viral growth without killing the host. Since that time, however, some molecular events unique to viral replication have been identified and exploited in the development of selective antiviral agents. Potential points of attack include virus-encoded enzymes and other proteins that appear during viral replication and are different from corresponding cellular enzymes in noninfected cells. Endogenous mediators of antiviral immunity are another potential source of antiviral compounds. Thus, although the issue of selective toxicity of antiviral agents remains a major challenge, there is now considerable optimism for the future of viral therapeutics.

More than three dozen antiviral agents have been approved for clinical use by the FDA. These drugs, reviewed in Table 40-2, include (1) amantadine and rimantadine for prophylaxis and treatment of influenza A infections; (2) idoxuridine, vidarabine, and trifluridine for ocular herpetic diseases; (3) acyclovir, ganciclovir, and foscarnet for various systemic and localized herpes group infections; (4) ribavirin, a broad-spectrum agent used to treat respiratory syncytial bronchitis and pneumonia; (5) interferons for the treatment of human papillomavirus and chronic hepatitis infections; and (6) three classes of antiviral agents for the control of HIV infection.

Amantadine and Rimantadine

Amantadine and rimantadine are synthetic tricyclic amines (Figure 40-5). In 1966, amantadine became the first antiviral agent to be licensed for general use in the United States. Rimantadine is a close structural analogue of amantadine in which the amino moiety is replaced with an α-aminoethyl group. It also shares a similar pharmacologic profile.

Amantadine inhibits the replication of the influenza A virus, influenza C virus, Sendai virus, and pseudorabies virus. However, no inhibition is observed with the influenza B virus, parainfluenza virus types 1 through 3, mumps virus, and Newcastle disease virus. Different strains of influenza A virus display sensitivities to amantadine that vary by 100-fold.[35]

Table • 40-2

Antiviral Spectrum, Mechanisms of Action, and Clinical Uses of Antiviral Agents

AGENT	ANTIVIRAL SPECTRUM	MECHANISM OF ACTION	CLINICAL USES
Amantadine, rimantadine	Influenza A virus	Blockade of uncoating process	Prophylaxis of influenza A infection
Idoxuridine	HSV	Inhibition of DNA synthesis	Topical treatment of herpetic keratitis
Vidarabine, trifluridine	HSV	Inhibition of DNA synthesis	Topical treatment of herpetic keratitis and keratoconjunctivitis
Acyclovir, valacyclovir	HSV and VZV	Inhibition of DNA synthesis	Treatment of primary and recurrent herpes genitalis, herpetic encephalitis, mucocutaneous herpetic infections in immunocompromised patients, neonatal herpetic infection, and VZV infection, CMV prophylaxis
Famciclovir, penciclovir	HSV and VZV	Inhibition of DNA synthesis	Treatment of acute VZV infection and recurrent herpes infections
Cidofovir	CMV and HSV	Inhibition of DNA synthesis	Treatment of CMV keratitis and HSV lesions
Foscarnet	HSV, VZV, and CMV	Inhibition of DNA synthesis	Treatment of CMV retinitis and acyclovir-resistant HSV and VZV infections
Ganciclovir	CMV	Inhibition of DNA synthesis	Treatment of CMV retinitis and prevention of CMV disease
Interferon α and α_{2b}	HCV and HPV	Stimulation of synthesis of antiviral proteins	Treatment of HBV and HCV and refractory genital warts
Ribavirin	RSV	Inhibition of mRNA synthesis, inhibits purine synthesis	Treatment of RSV pneumonia and bronchitis
Reverse transcriptase inhibitors*	HIV	Inhibition of viral DNA synthesis	Treatment of HIV infection and AIDS
Protease inhibitors†	HIV	Blockade of HIV protease	Treatment of HIV infection and AIDS

*Includes both nucleoside (e.g., zidovudine, didanosine, lamivudine) and nonnucleoside (e.g., nevirapine) inhibitors.
†Includes such drugs as saquinavir, indinavir, and ritonavir.
AIDS, Acquired immune deficiency syndrome; *CMV,* cytomegalovirus; *HBV,* hepatitis B virus; *HCV,* hepatitis C virus; *HIV,* human immunodificiency virus; *HPV,* human papillomavirus; *HSV,* herper simplex virus; *RSV,* respiratory syncytial virus; *VZV,* varicella-zoster virus.

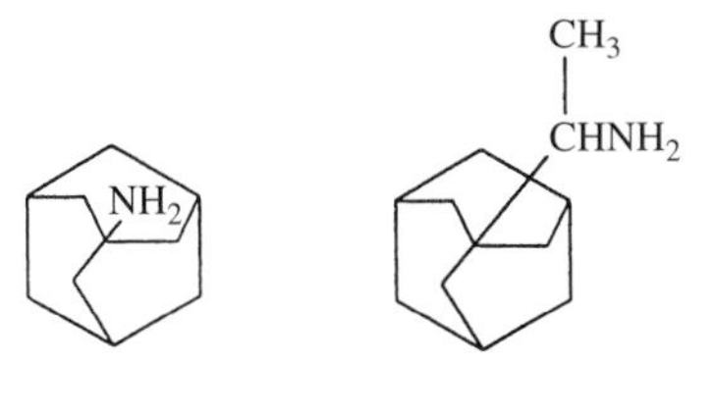

Amantadine Rimantadine

Fig. 40-5 Structural formulas of amantadine and rimantadine.

Although the mechanism by which amantadine inhibits virus replication has not been fully determined, it has been suggested that amantadine inhibits or delays the uncoating process that precedes primary transcription. Specifically, it blocks the action of the M2 viral protein that facilitates dissociation of the ribonucleoprotein complex preceding replication and the conformational changes in viral hemagglutinin that follow translation. Amantadine has no effect on the virus-specific RNA-dependent RNA polymerase activity of the influenza A virus.

Amantadine hydrochloride is a water-soluble compound and is rapidly absorbed from the gastrointestinal tract. Peak plasma concentrations are reached within 2 to 4 hours; the pulmonary concentration is approximately two thirds that of the plasma. Amantadine is excreted in the urine with an elimination half-life of approximately 15 hours.

Amantadine is available in capsules or syrup and is administered orally for the prevention of influenza A virus infection. Amantadine prophylaxis reduces infection rates by at least 50% and illness rates by at least 60%. The effectiveness of amantadine after the onset of influenza symptoms is not as convincing as that related to its prophylactic use. More recently, an aerosol mist of amantadine has been used for the treatment of influenza virus. Although such use significantly reduces certain respiratory symptoms of influenza, no effect is observed on fever, other constitutional symptoms, or pulmonary function measurements.

Dose-dependent side effects of amantadine are observed in 3% to 30% of patients. These effects include nervousness, drowsiness, difficulty in concentration, insomnia, and depression. Symptoms usually appear within 48 hours after the initiation of drug use and disappear quickly after drug administration is terminated. The ability of amantadine to affect CNS dopaminergic transmission (see Chapter 15) is largely responsible for the CNS disturbances.

Oseltamivir and Zanamivir

These are neuraminidase inhibitors effective against the symptoms related to infection with influenza A or B. Taken orally, oseltamivir can reduce the severity and duration of the symptoms caused by influenza viruses and decrease the incidence of upper respiratory complications. Zanamivir can be orally inhaled and is used for treatment of acute uncomplicated influenza A or B infection. These drugs are effective when taken within 30 to 36 hours after the onset of symptoms. Oseltamivir or zanamivir taken once or twice daily for prophylaxis appears to be effective against influenza-related illnesses. The common side effects include nausea and vomiting for oseltamivir and nasal discomfort or bronchospasm for zanamivir.

Antiherpetic Agents

With the exception of foscarnet, drugs effective against the herpes group of viruses are purine or pyrimidine analogues that are converted to active nucleotides either by cellular or virus-specific enzymes. Drugs that are activated by virus-encoded enzymes and inhibit a specific molecular event in viral replication are the most selective agents currently available.

Idoxuridine

Idoxuridine was synthesized in 1959 as part of an anticancer program and was soon found to possess antiviral activity against herpes simplex virus (HSV). Idoxuridine is a thymidine analogue with an iodine atom replacing the methyl group on the carbon 5 atom (Figure 40-6). Because iodine has almost the same radius as the methyl moiety, idoxuridine is readily phosphorylated to idoxuridine monophosphate by thymidine kinase. Idoxuridine monophosphate is further metabolized to the triphosphate form and is incorporated into viral and cellular DNA. Several enzymes involved in the biosynthesis of DNA, such as thymidine kinase, thymidylate kinase, and DNA polymerase, are inhibited by idoxuridine and its phosphorylated forms. However, the antiviral effect of idoxuridine is most likely related to the adverse biologic consequences of incorporating idoxuridine into viral DNA: chromosomal breakage and altered synthesis of viral proteins. The incorporation of idoxuridine into the DNA of normal uninfected cells is similarly responsible for the drug's toxicity.

Idoxuridine in vitro shows antiviral activity against a variety of DNA-dependent viruses, but the clinical use of idoxuridine solution and ointment is limited to the treatment of keratitis caused by herpes simplex virus (HSV) and vaccinia virus, the latter without specific FDA approval. Viral resistance commonly develops during therapy; idoxuridine is rapidly inactivated by deaminase or nucleotidase enzymes.

Topical application of idoxuridine to the conjunctiva can cause local irritation, contact dermatitis, punctate keratopathy (which may be more closely associated with the disease process than the drug), corneal clouding, photophobia, and lacrimation. In addition to these undesirable effects, idoxuridine causes chromosomal damage in cell culture and has disturbed embryonic development in animals after topical administration to the eye.

Vidarabine

Vidarabine (adenosine arabinoside or ara-A) is an analogue of adenosine originally synthesized but subsequently found in cultures of *Streptomyces antibioticus.* In vidarabine, the D-ribose moiety is replaced with arabinose (see Figure 40-6). Vidarabine exhibits a spectrum of antiviral activity in vitro against many DNA viruses (e.g., herpesvirus group and poxviruses) and some oncogenic RNA viruses (oncornaviruses). Studies indicate that the biologic activity of vidarabine can be attributed to phosphorylated derivatives, as shown in Figure 40-7, which inhibit viral DNA polymerases. However, the percentage of phosphorylated vidarabine is limited after intravenous infusion, and most of the drug is rapidly metabolized (plasma half-life is 3.5 hours) by adenosine deaminase to arabinosyl hypoxanthine, which is 60 times less potent than vidarabine. Because of the compound's low water solubility and poor gastrointestinal absorption, vidarabine must be administered by prolonged intravenous infusion of dilute solutions.

Topical treatment with vidarabine ointment is useful for keratitis caused by HSV and is the drug's main use.[56] It appears to be superior to idoxuridine in that it is at least as effective and is less allergenic, less irritating to the eye, and less likely to encounter viral resistance. Intravenous infusion of vidarabine is effective for the treatment of herpes encephalitis and useful for the control of varicella-zoster virus (VZV) infections in immunocompromised patients; however, acyclovir has essentially replaced vidarabine for these uses. Topical application of vidarabine for recurrent herpes labialis and herpes genitalis has been reported to have no significant therapeutic effect.

PURINES

Deoxyadenosine **Vidarabine** **Acyclovir** **Ribavirin**

PYRIMIDINES

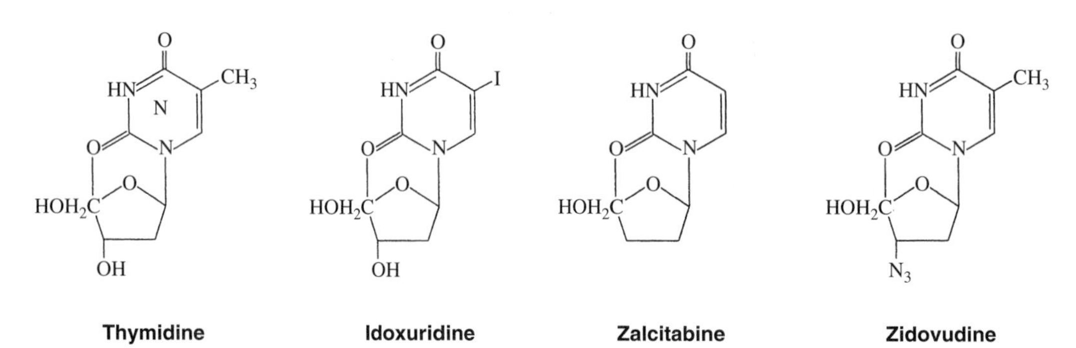

Fig. 40-6 Structural formulas of deoxyadenosine, thymidine, and several nucleoside antiviral drugs.

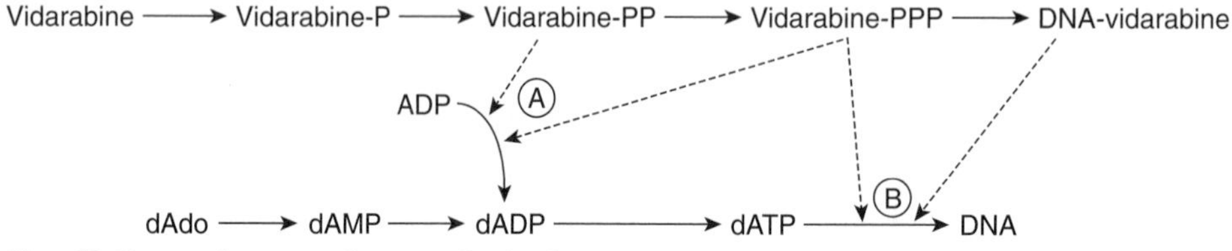

Fig. 40-7 Mechanisms of action of vidarabine. *Top,* Sequential phosphorylation of vidarabine by cellular enzymes and its incorporation into viral DNA; *bottom,* the conversion of deoxyadenosine *(dAdo)* to deoxyadenosine monophosphate *(dAMP)*, diphosphate *(dADP)*, and triphosphate *(dATP)* and the synthesis of normal viral DNA. *A,* Vidarabine diphosphates *(–PP)* and triphosphates *(–PPP)* inhibit ribonucleotide reductase–dependent production of dADP. *B,* Vidarabine triphosphate and vidarabine incorporated into DNA block further DNA synthesis by inhibiting the activity of DNA polymerases and terminal deoxynucleotidyl transferase.

Major toxic effects of vidarabine are for the most part associated with the phosphorylated derivatives and their effects on DNA synthesis. Adverse responses to parenteral vidarabine include gastrointestinal disturbance (nausea, vomiting, diarrhea), CNS manifestations (dizziness, confusion, ataxia), and hematologic disorders (hyperbilirubinemia, leukopenia). As with other drugs affecting DNA synthesis, vidarabine is potentially teratogenic and carcinogenic. The side effects of topical application are similar to those described for idoxuridine.

Trifluridine

Trifluridine (trifluorothymidine) is a derivative of idoxuridine in which the iodine atom (see Figure 40-6) is replaced with a trifluoromethyl group. Trifluridine exhibits antiviral activity against a number of DNA viruses, including HSV, vaccinia, and adenoviruses. The advantages of trifluridine over idoxuridine are its tenfold greater potency against herpetic keratitis and tenfold greater solubility in aqueous solution. Recent studies also suggest that trifluridine is often effective in patients who have previously not responded to idoxuridine or vidarabine.

The mechanism of antiviral action of trifluridine has primarily been studied regarding its effects against the vaccinia virus. Trifluridine is phosphorylated to trifluridine monophosphate, diphosphate, and triphosphate by viral or cellular thymidine kinase and thymidylate kinase. Trifluridine triphosphate is preferentially incorporated into viral DNA and produces effects similar to those of idoxuridine. Major cytotoxic reactions, however, are more closely associated with the inhibition of cellular thymidine synthetase by trifluridine monophosphate.[29]

Trifluridine, marketed as a 1% ophthalmic solution, is the drug of choice for superficial herpes keratitis. Toxic reactions to trifluridine are infrequent and generally mild, consisting of a burning sensation on instillation and palpebral edema. Allergic reactions are rare. Trifluridine is potentially mutagenic and carcinogenic; however, the risk from conjunctival application is minute.

Acyclovir and valacyclovir

Acyclovir is a product of research revolving around the synthesis of compounds designed to mimic substrates for adenosine deaminase, an enzyme essential to nucleic acid metabolism. (Although acyclovir proved not to act through inhibition of this enzyme, experimental drugs have been devised that do.) Acyclovir is an analogue of guanosine, or deoxyguanosine, in which two carbon atoms are missing from the ribose constituent (see Figure 40-6). Acyclovir is effective against herpesviruses such as HSV, VZV, and cytomegalovirus (CMV). As an antherpetic agent, acyclovir is 160 times as potent as vidarabine and 10 times as potent as idoxuridine.

Valacyclovir is the L-valyl ester of acyclovir. A prodrug, valacyclovir is rapidly absorbed after oral ingestion and converted to acyclovir during its first pass through the intestine and liver. Thus the pharmacologic actions and effects of valacyclovir and acyclovir are essentially identical.

The mechanisms of antiviral action of acyclovir are well known (Figure 40-8). The nucleoside analogue is phosphorylated to form acyclovir monophosphate by herpesvirus-encoded thymidine kinase and further phosphorylated by other enzymes to acyclovir diphosphate and triphosphate. Acyclovir triphosphate acts to inhibit viral DNA polymerase and to terminate elongation of the viral DNA chain as spurious nucleotide is incorporated into DNA (see Figure 40-8). In the noninfected host cell, phosphorylation of acyclovir occurs to a limited extent. Moreover, acyclovir triphosphate inhibits HSV DNA polymerase 10 to 30 times more effectively than it does cellular DNA polymerase.[22]

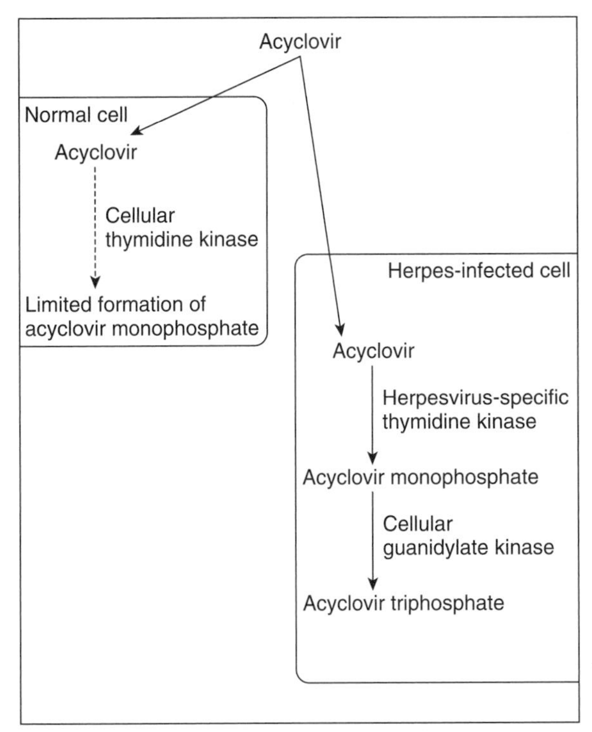

Fig. 40-8 Selective phosphorylation of acyclovir by herpesvirus-specific thymidine kinase and subsequent phosphorylation to acyclovir triphosphate by cellular guanidylate kinase. The preferential phosphorylation of acyclovir in herpesvirus-infected cells and selective inhibition of viral DNA polymerase by acyclovir triphosphate provide for the drug's selectivity; inhibition of the growth of uninfected cells requires up to a 3000-fold greater concentration of drug than does the inhibition of viral multiplication.

The bioavailability of acyclovir after oral administration is only approximately 20%. Peak plasma concentrations, which occur 2 hours after ingestion, are sufficient only for prophylaxis and treatment of highly susceptible infections such as genital herpes. Intravenous infusion can produce the much higher blood titers required for more resistant infections. The plasma half-life of acyclovir ranges from 2 to 5 hours in normal persons but is approximately 20 hours in patients with renal failure. Acyclovir is mostly eliminated through glomerular filtration and tubular secretion, with up to 90% of the excreted dose recovered as the parent molecule.

The FDA has approved the use of acyclovir ointment for the treatment of primary herpes genitalis and, in immunocompromised patients, for treatment of initial and recurrent mucocutaneous herpetic lesions that are not life threatening. Although physicians and dentists have used topical acyclovir for symptomatic relief of recurrent herpes labialis in patients with normal immune systems, there is little evidence of this practice providing real benefits.[49] Oral acyclovir is used for the prevention of recurrent herpes genitalis and treatment of primary and recurrent herpes genitalis and VZV infections. Oral therapy has also been shown to be effective in preventing reactivation of HSV in immunosuppressed patients.[4] Parenteral acyclovir has proved to be effective in the treatment of chronic and recurrent mucocutaneous HSV infections in immunocompromised patients, VZV infections, and herpes encephalitis.[18,55,57,58] Valacyclovir is currently indicated for treatment of VZV infections and recurrent genital herpes.

Because acyclovir is in extensive clinical use, reports concerning the facile emergence of acyclovir-resistant HSV mutants have received much attention.[14,25] The specific mechanisms of viral resistance against acyclovir include (1) loss of viral thymidine kinase activity, (2) elaboration of a viral thymidine kinase with altered substrate specificity, and (3) expression of altered DNA polymerase activity. The first two mechanisms account for the majority of resistant strains isolated in the laboratory; however, virulence is decreased by alterations in thymidine kinase activity. Full infectivity appears to be retained by mutant strains with DNA polymerase resistant to acyclovir binding.

No serious toxicity has been reported with topical or oral acyclovir therapy. The most frequent side effects during 3 to 6 months of oral use are headache, diarrhea, nausea and vomiting, arthralgias, and vertigo. Intravenous injection of acyclovir can induce local phlebitis, nausea and vomiting, diaphoresis, rash, and hypotension. Serious adverse effects such as nephrotoxicity or encephalopathy occasionally occur after the intravenous administration of acyclovir.

Ganciclovir and valganciclovir

Ganciclovir (9-[1,3-dihydroxy-2-propoxymethyl]-guanine) is a hydroxymethylated analogue of acyclovir. Valganciclovir is a prodrug of ganciclovir. Like acyclovir, ganciclovir is phosphorylated to the monophosphate form by herpesvirus-specific thymidine kinase and further phosphorylated to the triphosphate form.[13,48] Ganciclovir triphosphate inhibits viral DNA polymerase. The agent is more potent than acyclovir against HSV, CMV, and VZV, but the cytotoxicity of ganciclovir is also much greater.

Systemic ganciclovir is indicated for the treatment of life- and sight-threatening CMV infections, especially CMV retinitis in immunocompromised patients.[39] Ganciclovir is also effective for the treatment of some acyclovir-resistant HSV (DNA polymerase mutant) infections. The drug can cause aspermatogenesis in animals and is potentially carcinogenic and teratogenic. The most common serious side effects of ganciclovir are granulocytopenia and thrombocytopenia, and these toxicities are not always reversible after the cessation of drug administration.

Because of its poor oral bioavailability (less than 10%), ganciclovir is administered intravenously for treatment of active disease; oral administration may be used to prevent relapse after the infection has been suppressed. Recent studies showed that valganciclovir exhibited greater than tenfold oral bioavailability compared with ganciclovir, making it possible to replace intravenous ganciclovir with this drug.[46] The plasma half-life of ganciclovir is approximately 3 hours, with renal excretion of unchanged drug as the primary method of elimination.

Famciclovir and penciclovir

Famciclovir is an ester prodrug that is converted to penciclovir during its passage from the gut to the systemic circulation. Penciclovir is a guanine nucleoside analogue structurally related to acyclovir. It is less potent than acyclovir as an inhibitor of DNA polymerase, but the triphosphate form attains much higher concentrations than those of acyclovir and persists intracellularly for a longer period of time (half-life 7 to 20 hours). The spectrum of action is similar to acyclovir; herpesviruses that are resistant to acyclovir because of reduced thymidine kinase activity are also resistant to penciclovir. Famciclovir is currently approved for the treatment of acute, localized VZV infection; penciclovir is available as a topical agent for recurrent herpes labialis. Clinical trials involving additional uses of famciclovir and penciclovir are underway.

Foscarnet

Foscarnet is a phosphonoformate analogue of pyrophosphate. It is strongly active against HSV, CMV, other herpesviruses, and HIV-1. The drug inhibits herpetic DNA polymerase activity by blocking the pyrophosphate binding site on the enzyme. It inhibits the synthesis of DNA complementary to HIV-1 RNA by similarly suppressing the activity of reverse transcriptase. Foscarnet is approximately 100 times more selective for herpesvirus DNA polymerase than for mammalian DNA polymerase.

Foscarnet has been approved by the FDA for the treatment of acyclovir-resistant HSV infections in AIDS patients and CMV retinitis in immunocompromised patients.[20] The drug is also effective clinically against acyclovir-resistant VZV infection and against HIV-1 infection. The drug is highly ionized and must be given by slow (1 hour minimum) intravenous infusion every 8 hours.

Foscarnet has two major problems: renal toxicity and electrolyte disturbances. Nephrotoxicity occurs to some degree in most patients receiving foscarnet. Renal impairment is often reversible, but nephritis and necrosis may lead to permanent loss of renal function. Foscarnet binds divalent cations and causes a dose-dependent hypocalcemia, with possible paresthesias, muscle spasms, tetany, and seizures. Hypomagnesemia and disturbances in phosphate concentrations also occur. Malaise, nausea and vomiting, fatigue, headache, genital ulcers, CNS disturbances, anemia, leukopenia, and liver dysfunction are additional manifestations of foscarnet toxicity.

Cidofovir

Cidofovir is an analogue of cytidine that gets converted to cidofovir diphosphate, which inhibits DNA polymerase. The diphosphate form of the drug persists in the cell. This permits infrequent dosing intervals. Cidofovir is poorly absorbed orally and is given topically or intravenously. It is used to treat CMV retinitis and HSV mucocutaneous lesions.

Docosanol

Docosanol is a long-chain saturated alcohol and has been approved by the FDA for over-the-counter treatment of herpes labialis. In vitro, it prevents infection by lipid-enveloped viruses by inhibiting fusion between the viral envelope and the plasma membrane of the host cells. In clinical trials, docosanol, available in 10% cream, allowed for faster healing from recurrent herpes labialis compared with placebo, when docosanol was placed topically at the first sign of recurrence.

Ribavirin

Ribavirin is a synthetic triazole nucleoside analogue of guanosine (see Figure 40-6) with a broad spectrum of antiviral activity (including both DNA viruses and RNA viruses). Ribavirin exerts multiple actions. It directly inhibits guanine deaminase, and its metabolite, ribavirin 5′-phosphate, inhibits inosine monophosphate dehydrogenase and the formation of guanosine triphosphate. The triphosphate form of ribavirin, which is the predominant form intracellularly, interferes with viral messenger RNA transcriptase activity.

Although ribavirin shows broad antiviral spectrum in vitro, it is only approved in the United States as an aerosol for the treatment of respiratory syncytial virus bronchitis and pneumonia in children. Ribavirin administered by aerosolization to hospitalized infants and young children with respiratory syncytial virus infections produces significant reductions in fever and severity of systemic illness. It holds promise as an aerosol and oral medication for treatment of influenza, measles, acute and chronic hepatitis, Lassa fever, and a variety of RNA viral infections not commonly seen in the United States.[21]

The pharmacokinetics of ribavirin are complex. Systemic absorption occurs after inhalation, and plasma concentrations increase with long-term therapy. Ribavirin has a terminal half-life of 18 to 36 hours; however, the triphosphate derivative in red blood cells persists for several months after cessation of therapy.

A variety of serious toxic reactions have been attributed to its use, particularly in severely ill patients. Respiration may be worsened after inhalation, especially if the patient has preexisting chronic obstructive pulmonary disease. Anemia, hypotension, and cardiac arrest are possible side effects. Inasmuch as ribavirin is a nucleoside analogue and nonselective antiviral agent, it is potentially mutagenic, carcinogenic, and teratogenic.

Human Interferons

Interferons are glycoproteins secreted by virus-infected cells that promote the establishment of an antiviral state in uninfected cells. In addition to their antiviral activity, interferons regulate cellular functions dealing with cell proliferation and immunologic responses. Although all tissues appear to be capable of synthesizing interferons, cells that are derived from the hematopoietic system (e.g., lymphocytes and macrophages) may be the most significant in contributing to the total interferon synthesis of the body. All DNA and RNA viruses, single or double stranded, enveloped or not, with or without virion-associated polymerase, and replicating in the cytoplasm or nucleus, are sensitive to interferons to a greater or lesser degree.

Interferons can be classified according to three major groups: α, β, and γ. These are produced by induction of synthesis in human leukocytes, fibroblasts, or lymphoblastoid cells and, in larger amounts, by recombinant DNA techniques in bacteria. The mechanisms of action of interferons are complex; two important responses to interferon are reviewed in Figure 40-9. After binding to specific plasma-membrane receptors and being taken up by infected cells, interferon induces the synthesis of two enzymes: an oligonucleotide polymerase that synthesizes from adenosine triphosphate a series of oligonucleotides containing 2′,5′-phosphodiester bonds, and a protein kinase that phosphorylates and inactivates eukaryotic initiation factor. The oligonucleotides in turn stimulate cellular endonucleases to cleave viral messenger RNA, whereas the inactivated eukaryotic initiation factor no longer supports protein synthesis.[24,31] Additional antiviral effects may result from activation of macrophages and natural killer cells and modulation of cell-surface proteins to facilitate immune recognition.

For prophylaxis of viral infection or for early treatment, interferons may have certain advantages over more narrow-spectrum antiviral agents. In other circumstances, a specific antiviral agent may be preferable to interferons on the grounds of convenience of administration, a quicker onset of antiviral action, or a lack of side effects. Interferons can cause increases in pulse rate and temperature, decreases in white blood cell counts, and headache, somnolence, and malaise. Interferons are currently undergoing clinical trials for a variety of viral diseases, including AIDS. Interferon α_{2b} and mixed interferon α preparations are currently approved for use against chronic hepatitis B and C infections, condyloma acuminata (anogenital warts) caused by human papillomavirus infection, multiple sclerosis, and Kaposi's sarcoma in patients with HIV infection. The approved uses of interferons in the treatment of cancer are reviewed in Chapter 42. Interferons β_{1a} and β_{1b} have been approved for the management of multiple sclerosis, and interferon γ_{1b} has been approved for chronic granulomatous disease.

Antiretroviral Agents

Since AIDS was first characterized in the early 1980s and attributed to HIV, a retrovirus, tremendous efforts have been made to develop effective therapies against the disease. Although numerous anti-AIDS drugs have been tested, many have proved to be of dubious worth. However, three groups of drugs—nucleoside reverse transcriptase inhibitors, nonnucleoside reverse transcriptase inhibitors, and HIV protease inhibitors—are now available for clinical use. Because of the rapidity with which some of these drugs have been developed and approved for marketing, research is ongoing regarding the therapeutic uses and toxic profiles of these agents. An especially promising development from these studies has been the dramatic therapeutic benefits obtained with multiple drug therapy. Adverse effects of nucleoside reverse transcriptase inhibitors include lactic acidosis, headaches, gastrointestinal disorders such as nausea and vomiting, and hepatomegaly.

Zidovudine

Zidovudine (azidothymidine) was the first antiviral agent to be sufficiently safe and effective to receive FDA approval for the treatment of AIDS. Zidovudine is a thymidine analogue in which the 3′-hydroxyl group is replaced by an azido group (—N_3; see Figure 40-6).

Zidovudine is phosphorylated by cellular enzymes to zidovudine triphosphate, which is incorporated into viral complementary DNA (cDNA) by the reverse transcription of HIV RNA. The 3′ substitution of the zidovudine prevents further 5′-3′-phosphodiester linkages and terminates chain elongation. HIV-1 reverse transcriptase is approximately 100 times more susceptible to inhibition by zidovudine than is DNA polymerase of mammalian cells. Zidovudine seems not only to block replication of the virus but also promotes regeneration of CD4+ lymphocytes. The agent also delays progression of AIDS in HIV-infected individuals with CD4+ lymphocytes counts less than 500 cells/mm^3 and in individuals with no symptoms or early symptoms of AIDS-related

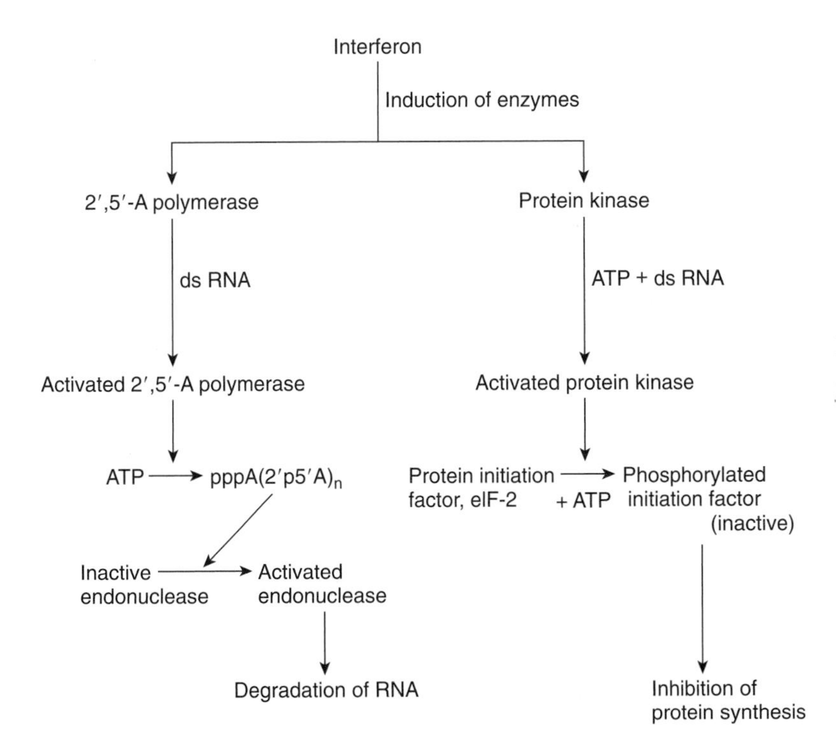

Fig. 40-9 Mechanisms of action of interferon. After incorporation into the cell, interferon induces the synthesis of two enzymes, an oligonucleotide polymerase (2′,5′-A polymerase) and a protein kinase, which in the presence of double-stranded RNA *(ds RNA)* lead to a cascade of reactions that inhibit viral replication.

illness. Zidovudine provides palliative treatment only; it does not cure AIDS and cannot eliminate HIV from the body. However, as a preventive measure, zidovudine significantly reduces the incidence of neonatal infection when the HIV-infected mother begins taking the drug orally after 14 weeks of gestation and continues until birth (at which time intravenous zidovudine is administered). The efficacy of zidovudine for postexposure prophylaxis is controversial. A case-controlled study indicated that zidovudine reduced the risk of HIV infection in exposed health care workers by 79%.[12] Preliminary guidelines at this time recommend the basic 4-week regimen of two drugs (zidovudine and lamivudine or didanosine and stavudine) for most HIV exposures.[50] For HIV exposures that pose an increased risk for transmission, an expanded regimen that includes the addition of a third drug is recommended.

Many HIV strains resistant to zidovudine have been isolated from clinical specimens. Although HIV strains from individuals not receiving zidovudine are very susceptible to zidovudine, the sensitivity of HIV from patients receiving zidovudine for 6 months is significantly decreased. Zidovudine-resistant strains are susceptible to other anti-HIV agents such as didanosine, zalcitabine, and foscarnet in vitro.

Zidovudine is given orally on a rigid 4-hour schedule. The drug is rapidly absorbed, quickly metabolized in the liver, and excreted in the urine. The mean elimination half-life is approximately 1 hour. Intracellular zidovudine triphosphate persists for several hours. Common side effects are nausea, headache, and bone marrow depression.[20] On occasion, transfusion may be required to correct the granulocytopenia and anemia. Other side effects of zidovudine include asthenia, dizziness, insomnia, malaise, and myalgia. Long-term use of this drug is infrequently associated with a toxic myopathy. Although zidovudine can induce cell transformation in vitro and tumors in animals, the teratogenic potential in human beings is unknown.

Didanosine

Didanosine (dideoxyinosine) is active against HIV, including zidovudine-resistant strains, and was approved for human use in 1991. Similar to zidovudine, didanosine, once converted to the triphosphate form, inhibits the activity of reverse transcriptase, and by so doing, blocks the synthesis of HIV cDNA. Oral didanosine increases the number of CD4+ lymphocytes, decreases viral antigen titers, and decreases symptoms of AIDS-related illness. So far, cross-resistance between didanosine and zidovudine has not been reported. Major side effects include peripheral neuropathy and potentially fatal pancreatitis.

Didanosine is well absorbed at neutral pH and should thus be taken on an empty stomach. The chewable didanosine tablet contains an antacid to neutralize the pH of the stomach. It should not be taken with medications that require an acidic pH for absorption, such as ketoconazole, itraconazole, and quinolone antibiotics. Although the drug is quickly eliminated in the urine (elimination half-life of approximately 1 hour), persistence of intracellular didanosine triphosphate permits twice daily dosing.

Didanosine was originally reserved for patients with advanced HIV infection who were intolerant to zidovudine or showed clinical or immunologic deterioration. It is now commonly used in combination with zidovudine and a protease inhibitor. Resistance to didanosine is progressive, with resistant strains appearing in the majority of patients after 6 months of monotherapy.

Zalcitabine

Zalcitabine is the 2′-3′-dideoxy analogue of cytidine (see Figure 40-6). Its mechanism of action and pharmacologic profile are similar to zidovudine. Zalcitabine was initially approved for the control of HIV infection in 1992, but it is inferior to zidovudine for monotherapy when used as the initial treatment modality. Zalcitabine shows therapeutic efficacy in patients who are resistant to zidovudine and is comparable to didanosine in patients intolerant to zidovudine.[2,3] Cross-resistance is common between didanosine and zalcitabine. The drug is often administered in combination with zidovudine and a protease inhibitor.

Stavudine

Stavudine, approved in 1994, is the 2′-3′-dideoxy analogue of thymidine. Its mechanism of action and clinical pharmacologic features are similar to those of the previously discussed antiretroviral agents. Studies have shown that stavudine therapy increases the number of CD4+ cells in patients who did not respond to zidovudine therapy. Occasionally, development of resistance to stavudine also confers resistance to zidovudine and didanosine. As with other retrovirals, stavudine is used in combination drug therapy.

Abacavir

Abacavir is a nucleoside analogue reverse transcriptase inhibitor that is useful in combination (see below) for treating HIV infections. It was approved for clinical use in 1998. Abacavir can cause adverse effects common to other nucleoside reverse transcriptase inhibitors and has been associated with fatal hypersensitivity reactions.

Lamivudine

Lamivudine is another nucleoside analogue introduced into clinical practice in 1995. It is the (—) enantiomer of 2′-deoxy-3′-thiacytidine. Conversion intracellularly to the triphosphate form inhibits chain elongation of the viral cDNA by inhibiting reverse transcriptase. Poorly effective as monotherapy, lamivudine is approved for the control of infection in combination with zidovudine. Clinical studies indicate that the combination synergistically inhibits HIV replication and strongly enhances CD4+ cell counts.[23] As with the other retroviral agents, the persistence of lamivudine triphosphate intracellularly effectively counteracts the rapid elimination of the parent drug. Side effects of lamivudine are generally mild and include nausea and headache.

Trizivir is a single tablet combination regimen of lamivudine, zidovudine, and abacavir for treatment of HIV. Trizivir should only be used for patients whose treatment regimens would otherwise include all three of the nucleoside analogues. It is not recommended for patients weighing less than 40 kg because it is a fixed-dose tablet. Because trizivir combines three drugs in a single tablet, it may help patients with compliance. The most notable side effect of trizivir is associated with the hypersensitivity reaction to abacavir, which has been observed in 5% of HIV patients.

Nevirapine, efavirenz, and delavirdine

Nevirapine, a dipyridodiazepinone (Figure 40-10), is the first nonnucleoside inhibitor of reverse transcriptase. The drug requires no activation; it binds directly to reverse transcriptase of HIV-1 and noncompetitively inhibits cDNA synthesis. Rapid development of drug resistance is the major limitation of this compound, which should never be used as monotherapy.

In contrast to the nucleoside analogues, nevirapine is lipid soluble, very well absorbed, and extensively metabolized by cytochrome P450 (CYP3A family). The elimination half-life decreases from 2 days to 1 day as nevirapine induces its own metabolism. The drug also induces the breakdown of estrogens and HIV protease inhibitors (described below). Nevirapine may cause rash, diarrhea, and drug fever.

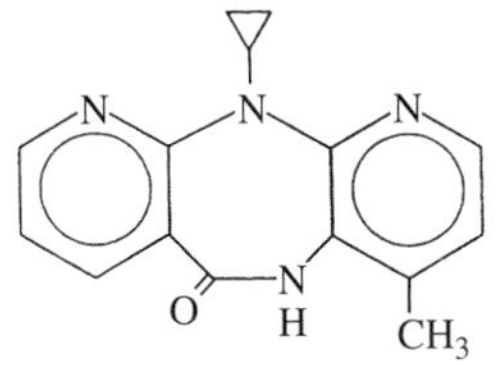

Nevirapine

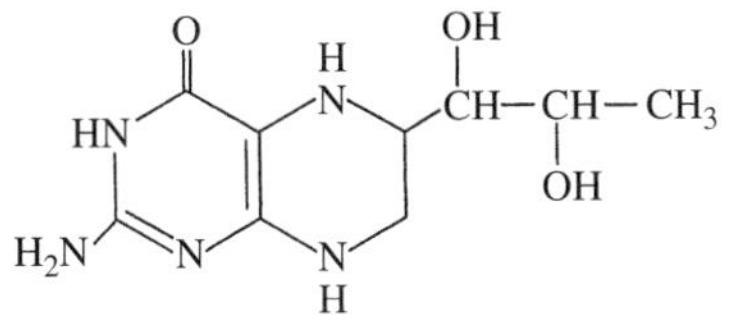

Saquinavir

Fig. 40-10 Structural formulas of nevirapine and saquinavir.

Two other nonnucleoside inhibitors of reverse transcriptase, efavirenz and delavirdine, are available. These drugs are used to treat HIV-1 infections.

Protease Inhibitors

HIV protease is a viral enzyme responsible for the cleavage of the Gag and Gag-Pol polyproteins into the enzymes and structural proteins that are required for the final assembly of new infectious virions.[8] In patients with advanced HIV infection, use of a protease inhibitor in combination therapy with other classes of antiretroviral agents significantly improved the survival of patients. After sustained exposure to antiviral agents, viral isolates may develop resistance to one class of drugs and remain susceptible to others. It is therefore preferred to use new protease inhibitors combined with other drugs when the drug resistance has occurred. All protease inhibitors exhibit similar side effects after prolonged exposure. Most commonly, patients may experience hyperglycemia, increased aminotransferase activity, and gastrointestinal dysfunction.[11] Fat redistribution and hyperlipidemia have also been noted.

Saquinavir

Saquinavir (see Figure 40-10) was the first drug approved by the FDA to inhibit HIV protease. Saquinavir has shown selective and potent anti-HIV activity; however, saquinavir monotherapy rapidly induces viral resistance. Similar to combination therapy involving nucleoside and nonnucleoside antiretrovirals, the use of protease inhibitors in conjunction with nucleoside analogues has shown improved clinical efficacy over single drugs or two-drug combinations. For example, the combination of saquinavir, zidovudine, and zalcitabine greatly reduced the viral load without causing any increased toxicity compared with two-drug therapy.[15] The side effects of saquinavir include gastrointestinal disturbances such as nausea and vomiting. Because saquinavir is both metabolized by and an inhibitor of hepatic CYP3A isoenzymes, interactions are possible with other drugs that rely on the same P450 enzymes for inactivation. Thus saquinavir may accumulate in patients taking ketoconazole and inhibit the metabolism of drugs such as verapamil and triazolam. Drugs that induce CYP3A enzymes, such as rifampin and nevirapine, may reduce the effectiveness of saquinavir.

Indinavir and ritonavir

Indinavir and ritonavir are HIV protease inhibitors. They were released for use in 1996 by the FDA under a special program for drugs with promising anti-HIV activity (as have several other drugs discussed in this chapter).[10] The triple-drug combination of ritonavir and two nucleoside analogues significantly increased the number of CD4+ lymphocytes and reduced the mortality rate of advanced AIDS patients,[23] and the combination of indinavir with zidovudine and lamivudine resulted in sustained undetectable viral titers for a year in more than 80% of patients receiving the therapy. A recent study evaluated the therapeutic efficacy of combination therapy with indinavir for pediatric patients seropositive for HIV-1.[51] The initial 2-year therapy showed HIV-1 RNA load below the detectable limit and increase in CD4+ cell counts to 94% of the age-matched normal value in the majority of the treated patients.

The major side effects of indinavir include hyperbilirubinemia and nephrolithiasis. Because 3% of patients receiving indinavir develop kidney stones, drinking at least 48 ounces of water per day is recommended. Ritonavir induces gastrointestinal disturbances, altered taste, and perioral paresthesia. Potential drug interactions for both drugs are similar to those mentioned for saquinavir.

Nelfinavir and lopinavir

Nelfinavir is probably the most commonly used protease inhibitor because of its relatively low toxicity. Its side effects include hyperglycemia, abnormal fat distribution, and diarrhea, often controllable with loperamide. Lopinavir is a new protease inhibitor that became available through clinical trials and shows high potency in vitro, especially when given in combination with ritonavir. The lopinavir/ritonavir combination causes mild gastrointestinal side effects and headache.

Amprenavir

Amprenavir is the most recent protease inhibitor to become available for treatment of HIV infection. It can be used for HIV-infected adults and children more than 4 years old. Amprenavir is available in large capsules (150 mg and 50 mg) and in oral solution (15 mg/ml). Amprenavir capsules contain vitamin E. The vitamin E facilitates the drug absorption. Each 150-mg capsule contains 109 IU of vitamin E, which exceeds the recommended daily allowance. Thus patients taking amprenavir should stop daily vitamin E supplements. In a 24-week study, combination therapy with amprenavir/zidovudine/lamivudine reduced the viral load to below 500 copies/ml.[41] The side effects of amprenavir include nausea, vomiting, diarrhea, oral and perioral paresthesias, and rash. Like other protease inhibitors, altered body fat distribution, hyperglycemia, and increased aminotransferase activity have been reported with amprenavir.

ANTIVIRAL THERAPY IN THE ORAL CAVITY

HSV causes a variety of oral mucosal lesions, including herpetic gingivostomatitis, recurrent intraoral herpes simplex, herpes labialis, herpes zoster, or the life-threatening eczema herpeticum. Herpetic gingivostomatitis can also manifest in weakened hosts as aphthoid of Pospischill-Feyrter, characterized by rapid expansion of the lesion to the throat and perioral skin. The majority of the HSV-associated viral lesions are routinely treated by oral acyclovir, with intravenous administration in some severe cases.

Acyclovir is best used as soon as the symptoms begin to appear. The intravenous dosage is based on body weight and the type of the lesion. Generally, 5 to 10 mg/kg of body weight is administered intravenously for a 1-hour period and repeated every 8 hours for 5 to 10 days. Long-term suppressive acyclovir therapy is recommended for patients with eczema herpeticum at 200 to 400 mg orally two to three times per day. In addition, supportive therapies for herpetic lesions include antipyretic analgesics, antibiotics, and antifungals that help control secondary infections.

HSV infection can develop into a more severe and generalized form in AIDS patients. Recurrent herpetic lesions become chronic in these patients and HSV strains resistant to acyclovir could arise, in which case other antherpetic agents, such as ganciclovir and foscarnet, may be effective. In AIDS patients, numerous concomitant oral lesions of different viral origins are not uncommon. Human papillomavirus infection is almost always noted in these patients, resulting in variants of papillomas, condylomas, and focal epithelial hyperplasia in the oral cavity. Also, CMV is associated with aphthae-like ulcerations in the oral mucosa. Oral hairy leukoplakia is an early sign of HIV infection, presumably caused by Epstein-Barr virus in immunocompromised patients. Treatment of oral hairy leukoplakia is rendered only in symptomatic patients and usually involves topical application of a solution of podophyllin resin 25% and acyclovir 800 mg four times daily. Systemic antiretroviral therapy is also provided as described above. Oral hairy leukoplakia disappears after the drug therapy but normally recurs when the medication is discontinued.

Antifungal and Antiviral Agents

Nonproprietary (generic) name	*Proprietary (trade) name*
Antifungal agents	
Amphotericin B	Abelcet, Amphotec, Fungizone
Butenafine	Mentax
Butoconazole	Femstat
Caspofungin	Cancidas
Ciclopirox	Loprox
Clioquinol	Vioform
Clotrimazole	Lotrimin, Mycelex
Econazole	Spectazole
Fluconazole	Diflucan
Flucytosine	Ancobon
Gentian violet	—
Griseofulvin	Fulvicin, Grifulvin V, Grisactin
Haloprogin	Halotex
Itraconazole	Sporanox
Ketoconazole	Nizoral
Miconazole	Micatin, Monistat-Derm, Monistat i.v.
Naftifine	Naftin
Natamycin	Natacyn
Nystatin	Mycostatin, Nilstat, Nystex
Oxiconazole	Oxistat
Sulconazole	Exelderm
Terbinafine	Lamisil
Terconazole	Terazol
Tioconazole	Vagistat-1
Tolnaftate	Aftate, Tinactin
Triacetin	in Fungoid
Undecylenic acid (and derivatives)	Crex, Desenex, Fungoid AF
Antiviral agents	
Abacavir	Ziagen
Abacavir, zidovudine, and lamivudine (combination)	Trizivir
Acyclovir	Zovirax
Amantadine	Symmetrel
Amprenavir	Agenerase
Cidofovir	Vistide
Delavirdine	Rescriptor
Didanosine	Videx
Docosanol	Abreva
Efavirenz	Sustiva
Famciclovir	Famvir
Fomivirsen	Vitravene
Foscarnet	Foscavir
Ganciclovir	Cytovene
Idoxuridine	Herplex
Imiquimod	Aldara
Indinavir	Crixivan
Interferon α_{2a}	Referon-A
Interferon α_{2b}	Intron A
Interferon α_{n3}	Alferon
Lamivudine	Epivir
Lopinavir	Kaletra
Nelfinavir	Viracept
Nevirapine	Viramune
Oseltamivir	Tamiflu
Penciclovir	Denavir
Ribavirin	Virazole
Rimantadine	Flumadine
Ritonavir	Norvir
Saquinavir	Invirase
Stavudine	Zerit
Tenofovir disoproxil fumarate	Viread
Trifluridine	Viroptic
Valacyclovir	Valtrex
Valganciclovir	Cymeval, Valcyte
Vidarabine	Vira-A
Zalcitabine	Hivid
Zanamivir	Relenza
Zidovudine	Retrovir

Cited References

1. Abernathy RS: Treatment of systemic mycoses, *Medicine* [Baltimore] 52:385-394, 1973.
2. Abrams DI, Goldman AI, Launer C, et al: A comparative trial of didanosine or zalcitabine after treatment with zidovudine in patients with human immunodeficiency virus infection, *N Engl J Med* 330:657-662, 1994.
3. Adkins JC, Peters DH, Faulds D: Zalcitabine. An update of its pharmacodynamic and pharmacokinetic properties and clinical efficacy in the management of HIV infection, *Drugs* 53:1054-1080, 1997.
4. Aoki FY: Management of genital herpes in HIV-infected patients, *Herpes* 8:41-45, 2001.

5. Arathoon EG, Gotuzzo E, Noriega LM, et al: Randomized, double-blind, multicenter study of caspofungin versus amphotericin B for treatment of oropharyngeal and esophageal candidiasis, *Antimicrob Agents Chemother* 46:451-457, 2002.
6. Arikan S, Rex JH: Nystatin LF (Aronex/Abbott), *Curr Opin Investig Drugs* 2:488-495, 2001.
7. Barchiesi F, Giacometti A, Arzeni D, et al: Fluconazole and ketoconazole in the treatment of oral and esophageal candidiasis in AIDS patients, *J Chemother* 4:381-386, 1992.
8. Bartlett JG: Protease inhibitors for HIV infection, *Ann Intern Med* 124:1086-1088, 1996.
9. Brajtburg J, Powderly WG, Kobayashi GS, et al: Amphotericin B: current understanding of mechanisms of action, *Antimicrob Agents Chemother* 34:183-188, 1990.
10. Carpenter CC, Cooper DA, Fischl MA, et al: Antiretroviral therapy in adults: updated recommendations of the International AIDS Society—USA panel, *JAMA* 283:381-390, 2000.
11. Carr A, Morey A, Mallon P, et al: Fatal portal hypertension, liver failure, and mitochondrial dysfunction after HIV-1 nucleoside analogue-induced hepatitis and lactic acidaemia, *Lancet* 357:1412-1414, 2001.
12. Case-control study of HIV seroconversion in health-care workers after percutaneous exposure to HIV-infected blood—France, United Kingdom, and United States, January 1988-August 1994, *MMWR Morb Mortal Wkly Rep* 44:929-933, 1995.
13. Chun Y-S, Park N-H: Effect of ganciclovir [9-(1,3-dihydroxy-2-propoxymethyl)-guanine] on viral DNA and protein synthesis in cells infected with herpes simplex virus, *Antimicrob Agents Chemother* 31:349-351, 1987.
14. Coen DM, Schaffer PA: Two distinct loci confer resistance to acyclo-guanosine in herpes simplex virus type 1, *Proc Natl Acad Sci USA* 77:2265-2269, 1980.
15. Collier AC, Cooms RW, Schoenfeld DA, et al: Treatment of human immunodeficiency virus infection with saquinavir, zidovudine, and zalcitabine. AIDS Clinical Trials Group, *N Engl J Med* 334:1011-1107, 1996.
16. Como JA, Dismukes WE: Oral azole drugs as systemic antifungal therapy, *N Engl J Med* 330:263-272, 1994.
17. Cupp-Vickery JR, Garcia C, Hofacre A: Ketoconazole-induced conformational changes in the active site of cytochrome P450eryF, *J Mol Biol* 311:101-110, 2001.
18. De Clercq E: Antivirals for the treatment of herpesvirus infections, *J Antimicrob Chemother* 32(suppl A):121-132, 1993.
19. Del Poeta M, Cruz MC, Cardenas ME, et al: Synergistic antifungal activities of bafilomycin A_1, fluconazole, and the pneumocandin MK-0991/caspofungin acetate (L-743,873) with calcineurin inhibitors FK506 and L-685,818 against *Cryptococcus neoformans*, *Antimicrob Agents Chemother* 44:739-746, 2000.
20. Drugs for HIV infections, *Med Lett Drugs Ther Handbook* 16:88-97, 2002.
21. Drugs for non-HIV viral infections, *Med Lett Drugs Ther* 44:9-16, 2002.
22. Elion GB: Mechanism of action and selectivity of acyclovir (Acyclovir Symposium), *Am J Med* 73(IA):7-13, 1982.
23. Eron JJ, Benoit SL, Jemsek J, et al: Treatment with lamivudine, zidovudine, or both in HIV-positive patients with 200 to 500 CD4+ cells per cubic millimeter, *N Engl J Med* 333:1662-1669, 1995.
24. Farrell PJ, Sen GC, Dubois MF, et al: Interferon action: two distinct pathways for inhibition of protein synthesis by double-stranded RNA, *Proc Natl Acad Sci USA* 75:5893-5897, 1978.
25. Field HJ, Larder BA, Darby G: Isolation and characterization of acyclovir-resistant strains of herpes simplex virus (Acyclovir Symposium), *Am J Med* 73(1A):369-371, 1982.
26. Flynn PM, Cunningham CK, Kerkering T, et al: Oropharyngeal candidiasis in immunocompromised children: a randomized, multicenter study of orally administered fluconazole suspension versus nystatin. The Multicenter Fluconazole Study Group, *J Pediatr* 127:322-328, 1995.
27. Gigolashvili T: Update on antifungal therapy, *Cancer Pract* 7:157-159, 1999.
28. Guo LS: Amphotericin B colloidal dispersion: an improved antifungal therapy, *Adv Drug Deliv Rev* 47:149-163, 2001.
29. Heidelberger C, King DH: Trifluorothymidine, *Pharmacol Ther* 6:427-442, 1979.
30. Hoang A: Caspofungin acetate: an antifungal agent, *Am J Health Syst Pharm* 58:1206-1214, 2001.
31. Hovanessian AG, Brown RE, Kerr IM: Synthesis of low molecular weight inhibitor of protein synthesis with enzyme from interferon-treated cells, *Nature* 268:537-540, 1977.
32. Irizarry L: Cryptococcal meningitis, *Curr Treat Options Neurol* 3:413-426, 2001.
33. Kerridge D: Mode of action of clinically important antifungal drugs, *Adv Microb Physiol* 27:1-72, 1986.
34. Knoppert DC, Salama HE, Lee DS: Eradication of severe neonatal systemic candidiasis with amphotericin B lipid complex, *Ann Pharmacother* 35:1032-1036, 2001.
35. Koff WC, Knight V: Effect of rimantadine on influenza virus replication, *Proc Soc Exp Bioi Med* 160:246-253, 1979.
36. Lake-Bakaar G, Tom W, Lake-Bakaar D, et al: Gastropathy and ketoconazole malabsorption in the acquired immunodeficiency syndrome (AIDS), *Ann Intern Med* 109:471-473, 1988.
37. Laochumroonvorapong P, Diconstanzo DP, Wu H, et al: Disseminated histoplasmosis presenting as pyoderma gangrenosum-like lesions in a patient with acquired immunodeficiency syndrome, *Int J Dermatol* 40:518-521, 2001.
38. Lucatorto FM, Franken C, Hardy WD, et al: Treatment of refractory oral candidiasis with fluconazole. A case report, *Oral Surg Oral Med Oral Pathol* 71:42-44, 1991.
39. Martin DF, Sierra-Madero J, Walmsley S, et al: A controlled trial of valganciclovir as induction therapy for cytomegalovirus retinitis, *N Engl J Med* 346:1119-1126, 2002.
40. Medoff G, Dismukes WE, Pappagianis D, et al: Evaluation of new antifungal drugs for the treatment of systemic fungal infections, *Clin Infect Dis* 15(suppl 1):S274-S281, 1992.
41. Murphy RL, Sommadossi JP, Lamson M, et al: Antiviral effect and pharmacokinetic interaction between nevirapine and indinavir in persons infected with human immunodeficiency virus type 1, *J Infect Dis* 179:1116-1123, 1999.
42. Octcenasek M: Susceptibility of clinical isolates of fungi to saperconazole, *Mycopathologia* 118:179-183, 1992.

43. Patton LL, Bonito AJ, Shugars DA: A systematic review of the effectiveness of antifungal drugs for the prevention and treatment of oropharyngeal candidiasis in HIV-positive patients, *Oral Surg Oral Med Oral Pathol Oral Radiol Endod* 92:170-179, 2001.
44. Pelletier R, Peter J, Antin C, et al: Emergence of resistance of *Candida albicans* to clotrimazole in human immunodeficiency virus-infected children: in vitro and clinical correlations, *J Clin Microbiol* 38:1563-1568, 2000.
45. Petersen EA, Ailing DW, Kirkpatrick CH: Treatment of chronic mucocutaneous candidiasis with ketoconazole: a controlled clinical trial, *Ann Intern Med* 93:791-795, 1980.
46. Reusser P: Oral valganciclovir: a new option for treatment of cytomegalovirus infection and disease in immunocompromised hosts, *Expert Opin Investig Drugs* 10:1745-1753, 2001.
47. Schuman P, Capps L, Peng G, et al: Weekly fluconazole for the prevention of mucosal candidiasis in women with HIV infection. A randomized, double-blind, placebo-controlled trial, *Ann Intern Med* 126:689-696, 1997.
48. Smee DF, Martin JC, Verheyden JP, et al: Anti-herpesvirus activity of the acyclic nucleoside 9-(1,3-dihydroxy-2-propoxymethyl)guanine, *Antimicrob Agents Chemother* 23:676-682, 1983.
49. Spruance SL, Crumpacker CS: Topical 5 percent acyclovir in polyethylene glycol for herpes simplex labialis: antiviral effect without clinical benefit (Acyclovir Symposium), *Am J Med* 73(IA):315-319, 1982.
50. US Public Health Service: Updated U.S. Public Health Service guidelines for the management of occupational exposures to HBV, HCV, and HIV and recommendations for postexposure prophylaxis, *MMWR* 50(RR-11):1-52, 2001.
51. van Rossum AMC, Geelen SPM, Hartwig NG, et al: Results of 2 years of treatment with protease-inhibitor containing antiretroviral therapy in dutch children infected with human immunodeficiency virus type 1, *Clin Infect Dis* 34:1008-1016, 2002.
52. Vazquez JA: Therapeutic options for the management of oropharyngeal and esophageal candidiasis in HIV/AIDS patients, *HIV Clin Trials* 1:47-59, 2000.
53. Warnock DW, Johnson EM, Richardson MD, et al: Modified response to ketoconazole of *Candida albicans* from a treatment failure, *Lancet* 1:642-643, 1983.
54. Wheat J, Hafner R, Korzun AH, et al: AIDS Clinical Trial Group. Itraconazole treatment of disseminated histoplasmosis in patients with the acquired immunodeficiency syndrome, *Am J Med* 98:336-342, 1995.
55. Whitley RJ and the NIAID Collaborative Antiviral Study Group: Interim summary of mortality in herpes simplex encephalitis and neonatal herpes simplex virus infections: vidarabine versus acyclovir, *J Antimicrob Chemother* 12(suppl B):105-112, 1983.
56. Wilhelmus KR: The treatment of herpes simplex virus epithelial keratitis, *Trans Am Ophthalmol Soc* 98:505-532, 2000.
57. Wutzler P: Antiviral therapy of herpes simplex and varicella-zoster virus infections, *Intervirology* 40:343-356, 1997.
58. Yamaguchi H, Abe S, Tokuda Y: Immunomodulating activity of antifungal drugs, *Ann NY Acad Sci* 685:447-457, 1993.
59. Zegarelli DJ: Fungal infections of the oral cavity, *Otolaryngol Clin North Am* 26:1069-1089, 1993.

General References

Brown TJ, Vander-Straten M, Tyring SK: Antiviral agents, *Dermatol Clin* 19:23-34, 2001.

Goldschmidt RH, Moy A: Antiretroviral drug treatment for HIV/AIDS, *Am Fam Phys* 54:574-580, 1996.

Kirkpatrick CH: Chronic mucocutaneous candidiasis, *Pediatr Infect Dis J* 20:197-206, 2001.

Lewis RE, Kontoyiannis DP: Rationale for combination antifungal therapy, *Pharmacotherapy* 21:149S-164S, 2001.

CHAPTER • 41

Immunotherapy

John A. Yagiela and Kenneth T. Miyasaki

Immunopharmacology is the study of the interaction between drugs and the immune system. Immunotherapy is the application of clinical strategies—based partly on this discipline and partly on other disciplines, such as radiology and gene therapy—to modulate the activities of certain components of the immune system. This chapter reviews the immune system with regard to the pathways toward adaptive, specific immunity that are or can be targeted for immunotherapy and discusses immunotherapeutic strategies that are of clinical importance today or show promise for the future. The pharmacologic manipulation of innate immune mechanisms involved in inflammation is covered in Chapters 21 and 35.

OVERVIEW OF SPECIFIC IMMUNITY

Components of the Immune System

Research in immunology has progressed rapidly over the last three decades. Spanning this period, major technologic feats (such as the development of hybridomas for the production of monoclonal antibodies) and major strides in our understanding of the immune system (including elucidation of cytokines and intracellular signaling) have resulted in significant advances in immunotherapeutics. Today immunopharmacologists use these new insights to pinpoint therapeutic targets among (1) a constellation of cytokines and other factors that influence cellular growth, differentiation, and function and (2) a myriad of receptors responsive to these mediators, specific antigens, or ligands found on other cells.

Cells

Although immunity involves almost every cell of the body, immunology focuses on the myeloid and lymphoid cells, which arise from a common pluripotent stem cell precursor in the bone marrow (Figure 41-1). In the bone marrow, myeloid progenitors differentiate into red blood cells, platelets, eosinophils, basophils, neutrophils, monocytes, and dendritic cells. Lymphoid progenitors differentiate into natural killer (NK) cells, (pre-)T cells, and B cells. The various cell types exit the bone marrow at different levels of maturation, circulate through the bloodstream, and may take up residence in specific tissues. Well-differentiated cells involved in the body's defense system provide rapid responses, whereas less mature cells support slower, adaptive responses. Neutrophils and NK cells exit the bone marrow in a relatively mature state and require very little time to respond to extracellular and intracellular changes, respectively. In contrast, monocytes, dendritic cells, and most lymphoid cells leave the bone marrow in a relatively "youthful" state and complete their maturation at some other tissue site, where they can adapt to local cues.

T cells exit the bone marrow as "pre-T" cells before entering the thymus. The large majority of T cells die in the thymus, where they are believed to undergo apoptosis. Initially, T cells that cannot express functional T-cell antigen receptors (TCRs) die. Surviving T cells differentiate into two major T-cell subpopulations expressing different surface proteins designated as *CD4* and *CD8* according to the cluster of differentiation (CD) classification of leukocyte antigens. Subsequently, those T cells that bind and react too strongly to self-antigens are also culled. The remaining T cells (both CD4+ and CD8+ subtypes) differentiate further outside the thymus into several phenotypes: TH1, TH2, and TH3. (The descriptor "TH0" is used to indicate activated T cells that have yet to differentiate.) These cell types are functionally distinguished by the different cytokines they synthesize. TH1 T cells produce cytokines that stimulate the proliferation and differentiation of lymphocytes (including T, B, and NK cells) important in immunity against intracellular changes, referred to inaccurately as "cell-mediated immunity" (CMI). Cytokines released by TH2 T cells stimulate lymphocytes important in immunity against extracellular changes, referred to inaccurately as "humoral immunity." TH3 T cells play an important role in the quiescence of the immune response and production of antiinflammatory immunoglobulin (Ig) A antibodies important in secretory immunity. TH0 T cells produce TH1, TH2, and TH3 cytokines.

Receptors and other cell-surface proteins

Cells involved in specific immunity express a variety of surface glycoproteins to help coordinate their functions and interactions. These glycoproteins include receptors that respond to specific antigens and receptors that combine with other environmental cues, including co-receptors and costimulatory receptors expressed by other cells.

Clonally distributed antigen-specific receptors Adaptive immune responses involve cellular differentiation (occasionally with cellular proliferation) in response to local factors. Imprecisely, immunologists use the term *adaptive immunologic responses* interchangeably with *specific responses.* The hallmark of a specific response is immunologic memory, which forms the basis of vaccinations. Immunologic memory results from clonal expansion (and the long-term maintenance of antigenic challenge by certain cells in the lymph nodes); that is, the cells that proliferate (and increase their numbers approximately 100- to 5000-fold) in response to an antigen possess clonally distributed receptors specific against that antigen. Clonal

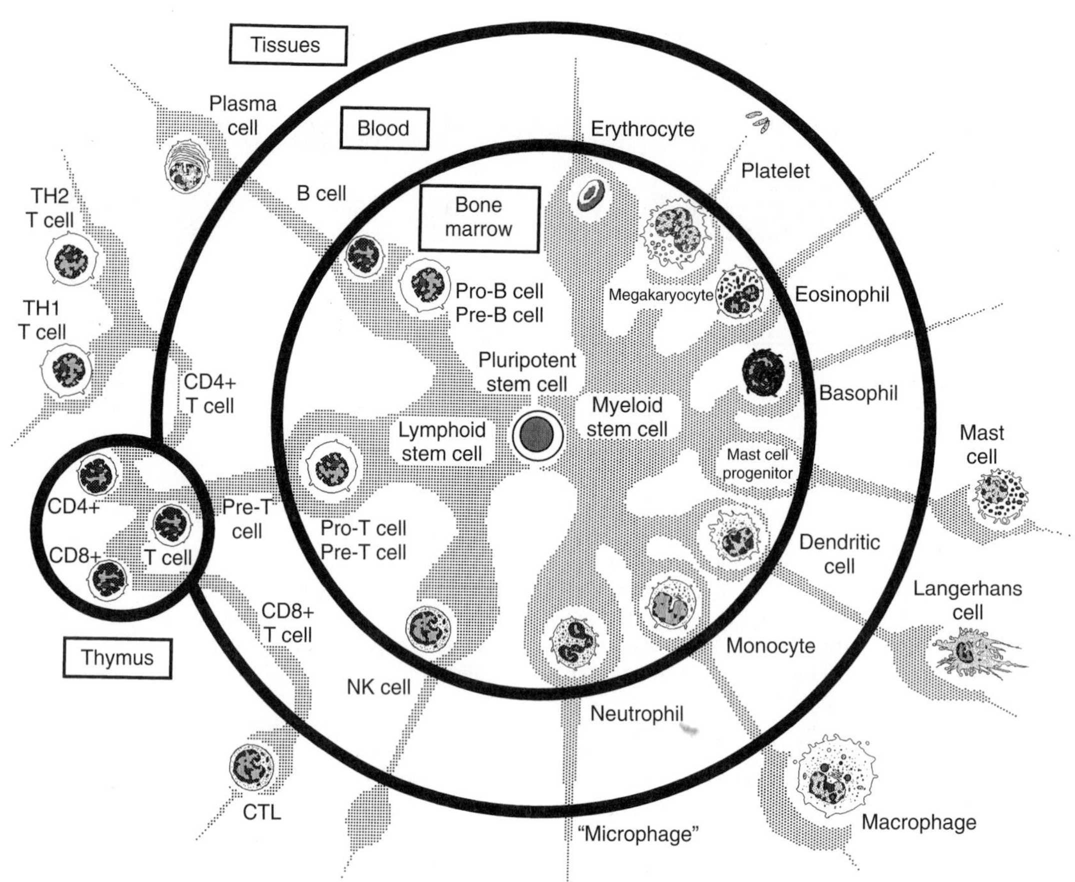

Fig. 41-1 Lineage and location of blood cells and other cells involved in the immune response. Differentiative and proliferative events are indicated by shading.

distribution means that only a small fraction of cells exhibit the antigen-specific receptor.

Only T cells and B cells possess receptors that specifically recognize the antigen and are distributed in a clonal manner. These receptors, both members of the immunoglobulin superfamily are, respectively, the TCR mentioned previously and the B-cell antigen receptor (BCR). Modified versions of the BCR constitute the immunoglobulins found in plasma, extracellular fluid, and secretions. Both the BCR and TCR recognize short oligomeric sequences of a molecule and thus exhibit primary sequence specificity. Additionally, the BCR (but not the TCR), which is designed to react with unprocessed antigen, may recognize secondary, tertiary, and quaternary structural features.

Nonclonally distributed antigen-binding receptors Most cells possess receptors that bind antigen specifically but are not clonally distributed. These receptors are members of the immunoglobulin superfamily and include two classes of proteins encoded within the major histocompatability gene complex (MHC). The MHC class I and MHC class II molecules recognize oligomeric peptides derived from proteins that have been processed. MHC class I and class II molecules do not discriminate the entire primary structure of the peptide, but instead recognize two (or more) "anchor" positions in the peptide separated by a short sequence of amino acids of virtually any composition or sequence. The term *human leukocyte antigen (HLA)* is used to indicate human MHC class I and class II molecules. HLA-A, HLA-B, and HLA-C, important determinants in tissue typing for organ transplantation, are MHC class I molecules; HLA-DR, HLA-DP, and HLA-DQ are MHC class II molecules.

Other cell surface glycoproteins Lymphocytes express various cell-surface glycoproteins depending on their lineage and maturation. Many of these glycoproteins, such as CD4 and CD8, also belong to the immunoglobulin superfamily; others are integrins or other glycoproteins. Some members of the immunoglobulin superfamily (e.g., CD3) support signal transduction after antigen recognition by T cells and B cells; others, including intercellular adhesion molecule-1, are present on endothelium and on antigen-presenting cells and participate in important activities such as transendothelial migration and "immune synapse" formation.

Mediators

Numerous water-soluble proteins affect or create specific immune reactions. Two principal groups of interest in immunotherapy are the cytokines and humoral antibodies.

Cytokines Cytokines are produced by a wide variety of cells. They play crucial roles in stimulating the production of blood cells of all types and in regulating the differentiation, activation, and suppression of cells involved in specific immunity. Some cytokines are referred to as *interleukins;* cytokines also include the chemokines, interferons, and blood cell colony–stimulating factors.

An important feature of cytokine action is that multiple cytokines often work in concert to foster a particular change in cellular activity. For example, the proliferation and differentiation of effector T cells important in CMI depend on the interplay of TH1 cytokines such as interleukin (IL)-2, IL-12, and interferon-γ (IFN-γ). Activation of B cells for humoral immunity is based on the release of several interleukins (IL-4, IL-5, IL-10, and IL-13) by TH2 T cells. TH3 T cells release transforming growth factor γ (TGF-γ). Note that TH1 cytokines are important in stimulating B-cell differentiation leading to the production of immunoglobulins IgG1, IgG2, and IgG3. TH2 cytokines stimulate IgE and IgG4 production, and the TH3 cytokine TGF-γ is important for IgA. The actions of selected cytokines are summarized in Table 41-1.

Humoral antibodies Immunoglobulin antibodies synthesized and released by plasma cells directly mediate humoral immunity. As shown in Figure 41-2, the basic immunoglobulin structure consists of two heavy and two light chains covalently linked by interchain disulfide bonds. Both chains consist of two or more domains, each defined by a single intrachain disulfide bond. The heavy chain is composed of three or four constant domains and one variable domain. The light chain incorporates one constant and one variable domain. The relatively flexible hinge regions found in certain immunoglobulins are believed to be remnants of primordial constant domains. Terminal sequences on the amino end of each chain make up the variable regions of the molecule. Within each variable region are hypervariable sequences that are responsible for specific antigen binding.

Immunoglobulins are classified into nine isotypes—IgM, IgD, IgG1, IgG2, IgG3, IgG4, IgE, IgA1, and IgA2—based on differences within the carboxyl terminal domains of the heavy chains. These domains form the Fc region of the molecule (Fc is the "crystallizable fragment" of a polyclonal immunoglobulin). The Fc region dictates the specific binding of each isotype to the different Fc receptors on phagocytes, mast cells, and other cells involved in inflammatory reactions. The Fc region also dictates complement activation by IgG and IgM.

IgM predominates in neonates and during initial, or primary, immune responses to antigenic challenges. IgG, IgA, and IgE are important in responses to antigens on secondary exposure. Because of an extended half-life (approximately 21 days), IgG comprises approximately 75% of circulating immunoglobulins. IgG is the principal opsonic antibody important for phagocytosis; thus it plays a central role in immune responses against submucosal antigens. Fc receptors for IgG are found on neutrophils, monocytes, and dendritic cells.

On a daily basis, approximately three times more IgA is produced than all other immunoglobulins combined. The IgA isotype predominates in salivary and mucous secretions, is important in mucosal immunity, and caries immunology. IgA and IgM are bound by the polymeric immunoglobulin receptor (pIgR), which is not within the Fc receptor family. Found on the basolateral surface of ductal epithelial and intestinal epithelial cells, the pIgR enables the two immunoglobulins to be transported by transcytosis across the epithelium and into secretions. IgA is important in specific immunity against supramucosal antigens and in antiinflammatory reactions below the mucosa. Although circulatory IgA production is equal to that of IgG, it has a shorter half-life (approximately 7 days) than IgG and thus a lower plasma concentration.

IgE is evolutionarily related to IgG in that both trace their immediate ancestry to IgY, the predominating inflammatory immunoglobulin found in all vertebrates except mammals. IgE is bound with extremely high affinity by Fc receptors found on mast cells and basophils; it is important in immediate inflammation (which, in turn, is important in initiating acute and chronic inflammation). IgE is also bound by low-affinity receptors present on eosinophils and enables these cells to exert antihelmintic and antiparasitic effects. IgE production is tightly controlled.

The role of IgD is less clear; it is not a secondary response antibody because it can be coexpressed with IgM on a single B cell. IgD and IgM mRNA is produced as a single transcript. Posttranscriptional modifications dictate whether IgM or IgD will be translated. IgD is believed to prevent the induction of B-cell tolerance, which can occur in B cells expressing IgM alone. Fc receptors for IgD have been found on T cells.

Each plasma cell produces a unique antibody because of the clonal distribution of the BCR. Initially, the differentiation

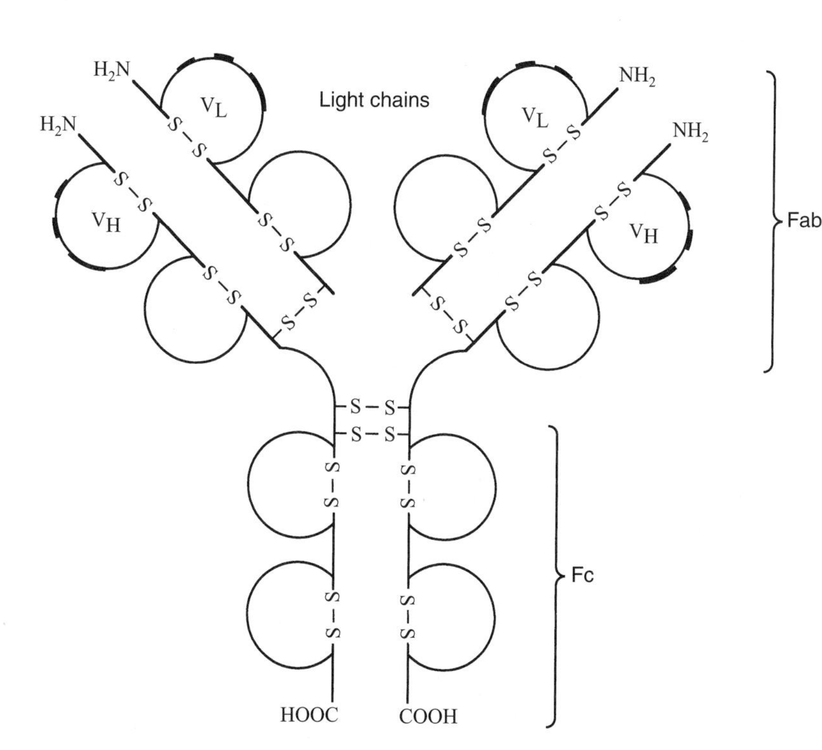

Fig. 41-2 Diagram of an IgG antibody, including disulfide linkages. The "crystallization fragment" *(Fc)* of the molecule, formed by portions of the two heavy chains, contains the binding sites for specific cells and for complement; the "antibody fragment" *(Fab)*, which consists of the two light chains and the remaining portions of the heavy chains, includes the variable regions (V_L and V_H, respectively) that participate in antibody binding. The hypervariable sequences of the variable regions are shown as thickened segments.

Table • 41-1

Selected Cytokines and Their Functional Relationships

CYTOKINE	SECRETED BY	FUNCTIONS
Lymphoid Hematopoiesis		
IL-7	SC	Lymphopoietin-1 Growth of pro-B and pre-B cells Growth of $CD4^-$ and $CD8^-$ T cells
T-Cell—Stimulating Factors		
IL-1 (α and β)	APC, B, Ep, En	Upregulation of IL-2 receptors on T cells Fever (endogenous pyrogen) Bone resorption (OAF)
IFN-α	B, Ma	Death of virus-infected cells Isotype switching Upregulation of MHC class II Ag
IFN-β	Fb, Ep	Same as for IFN-α
IFN-γ	T	Same as for IFN-α Upregulation of IL-2 receptors
IL-2	T	T-cell proliferation and formation of cytotoxic T lymphocytes
IL-10	T, B	T-cell proliferation Inhibition of cytokine synthesis by TH1 cells Cofactor for mast cell growth Increased B-cell expression of MHC class II molecules
B-Cell—Stimulating Factors		
IL-4	T	Activation of resting B cells Isotype switching (IgG1 and IgE)
IL-5	T	B-cell proliferation Isotype switching (IgA, IgM) Eosinophil differentiation factor
IL-6	T, M, Fb	B-cell proliferation Death of virus-infected cells
IL-13	CD4+ T	Monocytes assume dendritic features Stimulation of B-cell differentiation
Tumor Killers and Cell-Mediated Immunity		
TNF-α	Ma	Death of tumor cells Related to IFN-γ and TNF-β Promotion of healing Angiogenesis
TNF-β	T	Death of tumor cells (lymphotoxin)
IL-12β		Stimulation of TH1 cells and CMI Inhibition of TH2 cells and IgE production
Myeloid Factors		
IL-3	L, My	Multiple granulocytic cell type CSF
IL-8	Ma, En	Neutrophil (and lymphocyte) chemotaxis Granulocyte differentiation cofactor
IL-9	T	Erythroid cell precursor growth Mast cell growth
IL-11	SC	Megakaryocyte growth and differentiation
GM-CSF	L, My	Granulocyte/monocyte CSF
M-CSF	L, My	Monocyte CSF
G-CSF	L, My	Granulocyte/erythroid cell CSF
Erythropoietin	RC	Erythroid growth and differentiation

This summary table is not intended to provide a complete listing of all the biologic functions of the cytokines, but rather to point out the relationships among them.
APC, Antigen-presenting cell; *B,* B cell; *CSF,* colony-stimulating factor; *En,* endothelial cell; *Ep,* epithelial cell; *Fb,* fibroblast; *G,* granulocyte; *L,* lymphoid cell; *M,* monocyte; *Ma,* macrophage; *My,* myeloid cell; *OAF,* osteoclast-activating factor; *RC,* renal cortex; *SC,* stromal cell; *T,* T cell; *TNF,* tumor necrosis factor.

of B cells to plasma cells results in the production of IgM antibodies. If antigen has also been presented to CD4+ T cells by the B cells, the T cells can then guide B-cell differentiation along the memory pathway as opposed to the plasma cell differentiation pathway. In the memory pathway, the isotype may change. Thus secondary antigen exposure can elicit IgA, IgG, or IgE production. This process of isotype switching promotes a more appropriate interplay of antibodies with complement and with myeloid immune cells (e.g., neutrophils, monocytes, mast cells, and eosinophils).

B cells can also undergo somatic hypermutation along the memory pathway. This process results in point mutations within the variable domains of the BCR of a single B-cell clone. As the antigen concentration diminishes, B-cell clones possessing antibodies of the highest affinity are selected. Thus secondary exposure to the same antigen elicits antibodies that can be effective at greatly reduced concentrations.

Initiation, Progression, and Termination of Specific Immune Responses

The immune system is normally engaged in the homeostatic regulation of host-derived antigens. In addition, the immune system occasionally participates in its more widely appreciated inflammatory function known as the *immune response.* Immune responses are the measurable alterations in immune system activity after an antigenic perturbation. They are usually initiated by an immediate inflammatory reaction resulting from the activation of soluble factors (such as complement) found within the extracellular fluid or mediators released by resident leukocytes, especially the mast cell. The immediate inflammatory response signals postcapillary venule endothelial cells to recruit the appropriate acute- or chronic-phase leukocytes from the blood. Initially recruited are cells that do not need to progress through proliferation or differentiation to exert an effect, such as neutrophils. Hence, neutrophils are the predominant cell in acute inflammation. Acute inflammation may be followed by slower, chronic inflammation involving less mature cells capable of adaptive cellular differentiation (with or without proliferation). The proliferation and differentiation of clones of cells that recognize the antigen specifically constitute the specific immune response.

Specific immune responses involve a series of events (Figure 41-3), each of which offers a potential site for immunotherapeutic intervention. Included in this series are antigen processing and presentation, T-cell selection, lymphocyte differentiation, effector function, and shutdown. These events occur in response to changes in the concentrations of antigens both intracellularly and extracellularly.

Antigen processing

Antigen processing is the partial degradation of polymeric antigens into oligomeric units (especially the degradation of a protein into small peptides), which are subsequently bound by MHC class I or class II molecules. Various hydrophobic peptides and glycolipids can be bound by CD1 antigens, which are related to the MHC class I and II molecules.

Intracellular antigens Processing of intracellular antigens generated within the endoplasmic reticulum or cytosol occurs continuously in all cells. Processing is initiated within cytosolic structures called *proteasomes* or within the endoplasmic reticulum by proteases such as signal peptidase. Some proteasomes accept proteins for degradation only if they are tagged by small polypeptides called *ubiquitin.* The peptides generated in the cytosol are transported into the endoplasmic reticulum where they are bound by nascent MHC class I molecules.

Extracellular antigens Extracellular antigens are first ingested by endocytosis before processing. The three main cells that ingest antigens are macrophages, dendritic cells, and B lymphocytes. Macrophages ingest particulate antigens, dendritic cells ingest soluble antigens, and B cells ingest soluble antigens in an antigen-specific manner. Processing occurs when lysosomes (which store hydrolytic enzymes and MHC class II molecules) fuse with endosomes to form endolysosomes. Peptides from the cleaved antigens are bound by MHC class II molecules within the endolysosomes.

Antigen presentation

Vesicles formed by the Golgi apparatus (for intracellular antigens) or by remnants of the endolysosomes (for extracellular antigens) fuse with the cell membrane. As a result, oligomeric antigens bound by MHC class I or class II molecules are expressed on the surface of the antigen-presenting cell. This process of antigen presentation is the means by which changes in the antigenic environment, either extracellular or intracellular, are shown to responsive lymphocytes.

MHC class I and class II molecules require a bound peptide antigen to be expressed in a stable manner on the cell surface. Because all nucleated cells display MHC class I molecules in the absence of obvious infection, they must generally present self-derived intracellular antigens.

T-cell selection

The recognition of antigen by T cells is initiated by the adhesion of the T cell to the antigen-presenting cell. Adhesion involves several coordinated receptors, such as leukocyte function antigen-1 of the T cell and its natural ligand intercellular adhesion molecule-1 on the presenting cell. After initial binding, the T cell's CD4 or CD8 co-receptors determine the respective presence of MHC class II or MHC class I molecules. Recognition of appropriate MHC protein permits the T cell's TCRs to scan the surface of the antigen-presenting cell for peptide antigens associated with the MHC molecules. Thus CD8+ T cells recognize specific antigens associated with MHC class I molecules, and CD4+ T cells recognize specific antigens associated with MHC class II molecules. The CD4 and CD8 co-receptors also send important signals into the cell, which promote TCR signal transduction.

The actual recognition of antigen by the T-cell TCR is a low-affinity reaction. This characteristic enables many TCRs of a given T cell to interact with the few specific antigens actually presented by the antigen-presenting cell. Multiple interactions are important because T-cell activation depends on the number of TCRs that interact with antigen over time.[42] Therefore the factors that influence T-cell activation include the number of antigen molecules presented by the antigen-presenting cell, the affinity of the TCR for the antigen, and the number of TCRs. If the interaction with peptide antigen by TCRs is sufficient, the TCRs cluster on the T-cell surface and downregulate (the TCRs are probably internalized). With costimulation (described below), downregulation of approximately 4250 TCRs leads to T-cell activation.

T cells need to "see" antigen in the context of the environment to permit them to decide whether the antigen they detect is an appropriate stimulus or not. If the antigen is not presented with the proper cues, the T cell may choose to die by apoptosis. This need for "cognate recognition" is referred to as *costimulation* and involves the increased expression of relatives of the immunoglobulin superfamily, including B7-1 and B7-2 (i.e., CD80 and CD86) on the surface of the antigen-presenting cell. The immunoglobulin-like T-cell receptors for B7 molecules are CD28, which interacts initially and the closely related cytotoxic T-lymphocyte–associated antigen-4 (CTLA-4 or CD152), which is expressed after T-cell activation. In early stages of exposure to antigen, costimulatory

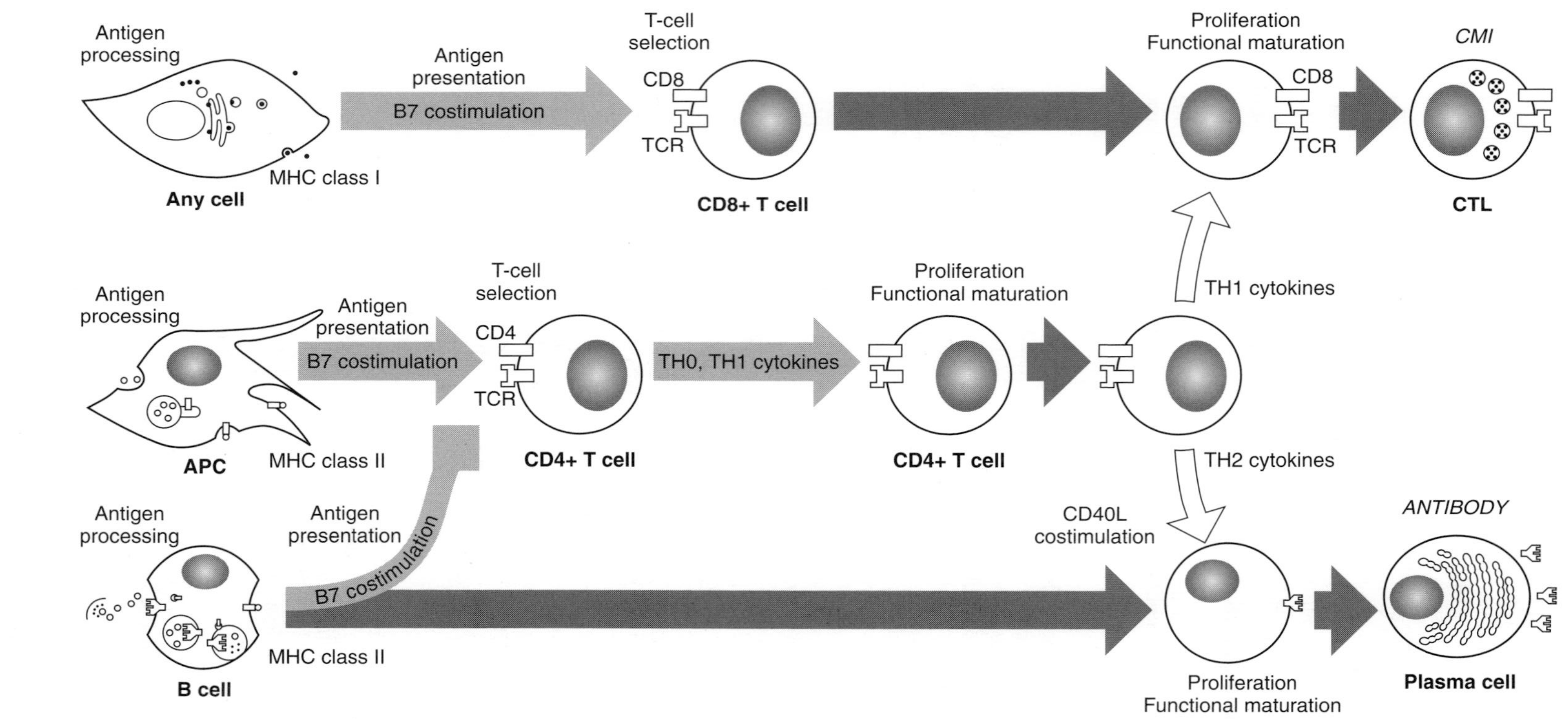

Fig. 41-3 Overview of specific immune responses. *APC,* Antigen-presenting cell; *CTL,* cytotoxic T lymphocyte.

signals permit T cells to become receptive to differentiative signals, allowing them to proliferate or mature in functionality. These signals also block apoptosis. Importantly, at later stages, the same signals can permit T cells to differentiate terminally, even to the point of death.

Differentiation

After TCR activation and costimulation, certain intracellular events allow the T cell to differentiate into either proliferative or functionally mature states (Figure 41-4). Much of present-day immunotherapy is aimed at this stage of the specific immune response. Membrane phospholipase C is activated, which leads to the production of inositol 1,4,5-trisphosphate (IP_3) and diacylglycerol. IP_3 stimulates calcium ion (Ca^{++} flux into the cytosol from the endoplasmic reticulum. A phosphorylated metabolite of IP_3 also promotes Ca^{++} entry from the external environment. In response to increases in Ca^{++}, a "calcineurin complex" is formed. It consists of three polypeptides: calcineurin A, calcineurin B, and calmodulin. The calcineurin complex dephosphorylates certain transcription-activating factors, especially the cytoplasmic component of nuclear factor of activated T cells (NF-ATc). This reaction permits the translocation of NF-ATc from the cytosol into the nucleus. Diacylglycerol meanwhile activates the cytosolic enzyme protein kinase C. Protein kinase C stimulates an increase in cytosolic pH, which ultimately leads to activation of the nuclear component of nuclear factor of activated T cells (NF-ATn). NF-ATc and NF-ATn combine to form NF-AT. In the nucleus, activating factors such as NF-AT bind to gene promoters and enhancers for a variety of cytokines.

Another nuclear factor of importance is nuclear factor κβ (NF-κβ). It is usually complexed with inhibitor proteins, called I-κβ, which prevent its translocation to the nucleus. NF-κβ is an important transcription factor for a variety of inflammatory cytokines and thus supports inflammatory aspects of the specific immune response. Tumor necrosis factor α (TNF-α), one of the cytokines whose synthesis is stimulated by both NF-AT and NF-κβ, increases the transcription of NF-κβ and its dissociation from I-κβ.

Proliferative signals stimulate the T cell to undergo "blast transformation" and proliferate and eventually to differentiate into effector cells.

Effector aspects of cell-mediated immunity

In specific CMI, both CD4+ and CD8+ T cells play important roles. CD4+ TH1 T cells receive antigen stimulation and costimulation from dendritic cells (such as the Langerhans cells). CD8+ T cells receive antigen stimulation and costimulation from infected or neoplastic cells and become primed to receive proliferative and differentiative signals from CD4+ T cells. CD8+ T cells proliferate and differentiate into cytotoxic T lymphocytes in the presence of TH1 cytokines, such as IL-2, IL-12, and IFN-γ.

Apoptosis When a cytotoxic T lymphocyte recognizes antigen in association with MHC class I molecules, it may "ask" the cell bearing the target antigen (for example, peptides derived from early viral proteins) to choose apoptosis, the pathway of death. The cytotoxic T lymphocyte does this by presenting the target cell with specific membrane-bound signals, such as Fas ligand and lymphotoxin, both of which are

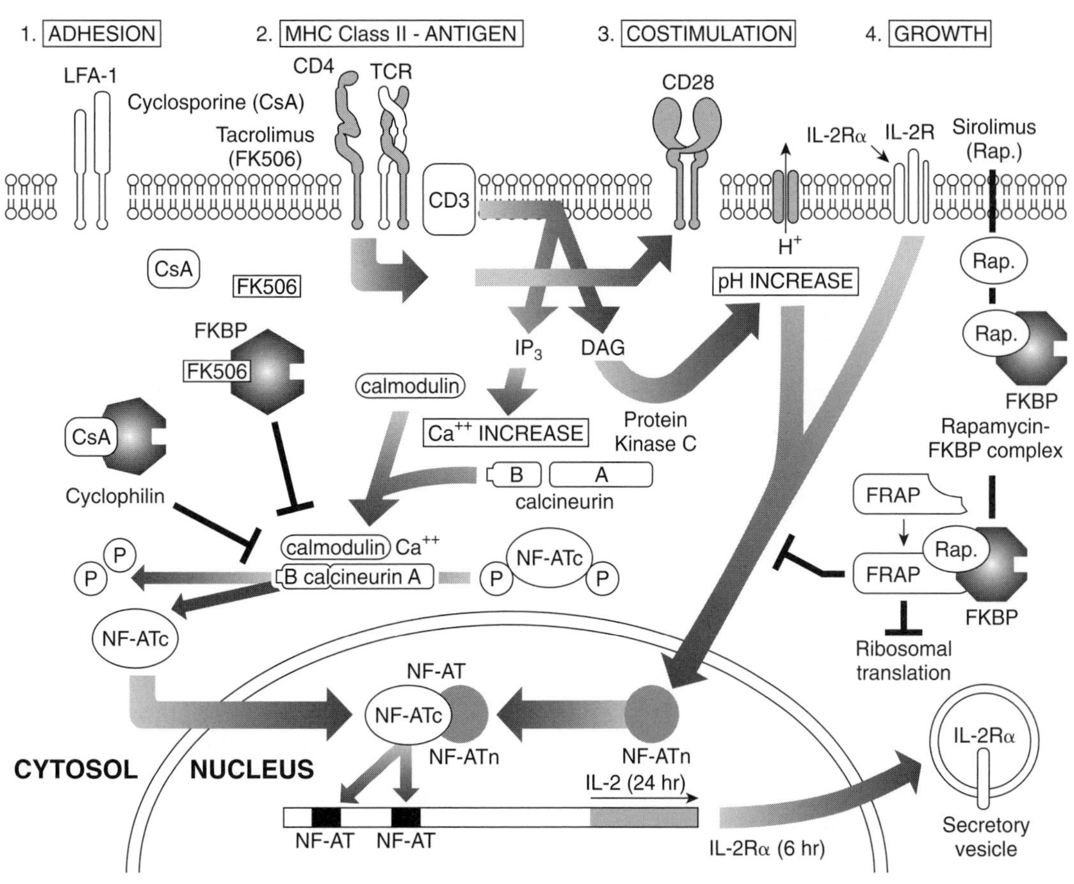

Fig. 41-4 Intracellular mediators of T-cell differentiation and its inhibition by immunosuppressant drugs. *CsA*, Cyclosporine; *DAG*, diacylglycerol; *Rap.*, sirolimus.

members of the TNF family.[22] If the signals are effective, the target cell will agree to die (for example, before the virus has a chance to express late proteins necessary for the completion of replication). Target cells express specific TNF-family receptors (TNFRs) for these signals. Apoptosis, as summarized in Figure 41-5, involves several steps that may be targeted for therapeutic intervention.

Cells possess mechanisms for preventing their untimely death by using small, integral membrane proteins, such as Bcl-2, and several inhibitor of apoptosis proteins (IAPs).[23] Bcl-2 is expressed on the membranes of intracellular organelles, including the mitochondria, nucleus, and smooth endoplasmic reticulum. Bcl-2 and IAPs delay or prevent apoptosis by inhibiting proteolysis mediated by cysteine proteases, termed *caspases*, that are responsive to apoptotic signals.[31] Several viruses (including the Epstein-Barr virus, adenovirus, the African swine fever virus, and cowpox) produce substances like Bcl-2 and IAP, which may help them evade host defenses by preventing apoptosis. Also, B-cell lymphomas have been associated with Bcl-2 overexpression. Costimulation of T cells and B cells induces the expression of apoptosis-inhibiting molecules after antigen stimulation.[7]

Cytolytic activities It is possible that a target cell will refuse to die, especially if the cell is infected by a virus that produces apoptotic inhibitors. In this case, the NK cell and the cytotoxic T lymphocyte must depend on apoptotic and cytolytic factors within their cytotoxic granules. Within the vesicular components and dense cores of these granules are numerous potentially cytocidal proteins, including perforin and granzymes A, B, and C. The vesicles and dense cores are discharged when the cytotoxic granules fuse with the plasma membrane of the NK cell or cytotoxic T lymphocyte.

Granule exocytosis can trigger several possible lethal events. One lethal mechanism is cytolysis of the target cell. Perforin can form polymeric channels in cell membranes.[26] Affected membranes lose their structural integrity, and lysis of the cell soon follows. A second possibility is circumvention of the apoptotic blockade. This outcome may occur when granzymes gain access to the target cell, either directly by fusion of the granule vesicles or dense core with the membrane of the target cell, or because a sublytic quantity of perforin allows granzymes to gain access to the cytosol of the target cell.[26] Once in the cytosol, granzyme B can activate apoptotic proteolysis.

Humoral immunity

Specific humoral immunity is initiated by the activation of antigen-specific CD4+ T cells responding to the presentation of partially digested antigen in association with MHC class II molecules and a costimulatory signal, as previously described. Once activated, CD4+ cells synthesize and release cytokines that stimulate proliferation and differentiation of antigen-specific B cells.

The BCRs of B cells bind antigens without associated MHC class I or class II molecules. B cells receive second signals that permit them to associate antigen recognition with an environmental cue. These signals have been referred to as *activators*, a vague term that includes various microbial substances (e.g., dextrans), IL-5, and a TNF family molecule called *CD40 ligand* (or *CD40L*). CD40L is expressed by activated T cells, and B cells recognize this costimulatory signal with CD40, a type of TNFR. Once the CD40-CD40L interaction has occurred, the B cell becomes receptive to memory pathway differentiative signals (i.e., T-cell-derived cytokines). Other activators can send B cells into the plasma cell differentiation pathway. Because isotype switching occurs along the memory pathway, CD40L is an important signal for isotype switching, and individuals with CD40L deficiency have hyperimmunoglobulinemia M, a disease characterized by an elevation

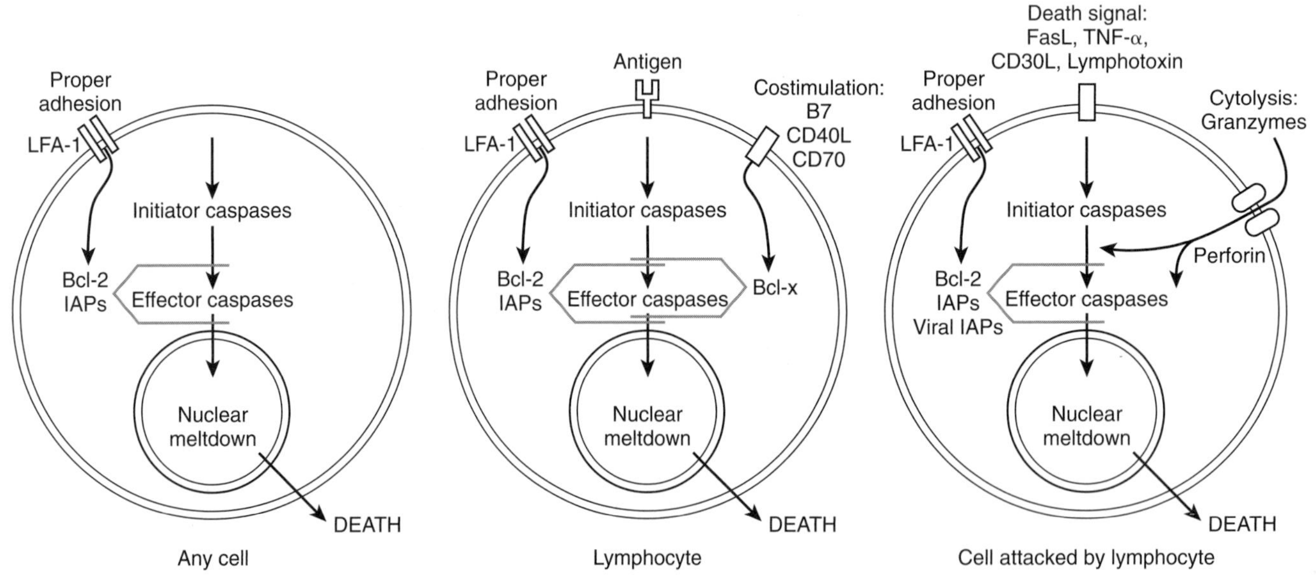

Fig. 41-5 Apoptosis and lymphocyte-induced cytolysis. Apoptosis, indicated by the sequence of *arrows*, involves the activation of initiator caspases (e.g., caspase 8), which then promotes proteolytic activation of other effector caspases involved in apoptosis. Environmental cues, such as cellular adhesion to leukocyte function antigen-1 *(LFA-1)*, help prevent programmed cellular death by invoking the blocking action of Bcl-2 and/or specific IAPs. Similar molecules (e.g., Bcl-x) inhibit apoptosis in lymphocytes costimulated by members of the tumor necrosis factor family (B7, CD40L, and CD70) and in virally infected cells. Cytotoxic lymphocytes destroy targeted cells either by (1) signaling for apoptosis to occur or (2) releasing perforins and granzymes that activate proteolysis directly. *FasL*, Fas ligand.

of IgM and a severe deficiency of almost all other isotypes. After CD40L activation, TH2 cytokines stimulate production of memory cells that express a highly inflammatory isotype, IgE (as well as IgG4). TH1 cytokines promote certain moderately inflammatory isotypes (IgG1, IgG2, and IgG3). The TH3 cytokine TGF-α results in the production of the anti-inflammatory IgA.

Differentiation along the plasma cell pathway causes the loss of the BCR, development of an extensive rough endoplasmic reticulum, and expression of soluble immunoglobulin antibodies. Soluble antibodies can neutralize microbial toxins and enzymes, prevent microbial adherence to and invasion of tissues, and lead to the clearance of microbes by activating complement or serving as an opsonin for phagocytic ingestion. Antibodies of the IgA subclass are particularly important in conferring protection to the mucosa and in the prevention of potentially deleterious "overkill" responses mediated by IgG or IgE. IgG and IgM are important in antibacterial and antifungal host defense but can also lead to type II (cytotoxic) and type III (immune complex) immunopathologic reactions (see Chapter 3). Antibodies of the IgE subclass provide host defense against parasites and worms but can also lead to type I immunopathologic reactions (anaphylaxis). On rare occasions, IgA has been associated with type II immunopathologic conditions.

The distinct functional and immunopathogenic attributes of the immunoglobulin isotypes provide another area of potential immunotherapeutic intervention.

Shutdown

Mechanisms exist to terminate immune responses when they are no longer required. These mechanisms involve the removal of effector cells that are no longer needed and the suppression of activity of remaining cells.

Propriocidal apoptosis In the later stages of antigen exposure, when the concentrations of proinflammatory cytokines are high, T cells may undergo a form of antigen-induced cell death known as *propriocidal apoptosis.* It may occur as a result of T-cell expression of different costimulatory receptors for factors such as B7 proteins. As previously mentioned, the interaction between B7 and CD28 may serve to prepare a cell for early differentiative events in the immune response (resulting in proliferation and functional maturation), but the interaction between B7 and CTLA-4 may prepare a cell for more terminal events (such as differentiation leading to death).

Suppression Suppression is involved in regulating the balance between humoral and CMI responses and in terminating these responses. The former form of suppression appears to relate to the activities of CD4+ T cells, whereas the latter form involves CD8+ T cells. CD4+ T cells of the TH1 phenotype suppress CD4+ T cells of the TH2 phenotype and directly suppress B-cell activity. CD4+ T cells of the TH2 phenotype suppress TH1 activities. CD4+ TH1 T cells also stimulate CD8+ T cells, which has been referred to as *suppressor induction*.

Classically, the CD8+ phenotype has been associated with both cytotoxicity and suppressor activity. It is becoming apparent that the CD8+ T cell's suppression mechanism can resemble its cytotoxic action. CD8+ T-cell suppression of specific humoral immunity and the termination of CMI may be accomplished with the CD30 ligand (CD30L). CD30L is a member of the TNF family recognized by CD30 (a member of the TNFR family) found on T cells. In this case, suppression results from the programmed death of the CD4+ T cell.

If there is an imbalance between TH1 and TH2 activities, or if CD8+ T-cell suppression is excessively active, immunodeficiency may occur. If suppression is insufficient, immunopathologic reactions, including autoimmunity, may ensue. Thus suppression pathways may play a role in two widely differing defective immune states often considered for immunotherapy: immunodeficiency and autoimmunity.

IMMUNOTHERAPEUTIC AGENTS

Therapies designed to stimulate or replicate endogenous immune reactions have long been used to prevent infectious disease and treat immunodeficiencies. More recently, attempts have been made to provoke immune responses to cancer, and specific antibodies have been developed for a wide range of applications.

In certain clinical situations, it is advantageous to suppress the inflammatory activities of the specific immune system temporarily. Organ transplantation is the best example of an instance in which immunosuppression is beneficial. Immunosuppression is also helpful in the treatment of autoimmune diseases and other immunopathologic conditions.

Vaccination

By far, the most successful area of immunotherapy has been vaccination, or "active immunization." It was first introduced to Western culture by Jenner in the eighteenth century, who injected individuals with the cowpox virus to protect them against smallpox. Vaccination is a procedure in which the immune system is exposed to an antigen, such as an inactivated toxin or attenuated pathogen, to elicit antigen-specific clonal expansion (i.e., the proliferation of T cells and B cells that recognize the antigen). Active immunization uses the host's immune system itself to generate antigen-specific immunotherapeutic agents (e.g., antibodies). On subsequent exposure to the actual pathogen, the immune response is of sufficient speed, magnitude, duration, and specificity to prevent the pathogen from causing disease (the secondary or anamnestic response). Clinically, most success has been observed with vaccination designed to elicit humoral immunity rather than CMI. The composition, recommended dosage, and schedule of administration of standard vaccines may be found in several references.[6,14]

Caries vaccines

One of the diseases of special interest to dentistry is dental caries. Vaccines directed against *Streptococcus mutans* and *S. sobrinus*—lactic acid bacteria long suspected of being the major cause of dental caries—have been investigated by several laboratories.[29] Their purpose was to induce an immune response that would prevent the adherence or metabolism by these bacteria on the tooth surface. Several types of vaccines have been considered, including (1) oral immunization by whole bacteria or live enteric bacteria that bear antigens of *S. mutans* as a result of recombinant DNA procedures, and (2) immunization by various routes using "subunit" vaccines containing isolated antigens (adhesins, glucosyltransferases, dextranases) believed to be involved in cell adherence and plaque formation. Whole-cell vaccines are anticariogenic in many laboratory animals, including primates.

In human beings, oral immunization results in the generation of secretory IgA antibodies in salivary secretions. Ingested antigens are subjected to partial breakdown within the stomach and small intestine. Specialized enterocytes in the gut transcytose macromolecular antigens to unencapsulated lymphoid structures known as *Peyer's patches.* Here, in the presence of TH3 T cells, antigen-specific B cells are selected to undergo IgA isotype switching. They eventually migrate to the regional lymph nodes, where they proliferate. IgA-committed progeny then enter the blood and are distributed to effector sites, such as the salivary glands, where they produce IgA antibodies for secretion.

Parenteral routes of administration usually lead to IgG antibodies that can gain access to the tooth by way of the gingival crevicular fluid. For parenteral administration, subunit vaccines are preferred because antibodies directed against lipoteichoic acid in the cell wall of *S. mutans* may cross-react with human heart muscle. Although purified antigens are effective in preventing caries in gnotobiotic rodents and lower primates, the actual antigenic components, dosage, route of administration, and potential benefits, costs, and adverse effects in human beings must be determined before a vaccine can be considered for routine use.

There are several modifications to the subunit vaccine approach that embellish traditional methods with purified bacterial antigens. For example, synthetic pieces of a larger antigen, such as glucosyltransferase, have been used as an immunogen.[37,38] Synthetic peptides derived from a glucan-binding domain of glucosyltransferase or from the amino terminus have also been used. Antisera or monoclonal antibodies raised in laboratory animals against these synthetic domains inhibit glucosyltransferase by 30% to 80%.

Antigen-delivery strategies Local immune responses can be elicited within the gingiva. The swabbing of gingiva with a 3800 da component of *S. mutans* in monkeys elicits increases in IgG in the crevicular fluid and secretory IgA in the saliva.[24] From a theoretical point of view, it is difficult to ascribe the IgA response to local (gingival) immunization rather than systemic (enteric), because some antigen must be ingested. From a therapeutic point of view, the method itself may be useful because the swabbing was administered only 10 times over the course of a year and resulted in a reduction in both *S. mutans* and caries activity.

Liposomes are artificial membrane vesicles that can be prepared to contain both hydrophilic solutes internally and hydrophobic molecules within the membrane. One method of increasing antibody responses by gingival immunization has been the sequestration of candidate antigens (i.e., glucosyltransferase) into liposomes, permitting the liposomes to desiccate, and administering the dehydrated liposomes to human beings. This technique resulted in salivary IgA2 antibodies against glucosyltransferase, suggesting that dehydrated liposomes may be useful in generating specific salivary immunity against target antigens in the oral cavity.[8]

Genetic engineering provides an especially efficient possibility for delivering a subunit vaccine. A major problem with subunit vaccines has been the inability to maintain sufficiently high amounts of antigen in the gut to stimulate antibody production in a cost-effective manner. Genes for candidate antigens of *S. mutans* have been introduced into "harmless" enteric bacteria. These bacteria can proliferate in the gut, elaborating antigen for a prolonged period of time compared with a conventional dosage form (e.g., gelatin capsules).

Antiidiotypic antibodies During an infection, the body commonly produces antibodies to its own immunoglobulins used to ward off the offending organism. These antibodies, called *antiidiotypic antibodies*, contain in their hypervariable regions a peptide sequence (idiotope) that is identical with or structurally analogous to an antigenic determinant (epitope) of the infecting microorganism. Injection of these antibodies into a host generates a second set of antiidiotypic antibodies directed against them. If the injected antibodies are the same allotype as the host, the host forms antiidiotypic antibodies against only the idiotope. These antibodies also bind to the bacterial epitope. This method can be used to elicit antibodies against virtually any antigenic target. A vaccine containing antiidiotypic antibodies with idiotopes equivalent to epitopes of streptococcal antigens has reduced caries in the gnotobiotic rat model.[21]

Adjuvants

The effects of a vaccine may be enhanced by incorporation of adjuvants, substances that increase the immune response. The mechanism of action of some adjuvants, such as alum (aluminum-containing hydroxides or phosphates), is simply to retard removal of the antigen and to attract lymphoid cells by increasing the inflammatory response (often quite severely) in the immediate area of the vaccine. Many adjuvants, such as complete Freund's adjuvant, that are effective in laboratory tests have not been cleared for routine use in human beings because they induce long-lasting necrotic lesions in the area of injection. Alum is the only adjuvant currently approved for use with vaccines (such as diphtheria and tetanus toxoids) in human beings; however, it is not active with all antigens and elicits only humoral responses. In mice, alum adjuvants selectively activate TH2 CD4+ T cells; one of the problems facing immunostimulant therapy has been devising methods to stimulate TH1 and CMI responses.

Bacillus Calmette-Guérin (BCG) is a live attenuated strain of *Mycobacterium bovis* that has been used as a vaccine against tuberculosis since the early part of the twentieth century. Like complete Freund's adjuvant, it contains mycobacterial derivatives and appears to stimulate CMI. BCG has been shown to stimulate specific tumor immunity in experimental animals, to induce responses in immunodeficient individuals, and to reverse the effects of immunosuppressive drugs. It activates macrophages that produce IL-1. In turn, IL-1 stimulates the maturation of CD4+ TH0 T cells. BCG has been used experimentally in the treatment of melanoma, hepatoma, leukemia, and bladder cancer; it may also have potential against chronic infections involving immunodeficiency. Severe allergic reactions and shock have occurred infrequently during BCG treatments. Other microbially derived immunostimulants that activate macrophages and should help trigger TH1 responses include extracts of pathogenic bacteria and fungal polysaccharides.

Quil-A is a partially purified saponin extract from plants. It forms immunostimulating complexes with cholesterol and various antigens. The complex may then intercalate into the membranes of cells, thereby introducing antigen into the cell cytosol. Both humoral immunity and CMI are stimulated by increased MHC presentation.

Enhancement of Costimulation

Because the presentation and recognition of antigen alone is not sufficient to initiate an immune response, immunotherapy has also focused on enhancement of costimulation. One method includes the antibody-mediated cross-linking of costimulatory receptors (such as CD28 and CTLA-4). It has been shown to enhance T-cell activity against tumor targets as measured by increased cytokine output. A second method involves immunization of an individual with tumor cells that have been transfected with a B7 gene plus an MHC class II gene, causing the cells to express these protein products constitutively. Such immunization has led to rejection of the tumor at a site distant from the immunization site.[5]

Immunostimulants

Thymic extracts

Primary CMI deficiencies may result from absence of the thymus gland or a defect in its function. Treatment has been directed toward inducing maturation of T cells by using thymic tissue or extracts. In several cases, thymus transplants in human beings have corrected CMI deficiencies, with sub-

sequent development of immunocompetence. Immunologically immature fetal thymic tissues are used to prevent graft-versus-host reactions.

Thymic extracts have been used nonspecifically to induce CMI competence.[3] These extracts, including thymosin, are usually extracted from calf thymus glands. They consist of a family of nonimmunogenic polypeptide hormones. Certain tumors, chronic mucocutaneous candidiasis, and several other diseases caused by primary CMI immunodeficiency have responded favorably to thymosin therapy. Thymic extracts must be administered continually. Although thymosin administration has been found to be of therapeutic benefit, it is still experimental, and routine use awaits further development.

In Europe, several peptides have been purified or synthesized for experimental use in human beings,[17] including thymostimulin, which has proved beneficial in the treatment of hepatocellular carcinoma and chronic obstructive pulmonary disease. These hormones function at different stages of CMI development, inducing the maturation of T cells or differentiation of T cells into functional effectors, such as cytotoxic or suppressor cells.

Levamisole

Levamisole is an antihelmintic drug that possesses nonspecific immunostimulatory properties. In deficient animals and human beings, it restores many different immunologic functions, suggesting that it acts on multiple populations of cells, including neutrophils, macrophages, and T cells (but not B cells). Its effects on the immune response and its pharmacologic activity indicate that levamisole is a thymomimetic agent.

Levamisole has been used in the treatment of tumors and other diseases in which there are manifestations of immune dysfunction, including rheumatoid arthritis and Crohn's disease. Several investigators have used it successfully in the treatment of recurrent aphthous stomatitis and herpes labialis. It has been suggested that the therapeutic effect of levamisole in aphthous stomatitis, which may have an autoimmune etiology, results from enhancement of suppressor T cells that normally prevent autoimmune responses.[25] It is currently approved for use in the United States as an adjunct to fluorouracil in the treatment of colorectal carcinoma.

Polyclonal Antibody Preparations

Human immune globulins

Deficiencies in humoral immunity may result from congenital defects in the production of all or selected immunoglobulin classes, or they may be acquired, as occurs with multiple myeloma. Severe deficiencies in humoral immunity, or hypogammaglobulinemias, require "replacement therapy" consisting of weekly or monthly injections of pooled human immunoglobulins, the dose and frequency depending on the patient's status. These treatments are often accompanied by antibiotics. Selective isotype deficiencies involving individual classes of immunoglobulins are usually less severe because the body may compensate by increased production of other immunoglobulin classes. Selective isotype deficiencies also can be treated with immunoglobulins.

Human immune globulin is effective against many common diseases, such as measles and infectious hepatitis, because it is derived from the pooled sera of many individuals, including some who would have contracted these infections in the past and produced protective antibodies against them. Although immunopathologic reactions are possible with allogenic human immunoglobulins, they are much less a problem than with xenogeneic immunoglobulins, and the risk is greatly minimized by using purified or partially purified IgG. In contrast to most other pooled blood products, human immune globulin carries no known risk of human immunodeficiency virus (HIV) or hepatitis B transmission. Intravenous, rather than intramuscular, administration of immunoglobulins is preferable because much larger doses can be infused.[34]

Antisera or purified immunoglobulins may be administered to prevent or treat specific diseases. In some cases, this is referred to as *passive immunization*, a classic term in immunology used to indicate that a donor was immunized with an antigen and that a recipient host was then injected with the protective antibodies generated by the donor. The injection of antibody obtained from an immune donor into a nonimmune recipient has the advantage of conferring almost instantaneous protection, as opposed to vaccines, which require days or weeks to stimulate a sufficient protective effect. However, the effects of passive immunization last only 4 to 6 weeks (equivalent to one to two half-lives of IgG in vivo). Human immune globulin preparations specifically directed against hepatitis B, cytomegalovirus, rabies, tetanus, infant botulism, respiratory syncytial virus, and varicella-zoster virus are available.

Rho(D) immune globulin

Rho(D) immune globulin represents a special case in which passive immunization is used to induce specific immunosuppression for the prevention of Rh disease. Rh disease occurs when an Rh-negative woman—one whose red blood cells do not contain the $Rh_o(D)$ antigen—becomes sensitized to the antigen by exposure to the blood of her Rh-positive fetus. On subsequent pregnancies, the mother's anti-Rh antibody passes through the placenta and causes massive destruction of fetal erythrocytes, resulting in hemolytic disease of the newborn.

The injection of anti-Rh antibody into Rh-negative mothers who will give birth to Rh-positive children is effective in preventing the disorder. The goal of treatment is to prevent mothers from generating anti-$Rh_o(D)$ antibodies. High titers of specific antibody against an antigen specifically inhibit the immune response to that antigen, but the mechanism may be more involved than simple binding of the antigenic stimulus. For example, the injection of anti-$Rh_o(D)$ antibodies may induce the mother to generate a set of antibodies against the variable domains of the injected antibodies. This second set of anti-idiotypic antibodies may impede the interaction of B cells with Rh antigen, cause B-cell inactivation or death, or neutralize anti-$Rh_o(D)$–specific antibodies as they are generated. Such idiotypic-antiidiotypic inhibitory effects have been demonstrated in laboratory animals. Alternatively, anti-$Rh_o(D)$ antibody may lead to rapid clearance of fetal red blood cells from the mother's circulation by liver macrophages, which would prevent the elicitation of chronic inflammatory reactions necessary for antibody responses.

Antiserum to the Rh antigen is produced in Rh-negative male volunteers. The γ-globulin fraction containing anti-Rh antibody, in the form of $Rh_o(D)$ immune globulin (human), must be given within hours of parturition because the fetal erythrocytes carrying the Rh antigen enter the mother's body at this time and induce the immune response that will cause problems in subsequent pregnancies. This specific immunosuppressive treatment has been very successful in preventing Rh disease, and it is now used routinely.

Antitoxins and antivenins

Immunoglobulin preparations that neutralize toxic compounds, such as rattlesnake venom and diphtheria toxin, are commonly derived from the sera of horses actively immunized against the noxious substances. The regional availability of these xenogeneic antibody products varies widely depending on the perceived risk of exposure. Therefore being bitten by

a poisonous animal outside its normal geographic range can delay the administration of the immunoglobulin antidote and increase the risk of injury or death.

If administered parenterally, xenogeneic (or even allogenic) sera or immunoglobulins may induce immunity in the recipient against animal (or human, respectively) serum antigens. Not only would this lead to rapid clearance of the antibodies—and therefore circumvent their therapeutic effect—it can induce type III immunopathologic reactions such as serum sickness or immune complex disease.

Oral administration of xenogeneic antibodies

The oral administration of xenogeneic antibodies offers one possible strategy for highly precise, cost-effective immunotherapeutics. For example, cows immunized against cariogenic bacteria exhibit antibodies against those bacteria in their milk. The milk (or whey) can confer protection to individuals consuming that milk in a passive manner. In cows' milk and colostrum, the antibodies are of the IgG1 subclass. Both *S. mutans* and caries scores can be reduced in this manner in gnotobiotic animals.[29] Whey from immunized cows also appears to decrease *S. mutans* in human volunteers when it is used as a mouth rinse.

Antithymocyte globulin

Antithymocyte globulin is produced in rabbits and horses by immunization with human thymocytes. It lyses or agglutinates human lymphocytes in vitro and produces lymphocytopenia in vivo. CMI responses are decreased and allograft survival is prolonged. Antithymocyte globulin is rich in cytotoxic antibodies directed against a number of antigens expressed by T cells, including CD2, CD3, CD4, CD8, CD11a, CD18, CD25, CD44, CD45, and HLA class I and II molecules. The immunosuppressive effects are transient, and antithymocyte globulin must be given repeatedly. However, because the preparation is itself antigenic, it can induce an immune response leading to serum sickness. The agent's primary indication is suppression of acute transplant rejection reactions.

Monoclonal Antibody Preparations

A monoclonal antibody (MAb) is an antibody of a single specificity produced by cells derived from a single B-cell clone. In most cases, the MAb is derived from mice (and is therefore xenogeneic). Fusion of a normal mouse plasma cell and a myeloma cell results in the formation of a hybridoma with the antibody-forming properties of the plasma cell and the proliferative properties of the myeloma cell.[16] When grown in tissue culture, hybridomas are capable of almost unlimited production of MAb. MAbs are increasingly being used diagnostically to assess immunocompetence, to identify infectious diseases, and to monitor the concentrations of hormones and chemotherapeutic agents in the plasma. Some are used as immunosuppressive agents. Their exquisite specificity also makes them ideal guidance systems as carriers for cytotoxic agents (described below). Table 41-2 lists clinically available MAbs and derivatives, their target antigens, and their principal therapeutic indications.

Muromonab-CD3, the first monoclonal antibody to be approved for human use (in 1986), is a mouse MAb that reacts with CD3, a component of the TCR complex (see Figure 41-4). Antibody binding induces internalization of the TCR. Sensitive T cells die in response to complement activation; other T cells redistribute to nonlymphoid tissues and become significantly less responsive to antigenic challenge. Muromonab-CD3 is highly effective in terminating acute cellular rejection episodes. The major adverse effect of therapy, known as the *cytokine release syndrome,* develops from the stimulation of Fc receptors by CD3-bound MAb. Affected T cells release TNF-α, IL-2, and other cytokines, causing high fever, chills, nausea and vomiting, malaise, weakness, and

Table • 41-2

Monoclonal Antibodies and Related Agents in Clinical Use

NONPROPRIETARY (GENERIC) NAME	PROPRIETARY (TRADE) NAME	RECEPTOR/TARGET	THERAPEUTIC INDICATION
Abciximab	ReoPro	GPIIb/IIIa	Prevent platelet aggregation in unstable angina or percutaneous cutaneous intervention
Adalimumab	Humira	TNF-α	Refractory rheumatoid arthritis
Alefacept	Amevive	CD2	Chronic plaque psoriasis (moderate-severe)
Alemtuzumab	Campath	CD52	B-cell chronic lymphocytic leukemia
Basiliximab	Simulect	IL-2	Prevention of renal allograft rejection
Daclizumab	Zenapax	IL-2	Prevention of renal allograft rejection
Digoxin immune Fab	Digibind	Digoxin	Serious digoxin toxicity
Efalizumab	Raptiva	CD11a	Plaque psoriasis (moderate-severe)
Etanercept	Enbrel	TNF	Refractory rheumatoid arthritis Psoriatic arthritis
Gemtuzumab ozogamicin	Mylotarg	CD33	Relapsed acute myeloid leukemia
Ibritumomab tiuxetan	Zevalin	CD20	Non-Hodgkin's lymphoma
Infliximab	Remicade		Refractory rheumatoid arthritis Refractory Crohn's disease
Muromonab-CD3	Orthoclone OKT3	CD3	Acute graft rejection
Palivizumab	Synagis	RSV F protein	Prevention of RSV disease
Rituximab	Rituxan	CD20	Non-Hodgkin's lymphoma
Tositumomab and iodine I 131 tositumomab	Bexxar	CD20	Non-Hodgkin's lymphoma
Trastuzumab	Herceptin	HER2	Metastatic breast cancer

RSV, Respiratory syncytial virus.

generalized pain. The syndrome usually begins within 30 minutes of drug injection, lasts for hours, and rarely may produce life-threatening cardiovascular and pulmonary disturbances. Repeated MAb treatment may lead to the development of human antimouse antibodies that block the therapeutic effect or sensitize the patient to the drug.

Chimeric antibodies

The most important factor that limits the therapeutic potential of MAbs as a group is their xenogeneic origin, and clinical testing of these reagents has led to some disappointment. One approach to circumvent this problem has been to combine the antigen-specific portions of mouse MAbs with human constant or framework domains. Chimeric MAbs, which represent the second generation of MAbs, are produced by the grafting of the variable regions of rodent immunoglobulin to the constant regions of human immunoglobulin (see Figure 41-2). Because the constant region of an immunoglobulin also confers function to an antibody, chimeric MAb engineering permits the selection of functional attributes. For example, a chimeric MAb possessing an IgG1 isotype constant region will be most effective in complement activation and antibody-dependent cell-mediated cytotoxicity, whereas a chimeric antibody of the IgA subclass may exhibit antiinflammatory effects.

Basiliximab is a chimeric MAb used to prevent allograft rejection in patients receiving other immunosuppressants. It is directed against the α subunit of the IL-2 receptor on activated T cells (see Figure 41-4). IL-2 is a major cytokine supporting CMI and organ rejection. In general, the drug is only administered twice; the first dose is infused intravenously within 2 hours before transplantation surgery and the second is given 4 days later. The only adverse events attributable to basiliximab used in this manner are rare cases of allergic reactions and cytokine release syndrome.

Complementarity-defining region-grafted (humanized) antibodies

Although chimeric MAbs may seem rather exotic, they are being replaced by a third-generation MAb, the complementarity-defining region (CDR)–grafted MAb, more simply known as the "humanized" MAb. *CDR* refers to the hypervariable peptide sequences of an antibody that actually bind to an antigen. These hypervariable regions are joined by intervening framework sequences. A CDR-grafted MAb contains rodent hypervariable sequences, human framework sequences, and human constant regions. There is some loss of affinity in humanized MAbs, but it is usually an acceptable tradeoff for the reduced allergenicity. Humanized MAbs are used clinically to prevent rejection of organ transplants. Other diseases in which CDR-grafted MAbs have been used include rheumatoid arthritis, Crohn's disease, systemic vasculitis, septic shock, various neoplasms, and viral infections.[44]

Daclizumab is a humanized variant of basiliximab. As expected daclizumab is somewhat less potent than basiliximab in binding to the α subunit of the IL-2 receptor. A one-time five-dose regimen is used, with the first dose given within 24 hours before transplantation surgery and subsequent doses every 14 days thereafter. As yet, no adverse reactions have been reported for this use of daclizumab.

Immunotoxins and radioimmunotherapy

Immunotoxins are antibodies coupled with a poison (toxin). Toxins may be derived from a number of sources, including plants and microbes (e.g., the lectin ricin, *Pseudomonas* exotoxin, diphtheria toxin). The therapeutic strategy is to have the antibody selectively deliver the toxin to undesirable cells, such as those infected by HIV-1, or participate in immunopathologic reactions. Immunotoxins have also been explored for their potential in cancer immunotherapy (including metastatic melanoma; colorectal, ovarian, and breast carcinomas; non-Hodgkin's lymphoma; Hodgkin's disease; B-cell leukemia; and T-cell lymphoma) and immune suppression in steroid-resistant graft-versus-host disease. Although immunotoxins have been called "magic bullets" capable of pinpoint target destruction, it has become clear that most of these bullets are not as accurate as desired and have significant side effects, including vascular leak syndrome, myalgia, aphasia, paresthesia, encephalopathy, neuropathy, thrombocytopenia, liver destruction, renal insufficiency, proteinuria, hypoalbuminemia, dyspnea, hematuria, and tremors. Moreover, the toxins themselves have proved quite antigenic, eliciting immune reactions in most cases. Gemtuzumab ozogamicin is the first immunotoxin to be approved for clinical use. It combines the anti-CD33 antibody gemtuzumab with the anticancer agent ozogamicin.[1] When the agent binds its antigen receptor, it is internalized. The active agent is then released to kill the cell. The drug is approved for treatment of acute myeloid leukemia.

Immunotoxins have not been explored aggressively as therapeutic agents delivered locally in the oral cavity. Such a strategy might be used to eliminate pathogens selectively or reduce inflammatory activities of the host immune system and may not result in the same degree of toxicity observed in systemic administration.

Radioimmunotherapy relies on a similar strategy to deliver radioactive substances in a selective manner for diagnostic or therapeutic purposes. In this case, the potential for tissue damage by the toxin has been replaced by the potential for radiation injury. Inasmuch as several radioimmunotherapeutic agents have been approved for human use, the tradeoff appears favorable.

Ibritumomab tiuxetan, approved in 2002, is a covalently linked conjugate of the MAb ibritumomab and the linker-chelater tiuxetan. Ibritumomab is selective for CD20, a cell-surface antigen expressed by normal B cells and more than 90% of B-cell non-Hodgkin's lymphomas. Tiuxetan contains a high-affinity binding site that can accommodate either indium-111 (used for diagnostic imaging) or yttrium-90 (used for target cell destruction). A complex administration schedule involving the prior administration of radiation-free MAb is used to limit damage of healthy lymphoid tissue and maximize destruction of lymphoma cells.[19] Common adverse effects include neutropenia and thrombocytopenia. Infection, hemorrhage, allergic reactions, and new malignancies are potentially life-threatening reactions.

Immunophilin Ligands

Cyclosporine (cyclosporin A), tacrolimus (FK506), and sirolimus (rapamycin) are microbial derivatives now classified as immunophilin ligands because they all initially form a complex with cytosolic receptors of the immunophilin family. These drugs appear to have similar (but not identical) mechanisms of action. Cyclosporine, the first of these agents to gain approval for human use, revolutionized the field of organ transplantation.

Cyclosporine

Cyclosporine was originally isolated from a fungus, *Beauveria nivea*. It is a neutral hydrophobic macrocyclic undecapeptide (Figure 41-6). Cyclosporine binds immunophilins called *cyclophyllins*. The cyclosporine-cyclophyllin complex interacts with calcineurin, a Ca^{++}-dependent protein phosphatase (see Figure 41-4).[27] The calcineurin complex is then inhibited from dephosphorylating NF-ATc, thus impeding its translocation into the nucleus and impairing transcription important in the earlier phases of immune responses. The immunosuppressive activity of cyclosporine is usually ascribed to its ability to

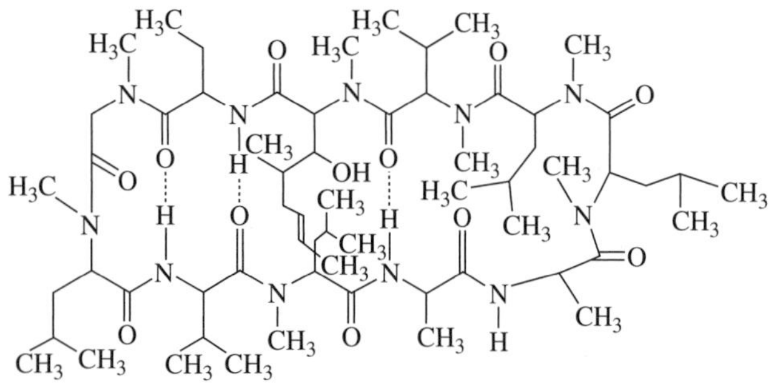

Cyclosporine

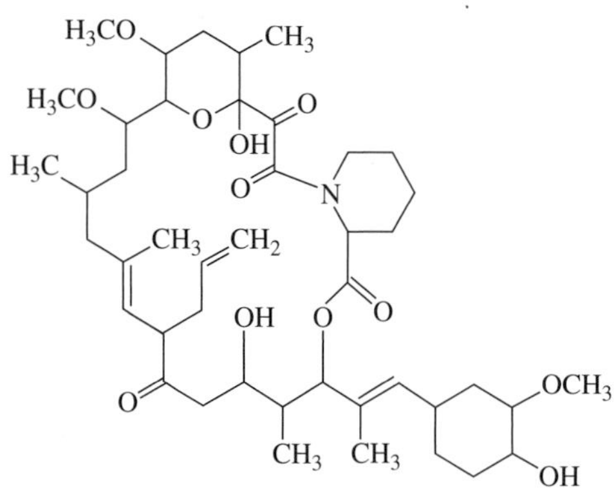

Tacrolimus

Fig. 41-6 Structural formulas of cyclosporine and tacrolimus.

block IL-2 synthesis, but the drug also suppresses macrophage activation and the release of IL-1, prevents the formation of IL-1 receptors on CD4+ T cells, and blocks the expression of IL-2 receptors on naive T cells.[11] Increased synthesis of TGF-β inhibits IL-2 activity. The primary outcome is that CD4+ T cells are not stimulated to proliferate in response to an antigenic challenge. B-cell function is also impaired by the reduced synthesis of TNF-α, and mast cell degranulation is blocked.

Cyclosporine is commonly used as an immunosuppressive agent to promote graft survival. It has proved successful in preventing rejections of nonmatched kidney, liver, heart, heart-lung, bone marrow, and pancreas transplants. The first-year survival of liver transplants rose from 35% to 70% after the introduction of cyclosporine. Cyclosporine is also effective as a topical agent in the treatment of oral lichen planus,[15] and it has been used systemically to treat other autoimmune diseases that may affect oral (bullous pemphigoid, pemphigus) and nonoral (psoriasis, rheumatoid arthritis) tissues. Lastly, cyclosporine has proved effective in the treatment of Behçet's syndrome (a vasculitis that almost always includes oral aphthous ulcers and uveitis), nephrotic syndrome, inflammatory bowel disease, atopic dermatitis, and endogenous uveitis. Cyclosporine is better tolerated than less selective immunosuppressant drugs. However, the drug is potentially dangerous. The two major adverse side effects associated with long-term use are (1) dose-related renal toxicity, which, including mild forms, may occur in up to 75% of patients; and (2) hypertension, which is not apparently dose related and occurs in 50% of all renal transplant patients (and is especially common in children). Other side effects include central nervous system toxicity (headache, confusion, depression, seizures), gingival hyperplasia, hirsutism, mild tremor, and hepatotoxicity. The risk of lymphoma and other neoplasias is increased.

The precise mechanism of cyclosporine-induced gingival hyperplasia is unknown; corrective procedures involve mainly drug titration and surgical intervention. Some studies indicate that cyclosporine therapy results in the selection of fibroblasts with cyclosporine receptors, and it has been proposed that there is an associated immunologic cytokine imbalance.[18]

The absorption of cyclosporine is incomplete and variable among patients. Because interstitial fibrosis of the kidney has been associated with sustained high concentrations of cyclosporine, monitoring of plasma cyclosporine concentrations is necessary. A microemulsion form offers higher and more reliable absorption than the original product. Cyclosporine is metabolized by CYP3A enzymes; thus drugs that induce these enzymes (e.g., carbamazepine, phenobarbital, rifampin) reduce plasma concentrations of cyclosporine, whereas drugs that inhibit them (e.g., erythromycin, ketoconazole, prednisolone) have the opposite effect. Nonsteroidal antiinflammatory drugs, aminoglycosides, and other drugs that cause nephrotoxicity are contraindicated in patients receiving cyclosporine.

Tacrolimus

Tacrolimus is a macrolide antibiotic originally isolated from *Streptomyces tsukubaensis.* Tacrolimus binds to immunophilins known as *FK506-binding proteins (FKBPs)*. The resulting tacrolimus-immunophilin complex produces the same action and effects as described for cyclosporine. However, tacrolimus is approximately 100 times more potent than cyclosporine. Tacrolimus is approved for prophylaxis against rejection of allogenic liver transplants. The drug is also potentially as useful as cyclosporine for other conditions. For instance, tacrolimus has been shown to exert profound antipsoriatic effects, probably by direct interaction with keratinocytes.[30] Adverse effects of tacrolimus are qualitatively similar to those of cyclosporine, except that gingival overgrowth and hirsutism are not observed. Drug interactions are also similar because tacrolimus is metabolized by CYP3A.

Sirolimus

Sirolimus, originally known as *rapamycin,* was originally detected in the fermentation broth of *Streptomyces hygroscopicus.* A structural analogue of tacrolimus, sirolimus binds to the same FKBP receptors (see Figure 41-4) and is approved for a similar therapeutic indication. However, the sirolimus-immunophilin complex binds, not to calcineurin, but to a serine-threonine kinase often referred to as *FKBP-rapamycin–associated protein (FRAP)*.[9] The FRAP-sirolimus-FKBP complex cannot phosphorylate a set of proteins involved in protein translation important in later stages of the T cell's immune response (i.e., its response to growth factors, IL-2 in particular).[43] Thus it is believed that sirolimus interferes with signals from growth factor receptors, such as the IL-2 receptor (IL-2R) rather than with signals generated by the TCR. In addition to blocking proliferation of T cells, sirolimus affects nonhematopoietic cells and therefore may find applications different from those of cyclosporine or tacrolimus.

Sirolimus is free of nephrotoxicity and neurotoxicity, and it does not promote hypertension. Hyperlipidemia is a common dose-dependent side effect. Anemia, thrombocytopenia, and leukopenia may occur. Combined use of sirolimus with cyclosporine significantly worsens renal function, but a positive drug interaction permits use of reduced cyclosporine doses.

Glucocorticoids

Glucocorticoids such as prednisone and dexamethasone have long been used as immunosuppressive agents, but their mechanism of action has only recently been defined. As discussed in Chapter 35, glucocorticoids bind to a soluble intracellular receptor and then enter the nucleus of the cell. Specific glucocorticoid response elements on DNA interact with the glucocorticoid receptor, and transcription of specific genes is promoted or inhibited. Several cytokines and other proteins involved in inflammatory reactions are affected. Dexamethasone has also been shown to induce transcription of the I-κβ gene. The subsequent increased synthesis of I-κβ prevents the translocation of NF-κβ from the cytosol to the nucleus.[33] Because NF-κβ promotes IL-6 and IL-8 transcription, glucocorticoids are important both as antiinflammatory agents and immunosuppressants. Apoptosis contributes to the rapid decline in peripheral lymphocytes.

Corticosteroids alone or with other immunosuppressive agents that inhibit antibody production and phagocytosis are often used to treat severe type II autoimmune reactions. Corticosteroids are also useful in the treatment of type III immune complex immunopathologic conditions, primarily because of their antiinflammatory properties. In severe cases, another immunosuppressant may be added to block the immune response and allow use of reduced quantities of steroids. The steroids mainly act on CMI. In addition to their lympholytic effects, steroids may interfere with macrophage processing by stabilization of macrophage cell membranes.

Thalidomide

Thalidomide, a sedative agent briefly available in Europe more than 4 decades ago but quickly withdrawn because of its powerful teratogenic effects (see Chapter 3), was approved in 1998 for restricted use by the Food and Drug Administration in the treatment of erythema nodosum leprosum. Although its mechanism of action is unknown, thalidomide decreases excessive production of TNF-α in target patients and downregulates certain surface adhesion molecules involved in leukocyte migration. TH2 cell responses are favored over TH1, yielding increases in IL-4 and IL-5. The drug can only be sold by registered pharmacies, which must obtain informed consent about its use from all patients. Thalidomide should never be used by women who are or may become pregnant; it is also contraindicated in men who are sexually mature and will not agree in writing to the need for using latex condoms when having sexual intercourse with women of childbearing potential. Peripheral neuropathy is an important side effect of the drug.

Cytotoxic Drugs

Cytotoxic drugs are of two classes: the first kills lymphocytes, and the second interferes with the proliferative stage of the immune response. The lympholytic drugs are most effective if given before antigen administration. They include the alkylating agents such as cyclophosphamide and phenylalanine mustard. Drugs that impede cellular proliferation include various metabolite analogues that inhibit DNA synthesis. The general pharmacologic characteristics of most of these drugs are covered in Chapter 42.

Cyclophosphamide

Cyclophosphamide was originally developed for cancer chemotherapy and has been adapted for immunotherapy in the prevention of allograft rejection, control of autoimmune and rheumatoid diseases mediated by antibody, and control of T-cell–mediated diseases. Although considered an alkylating agent, cyclophosphamide is inactive until it is metabolized within the liver microsomes (the phosphamide ring is hydrolyzed). Cyclophosphamide metabolites are eliminated by the kidney. Thus both liver and kidney function should be considered in the use of this drug. The metabolites of cyclophosphamide exert their effect by alkylating and cross-linking cellular macromolecules, including DNA, ribonucleic acid (RNA), and proteins. Damage to DNA can occur at all stages of the cell cycle, but lethal hits occur mainly in the S phase.

The daily, long-term administration of cyclophosphamide at low therapeutic doses leads to a progressive reduction in circulating lymphocytes, with minimal effect on myeloid cell populations. Within 7 days, B cells, CD4+ T cells, and CD8+ T cells show a 30% to 40% reduction in numbers. Cessation of cyclophosphamide therapy results in a differential rate of recovery of lymphocyte populations. CD8+ T cells recover first, followed by B cells and, finally, CD4+ T cells. Interestingly, intermittent low-dose administration appears to affect antibody production, but long-term low-dose administration diminishes CMI as assessed by decreased delayed-type allergic reactions. Paradoxic increases in immune activity have also been observed after low-dose cyclophosphamide therapy, attributable to selective depression of T-suppressor cell activity. Cyclophosphamide also depresses myeloid hematopoiesis in the bone marrow and has been associated with both neutropenia and thrombocytopenia.

Metabolite analogues

The purine, pyrimidine, and folate antagonists represent a second group of cytotoxic drugs active against rapidly dividing or metabolizing cells. Included among these are the purine antagonists azathioprine and 6-mercaptopurine, the pyrimidine antagonist floxuridine, and the folate antagonist methotrexate. These agents are given with, or within 48 hours of, antigen administration and inhibit cellular proliferation and initial differentiation, usually through inhibition of DNA and/or RNA synthesis. They all appear to impair both CMI and humoral immunity. Originally developed for cancer therapy, these drugs can affect any group of rapidly proliferating cells. Because they are particularly toxic to hematopoietic tissues, they may induce leukopenia (especially neutropenia), thrombocytopenia, and anemia.

Azathioprine Azathioprine deserves special mention because it is used solely as an immunosuppressant. Azathioprine is a prodrug that yields 6-mercaptopurine on intracellular exposure to glutathione and other nucleophilic reactants. Although the pharmacologic features of azathioprine are essentially identical to that of 6-mercaptopurine (see Chapter 42), azathioprine is believed to be a more selective immunosuppressant. This advantage may stem from an enhanced uptake or metabolic activation of azathioprine in T cells.

Mycophenolate Mycophenolate mofetil is an ester that is rapidly hydrolyzed to mycophenolic acid, the active form of the drug. Mycophenolate is an inhibitor of inosine monophosphate dehydrogenase, an important enzyme in purine synthesis. Because lymphocytes are more dependent on the de novo synthesis of purines than are other cells, which can reclaim purines by the salvage pathway, mycophenolate is a more selective immunosuppressant than are other cytotoxic agents. CMI and humoral immunity are suppressed, and leukocyte recruitment to inflammatory sites is inhibited.

Slow-Acting, Disease-Modifying Antirheumatic Drugs

One potential immunosuppressive strategy involves the inhibition of selected aspects of antigen processing within the endolysosome or by the proteasome. The antimalarial disease-modifying antirheumatic drugs (DMARDs) chloroquine and hydrochloroquine appear to have several effects on the immune system, including inhibition of endolysosomal antigen processing. It has been suggested that these weak bases may impair endolysosomal acidification. As a result, individuals treated with chloroquine or hydrochloroquine exhibit diminished antibody formation (including decreased formation of rheumatoid factor, decreased autoantibodies, and decreased total serum IgG and IgA), which is one of the main rationales for their use in Sjögren's syndrome and other autoimmune rheumatic diseases.

Gold compounds—gold sodium thiomalate, aurothioglucose, and auranofin—function in part by inhibiting transcription activation. Gold compounds may be active against protein kinase C. As a result, not only are various lymphocyte functions diminished, but also the induction of immune function in nonhematopoietic cells is impaired. In the latter situation, it has been demonstrated that the expression of MHC class II molecules by endothelial cells can be inhibited by gold compounds.

Penicillamine and sulfasalazine are DMARDs that inhibit proliferation through unknown mechanisms. Penicillamine blocks T-cell proliferation in response to IL-1 and blocks IL-1 production by monocytes; sulfasalazine blocks both T-mitogen–induced and B-mitogen–induced proliferation of peripheral blood lymphocytes.[10]

Cytokine Therapy

Therapeutics based on the administration of hormones is not new. As more is learned about the activities of immunologic hormones, loosely referred to as *cytokines*, new therapies to increase or decrease immunologic activities will be developed. Currently, several cytokines have been approved for human use, and others are in clinical trials. In the discussion that follows, cytokines and soluble cytokine receptors are reviewed in accordance with their principal biologic activities (see Table 41-1).

Hematopoietic growth factors

The hematopoietic growth factors, also referred to as *colony-stimulating factors*, include granulocyte colony-stimulating factor, granulocyte/macrophage colony-stimulating factor, monocyte/macrophage colony-stimulating factor, stem cell factor, erythropoietin, and a number of interleukins. Although it is beyond the scope of this chapter to discuss these growth factors, they are used clinically in the treatment of various hematopoietic deficiencies, including neutropenia, anemia, and thrombocytopenia, and are reviewed in Chapter 30.

Interleukin-1 family

IL-1 occupies the borderland between adaptive, nonspecific immune responses and adaptive, specific immune responses. Several related molecules, including IL-1α, IL-1β, IL-1 receptor antagonist (IL-1Ra) and their receptors in soluble form, are under consideration for use in immunotherapeutics.[13] IL-1 is produced by many cells, but mainly monocytes/macrophages, in the form of precursor molecules lacking a signal sequence. A large fraction of IL-1α remains inactive in the cytosol of the cell. In contrast, IL-1β is rapidly converted to its active form and released extracellularly in large quantities.

IL-1 can exist in both soluble and membrane-associated forms. As a soluble molecule, IL-1 is a hormone with wide-ranging systemic effects involving the CNS, liver, kidney, hematopoietic system (including neutrophilia and lymphopenia), and vascular system (promotes leukocyte adherence, for one). The membrane-associated form may be a partially degraded version of IL-1α, which can function as a costimulatory factor for naive T cells. Some immunologic effects of IL-1 are listed in Table 41-3. In addition, IL-1β is important as an osteoclast-activating factor and is believed to be involved in periodontal bone destruction. IL-1 has cytotoxic activities; it kills melanoma cells, thyrocytes, and β-islet (insulin-producing) cells. IL-1 also induces fever, and as such it is one of the more important endogenous pyrogens. The pyrogenic effect of IL-1 is blocked by nonsteroidal antiinflammatory drugs, suggesting that it depends on the elaboration of cyclooxygenase products.

IL-1Ra, a protein with structural homology to IL-1α and IL-1β, is secreted by monocytes. It is found in the urine of patients with fever or monocytic leukemia. The molecule binds to the IL-1 receptor in competition with IL-1α and IL-1β, but it does not trigger the cellular responses typical of IL-1. IL-1Ra is considered a natural means of blocking excessive IL-1 inflammatory events, which can lead to shock, arthritis, osteoporosis, colitis, leukemia, diabetes, wasting, and atherosclerosis. IL-1Ra has potential therapeutic application in human beings, and clinical trials have demonstrated some efficacy in septic shock syndrome and more consistent benefits in rheumatoid arthritis.[12]

Table • 41-3

Effects of Interleukin-1 on Immune Cells

TARGET CELLS	EFFECTS
Lymphoid Cells	
T cells	Growth factor (primarily due to its ability to stimulate IL-2)
	Increased IL-2 receptors
	Induction of cytokine synthesis (IL-2, IL-3, others)
	Induction of IFN-γ synthesis
	Chemoattractant
B cells	Growth factor for transformed B cells (B blasts)
	Potentiates B-cell growth and differentiation factors (IL-4, IL-6)
	Chemoattractant
NK cells	Facilitates IL-2 and IFN enhancement of tumor cell lysis
	Increases binding of NK cells to targets
	Induces cytokine synthesis (IL-1)
Myeloid Cells	
Neutrophils	Thromboxane synthesis
	Degranulation (secretion)
Monocytes/macrophages	Induces synthesis of PGE_2, IL-1, and other cytokines
	Induces cytotoxicity
	Colony-stimulating factors
	Stimulates migration

IFN, Interferon; *PGE_2*, prostaglandin E_2.

Interleukin-1 receptors
The IL-1 receptor (IL-1R) is a member of the immunoglobulin superfamily. There are two subtypes of IL-1R. Subtype 1 (IL-1RI) binds IL-1α preferentially and is found on T cells, endothelial cells, keratinocytes, hepatocytes, and fibroblasts. Subtype 2 (IL-1RII) is expressed by neutrophils, monocytes, B cells, and bone marrow cells, and it binds IL-1β preferentially. IL-1RI is more sensitive to inhibition by IL-1Ra than is IL-1RII. IL-RII exhibits a very short cytoplasmic domain compared with IL-1RI, suggesting that it may serve as a "decoy" receptor. IL-1R can exist in either a transmembranous form or a soluble form. Soluble receptors exert an antagonistic effect by binding to IL-1. (Because both IL-1 and the IL-1R can be either membrane-bound or soluble, the distinction between ligand and receptor blurs.) Experiments in mice have shown that recombinant soluble IL-1RI can prolong the survival of cardiac allografts. Much of this survival is attributable to decreased inflammation rather than to specific immunosuppression. Anakinra, a recombinant form of IL-1RI, has recently been marketed for the treatment of rheumatoid arthritis not responding to more traditional DMARDs.

Interleukin-2
Lymphocytotrophic hormone, or IL-2, is a glycoprotein produced by TH0 and TH1 T cells in the presence of antigen-presenting cells. IL-2 abrogates suppressor T-cell activity and is required for IFN-γ production. In specific immune responses, the main function of IL-2 is to induce T-cell proliferative differentiation; as such, IL-2 enhances the growth of TH0 CD4+ T cells, TH1 CD4+ T cells, and CD8+ T cells. In nonspecific, innate responses, IL-2 can activate NK cells to form more aggressive lymphokine-activated killer (LAK) cells. Most immunotherapies involving IL-2 are based on its ability to alter NK cell activity.

The IL-2 receptor is a collection of isoforms designated by their relative affinities for IL-2. These isoforms result from unique combinations of three different IL-2R subunits.[40] The high-affinity form is usually present on less than 1% of the circulating mononuclear cells.

IL-2 therapy has been explored in a variety of immunodeficiency diseases and cancer, and IL-2 replacement has been effective in treating patients with IL-2 deficiency. The cytokine has been given the nonproprietary name of *aldesleukin* and marketed for the treatment of metastatic renal cell carcinoma (see Chapter 42).

The NK cell is believed to be the most important target for IL-2 therapy because depletion of this cell type can negate the protective effects of IL-2 in animal models.[4] The high doses used in cancer chemotherapy are believed to completely saturate the intermediate-affinity IL-2 receptors of NK cells.[39] In animal models, transplanted tumor micrometastases appear to regress when IL-2 is used alone or in combination with LAK cells. In human clinical trials involving advanced melanoma, the coadministration of IL-2 and LAK cells resulted in the complete regression of tumors in approximately 5% of cases, and the partial regression (more than a 50% reduction in tumor mass) in 15% of cases. Comparative values for metastatic renal cancer were 4% and 11%. IL-2 therapy has certain inherent problems not found in classic hormone therapy. IL-2 is a short-range hormone designed to influence cells in an extremely local manner. Furthermore, high-dose IL-2 therapy is toxic, and complications lead to a mortality rate of approximately 4%. Adverse effects include capillary leak syndrome (resulting in edema, reduced organ perfusion, and hypotension), cardiac arrhythmias, myocardial infarction, respiratory insufficiency, mental disturbances, and increased infections.[43]

Experimentation with lower dosages has greatly influenced IL-2 immunotherapy. Lower dosages are based on the observation that 10% of NK cells express high-affinity receptors for IL-2; therefore a 500-fold decrease in the IL-2 dose (administered as a continuous intravenous infusion) would still be sufficient to saturate all these high-affinity receptors. The low-dose regimen was found to produce a gradual, 10-fold increase in circulating NK cells without causing significant toxicity.[39] Such low-dose administration of IL-2 has also been used to raise the number of NK cells in patients with HIV infection or advanced cancer.[4,39]

Subcutaneous administration of IL-2 has been tested as an immunostimulant in individuals with asymptomatic HIV infection. This route leads to an increase in the proportion of T cells expressing IL-2Rs without increasing NK cells or viral proliferation.[39]

Interferons
There are two major classes of interferons, type 1 interferons (IFN-α, IFN-β, and IFN-ω), and type 2 interferon (IFN-γ). Type 1 interferons are produced by most nucleated cells. IFN-γ is mainly a product of TH1 T cells and activated NK cells.[20]

Type 1 interferons act by stimulating the phosphorylation of cytosolic proteins termed *signal transducers and activators of transcription (STAT)*. These STAT proteins then form a complex with a specific nonphosphorylated protein; the complex then enters the nucleus, binds to its designated response element on DNA, and promotes transcription.[36] Only the nonphosphorylated protein constituent actually binds to DNA.

Recombinant forms of IFN-α (interferon alpha-2a, interferon alpha-2b, interferon alphacon-1) and IFN-β (interferon beta-1a, interferon beta-1b) and a purified form from human leukocytes (interferon alpha-N3) have received approval by the Food and Drug Administration (FDA) for use in the clinical setting, as described in Chapters 40 and 42.[35] IFN-α preparations are indicated in the treatment of numerous diseases, including hairy cell leukemia, chronic myelogenous leukemia, condyloma acuminata, AIDS-related Kaposi's sarcoma, chronic hepatitis B and C, and malignant melanoma. IFN-β preparations are approved for the treatment of remitting and recurring multiple sclerosis. Additionally, trials are ongoing for the use of type 1 interferons in a number of other cancers, acquired immune deficiency syndrome, viral infections, papillomas, and angiogenic disorders.

IFN-γ was initially discovered as a result of its antiviral properties, but it also displays antiproliferative effects against tumors. IFN-γ is a glycosylated protein that exists exclusively as a covalently coupled homodimer. It shares very little DNA sequence homology with either IFN-α or IFN-β, and IFN-γ is, in fact, more accurately classified as an interleukin. The mechanism by which IFN-γ stimulates transcription, however, is similar to that of the type 1 interferons. The resultant effects of its action include (1) stimulation of CD4+ TH1 T cells and macrophages; (2) suppression of antibody production (IFN-γ antagonizes CD4+ TH2 T cells); (3) induction of immunoglobulin class switching; (4) upregulation of MHC class II molecule expression by epithelial tumor cells and macrophages (an effect antagonized by prostaglandin E_2); and (5) alteration of antigen processing by changing the mix of peptide products produced by the proteasome.[2] IFN-γ, in the form of a single polypeptide chain designated *interferon γ-1b*, is approved for managing serious infections associated with granulomatous disease and delaying the progression of malignant osteopetrosis. It is also useful in the management of rheumatoid arthritis.

TH1 and TH2 Cytokines
In later phases of specific immune responses, one function of cytokines is to regulate the nature of the immune response. TH1 cytokines help guide specific immunity against changes

in intracellular, cytosolic antigens, and TH2 cytokines help direct specific immunity against changes in extracellular antigens. Moreover, these TH1 and TH2 responses are mutually inhibitory: the TH1 cytokines IFN-γ and IL-12 inhibit TH2 responses, and the TH2 cytokines IL-4 and IL-10 inhibit TH1 responses. As such, pharmacologic regulation of the relative proportions of TH1 and TH2 cytokines may provide a way to treat diseases in which an inappropriate TH1 or TH2 response is a component of the disease process (in contrast to the problem of simply too much or too little immune response).

The types of disorders that may be amenable to cytokine intervention in these later stages include infectious diseases in which there is an inappropriate type of immune response, inflammatory autoimmune diseases, and IgE-mediated allergic diseases.[32] Lepromatous leprosy, nonhealing forms of leishmaniasis, tuberculosis, trypanosomiasis, and certain fungal diseases are infections that may be exacerbated by an inappropriately strong TH2 response. The administration of the TH1 cytokine IFN-γ, as mentioned previously, is approved for this indication.

Experimental allergic encephalomyelitis, a potential animal model for multiple sclerosis, appears to involve an overzealous TH1 response and can be transferred by T cells with the TH1 phenotype. In animals, spontaneous recovery from the disease is associated with an expansion of T cells with the TH2 phenotype; a study in human beings with multiple sclerosis suggests that the administration of IFN-γ exacerbates the disease process (to the point where the research had to be terminated). Opposite effects occur with IFN-β,[41] which has FDA approval for the treatment of this form of the disease. The destruction of β-islet cells in insulin-dependent diabetes mellitus has been associated with tissue infiltration by T cells of the TH1 phenotype. For such TH1-mediated disease, it is possible that the administration of TH2 cytokines IL-4 and IL-10 may be of benefit.

IgE-mediated allergic diseases are consistent with the overactivity of TH2 T cells. Well-known examples include allergic rhinitis, immediate drug allergies, and life-threatening anaphylaxis resulting from insect stings. The successful long-term treatment of IgE-mediated allergies empirically corresponds with a shift in antibody isotypes from IgE to IgG; hence it is widely believed that various desensitization procedures in which the allergen is injected into the allergic host owe their success to the generation of "blocking antibodies" of the IgG subclass. Bee venom immunotherapy is a good model for such procedures; it is associated with a TH2-to-TH1 shift.[28] The TH1 cytokine profile favors production of IgG rather than IgE. In local tissues, mast cells and basophils are important sources of IL-4. Local therapies currently being explored include anti-IL-4 antibodies and IFN-α.

There are also short-term desensitization procedures for dealing with IgE-mediated allergies. On occasion it may be essential to treat a patient with a certain drug despite a known allergy to that drug (for example, using penicillin to treat an infection in an individual with a positive skin test indicative of penicillin allergy). Actually, most individuals are not allergic to penicillin itself, but rather to antigens that form by the covalent linkage between the β-lactam ring of penicillin metabolites and certain proteins. In acute desensitization, penicillin is administered in incrementally increasing dosages over a period of 4 to 6 hours. The goal of these therapies is not to cause a permanent reduction in antipenicillin IgE, but instead to induce rapidly a state of clinical tolerance. The actual mechanism of clinical tolerance is unclear (possible Fc receptor downregulation in mast cells); the end result, however, is a diminished risk of anaphylaxis with only minor urticarial side effects.

Drugs Used in Immunotherapy

Nonproprietary (generic) name	*Proprietary (trade) name*
Agents for active immunization	
See references 6 and 14	
Agents for passive immunization	
Botulism immune globulin (human)	BabyBIG
Cytomegalovirus immune globulin (human)	CytoGam
Hepatitis B immune globulin (human)	BayHep B, Nabi-HB
Immune globulin (human)	BayGam, Gamimune N
Rabies immune globulin (human)	BayRab
Respiratory syncytial virus immune globulin (human)	RespiGam
Rho(D) immune globulin (human)	RhoGAM, Winrho SDF
Tetanus immune globulin	BayTet
Varicella-zoster immune globulin	—
Antitoxins	
Antivenin (Crotalidae), polyvalent	—
Antivenin *(Latrodectus mactans)*	—
Antivenin *(Micrurus fulvius)*	—
Crotalidae polyvalent immune fab	CroFab
Rabies immune globulin (human)	Hyperab, Imogam
Immunostimulants	
Thymosin	—
Levamisole	Ergamisol
Immunomodulators	
Mitoxantrone	Novantrone
Thalidomide	Thalomid
Monoclonal antibodies	
See Table 41-2	
Immunosuppressants	
Azathioprine	Imuran
Cyclophosphamide	Cytoxan
Cyclosporine	Gengraf, Neoral, Sandimmune
Glatiramer	Copaxone
Lymphocyte immune globulin, antithymocyte globulin (equine)	Atgam
Antithymocyte globulin (rabbit)	—
Melphalan	Alkeran
Mercaptopurine	Purinethol
Methotrexate	Rheumatrex Dose Pack

Drugs Used in Immunotherapy—cont'd

Nonproprietary (generic) name	*Proprietary (trade) name*
Muromonab-CD3	Orthoclone OKT3
Mycophenolate mofetil	CellCept
Prednisone	Deltasone, Sterapred
Sirolimus	Rapamune
Tacrolimus	Prograf
Slow-acting disease-modifying antirheumatic drugs	
See Chapter 21	
Cytokines	
Aldesleukin (IL-2)	Proleukin
Anakinra	Kineret
Denileukin diftitox	Ontak
Interferon α-2a	Roferon-A
Interferon α-2b	Intron A
Interferon α-N3	Alferon N
Interferon alfacon-1	Infergen
Interferon β-1a	Avonex, Rebif
Interferon β-1b	Betaseron
Interferon γ-1b	Actimmune
Peginterferon α-2a	Pegasys
Peginterferon α-2b	PEG-Intron
Hematopoietic growth factors	
See Chapter 30	
Therapy for allergic reactions	
See Chapters 22, 32, and 35	

CITED REFERENCES

1. Abou-Jawde R, Choueiri T, Alemany C, et al: An overview of targeted treatments in cancer, *Clin Ther* 25:2122-2137, 2003.
2. Akiyama K, Yokota K, Kagawa S, et al: cDNA cloning and interferon γ down-regulation of proteasomal subunits X and Y, *Science* 265:1231-1234, 1994.
3. Bach JF, Bach MA, Charreire J, et al: The mode of action of thymic hormones, *Ann N Y Acad Sci* 332:23-32, 1979.
4. Baiocchi RA, Caligiuri MA: Low-dose interleukin 2 prevents the development of Epstein-Barr virus (EBV)-associated lymphoproliferative disease in scid/scid mice reconstituted i.p. with EBV-seropositive human peripheral blood lymphocytes, *Proc Natl Acad Sci USA* 91:5577-5581, 1994.
5. Baskar S, Ostrand-Rosenberg S, Nabavi N, et al: Constitutive expression of B7 restores immunogenicity of tumor cells expressing truncated major histocompatibility complex class II molecules, *Proc Natl Acad Sci USA* 90:5687-5690, 1993.
6. Benenson AS, editor: *Control of communicable diseases manual: an official report of the American Public Health Association,* ed 16, Washington, DC, 1995, American Public Health Association.
7. Boise LH, Thompson CB: Hierarchical control of lymphocyte survival, *Science* 274:67-68, 1996.
8. Childers NK, Zhang SS, Michalek SM: Oral immunization of humans with dehydrated liposomes containing *Streptococcus mutans* glucosyltransferase induces salivary immunoglobulin A_2 antibody responses, *Oral Microbiol Immunol* 9:146-153, 1994.
9. Choi J, Chen J, Schreiber SL, et al: Structure of the FKBP12-rapamycin complex interacting with the binding domain of human FRAP, *Science* 273:239-242, 1996.
10. Cronstein BN: Second-line antirheumatic drugs. In Gallin JI, Snyderman R, eds: *Inflammation: basic principles and clinical correlates,* ed 3, Philadelphia, 1999, Lippincott Williams & Wilkins.
11. de Camargo PM: Cyclosporin- and nifedipine-induced gingival enlargement: an overview, *J West Soc Periodontol* 37:57-64, 1989.
12. Dinarello CA: Interleukin-1: a proinflammatory cytokine. In Gallin JI, Snyderman R, eds: *Inflammation: basic principles and clinical correlates,* ed 3, Philadelphia, 1999, Lippincott Williams & Wilkins.
13. Dinarello CA: Modalities for reducing interleukin 1 activity in disease, *Immunol Today* 14:260-264, 1993.
14. *Drug facts and comparisons, 2004,* ed 58, St Louis, 2003, Facts and Comparisons.
15. Eisen D, Ellis CN, Duell EA, et al: Effect of topical cyclosporine rinse on oral lichen planus. A double-blind analysis, *N Engl J Med* 323:290-294, 1990.
16. Ferrone S, Dierich MP, eds: *Handbook of monoclonal antibodies: applications in biology and medicine,* Park Ridge, NJ, 1985, Noyes.
17. Goldstein AL, Low TL, McAdoo M, et al: Thymosin α_1: isolation and sequence analysis of an immunologically active thymic polypeptide, *Proc Natl Acad Sci USA* 74:725-729, 1977.
18. Hassell TM, Hefti AF: Drug-induced gingival overgrowth: old problem, new problem, *Crit Rev Oral Biol Med* 2:103-137, 1991.
19. Horning SJ: Future directions in radioimmunotherapy for B-cell lymphoma. *Semin Oncol* 30(suppl 17):29-34, 2003.
20. Hsu DH, de Waal Malefyt R, Fiorentino DF, et al: Expression of interleukin-10 activity by Epstein-Barr virus protein BCRF1, *Science* 250:830-832, 1990.
21. Jackson S, Mestecky J, Childers NK, et al: Liposomes containing anti-idiotypic antibodies: an oral vaccine to induce protective secretory immune responses specific for pathogens of mucosal surfaces, *Infect Immun* 58:1932-1936, 1990.
22. Kiechle FL, Zhang X: Apoptosis: biochemical aspects and clinical implications, *Clin Chim Acta* 326:27-45, 2002.
23. LeBlanc AC: Natural cellular inhibitors of caspases, *Prog Neuropsychopharmacol Biol Psychiatr* 27:215-229, 2003.
24. Lehner T, Mehlert A, Caldwell J: Local active gingival immunization by a 3,800-molecular-weight streptococcal antigen in protection against dental caries, *Infect Immun* 52:682-687, 1986.
25. Lehner T, Wilton JMA, Ivanyi L: Double blind crossover trial of levamisole in recurrent aphthous ulceration, *Lancet* 2:926-929, 1976.
26. Liu C-C, Walsh CM, Young JD-E: Perforin: structure and function, *Immunol Today* 16:194-201, 1995.
27. Liu J, Farmer JD, Jr, Lane WS, et al: Calcineurin is a common target of cyclophilin-cyclosporin A and FKBP-FK506 complexes, *Cell* 66:807-815, 1991.

28. McHugh SM, Deighton J, Stewart AG, et al: Bee venom immunotherapy induces a shift in cytokine responses from a TH-2 to a TH-1 dominant pattern: comparison of rush and conventional immunotherapy, *Clin Exp Allergy* 25:828-838, 1995.
29. Michalek SM, Childers NK: Development and outlook for a caries vaccine, *Crit Rev Oral Biol Med* 1:37-54, 1990.
30. Michel G, Kemeny L, Homey B, et al: FK506 in the treatment of inflammatory skin disease: promises and perspectives, *Immunol Today* 17:106-108, 1996.
31. Mitsiades CS, Poulaki V, Mitsiades N: The role of apoptosis-inducing receptors of the tumor necrosis factor family in thyroid cancer, *J Endocrinol* 178:205-216, 2003.
32. Powrie F, Coffman RL: Cytokine regulation of T-cell function: potential for therapeutic intervention, *Trends Pharmacol Sci* 14:164-168, 1993.
33. Scheinman RI, Cogswell PC, Lofquist AK, et al: Role of transcriptional activation of I-κβα in mediation of immunosuppression by glucocorticoids, *Science* 270:283-290, 1995.
34. Schiff RI, Rudd C, Johnson R, et al: Use of a chemically modified intravenous IgG preparation in severe primary humoral immunodeficiency: clinical efficacy and attempts to individualize dosage, *Clin Immunol Immunopathol* 31:13-23, 1984.
35. Shankaran V, Schreiber RD: The interferons: basic biology and therapeutic potential. In Austen KF, Burakoff SJ, Rosen FS, et al, eds: *Therapeutic immunology,* ed 2, Cambridge, MA, 2001, Blackwell Science.
36. Shuai K, Schindler C, Prezioso VR, et al: Activation of transcription of IFN-γ: tyrosine phosphorylation of a 91-kD DNA binding protein, *Science* 258:1808-1812, 1992.
37. Smith DJ, Taubman MA, Holmberg CF, et al: Antigenicity and immunogenicity of a synthetic peptide derived from a glucan-binding domain of mutans streptococcal glucosyltransferase, *Infect Immun* 61:2899-2905, 1993.
38. Smith DJ, Taubman MA, King WF, et al: Immunological characteristics of a synthetic peptide associated with a catalytic domain of mutans streptococcal glucosyltransferase, *Infect Immun* 62:5470-5476, 1994.
39. Smith KA: Interleukin-2 immunostimulation. In Austen KF, Burakoff SJ, Rosen FS, et al, eds: *Therapeutic immunology,* ed 2, Cambridge, MA, 2001, Blackwell Science.
40. Taniguchi T, Minami Y: The IL-2/IL-2 receptor system: a current overview, *Cell* 73:5-8, 1993.
41. The IFNB Multiple Sclerosis Study Group: Interferon beta-1b is effective in relapsing-remitting multiple sclerosis. I. Clinical results of a multicenter, randomized, double-blind, placebo-controlled trial, *Neurology* 43:655-661, 1993.
42. Viola A, Lanzavecchia A: T cell activation determined by T cell receptor number and tunable thresholds, *Science* 273:104-106, 1996.
43. Waldmann TA: The IL-2/IL-2 receptor system: a target for rational immune intervention, *Immunol Today* 14:264-270, 1993.
44. Winter G, Harris WJ: Humanized antibodies, *Immunol Today* 14:243-246, 1993.

General References

Alberts B, Johnson A, Lewis J, et al: *Molecular biology of the cell,* ed 4, New York, 2002, Garland.

Austen KF, Burakoff SJ, Rosen FS, et al, eds: *Therapeutic immunology,* ed 2, Cambridge, MA, 2001, Blackwell Science.

Gallin JI, Snyderman R, eds: *Inflammation: basic principles and clinical correlates,* ed 3, Philadelphia, 1999, Lippincott Williams & Wilkins.

Rich RR, Fleisher TA, Shearer WT, et al, eds: *Clinical immunology: principles and practice,* ed 2, London, 2001, Mosby International.

CHAPTER • 42

Antineoplastic Drugs

Karl K. Kwok, Ania U. Sweet, and Mark M. Schubert

The role of antineoplastic drugs in the fight against cancer has greatly expanded in the past few decades. These drugs can cure a number of advanced tumors and are the treatment of choice for many widely disseminated malignancies that cannot be reached by surgery or are beyond the limits of safety of radiotherapy. They are also used as adjuncts to surgery and irradiation in the prevention of metastasis from locally treated primary tumors. Research has brought the development of new agents, more effective application of existing agents, and the use of adjunctive drugs to overcome resistance and minimize drug toxicity. The past decade has also brought about a greater depth of research and understanding of the molecular biology of cancer cell growth. Many mechanisms of growth stimulation and retardation and the actions of growth modulators have been discovered. Gene rearrangements and mutations and their resultant influences on cell growth are being elucidated. These discoveries provide a number of new targets for the management of abnormal cell growth. The traditional agents that contribute to the goal of eliminating and destroying neoplastic cells are covered under the broad heading of antineoplastic agents and include traditional chemotherapeutic drugs (i.e., alkylators, antimetabolites, antibiotics, steroids, plant alkaloids, other agents), biologic response modifiers, and agents used specifically to protect the patient from the toxic effects of these drugs. A number of newer chemotherapy drugs such as oxaliplatin, irinotecan, and others joins this group of antineoplastic agents along with some older therapeutic agents such as arsenic trioxide and thalidomide. Also new are more specific hormonal agents such as letrozole, anastrozole, and fulvestrant; differentiating agents such as tretinoid; and monoclonal antibodies, which have a variety of different targets and potential mechanisms of actions. Newer classes of drugs used in oncology are drugs that target signal transduction such as imatinib mesylate; drugs that block crucial cellular receptors, including epidermal growth factor receptors such as gefitinib; and drugs that inhibit angiogenesis such as bevacizumab, a monoclonal antibody that blocks vascular endothelial growth factor. Additional newer targets include proteasome inhibitors such as bortezomib; drugs that inhibit matrix metalloproteinase and cyclin-dependent kinase; and drugs that may enhance or remove blocks to apoptosis (programmed cell death).

HISTORY OF CANCER CHEMOTHERAPY

The cytotoxic effects of drugs were observed well before the turn of the century, but it was not until the mid-1940s that their usefulness in the treatment of disease was appreciated. Chemical warfare with sulfur mustard gas in World War I resulted in shrinkage of lymph nodes and myeloid tissues in the victims. The application of these nitrogen mustard compounds for the medical treatment of Hodgkin's disease, malignant lymphomas, and chronic leukemia followed these observations but was not reported until the end of World War II. In 1944 the glucocorticoids were shown to have a profound effect on the volume, structure, and function of lymphoid tissue.[17] Subsequently, this effect was used in the control of human leukemia, and since then prednisone and prednisolone have been incorporated in drug protocols designed to ablate lymphoproliferative and myeloproliferative diseases.

In 1948, Farber et al[20] obtained temporary remissions in children with acute leukemia who were given the folic acid antagonist 4-aminopteroylglutamic acid (aminopterin). This specially tailored molecule was the first antimetabolite to produce unequivocally beneficial results in a human neoplastic disease.

The folate antagonist approach led to the development of competitive inhibitors of purines and pyrimidines that interfered with the synthesis of nucleic acids in rapidly multiplying neoplastic cells. Observations in animal tumor models of selective uptake of uracil by colon tumor cells resulted in the development of a "designer" antimetabolite, 5-fluorouracil.

The first antibiotic with activity against human tumors was actinomycin D. Introduced as an anticancer agent in 1952, dactinomycin (actinomycin D) is curative in many patients with Wilms' tumor and uterine choriocarcinoma.[23] The anticancer effects of the *Vinca* alkaloids, extracted from the periwinkle plant *(Vinca rosea)*, were initially demonstrated in animals with experimental leukemia in 1960.[40] In the same year, vinblastine was found to be of value in the treatment of acute forms of leukemia, Hodgkin's disease, and adenocarcinoma of the colon.[35] The earliest reports of the use of carmustine, the prototype of the nitrosourea group of cytotoxic compounds, against human malignancies appeared in 1966.[38]

In 1967 the enzyme L-asparaginase was found to produce remissions in some patients with acute leukemia.[50] The first of the heavy metal complexes to have significant success in the treatment of human cancer was cisplatin, introduced in 1969.[57] While the 1950s and 1960s brought rapid development of new agents, continued refinements in their use occurred in the 1970s and early 1980s with additional combination chemotherapy regimens and a better understanding of the cytokinetics of tumor cells and the pharmacokinetics of the drugs.[13,15] The late 1980s and early 1990s have contributed several new agents such as the taxenes, topoisomerase I inhibitors, and others with measurable efficacy and decreased toxicity; the biologic response modifiers such as interferon and interleukin-2; and chemoprotective agents and newer technologies for the application of these antineoplastic agents. The late 1990s brought the commercial availability of monoclonal antibodies for the treatment of several cancers and further research on the role of angiogenesis, which had started in the 1960s.

Angiogenesis, which is the formation of new blood vessels, plays a role in supporting existing tumors with required nutrients and oxygen and in forming metastatic tumors. The identification of angiogenic factors such as vascular endothelial growth factor (VEGF), basic fibroblastic growth factor (bFGF), and other regulators and inhibitors of angiogenesis is leading to the development of new drugs to target these factors and evaluate their role in starving cancer cells and preventing the formation of metastatic disease.[44]

Several novel strategies are being considered in clinical trials, applying newer drug entities for newly identified targets. The drugs being studied include angiogenesis factors; drugs that inhibit matrix metalloproteinase; and drugs that affect intracellular signaling pathways (e.g., tyrosine kinase inhibitors). Many drugs have been developed that can promote apoptosis; target the cyclin-dependent kinases (CDK), and inhibit the family of enzymes that plays a role in cell cycle progression. The challenge of these clinical trials will be to identify agents specific to the cancer cell process and determine the appropriate role of these agents, combined with existing therapies, in enhancing cancer treatment responses and minimizing side effects.[59]

PRINCIPLES OF CANCER CHEMOTHERAPY

The goal of chemotherapy is to eradicate every viable tumor cell without significantly damaging normal host tissue. This requires that the tumor be inherently sensitive to the chemotherapy agents, that the tumor receptor sites be exposed to adequate concentrations of active drug for sufficient periods of time, and that the host cells be resistant to the effects of the chemotherapy drugs. Chemotherapy agents unfortunately are not tumor cell–specific and will kill all cells actively undergoing cell division. These include the normal cells in the gastrointestinal tract, bone marrow, and hair follicles as well as the abnormal or malignant cells. The chemotherapy drugs kill or impair susceptible tumor cells by blocking a drug-sensitive biochemical or metabolic pathway. Some, such as the cell cycle phase–specific antimetabolites, act by inhibiting DNA synthesis and are most effective against rapidly dividing cells. Others, including the alkylating agents, act by interfering with nucleic acid function and protein production throughout the cell division cycle and are thus effective against both proliferating and resting cells (Figures 42-1 and 42-2). All are extremely cytotoxic and have low margins of safety. With the current understanding of tumor biology, the patient's physiologic status, and the drug's pharmacologic features, the principles that govern the useful application of cancer chemotherapy include the following:

1. The tumor must be susceptible to the drugs selected for treatment. Not all tumors are responsive to the same agents.
2. The drugs or methods of administration must not have intolerable local or systemic toxicity that would prevent the completion of an adequate course of treatment.
3. The dosages and schedules for the drugs must be calculated to maximize the contact with the tumor cells, and the drugs must be present in sufficient concentration during the crucial periods of the cell's metabolic cycle.
4. Cancer chemotherapy is more effective when the tumor mass is small than when the tumor cell burden is high. A larger fraction of the tumor cell population is undergoing active division in a small tumor mass, and the blood supply is more plentiful, allowing for increased sensitivity and delivery of the drugs. Debulking by surgery or irradiation reduces tumor cell burden and can induce

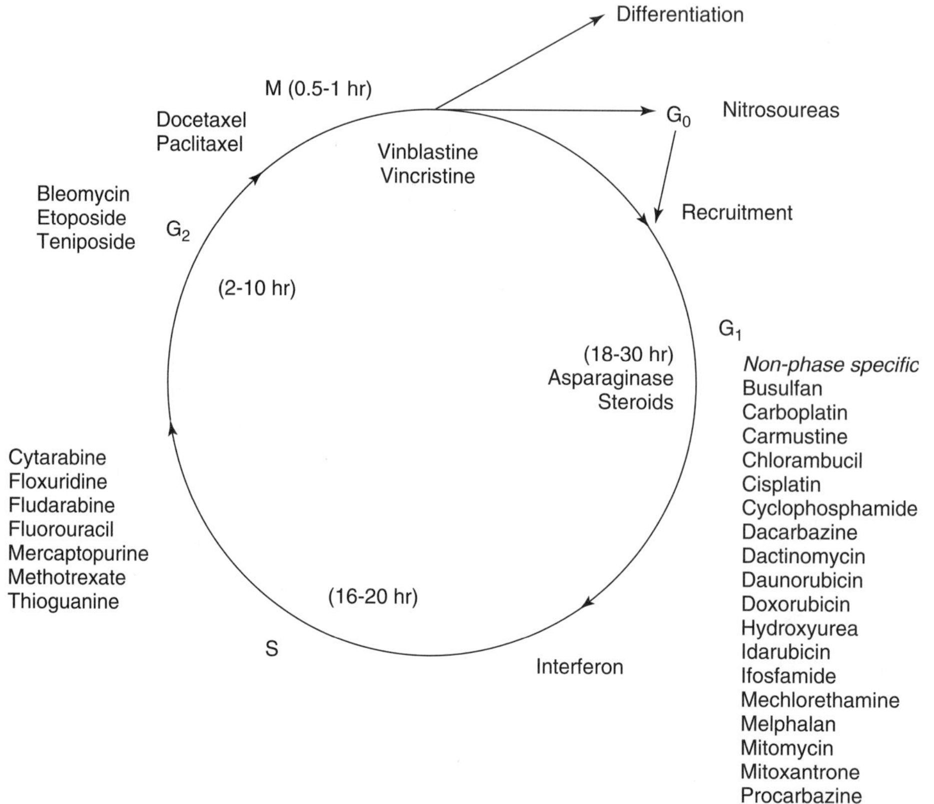

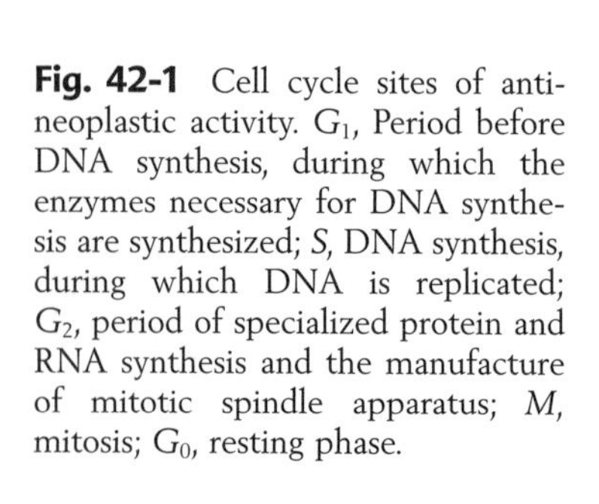
Fig. 42-1 Cell cycle sites of antineoplastic activity. G_1, Period before DNA synthesis, during which the enzymes necessary for DNA synthesis are synthesized; *S*, DNA synthesis, during which DNA is replicated; G_2, period of specialized protein and RNA synthesis and the manufacture of mitotic spindle apparatus; *M*, mitosis; G_0, resting phase.

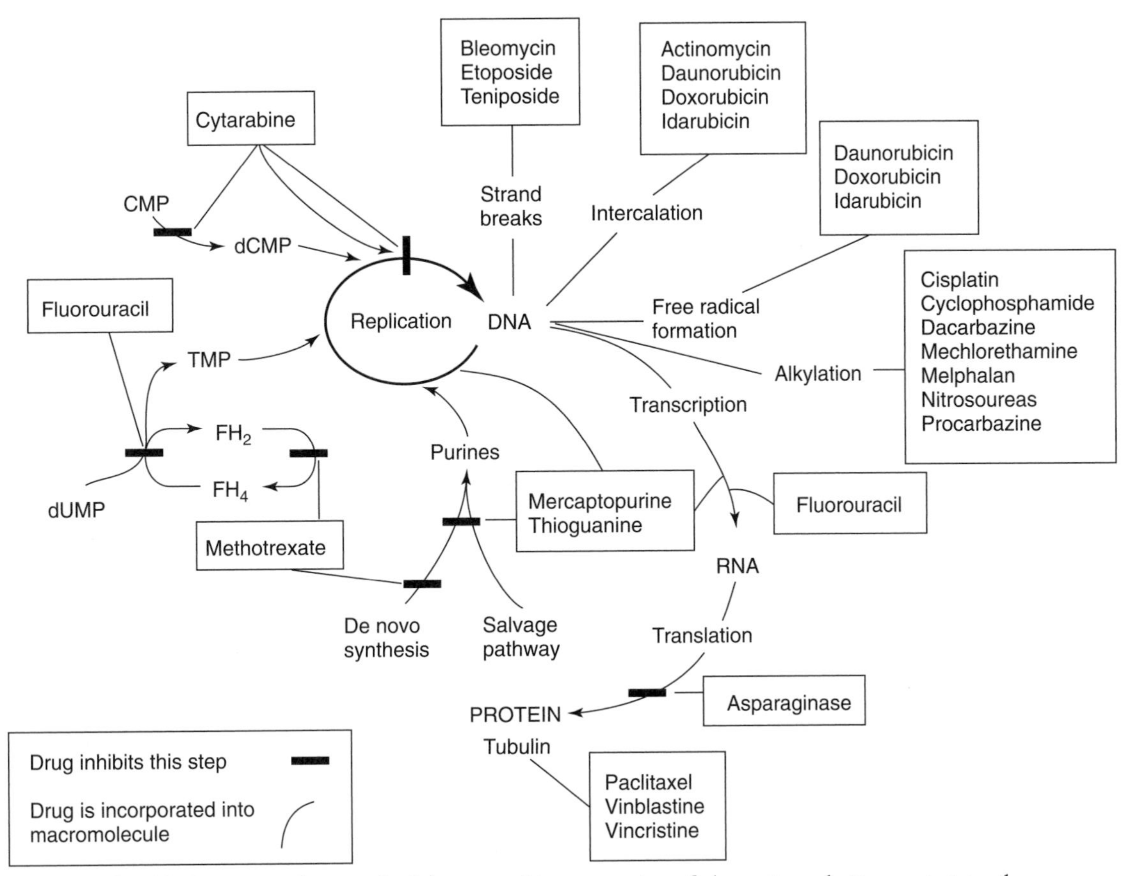

Fig. 42-2 Potential sites of inhibition and incorporation of the antineoplastic agents into the biosynthetic pathways of nucleic acids and proteins. *CMP,* Cytosine monophosphate; *dCMP,* deoxycytosine monophosphate; *dUMP,* deoxyuridine monophosphate; *FH_2,* dihydrofolate; *FH_4,* tetrahydrofolate; *TMP,* thymidine monophosphate.

resting cell populations into active cell division, increasing the growth fraction of the tumor.

5. Anticancer drugs kill cells according to first-order kinetics. Even a drug that destroys 99.99% of the tumor cells will leave a substantial number of tumor cells intact if the initial quantity was large. Because survival of a few or perhaps even a single malignant cell may lead to tumor regrowth, chemotherapy is generally given in cycles to maximize tumor cell reduction. The optimal interval between cycles is determined by the time required to allow for sufficient bone marrow recovery without allowing significant tumor regrowth.
6. The administration of combinations of antineoplastic drugs takes advantage of the different mechanisms of action. By using agents that act at different phases of the cell cycle, synergistic effects may be obtained as well as an increase in the collective antitumor effect without a concomitant increase in undesirable side effects. Combination chemotherapy may prevent or slow the development of resistant strains.
7. Cancer cells may build up resistance to a previously effective drug, which then becomes ineffective. Such resistance has been ascribed to a variety of causes, including decreased drug penetration resulting from a reduction in tumor blood supply, drug-provoked mutations, enzyme alterations, and acquired resistance through natural selection of tumor cells insensitive to the drug. The therapeutic potential of the antineoplastic drugs may be enhanced by active antitumor defense mechanisms in the host. Immunotherapy given with chemotherapy, either concurrently or sequentially, may boost the tumoricidal effect of the drugs.

CHEMOTHERAPEUTIC DRUGS

Antineoplastic Alkylating Agents

The alkylating agents (Table 42-1) are composed of six major chemical classes: (1) the nitrogen mustards (including chlorambucil, cyclophosphamide, estramustine, ifosfamide, mechlorethamine, and melphalan), (2) the alkyl sulfonates (busulfan), (3) the ethylenimines (thiotepa), (4) the triazines (dacarbazine), (5) the tetrazines (temozolomide), and (6) the nitrosoureas (carmustine, lomustine, and streptozocin). They all share the common chemical characteristic of forming alkyl radicals, which form covalent linkages with nucleophilic moieties such as the phosphate, sulfhydryl, hydroxyl, carboxyl, amino, and imidazole groups.[9] They react with organic compounds such as DNA and RNA as well as proteins essential for cell metabolism and protein synthesis and prevent cell division by cross-linking strands of DNA. The alkylating agents are not cell cycle specific, although they are most destructive to rapidly proliferating tissues and appear to cause cellular death only when the cell attempts to divide. Because they produce irreversible changes in the DNA molecule, the alkylating agents are mutagenic, teratogenic, and carcinogenic in addition to being oncolytic. The alkylating agents are also radiomimetic because they produce morphologic damage in cells similar to that caused by radiation injury. Because most of these agents are myelosuppressive, immunosuppression and susceptibility to infection are common outcomes. They vary greatly in lipid solubility, membrane transport, and pharmacokinetic properties and therefore differ in clinical use. The molecular structures of representative alkylating agents are shown in Figure 42-3; adverse effects and clinical applications are listed in Table 42-1.

Mechlorethamine

Mechlorethamine was the first nitrogen mustard introduced in clinical practice and the progenitor of the antineoplastic alkylating agents.[25] It is still used systemically in the treatment of Hodgkin's disease, in combination with vincristine, procarbazine, and prednisone, and topically to treat mycosis fungoides. The drug is a vesicant that produces severe local tissue necrosis unless administered through a running intravenous infusion. This irritant effect is used to control intractable pleural effusions caused by intrapleural malignancies. In such instances, the drug is injected intracavitarily. Usually given intravenously, this drug is highly reactive and has a short stability and biologic half-life. The acute side effects of nitrogen mustard are nausea and vomiting, and these usually begin within 30 minutes after injection and persist for up to 8 hours.

Busulfan

Busulfan is used almost exclusively in the control of chronic myelogenous leukemia. A slow-acting sulfur mustard that is well absorbed after oral administration, busulfan is rapidly cleared from the blood and excreted in the urine as inactive metabolites. It has bone marrow suppressive effects similar to other antineoplastic alkylating drugs; however, with busulfan the myelosuppression can be quite prolonged.

Chlorambucil

Chlorambucil is given orally for chronic lymphocytic leukemia, indolent non-Hodgkin's lymphomas (NHL), carcinoma of the ovary and breast, and multiple myeloma. The drug is well absorbed and rapidly metabolized, but its route of excretion is uncertain. Chlorambucil is generally well tolerated with minimal gastrointestinal toxicity in the usual doses.

Cyclophosphamide

Cyclophosphamide is a cyclic mustard that resulted from attempts to produce an alkylating agent with greater selectivity for neoplastic tissues than the original nitrogen mustard mechlorethamine. Cyclophosphamide is a broad-spectrum agent and is of value in induction, maintenance, and remission therapy for NHL; leukemia; and prostate, lung, breast, and ovarian cancers. It is also used in high doses as part of the conditioning regimen for bone marrow transplants. Cyclophosphamide also has excellent immunosuppressive properties and finds use in severe rheumatoid arthritis, allograft rejection, and other immune disorders. The drug may be administered orally or intravenously and is metabolized to the active compounds phosphoramide mustard and acrolein by the liver. Acrolein is toxic to the bladder, producing hemorrhagic cystitis and dysuria that can be minimized by vigorous hydration and frequent bladder emptying. Cyclophosphamide is a powerful myelosuppressant manifested primarily as leukopenia.

Ifosfamide

Ifosfamide is a nitrogen mustard differing from cyclophosphamide only in the location of a chloroethyl moiety. This intravenous drug is also a prodrug that must be metabolized by the liver cytochrome P450 (CYP) system to the active alkylating agent ifosfamide mustard and other toxic metabolites (acrolein and chloroacetic acid). Ifosfamide has a broad spectrum of antineoplastic activity. Although ifosfamide has significant toxic effects, the dose-limiting toxicity of this newest alkylator is hemorrhagic cystitis. The high incidence of this toxicity requires uroprotection with adequate hydration, frequent bladder emptying, and the concurrent use of mesna, a uroprotective agent. Mesna contains a free sulfhydryl group that reacts with and inactivates the toxic metabolites.

Melphalan

Melphalan is a phenylalanine mustard that is available orally for the treatment of multiple myeloma and carcinomas of the ovaries and breast. Melphalan is erratically absorbed from the gastrointestinal tract, and intravenous melphalan is available for use in high doses for bone marrow transplant conditioning regimens.

Thiotepa

Thiotepa (triethylenethiophosphoramide) is an alkylating agent that has produced favorable results in breast and ovarian cancers, lymphoma, and rhabdomyosarcoma. It is clinically used in standard doses for the treatment of superficial bladder cancer, where it is directly instilled into the bladder lumen. This agent has also been used for the control of malignant effusions, and high doses are used in the treatment of refractory cancer and in bone marrow transplants. After intravenous infusion, most of the drug is excreted unchanged in the urine.

Dacarbazine

Dacarbazine (DTIC) is an artificially synthesized congener of the naturally occurring purine precursor 5-aminoimidazole-4-carboxamide. Originally developed as an antimetabolite, DTIC is N-demethylated in the liver to yield an effective alkylating derivative. After intravenous administration, the drug is extensively metabolized and renally excreted. DTIC has an elimination half-life of approximately 5 hours. The drug is most effective in the management of malignant melanoma, soft tissue sarcomas, and Hodgkin's disease. Nausea and vomiting are the predominant side effects, with an onset in the

Text continued on p. 707.

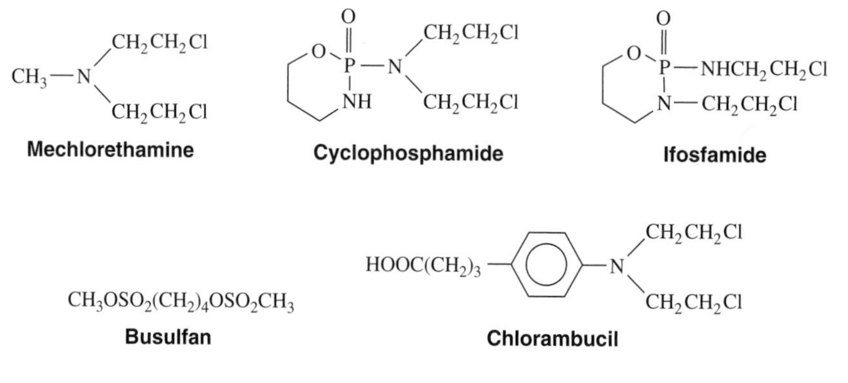

$CH_3-N(CH_2CH_2Cl)_2$

Mechlorethamine

Cyclophosphamide

Ifosfamide

$CH_3OSO_2(CH_2)_4OSO_2CH_3$

Busulfan

$HOOC(CH_2)_3-C_6H_4-N(CH_2CH_2Cl)_2$

Chlorambucil

Fig. 42-3 Structural formulas of representative alkylating agents.

Table • 42-1

Classification of Available Antineoplastic and Associated Drugs

CLASS OR TYPE OF AGENT(S)	NONPROPRIETARY (GENERIC) NAME	PROPRIETARY (TRADE) NAME	ADVERSE EFFECTS	STOMATITIS*	CLINICAL APPLICATIONS
Alkylating Agents					
Nitrogen mustards	Chlorambucil	Leukeran	*Myelosuppression,* pulmonary fibrosis, dermatotoxicity, hepatotoxicity	0	Chronic lymphocytic leukemia, Hodgkin's disease, lymphosarcoma, ovarian cancer, seminoma
	Cyclophosphamide	Cytoxan	Immunosuppression, *myelosuppression,* dermatotoxicity, hemorrhagic cystitis, *gastrointestinal enterotoxicity,* hepatotoxicity, alopecia, SIADH	+	Hodgkin's disease; lymphoma; leukemia; multiple myeloma; sarcoma; testicular, prostate, lung, breast, and ovarian carcinoma
	Estramustine	Emcyt	*Myelosuppression,* cardiovascular toxicity, gastrointestinal enterotoxicity, gynecomastia	+	Prostate cancer
	Ifosfamide	IFEX	*Myelosuppression,* nausea and vomiting, *hemorrhagic cystitis,* lethargy, confusion	+	Testicular carcinoma, sarcoma, ovarian carcinoma
	Mechlorethamine	Mustargen	*Myelosuppression, nausea and vomiting,* tissue necrosis, alopecia, neurotoxicity	0	Hodgkin's disease, lymphoma, mycosis fungoides
	Melphalan	Alkeran	*Myelosuppression,* gastrointestinal enterotoxicity, pulmonary fibrosis, dermatotoxicity, teratogenicity, SIADH	0	Multiple myeloma, ovarian carcinoma
Alkyl sulfonate	Busulfan	Myleran	*Myelosuppression, nausea and vomiting, pulmonary fibrosis,* dermatotoxicity, cataract formation, gynecomastia	0	Chronic myelocytic leukemia, polycythemia vera
Ethylenimine derivative	Thiotepa	Thioplex	*Myelosuppression,* infertility, dermatotoxicity, nausea and vomiting	0	Carcinoma of breast, ovary, and bladder; rhabdomyosarcoma
Triazene derivative	Dacarbazine	DTIC	*Nausea and vomiting,* fever, *myelosuppression,* alopecia, hepatotoxicity, dermatotoxicity	0	Melanoma, Hodgkin's disease, sarcoma
Tetrazine derivative	Temozolomide	Temodar	*Myelosuppression, gastrointestinal enterotoxicity*	+	Brain tumor, melanoma
Nitrosoureas	Carmustine	BiCNU	*Myelosuppression, gastrointestinal enterotoxicity,* hepatotoxicity, nephrotoxicity, pulmonary fibrosis	0	Hodgkin's disease, brain tumor, lymphoma, melanoma, multiple myeloma
	Lomustine	CeeNU	*Myelosuppression,* gastrointestinal enterotoxicity, hepatotoxicity, nephrotoxicity, pulmonary fibrosis	0	Hodgkin's disease, lung and brain tumors, multiple myeloma, melanoma
	Streptozocin	Zanosar	*Nausea and vomiting, nephrotoxicity,* hypoglycemia, hepatotoxicity, fever, myelosuppression	0	Islet cell carcinoma of the pancreas
Antimetabolites					
Folic acid analogue	Methotrexate	Trexall	*Myelosuppression, mucositis,* nausea and vomiting, pulmonary fibrosis, nephrotoxicity, nephrotoxicity, neurotoxicity	++	Choriocarcinoma; carcinomas of head, neck, breast, and lung; lymphocytic leukemia; sarcoma; trophoblastic tumor; testicular and bladder tumors; psoriasis

Continued

Table • 42-1

Classification of Available Antineoplastic and Associated Drugs—cont'd

CLASS OR TYPE OF AGENT(S)	NONPROPRIETARY (GENERIC) NAME	PROPRIETARY (TRADE) NAME	ADVERSE EFFECTS	STOMATITIS*	CLINICAL APPLICATIONS
Antimetabolites—cont'd					
Purine analogues	Mercaptopurine	Purinethol	*Myelosuppression,* nausea and vomiting, hepatotoxicity, immunosuppression	++	Acute leukemia, chronic myelogenous leukemia
	Thioguanine	Tabloid	*Myelosuppression,* hepatotoxicity, nausea and vomiting	++	Acute leukemia, chronic myelogenous leukemia
	Fludarabine	Fludara	*Myelosuppression,* nausea and vomiting, alopecia	++	Chronic lymphocytic leukemia
	Pentostatin (2′-deoxycorformycin)	Nipent	*Nephrotoxicity, CNS depression,* nausea and vomiting	0	Hairy cell leukemia
	Cladribine (2-CDA, 2-chloro-deoxyadenosine)	Leustatin	*Myelosuppression*	0	Hairy cell leukemia
Pyrimidine analogues	Cytarabine	Cytosar-U	*Myelosuppression,* nausea and vomiting, hepatotoxicity, dermatotoxicity, CNS, conjunctivitis	++	Acute leukemia, lymphoma, chronic myelogenous leukemia
	Capecitabine	Xeloda	*Gastrointestinal enterotoxicity, myelosuppression,* dermatotoxicity, neurotoxicity, hepatotoxicity	++	Colorectal cancer, metastatic breast cancer
	Fluorouracil	Adrucil	*Gastrointestinal enterotoxicity,* myelosuppression, dermatotoxicity, neurotoxicity	++	Gastrointestinal adenocarcinoma; carcinoma of lung, breast, ovary, prostate, cervix, bladder, head and neck
	Floxuridine	FUDR	*Gastrointestinal enterotoxicity,* myelosuppression, dermatotoxicity, hepatotoxicity, neurotoxicity	++	Hepatic metastases from gastrointestinal adenocarcinomas, carcinomas of head and neck
	Gemcitabine	Gemzar	*Myelosuppression,* fever and flulike symptoms	0	Adenocarcinoma of the pancreas
Vinca Alkaloids					
	Vincristine	Oncovin	*Neurotoxicity,* SIADH, dermatotoxicity, gastrointestinal enterotoxicity, alopecia	+	Hodgkin's disease; lymphocytic leukemia; chronic myelogenous leukemia; Wilm's tumor; sarcoma; multiple myeloma; cancer of breast, cervix, lung, and ovary
	Vinblastine	Velban	*Myelosuppression,* gastrointestinal enterotoxicity, neurotoxicity, SIADH	+	Hodgkin's disease; lymphoma; cancer of breast, bladder, and testis; Kaposi's sarcoma
	Vinorelbine	Navelbine	*Myelosuppression,* gastrointestinal enterotoxicity, neurotoxicity	+	Non–small-cell lung carcinoma, breast carcinoma
Antibiotics					
	Bleomycin	Blenoxane	*Pulmonary toxicity,* gastrointestinal enterotoxicity, skin reactions, anaphylaxis, fever	+	Testicular cancer, Hodgkin's disease, lymphoma, sarcoma, squamous cell carcinoma of head and neck, gastrointestinal tumors

	Dactinomycin (actinomycin D)	Cosmegen	*Myelosuppression,* gastrointestinal enterotoxicity, dermatotoxicity, tissue necrosis	+	Wilm's tumor, rhabdomyosarcoma, Ewing's sarcoma, neuroblastoma, testicular carcinoma, osteosarcoma, choriocarcinoma
	Daunorubicin, liposomal daunorubicin	Cerubidine, DaunoXome	*Myelosuppression, cardiotoxicity,* gastrointestinal enterotoxicity, alopecia, *tissue necrosis,* radiation recall reaction	+	Acute leukemia
	Doxorubicin, liposomal doxorubicin	Adriamycin, Doxil	*Myelosuppression, cardiotoxicity,* gastrointestinal enterotoxicity, alopecia, *tissue necrosis,* radiation recall reaction	++	Acute leukemia; sarcoma; Hodgkin's disease; neuroblastoma; bladder cancer; carcinoma of lung, gastrointestinal tract, endometrium, ovary, thyroid, and breast; Wilm's tumor, multiple myeloma
	Epirubicin	Ellence	*Myelosuppression, cardiotoxicity,* gastrointestinal enterotoxicity, dermatotoxicity	++	Breast cancer
	Idarubicin	Idamycin	*Myelosuppression,* alopecia, cardiotoxicity, nausea and vomiting	+	Acute leukemia
	Plicamycin	Mithracin	*Myelosuppression,* fever, gastrointestinal enterotoxicity, hepatotoxicity, nephrotoxicity, dermatotoxicity, *hypocalcemia*	+	Testicular carcinoma, tumor-associated hypercalcemia
	Mitomycin	Mutamycin	*Myelosuppression,* pulmonary toxicity, alopecia, tissue necrosis, gastrointestinal enterotoxicity	+	Carcinoma of head, neck, lung, gastrointestinal tract, breast, cervix, and bladder
	Mitoxantrone	Novantrone	*Myelosuppression,* hepatotoxicity, gastrointestinal enterotoxicity, cardiac toxicity	+	Acute leukemia, chronic myelogenous leukemia, lymphoma, breast and ovarian cancer
Hormone Agonists and Antagonists					
Adrenal corticosteroids	Prednisone, prednisolone	Deltasone, Delta-Cortef	Peptic ulcer, hypokalemia, hyperglycemia, psychosis, osteoporosis, infections, fluid retention	0	Hodgkin's disease, lymphocytic leukemia, multiple myeloma, breast cancer, hypercalcemia
Androgens	Fluoxymesterone, testolactone	Halotestin, Teslac	Masculinization, edema, alopecia, acne, hypercalcemia	0	Metastatic breast cancer
Estrogens	Chlorotrianisene, diethylstilbestrol, ethinyl estradiol	TACE, Stilphostrol, Estinyl	Gynecomastia, breast tenderness, edema, thrombosis, depression	0	Postmenopausal carcinoma of breast, carcinoma of prostate
Progestins	Hydroxyprogesterone, medroxyprogesterone, megestrol	Delalutin, Depo-Provera, Megace	Edema, alopecia, hirsutism, genitourinary toxicity, neurotoxicity	0	Metastatic endometrial carcinoma, renal and breast carcinoma
Adrenal suppressant	Aminoglutethimide	Cytadren	Hypotension, fever, myelosuppression, neurotoxicity, masculinization	0	Carcinoma of the adrenal cortex and breast, Cushing's syndrome

Continued

Table • 42-1

Classification of Available Antineoplastic and Associated Drugs—cont'd

CLASS OR TYPE OF AGENT(S)	NONPROPRIETARY (GENERIC) NAME	PROPRIETARY (TRADE) NAME	ADVERSE EFFECTS	STOMATITIS*	CLINICAL APPLICATIONS
Hormone Agonists and Antagonists—cont'd					
Anastrozole, inhibitors	Arimidex, exemestane, letrozole	Aromasin, Femara	Nausea, vomiting, hot flashes, gastrointestinal enterotoxicity, hepatotoxicity, hypertension	0	Advanced carcinoma of the breast
Gonadotropin-releasing hormone analogues (agonists-antagonists)	Goserelin, leuprolide	Zoladex, Lupron	Hot flashes, tumor flares, impotence, amenorrhea, vaginal bleeding	0	Carcinoma of prostate and breast
Antiestrogen	Tamoxifen, toremifene	Nolvadex, Fareston	Gastrointestinal enterotoxicity, hot flashes, tumor flare, vaginal discharge, ocular toxicity	0	Postmenopausal carcinoma of breast, metastatic melanoma
	Raloxifene	Evista	Hot flashes, gastrointestinal enterotoxicity	0	Breast cancer, osteoporosis
Antiandrogen	Bicalutamide	Casodex	Gynecomastia, nausea, hot flashes	0	Carcinoma of prostate
	Flutamide, nilutamide	Eulexin, Nilandron	Gynecomastia, nausea	0	Carcinoma of prostate
Miscellaneous Classes					
Enzymes	L-Asparaginase, PEG-L-asparaginase	Elspar, Oncaspar	Acute hypersensitivity reaction, fever, hepatotoxicity, coagulation defects, gastrointestinal enterotoxicity	0	Acute lymphocytic leukemia
Platinum complexes	Cisplatin	Platinol	*Nephrotoxicity,* ototoxicity, *nausea and vomiting,* gastrointestinal enterotoxicity, neurotoxicity, acute allergic reactions	0	Carcinoma of testis, prostate, cervix, ovary, endometrium, lung, bladder, head and neck; sarcoma; neuroblastoma
	Carboplatin	Paraplatin	*Myelosuppression,* gastrointestinal enterotoxicity, neurotoxicity	0	Testicular and ovarian carcinoma, head and neck cancers, lung cancer
	Oxaliplatin	Eloxatin	*Pharyngolaryngeal dysesthesia, paresthesias,* peripheral neuropathy, diarrhea, myelosuppression	0	Colorectal cancer
Other Drugs					
	Altretamine	Hexalen	*Gastrointestinal enterotoxicity,* neurotoxicity, myelosuppression	0	Ovarian cancer
	Arsenic trioxide	Trisenox	*Gastrointestinal enterotoxicity, dermatotoxicity,* cardiotoxicity, leukocytosis, retinoic acid syndrome	0	Acute promyelocytic leukemia
	Bexarotene	Targretin	Rash, headaches, hypothyroidism, photosensitivity, hypertriglyceridemia, hypercholesterolemia	0	Cutaneous T-cell lymphoma

	BCG, intravesical	TheraCys	Cystitis, flulike symptoms, infections	0	Superficial bladder cancer
	Hydroxyurea	Hydrea	Myelosuppression, alopecia, gastrointestinal enterotoxicity, rare neurologic disturbances	+	Chronic myelogenous leukemia, sickle cell anemia, polycythemia vera
	Mitotane	Lysodren	Gastrointestinal enterotoxicity, neurotoxicity, hematuria, cystitis, dermatotoxicity, adrenal insufficiency	0	Carcinoma of adrenal cortex
	Porfimer	Photofrin	Photosensitivity, gastrointestinal enterotoxicity, cardiotoxicity, anemia, fever	0	Endobronchial cancer, esophageal cancer
	Procarbazine	Matulane	Gastrointestinal enterotoxicity, myelosuppression, CNS depression, dermatotoxicity, disulfiram reactions	+	Hodgkin's disease, lymphoma, multiple myeloma
	Thalidomide	Thalomid	*Neurotoxicity, dermatotoxicity,* fever, gastrointestinal enterotoxicity, tooth pain, dry mouth, tongue discoloration, taste changes	0/+	Melanoma, multiple myeloma, renal cell carcinoma, erythema nodosum leprosum
	Tretinoin	Vesanoid	*Headache, xerosis, cheilitis, teratogenicity,* arthralgia, myalgia, leukocytosis, retinoic acid syndrome	0	Acute promyelocytic leukemia
Natural Products					
	Paclitaxel	Taxol	*Myelosuppression,* alopecia, hypersensitivity reaction, neuropathy, bradycardia	0	Metastatic carcinoma of ovary and breast
	Docetaxel	Taxotere	*Myelosuppression,* hypersensitivity reaction, neurologic toxicity	0	Advanced breast carcinoma
	Etoposide	VePesid	*Myelosuppression,* nausea and vomiting, hypersensitivity reaction	0	Carcinoma of testis and lung, Hodgkin's disease, lymphoma, lung cancer, sarcoma
	Teniposide	Vumon	*Myelosuppression,* alopecia, neuropathy, nausea and vomiting	0	Acute lymphocytic leukemia, lymphoma, carcinoma of lung and breast
	Irinotecan	Camptosar	*Diarrhea, myelosuppression,* nausea and vomiting	0	Metastatic carcinoma of the colon or rectum
	Topotecan	Hycamtin	*Myelosuppression,* nausea and vomiting, flulike symptoms	0	Metastatic carcinoma of the ovary
Monoclonal Antibodies and other targeted drug therapies					
	Alemtuzumab	Campath	*Infusion-related reactions, severe immunosuppression, and infections*	0	Chronic B-cell lymphocytic leukemia
	Bevacizumab	Avastin	Hypertension, tumor-related bleeding, mild neutropenia	0	Renal cell carcinoma, in combination wth chemotherapy for colorectal and breast cancers
	Bortezomib	Velcade	Diarrhea, fatigue, peripheral neuropathy	0	Refractory and relapsed multiple myeloma
	Gefitinib	Iressa	Diarrhea, acneiform rash	0	Metastatic non—small cell lung cancer, other solid tumors
	Gemtuzumab ozogamicin	Mylotarg	*Myelosuppression, hepatotoxicity, infusion-related adverse effects, hypertension/hypotension*	+	Acute myeloid leukemia

Continued

Table 42-1

Classification of Available Antineoplastic and Associated Drugs—cont'd

CLASS OR TYPE OF AGENT(S)	NONPROPRIETARY (GENERIC) NAME	PROPRIETARY (TRADE) NAME	ADVERSE EFFECTS	STOMATITIS*	CLINICAL APPLICATIONS
Monoclonal Antibodies and other targeted drug therapies—cont'd					
	Ibritumomab tiuxetan	Zevalin	*Infusion related reactions, neutropenia, thrombocytopenia*	0	B-cell low grade or follicular non-Hodgkin's lymphoma
	Imatinib	Gleevec	Edema, nausea and vomiting, muscle cramps, liver function test abnormalities	0	Chronic myelogenous leukemia
	Rituximab	Rituxan	*Hypersensitivity, infusion-related adverse effects*	+	Lymphomas
	Trastuzumab	Herceptin	*Hypersensitivity, infusion-related adverse effects,* gastrointestinal enterotoxicity	0	Breast cancer
	Tositumomab/^{131}I-tositumomab	Bexxar	*Infusion-related reactions,* neutropenia, thrombocytopenia, nausea and vomiting, potential hypothyroidism	0	Follicular low grade non-Hodgkin's lymphoma, transformed or relapse non-Hodgkin's lymphoma
Biologic Response Modifiers					
	Interferon α_{2a}, interferon α_{2b}, interferon α_{n3}	Roferon-A, Intron-A, Alferon-N	*Fever,* myalgia, gastrointestinal enterotoxicity, neurotoxicity, myelosuppression	0	Hairy cell leukemia, chronic myelogenous leukemia, Kaposi's sarcoma, chronic hepatitis
	Aldesleukin (IL-2)	Proleukin	*Fever,* fluid retention, hypotension, respiratory distress, *capillary leak syndrome,* nephrotoxicity, rashes	0	Metastatic renal cell carcinoma
	Levamisole	Ergamisol	Flulike symptoms, nausea and vomiting	0	In combination with fluorouracil for colorectal cancer
Protectants					
	Amifostine	Ethyol	*Hypotension,* nausea and vomiting	0	Administered before cisplatin to reduce incidence of nephrotoxicity, before radiation therapy for head and neck cancer to reduce xerostomia
	Dexrazoxane	Zinecard	Abnormalities in liver and renal function test results, additive myelosuppression	0	In combination with doxorubicin therapy in breast carcinoma to reduce incidence of cardiomyopathy
	Filgrastim, sargramostim	Neupogen, Leukine	Fever, myalgia, bone pain, pericardial effusions	0	Prevent chemotherapy-induced neutropenia, to increase neutrophil counts and prevent infections
	Leucovorin	Wellcovorin	Hypocalcemia	0	Methotrexate rescue, used with fluorouracil to increase activity of chemotherapy agent
	Oprelvekin	Neumega	Edema, dizziness, dyspnea, fatigue, arthralgia, myalgia, palpitations	0	Prevention of chemotherapy-induced thrombocytopenia
	Mesna	Mesnex	Nausea and vomiting	0	In combination with ifosfamide or with cyclophosphamide to prevent hemorrhagic cystitis

*Stomatitis: *0,* rare; +, occasional; ++, frequent or common.
Italic type indicates a frequent or dose-limiting toxicity.
Myelosuppression includes suppression of blood cell–forming elements resulting in leukopenia, thrombocytopenia, and anemia. Gastrointestinal enterotoxicity includes nausea, vomiting, diarrhea, and mucosal damage. Dermatotoxicity includes cutaneous toxicities such as pigmentation, rashes, erythema, and exfoliation. Neurotoxicity includes peripheral neuropathy, pain, paresthesias, altered sensorium, decrease in sensory and motor acuity, and paralytic ileus. Hepatotoxicity includes liver dysfunction such as drug-induced hepatitis, transient elevation of transaminases, bile stasis, cholangitis, and veno-occlusive disease. Cardiotoxicity includes myocardial damage, congestive heart failure, and arrhythmias. Nephrotoxicity may present as renal insufficiency or acute renal tubular necrosis.
SIADH, Syndrome of inappropriate antidiuretic hormone.

first few hours that may persist for several days. Fatal hepatic damage has occurred rarely.

Temozolomide

Temozolomide is the first imidazotetrazinone derivative used in clinical practice. Similarly to DTIC, temozolomide is metabolized to monomethyl 5-triazinoimidazole carboxamide (MTIC), which is ultimately converted to the cytotoxic methyldiazonium ion. Temozolomide has several advantages over DTIC: it can be administered orally, and it does not require hepatic conversion to MTIC because temozolomide is spontaneously converted to the active metabolite at physiologic pH.[29] Temozolomide penetrates tissues well and is able to cross the blood-brain barrier. Therefore it has been used to treat brain tumors such as astrocytoma.[68] Temozolomide has also been used to treat malignant melanoma. The major toxic effects associated with this alkylating agent include myelosuppression, nausea, vomiting, headache, and fatigue.

Nitrosoureas

Two of the nitrosoureas, carmustine and lomustine, decompose in the body to yield reactive intermediates that act as classic alkylating agents in causing strand breaks and cross-links in DNA. They also produce isocyanates that inhibit DNA repair and RNA synthesis. Carmustine is administered intravenously, whereas lomustine is given orally. Both are rapidly metabolized and slowly excreted in the urine. The nitrosoureas are characterized by their lipophilicity and their ability to cross the blood-brain barrier. This property is useful in the treatment of brain tumors. Each produces nausea and vomiting within 2 to 6 hours after administration and delayed bone marrow depression that becomes apparent in 3 to 6 weeks and lasts for 2 to 3 weeks.

Streptozocin

Streptozocin is a naturally occurring antibiotic that has a mode of action similar to that of the nitrosoureas. Unlike carmustine and lomustine, however, streptozocin does not readily cross the blood-brain barrier, and it is not strongly myelosuppressive. Streptozocin is unique in its special affinity for the islet cells of the pancreas. The drug is diabetogenic in animals and effective against metastatic insulinomas in human beings. Streptozocin should be administered intravenously with care because it is a vesicant. It is one of the most emetogenic agents and requires adequate premedication with antiemetics. Potentially fatal renal toxicity and hepatotoxicity have occurred.[66]

Antimetabolites

The antimetabolites bear a marked structural resemblance to folic acid and to the purine and pyrimidine bases involved in the synthesis of DNA, RNA, and certain coenzymes (Figure 42-4). They differ in molecular arrangement from the corresponding metabolite to a degree sufficient to serve as fraudulent substrates for biochemical reactions, either inhibiting synthetic steps or becoming incorporated into molecules and interfering with cellular function or replication. The antimetabolites characteristically exert their major effects during the S (DNA synthesis) phase of the cell cycle. This interferes with the growth of rapidly proliferating cells throughout the body—the bone marrow, germinal cells, hair follicles, and lining of the alimentary tract. Oral manifestations are an especially prominent feature of the toxicity of these agents. Three classes of antimetabolites exist: the folic acid analogues, the purine analogues, and the pyrimidine analogues.

Folic acid analogues

Folic acid is an essential vitamin that is converted into metabolically active tetrahydrofolic acid by the enzyme dihydrofolate reductase. Tetrahydrofolic acid participates in the synthesis of purines, thymidylate, and ultimately nucleic acids by transferring one-carbon units to the nucleotide precursors.

Methotrexate is the 4-amino, 10-methyl analogue of folic acid and a potent inhibitor of dihydrofolate reductase. This inhibition results in the decreased conversion of dihydrofolate to tetrahydrofolate and impaired synthesis of thymidylic acid and inosinic acid. Deficiencies of these acids retard DNA and RNA synthesis. Protein synthesis is also inhibited because reduced folates are cofactors in the conversion of glycine to serine and homocysteine to methionine.

Methotrexate is readily absorbed from the gastrointestinal tract and is primarily excreted in the urine. There is some enterohepatic recycling of methotrexate, which extends the elimination half-life of the drug and is responsible for most of the marrow and gastrointestinal toxicity. Methotrexate tends

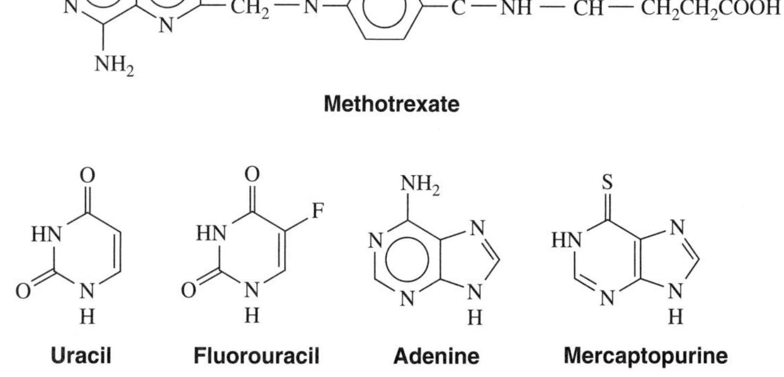

Fig. 42-4 Structural relationships between several antimetabolites and their respective analogues.

to distribute into "third spaces," such as ascitic, pleural, or peritoneal fluid and can potentially act as drug reservoirs. The presence of these clinical features or renal failure contributes to increased toxicity. Depending on the indication, methotrexate may be administered by many different routes with a variable dosing range. Administered orally, the drug is often used to treat rheumatoid arthritis and psoriasis. Intrathecal administration is used to treat CNS tumors, and intraarterial administration is used for regional therapy of head and neck cancers. Given intravenously and intramuscularly, methotrexate is a valuable therapeutic agent in some forms of leukemia, choriocarcinoma, lymphoma, sarcoma, testicular tumors, and carcinoma of the breast and lung. The drug is also used in very high doses for adjuvant and salvage therapies for osteosarcoma and leukemia.

High-dose therapy with methotrexate requires monitoring of serum blood concentrations and the use of folinic acid "rescue." The folinic acid (citrovorum factor, calcium folinate, leucovorin) bypasses the blockade of dihydrofolate reductase in normal cells and may reduce the incidence and severity of mucositis and myelosuppression. Other nontumoricidal applications of methotrexate include its use after allogenic bone marrow transplants to prevent graft-versus-host disease and in steroid-dependent asthmatic patients to decrease asthmatic symptoms.

Methotrexate is subject to a number of important drug interactions. Highly plasma protein–bound drugs such as salicylates, sulfonamides, and phenytoin may displace methotrexate from its protein-binding sites and result in greater toxicity. Organic acids such as salicylate and probenecid inhibit the tubular secretion of methotrexate, resulting in increased concentrations of methotrexate and toxicity. Penicillins can also compete with methotrexate for renal tubular secretion.[33] In patients receiving large gram doses of methotrexate, the concurrent use of NSAIDs should be avoided because this drug class can also reduce renal blood flow and increase the risk of nephrotoxicity.

Dose-limiting toxic effects of methotrexate include bone marrow depression manifested by leukopenia and thrombocytopenia, which are conducive to secondary infection and hemorrhage, a very painful stomatitis with mucosal and epithelial ulceration, pharyngitis and dysphagia, esophagitis, gastroenterocolitis, and proctitis with associated watery and bloody diarrhea. Large doses can be nephrotoxic and chronic dosing can lead to changes in hepatic function.

Purine analogues

Historically, the most commonly used purine analogues in cancer chemotherapy have been mercaptopurine and thioguanine. Newer agents include fludarabine, pentostatin, and cladribine.

Mercaptopurine and thioguanine The mechanisms of action of these thiopurines have not yet been fully established. Presumably, they affect the incorporation of purine derivatives into nucleic acids. The analogues are converted in the body to the ribonucleotide form, which interferes with the conversion of inosinic acid to the nucleotides of adenine and guanine, resulting in the inhibition of DNA and RNA synthesis. They also inhibit de novo biosynthesis of purines from the small molecule precursors (glycine, formate, and phosphate) and are incorporated into fraudulent DNA.

Orally administered mercaptopurine is readily absorbed but undergoes extensive first-pass metabolism by the liver. After intravenous injection, the plasma half-life is approximately 90 minutes. The drug is metabolized by methylation in the liver and by the hepatic enzyme xanthine oxidase. Concurrent administration with allopurinol, a xanthine oxidase inhibitor originally developed to increase the anticancer effect of mercaptopurine, requires a 50% reduction in the dose of mercaptopurine. Allopurinol is of little clinical value in this setting because it also increases the toxicity of mercaptopurine. The use of allopurinol in the treatment of gout is described in Chapter 21. Currently, mercaptopurine is used mainly for remission maintenance in acute lymphocytic leukemia. The chief toxic effect is myelosuppression. Pulmonary fibrosis and pancreatitis may also occur. Thioguanine has activity, toxicity, and clinical applications similar to those of mercaptopurine.

Fludarabine Fludarabine (2-fluoro-ara-AMP) is an analogue of adenosine. This injectable purine antagonist is quickly dephosphorylated in the plasma, enters the cell, and is converted to the triphosphate form. This false nucleotide inhibits ribonucleotide reductase and DNA polymerase, which results in the inhibition of DNA synthesis.[37] Fludarabine is indicated for the treatment of B-cell chronic lymphocytic leukemia in patients who have not responded to traditional therapy with an alkylating agent. Fludarabine is primarily excreted by the kidneys and has a long plasma half-life of approximately 10 hours. Transient myelosuppression and immunosuppression, with an increased risk of opportunistic infection, appears to be the major toxicity at current doses. Fludarabine has also been used for NHL, haircell leukemia, and cutaneous T-cell lymphoma.

Pentostatin Pentostatin is a newer antimetabolite isolated from *Streptomyces antibioticus.* This purine analogue is an inhibitor of adenosine deaminase, which converts adenosine to inosine. This inhibition apparently leads to inhibition of methylation and other reactions. Cytotoxic treatment with pentostatin results in the accumulation of deoxyadenosine triphosphate. The drug exhibits activity in both nonreplicating and dividing cells. Pentostatin is quickly distributed to all body tissues after administration; the plasma half-life is 2.6 to 9.4 hours, with the major portion of the drug recovered in the urine unchanged. Pentostatin has been most active in the treatment of hairy cell leukemia; it also has activity in patients with chronic lymphocytic leukemia. Toxicity is dose dependent, with acute renal failure and CNS side effects being the most severe.

Cladribine Cladribine is an adenosine deaminase–resistant purine substrate analogue toxic to lymphocytes and monocytes. It is undergoing clinical trials against hematologic malignancies and is available for the treatment of hairy cell leukemia. The major limiting toxicity is myelosuppression.

Pyrimidine analogues

Several pyrimidine congeners have been examined for antineoplastic activity. These drugs exert multiple effects on cellular growth and are among the most useful of agents for both solid tumors and leukemia.

Fluorouracil and floxuridine The fluorinated pyrimidines fluorouracil and floxuridine are prepared by substituting a stable fluorine atom for hydrogen in position 5 of the uracil and deoxyuridine molecules, respectively. These compounds, after intracellular conversion to 5-fluoro-2′-deoxyuridine monophosphate, are potent antimetabolites that bind to and inhibit thymidylate synthetase, inhibiting formation of thymidylic acid and impairing DNA synthesis. Fluorouracil metabolism also produces a critical intermediate, 5-fluorouridine triphosphate, which is incorporated into RNA and interferes with its function. 5-Fluoro-deoxyuridine triphosphate (5-FdUTP) may also be incorporated into

DNA, producing single-strand breaks contributing to the cytotoxicity.[53]

Fluorouracil is used most often in the treatment of gastrointestinal adenocarcinomas, breast cancer, and ovarian cancer. Activity has also been reported in bladder and prostate cancer. The drug is usually given intravenously as a bolus or short infusion or as a prolonged continuous infusion daily, over several days, or for months. Continuous infusion is advantageous because the plasma half-life of the drug is short (10 to 20 minutes), and the drug, like other antimetabolites, works primarily in the S phase of the cell cycle. Continuous infusion provides for prolonged exposure of the cells to the drug and the opportunity for cell populations not in the S phase to cycle into that sensitive phase. Interestingly, the toxicity profile of fluorouracil depends on the method of administration. Given as a continuous infusion over a 96-hour period, the dose-limiting toxicity is mucositis, whereas intravenous bolus results in bone marrow suppression. Fluorouracil can be administered topically to treat actinic keratoses and noninvasive skin cancers and, commonly, to improve efficacy of radiation therapy in head and neck cancers by working as a radiosensitizer. Folinic acid (leucovorin) has been combined with fluorouracil to enhance the thymidylate synthetase inhibition in resistant disease.

Floxuridine, the deoxyribonucleoside of fluorouracil, exerts a more direct inhibition of thymidylate synthetase than does fluorouracil. The drug must be given by continuous infusion because it is rapidly catabolized in vivo. Floxuridine administered intraarterially is indicated for gastrointestinal adenocarcinomas metastatic to the liver and has produced beneficial results in the treatment of head and neck carcinoma, although fluorouracil is now the preferred agent. The adverse effects of the fluorinated pyrimidines may be quite severe. Stomatitis, pharyngitis, dysphagia, enteritis, and diarrhea can be life threatening. Myocardial ischemia caused by coronary artery vasospasm has been described with fluorouracil.

Capecitabine Capecitabine (5′-dexoy-5-fluoro-N-[(pentuloxy)carbonyl]-cytidine) is a newer oral agent used in the treatment of advanced breast and colorectal cancers. Capecitabine is hydrolyzed in the liver and ultimately converted to the active drug 5-fluorouracil. Its activity profile and pharmacokinetic profile are similar to infusional fluorouracil. Capecitabine's side effect profile includes severe diarrhea, stomatitis, and some mild nausea and vomiting. Severe hand-foot syndrome (palmar/plantar erythrodysesthesia) and other dermatologic changes have been reported.[16]

Cytarabine Cytarabine (cytosine arabinoside) is an analogue of 2′-deoxycytidine that can inhibit DNA synthesis by inhibiting DNA polymerase activity as a result of its incorporation into DNA and the formation of fraudulent DNA. This results in premature DNA chain termination. Cytarabine is primarily a cell cycle S–phase-specific agent. When given intravenously, the drug is rapidly cleared from the blood by deamination in the liver, with a plasma half-life of 5 to 20 minutes. With these properties, continuous infusion is often the preferred route of administration. Cytarabine crosses the blood-brain barrier, achieving cerebrospinal fluid concentrations of 40% to 50% of those of plasma. This features allows for the treatment of CNS disease with systemic high-dose therapy. Cytarabine may be administered intrathecally and will produce high concentrations that decline slowly because of the absence of cytidine deaminase in the CNS.[1] Cytarabine is the most active single drug available for the treatment of acute myelogenous leukemia in adults, producing about a 25% incidence of complete remission. It is often used in combination with other agents. It has some modest activity against lymphomas. The major side effect is myelosuppression. High doses produce severe nausea and vomiting, severe diarrhea, cerebellar toxicity, and keratoconjuctivitis.[26]

Gemcitabine Gemcitabine (difluorodeoxycytidine) is a newer antimetabolite useful in a number of experimental tumor models, with clinical responses in non–small-cell lung cancer (NSCLC) and breast cancer. It has a current indication for first-line treatment of patients with locally advanced or metastatic adenocarcinoma of the pancreas.[32] Recent trials support the use of gemcitabine in combination with cisplatin to treat metastatic NSCLC. Its dose-limiting side effect is myelosuppression characterized by thrombocytopenia. Transient febrile episodes and a flulike syndrome have been commonly reported.

Antibiotics

A number of substances originally isolated as antibiotics have been found to exert antineoplastic activity because of their cytotoxic properties. These substances, produced naturally by various *Streptomyces* species, operate by binding with DNA to produce irreversible complexes that inhibit cell division. Various other possible mechanisms for cytotoxicity have been proposed for these agents. Antibiotics can work on cells in different phases of the cell cycle, behaving as non–phase-specific agents. Semisynthetic derivatives of some of the antibiotics are being prepared and tested clinically in an effort to reduce toxicity but retain the oncolytic potency of the parent compound.

Dactinomycin

Dactinomycin (actinomycin D) is a crystalline antibiotic composed of a phenoxazone chromophore and two cyclic peptide chains obtained as a product of fermentation by *Streptomyces parvulus.* The drug intercalates into DNA between adjacent guanine-cytosine base pairs and inhibits DNA-directed RNA synthesis. Dactinomycin is rapidly distributed into tissues and has a prolonged terminal half-life. The drug does not appear to be metabolized, but is primarily excreted in the bile. Dactinomycin is the main agent for the treatment of pediatric tumors, such as Wilms' tumor, Ewing's sarcoma, and embryonal rhabdomyosarcoma, and is of considerable value against choriocarcinoma and testicular tumors. Mucositis characterized by oral ulcerations and diarrhea often necessitates limiting the dose. Extravasation from the vein causes severe tissue necrosis.

Daunorubicin

Daunorubicin is a cytotoxic anthracycline antibiotic produced by *Streptomyces peucetius* subsp. *caesius,* which is also the source of doxorubicin and idarubicin (Figure 42-5). The drug combines with DNA in an intercalative mode by slipping into the helical structure between stacked bases. Both DNA and RNA synthesis are inhibited, and preformed DNA is damaged. Other possible mechanisms are postulated, including metabolism to form cytotoxic free radicals, a cell membrane surface cytotoxic action, and inhibition of topoisomerase II. The killing effect of daunorubicin is at a maximum in the DNA-synthesis S phase of the cell cycle, but damage is not phase specific. Experimental evidence exists for synergy between these antibiotics and drugs such as etoposide.

The drug is most useful in the treatment of acute myelogenous leukemia and acute lymphocytic leukemia. Daunorubicin is extensively tissue bound with a long elimination half-life. The major route of elimination is through biliary excretion, with some urinary excretion. Patients should

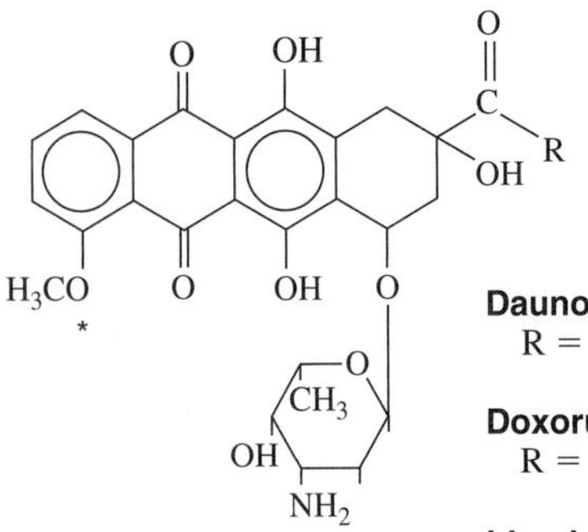

Daunorubicin
$R = CH_3$

Doxorubicin
$R = CH_2OH$

Idarubicin
*Differs from daunorubicin in the substitution of a proton for the methoxy (—OCH_3) on the "D" ring.

Fig. 42-5 Structural formulas of the anthracycline antibiotics. $R = CH_3$ for daunorubicin; $R = CH_2OH$ for doxorubicin.

be warned about red-colored urine a few days after a dose of daunorubicin. Cardiomyopathy, manifested by acute congestive heart failure, as well as acute cardiac arrhythmias, radiation recall dermatitis, and local necrosis from extravasation at the injection site are associated with cumulative doses of daunorubicin exceeding total lifetime limits of 450 to 550 mg/m^2.

Doxorubicin

Doxorubicin differs from daunorubicin by one hydroxy group (see Figure 42-5). This anthracycline glycoside acts by intercalating into DNA and shares other mechanisms of action with daunorubicin. Doxorubicin has a much broader spectrum of antineoplastic activity than daunorubicin.

Doxorubicin is a vesicant that is always given intravenously. It is rapidly cleared from the plasma and concentrated in the tissues. Urinary excretion is low, rarely accounting for more than 10% of the administered dose; in contrast, biliary excretion is high. Plasma concentrations of doxorubicin and its metabolites are markedly elevated, and the rate of elimination is greatly prolonged in the presence of severely impaired liver function.

The major toxic effects begin shortly after drug administration and last 2 to 3 days. Extravasation of the drug produces soft tissue necrosis. Myelosuppression, primarily granulocytopenia, is maximal 10 to 14 days after drug administration. Mucositis manifested mainly as soreness of the mouth with ulcerations occurs in almost all patients. Cardiomyopathy expressed as congestive heart failure becomes a serious risk in patients given a total dose exceeding 550 mg/m^2. Concurrent administration with dexrazoxane may help reduce the incidence of cardiomyopathy associated with doxorubicin therapy.[12] New liposomal encapsulated forms of doxorubicin and daunorubicin are now available. They allow for increased circulation time and the possibility of enhanced antitumor activity and decreased cardiomyopathy in the treatment of AIDS-related Kaposi's sarcoma, advanced breast and ovarian cancers, and others.[43]

Epirubicin is a semisynthetic derivative of doxorubicin, which has been extensively evaluated in patients with breast cancer.[52] Epirubicin is also being evaluated for its intravesical use in superficial bladder cancer.[51] The major dose-limiting adverse effects include hematologic and cumulative dose-related cardiotoxicity. Other important side effects include mucositis, nausea and vomiting, alopecia, and local cutaneous reactions.

Idarubicin

Idarubicin is an analogue of daunorubicin lacking the methoxy group on the C_4 position of the aglycone (see Figure 42-5). This antibiotic is used for the treatment of acute myelogenous leukemia, breast cancer, and some lymphomas. Oral idarubicin is not currently available. The toxicity of idarubicin appears less severe than that of either daunorubicin or doxorubicin, and it may have a lower risk of cardiotoxicity. Nausea, vomiting, and mucositis appear equivalent to the other anthracyclines.

Mitoxantrone

Mitoxantrone, an anthraquinone antibiotic, is a synthesized drug with antibacterial, antiviral, antiprotozoal, and immunomodulating activities. Its antineoplastic activity results from intercalation to DNA and inhibition of topoisomerase II, producing DNA strand breaks. Mitoxantrone is not phase specific. It is clinically active against breast carcinomas, acute leukemias, and lymphomas. Mitoxantrone has recently been approved for patients with progressive multiple sclerosis and is recognized for its potential use as first-line therapy in acute myelogenous leukemia.[39,64] Mitoxantrone exhibits perhaps less cumulative cardiac toxicity than do the anthracyclines. The drug can impart a blue-green color to the urine 24 hours after administration; bluish discoloration of the sclera may also occur.

Bleomycin

Bleomycin is an antibiotic complex of several glycopeptides derived from *Streptomyces verticillus.* The cytotoxic action of bleomycin has been attributed to DNA scission and fragmentation with inhibition of the usual DNA repair mechanisms. RNA and protein synthesis appear inhibited as well. Bleomycin is rapidly cleared from the blood and concentrated in the liver, lungs, spleen, kidneys, and epithelial tissue. Approximately 80% is excreted in the urine within 24 hours. Bleomycin is cell phase specific, having its major effects on those cells in the G_2 and M phases of the cell cycle.[2]

The main clinical applications of bleomycin are in the treatment of squamous cell carcinoma, testicular tumors, and lymphomas. Bleomycin is also used to treat malignant pleural effusions by direct instillation into the pleural space. The major attractive features of bleomycin include minimal nausea and vomiting, almost no myelosuppression, and the lack of local tissue toxicities. This improved toxicity profile accounts for the inclusion of bleomycin into many combination chemotherapy protocols. The major dose-limiting toxicity is pulmonary, manifesting as interstitial pneumonitis that might progress to pulmonary fibrosis and fatal pulmonary insufficiency. This toxicity is associated with a cumulative dose of more than 400 U, age greater than 70 years, underlying pulmonary disease, chest irradiation, and high oxygen exposure. Some reports suggest an increase in oxygen-induced pulmonary complications in patients previously treated with bleomycin. For anesthesia and postoperative periods, it is recommended that elevated inspired oxygen concentrations should be administered only when clearly indicated.

Plicamycin

Plicamycin (formerly mithramycin), an antibiotic produced by *Streptomyces plicatus,* intercalates with DNA to interfere with the production of RNA. Plicamycin was effectively used in the past against cancer of the testis, but it is now used to treat tumor-associated hypercalcemia because of its osteoblast-inhibiting activity.

Mitomycin

Mitomycin is derived from *Streptomyces caespitosus.* After intracellular activation, mitomycin inhibits DNA synthesis by reacting with DNA in the manner of the alkylating agents. When combined with fluorouracil or the nitrosoureas, mitomycin has been effective against gastrointestinal, head and neck, breast, cervix, and lung carcinomas. Severe toxicity to the bone marrow (neutropenia and thrombocytopenia), reaching a maximum in about 3 to 4 weeks, and to the alimentary tract (nausea, vomiting, oral ulceration, and diarrhea) is the limiting factor in the use of this drug. Pulmonary toxicity and adult hemolytic uremic syndrome are dose related.

Vinca Alkaloids

Vinblastine and vincristine, the two older alkaloids in clinical use, are derived from asymmetrical dimeric compounds extracted from the shrub *Vinca rosea;* they are almost identical in structure (Figure 42-6). Vinblastine contains a methyl group and vincristine a formyl group attached to the nitrogen in the dihydroindole portion of the molecule. Vinorelbine, a newer third vinca alkaloid, is a semisynthetic derivative of vinblastine.[65] The antineoplastic activity of the vinca alkaloids has been attributed to their capacity to arrest cell division in metaphase by binding to the microtubular protein tubulin that forms the mitotic spindle.

These drugs are metabolized in the liver and excreted mainly by the biliary and intestinal tracts. Vinblastine and vincristine are of major value in treating Hodgkin's disease and other lymphomas. Vinorelbine is used in the treatment of NSCLC and may have future roles in the treatment of other carcinomas such as those of the breast.[67] The most common toxic manifestation of vinblastine is leukopenia. High doses induce gastrointestinal disturbances, including nausea, vomiting, diarrhea, and anorexia. Partial alopecia, headache, paresthesias, mental depression, mild peripheral neuropathy, and phlebitis at the injection site are other side effects of this drug. Vincristine produces neurotoxicity that is dose related. Hyponatremia associated with the syndrome of inappropriate antidiuretic hormone secretion has been reported. Tissue damage from extravasated drug requires immediate attention. Dose-limiting toxic effects of vinorelbine appear to be myelosuppression and neurotoxicity manifested by decreased deep tendon reflexes.

Hormone Agonists and Antagonists

The role of hormonal manipulation for cancer therapy was explored as early as 1896, when ovariectomy was first used in the treatment of breast cancer. Adrenocorticosteroids, estrogens, antiestrogens, androgens, progestational agents, and gonadotropin-releasing factors each have a role in cancer control.

Drugs affecting corticosteroid status

Prednisone is widely used in combination with other antineoplastic drugs in acute and chronic lymphocytic leukemia, Hodgkin's disease, lymphoma, and multiple myeloma; it is also helpful in reducing hypercalcemia associated with bony metastases.[21] The estrogens are useful in the treatment of advanced prostatic carcinoma and as adjunctive treatment in select patients with postmenopausal carcinoma of the breast. Although the mode of action is unknown, the therapeutic response in breast cancer is correlated with the presence of estrogen-binding receptor sites in the tumor. The antiestrogen tamoxifen is beneficial in patients whose adenocarcinoma of the breast depends on estrogen for growth, as demonstrated by positive estrogen and progesterone receptor status. It has also been used in endometrial carcinoma and malignant melanoma. The side effects seen with this oral agent include initially a flare-up in disease activity, bone pain, or hypercalcemia. This is associated with efficacy of the medication. Additional side effects include hot flashes, sweating, nausea and vomiting, and increased risk for blood clot formation. Toremifene is a chlorinated derivative of tamoxifen and has demonstrated a similar efficacy and tolerability profile as tamoxifen.[4] Androgens are effective in some cases of metastatic breast cancer. The progestational agents such as megestrol are effective in metastatic endometrial, breast, and renal cell carcinoma. The pharmacologic characteristics of the steroid hormones are detailed in Chapters 35 and 37.

Adrenocortical secretion is suppressed by the agents mitotane and aminoglutethimide. Mitotane causes atrophy of the adrenal cortex by inhibiting mitochondrial function. Aminoglutethimide, an inhibitor of several CYP450 enzymes, inhibits the conversion of cholesterol to pregnenolone, thereby reducing the synthesis of corticosteroids and the sex steroids. It also blocks the conversion of androgens to estrogens. These agents are used in patients with adrenal tumors and occasionally in breast cancer patients.[5]

Drugs affecting sex hormone status

Anastrozole and letrozole are nonsteroidal, selective aromatase inhibitors that do not reduce mineralocorticoid or glucocorticoid activity. Their structure and site of action are seen in Figures 42-7 and 42-8. These agents are indicated for use in postmenopausal women with advanced breast cancer that has progressed during therapy with tamoxifen. The randomized clinical trials comparing anastrozole and letrozole with megestrol acetate showed at least similar, if not superior, response rates and duration of response. The selective aromatase inhibitors are generally well tolerated. Adverse effects include nausea, vomiting, and hot flashes. Letrozole is currently being evaluated in comparison with tamoxifen as a first-line therapy for advanced breast cancer[47] and may be useful

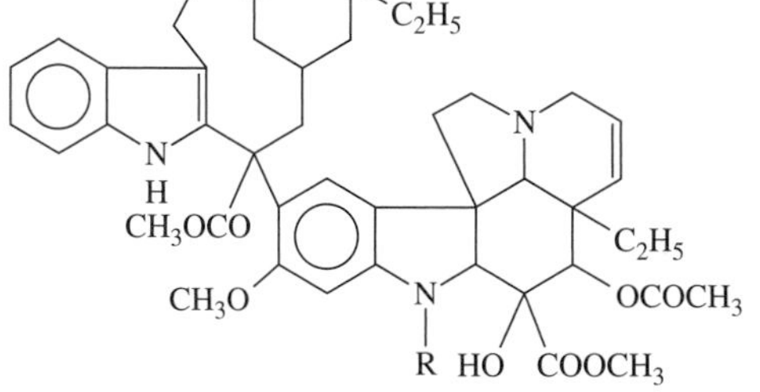

R = $—CH_3$ **Vinblastine**
R = —CHO **Vincristine**

Fig. 42-6 Structural formulas of vinca alkaloids.

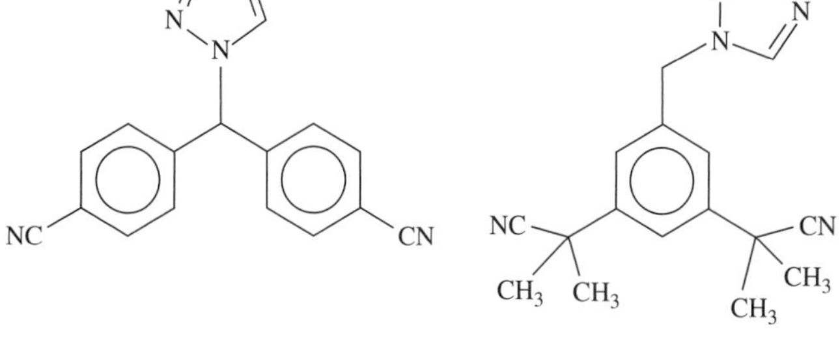

Letrozole **Anastrozole**

Fig. 42-7 Structural formulas of representative nonsteroidal aromatase inhibitors.

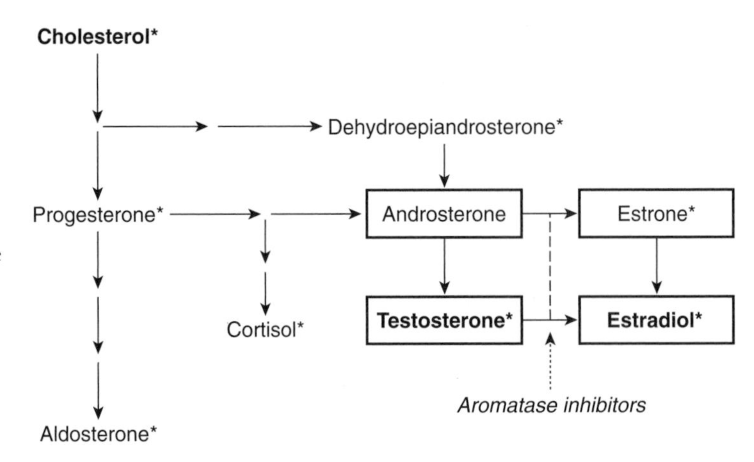

Fig. 42-8 Aromatase inhibitor site of activity in the steroidogenic pathway.

in preventing recurrence when used as adjuvant therapy for estrogen receptor/progesterone receptor (ER/PR) positive breast cancer after tamoxifen therapy. Exemestane is an orally irreversible steroidal aromatase inhibitor or inactivator. Clinical trials demonstrate its effective antitumor activity in postmenopausal breast cancer patients with similar side effect profiles as the other aromatase inhibitors.[8]

Leuprolide (a nonapeptide) and goserelin (a decapeptide) are synthetic analogues of the naturally occurring gonadotropin-releasing hormone (GnRH). They have potent GnRH-agonist properties during short-term or pulsatile therapy, but paradoxically inhibit gonadotropin secretion and suppress ovarian and testicular steroidogenesis during long-term administration. The drugs act principally on the pituitary gland in human beings to limit the release of follicle-stimulating hormone and luteinizing hormone. Because of these inhibitory effects, these agents may interfere with the growth of hormone-dependent tumors. The drugs are used clinically for the palliative treatment of advanced carcinoma of the prostate and may have value in the control of breast cancer. They are also used to treat endometriosis. Even with continued treatment, acute flare-ups in the diseases are also possible, with pain and hypercalcemia.

Flutamide is a nonsteroidal antiandrogen that competes directly for testosterone receptor binding sites in the prostate cells. This agent, used orally for prostate cancer, can help prevent flare-ups when used with a GnRH agonist such as leuprolide. Adverse reactions include gynecomastia and decreased libido. Bicalutamide is a new nonsteroidal antiandrogen agent similar to flutamide and is used in combination with leuprolide for advanced prostate cancer.

Enzymes

Asparaginase

Asparaginase is an enzyme that catalyzes the hydrolysis of L-asparagine to L-aspartic acid and ammonia. The therapeutic drug is one of the isozymes elaborated by *Escherichia coli.* It inhibits protein synthesis in tumor cells by depriving them of the amino acid asparagine. This drug is phase specific, with the greatest activity in the G_1 phase of the cell cycle. Timing and scheduling of asparaginase with other chemotherapy agents is important to prevent the antagonism of the effects of the other agents. Clinical use is confined at present to acute lymphocytic leukemia. The drug may produce acute anaphylaxis with hypotension, sweating, bronchospasm, and urticaria, and test doses are usually administered to help detect the possibility of a hypersensitivity reaction.

Platinum Complexes

Cisplatin

Cisplatin (*cis*-diamminedichloroplatinum) is a heavy metal complex containing a central atom of platinum surrounded by two chloride ions and two amino groups in the *cis* position (Figure 42-9). The compound has biochemical properties similar to bifunctional alkylating agents in that it produces interstrand and intrastrand cross-links in DNA, thereby inhibiting its synthesis. Cisplatin is not a cell cycle phase–specific agent. The drug has proved most effective in the treatment of carcinoma of the testis and ovary, transitional cell bladder neoplasia, and head and neck cancer. It also has activity in small-cell lung cancer in combination with etoposide. After intravenous injection, cisplatin is excreted primarily in the urine; the other excretory pathways are undetermined. Severe emesis is the dose-limiting toxicity. Newer antiemetic agents and protocols allow for the completion of therapy. Nephrotoxicity expressed as renal tubular necrosis is another major dose-limiting side effect. The agent is also ototoxic, causing initially high frequency and later complete hearing loss, and long-term use produces peripheral neuropathy. Bone marrow suppression is rare in usual doses; high doses can cause leukopenia. Concurrent administration of amifostine with cisplatin may reduce the cumulative renal toxicity associated with repeated administration in patients with advanced carcinoma of the ovary and NSCLC. Other toxic effects associated with cisplatin in combination with other chemotherapy agents may also be reduced by pretreatment with amifostine.[42]

Carboplatin

Carboplatin is a second-generation platinum complex designed to maintain antitumor efficacy while decreasing nephrotoxicity, ototoxicity, and neurotoxic effects. The emetogenic potential of carboplatin is less than that of cisplatin. The major dose-limiting side effect is myelosuppression, with

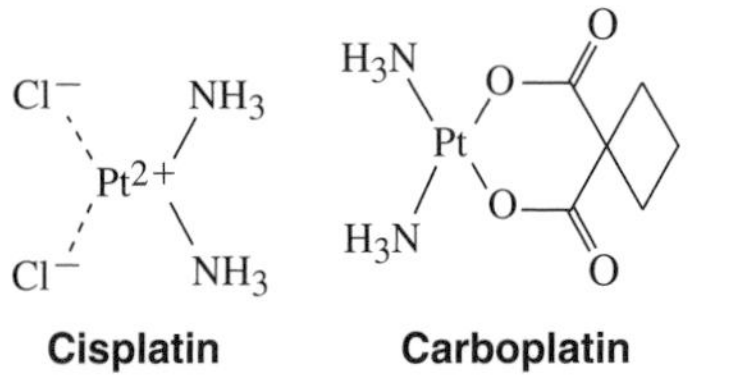

Cisplatin Carboplatin

Fig. 42-9 Structural formulas of the platinum compounds.

thrombocytopenia being more significant than leukopenia. Carboplatin is active in small-cell lung cancer, ovarian carcinoma, and head and neck carcinomas.

Oxaliplatin

Oxaliplatin is a third-generation platinum derivative with a novel mechanism of action. Oxaliplatin may exert its cytotoxic effects by blocking DNA replication and transcription. It is more potent than the other platinums and has activity against tumors resistant to cisplatin and carboplatin. Early trials suggest synergistic activity in colorectal cancer when used with fluorouracil.[7] Oxaliplatin has been approved recently for the treatment of patients with advanced colorectal cancer when administered in combination with fluorouracil and leucovorin. The toxicity profile of oxaliplatin includes some unique neurotoxic effects. There is both an acute and chronic presentation of the toxicity. The acute symptoms include paresthesia of the hands, feet, and perioral area; jaw tightness; and laryngopharyngeal dysesthesia. These symptoms can occur with the infusion or within hours after administration and may be triggered by exposure to cold temperatures or cold objects such as ice used for mucositis prophylaxis. Chronic symptoms of peripheral neuropathy may be aggravated by exposure to cold.

Podophyllotoxins

Etoposide

Etoposide, a semisynthetic derivative of the mandrake plant substance podophyllotoxin (Figure 42-10), is indicated for the treatment of advanced testicular cancer. It is also active against Kaposi's sarcoma, small-cell lung cancer, NSCLC, and lymphomas. A cell cycle–specific drug, etoposide is unique in that it is most active in the G_2 phase of the cycle. The drug appears to prevent cell division by damaging DNA, by topoisomerase II inhibition, or by the formation of free radicals. Oral etoposide is commercially available and is approximately 50% bioavailable. However, the drug is typically given intravenously (and slowly to avoid hypotension). Myelosuppression and nausea and vomiting are the most common adverse effects. Etopophos is a prodrug formulation of etoposide. This formulation has greater solubility, allowing for more rapid infusion with less hypersensitivity and hypotensive reactions.[30]

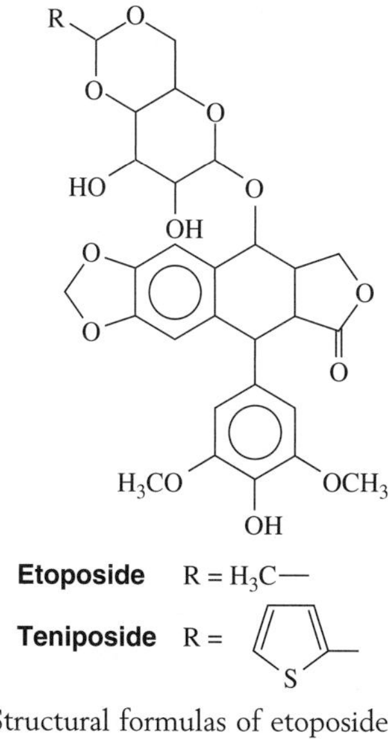

Fig. 42-10 Structural formulas of etoposide and teniposide.

Teniposide

Teniposide is similar to etoposide, differing in the substitution of a thenylidene group for a methyl group on the carbohydrate moiety (see Figure 42-10). Although the mechanism of action is similar to that of etoposide, its cytotoxic properties are more potent. Current uses include treatment of refractory childhood leukemias and neuroblastoma. Myelosuppression is dose limiting; allergic reactions have been reported.

Camptothecins

Topotecan

Topotecan is a semisynthetic analogue of camptothecin. Camptothecin is isolated from an ornamental tree, *Camptotheca acuminata*, found in China. The mechanism of action is the inhibition of topoisomerase I, which causes single-strand breaks in DNA. The current indication for topotecan is for the treatment of metastatic ovarian carcinoma. Topotecan in combination with cytarabine is also used in the treatment of advanced myelodysplastic syndromes and acute myelogenous leukemia.[3] The major dose-limiting side effect is myelosuppression. Irinotecan, another derivative of camptothecin, is indicated for use in colorectal carcinomas that have not responded to fluorouracil therapy. Irinotecan in combination with fluorouracil/leucovorin has been shown to increase survival in colorectal cancer patients and may move to first-line therapy for this disease.[58,60] Its major side effects include myelosuppression and diarrhea requiring aggressive medical management.

Taxoids

Paclitaxel

Paclitaxel is another naturally derived product. Originally extracted from the bark of the western yew tree, *Taxus brevifolia*, paclitaxel induces polymerization and stabilization of microtubules. The development of paclitaxel has been slow because of the laborious process for extracting the active drug and the lack of success in synthesizing it because of its complex chemical structure (Figure 42-11). It is poorly soluble in water and is formulated in a Cremophor El (polyoxyethylated castor oil) and alcohol vehicle. This vehicle may contribute to the high incidence of allergic reactions to the injectable drug. These severe reactions result in dyspnea, hypotension, bronchospasm, urticaria, and erythematous rashes, and they must be managed prophylactically by premedication with steroids or H_1 and H_2 antihistamines and by prolonging the infusion. The antineoplastic activity is broad, and the current approved use of paclitaxel includes the treatment of metastatic carcinoma of the ovaries and breast.

Docetaxel

Docetaxel is an antineoplastic agent belonging to the taxoid family. Its semisynthetic preparation starts from the needles of yew plants. It works like paclitaxel by binding to free

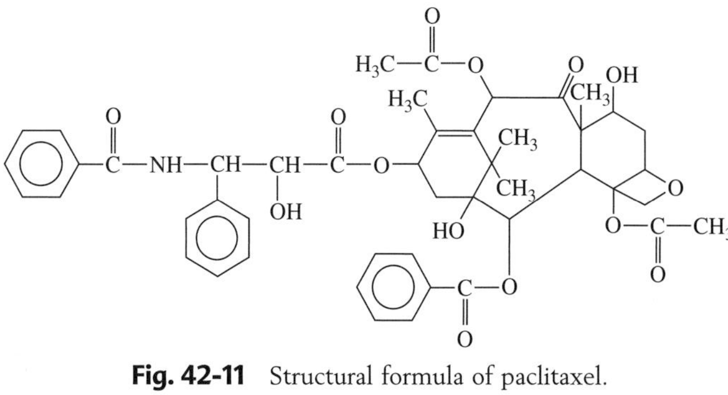

Fig. 42-11 Structural formula of paclitaxel.

tubulin, promoting the assembly of tubulin and inhibiting its disassembly. Docetaxel is indicated for the treatment of locally advanced breast cancer. Docetaxel has moved rapidly from second-line treatment of breast cancer to current evaluations in large, adjuvant trials in breast cancer and use in NSCLC.[10,22] Docetaxel has a toxicity profile similar to that of paclitaxel, with allergic reactions requiring premedication with dexamethasone starting 1 day before therapy. Fluid retention and cutaneous toxicity occur more frequently than with paclitaxel, but there are fewer cardiac arrhythmias and myalgias.

Other Agents

Hydroxyurea

Hydroxyurea inhibits DNA synthesis by blocking the action of ribonucleoside diphosphate reductase. Hydroxyurea is readily absorbed from the alimentary tract; tissue distribution includes the CNS, and elimination is mainly by urinary excretion. Hydroxyurea is used principally to treat busulfan-resistant chronic myelogenous leukemia and to lower rapidly rising peripheral blast counts in acute leukemia. Hydroxyurea is also used in sickle cell disease and for other myeloproliferative disorders such as polycythemia vera. High doses most often produce myelosuppression and megaloblastic anemia.

Procarbazine

Procarbazine, a derivative of methylhydrazine, was originally synthesized for its use as an antidepressant. It suppresses mitosis and produces chromosomal defects. It is a monoamine oxidase inhibitor that possesses teratogenic and carcinogenic properties in addition to antineoplastic activity. Procarbazine is rapidly absorbed from the alimentary tract, quickly metabolized by the liver, and excreted in the urine mainly in the form of a metabolic breakdown product. Procarbazine is most active against Hodgkin's disease and is modestly effective in other lymphomas and multiple myeloma when given in combination with alkylating agents and *Vinca* alkaloids. Nausea and vomiting occur with high doses, and hematologic toxicity in the form of leukopenia and thrombocytopenia appears within 3 to 4 weeks. Because procarbazine is a mild monoamine oxidase inhibitor, patients should be warned about concurrent use of tyramine-rich foods, antidepressants, CNS depressants, and other drugs that are known to interact significantly with monoamine oxidase inhibitors. Procarbazine is reported to have some degree of disulfiram-like activity, so alcoholic beverages should be avoided.

Thalidomide

Thalidomide (Figure 42-12) was used in Europe and Canada in the 1950s as an anxiolytic, antiemetic, and sedative drug until it was discovered to cause major teratogenic effects. This agent was not approved for use in the United States at that time because of a potential for irreversible neurotoxicity after long-term use. In the late 1990s, thalidomide was approved by the FDA for the treatment of Hansen's disease (leprosy). Since then, many additional conditions and disease states, such as AIDS-related cachexia, rheumatoid arthritis, graft-versus-host disease, and cancers such as multiple myeloma, have been treated with thalidomide.[6,63] The mechanism of thalidomide activity is complex and still not well understood, but it involves two major effects, antiangiogenesis and immune system modulation. Angiogenesis, as stated previously, is an important mechanism for tumor growth and formation of metastases. On inhibition of angiogenesis, the tumor cells will starve without the necessary nutrient supply. In addition, thalidomide can inhibit tumor necrosis factor–α production, stimulate T-cell proliferation, and increase interferon and interleukin-2 release. The role of each of these mechanisms in its antineoplastic effect is not known. The success rates in multiple myeloma as a single agent range from 25% to 75%. The most frequent dose-dependent adverse effects include sedation, rash, fatigue, and constipation.

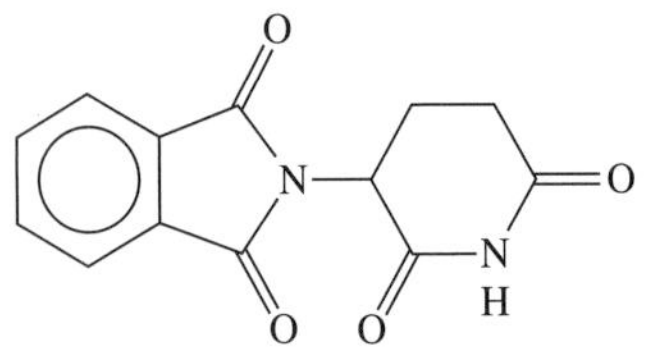

O
N
O
N
H
O
O

Fig. 42-12 Structural formula of thalidomide.

Arsenic trioxide

Arsenic trioxide (As_2O_3) has been recently investigated in clinical trials for treatment of acute promyelocytic leukemia in patients who relapsed after standard treatment with chemotherapy and all-*trans*-retinoic acid or after a bone marrow transplant. The rates of complete remission with low-dose arsenic were impressive in this refractory patient population. The proposed mechanisms of activity of this arsenical compound include induction of apoptosis by activation of cysteine proteases (caspases) and initiation of cytodifferentiation. The adverse effects linked to low-dose arsenic trioxide in clinical trials consisted of lightheadedness during infusion, fatigue, musculoskeletal pain, hyperglycemia, and peripheral neuropathy.[62] The frequency of oral complications from this treatment is low and includes sore throat, oral blisters, and dry mouth. More serious but rare side effects include a "retinoic acid syndrome" similar in presentation after the administration of all-*trans*-retinoic acid observed in patients with acute promyelocytic leukemia receiving arsenic trioxide. Cardiac side effects include QTc interval prolongation on electrocardiogram.[49]

Differentiating Agents: Retinoids

Several classes of compounds have the potential in vitro and in vivo to have a differentiating effect on the malignant clone, thereby inhibiting growth and proliferation. Among these compounds are the retinoids, including some commercially available and experimental agents such as isotretinoic acid (13-cis-retinoic acid), 9-cis-retinoic acid, all-*trans*-retinoic acid, bexarotene, etretinate, and arotinoid. Retinoid effects appear to result from changes in gene expression mediated through specific intracellular receptors. There are two subfamilies of retinoid intracellular receptors: the retinoid acid receptors (RARs) and the retinoid X receptors (RXRs). These retinoid receptors each have three subtypes, designated *RARα, RARβ, RARγ, RXRα, RXRβ,* and *RXRγ.* These receptors may form dimers with each other or other receptors, and each receptor subtype or combination is thought to control unique and overlapping target genes, regulating their transcription. Retinoids play crucial roles in normal development and physiologic functioning. They are also capable of inhibiting cell growth, inducing differentiation, and inducing apoptosis in a variety of tumor cell lines.

Tretinoin

Tretinoin is the commercial formulation of all-*trans*-retinoic acid. This agent has been the most successful differentiating agent used in the treatment of acute promyelocytic leukemia. Genotypically, these leukemic clones have a characteristic translocation between the long arms of chromosome 15 and 17, which results in fusion between a gene that encodes a specific RAR (RARα) and a gene known as *pml.* The *pml*/RAR fusion protein functions as an oncogene and blocks differentiation of the myelocytes at the promyelocyte stage. The orally administered tretinoin induces differentiation and apoptosis of malignant promyelocytes. Tretinoin is metabolized in the liver and can induce its own metabolism, leading to decreased levels and clinical effects with continued administration. Tretinoin, like most retinoids, is teratogenic. Common side effects include dry skin, exfoliation, xerostomia, and cheilitis. A rare but potentially lethal dose-limiting toxicity is known as the *retinoic acid syndrome,* which consists of fever, chest pain, dyspnea, hypoxia, pulmonary infiltrates, and pleural or pericardial effusions.[14]

Bexarotene

Bexarotene is a retinoid that selectively activates RXRs. The approved indication for bexarotene is for the treatment of cutaneous T-cell lymphoma. In vitro and animal testing suggest potential applications of bexarotene in other malignancies. This oral retinoid is hepatically metabolized and primarily eliminated through the hepatobiliary system. Bexarotene can cause major lipid abnormalities in patients and may require monitoring and treatment. Other side effects include headache, asthenia, hypothyroidism, rash, dry skin, leukopenia, and nausea.

Other retinoids

Of all the retinoids, isotretinoic acid (13-cis retinoic acid) has undergone the most extensive clinical examination. The activity of this agent alone in established cancers is limited. This agent has been used to reverse oral leukoplakia in heavy tobacco users.[36] The duration of clinical response is brief and most patients have a relapse if the drug is stopped. Other retinoids, such as 9-cis-retinoic acid, which is a pan-agonist for both RAR and RXR, are undergoing clinical evaluations for roles in the treatment of other tumors.

Biologic Response Modifiers

The continuing evolution of recombinant technology beginning in the early 1970s has resulted in the availability of agents used clinically, by themselves and in combination with other cytotoxic agents, to modify host responses and aid in killing cancer cells. Known as the *fourth modality of cancer therapy,* biologic response modifiers are used to assist in the killing of cancer cells or in minimizing adverse effects on normal cells.

Interferons

Two types of human interferon, interferon α_{2a} and interferon α_{2b}, have been produced by recombinant DNA techniques and marketed for cancer chemotherapy. Each agent is a protein chain of 165 amino acids, differing from the other only at a single amino acid residue. A purified form of interferon α, prepared from human plasma, is also available under the nonproprietary name of *interferon alfa-n3.*

These agents exert antiviral, immunostimulant, and antiproliferative properties by binding to specific cell membrane receptors; however, the exact mechanism of action remains to be elucidated. They are currently being used to treat hairy cell leukemia, Kaposi's sarcoma, chronic hepatitis, chronic myelogenous leukemia, melanoma, and other malignancies in combination with chemotherapy and as biologic response modifiers in other situations.[41]

The interferons are given by subcutaneous or intramuscular injection and have plasma half-lives of 4 to 8 hours. They are hydrolyzed in the kidney, and metabolites are largely reabsorbed from the glomerular filtrate. Interferons have the ability to depress the activity of the hepatic CYP450 system. A number of side effects have been associated with their use. Most patients have a flulike syndrome with fever, chills, myalgia, fatigue, and headache. Loss of appetite is also common, and patients may have nausea, vomiting, and diarrhea. Dermatologic and CNS disturbances (e.g., ataxia, confusion) occur in a minority of patients.[41]

Aldesleukin

Aldesleukin (interleukin-2 [IL-2]) is a recombinant product produced by a genetically engineered *Escherichia coli* strain. IL-2 has a number of immunoregulatory properties, including enhancement of lymphocyte mitogenesis, lymphocyte cytotoxicity, induction of killer cells (natural and lymphokine activated), and induction of interferon-γ production. IL-2 is administered by intravenous infusion and is metabolized and eliminated by the kidneys. The plasma half-life of IL-2 is short, approximately 90 minutes. Currently, IL-2 is used for the treatment of adults with metastatic renal cell carcinoma. In addition, high-dose IL-2 treatment has produced some long-lasting complete responses or partial remissions in metastatic melanoma patients. The major toxicities of IL-2 are associated with the capillary leak syndrome, resulting in clinically significant hypotension, weight gain, fluid retention and accumulation, pulmonary edema, and acute renal dysfunction with oliguria or anuria. Some of the common side effects (e.g., chills and fevers) can be reduced with appropriate premedication. Pruritic rashes are common.

Oprelvekin

Interleukin-11 (IL-11) is a cytokine that occurs in vivo in a number of tissues such as bone marrow, brain, kidneys, heart, lungs, spleen, uterus, and the intestines. IL-11 participates in stimulating megakaryocytes and their precursors in the bone marrow. Other important growth factors and cytokines are necessary for megakaryocyte production and maturation. For instance, interleukin-3 (IL-3) acts synergistically with IL-11. Oprelvekin is a recombinant IL-11 produced similarly to aldesleukin. Thrombocytopenia and neutropenia are important dose-limiting toxicities of chemotherapy that will potentially delay treatment or require reduction in the total dose delivered to the patient. Prevention and reduction in duration and severity of bone marrow toxicity will enable the patient to receive a planned chemotherapeutic regimen. To that end, IL-11 reduces bone marrow toxicity occurring during chemotherapy. As discussed above, filgrastim and sargramostim stimulate white blood cell production but they do not have any effects on increasing platelet and red blood cell production. Oprelvekin was found to prevent severe thrombocytopenia and decrease the need for platelet transfusions in several double-blind, randomized clinical trials in cancer patients receiving highly myelosuppressive chemotherapeutic regimens.[56] However, the widespread use of oprelvekin is limited by its adverse effects profile and cost. Administration of oprelvekin leads to significant fluid retention that may cause other important complications such as peripheral edema, dilutional anemia, palpitations, dyspnea, headache, and atrial arrhythmias. Headache, myalgia, arthralgia, and fatigue are also reported frequently.

Filgrastim and sargramostim

Colony-stimulating factors represent a third group of biologics (in addition to interferons and interleukins) that has had a clinical effect in the treatment of neoplastic disease. These agents—filgrastim (granulocyte colony-stimulating factor) and sargramostim (granulocyte macrophage colony-stimulating factor)—are not cytotoxic. They offer the benefit of ameliorating the hematologic toxicity induced by the chemotherapeutic agents. Injected subcutaneously or intravenously, the colony-stimulating factors are approved for the treatment of chemotherapy- and transplant-related neutropenia in bone marrow transplant patients. The growth factors can shorten the overall period of neutropenia, reduce the number of febrile episodes, and decrease the need for broad-spectrum antibiotics. They are used investigationally for other clinical conditions of neutropenia. They also can mobilize stem cells into the peripheral blood for collection by cell separation for stem cell transplants after high-dose chemotherapy and radiation therapy. The value of the growth factors may be ultimately to allow more chemotherapy to be administered, with less need for dose reductions because of side effects. Predictably, other adverse effects, such as mucositis, may become dose limiting as dosages are escalated. Adverse effects of these agents are usually flulike symptoms, fever, chills, bone pain, and myalgia. Pleuritis and pericarditis have been reported.

Many other biologic response-modifying approaches are being explored in clinical trials. Levamisole, an anthelmintic agent, has found a role with fluorouracil for the treatment of Dukes C colon cancer by virtue of its immunomodulating effects. Vaccines, new cytokines, additional interleukins and colony-stimulating factors, and interferon-α are all being evaluated both alone and in combination with chemotherapy to increase responses against these neoplastic diseases.

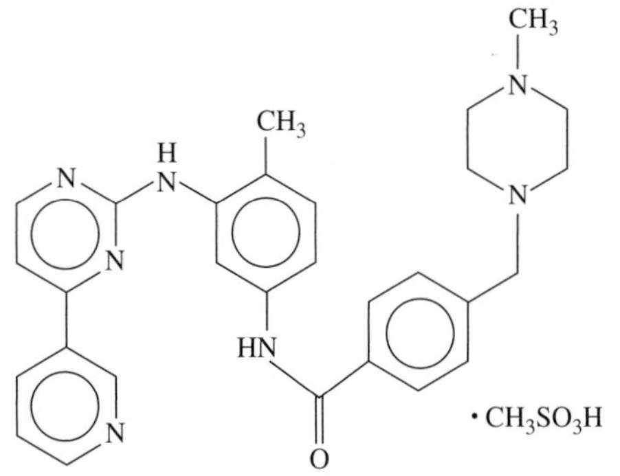

TARGETED ANTINEOPLASTIC THERAPY

Researchers constantly strive to find the "magic bullet" to cure cancer. In the process of discovering new molecules with anticancer activity, the molecular mechanisms and cellular processes are better understood. The idea of targeting a specific molecular pathway in the tumor cell cycle originated from the limitations of traditional antineoplastic drugs such as nonselective toxicity, drug resistance, and suboptimal success rates. The monoclonal antibodies have been used in clinical practice for several years, representing a form of targeted therapy. Newer drug classes are being evaluated. The members of two new drug classes, tyrosine kinase inhibitors and matrix metalloproteinase inhibitors, most likely will be used clinically in combination with standard antineoplastic drugs to eradicate a variety of tumors and to increase the response rates.[59]

Tyrosine Kinase Inhibitors

The overexpression of epidermal growth factor receptor tyrosine kinase (EGFR-TK) has been identified in malignant cells. This glycoprotein spans the cellular membrane and transduces extracellular stimuli into intracellular responses. An abnormally high activity of EGFR-TK has been linked to induction, growth, and metastatic potential of malignant cells. Inhibition of the EGFR-TK–mediated signaling pathway has been shown to result in suppression of tumor growth. The most effective drugs target the extracellular ligand–receptor binding or the intracellular phosphorylation step. The former task is accomplished with the use of monoclonal antibodies that target specific EGFR-TK.[55] Trastuzumab, described below, is already being used in clinical practice to treat breast cancer patients. Small molecules, called *tyrosine kinase inhibitors,* are currently in phase I, II, and III clinical trials.[48] Imatinib mesylate is the first of this new class of therapeutic agents approved by the Food and Drug Administration (FDA); its structure is seen in Figure 42-13. Imatinib is an effective agent used to halt the progression of chronic myeloid leukemia (CML). A characteristic of this type of leukemia is a translocation between two chromosomes to form the Philadelphia (Ph) chromosome. This translocation occurs at the breakpoint cluster region (Bcr) gene on chromosome 22 and the protocogene on chromosome 9 identified by Dr. Abelson known as *Abl.* This translocation forms the Bcr-Abl fusion gene, which codes for the Bcr-Abl tyrosine kinase present in most patients with CML. Imatinib inhibits the signal transduction of the oncoprotein Bcr-Abl tyrosine kinase. Trial results in patients with CML demonstrate greater than 90% hematologic response that appears to persist. This oral agent has only mild to moderate adverse effects, with nausea and vomiting, myalgia, fluid retention, and edema occurring most frequently. Potentially severe side effects include elevation of liver function tests (1% to 3.5%) and hemorrhage.[18] This drug also binds to other receptors, including c-Kit (stem-cell factor), and is being studied for use in patients with gastrointestinal stromal tumor.

Fig. 42-13 Structural formula of imatinib mesylate.

A newly FDA-approved tyrosine kinase inhibitor that targets epidermal growth factor receptor (EGFR) is gefitinib. A number of tumors overexpress EGFR, including NSCLC, for which the use of oral gefitinib has demonstrated modest objective response in a small number of patients and disease stabilization in about one third of the study participants. The toxicity of this agent is common to the inhibition of EGFR and includes acneiform rashes in more than 50% of the patients, as well as diarrhea in about 40%. Mouth ulcerations are rare, accounting for less than 1% of the adverse reactions.

Other sites for signal transduction inhibition are being identified. One agent in clinical trial is a farnesyltransferase inhibitor, which targets RAS, an oncogene implicated in a number of cancers.

Proteasome Inhibitors

The proteasome is a ubiquitous and essential intracellular enzyme that degrades many proteins regulating the cell cycle, apoptosis, transcription, cell adhesion, angiogenesis, and antigen presentation. Bortezomib is a newly approved proteasome inhibitor indicated for the treatment of relapsed or refractory multiple myeloma. Bortezomib's inhibition of proteasome prevents the degradation of intracellular proteins, leading to activation of signaling cascades, cell-cycle arrest, and apoptosis. The major side effects reported include fatigue, malaise, some peripheral neuropathy, and bone marrow suppression.

Matrix Metalloprotease Inhibitors

Matrix metalloproteases consist of a family of 16 enzymes. Inhibitors of these enzymes in animal tumor models have been shown to inhibit tumor progression and prevent spread of cancer cells to distant sites. MMPIs have important physiologic roles under normal conditions and participate in normal bone growth and resorption, ovulation, and thromboblast implantation. However, overexpression of certain MMP types has been identified in rheumatoid arthritis, osteoarthritis, inflammatory bowel disease, chronic liver disease, abdominal aortic aneurysm, breast cancer, lung cancer, head and neck cancer, melanoma, and gastrointestinal, genitourinary, and gynecologic tumors. The targets of MMPI include several enzymes such as collagenases, stromelysins, and gelatinases. These enzymes are present in the extracellular matrix in a proenzyme form and, on activation, damage the basement membrane and the stroma of the extracellular matrix. This degradation is a first step to opening the gates to the general circulation for the neoplastic cells. Currently, several agents are being evaluated in clinical trials as single agents or in combination with standard chemotherapeutic drugs. The limitations of these studies include small patient samples and lack of validated biologic end points (i.e., levels of MMP expression). So far, the major adverse effects associated with MMPI are related to the musculoskeletal system, including joint stiffness and pain seen with prolonged administration.[31]

Monoclonal Antibodies

Malignant cells often have unique antigens expressed on their surfaces known as *tumor-associated antigens.* Monoclonal antibodies (MoAbs) are single immunoglobulin antibodies or fragments specific to a targeted surface antigen. These antibodies are produced in vitro in large quantities by an immortalized plasma cell clone. Some of these antibodies have been made in the human form by DNA recombinant technology to reduce the formation of human anti-mouse antibodies against the MoAbs. Interactions between human anti-mouse antibodies and MoAbs may reduce the effectiveness of the MoAbs and may initiate an allergic reaction. The human sequence, such as the Fc portion, may provide sites of interactions for the human immune system to initiate complement and other immune-mediated lysis of the targeted cells. The binding of these MoAbs to the targeted surface antigen may lead to complement-mediated lysis, antibody-dependent cellular cytotoxicity, or signal transduction–mediated apoptosis. Cytotoxins and radioisotopes may also be attached to these MoAbs, providing additional mechanisms of action by which these antibodies can target and kill malignant cells. Many of the MoAbs are in clinical trials, and some have been recently approved by the FDA.[28]

Rituximab

Rituximab is a chimeric MoAb consisting of a human and mouse portion, and its target is an antigen CD-20 present on mature B cells. The CD-20 antigen makes an excellent target for a therapeutic approach because this hydrophobic phosphoprotein is present on mature B cells but not on stem cells, plasma cells, or pre-B cells.[27] This antigen also participates in cell cycle initiation and differentiation. Rituximab was approved by the FDA in 1997, and it was the first MoAb on the market with an indication for treatment of cancer. This MoAb is used to treat low-grade and follicular lymphomas expressing CD-20 antigen. In clinical trails rituximab was effective as a single agent and in combination with standard chemotherapy; overall response rates were 48% and 100%, respectively.[27] The rationale for use of this MoAb in combination with chemotherapy is its unique mechanism of action and its adverse effects profile. On binding of rituximab to the CD-20 antigen, the cascade of complement-dependent cell lysis is initiated and the antibody-dependent cellular cytotoxicity takes place. In addition, rituximab has the ability to sensitize resistant human lymphoma cells. In contrast to chemotherapy-induced adverse effects (e.g., bone marrow suppression, mucositis), the most common adverse effects seen with rituximab are infusion related and include chills, fever, flushing, nausea, fatigue, pruritus, and angioedema. The severity of these infusion-related adverse effects subsides significantly with subsequent infusions.[27,46]

Trastuzumab

Trastuzumab is a human MoAb against human EGFR-2 that is overexpressed in 25% to 30% of patients with breast cancer.[61] The overexpression of this receptor has been associated with more aggressive tumors, lower response rates to standard chemotherapy regimens, and ultimately decreased survival. The mechanism of action of this MoAb consists of at least three major effects: alteration of the signaling potential between the receptor and the nucleus, stimulation of the immune system components that will attack and kill the tumor cells, and augmentation of the cytotoxic activity of antineoplastic drugs. Trastuzumab is given intravenously in weekly intervals for prolonged periods. Infusion-related chills, fever, and rigidity can occur frequently with trastuzumab, especially during the first dose. Other common adverse effects include headache, nausea, diarrhea, vomiting, cough, shortness of breath, and rash.[61]

Gemtuzumab ozogamicin

Gemtuzumab ozogamicin is a conjugate of a MoAb against CD-33 antigen and a potent antineoplastic agent, calicheamicin. This novel agent has been recently approved by the FDA for the management of acute myeloid leukemia in elderly patients who are unlikely to tolerate standard induction regimens. The CD-33 antigen is a glycoprotein present on most of the acute myeloid leukemia cells; however, it is not present on normal stem cells that are necessary for bone marrow recovery. The discovery of a MoAb against this leukemic antigen made possible the use of a highly cytotoxic antibiotic, calicheamicin. Calicheamicin is a small molecule that contains two domains, the enediyne portion and the carbohydrate tail, and it binds to the minor groove of the DNA. This binding results in DNA double-stranded breaks. This potent group of agents has been studied in vitro and in animal trials since the 1970s but could not be used in clinical practice because of severe, nonselective toxicity. The role of the MoAb is to deliver this potent antineoplastic drug to the leukemic cell, which, on binding the drug, will subsequently engulf the molecule. Once inside the cell, calicheamicin finds its way into the nucleus and binds to the DNA. This activity is illustrated in Figure 42-14. The majority of patients have infusion-related adverse effects such as chills, fevers, changes in blood pressure, and shortness of breath. Additional adverse effects that occur days after this drug is administered include hepatotoxicity and severe bone marrow toxicity that can last for 4 to 6 weeks. The incidence of severe mucositis is approximately 4% in clinical trials to date.[34]

Ibritumomab and tositumomab

Two radioimmunoconjugates are available for the treatment of lymphoid malignancies. Tositumomab and ibritumomab are anti–CD-20 murine MoAbs that target the same antigen as rituximab. The radionucleotide iodine131, conjugated to tosi-

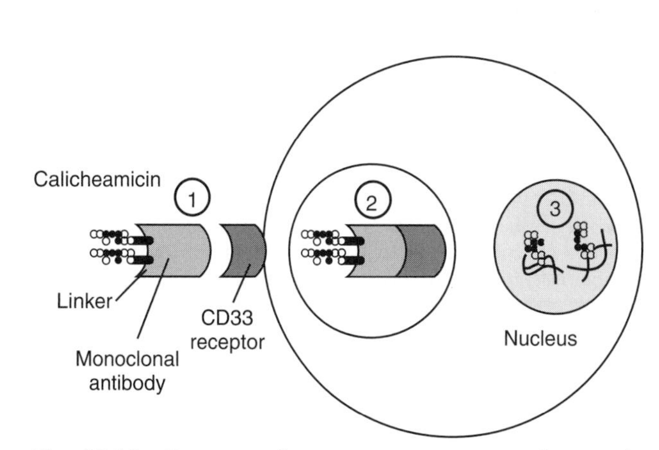

Fig. 42-14 Gemtuzumab ozogamicin conjugate and its mechanism of action. The major three steps are *(1)* CD33 receptor binding and receptor complex internalization, *(2)* calicheamicin transport to the nucleus, and *(3)* calicheamicin binding to DNA, which causes DNA strand breaks.

tumomab, and yttrium-90, conjugated to ibritumomab, provide an additional mechanism of cytotoxicity. The radiation source also allows for greater crossfire effect, radiating nearby malignant lymphoma cells that may not express the CD-20 antigen as well as large tumor clusters in which the blood circulation is unable to deliver the MoAbs. Both have been used in refractory indolent NHL with good overall response rates. The toxicity profiles of these radioimmunoconjugates are similar, with the most common toxicity being hematologic (i.e., thrombocytopenia, neutropenia). The onset of myelosuppression is delayed, with a nadir in bone marrow function at 30 to 40 days. The advantages of the ibritumomab-^{90}Y are the shorter half-life of the ^{90}Y, allowing easier use in the outpatient setting and greater radiation penetration for the treatment of bulky lymphomas over rituximab alone.[54] The radioisotope I-131 associated with tositumomab requires more radiation safety precautions as it emits both β and γ radiation.

Alemtuzumab

Alemtuzumab is a human MoAb that targets the CD-52 antigen found on B and T lymphocytes, inducing complement fixation, cell-mediated cytotoxicity, and apoptosis. This antigen CD-52 is not present in progenitor cells. Infectious complications are the most significant side effect associated with this infusional therapy; the most common are fever, chills, nausea, and vomiting. Alemtuzumab may provide a third-line therapy for chronic lymphocytic leukemia for patients who have been treated with alkylating agents and have not responded to fludarabine therapy.[19]

Bevacizumab

Bevacizumab is a recombinant human monoclonal antibody against vascular endothelial growth factor (VEGF). VEGF is required for blood vessel formation and is produced by many malignant cells. Bevacizumab is being studied for use in renal cell carcinoma and in combination with chemotherapy for the treatment of breast and colorectal carcinomas.

COMBINATION THERAPY

The previously discussed drugs are rarely used as single entities for the treatment of a specific tumor. Choriocarcinoma is one of a few malignancies that can be cured with a single agent (doxorubicin). Resistance of tumor cells to chemotherapy may explain poor initial responses and relapses during treatment. A hypothesis for tumor resistance has been proposed by Goldie and Coldman.[24] Resistant tumors exhibit either inherent resistance or acquired resistance. The possible mechanisms of acquired resistance include defects in the resistant cells, transport, and activation of the chemotherapeutic prodrug to the active species. Also involved may be an alteration of the DNA repair, gene amplification, altered nucleotide pool, increased salvage pathways, and the development of pleiotropic drug resistance or multidrug resistance. Research is in progress to better understand and overcome tumor resistance. The current chemotherapeutic approach to prevent resistance is similar to that described for combination chemotherapy: (1) use agents with different cell cycle specificity, mechanisms of actions, toxicities, and potential combinations for synergy; and (2) administer the drugs in intermittent courses and at maximal tolerated doses to maximize cell kill, allow for host recovery, and avoid prolonged drug-free intervals. The dose intensity of a regimen is a well-recognized variable for response and cure in sensitive tumors. The use of alternating non–cross-resistant regimens may further improve outcome, as seen with the ABVD regimen (*a*driamycin [doxorubicin], *b*leomycin, *v*inblastine, and *d*acarbazine), alternating monthly with the traditional MOPP regimen (*m*echlorethamine, *o*ncovin [vincristine], *p*rocarbazine, *p*rednisone) for the treatment of advanced Hodgkin's disease. This regimen had been further dose intensified by combining the two regimens into a monthly cycle MOPP/ABV hybrid program.[11] The ultimate dose-intensive regimens include high-dose chemotherapy, with or without irradiation, requiring bone marrow transplantation or peripheral stem cell reinfusion to rescue the host from total marrow aplasia. The antineoplastic agents are also finding increasing success when used in combination with radiation therapy and surgery for the treatment of tumors such as head and neck carcinomas. Combination regimens containing cisplatin and fluorouracil are being used simultaneously with radiotherapy to render the tissue radiosensitive and as a postoperative adjunct to destroy micrometastases that may have been missed during local surgery.

Potential Drug Interactions and Relative Contraindications

Most antineoplastic drugs have a narrow therapeutic index. Therefore, although drug interactions may enhance or diminish the antitumor effects and result in improvement or treatment failure, drug interactions may also increase or decrease the side effect profile of the antineoplastic drug. Caution should be used when adding other therapeutic agents in patients undergoing active therapy. Interactions may occur between antineoplastic drugs and drugs that have no antineoplastic effects. One example is the relative contraindication for the use of NSAIDs such as ibuprofen, aspirin, and others in patients who may be thrombocytopenic from myelosuppressive antineoplastic agents. NSAIDs may affect platelet function and increase gastrointestinal irritation, increasing the bleeding risk in patients with a low platelet count. Other drug-drug interactions may occur from changes in absorption, clearance, or excretion of the antineoplastic drugs; from changes in protein binding; or through the induction or inhibition of isoenzymes of the CYP450 system that metabolize the particular antineoplastic substrate or its metabolites.

Unfortunately, not all the metabolic pathways and interactions for antineoplastic agents have been identified. Many of the antineoplastic agents are substrates for metabolism by the CYP3A4, CYP2B6, and CYP2D6 isoenzymes. Concurrent use of an antineoplastic agent and the inhibitors of these and other hepatic isoenzymes may potentially cause delayed elimination of an antineoplastic agent and enhance its activity or toxicity. Examples of inhibitors of the CYP3A4 isoenzyme are the commonly used antifungal drugs, fluconazole and ketoconazole, which may possibly increase blood levels of cyclophosphamide, a substrate of a CYP3A4 isoenzyme. Fortunately, this antineoplastic agent is also metabolized by the CYP2B6 isoenzyme, so the metabolism of cyclophosphamide is only partially affected by the inhibitory effects of these antifungal agents. The antibiotic erythromycin can increase the toxicities of vincristine, possibly through inhibition of vincristine metabolism by CYP3A4. Although many analgesics are substrates for metabolism by CYP isoenzymes, no clinically significant drug interactions from CYP isoenzyme effects on these analgesics and antineoplastic drugs have been reported.

Many of the antineoplastic drugs are excreted by the kidney. Nephrotoxic drugs may increase the toxicity of these agents by delaying drug elimination. Methotrexate is an antifolate antimetabolite with a wide spectrum of activity. Methotrexate is a weak acid and is eliminated by tubular secretion in the kidney. The renal clearance may be decreased by drugs that inhibit the tubular secretion of methotrexate and compete for secretion or by reduced renal blood flow resulting from inhibited prostaglandin synthesis. Drugs that decrease methotrexate elimination include salicylates, some NSAIDs, probenecid, sulfonamides, and penicillins. The toxic effects associated with delayed elimination of methotrexate include pancytopenia and mucositis. The risk of this interaction is lower with low-dose methotrexate used for arthritis. During methotrexate therapy, acetaminophen or the newer cyclooxygenase-2 inhibitors, celecoxib and rofecoxib, should be considered as alternatives to salicylates or other NSAIDs for use as nonnarcotic analgesic agents.

Some interactions result from pharmacodynamic mechanisms. Procarbazine is a weak monoamine oxidase inhibitor. Caution should be taken in the administration of indirect-acting sympathomimetics while the patient is taking procarbazine to prevent potentially dangerous hypertensive episodes. Direct-acting sympathomimetics such as epinephrine, isoproterenol, and norepinephrine do not appear to interact to the same degree. A case has been reported of a patient who was receiving procarbazine and had a manic reaction after the administration of lidocaine plus epinephrine for the extraction of three teeth.[45] While receiving procarbazine, the ingestion of ethanol may result in a disulfiram-like reaction: flushing, headaches, nausea, and hypotension.

Other drugs with harmful interactions include warfarin and antineoplastic agents such as 5-fluorouracil, capecitabine, and ifosfamide; close monitoring of the prothrombin time is necessary to prevent life-threatening bleeding.

Many interactions have been reported and consideration should be given to those that can result in clinically significant reactions. Not all drug-drug interactions require avoidance of such therapeutic agents. In some cases, dosages may be titrated and patients monitored to minimize the risk.

IMPLICATIONS FOR DENTISTRY

Currently available antitumor drugs cannot distinguish between malignant cells and dividing normal cells and are thus potentially damaging to both. The mouth, by virtue of the rapid cellular turnover of the oral mucosa, the daily exposure of oral tissues to minor trauma, and the presence of an extensive and potentially infective microflora, is at special risk of developing drug-induced toxicity. Adverse reactions include stomatitis, hemorrhage, acute and chronic infection, and rapid progression of caries and periodontal bone loss. Additionally, the pain associated with these conditions can impair nutrition. These issues and their management are discussed in detail in Chapter 50.

CITED REFERENCES

1. Balis FM, Poplack DG: Central nervous system pharmacology of antileukemic drugs, *Am J Pediatr Hematol Oncol* 11:74-86, 1989.
2. Bennett JM, Reich SD: Bleomycin, *Ann Intern Med* 90:945-948, 1979.
3. Beran M, Kantarjian H: Results of topotecan-based combination therapy in patients with myelodysplastic syndrome and chronic myelomonocytic leukemia, *Semin Hematol* 36:3-10, 1999.
4. Buzdar AU, Hortobagyi GN: Tamoxifen and toremifene in breast cancer: comparison of safety and efficacy, *J Clin Oncol* 16:348-353, 1998.
5. Buzdar AU, Powell KC, Legha SS, et al: Treatment of advanced breast cancer with aminoglutethimide after therapy with tamoxifen, *Cancer* 50:1708-1712, 1982.
6. Calabrese L, Fleischer AB: Thalidomide: current and potential clinical applications, *Am J Med* 108:487-496, 2000.
7. Cassidy J: Review of oxaliplatin: an active platinum agent in colorectal cancer, *Int J Clin Pract* 54:399-402, 2000.
8. Clemett D, Lamb HM: Exemestane: a review of its use in postmenopausal women with advanced breast cancer, *Drugs* 59:1279-1296, 2000.
9. Colvin M, Chabner BA: Alkylating agents. In Chabner BA, Collins JM, eds: *Cancer chemotherapy: principles and practice*, Philadelphia, 1990, JB Lippincott.
10. Comer AM, Goa KL: Docetaxel: a review of its use in non-small cell lung cancer, *Drugs Aging* 17:53-80, 2000.
11. Connors JM, Klimo P: MOPP/ABV hybrid chemotherapy for advanced Hodgkin's disease, *Semin Hematol* 24(2 suppl 1):35-40, 1987.
12. Curran CF, Narang PK, Reynolds RD: Toxicity profile of dexrazoxane (Zinecard, ICRF-187, ADR-529, NSC-169780), a modulator of doxorubicin cardiotoxicity, *Cancer Treat Rev* 18:241-252, 1991.
13. Damon LE, Cadman EC: The metabolic basis for combination chemotherapy, *Pharmacol Ther* 38:73-127, 1988.
14. Degos L, Dombret H, Chomienne C, et al: All-trans-retinoic acid as a differentiating agent in the treatment of acute promyelocytic leukemia, *Blood* 85:2643-2653, 1995.
15. DeVita VT, Jr, Young RC, Canellos GP: Combination versus single agent chemotherapy: a review of the basis for selection of drug treatment of cancer, *Cancer* 35:98-110, 1975.
16. Dooley M, Goa KL: Capecitabine, *Drugs* 58:69-76, 1999.
17. Dougherty TE, White A: Influence of hormones on lymphoid tissue structure and function: the role of the pituitary adrenotrophic hormone in the regulation of the lymphocytes and other cellular elements of the blood, *Endocrinology* 35:1-14, 1944.
18. Druker BJ, Talpaz M, Resta DJ, et al: Efficacy and safety of a specific inhibitor of the BCR-ABL tyrosine kinase chronic myeloid leukemia, *N Engl J Med* 344:1031-1037, 2001.
19. Dyer MJ: The role of CAMPATH-1 antibodies in the treatment of lymphoid malignancies, *Semin Oncol* 26(suppl 14):52-57, 1999.
20. Farber S, Diamond LK, Mercer RD, et al: Temporary remissions in acute leukemia in children produced by folic acid antagonist, 4-aminopteroyl-glutamic acid (aminopterin), *N Engl J Med* 238:787-793, 1948.
21. Fessas P, Wintrobe M, Thompson R, et al: Treatment of acute leukemia with cortisone and corticotropin, *Arch Intern Med* 94:384-401, 1954.
22. Figgitt DP, Wiseman LR; Docetaxel: an update of its use in advanced breast cancer, *Drugs* 59:621-651, 2000.
23. Frei E, III: The clinical use of actinomycin, *Cancer Chemother Rep* 58:49-54, 1974.
24. Goldie JH, Coldman AJ: The genetic origin of drug resistance in neoplasms: implications for systemic therapy, *Cancer Res* 44:3643-3653, 1984.
25. Goodman LS, Wintrobe M, Dameshek W, et al: Nitrogen mustard therapy: use of methyl-bis (beta-chloroethyl) amine hydrochloride and tris (beta-chloroethyl) amine hydrochloride for Hodgkin's disease, lymphosarcoma, leukemia and certain allied and miscellaneous disorders, *JAMA* 132:126-132, 1946.

26. Graves T, Hooks MA: Drug-induced toxicities associated with high dose cytosine arabinoside infusions, *Pharmacotherapy* 9:23-28, 1989.

27. Grillo-Lopez AJ, White CA, Varns C, et al: Overview of the clinical development of rituximab: first monoclonal antibody approved for the treatment of lymphoma, *Semin Oncol* 26(suppl 14):66-73, 1999.

28. Hainsworth JD: Monoclonal antibody therapy in lymphoid malignancies, *Oncologist* 5:376-384, 2000.

29. Hammond LA, Eckardt JR, Baker SD, et al: Phase I and pharmacokinetic study of temozolomide on a daily-for-5-days schedule in patients with advanced solid malignancies, *J Clin Oncol* 17:2604-2613, 1999.

30. Hande KR: Etoposide: four decades of development of a topoisomerase II inhibitor, *Eur J Cancer* 34:1514-1521, 1998.

31. Heath EI, Grochow LB: Clinical potential of matrix metalloprotease inhibitors in cancer therapy, *Drugs* 59:1043-1055, 2000.

32. Heinemann V: Gemcitabine: progress in the treatment of pancreatic cancer, *Oncology* 60:818, 2001.

33. Henriksson R, Grankvist K: Interactions between anticancer drugs and other clinically used pharmaceuticals. A review, *Acta Oncol* 28:451-462, 1989.

34. Hinman LM, Hamann PR, Wallace R, et al: Preparation and characterization of monoclonal antibody conjugates of the calicheamicins: a novel and potent family of antitumor antibiotics, *Cancer Res* 53:3336-3342, 1993.

35. Hodes ME, Rohn RJ, Bond WH: Vincaleukoblastine. I. Preliminary clinical studies, *Cancer Res* 20:1041-1049, 1960.

36. Hong WK, Endicott J, Itri LM, et al: 13-Cis-retinoic acid in the treatment of oral leukoplakia, *N Engl J Med* 315:1501-1505, 1986.

37. Hood MA, Finley RS: Fludarabine: a review, *DICP Ann Pharmacother* 25:518-524, 1991.

38. Iriarte PV, Hananian J, Cortner JA: Central nervous system leukemia and solid tumors of childhood: treatment with 1,3-bis (2-chloroethyl)-1-nitrosourea (BCNU), *Cancer* 19:1187-1194, 1966.

39. Jain KK: Evaluation of mitoxantrone for the treatment of multiple sclerosis, *Expert Opin Investig Drugs* 9:1139-1149, 2000.

40. Johnson IS, Wright H, Svoboba G, et al: Antitumor principles derived from *Vinca rosea* Linn. I. Vincaleukoblastine and leurosine, *Cancer Res* 20:1016-1022, 1960.

41. Jonasch E, Haluska FG: Interferon in oncological practice: review of interferon biology, clinical applications, and toxicities, *Oncologist* 6:34-55, 2001.

42. Kemp G, Rose P, Lurain J, et al: Amifostine pretreatment for protection against cyclophosphamide-induced and cisplatin-induced toxicities: results of a randomized control trial in patients with advanced ovarian cancer, *J Clin Oncol* 14:2101-2112, 1996.

43. Lasic DD: Doxorubicin in sterically stabilized liposomes, *Nature* 380:561-562, 1996.

44. Liekens S, Clercq ED, Neyts J: Angiogenesis: regulators and clinical applications, *Biochem Pharmacol* 61:253-270, 2001.

45. Mann AM, Hutchison JL: Manic reaction associated with procarbazine hydrochloride therapy of Hodgkin's disease, *Can Med Assoc J* 97:1350-1353, 1967.

46. Mathews DC: Immunotherapy in acute myelogenous leukemia and myelodysplastic syndrome, *Leukemia* 12(suppl 1):S33-S36, 1998.

47. Njar VC, Brodie AM: Comprehensive pharmacology and clinical efficacy of aromatase inhibitors, *Drugs* 58:233-255, 1999.

48. Noonberg SB, Benz CC: Tyrosine kinase inhibitors targeted to the epidermal growth factor receptor subfamily: role as anticancer agents, *Drugs* 59:753-767, 2000.

49. Novick SC, Warrell RP, Jr: Arsenicals in hematologic cancers, *Semin Oncol* 27:495-501, 2000.

50. Oettgen HF, Old LJ, Boyse EA, et al: Inhibition of leukemias in man by L-asparaginase, *Cancer Res* 27:2619-2631, 1967.

51. Onrust SV, Wiseman LR, Goa KL: Epirubicin: a review of its intravesical use in superficial bladder cancer, *Drugs Aging* 15:307-333, 1999.

52. Ormrod D, Holm K, Goa K, et al: Epirubicin: a review of its efficacy as adjuvant therapy and in the treatment of metastatic disease in breast cancer, *Drugs Aging* 15:389-416, 1999.

53. Pinedo HM, Peters GFJ: Fluorouracil: biochemistry and pharmacology, *J Clin Oncol* 6:1653-1664, 1988.

54. Press OW: Radiolabeled antibody therapy of B-cell lymphomas, *Semin Oncol* 26(suppl 14):58-65, 1999.

55. Raymond E, Faivre S, Armand JP: Epidermal growth factor receptor tyrosine kinase as a target for anticancer therapy, *Drugs* 60(suppl 1):15-23, 2000.

56. Reynolds CH: Clinical efficacy of rhIL-11, *Oncology* 14(suppl 8):32-40, 2000.

57. Rosenberg B, VanCamp L, Trosko JE, et al: Platinum compounds: a new class of potent antitumour agents, *Nature* 222:385-386, 1969.

58. Rothenberg ML: Irinotecan (CPT-11): Recent developments and future directions-colorectal cancer and beyond, *Oncologist* 6:66-80, 2001.

59. Rowinsky EK: The pursuit of optimal outcomes in cancer therapy in a new age of rationally designed target-based anticancer agents, *Drugs* 60(suppl 1):1-14, 2000.

60. Saltz LB, Douillard JY, Pirotta N, et al: Irinotecan plus fluorouracil/leucovorin for metastatic colorectal cancer: a new survival standard, *Oncologist* 6:81-91, 2001.

61. Shak S: Overview of the trastuzumab (Herceptin) anti-HER2 monoclonal antibody clinical program in HER2 overexpressing metastatic breast cancer, *Semin Oncol* 26(suppl 12):71-77, 1999.

62. Soignet SL, Maslak P, Wang ZG, et al: Complete remission after treatment of acute promyelocytic leukemia with arsenic trioxide, *N Engl J Med* 339:1341-1348, 1998.

63. Thomas DA, Kantarjian HM: Current role of thalidomide in cancer treatment, *Curr Opin Oncol* :12:564-573, 2000.

64. Thomas X, Archimbaud E: Mitoxantrone in the treatment of acute myelogenous leukemia: a review, *Hematol Cell Ther* 39:63-74, 1997.

65. Toso C, Lindley C: Vinorelbine: a novel vinca alkaloid, *Am J Health-System Pharm* 52:1287-1304, 1995.

66. Weiss RB: Streptozocin: a review of its pharmacology, efficacy, and toxicity, *Cancer Treat Rep* 66:427-438, 1982.

67. Wozniak AJ. Single-agent vinorelbine in the treatment of non-small cell lung cancer, *Semin Oncol* 26(suppl 16):62-66, 1999.

68. Yung AW, Prados MD, Yaya-Tur R, et al: Multicenter phase II trial of temozolomide in patients with anaplastic astrocytoma or anaplastic oligoastrocytoma at first relapse, *J Clin Oncol* 17:2762-2771, 1999.

General References

Abeloff MD, Armitage JO, Lichter AS, et al, eds: *Clinical oncology,* ed 2, Philadelphia, 2000, Churchill Livingstone.

Bast RC, Gansler TS, Holland JF, et al, eds: *Cancer medicine,* ed 5, Hamilton, Ont, 2000, Decker.

Chabner BA, Longo DL, eds: *Cancer chemotherapy and biotherapy: principles and practice,* ed 3, Philadelphia, 2001, Lippincott-Williams & Wilkins.

DeVita VT, Jr, Hellman S, Rosenberg SA, eds: *Cancer: principles and practice of oncology,* ed 6, Philadelphia, 2001, Lippincott Williams & Wilkins.

Dorr RT, Von Hoff DD: *Cancer chemotherapy handbook,* ed 2, Norwalk, CT, 1994, Appleton & Lange.

Drugs of choice for cancer chemotherapy, *Med Lett Drugs Ther* 42:83-92, 2000

Fischer DS, Knobf MT, Durivage HJ, et al, eds: *The cancer chemotherapy handbook,* ed 6, Philadelphia, 2003, Mosby.

Perry MC, ed: *The chemotherapy source book,* ed 3, Baltimore, 2001, Williams & Wilkins.

CHAPTER • 43

Aliphatic Alcohols

Frank J. Dowd

The aliphatic alcohols of therapeutic value are ethyl alcohol (ethanol) and isopropyl alcohol. Methanol and ethylene glycol, the latter a dihydroxy alcohol, are mainly of toxicologic interest. Propylene glycol, another dihydroxy alcohol, is useful as a food additive and in drug compounding. Isopentanol is one of the longer-chain alcohols found in small concentrations in alcoholic beverages. The principal medical use of ethyl and isopropyl alcohol is topical disinfection, as discussed in Chapter 46. Although ethanol has limited clinical application, as the most common intoxicant in Western civilization it is of immense importance because of its potential for abuse and dependence and because it is a major contributing factor to both individual and social ills in the United States and other nations.

Alcohols are hydroxyl derivatives of aliphatic hydrocarbons (Table 43-1). They are clear, colorless, flammable liquids that are completely miscible with water and most organic solvents. The aliphatic monohydroxy alcohols form a homologous series and, with increasing numbers of carbon atoms, display increasing potency as nonselective central nervous system (CNS) depressants. Dihydroxy alcohols (glycols) have similar CNS properties, whereas trihydroxy derivatives lack depressant effects.

ETHANOL

Ethanol can be obtained as anhydrous alcohol (100% ethanol), as neutral spirits (95% ethanol), and as denatured alcohol. Denatured alcohol, intended primarily for industrial use, is ethanol with a substance added to render it unfit for consumption, such as methanol, benzene, diethyl ether, or kerosene.

The social costs of ethanol abuse are staggering. Ethanol-related industrial losses, caused by absenteeism and job inefficiency, welfare costs, and property damage related to ethanol exceed $40 billion annually. Approximately 50% of all fatal traffic accidents are related to the use of ethanol. Drinking aggravates criminal behavior. Ethanol is involved in approximately one third of suicides and rapes, half of assaults, and one half to two thirds of homicides.

Mechanism of Action

It has long been held that the effects of ethanol on the CNS are mediated by an increase in membrane fluidity, leading to disorder of the membrane lipids and resulting in abnormal activity of ion channels and other proteins. Although there is evidence to support this mechanism, the focus has more recently been on the effect of ethanol on excitatory and inhibitory amino acids in the brain. Ethanol potentiates the effect of γ-aminobutyric acid (GABA) at $GABA_A$ receptors. Its mechanism in this respect is similar to that of other sedatives, such as the benzodiazepines, which also enhance the effect of GABA at $GABA_A$ receptors and thereby increase Cl^- conductance.[18,32] In addition, ethanol exerts an inhibitory effect on the CNS by reducing glutamate activation of excitatory ion channels. More specifically, ethanol inhibits the response of the N-methyl-D-aspartate (NMDA) receptor to glutamate.[30,32] Long-term ethanol abuse may cause a change in the subunit structure of the NMDA receptor, leading to an excitatory toxic effect when ethanol is withdrawn acutely. It may also be possible to attribute other side effects, such as chronic CNS effects, to actions on the NMDA receptor. Consistent with this notion is the observation that certain NMDA receptor antagonists can reduce the intake of ethanol in a chronically treated animal model.[12] This has led to the search for NMDA receptor antagonists as potential therapeutic agents in treating alcohol dependence.

Biochemical mechanisms involved in the CNS effects of ethanol also appear to involve, among others, dopaminergic, adrenergic, serotonergic, and opioid pathways.[15,23] Reward mechanisms are enhanced by dopaminergic stimulation and also by opioid peptides.[5] Naltrexone, an opioid receptor antagonist, inhibits the desire for alcohol intake, as do dopamine-receptor antagonists. Agonists at these respective receptors have the opposite effect. Ethanol can deplete the neurotransmitter 5-hydroxytryptamine, which is consistent with aggressive behavior in the alcohol abuser. Although ethanol obviously has a wide range of effects on neurotransmitters and receptors in the CNS, the exact contributions of these systems to the pharmacologic features of ethanol are not known at this time. Furthermore, the mechanisms by which these receptors and neurotransmitters are affected are not well described.

Several actions of ethanol appear attributable to the drug itself but, in many instances, ethanol's effects may result from its primary oxidative metabolite, acetaldehyde.

Pharmacologic Effects

Central nervous system

There is a common but mistaken notion that ethanol is a CNS stimulant. To the contrary, ethanol is a sedative-hypnotic that depresses the CNS in a dose-dependent fashion. Much of the apparent stimulation resulting from ethanol use results from disinhibition of CNS function because of selective depression of inhibitory pathways at lower concentrations of ethanol. Thus, although mental processes, memory, and concentration are reduced, the individual may feel euphoric, confident, and socially uninhibited. Higher doses (intoxication) lead to overall depression of the CNS. As with other CNS depres-

Table • 43-1

Aliphatic Alcohols

	SYNONYMS	CHEMICAL FORMULA
Methyl alcohol	Methanol, carbinol, wood alcohol, wood spirit	CH_3OH
Ethyl alcohol	Ethanol, grain alcohol	CH_3CH_2OH
Isopropyl alcohol	Isopropanol, 2-propanol, secondary propyl alcohol	$(H_3C)_2CHOH$

Table • 43-2

Correlates of the BAC

BAC (mg/dl)	CLINICAL STATE*
50	Dizzy
100	Drunk (legally)†
150	Drunk and disorderly
300	Dazed and dejected
400	Dead drunk
500	Dead

*Classification modified from Gaddum JH: *Pharmacology*, ed 5, New York, 1968, Oxford University Press.
†In some states, 80 mg/dl.

sants, the major acute toxicity of ethanol is respiratory depression from inhibition of the medullary respiratory center.

The concentration of ethanol in alcoholic beverages is often listed as the "proof." The actual concentration of ethanol, in percent by volume, is half the proof number. Thus 80 proof equals 40% ethanol by volume. Because of the variability of absorption of different alcoholic beverages, the effects of ethanol are most commonly correlated with the blood alcohol concentration (BAC), as illustrated in Table 43-2. Ethanol's effects are dose related and progress through the typical sequence of anxiolysis, sedation, hypnosis, anesthesia, and death. Ethanol is a soporific, increasing the time spent in sleep and decreasing the time it takes to get to sleep. With low doses of alcohol, the electroencephalogram displays a reduced frequency and increased amplitude of α waves and, with high doses, an enhanced δ activity similar to a pattern of deep sleep. At a BAC of approximately 150 mg/dl, there is a reduction in the length, although not in the number, of episodes of rapid eye movement sleep throughout the night, together with reduced movement during sleep. Sleep patterns are disturbed with repeated ingestion, however, so that sleep comes in short segments, and the wake time is actually increased.

Even at a BAC less than 50 mg/dl, binocular fusion is impaired and blurred vision occurs. Handwriting deteriorates, fine motor coordination is reduced, and complex sensorimotor tasks begin to show impairment. The Romberg "standing steadiness" test reveals marked unsteadiness and increased body sway at a BAC of as little as 30 mg/dl. At a BAC between 50 and 100 mg/dl, a drinker displays reductions in anxiety, critical judgment, and self-criticism, with enhanced sociability and self-esteem in group situations. Disinhibition, with talkativeness and a feeling of elation, occurs at the same time that mild sedation is produced, along with relaxation, drowsiness, and reduced alertness. Speech, movement, and simple reaction times are slowed. Fear is reduced, and impulsive risk-taking behavior becomes evident. Many performance tasks are unaltered at a BAC of 50 mg/dl, but most are impaired at 100 mg/dl. Sexual motivation may be enhanced at lower BACs through a reduction in anxiety and muscular tension, and maximum penile diameter, in response to visual stimulation, is increased at a BAC of 25 mg/dl but is reduced at concentrations greater than 50 mg/dl.

At a BAC of 100 to 200 mg/dl, nausea, vomiting, and loss of self-control are common in an inexperienced drinker, whereas the experienced inebriate speaks and moves with exaggerated care. Subjective time passes more slowly. Speech becomes slurred, and ataxia with staggering gait occurs. A unique positional alcohol nystagmus is produced in which, with the head tilted to the side, the eyes drift slowly upward and then jerk rapidly downward. Ethanol produces deficits in both short-term and long-term memory, and amnesia ("blackouts") may occur. Ethanol increases assertive or aggressive behavior and may precipitate a rage-release reaction, especially if the initial mood of the drinker is unpleasant. Significant analgesia is also produced.

In the range of 300 mg/dl of ethanol, intoxication is severe and is accompanied by a loss of consciousness. There may be mydriasis, sweating, hypotension, and hypothermia. At a BAC of 400 to 500 mg/dl, medullary paralysis, cardiovascular depression, and death are likely to occur.

Drivers with a BAC of 100 mg/dl or greater are considered legally intoxicated; usually if the BAC is 50 mg/dl or less, the person is considered not intoxicated. In some states, 80 mg/dl constitutes legal intoxication. Certain conditions such as sleepiness may make individuals susceptible to the effects of small amounts of ethanol or to the effects of previous exposure to alcohol even when the BAC is undetectable.[22]

Cardiovascular system

Acute alcohol administration results in an elevated catecholamine concentration in blood and urine. Adrenal monoamine release is accompanied by compensatory increases in the activity of medullary tyrosine hydroxylase, dopamine β-hydroxylase, and phenylethanolamine-N-methyl transferase. Vascular smooth muscle exhibits hyperreactivity to norepinephrine at low ethanol concentrations and hyporeactivity at high concentrations. The latter effect may be caused by ethanol-induced facilitation of neuronal monoamine uptake. The direct actions of ethanol on vasomotor tone, coupled with its complex adrenergic effects and centrally mediated influences, produce variable cardiovascular responses. In general, coronary blood flow is slightly enhanced, but there is no concomitant increase in myocardial oxygen uptake. Indeed, myocardial contractility is depressed by ethanol. Direct vasoconstriction has been observed in cerebral and renal vascular beds in vitro, but in vivo the effect of ethanol, occurring only at large doses, is an increase in blood flow to the brain and kidneys. Mesenteric blood flow also appears to be increased. One of the more consistent cardiovascular effects of alcohol ingestion is cutaneous vasodilation. The increased blood flow to the skin provides a feeling of warmth. In cold environments, heat loss may be greatly accentuated, and alcohol is generally to be avoided in treating the hypothermic person. Furthermore, at low ambient temperatures individuals under the influence of ethanol have a high risk of hypothermia. The ethanol metabolite acetaldehyde causes catecholamine release and produces tachycardia, increased cardiac output, and increased arterial blood pressure in human beings, effects that are abolished by adrenoceptor blockade. However, the concentrations of acetaldehyde normally resulting from low amounts of ingested ethanol have little acute effect on the cardiovascular system. Long-term effects of ethanol are different from its short-term effects. Ethanol, when ingested in excess on a long-term basis, increases the risk of hypertension and adverse cardiac effects. Long-term ethanol abuse can cause a cardiomyopathy characterized by a decreased ventricular ejection fraction and even heart failure.[24] Fibrosis of the myocardium may also occur.

Liver

A number of effects of ethanol on the liver have been documented. Acute ingestion of intoxicating amounts of ethanol leads to a reduced liver-metabolizing activity. This effect is reversed once the ethanol is eliminated. In the long-term alcoholic, induction of liver microsomal enzymes is common; if the individual is not intoxicated, drug metabolism may be enhanced. If cirrhosis of the liver occurs, overall metabolism is reduced because of impaired hepatic blood flow and destruction of liver tissue. Thus the use of ethanol has several implications for drug metabolism.

Ethanol can also influence nutritional status. Ethanol inhibits the activation of vitamins A and D and causes depletion of pyridoxine.[19] Trace metals, such as zinc and selenium, are also depleted. Cirrhosis of the liver leads to further reduction in nutritional status. Nutritional deficiencies are also common because ethanol can marginally meet an alcoholic's caloric needs without supplying other nutritional requirements. Other long-term effects are discussed later in the chapter.

Kidney

Ethanol has a diuretic effect resulting from inhibition of antidiuretic hormone (ADH) secretion by the posterior pituitary. Urinary Na^+, K^+, and Cl^- concentrations are reduced, whereas Mg^{++} and norepinephrine are increased.

Sexual function

Ethanol interferes with sexual function in both men and women. It can cause temporary impotence even though overall aggressiveness may be enhanced. Long-term alcoholism may lead to more lasting impotence and sterility. Testosterone production may be depressed and testosterone metabolism enhanced, the latter as a result of induction of liver microsomal enzymes. Feminization in men is a possible outcome.

Blood lipids

One of the potential salutary effects of moderate consumption of ethanol is its influence on lipid metabolism. Intake on the order of one to two drinks a day increases the ratio of high-density to low-density lipoproteins in the plasma, an effect inversely correlated with the incidence of coronary heart disease and myocardial infarction.[28] Other effects such as reduced platelet aggregation may also provide a cardioprotective effect. In one study, men who were homozygous for the "slow" form of one of the isozymes of alcohol dehydrogenase ADH3 had an especially enhanced increase in high-density lipoprotein and decreased risk of myocardial infarction.[10] Nevertheless, controlling ethanol intake is a much more crucial need facing society as a whole.

Other effects

Small oral doses of ethanol temporarily enhance both salivary and gastric acid secretion, the increased salivation probably by a conditioned reflex. Large doses of alcohol reduce salivation. Ethanol is a gastric irritant, producing inflammation of the stomach wall in concentrations greater than 15%. Ingestion of solutions of more than 20% ethanol results in increased gastric mucus secretion and in petechial hemorrhage and ulceration. Ethanol retards intestinal absorption of glucose, amino acids, folic acid, thiamine, and vitamin B_{12}. Adrenal gland activation results in increased blood concentrations of corticosteroids, epinephrine, and glucose.

The effects of ethanol on the peripheral vasculature, CNS, ADH secretion, and sexual function are summarized in this exchange between Macduff and the porter in Shakespeare's *Macbeth:*

Macduff: What three things does drink especially provoke?
Porter: Marry, Sir, nose-painting, sleep, and urine. Lechery, sir, it provokes and unprovokes: it provokes the desire but not the performance.[25]

Absorption, Fate, and Excretion

Ethanol is rapidly absorbed from the stomach and small intestine. After oral ingestion, the rate of absorption largely depends on the gastric emptying time because 75% of a dose is rapidly and completely taken up from the small intestine. Indeed, gastrectomized patients often note enhanced effects of ethanol. The rate of gastric absorption is reduced by the presence of food. Concentrations of ethanol greater than 20% retard absorption by inducing both gastric mucosal irritation and pylorospasm.

Approximately 60% of inspired ethanol vapor is absorbed through the lungs, and intoxication can be achieved by this route. Percutaneous absorption can also occur and has led to death when infants were wrapped in ethanol-soaked cloth to treat hyperthermia.

After intravenous ethanol administration, the BAC exhibits an abrupt curvilinear decline, lasting from 10 to 30 minutes, caused by distribution throughout total body water.[11] This distributional phase is not noted in serial drinking situations, in which distributional equilibrium occurs in concert with gastrointestinal absorption.

After oral intake, the arterial BAC exceeds the venous BAC because of rapid tissue uptake of alcohol from capillary blood. Maximum electroencephalogram changes occur approximately 25 minutes before the maximum venous BAC is achieved. The BAC after ingestion of a fixed amount of alcohol is a function of sex, age, and adiposity as well as the nature of the beverage and the time over which it is ingested. In Table 43-3, which shows the influence of alcoholic beverage, age, and sex on BAC, the BAC has been calculated on the basis of reported age- and sex-corrected values for total body water and blood water content. The tissue alcohol concentration is proportional to both lean body weight and tissue water content. Considering the BAC as unity, the relative concentration of ethanol at equilibrium is 1.35 in urine, 1.17 in brain, 1.16 in blood plasma, 1.12 in saliva, 0.05 in alveolar air, and 0.02 in fat.

More than 95% of ingested ethanol is metabolized under normal circumstances. High doses of ethanol, however, are associated with lower metabolism (approaching 90%). Metabolism takes place mostly by a three-phase hepatic oxidation (Figure 43-1). Ethanol is initially converted to acetaldehyde by alcohol dehydrogenase, which requires nicotinamide adenine dinucleotide (NAD) as the hydrogen acceptor:

$$CH_3CH_2OH + NAD^+ \leftrightarrow CH_3CHO + NADH + H^+$$

The binding of substrate and coenzyme to alcohol dehydrogenase involves sites on the enzyme containing zinc and sulfhydryl groups. Human alcohol dehydrogenase also oxidizes methanol, isopropyl alcohol, and ethylene glycol. This dehydrogenase reaction is the rate-limiting step in the metabolism of alcohol except in those individuals who have a deficiency in the subsequent enzyme.[6,11]

The second phase, conversion of acetaldehyde to acetate, occurs in liver and other tissues and is catalyzed by aldehyde

Table • 43-3

Equivalents of Alcoholic Beverages

	CLASSIFICATION OF DRINKER		
FORM OF ALCOHOL	SEX	AGE (YEARS)	POTENTIAL RESULTING BAC (mg/dl)*
Regular beer (12 ounces, 3.5% ethanol)	Male	17 to 34	22.7
		57 to 86	25.5
	Female	20 to 31	27.7
		60 to 82	30.7
Distilled spirits (1 ounce, 40% ethanol)†	Male	17 to 34	17.1
		57 to 86	19.3
	Female	20 to 31	21.0
		60 to 82	23.2

*Calculated on the basis of a lean body mass of 153.4 lb (70 kg).
†American proof number is twice the percentage of ethanol by volume.

dehydrogenase, which has a much greater affinity for acetaldehyde than does alcohol dehydrogenase:

$$CH_3CHO + NAD + OH^+ \leftrightarrow CH_3CHOO^- + NADH + H^+$$

In the third step, acetate, as acetyl coenzyme A, is further oxidized through the Krebs cycle to carbon dioxide and water.

The reductive environment resulting from ethanol oxidation upsets hepatic chemistry and results in reduced gluconeogenesis and enhanced triglyceride and lactate formation. Heavy bouts of drinking can cause hypoglycemia, lactic acidosis, and hyperuricemia (because acetate and lactate, respectively, stimulate the synthesis of uric acid and inhibit its renal excretion), which can precipitate gout, hyperlipidemia, and fatty liver.

An alternate oxidative pathway for alcohol involving the microsomal enzyme oxidation system (MEOS) becomes an important factor in alcohol elimination at high BACs, during which it may account for 10% to 20% of ethanol metabolism. This pathway also yields acetaldehyde. The MEOS pathway is inducible and therefore may account for the somewhat higher metabolic inactivation of ethanol seen in individuals who abuse ethanol over the long term.

Ethanol elimination appears to follow zero-order kinetics (it is pseudolinear regarding time) down to a certain BAC, where it assumes a curvilinear, first-order decline. The reported point at which this change occurs varies according to the study. Such elimination kinetics are best described by modified Michaelis-Menten models because the rate of pseudolinear elimination is dose dependent, ranging from 16 to 25 mg/dl per hour as the peak BAC increases from 50 to 185 mg/dl. After low-to-moderate doses of ethanol, the rate of ethanol metabolism is approximately 80 mg/kg per hour, or roughly 5.6 g or 0.2 oz (of 100% ethanol) per hour for a 70-kg adult.[11] Approximately 2% to 10% of absorbed alcohol is excreted unchanged, largely through the lungs and kidneys. Minor amounts are detectable in saliva, tears, sweat, and feces. Because ethanol is metabolized to acetate, it can provide calories (a maximum of approximately 1200 kcal/day). However, it provides no other essential nutrients, such as vitamins, amino acids, or fatty acids.

Drug Interactions

Ethanol produces additive effects with all CNS depressants and increases the hypotensive effects of most vasodilators. Long-acting drugs such as diazepam may cause increased depression with ingested alcohol for up to 24 hours after the drug was given. The benzodiazepine-ethanol combination, in fact, seems to pose a particular risk. At high BACs, ethanol many inhibit the metabolism of, and therefore potentiate the effects of, benzodiazepines and some other CNS depressants. Short-term alcohol ingestion may also result in exaggerated clinical responses to oral anticoagulants and hypoglycemic agents.

The use of ethanol influences the in vivo absorption of certain drugs. For example, short-term ethanol ingestion increases, although long-term alcoholism reduces, the oral absorption rate of diazepam. Ethanol also inhibits the absorption and enhances the breakdown of penicillins in the stomach for up to 3 hours after ethanol intake. Aspirin and other nonsteroidal antiinflammatory drugs (NSAIDs) promote gastric

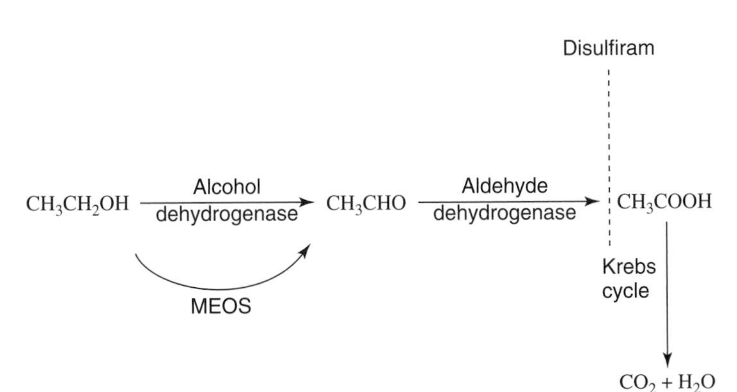

Fig. 43-1 Metabolism of ethanol and its blockade by disulfiram. Disulfiram inhibits both the mitochondrial and cytoplasmic forms of aldehyde dehydrogenase. *MEOS*, Microsomal enzyme oxidizing system.

bleeding when combined with ethanol and can cause gastric hemorrhage in alcoholics who have alcoholic gastritis.

In the long-term alcoholic without liver damage, induction of MEOS activity takes place. Increased enzyme activity appears after approximately 3 weeks of heavy drinking and lasts 4 to 9 weeks after the cessation of drinking. A significant reduction in plasma half-life of, and clinical response to, many drugs occurs (e.g., intravenous anesthetics, barbiturates, antianxiety drugs). In long-term alcoholism, however, the development of hepatic damage offsets the effects of enzyme induction, and drug sensitivity may return to normal. Eventually, cirrhosis leads to significantly reduced drug metabolism. The induction of liver microsomal enzymes with long-term ethanol ingestion is the basis for the enhanced toxicity of acetaminophen in long-term alcohol abusers. Induction, particularly of cytochrome P4503A, favors the production of reactive and hepatotoxic metabolites of acetaminophen (see Chapter 21).[26] Interestingly, acute ingestion of ethanol, under certain circumstances, can actually protect against acetaminophen toxicity because at higher blood alcohol levels the metabolism of acetaminophen to toxic metabolites is inhibited despite a concurrent long-term inductive effect of ethanol.

Drugs that inhibit aldehyde dehydrogenase can lead to unpleasant and even potentially life-threatening symptoms after ethanol ingestion. These inhibitors include disulfiram, which is given to prevent the use of ethanol by abusers, metronidazole, certain cephalosporins, and oral hypoglycemics. Acutely, acetaldehyde can cause flushing and headache, nausea and vomiting, hypotension, blurred vision, and mental confusion. Because acetaldehyde concentrations vary directly with ethanol intake, high doses of ethanol alone may lead to these symptoms. If aldehyde dehydrogenase is inhibited by drugs such as disulfiram, even low and moderate amounts of ethanol can lead to adverse reactions because of acetaldehyde accumulation.[33] Individuals with a genetic deficiency in aldehyde dehydrogenase, which is common in certain races, also experience the accumulation of acetaldehyde and have alcohol intolerance.[3]

General Therapeutic Uses

Topically applied 70% ethanol is used as a rubefacient, anhidrotic, and antiseptic and as a means to cool the skin in cases of fever. Ethanol hardens the skin by protein precipitation and is used to prevent decubitus ulcers in bedridden patients. Ethanol is a solvent for the irritating principle of poison ivy, and its early use on affected skin can markedly reduce resulting dermatitis.

Absolute ethanol has been injected to destroy nerves or ganglia in treating intractable pain arising from conditions such as trigeminal neuralgia and inoperable cancer. However, other treatment modalities are usually more desirable. Inhalation of ethanol vapor is of value in attacks of acute pulmonary edema because of its antifoaming action.

Ethanol is also used to treat poisoning by methanol, isopropyl alcohol, and ethylene glycol.

Therapeutic Uses and Implications for Dentistry

The dental uses of ethanol as an antiseptic and disinfectant are discussed in Chapter 46. The dentist can expect to encounter alcoholic patients in everyday practice. Alcoholics usually exhibit signs of deficient oral hygiene, such as coated tongue and heavy plaque and calculus deposits. They have twice the rate of tooth loss of the general population, commonly lack the mandibular and maxillary first molars, and frequently have advanced chronic periodontitis. Chronic asymptomatic enlargement of the parotid, and sometimes submandibular, glands may be observed. The dentist should be aware of the increased incidence of oral leukoplakia in alcoholics and be familiar with its appearance, particularly the erosive form, because 6% of such persons develop carcinoma, especially of the tongue, within 9 years of diagnosis of the lesion. Postoperative healing time is prolonged in alcoholics. This may be related to a marked increase in collagenase activity, which has been observed in the liver of alcoholics. Long-term ethanol use may reduce the analgesic potency of nitrous oxide[9] specifically and the efficacy of conscious sedation in general. The potential interactions of ethanol with acetaminophen and NSAIDs should be kept in mind. Large therapeutic doses of acetaminophen should be avoided in moderate to heavy drinkers. Concurrent intake of NSAIDs and ethanol should be avoided.

Alcohol Dependence

Abuse characteristics

Alcoholism is similar to dependence on CNS depressants, except that ethanol produces unique direct neurologic, hepatic, and muscular toxicity. Because ethanol can provide a major source of dietary calories, it also promotes malnutrition in the chronic drinker. Ethanol dependence is characterized by marked psychic and physical dependence, moderate tolerance, and a wide range of pathologic sequelae.

Emotional dependence on alcohol is severe. The alcoholic develops a compulsion to obtain and use the drug to the extent that all other activities become secondary, and deterioration of personal and social concerns ensues. Personal, social, and medical problems appear early in life, and life expectancy is decreased. Alcoholism has a partial genetic basis, with a degree of heritability approximately that of diabetes mellitus.

Tolerance develops to ethanol after long-term abuse, but the degree of tolerance, as with other sedative hypnotics, is much less than that which occurs with the opioids.[13] Tolerance to ethanol is partly a result of behavioral adaptation to the effects of ethanol. Adaptive changes by receptor mechanisms and membrane fluidity may also play a role. Furthermore, induction of the MEOS somewhat increases the rate of ethanol metabolism.[11] The acute lethal dose of ethanol, however, is not greatly increased over that for the nonalcoholic.[13] Cross-tolerance also occurs with other sedative-hypnotics.

Alcohol abstinence syndrome

The severity of the acute alcohol abstinence syndrome correlates with the amount and duration of preabstinent ethanol intake. The mildest form is the tremulousness and nausea experienced "the morning after," which is readily reversed by "taking a hair of the dog" (i.e., a small amount of ethanol). The most severe abstinence syndrome is delirium tremens. Severe withdrawal symptoms appear 6 to 8 hours after drinking ceases, peak at 48 to 96 hours, and generally resolve in approximately 2 weeks.

Moderate abstinence results in anorexia, nausea, epigastric upset, tremulousness, sweating, apprehension, and insomnia. In more severe abstinence, additional symptoms of diarrhea, vomiting, nightmares, and agitation occur, together with autonomic signs of tachycardia, hyperpnea, and fever. Delirium tremens, if it occurs, is manifested by all the preceding symptoms together with possible psychosis, seizures, and hyperthermia. Psychotic manifestations include muttering, delirium, paranoia, delusions, and auditory, visual, and tactile hallucinations of a threatening nature. The person usually displays agitation, confusion, disorientation, and panic. The hallucinatory symptoms appear to be at least partially the result of excessive rebound rapid eye movement sleep that, suppressed during the drinking phase, spills over into the waking state during withdrawal. Neuromuscular hyperexcitability is manifested by gross tremors and grand mal convulsions (with a marked sensitivity to stroboscopically induced seizures), both of which correlate with a rapid urinary excretion of Mg^{++} and a resultant hypomagnesemia during withdrawal. Abstinence may also lead to hyperthermia and circulatory collapse.

Pathologic sequelae of alcoholism

Chronic alcoholism is associated with a number of severe physical complications, primarily of the nervous and gastrointestinal systems and of skeletal and cardiac muscle. These complications are summarized in Table 43-4. Alcohol damage to the liver, in which extensive oxidative ethanol metabolism occurs, results from direct acetaldehyde and ethanol toxicity and the reductive environment brought on by ethanol metabolism. Ethanol metabolism by alcohol dehydrogenase and MEOS activity leads to acetaldehyde production. Acetaldehyde has several adverse effects, both short and long term. The short-term effects have been previously reviewed. Over the long term, acetaldehyde is responsible for nutritional depletion in the liver and depletion of glutathione. It enhances lipid peroxidation and membrane damage.[21] Triglyceride accumulation is also favored by the reductive environment from excess NADH production resulting from ethanol oxidation. The incidence of liver cancer is higher in alcoholics.[21]

Ethanol has also been shown to change the flora in the gastrointestinal tract, favoring the growth of certain gram-negative bacteria. This in turn leads to the production of more bacterial endotoxins (lipopolysaccharides).[29] Evidence is accumulating that the endotoxins stimulate liver Kupffer cells that produce inflammatory mediators and oxygen radicals that cause apoptotic changes in hepatic parenchymal cells (Figure 43-2).[8] Damage by this mechanism may account in part for both short- and long-term changes.[16] Free radical production in parenchymal cells may also occur that could contribute to overall liver damage. Apoptosis may also be favored by ethanol's ability to inhibit insulin-like growth factor receptor signaling.[7] Alcoholic liver damage is heralded by the appearance of steatosis, or fatty liver, which is a benign and reversible syndrome seen almost universally among heavy drinkers. Hepatomegaly, associated with this early phase of liver disease, is caused by lipid accumulation and water retention, resulting in "ballooning" of hepatocytes. The fatty liver phase of liver damage can progress to generalized hepatic inflammation and

Table • 43-4

Pathologic Sequelae of Alcoholism

SYSTEM OF ORIGIN	SYNDROME	CAUSES	SIGNS AND SYMPTOMS
Nervous system	Wernicke's syndrome	Ethanol toxicity, malnutrition	Confusion, amnesia, confabulation, peripheral neuropathy, diplopia, nystagmus, tremor, ataxia
	Korsakoff's psychosis	Ethanol toxicity, malnutrition	Disorientation, amnesia, confabulation, peripheral neuritis
	Cerebral atrophy	Ethanol toxicity, malnutrition	Irreversible degeneration of frontal lobe cortical cells with premature senility, dementia, personality disintegration
	Cerebellar atrophy	Ethanol toxicity, malnutrition	Irreversible ataxia
	Peripheral neuropathy	Thiamine deficiency	Diminished tendon reflexes, sensory loss in feet or legs, muscle atrophy
Gastrointestinal tract	Esophagitis and gastritis	Secretory and inflammatory effects of ethanol	Heartburn, vomiting, gastric ulceration, hematemesis
	Peptic ulcers	Secretory and inflammatory effects of ethanol	Epigastric pain, anorexia, vomiting
	Pancreatitis	Secretory effect of ethanol, obstruction of pancreatic duct	Weight loss, abdominal pain, blood loss, shock
Liver	Steatosis or fatty liver	Direct toxicity of acetaldehyde and ethanol, reductive environment	Enlarged liver
	Alcoholic hepatitis	Direct toxicity of acetaldehyde and ethanol, reductive environment	Anorexia, vomiting, weakness, jaundice, ascites, enlarged spleen and liver
	Laennec's cirrhosis	Direct toxicity of acetaldehyde and ethanol, reductive environment	Jaundice, portal hypertension, mental deterioration, renal failure, coma
Skeletal muscle	Alcoholic myopathy	Ethanol toxicity	Cramping, weakness, edema, atrophy of muscle
Cardiac muscle	Alcoholic heart muscle disease	Direct toxicity of ethanol and acetaldehyde	Weakness, shortness of breath, congestive heart failure, pulmonary congestion
Fetus	Fetal alcohol syndrome	Ethanol toxicity	Microcephaly; reduced IQ; facial, cardiac, and genital defects

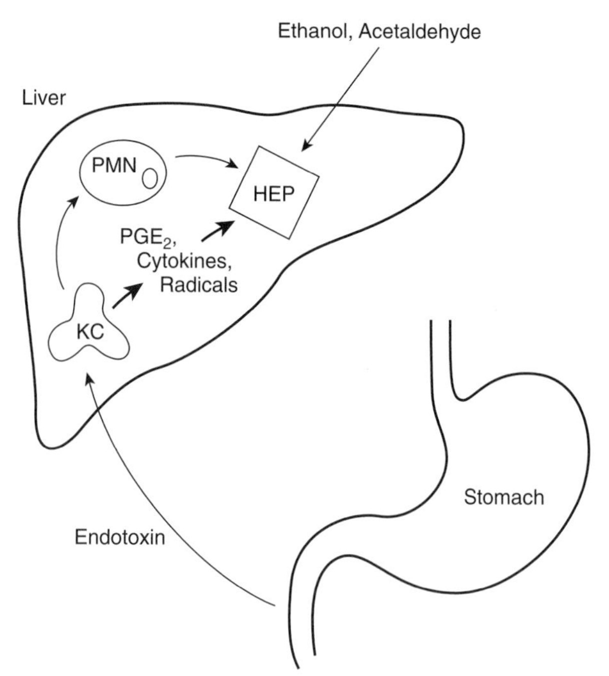

Fig. 43-2 Mechanism of liver damage from ethanol. Use of ethanol leads to an increase in certain intestinal gram-negative organisms, resulting in an increase in endotoxins. These in turn stimulate Kupffer cells *(KC)* in the liver to produce mediators, including prostaglandin E_2 (PGE_2), cytokines, and free radicals, that damage hepatocytes *(HEP)*. Effects on Kupffer cells lead to stimulation of polymorphonuclear leukocytes *(PMN)* that also release mediators that damage liver cells. Ethanol or acetaldehyde may also act directly on hepatocytes to alter lipid metabolism, damage cell macromolecules, or block the effect of insulinlike growth factor. (Modified from Thurman RG: Mechanisms of hepatic toxicity II. Alcoholic liver injury involves activation of Kupffer cells by endotoxin, *Am J Physiol* 275:G605-G611, 1998.)

"florid" alcoholic hepatitis, a condition that has a 10% to 30% fatality rate. In 10% to 15% of heavy drinkers, fatty liver progresses to Laennec's cirrhosis. The toxic effects of long-term abuse of ethanol are summarized in Figure 43-2.

Ethanol-induced damage in organs lacking significant ethanol oxidative capacity may result from enzyme-catalyzed esterification of fatty acids with ethanol.[1,17] Transient accumulation of such fatty acid ethyl esters, or their fatty acid metabolites, appears to inhibit oxidative phosphorylation and may alter plasma membranes, leading to damage in organs such as the heart,[2] pancreas, and brain.[1]

Cardiovascular complications of alcoholism include cardiac disease, hypertension, and atrial arrhythmias, the first accounting for one third of deaths among heavy drinkers.[31] Alcoholic heart muscle disease results from long-term intake of ethanol. This disease is characterized by cardiomegaly (heart weight doubles in 28% of heavy drinkers), biventricular congestive failure (with pulmonary and peripheral edema), breathlessness, and sometimes arrhythmias. Treatment is the same as for other types of congestive heart failure, coupled with permanent abstinence from ethanol. Alcoholic hypertension is exhibited, especially in white men, as a reversible dose-dependent increase in systolic and diastolic blood pressures and can be associated with only moderately heavy ethanol consumption. The "holiday heart syndrome" refers to severe atrial arrhythmias precipitated by bouts of periodic heavy drinking.

The inflammatory effects of alcohol on the gastrointestinal tract lead to esophagitis and chronic gastritis frequently associated with intense episodes of vomiting, which may lead to gastric laceration and hematemesis. There is a high correlation between heavy drinking and cancer of the mouth and throat. Peptic ulcers and pancreatitis are common among alcoholics.[27]

Effects of alcohol on skeletal muscle may produce acute alcoholic myopathy characterized by muscle cramps, weakness, and swelling, which resolve after a few weeks of alcohol abstinence. In severe cases, extensive muscle degeneration results in myoglobinemia, hyperkalemia, and renal failure. A chronic form of alcoholic myopathy ultimately produces marked muscular atrophy, usually of the pelvic girdle and thighs.

Fetal alcohol syndrome is a cluster of physical and mental defects occurring in children of women who consume ethanol during pregnancy. In more than 90% of cases of fetal alcohol syndrome, there is growth deficiency, microcephaly, and short palpebral fissures. Also common are midfacial hypoplasia, mental retardation, and deficiencies in coordination and fine motor skills. The mental and motor deficiencies may be causally related to the developmental abnormalities of cortical neurons, as observed in rats prenatally exposed to ethanol.[20] The degree of dysmorphogenesis correlates with mental deficiency, with IQs ranging from 55 to 82. Neither the dysmorphic nor the intellectual aspects of the syndrome improve with age. Pregnant patients should be advised to avoid alcoholic beverages and to be aware of the alcoholic content of food and drugs.

Both central and peripheral nerve degeneration occur, resulting in a wide range of neurologic disorders involving psychologic and personality changes as well as peripheral neuritis, sensory loss, and muscle atrophy. Changes in the nervous system are related in part to malnutrition, and most respond to thiamine administration, indicating a thiamine deficiency.[19]

Ethanol changes plasma membranes and their component lipids and alters protein and DNA synthesis. The mechanism(s) accounting for these changes may be at the receptor and/or signal transduction level and may be one result of producing reactive oxygen species. Ethanol has also been shown to inhibit the proliferation and growth of both glial and neuronal cells resulting from muscarinic receptor stimulation.[4] Muscarinic receptors have been proposed to play a crucial role in synaptogenesis in the developing brain. Ethanol may disrupt this process by inhibiting signaling at the G protein level.[4] Changes in vitamin A metabolism and the previously mentioned inhibition of the insulin-like growth factor receptor are also potential mechanisms of fetal damage. It has also been reported that ethanol can cause an apoptotic pattern in the developing rat brain that is consistent with its ability to block NMDA receptors[14] (see Chapter 11) and to stimulate $GABA_A$ receptors (see Chapter 13). Toxic effects of ethanol on the brain are summarized in Figure 43-3.

Women are more susceptible to the toxic effects of ethanol than are men. The smaller average size of the individual is part of the reason blood alcohol levels are higher than men for comparable alcohol intakes. However, women also have higher levels of alcohol dehydrogenase and therefore produce higher levels of tissue and plasma acetaldehyde. In addition, estrogens enhance the toxic effect of ethanol on the liver. Tissue hypoxia, fibrosis, extent of fat distribution, and level of endotoxin are all elevated in women compared with men, and estrogen appears to be a major factor.[24]

Treatment of alcoholism

The treatment of alcoholism involves the detoxification of the acutely inebriated individual, medication to prevent severe symptoms of abstinence, and long-term rehabilitation. To a

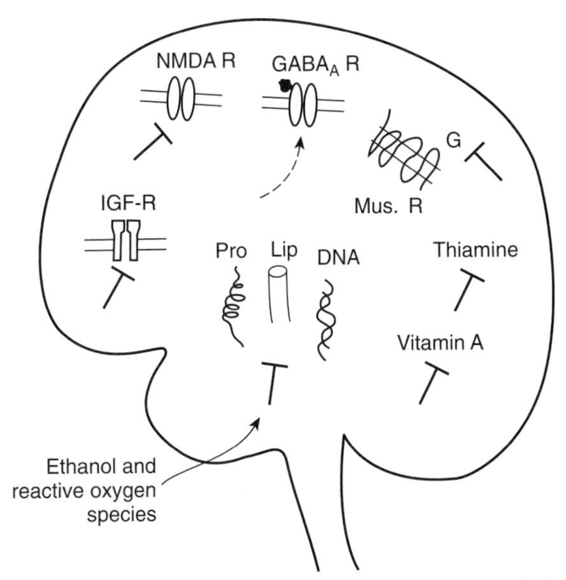

Fig. 43-3 Mechanisms by which ethanol may damage the brain. Ethanol inhibits NMDA receptor *(R)* function initially, followed by supersensitivity of the receptor; stimulates GABA$_A$ receptor function *(arrow)*; inhibits muscarinic receptor function *(Mus. R)*, inhibits insulinlike growth factor receptor function; depletes thiamine; and alters the metabolism of vitamin A. In addition, cell toxicity may result from ethanol itself or from reactive oxidative species that alter membrane lipids, proteins, and DNA. *Lip*, Lipid; *Pro*, protein.

large extent, the rate of detoxification is determined by the rate at which the liver disposes of the ethanol, but the nature of the withdrawal period also depends on the degree of dependence, the environment, and the nutritional status of the patient. The symptoms associated with abstinence are usually treated with a long-acting benzodiazepine (e.g., diazepam). Supplemental dietary thiamine and other vitamins may be given.

Disulfiram (Antabuse) is used in avoidance therapy for alcoholics.[33] Disulfiram is rapidly converted to metabolites such as diethyldithiocarbamate and diethylthiomethylcarbamate. These and possible other metabolites probably account for the action of the drug (see Figure 43-1). Disulfiram inhibits aldehyde dehydrogenase through the formation of a covalent disulfide bond between an enzymic thiol group and an active drug metabolite. The enzyme is inhibited irreversibly. Disulfiram also inhibits other enzymes, notably dopamine β-hydroxylase and oxidases of the MEOS.

Oral doses of disulfiram have an onset of action of approximately 12 hours, and the effects are evident for up to 2 weeks after treatment is stopped. The protracted duration of action is based on the irreversible nature of the binding of disulfiram metabolites. Only with the synthesis of new enzyme does the metabolism of ethanol return to normal. Disulfiram itself commonly produces drowsiness, and, in large daily doses, it may cause paresthesias and muscle weakness. The drug may exaggerate schizophrenia or depression, possibly through alteration of central monoamine concentrations caused by the inhibition of dopamine β-hydroxylase.

If ethanol is ingested during disulfiram treatment, symptoms of acetaldehyde poisoning develop.[33] Drinking 1.2 ounces of 80 proof liquor causes flushing, tachycardia, palpitation, and tachypnea, all lasting approximately 30 minutes. Ingestion of more than 1.6 ounces of 80 proof liquor produces intense palpitation and dyspnea, nausea, vomiting, and headache lasting up to 90 minutes. Unconsciousness, hypotensive shock, and sudden myocardial infarction may occur. For this reason, the drug must be used only under strict medical supervision.

Disulfiram inhibits oxidative biotransformation but not glucuronide conjugation of benzodiazepines (see Chapter 13). Hypotensive episodes may occur during general anesthesia as a result of dopamine β-hydroxylase inhibition and depletion of neuronal norepinephrine. However, even large therapeutic doses fail to alter the cardiovascular response to pressor amines of either the direct- or indirect-acting variety. Paraldehyde, because of its metabolic conversion to acetaldehyde, produces toxic reactions in patients taking disulfiram.

Acamprosate (calcium acetylhomotaurine) offers promise for reducing relapse in alcoholics. Acamprosate appears to have effects on both NMDA and GABA$_A$ receptor–mediated events.

METHANOL

Methanol is widely used as an industrial solvent, as a denaturing agent for ethanol, and in "canned heat." Poisoning occurs when substances containing methanol are used as beverages in place of alcohol or when industrial workers are exposed to atmospheres containing methanol vapor. The metabolism of methanol involves the same enzyme systems as that of ethanol. Its elimination follows zero-order kinetics, but at a much slower rate than ethanol. This slow metabolism accounts for the delay in symptoms of methanol poisoning, which are caused by its oxidized metabolites formaldehyde and formic acid.

Symptoms of methanol poisoning include early mild inebriation followed in 6 to 30 hours by dizziness, headache, vertigo, and occasional nausea and vomiting. As acidosis is produced by the accumulation of formic acid, extreme abdominal pain develops, respirations increase in depth and frequency, and the patient lapses into coma. Visual symptoms are characteristic of methanol intoxication. Blurred vision, with spots or gray mist, photophobia, and eye tenderness, commonly occurs. The pupils are dilated, and the light reflex becomes sluggish. Permanent blindness is not uncommon even if the victim completely recovers. Visual damage develops because of the high rate of retinal oxidation of methanol, leading to formaldehyde and formic acid accumulation with edema and permanent damage to ganglion cells.

Death follows the ingestion of 2 to 8 ounces of methanol and is associated with blood concentrations of 74 to 110 mg/dl of methanol and 9 to 68 mg/dl of formic acid. The urinary methanol concentration is approximately twice that in blood and is diagnostic of methanol poisoning. The direct cause of death is cessation of respiration. Breathing becomes shallow and slow, tonic seizures develop, and the victim dies with a marked terminal inspiratory gasp.

The treatment of choice is hemodialysis, which provides rapid recovery without residual effects. Peritoneal dialysis, although also indicated, is less efficient. Acidosis is treated with intravenous infusions of sodium bicarbonate solution. Because ethanol is the preferred substrate for alcohol dehydrogenase, the administration of ethanol can be used to inhibit the formation of toxic methanol metabolites. For this purpose, ethanol should be administered intravenously or given orally to maintain a BAC of 100 mg/dl.

ISOPENTANOL

Isopentanol is also present in alcoholic beverages, albeit typically at concentrations less than 0.5%. At least some effects of ethanol are shared by isopentanol, including induction of liver microsomal enzymes and enhancement of acetaminophen toxicity.[26] The combination of isopentanol and ethanol may constitute a synergistic combination for some responses.

ISOPROPYL ALCOHOL

Isopropyl alcohol is used as an antiseptic and disinfectant in dentistry. In a concentration of 70%, it is used as rubbing alcohol, and it is present in many hand lotions. Isopropyl alcohol is oxidized in vivo to acetone, which is largely excreted in expired air at 10 times the rate of ethanol.

Toxicity arises if isopropyl alcohol is ingested. Symptoms are similar to those of ethanol intoxication but are marked by nausea, vomiting, abdominal pain, hematemesis, and melena. Severe renal dysfunction for 2 to 3 weeks is seen in survivors. Extensive hemorrhagic inflammation and edema of the bronchopulmonary tree are observed in fatal cases. Hemodialysis is the treatment of choice in isopropyl alcohol poisoning. Ethanol appears to increase, rather than reduce, the toxic effects of isopropyl alcohol.

ETHYLENE GLYCOL

Ethylene glycol is used as an antifreeze and is highly toxic if ingested. Ethylene glycol is a CNS depressant. It is metabolized by alcohol dehydrogenase to glycoaldehyde and then by aldehyde dehydrogenase to glycolic acid. Glycolic acid is converted to oxalic acid. Metabolites appear to be largely responsible for the acute renal toxicity seen with ethylene glycol. This finding may be particularly true for oxalic acid, which forms crystals in the renal tubules.

Toxicity caused by ethylene glycol is treated by correcting the metabolic acidosis with sodium bicarbonate. Ethanol is also used to prevent the conversion of ethylene glycol to its metabolites by competing for alcohol dehydrogenase. 4-Methylpyrazole, a potent inhibitor of alcohol dehydrogenase, is used to treat ethylene glycol toxicity.

PROPYLENE GLYCOL

Propylene glycol is used as a replacement for ethylene glycol. It is an effective antifreeze and is much less toxic than ethylene glycol. In fact, propylene glycol is also used as a solvent for drugs and in food. Although it can depress the CNS, little effect is seen at concentrations normally encountered.

CITED REFERENCES

1. Baker RC, Kramer RE: Cytotoxicity of short-chain alcohols, *Annu Rev Pharmacol Toxicol* 39:127-150, 1999.
2. Beckemeier ME, Bora PS: Fatty acid ethyl esters: potentially toxic products of myocardial ethanol metabolism, *J Mol Cell Cardiol* 30:2487-2494, 1998.
3. Bosron WF, Lumeng L, Li TK: Genetic polymorphism of enzymes of alcohol metabolism and susceptibility to alcoholic liver disease, *Mol Aspects Med* 10:147-158, 1988.
4. Costa LG, Guizzetti M: Muscarinic cholinergic receptor signal transduction as a potential target for the developmental neurotoxicity of ethanol, *Biochem Pharmacol* 57: 721-726, 1999.
5. Cowen MS, Lawrence AJ: The role of opioid-dopamine interactions in the induction and maintenance of ethanol consumption, *Prog Neuropsychopharm Biol Psych* 23: 1171-1212, 1999.
6. Crabb DW, Bosron WF, Li TK: Ethanol metabolism, *Pharmacol Ther* 34:59-73, 1987.
7. Cui SJ, Tewari M, Schneider T, et al: Ethanol promotes cell death by inhibition of the insulin-like growth factor I receptor, *Alcohol Clin Exp Res* 21:1121-1127, 1997.
8. Enomoto N, Ikejima K, Yamashima S, et al: Kupffer cell-derived prostaglandin E_2 is involved in alcohol-induced fat accumulation in rat liver, *Am J Physiol* 279:G100-G106, 2000.
9. Henry RJ, Ishii MM, Quock RM: Influence of chronic ethanol exposure on nitrous oxide analgesia in mice, *J Dent Res* 69:1674-1677, 1990.
10. Hines LM, Stampfer MJ, Ma J, et al: Genetic variation in alcohol dehydrogenase and the beneficial effect of moderate alcohol consumption on myocardial infarction, *N Engl J Med* 344:549-555, 2001.
11. Holford NHG: Clinical pharmacokinetics of ethanol, *Clin Pharmacokinet* 13:273-292, 1987.
12. Hölter SM, Danysz W, Spanagel R: Novel uncompetitive N-methyl-D-aspartate (NMDA)-receptor antagonist MRZ 2/579 suppresses ethanol intake in long-term ethanol-experienced rats and generalizes to ethanol cue in drug discrimination procedure, *J Pharmacol Exp Ther* 292:545-552, 2000.
13. Holtzman JL, Gebhard RL, Eckfeldt JH, et al: The effects of several weeks of ethanol consumption on ethanol kinetics in normal men and women, *Clin Pharmacol Ther* 38:157-163, 1985.
14. Ikonomidou C, Bittagu P, Ishimaru MJ, et al: Ethanol-induced apoptotic neurodegeneration and fetal alcohol syndrome, *Science* 287:1056-1060, 2000.
15. Koob GF: Drugs of abuse: anatomy, pharmacology and functions of reward pathways, *Trends Pharmacol Sci* 13:177-184, 1992.
16. Koop DR, Klopfenstein B, Imuro Y, et al: Gadolinium chloride blocks alcohol-dependent liver toxicity in rats treated chronically with intragastric alcohol despite the induction of CYP2E1, *Mol Pharmacol* 51:944-950, 1997.
17. Laposata EA, Lange LG: Presence of nonoxidative ethanol metabolism in human organs commonly damaged by ethanol abuse, *Science* 231:497-499, 1986.
18. Lister RG, Linnoila M: Alcohol, the chloride ionophore and endogenous ligands for benzodiazepine receptors, *Neuropharmacology* 30:1435-1440, 1991.
19. Manzo L, Locatelli C, Candura SM, et al: Nutrition and alcohol neurotoxicity, *Neurotoxicology* 15:555-565, 1994.
20. Miller MW: Effects of alcohol on the generation and migration of cerebral cortical neurons, *Science* 233:1308-1311, 1986.
21. Mufti SI, Eskelson CD, Odeleye OE, et al: Alcohol-associated generation of oxygen free radicals and tumor production, *Alcohol Alcohol* 28:621-628, 1993.
22. Roehrs T, Beare D, Zorick F, et al: Sleepiness and ethanol effects on simulated driving, *Alcohol Clin Exp Res* 18:154-158, 1994.
23. Samson HH, Tolliver GA, Haraguchi M, et al: Alcohol self-administration: role of mesolimbic dopamine, *Ann NY Acad Sci* 654:242-253, 1992.
24. Schenker S, Bay MK: Medical problems associated with alcoholism, *Adv Intern Med* 43:27-78, 1998.
25. Shakespeare W: Macbeth. In Wells S, Taylor G, eds: *William Shakespeare, the complete works*, Oxford, 1986, Clarendon Press.

26. Sinclair J, Jeffrey E, Wrighton S, et al: Alcohol-mediated increases in acetaminophen hepatotoxicity: role of CYP2E and CYP3A, *Biochem Pharmacol* 55:1557-1565, 1998.
27. Steinberg W, Tenner S: Acute pancreatitis, *N Engl J Med* 330:1198-1210, 1994.
28. Suh I, Shaten BJ, Cutler JA, et al: Alcohol use and mortality from coronary heart disease: the role of high-density lipoprotein cholesterol, *Ann Intern Med* 116:881-887, 1992.
29. Thurman RG: Mechanisms of hepatic toxicity II. Alcoholic liver injury involves activation of Kupffer cells by endotoxin, *Am J Physiol* 275:G605-G611, 1998.
30. Tsai G, Gastfriend DR, Coyle JT: The glutamatergic basis of human alcoholism, *Am J Psychiatry* 152:332-340, 1995.
31. Waldenstrom A: Alcohol and congestive heart failure, *Alcohol Clin Exp Res* 22:315S-317S, 1998.
32. Weight FF, Aguayo LG, White G, et al: GABA- and glutamate-gated ion channels as molecular sites of alcohol and anesthetic action, *Adv Biochem Psychopharmacol* 47:335-347, 1992.
33. Wright C, Moore RD: Disulfiram treatment of alcoholism, *Am J Med* 88:647-655, 1990.

General References

Agarwal DP, Goedde HW, eds: *Alcohol metabolism, alcohol intolerance, and alcoholism: biochemical and pharmacogenetic approaches,* New York, 1990, Springer-Verlag.

Deitrich RA, Erwin VG, eds: *Pharmacological effects of ethanol on the nervous system,* Boca Raton, FL, 1996, CRC Press.

Nutt DJ, Peters TJ: Alcohol: the drug, *Br Med Bull* 50:5-17, 1994.

Rapaka RS, Chiang CN, Martin BR, eds: *Pharmacokinetics, metabolism, and pharmaceutics of drugs of abuse,* Bethesda, MD, 1997, US Department of Health and Human Services, Public Health Service, National Institutes of Health.

Wood A: Drug therapy for alcohol dependence, *N Engl J Med* 340:1482:1490, 1999.

CHAPTER • 44

Anticaries Agents

Ernest Newbrun

Dental caries is a pathologic process of microbial etiology that results in localized destruction of tooth tissues. From an anatomic and microbiologic perspective there are several different types: pit and fissure caries, smooth surface caries, root caries, and deep dentinal caries. The process of tooth destruction involves dissolution of the mineral phase, consisting primarily of hydroxyapatite crystals, by organic acids produced by bacterial fermentation. Dental caries is a multifactorial disease involving three principal factors: the host, particularly the saliva and teeth; the microflora; and their substrate, the diet. In addition, a fourth factor, time, must be considered in any discussion of the causes of caries. These factors can be portrayed as four overlapping circles (Figure 44-1).

For caries to occur, conditions within each of these factors must be favorable. Caries requires a susceptible host, a cariogenic oral flora, and a suitable substrate, all of which must be present together for a sufficient length of time. Caries prevention is based on attempts to (1) increase the resistance of the host (fluoride therapy, occlusal sealants, immunization), (2) lower the number of cariogenic microorganisms in contact with the tooth (plaque control and antiplaque agents), (3) modify the substrate by selecting noncariogenic foods, and (4) reduce the time that the microflora is provided with substrate by limiting the frequency of intake of fermentable substrate. Consideration of all four factors is beyond the scope of this chapter. Dietary factors, caries immunization, and occlusal sealants are discussed in detail in textbooks on nutrition and cariology. Concerning host factors, an adequate flow of saliva is a well-recognized protective mechanism. Problems of xerostomia, particularly as a side effect of various drugs, are discussed elsewhere in this book. In this chapter, fluorides are covered as the anticaries agents par excellence for increasing host resistance to decay and also as antibacterial agents.

Fluorine is a member of the halogen family. It is the most electronegative of all the elements, which makes it extremely reactive. Fluorine combines with almost every element. It is also reactive with organic radicals. It is rarely found in the free state in nature but is widely distributed as fluorides* in the earth's crust, ranking seventeenth in abundance (0.06% to 0.09%). It usually occurs in minerals such as fluorspar (CaF_2), cryolite (Na_3AlF_6), or fluorosilicates (Na_2SiF_6) and in rocks in the form of mica, hornblende, and pegmatite. In biologic mineralized tissues, such as bones and teeth, it occurs as an impure apatite crystal, not as fluorapatite ($Ca_{10}[PO_4]_6F_2$). The lattice of biologic apatite crystals contains many impurities, either in the lattice itself or adsorbed on the surface.[72] Carbonate ions (2% to 5%) substitute for some phosphate ions; some Ca^{++} is substituted by other ions, such as Na^+, K^+, Mg^{++}, and Zn^{++}; and some hydroxyl ions are substituted by fluoride. Therefore the approximate representation of the formula of this apatite is $Ca_{10-x}(Na)_x(PO_4)_{6-y}(CO_3)_z(OH)_{2-u}(F)_u$. Although only some of the hydroxyls of the apatite lattice are substituted by fluoride (i.e., u is much smaller than 2), this change profoundly alters the resistance of enamel to demineralization.

In this discussion, fluoride therapy for the prevention of dental caries is considered under two main headings: systemic fluoride and topical fluoride. Although such a division is convenient for didactic purposes and serves to distinguish between the very low dosages used systemically and the somewhat higher concentrations of fluoride used topically, it has become increasingly evident that such a separation is not absolute and that fluorides, while being ingested for their systemic effect, also have a topical benefit even at low concentrations on teeth that are already erupted. This topical effect can be direct while the fluoride-containing water, tablets, or drops are being ingested, or indirect from the slight elevation in salivary fluoride concentration after ingestion. Conversely, topical fluoride agents may be swallowed, particularly by

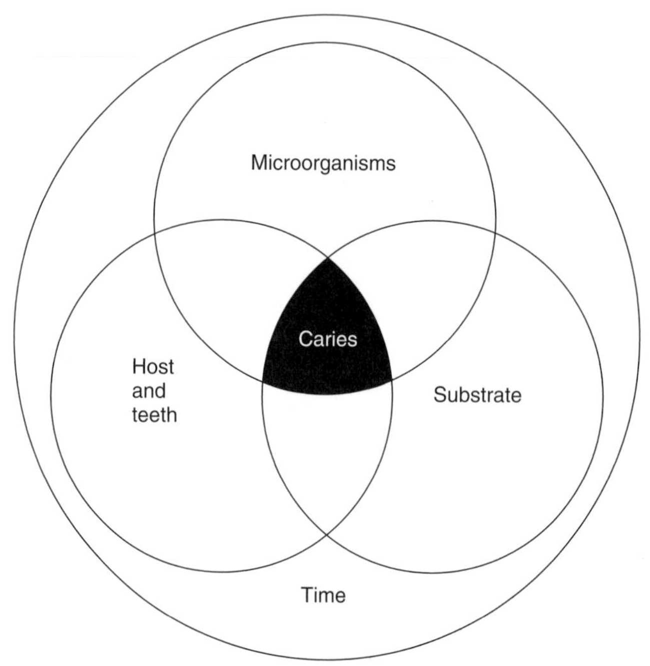

Fig. 44-1 Etiology of dental caries. The three *inner circles* represent the factors involved in the carious process; all three must be acting concurrently for caries to occur. The fourth *all-inclusive circle* represents time, which affects each of the individual factors.

*In this chapter, the term *fluoride* is used to indicate the element as the free anion or as linked to other elements in molecular form.

young children, and thereby exert a systemic effect on teeth that are still undergoing mineralization.

Previous theories held that systemically acquired fluoride (pre-eruptive) was of prime importance in caries prevention and that it was not necessary to continue the use of fluoridated water after the enamel had calcified.[45] However, subsequent findings clearly showed a benefit of posteruptive or topical fluoride exposure; indeed, in some communities that stopped fluoridating the water or in children that moved away from fluoridated communities, caries rates increased. Recently, some have argued that posteruptive or topical fluoride effects are of sole importance in caries prevention and that systemic benefits are minimal.[20,40] However, careful analyses of caries epidemiology in teeth according to their eruption time, as related to the onset of water fluoridation, have revealed significant pre-eruptive and posteruptive beneficial effects.[25,69] Approximately two thirds of the greatest reductions in pit and fissure caries came from preeruptive fluoride, whereas in smooth surfaces the decrease was only 25%. In approximal surfaces, half the reduction was from pre-eruptive fluoride and half was posteruptive fluoride.[25] Maximum caries-preventive effects of fluoridated water were achieved by optimum pre-eruptive and posteruptive exposure of all surfaces types.[69]

SYSTEMIC FLUORIDE

Fluoridation of Communal Water Supplies

Classic epidemiologic surveys of the prevalence of dental caries, carried out by Dean and others during the late 1930s and early 1940s, demonstrated an inverse relationship between caries prevalence and fluoride concentration in drinking water. Initially, these surveys were limited to school-age children residing in different cities with naturally high or low fluoride levels in the public water supplies (Figure 44-2). Subsequently, it was shown that adults as well as children who have continually consumed fluoridated water lose fewer teeth and have lower incidences of decayed, missing, and filled teeth. Of increasing importance regarding geriatric dentistry is the finding that lifelong residence in communities with naturally occurring fluorides is associated with a significant reduction in the prevalence of root caries or root fillings in the population.[3,70]

Dental fluorosis (discussed later) has been directly related to the concentration of fluoride in the drinking water. An optimal level of fluoride in the water supply provides significant protection against caries yet entails minimal risk of fluorosis. The optimal concentration depends on the annual average maximum daily air temperature in the community (temperature influences the amount of water ingested). In temperate climates, where the annual average maximum daily air temperature ranges between 14.7° and 17.7° C (58.4° and 63.8° F), the optimal level of fluoride is 1.0 ppm. Carefully controlled independent studies conducted during the 1940s to the 1960s have shown that if fluoride is added to the domestic water supply to bring it up to optimal levels (controlled water fluoridation), decay could be reduced by 50% to 60% (Figure 44-3). These clinical trials were conducted in the United States and Canada, which were the first countries to initiate such programs, as well as in diverse populations in Australia, Hong Kong, Ireland, Germany, The Netherlands, New Zealand, and the United Kingdom. More recently,

Number of cities studied	Number of children examined	Number of DMF teeth per 100 examinees (0 100 200 300 400 500 600 700)	Fluoride content of water (ppm)
11	3867		<0.5
3	1140		0.5-0.9
4	1403		1.0-1.4
3	847		>1.4

Fig. 44-2 Data from 21 US cities grouped according to fluoride content of the drinking water. An inverse relationship between caries prevalence and fluoride content of the water is illustrated. *DMF,* Decayed, missing, and filled teeth. (From Newbrun E, ed: *Fluorides and dental caries,* ed 3, Springfield, IL, 1986, Charles C. Thomas.)

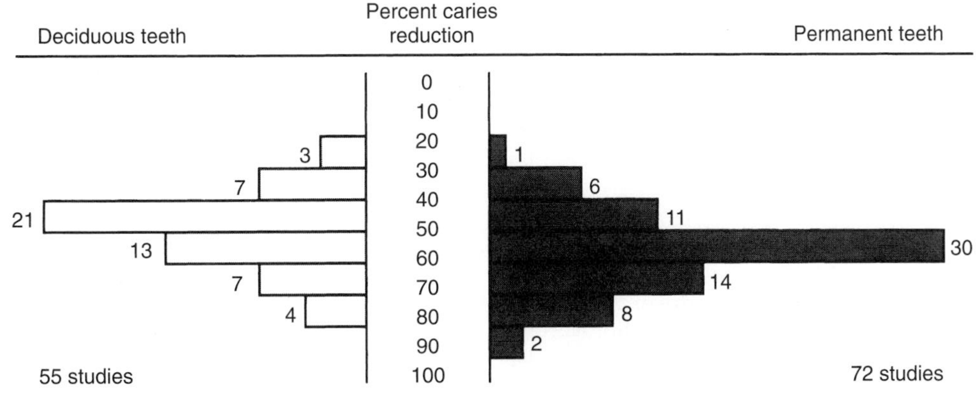

Fig. 44-3 Caries reductions (percentage) observed in 55 studies on the effectiveness of controlled fluoridation in 20 countries. Fifty-five studies gave results for the deciduous dentition and 72 for the permanent dentition. (From Murray JJ, Rugg-Gunn AJ: *Fluorides in caries prevention,* ed 2, Bristol, 1982, John Wright & Sons.)

because of the widespread daily use of topical fluoride and the ingestion of fluoride-containing foods and beverages made in fluoridated communities, the difference in caries prevalence between fluoridated and nonfluoridated communities has been observed to be 15% to 40% depending on the age group and area examined.[52] In some regions of the United States, a high proportion of the population is living in optimally fluoridated communities, so that the minority of the population where the water fluoride is suboptimal may be getting significant amounts of fluoride from food and beverage products processed in the optimally fluoridated areas, yielding a "diffusion" or "halo" effect on caries reduction. Failure to account for the diffusion effect may result in underestimation of the total benefit of water fluoridation, especially in high-diffusion exposure regions.[24] Studies in Canada have documented the processing of beverages, especially soft drinks, in fluoridated communities and their distribution in nonfluoridated areas.[10] However, the halo effect does not uniformly apply throughout the United States. Marked regional differences exist, for example, between the Midwest, which is 74% fluoridated, and the Pacific Coast, where 19% of the population is provided with optimally fluoridated water supplies.[77] The benefits of water fluoridation in caries prevention are inversely related to the extent of communal water fluoridation in the region (Figure 44-4).[6] In the United States, approximately 162 million persons (65.8% of the population served by public water supplies) were provided with optimally fluoridated drinking water.[2] Worldwide, more than 300 million persons are now consuming water that either is adjusted to or naturally contains an optimal concentration of fluoride.

Opponents of water fluoridation have questioned its safety, yet careful comparisons of communities with optimal versus suboptimal concentrations of fluoride in water supplies have found no significant difference in the frequency of birth defects or in mortality statistics (including deaths from heart disease, cancer, and stroke). Optimal fluoridation of drinking water does not pose a detectable cancer risk to human beings, as evidenced by extensive human epidemiologic data.[78] Thorough medical examinations of children in fluoridated and nonfluoridated communities were undertaken in some of the initial studies of controlled water fluoridation; no significant differences in health or in growth and development were found. One study was quite detailed and included tonsillectomy rates; height and weight; onset of menstruation; bone density by x-ray examination of hands and knees; skeletal maturation; blood hemoglobin titer; erythrocyte and leukocyte count; urinalysis; and skin moisture, texture, color, and eruptions.[66] The conclusion of this long-term pediatric study was that the reduction in caries was accompanied by no indication of any adverse effect from the use of fluoridated water.

Some concern has been raised about a possible relation between fluoride in the water supply and frequency of hip fractures. Of the several studies, two showed a protective relation, four found no relation, and three reported an increased relative risk. These conflicting findings are caused by the multifactorial pathogenesis of osteoporotic fractures (cigarette smoking, having a small thin frame, history of previous fracture, excessive alcohol intake, estrogen deficiency, physical inactivity) and may prove impossible to resolve by current epidemiologic-ecologic methods.[37] The collective results of all these studies on hip fracture rates have yielded relatively small or no associations or have had weak statistical power and do not provide a basis for altering public health policy regarding water fluoridation.[22] Indeed, an expert committee of the World Health Organization concluded, "With respect to hip fracture and bone health, there is no scientific evidence for altering current public health policy on the use of fluorides for caries prevention."[19] Finally, a recent meta-analysis of papers on fluoridation and bone fracture published between 1966 and 1997 found that the relative risk was 1.02. It concluded that water fluoridation has little effect on fracture risk, either protective or deleterious.[34]

More detailed discussion of some of the claimed health risks of water fluoridation can be found elsewhere.[29,53] Recently, opponents have focused on the use of fluorosilicic acid and its sodium salt, which together account for 91% of the fluoridating agents used by American water works.[75] They have asserted that the fluorosilicate ion (SiF_6^-) promotes the solubilization of lead from the distribution system, thereby increasing the lead concentration in the tap. In addition, they believe that residual fluorosilicate is responsible for lowering gastric pH and therefore converting particulate lead to bioavailable lead ion, thereby increasing its uptake in the bloodstream.[43,44] Supposedly such higher blood lead levels account for aggressive and violent behavior. Although the kinetics of the dissociation and hydrolysis of fluorosilicate are poorly understood, all the rate data suggest that equilibrium should have been achieved by the time water reaches the consumer's tap if not by the time it leaves the water plant.[75,76] There is no proof that the ingestion of lead or its bioavailability is increased.

Communal water fluoridation continues to be the cornerstone of an ideal caries prevention program. Its efficacy in reducing caries prevalence has been amply demonstrated. Its safety has also been well established. The cost benefits are impressive, but even more important are the value of teeth saved from extraction and the avoidance of pain and discomfort from carious lesions and of time lost from school or work.

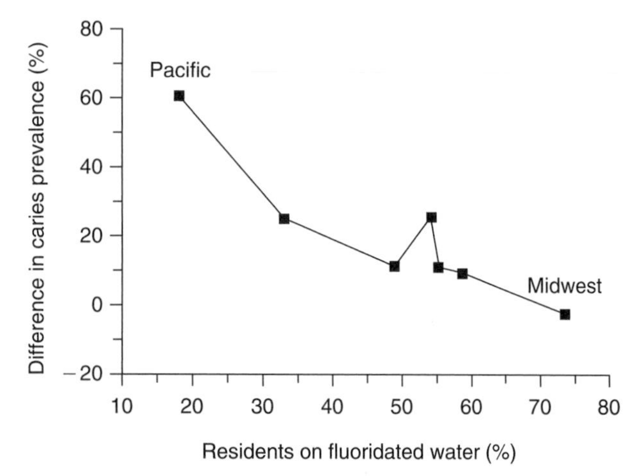

Fig. 44-4 Percentage difference in caries prevalence between children with life-long water fluoride exposure and those with deficient water fluoride exposure *(y axis)* plotted against the percentage of the population served by fluoridated water in each of the seven US regions *(x axis)*. The large difference in the Pacific Coast region (Washington, Oregon, California, Hawaii), where only 19% of the population are served by optimally fluoridated water, is in strong contrast to the negligible difference in the Midwest, where 74% of the population is served by optimally fluoridated water. (Data from Brunelle JA, Carlos JP: Recent trends in dental caries in U.S. children and the effect of water fluoridation, *J Dent Res* 69[special issue]:723-727, 1990.)

Fluoridation of School Water Supplies

Because central water supplies are not available to large segments of the world's population, other methods of caries prevention have been sought. Research has shown that adjusting the fluoride content of a school's water supply produces a reduction in dental caries with no objectionable dental fluorosis. Children spend from 20% to 25% of their total waking hours in school annually. To compensate for this part-time exposure to fluoride, the currently recommended concentration for school water fluoridation is 4.5 times the optimal value recommended for community water fluoridation in the same geographic area. One disadvantage of school fluoridation is that children are 5 to 6 years old before they begin attending school and drinking the water. Maximum caries prevention accrues when fluoridated water is consumed from birth. Moreover, continued protection is not provided when the children leave school. Operating and maintaining small fluoridation systems (i.e., those serving fewer than 500 persons) creates practical and logistic difficulties.

Fluoride Supplements

Communal water fluoridation is the best method for providing systemic fluoride because the benefits accrue automatically without any conscious effort required. Where water fluoridation is not feasible because of individual wells (approximately 20% of the US population), or where political opposition, apathy, or lack of funds prevent its implementation (approximately 30% of the US population), supplements offer an alternative source of systemic fluoride. Fluoride tablets, drops, and lozenges have been proved unequivocally to be effective cariostatic agents, provided such supplements are taken on a daily basis continuously from birth to approximately 16 years of age. The cariostatic effects of fluoride supplements have ranged from less than 10% to more than 80%, generally depending on how soon after birth supplementation starts and on the degree of compliance.[15] The highest caries reductions have been reported in private pediatric practices in which there is a high degree of motivation on the part of the professionals who prescribe the supplements, the parents who give the supplements to their young children, and the children themselves as they get older and become responsible for taking the supplements. When distribution of fluoride supplements has been attempted on a large scale, such as by community health centers, well-baby clinics, and county health departments, long-term compliance has been poor. An estimated 16% of US children younger than 2 years used fluoride supplements in 1986,[54] but compliance tends to decrease in older children.

The correct dosage in prescribing fluoride supplements depends on two factors: the age of the child and the existing fluoride concentration in the water supply (Table 44-1). The latter information can be obtained from the local water supply authority (except in the case of private well water). Failure to determine the fluoride concentration in the communal water source can result in a fluoride overdosage and consequent dental fluorosis. For young infants, drops are more convenient than tablets because they can be directly dispensed into the child's mouth with a medicine dropper or added to foods (such as cereals) or beverages (such as milk, formula, or juices). For older children whose primary teeth have erupted, fluoride tablets or lozenges are indicated, which provide both systemic benefits when swallowed and topical benefits as they are chewed and swished around the teeth. Fluoride tablets or lozenges are available in 0.25, 0.5, and 1 mg strengths. No more than 120 mg of fluoride (264 mg of sodium fluoride) should be dispensed in any one container, which should be provided with a childproof top and labeled: "Caution—Store out of reach of children." A sample prescription of a fluoride supplement for a 2-year-old residing in a community with 0.1 ppm of fluoride in the water supply is shown in Figure 55-5.

Because fluoride supplements are taken as a single bolus that causes a rapid elevation in blood fluoride levels, most studies have identified them as a major risk factor for dental fluorosis.[65] Accordingly, current fluoride prescription practices have undergone close scrutiny, and it is generally agreed that a reduction in dosage is indicated in the age period from birth to 6 years because this is the period when the permanent anterior teeth are vulnerable to dental fluorosis (the "window of vulnerability"). A lowered dosage schedule of fluoride supplements has been accepted by the American Dental Association, the American Academy of Pediatric Dentistry, and the American Academy of Pediatrics, as shown in Table 44-1.[1] In the youngest age group, it is recommended that fluoride drops be prepared in a more dilute form, such as containing 0.25 mg fluoride in 0.25 ml (instead of in a single drop), to minimize overdispensing errors at home. In Canada, a more drastic reduction in dosage—with no supplements until age 3 years; 0.25 mg at ages 3, 4, and 5 years; and 1 mg from age 6 years—has been recommended.[9]

Insufficient data exist to establish the efficacy of prenatal supplements given to the pregnant mother in reducing caries in offspring. Accordingly, the Food and Drug Administration (FDA) does not permit any fluoride preparation to be labeled, represented, or advertised for prenatal use. Only a small portion of the enamel of some of the primary teeth (mostly of the incisors) has entered the stage of secondary mineralization (maturating stage) at birth, and almost no permanent teeth, except the tips of the first molars (which are at the formative stage).[13] It is more important to ensure that adequate fluoride supplements are taken regularly after birth. The concentration of total fluoride in human milk is approximately 0.05 ppm and of cow's milk approximately 0.1 ppm. Hence, both types of milk are negligible sources of fluoride. Although the infant gets very little fluoride from the mother's milk, in most cases there is no need to supplement breast-fed children who reside in optimally fluoridated communities. Because the average duration of nursing in the United States is only 4 months, the amount of fluoride obtained from optimally fluoridated water supplies, used in preparing formula and baby food, will suffice. If the infant resides in a suboptimally fluoridated community, the dosage schedule shown in Table 44-1 should be followed. Vitamins neither interfere with nor potentiate the caries-preventive effects of fluoride supplements, but they do increase the cost to the patient. If the child needs vitamins, a fluoride-vitamin combination may be more convenient, but children are unlikely to require vitamins from birth to teens. Moreover, some fluoride-vitamin preparations contain as much as 60% total sugar as a sweetener to mask the taste of some of the B vitamins. Such products are contraindicated for caries prevention.

Table • 44-1

American Dental Association Dosage Schedule (mg/Day) for Fluoride Supplements*

	FLUORIDE CONCENTRATION (ppm) IN PRIMARY DRINKING WATER		
AGE (YEARS)	<0.3	0.3 TO 0.6	>0.6
0.5 to 3	0.25	0	0
3 to 6	0.5	0.25	0
6 to at least 16	1.0	0.5	0

*Council on Dental Therapeutics, 1994.

TOPICAL FLUORIDE

Not all fluoride agents and treatments are equal. Different fluoride compounds, different vehicles, and vastly different concentrations of fluoride, ranging nearly 100-fold, have been used with different frequency and duration of application (Table 44-2). All these variables can influence the clinical outcome regarding caries prevention and management. The efficacy of topical fluoride in caries prevention depends on the concentration of fluoride used, the frequency with which it is applied and probably the duration of application, and, to some extent, the specific fluoride compound used.[41,50,51]

Regarding the concentration of fluoride used, the preponderance of fluoride dentifrice studies have shown a dose-response effect[50,62] and the trend in clinical effectiveness of professionally applied topical fluoride agents is similar (Table 44-3).[27,32,79] Regarding the frequency of topical fluoride application, in studies of the same commercial stannous fluoride dentifrice, the efficacy of unsupervised once per day or *ad libitum* use was an approximate 21% caries reduction,[33,35] whereas the efficacy of supervised thrice per day use was an approximate 45% caries reduction (Table 44-4).[5,56]

No controlled clinical trials have been reported in which the same concentration of a topical fluoride agent has been tested for varying durations of application. In vitro testing of both sodium fluoride and acidulated phosphate fluoride (APF) solutions has shown that fluoride uptake is time related, and in the case of APF solutions the most rapid uptake occurs during the first 4 minutes.[36] However, it is not known whether more rapid fluoride uptake means greater caries reduction.

Table • 44-2

Range of Therapeutic Fluoride Concentrations in Topical Agents Used to Prevent Caries

METHOD/VEHICLE	FLUORIDE CONCENTRATION (ppm)
Mouth rinse, daily	230
Dentifrices, children	250 to 500
Mouth rinse, weekly	920
Dentifrices, adult	1000 to 1500
Self-applied gels or rinses, prescription	5000
Professionally applied sodium fluoride solutions	9200
Professionally applied APF solutions, gels, foams	12,300
Professionally applied stannous fluoride solutions	19,500
Professionally applied varnishes	22,600

Table • 44-3

Comparative Effectiveness of Professionally Applied Topical Fluoride Agents

AGENT	FLUORIDE CONCENTRATION (ppm)	AVERAGE EFFECTIVENESS (% CARIES REDUCTION)*
2% Sodium fluoride	9200	29
APF (1.2% fluoride)	12,300	22
8% Stannous fluoride	19,500	32
Fluoride varnish (5% sodium fluoride)	22,600	38

*Effectiveness estimates from several sources.[32,79,27]

Professional Topical Application of Fluorides: Solutions, Gels, and Foams

Semiannual topical application of concentrated fluoride (2% sodium fluoride, 8% stannous fluoride, or APF containing 1.23% fluoride) by a dentist or dental hygienist provides an average 26% reduction of decay of permanent teeth of children living in nonfluoridated areas.[61] Neutral sodium fluoride solutions (2%) were first tested in the early 1940s and were shown to reduce caries. Teeth were first cleaned with pumice paste, and the solution was applied to the teeth for 3 minutes. The application, but not the pumicing, was repeated at weekly intervals for a total of four applications at ages 3, 7, 11, and 13 years.[38] This sequence of application was used more widely in public health programs than in private practice. In 1958, 8% stannous fluoride was also shown to be an anticaries agent.[48] The procedure again involved coronal polishing, and the stannous fluoride was applied for 4 minutes semiannually. Aqueous stannous fluoride solutions have the disadvantages of undergoing rapid hydrolysis and oxidation; because of this instability, they must be freshly prepared for each treatment. Stannous fluoride has a low pH (approximately 2.7) and has a disagreeable acidic and metallic taste. Many investigators have also reported that teeth stain (from light brown to black) at carious lesions, hypocalcified areas, and around the margins of restorations after stannous fluoride application.[47] This discoloration is caused by the conversion of tin phosphates, which form on the enamel, to tin sulfides, which have the characteristic dark brown or black color.

In the United States, the most popular form of office fluoride therapy is the application of APF in the form of a solution, gel, or foam. APF agents should have a pH of

Table • 44-4

Frequency of Supervised Toothbrushing with a Stannous Fluoride Dentifrice (Crest) and Caries Reduction

STUDY	BRUSHING FREQUENCY	SUBJECT AGES (YEARS)	STUDY LENGTH	DMF REDUCTION
Jordan and Peterson, 1959[35]	1× day	8 to 12	2 years	21%
Horowitz et al, 1966[33]	1 × day + ad libitum home use	6 to 10	2 years	21%
Peffley and Muhler, 1960[56]	3× day	10 to 15	2 years	46%
Bixler and Muhler, 1962[5]	3× day	12 to 16	8 months	45%

DMFS, Decayed, missing, and filled teeth.

Box • 44-1

Recommended Procedures To Reduce Fluoride Ingestion from Professional Gel Tray Applications

Place patient in an upright position.
Warn patient not to swallow the gel.
Use small amounts (no more than 2.5 ml per tray).
Use custom-fitted or stock trays with absorptive liners.
Use suction.
Remove excess gel from teeth and gingiva with gauze.
Have patient expectorate thoroughly after treatment.

approximately 3.0 and contain 1.23% fluoride and 0.1 mol/L of orthophosphoric acid. The low pH of this agent favors more rapid fluoride uptake by enamel, and the presence of the orthophosphate prevents enamel dissolution by the common ion effect. Application of one of these solutions or gels is preceded by a coronal polishing, and the agent should be applied for 4 minutes, usually in a disposable tray applicator. The procedure should be repeated semiannually. The need for coronal polishing preceding application of APF gels has been called into question, and clinical trials indicate that the efficacy of the gels is similar regardless of whether coronal polishing is performed.[63] Some commercial products have been promoted on the basis of claims that they need to be applied for only 1 minute instead of 4 minutes. These claims have not been supported by clinical trials demonstrating caries reductions; until they are, a 4-minute application of the agent should be the designated method.

Because these agents used in the dental office contain relatively high concentrations of fluoride, the operator should observe certain precautions to prevent inadvertent ingestion of them by the patient, who should be in an upright position in the chair.[26] If solutions are used, the teeth should be carefully isolated with cotton rolls or gauze swabs and only sufficient solution applied to wet the surfaces of the teeth and keep them wet. If gels in trays are to be used, only a minimum amount of gel should be dispensed in the tray, sufficient to cover the teeth but not to exude from the tray. A saliva ejector, or better still high-vacuum suction, should be used during the 4-minute application of the agent. On removal of the tray, any excess gel should be wiped away from the teeth and gingiva with gauze, and the patient should be instructed to expectorate thoroughly. The recommended procedures to reduce fluoride ingestion from professional gel tray applications are summarized in Box 44-1.

Professional Topical Application of Fluorides: Varnishes

The previously discussed agents (sodium fluoride, stannous fluoride, and APF) are all aqueous preparations, but other research has involved nonaqueous solutions that are applied as varnishes with longer retention time on the tooth surface. In 1964, Schmidt[68] tested the practicality of a 2% sodium fluoride lacquer in an alcoholic solution of natural resins. After clinical trials of this fluoride varnish demonstrated its efficacy as an anticaries agent,[28] it was marketed in Germany as a 5% sodium fluoride preparation under the brand name of Duraphat. This product is now widely used for office topical applications throughout Europe, the Middle East, Australia, New Zealand, and Asia; in fact, it is currently used in more than 40 different countries throughout the world.

In the mid-1970s, a difluorosilane agent containing 0.7% fluoride in a polyurethane varnish was introduced for caries prevention in Europe as Fluor Protector. This agent boasts a high fluoride uptake by enamel.[60] It is available in the United States as a cavity varnish to seal and prevent the permeation of fluids and metal ions.

In 1994, a 5% sodium fluoride varnish under the name of Duraflor obtained FDA approval for its use in the United States as a cavity liner. Subsequently, the Duraphat formulation of 5% sodium fluoride varnish received FDA approval as a dentin-desensitizing agent and as a cavity liner "medical device." A practitioner can use fluoride varnish for caries prevention as an off-label use on the basis of professional judgment.[80] An extensive literature exists on the clinical efficacy of Duraphat varnish as a safe and effective anticaries agent for use in children.[4,58] One advantage of fluoride varnishes is that they adhere to tooth surfaces, thereby permitting prolonged fluoride exposure and uptake. In a meta-analysis of the efficacy of fluoride varnishes[27] using rigid criteria for inclusion of data, a mean caries reduction of 38% for fluoride varnishes was obtained (see Table 44-3).

Self-Applied Topical Fluoride in the Home

One of the most effective means of caries reduction involves the daily (on school days) self-application of 1.1% sodium fluoride gel (about 40% of the concentration of fluoride used for professional office applications) in custom-fitted trays for 5 minutes daily. The custom-fitted maxillary and mandibular trays ("toplicators") are fashioned by vacuum-drawing heat-treated sheets of polyvinyl over plaster models of the teeth. This procedure, first demonstrated in supervised school programs, reduced decay by approximately 75% after 2 years in nonfluoridated communities[18] and by approximately 30% in fluoridated communities.[17] This form of self-therapy is best suited only for high-risk caries patients who are sufficiently motivated to conform with the daily regimen. It is not intended for very young children but is appropriate for those of school age and has also been found to be effective for adults with xerostomia after radiation therapy to the head and neck region.[14] The advantage of the technique is that fluoride preparations are held in intimate contact with the teeth daily for 5 minutes. Saliva is excluded from the field of application so that it cannot dilute the effective concentration of the active agent in the gel. Intermittent biting pressure on the plastic trays tends to pump the fluoride into pits, fissures, and interproximal spaces. Because the trays are custom-made, a minimum amount of gel (usually 0.5 ml) is required in each tray. The main disadvantage is the relatively high cost of fabricating individual trays for each patient, which renders it impractical for school-based programs.

Self-application by brushing with a fluoride gel (0.4% stannous fluoride) has been used as an alternative to the custom-fitted tray method and has been actively promoted by several commercial manufacturers of these products. Although published clinical data have not been provided to support the efficacy of these agents, many of the stannous fluoride gels have been accepted by the Council on Scientific Affairs of the American Dental Association, presumably based on the findings with stannous fluoride dentifrices. The gels vary considerably in the amount of available tin ion.[73] The original formulation, developed at the Veterans Administration Hospitals, had an unpleasant taste, so many of the high-risk caries patients either refused to use the gel or used it only sporadically. The commercial products have been formulated with more acceptable flavors to encourage better compliance. Because the fluoride uptake is time dependent, applying a gel containing 1000 ppm of fluoride for approximately 1 minute by brushing does not provide as much fluoride uptake as from a gel in a custom-fitted tray containing 5000 ppm applied for 5 minutes. No direct comparisons are available to determine the clinical efficacy of these two techniques for caries prevention.

Fluoride Mouth Rinses

In the mid-1960s, Scandinavian researchers showed that a biweekly rinse for 1 minute with a solution of 0.2% sodium fluoride (920 ppm of fluoride) was more effective in reducing decay than an annual treatment with 10% stannous fluoride professionally applied, equally effective as four professional treatments with 2% sodium fluoride applied every 3 years, and approximately as effective as the daily use of the fluoride dentifrices then available.[74] Furthermore, it was also shown that daily rinsing for 1 minute with an even more dilute solution containing 0.05% sodium fluoride (230 ppm of fluoride) gave even greater caries protection. The benefits from fluoride mouth rinsing are approximately 30% less decay.[64] The original Scandinavian findings have since been reproduced in many different countries around the world, so that now a weekly fluoride rinse has become widely adopted in many school-based preventive dentistry programs. Its popularity is based on the fact that it is safe, effective, relatively inexpensive, easy to learn, requires little time (approximately 5 minutes of class time weekly), and can be supervised by nondental personnel. Compliance may vary and is generally better in elementary schools than in junior and senior high schools. Compliance depends on successfully motivating and interesting classroom teachers, as well as the school administrators, in the preventive dentistry program. Fluoride mouth rinses were prescription items when originally introduced, and the 0.2% sodium fluoride rinse still is. In 1983, the FDA approved the sale of 0.05% sodium fluoride mouth rinses, 0.1% stannous fluoride mouth rinses, and 0.4% stannous fluoride gels as over-the-counter products. In the case of the 0.05% sodium fluoride rinse, 10 ml of the solution (the recommended dosage) contains only 2.3 mg of fluoride. The products are packaged with childproof caps, and their labels state that use is restricted to persons 6 years of age and older. The rinse should be vigorously swished around the mouth for 1 minute and then expectorated. The dentist needs to advise the patient, or parent, of these instructions, both to ensure that the agent is present for enough time to ensure efficacy and also to avoid unnecessary ingestion of the rinse.

Fluoride Dentifrices

In the 1940s, the first clinical evaluations of dentifrices containing fluoride were undertaken with products in which fluoride was simply incorporated into existing dentifrice formulations. Because the abrasive systems used in these early dentifrices contained Ca^{++} salts that interfered with the availability of fluoride, these products were ineffective or less than fully effective in reducing decay. The first report of a clinical decrease in the incidence of caries with a fluoride-containing dentifrice, compared with the similar use of a nonfluoride dentifrice, involved a dentifrice system containing stannous fluoride (0.4%) with an abrasive, calcium pyrophosphate, that had been heat-treated to increase its compatibility with fluoride.[49] In 1960, this dentifrice was given provisional acceptance, and in 1964 full acceptance, by the ADA's Council on Dental Therapeutics. This acceptance stimulated other manufacturers to develop and test various fluoride formulations and abrasive systems. Currently, the sale of these products exceeds $1 billion annually in the United States, and approximately 98% of all toothpastes sold contain some form of fluoride. With few exceptions, fluoride toothpastes dominate dentifrice markets in most Western industrialized countries. The original stannous fluoride formulation has been superseded by more compatible and effective formulations.

Sodium monofluorophosphate (MFP; Figure 44-5) was first tested as a therapeutic agent in dentifrices in the early 1960s. Numerous clinical trials of dentifrices containing 0.76% or 0.8% MFP have since been conducted by different groups in various countries. In almost all these trials, some degree of effectiveness (i.e., approximately 25% caries reduction) has been demonstrated after 1 to 3 years of use.[12] In the United States, MFP of 0.76%, or 1000 ppm of fluoride, is the most commonly used therapeutic ingredient in commercial toothpastes. A dose-response effect has been shown; dentifrices with less MFP are less effective,[39,46] and dentifrices with more MFP (1500, 2000, and 2500 ppm of fluoride) are more effective.[7,11,21,30,41,71] Sodium fluoride was the first fluoride to be tested in a toothpaste and was originally found ineffective because of incompatibility with the earlier abrasive systems used. Later, when tested with acrylic particles or hydrated silica as the abrasive, sodium fluoride–containing dentifrices were found to give significant cariostatic benefits. A dose-response relation has been reported with sodium fluoride toothpaste tested at 0, 250, 500, and 1000 ppm of fluoride.[59] A sodium fluoride formulation (1100 ppm fluoride) with silica abrasive has been found to be more effective than the earlier stannous fluoride–calcium pyrophosphate dentifrice, undoubtedly because of the greater availability of fluoride in this newer system.[67,83] Several commercial products now use sodium fluoride as the active therapeutic ingredient. The original stannous fluoride formulation has been superseded by more compatible and effective formulations. Clinically effective fluoride toothpastes with compatible abrasive systems are summarized in Table 44-5.

In Europe, an amine fluoride dentifrice containing two compounds—diethanol aminopropyl-N-ethanol octadecylamine-dihydrofluoride and cetylamine hydrofluoride (see Figure 44-5) at a concentration providing 1250 ppm of fluoride—has been used for many years. Both substances have a long aliphatic chain, containing 16 or 18 carbon atoms, which is responsible for the dentifrice's property of lowering surface tension. This dentifrice has also been shown to be effective in reducing dental decay.[67]

Without doubt the widespread use, most commonly twice a day, of fluoride-containing dentifrices has had a profound effect in reducing caries in many developed countries and accounts for some of the secular decline in caries observed in communities lacking optimal fluoride concentrations in the

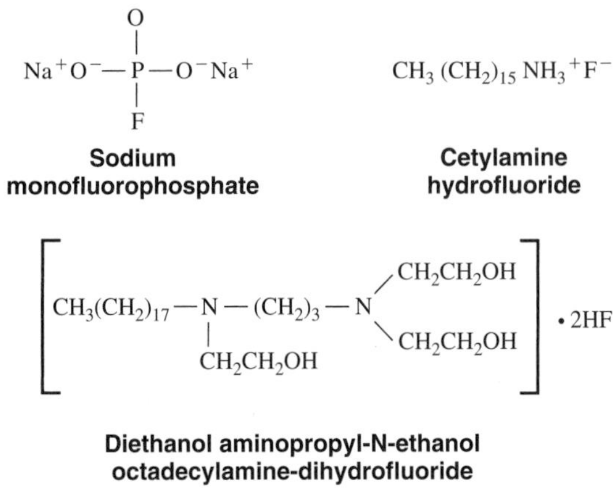

$Na^+O^-—P(=O)(F)—O^-Na^+$

Sodium monofluorophosphate

$CH_3(CH_2)_{15}NH_3^+F^-$

Cetylamine hydrofluoride

$[CH_3(CH_2)_{17}—N(CH_2CH_2OH)—(CH_2)_3—N(CH_2CH_2OH)_2] \cdot 2HF$

Diethanol aminopropyl-N-ethanol octadecylamine-dihydrofluoride

Fig. 44-5 Structural formulas of sodium monofluorophosphate and the active ingredients in amine fluoride dentifrices.

Table • 44-5

Clinically Effective Fluoride Abrasive Systems in Dentifrices

FLUORIDE COMPOUND	ABRASIVE SYSTEM	FORMULA
Stannous fluoride (SnF_2)	Calcium pyrophosphate	$Ca_2P_2O_7$
	Insoluble sodium metaphosphate	$(NaPO_3)_x$
	Silica	SiO_2
Sodium fluoride (NaF)	Calcium pyrophosphate	$Ca_2P_2O_7$
	Insoluble sodium metaphosphate	$(NaPO_3)_x$
	Polymethylmethacrylate	*
	Silica	SiO_2
Sodium monofluorophosphate (Na_2PO_3F)	Calcium carbonate	$CaCO_3$
	Aluminum oxide	Al_2O_3
	Insoluble sodium metaphosphate	$(Na_2PO_3)_x$
	Silica	SiO_2
	Dibasic calcium phosphate	$CaHPO_4$
	Calcium pyrophosphate	$Ca_2P_2O_7$
Amine fluoride	Insoluble sodium metaphosphate	$(Na_2PO_3)_x$

x, 2 or more.
*Composed of repeating units of methylmethacrylate:

```
        CH3
        |
 —CH2—C—
        |
   O=C—O—CH3
```

water supply. The degree of effectiveness may vary with different dentifrice formulations.

As a response to concerns about fluorosis, low-concentration (250, 400, and 500 ppm fluoride) toothpastes are available in Austria, Belgium, Czechoslovakia, Finland, France, Germany, Israel, Luxembourg, The Netherlands, New Zealand, Portugal, Sweden, Switzerland, and the United Kingdom. However, dose-response efficacy data indicate that a dentifrice with a lower fluoride concentration provides less caries protection. From the growing literature on dentifrice retention and ingestion, it has been estimated that for children younger than 6 years the average retention was 27% of the amount placed on the brush.[62] Because most children brush twice daily, this could contribute between 0.3 to 0.6 mg to total fluoride intake, depending on how much toothpaste (0.5 to 1.0 g) is used habitually. Although several of the early studies that looked at the dentifrice-fluorosis relationship have not found an association, they have generally been small and lacked sufficient statistical power to demonstrate such an association if there were one.[55] Several recent studies have attributed much of the increase in fluorosis prevalence to early use of fluoride dentifrice, especially before 2 years of age.[31,42,55,57,82] To avoid unintentional ingestion of fluoride from dentifrices, the following guidelines should be followed:

1. Parents should brush preschool children's teeth until they can do it properly by themselves.
2. Parents should apply the dentifrice to the toothbrush of preschool children until they can do it properly by themselves.
3. Parents of preschool children should supervise their toothbrushing activity, and dentifrices should be stored out of the reach of toddlers.
4. Preschool children should use a child's-size toothbrush.
5. Only a dab or pea-sized amount of dentifrice should be applied to the toothbrush bristles.
6. Children should be taught to spit out and rinse thoroughly after toothbrushing.

FLUORIDE TOXICOLOGY

Acute Toxicity

Paracelsus said that "all substances are poison; there is none which is not a poison. The right dose differentiates a poison and a remedy." Fluoride is no exception to this historic observation. When ingested in amounts of 1 to 3 mg/day, as would be the case in optimally fluoridated communities, it is perfectly safe. However, 5 to 10 g of sodium fluoride (approximately 2.5 to 5 g of fluoride) is a certain fatal dosage for an adult, and lesser amounts are lethal to children. Incidents of acute fluoride poisoning have been recorded, such as industrial accidents, fumigant inhalation, ingestion of household insecticides containing fluoride, or deliberate attempts at suicide.

Patients with severe fluoride poisoning characteristically exhibit nausea, vomiting, and diarrhea; progressive hypotension, pronounced hypocalcemia and hypomagnesemia, and acidosis; and cardiac irregularities, including ventricular tachycardia and sometimes fibrillation and asystole. Successful treatment is based on early initiation of the following procedures:

1. Steps to prevent further systemic absorption of fluoride (e.g., administration of emetics to induce vomiting, gastric lavage with fluids containing Ca^{++})
2. Cardiopulmonary monitoring and preparation for endotracheal intubation and direct-current cardioversion
3. Prompt and frequent blood analyses, especially for plasma Ca^{++}, Mg^{++}, K^{+}, and pH
4. Intravenous infusion of salt solutions as needed to correct acid-base imbalances and restore plasma electrolytes to the normal range

5. Alkaline diuresis to enhance fluoride excretion
6. Appropriate treatment of severe cardiac arrhythmias

Only three incidents of dentally related fluoride fatalities have been recorded. One case followed office topical therapy in which inappropriate agents and procedures were used and adequate treatment was not provided for management of the overdose.[8] The other two cases resulted from ingesting fluoride tablets from containers that were not equipped with a childproof cap.[16,81] However, there have been numerous occasions, both reported and unreported, when patients have had transitory nausea from unintentional swallowing of concentrated fluoride topical agents used in the dental office. When recommended procedures are followed, as listed in Box 44-1, the topical application of fluoride agents in the office or the self-application of fluoride agents in the home does not pose a risk of acute toxicity.

Chronic Toxicity

At one time chronic fluoride inhalation was an industrial hazard of cryolite workers handling crushed sodium aluminum fluoride in aluminum refineries. It resulted in crippling skeletal changes with calcification of ligaments, kyphosis, and limitation of motility in the spinal column and thorax. Modern regulations of industrial hygiene require air scrubbers to remove fluoride particles. Crippling skeletal fluorosis is not a public health problem in the United States, as evidenced by the reports of only five cases in 30 years. Of greater concern is fluorosis of the dentition.

Dental fluorosis is a hypomineralization of enamel produced by chronic ingestion of excessive amounts of fluoride during tooth development. Fluorosis may range in severity from a few white flecks to extensive brown staining and pitting. Pits are secondarily produced defects of posteruptive origin rather than true hypoplasias. The hypomineralization is mostly in the outer third of enamel. The secretory stage of enamel development is a crucial time for fluorosis to occur. Ameloblasts are more sensitive to fluoride than are other cells. The mineralization phase is also affected. In excess, fluoride interferes with the normal postsecretory, pre-eruptive development of enamel. Chronically high levels of fluoride interfere with deposition of mineral, degradation of matrix proteins (amelogenin and enamelin), and withdrawal of water during enamel maturation.

The prevalence and severity of fluorosis depend on the amount or concentration of fluoride, the duration of exposure, the state of tooth development (i.e., age when exposed), and individual variations in susceptibility (e.g., body weight). In the oral health survey of US school children sponsored by the National Institute of Dental Research in 1987, 52% were found to have questionable, very mild, or mild fluorosis—forms that are not a serious cosmetic problem. Only 1.3% had moderate or severe fluorosis involving pitting or brown staining. Approximately 2% of US schoolchildren may have perceived esthetic problems that could be attributed to currently recommended levels of fluoride in the drinking water.[23] If the natural water supply contains in excess of 2 ppm fluoride, the prevalence of fluorosis can be reduced by changing the source of the water supply or by defluoridation with activated alumina or bone char for adsorption. Some fluorosis can also be prevented by stopping the use of fluoride supplements in communities that already provide optimal levels in the water supply. Because supplements require a prescription, there is clearly a need to educate dentists, physicians (particularly pediatricians), and pharmacists better on when supplementation is indicated and when it is not. Finally, some fluorosis can be prevented by decreasing the unintentional ingestion of fluoride from dentifrices by young children. Children younger than 6 years need to be instructed to use only a pea-size portion of paste, to spit out thoroughly after brushing, and to avoid swallowing the paste. Dentifrice manufacturers have a responsibility to provide better and more conspicuous labeling in this regard.

Cited References

1. Anonymous: Dosage schedule for dietary fluoride supplements, *J Public Health Dent* 59:203-204, 1999.
2. Apanian D, Malvitz D, Presson S: Populations receiving optimally fluoridated public drinking water—United States, 2000, *MMWR* 51:144-147, 2002.
3. Banting DW: Dental caries in the elderly, *Gerodontology* 3:55-61, 1984.
4. Beltrán-Aquilar ED, Goldstein JW, Lockwood SA: Fluoride varnishes: a review of their clinical use, cariostatic mechanism, efficacy, and safety, *J Am Dent Assoc* 131:589-596, 2000.
5. Bixler D, Muhler JC: Experimental clinical human caries test design and interpretation, *J Am Dent Assoc* 65:482-490, 1962.
6. Brunelle JA, Carlos JP: Recent trends in dental caries in US children and the effect of water fluoridation, *J Dent Res* 69:723-727, 1990.
7. Chesters R, Pitts N, Matuliene G, et al: An abbreviated caries clinical trial design validated over 24 months, *J Dent Res* 81:637-640, 2002.
8. Church LE: Fluorides—use with caution, *J Maryland State Dent Assoc* 19:106, 1976.
9. Clark DC: Appropriate uses of fluorides for children: guidelines from the Canadian Workshop on the Evaluation of Current Recommendations Concerning Fluorides, *Can Med Assoc J* 149:1787-1793, 1993.
10. Clovis J, Hargreaves JA, Thomson GW: Caries prevalence and the length of residency in fluoridated and non-fluoridated communities, *Caries Res* 22:311-315, 1988.
11. Conti AJ, Lotzkar S, Daley R, et al: A 3-year clinical trial to compare efficacy of dentifrices containing 1.14% and 0.76% sodium monofluorophosphate, *Community Dent Oral Epidemiol* 16:135-138, 1988.
12. DePaola PF: Clinical studies of monofluorophosphate dentifrices, *Caries Res* 17(suppl 1):119-135, 1983.
13. Deutsch D, Pe'er E: Development of enamel in human fetal teeth, *J Dent Res* 61:1543-1551, 1982.
14. Dreizen S, Brown LR, Daly TE, et al: Prevention of xerostomia-related dental caries in irradiated cancer patients, *J Dent Res* 56:99-104, 1977.
15. Driscoll W: The use of fluoride tablets for the prevention of dental caries, In Forrester D, Schulz E, eds: *International workshop on fluorides and dental caries reduction*, Baltimore, 1974, University of Maryland.
16. Eichler HG, Lenz K, Fuhrmann M, et al: Accidental ingestion of NaF tablets by children—report of a poison control center and one case, *Int J Clin Pharmacol Ther Toxicol* 20:334-338, 1982.
17. Englander HA, Sherrill LT, Miller BG, et al: Incremental rates of dental caries after repeated topical sodium fluoride applications in children with lifelong consumption of fluoridated water, *J Am Dent Assoc* 82:354-358, 1971.
18. Englander HR, Keyes PH, Gestwicki M, et al: Clinical anticaries effect of repeated topical sodium fluoride applications by mouthpieces, *J Am Dent Assoc* 78:354-358, 1967.

19. Expert committee on oral health status and fluoride use, World Health Organization: *Fluorides and oral health,* Geneva, 1994, World Health Organization.
20. Featherstone JDB: Prevention and reversal of dental caries: role of low level fluoride, *Community Dent Oral Epidemiol* 27:31-40, 1999.
21. Fogels HR, Meade JJ, Griffith J, et al: A clinical investigation of a high-level fluoride dentifrice, *J Dent Child* 55: 210-215, 1988.
22. Gordon SL, Corbin SB: Summary of workshop on drinking water fluoride influence on hip fracture on bone health (National Institutes of Health, 10 April, 1991), *Osteoporos Int* 2:109-117, 1992.
23. Griffin S, Beltran E, Lockwood S, et al: Esthetically objectionable fluorosis attributable to water fluoridation, *Community Dent Oral Epidemiol* 30:199-209, 2002.
24. Griffin SO, Gooch BF, Lockwood SA, et al: Quantifying the diffused benefit from water fluoridation in the United States, *Community Dent Oral Epidemiol* 29:120-129, 2001.
25. Groeneveld A, van Eck AAJM, Backer Dirks O: Fluoride in caries prevention: is the effect pre- or post-eruptive? *J Dent Res* 69(special issue):751-755, 1990.
26. Heifetz SB, Horowitz HS: The amounts of fluoride in current fluoride therapies: safety considerations for children, *J Dent Child* 51:257-269, 1984.
27. Helfenstein U, Steiner M: Fluoride varnishes (Duraphat): a meta-analysis, *Community Dent Oral Epidemiol* 22:1-5, 1994.
28. Heuser H, Schmidt HF: Zahnkariesprophylaxe durch tiefenimprägnierung des zahnschmelzes mit Fluor-Lack, *Stoma* 21:91-100, 1968.
29. Hodge HC: Evaluation of some of the objections to water fluoridation. In Newbrun E, ed: *Fluorides and dental caries,* ed 3, Springfield, IL, 1986, Charles C. Thomas.
30. Hodge HC, Holloway PJ, Davies TGH, et al: Caries prevention by dentifrices containing a combination of sodium monofluorophosphate and sodium fluoride, *Br Dent J* 149:201-204, 1980.
31. Horowitz HS: The need for toothpastes with lower than conventional fluoride concentrations for preschool-aged children, *J Public Health Dent* 52:216-221, 1992.
32. Horowitz HS, Heifetz SB: Topically applied fluorides. In Newbrun E, ed: *Fluorides and dental caries,* ed 3, Springfield, IL, 1986, Charles C. Thomas.
33. Horowitz HS, Law FE, Thompson MP, et al: Evaluation of a stannous fluoride dentifrice for use in dental public health programs. I. Basic findings, *J Am Dent Assoc* 72:408-422, 1966.
34. Jones G, Riley M, Couper D, et al: Water fluoridation, bone mass and fracture: a quantitative overview of the literature, *Aust N Z J Public Health* 23:34-40, 1999.
35. Jordan WA, Peterson JK: Caries-inhibiting value of a dentifrice containing stannous fluoride. Final report of a two-year study, *J Am Dent Assoc* 58:42-46, 1959.
36. Joyston-Bechal S, Duckworth R, Braden M: The mechanism of uptake of ^{18}F by enamel from sodium fluoride and acidulated phosphate fluoride solution labeled with ^{18}F, *Arch Oral Biol* 18:1077-1089, 1973.
37. Kleerekoper M: Fluoride and the skeleton. In Bilezikian JP, Raisz LG, Rodan GA, eds: *Principles of bone biology,* San Diego, 1996, Academic Press.
38. Knutson JW: Sodium fluoride solutions: technic for application to the teeth, *J Am Dent Assoc* 36:37-39, 1948.
39. Koch G, Bergmann-Arnadottir S, Bjarnason S, et al: Caries-preventive effect of fluoride dentifrices with and without anticalculus agents: a 3-year controlled clinical trial, *Caries Res* 24:72-79, 1990.
40. Limeback H: A re-examination of the pre-eruptive and post-eruptive mechanism of the anti-caries effects of fluoride: is there any anti-caries benefit from swallowing fluoride? *Community Dent Oral Epidemiol* 27:62-71, 1999.
41. Marks RG, Conti AJ, Moorhead JE, et al: Results from a three-year clinical trial comparing NaF and SMFP fluoride formulations, *Int Dent J* 44:275-285, 1994.
42. Mascarenhas AK, Burt BA: Fluorosis risk from early exposure to fluoride toothpaste, *Community Dent Oral Epidemiol* 26:241-248, 1998.
43. Masters RJ, Coplan MJ: Water treatment with silicofluorides and lead toxicity, *Int J Environ Studies* 56:435-449, 1999.
44. Masters RJ, Coplan MJ, Hone BT, et al: Association of silicofluoride treated water with elevated blood lead, *Neurotoxicity* 21:1091-1100, 2000.
45. McCay FS: The study of mottled enamel (dental fluorosis), *J Am Dent Assoc* 44:133-137, 1952.
46. Mitropoulos CM, Holloway PJ, Davies TGH, et al: Relative efficacy of dentifrices containing 250 to 1000 ppm F^- in preventing dental caries—report of a 32-month clinical trial, *Community Dent Health* 1:193-200, 1984.
47. Muhler JC: Effect on gingiva and occurrence of pigmentation on teeth following the topical application of stannous fluoride or stannous chlorofluoride, *J Periodontol* 28:281-286, 1957.
48. Muhler JC: The effect of a single topical application of stannous fluoride on the incidence of dental caries in adults, *J Dent Res* 37:415-416, 1958.
49. Muhler JC, Radike AW, Nebergall WH, et al: The effect of stannous fluoride-containing dentifrice on caries reduction in children, *J Dent Res* 33:606-612, 1954.
50. Newbrun E: Current regulations and recommendations concerning water fluoridation, fluoride supplements and topical fluoride agents, *J Dent Res* 71(special issue):1255-1265, 1992.
51. Newbrun E: Current treatment modalities of oral problems of patients with Sjögren's syndrome: caries prevention, *Adv Dent Res* 10:29-34, 1996.
52. Newbrun E: Effectiveness of water fluoridation, *J Public Health Dent* 49:279-289, 1989.
53. Newbrun E, Horowitz H: Why we have not changed our minds about the safety and efficacy of water fluoridation, *Perspect Biol Med* 42:526-543, 1999.
54. Nourjah P, Horowitz A, Wagener D: Factors associated with the use of fluoride supplements and fluoride dentifrice by infants and toddlers, *J Public Health Dent* 54:47-54, 1994.
55. Osuji OO, Leake JL, Chipman ML, et al: Risk factors for dental fluorosis in a fluoridated community, *J Dent Res* 67:1488-1492, 1988.
56. Peffley GE, Muhler JC: The effect of a commercially available stannous fluoride dentifrice under controlled brushing habits on dental caries incidence in children: preliminary report, *J Dent Res* 39:871-875, 1960.

57. Pendrys DG, Katz RV, Morse DE: Risk factors for enamel fluorosis in a nonfluoridated population, *Am J Epidemiol* 143:808-815, 1996.

58. Petersson L, Twetman S, Pakhomov GN: *Fluoride varnish for community-based caries prevention in children*, Geneva, 1997, World Health Organization.

59. Reed MW: Clinical evaluation of three concentrations of sodium fluoride in dentifrices, *J Am Dent Assoc* 87:1401-1403, 1973.

60. Retief DH, Bradley EL, Holbrook M, et al: Enamel fluoride uptake, distribution and retention from topical fluoride agents, *Caries Res* 17:44-51, 1983.

61. Ripa L: An evaluation of the use of professionally (operator-applied) topical fluorides, *J Dent Res* 69:786-796, 1990.

62. Ripa LW: Clinical studies of high-potency fluoride dentifrices: a review, *J Am Dent Assoc* 118:85-91, 1989.

63. Ripa LW: Need for prior toothcleaning when performing a professional topical fluoride application: review and recommendations for change, *J Am Dent Assoc* 109:281-285, 1984.

64. Ripa LW: Rinses for the control of dental decay, *Int Dent J* 42:263-269, 1992.

65. Rozier RG, Beck JD: Epidemiology of oral diseases, *Curr Opin Dent* 1:308-315, 1991.

66. Schlesinger ER, Overton DE, Chase HC: A long-term medical study of children in a community with fluoridated water supply, In Shaw JH, ed: *Fluoridation as a public health measure*, Washington, DC, 1954, American Association for the Advancement of Science.

67. Schmid R, Barbakow F, Mühlemann H, et al: Amine fluoride and monofluorophosphate: I. Historical review of fluoride dentifrices, *ASDC J Dent Child* 51:99-103, 1984.

68. Schmidt HF: Ein neues tauchierungsmittel mit besonders lang anhaltendem intensivem fluoridierungseffekt, *Stoma* 17:14-20, 1964.

69. Singh KA, Spencer AJ, Armfield JM: Pre- and post-eruption fluoride exposure and caries by surface type, *J Dent Res* 79:159, 2000.

70. Stamm JW, Banting DW, Imrey PB: Adult root caries survey of two similar communities with contrasting natural water fluoride levels, *J Am Dent Assoc* 120:143-149, 1990.

71. Stephen KW, Creanor SL, Russell JI, et al: A 3-year oral health dose-response study of sodium monofluorophosphate dentifrices with and without zinc citrate: anti-caries results, *Community Dent Oral Epidemiol* 16:321-325, 1988.

72. ten Cate JM, Featherstone JDB: Physicochemical aspects of fluoride-enamel interactions. In Fejerskov O, Ekstrand J, Burt, BA, eds: *Fluoride in dentistry*, Copenhagen, 1996, Munksgaard.

73. Tinanoff N: Stannous fluoride in clinical dentistry. In Wei SHY, ed: *Clinical uses of fluorides*, Philadelphia, 1985, Lea & Febiger.

74. Torell P, Ericsson Y: Two-year clinical tests with different methods of local caries-preventive fluorine application in Swedish schoolchildren, *Acta Odontol Scand* 23:287-322, 1965.

75. Urbansky ET: Fate of fluorosilicate drinking water additives, *Chem Rev* 102:2837-2854, 2002.

76. Urbansky ET, Schock MR: Can fluoridation affect lead (II) in potable water? Hexafluorosilicate and fluoride equilibria in aqueous solution, *Int J Environ Studies* 57:597-637, 2000.

77. US Department of Health and Human Services: *Fluoridation census 1988—summary*, Atlanta, 1988, US Government Printing Office.

78. US Department of Health and Human Services: *Review of fluoride benefits and risks: report of the Ad Hoc Subcommittee on Fluoride of the Committee to Coordinate Environmental Health and Related Programs, US Public Health Service*, Washington, DC, 1991, US Government Printing Office.

79. van Rijkom HM, Truin GJ, van't Hof MA: A meta-analysis of clinical studies on the caries inhibiting effect of fluoride gel treatment, *Caries Res* 32:83-92, 1998.

80. Wakeen L: Legal implications of using drugs and devices in the dental office, *J Public Health Dent* 52:403-408, 1992.

81. Waldbott GL: Another fluoride fatality: a physician's dilemma, *Fluoride* 12:55-57, 1979.

82. Warren JJ, Levy S: A review of fluoride dentifrice related to dental fluorosis, *Pediatr Dent* 21:265-271, 1999.

83. Zacherl WA: A three-year clinical caries evaluation of the effect of a sodium fluoride-silica abrasive dentifrice, *Pharmacol Ther Dent* 6:1-7, 1981.

General References

Centers for Disease Control and Prevention: Recommendations for using fluoride to prevent and control dental caries in the United States, *MMWR* 50:1-42, 2001.

Ciancio SG, ed: *ADA Guide to dental therapeutics*, ed 3, Chicago, 2003, American Dental Association.

McClure FJ: *Fluoride drinking waters*, Public Health Service Publication No 825, Washington, DC, 1962, US Government Printing Office.

Mellberg JR, Ripa LW: Fluoride in preventive dentistry, *Quintessence Int* 14:733-736, 1983.

Murray JJ, Rugg-Gunn AJ: *Fluorides in caries prevention*, ed 2, Bristol, 1982, John Wright & Sons.

Naylor MN, Pindborg JJ, eds: The contribution of dentifrices to oral health, *Community Dent Oral Epidemiol* 8:217-285, 1980.

Newbrun E, ed: *Fluorides and dental caries: contemporary concepts for practitioners and students*, ed 3, Springfield, IL, 1986, Charles C Thomas.

Ripa LW, ed: *A guide to the use of fluorides for the prevention of dental caries*, ed 2, Chicago, 1986, American Dental Association.

Wei SHY, ed: *Clinical uses of fluorides: a state of the art conference on the uses of fluorides in dentistry*, Philadelphia, 1985, Lea & Febiger.

CHAPTER • 45

Antiplaque/Antigingivitis Agents

Ernest Newbrun

Dental plaque is the soft, nonmineralized bacterial deposit that forms on teeth that are not adequately cleaned. Much attention has been devoted to the testing of antimicrobial agents for efficacy in reducing plaque, preventing gingivitis, and suppressing or even eliminating periodontopathic or cariogenic microflora of the oral cavity.

Antibacterial agents, particularly antibiotics, and their therapeutic uses in dentistry for the treatment of common oral infections are discussed in Chapters 39 and 49. Antiseptics and disinfectants are considered in Chapter 46. In this chapter these compounds are examined more specifically regarding their ability to act as antiplaque/antigingivitis agents and their possible role in suppressing or eliminating odontopathic microflora. Because antimicrobial oral rinses do not penetrate to the base of periodontal pockets, they are considered to act against gingivitis. Controlled local drug delivery devices that release antimicrobial agents at the base of periodontal pockets constitute antiperiodontitis therapy.

EARLY TESTS OF ANTISEPTIC AGENTS

In 1890, Miller[73] recognized that, in addition to practicing oral hygiene and limiting the consumption of carbohydrate foods and "luxuries," caries could be prevented "by the proper and intelligent use of antiseptics to destroy the bacteria, or at least to limit their number and activity." However, he also realized that nearly all the antiseptics then available were contraindicated because of their toxicity. For example, one of his most effective antiseptic mixtures, which almost completely "sterilized" the mouth in 1 minute, contained mercuric chloride ($HgCl_2$), a highly toxic chemical that can be fatal if swallowed. Miller mentioned that this mouthrinse discolored the teeth but that the exogenous stain could readily be removed. He noted that $HgCl_2$ had an exceedingly disagreeable taste that could be disguised to a certain extent by rosewater flavoring. He astutely perceived that 1 minute was the maximum duration for mouth rinsing. Other investigators applied less toxic agents, such as metaphen and aniline dyes, to the teeth to control bacterial growth. An organic mercurial, sodium parahydroxymercurobenzoate, used twice daily for rinsing was also found to be an effective antiplaque agent.

RATIONALE FOR PLAQUE CHEMOTHERAPY

Why are antiplaque agents of interest to the dental profession? The answer is that dental plaque, or more correctly the microflora of the plaque, is the source of numerous noxious products that are deleterious either to the teeth (such as organic acids) or to the periodontium (such as ammonia, hydrogen sulfide, methyl mercaptan, toxic amines, proteases, hyaluronidases, chondroitin sulfatase, and β-glucuronidase). In addition, plaque bacteria produce inflammation-inducing substances and release endotoxin and bacterial antigens, which indirectly cause tissue damage. Accordingly, dental plaque has been considered the common denominator in caries and periodontal diseases. This concept, however, is a gross oversimplification because there are different types of plaque, some of which may be cariogenic, some of which may be periodontopathic (with subsets leading to different forms of periodontal diseases), and some of which may be relatively innocuous and cause only low-grade dental disease. For many years, prophylaxis or therapy of plaque-related dental diseases has been based on what Loesche[69] has called the *nonspecific plaque hypothesis.* The correct treatment, according to the hypothesis, is to remove all plaque as quickly and as completely as possible. On the other hand, according to the *specific plaque hypothesis,* only certain organisms within the total plaque flora are associated with disease. In the case of caries, *Streptococcus mutans* and *Streptococcus sobrinus* have been strongly implicated as the most virulent organisms. In the various forms of periodontal diseases, organisms such as *Treponema denticola, Eubacterium saphenum, Porphyromonas endontalis, Porphyromonas gingivalis, Prevotella denticolla, Tannerella forsythensis (Bacteroides forsythus), Filifactor alocis, Cryptobacterium curtum, Treponema medium, Treponema socranskii, Eikenella corrodens, Fusobacterium nucleatum, Actinobacillus actinomycetemcomitans, Micromonas micros (Peptostreptococcus micros), Campylobacter rectus,* and several uncultivated phylotypes are currently considered to be pathogenic and strongly related to disease.[56,111] Ideally, according to the specific plaque hypothesis, a chemotherapeutic agent would be targeted to eliminate or suppress these pathogens without affecting the commensal plaque flora. Currently no "magic bullet" exists that provides such specificity against plaque pathogens.

The current therapeutic measures for controlling plaque can be classified as follows: (1) agents acting against the microflora per se, (2) agents interfering with bacterial attachment by attacking plaque matrix components or altering the tooth surface, and (3) mechanical removal of plaque. Mechanical plaque removal has been the traditional method since time immemorial. Discussion of such techniques is beyond the scope of this chapter, but excellent comprehensive reviews on mechanical plaque control can be found elsewhere.[13,31,78]

PROBLEMS IN THE ANTIPLAQUE USE OF CHEMOTHERAPEUTIC AGENTS

Before considering specific chemotherapeutic agents, several problems common to their general use need to be considered. Effective therapy requires that an adequate amount of the drug remain at the plaque site long enough for the drug to exert a therapeutic effect. This principle has been largely ignored by many who have tried to prevent or treat bacterial infections of tooth surfaces with antimicrobial agents. Most compounds have been tested as topical agents in such vehicles as mouthrinses, dentifrices, chewing gums, and gels, all requiring repeated application.[116] Investigators have usually performed these studies without knowing the concentration of the drug necessary to inhibit the growth of the odontopathic plaque microorganisms. Such highly empirical modes of administration may not accurately reflect a given drug's therapeutic potential. As might be expected, the results have been variable.

In most cases, in vitro tests have been conducted on planktonic plaque organisms (freely floating in a tube of culture medium) to determine the minimal inhibitory and bactericidal concentration of an active agent used in topically applied products.[79] Although these measurements provide important information about the antimicrobial spectrum and potency of a formulation, by themselves they are not predictive of clinical effectiveness.[8] This is because plaque microbiota exist not just as planktonic organisms in saliva but as a biofilm of densely packed bacteria, often in an extracellular matrix. Biofilm experiments indicate that the necessary minimum inhibitory concentrations of antimicrobial agents are at least 50 times higher than for bacteria growing under planktonic conditions.[89] Laboratory tests with biofilm models have been developed that may be more predictive of clinical effectiveness.[106] However, such tests still do not include potential interactions between salivary components or other oral hygiene products and the active ingredient. Such interactions can only be tested by a clinical trial.

A relationship between dental plaque accumulation and gingivitis has been well established by the gingivitis that develops when volunteers cease all oral hygiene.[66] Generally, when such subjects resume cleaning their teeth, the gingivitis resolves. However, in studies in which various mouthrinses or dentifrices are used as the vehicle to deliver chemotherapeutic agents, a reduction in plaque scores is not always accompanied by a parallel decrease in the gingival index.[113] No convincing evidence supports a linear relationship between the quantity of plaque and the extent of oral disease.[53] There are three explanations for this apparent paradox. First, plaque scoring does not consider the specific periodontal pathogenic components of that plaque. Second, the indexes that have been used for measuring oral hygiene are based on plaque surface area score[38,88] or on plaque thickness[109] and depend on the amount of plaque on the buccal or lingual surfaces. They do not emphasize fissure or interproximal plaque, although a modification of the Navy plaque index has attempted to give more emphasis to interproximal areas.[95] Similarly, the plaque thickness index[109] can be adapted to score interproximal areas. Third, current plaque indexes do not consider subgingival extension, only supragingival sites. Hence most of these standard methods for measuring the efficacy of chemotherapeutic antiplaque agents ignore the sites that are most likely to be involved in periodontal diseases and caries.

Another important problem in the topical use of chemotherapeutic antiplaque agents is their continuous dilution and elimination by saliva. Even if the minimal inhibitory concentration of a drug were initially used, rapid clearance from the oral cavity may prevent maintenance of an effective concentration. The failure or limited success of many agents in preventing caries or periodontal diseases can be attributed to their transitory presence in the mouth. It is not that they cannot kill plaque microflora or hydrolyze plaque matrixes; many of them do so in the test tube. It is primarily a problem of effective delivery. To overcome this limitation, agents with substantivity have been sought. *Substantivity* refers to an association between the drug and a substrate that is greater or more prolonged than would be expected with simple mechanical deposition. It involves mechanisms such as adsorption, ion exchange, and chemical interaction. Examples of such agents are the bis-biguanides and fluoride, which are able to adsorb to, or chemically interact with, either the tooth surface or the plaque itself. Accordingly, investigators have explored the use of controlled-release devices for delivering chemotherapeutic drugs into the periodontal pocket, thereby overcoming the problem of salivary dilution. The agent is either embedded in a polymer matrix that permits gradual local release for days or weeks after insertion or is incorporated into a biodegradable matrix. Extensive animal and clinical trials are necessary to determine which drugs and concentrations will be most effective.

Box • 45-1

Properties of an Ideal Antiplaque Agent

- Safety (nontoxic, nonallergenic, nonirritating)
- Efficacy (statistically and clinically meaningful reduction of plaque and gingivitis)
- Specificity (affects only the pathogenic flora)
- Substantivity (binds to and slowly releases from the tooth surface)
- No induced drug resistance
- Acceptable taste
- Low cost

IDEAL PROPERTIES OF ANTIPLAQUE/ANTIGINGIVITIS AGENTS

The properties of an ideal antiplaque agent are listed in Box 45-1. Clearly, an antiplaque agent must be safe, with no untoward systemic or local side effects such as irritation, injury, or host sensitization. It must be more effective than a placebo in reducing plaque and gingivitis to a clinically meaningful degree. It should eliminate or suppress the specific plaque pathogens and must prevent or cure the disease caused by them. It should be stable and have substantivity so that it will act over a prolonged period. It should not allow the overgrowth of resistant organisms, and preferably it should be palatable and relatively inexpensive. Needless to say, no such perfect antiplaque agent exists.

At a workshop on dental plaque control measures and oral hygiene practices, Kornman[53] proposed classifying plaque control agents into two categories: clearly effective and possibly effective. Agents are to be tested in a short-term experimental gingivitis model in which subjects would refrain from any means of plaque control during a 7- to 21-day period. The criteria for this classification scheme are listed in Box 45-2.

At present, the only agents that fulfill the "clearly effective" criteria are the bis-biguanides, such as chlorhexidine. Several commercially available mouthrinses containing essential oils and phenols, quaternary ammonium compounds, sanguinarine or triclosan and zinc chloride, or stannous fluoride have demonstrated possible efficacy.[70]

Box • 45-2

Criteria for Classifying Plaque-Control Agents According to Efficacy

Clearly Effective

Prevent most detectable plaque (plaque scores reduced by 80% or more compared with placebo) *or*
Prevent most clinically detectable gingivitis (gingivitis scores reduced by 80% or more compared with placebo) *or*
Prevent the development of white-spot lesions during sucrose challenge *or*
Prevent the development of bacterial shifts associated with gingivitis or caries

Possibly Effective

Agent does not fulfill clearly effective criteria *but*
Agent substantially reduces plaque accumulation, compared with a placebo, in multiple clinical trials

In contrast to these criteria for short-term clinical trials, the American Dental Association (ADA) Council on Scientific Affairs[24] has developed guidelines for testing chemotherapeutic products for control of supragingival dental plaque and gingivitis that require long-term proof of efficacy. The requirements of these guidelines are summarized in Box 45-3 and have been adopted, in some cases with modifications, by the FDA, the Canadian Dental Association, and the British Dental Association. Subsequent modifications deal with issues of study design, such as making the need for randomization and blinding explicit, requiring a gingival bleeding component in the assessment of gingivitis; indicating methods for standardization of examiners; specifying elements to be included in the statistical analyses, and establishing a minimum acceptable effect level.[44] To be considered acceptable, a product should be tested in two independently conducted trials that use either a crossover or a parallel study design and last a minimum of 6 months. The Council has set a 20% reduction in gingivitis for establishing definite improvement of mean gingivitis scores, measured against a placebo agent or inactive control treatment. This last requirement is important because participants in studies that use a placebo agent often show improvement simply because they are in a dental study, have had their teeth, plaque, and gingivae examined, and subsequently are more dentally aware (Hawthorne effect). The Council also recommends that, in addition to measuring plaque quantitatively by any of the traditional indexes, investigators should obtain microbiologic samples from several supragingival sites and should clearly characterize the oral flora in a control group as well as in the test group. In evaluating the efficacy of a chemotherapeutic agent on gingivitis, the Council recommends that both subjective scoring of gingivae, based on tissue color or estimated degree of swelling, and objective measures, such as extent of gingival bleeding on probing or the amount of crevicular fluid flow, should be made. Revision of some aspects of these guidelines has been proposed.[84] Because all dentifrices contain abrasives and detergents, they are able to facilitate the removal of plaque and thereby help reduce plaque and gingivitis. This mechanical reduction of plaque is distinct from any decrease that might be caused by the presence of therapeutic agents.

Box • 45-3

Guidelines for Evaluating Chemotherapeutic Products for the Control of Supragingival Plaque and Gingivitis

- Characteristics of the study population should represent typical product users.
- Active products should be used in a normal regimen and compared with a placebo control or, where applicable, an active control.
- Crossover or parallel-designed studies are acceptable.
- Studies should be a minimum of 6 months in duration.
- Two studies conducted by independent investigators are required.
- Microbiologic sampling should estimate plaque qualitatively to complement indexes that measure plaque quantitatively.
- Plaque and gingivitis scoring and microbiologic sampling should be conducted at baseline, 6 months, and an intermediate period.
- Microbiologic profile should demonstrate that pathogenic or opportunistic microorganisms do not develop over the course of the study.
- The toxicologic profile of products should include carcinogenicity and mutagenicity assays in addition to generally recognized tests for drug safety.

From Council on Dental Therapeutics: Guidelines for acceptance and chemotherapeutic products for the control of supragingival dental plaque and gingivitis, *J Am Dent Assoc* 112:529-532, 1986.

The dental plaque literature is replete with clinical trials of antimicrobial agents. Table 45-1 lists some of these agents by category and antibacterial spectrum. Proprietary products for oral use and their corresponding active antimicrobial ingredients are shown in Table 45-2.

TYPES OF CHEMOTHERAPEUTIC AGENTS

Antibiotics

Antibiotics are antimicrobial substances produced by microorganisms, or semisynthetic derivatives thereof, that are capable of inhibiting or killing other specific microorganisms. Penicillin, erythromycin, and tetracycline, when administered in the diet of experimental rodents, can be highly effective in controlling plaque and dental caries. Although some studies with human beings have demonstrated plaque reductions after administration of penicillin and erythromycin, these antibiotics are not indicated for plaque control because their use may result in the emergence of drug-resistant microorganisms. Topical tetracycline rinses can reduce the amount of plaque formed during a nonbrushing period and can inhibit the development of gingivitis. However, the greatest promise of this antibiotic is in its use in controlled delivery systems (in which the drug is embedded in a polymer matrix or in a biodegradable carrier) suitable for intrapocket insertion to suppress or eliminate periodontal pathogens of the subgingival plaque microflora.[35]

Vancomycin, bacitracin, kanamycin, niddamycin, and polymyxin B, agents that are not absorbed from the gastrointestinal tract, have been used as topical antibiotics in

Table • 45-1

Antimicrobial Agents Tested for Plaque Prevention or Reduction

CATEGORY	ANTIBACTERIAL SPECTRUM*	AGENT
Antibiotics	Broad	Actinobolin†
		Chlortetracycline
		Tetracycline
		Streptomycin†
		Kanamycin†
		Neomycin†
		Niddamycin†
	Gram-positive	Bacitracin†
		Erythromycin
		Penicillin V
		Vancomycin†
		Gramicidin†
		Spiramycin‡
	Gram-negative	Polymyxin B†
Benzophenanthridines	Broad	Sanguinarine
Bis-biguanides		Alexidine†
		Chlorhexidine†
Bispyridines		Octenidine
Phenolic compounds		Phenol
		β-Naphthol
		Hexylresorcinol
		Triclosan
Halogens		Iodine and iodophors
		Chlorine dioxide
		Oxychlorosene
		Chloramine-T
		Fluoride
Oxygenating agents		Peroxide
		Perborate
Imidazoles	Anaerobic	Metronidazole
Quaternary ammonium compounds	Mostly gram-positive	Cetylpyridinium chloride
		Benzethonium chloride
		Domiphen bromide

*See Chapter 39 for more specific information on sensitive organisms.
†Not absorbed or poorly absorbed from the gastrointestinal tract.
‡Also effective against some gram-negative bacteria.

mouthrinses or gels for plaque control and treatment of gingivitis. Vancomycin is a polypeptide inhibitor of cell-wall synthesis and is primarily active against gram-positive organisms in the oral cavity. Kanamycin is an aminoglycoside that inhibits synthesis of bacterial protein and has a broader spectrum of activity. Niddamycin is a macrolide broad-spectrum antibiotic with antimicrobial activity similar to that of spiramycin and erythromycin. Vancomycin has been used in several studies for the prevention of plaque formation, caries, and gingivitis, but results have been inconclusive. Kanamycin (5% topical paste) reduced but did not eliminate gingivitis. When applied twice daily for 1 week in children with rampant caries, it also reduced subsequent development of caries. Rinsing with vancomycin or polymyxin B (three times daily) produced, respectively, a predominantly gram-negative or a predominantly gram-positive bacterial plaque, but both treatment groups developed gingivitis.[67] The long-term use of antibiotics for inhibition of plaque formation is imprudent because of the high risk/benefit ratio.

Oxygenating Agents

Agents such as peroxides and perborates release molecular oxygen. Periodontal pathogenic bacteria can be killed by peroxides in vitro.[74] Hydrogen peroxide has been used in aqueous form, in gels, in dentifrices, and in a paste with sodium bicarbonate[50] for the treatment of periodontal disease. Some studies have reported that the salt and peroxide regimen is effective in changing clinical measures of periodontal disease when combined with professional care,[93,120] but it is generally no more effective than conventional oral hygiene. Mouthrinses with hydrogen peroxide have been reported to reduce plaque formation and gingivitis and arrest ulcerative gingivitis. In one long-term study (18 months) of orthodontic patients with fixed appliances, a once-daily rinse with 1.5% hydrogen peroxide and 0.05% sodium fluoride (Orthoflur) as an adjuvant to normal oral hygiene prevented the increase in gingival indexes and bleeding tendency scores seen in the control group that used 0.05% sodium fluoride only.[16] However, in a short-term study (7 days) with no toothbrush-

Table • 45-2

Antimicrobial Agents Used in Proprietary Mouth Rinses and Oral Products

TYPE	AGENT	PROPRIETARY (TRADE) NAMES
Phenolic compounds	Phenol	Chloraseptic, Phenaseptic, Cepastat
	Thymol	Listerine,* other private-label products*
	Chlorothymol	Dalidyne
	Hexylresorcinol	ST-37
	Triclosan	ActiBrush†, Colgate Plax†, Total*
Oxygenating agents	Sodium peroxyborate	Amosan
	Carbamide peroxide	Gly-Oxide
	Hydrogen peroxide	Peroxyl, Orajel
Halogens	Chloramine-T	Chlorazene
	Chlorine dioxide	Oxyfresh, RetarDENT
	Oxychlorosene	Kasdenol
	Iodine	Ora5
	Povidone-iodine	Betadine
Quaternary ammonium compounds	Cetylpyridinium chloride	Advanced Breath Care, Cepacol, Clear Choice, Scope, Viadent Advanced Care, Oral
	Domiphen bromide	Clear Choice, Scope
Benzophenanthridines	Sanguinarine	Herbal Mouth & Gum Therapy
Bis-biguanides	Chlorhexidine	Corsodyl†, Peridex*, PerioGard, generic chlorhexidine products

*Accepted by the Council on Scientific Affairs of the ADA.
†Not currently available in the United States.

ing, 1.5% hydrogen peroxide, used as a mouthrinse or in an oral irrigator, was of no therapeutic value in the prevention or the treatment of experimental gingivitis.[47]

Antiplaque and antigingivitis claims have been made for some commercial products, but because of their rapid breakdown in the presence of organic material and bacterial catalase, their effects are at best transient. The oxygenating cleansers approved by the FDA for OTC use include (1) hydrogen peroxide, 3%, applied full strength or diluted to half strength for use as an oral rinse; (2) carbamide peroxide, 10 to 11%, applied directly or swished as a rinse; and (3) sodium perborate monohydrate, 1 to 2 g in 30 ml of warm water, as an oral rinse. These products should not be swallowed. Occasionally, patients have oral ulceration after frequent use (three times per day) of 3% hydrogen peroxide mouthrinse.[91]

Halogens

Chlorophors and iodophors are halogen-releasing compounds (chlorine and iodine, respectively). They are the active ingredients in several antiseptic mouthwashes that have been promoted for plaque control and the treatment of gingivitis. Oxychlorosene, a buffered hypochlorous acid derivative, and chlorine dioxide are used in mouthwashes; chloramine-T (1% solution) is used as a subgingival irrigant for office use.[90]

Povidone-iodine, an iodine-polyvinylpyrrolidone complex, exerts antibacterial activity by oxidation of amino (NH^-), thiol (SH^-), and phenolic hydroxy (OH^-) groups in amino acids and nucleotides and its interaction with unsaturated fatty acids in cell walls and organelle membranes. Povidone-iodine is microbiocidal for gram-positive and gram-negative bacteria, fungi, mycobacteria, viruses, and protozoans. It has been used in a number of mouthwashes that claim therapeutic benefit in the treatment of gingivitis. One discontinued product, Perimed, provided povidone-iodine and hydrogen peroxide in separate packages that were combined immediately before use. Data from a supervised long-term study indicated reductions in gingivitis and bleeding scores.[19] However, these products have a disagreeable taste and may stain teeth and tongue, which would discourage compliance during long-term unsupervised use.

Fluorides

At sufficiently high concentrations, fluorides act as antibacterial agents by their ability to inhibit many enzymatic reactions involved in glycolysis and in glucose transport into cells. The antimicrobial activity varies with the particular organism and type of compound as well as with the F^- concentration, pH, and length of exposure.

When the antimicrobial potencies of sodium fluoride and stannous fluoride were compared directly in vitro, stannous fluoride was the more effective agent, suggesting an additive effect of the stannous ion. Several short-term in vivo studies[10,83,114] have shown that rinsing with stannous fluoride or using a toothpaste with stannous fluoride diminishes the formation of plaque. Daily rinsing with stannous fluoride (0.3%) for 1 minute resulted in less plaque, measured by both tooth surface area and plaque thickness, than daily rinsing with sodium fluoride (0.2%).[9] When all oral hygiene was stopped (no brushing) and only rinsing was permitted, subjects using a stannous fluoride solution formed significantly less plaque than did those using a placebo rinse. Several studies have also shown that rinsing with stannous fluoride solutions or application of stannous fluoride gels improved gingival health; the benefits were not as great as with chlorhexidine,[42] and other studies have not found the improvement to be statistically significant.[58,60,83,119] In a long-term (18 months) clinical trial, no differences were observed in gingivitis, bleeding, or mean proportions of microbial forms in the stannous fluoride (0.4%) or sodium fluoride (0.22%) groups when compared with the placebo group. Furthermore, daily rinsing with stannous fluoride resulted in more exogenous staining of the teeth than did sodium fluoride or placebo rinses.[119]

Fluorides, when used as topical agents, clearly exert antibacterial effects. Their efficacy in clinical trials in reducing plaque and gingivitis remains unproved. The lack of statistically significant effects may result from too brief an application. Commercially available 0.4% stannous fluoride gels vary considerably (from 21% to 102% of what is theoretically claimed) in the availability of the stannous ion.[115] Clinical studies to test the benefits of stannous fluoride as an adjunct to plaque control and reduction of gingivitis should ensure that the agent contains the maximal available stannous and fluoride ions, that it is applied for an adequate period, and that there is good patient compliance with the regimen.

Quaternary Ammonium Compounds

Surface-active compounds characteristically have hydrophobic and hydrophilic groups in each molecule. They are classified as anionic (e.g., detergents such as sodium lauryl sulfate), cationic (e.g., quaternary ammonium compounds), and nonionic (e.g., polysorbate). Generally they exert their bactericidal effect by inactivating membrane-associated enzymes or by physically disorganizing the membrane itself.

Quaternary ammonium compounds are represented by cetylpyridinium chloride (Figure 45-1). Quaternary ammonium compounds are capable of reducing surface tension and adsorbing to negatively charged surfaces. They have greater activity against gram-positive bacteria than against gram-negative bacteria and are inactivated by the presence of organic matter; by low pH; and by anionic compounds, soaps, and metallic ions. Several over-the-counter (OTC) mouthrinses contain cetylpyridinium chloride, benzethonium chloride, or domiphen bromide at concentrations of 0.025% to 0.075%. Studies of these agents have reported modest plaque reductions compared with placebo rinses.[15,61] Occasional side effects of quaternary ammonium compounds include oral ulceration and discomfort and a mild burning sensation of the tongue. Quaternary ammonium compounds have a lingering bitter and unpleasant taste. Judicious flavoring can overcome this limitation. As a group, the quaternary ammonium compounds are moderately effective antiplaque agents.

Phenolic Compounds

Phenol and its derivatives, thymol, chlorothymol, and hexylresorcinol, although used in a number of mouthrinses, have several limitations. These include objectionable taste, poor water solubility, rapid discoloration, and toxicologic and allergenic properties. Phenolic compounds used in clinical trials have demonstrated mixed results as antiplaque agents, with some studies reporting no reduction compared with placebo and others claiming reduced plaque and gingivitis scores.[4,30] In several studies of long-term twice-daily use of a rinse containing thymol and essential oils, in combination with normal oral hygiene, plaque and gingivitis were reduced below levels seen with a placebo rinse.[26,29,94] However, in one long-term study of this agent, the observed reductions in plaque and gingivitis scores were not impressive.[37] No adverse reactions have been reported and Listerine (Antiseptic, Cool Mint, Fresh Burst, Tartar Control) containing a combination of these essential oils (thymol, 0.064%; menthol, 0.042%; eucalyptol, 0.092%; methyl salicylate, 0.06%; plus alcohol, 26.9%) has received the ADA Council on Scientific Affairs Seal of Acceptance as a safe and effective adjunct to brushing and flossing and regular professional care in helping to reduce supragingival plaque and gingivitis.[22] A number of private-label amber antiseptic rinses of the same formulation have been granted acceptance by the Council based on in vitro equivalency data and studies showing lack of oral irritation.

Triclosan (2,4,4′-trichloro-2′-hydroxydiphenyl ether), a broad-spectrum noncharged antimicrobial agent, has been used extensively in consumer products, principally in deodorants, soaps, and other dermatologic preparations. In vitro data indicate that triclosan inhibits growth of certain gram-negative oral species and *Streptococcus mutans*, whereas other oral streptococci are relatively unaffected.[17] In 1973, Mühlemann[77] was the first to report that triclosan applied in a hydroxyethyl cellulose gel reduced plaque in rats. However, in the same study chlorhexidine was twice as effective. Several studies[1,25,62,96,110] have tested a mouthrinse containing 0.03% triclosan together with 0.125% or 0.25% of a copolymer of methoxylene and maleic acid (Gantrez) used to increase triclosan uptake and retention by plaque. In short-term clinical trials this combination resulted in a 20% to 30% reduction of supragingival plaque. Numerous studies, both short and long term, have also found reductions in plaque and gingivitis when triclosan, together with a copolymer or zinc salts, is incorporated into dentifrice formulations.

Sanguinarine

Sanguinarine is a component of an alkaloid extract obtained from the dried rhizome of the bloodroot plant, *Sanguinaria canadensis*. The extract is principally a mixture of benzophenanthridine alkaloids, the main constituent (approximately 33% by weight) being sanguinarine (Figure 45-2). This extract has been used for many years in a variety of medications as an expectorant and as a topical treatment for chronic eczema. It has been incorporated in a dentifrice as an antiplaque and antigingivitis agent. Sanguinarine exists in an iminium ion form (see Figure 45-2) below pH 6.0 or in an

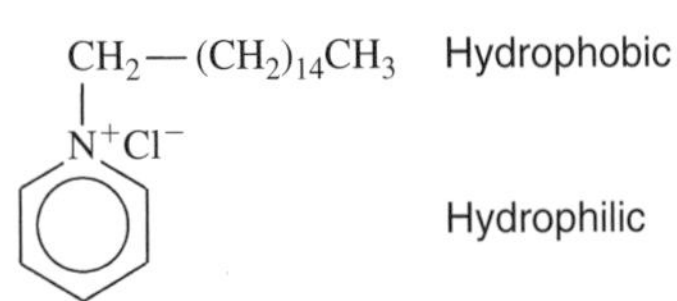

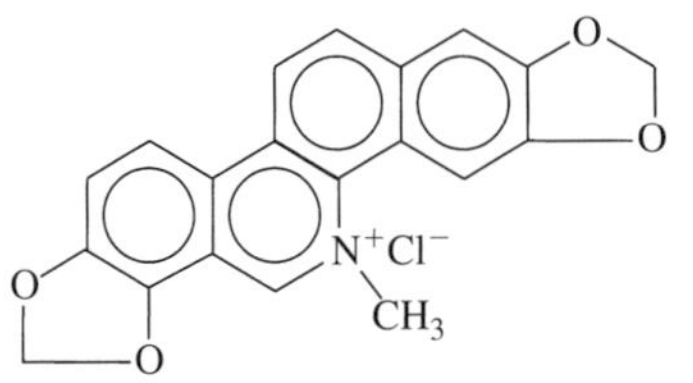

Fig. 45-1 Structural formula of cetylpyridinium chloride showing the hydrophobic and hydrophilic substituents characteristic of the quaternary ammonium disinfectants.

Fig. 45-2 Structural formula of sanguinarine chloride.

alkanolamine form above pH 7.0.[48] The sanguinarine-containing dentifrice and mouthrinse had pH values of 5.2 and 3.2, respectively. The antibacterial activity of sanguinarine is thought to be caused by its ability to inhibit sulfhydryl group–dependent enzymes.

Bis-Biguanides

The bis-biguanides chlorhexidine and alexidine are cationic agents with fungicidal activity and bactericidal action against gram-positive and gram-negative organisms. Chlorhexidine is a chlorophenyl biguanide (Figure 45-3) that has been used as the acetate and, more commonly, the gluconate salt (which is more soluble) in mouthrinses, gels, and dentifrices for control of plaque and gingivitis. It binds to anionic groups on the bacterial surface, probably the phosphate groups of teichoic acid in gram-positive bacteria and the phosphate groups of lipopolysaccharides in gram-negative bacteria. When the bis-biguanide binds to the organism, the cell's membrane becomes permeable, allowing the cytoplasmic contents to leak. At higher concentrations, chlorhexidine causes precipitation of cytoplasmic proteins. By virtue of their cationic properties, the bis-biguanides also bind electrostatically to hydroxyapatite of teeth, to acquired pellicle, to plaque, and to buccal mucosa.

In one of the earliest studies on the dental applications of chlorhexidine, Schroeder[104] showed a 73% reduction of supragingival calculus plaques formed on carrier foils in short-term (3-day) tests. Subsequently, Löe and Rindom Schiøtt[65] clearly documented that chlorhexidine was the most effective antiplaque and antigingivitis agent that had been tested until that time. In short-term trials with an experimental gingivitis model, a twice-daily rinse with 0.2% chlorhexidine gluconate completely prevented accumulation of plaque and the onset of gingivitis. These observations have been confirmed in numerous trials in human beings and animals. Furthermore, chlorhexidine mouthrinse in this experimental model prevented the development of white-spot lesions associated with incipient caries.[68]

The efficacy of chlorhexidine mouth rinse as an antiplaque/antigingivitis agent is dose dependent in the range of 0.03% to 0.2%.[4,57] The volume and frequency of use as well as the concentration are important in determining the clinical response.[59] Accordingly, although no significant difference in response was found between a 0.2% and a 0.12% chlorhexidine mouthrinse when administered in a 15-ml dose twice daily (delivering a total of 60 and 36 mg of the agent, respectively),[105] a significant difference in response was found between a 0.2% and a 0.1% chlorhexidine mouthrinse when administered in a 10-ml dose twice daily (providing 40 or 20 mg of the agent, respectively).[4] Additional factors, such as bioavailability of the formulation, may also affect the dose response. Long-term use (up to 6 months) of chlorhexidine mouthrinses has shown plaque reduction and significant prevention of gingivitis in both children[59] and adults.[40] In a short-term study (21 days), 0.12% chlorhexidine mouth rinse used twice daily was clearly effective in reducing plaque (62% to 99%) compared with placebo, whereas rinsing with a phenolic compound containing essential oils, or sanguinarine with zinc chloride, gave no significant reduction in plaque.[108] Furthermore, the chlorhexidine rinse was superior to the other agents in its ability to maintain optimum gingival health during the entire 3 weeks the mouthrinses were used. Similarly, a 0.2% chlorhexidine rinse was approximately twice as effective as a sanguinarine rinse in a 19-day nonbrushing study in which both plaque and gingivitis scores were assessed.[75] Fluoride (100 ppm), when combined with chlorhexidine (0.12%), does not interfere with the antiplaque/antigingivitis activity of a mouthwash.[46] The ADA Council on Scientific Affairs has accepted a mouthrinse (Peridex) containing 0.12% chlorhexidine gluconate as a safe and effective adjunct to brushing and flossing and regular professional care in helping prevent and reduce supragingival plaque and gingivitis.[23]

Chlorhexidine rinses occasionally give rise to some undesirable side effects, the most conspicuous being the development of yellow-brown stains on the teeth, anterior restorations, and the dorsum of the tongue. Although the stain is extrinsic, it cannot be removed by brushing with a normal toothpaste; mechanical polishing is necessary for its removal. Chlorhexidine also tends to promote supragingival calculus formation. A few persons have had mucosal desquamation and soreness. Solutions containing bis-biguanides have a disagreeable, bitter taste that requires masking by compatible flavoring agents to be palatable. Some patients have a persistent aftertaste or disturbed taste sensation. Extensive safety testing of both the short- and long-term effects of these compounds shows extremely low levels of toxicity both locally and systemically. No teratogenic or reproductive changes have been found.

The bis-biguanides are clearly effective as antiplaque and antigingivitis agents. They should not be used prophylactically but as therapeutic agents for patients with active disease. This use requires proper diagnosis and supervised care until the disease is controlled. Accordingly, in the United States these agents are for prescription use only. Chlorhexidine mouthrinses can serve as an important adjunct to regular oral hygiene for short-term application, particularly for patients in the healing phase after periodontal surgery, oral surgery, and insertion of immediate dentures and for the treatment of acute necrotizing ulcerative gingivitis.[57] Chlorhexidine rinses can also be used for intermittent short-term application three to four times a year to prevent repeated denture stomatitis, limit plaque and gingivitis in patients with dental implants, and suppress the salivary titers of *S. mutans* in patients with high caries activity. Finally, long-term use of such a mouthrinse on a daily, weekly, or biweekly basis may benefit special patients with agranulocytosis, leukemia, hemophilia, thrombocytopenia, kidney disease, bone marrow transplantation, or AIDS; those being treated with cytotoxic or immunosuppressive drugs or radiation therapy; and those who are physically handicapped or mentally retarded (Box 45-4).

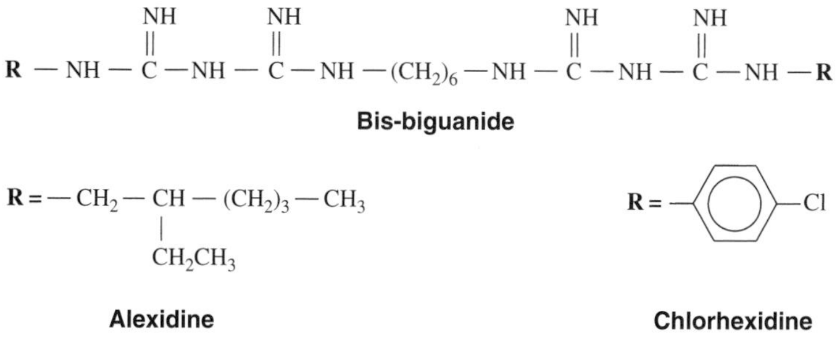

$$\mathbf{R}-NH-\underset{\|}{\overset{NH}{C}}-NH-\underset{\|}{\overset{NH}{C}}-NH-(CH_2)_6-NH-\underset{\|}{\overset{NH}{C}}-NH-\underset{\|}{\overset{NH}{C}}-NH-\mathbf{R}$$

Bis-biguanide

$$\mathbf{R} = -CH_2-\underset{CH_2CH_3}{\underset{|}{CH}}-(CH_2)_3-CH_3$$

Alexidine

$$\mathbf{R} = -C_6H_4-Cl$$

Chlorhexidine

Fig. 45-3 Structural formulas of the bis-biguanides.

Box • 45-4

Clinical Indications for Chlorhexidine

Short-Term Applications
Healing phase in periodontal surgery
Healing phase in oral surgery
Mandibular fracture, third molar extraction, immediate denture
Presurgical use to reduce bacteremia
Therapy for aphthous ulcerations
Therapy for denture stomatitis
Therapy for acute necrotizing ulcerative gingivitis

Intermittent Short-Term Application (3- to 4-Month Cycle)
Repeated denture stomatitis
Adjunct to periodontal maintenance care
High caries activity
Dental implants

Long-Term Application
Medically compromised patient
Agranulocytosis, leukemia, hemophilia, thrombocytopenia, kidney disease, allergies, bone marrow transplant, AIDS
Iatrogenic risk patient
Cytotoxic drugs, immunosuppressive agents, radiation therapy
Physically handicapped patient
Arthritis, scleroderma, disturbed motor capacity or muscle function
Mentally handicapped patient

Adapted from Lang NP, Brecx MC: Chlorhexidine digluconate—an agent for chemical plaque control and prevention of gingival inflammation, *J Periodont Res* 21(suppl 16):74-89, 1986.

Investigators have tested more intensive, professionally applied antimicrobial treatment with varnishes containing high concentrations of chlorhexidine compounds: 5%, 10%, 20%, and even 40%.[54,97-103] The goals were to suppress *S. mutans* for an extended period, to prevent the increase of *S. mutans* normally accompanying placement of fixed orthodontic appliances, and possibly to eliminate them from the mouth. In these studies *S. mutans* was successfully suppressed and in some cases eliminated for periods up to 22 months. However, there was no long-term effect on *Actinomyces* species or *Streptococcus sanguis.* A 40% chlorhexidine varnish, applied to exposed root surfaces of patients who had had periodontal surgery, was as effective as a fluoride varnish (Duraphat) in preventing root caries.[100]

In summary, the bis-biguanides are useful adjuncts in the treatment of periodontal disease or rampant caries. They are not a panacea or magic bullet; in the absence of conventional therapeutic and preventive measures, the bis-biguanides alone have not been able to cure periodontal disease or prevent caries.

Miscellaneous Agents

A prebrushing rinse, Plax, consists of a mixture of allantoin (a topical vulnerary used to stimulate healing of suppurative wounds), sodium benzoate (a food preservative and antifungal agent), sodium bicarbonate (an antacid and weak antibacterial agent), sodium borate (an astringent and feeble antiseptic), polysorbate 20 (an ester of sorbitol and its anhydrides, used as an emulsifier and nonionic surfactant), xanthan gum (a polysaccharide used in foods and cosmetics as a stabilizer and emulsifier), sodium salicylate (a systemic analgesic and antipyretic, also used as a preservative), sodium saccharin (a sweetener), sodium lauryl sulfate (a strong anionic detergent, used commonly in dentifrices), glycerin, and ethyl alcohol (7.5%) in a colored flavored aqueous solution. Extravagant advertising claims were made regarding the ability of Plax to remove plaque, but no single active ingredient was identified.

Initial short-term studies reported significant reductions in plaque scores when used before brushing or alone.[5,6,28,63,92] Several of these studies used an identical protocol of supervised brushing for only 15 seconds and without a dentifrice, conditions unlike those of normal brushing, which averages 60 seconds and is done with a dentifrice. The longer the brushing time, the more plaque is removed; brushing with a dentifrice also removes more plaque than brushing without one. Subsequent short-term studies[12,49,107] and several extending up to 5 weeks[18,39,52,87] found Plax to be no more effective than a placebo rinse. In long-term unsupervised studies (6 months), Plax was also found to be no more effective than a control rinse in reducing plaque, gingivitis, calculus, and stain. Microbiologic studies of plaque samples from Plax and control groups revealed overall similarity at baseline and each examination period.[64] In another long-term (6 months) unsupervised study no significant difference in gingivitis was found in persons using Plax compared with those using normal oral hygiene.[81] Although additional studies have reported plaque reduction with the use of Plax,[81,82,86] a larger number have not found any significant difference between test and control subjects.* Plax inhibits the in vitro uptake of fluoride by enamel powder.[72] On the basis of currently accepted standards, Plax cannot be considered to be a beneficial agent either alone or as part of a therapeutic regimen.

Several other agents have been tested for antiplaque/antigingivitis activity. These include the antiseptic octenidine, a bispyridine,[85] and delmopinol (decapinol), a low- molecular-weight morpholinoethanol derivative.[43] In two long-term supervised studies (6 months) delmopinol (0.2%), when used as a 60-second rinse twice a day (as a supplement to normal mechanical oral hygiene), reduced plaque, gingivitis, and bleeding sites when compared with a placebo rinse, but caused significantly higher staining of the teeth and transient anesthesia of the oral mucosa.[41,58] In both studies chlorhexidine was more effective than delmopinol in limiting plaque formation and gingivitis, but was considered less tolerable by the patients because of the tooth discoloration. In another long-term study (3 months) octenidine (0.1%), when used as a 30-second rinse twice a day, reduced plaque, gingivitis, and bleeding sites when compared with a placebo rinse, but caused significantly higher staining.[11] In short-term studies, mouthrinses containing delmopinol (0.2%) reduced plaque formation and gingivitis.[3,20,21,51,76] Rinses containing these active ingredients are not commercially available.

Most mouthrinses contain ethanol at a concentration between 5% to 27%, primarily to dissolve organic ingredients (flavoring agents, essential oils) and prevent their separation. It should be noted that ethanol at these concentrations is not an effective antibacterial agent. As a result of concerns about possible ingestion of alcohol-containing products by children, it is likely that mouthrinses will eventually be packaged with child-proof caps.

*References 7, 14, 18, 32, 33, 55, 71, 117.

Table • 45-3

Controlled Local Drug Delivery Products

PRODUCT	ACTIVE INGREDIENT	AMOUNT	DESCRIPTION	FDA APPROVED	RESERVOIR DURATION
Actisite	Tetracycline	0.55 mg/cm of filament, 12.7 mg/dose	Nonresorbable ethyl-vinyl acetate monofilament	Yes, but no longer available	>240 hr
Arestin	Minocycline	1 mg/dose	Biodegradable polyglycolide-lactide polymer microspheres	Yes	>14 days
Atridox	Doxycycline	42.5 mg/dose	Biodegradable polymer	Yes	>7 days
Elysol	Metronidazole	25%	Bioresorbable glyceryl monooleate + sesame oil gel	No, sold only in Europe, Asia	<12 hr
Periochip	Chlorhexidine	2.5 mg/dose	Bioabsorbable cross-linked gelatin wafer	Yes	>200 hr

CONTROLLED LOCAL DRUG DELIVERY

Controlled drug delivery in the mouth allows sustained local availability of high concentrations of chemotherapeutic agents such as tetracyclines (minocycline, doxycycline) or chlorhexidine or metronidazole. Intraperiodontal pocket devices permit the release of agents into the crevicular fluid at bactericidal concentrations while avoiding wasteful and potentially toxic systemic administration. Local delivery devices, originally consisting of drug-filled cellulose hollow fibers containing tetracycline, were pioneered by Goodson in the late 1970s.[35] In the past 30 years improved products have been developed and marketed (Table 45-3) such as Actisite (nonresorbable monolithic fiber of ethylene-vinyl acetate impregnated with tetracycline), Periochip (bioabsorbable wafer of cross-linked gelatin containing 2.5 mg chlorhexidine), Arestin (bioresorbable polymer microspheres containing 1 mg minocycline), Atridox (bioabsorbable polymer gel containing 42.5 mg doxycycline hyclate), and Elysol (glycerol monooleate and sesame oil containing 25% metronidazole). The FDA has approved Actisite, Periochip, and Arestin as adjuncts to scaling and root planing. Atridox has FDA approval as a stand-alone therapy for the reduction of probing depths, bleeding on probing, and gain of clinical attachment. Although Actisite was the first of the controlled-release antimicrobial products to be made commercially available (1994), it is no longer marketed. Because it was nonresorbable, it needed to be removed at the end of therapy. It was also time consuming and tedious to insert into pockets and had a tendency to dislodge. Elysol is not available in the United States; it is marketed in Asia and Europe.

The pharmacokinetics of release of all these products indicates antimicrobial concentrations at levels in excess of the minimum inhibitory concentrations for periodontal pathogens.[36,89] Their efficacy in clinical studies is similar, with an average greater reduction of 0.5 mm or less in probable pocket depth compared with scaling and root planing alone.[27,45,80,112,118] Some consider the clinical benefits of most slow-release devices, even when showing statistical significance, as not impressive and do not recommend their routine use.[89] Local delivery systems have potential limitations and benefits. If used as a monotherapy[34] (e.g., Atridox), problems can include failure to remove calculus. The benefits include the ease of application, selectivity in targeting a limited number of diseased sites that were unresponsive to conventional therapy, and possible enhanced treatment results at specific locations.[2] Limited data also suggest that local delivery of antibiotics may be beneficial in preventing recurrent attachment loss in the absence of maintenance therapy. There are no current head-to-head studies comparing one controlled-release antimicrobial product with another. Because their efficacy in clinical studies is similar, ultimately the choice may hinge on an agent's handling characteristics. In this respect Arestin is superior to the others; the simplicity of placement of the cannula and the short, swift injecting movement is easier than the more time-consuming and intensive placement of Periochip or Atridox.

CITED REFERENCES

1. Abello R, Buitrago C, Prate CM, et al: Effect of a mouthrinse containing triclosan and a copolymer on plaque formation in the absence of oral hygiene, *Am J Dent* 3:S57-S61, 1990.
2. American Academy of Periodontology: Treatment of plaque-induced gingivitis, chronic periodontitis, and other clinical conditions, *J Periodontol* 72:1790-1800, 2001.
3. Attström R, Collaert B, De Bruyn H, et al: Effect of decapinol on plaque development and gingivitis healing [abstract], *J Dent Res* 68:837, 1989.
4. Axelsson P, Lindhe J: Efficacy of mouthrinses in inhibiting dental plaque and gingivitis in man, *J Clin Periodontol* 14:205-212, 1987.
5. Bailey L: Direct plaque removal by a pre-brushing dental rinse, *Clin Prev Dent* 3:21-27, 1989.
6. Bailey L, Pader M: Plaque reduction by a detergent rinse used prior to toothbrushing [abstract], *J Dent Res* 69:451, 1990.
7. Balanyk T, Sharma N, Galustians J: Antiplaque efficacy of Plax prebrushing rinse; plaque mass/area analysis [abstract], *J Dent Res* 70:869, 1991.
8. Barnett ML: The role of therapeutic antimicrobial mouthrinses in clinical practice: control of supragingival plaque and gingivitis, *J Am Dent Assoc* 134:699-704, 2003.
9. Bay I, Rølla G: Morphological studies of plaque formation and growth after NaF and SnF_2 rinses. In Rølla G, Sonju T, Embery G, eds: *Tooth surface interactions and preventive dentistry*, London, 1981, IRL Press.

10. Bay I, Rølla G: Plaque inhibition and improved gingival condition by the use of stannous fluoride toothpaste, *Scand J Dent Res* 88:313-315, 1982.
11. Beiswanger BB, Mallalt ME, Mau MS, et al: The clinical effects of a mouthrinse containing 0.1% octenidine, *J Dent Res* 69:454-457, 1990.
12. Beiswanger BB, Mallalt ME, Mau MS, et al: The relative plaque removal effect of a prebrushing mouthrinse, *J Am Dent Assoc* 120:190-192, 1990.
13. Bergenholtz A: Mechanical cleaning. In Frandsen A, ed: *Oral hygiene,* Aalborg, Denmark, 1972, Munksgaard.
14. Binney A, Addy M, Newcombe RG: The plaque removal effects of single rinsings and brushings, *J Periodontol* 64:181-185, 1993.
15. Bonesvol P, Gjermo P: A comparison between chlorhexidine and some quaternary ammonium compounds with regard to retention, salivary concentration and plaque-inhibiting effect in the human mouth after mouthrinses, *Arch Oral Biol* 23:289-294, 1978.
16. Boyd RL: Effects on gingivitis of daily rinsing with 1.5% H_2O_2, *J Clin Periodontol* 16:557-562, 1989.
17. Bradshaw DJ, Marsh PD, Cummins D: The effects of triclosan and zinc citrate, alone and in combination, on a community of oral bacteria grown in vitro, *J Dent Res* 72:25-30, 1993.
18. Chung L, Smith SR, Joyston-Bechal S: The effect of using a pre-brushing mouthwash (Plax) on oral hygiene in man, *J Clin Periodontol* 19:679-681, 1992.
19. Clark WB, Magnusson I, Walker CB, et al: Efficacy of Perimed antibacterial system on established gingivitis. Clinical results, *J Clin Periodontol* 16:630-635, 1989.
20. Collaert B, Attstrom R, De Bruyn H, et al: The effect of delmopinol rinsing on dental plaque formation and gingivitis healing, *J Clin Periodontol* 19:274-280, 1992.
21. Collaert B, Attström R, Hase JC, et al: Rinsing with delmopinol 0.2% and chlorhexidine 0.2%: short-term effect on salivary microbiology, plaque, and gingivitis, *J Periodontol* 63:618-625, 1992.
22. Council on Dental Therapeutics: Council on Dental Therapeutics accepts Listerine, *J Am Dent Assoc* 117:515-516, 1988.
23. Council on Dental Therapeutics: Council on Dental Therapeutics accepts Peridex, *J Am Dent Assoc* 117:516-517, 1988.
24. Council on Dental Therapeutics: Guidelines for acceptance of chemotherapeutic products for the control of supragingival dental plaque and gingivitis, *J Am Dent Assoc* 112:529-532, 1986.
25. Deasy MJ, Battista G, Rustogi KN, et al: Antiplaque efficacy of a triclosan/copolymer prebrush rinse: a plaque prevention study, *Am J Dent* 5:91-94, 1992.
26. DePaola LG, Overholser CD, Meiller TF, et al: Chemotherapeutic inhibition of supragingival plaque and gingivitis development, *J Clin Periodontol* 16:311-315, 1989.
27. Drisko CH, Cobb CM, et al: Evaluation of periodontal treatments using controlled release tetracycline fibers: clinical response, *J Periodontol* 66:692-699, 1995.
28. Emling RC, Yankell SL: First clinical studies of a new prebrushing mouthrinse, *Compend Continuing Ed Dent* 6:636-646, 1985.
29. Fine DH, Letizia J, Mandel I: The effect of rinsing with Listerine antiseptic on the properties of developing dental plaque, *J Clin Periodontol* 12:660-666, 1985.
30. Fornell J, Sundin Y, Lindhe J: Effect of Listerine on dental plaque and gingivitis, *Scand J Dent Res* 83:18-25, 1975.
31. Frandsen A: Mechanical oral hygiene practices. In Loe H, Kleinman DV: *Dental plaque control measures and oral hygiene practices,* Oxford, 1986, IRL Press.
32. Freitas BL, Collaert B, Attström R: Effect of prebrushing rinse, Plax, on dental plaque formation, *J Clin Periodontol* 18:713-715, 1991.
33. Frostmar G, Olsson A, Collaert B: Muskoljningsmedelet Plax-effekten pa gingivet och plack, *Tandläkartidingen* 22:1172-1176, 1990.
34. Garrett S, Johnson L, Drisko CH, et al: Two multicenter studies evaluating locally delivered doxycycline hyclate, placebo control, oral hygiene, and scaling and root planing in the treatment of periodontitis, *J Periodontol* 70:490-503, 1999.
35. Goodson JM, Holborow D, Dunn RL, et al: Monolithic tetracycline-containing fibers for controlled delivery to periodontal pockets, *J Periodontol* 54:575-579, 1983.
36. Goodson JM, Tanner A, McArdle S, et al: Multicenter evaluation of tetracycline fiber therapy: III. Microbiological response, *J Periodont Res* 26:440-451, 1991.
37. Gordon JM, Lamster IB, Seiger MC: Efficacy of Listerine antiseptic in inhibiting the growth of plaque and gingivitis, *J Clin Periodontol* 12:697-704, 1985.
38. Greene JC, Vermillion JR: The simplified oral hygiene index, *J Am Dent Assoc* 68:7-13, 1964.
39. Grossman E: Effectiveness of a prebrushing mouthrinse under single trial and home use conditions, *Clin Prev Dent* 10:3-6, 1988.
40. Grossman E, Reiter G, Sturzenberger OP, et al: Six-month study of the effects of a chlorhexidine mouthrinse on gingivitis in adults, *J Periodont Res* 21:33-43, 1986.
41. Hase JC, Attström R, Edwardsson S, et al: 6-month use of 0.2% delmopinol hydrochloride in comparison with 0.2% chlorhexidine digluconate and placebo. I. Effect on plaque formation and gingivitis, *J Clin Periodontol* 25:746-753, 1998.
42. Helldén L, Camosci D, Hock J, et al: Clinical study to compare the effect of stannous fluoride and chlorhexidine mouthrinses on plaque formation, *J Clin Periodontol* 8:12-16, 1981.
43. Hernestam SE, Nilsson NA, Willard L-O: *Morpholino compounds and compositions,* U.S. Patent # 4,636,382, Jan 13, 1987, AB Ferrosan.
44. Imrey PB, Chilton NW, Pihlstrom BL: Recommended revisions to the American Dental Association guidelines for acceptance of chemotherapeutic products for gingivitis control: report of the Task Force on Design and Analysis in Dental and Oral Research to the Council on Therapeutics of the American Dental Association, *J Periodont Res* 29:299-304, 1994.
45. Jeffcoat MK, Bray KS, Ciancio SG: Adjunctive use of a subgingival controlled-release chlorhexidine chip reduces probing depth and improves attachment level compared with scaling and root planing alone, *J Periodontol* 69:989-997, 1998.

46. Jenkins S, Addy M, Newcombe R: Evaluation of a mouthrinse containing chlorhexidine and fluoride as an adjunct to oral hygiene, *J Clin Periodontol* 20:20-25, 1993.
47. Jones CM, Blinkhorn AS, White E: Hydrogen peroxide, the effect on plaque and gingivitis when used in an oral irrigator, *Clin Prev Dent* 12:15-18, 1990.
48. Jones RR, Harkrader RJ, Southard GL: The effect of pH on sanguinarine iminium ion form, *J Natural Products* 49:1109-1111, 1986.
49. Kazmierczak M, Ciancio S, Mather M: Clinical evaluation of Plax as a prebrushing rinse [abstract], *J Dent Res* 68:1474, 1989.
50. Keyes P, Wright WE, Howard SA: The use of phase-contrast microscopy and chemotherapy in the diagnosis and treatment of periodontal lesions—an initial report (I), *Quintessence Int* 9:51-56, 1978.
51. Klinge B, Matsson L, Attström R, et al: Effect of local application of decapinol on developing and early established plaque in humans [abstract], *J Dent Res* 68:829, 1989.
52. Kohut BE, Mankodi S: The effectiveness of a prebrushing mouthrinse in reducing supragingival plaque and gingivitis in single-use and extended-use trials, *Am J Dent* 2:157-160, 1989.
53. Kornman KS, *Antimicrobial agents,* Oxford, 1986, IRL Press.
54. Kozai K, Wang DS, Sandham HJ, et al: Changes in strains of mutans streptococci induced by treatment with chlorhexidine varnish, *J Dent Res* 70:1252-1257, 1991.
55. Kozlovsky A, Zuberty Y: The efficacy of Plax prebrushing rinse: a review of the literature, *Quintessence Int* 24:141-144, 1993.
56. Kumar PS, Griffen AL, Barton JA, et al: New bacterial species associated with chronic periodontitis, *J Dent Res* 82:338-344, 2003.
57. Lang NP, Brecx MC: Chlorhexidine digluconate—an agent for chemical plaque control and prevention of gingival inflammation, *J Periodont Res* 21:74-89, 1986.
58. Lang NP, Hase JC, Grassi M, et al: Plaque formation and gingivitis after supervised mouthrinsing with 0.2% delmopinol hydrochloride, 0.2% chlorhexidine digluconate and placebo for 6 months, *Oral Dis* 4:105-113, 1998.
59. Lang NP, Hotz P, Graf H, et al: Effects of supervised chlorhexidine mouthrinses in children, *J Periodont Res* 17:101-111, 1982.
60. Larson LC, Allen JM, Hyman JJ, et al: Effect of a 0.2% SnF_2 mouthrinse on gingival tissues and associated microflora, *Clin Prev Dent* 7:5-8, 1985.
61. Llewelyn J: A double-blind crossover trial on the effect of cetylpyridinium chloride 0.05 per cent (Merocet) on plaque accumulation, *Br Dent J* 148:103-104, 1980.
62. Lobene RR, Singh SM, Garcia L, et al: Clinical efficacy of a triclosan/copolymer pre-brush rinse: a plaque removal clinical study, *J Clin Dent* 3:54-58, 1992.
63. Lobene RR, Sopakar PM, Emling RC, et al: Plaque removal with a prebrushing mouthrinse [abstract], *J Dent Res* 65:771, 1986.
64. Lobene RR, Sopakar PM, Newman MB: Long-term evaluation of a prebrushing dental rinse for the control of dental plaque and gingivitis, *Clin Prev Dent* 12:26-30, 1990.
65. Löe H, Rindom Schiøtt C: The effect of mouthrinses and topical applications of chlorhexidine on the development of dental plaque and gingivitis in man, *J Periodont Res* 5:79-83, 1970.
66. Löe H, Theilade E, Borglum Jensen S: Experimental gingivitis in man, *J Periodontol* 36:177-187, 1965.
67. Löe H, Theilade E, Borglum Jenson S, et al: Experimental gingivitis in man. III. The influence of antibiotics on gingival plaque development, *J Periodont Res* 2:282-289, 1967.
68. Löe H, Von der Fehr FR, Rindom Schiott C: Inhibition of experimental caries by plaque prevention: the effect of chlorhexidine mouthrinses, *Scand J Dent Res* 80:1-9, 1972.
69. Loesche WJ: Chemotherapy of dental plaque infections, *Oral Sci Rev* 9:65-107, 1976.
70. Mandel ID: Chemotherapeutic agents for controlling plaque and gingivitis, *J Clin Periodontol* 15:488-498, 1988.
71. McCarthy R, Naylor MN, Wilson RF: The efficacy of a prebrushing mouthrinse used on a single occasion [abstract], *J Dent Res* 70:106, 1991.
72. Melo Franco E, Cury JA: Effect of prebrushing rinse (Plax) on the deposition of fluoride on enamel in vitro [abstract], *J Dent Res* 72:2316, 1993.
73. Miller WD, *The micro-organisms of the human mouth,* Philadelphia, 1890, SS White Dental Mfg. Co.
74. Miyasaki KT, Genco RJ, Wilson M: Antimicrobial properties of hydrogen peroxide and sodium bicarbonate individually and in combination against selected oral gram-negative facultative bacteria, *J Dent Res* 65:1142-1148, 1986.
75. Moran J, Addy M: Comparison between chlorhexidine and sanguinarine mouthrinses on plaque and gingivitis [abstract], *J Dent Res* 66:1381, 1987.
76. Moran J, Addy M, Wade WG, et al: A comparison of delmopinol and chlorhexidine on plaque regrowth over a 4-day period and salivary counts, *J Clin Periodontol* 19:749-753, 1992.
77. Muhlemann HR: Chlorhexidine, Vantocil, Fluorphene and antimycotic agents in an animal caries test, *Helv Odontol Acta* 17:99-103, 1973.
78. Newbrun E: Chemical and mechanical removal of plaque, *Compend Contin Educ Dent* 6:S110-S116, 1985.
79. Newbrun E, Felton RA, Bulkacz J: Susceptibility of some plaque microorganisms to chemotherapeutic agents, *J Dent Res* 55:574-579, 1976.
80. Newman MG, Kornman KS, Doherty FM: A 6-month multicenter evaluation of adjunctive tetracycline fiber therapy used in conjunction with scaling and root planing in maintenance patients: clinical results, *J Periodontol* 65:685-691, 1994.
81. O'Mahony G, O'Mullane DM: Evaluation or a prebrushing mouthrinse in controlling dental plaque, *J Irish Dent Assoc* 37:44-47, 1991.
82. O'Mullane DM, Whelton H, Galvin N, et al: A 12-month study of the efficacy of a prebrushing rinse in plaque removal, *J Dent Res* 72:278, 1993.
83. Ogaard B, Gjermo P, Rolla G: Plaque-inhibiting effect in orthodontic patients of a dentifrice containing stannous fluoride, *Am J Orthod* 78:266-272, 1980.
84. Page RC: Review of the guidelines for acceptance of chemotherapeutic products for the control of supragingival dental plaque and gingivitis, *J Dent Res* 68:1640-1644, 1989.

85. Patters MR, Nalbandian J, Nichols FC, et al: Effects of octenidine mouthrinse on plaque formation and gingivitis in humans, *J Periodont Res* 21:154-162, 1986.
86. Patters MR, Shiloah J: A method for evaluating the effect of a pre-brushing oral rinse [abstract], *J Dent Res* 70:463, 1991.
87. Pontier J-P, Pine C, Jackson DL, et al: Efficacy of a pre-brushing rinse for orthodontic patients, *Clin Prev Dent* 12:12-16, 1990.
88. Quigley G, Hein J: Comparative cleansing efficiency of manual and power brushing, *J Am Dent Assoc* 65:26-29, 1962.
89. Quirynen M, Teughels W, De Soete M, et al: Topical antiseptics and antibiotics in the initial therapy of chronic adult periodontitis: microbiological aspects, *Periodont 2000* 28:72-90, 2002.
90. Rams TE, Wright WE, Keyes PH, et al: Long-term effects of microbiologically modulated periodontal therapy on advanced adult periodontitis, *J Am Dent Assoc* 111:429-441, 1985.
91. Rees TD, Orth CF: Oral ulceration with use of hydrogen peroxide, *J Periodontol* 57:689-692, 1986.
92. Robertson P, Walsh M, Armitage G, et al: Clinical plaque efficacy study of a prebrushing mouthrinse [abstract], *J Dent Res* 65:405, 1986.
93. Rosling BG, Slots J, Webber RL, et al: Microbiological and clinical effect of topical subgingival antimicrobial treatment of human periodontal disease, *J Clin Periodontol* 10:487-514, 1983.
94. Ross NM, Charles CH, Dills SS: Long-term effects of Listerine antiseptic on dental plaque and gingivitis, *J Clin Dent* 1:92-95, 1989.
95. Rustogi KN, Curtis JP, Volpe AR, et al: Refinement of the modified Navy plaque index to increase plaque scoring efficiency in gumline and interproximal tooth areas, *J Clin Dent* 3:C9-C12, 1992.
96. Rustogi KN, Petrone DM, Singh SM, et al: Clinical study of a pre-brush rinse and a triclosan/copolymer mouthrinse: effect on plaque formation, *Am J Dent* 3:S67-S69, 1990.
97. Sandham HJ, Brown J, Chan KH, et al: Clinical trial in adults of an antimicrobial varnish for reducing mutans streptococci, *J Dent Res* 70:1401-1408, 1991.
98. Sandham HJ, Brown J, Phillips HI, et al: A preliminary report of long-term elimination of detectable mutans streptococci in man, *J Dent Res* 67:9-14, 1988.
99. Sandham HJ, Nadeau L, Phillips HI: The effect of chlorhexidine varnish treatment on salivary mutans streptococcal levels in child orthodontic patients, *J Dent Res* 71:32-35, 1992.
100. Schaeken MJM, Keltjens HMAM, Van Der Hoeven JS: Effects of fluoride and chlorhexidine on the microflora of dental root-surface caries, *J Dent Res* 70:150-153, 1991.
101. Schaeken MJM, de Jong MH, Franken HCM, et al: Effect of chlorhexidine and iodine on the composition of the human dental plaque flora, *Caries Res* 18:404-407, 1984.
102. Schaeken MJM, van der Hoeven JS, Franken HCM: Comparative recovery of *Streptococcus mutans* on five isolation media, including a new simple selective medium, *J Dent Res* 65:906-908, 1986.
103. Schaeken MJM, van der Hoeven JS, Hendricks JCM: Effects of varnishes containing chlorhexidine on the human dental plaque flora, *J Dent Res* 68:1786-1789, 1989.
104. Schroeder HE: Quantitative in-vivo-Studie mit Zahnsteinhemmstoffen, *Schweiz Monatsschr Zahnheilkunde* 72:294-312, 1962.
105. Segreto VA, Collins EM, Beiswanger BB, et al: A comparison of mouthrinses containing two concentrations of chlorhexidine, *J Periodont Res* 21:23-32, 1986.
106. Shapiro S, Giertsen E, Guggenheim B: An in vitro biofilm model for comparing the efficacy of antimicrobial mouthrinses, *Caries Res* 36:93-100, 2002.
107. Sharma N: Efficacy of Plax prebrushing mouthrinse under single trial and home use conditions [abstract], *J Dent Res* 68:1473, 1989.
108. Siegrist BE, Gusberti FA, Brecx MC, et al: Efficacy of supervised rinsing with chlorhexidine digluconate in comparison to phenolic and plant alkaloid compounds, *J Periodont Res* 21:60-73, 1986.
109. Silness J, Löe H: Periodontal disease in pregnancy. II. Correlation between oral hygiene and periodontal condition, *Acta Odont Scand* 22:121-135, 1964.
110. Singh SM, Rustogi KN, Volpe AR, et al: Effect of a mouthrinse containing triclosan and a copolymer on plaque formation in a normal oral hygiene regimen, *Am J Dent* 3:S63-S65, 1990.
111. Socransky SS, Haffajee AD, Cugini MA, et al: Microbial complexes in subgingival plaque, *J Clin Periodontol* 25:133-144, 1998.
112. Soskolne WA, Heasman PA, Stabholz A, et al: Sustained local delivery of chlorhexidine in the treatment of periodontitis: a multicenter study, *J Periodontol* 68:32-38, 1997.
113. Spindel LM, Chauncey HH, Person P: Plaque reduction unaccompanied by gingivitis reduction, *J Periodontol* 57:551-554, 1986.
114. Svantun B, Gjermo P, Eriksen HM, et al: A comparison of the plaque-inhibiting effect of stannous fluoride and chlorhexidine, *Acta Odont Scand* 35:247-250, 1977.
115. Tinanoff N: Stannous fluoride in clinical dentistry. In Wei SHY, ed: *Clinical uses of fluorides,* Philadelphia, 1985, Lea and Febiger.
116. Van der Ouderaa FJG: Anti-plaque agents. Rationale and prospects for prevention of gingivitis and periodontal disease, *J Clin Periodontol* 18:447-454, 1991.
117. Wilder RS, Mitchell SC, Hamilton SA: Clinical evaluation of a prebrushing mouthrinse, *J Dent Res* 72:336, 1993.
118. Williams RC, Paquette DW, Offenbacher S, et al: Treatment of periodontitis by local administration of minocycline microspheres: a controlled clinical trial, *J Periodontol* 72:1535-1544, 2001.
119. Wolff LF, Pihlstrom BL, Bakdash MB, et al: Effect of toothbrushing with 0.4% stannous fluoride and 0.22% sodium fluoride gel on gingivitis for 18 months, *J Am Dent Assoc* 119:283-289, 1989.
120. Wolff LF, Pihlstrom BL, Bakdash MB, et al: Four-year investigation of salt and peroxide regimen compared with conventional oral hygiene, *J Am Dent Assoc* 118:67-72, 1989.

General References

American Academy of Periodontology: *Chemical agents for the control of plaque,* Chicago, 1989, American Academy of Periodontology.

American Academy of Periodontology: *Perspectives on antimicrobial therapeutics,* Littleton, MA, 1987, PSG.

American Academy of Periodontology: The role of controlled drug delivery for periodontitis [position paper], *J Periodontol* 71:125-140, 2000.

Ciancio SG, ed: *ADA Guide to dental therapeutics,* ed 3, Chicago, 2003, American Dental Association.

Drisko CH: Non-surgical pocket therapy: pharmacotherapeutics, *Ann Periodontol* 1:491-566, 1996.

Joyston-Bechal S: Topical and systemic antimicrobial agents in the treatment of chronic gingivitis and periodontitis, *Int Dent J* 37:52-62, 1987.

Löe H: Chlorhexidine in the prevention of gingivitis, *J Periodont Res* 21(suppl 16), 1986.

Löe H, Kleinman DV, eds: *Dental plaque control measures and oral hygiene practices,* Oxford, 1986, IRL Press.

Parsons JC: Chemotherapy of dental plaque—a review, *J Periodontol* 45:177-186, 1974.

Schonfeld SE: Current status of antiplaque agents, *CDA* 13:53-57, 1985.

Strølfors A: Disinfection of dental plaques in man, *Odontologisk Tidskrift* 70:183-203, 1962.

CHAPTER • 46

Antiseptics and Disinfectants

Michael J. Gleason and John A. Molinari

Numerous treatment area surfaces can become contaminated with saliva, blood, and other potentially infectious substances during provision of care. The routine use of chemical disinfectants and disposable supplies has thus become very important because it is neither possible nor necessary to sterilize all contaminated items or surfaces. This trend is especially applicable in dentistry, where many instruments and environmental surfaces become contaminated with saliva and blood during routine procedures.[7] Organisms contained in these fluids include staphylococci, streptococci, *Mycobacterium tuberculosis*, cytomegalovirus, herpes simplex virus types 1 and 2, hepatitis B virus, hepatitis C virus, human immunodeficiency virus (HIV), and a number of upper respiratory tract viruses.

The importance of routine infection control procedures was underscored by the estimate that an office treating 20 patients a day would encounter one active carrier of hepatitis B every 7 days.[8] This early finding, coupled with the fact that all viral infections, including hepatitis B virus, hepatitis C virus, and HIV, appear to be infectious before distinct signs and symptoms appear, makes the likelihood of unknowingly treating an infectious patient a certainty. Failure to treat every patient as potentially infectious—that is, with "standard precautions," previously termed *universal precautions*—places both the health care worker and all patients at avoidably increased risk of infection.

The overall goals of infection control programs are as follows: (1) to reduce the numbers of pathogenic microorganisms to levels where patients' normal defense mechanisms can prevent infection; (2) to break the cycle of infection and eliminate cross-contamination; (3) to treat every patient and instrument as capable of transmitting infectious disease; and (4) to protect patients and health care workers from infection and its consequences.[6,14] The proper use of barrier techniques (gloves, mask, gown, eye protection, rubber dam) combined with proper sterilization, disinfection, and antisepsis protocols will accomplish these goals.

It is important to understand the differences between the terms *sterilization*, *disinfection*, and *antisepsis*.[26] *Sterilization* is the ultimate goal of any infection control protocol because it is the killing of all forms of microorganisms. To eradicate resistant viruses and bacterial endospores effectively requires the application of high heat and/or chemicals for a sufficient time. The most widely used means of attaining this objective in a dental office are dry heat, steam, and chemical vapor sterilization units. In medicine and industry, other forms of sterilization include ethylene oxide and formaldehyde gases, ultraviolet and gamma radiation, and filtration. *Disinfection* is the application of chemicals to destroy most pathogenic organisms on inanimate surfaces. Although some chemicals used for disinfection are capable of achieving sterilization given sufficient time of exposure, their use to effect sterilization is discouraged because of the number of conditions that can lead to failure in this application. *Antisepsis* is the use of chemicals to destroy most pathogenic organisms on animate surfaces. The difference between disinfection and antisepsis may seem small, but it leads to a wide divergence in the products used and the regulation of the products.

Disinfectants fall under the regulatory authority of the Environmental Protection Agency and are thus subject to that agency's rules for demonstration of effectiveness and safety in the workplace. Antiseptics, because they are intended for application on living tissue, fall under the regulations of the Food and Drug Administration (FDA) regarding effectiveness and clinical use.

The ideal disinfectant would be a chemical with the following advantageous properties: the ability to kill the vegetative form of all pathogenic organisms; effectiveness with limited time of exposure; and effectiveness at room temperature. It should also be noncorrosive, nontoxic to human beings, and inexpensive. Given the numerous similarities in chemical composition and metabolism between human beings and microorganisms, this ideal is unlikely to be achieved. In practice, however, proper use of the available chemical disinfectants reduces the numbers of viable pathogenic organisms on surfaces to levels that will allow a healthy person's natural defenses to prevent infection.

The ideal antiseptic would have properties similar to those of an ideal disinfectant. However, selective toxicity (toxicity to microorganisms but not to human cells) is of primary importance for antiseptics. The degree of selectivity of the antiseptic agents can vary depending on the tissues with which they come in contact. An antiseptic intended for handwashing can be less selective than one used in an oral rinse because the highly keratinized epithelium of the skin affords a greater degree of protection from the antiseptic than does the oral epithelium.

The various antiseptics and disinfectants can be classified according to mechanism of action: those that denature proteins, those that cause osmotic disruption of the cell, and those that interfere with specific metabolic processes. Agents that cause protein denaturation or osmotic disruption tend to kill the organisms and are described as *bactericidal*, *virucidal*, or *fungicidal* in nature. Interference with specific metabolic processes usually affects cell growth and reproduction without killing the cell, causing a bacteriostatic effect.

Table 46-1 lists representative classes of compounds used as disinfectants or antiseptics with their effectiveness against various representative organisms. The aldehyde and certain halogen-based and oxidizing compounds have the broadest

Table • 46-1

Antimicrobial Activity of Different Classes of Disinfectants and Antiseptics

CLASS OR AGENT	GRAM-POSITIVE BACTERIA	GRAM-NEGATIVE BACTERIA	BACTERIAL SPORES	TUBERCLE BACILLI	VIRUSES HBV	VIRUSES HIV	FUNGI
Halogens	+	+	±	±	+	+	+
Aldehydes	+	+	+	+	+	+	+
Phenols	+	+	−	+	−	+	+
Alcohols	+	+	−	+	±	+	±
Chlorhexidine	+	+	−	−	−	+	±
Surface-active agents							
Anionic	+	−	−	−	−		−
Cationic	+	±	−	−	−		+
Oxidizing agents	+	+	+	+	+	+	+
Heavy metals	+	±	−	−	±		+

HBV, Hepatitis B virus; *HIV*, human immunodeficiency virus.

range of effectiveness. Unfortunately, these agents also tend to be the most toxic to human tissue. As a consequence, their use has been primarily limited to disinfection. The other chemical classes are less effective antimicrobial agents but also tend to be less harmful to human tissue and find use both in disinfectants and antiseptics. Some distinguishing features of the chemical groups are listed in Table 46-2.

HALOGENS AND HALOGEN-RELEASING COMPOUNDS

The halogens and halogen-releasing compounds include some of the most effective antimicrobial compounds used for disinfection and antisepsis. Their primary mode of action appears to depend on the free halogen reacting covalently with key enzyme systems.[9] Despite many years of research and use, the exact mechanism is not known, although reactions with sulfhydryls and disulfides within proteins appear to be the most likely sites of action. Iodine and chlorine are the most effective halogens.

The salts (sodium, calcium, and lithium) of hypochlorite, in the form of chloride lime, have been used since the mid-1800s as a source of chlorine for disinfection and as an antiseptic. Because of the irritating nature of the products of sodium hypochlorite, it is currently used primarily as a disinfectant. Standard household bleach is a 5.25% solution of sodium hypochlorite with a strong base added. The presence of the base helps to stabilize the hypochlorite, which must first be converted to hypochlorous acid before it can release the chlorine. Useful dilutions for surface disinfection range from 1:10 to 1:100 parts bleach to water, with exposure times of 10 to 30 minutes.[5] The main disadvantages of bleach solutions are their tendency to corrode metals, an odor that some people find offensive, and the need for diluted disinfectant solution to be prepared fresh daily. Even though they are destroyed during disinfection, tubercle bacilli appear to be somewhat resistant to hypochlorite compared with other common pathogens.[25]

Iodine compounds have a long history, dating from the early 1800s, of use as antiseptics and disinfectants. Iodine is relatively nontoxic and noncorrosive, its activity is not inhib-

Table • 46-2

Characteristics of Common Chemical Disinfectants

AGENT	ACTIVITY	LIABILITIES
Chlorine dioxide	Rapid disinfection activity; can be used for sterilization with 6 hours of exposure	Corrosive; activity greatly reduced in the presence of protein and organic debris; requires good ventilation
Glutaraldehyde	As 2.0% to 3.2% immersion preparation, broad-spectrum antimicrobial activity; sporicidal after 10 hours of contact; long use life	Very irritating to skin and mucous membranes; allergenic with repeated exposures
Hypochlorite	Rapidly-acting, broad-spectrum bactericidal, sporicidal, virucidal disinfectant	Irritating to skin; corrosive; can degrade some plastics
Iodophors	Rapidly-acting, broad-spectrum bactericidal disinfectant; residual antimicrobial activity remains on surface after drying	Corrosive to some metals; may discolor some surfaces; inactivated by hard water
Phenols	Broad-spectrum antimicrobial activity; effective in presence of detergents	Can degrade plastics; irritating to skin and eyes; inactivated by hard water and organic debris

ited by the presence of organic compounds, and it possesses a broad spectrum of activity. Thus iodine makes a nearly ideal antimicrobial agent. Originally used as elemental iodine (with potassium iodide or sodium iodide added for increased solubility) in aqueous solutions or in tinctures (alcohol solutions), iodine has the disadvantages of discoloring skin and other material, having an odor, and being painful on open wounds. The development of iodophors—iodine or triiodide complexed with natural polymers such as polyvinyl pyrrolidone or polyether glycols—has led to the wide acceptance of iodine as a disinfectant. Iodophors have little or no odor, increase the solubility of iodine, reduce discoloration of surfaces, and provide a reservoir for sustained release. The concentration of free molecular iodine, the active antimicrobial agent, is lower in iodophor preparations compared with aqueous solutions with the same total iodine concentration. This liability is offset by the release of iodine from the polymer complex as the free iodine reacts with the microorganism. When used with the spray-wipe-spray technique, iodophors are efficient cleaning agents and effective surface disinfectants.[7]

Within the last few years, a combination of sodium chloride and sodium bromide has been demonstrated to be an effective tuberculocidal surface disinfectant. Currently, only one product is commercially available for dentistry. The active ingredients are prepared separately in tablet form (one containing sodium chloride and the other containing sodium bromide). After the tablets are dissolved in water, the resultant solution provides an appropriate broad-spectrum antimicrobial effect and is compatible with most dental equipment surfaces.

ALDEHYDES

Glutaraldehyde (1,5-pentanedial) was first proposed as an antimicrobial in the early 1960s. Since then, it has achieved wide use in dentistry and medicine as an immersion disinfectant.[27] The antimicrobial action appears to be the result of the cross-linking of proteins, both in the organism's cell wall and intracellularly. Glutaraldehyde is not significantly affected by the presence of organic material and is relatively nonirritating, nonallergenic, and noncorrosive when proper safeguards are used.[15] Caution should still be used with glutaraldehyde because repeated exposure of skin and mucous membranes can cause sensitization, irritation, and damage. At least 10 cases of occupational asthma have been reported from the use of glutaraldehyde, which underscores the importance of using it only in well-ventilated areas and never using it as a surface disinfectant.[11] Marketed as an acidic or alkaline 2% to 3.2% aqueous solution, it retains activity against tubercle bacilli, spores, viruses, and fungi when stored for up to 30 days after activation. Activation takes place by alkalization of the glutaraldehyde solution. Alkalization also reduces the stability of the solution. The reuse life of a glutaraldehyde solution (i.e., the length of time the solution remains effective when challenged by dirty instruments, dilution, and evaporation) may therefore be considerably shorter than 30 days.[22] The use of glutaraldehyde in dentistry as a "cold sterilant" has declined considerably in recent years. At best, its use should be limited to those few instruments and small items that should be sterilized but cannot withstand the high heat required by sterilization methods available in a dental office. Such use requires at least 10 hours' immersion in the solution after initial cleaning to remove solid debris.

Formaldehyde, once widely used, is now rarely used because of its toxicity and tendency to cause sensitization with repeated contact.[11] The relative risk of formaldehyde as a human carcinogen when used as a disinfectant remains unknown.[23]

PHENOLS AND RELATED COMPOUNDS

Sir Joseph Lister introduced phenol as a surgical disinfectant in the mid-1800s, but its irritating and toxic nature led to its replacement by a number of substituted phenolic compounds. These substitutions have increased the antimicrobial effect of phenol without significantly increasing its human toxicity. Many of the phenolic compounds also have a local anesthetic effect, making them useful as antiseptics, particularly when pain is associated with an infection.

Generally, the phenols have the advantage of retaining their antimicrobial effectiveness in the presence of organic material, which makes them useful when the complete removal of tissue and debris is impossible or impractical.

Cresol, the active ingredient in coal-tar disinfectants, is a mixture of the three isomers of methylphenol. It has three to 10 times the antimicrobial activity of phenol but approximately the same human toxicity. Mixtures of cresol with detergents formed by the saponification of various vegetable oils have been used as surface disinfectants since the early 1900s.[13] The original proprietary formulation of Lysol was a 50% mixture of cresol in saponified vegetable oil. (More recently, Lysol has been composed of other disinfectants such as ethanol and quaternary ammonium compounds.)

Eugenol (2-methoxy-4-allylphenol) and guaiacol (*o*-methoxyphenol) have weak antimicrobial activity but are useful for their rapid analgesic properties. Eugenol is common in many sedative pastes used in dentistry and is the active phenolic component in oil of cloves. Prolonged contact of eugenol with tissue, as when sealed in a root canal preparation, can lead to severe tissue damage without pain because of the agent's analgesic properties.[4]

Bisphenols, especially hexachlorophene (2,2′-methylene-bis[3,4,6-trichlorophenol]), have proved to be effective antimicrobials when used with detergents. Hexachlorophene was shown to accumulate on the skin with repeated use, reaching a maximum level in 3 to 4 days, at which time the resident bacterial count on the skin was reduced by 95% to 99%. It was shown to be most effective against gram-positive organisms, which constitute the most common components of the bacterial skin flora, and remain major potential pathogens for cross-infection. The substantivity and effectiveness of hexachlorophene made it a widely used component in surgical soaps. (*Substantivity* is the ability of an antiseptic to remain on the skin and, as a result, to extend the period of the antimicrobial effect.) Available over the counter for many years, soaps containing greater than 0.1% hexachlorophene were banned by the FDA in the 1970s after concerns about cutaneous absorption and neural toxicity.[16]

Triclosan (2,4,4′-trichloro-2′-hydroxydiphenyl ether) has been used in antimicrobial soaps (as a 0.3% solution) and investigated in a number of mouthrinses and dentifrices as an antiplaque agent.[18,21] Triclosan is bacteriostatic and fungistatic, with a reasonably broad-spectrum range of antimicrobial activity. A relatively low toxicity effect on *Pseudomonas aeruginosa* strains diminishes some of its clinical usefulness, but its epithelial substantivity has allowed inclusion of triclosan in a number of medicated hand soaps, antiperspirants, and dentifrices. In dental products, it is frequently formulated in combination with retentive agents such as Gantrez, a proprietary copolymer of methoxyethylene and maleic acid. In addition to its antimicrobial activity, triclosan appears to have a direct antiinflammatory effect. This effect may result from the inhibition of a portion of the histamine cascade.[17]

Parachlorometaxylenol (PCMX) is a halogen-substituted phenolic compound that has found widespread usefulness as an effective hand wash antiseptic. Its antimicrobial activity against susceptible bacteria occurs from disruption of the microbial cell wall and enzyme inactivation. PCMX is more active than chlorhexidine as a broad-spectrum antiseptic because it is most effective against gram-positive bacteria, somewhat less active against gram-negative organisms, and exerts some antifungal effects. Of special importance in health care settings, however, is the ability of PCMX to kill *Pseudomonas* species. Because it can penetrate epithelial surfaces, PCMX has been shown to be an effective alternative to chlorhexidine gluconate in many hand wash preparations, with little reported allergic sensitization potential.[20]

The introduction and subsequent widespread use of phenolic surface disinfectants that are synthetic mixtures of two or three phenolic compounds have led to the commercial availability of numerous similar products. The phenols are chosen to act synergistically, yielding a product that is a more effective disinfectant than a comparable concentration of its individual components. In addition, many of the synthetic mixtures are diluted with water before use, which enhances their cleaning effectiveness relative to alcohol-phenol-based products.[24] One common example is the combination of *o*-phenylphenol and *o*-benzyl-*p*-chlorophenol.

ALCOHOLS

The alcohols (see Chapter 43), especially ethanol and isopropanol, have been used for many years as antimicrobials and as carriers for other water-insoluble antimicrobials such as iodine and phenols. Their low cost, rapid evaporation, and lack of residue make them useful for disinfecting inanimate objects. However, their ability to denature and precipitate proteins greatly decreases their antimicrobial effectiveness in the presence of a bioburden (blood and saliva), in addition to their detrimental effect on dental equipment surfaces, such as leather-like chair coverings and plastic items. The precipitated proteins coat the microorganisms, protecting them from direct exposure to the alcohols. The ineffectiveness of alcohols against many bacterial spores, viruses, and fungi further reduces their usefulness as disinfectants for surfaces or instruments.

The historic use of alcohols as topical antiseptics in addition to disinfection has also been documented for well over 100 years. The use of either isopropanol, ethanol, or *n*-propanol in combination with other antimicrobials such as chlorhexidine gluconate, iodine, or quaternary ammonium compounds can effectively reduce bacterial concentration on hands.[2,20] Their rapid, broad-spectrum antimicrobial activity against gram-positive and gram-negative bacteria, tubercle bacilli, and a wide array of viruses is augmented by the fact that regrowth of bacteria on washed hands occurs only slowly. In recent years an increasing number of studies have investigated the clinical use of waterless, alcohol-based hand sanitizers in gel or rub delivery systems. These products were developed in part to overcome the longer times required for soap and water handwashing procedures and an observed lack of washing compliance by health care workers in clinical facilities. Investigation of these formulations in medical settings continues to be expanded and has shown promise in both improving compliance and decreasing observed infection rates.[10]

CHLORHEXIDINE

Chlorhexidine (see Chapter 45) was approved for use in surgical scrubs by the FDA in the mid-1970s and as a 0.12% oral rinse in the late 1980s. As a surgical scrub, 4% chlorhexidine solutions are fast acting like the iodophors and have the substantivity of hexachlorophene.[20] Chlorhexidine is highly effective against gram-positive organisms, less so against gram-negative organisms, and ineffective against tubercle bacilli, spores, and many viruses.

In Europe, 0.2% solutions of chlorhexidine have been used as oral rinses since the 1970s.[12] The effectiveness of chlorhexidine in oral rinses results primarily from its substantivity. The cationic nature of chlorhexidine allows it to bind to both hard and soft tissues within the oral cavity; it is then released over time to provide a continuing bacteriostatic effect. Used twice daily, these solutions have been shown to be effective in reducing plaque formation and gingivitis. The major side effects are staining of the teeth, an increase in calculus formation, and alteration in taste perception.[3] Two 0.12% chlorhexidine oral rinses have been approved by the FDA and are as clinically effective as the stronger 0.2% solution but with a significantly reduced incidence of side effects.[1]

SURFACE-ACTIVE AGENTS

Surface-active agents are compounds that produce a detergent effect because of their ability to interact noncovalently with membrane proteins and lipids. Anionic agents such as common soaps and dodecylsulfate phosphate detergents appear to be effective primarily because of their cleaning and emulsifying ability. Agents that possess specific antimicrobial activity are almost exclusively effective against only gram-positive bacteria.

Cationic agents, as exemplified by the quaternary ammonium compounds (e.g., benzalkonium chloride), were used for many years as cold sterilization solutions. Referring to them as *sterilizing solutions* was a grave misnomer because they are totally ineffective against bacterial spores, tubercle bacilli, many gram-negative bacteria, fungi, and viruses. Bioburden, hard water, and time reduce the effectiveness of these solutions against even gram-positive bacteria. As a result of these limitations, the Council on Dental Therapeutics of the American Dental Association (ADA) eliminated these compounds in 1978 as disinfectants from the ADA's Accepted Product List. Despite these drawbacks, a variety of surface disinfectant solutions and impregnated cloth wipes containing quaternary ammoniums are marketed. These preparations are good cleaning agents, are still marketed for their cleaning ability, and are often formulated with other agents serving as the primary broad-spectrum disinfectants. The cationic agents used in mouthrinses are discussed in Chapter 45. Cationic agents are also used as sore throat remedies.

OXIDIZING COMPOUNDS

Hydrogen peroxide is the most common of a number of oxidizing compounds that have been used as antiseptics in dentistry. Hydroxyl radicals released during decomposition of the parent molecule are believed to be primarily responsible for the microbicidal effect. Concentrations potentially useful for antisepsis (e.g., 3%) are active against vegetative bacteria; higher concentrations (10% to 30%) are sporicidal. These agents are also referred to as *oxygenating compounds* because they release molecular oxygen.

In combination with sodium bicarbonate, hydrogen peroxide was advocated for use against the anaerobic bacteria prevalent in periodontal disease. The basis for this use was the assumption that the oxygen released by the peroxide would be toxic to the anaerobic bacteria. The ubiquitous presence of peroxidase enzymes in the periodontal tissues and fluids quickly destroys any peroxide, resulting in little if any toxicity to the microorganisms present. The effervescent oxygen released, however, may assist in the debridement of soft tissue wounds.

Table • 46-3

Miscellaneous Uses of Disinfectants and Antiseptics

AGENT	FORMULATION (WT/VOLUME)	USE
Alcohol	70%	Solvent and adjuvant for other agents; prevention of bedsores
Parachlorophenol	Variable	Root canal debridement
Phenol	0.5% to 1.4%	Relief of sore throat
Eugenol	Variable	Relief of pulpal pain
Guaiacol	Variable	Relief of pupal pain
Sodium hypochlorite	5% solution	Root canal debridement
Iodine solution	8% to 9% iodine	Plaque-disclosing solution
Povidone-iodine	Solution with 1% available iodine	Plaque-disclosing solution
Formaldehyde	4% (10% formalin)	Fixative for biopsied tissue
Hydrogen peroxide	3%	Wound cleaning
	30%	Tooth bleaching

HEAVY METALS

Heavy metals, particularly mercury and silver compounds, have a long history as antimicrobial agents. Organic mercurials are still used in some countries as fumigants, but they have been replaced by more effective and less toxic compounds in dentistry and medicine. Silver nitrate was commonly used in dentistry to treat oral ulcers but is no longer used because it delays healing and alters cellular morphology. Silver nitrate eye drops remain useful in the prophylaxis of gonococcal infection in the newborn.

Tin, the stannous ion, is an effective antimicrobial. As a disinfectant, it is complexed with organic anions, forming triorganotins. The primary applications of these compounds are in industry and agriculture. In dentistry, stannous fluoride has once again become popular as a fluoride source in dentifrices, particularly in those marketed for their effect on gingival health. The ability of tin to inhibit both bacterial growth[15] and plaque formation[19] supported its initial use in dentifrices and as a topical fluorine salt. Subsequently, problems with stability, taste, and staining led to its replacement for a time by sodium fluoride and monofluorophosphate as a source of fluoride.

USES IN DENTISTRY

The importance of the role played by antiseptics and disinfectants in the practice of modern dentistry has never been greater. The battle to prevent cross-contamination and cross-infection by microbial pathogens must be pursued by all available means. The dental team can do much to reduce the presence of pathogenic organisms and thereby greatly enhance the potential for an uneventful recovery from dental procedures. Effective infection control protocols include thorough handwashing techniques with appropriate antiseptics, combined with appropriate barrier techniques (gloves, masks, eye protection, rubber dam), disposable covers for surfaces, disinfection of nonsterilizable surfaces and equipment, and heat sterilization of all compatible equipment. Disinfectants are an important tool in achieving effective infection control.

The range of antiseptics for home use in the control of oral microorganisms, plaque reduction, and the prevention of gingivitis has mushroomed in the last few years. New prerinses, dentifrices, and mouthrinses appear every day using new antiseptic compounds and reformulations of old ones. These agents and their uses are considered in Chapter 45.

Although this is not the focus of this chapter, compounds used for disinfection and antisepsis also find application in dentistry for purposes unrelated, in many cases, to their antimicrobial actions. These uses, some of which have been mentioned previously, are listed in Table 46-3.

Representative Antiseptics and Disinfectants

Nonproprietary (generic) name	*Proprietary (trade) name*
Halogens and Halogen-Releasing Compounds	
Chlorine-based	
Chlorine dioxide	Dent-A-Gene
Hypochlorite solution	Dispatch
Iodine-based	
Iodine solution	—
Iodine tincture	—
Iodoform gauze	NuGauze
Oxychlorosene	Clorpactin WCS-90
Povidone-iodine	Betadine, ACU-dyne, Aerodyne
Miscellaneous iodophors	Biocide, Iodo-Five, Surf-A-Cide, Wescodyne
Aldehydes	
Formaldehyde	Formalhyde-10
Glutaraldehyde	Banicide, Cidex 7, Cidex Plus, Multicide Plus, Omnicide, ProCide, Sterall, Vital Defense-D
Phenols	
Combined phenols in 57% ethanol	ProCide ES Spray, Coe Spray
Eugenol	—
Formocresol	Buckley's Formo Cresol
Hexachlorophene	pHisoHex, Septisol
Parachlorometaxylenol	Medical Lotion Soap
Phenol	Vicks Chloraseptic

Representative Antiseptics and Disinfectants—cont'd

Nonproprietary (generic) name	*Proprietary (trade) name*
o-Phenylphenol and *o*-benzyl-*p*-chlorophenol	Birex, Multicide, Omni II, Vital Defense
Phenylphenol in 67% to 79% ethanol or isopropanol	Lysol IC spray, MSD Surface Disinfectant
Triclosan	Septi-Soft, Septisol, Stridex Face Wash
Alcohols	
Ethanol	Alcare, Alco-Gel
Isopropyl alcohol	Stat-One Isopropyl Rubbing Alcohol
Alcohols and quaternary ammonium compounds	
Aseptic wipes	Metriwipes, Discide Ultra Wipes, Sani-Cloths
Biguanides	
Chlorhexidine	Dyna-Hex, Hibistat, Hibiclens, Peridex, PerioGard
Surface-active agents (cationic)	
Benzalkonium chloride	Benza, Mycocide, Zephiran
Benzethonium chloride	Critic-Aid, Puri-Clens
Cetyldimethylethyl ammonium bromide	Cetylcide
Cetylpyridinium chloride	Bactalin
Cetyltrimethyl ammonium bromide	Cetrimide B.P., Cetavlon
Methylbenzethonium chloride	in Orasept
Oxidizing compounds	
Hydrogen peroxide	Stat-One Hydrogen Peroxide
Carbamide peroxide (urea peroxide)	Cankaid, Gly-Oxide, Proxigel
Heavy metals	
Organic mercurials	
Merbromin	Mercurochrome
Nitromersol	Metaphen
Thimerosal	Aeroaid, Mersol
Silver compounds	
Silver nitrate	—
Silver protein	Argyrol S.S. 10%

CITED REFERENCES

1. Adams D, Addy M: Mouthrinses, *Adv Dent Res* 8:291-301, 1994.
2. Ali Y, Dolan MJ, Fendler EJ, et al: Alcohols. In Block SS, ed: *Disinfection, sterilization, and preservation*, ed 5, Philadelphia, 2001, Lippincott, Williams & Wilkins.
3. al-Tannir MA, Goodman HS: A review of chlorhexidine and its use in special populations, *Spec Care Dent* 14:116-122, 1994.
4. Araki K, Suda H, Barbosa SV, et al: Reduced cytotoxicity of a root canal sealer through eugenol substitution, *J Endod* 19:554-557, 1993.
5. Centers for Disease Control and Prevention: Recommended infection-control practices for dentistry, 1993, *MMWR* 42(RR-8):1-12, 1993.
6. Cleveland JL, Gooch BF, Bolyard EA, et al: TB infection control recommendations from the CDC, 1994: considerations for dentistry. United States Centers for Disease Control and Prevention, *J Am Dent Assoc* 126:593-599, 1995.
7. Cottone JA, Terezhalmy GZ, Molinari JA: *Practical infection control in dentistry*, ed 2, Baltimore, 1996, Williams & Wilkins.
8. Crawford JJ: State-of-the-art: practical infection control in dentistry, *J Am Dent Assoc* 110:629-633, 1985.
9. Dychdala GR: Chlorine and chlorine compounds. In Block SS, ed: *Disinfection, sterilization, and preservation*, ed 5, Philadelphia, 2001, Lippincott, Williams & Wilkins.
10. Fendler EJ, Ali Y, Hammond BS, et al: The impact of alcohol hand sanitizer use on infection rates in an extended care facility, *Am J Infect Control* 30:226-233, 2002.
11. Gannon PF, Bright P, Campbell M, et al: Occupational asthma due to glutaraldehyde and formaldehyde in endoscopy and x-ray departments, *Thorax* 50:156-159, 1995.
12. Gjermo P, Bonesvoll P, Rølla G: Relationship between plaque-inhibiting effect and retention of chlorhexidine in the human oral cavity, *Arch Oral Biol* 19:1031-1034, 1974.
13. Goddard PA, McCue KA: Phenolic compounds. In Block SS, ed: *Disinfection, sterilization, and preservation*, ed 5, Philadelphia, 2001, Lippincott, Williams & Wilkins.
14. Infection control: its evolution to the current standard precautions, *J Am Dent Assoc* 134:569-574, 2003.
15. Jordan SL: The correct use of glutaraldehyde in the healthcare environment, *Gastroenterol Nurs* 18:143-145, 1995.
16. Kimbrough RD: Review of the toxicity of hexachlorophene, including its neurotoxicity, *J Clin Pharmacol* 13:439-444, 1973.
17. Kjaerheim V, Barkvoll P, Waaler SM, et al: Triclosan inhibits histamine-induced inflammation in human skin, *J Clin Periodontol* 22:423-426, 1995.
18. Kjaerheim V, Waaler SM, Kalvik A: Experiments with two-phase plaque-inhibiting mouthrinses, *Eur J Oral Sci* 103:179-181, 1995.
19. Larson EL: APIC guideline for handwashing and hand antisepsis in health care settings, *Am J Infect Control* 23:251-269, 1995.
20. Lowbury EJL, Lilly HA: Use of 4% chlorhexidine detergent solution (Hibiclens) and other methods of skin disinfection, *Br Med J* 1:510-515, 1973.
21. Mandel ID: Antimicrobial mouthrinses: overview and update, *J Am Dent Assoc* 125(suppl 2):2S-10S, 1994.
22. Mbithi JN, Springthorpe VS, Satar SA, et al: Bactericidal, virucidal, and mycobactericidal activities of reused alkaline glutaraldehyde in an endoscopy unit, *J Clin Microbiol* 31:2988-2995, 1993.

23. McLaughlin JK: Formaldehyde and cancer: a critical review, *Int Arch Occup Environ Health* 66:295-301, 1994.
24. Molinari JA, Gleason MJ, Cottone JA, et al: Cleaning and disinfectant properties of dental surface disinfectants, *J Am Dent Assoc* 117:179-182, 1988.
25. Piskin B, Turkun M: Stability of various sodium hypochlorite solutions, *J Endod* 21:253-255, 1995.
26. Rutala WA: APIC guideline for selection and use of disinfectants, *Am J Infect Control* 24:313-342, 1996.
27. Stonehill AA, Krop S, Borick PM: Buffered glutaraldehyde: a new chemical sterilizing solution, *Am J Hosp Pharm* 20:458-465, 1963.

PART III

Special Subjects in Pharmacology and Therapeutics

CHAPTER • 47

Analgesic Use for Effective Pain Control*

Paul J. Desjardins and Elliot V. Hersh

Fear of pain is a significant reason why many people avoid seeking dental care. No matter how successful or how effectively performed, most dental surgical procedures produce tissue trauma and release potent mediators of inflammation and pain. In the past, postoperative pain was thought to be inevitable and harmless. We now know that unrelieved pain after surgery or trauma has negative physical and psychologic consequences. Acute pain is often associated with a reactive anxiety and an increase in sympathetic nervous system activity, resulting in tachycardia, hypertension, diaphoresis, mydriasis, and pallor. A patient with severe tooth or jaw pain may avoid eating or drinking and may become malnourished and dehydrated. Severe chest, abdominal, or back pain may lead to shallow breathing and cough suppression in an attempt to "splint" the injured site, followed by retained pulmonary secretions and pneumonia.[13,28] Unrelieved pain may also delay the return of normal gastric and bowel function in the postoperative patient.[31] Fortunately, pain is preventable or controllable in an overwhelming majority of cases if managed aggressively.

Undertreatment of pain is a significant medical problem. Numerous clinical surveys have shown that postoperative pain is often inadequately treated because of undermedication, leaving patients to suffer needlessly.[11,24] Recognition of the widespread inadequacy of pain management and the detrimental effects of untreated pain has led to corrective efforts in numerous health care disciplines involved with pain management. These efforts culminated in 1992, when the Agency for Health Care Policy and Research, a division of the United States Public Health Service, published its *Clinical Practice Guideline* [for] *Acute Pain Management: Operative or Medical Procedures and Trauma*.[2] This guideline represents the efforts of a multidisciplinary panel of expert clinicians and researchers. It provides an excellent framework for the care of patients with acute pain and includes a section on pain control specifically for dental surgery.

PAIN CLASSIFICATION

Successful treatment of painful conditions with analgesics requires a basic understanding of their pathophysiologic characteristics. Painful conditions can be divided into two basic categories: nociceptive pain and neuropathic pain, categories based on the condition's underlying pathophysiologic features. *Nociceptive pain* is a result of mechanical, thermal, or chemical activation of nociceptive afferent receptors and can be classified as either somatic or visceral in origin. Somatic nociception involves pathologic conditions of the skin, muscles, fascia, and bones and is well localized. Examples include the pain associated with cavity preparation or periodontitis. In both conditions, inflammatory mediators may sensitize or activate nociceptive receptors, resulting in transduction of the noxious stimulus into electrical and biochemical signals between neurons. The electrical signal is then conducted to the brain for interpretation. Visceral nociceptive pain is poorly localized, may be referred to superficial somatic regions, and involves pathologic conditions in deep, visceral tissues. An example is angina resulting from myocardial ischemia, which can be referred to the jaw, neck, or arm.

Neuropathic pain is thought to be a result of aberrant somatosensory activity either in the peripheral nervous system or the central nervous system (CNS) (see Chapter 23). It is frequently characterized by paroxysmal shooting or electrical shocklike pains, often on a background of burning or constricting sensation. Examples of neuropathic pain encountered in the orofacial region include trigeminal neuralgia and postherpetic neuralgia. Orofacial pain of neuropathic origin generally requires more sophisticated diagnostic testing and management; this sort of care is frequently available at specialized clinical practices.

Pain may also be characterized as acute or chronic based on its temporal and other characteristics. Acute pain frequently has a known cause, has identifiable tissue damage, usually subsides as healing takes place, and has a predictable endpoint. Acute pain is associated with anxiety and the physiologic "flight or fight" responses of increased pulse and respiratory rate. In contrast, chronic pain is of greater than 3 to 6 months' duration, and patients with chronic pain do not usually manifest the physiologic arousal seen with acute pain because the body has adapted to the pain state. However, they may exhibit reactive depression and decreased function.

PAIN ASSESSMENT

Successful assessment and control of pain depend, in part, on establishing effective communication between the dentist and the patient. Patients should be informed that pain relief is an important part of their health care. Because pain is a subjective phenomenon, the care provider must accept that the patient's self-report is the single most accurate and reliable indicator of the existence and intensity of pain and any resultant distress.[2] This orientation is reflected in a commonly cited definition of pain: *Pain is whatever the experiencing person says it is and exists whenever he says it does.*[20] Self-report measurement tools such as adjective or numerical rating scales or visual analogue scales can assist the patient in quantifying and characterizing the pain (Figure 47-1).

*The authors with to recognize Dr. Warren Vallerand for his past contributions to this chapter. See the Acknowledgments.

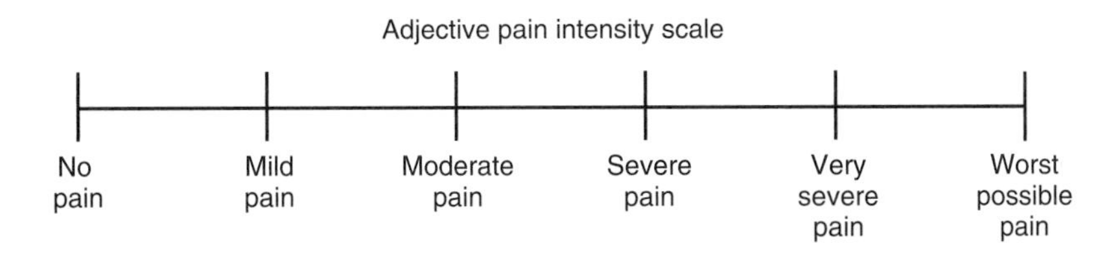

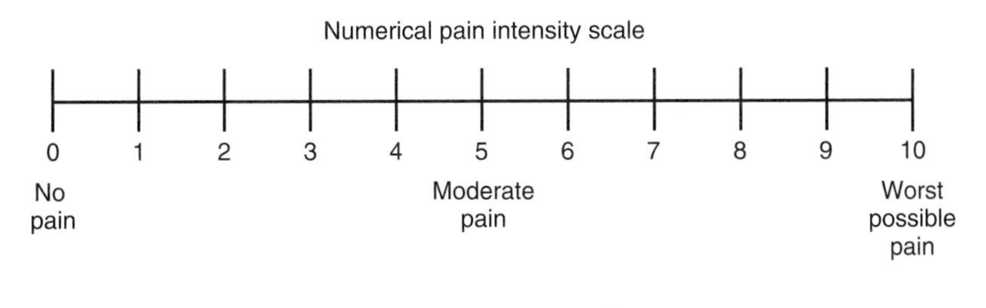

Visual analog scale (VAS)

No pain

Worst possible pain

Fig. 47-1 Pain intensity scales. A 10-cm baseline is recommended for the visual analog scale and for the other scales if used for graphic rating (i.e., linear measurement of patient responses).

These tools are reliable, valid, and easy for the patient and the dentist or assistant to use. They may be administered by showing a diagram to the patient and asking the patient to indicate the appropriate rating. Some tools may also be used by simply asking the patient for a verbal response (e.g., "On a scale of 0 to 10, with 0 as no pain and 10 as the worst pain possible, how would you rate your pain?"). Patients who may have difficulty communicating require particular attention. This group includes patients who are cognitively impaired; psychologically or severely emotionally disturbed patients; young children and the very old; and patients whose language, level of education, or cultural background differs significantly from that of the health care team.

Assessment of the patient's pain is a crucial part of initial evaluation to estimate analgesic requirements. To determine the adequacy of the chosen analgesic regimen, the clinician must also assess pain intensity and pain relief at the peak of the analgesic effect and at regular intervals after the initiation of analgesic treatment.[7]

MISCONCEPTIONS REGARDING PAIN AND ANALGESICS

A significant barrier to the effective use of analgesics in managing pain involves several misconceptions regarding pain and analgesia held by both patients and health care providers.

Misconception 1: Patients who are in pain always have observable signs. Although many patients in acute pain exhibit evidence of anxiety, distress, or decreased function, many do not. Such overt pain behaviors also may not be seen at all in patients attempting to adapt to, and cope with, persistent pain. Expecting patients to display these pain behaviors in order to believe the patient's complaint of pain and making the decision to dispense analgesics contingent on the display of these behaviors only serve to reinforce pain behaviors that may actually interfere with recovery. To treat the pain effectively, the clinician must first believe the patient's complaint of pain.

Misconception 2: Obvious pathology, test results, and the type of surgery determine the existence and the intensity of pain. Although the ability to identify a pathologic process underlying a patient's pain complaint is a key element in planning and initiating definitive treatment, failure to identify the source of a patient's pain does not necessarily mean that it does not exist. Patients with chronic, neuropathic pain frequently present such diagnostic challenges. As medical and diagnostic technology progresses, we are better able to understand the mechanisms underlying disease processes that might have gone undiagnosed, or misdiagnosed, in the past. Failure to identify an organic source for a patient's pain does not mean that the pain does not exist.

Misconception 3: Patients should wait as long as possible before taking a pain medication. This period of abstinence will teach them to have a better tolerance for pain. Pain that is untreated often escalates in severity and disability. Without treatment, sensory input from injured tissue reaches spinal cord neurons and causes subsequent responses to be enhanced. Pain receptors in the periphery also become more sensitive after injury. Studies have demonstrated long-lasting changes in cells within the spinal cord pain pathways after brief painful stimuli.[5] These physiologic studies confirm long-standing clinical impressions that established pain is more difficult to suppress.[2,5,12] Aggressive pain prevention and control that occurs before, during, and after a painful event such as dental surgery can yield both short- and long-term benefits. Patients should be encouraged to use analgesics before pain becomes severe and difficult to control.

CHOICE OF ANALGESIC REGIMEN

Pharmacologic control of pain can be directed at any of three nociceptive processes: the initiation of impulses, propagation of those impulses, and perception of painful stimuli.

Nonsteroidal antiinflammatory drugs (NSAIDs) are thought to act primarily at the site of initiation of nociceptive impulses. Although separating their antiinflammatory effects from their analgesic effects is difficult, nonopioid drugs such as the salicylates, other NSAIDs, and cyclooxygenase (COX)-2 inhibitors work predominantly in the periphery by preventing the synthesis and release of inflammatory mediators that sensitize nociceptive receptors to other algesic mediators, such as bradykinin, and to physical forces. Recent studies suggest that NSAIDs may also have central effects.[4,17] Acetaminophen has been shown to have analgesic and antipyretic properties, but it lacks significant antiinflammatory effects. Acetaminophen appears to exert its effects both in the CNS and in the periphery.[1,21,29]

Local anesthetics can be administered topically or parenterally to block the propagation of nerve impulses originating from nociceptive stimuli at a peripheral site so that they do not reach the spinal cord or brain. Administration of long-acting local anesthetics can have significant value in delaying the onset of pain after oral surgery procedures and decreasing the overall level of discomfort in the immediate recovery period. The systemic use of local anesthetics also has some use in the management of chronic pain.

Opioids decrease the perception of pain in the CNS. The opioid analgesics act in the CNS at receptors in the spinal cord, rostroventral medulla, and periaqueductal gray matter. These anatomic loci are considered important to the perception of pain (see Chapter 20). Laboratory studies have also identified and characterized opioid receptors in peripheral tissue. This finding has, in turn, led to clinical studies that have identified opioids as contributors to antinociceptive responses in the peripheral nervous system.[16,22]

Analgesic Selection

Before initiating treatment with analgesics, the practitioner must choose a specific drug or drugs, each with its own route of administration, dose, and frequency. Given the myriad of analgesics available to choose from, how does one select the most effective analgesic? It is important to analyze each situation and individualize the analgesic regimen to best fit each patient's current condition.

The cause of the pain and the pain severity are the most important pieces of information in choosing an analgesic regimen. Equally important, and often overlooked, is the patient's recent and past history of painful conditions and how they were treated. A patient who has had episodes of pain treated with analgesics in the past may be acutely aware of which analgesics are likely to be most effective in a new situation and which are not, so asking the patient which analgesic has worked best in the past and which they would prefer is appropriate. Some practitioners may not be comfortable with this approach because they believe that it amounts to the patient dictating treatment and may arouse suspicion regarding drug-seeking behavior. However, it is important to remember that the patient is considered the authority on his or her pain.[2] Unless the requested drug is inappropriate, the patient's judgment and preference should be taken into account. This strategy increases the likelihood of compliance with the prescribed regimen.

In considering the choice of analgesic, it is reasonable to estimate the degree of pain that might be anticipated after a certain procedure based on the clinical and personal experience of the practitioner and to base the choice of analgesic on that estimate. Of course, the empirical nature of this approach must always be kept in mind. Inadequate pain relief may indicate the need for an increase in dose, more frequent administration, or a different drug. A common misconception is that a given stimulus will produce the same amount of pain in different patients. No data support this assumption. Pain threshold and tolerance and analgesic requirements vary widely among patients.

Local anesthetics

In addition to providing the pain control required to carry out most operative dentistry or dentoalveolar surgery, local anesthetics may also decrease pain after treatment. The perioperative administration of a long-acting anesthetic agent (such as etidocaine or bupivacaine) as an addition to or substitute for an agent with shorter duration (such as lidocaine) can delay the onset of postprocedural pain after dental surgery. Because of the potential for self-inflicted injury and a lack of relevant clinical data, the long-acting agents should not be used in children younger than 10 years.

Nonopioid analgesics

This category is composed of various drugs (e.g., NSAIDs, COX-2 inhibitors, acetaminophen) that have a similar mechanism of action and share clinically important analgesic, antiinflammatory, and antipyretic properties. These agents differ from opioid analgesics in the following ways: (1) there is a ceiling effect to the analgesia; (2) they do not produce tolerance or physical dependence; (3) they are antipyretic; and (4) they possess both antiinflammatory as well as analgesic properties, except for acetaminophen, which has minimal antiinflammatory activity. Pharmacologic management of mild to moderate dental and orofacial pain should begin, unless there is a contraindication, with a nonopioid analgesic drug. As a general rule, any analgesic regimen should include a nonopioid drug, even if pain is severe enough to require the addition of an opioid. Most controlled clinical trials in postoperative dental pain directly comparing full doses of aspirin, acetaminophen, ibuprofen, and other NSAIDs with oral doses of single-entity opioids such as codeine 60 mg or oxycodone 5 mg have demonstrated the superiority of the nonopioids in analgesic efficacy.

Nonopioids are most effective in treating postprocedural pain when given before the procedure or immediately after a short procedure, thus preventing the synthesis of prostaglandins that quickly follow the surgical insult. The delayed use of NSAIDs postoperatively inhibits the subsequent prostaglandin synthesis and provides analgesia, but it does not interfere with the effects of those prostaglandins already produced. Preoperative administration of NSAIDs or COX-2 inhibitors delays the onset of postoperative dental pain and lessens its severity and subsequent analgesic requirements (Figure 47-2).[8,9,15]

The NSAIDs all share a qualitatively similar side-effect profile. However, with the exception of true allergic reactions; bronchoconstriction in asthmatics (see Chapter 21); and prior gastrointestinal perforations, ulcerations, or serious bleeding reactions, a patient's inability to tolerate one specific NSAID or COX-II inhibitor does not mean the patient will be intolerant of all other NSAIDs. Also, patients may vary in their relative analgesic response to various NSAIDs. Therefore if a patient does not respond to a particular drug at the maximum therapeutic dose, an alternative NSAID should be considered.

The oral route of administration is preferred for nonopioids. Some patients, such as young children or patients with intermaxillary fixation after maxillofacial surgery or trauma, are unable to swallow tablets or capsules. For these patients, liquid formulations of acetaminophen or ibuprofen should be considered. For the rare dental patient who is unable to take any medications by mouth, parenteral (ketorolac) or rectal (acetaminophen, aspirin) dosage forms are available. Injectable formulations of novel COX-2 inhibitors are under development.

Distinct advantages for the COX-2 inhibitors over traditional NSAIDs include a lower incidence of serious upper gastrointestinal toxicity (symptomatic ulcers, bleeding, and perforation), decreased nephrotoxicity, and a lack of effect on platelet aggregation. This improved therapeutic index

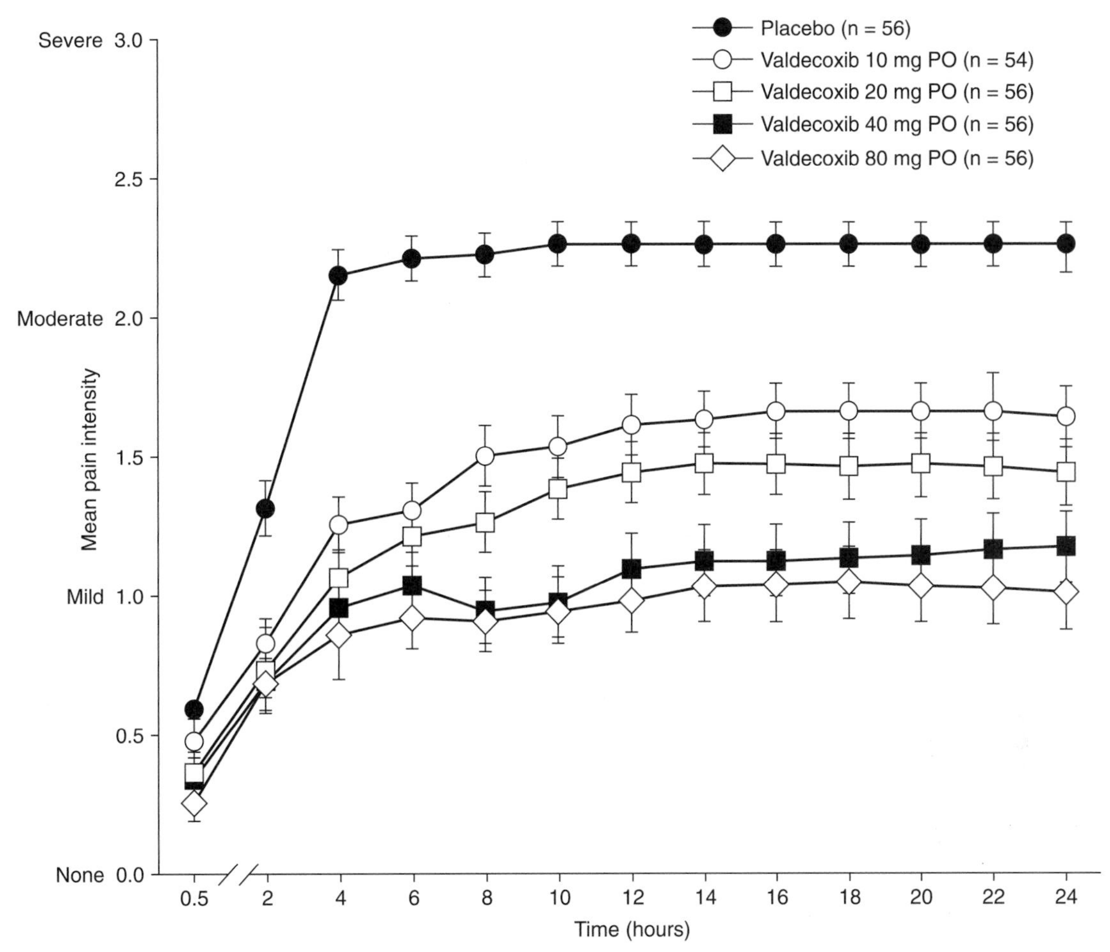

Fig. 47-2 Effect of single preoperative doses of the COX-2 inhibitor valdecoxib on mean pain intensity after dental impaction surgery. *Brackets* indicate the standard error. (From Desjardins PJ, Shu VS, Recker DP, et al: A single preoperative oral dose of valdecoxib, a new cyclooxygenase-2 specific inhibitor, relieves post-oral surgery or bunionectomy pain, *Anesthesiology* 97:565-575, 2002.)

accounts for a significant increase in their prescribing, especially for chronic inflammatory diseases. Full adult doses of rofecoxib have been demonstrated to be at least as effective as full adult doses of traditional NSAIDs (see Chapter 21).

Opioid analgesics

Opioid analgesics are added to nonopioids to manage pain that is moderate to severe or that does not respond to nonopioids alone. Opioids differ from the nonopioids in that there is no ceiling effect on their analgesic response. The only dosing limitation is based on side effects. Although injectable opioids and oral opioid combinations are quite effective for management of moderate to severe acute pain, they are frequently underutilized and prescribed at subtherapeutic doses as a result of misconceptions and fears regarding their use. Fear of possible sedation or respiratory depression causes some practitioners to underprescribe and underdose opioids. These adverse events rarely occur when appropriate starting doses are used and then titrated to effect based on the patient's analgesic response and side effects. Patients vary greatly in their analgesic dose requirements and responses to opioid analgesics. Relative potency estimates provide a rational basis for selecting the appropriate dose to initiate analgesic therapy or when switching from one opioid to another or from one route of administration to another.

Physical dependence and tolerance can occur in virtually all patients taking opioid analgesics for a prolonged period. Fortunately, in the overwhelming majority of instances in which opioids or opioid combinations are used in dentistry, the duration of therapy is so short (generally 7 days or less) that these clinical phenomena are not seen. Tolerance is managed with careful upward titration of the dose until adequate pain relief is reobtained. The effects of physical dependence are easily avoided by the gradual tapering of opioids on discontinuation of therapy as opposed to abrupt withdrawal. Addiction is a phenomenon that rarely occurs in patients taking opioid analgesics for pain (see Chapter 51).[30] The overwhelming majority of patients taking pain medication stop taking the medication when the pain stops. Early reports on the incidence of medical patients with addiction problems were fraught with methodologic flaws and significantly overestimated the risk.[19,27] Recent studies provide a more accurate estimate. In 1980, the Boston Collaborative Drug Surveillance Project identified only four cases of addiction among 11,882 hospitalized patients with no history of substance abuse who received at least one dose of an opioid.[26] A national survey of burn units found no cases of addiction in close to 10,000 patients treated for burn pain.[25] Another study surveying patients attending a headache clinic revealed that only three of 2369 patients had a management problem with analgesics used to treat intermittent headaches.[23]

Opioid analgesics include both pure agonists, such as codeine and oxycodone, and agonist/antagonists, such as pentazocine and butorphanol. As a general rule, the agonist/antagonists should not be used as first-line therapy. There is no convincing evidence that these drugs offer any advantage over the pure opioid agonists. Agonist/antagonists become less effective at high doses because they have a ceiling effect (see Chapter 20), frequently cause dysphoria, and may cause confusion and hallucinations. In addition, they may cause withdrawal symptoms when given to patients physically dependent on opioid agonists. On occasion, they may be useful in treating individuals unable to tolerate other opioids.[3]

In 1990, the World Health Organization proposed a stepwise approach for the management of cancer pain.[7] This approach (Figure 47-3) has subsequently come to be recommended for the treatment of noncancer pain as well. The first step, representing treatment of mild pain, is to administer a nonopioid drug. In many dental surgical procedures, NSAIDs alone can achieve excellent pain control.[6,10] Nonopioid therapy should be considered the cornerstone for management of acute dental pain. Pain that does not respond adequately to nonopioid agents should be treated with the combination of a nonopioid and an opioid such as codeine, hydrocodone, or oxycodone. Even when insufficient alone to control pain, NSAIDs can reduce the dose of opioid required to achieve relief.[14,18] More severe pain, or pain that persists, should be treated with a combination of a nonopioid and a more potent opioid, such as morphine or hydromorphone. Adjuvant agents such as certain anticonvulsants or tricyclic antidepressants may be added when indicated. Common indications in dentistry include the treatment of neuropathic pain and some chronic orofacial pain conditions (see Chapter 23).

Because most dental care is provided to ambulatory dental outpatients, the oral administration of opioid analgesics is preferred whenever possible. It is convenient and inexpensive. Even severe postsurgical pain can be effectively treated with orally administered opioids in the proper doses. For the patient who is unable to swallow a tablet or capsule, numerous liquid formulations of opioids are available (e.g., codeine, hydrocodone, oxycodone). Peak drug effects (including side effects) occur 1.5 to 2 hours after the oral administration of most opioids (sustained-release tablets excepted). Therefore patients may take a second opioid dose safely 2 hours after the first dose if the pain persists and side effects are mild at that time.[3,7] For patients unable to take medications by mouth, the intravenous, intramuscular, or rectal routes of administration can be considered. Use of the intravenous or intramuscular route to deliver analgesics is almost exclusively limited to inpatient hospital settings. Of the two routes, intravenous administration is preferred. Intravenous bolus administration provides the most rapid and predictable onset of effect. Time to peak effect varies with drug lipid solubility, ranging from 1 to 5 minutes for fentanyl to 15 to 30 minutes for morphine. Although commonly used, intramuscular injections can themselves cause pain and trauma and may deter patients from requesting pain medication. Also, absorption from intramuscular sites can be erratic and variable. Several opioids are available in rectal suppository form (e.g., hydromorphone, morphine). Sustained-release opioids (e.g., controlled-release morphine and oxycodone) appear to have little role in the management of acute dental pain.

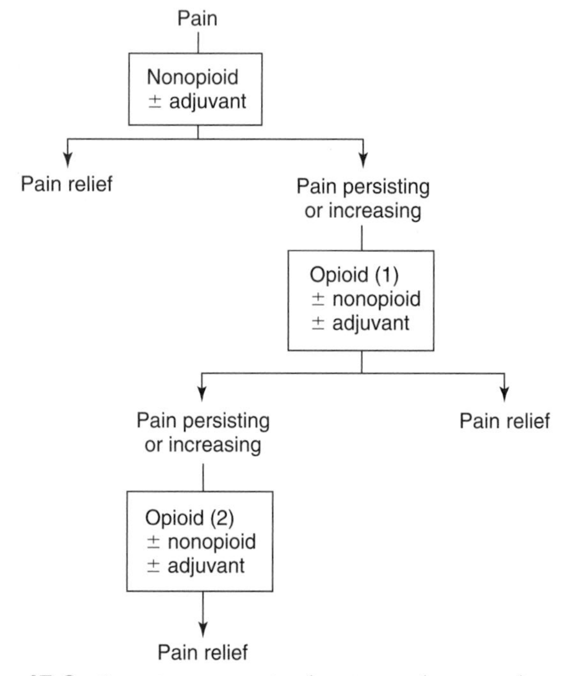

Fig. 47-3 Stepwise process in choosing analgesic medication. Opioid *(1)* indicates a standard oral opioid in a conventional dose; *(2)* indicates increasing doses or a change in opioid to increase the analgesic effect. (Based on recommendations of the World Health Organization as described in Deglin JH, Vallerand AH: *Davis's Drug guide for nurses,* ed 5, Philadelphia, 1997, FA Davis.)

As mentioned previously, opioids should almost always be administered with nonopioids for maximum pain relief in dental pain. Many opioids are marketed in combination with a nonopioid, and it is the latter component that limits the dose. For example, the upper dose limit for acetaminophen is 4000 mg/day. Therefore for combinations containing 325 mg of acetaminophen, the maximum number of tablets per day is 12. For combinations containing 500 mg of acetaminophen, the maximum number of tablets per day is eight. In children who weigh less than 45 kg, the limit is 90 mg/kg of acetaminophen.

One controversial area of change in pain therapeutics is in the use of potent opioids in patients with severe or unremitting chronic pain from either malignant or nonmalignant disease. Pain specialists have advocated the use of potent opioids in such patients when all other reasonable therapeutic approaches have failed. Special considerations and management approaches, including documenting failed approaches, closely monitoring refill records, and having patients sign contracts with the health care provider, are thought to be essential to avoid future medical and legal challenges to the patient and provider.

Principles of Analgesic Use

Analgesics should be administered initially on a regular time schedule. For example, if the patient is likely to have pain requiring analgesics for 48 hours after dental surgery, analgesics might be ordered every 4 hours while awake, not as needed, for the first 36 hours. This schedule provides more stable plasma concentrations of the agent with less breakthrough pain. If only as-needed medications are used, several hours and higher doses may be required to relieve pain, leading to a cycle of undermedication and pain alternating with periods of overmedication and unnecessary adverse effects. Later in the postoperative course, as the patient's analgesic dose requirement diminishes, dosing may be switched to an as-needed basis.

Children should also be given adequate doses of analgesics. Children may not communicate their pain effectively and are frequently undermedicated for pain. The clinical effects and pharmacokinetics of opioids in children older than 6 months are approximately the same as in adults. Starting doses of opioids and nonopioids may be calculated according to weight. Aspirin should not be used in children because of the potential for Reye's syndrome.

Dentists should be familiar with several analgesics in both the opioid and nonopioid categories. Different patients vary greatly in their response to, and ability to tolerate, different agents. For this reason, it is important to be familiar with the recommended dose, side-effect profile, and time course of several agents in each category.

Patients should be followed closely, particularly when beginning or changing analgesic regimens. Analgesics are more beneficial if the clinician monitors pain relief and adverse effects frequently and adjusts the regimen as needed to optimize therapy. This monitoring is particularly important when using an agent or combination with which the doctor has little or no experience or when changing from one analgesic to another.

Although pain is a common occurrence in patients seeking or undergoing dental care, it is generally manageable and often avoidable. Accurate assessment, methodical preventive regimens, and aggressive treatment are the tools required to keep pain at a minimum. Rational clinical practice guidelines[2] and equianalgesic charts allow practitioners to determine the appropriate analgesic regimen and dose for each patient.

Cited References

1. Abbadie JC, Besson JM: Chronic treatment with aspirin or acetaminophen reduce both the development of polyarthritis and Fos-like immunoreactivity in rat lumbar spinal cord, *Pain* 57:45-54, 1994.
2. Acute Pain Management Guideline Panel: *Acute pain management: operative or medical procedures and trauma. Clinical practice guideline, no. 1*, AHCPR Pub No 92-0032, Rockville, MD, 1992, U.S. Department of Health and Human Services, Public Health Service, Agency for Health Care Policy and Research.
3. American Pain Society: *Principles of analgesic use in the treatment of acute pain and cancer pain*, ed 3, Skokie, IL, 1992, American Pain Society.
4. Chapman V, Dickenson AH: The spinal and peripheral roles of bradykinin and prostaglandins in nociceptive processing in the rat, *Eur J Pharmacol* 219:427-433, 1992.
5. Coderre TJ, Katz J, Vaccarino AL, et al: Contribution of central neuroplasticity to pathological pain: review of clinical and experimental evidence, *Pain* 52:259-285, 1993.
6. Davie IT, Slawson KB, Burt RA: A double-blind comparison of parenteral morphine, placebo, and oral fenoprofen in management of postoperative pain, *Anesth Analg* 61:1002-1005, 1982.
7. Deglin JH, Vallerand AH: *Davis's Drug guide for nurses*, ed 5, Philadelphia, 1997, FA Davis.
8. Desjardins PJ, Dhadda S, Hubbard RC, et al: Preoperative valdecoxib, a COX-2 specific inhibitor, provides effective and long lasting analgesia following bunionectomy surgery [abstract], *Anesthesiology* 95:A811, 2001.
9. Desjardins PJ, Vincent SS, Recker DP, et al: A single preoperative oral dose of valdecoxib, a new cyclooxygenase-2 specific inhibitor relieves post-oral surgery or bunionectomy pain, *Anesthesiology* 97:565-575, 2002.
10. Dionne RA, Berthold CW: Therapeutic uses of nonsteroidal anti-inflammatory drugs in dentistry, *Crit Rev Oral Biol Med* 12:315-330, 2001.
11. Donovan M, Dillon P, McGuire L: Incidence and characteristics of pain in a sample of medical-surgical inpatients, *Pain* 30:69-78, 1987.
12. Gordon SM, Dionne RA, Brahim J, et al: Blockade of peripheral neuronal barrages reduces post-operative pain, *Pain* 70:209-215, 1997.
13. Hewlett AM, Branthwaite MA: Postoperative pulmonary function, *Br J Anaesth* 47:102-107, 1975.
14. Hodsman NB, Burns J, Blyth A, et al: The morphine sparing effects of diclofenac sodium following abdominal surgery, *Anaesthesia* 42:1005-1008, 1987.
15. Jackson DL, Moore PA, Hargreaves KM: Preoperative nonsteroidal anti-inflammatory medication for the prevention of postoperative dental pain, *J Am Dent Assoc* 119:641-647, 1989.
16. Joshi GP, McCarroll SM, O'Brien TM, et al: Intraarticular analgesia following knee arthroscopy, *Anesth Analg* 76:333-336, 1993.
17. Malmberg AB, Yaksh TL: Antinociceptive actions of spinal nonsteroidal anti-inflammatory agents on the formalin test in the rat, *J Pharmacol Exp Ther* 263:136-146, 1992.
18. Martens M: A significant decrease of narcotic drug dosage after orthopaedic surgery. A double-blind study with naproxen, *Acta Orthop Belg* 48:900-906, 1982.
19. Maruta T, Swanson DW, Finlayson RE: Drug abuse and dependency in patients with chronic pain, *Mayo Clin Proc* 54:241-244, 1979.
20. McCaffery M, Beebe A: *Pain: clinical manual for nursing practice*, St Louis, 1989, Mosby.
21. McQueen DS, Iggo A, Birrel GJ, et al: Effects of paracetamol and aspirin on neural activity of joint mechanonociceptors in adjuvant arthritis, *Br J Pharmacol* 104:178-182, 1991.
22. McSwiney MM, Joshi GP, Kenny P, et al: Analgesia following arthroscopic knee surgery. A controlled study of intra-articular morphine, bupivacaine or both combined, *Anaesth Intensive Care* 21:201-203, 1993.
23. Medina JL, Diamond S: Drug dependency in patients with chronic headaches, *Headache* 17:12-14, 1977.
24. Oden R: Acute postoperative pain: incidence, severity, and the etiology of inadequate treatment, *Anesthesiol Clin North Am* 7:1-15, 1989.
25. Perry S, Heidrich G: Management of pain during debridement: a survey of U.S. burn units, *Pain* 13:267-280, 1982.
26. Porter J, Jick H: Addiction rare in patients treated with narcotics, *N Engl J Med* 302:123, 1980.
27. Rayport M: Experience in the management of patients medically addicted to narcotics, *JAMA* 156:684-691, 1954.
28. Sydow F-W: The influence of anesthesia and postoperative analgesic management of lung function, *Acta Chir Scand* 550(suppl):159-165, 1989.
29. Tjølsen A, Lund A, Hole K: Antinociceptive effect of paracetamol in rats is partly dependent on spinal serotonergic systems, *Eur J Pharmacol* 193:193-201, 1991.
30. Vallerand AH: Street addicts and patients with pain: similarities and differences, *Clin Nurse Spec* 8:11-15, 1994.
31. Wattwil M: Postoperative pain relief and gastrointestinal motility, *Acta Chir Scand* 550(suppl):140-145, 1989.

CHAPTER • 48

Management of Fear and Anxiety

Daniel A. Haas

Fear and anxiety of dental procedures are common emotions. The severity ranges widely, with mild apprehension being reported by as many as 75% of the population[62] and severe anxiety, leading to avoidance of dental treatment, affecting 6% to 20%.[23,25,26,44,52] Although mild fear may have only a minor effect on oral health, true phobia can cause patients to avoid treatment in spite of significant symptoms and to have detrimental consequences for their overall health.[9] Approximately 40% of the population do not receive routine dental care, with apprehension being cited as the most common reason.[5] These patients often require special nonpharmacologic or pharmacologic approaches to allow dental procedures to be carried out. These pharmacologic approaches involve drugs that produce effects ranging from sedation to anesthesia.

Dentistry has historically been at the forefront in the development of anesthetic techniques to manage fear and anxiety. As described in Chapter 17, two dentists, Horace Wells and William Morton, were largely responsible for the clinical introduction of general anesthesia. The first description of nitrous oxide (N_2O) as a sedative, as opposed to a general anesthetic, appeared in a textbook on anesthesia for dentistry published in 1908.[18] The modern form of N_2O and oxygen sedation evolved in the 1940s and 1950s, and this practice has become a standard component of the predoctoral dental curriculum.[4] Intravenous anesthesia with hexobarbital was pioneered by the English dentist S.L. Drummond-Jackson in the 1930s. Shortly after World War II, Harold Krogh and Adrian Hubbell developed the use of thiopental for oral surgery. Intravenous conscious sedation was introduced by Niels Jorgensen in 1945.

Behavioral or psychologic techniques to manage anxiety in the dental patient are unquestionably important, but their detailed description lies beyond the scope of this textbook. The purpose of this chapter is to provide a summary of the pharmacologic approaches to the management of fear and anxiety in the dental patient, with emphasis on the administration of conscious sedation. Complete understanding of this subject requires comprehension of the pharmacologic features of the specific drugs, as described in other chapters.

GENERAL PRINCIPLES

Indications for Use

The primary indication for pharmacologic methods of patient management is the presence of anxiety, fear, or phobia sufficient to prevent the delivery of needed dental care. *Anxiety* may be defined as a stress response to an ill-defined or anticipated situation[49] and may consist of patterns of autonomic arousal with thoughts of fear and feelings of threat.[57] Dental anxiety may be related to specific dental procedures or may be precipitated by a mere visit to the dentist's office. Although anxiety of dentistry usually originates from past experiences as a child,[42] it may develop in adulthood and not be associated with any previous adverse event.[69]

Fear is defined as an emotional response to a perceived immediate threat.[27,60] Fear of dentistry may evolve from many sources, including past traumatic experiences, concerns about physical loss and disfigurement, observation of anxiety or fear in others, and exposure to frightening anecdotes by friends or the mass media.[62] Specifically, fears of the anesthetic "shot" and dental "drill" are the most common.[38,51] A *phobia* is a persistent and irrational fear that results in a compulsion to avoid a specific object, activity, or situation.

A strong relationship exists between anxiety and pain. Expectation of pain contributes significantly to dental anxiety, and anxiety can lower pain tolerance[62] to the extent that normally innocuous stimuli such as touch may be interpreted as pain. Many cases of failed mandibular block are a result of patient anxiety.[70] Anxiety can also contribute to adverse reactions in the dental chair; these are then unfortunately but commonly misdiagnosed as either allergic or toxic reactions to the local anesthetic or vasoconstrictor. Therefore comprehensive pain control requires an ability to manage fear and anxiety.

Other potential indications for the use of pharmacologic methods for patient management include cognitive impairment such as that found with mentally challenged patients or those with Alzheimer's dementia. These patients may be unable to cooperate sufficiently to permit treatment or perhaps even an adequate intraoral examination. Another legitimate indication is the presence of motor dysfunction, such as that found in patients with cerebral palsy or Parkinson's disease, whose tremor or uncoordinated movements may be exacerbated by the anxiety of being in the dental office. Pharmacologic management may also be required for the pediatric patient who may not understand the treatment and is reacting normally for a young child. Traumatic or extensive dental procedures are additional potential indications when coupled with a level of anxiety. Finally, some patients cannot physiologically tolerate the stress that even a minimal amount of anxiety may induce; they include patients with ischemic heart disease, labile hypertension, or stress-induced asthma. Any of the modalities defined below, namely conscious sedation, deep sedation, or general anesthesia, may be used to treat these patients.

Identification of the Fearful or Anxious Patient

To address the needs of the fearful or anxious patient, the dentist must first be able to recognize or diagnose anxiety and fear. Discussion of how to identify these patients accurately is beyond the scope of this chapter but can be found in a number of excellent sources.[27,53] The degree of anxiety should be determined as part of an appropriate history and patient evaluation. Observation of the patient and questions addressing possible anxiety caused by dentistry may aid in diagnosis. Such interviews can identify specific concerns, such as fear of the injection of local anesthetic, the sound of the handpiece, or certain surgical procedures. Standardized measures of anxiety, such as the Corah scale,[13,14] may be of use in quantifying the severity of anxiety.

Treatment Planning

After identifying the anxious, fearful, or phobic patient, thought should be given to the optimal method of managing this patient. Initially, nonpharmacologic methods of anxiety reduction should be considered.[43,57,60] Appropriate chairside manner is often all that is required; it includes use of basic behavioral modification, positive suggestion, and reassurance. This approach is of value not only when used alone but also when used with more specific therapies for anxiety reduction. Specific psychologic interventions that may be helpful include desensitization and hypnosis. Although these techniques will not overcome poor chairside manner, they can effectively aid the dentist in achieving patient comfort.

In spite of effective chairside manner, many patients still wish to receive sedation or anesthesia. It has been reported that more than 50% of those patients classified as having high fear or anxiety preferred sedation for their dentistry.[23] The same study showed that three times as many subjects reported a preference for parenteral sedation or general anesthesia when undergoing dental treatment than were actually receiving these modalities.[23] This suggests a distinct need for these services within dentistry.

An absolute requirement basic to the success of patient management is effective local anesthesia. One cannot avoid this necessity in most invasive dental procedures unless complete general anesthesia is being administered. Even then there may be benefits to the so-called preemptive local anesthetic use.[36,48,71] Therefore the dentist should not be misled into thinking that poor local anesthetic technique can be overcome by administering a sedative. Only when the failure is strictly caused by anxiety[70] will conscious or deep sedation be effective.

The approach to anxiety control should be individualized. As an example, it is as faulty to assume that every patient requires general anesthesia for the removal of impacted teeth as it is to assume that no patient requires anxiety control for a simple dental procedure or examination.

The ability to use a particular pharmacologic approach depends on the level of training of the dentist and the applicable laws and regulations.[4] Education for the simple forms of conscious sedation—inhalation and oral administration—is within the realm of the predoctoral dental curriculum. More advanced forms, such as intravenous conscious sedation, usually require training at a postdoctoral or continuing education level, although some dental schools have demonstrated that it can be part of a predoctoral program. The most advanced modalities, deep sedation and general anesthesia, require the most formal training. Here, education entails a specific postgraduate program devoted to anesthesia or an oral and maxillofacial surgery residency, which includes advanced training in anesthesia.

Patient Selection

Before choosing pharmacologic adjuncts for patient management, the dentist should carefully review the patient's medical history. In this context, the American Society of Anesthesiologists' (ASA) Physical Status Classification System, which is summarized in Box 48-1, can be helpful. This risk assessment tool can be used to estimate the patient's overall ability to tolerate the stress of a planned procedure. It can also help determine the need for further patient evaluation and the degree of monitoring required for the procedure.

ASA I and II patients are often suitable candidates for sedation or general anesthesia in the outpatient setting. Although outpatient general anesthesia is often not suitable for ASA III patients, these same patients are at increased risk during stressful procedures when the practitioner has neglected to control fear or anxiety. In fact, anxiety-control techniques with conscious or even deep sedation may be particularly valuable to the ASA III patient because they reduce the release of endogenous catecholamines.[20,22]

PHARMACOLOGIC APPROACHES

Several pharmacologic approaches can be used to manage fear and anxiety in the dental patient. These are commonly referred to collectively as the *spectrum of pain and anxiety control*, which incorporates all major routes of administration and levels of CNS depression.[46,65] However, the route of administration is not synonymous with the level of depression. In Figure 48-1, a spectrum of fear and anxiety control shows the range of sedation or anesthesia normally sought from the various routes and techniques of administration. In its simplest form, this spectrum is divided into techniques expected to leave the patient awake or to render the patient unconscious. These modalities correspond to conscious sedation and general anesthesia, respectively. However, an intermediate state of deep sedation exists and is an important anesthetic level in dentistry. The characteristics of these states are compared in Table 48-1. The American Dental Association has defined them as follows[4]:

Conscious sedation is a minimally depressed level of consciousness that retains the patient's ability independently and continuously maintain an airway and respond appropriately to physical stimulation or verbal command and that is produced by a pharmacologic or nonpharmacologic method or a combination thereof.

Box 48-1

ASA* Physical Status Classification System

Class	Description
I	A normal, healthy patient
II	A patient with mild systemic disease
III	A patient with severe systemic disease that limits activity but is not incapacitating
IV	A patient with incapacitating systemic disease that is a constant threat to life
V	A moribund patient not expected to survive 24 hours with or without operation
E	Emergency operation of any variety; E is appended to the patient's physical status

*American Society of Anesthesiologists.

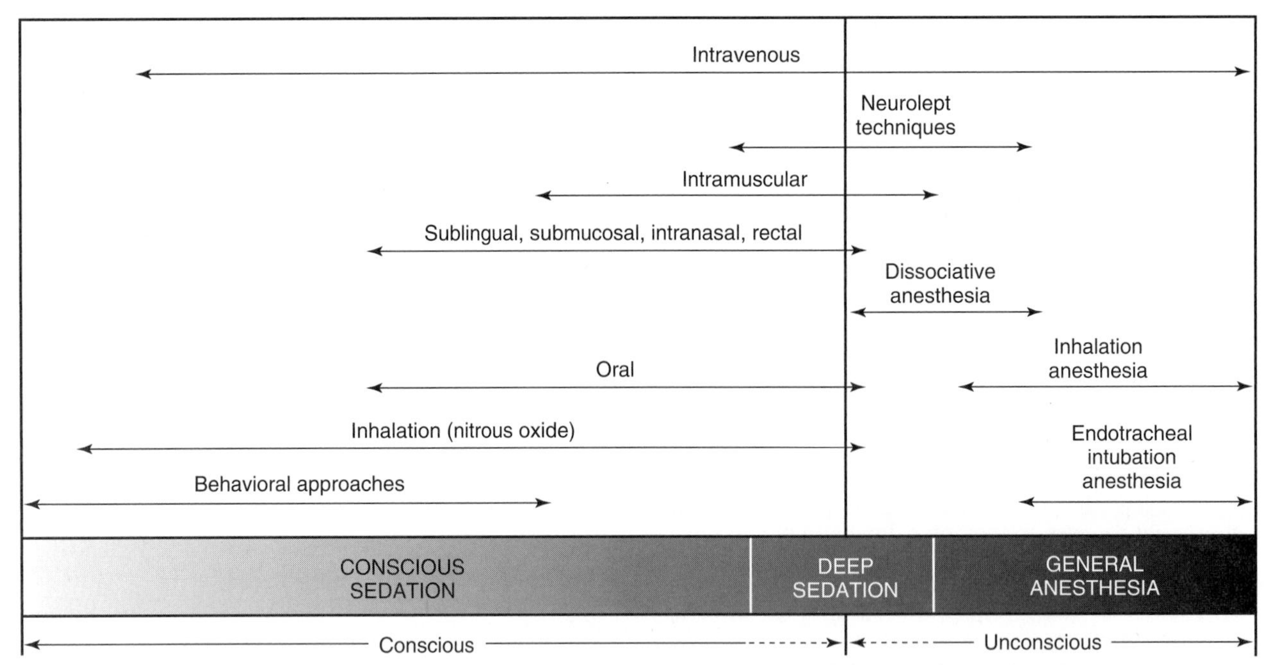

Fig. 48-1 The spectrum of fear and anxiety control in dentistry. The range of CNS depression normally achieved by various techniques is illustrated by *arrows*. The depth of sedation or anesthesia induced by a given drug primarily depends on the dose used and the susceptibility of the patient.

Deep sedation is an induced state of depressed consciousness accompanied by partial loss of protective reflexes, including the inability to continually maintain an airway independently and/or to respond purposefully to physical stimulation *or* verbal command, and is produced by a pharmacologic or nonpharmacologic method or a combination thereof.

General anesthesia is an induced state of unconsciousness accompanied by partial or complete loss of protective reflexes, including the inability to continually maintain an airway independently and respond purposefully to physical stimulation or verbal command, and is produced by a pharmacologic or nonpharmacologic method or a combination thereof.

Conscious sedation is not a substitute for appropriate chairside manner and use of behavioral techniques but is used to reinforce positive suggestion and reassurance in a way that allows dental treatment to be performed with minimal physiologic and psychologic stress. The technique should carry a margin of safety wide enough to render unintended loss of consciousness unlikely.[58] Deep sedation or general anesthesia can be induced by many of the same drugs that induce conscious sedation. The resulting state depends on patient susceptibility, age, medical status, and degree of anxiety as well as the drug or drugs used and doses administered. Either deep sedation or general anesthesia may be indicated when conscious sedation techniques are insufficient to permit treatment.

Table • 48-1

Comparison of Conscious Sedation, Deep Sedation, and General Anesthesia

CHARACTERISTICS	CONSCIOUS SEDATION	DEEP SEDATION	GENERAL ANESTHESIA
Consciousness	Maintained	Obtunded	Unconscious
Protective reflexes	Intact	Depressed	Absent
Unassisted airway maintenance	Present	May be absent	Absent
Response to verbal command	May be obtunded	May be absent	Absent
Vital signs	Stable	Usually stable	May be labile
Anxiety	Decreased	Absent	Absent
Amnesia	Dependent on drug and dosage	Marked	Total
Monitoring required	Basic or intermediate	Advanced	Advanced
Efficacy	Mild to moderate anxiety	Most anxiety, fear, and phobia	All levels of phobia
Relative risk	Low	Intermediate	High
Recovery time	Usually rapid	Intermediate	May be prolonged
Postoperative sequelae	Uncommon	Uncommon	More common

If a separate trained anesthesia provider is not used to administer deep sedation or general anesthesia, then a team approach is indicated. For this approach, at least three individuals must be in the operatory: the dentist (trained in anesthesia), the anesthetic assistant, and the operative assistant. Under the direction of the dentist, the anesthetic assistant's primary function is to assess the patient, monitor vital signs, record appropriate information, and (as required and permitted by relevant laws and regulations) assist in the maintenance of a patent airway, establish intravenous access, administer medications, monitor recovery, and assist in any emergency procedures. The operative assistant's primary function is to keep the operative field free of blood, mucus, and debris and to assist in the management of the dental procedure.

Reliable morbidity and mortality data for the different forms of sedation or general anesthesia are scarce, but several studies have shown that, overall, the techniques used in dentistry should be considered safe.[24,41,45,55,72] Increased mortality is usually associated with inadequate training or inadequate monitoring of the patient.[28,35,40] If the goal is conscious sedation, one must avoid administering excessive doses of a sedative to the patient who remains uncooperative while conscious because it could easily lead to a deepening of sedation in which airway patency and protective reflexes may be lost. Any subsequent lack of oxygenation can rapidly lead to a tragic result. Although the progression from conscious to deep sedation can be accomplished easily, it requires a significantly increased degree of practitioner training, patient monitoring, and physical resources (e.g., anesthetic equipment and supplies) to be performed safely.

CONSCIOUS SEDATION

Numerous routes of administration can be used to achieve conscious sedation: inhalational, oral, intramuscular, intravenous, submucosal, sublingual, rectal, and intranasal. The first four are commonly used and are discussed in detail below, whereas the latter four are used less frequently. The submucosal route is analogous to a subcutaneous injection given intraorally and shares many of the same characteristics as the intramuscular route. The submucosal route has no apparent advantage over any of the others. Furthermore, a patient who accepts an intraoral injection for a sedative could likely accept a local anesthetic injection. The sublingual (or transmucosal) route, restricted to those drugs with high lipid solubility and available in suitable formulations, is similar to the oral route except that there is a more rapid absorption and no first-pass effect. Therefore the difference in recommended dosages can be large when comparing oral with sublingual absorption depending on the extent of this first-pass effect. An advantage with sublingual administration is that the onset of action is more rapid than with oral administration, often in the order of minutes. The rectal route is not often used in dentistry, with the exception of pediatric patients. Disadvantages of this route include inability to titrate, inconsistencies in absorption, often poor patient acceptance, and inconvenience. The intranasal route is a topical application to the nasal mucosa and as such has rapid absorption and should have a rapid onset of action. However, this benefit is diminished by the disadvantages of discomfort, difficulty in making dose determination because of variable absorption, and the potential for damage to the nasal mucosa. The intranasal route has no apparent advantage over any of the others. These latter four routes are not discussed in detail in this chapter.

Management of the anxious patient can be discussed according to route of administration because the inhalational and oral routes are most commonly used for conscious sedation and are normally the first to be considered for use. Parenteral routes are more likely to be selected to induce a greater range of effect, from conscious sedation to deep sedation to general anesthesia. Again, however, the clinician must understand that any route has the potential to induce any degree of sedation or anesthesia. A brief comparison of the routes of administration for conscious sedation is provided in Table 48-2. The commonly used drugs, their routes of administration, and doses for conscious sedation are summarized in Table 48-3.

Inhalation Sedation

Inhalation sedation refers to the administration of N_2O and oxygen (N_2O-O_2), the pharmacologic features of which are described in Chapters 17 and 18. N_2O-O_2 inhalation is a technique of choice for dental procedures that require conscious sedation, regardless of their length. The analgesia produced by N_2O-O_2 ameliorates the incidental discomforts associated with dental treatment. However, as with other modalities of conscious sedation, N_2O-O_2 is not a substitute for effective local anesthesia.

Inhalation sedation units must meet stringent safety standards, including color coding of compressed gas cylinders, a pin-indexed or diameter-indexed safety system to prevent incorrect connection of gas cylinders, minimum O_2 flow, and an O_2 fail-safe valve to shut off the N_2O if O_2 delivery is interrupted. However, all mechanical devices can fail, and careful

Table • 48-2

Comparison of Routes of Administration for Conscious Sedation

CHARACTERISTIC	INHALATION	ORAL	INTRAMUSCULAR	INTRAVENOUS
Ability to titrate	Excellent	Minimal	Minimal	Excellent
Technique difficulty	Easy	Very easy	Easy	Moderate
Ability to reverse	Excellent	Difficult*	Difficult*	Difficult*
Onset	Rapid	Slow	Intermediate	Rapid
Duration	Controlled	Prolonged	Prolonged	Variable
Patient acceptance	Good	Very good	Fair	Fair
Training†	Predoctoral	Predoctoral	Postdoctoral	Postdoctoral
Efficacy	Moderate	Moderate	Moderate	Very good
Need for escort home	No	Yes	Yes	Yes

*Varies with the availability of reversal agents.
†Educational level at which training is usually provided.

Table • 48-3

Drugs, Routes, and Doses for Conscious Sedation

DRUG	ROUTE OF ADMINISTRATION	APPROXIMATE DOSE (mg/kg, UNLESS MARKED OTHERWISE)
Nitrous oxide	Inhalational	20% to 50%
Diazepam	PO, IV	0.05 to 0.3
Midazolam	PO, IM, IV	0.03 to 0.1 (IM or IV), 0.5 (PO)
Triazolam	PO	0.002 to 0.007
Lorazepam	PO	0.01 to 0.04
Promethazine	PO, IM	0.5 to 1.0
Hydroxyzine	PO, IM	0.5 to 1.0
Chloral hydrate	PO	40 to 50
Meperidine	IV	0.5 to 1.0
Fentanyl	IV	0.0006 to 0.0015
Nalbuphine	IV	0.05 to 0.1
Propofol	IV infusion	0.025 to 0.1/min

PO, Oral; *IM,* intramuscular; *IV,* intravenous.

technique and continuous observation of the patient are more effective in preventing accidents than simple reliance on mechanical safeguards.[66] The reader is referred elsewhere for a thorough discussion of the safety and design features of inhalation equipment.[12,25,46,65]

Advantages

The advantages and disadvantages of the inhalation route are summarized in Table 48-2. Because of its relative insolubility in blood, N_2O has a rapid onset of action, with clinical effects becoming apparent within a few minutes. This property of N_2O allows for titration to effect. In this context, *titration* is defined as the incremental administration of small amounts of a drug until a desired clinical effect is observed. The ability to titrate a drug enables the dentist to control its ultimate effect and eliminates the need to guess the correct dose for a particular patient. This characteristic is a major reason why N_2O-O_2 is considered a near ideal technique for conscious sedation. Moreover, in the event that a patient inadvertently receives too much drug, the effect can be rapidly decreased by reducing the concentration administered. The inhalation route is the only one in which the actions of a drug can be quickly adjusted in either direction.

Another major advantage of N_2O-O_2 inhalation is that recovery is rapid. Normally, there is no residual effect on the patient's psychomotor skills and ability to operate a motor vehicle after termination of N_2O-O_2 inhalation.[33,39] When it is not combined with any other sedative agent, N_2O-O_2 is the only sedation technique in which a patient may be discharged home alone; all other conscious sedation techniques require that the patient be discharged in the care of a responsible adult.

Disadvantages

N_2O-O_2 sedation has relatively few disadvantages. The maximum efficacy may be considered only moderate because in a small number of patients this method will be ineffective. However, the majority of patients will have the desired clinical effect between 20% and 50% N_2O. Another disadvantage is the requirement for patient cooperation. Success with this technique requires the patient to breathe through the nose and to leave a nasal hood in place throughout the procedure. Claustrophobic patients and certain apprehensive children may be unable to tolerate the nasal hood.

Nasal obstruction, acute or chronic, precludes the use of N_2O-O_2 because the patient is unable to inhale the administered gases. Patients who are mouth breathers for other reasons are also not suitable candidates. Because of a risk of expansion and rupture of enclosed gas spaces, contraindications include recent vitreoretinal surgery with intraocular gas infusion, pulmonary bullae, pneumothorax, intestinal obstruction, or an obstructed middle ear. Pregnancy is a relative contraindication because of the usual preference to avoid the administration of any drug during pregnancy. Nevertheless, if drug-induced sedation is to be carried out for a pregnant patient, N_2O-O_2 is preferred over the benzodiazepines and may be the technique of choice for a short procedure. Two minor disadvantages are the cost and space needed for the N_2O-O_2 equipment. A final disadvantage is the occupational health hazards from trace anesthetic gases, as discussed in Chapters 17 and 18.

For two groups of patients, it is not the N_2O that is the concern but the high inspired O_2. First, those with severe chronic obstructive pulmonary disease may have chronically elevated carbon dioxide tensions and depend on the hypoxic drive to stimulate breathing. When elevated O_2 concentrations occur, as during N_2O-O_2 administration, the stimulus for involuntary breathing may be removed, leading to respiratory depression and a worsening of respiratory acidosis. Second, patients who have had bleomycin chemotherapy within the past year may be predisposed to pulmonary fibrosis after exposure to high O_2 concentrations.[6]

Clinical application

Administration begins with 100% O_2 at an appropriate flow rate, approximately 6 L/min for most adults. With the reservoir bag filled and O_2 flowing, the mask is placed on the patient. The operator initially administers a 20% concentration of N_2O to the patient and waits 1 to 2 minutes to judge clinical effectiveness. Then, as necessary, the operator increases the N_2O concentration in 5% to 10% increments until the patient demonstrates the desired clinical signs and symptoms. In a few patients, doses of 20% or even less may be all that is required.

The dentist should advise the patient of the symptoms that may be experienced and that the goal is to feel comfortable. Symptoms occurring during inhalation sedation may include lightheadedness; tingling of the fingers, toes, or lips; warmth; and euphoria. The clinician should not be dogmatic in describing potential symptoms because failure to experience one or more of them may be misinterpreted by the patient as a failure of the technique. Once the patient reports being comfortable, the dentist then stops increasing the N_2O percentage and begins treatment. Oversedation may be indicated by excessive drowsiness, loss of response to verbal command, inappropriate movement, hearing abnormalities, visual disturbances, sweating, or nausea. Patients should be monitored by clinical assessment of level of consciousness and adequacy of respiration as well as heart rate and blood pressure.

Recovery is accomplished by terminating N_2O flow and administering 100% O_2 at the previously established flow rate for approximately 5 minutes (to allow for scavenging of exhaled N_2O) or longer if clinical signs and symptoms warrant. Recovery should be evaluated by visual observation, patient report, and, if necessary, assessment of the postoperative vital signs relative to baseline values.

Oral Sedation

The oral route is the second most frequently used route to accomplish conscious sedation in dentistry. It has a number of advantages and disadvantages, as summarized in Table 48-2.

Advantages

The oral route is commonly used to achieve conscious sedation because of the ease of administration. Most adults readily accept oral medication; however, the young child, the mentally challenged patient, or the demented patient may not willingly swallow drugs, particularly in tablet or capsule form. Problems such as overdose, idiosyncratic reactions, allergy, and other adverse events may occur whenever drugs are administered, but such reactions are less likely to arise when drugs are given orally, and, if they do develop, they are often less intense. Nevertheless, careful administration of any drug by any route is required because fatal reactions have resulted from oral sedation.[16,17,34]

Disadvantages

The major disadvantage of oral sedation is the inability to titrate, so the dentist cannot adjust for individual patient response. After a drug is taken orally, it is impractical to provide an additional dose because of the delay in absorption and onset of action. A predetermined dose must be administered, with the risk of an excessive dose leading to prolonged action or inadvertent deep sedation, or with the risk of an insufficient dose, in which case the patient will not be sufficiently sedated to allow dental treatment.

A further disadvantage of oral sedation is the potential for a prolonged duration of action. The patient can remain under the influence of the drug postoperatively and therefore should not leave the dental office unescorted. Specific contraindications to oral sedation depend on the drug used.

Clinical application

The oral route may be used the night before the dental procedure, when the patient may not be able to obtain adequate sleep otherwise. Preoperative anxiety reduction may be a second indication for the patient to be transported to the dental office. Dosages for these two indications should be kept low enough to minimize the likelihood of oversedation because the dentist is not present to deal with any potential adverse event. The third indication is the most common one—the administration of an oral drug for conscious sedation during the dental procedure. Ideally, a dose used to induce conscious sedation should be administered to the patient in the dental office, taking into account the time required for drug absorption. Although great variability exists, initial clinical effects are often evident approximately 30 minutes after ingestion, with peak effects occurring at approximately 60 minutes. Patients should be monitored by clinical assessment of level of consciousness and adequacy of respiration as well as heart rate and blood pressure as necessary. At the end of the case, patients should be discharged to the care of a responsible adult only when they are oriented and ambulatory, have stable vital signs, and show signs of increasing alertness. The patient should be instructed not to drive a vehicle, operate hazardous machinery, or consume alcohol for the remainder of the day.

Determinants of dose The suggested doses for sedation recommended in this chapter apply to the typical 70-kg, healthy adult. Some factors modify these recommendations. The first consideration is the patient's weight. Determining a dose based on body surface area is theoretically more accurate, but using body weight has the advantage of simplicity. Extremes of age are a further consideration. The dosage regimens for pediatric patients may often be determined by body weight or surface area calculations. However, specific doses for certain drugs may differ in young children for reasons other than body size.[15] Geriatric patients may react much more profoundly to central nervous system (CNS) depressants with respect to both depth and duration of action. Thus, as a general recommendation, one should consider an initial dose for the elderly patient of half that usually administered for a typical adult of the same body size.

Medical history and concurrent medication may influence the dose to be used. In particular, drugs affecting the CNS must be assessed, not only regarding interactive potential leading to excessive CNS depression and subsequent respiratory and cardiovascular depression, but also regarding the possibility of cross-tolerance and therefore decreased effect of the planned medications. History of the patient's response to mood-altering drugs such as alcohol may indicate an altered dose requirement.

Chemically dependent patients require special consideration. Patients who depend on alcohol, opioids, or other mood-altering drugs may require an increased dose of sedative because of tolerance. A patient who is recovering from chemical dependency should ideally only have an oral sedative administered after thorough consultation with both the patient and the health professional treating the dependency.

Finally, increased anxiety often correlates with increased dose requirement. Thus larger doses (although still within the acceptable range) are generally indicated for patients with an increased need for pharmacologic sedation.

Specific drugs

Numerous drugs are available for oral sedation. The following is a summary of those commonly used in dentistry.

Benzodiazepines Benzodiazepines are typically the drugs of choice for oral sedation. As described in Chapter 13, benzodiazepines have a relatively wide margin of safety when compared with other antianxiety and sedative drugs. They are well absorbed, and most have a rapid onset of action. Contraindications to the use of benzodiazepines include myasthenia gravis, sleep apnea, angle-closure glaucoma, and the first trimester of pregnancy. Concurrent use of cimetidine, erythromycin, disulfiram, or oral contraceptives may result in prolonged action of diazepam and related benzodiazepines that are similarly biotransformed.

Diazepam is the prototypic benzodiazepine and has a long history of use in dentistry. It is efficacious, but it has active metabolites and may therefore have a prolonged duration of action. It may be administered orally for use in conscious sedation in adults in doses ranging from 5 to 20 mg. For children, doses from 0.3 to 0.6 mg/kg have been suggested.[54,64] It is available in tablets (2, 5, and 10 mg) and as a syrup (5 and 25 mg/5 ml).

Triazolam is an effective anxiolytic and amnestic agent; it possesses a rapid onset of action and has a short elimination half-life. This short duration of action is ideally suited to dentistry, allowing for rapid recovery, which is important for outpatient procedures.[10] It has also been shown to be as effective as intravenous diazepam for conscious sedation.[37] Significant adverse reactions of triazolam (e.g., behavioral abnormalities), widely publicized in the lay press, are associated with repeated use of high doses, particularly in the elderly.[29,59] A significant interaction can occur with erythromycin, which inhibits triazolam's hepatic breakdown, leading to increased plasma concentrations.[32] Erythromycin may therefore potentiate the magnitude and duration of triazolam's sedative effect. Overall, triazolam's pharmacologic advantages make it a drug of choice for oral sedation in dentistry. The adult dose range is 0.125 to 0.5 mg, and it is available in 0.125- or 0.25-mg tablets.

Lorazepam is an effective premedicant. Although it can elicit satisfactory sedation for dental procedures, it has the drawbacks of profound anterograde amnesia and an unnecessarily long duration of action. Furthermore, peak effects may occur 1 to 6 hours after administration,[67] making appropriate scheduling difficult. It is available as 0.5-, 1-, or 2-mg tablets, and doses of 0.5 to 3 mg are suggested for adults.

Midazolam, widely used parenterally, is also available as an oral formulation for use in pediatrics. It is not normally used orally in adults. It has a rapid onset and short duration of action. Similar to triazolam, oral midazolam is contraindicated for the patient taking erythromycin because this interaction can lead to increased plasma levels of midazolam with subsequent increased and prolonged sedation.[32] Midazolam's high first-pass effect leads to large differences in the parenteral/oral dosing recommendations. For oral midazolam, doses approximating 0.5 mg/kg appear appropriate,[31] to a maximum of 20 mg.

Other benzodiazepines such as flurazepam, oxazepam, alprazolam, temazepam, and nitrazepam may also be considered for use in conscious sedation.

Zolpidem Zolpidem, an imidazopyridine sedative-hypnotic, is similar pharmacologically to the benzodiazepines because it interacts with a subtype of benzodiazepine receptors (see Chapter 13). Regarding conscious sedation, zolpidem offers several advantages over diazepam. The onset of action is quite fast, with peak effects occurring in as little as 30 minutes. Prolonged sedation is not a problem because the drug has a metabolic half-life of approximately 2.6 hours and is converted to inactive derivatives. Zolpidem is not contraindicated in pregnant women or in patients with angle-closure glaucoma. Possible disadvantages are the drug's relative lack of anticonvulsant and muscle relaxant properties. Some question remains regarding whether zolpidem produces specific anxiolytic effects common to the benzodiazepines. The average adult dose is 10 mg; zolpidem is available in 5- and 10-mg tablets.

Barbiturates The use of oral barbiturates to induce sedation is principally of historic interest because they have been superseded by superior drugs, primarily the benzodiazepines. Representative drugs from this group are secobarbital and pentobarbital, which have an onset of action of approximately 1 hour and a duration of 3 to 6 hours. Recommended doses for preoperative sedation approximate 100 mg. The major drawbacks to barbiturates are prolonged action leading to a residual CNS depression, also known as a "hangover" effect; antianalgesic action; increased tendency to produce dependence; paradoxical excitation; and adverse drug interactions. Whereas benzodiazepine overdose alone is unlikely to cause death, barbiturates are more likely to depress respiration and cardiovascular function severely, whether ingested alone or in combination with other CNS depressants. They are also contraindicated in certain forms of porphyria (see Chapter 13).

Alcohols Chloral hydrate has been widely used as a conscious sedation agent in pediatric dentistry.[17] It is usually administered in the form of an elixir, with the recommended dose of 40 to 50 mg/kg when administered alone, not to exceed 1000 mg. Although commonly considered to be safe,[3] it should be administered to the patient in the dental office, not at home. It is available as either 250- or 500-mg capsules or as a syrup (250 or 500 mg/5 ml).

Antihistamines Promethazine is a phenothiazine derivative with antihistaminic properties that is used for conscious sedation, particularly in the pediatric patient. In addition to causing sedation, it is also noted for having anticholinergic and antiemetic effects. It may also have modest antidopaminergic effects that can lead to dyskinesia in sensitive individuals. The recommended dose for conscious sedation is 25 to 50 mg in adults and 0.5 to 1 mg/kg in children if administered alone. Promethazine has been used in combination with opioids, in which case doses should be reduced. It is available in tablet form (12.5, 25, and 50 mg) and as a syrup in a concentration of 6.25 or 25 mg/5 ml.

Hydroxyzine is similar to promethazine in that it is an antihistamine and induces sedation and has anticholinergic and antiemetic effects. Recommended doses range from 50 to 100 mg for adults, if given alone, and 0.6 mg/kg for children. If it is combined with either chloral hydrate or an opioid, dosages should be reduced. It is available in tablet (10, 25, 50, and 100 mg), capsule (25, 50, and 100 mg), and syrup (10 and 25 mg/5 ml) formulations.

Ketamine Ketamine is discussed in more detail below because it is primarily used intramuscularly or intravenously to induce dissociative anesthesia, an anesthetic state deeper than conscious sedation. It has been used orally in doses approximating 6 mg/kg as a premedicant (see Chapter 18).[1,2,30,63]

Opioids As described in Chapter 18, opioids are important in sedation and anesthesia but are much more effective when used intravenously compared with orally because of their high first-pass metabolism.

Intramuscular Sedation

Intramuscular administration is the least used of the four routes discussed in this chapter. Compared with the oral and inhalation routes, this parenteral technique generally requires additional training beyond that typically provided at the predoctoral level. Several anatomic locations are available for intramuscular injection, including the mid-deltoid region (the most commonly used site in adults), the superolateral quadrant of the gluteal region, and the anterolateral aspect of the thigh.

Advantages

Compared with the oral route, the absorption of drugs into the circulation tends to be faster and more predictable. Patient cooperation is not as essential as it is with other techniques described in this chapter. This advantage is important in the management of patients who are mentally challenged, have disruptive movement disorders, or are too young to cooperate with care. After appropriate informed consent is obtained, the patient need only be carefully restrained momentarily while the drug is administered. The advantages and disadvantages of the intramuscular route are summarized in Table 48-2.

Disadvantages

The disadvantages of intramuscular injection include pain on injection, a prolonged duration of action, and a necessity for the patient to be accompanied home. Titration is not practical. Intramuscular injections also have the potential for local tissue damage.

Clinical applications

The disadvantages of the intramuscular route have restricted its use in dentistry.[7] Although few indications exist for giving drugs intramuscularly to adult patients, this route may be the only effective means of conscious sedation available for cognitively impaired patients or uncooperative children. Thus the technique is indicated for patients who cannot take oral medication or accept the mask for inhalation sedation. It is also used to facilitate venipuncture for intravenous conscious sedation, deep sedation, or general anesthesia. Contraindications to this route would include patients on anticoagulant therapy and extremes in body weight—the emaciated or very obese. These latter patients may exhibit unusual patterns of absorption. Ideally, monitoring should include oxyhemoglobin saturation, heart rate, blood pressure, and adequacy of respiration.

Specific agents

Several agents may be considered for intramuscular injection.

Benzodiazepines Diazepam is not recommended for intramuscular administration because tissue irritation may occur and because it is one of the few drugs that is less effective and less reliable clinically after intramuscular injection than after oral administration. Intramuscular administration leads to a peak plasma concentration in 30 to 90 minutes.[67]

Midazolam is the benzodiazepine of choice, and may be the drug of choice, for intramuscular sedation. It is water soluble and devoid of irritating effects. Given in a dose up to 0.075 mg/kg in adults (and 0.1 to 0.15 mg/kg for children), midazolam has an onset time of 15 minutes, peaks within 15 to 60 minutes, and lasts for 2 to 3 hours. The 5 mg/ml formulation is useful for intramuscular administration.

Lorazepam can be used for intramuscular sedation. By this route, the peak effect may occur in 1 to 1.5 hours. It offers no advantages over midazolam.

Antihistamines Promethazine can be administered to children in a dose of 1 mg/kg and to adults in a dose of 25 to 50 mg. It is available in strengths of 25 and 50 mg/ml for parenteral administration. Hydroxyzine can also be administered to children in a dose of 1 mg/kg and, for adults, in a dose of 25 to 100 mg. It is also available in 25 and 50 mg/ml solutions for intramuscular injection.

Opioids Meperidine is often combined with one or more CNS depressants for sedation. The usual precautions with opioid administration, as described elsewhere, apply. The normal dose approximates 1 mg/kg.

Ketamine As described in detail in Chapter 18, ketamine induces a state known as *dissociative anesthesia;* therefore it is not appropriate to consider this truly conscious sedation. Ketamine should only be administered by those trained in deep sedation and general anesthesia. It is effective for intramuscular administration in the uncooperative patient who will not permit venipuncture or inhalation sedation. An antimuscarinic is generally administered with or before the ketamine to reduce salivary secretions, and a benzodiazepine is often coadministered to reduce emergence effects (hallucinations).

Intravenous Sedation

The intravenous route is the most effective method to achieve conscious sedation. The advantages and disadvantages of this route of administration are summarized in Table 48-2.

Advantages

The intravenous route makes possible the rapid attainment of blood concentrations at which drugs are clinically effective. Intravenous injection leads to a very short latent period, which ranges from as little as 10 seconds, the time it may take to go from the intravenous site to the site of action in the brain, to a few minutes. The ability to titrate drugs, and thereby minimize the likelihood of overdosage, and to enhance drug action rapidly are other advantages. In clinical practice, the operator requires 2 to 15 minutes to titrate a drug to a desired clinical endpoint. One more advantage is that a patent intravenous line provides the ideal route for drug administration in the event of an emergency.

Disadvantages

Patients must be somewhat cooperative to permit venipuncture. Many children will actively resist, and therefore intravenous sedation for children is often not desirable or even possible. Another disadvantage of this route is that the rapid onset of action and the accentuated drug effects likely to be observed tend to magnify problems associated with drug overdosage or side effects. As stated earlier in this chapter, administering intravenous sedation requires advanced training, in part because adverse effects may occur more readily and with more severe consequences.

Clinical applications

For intravenous conscious sedation, monitoring should include oxyhemoglobin saturation, heart rate, blood pressure, and adequacy of respiration.

Benzodiazepines As with the oral route, benzodiazepines are the ideal drugs to induce intravenous conscious sedation. Diazepam is lipid soluble and water insoluble and therefore is formulated dissolved in propylene glycol. This vehicle can be irritating on intravenous administration and may lead to thrombophlebitis.[61] Irritation may be minimized by slow administration into large-caliber veins or by use of the formulation of diazepam dissolved in an injectable emulsion. Diazepam is prepared as a 5 mg/ml solution. The drug must be titrated slowly, with sedative and anxiolytic effects usually beginning at doses of 2 to 10 mg, although great interpatient variability is possible. Appropriate sedation often corresponds with ptosis. By this route, diazepam has a rapid onset of 30 to 60 seconds, with peak effects occurring after approximately 3 minutes. The duration of sedation is somewhat dependent, but averages approximately 45 to 60 minutes for sedative doses. Overall, diazepam is an effective agent for intravenous conscious sedation, but it possesses the disadvantages of active metabolites and the potential for thrombophlebitis.

Midazolam injection is water soluble and, when administered intravenously, does not cause venous irritation. Midazolam is rapidly eliminated and is converted to essentially inactive metabolites. After intravenous administration, it has a rapid onset of 30 to 60 seconds, with peak effects reported to occur after 3 to 5 minutes, which is slightly slower than with diazepam. The distributional half-life is very short, 6 to 15 minutes, leading to a short duration of action of approximately 45 minutes. Again, the duration of action is somewhat dose dependent. It has been suggested that midazolam is twice as potent as diazepam in low doses and up to four times as potent at high doses. Conscious sedation is achieved by doses approximating 0.07 mg/kg, titrated slowly in 1-mg increments. Midazolam is provided in strengths of 1 and 5 mg/ml. A 1 mg/ml solution is recommended for conscious sedation to facilitate accurate titration.

Barbiturates As discussed in Chapter 18, the barbiturates have important application in general anesthetic induction, but they are inferior to the benzodiazepines for conscious sedation. Pentobarbital, which is used parenterally as part of the Jorgensen technique, may be administered in doses usually up to 100 mg. When administered intravenously, it has a clinical action lasting from 2 to 3 hours. It may be useful, therefore, for long dental procedures.

Opioids The pharmacologic characteristics of the opioids are discussed in Chapter 20. These drugs are not used alone for sedation but are commonly given to supplement the benzodiazepines or other sedatives to either facilitate conscious sedation or, with increasing doses, to induce deep sedation or general anesthesia. They are useful for painful procedures such as those common in dentistry and oral surgery. Opioids typically provide the advantages of profound analgesia and sedation with minimal cardiovascular effects. The duration of action varies with the drug. Administration of the opioid should be timed so that the peak effect coincides with the most painful part of the procedure.

Generally, ASA III patients, such as those with significant cardiovascular disease, and the elderly require lower doses of opioids than do younger ASA class I or II patients. Specific concerns with opioids include respiratory depression and chest wall rigidity. This latter syndrome is characterized by an increase in muscle tone leading to severe truncal stiffness. It appears to be more prevalent with high doses, in the elderly, and when N_2O is coadministered. Rapid or bolus administration increases the severity. Treatment consists of the administration of either naloxone or a neuromuscular blocker.

Opioids commonly used for sedation include meperidine, fentanyl, pentazocine, nalbuphine, and butorphanol. Meperidine is administered for sedation in doses of 0.5 to 1 mg/kg, usually not exceeding 100 mg. At these doses, meperidine can be expected to have a duration of action of 1 to 2 hours. In addition to its expected actions of analgesia and sedation, meperidine is noted for its antisialagogue effect and potential to induce tachycardia. It is contraindicated in patients taking monoamine oxidase inhibitors or amphetamines and should be used cautiously, or not at all, in patients with asthma because of the potential for histamine release.

Fentanyl is particularly suited for procedures of short duration. The dose for sedation is on the order of 1 μg/kg. At this dose, it can be expected to have a duration of action of 30 to 60 minutes. Advantages of fentanyl over other opioids include cardiovascular stability, a relatively short duration of action, and lack of histamine release. On the other hand, fentanyl is more likely to produce chest wall rigidity.[68] Related to fentanyl is remifentanil, which is given by intravenous infusion. Its advantages are its rapid onset and its very short duration of action.

Pentazocine is a mixed agonist-antagonist, which results in a ceiling effect regarding analgesia and respiratory depression. Adverse reactions include a potential for psychotomimetic effects, such as disorientation, confusion, depression, hallucinations, and dysphoria, as well as diaphoresis and dizziness. In doses approximating 0.5 mg/kg, to a maximum of 30 mg, it can be expected to have a duration of action of 1 to 2 hours.

Nalbuphine is also a mixed agonist-antagonist used for sedation. A dose of 0.1 mg/kg, up to a maximum of 10 mg, may be considered. A third agonist-antagonist, butorphanol, has been used for sedation in doses of 0.02 mg/kg, usually to a maximum of 2 mg.

Jorgensen technique The Jorgensen technique, also known as the *Loma Linda technique,* has a long history of safe use. It involves the titration of pentobarbital incrementally until the patient is minimally sedated. At this point, a solution containing 25 mg of meperidine and 0.32 mg of scopolamine is administered in a ratio of 1 ml solution per 20 mg pentobarbital up to a maximum of 5 ml. An additional 10% of the baseline barbiturate dose is also given.

Propofol Propofol, an intravenous general anesthetic, is described in Chapter 18. In low doses, propofol can be used for conscious sedation or deep sedation.[56] This use requires careful infusion at a rate of 25 to 100 μg/kg per minute.

DEEP SEDATION OR GENERAL ANESTHESIA

Many of the drugs described for intravenous conscious sedation can also induce deep sedation or general anesthesia. The characteristics of these deeper levels of CNS depression are summarized in Table 48-1. Drugs used only for general anesthesia, such as the volatile anesthetics, are described in Chapter 18. These techniques require more advanced monitoring than does conscious sedation. Techniques used for deep sedation are described below.

Benzodiazepine-Opioid Combinations

The combination of midazolam with fentanyl has been shown to be effective and safe for the induction of conscious sedation.[19,21,24,50,73] These same drug combinations, when administered in higher doses or in more susceptible patients, are also effective in inducing deep sedation. Use of either diazepam or midazolam with an opioid such as fentanyl, meperidine, or nalbuphine can provide effective deep sedation. These drugs are often further combined with N_2O-O_2, propofol, or methohexital.

Neuroleptanalgesia/anesthesia

This is a state of sedation that was commonly used in the past.[11] In its strictest sense it is rarely used today, but it was the forerunner of deep sedation techniques now practiced. Classically, neuroleptanalgesia was induced by using droperidol, a butyrophenone antipsychotic, in combination with an opioid, usually fentanyl. This state is characterized by somnolence without total unconsciousness, psychologic indifference, good analgesia, amnesia, and decreased motor activity. When droperidol and fentanyl were combined with N_2O-O_2 the effect was referred to as *neuroleptanesthesia*. Droperidol, which also had wide use as an antiemetic, is used much less commonly today because of concerns regarding its potential to induce serious cardiac dysrhythmias, including QT prolongation and torsades de pointes.

Methohexital

The ultrashort-acting barbiturate methohexital is used widely in outpatient deep sedation and general anesthesia in dentistry.[47] It may be administered alone for procedures of short duration, although it is more commonly administered in combination with other agents, such as the benzodiazepines, opioids, and N_2O-O_2.[24] A dose of 1 to 1.5 mg/kg is used for the induction of general anesthesia, whereas increments of 10 mg can be used for maintenance of deep sedation. The use of methohexital is characterized by a more rapid induction, more rapid recovery, and increased heart rate compared with thiopental. Its disadvantages include the potential for respiratory depression, apnea, hiccough, and coughing. It is contraindicated in patients with certain forms of porphyria, as described in Chapter 13.

Propofol

Propofol (see Chapter 18) is characterized by its uniquely short duration of action. The rapid recovery makes it advantageous for ambulatory sedation and general anesthesia in the dental office. Propofol compares favorably to methohexital for providing sedation and anesthesia for regional blockade, dentistry, and other short procedures. The most frequent adverse effects of propofol include pain on injection as well as apnea and hypotension in higher doses.

Propofol has been administered by continuous infusion specifically for conscious sedation in dentistry.[56] However, because of the increased likelihood of inducing deep sedation or general anesthesia, it is best to monitor the patient with these deeper states in mind. The dose for induction of general anesthesia is 2 to 2.5 mg/kg. If used alone, an infused dose of 25 to 100 μg/kg per minute should accomplish conscious sedation in healthy adults.

Ketamine

In addition to its use as an intramuscular agent, ketamine can be administered intravenously as an adjunct for deep sedation or general anesthesia. It has been suggested that administering ketamine as a sole agent by low-dose intravenous infusion may provide analgesia, amnesia, and sedation.[8] For use as a general anesthetic agent, ketamine is administered in a dose of 1 to 2 mg/kg intravenously or 5 to 10 mg/kg intramuscularly. For use in sedation or analgesia only, the suggested doses are 200 to 750 μg/kg intravenously, followed by 5 to 20 μg/kg per minute as a continuous infusion, or 2 to 4 mg/kg if given intramuscularly.

REVERSAL AGENTS

Specific antagonists are available for opioids and benzodiazepines. A brief summary follows.

Naloxone

As described in Chapters 18 and 20, naloxone is a reversal agent for the opioid analgesics. Its primary indication is in the treatment of opioid-induced respiratory depression, chest wall rigidity, or overly deep sedation. The drug has a peak effect in 5 to 15 minutes, with a duration of action of as little as 45 minutes. Naloxone should be used with caution. Particular concern should be given to patients with cardiac irritability or opioid dependency. Convulsions have been reported to occur, as well as alterations in blood pressure, ventricular tachycardia, and ventricular fibrillation. Therapeutic doses are best administered by titrating slowly in 0.1-mg increments to effect, often to a final dose of 0.4 to 0.8 mg in cases of true opioid overdosage. The duration of action is short, so there is a danger that the antagonistic effect of naloxone will wear off before the agonistic effect of the opioid, resulting in a return of respiratory difficulties. Therefore after the administration of naloxone, the patient should be carefully monitored for 1 hour or more, depending on the opioid being antagonized.

Flumazenil

Flumazenil, a specific benzodiazepine receptor antagonist, exerts little effect by itself. However, when administered to reverse benzodiazepine-induced CNS depression, it causes a rapid reversal of unconsciousness, sedation, amnesia, and psychomotor dysfunction. In the presence of a high dose of agonist, flumazenil will first reverse the loss of consciousness and respiratory depression, but drowsiness and amnesia may persist. These latter two signs will diminish after higher doses of flumazenil. Onset is rapid, with the peak effect occurring in 1 to 3 minutes. The duration of action is dose dependent, depending on the specific agonist being reversed and how much of it was administered. Incremental doses of 0.1 to 0.2 mg flumazenil intravenously, up to 3 mg, can be used. Reports indicate that 3 mg may provide 45 to 90 minutes of antagonism.

Flumazenil apparently has relatively few adverse effects other than the important possibility of resedation. The adverse cardiovascular sequelae sometimes seen with naloxone after reversal of opioid overdosage do not occur with flumazenil. Agitation and headache have been reported. Convulsions have occurred in epileptic patients taking benzodiazepines for their condition. Patients taking seizureogenic medications, such as tricyclic antidepressants, may also be susceptible to convulsions. Flumazenil is indicated whenever rapid reversal of benzodiazepine agonist action is required. As with any reversal agent, the potential for resedation demands that whenever this agent is used to treat an emergency, the patient must be monitored in recovery beyond the duration of action of flumazenil.

SUMMARY

Significant progress in the science of dentistry has resulted in important advances in the prevention and treatment of caries and periodontal disease. However, many patients fail to benefit from modern dentistry because of fear and anxiety regarding dental treatment. Dentists who gain the ability to use the techniques discussed in this chapter will be able to carry out dentistry in a compassionate manner for all patients. Patients deserve and expect to be treated as atraumatically as possible, and the administration of judiciously selected drugs can help achieve this goal. This, in turn, will allow dentists to optimize the oral health of their patients.

CITED REFERENCES

1. Alderson PJ, Lerman J: Oral premedication for paediatric ambulatory anaesthesia: a comparison of midazolam and ketamine, *Can J Anaesth* 41:221-226, 1994.
2. Alfonzo-Echeverri EC, Berg JH, Wild TW, et al: Oral ketamine for pediatric outpatient dental surgery sedation, *Pediatr Dent* 15:182-185, 1993.
3. American Academy of Pediatrics Committee on Drugs and Committee on Environmental Health: Use of chloral hydrate for sedation in children, *Pediatrics* 92:471-473, 1993.
4. American Dental Association: *Guidelines for teaching the comprehensive control of anxiety and pain in dentistry,* Chicago, 2002, American Dental Association.
5. Ayer WA, Jr, Domoto PK, Gale EN, et al: Overcoming dental fear: strategies for its prevention and management, *J Am Dent Assoc* 107:18-27, 1983.
6. Barash PG, Cullen BF, Stoelting RK, eds: *Handbook of clinical anesthesia,* ed 2, Philadelphia, 1992, JB Lippincott.
7. Becker DE, Bennett CR: Intravenous and intramuscular sedation. In Dionne RA, Phero JC, Becker DE, eds: *Management of pain and anxiety in the dental office,* Philadelphia, 2002, WB Saunders.
8. Bennett CR: Dissociative-sedation: a new concept, *Compendium* 11:34, 36-38, 1990.

9. Berggren U, Meynert G: Dental fear and avoidance: causes, symptoms, and consequences, *J Am Dent Assoc* 109:247-251, 1984.
10. Berthold CW, Schneider A, Dionne RA: Using triazolam to reduce dental anxiety, *J Am Dent Assoc* 124:58-64, 1993.
11. Bissonnette B, Swan H, Ravussin P, et al: Neuroleptanesthesia: current status, *Can J Anesth* 46:154-168, 1999.
12. Clark M, Brunick A: *Handbook of nitrous oxide and oxygen sedation,* ed 2, St Louis, 2003, Mosby.
13. Corah NL: Development of a dental anxiety scale, *J Dent Res* 48:596, 1969.
14. Corah NL, Gale EN, Illig SJ: Assessment of a dental anxiety scale, *J Am Dent Assoc* 97:816-819, 1978.
15. Coté CJ: Sedation for the pediatric patient. A review, *Pediatr Clin North Am* 41:31-58, 1994.
16. Coté CJ, Karl HW, Notterman DA, et al: Adverse sedation events in pediatrics: analysis of medications used for sedation, *Pediatrics* 106:633-644, 2000.
17. Coté CJ, Notterman DA, Karl HW, et al: Adverse sedation events in pediatrics: a critical incident analysis of contributing factors, *Pediatrics* 105:805-814, 2000.
18. DeFord WH: *Lectures on general anesthetics in dentistry,* Kansas City, MO, 1908, John T Nolde.
19. Dionne RA: Scientific basis for the use of anesthesia and sedation in dentistry, *Oral Maxillofac Surg Clin North Am* 4:887-901, 1992.
20. Dionne RA, Driscoll EJ, Gelfman SS, et al: Cardiovascular and respiratory response to intravenous diazepam, fentanyl, and methohexital in dental outpatients, *J Oral Surg* 39:343-349, 1981.
21. Dionne RA, Gift HC: Drugs used for parenteral sedation in dental practice, *Anesth Prog* 35:199-205, 1988.
22. Dionne RA, Goldstein DS, Wirdzek PR: Effects of diazepam premedication and epinephrine-containing local anesthetic on cardiovascular and plasma catecholamine responses to oral surgery, *Anesth Analg* 63:640-646, 1984.
23. Dionne RA, Gordon SM, McCullagh LM, et al: Assessing the need for anesthesia and sedation in the general population, *J Am Dent Assoc* 129:167-173, 1998.
24. Dionne RA, Yagiela JA, Moore PA, et al: Comparing efficacy and safety of four intravenous sedation regimens in dental outpatients, *J Am Dent Assoc* 132:740-751, 2001.
25. Garrison RS, Holliday SR, Kretzchmar DP: Nitrous oxide sedation. In Dionne RA, Phero JC, Becker DE, eds: *Management of pain and anxiety in the dental office,* Philadelphia, 2002, WB Saunders.
26. Gatchel RJ: The prevalence of dental fear and avoidance: expanded adult and recent adolescent surveys, *J Am Dent Assoc* 118:591-593, 1989.
27. Gift H: Issues to consider in the control of acute pain, fear and anxiety. In Dionne RA, Phero JC, eds: *Management of pain and anxiety in dental practice,* New York, 1991, Elsevier Science.
28. Goodson JM, Moore PA: Life-threatening reactions after pedodontic sedation: an assessment of narcotic, local anesthetic, and antiemetic drug interaction, *J Am Dent Assoc* 107:239-245, 1983.
29. Greenblatt DJ, Harmatz JS, Shapiro L, et al: Sensitivity to triazolam in the elderly, *N Engl J Med* 324:1691-1698, 1991.
30. Haas DA, Harper DG: Ketamine: a review of its pharmacologic properties and use in ambulatory anesthesia, *Anesth Prog* 39:61-68, 1992.
31. Haas DA, Nenniger SA, Yacobi R, et al: A pilot study of the efficacy of oral midazolam for sedation in paediatric dental patients, *Anesth Prog* 43:1-8, 1996.
32. Hersh EV: Adverse drug interactions in dental practice: interactions involving antibiotics, *J Am Dent Assoc* 130:236-251, 1999.
33. Jastak JT, Orendurff D: Recovery from nitrous sedation, *Anesth Prog* 22:113-116, 1975.
34. Jastak JT, Pallasch T: Death after chloral hydrate sedation: report of case, *J Am Dent Assoc* 116:345-348, 1988.
35. Jastak JT, Peskin RM: Major morbidity or mortality from office anesthetic procedures: a closed-claim analysis of 13 cases, *Anesth Prog* 38:39-44, 1991.
36. Katz J, Kavanagh BP, Sandler AN, et al: Preemptive analgesia. Clinical evidence of neuroplasticity contributing to postoperative pain, *Anesthesiology* 77:439-446, 1992.
37. Kaufman E, Hargreaves KM, Dionne RA: Comparison of oral triazolam and nitrous oxide with placebo and intravenous diazepam for outpatient premedication, *Oral Surg Oral Med Oral Pathol* 75:156-164, 1993.
38. Kleinknecht RA, Thorndike RM, McGlynn FD, et al: Factor analysis of the dental fear survey with cross-validation, *J Am Dent Assoc* 108:59-61, 1984.
39. Korttila K, Ghoneim MM, Jacobs L, et al: Time course of mental and psychomotor effects of 30 per cent N_2O during inhalation and recovery, *Anesthesiology* 54:220-226, 1981.
40. Krippaehne JA, Montgomery MT: Morbidity and mortality from pharmacosedation and general anesthesia in the dental office, *J Oral Maxillofac Surg* 50:691-698, 1992.
41. Leelataweedwud P, Vann WF: Adverse events and outcomes of conscious sedation for pediatric patients. Study of an oral sedation regimen, *J Am Dent Assoc* 132:1531-1539, 2001.
42. Liddell A: Personality characteristics versus medical and dental experiences of dentally anxious children, *J Behav Med* 13:183-194, 1990.
43. Liddell A, Ackerman C, Locker D: What dental phobics say about their dental experiences, *J Can Dent Assoc* 56:863-866, 1990.
44. Lindsay SJ, Humphris G, Barnby GJ: Expectations and preferences for routine dentistry in anxious adult patients, *Br Dent J* 163:120-124, 1987.
45. Lytle JJ, Stamper EP: The 1988 survey of the Southern California Society of Oral and Maxillofacial Surgeons, *J Oral Maxillofac Surg* 47:834-842, 1989.
46. Malamed SF: *Sedation: a guide to patient management,* ed 4, St Louis, 2003, Mosby.
47. Martone CH, Nagelhout J, Wolf SM: Methohexital: a practical review for outpatient dental anesthesia, *Anesth Prog* 38:195-199, 1991.
48. McQuay HJ, Carroll D, Moore RA: Postoperative orthopaedic pain—the effect of opiate premedication and local anaesthetic blocks, *Pain* 33:291-295, 1988.
49. Merskey H: Pain terms: a list with definitions and notes on usage, *Pain* 6:249-252, 1979.
50. Milgrom P, Beirne OR, Fiset L, et al: The safety and efficacy of outpatient midazolam intravenous sedation for oral surgery with and without fentanyl, *Anesth Prog* 40:57-62, 1993.

51. Milgrom P, Coldwell SE, Getz T, et al: Four dimensions of fear of dental injections, *J Am Dent Assoc* 128:756-762, 1997.
52. Milgrom P, Fiset L, Melnick S, et al: The prevalence and practice management consequences of dental fear in a major US city, *J Am Dent Assoc* 116:641-647, 1988.
53. Milgrom P, Weinstein P, Kleinknecht R, et al: *Treating fearful dental patients: a patient management handbook,* Reston, VA 1995, Reston.
54. Moore PA, Houpt M: Sedative drug therapy in pediatric dentistry. In Dionne RA, Phero JC, eds: *Management of pain and anxiety in dental practice,* New York, 1991, Elsevier Science.
55. Nkansah PJ, Haas DA, Saso JA: Mortality incidence in outpatient anesthesia for dentistry in Ontario, *Oral Surg Oral Med Oral Pathol Oral Radiol Endod* 83:646-651, 1997.
56. Oei-Lim LB, Vermeulen-Cranch DME, Bouvy-Berends ECM: Conscious sedation with propofol in dentistry, *Br Dent J* 170:340-342, 1991.
57. Pawlicki RE: Psychological/behavioral techniques in managing pain and anxiety in the dental patient. In Dionne RA, Phero JC, eds: *Management of pain and anxiety in dental practice,* New York, 1991, Elsevier Science.
58. Poswillo DE: *General anaesthesia, sedation and resuscitation in dentistry. Report of an expert working party,* London, 1990, Standing Dental Advisory Committee.
59. Rothschild AJ: Disinhibition, amnestic reactions, and other adverse reactions secondary to triazolam: a review of the literature, *J Clin Psychiatry* 53(suppl):69-79, 1992.
60. Rubin JG, Slovin M, Krochak M: The psychodynamics of dental anxiety and dental phobia, *Dent Clin North Am* 32:647-656, 1988.
61. Schou Olesen A, Hüttel MS: Local reactions to i.v. diazepam in three different formulations, *Br J Anaesth* 52:609-611, 1980.
62. Scott DS, Hirschman R: Psychological aspects of dental anxiety in adults, *J Am Dent Assoc* 104:27-31, 1982.
63. Stewart KG, Rowbottom SJ, Aitken AW, et al: Oral ketamine premedication for paediatric cardiac surgery—a comparison with intramuscular morphine (both after oral trimeprazine), *Anaesth Intensive Care* 18:11-14, 1990.
64. Trapp LD: Pharmacologic management of pain and anxiety. In Stewart RE, et al, eds: *Pediatric dentistry: scientific foundations and clinical practice,* St Louis, 1982, Mosby.
65. Trieger N: *Pain control,* ed 2, St Louis, 1994, Mosby.
66. Upton LG, Robert RC, Jr: Hazard in administering nitrous oxide analgesia: report of case, *J Am Dent Assoc* 94:696-697, 1977.
67. *USP Dispensing information (USP DI). Vol 1.—Drug information for the health care professional,* ed 24, Greenwood Village, CO, 2004, Thomson MICROMEDEX.
68. Vaughn RL, Bennett CR: Fentanyl chest wall rigidity syndrome—a case report, *Anesth Prog* 28:50-51, 1981.
69. Weiner AA: Dental anxiety: differentiation, identification and behavioral management, *J Can Dent Assoc* 58:580-585, 1992.
70. Wong MKS, Jacobsen PL: Reasons for local anesthesia failures, *J Am Dent Assoc* 123:69-73, 1992.
71. Woolf CJ, Chong M-S: Preemptive analgesia—treating postoperative pain by preventing the establishment of central sensitization, *Anesth Analg* 77:362-379, 1993.
72. Yagiela JA: Making patients safe and comfortable for a lifetime of dentistry: frontiers in office-based sedation, *J Dent Educ* 65:1348-1356, 2001.
73. Yagiela JA, Quinn CL, Graff JR, et al: Enhanced efficacy of conscious sedation using multidrug therapy, *J Dent Res* 73(special issue):873, 1994.

General References

Clark M, Brunick A: *Handbook of nitrous oxide and oxygen sedation,* ed 2, St Louis, 2003, Mosby.

Dionne RA, Phero JC, Becker DE: *Management of pain and anxiety in the dental office,* Philadelphia, 2002, WB Saunders.

Malamed SF: *Sedation: a guide to patient management,* ed 4, St Louis, 2003, Mosby.

CHAPTER • 49

Antibiotic Prophylaxis*†

Thomas J. Pallasch

Antibiotic prophylaxis is the use of antibiotics to prevent infections and is based on the assumption that if antibiotics are useful in treating infections, then they will prevent infections. Because treating infections and preventing them entail two entirely different biologic processes, the latter assumption may be false in most instances. Antibiotic prophylaxis is used in three situations: (1) to prevent metastatic bacteremias that originate in one body part and move in blood (metastasize) to infect another body area, (2) to reduce infections associated with surgery, and (3) as "drugs of fear" in an attempt to prevent claims of negligence.[53] In the latter case, no medical justification exists for antibiotic prophylaxis, but it is used to prevent malpractice litigation by enabling the claim that "everything was done" to treat the patient properly.

Antibiotic prophylaxis is unlike most public health measures that affect millions of people because prophylaxis must be given to large numbers of individuals to prevent very few infections. In virtually all situations in which antibiotic prophylaxis is used, the infection to be prevented is rare and almost all individuals exposed to the antibiotic would never have needed it in any case. This is in contrast to other public health measures (immunization, fluoridation) in which virtually all persons exposed to the prevention will benefit. Even in the best documented efficacious use of antibiotic prophylaxis (perioperatively in clean-clean and clean-contaminated surgery), the reduction of infection rates from 2% to 1% still means that 99% of patients did not benefit from prophylaxis. With the use of antibiotic prophylaxis to prevent bacterial endocarditis from dental treatment procedures, only one in more than 100,000 patients is likely to benefit (assuming that such prophylaxis is effective).

The unsolved problems associated with antibiotic prophylaxis, particularly regarding dentistry, have recently been reviewed: (1) the high financial costs of antibiotic prophylaxis (literally hundreds of thousands to millions of dollars to prevent one case of infective endocarditis); (2) the realization that the risk of a bacteremia from activities of daily living (oral hygiene procedures, mastication) are greater than those associated with many dental treatment procedures; (3) the extreme rarity of endocarditis caused by periodontal pathogens (less than 150 cases in the literature); (4) the extremely low absolute risk rate for bacterial endocarditis from a single dental treatment procedure; (5) recent studies indicating that dental treatment procedures are rarely if ever a cause of bacterial endocarditis, (6) the likelihood that antibiotic prophylaxis does not significantly reduce bacteremias, prompting speculation that it may not work or does so by different mechanisms; (7) the contribution of antibiotic prophylaxis practices to the global epidemic of antibiotic-resistant bacteria; and (8) the possibility that the mortality rate from penicillin anaphylaxis may be greater than that from viridans group streptococcal (VGS) bacterial endocarditis.[54,57,61] Despite these questions that require clarification, dental practitioners should not take it on themselves to modify established guidelines. As of now the recommendations of the American Heart Association (AHA) are reasonable and prudent regarding endocarditis prophylaxis, as are those of the American Dental Association/American Academy of Orthopedic Surgeons regarding dental patients with prosthetic joints.

In view of the fact that antibiotic prophylaxis has legitimately been called into question, the following discussion uses evidence-based medicine and concentrates on two objectives: (1) to present the biologic basis of this practice and (2) to dissect pragmatically various clinical situations for which antibiotic prophylaxis is used, suggested, or not indicated.

PRINCIPLES OF ANTIBIOTIC PROPHYLAXIS

Antibiotic prophylaxis may be indicated if the infection to be prevented is common but not fatal or if it is rare but carries an unacceptably high mortality rate.[3] The principles of antibiotic prophylaxis were established 30 to 40 years ago but have not often been appreciated.[53,64,82,94] These include the following: (1) satisfactory risk and cost-benefit ratios should exist in which benefit to the patient significantly outweighs medical and financial risks, (2) the antibiotic must be in high concentrations at the target site (blood or tissue) before the onset of the bacteremia or surgery, (3) an antibiotic loading dose (two to four times the maintenance dose) must be used, (4) the antibiotic chosen should be active against the single most likely microorganism to cause the infection (antibiotic prophylaxis is not effective against polymicrobial infections), and (5) the antibiotic is continued only as long as microbial contamination of or from an operative site continues.[53,57,61,82,94]

The adverse effects of antibiotic prophylaxis include (1) antibiotic allergy and toxicity, (2) superinfection (onset of a new infection while treating another infection), (3) selection of antibiotic-resistant microorganisms, and (4) induction of resistance gene expression or transfer.[56,57,61] The contraindications to antibiotic prophylaxis include (1) an at-risk group that cannot be sufficiently defined to prevent overuse or abuse of antibiotic prophylaxis, (2) efficacy of prophylaxis is too

*The opinions and conclusions contained herein are those of the author and not necessarily of the American Heart Association or the American Dental Association.

†The authors wish to recognize Dr. Edward Montgomery for his past contributions to this chapter. See the Acknowledgments.

limited or unreliable, (3) the bacteremia to be prevented is too seldom a cause of infection, or (4) prophylaxis is directed at any or all potential microbial pathogens rather than the colonization of a single pathogen.[56,57,61] Justification for antibiotic prophylaxis includes situations in which there is a high risk of infection or where an infection represents a high risk to the patient, and when certain prosthetic devices are being placed.[54]

Antibiotic prophylaxis is primarily intended for two clinical situations: to prevent metastatic bacteremias or postsurgical infectious sequelae. The science to support either of these indications is limited, but in certain situations antibiotic prophylaxis is or may be reasonable.

PREVENTION OF METASTATIC INFECTIONS

The most prominent and important use of antibiotic prophylaxis is to attempt to prevent infective endocarditis (IE), principally bacterial endocarditis (BE). *IE* is an all-inclusive term for all microorganisms (bacteria, fungi, rickettsia, mycoplasma) that can cause an infection of the cardiac valves or mural endocardium, whereas the term *BE* is limited only to bacteria. Pragmatically, antibiotic prophylaxis is only employed to attempt prevention of BE and not all possible microbial causes of IE. Most of what is known about antibiotic prophylaxis is derived from animal and some clinical studies on endocarditis. Unfortunately, unwarranted extrapolations have been made from these data to clinical situations that are not comparable.

Bacterial Endocarditis: Causes and Diagnosis

The rationale for the use of antibiotic prophylaxis to prevent infections in patients with cardiac valvulopathy is that: (1) certain cardiac defects predispose to endocarditis, (2) the majority of microbes causing BE are routinely susceptible to antibiotics, (3) the risk of bacteremia is increased by certain medical and dental invasive procedures, (4) antibiotic prophylaxis reduces the incidence and magnitude of such bacteremias, and (5) antibiotic prophylaxis prevents microbial attachment to the damaged valves or inhibits their multiplication once attached.[37] Certain cardiac defects (valvulopathy, prosthetic cardiac valves) and other disorders (Box 49-1) predispose to BE, and antibiotic prophylaxis may prevent bacterial attachment to these cardiac defects or inhibit their growth. However, the majority of microorganisms causing BE are not routinely susceptible to common antibiotics because most are now caused by multiply antibiotic resistant staphylococci. Moreover, dental procedures are not a significant cause of BE and antibiotic prophylaxis may not necessarily reduce bacteremia.[57]

Oral bacteremias

The magnitude of bacteremia after various oral manipulations (oral hygiene, mastication, dental treatment) is of a low-grade intensity (1 to 12 cfu/ml of blood),[46] with the blood returning to sterility usually within 15 minutes and in many cases much sooner because the lungs, liver, spleen, and reticuloendothelial system are very efficient in clearing bacteria from the blood. It is commonly assumed that the blood is sterile before oral manipulations, but this does not always appear to be the case; two studies have indicated an 80% incidence of bacteremia at 1.5 cfu/ml before dental extractions versus 90% after extractions at 2.1 cfu/ml[31] and a preextraction bacteremia incidence of 31% at 3.6 cfu/ml versus 42.9% at 5.9 cfu/ml after the extractions.[46]

That bacteremias arise from the oral cavity and elsewhere in the body on a daily basis is well established. According to the principles of antibiotic prophylaxis, the drug chosen should be directed at the single most likely microorganism to be responsible for the infection. In the oral cavity these are viridans group streptococci (VGS) composed of *Streptococcus mitis, S. mutans, S. sanguis, S. parasanguis, S. oralis, S. crista, S. gordonii, S. anginosus, S. constellatus, S. intermedius, S. salivarius,* and *S. vestibularis.*[74] Nutritionally variant streptococci are now classified as a separate species, the *Abiotrophia. S. mutans* and *S. sanguis* are ubiquitous in the oral cavity, *S. salivarius* is primarily confined to the pharynx, *S. oralis* is almost exclusively in early dental plaque, and *S. anginosus* is primarily in subgingival plaque.[19] The importance of periodontopathic bacteria in the etiology of BE has been greatly exaggerated; fewer than 150 cases caused by these microbes have been reported in the medical literature: 102 cases from *Actinobacillus actinomycetemcomitans,* two from *Prevotella oralis,* one each from *P. bivia* and *Bacteroides melaninogenicus,* five from *Veillonella* and very rare reports of *Peptostreptococcus,* 10 from *Actinomyces,* and approximately 50 from *Lactobacillus.*[57] Periodontopathic obligate anaerobes are not likely to survive in the highly oxygenated blood of the heart and arterial system and also do not possess the surface adhesion factors that are a major factor in the propensity of streptococci and staphylococci to attach to surfaces (damaged cardiac valves).

Streptococci and staphylococci cause approximately 80% of all BE for two major reasons: (1) their ability to use various surface adhesive factors such as dextrans, glucans, selectins, fibronectin, integrins, and cadherins along with adhesion genes to attach strongly to surfaces and (2) their common location on skin and mucosa, giving them ready entry into blood as induced by trauma.

The incidence of bacteremia from various dental treatment procedures with prophylactic implications (Box 49-2) has been estimated to include tooth extraction (40% to 89%); periodontal surgery (36% to 88%); scaling and root planing (8% to 80%); simple prophylaxis (up to 40%); buccal local anesthetic injection (16%); intraligamentary injection (97%); rubber dam/matrix and wedge placement (9% to 32%); and nonsurgical endodontic treatment (up to 15%) versus those of oral hygiene procedures and mastication: tooth brushing (up to 26%), dental flossing (20% to 58%), wooden cleansing devices (20% to 40%), water irrigation devices (7% to 50%), and mastication (17% to 51%).[57,61] The pressure gradient is outward in severed blood vessels and this retards vascular uptake; therefore lymphatics may be the primary mechanism for uptake of bacteria into the blood with mastication as the major impetus.[25,57]

The studies of Guntheroth[25] and Roberts[72] indicate that the likelihood of a bacteremia arising from normal activities of daily living is 1000 to 8000 times greater than from a dental treatment procedure, if only because daily activities are so much more common than dental treatment. It is widely believed that the incidence and magnitude of oral bacteremia are directly proportional to the amount of oral inflammation present and the degree of trauma inflicted, but this concept has been challenged with significant documentation that the presence or absence of dental disease may have little to do with the advent of positive blood cultures.[45] Moreover VGS are ubiquitous in the human body as natural commensals and opportunists on the skin and conjunctiva and in the mouth, oropharynx, and gastrointestinal and genitourinary tracts.

Another consideration that requires future study is the observation that periodontal pathogens are rarely a cause of BE and that VGS are antagonistic to periodontal pathogens and dominate in a healthy mouth.[30] It is then possible that a healthy mouth may be a greater risk for endocarditis than one afflicted with periodontitis, particularly if the lymphatics are the route to the systemic circulation (oral lymphatic flow is best stimulated by mastication).

Given these data, determining causality in any case of endocarditis (or any other oral metastatic infection) allegedly

Box • 49-1

Antibiotic Prophylaxis for Various Medical Conditions

Prophylaxis Recommended
Previous IE
Cardiac valve prosthesis
Rheumatic heart disease
Hypertrophic cardiomyopathy
Solid organ transplants with valvulopathy
Mitral valve prolapse with regurgitation
Congenital heart disease*
Kawasaki disease with valvulopathy
VA shunt for hydrocephalus
Collagen disorders with valvulopathy†
Indwelling catheter (right heart)
Myeloproliferative disorders with valvulopathy‡
Mitral and aortic valve stenosis/regurgitation
Idiopathic hypertrophic aortic stenosis
Surgically repaired intracardiac CHD with residua with hemodynamic defects
Mitral and aortic valve stenosis/regurgitation§
WBC count less than 500 to 1000

Prophylaxis Not Recommended
Coronary bypass surgery
Previous rheumatic fever without RHD
Isolated secundum atrial-septal defect
Solid organ transplants without valvulopathy
Coronary artery disease
Mitral valve prolapse without regurgitation
Cardiac pacemakers and implanted defibrillators
Kawasaki disease without valvulopathy
Physiologic, functional heart murmurs
Arterial grafts
Peripheral and coronary stents
HIV/AIDS
Asplenia
Surgically repaired intracardiac CHD without residual hemodynamic defects
Orthopedic pins and screws
Orthopedic prosthetic joints¶
Dacron carotid patches
Diabetes
Left ventricular assist devices
Artificial hearts
Hemodialysis
Breast and penile implants

Prophylaxis Undecided
Intravenous drug abusers
Congenital pulmonary stenosis
Head and neck radiation
Libman-Sacks (marantic) endocarditis‖
Calcific aortic stenosis

From Osmon DR: Antimicrobial prophylaxis in adults, *Mayo Clin Proc* 75:98-109, 2000; Pallasch TJ: Antibiotic prophylaxis, *Endod Topics* 4:46-59, 2003; Pallasch TJ: Antibiotic prophylaxis: the clinical significance of its recent evolution, *J Calif Dent Assoc* 25:619-624, 626-632, 1997; Pallasch TJ, Slots J: Antibiotic prophylaxis and the medically compromised patient, *Periodontol 2000* 10:107-138, 1996.
*Includes bicuspid/unicuspid aortic valve, coarctation of the aorta, patent ductus arteriosus, atrial septal defect, ventricular septal defect, complex cyanotic heart disease, tetralogy of Fallot, transposition of the great vessels, and systemic pulmonary artery shunt.
†Includes systemic lupus erythematosus, rheumatoid arthritis, osteogenesis imperfecta, Marfan syndrome, Ehlers-Danlos syndrome, Hurler's syndrome, pseudoxanthoma elasticum with possible valvulopathy, and Libman-Sacks endocarditis.
‡Includes polycythemia vera, essential thrombocytopenia, anogenic myeloid metaplasia with possible valvulopathy, and Libman-Sacks endocarditis.
§Depends on severity; physician consult may be advisable.
¶Should be considered but not mandatory for patients with inflammatory arthropathies (systemic lupus erythematosus, rheumatoid arthritis); disease-, drug-, or radiation-induced immunosuppression; type 1 diabetes; hemophilia; malnourishment; 2 years or less after joint replacement; previous joint infection.
‖Includes patients with heart and other solid organ transplants, cancer, collagen and myeloproliferative disorders, and primary antiphospholipid syndrome. Valvulopathy may or may not be present; physician consultation may be in order.
VA, Ventricular atrial; *CHD*, congenital heart disease; *WBC*, white blood cell; *RHD*, rheumatoid heart disease.

from dental treatment is impossible unless the microbe is determined to be genetically identical to that in the infected body part. Even then, determining whether the VGS originated from the specific dental procedure, as a result of daily living bacteremias before or after the treatment, or from a distant source makes attribution of BE to a specific dental procedure very difficult. The advent of recent clinical data that dental treatment procedures are likely not associated with endocarditis[39,84] should greatly reduce the involvement and blame of dental health professionals as the proximate cause of BE.[62]

Microbial Causation of Infective Endocarditis (IE)

Virtually any microbial pathogen can or has caused IE, but 80% to 85% are associated with streptococci and staphylococci. Since 1992 certain trends have become apparent: (1) rates of BE from VGS have decreased from 40% of the total IE percentage to approximately 25%; (2) the incidence of *S. aureus* endocarditis has significantly increased, whereas coagulase-negative staphylococcal (CoNS) BE has remained static; (3) rates of non-VGS streptococcal BE have doubled; (4) cases of fungal IE have increased; and (5) the incidence of culture-negative IE has declined.[8] Most left-sided acute endocarditis is caused by *S. aureus* (with a 40% mortality rate); however, *S. pneumoniae, Neisseria gonorrhoeae,* and fungi are also highly virulent. Rare organisms include *Staphylococcus lugdunensis, Rothia dentocariosa, Clostridium perfringens, Acinetobacter baumanii, Yersinia pestis,* and *Erysipelothrix rhusiopathiae.* Nosocomial (hospital-acquired) endocarditis accounts for 10% to 29% of all IE cases and is almost exclusively caused by gram-positive aerobes such as staphylococci and enterococci as well as fungi.[8]

Culture-negative endocarditis accounts for 5% to 8% of cases and is commonly caused by fastidious, slow-growing

Box • 49-2

Relative Bacteremia Incidence with Dental Treatment Procedures versus Activities of Daily Living

Dental Treatment Bacteremias

Tooth extraction: 40% to 89%
Periodontal surgery: 36% to 88%
Simple prophylaxis: 0% to 40%
Buccal anesthetic injection: 16%
Intraligamentary injection: 97%
Rubber dam/matrix/wedge: 9% to 32%
Nonsurgical endodontic treatment: 0% to 15%

Activities of Daily Living

Tooth brushing: 0% to 26%
Dental flossing: 20% to 58%
Wooden cleansing devices: 20% to 40%
Water irrigation devices: 7% to 50%
Mastication: 17% to 51%

From Pallasch TJ: Antibiotic prophylaxis: problems in paradise, *Dent Clin North Am* 47:665-679, 2003; Pallasch TJ, Slots J: Antibiotic prophylaxis and the medically compromised patient, *Periodontol 2000* 10:107-138, 1996.

microorganisms such as the HACEK group (*Haemophilus influenzae*, *A. actinomycetemcomitans*, *Cardiobacterium hominis*, *Eikenella corrodens*, *Kingella kingae*), *Bartonella*, *Brucella*, *Chlamydia*, *Legionella*, *Neisseria*, *Abiotrophia*, *Corynebacterium*, *Aspergillus*, *Candida*, and *Coxiella burnetii* (Q fever). A major factor in culture-negative IE is the common use of antibiotics to treat the early symptoms of endocarditis, since these closely resemble influenza. Such faulty use of antibiotics doubles the time to diagnosis and hospitalization that is crucial in the successful treatment of IE.[61]

Incidence of infective endocarditis

IE is a rare disease estimated to occur at a rate of 11 to 50 per 1 million population per year (11,200 annual cases in the United States, 1500 cases in Britain), which equates to 1.7 to 4.9 per 100,000 person-years in the United States. Because the incidence of IE has not declined since the advent of antibiotic prophylaxis in the 1950s,[56] it may be that antibiotic prophylaxis is ineffective or poorly applied, that the nature and risks of the disease have changed, or that endocarditis is a disease resulting from a confluence of events not under control of either the patient or health care professional. These events may include random spontaneous bacteremias with virulent and adhesive microbes encountering damaged cardiac valves and a failed host defense system. Harmless bacteremias occur daily, making bacteremias very common but endocarditis very rare. BE is one of the few documented examples of focal infection, a topic that has undergone recent extensive review and is of considerable current interest.[62,63]

Risk Factors for Infective Endocarditis

Cardiovascular abnormalities predisposing to IE are either congenital or acquired (see Box 49-1). Congenital heart disease includes atrial septal defect, ventricular septal defect, patent ductus arteriosus, coarctation of the aorta, bicuspid or unicuspid aortic valve, complex cyanotic heart disease, and transposition of the great vessels. Acquired valvular disease includes rheumatic heart disease; mitral valve prolapse; previous endocarditis; and varying degrees of mitral and aortic valve stenosis, calcification, and regurgitation.

Most acquired valve disease is caused by high-velocity turbulent blood flow (jet streams) that are detected as cardiac murmurs and over time damage the endothelium of the valve surfaces (wear and tear), promoting the deposition of fibrin and platelets in the form of a nonbacterial thrombotic endocarditis or vegetation. This progressive valvular damage over time explains why IE is now primarily a disease of older individuals.

The classic study by Steckelberg and Wilson[78] established the risk of acquiring IE based on certain cardiac risk factors. The incidence of IE in the general population is 1.7 to 4.9 per 100,000 person-years but rises to 300 to 740 per 100,000 with previous endocarditis, 308 to 630 per 100,000 with a cardiac valve prosthesis, 380 to 440 per 100,000 with rheumatic heart disease, 120 per 100,000 for congenital heart disease, 60 per 100,000 for corrected congenital heart disease, and 52 per 100,000 for mitral valve prolapse with regurgitation. For mitral valve prolapse without regurgitation the risk is the same as for the general population.

The risk for endocarditis in intravenous drug abusers is 2% to 5% per year, with 40% of recurrent endocarditis occurring in this population.[75] Between 20% and 40% of intravenous drug users have valve damage either from previous IE or contaminants of street drugs, and these patients should receive IE antibiotic prophylaxis[24] even though most BE in drug abusers is right sided (tricuspid valve) and associated with staphylococci.

As the population grows older, concerns have arisen regarding calcification of the mitral and aortic valves and the potential risk for endocarditis. Calcific aortic stenosis is the most common valvular lesion in the United States and a major risk for aortic valve replacement, whereas mitral annular calcification can lead to mitral regurgitation. In a study of 5201 patients older than 65 years, aortic valve stenosis was found in 26% and aortic valve sclerosis in 37% older than 75 years.[81] Aortic valve disease is common in the elderly and its relation to endocarditis will be addressed in the future by the American Heart Association.

One of the highest risks for endocarditis is the patient with a prosthetic heart valve with a 1% to 4% lifetime risk of endocarditis,[78] resulting in 9.5% to 16% of all endocarditis cases.[50] The incidence of IE is similar with either the bioprosthetic or mechanical valve and the mortality rate is 5% for BE from VGS and 65% from *S. aureus*,[84] with approximately 15% of cases caused by VGS.

Recent general agreement on case definitions for mitral valve prolapse has led to an estimated incidence in the general population of 1.6% to 2.4%, with an equal prevalence in men and women.[14,20] This disorder is much more serious in men than women, with the risk for valve degeneration leading to valve repair or replacement being two to four times greater in men.[76]

Mitral valve prolapse is a cardiac valve disorder characterized by a midsystolic click or a late systolic murmur with a greater than 2 mm displacement of the mitral leaflet(s) into the atrial cavity during systole and more than 5 mm of leaflet thickness (classic mitral valve prolapse) or less than a 5-mm valve thickness (nonclassic mitral valve prolapse). It is now considered a spectrum of abnormalities ranging from a slight billowing of the valve to thick redundant leaflets with myxomatous degeneration, elongation of the chordae tendineae, and severe mitral regurgitation with eventual death without valve replacement or repair.[20] The severity of the mitral regurgitation can only be accurately determined by a two-dimensional color-flow Doppler echocardiogram.[67]

The risk of IE in mitral valve prolapse with regurgitation is relatively low at 52 per 100,000 person-years, with various estimates at 4.5 to 13 times greater than the normal population and an absolute risk rate of 140 per 1 million population per year.[61] The majority of people with mitral valve prolapse have a normal life span with no significant disability or acquisition of IE. A small subset gradually develops billowing mitral leaflets, myxomatous degeneration, floppy mitral valves, and flail leaflets over an average of 25 years of diagnosis of mitral valve prolapse, leading to severe mitral regurgitation necessitating valve surgery.[83]

In 1997, reports began to appear of cardiac valve abnormalities in patients taking serotonergic appetite suppressants (fenfluramine, dexfenfluramine), and considerable debate ensued regarding the actual incidence and prevalence of such pathology.[59] Guidelines for the management of these patients were formulated by the Department of Health and Human Services and the American College of Cardiology/AHA that are still in effect and have not been rescinded or modified.[59]

All recommendations require a physical examination and an echocardiogram when deemed appropriate. If valvulopathy is present, the 1997 AHA guidelines for the prevention of BE are to be used. If these individuals require emergency dental treatment before such tests can be performed, AHA antibiotic prophylaxis is used, with the tests to follow later. A prudent dentist should identify these patients with a written and dialogue medical history, advise the patient to seek this examination, and defer any elective dental treatment until a determination of any valvulopathy is made.[59]

In a study of 1142 patients at 17.5 to 18.7 months after fenfluramine (plus phentermine) or dexfenfluramine were discontinued, 95.6% had either no valve damage or no change whereas 4.4% got worse.[22] In a study of 1473 patients from 25 US medical centers having taken fenfluramine or dexfenfluramine (phentermine was never associated with valve damage) for a mean duration of 6 months, aortic regurgitation was detected in 8.9% with dexfenfluramine, 13.7% with fenfluramine/phentermine, and 4.1% of control subjects.[21] In most but not all reports the incidence and severity of the valvulopathy increased with dose and duration of use: a three times greater risk of valve damage if taken for 1 year versus 90 days and if doses were greater than 60 mg/day.[35]

The current understanding of this disorder associated with fenfluramine or dexfenfluramine indicates that (1) virtually all studies detect some incidence of valve pathology depending on dose and duration of drug use; (2) some lesions regress, some remain the same, and some progress over time; and (3) many studies were compromised by variations in echocardiographic technique, substantial referral bias (only the most serious cases sent to the centers where the studies were performed), and often a lack of predrug-exposure echocardiograms to compare with postdrug examinations. The histologic examination of valve specimens taken during valve replacement was consistent: valve thickening with chordae fusion, myxoid stroma, and dense fibroblastic tissue with the leaflets and chordae encased in plaque adherent to the valve.[92,93] As yet no data have appeared on the incidence of IE in such patients.

Innocent Heart Murmurs

One of the most perplexing questions on the health history is the determination of whether the "childhood murmur" indicated by the patient is an innocent (physiologic, functional) murmur of no current concern or an organic murmur requiring antibiotic prophylaxis. Not all murmurs are pathologic even in adulthood.

The incidence of heart murmurs in children is greater than 50%, with a reported range of 32% to 95% depending on how often the child is examined and the skill of the examiner,[26] whereas the incidence of cardiac malformations at birth is 6.0 to 9.3 per 1000 live births. Common innocent childhood murmurs include pulmonary flow murmur, vibratory Still's murmur, peripheral pulmonary arterial stenosis murmur, aortic systolic murmur, normal continuous murmur, and supraclavicular murmurs. All these are the result of the changing hemodynamics of the heart during growth.[66]

Many cardiac murmurs in adulthood are also nonpathologic and have certain characteristics: (1) a systolic murmur of short duration with a grade 1 or 2 intensity at the left sternal border, (2) normal intensity and splitting of the second heart sound, (3) no other abnormal sounds or murmurs, (4) no evidence of ventricular dysfunction, (5) no thrills, and (6) no increase in intensity with the Valsalva maneuver.[9] An astute pediatric or adult cardiologist can readily distinguish between physiologic and pathologic heart murmurs; the problem lies with internists and medical residents who, in a study of stethoscope skills, could only diagnose 20% of 12 common cardiac valve pathologic conditions with no improvement 1 year later in their training.[47] With reticence in managed care to incur the costs of specialist referral or an echocardiogram for diagnosis, dentists will likely employ antibiotic prophylaxis on many patients who do not actually require it.

Signs and Symptoms of Infective Endocarditis

One of the most important factors in the successful treatment of endocarditis is early detection. Unfortunately the early signs and symptoms are vague and resemble influenza: night chills, fever, malaise, myalgia, arthralgia, and anorexia.[6] Other signs and symptoms include back pain, polyarthritis, splenomegaly, anemic pallor, and a changing or new heart murmur. Immunologic phenomena are uncommon today: nail splinter hemorrhages, Osler's nodes (small, purple, tender nodules in the pulp of the fingers and toes), Janeway lesions (small erythematous maculae on the palms and the soles of the feet), and Roth spots (pale, oval retinal hemorrhages).[6] No laboratory tests are diagnostic for IE, but findings include normochromic normocytic anemia, elevated sedimentation rate, microscopic hematuria, increased C-reactive protein (CRP) level, and circulating immune complexes.[6]

Echocardiographic Diagnosis

The current standard for the diagnosis of IE is the reliance on the "Duke Criteria"; major criteria include positive blood cultures with common etiologic microorganisms and a positive echocardiogram for valve pathology.[6,17,40] Minor criteria include intravenous drug abusers or predisposing heart problems, fever, vascular or immunologic phenomena, consistent but not definitive echocardiographic findings, and consistent but not definitive serologic or bacteriologic findings.[17] The Duke Criteria for the diagnosis of endocarditis differ from the older Beth Israel (Von Reyn) criteria by a strong reliance on echocardiographic findings of an oscillating cardiac mass on a valve or supporting structures in the path of a regurgitant jet stream or implanted material, a valve ring abscess, a new prosthetic valve dehiscence, or a new valvular regurgitant murmur.[17,86] A definitive diagnosis is made on the basis of two major criteria, one major and three minor criteria, or five minor criteria.[17] Suggested additional minor criteria are newly diagnosed clubbing of fingers, splenomegaly, splinter hemorrhages, skin petechiae, high CRP level, microscopic hematuria, high erythrocyte sedimentation rate, and the presence of central or peripheral venous lines.[40]

Incubation Period and Time to Hospitalization

One of the most important criteria for attempting to determine the proximate cause of BE is the incubation period, the time from initiation of the bacteremia to the onset of the signs and symptoms of endocarditis. The resemblance of the early symptoms of IE to influenza can make this determination difficult.

Only one study has been performed to determine this incubation period and then only for VGS and enterococci.[77] The median incubation period for 76 cases was assessed to be 5 days for enterococci and 7 days for VGS, with 84% of cases displaying signs or symptoms within 14 days.[77] A Netherlands study determined a mean 14-day period between dental treatment and the onset of IE symptoms, but the range was so wide (0 to 175 days) that it cast doubt on the relevance of the data.[91] The AHA guidelines state that the incubation period is usually 14 days or less.[10]

In acute left-sided endocarditis from *S. aureus* and other highly virulent microorganisms (*S. pneumoniae* or *pyogenes, N. gonorrhoeae*), the incubation period is very short (usually 2 to 5 days).[61] With *S. epidermidis* and other CoNS, the incubation period is likely longer than that for VGS. For the HACEK group bacteria and other fastidious, slow-growing microorganisms, the period may be even longer than for CoNS.[61]

The time from onset of signs and symptoms to diagnosis and hospitalization is more variable than the incubation period because it depends on microorganism virulence, host resistance, patient reticence to seek medical care, and, importantly, any antibiotic therapy given for the initial flulike symptoms. In five clinical studies the time to hospitalization for native valve endocarditis was a mean 58 days (range 31 to 78 days) for VGS, 12 days (range 8 to 19 days) for *S. aureus*, and 37 to 41 days for *S. epidermidis*.[61] In The Netherlands the mean time to hospitalization for native valve endocarditis was 27 days and 11.5 days for prosthetic valve endocarditis.[90]

The use of antibiotics before diagnosis is associated with an increase in time (up to double) between diagnosis and treatment. At the Bergen University Hospital, the time to hospitalization for staphylococcal endocarditis was 2 to 8 days without prior antibiotics and 10 to 14 days with antibiotics and for streptococcal endocarditis was 26.6 days without antibiotics and 46.6 days with antibiotics.[41]

Complications of Infective Endocarditis

Before the advent of antibiotics IE was universally fatal, with the only distinction being the time taken to die: acute (less than 6 weeks), subacute (6 weeks to 3 months), and chronic (longer than 3 months). Because of early detection, antibiotic therapy, and valve replacement, the mortality rate now primarily depends on early diagnosis, response to treatment, and the particular etiologic microorganism (less than 10% for VGS, up to 50% for left-sided *S. aureus*, and up to 80% for fungal endocarditis).

The sequelae to IE are many and include congestive (left-sided) heart failure, peripheral embolization, perivalvular abscess, focal neurologic deficits, heart block, and metastatic septic emboli to virtually any organ but particularly the brain, heart, kidney, lungs, or spleen. Heart failure is the most ominous development, the most common cause of death, and the major reason for valve replacement. Systemic peripheral emboli occur in 22% to 50% of cases, mostly in the first 2 weeks, and up to 65% locate in the brain, with 90% of those along the course of the middle cerebral artery.[6] Brain mycotic infected aneurysms are very serious and commonly heralded by severe headache. Cardiac sequelae include bulky vegetations, valve and chordae destruction, and intracardiac abscesses. Neurologic complications include stroke (10% to 18%), seizures, and encephalitis.[6]

The management of IE critically depends on isolating the offending microorganism (IE is very rarely polymicrobial) and determining its antibiotic susceptibility profile. Various formulas for proper culturing include several positive cultures more than 12 hours apart, positive blood cultures in three of three sets, the majority of four or more sets (with the first and last 1 hour apart), or three positive blood cultures spaced 30 to 60 minutes apart, all reflecting persistent bacteria shed into the blood from infected vegetations.[87] Polymerase chain reaction (PCR) technology can identify any microorganism, particularly the fastidious microbes, and is now available in real time, providing microorganism identification in minutes. In a study of 116 patients with IE, only 60% had blood cultures taken before antibiotic treatment, 40% had an unnecessary delay in valve replacement, only 66% had an identifiable portal of entry for the inciting bacteremia, and only 38% complied with the established treatment guidelines for IE.[11] The trend is toward earlier valve replacement, particularly if multiple early embolizations and signs of heart failure are present.

Antibiotic Prevention of Bacterial Endocarditis

A summary of dental procedures for which endocarditis prophylaxis is either recommended or not required is given in Box 49-3. This classification is intended to indicate which are associated with significant bleeding and which are not. The AHA has published its recommendations for the prevention of BE at intervals dating back to 1955, with the most current dose recommendations listed in Table 49-1.[10] These current

Box • 49-3

Dental Procedures and Endocarditis Prophylaxis

Endocarditis Prophylaxis Recommended*

- Dental extractions
- Periodontal procedures, including surgery, scaling, root planing, probing, and recall maintenance
- Dental implant placement and reimplantation of avulsed teeth
- Endodontic (root canal) instrumentation or surgery only beyond the apex
- Subgingival placement of antibiotic fibers or strips
- Initial placement of orthodontic bands (but not brackets)
- Intraligamentary local anesthetic injections
- Prophylactic cleaning of teeth or implants where bleeding is anticipated

Endocarditis Prophylaxis Not Recommended

- Restorative dentistry† (operative and prosthodontic) with or without retraction cord‡
- Local anesthetic injections (nonintraligamentary)
- Intracanal endodontic treatment; post placement and build up
- Placement of rubber dams
- Postoperative suture removal
- Placement of removal prosthodontic or orthodontic appliances
- Fluoride treatments
- Taking of oral radiographs
- Orthodontic appliance adjustment
- Shedding of primary teeth

*Prophylaxis is recommended for patients with high- and moderate-risk cardiac conditions.
†This includes restoration of decayed teeth (filling cavities) and replacement of missing teeth.
‡Clinical judgment may indicate antibiotic use in selected circumstances that may create significant bleeding.

Table • 49-1

Antibiotic Prophylaxis Guidelines for the Prevention of BE

	DOSAGE FOR ADULTS	DOSAGE FOR CHILDREN*
Standard Regimen (Oral)†		
Amoxicillin	2 g 1 hour before procedure	50 mg/kg 1 hour before procedure
Penicillin Allergy (Oral)		
Clindamycin *or*	600 mg 1 hour before procedure	20 mg/kg 1 hour before procedure
Cephalexin or cefadroxil† *or*	2 g 1 hour before procedure	50 mg/kg 1 hour before procedure
Clarithromycin or azithromycin	500 mg 1 hour before procedure	15 mg/kg 1 hour before procedure
Unable To Take Oral Medications		
Ampicillin	2 g IM or IV 30 min before procedure	50 mg/kg IM or IV 30 min before procedure
Penicillin Allergy and Unable To Take Oral Medications		
Clindamycin	600 mg IV 30 min before procedure	20 mg/kg IV 30 min before procedure
Cefazolin†	1 g IM or IV 30 min before procedure	25 mg/kg IM or IV 30 min before procedure

Adapted from Dajani AS, Taubert KA, Wilson W, et al: Prevention of bacterial endocarditis: recommendations by the American Heart Association, *JAMA* 277:1794-1801, 1997; Pallasch TJ: Antibiotic prophylaxis: the clinical significance of its recent evolution, *J Calif Dent Assoc* 25:619-624, 626-632, 1997.
*Total children's dose should not exceed adult dose.
†Cephalosporins should not be used in patients with a history of immediate allergic reactions (urticaria, angioedema, anaphylaxis) to penicillin.
IM, Intramuscularly; *IV*, intravenously.

guidelines differ from those of the past primarily in antibiotic dosage, a more detailed discussion of at-risk patients, and a delineation of dental procedures into those with a significant risk for bleeding and those with minimal risk. This distinction, along with the stratification of risk patients, was formulated to reduce the use of antibiotic prophylaxis and its deleterious contribution to global microbial resistance to antibiotics in view of the limited evidence for the efficacy of such antibiotic prophylaxis in humans.

After the publication of these recommendations in 1997, a number of questions arose regarding some of the specifics that could not be included in the original document. These questions were answered in 1999,[60] and the major points are summarized as follows:

1. The guidelines provided the reader with dental procedures that were often considered associated with significant bleeding and should receive antibiotic prophylaxis versus those that were likely to be associated with little or no bleeding and did not require prophylaxis; previous guidelines suggested prophylaxis for all dental procedures associated with any bleeding of any magnitude.
2. Prophylaxis was not recommended for routine suture removal, but if a large number of sutures were present the clinical judgment of the dentist should prevail if significant bleeding would be involved.
3. Dental matrix bands and gingival retraction cord do not ordinarily produce significant bleeding, but if significant bleeding is anticipated, clinical judgment might suggest prophylaxis.
4. If dental patients forget to take their antibiotic before the appointment, they should reschedule the appointment or be given the drug and asked to wait 1 hour before beginning dental treatment. Antibiotic prophylaxis works best if the drug is in the system before the onset of bacteremia, and it would be difficult to defend giving the antibiotic and immediately beginning treatment if it were established that this was done to prevent the economic loss of a canceled appointment.
5. If the dentist did not anticipate significant bleeding and later in the appointment encountered such bleeding, she/he can administer the antibiotic prophylaxis and finish the treatment because research suggests that prophylaxis may be effective up to 2 hours after onset of the bacteremia. This recommendation was formed to encourage the dentist not to use prophylaxis for dental procedures with minimal risk for bacteremia but not to avoid patient rescheduling or a 1-hour wait.
6. A 9- to 14-day interval is advised between appointments because significant antibiotic resistance may be seen in oral bacteria even with a single antibiotic dose, and this interval will likely allow for a return to drug sensitivity.
7. If only a short interval occurs between appointments (e.g., 12 to 24 hours), significant selection of resistant strains is not likely to occur and the same antibiotic can be used.
8. If multiple appointments are necessary, with an interval shorter than 9 to 14 days, antibiotic prophylaxis should be alternated between amoxicillin and a drug of a different class, such as clindamycin.
9. Patients with ongoing poor gingival health likely have a greater risk for bacteremia than any associated with sporadic oral hygiene procedures; therefore any brief and temporary increase in bacteremia associated with initiating improved daily oral hygiene (brushing, flossing) in the presence of such inflammation is more than offset by the benefit of eliminating future inflammation via periodontal treatment by a dental health professional.
10. A second antibiotic dose could conceivably be useful if the patient has two appointments in the same day (e.g., early morning, then early evening); both appointments could employ the 2 g dose or alternately only 1 g as the second dose if the treatment takes longer than 4 to 6

hours (as in a dental school setting); amoxicillin, because of its longer half-life than penicillin V generally provides adequate prophylaxis for a 4- to 6-hour period.

The 1997 AHA endocarditis prevention guidelines are one standard of care and are not intended as *the* standard of care. The committee formulating these recommendations fully recognizes that they cannot cover all possible and conceivable clinical situations and that the clinical judgment of the dentist and physician is paramount because only these individuals have all the facts at hand. If the dentist thinks that, based on the clinical situation, these recommendations may need modification, she/he may wish to contact the AHA in Dallas for advice. It would be wise to make a note in the dental record that a course of treatment was undertaken "in my best clinical judgment" in unusual situations known to the dentist in order to deter later possible criticism if the records should be examined in hindsight by medicolegal experts or attorneys.

Oral Hygiene and Bacterial Endocarditis

Good oral hygiene is likely to reduce the incidence of daily, random, spontaneous bacteremia resulting from periodontal disease, but there are no data to indicate that good oral hygiene also reduces endocarditis incidence. Good oral health habits may only apply to gingivitis because periodontitis pathogens are rarely a cause of endocarditis. Subgingival inflammation could increase the likelihood of a VGS bacteremia but no data exist to support this contention. Flossing may reduce the risk of endocarditis,[85] but little direct evidence suggests that an increase in the magnitude and incidence of bacteremia results in an increase in endocarditis.[43,45,61] An additional difficulty is the association of VGS with gingival health:[30] the more VGS present, the healthier the mouth. Because VGS causes 25% of all BE, and periodontopathic bacteria are rarely a cause, it could be argued that a mouth diseased with periodontitis is less of a risk for BE than a healthy mouth. Alternately, a healthy mouth is less likely to bleed significantly, which could reduce the risk if blood vessels and not lymphatics are the avenue to the systemic circulation. It is hoped these issues can be clarified in the future. Good oral health remains a good idea but its relevance to the etiology of BE is not established.[56,57,62]

Antibiotic Prophylaxis and Bacteremia Reduction

Numerous studies have indicated that antibiotic prophylaxis reduces bacteremia,[61] but as yet no plausible biologic explanation has been found as to why drugs (antibiotics) that act so slowly (in hours) eliminate bacteremias so quickly (in seconds to minutes). The penicillins and cephalosporins require bacteria in the active process of cell division to prevent the final transpeptidation reaction leading to the formation of the rigid bacterial cell wall. If the microorganism is not dividing, β-lactams have no activity. Not all VGS in the blood will suddenly begin to divide as soon as the dentist places the forceps on the tooth to be extracted. Similarly, bacteriostatic antibiotics (macrolides, clindamycin) may take hours to inhibit bacterial ribosomal protein synthesis.

Studies in Sweden with sophisticated microbial culturing techniques document that neither penicillin V, amoxicillin, cefaclor, erythromycin, nor clindamycin given orally 1.0 to 1.5 hours before dental extractions significantly reduces bacteremia.[27-29] It has been suggested that antibiotic prophylaxis prevents endocarditis by either limiting or preventing microorganism adherence to the nonbacterial thrombotic endocarditis through an action on cell walls or by eliminating the organisms after they attach to the damaged wall.[15,52] An alteration in adhesion is not likely to apply to bacteriostatic agents, and, given the difficulties of antibiotic penetration into the vegetation during treatment of BE, antibiotic prophylaxis is not likely to inhibit or kill bacteria embedded in fibrin and platelets.

In a best case scenario, antibiotic prophylaxis may prevent only 10% of all endocarditis cases.[37] Studies in The Netherlands have indicated that antibiotic prophylaxis may prevent 5.7% of all native valve endocarditis and 3.8% of all prosthetic valve endocarditis, which would then prevent (assuming 49% efficacy) five cases per year in a population of 14.5 million in The Netherlands.[90,91] Optimal prophylaxis might prevent 240 to 280 cases out of 11,200 annually in the United States.[15]

Antibiotic Prophylaxis Failures

Few data support the efficacy of antibiotic prophylaxis in humans—such a study would need 6000 at-risk patients and would never be approved by an institutional review committee. In 1983 the AHA published a study of 52 apparent failures but 88% of these had not followed the 1977 AHA prevention regimen.[16] The clinical failures of the AHA regimen are not likely to ever be adequately documented because of patient noncompliance, fear of malpractice litigation, lack of attention to the incubation period, and the substantial role of random spontaneous bacteremias.

Risk-Benefit Ratio of Antibiotic Prophylaxis

It was not until the mid-1980s that attention was paid to the adverse effects of antibiotic prophylaxis, particularly regarding penicillin allergy.[61] One calculation indicates that the death rate from endocarditis exceeds that of penicillin anaphylaxis only when the highest incidence of IE (50 per 1 million population) and the highest death rate (40%) occurs.[55] Tzukert et al[88] determined that 1.36 persons per 1 million population are likely to die from penicillin anaphylaxis during endocarditis prevention, whereas only 0.26 deaths per 1 million population are the result of dental treatment–induced endocarditis.[88]

Economics of Antibiotic Prophylaxis

Antibiotic prophylaxis is expensive because the drugs must be given to so many to prevent only a few infections. The cost of preventing VGS endocarditis according to 1990 doses (3 g of amoxicillin initially, then 1.5 g 6 hours later) is $96 million to prevent 32 fatal cases, or $3 million per fatal case (or $300,000 for each nonfatal case).[61] This cost has been significantly reduced by the present 2 g dose but is still substantial. Other calculations have been (1) $20 million to prevent 35 BE cases in mitral valve prolapse patients with erythromycin and (2) $1 million per life saved with penicillin for mitral valve prolapse.[61]

The Absolute Risk Rate for Endocarditis from Dental Treatment

Estimates have appeared in the literature with no corroborating data that dental treatment or poor oral hygiene accounts for 8% to 30% of all endocarditis, with a risk of 1 in 3000 to 1 in 5000 dental procedures.[57] In contrast to these estimates, several evidence-based case-control studies strongly suggest that no association may exist between dental treatment and endocarditis causation.[39,84,85] Using the relative risk rates of Steckelberg and Wilson,[78] along with certain assumptions, the estimated absolute risk rate of acquiring endocarditis from a single dental treatment procedure can be calculated.[57,62]

If 250 million people in the United States visit a dentist on average of 1.6 times per year (400 million visits per year) and the incidence of IE is 11,200 cases per year, with 25% caused by VGS (2800 cases), the absolute risk rate is 1 in 142,258 in the general population if all VGS endocarditis is caused by dental treatment.[57,62] If only 1% is caused by dental treatment (28 cases), the absolute risk rate rises to 1 in 14,258,714 in the general population. The absolute risk rate by the Steckelberg and Wilson data[78] in people with cardiac risk factors rises substantially: 1 in 95,058 for previous endocarditis, 1 in 114,069 for cardiac valve prosthesis, 1 in 142,258 for rheumatic heart disease, 1 in 475,290 for congenital heart disease, and 1 in 1,096,824 for mitral valve prolapse with regurgitation.[57,62] Even in high-risk BE patients, the absolute risk rate is very low and will be addressed in future American Heart Association guidelines.

POTENTIAL ANTIBIOTIC PROPHYLAXIS SITUATIONS

The following sections discuss the evidence supporting or not supporting prophylactic antibiotic use in other clinical situations.

Orthopedic Prosthetic Joints

The 2003 Advisory Statement of the American Dental Association and the American Academy of Orthopedic Surgeons on antibiotic prophylaxis for dental patients with prosthetic joints (Box 49-4) concludes that "Presently, no scientific evidence supports the position that antibiotic prophylaxis to prevent hematogenous infections is required prior to dental treatment in patients with total joint prosthesis."[1] The guidelines suggest that with certain patients (as listed in Box 49-5) antibiotic prophylaxis should be considered.[58]

This has commonly been interpreted to mean that such patients *must* be given prophylaxis, which is inaccurate. Little evidence indicates that potentially immunocompromised total joint prosthesis patients are at a greater risk for infection. Some evidence suggests that oral sepsis (gross caries, periodontal inflammation, periapical abscesses) not associated with dental treatment can result in prosthetic joint infections; four cases have been reported to be caused by *S. sanguis,* with genetically identical organisms as in the septic oral cavity.[5] No such documented cases have been associated with dental treatment–induced bacteremia. Infection of prosthetic joints does occur with oral microorganisms, but as yet none have been scientifically linked to dental treatment. Data from the Mayo Clinic indicate that the incidence of late prosthetic joint infections rapidly decreases with time and reaches a low-level plateau at 2 years from placement.[54] In a study of the microbial contamination of prosthetic joint replacement sites *before* implantation, 12.8% were contaminated with streptococci, staphylococci, and gram-negative rods.[23]

As a worst-case scenario, dental treatment procedures may be associated with a 0.03% to 0.04% rate (30 to 40 cases per 100,000 person-years) of prosthetic joint infections.[61,62] If the risk of such infections is 1000 times greater from activities of daily living than from dental treatment, the absolute risk rate for dental treatment–induced prosthetic joint infections is 1 per 2.5 million procedures.[61,62] Penicillin prophylaxis for such patients would likely result in a net loss of life, mostly from penicillin allergies, with a potentially similar result with the cephalosporins. Proper screening of patients is important in reducing the risk of allergies to β-lactam antibiotics. No antibiotic prophylaxis is indicated for such dental patients undergoing dental procedures where there is minimal risk from bacteremia (as listed in Box 49-3) for patients with increased risk of BE.

These data must be tempered with the realization that up to 18% of prosthetic joint infections may be fatal.[61] This high death rate is very rarely associated with oral microorganisms and constitutes the only conceivable reason for antibiotic prophylaxis in dental patients with prosthetic joints (with the possible exception of less than 2 years since joint placement) in the face of substantial evidence that such prophylaxis is unnecessary, harmful (from antibiotic allergy and promotion of microbial antibiotic resistance), and likely ineffective (no clinical studies exist to support efficacy). In no clinical situation is antibiotic prophylaxis for dental patients

Box 49-4

Guidelines for Antibiotic Prophylaxis for Dental Patients with Prosthetic Joints

	DOSAGE REGIMEN
Standard Regimen (Oral)	
Cephalexin or cephradine or amoxicillin	2 g 1 hour before or procedure
Penicillin/Cephalosporin Allergy (Oral)	
Clindamycin procedure	600 mg 1 hour before
Unable To Take Oral Medications	
Cefazolin *or*	1 g IM or IV 1 hour before procedure
Ampicillin	2 g IM or IV 1 hour before procedure
Penicillin/Cephalosporin Allergy and Unable To Take Oral Medications	
Clindamycin	600 mg IV 1 hour before procedure

Adapted from American Dental Association, American Academy of Orthopaedic Surgeons: Antibiotic prophylaxis for dental patients with total joint replacements, *J Am Dent Assoc* 134:895–898, 2003; Pallasch TJ: Antibiotic prophylaxis: the clinical significance of its recent evolution, *J Calif Dent Assoc* 25:619-624, 626-632, 1997. *IM,* Intramuscularly; *IV,* intravenously.

Box 49-5

Patients with Potential Increased Risk of Hematogenous Total Joint Infection

All Patients

During the first 2 years after joint replacement

Immunocompromised/Immunosuppressed Patients

Inflammatory arthropathies such as rheumatoid arthritis and systemic lupus erythematosus

Drug- or radiation-induced immunosuppression

Patients with Other Conditions

Hemophilia

HIV infection

Insulin-dependent (type 1) diabetes

Malignancy

Malnourishment

Previous prosthetic joint infection

Adapted from the American Dental Association, American Academy of Orthopaedic Surgeons: Antibiotic prophylaxis for dental patients with total joint replacements, *J Am Dent Assoc* 134:895-898, 2003.

with orthopedic prostheses ever mandatory.[1] If such patients have an acute orofacial infection, then suitable incision and drainage and therapeutic antibiotics should be employed.

Breast and Penile Implants

No data support the contention by some plastic surgeons that dental treatment–induced bacteremias are a cause of postoperative infections in breast and penile implants. The risk of late (greater than 7 months) infections in breast implants is 1 in 10,000 cases.[7] In a survey of urologists, most were of the opinion that antibiotic prophylaxis for patients with penile implants before dental treatment was inappropriate.[42] If the physician requests antibiotic prophylaxis for either of these types of patients, the dentist can advise that no scientific data support such prophylaxis, that the harm will likely outweigh the benefit, and that, if the physician still insists, she/he prescribe the prophylactic antibiotics.[56]

Brain Abscess

Along with BE and joint infections, brain abscesses are the third metastatic infection likely to involve a dentist in negligence litigation. This derives from the observation that VGS are the most likely cause of brain abscesses and that most occur in the temporal and frontal lobes supplied by the middle cerebral artery. Microbes can reach the brain by direct contiguous spread (middle ear and sinuses), head trauma, or the hematogenous route.

Otitis media and sinusitis account for 50% to 60% of brain abscesses in the United States, with 20% having no known source of infection.[61,62] In the majority of clinical studies an oral focus of infection is not listed. The incubation period has been calculated to be 16 to 18 days, with a mean time to hospitalization of 12 days, making the mean time from onset of bacteremia to diagnosis and hospitalization approximately 30 days.

Brain abscesses are rare and are diagnosed at a rate of 1 per 10,000 hospital admissions. With an incidence of 1.3 to 12 per 1 million population per year possibly from oral hygiene or dental treatment procedures and with bacteremia 1000 to 8000 times more likely from activities of daily living, the absolute risk that a dental procedure causes a brain abscess is likely to be 1 in 1 million to 1 in 10 million.[61,62]

Nonvalvular Cardiovascular Devices

Considerable opinion has been expressed regarding whether certain cardiovascular devices require antibiotic prophylaxis before dental treatment: pacemakers, implantable cardioverter defibrillators, peripheral and cardiac vascular stents, prosthetic vascular grafts, and Dacron carotid patches.[4] Infections of these devices are rare except for pacemakers, which have an infection incidence between 0.13% and 19.9%—the vast majority of which are of the pacemaker pocket and associated with skin bacteria (staphylococci and *Corynebacterium*). The infection rate with peripheral vascular stents (femoral or renal arteries) is less than 1 in 10,000, and only five cases have been reported of infections of coronary artery stents, with three from *S. aureus* and two from *Pseudomonas aeruginosa*.

The infection rate with prosthetic vascular grafts is 1% to 6% after 5 years, with most occurring in the first 2 months after placement.[4] Very few infections of carotid Dacron patches have been reported, with a possible 1.8% rate on the basis of 10 cases, four of which were caused by VGS but all occurring within 32 days of placement, indicating a nosocomial origin.[71,80]

The evidence for hematogenous infection of these devices is extremely limited, with no documentation of dental treatment causation. No antibiotic prophylaxis risk-benefit determinations have been made. The AHA review[4] concludes that (1) currently no convincing evidence exists that microorganisms associated with dental procedures cause infection of nonvalvular vascular devices at any time after implantation, (2) these infections are mostly caused by staphylococci, gram-negative bacteria, or other microorganisms in association with implantation of the devices or resulting from wound or other active infections, (3) accordingly, antibiotic prophylaxis is not recommended after device placement for patients who undergo dental procedures, and (4) severely immunocompromised patients may have a risk of infection, but being immunocompromised is not an independent risk factor for nonvalvular device infection.

Hemodialysis

Controversy exists regarding the advisability of antibiotic prophylaxis for patients with indwelling catheters because no case-control studies have been performed. In a study of long-term hemodialysis patients from 1983 to 1997, 20 cases of IE occurred in 1559 patients, with three caused by VGS.[49] In 1455 patients receiving long-term hemodialysis, 63 cases of bacteremia occurred (0.7 per 100 patient-months), with two of the 63 caused by VGS.[38] In a 2002 study of IE hemodialysis patients, 3.3% were caused by VGS.[48] Virtually all these BE cases were caused by staphylococci, and antibiotic prophylaxis was recommended in none before dental treatment, and none listed dental treatment as causative. Some in the dental literature suggest that antibiotic prophylaxis be used in these patients;[12] however, no risk-benefit determinations have been made. If these patients have an acute orofacial infection, incision and drainage and appropriate antibiotic therapy are in order,[4] as with patients with orthopedic prosthetic devices.[1]

Splenectomy

Individuals without spleens have a small but significant lifelong susceptibility to infection, particularly with encapsulated microorganisms: *S. pneumoniae, H. influenzae,* and *N. meningitidis.* None of these is typical oral flora. In 5902 cases of postsplenectomy infection, 0.8% were caused by VGS.[33] In 77 recent cases, none was caused by VGS.[92] No data support antibiotic prophylaxis for asplenic patients before dental treatment.

Solid Organ Transplants

Antibiotic prophylaxis for IE prevention in heart transplant recipients is not generally recommended because no study has determined that such individuals are at risk for bacteremic infections.[68] Solid organ transplant patients may develop marantic (nonbacterial thrombotic endocarditis) valve lesions similar to those in patients with systemic lupus erythematosus, and a medical consultation may be in order to determine whether cardiac valve pathologic findings are present. In 46 solid organ transplant recipients, 4% (two cases) were associated with VGS without documentation of recent dental treatment.[65]

Diabetes

No data support the use of antibiotic prophylaxis in well-controlled, nonketonic diabetic dental patients.[2] Antibiotic prophylaxis may be used for emergency dental treatment in uncontrolled diabetics with a fasting glucose level of more than 250 mg/dl, but no controlled studies support this contention.[2] Only 2% of surveyed infectious disease specialists would recommend antibiotic prophylaxis in poorly controlled diabetics.[44]

Immunocompromised Patients

Dental patients with a suppressed granulocyte count (500 to 1000) may be at risk for bacteremia-induced infections, but no controlled studies support this concept or any risk-benefit determinations.[18] The risk for VGS infections is greatest in the early stages of blood and bone marrow transplantation (30 days before hospitalization) and is likely to be proportional to the prevalence and magnitude of the oral mucositis present.[89] Severely neutropenic patients should only receive emergency dental care, and the AHA regimen could be employed, although it is not designated by the AHA for this purpose.

There is a lack of consensus regarding the use of antibiotic prophylaxis in patients who have had radiation therapy for head and neck cancer requiring dental treatment and no data exist to support efficacy, any dosing schedules, or drugs used.[36] The risk for osteoradionecrosis is approximately 5.8% and greater in the mandibular arch than in the maxilla. In a survey of oral and maxillofacial surgeons in the United Kingdom concerning extractions after radiotherapy to the oral cavity, no consensus was found on the antibiotics or dosing schedules, and the lack of understanding of antibiotic prophylaxis principles with most antibiotics used postoperatively instead of perioperatively and for long durations (3 to 28 days) promoted selection of resistant oral microorganisms.

Dental patients with HIV/AIDS are not at greater risk from postoperative infectious dental complications than non-HIV/AIDS patients and therefore do not require antibiotic prophylaxis before dental treatment.[61] The risk for BE in HIV/AIDS patients who are not now or ever have been intravenous drug abusers is no greater than the general population, with no significant differences in mortality rate from BE than the general population.[70] Intravenous drug abusers with active BE demonstrate a 40% to 90% seropositivity for HIV.[51] The question is not whether the patient is HIV positive but whether the HIV was acquired by intravenous drug abuse because such patients have a 20% to 40% risk of cardiac valvulopathy.

Collagen Diseases and Other Disorders

A significant number of people with collagen diseases, particularly systemic lupus erythematosus, develop cardiac disorders, particularly marantic or Libman-Sacks endocarditis characterized by noninfected valvular vegetations (nonbacterial thrombotic endocarditis or nonbacterial thrombotic vegetations). In an echocardiographic study of 69 patients with systemic lupus erythematosus, 51% had cardiac valve thickening, 34% to 43% had marantic cardiac vegetations, 25% to 28% had valvular regurgitation, and 3% to 4% had valve stenosis.[73] Approximately 50% of persons with systemic lupus erythematosus have Libman-Sacks nonbacterial thrombotic endocarditis and 25% of these develop various cardiovascular complications such as IE, stroke, peripheral emboli, or heart failure or require valve replacement.[73]

Significant cardiac valvular pathology may also develop in patients with other collagen or myeloproliferative disorders: Marfan syndrome, Ehlers-Danlos syndrome, Hurler's syndrome, pseudoxanthoma elasticum, polycythemia vera, essential thrombocytopenia, and anogenic myeloid metaplasia.[69] Libman-Sacks/marantic endocarditis is also seen in patients with cancer, burns, septicemia, disseminated intravascular coagulation, rheumatoid arthritis, and primary antiphospholipid syndrome.[32,34,79] Libman-Sacks valve pathology and collagen disorder–associated valve pathology may predispose more to embolization than to IE. Not all patients are at risk for BE, but a consultation may be in order, with AHA antibiotic prophylaxis used if deemed appropriate.[13,61]

SURGICAL ANTIBIOTIC PROPHYLAXIS

Dentists commonly provide the patient with an antibiotic prescription after completing various dental procedures, with instructions to have it filled and take all the antibiotic. This practice in an otherwise healthy patient without evidence of an active orofacial infection likely constitutes the most common misuse of antibiotics in dentistry and may contribute significantly to microbial antibiotic resistance.

The use of postsurgical antibiotics has not been proved effective and in the majority of clinical studies does not reduce edema, pain, or trismus.[61] This practice violates several of the principles of antibiotic prophylaxis: not having the drug in the system before onset of surgery, not using a loading dose, directing the antibiotic at all potential pathogens rather than at the single most likely pathogen, and in many cases continuing the drug well beyond the period of infectivity. Antibiotic pharmacokinetics dictate that an antibiotic given without a loading dose and with the first dose likely taken hours after completion of the surgery (after the spouse has gone to the pharmacy for the drug and probably right before bedtime) will achieve steady-state blood levels at least 6 to 12 hours after the first several doses. Therefore potentially optimal blood levels will be reached, at the earliest, sometime the next day, when the issue of whether an infection is to occur has already been decided.[56,61] There is always the suspicion that much of this postsurgical antibiotic "prophylaxis" is done to prevent negligence claims.

Surgical prophylaxis is only indicated (1) to prevent contamination of a sterile area, (2) when infection is unlikely but is associated with high rates of morbidity or mortality, (3) in surgical procedures with a high infection rate, and (4) during implantation of prosthetic material.[3,56,61,64] The *Medical Letter* only recommends surgical antibiotic prophylaxis for procedures with a high infection rate, implantation of prosthetic material, and in head and neck surgery only if the incision passes into the pharynx.[3] Surgical antibiotic prophylaxis is properly reserved for clean-clean surgery (open heart, major vascular reconstruction, prosthetic joint, central nervous system), when the risk of infection is remote but its consequences are grave, or in clean-contaminated surgery (elective biliary, gastric, or colonic), when the likelihood of infection is great but seldom fatal.[53,57,61,82,94] In these situations hospital antibiotic prophylaxis is used perioperatively, begun shortly before the surgery (1 to 2 hours intravenously), and terminated no later than 24 to 48 hours after surgery (preferably with the last suture) because the likelihood of superinfection increases when antibiotic prophylaxis is used for more than 1 to 2 days postoperatively.[3,64,94] No adequate studies addressing the risks and benefits of perioperative surgical prophylaxis have been performed in dentistry.

Because the oral cavity is one of the most heavily contaminated regions of the body, oral surgical procedures of any type cannot be classified as clean-contaminated; the risk of serious postoperative sequelae is rare, and no adequate clinical studies that document risk and cost benefit have been performed. All we know for sure about prophylaxis for oral surgical procedures is that it is not very effective.

Antibiotic prophylaxis is often abused in health care and the principles of antibiotic prophylaxis are often not recognized, much less followed. The use of antibiotics in dentistry after dental procedures to prevent infections or postoperative sequelae of pain, edema, and trismus has been found ineffective in most studies, and no risk-benefit and cost-benefit determinations have been performed. Much antibiotic prophylaxis is employed as "drugs of fear," with a tendency to let lawyers dictate treatment for which they bear no shared responsibility. The contribution of this abuse of antibiotics to the problem of microbial resistance is likely significant. The present AHA guidelines for the potential prevention of BE with antibiotic prophylaxis in dental patients are currently reasonable but will undergo substantial revision in the future.

Cited References

1. Advisory statement: Antibiotic prophylaxis for dental patients with total joint replacements, *J Am Dent Assoc* 134:895-898, 2003.
2. Alexander RE: Routine prophylactic antibiotic use in diabetic dental patients, *J Calif Dent Assoc* 27:611-618, 1999.
3. Antimicrobial prophylaxis in surgery, *Med Lett Drugs Ther* 35:91-94, 1993.
4. Baddour LM, Bettman MA, Bolger AF, et al: Nonvalvular cardiovascular device-related infections, *Circulation* 108: 2015-2031, 2003.
5. Bartzokas CA, Johnson R, Jane M, et al: Relation between mouth and haematogenous infection in total joint replacements, *Br Med J* 309:506-508, 1994.
6. Bayer AS, Bolger AF, Taubert KA, et al: Diagnosis and management of infective endocarditis and its complications, *Circulation* 98:2936-2948, 1998.
7. Brand KG: Infection of mammary prostheses: a survey and the question of prevention, *Ann Plastic Surg* 30:289-295, 1993.
8. Cabell CH, Abrutyn E: Progress toward a global understanding of infective endocarditis: early lessons from the International Collaboration on Endocarditis investigation, *Infect Dis Clin North Am* 16:255-272, 2002.
9. Cheitlin MD, Alpert JS, Armstrong WF, et al: ACC/AHA guidelines for the clinical application of echocardiography, *Circulation* 95:1686-1744, 1997.
10. Dajani AS, Taubert KA, Wilson W, et al: Prevention of bacterial endocarditis: recommendations by the American Heart Association, *JAMA* 277:1794-1801, 1997.
11. Delahaye F, Rial MO, de Gevigney G, et al: A critical appraisal of the quality of the management of infective endocarditis, *J Am Coll Cardiol* 33:788-793, 1999.
12. DeRossi SS, Glick M: Dental considerations for the patient with renal disease receiving hemodialysis, *J Am Dent Assoc* 127:211-219, 1996.
13. DeRossi SS, Glick M: Lupus erythematosus: considerations for dentistry, *J Am Dent Assoc* 129:330-339, 1998.
14. Devereux RB, Jones EC, Roman MJ, et al: Prevalence and correlates of mitral valve prolapse in a population-based sample of American Indians: the Strong Heart Study, *Am J Med* 111:679-685, 2001.
15. Durack DT: Prevention of infective endocarditis, *N Engl J Med* 332:38-44, 1995.
16. Durack DT, Kaplan EL, Bisno AL: Apparent failures of endocarditis prophylaxis: an analysis of 52 cases submitted to a national registry, *JAMA* 250:2318-2322, 1983.
17. Durack DT, Lukes AS, Bright DK, et al: New criteria for diagnosis of infective endocarditis: utilization of specific echocardiographic findings, *Am J Med* 96:200-209, 1994.
18. Emmanouilides C, Glaspy J: Opportunistic infections in oncologic patients, *Hematol/Oncol Clin North Am* 10:841-860, 1996.
19. Frandsen EV, Pedrazzoli V, Kilian M: Ecology of viridans streptococci in the oral cavity and pharynx, *Oral Microbiol Immunol* 6:129-133, 1991.
20. Freed LA, Levy D, Levine RA, et al: Prevalence and clinical outcome of mitral-valve prolapse, *N Engl J Med* 341:1-7, 1999.
21. Gardin JM, Schumacher D, Constantine G, et al: Valvular abnormalities and cardiovascular status following exposure to dexfenfluramine or phentermine/fenfluramine, *JAMA* 283:1703-1709, 2000.
22. Gardin JM, Weissman NJ, Jeung C, et al. Clinical and echocardiographic followup of patients previously treated with dexfenfluramine or phentermine/fenfluramine, *JAMA* 286: 2011-2014, 2001.
23. Gill GS, Mills DM: Long-term follow-up evaluation of 1000 consecutive cemented total knee arthroplasties, *Clin Orthop Rel Res* 273:66-77, 1991.
24. Glick M: Intravenous drug users: a consideration for infective endocarditis in dentistry [editorial], *Oral Surg Oral Med Oral Pathol Oral Radiol Endod* 80:125, 1995.
25. Guntheroth WG: How important are dental procedures as a cause of infective endocarditis? *Am J Cardiol* 54:797-801, 1984.
26. Guntheroth WG: Initial evaluation of the child for heart disease, *Pediatr Clin North Am* 25:657-675, 1978.
27. Hall G, Hedstrom SA, Heimdah A, et al: Prophylactic administration of penicillins for endocarditis does not reduce the incidence of postextraction bacteremia, *Clin Infect Dis* 17:188-194, 1993.
28. Hall G, Heimdahl A, Nord CE: Effect of prophylactic administration of cefaclor on transient bacteremia after dental extraction, *Eur J Clin Microbiol Infect Dis* 15:646-649, 1996.
29. Hall, G, Nord CE, Heimdahl A: Elimination of bacteremia after dental extraction: comparison of erythromycin and clindamycin for prophylaxis of infective endocarditis, *J Antimicrob Chemother* 37:783-795, 1996.
30. Hillman JD, Socransky SS, Shivers M: The relationships between streptococcal species and periodontopathic bacteria in human dental plaque, *Arch Oral Biol* 30:791-795, 1985.
31. Hockett RN, Loesche WJ, Sodeman TM: Bacteremia in asymptomatic human subjects, *Arch Oral Biol* 22:91-98, 1977.
32. Hojnik M, George J, Ziporen L, et al: Heart valve involvement (Libman-Sacks endocarditis) in the antiphospholipid syndrome, *Circulation* 93:1579-1587, 1996.
33. Holdsworth RJ, Irving AD, Cuschieri A: Postsplenectomy sepsis and its mortality rate: actual versus perceived risks, *Br J Surg* 78:1031-1035, 1991.
34. Joffe IJ, Jacobs LE, Owen AN, et al: Noninfective valvular masses: review of the literature with emphasis on imaging techniques and management, *Am Heart J* 131:1175-1183, 1996.
35. Jollis JG, Landolfo CK, Kisslo J, et al: Fenfluramine and phentermine and cardiovascular findings: effect of treatment duration on prevalence of valve abnormalities, *Circulation* 101:2071-2077, 2000.
36. Kanatas AN, Rogers SN, Martin MV: A survey of antibiotic prescribing by maxillofacial consultants for dental extractions following radiotherapy to the oral cavity, *Br Dent J* 192:157-160, 2002.
37. Kaye D: Prophylaxis for infective endocarditis: an update, *Ann Intern Med* 104:419-423, 1986.
38. Kessler M, Hoen B, Mayeux D: Bacteremia in patients on chronic hemodialysis: a multicenter prospective survey, *Nephron* 64:95-100, 1993.

39. Lacassin F, Hoen B, Leport C, et al: Procedures associated with infective endocarditis in adults, a case control study, *Eur Heart J* 16:1968-1974, 1995.
40. Lamas CC, Eykyn SJ: Suggested modifications to the Duke criteria for the clinical diagnosis of native valve and prosthetic valve endocarditis: analysis of 118 pathologically proven cases, *Clin Infect Dis* 25:713-719, 1997.
41. Lien EA, Solberg CO, Kalager T: Infective endocarditis 1973-1984 at the Bergen University Hospital: clinical feature, treatment and prognosis, *Scand J Infect Dis* 20:239-246, 1988.
42. Little JW, Rhodus NL: The need for antibiotic prophylaxis of patients with penile implants during invasive dental procedures: a national survey of urologists, *J Urol* 148:1801-1804, 1992.
43. Lockhart PB: The risk for endocarditis in dental practice, *Periodontol 2000* 23:127-135, 2000.
44. Lockhart PB, Brennan MT, Fox PC, et al: Decision-making on the use of antimicrobial prophylaxis for dental procedures: a survey of infectious disease consultants and review, *Clin Infect Dis* 34:1621-1626, 2002.
45. Lockhart PB, Durack DT: Oral microflora as a cause of endocarditis and other distant site infections, *Infect Dis Clin North Am* 13:833-850, 1999.
46. Lucas VS, Lytra V, Hassan T, et al: Comparison of lysis filtration and an automated blood culture system (BACTEC) for detection, quantification, and identification of odontogenic bacteremia in children, *J Clin Microbiol* 40:3416-3420, 2002.
47. Mangione S, Nieman LZ: Cardiac auscultatory skills of internal medicine and family practice trainees: a comparison of diagnostic proficiency, *JAMA* 278:717-722, 1997.
48. Maraj S, Jacobs LE, Kung S-C, et al: Epidemiology and outcome of infective endocarditis in hemodialysis patients, *Am J Med Sci* 324:254-260, 2002.
49. McCarthy JT, Steckelberg JM: Infective endocarditis in patients receiving long-term hemodialysis, *Mayo Clin Proc* 75:1008-1014, 2000.
50. McFarland MM: Pathology of infective endocarditis. In Kaye D, ed: *Infective endocarditis*, ed 2, New York, 1992, Raven Press.
51. Miro JM, del Rio A, Mestres CA: Infective endocarditis in intravenous drug abusers and HIV-1 infected patients, *Infect Dis Clin North Am* 16:273-295, 2002.
52. Morellion P, Francioli P, Overholser D, et al: Mechanisms of successful amoxicillin prophylaxis of experimental endocarditis due to *Streptococcus intermedius*, *J Infect Dis* 154:801-807, 1986.
53. Neu HC: Prophylaxis—has it at last come of age? *J Antimicrob Chemother* 5:331-333, 1979.
54. Osmon DR: Antimicrobial prophylaxis in adults, *Mayo Clin Proc* 75:98-109, 2000.
55. Pallasch TJ: A critical appraisal of antibiotic prophylaxis, *Int Dent J* 39:183-196, 1989.
56. Pallasch TJ: Antibiotic prophylaxis, *Endod Topics* 4:46-59, 2003.
57. Pallasch TJ: Antibiotic prophylaxis: problems in paradise, *Dent Clin North Am* 47:665-679, 2003.
58. Pallasch TJ: Antibiotic prophylaxis: the clinical significance of its recent evolution, *Calif Dent Assoc J* 25:619-624, 626-632, 1997.
59. Pallasch TJ: Current status of fenfluramine/dexfenfluramine-induced cardiac valvulopathy, *Calif Dent Assoc J* 27:400-404, 1999.
60. Pallasch TJ, Gage TW, Taubert KA: The 1997 prevention of bacterial endocarditis recommendations by the American Heart Association: questions and answers, *Calif Dent Assoc J* 27:393-399, 1999.
61. Pallasch TJ, Slots J: Antibiotic prophylaxis and the medically compromised patient, *Periodontol 2000* 10:107-138, 1996.
62. Pallasch TJ, Wahl MJ: Focal infection: new age or ancient history, *Endod Topics* 4:32-59, 2003.
63. Pallasch TJ, Wahl MJ: The focal infection theory: appraisal and reappraisal, *Calif Dent Assoc J* 28:194-200, 2000.
64. Paluzzi RG: Antimicrobial prophylaxis for surgery, *Med Clin North Am* 77:427-441, 1993.
65. Paterson DL, Dominguez EA, Chang FY, et al: Infective endocarditis in solid organ transplant recipients, *Clin Infect Dis* 26:689-694, 1998.
66. Pelech AN: The cardiac murmur: when to refer? *Pediatr Clin North Am* 45:107-122, 1998.
67. Pellerin D, Brecker S, Veyrat C: Degenerative mitral valve disease with emphasis on mitral valve prolapse, *Heart* 88(Suppl 4):IV20-28, 2002.
68. Petri WA, Jr: Infections in heart transplant recipients, *Clin Infect Dis* 18:141-148, 1994.
69. Reisner SA, Rinkevich D, Mariewicz W, et al: Cardiac involvement in patients with myeloproliferative disorders, *Am J Med* 93:498-504, 1992.
70. Ribera E, Miro JM, Cortes E, et al: Influence of human immunodeficiency virus 1 infection and degree of immunosuppression in the clinical characteristics and outcome of infective endocarditis in intravenous drug users, *Arch Int Med* 158:2043-2050, 1998.
71. Rizzo A, Hertzer NR, O'Hara PJ, et al: Dacron carotid patch infections: a report of eight cases, *J Vasc Surg* 32:602-606, 2000.
72. Roberts GJ: Dentists are innocent! "Everyday" bacteremia is the real culprit: a review and assessment of the evidence that dental surgical procedures are a principal cause of bacterial endocarditis in children, *Pediatr Cardiol* 20:317-325, 1999.
73. Roldan CA, Shivley BK, Crawford MH: An echocardiographic study of valvular heart disease associated with systemic lupus erythematosus, *N Engl J Med* 335:1424-1430, 1996.
74. Ruoff KL, Whiley RA, Beighton D: Streptococcus. In Murray PR, Baron EJ, Pfaller MA, et al, eds: *Manual of clinical microbiology*, ed 7, Washington DC, 1999, American Society for Microbiology.
75. Sande MA, Lee BL, Mills J, et al: Endocarditis in intravenous drug users. In Kaye D, ed: *Infective endocarditis*, ed 2, New York, 1992, Raven Press.
76. Singh RG, Cappucci R, Kramer-Fox R, et al: Severe mitral regurgitation due to mitral valve prolapse: risk factors for development, progression, and need for mitral valve surgery, *Am J Cardiol* 85:193-198, 2000.
77. Starkebaum M, Durack D, Beeson P: The "incubation period" for subacute bacterial endocarditis, *Yale J Biol Med* 50:49-58, 1977.
78. Steckelberg JM, Wilson WR: Risk factors for infective endocarditis, *Infect Dis Clin North Am* 7:9-19, 1993.

79. Steiner I: Nonbacterial thrombotic versus infective endocarditis: a necropsy study of 320 cases, *Cardiovasc Pathol* 4:207-208, 1995.
80. Sternbergh WC III: Regarding "Dacron coated patch infection: a report of eight cases" [Letter], *J Vasc Surg* 33:663-664, 2001.
81. Stewart BF, Siscovick D, Lind BK, et al: Clinical factors associated with calcific aortic valve disease: Cardiovascular Heart Study, *J Am Coll Cardiol* 29:630-634, 1997.
82. Stone HH: Basic principles in the use of prophylactic antibiotics, *J Antimicrob Chemother* 14:33-37, 1984.
83. Stouffer GA, Sheahan RG, Lenihan DJ, et al: Mitral valve prolapse: a review of the literature, *Am J Med Sci* 321:401-410, 2001.
84. Strom BL, Abrutyn E, Berlin JA, et al: Dental and cardiac risk factors for infective endocarditis: a population-based, case-control study, *Ann Intern Med* 129:761-769, 1998.
85. Strom BL, Abrutyn E, Berlin JA, et al: Risk factors for infective endocarditis: oral hygiene and nondental exposures, *Circulation* 102:2842-2848, 2000.
86. Tornos P, Almilante B, Olona M, et al: Clinical outcome and long-term prognosis of late prosthetic valve endocarditis: a 20-year experience, *Clin Infect Dis* 24:381-386, 1997.
87. Towns ML, Reller LB: Diagnostic methods current best practices and guidelines for isolation of bacteria and fungi in infective endocarditis, *Infect Dis Clin North Am* 16:363-376, 2002.
88. Tzukert AA, Leviner E, Benoliel R, et al: Analysis of the American Heart Association's recommendations for the prevention of infective endocarditis, *Oral Surg Oral Med Oral Pathol* 62:276-279, 1986.
89. Van Burik JAH, Weisdorf DJ: Infections in recipients of blood and bone marrow transplants, *Hematol/Oncol Clin North Am* 13:1065-1069, 1999.
90. van der Meer JTM, Thompson J, Valkenburg HA, et al: Epidemiology of bacterial endocarditis in The Netherlands. I. Patient characteristics, *Arch Intern Med* 152:1863-1868, 1992.
91. van der Meer JTM, Thompson J, Valkenburg HA, et al: Epidemiology of bacterial endocarditis in The Netherlands. II. Antecedent procedures and use of prophylaxis, *Arch Intern Med* 152:1869-1873, 1992.
92. Waghorn DJ. Overwhelming infection in asplenic patients: current best practice preventive measures are not being followed, *J Clin Pathol* 54:214-228, 2001.
93. Volmar KE, Hutchins GM: Aortic and mitral fenfluramine-phentermine valvulopathy in 64 patients treated with anorectic agents, *Arch Pathol Lab Med* 125:1555-1561, 2001.
94. Waddell TK, Rotstein OD: Committee on Antimicrobial Agents, Canadian Infectious Disease Society: antimicrobial prophylaxis in surgery, *Can Med Assoc J* 151: 925-931, 1994.

CHAPTER • 50

Oral Complications of Cancer Therapy

Mark M. Schubert, Joel B. Epstein, and Douglas E. Peterson

The management of cancer has become increasingly complex with the expanding use of combined modalities of surgery, chemotherapy, and radiation therapy. Considerable attention is being paid to the medical significance of complications of cancer therapy as well as to the effect of these complications on the quality of life. Studies have demonstrated the effects of oral complications on cancer therapy and how they can significantly affect the course of therapy "medically," increase patient-related complaints during treatment, affect general quality of life, and influence the cost of care.[72] In addition, a number of chronic orofacial complications can significantly affect life-long quality of life and oral function. Protocols that use chemotherapy or chemoradiotherapy dose intensification followed by hematopoietic stem cell rescues are increasingly being used to treat a number of solid and disseminated forms of cancer. Changes in radiation protocols and combined chemotherapy and radiation therapy are used to increase control and cure. Oral complications resulting from these therapies can clearly influence the course and success of therapy. Successful prevention and treatment of the oral complications of cancer therapy can reduce pain, suffering, and disability and decrease the risk of complications that may interfere with ongoing cancer therapy or result in death.

Many factors make oral complications of chemotherapy and radiation therapy unique. Both treatment modalities cause complications such as oral mucositis, taste dysfunction, and salivary gland dysfunction. A significant difference exists between the two modalities relative to whether toxicity is transient (i.e., during chemotherapy) or progressive and permanent (as is often the case with radiation therapy). Furthermore, cancer chemotherapy is predominantly administered systemically, which further increases the risk that an oral complication (e.g., infection) may lead to systemic complications. In contrast, the effects of radiation are primarily limited to the irradiated tissues.

CHEMOTHERAPY

Generally stated, cancer chemotherapy's therapeutic effect comes through damage and toxicity directed toward rapidly dividing cells (see Chapter 42). Only a small number of agents can specifically target cancer cells (e.g., imatinib); most will inadvertently damage normal tissues of the body. However, because the growth fraction for cancers is so much higher than most normal tissue compartments, there is a "quantitative" difference in damage to the cancer compared with the rest of rapidly dividing cells. Systemic toxic effects of cancer chemotherapy usually result from damage to rapidly dividing cells; however, some toxic effects result from damage that is not directly related to cell division (Box 50-1). A number of factors affect the clinical expression of oral toxic effects of chemotherapy, the most prominent being which chemotherapeutic agent is administered, along with dose and schedule (see Chapter 42). The high turnover rate of oral mucosal tissues puts them at risk for the cytotoxic effects of antineoplastic agents. Direct mucosal damage may be accentuated by a number of factors, including (1) salivary gland dysfunction, which compromises the barrier and lubricating functions provided by saliva; (2) mucosal trauma/irritation (e.g., from normal oral function, medications, and mouth breathing); and (3) infection caused by indigenous oral flora (especially opportunistic oral pathogens), acquired pathogens, and the reactivation of latent herpesviruses that cause local and systemic complications in patients who are immunosuppressed.[52] Preexisting oral and dental diseases, oral hygiene, and oral infections can have a profound effect on the course of cancer therapy.

Oral complications of cancer therapy may directly result from the cytotoxic effects (direct toxic effects) of the drugs on oral tissues (including salivary glands) or from therapy involving distant tissues (indirect toxic effects). These oral complications are listed in Box 50-2.

Direct Oral Toxic Effects

The oral cavity is often affected by cytotoxic cancer chemotherapy, and although it is often convenient to think of various oral complications as resulting from either direct or indirect toxicity, the clinical presentation of complications generally represents the results of complex interactions among multiple factors.

Oral mucositis

Oral mucositis is virtually a universal oral complication in patients receiving high-dose chemotherapy or head/neck radiation therapy.[76] It is the single most significant patient-reported symptom. It can result in clinically and economically important adverse sequelae in selected cancer patient cohorts, including hematopoietic stem cell recipients.[72]

Severe oral toxic effects can compromise delivery of optimal cancer therapy protocols. For example, dose reduction or treatment schedule modifications may be necessary to allow for resolution of oral lesions. In cases of severe oral morbidity, the patient may no longer be able to continue cancer therapy; treatment is then usually discontinued. These disruptions in dosing from oral complications can thus directly affect patient survival.

The terms *oral mucositis* and *stomatitis* are often used interchangeably at the clinical level, but they do not reflect identical processes.[48] *Oral mucositis* refers to inflammation and breakdown of the oral mucosa resulting from chemotherapeutic agents or ionizing radiation. Mucositis typically manifests as erythema with or without ulcerations. It may be exacerbated by local factors. *Stomatitis* refers to any inflammatory condition of oral tissue, including mucosa, dentition/periapices, and periodontium. Stomatitis thus includes oral mucosal infections as well as mucositis, as defined above. Increasingly, the term *mucositis* is being used to represent the direct mucosal toxicity of cancer therapies.

The clinician should note the biologic and clinical context in which oral mucositis occurs as a cancer therapy–associated toxicity. The oral cavity is highly susceptible to the direct and indirect toxic effects of cancer chemotherapy and ionizing radiation. This risk is attributable to multiple factors, including high cellular turnover rates for the lining mucosa, a diverse and complex microflora, and trauma to oral tissues during normal oral function. Although oral complications may mimic selected systemic disorders, unique oral toxic effects may emerge in the context of specific oral anatomic structures and their functions (see Boxes 50-1 and 50-2).

Although many factors contribute to the clinical expression of *mucositis,* this term will be used to denote clinically evident changes that are ascribed to the direct damage caused by the cancer therapy to the mucosa.[65] The direct mucosal toxicity associated with chemotherapy is the primary cause of mucositis, but the mucositis noted clinically may be modified by the oral microflora. Chemotherapy-associated toxicity compromises the oral mucosa and impedes repair of the mucosal injury caused by normal oral functions. Emesis can increase mucosal damage because of exposure of the mucosa to acidic gastric fluid. Physical trauma, including dental abrasion of oral mucosa and traumatic diet, may initiate and aggravate tissue damage and repair. The compromised mucosal renewal reduces clearance of adherent oral microorganisms and increases the risk of penetration of chemical compounds into the epithelium. In addition, mucosal immune components, including neutrophils, macrophages, T and B lymphocytes, Langerhans cells, and mast cells, may be reduced in number and function as a result of drug-induced damage to these cells or myelosuppression.

The mucosal surfaces throughout the oral cavity have different cellular turnover rates, which can vary from 4 to 5 days for nonkeratinized buccal and labial mucosa to as many as 14 days for the orthokeratinized hard palate. The more rapid the cell division rate of the progenitor epithelial cells, the higher the susceptibility to damage from chemotherapy and radiotherapy. Histologically, the mucosal damage is characterized by mucosal atrophy, inflammatory cell infiltrates, collagen degradation, and edema.[42] Clinically, these changes are initially evident as mucosal redness. If damage increases, ulceration can present as isolated lesions and even progress to confluent ulcers.[53] The initial changes of oral mucositis generally become evident 3 to 6 days after the start of chemotherapy. Damage peaks 7 to 11 days after the last dose, and mucosal healing then proceeds over the next 7 to 28 days.

A major concern for the immunosuppressed patient with severe oral mucositis undergoing chemotherapy is that the disrupted mucosal surface may serve as a portal for infectious agents. The influence of indigenous oral flora on oral mucosi-

Box • **50-1**

Systemic Toxicity of Cancer Chemotherapy

Direct Toxicities
- Bone marrow
  - Neutropenia
  - Thrombocytopenia
  - Anemia
- Gastrointestinal mucosa
  - Mucositis
  - Nausea/vomiting/diarrhea
  - Nutritional disturbances
- Oral mucosa
- Skin
- Hair follicles
- Gonads

Other Toxicities
- Heart
- Liver
- Lung
- CNS
- Kidney

Box • **50-2**

Oral Complications of Cancer Chemotherapy

Direct Toxicities
- Oral mucositis
  - Mucosal inflammation
  - Cytotoxicity
  - Bacterial infection
- Salivary gland dysfunction
- Neurotoxicity
  - Trigeminal nerve neuropathies
  - Taste dysfunction
  - Dentinal hypersensitivity
- Temporomandibular dysfunction
  - Myofascial pain
  - Temporomandibular joint dysfunction
- Dental and skeletal growth and development (pediatric patients)
  - Abnormalities in dentition
  - Changes in jaw development

Indirect Toxicities
- Myelosuppression
  - Neutropenia
  - Immunosuppression
  - Anemia
  - Thrombocytopenia
- Infection
  - Viral (HSV, VZV, CMV, EBV, other)
  - Fungal (*Candida, Aspergillus,* other)
  - Bacterial
- Gastrointestinal mucositis
  - Nutritional disturbances
- Nausea and vomiting
  - Acidic damage to oral tissues
  - Heightened gag reflexes

CMV, Cytomegalovirus; *EBV,* Epstein-Barr virus; *HSV,* herpes simplex virus; *VZV,* varicella zoster virus.

tis has been investigated, and bacteria and fungi have been implicated as contributing factors. Improving the effectiveness of oral hygiene efforts has been associated with reduction of mucositis severity, presumably by reducing numbers of potential oral pathogens. A recent study of oral hygiene in immunocompromised patients demonstrated a statistically significant reduction in the severity of mucositis, and no evidence of bacteremia was seen.[5] Oral infections caused by organisms acquired during hospitalization as well as the reactivation of latent viruses (e.g., herpes simplex [HSV], cytomegalovirus [CMV], varicella-zoster [VZV]) can also influence the clinical presentation of mucositis.

Although predicting whether mucositis will develop in a patient during chemotherapy purely on the basis of which drugs will be administered is difficult, several drugs have a higher propensity to damage the oral mucosa. These include methotrexate, doxorubicin, fluorouracil, platinum derivatives, and aldesleukin (see Table 42-1). After a patient has had mucositis with a particular chemotherapy regimen, mucositis will likely occur with subsequent courses of therapy that use the same regimen.

Management of oral mucositis Mucositis should be assessed with reliable and validated measures.[70] The clinician should consider the purposes of the assessment so that appropriate selection of the instrument can be made. For example, the World Health Organization–based scales commonly used by the cooperative oncology groups in the United States provide estimates of severity of oral mucositis in the context of patient symptoms, signs, and functional disturbances. In contrast, scales that measure a specific component of clinical mucositis (e.g., erythema, ulceration) are typically more valid in a research setting.[72] As mucosal atrophy and breakdown progress, complaints of mild irritation and increasing oral pain often require the use of high-dose opioid medications. Management of mucositis currently remains focused on palliation of symptoms and efforts to reduce the influence of secondary factors on mucositis.

Protocols to manage mucositis topically should address efficacy, patient acceptance, and appropriate dosing. Many of the currently utilized treatment agents have not been scientifically tested to determine efficacy, and many are empirically accepted as being appropriate. For the most part, the goal of

Box • 50-3

Management of Oral Mucositis

Bland Oral Rinses	
0.9% Saline solution Sodium bicarbonate solution 0.9% Saline/sodium bicarbonate solution	Rinse with 12 to 16 oz; expectorate. Repeat every 15 minutes to 4 hours depending on severity of mucositis.
Topical Anesthetics	
Lidocaine viscous sprays/gels Benzocaine sprays/gels Diphenhydramine solutions Benzonatate	Rinse/hold anesthetic for 1 to 3 minutes; expectorate. Avoid posterior oropharynx anesthesia and do not attempt to eat while anesthetized. Do not swallow.
Topical Anesthetics/Analgesics	
Doxepin solution Benzydamine HCl solution	Rinse/hold solution in mouth for 1 to 2 minutes; expectorate.
Mucosal Coating Agents/Surface Protectants	
Amphojel solution Kaopectate solutions Zilactin (lidocaine plus film-forming agent)	Rinse/hold for 15 to 30 seconds; expectorate. Apply to ulcers every 2 to 6 hours as needed.
Systemic Analgesics/Opioids	
Nonnarcotic analgesics Fentanyl patches Morphine (oral, bolus, PCA) Codeine/codeine derivatives	
Experimental Agents Under Investigation	
Keratinocyte growth factors	Stimulation of mucosal cell division to counter mucosal atrophy
Low-energy laser therapy	Protection against damage/stimulate mucosal cell
Misoprostol	Modulation of inflammatory reactions
Antiinfectives: defensins/protegrins, topical antibacterial agents	Prevention of "infectious" component of mucositis
Transforming growth factor β_3	Stops/reduces cell division to reduce cytotoxicity during treatment
Interleukin-11	Modulates inflammation to reduce mucosal toxicity

PCA, Patient-controlled analgesia.

therapy is primarily palliative. A "stepped" approach is typically followed, with progression from one level to the next (Box 50-3):

1. Bland rinses (e.g., normal saline or sodium bicarbonate solutions)
2. Mucosal coating agents (e.g., antacid solutions, kaolin solutions)
3. Water-soluble lubricating agents, including artificial saliva for xerostomia
4. Topical anesthetics (e.g., viscous lidocaine, benzocaine sprays/gels, dyclonine rinses, diphenhydramine solutions)
5. Film-forming agents to cover localized ulcerative lesions (e.g., hydroxypropyl cellulose)

Normal saline solution can be prepared by adding approximately three quarters of a teaspoon of table salt to 1 quart of water. It can be kept at room temperature or refrigerated, depending on what is most comfortable for the patient. The patient can then rinse, hold, and expectorate as often as necessary to maintain oral comfort. Sodium bicarbonate (1 to 2 tablespoons/quart) can be added. In addition to providing a soothing rinse, saline solutions can stimulate salivary flow and thus provide an improved sensation of oral moistness.

Focal application of topical anesthetic agents is preferred over widespread oral administration for a number of reasons. Generalized oral mucosal anesthesia carries an increased risk of accidental mucosal trauma. When mucositis becomes extensive, generalized topical applications of anesthetics may be used to reduce pain. Generalized rinsing with anesthetics also may reduce or eliminate the gag reflex, which may increase the risk of aspiration pneumonia. Systemic absorption or swallowing of anesthetics from ulcerated mucosa can result in systemic toxicity, depending on the agent and the dose that is swallowed.

A common approach to managing oral mucositis is to use a combination solution that includes a number of different agents: topical anesthetics, coating agents, antifungal drugs, and even steroids. However, when using these rinses the clinician faces a number of considerations:

1. Are all the agents necessary? For instance, topical antifungals are not effective for prophylaxis. Is a topical coating agent necessary, or will a simple topical anesthetic suffice? Are the agents collectively compatible?
2. Are all the agents well tolerated? Diphenhydramine elixir contains alcohol, coloring, and flavoring agents, all of which can irritate damaged mucosa. Diphenhydramine formulated for intravenous injection can be substituted to provide topical anesthesia without the other irritating agents in the elixir.
3. Have the medications been compounded in the correct proportions, and is the patient using an adequate volume for appropriate dosing? Does compounding reduce the concentration of each agent to a less than optimal level?
4. What is the cost-benefit ratio for the rinse, and are the added pharmacy costs for compounding a combination rinse offset by significantly improved effectiveness and convenience compared with single agents? Since the primary goal of these rinses is to provide pain relief, this can be an important consideration.

When topical pain control strategies become inadequate for controlling pain, systemic analgesics are necessary. Nonsteroidal antiinflammatory drugs (NSAIDs) that affect platelet adhesion and damage gastric mucosa are contraindicated, especially in the presence of thrombocytopenia. Opioids are usually the drugs of choice. The combination of long-term indwelling venous catheters and computerized drug administration pumps to provide patient-controlled analgesia has significantly increased the ability to control severe mucositis pain while lowering the dose and side effects of opioid analgesics. In this setting, the use of protocols that provide continuous pain relief is preferred and should include delivery of pain medications in the manner most acceptable to the patient on a time contingency basis and doses titrated to effect. Alternative delivery systems such as time-release oral tablets, dermal patches, oral transmucosal agents, and suppositories can also be used to provide adequate pain relief. Additionally, managing clinicians should anticipate potential side effects of opioids (nausea, vomiting, constipation, etc.) and provide appropriate supportive care. Even after the patient is placed on systemic pain medications, the clinician should encourage the patient to continue routine oral care as best as possible.

Future directions in oral mucositis management The contemporary model of cancer therapy–associated oral mucositis involves four phases: the proinflammatory phase, epithelial cytotoxicity phase, bacteriologic phase, and wound healing.[68] More recently a fifth phase has been added, such that the phases are (1) initiation, (2) upregulation and message generation, (3) signaling and amplification, (4) ulceration, and (5) healing (S. Sonis, personal communication). Delineation of this model has permitted targeted interventions at the molecular level, with a goal of reducing the severity of or preventing the lesion.[53,56] Efforts to identify agents or techniques capable of reducing or eliminating oral mucositis are ongoing.[77]

Strategies that have been investigated to reduce the inflammatory phases of mucositis include benzydamine[25] and prostaglandins E_1 and E_2 (including the E_1 analogue misoprostol).[44] In contrast to earlier reports, several recent studies have suggested that oral sucralfate suspension is not effective in preventing or treating oral mucositis in cancer patients (see below).[43] Various therapies and agents that may have potential to reduce mucosal cytotoxicity and/or improve healing of mucosa are currently under study. They include the low-energy helium-neon laser,[11] epidermal growth factor,[69] transforming growth factor β_3,[71] α-interferon, and keratinocyte growth factors. Finally, antimicrobial strategies have included the use of chlorhexidine, povidone-iodine, polymyxin/tobramycin/amphotericin B lozenges, and antimicrobial proteins such as defensins. The new technologies could also provide the setting in which novel classes of chemotherapeutic drugs, used at increased doses, could be considered. These advances in turn could lead to enhanced cancer cure rates and durability of disease remission.[48]

Salivary gland dysfunction

Saliva plays an important role in maintaining oral health. Although the effects of ionizing radiation on salivary gland tissue have been well documented, the corresponding effects of cancer chemotherapy have not.[62] Overall results are inconsistent, with trials showing varied effects of various chemotherapy protocols on flow rate and sialochemistry.[36]

No histopathologic investigations of major salivary glands have been reported, but a postmortem study has shown minor salivary gland damage after the administration of various chemotherapeutic agents, with changes evident in the first 3 weeks after chemotherapy administration followed by gradual healing with minimal or no sequelae in the weeks to months after therapy. Clinical observations support the contention that alterations in salivary function associated with cancer chemotherapy are generally reversible, unlike those seen after salivary gland exposure to radiation therapy.

The clinician should determine whether patients are receiving other drugs that can alter salivary function (e.g., anticholinergic antiemetic drugs or tricyclic antidepressants). Oral dryness can also be worsened by mouth breathing or oxygen administration.

Attempts to manage salivary gland dysfunction can have a beneficial effect on the quality of life for cancer patients and improve oral health. Frequent rinsing with normal saline can help keep mucosal surfaces moist, clear debris, and stimulate salivary gland function for short periods. Saliva replacements (mouth-wetting agents) may provide temporary symptomatic relief. Other strategies to stimulate salivary glands include the use of "taste stimulation" with sugarless gum or candies and regimens that use cholinergic drugs. Bethanechol, cevimeline, and pilocarpine, which directly stimulate salivary glands, have been reported to be useful for treating xerostomia[39,78] (see Chapter 8). Increasing the ingestion of moist foods (e.g., flavored gelatins), sauces, and gravies can ameliorate the discomfort of eating. Dry or cracked lips should be kept lubricated with agents such as lanolin-based creams and nonperfumed, nonmedicated skin moisturizing agents.

Neurotoxicity

Direct neurotoxicity from cancer chemotherapy has been noted with the microtubular agents (vincristine, vinblastine, and taxol), and may result in severe, deep-seated, throbbing mandibular or maxillary pain that can mimic dental pathology (i.e., toothache). Neurotoxicity is generally considered a dose-limiting complication for these drugs, and thus prompt diagnosis is important.[45] Appropriate dental/periodontal examinations (including tooth vitality testing as necessary) must be performed to rule out pulpal or periodontal pathology. Opioid-containing analgesics may be useful in controlling pain, and the use of neurologically active medications may be considered. The neurotoxicity may be transient and generally subsides shortly after dose reduction or cessation of chemotherapy.

Tooth thermal hypersensitivity is occasionally reported by patients after chemotherapy. Symptoms usually resolve spontaneously within a few weeks to months of discontinuation of chemotherapy. Topical brush-on fluorides and desensitizing toothpastes are often helpful in reducing or eliminating symptoms.

Taste dysfunction is a neurosensory problem that can be associated with cancer chemotherapy.[35] Taste receptors are neuroepithelium-derived cells, with a turnover rate of approximately 10 days, that generally regenerate if not irreversibly damaged.[74] In addition, the damage to olfactory receptor cells must be considered when a patient has taste dysfunction.[3] Aberrations in taste perception can vary from hypergeusia to hypogeusia to dysgeusia. Some patients simultaneously report several different symptoms—hypergeusia with some tastes and dysgeusia with others. Patients receiving cancer chemotherapy occasionally report a bad taste that results from the diffusion of drug into the oral cavity, known as "venous taste phenomenon."

Temporomandibular joint disorders may present as facial pain, headache, temporomandibular joint dysfunction, and occasionally ear or throat pain. The myofascial-based complaints generally result from clenching or bruxing as a result of stress, sleep dysfunction, or occasionally CNS toxicity from certain medications. The short-term use of muscle relaxants or anxiety-reducing agents plus physical therapy (moist heat applications, massage, and gentle stretching) often resolves these problems. Occlusal splints to be used while sleeping may be of limited help for patients with more persistent clenching/bruxing tendencies.

Alterations in dental and skeletal growth and development

As the number of long-term survivors of childhood cancer has increased, the risk for damage to developing dental and skeletal structures from cancer therapies has become apparent.[14,15] Chemotherapy-related damage to developing teeth includes hypoplastic dentin and enamel, shortened and conical roots, taurodontic-like teeth, microdontia, incomplete enamel formation, and complete agenesis of teeth.[15] Eruption patterns may be altered, and changes in alveolar, mandibular, and maxillary bone growth and development can have orthodontic and cosmetic implications.[13] The addition of radiation to treatment protocols (e.g., cranial radiation for leukemia or total body irradiation for marrow stem cell transplants) significantly increases the risk for damage to developing teeth.

Indirect Oral Toxic Effects

Although direct oral toxic effects are generally the most visible oral complications of cancer chemotherapy, indirect oral effects can potentially be of more concern. The most important indirect effects are infections from myelosuppression and immunosuppression associated with damage of myelogenous stem cells and cellular elements of the immune system. Preexisting oral and dental infections can spread, with the oral cavity serving as the point of entry for organisms into deeper tissues and the systemic circulation. Other indirect toxic effects to the oral cavity are thrombocytopenia, anemia, and gastrointestinal toxicity (nausea, vomiting, and alteration in absorption of nutrients).

Oral mucosal infections

The risk for infection increases in concert with the degree and duration of immunosuppression. As immunosuppression worsens, the classic signs and symptoms of infection (redness, swelling, pain, etc.) may be reduced because of altered immune responses and thus alter the clinical presentation of oral infections. It is important to remember that patients who receive cancer therapy often have chronic low-grade oral infections (periodontal disease and endodontic infections) that can become serious infections when patients are immunocompromised. Many cancer patients are inappropriately instructed to stop tooth brushing and flossing during cancer therapy or specifically when blood counts drop, which only increases the risk of infection and bleeding.[5]

Fungal infections Superficial colonization by *Candida* species, especially *Candida albicans*, is the most frequently documented oral infection in cancer chemotherapy patients.[27,55] However, as the degree and duration of immunosuppression increases in patients receiving myelosuppressive/immunosuppressive therapy, there is a distinct risk for oral fungal infections such as aspergillosis and mucormycosis, as well as a large number of other invasive fungal organisms. Changes in the local or systemic factors that normally suppress or prevent oral fungal colonization (and invasion) are responsible for fungal infections.[65] The factors affecting colonization and growth rates are alterations in competing oral bacterial flora, xerostomia, use of systemic antimicrobials, and immunosuppression, especially involving neutropenia. Alteration in host oral bacterial flora in myelosuppressed cancer patients has supported increased candidal colonization.[55,63] However, as new strategies to prevent and treat fungal infections are developed, the types of *Candida* or other fungal organisms are changing. The widespread use of fluconazole prophylaxis has been associated with increasing numbers of *C. glabrata*, *C. torulopsis*, and *C. krusei* infections that may have altered sensitivity to fluconazole and other antifungal agents.

Oral candidal infections can have a variety of presentations: pseudomembranous, erythematous, hyperplastic, and invasive. The most common form is pseudomembranous candidiasis, in which mild to heavy surface colonization occurs with raised, white, curdlike masses of organisms. With hyphal invasion of the upper cellular layers of the mucosal epithelium, the mucosal surface can become atrophic, often with little or no evidence of pseudomembranous masses. Atrophic or erythematous candidiasis is particularly common on the dorsal tongue, where the only clinical evidence of infection may be a patchy loss of filiform papillae. With deeper mucosal invasion, a hyperplastic or ulcerative lesion can be noted. Invasive candidiasis is characterized usually by discrete, firm, almost leathery, white-yellow lesions with marginal erythema. These lesions are primarily noted in patients who are significantly immunocompromised and are at high risk of systemic dissemination. Candidal infections of the lip commissures usually present with cracking, pain, and varying degrees of erythema. Symptoms associated with candidiasis elsewhere in the oral cavity are variable and often occur with no overt signs. Although oral candidal infections are classically reported to be associated with symptoms of "metallic taste" and "increased sensitivity to spices," this is not frequently noted in infections associated with cancer therapy.

The diagnosis of *Candida* infection often requires correlation of the clinical presentation of lesions with laboratory tests. Clinical lesions are often nonspecific, and because *Candida* can be a normal inhabitant, reliance only on fungal cultures may lead to false-positive results. Using direct microscopic examination (with Gram's stain or potassium hydroxide to identify pseudo-branching hyphae) followed by culture to speciate the fungus can be helpful. Because different species of *Candida* can have different sensitivities to different antifungals, speciation becomes particularly important in cases in which the patient has not responded to therapy. For hyperplastic and invasive candidiasis, cultures from surface swabs and scrapings can produce false-negative results, and biopsy with specific stains for *Candida* may be required to establish a definitive diagnosis.

While the therapeutic efficacy of nystatin has been demonstrated, prophylaxis with nystatin has never been shown to be effective in preventing candidal infections. Additionally, nystatin oral rinses (swish and swallow regimens) can cause significant nausea and vomiting when swallowed; "swish and spit" regimens can sometimes diminish this problem, but not always.[27] Although prophylactic clotrimazole oral troches have been shown to reduce the rate of oral infection in some instances (renal transplant recipients and patients with solid malignant tumors), the drug's efficacy in other immunosuppressed hosts remains to be demonstrated.[27] More recently, the efficacy of systemic azole (e.g., fluconazole, itraconazole, ketoconazole) antifungal prophylaxis has clearly been demonstrated in a number of clinical settings, including hematopoietic cell transplantation (HCT) recipients, and these agents are generally considered the most effective way to prevent/reduce fungal colonization and subsequent infection.

After a fungal infection has been documented, appropriate therapy should be instituted. Topical therapy with nystatin or clotrimazole is useful for superficial oral infection. Persistent or locally invasive infection (including atrophic and erythematous candidiasis), especially when a risk exists for systemic spread, should be treated with appropriate systemic agents. Fluconazole and itraconazole have been reported to produce good responses in HCT patients.[31] The treatment of disseminated candidal infections remains difficult, and there is increasing evidence of infection from azole-resistant organisms. Amphotericin B remains the systemic antifungal of choice for severe deep mycoses, especially in immunocompromised patients. The frequency and range of fungal organisms causing serious oral infection in immunocompromised cancer patients have increased significantly and include infection by *Aspergillus*, *Mucor*, and *Rhizopus*. These infections often have a nonspecific appearance and can be confused with other oral toxic effects. Diagnosis depends on laboratory tests, and systemic therapy must be instituted immediately because these infections can spread systemically and are frequently fatal.

Viral Infections Herpes group viruses cause significant oral disease in patients receiving cancer chemotherapy.[7,41,66,67] Herpes simplex virus (HSV), varicella-zoster virus (VZV), cytomegalovirus (CMV), and Epstein-Barr virus (EBV) are recognized causes of oral lesions in cancer patients. Most infections with HSV, VZV, and EBV represent reactivation of latent virus, whereas CMV infections can result from either reactivation of latent virus or newly acquired virus. Other viruses causing oral lesions in cancer chemotherapy and HCT patients are adenovirus, Coxsackie viruses, and human herpes virus 6.

The diagnosis of oral virus lesions can be made through direct immunofluorescent examination and culture and, at times, examination of biopsy material with immunohistologic stains.

Herpes Simplex Virus The clinical presentation of oropharyngeal HSV infections can vary from localized herpes labialis to widespread oropharyngeal ulcerations. When they are superimposed on chemotherapy-induced mucositis, HSV lesions can be difficult to recognize clinically. A sudden and dramatic onset or worsening of mucositis often warrants investigation of a potential HSV cause in patients who are HSV antibody positive or who have possibly been exposed to HSV.

Acyclovir and valacyclovir prophylaxis for HSV is clearly effective, especially for HSV-seropositive HCT recipients. Oral dosing may be switched to parenteral if the patient is unable to tolerate oral administration because of nausea or oral/esophageal ulcerative mucositis or if gastrointestinal absorption is not adequate. Many cases of suspected acyclovir resistance may be caused by inadequate dosing or absorption of oral acyclovir. Acyclovir-resistant HSV is, however, a growing concern. Early diagnosis of HSV is important, because the infection is usually successfully managed with systemic acyclovir.[7] Topical therapy may have little effect in this setting.

Varicella-Zoster Virus The most frequent presentation of VZV infection is herpes zoster lesions characterized by vesicular eruptions that follow dermatomal distributions. In severe cases, VZV can involve multiple dermatomes, and a risk exists for dissemination that can result in a serious life-threatening disease.[66] In susceptible patients, primary VZV infection can occur with the typical skin lesions of chickenpox; in immunosuppressed patients, this represents a potentially fatal infection. Direct immunofluorescent examination of swab material and viral cultures are used to diagnose VZV infections. Acyclovir and famciclovir are currently the drugs of choice to treat these infections.

Cytomegalovirus CMV can cause oral lesions in immunosuppressed patients.[41,64] CMV lesions have a nonspecific appearance with a tendency for irregular ulcerations covered with a pseudomembranous fibrin exudate. Surface swabs for direct immunofluorescence have only a fair reliability for diagnosing CMV, possibly because the virus appears primarily to infect endothelial cells and fibroblasts (i.e., deep to the surface) and thus yields low numbers of free virus.[67] Cultures may improve the detection of CMV, but the most reliable technique to diagnose this disease appears to be biopsy with immunohistochemical stains specific for CMV.[41] Ganciclovir is the drug of choice.

Epstein-Barr Virus EBV-related hairy leukoplakia lesions have been described in non–HIV-infected immunosuppressed patients, including HCT patients. These lesions have no apparent clinical significance. However, EBV-related lymphomas and immunoblastic sarcomas can present with oral lesions and head and neck lymphadenopathy with a potentially fatal outcome. These lymphomas are generally responsive to radiation therapy.

Bacterial infections The different environmental niches of the oral cavity—mucosal surfaces, periodontal sulci, and tooth surfaces—harbor a wide array of organisms, and in the immunosuppressed patient the potential for acquisition of nonoral bacteria must also be considered. As infectious disease protocols and antibiotics have evolved, the pressures on the oral microflora have been constantly altered. Over the years, oral flora in cancer patients have demonstrated a shift from a risk for overgrowth by primarily gram-negative enteric bacilli (e.g., *Pseudomonas, Escherichia coli, Serratia,* and *Klebsiella*)[63] to the reemergence of a risk for infection primarily from gram-positive organisms, especially streptococcal and staphylococcal species. As with fungal and viral infections, the risk for bacterial infection increases as the severity and duration of immunosuppression increases. Neutropenia is the primary risk factor predisposing to bacterial infection, with risk increasing significantly when the neutrophil count decreases to less than 1000/mm.[3,55,59]

Mucositis and mechanical disruption in the oral mucosa can create a point of entry for oral bacteria, and oral colonization and secondary infection of the oral tissues increase the severity and course of oral mucositis.[32] Cancer patients have a wide range of chronic dental diseases that can adversely affect the course of treatment, which makes pretreatment oral and dental evaluations and disease stabilization extremely important.

Dental Plaque, Dental Caries, and Pulpal Infections Dental plaque can increase the risk of local and systemic infection, and efforts should be directed at keeping plaque accumulation as low as possible.[5] A growing body of research suggests that even the less virulent oral bacteria can exacerbate oral mucositis. Thus a clear need exists to maintain the highest compliance with oral hygiene protocols for mechanical plaque removal (brushing, flossing, etc.), augmented with topical antimicrobial regimens (e.g., chlorhexidine) as needed.

Dental decay threatening the pulp should be stabilized before therapy to prevent the risk of pulpal infection and pain during therapy. Temporary materials can be placed until the patient has recovered from cancer therapy. Incipient-to-minimal decay can be treated with fluorides and sealants until more definitive therapy can be completed.

Pulpal/periapical infections can have a significant effect on cancer chemotherapy and may be difficult to manage in patients receiving chemotherapy; considerable attention should be paid to stabilization before medical management. Careful and complete diagnostic tests should be performed to determine pulpal vitality and endodontic status.[52] The clinician should distinguish between osteolytic periapical infections and endodontic failures versus noninfectious periapical conditions such as apical scars, metastatic cancer lesions, or leukemic infiltrates that mimic periapical infection.[54] If an endodontic procedure is necessary, enough time must be allowed for assessment of treatment success before cancer chemotherapy begins. Prophylactic antibiotics may be indicated if the risk for subsequent infection is considered clinically significant. If the endodontic disease is associated with nonrestorable teeth, every effort should be made to extract these teeth as soon as possible and thus allow maximum time for healing before cancer treatment begins.

Invasive dental and surgical procedures should be undertaken only with a clear understanding of a patient's immune and coagulation status. Table 50-1 presents guidelines for antibiotic and platelet support. However, every case should be individually assessed, and the patient's physician and other appropriate specialists should be consulted before the clinician renders care. Extractions should be atraumatic, and efforts should be instituted to promote rapid stabilization and healing. Socket sites should be debrided and copiously irrigated. Some centers recommend against the use of hemostatic agents because of the concern that they may promote infection at the extraction site and delay healing. Attempts should be made to obtain primary closure with conservative alveolectomy. Generally stated, the most accepted time for initial healing before commencing chemotherapy is 10 to 14 days. If less time is available, more vigorous supportive care and more frequent follow-up evaluations may be necessary. If documented infection is associated with the teeth scheduled for extraction, antibiotics (ideally chosen with the benefit of sensitivity testing) should be administered for 7 to 10 days after the extraction.

If extraction is not possible for medical reasons, the clinician may consider providing initial endodontic therapy (open and broach, careful initial filing) and sealing antimicrobial medicaments in the root canal chamber. Antibiotics should be administered for 7 to 10 days. Extraction of the tooth can be performed after the patient's hematologic status has returned to normal. Appropriate treatment to eliminate the risk of infection is important because pathogens can readily disseminate directly from the dental pulp and periapical tissues into the systemic circulation.

Multiple topical and systemic approaches have been considered to prevent mucosal infection in the granulocytopenic patient.[52] Most bacterial infections in the compromised host are caused by organisms colonizing at or near the site of infection.[55,61] Substantial advances in cytokine research, including the discovery and synthesis of granulocyte colony-stimulating factor and granulocyte/macrophage colony-stimulating factor, have led to the use of such agents (in the form of filgrastim and sargramostim, respectively) to rejuvenate host defenses against these organisms by increasing neutrophil and macrophage counts.

Studies of topical chlorhexidine (0.12% to 0.2%) used to reduce bacterial colonization and infections have shown mixed results. The drug has been reported to diminish the severity and duration of mucositis in cancer patients in some studies[28] but has shown no benefit in others.[27,30] Chlorhexidine rinses can promote a decreased rate of colonization by bacteria in and around teeth and thus reduce gingival infections.

Poorly fitting removable prosthetic appliances can abrade oral mucosa and increase the risk of microbial invasion into deeper tissues. The dentist should adjust dentures before the start of chemotherapy and instruct patients to change soaking solutions daily. Denture-soaking cups can readily become colonized with a variety of pathogens, including *Pseudomonas aeruginosa, Escherichia coli, Enterobacter* species, *Staphylococcus aureus, Klebsiella* species, *T. glabrata,* and *C. albicans.* Routine cleaning of denture cups with a weak bleach solution can prevent contamination and reduce the risk for denture-associated oral infections. Chemotherapy patients may also choose to restrict or reduce denture use during chemotherapy to reduce the risk of mucosal trauma and irritation that may worsen oral mucositis.

Periodontal Infections Periodontal infection is a major concern for cancer chemotherapy patients. Approximately 25% of all acute infections in acute nonlymphocytic leukemia patients undergoing induction therapy may arise in a site of preexisting periodontal disease. Improved protocols for managing immunosuppressed patients may reduce this rate, and

Table • 50-1

Management Suggestions for Invasive Dental Procedures

MEDICAL SITUATION	MANAGEMENT SUGGESTIONS FOR INVASIVE DENTAL PROCEDURES	SUGGESTED INTERVENTION	NOTES
Patients with chronic indwelling venous access lines	American Heart Association prophylactic antibiotic recommendations		No clear scientific proof exists detailing infectious risk for these lines after dental procedures. This recommendation is empirical.
Neutropenia			Obtain current CBC to determine actual level.
>2000 mm^3	No prophylaxis indicated		
1000 to 2000 mm^3	American Heart Association prophylactic antibiotic recommendations		Clinical judgment is crucial; if infection is present or unclear, more aggressive antibiotic therapy may be indicated.
<1000 mm^3	Consultation with infectious disease specialists is indicated	Consideration for broad-spectrum IV antibiotics	If organisms are known or suspected, appropriate adjustments should be made based on sensitivities.
Thrombocytopenia*			Order platelet count and coagulation tests
>75,000/mm^3	No additional support needed		
40,000 to 75,000/mm^3	Platelet support is optional	If platelet transfusion is to be used, consider administering platelets preoperatively and 24 hours later. Further transfusions are based on clinical course.	Use techniques to promote control of bleeding (sutures, pressure packs, minimize trauma, etc.)
<40,000/mm^3		Platelets should be transfused 1 hour before procedure; obtain platelet counts during surgery; transfuse regularly to maintain counts greater than 30,000 to 40,000 mm^3 until initial healing has occurred.	Use all of the above. Consider using hemostatic agents (microfibrillar collagen, topical thrombin, etc.). If clots are friable and break down rapidly, consider use of aminocaproic acid. Monitor sites carefully.

*Assumes that all other coagulation parameters are within normal limits and that platelet counts will be maintained at or above the specified level until initial stabilization/healing has occurred.
CBC, Complete blood count; *IV*, intravenous.

acute periodontal flare-ups may be reduced in myelosuppressed cancer patients. The signs and symptoms of periodontal disease may be decreased in immunosuppressed patients or those with hematologic malignancies, which can lead to underrecognition of the degree of periodontal disease. In addition, extensive ulceration of sulcular epithelium, which may be present with periodontal disease, is not directly observable yet may represent a source for disseminated infection by a wide variety of organisms. Bacteremias from colonizing organisms have been noted to develop in these patients. In patients with leukemic gingival infiltrates, the enlargements will shrink with appropriate chemotherapy, which permits improved hygiene care. Chronic periodontal disease may develop into acute periodontal infections with associated systemic sequelae during granulocytopenia.[33,41,52] Dental disease prevention programs have been shown to reduce the risk of potential oral sequelae associated with cancer therapy, with complications being prevented, reduced in severity, or alleviated.[5] When acute periodontal infection is diagnosed, broad-spectrum antibiotic therapy should be considered while culture results are pending. Local therapy may include chlorhexidine rinsing, irrigation with effervescent agents (e.g., hydrogen peroxide) that may affect anaerobic bacteria colonizing the periodontal pocket, and gentle mechanical plaque removal (dental brushing and flossing); placement of periodontal antibacterials may also be considered. The key to reducing the risk of significant gingiva-associated infections (and bleeding) is to perform dental prophylaxis in advance of myelosuppression and to maintain excellent oral hygiene throughout treatment.

Oral hemorrhage

Hemorrhage from oral tissues in patients receiving cancer therapy can result from thrombocytopenia, loss of coagulation factors from disseminated intravascular coagulation or liver disease, and mucosal lesions such as gingivitis and periodontitis.[54] Spontaneous mucosal petechiae and gingival bleeding may be observed when the platelet count drops to less than 20,000 to 30,000/mm^3. Damage to mucosal tissues, such as that resulting from oral HSV infections, increases the risk of bleeding. Trauma associated with oral function can also induce minor hemorrhage.

Oral hemorrhage in cancer patients with thrombocytopenia is rarely a debilitating complication, although its occurrence can be alarming to patients, caregivers, and family. Local measures center on forming an adequate clot and protecting the clot until healing has occurred. Direct pressure applied by gauze soaked in topical thrombin can be used. A vasoconstrictor such as cocaine or epinephrine can help with initial control, but rebound vasodilation can occur as the drug's effect wears off. Clot-forming agents such as those made from microfibrillar collagen can also be used to organize and stabilize clots. Platelet transfusions are usually not required except for patients whose platelet counts are profoundly suppressed, resulting in insufficient clot formation and repeated significant bleeding episodes. Aprotinin or aminocaproic acid can be used adjunctively to promote coagulation, especially when platelet transfusions are marginally effective in controlling bleeding.

Gastrointestinal effects: nutritional disturbances, nausea, and emesis A frequent and often significant site of toxicity of cancer chemotherapy is the gastrointestinal tract. As it does with the oral mucosa, chemotherapy can damage the rapidly proliferating mucosal lining of the stomach and intestines. The resulting mucositis can lead to significant discomfort (cramping, pain), diarrhea, and disruption in the absorption of nutrients. Additionally, gastric injury plus CNS toxicity from chemotherapy can cause patients to have frequent and profound nausea and emesis. This complication is generally the second most frequent significant complication affecting the quality of life after cancer chemotherapy.[4,51]

In addition to the effect on the quality of life, however, is the negative influence on oral nutrition intake and the potential damage to oral tissues after emesis; the pH of oral tissues can fall to approximately 2. In the presence of mucositis, the exposure of compromised mucosa to this acidic fluid can potentially further damage tissues. Also, the vigorous tongue movements usually associated with chemotherapy-associated emesis can result in increased trauma to the tongue and floor of mouth as these tissues move against incisal and occlusal surfaces.

Protocols to reduce or prevent nausea and vomiting after chemotherapy have become remarkably more effective. Often initiated prophylactically, these therapies can minimize the problem and ensure patient comfort. Strategies often combine approaches that target both the gastrointestinal mucosa and the CNS nausea and vomiting centers.[2,49]

The nausea and vomiting associated with chemotherapy can result in adverse conditioning such that normal smells, tastes, and other associated stimuli can induce nausea and vomiting—even just driving by the clinic or hospital where the therapy was administered can be a trigger. Patients may even develop an aversion to swallowing their own saliva, toothbrushing, or wearing removable dental appliances. These simple "oral events" can trigger the response. A heightened gag reflex is usually associated with the triggering by the latter two. Systematic deconditioning strategies can generally help control or eliminate this problem and allow for the resumption of routine oral care.

HEMATOPOIETIC CELL TRANSPLANTATION (HCT)

HCT is one of the most intense forms of cancer therapy. Patients are given supralethal doses of chemotherapy with or without total body irradiation. The patient's stored hematopoietic stem cells or stem cells from the best available human leukocyte antigen–matched donor are infused into the patient so he or she survives the supralethal "conditioning" treatment. Oral complications frequently associated with HCT are similar to those noted in patients undergoing high-dose chemotherapy.[62] Mucositis, salivary gland dysfunction, infections, taste dysfunction, and bleeding are common acute oral complications in the first 4 weeks after transplantation. Risk of oral infection slowly declines over the next several months as neutrophil counts recover, although oral candidiasis and reactivation of HSV and VZV can occur in susceptible patients for many months after engraftment. Full immune recovery takes between 7 and 12 months after transplantation.

The severity of mucositis is clearly related to the type of conditioning regimen used.[62] Oral mucosal healing only partially depends on the rate of engraftment (especially neutrophils), with mucositis tending to heal more slowly in allogenic patients (versus autologous/syngeneic transplant recipients) because of posttransplantation prophylaxis for acute graft-versus-host disease (GVHD) with methotrexate or the potential emergence of acute GVHD (see below).

Oral infections noted in bone marrow transplant recipients are similar to those seen in immunosuppressed patients receiving high-dose chemotherapy without transplantation. Use of prophylactic fluconazole reduces the incidence of oral and disseminated candidal and other fungal infection. The risk for reactivation of latent HSV and the risk for reactivation or acquisition of CMV are very high in the early period after bone marrow transplant; however, prophylaxis with acyclovir for HSV and the use of CMV-negative blood products and ganciclovir for CMV have significantly reduced the frequency and effect of these infections. Risk of oral bacterial infection has decreased over the past decade, which may be attributable to oral hygiene protocols and improved antibiotic prophylactic and treatment protocols. Opportunistic gram-negative pathogens, such as *P. aeruginosa*, *Neisseria* species, and *E. coli*, as well as gram-positive cocci such as staphylococci and streptococci, remain a major concern.

GVHD represents an immune-mediated disease occurring after transplantation and results from immunologic reactions and damage mediated by donor lymphocytes against the patient's tissues. GVHD is potentially lethal.[62,64] In the oral cavity, GVHD mimics a number of naturally occurring autoimmune disorders (e.g., lichen planus, lupus, scleroderma, Sjögren's syndrome). Oral acute GVHD can become apparent as early as 18 to 21 days after transplantation and is characterized by mucosal erythema, atrophy, ulceration, and later hyperkeratotic striae and plaques. Chronic oral GVHD presents similarly and becomes apparent 100 days after transplantation. Topical steroid rinses, creams, and gels and topical azathioprine can help reduce symptoms and promote healing of ulcerations, but resolution generally depends on successful systemic therapy with prednisone, cyclosporine, mycophenolate, tacrolimus, and other immunosuppressive agents. Cutaneous GVHD has been shown to be responsive to treatment with psoralen plus ultraviolet-A (PUVA).[38] The use of extracorporeal PUVA therapy has shown promise for the treatment of refractory chronic GVHD.[60] Intraoral PUVA therapy with UV-A light sources that can directly expose oral mucosal surfaces has been reported to help manage oral GVHD lesions.[57]

GVHD can also damage salivary glands with resulting xerostomia and mucoceles involving major and minor salivary gland tissue.[47]

Chronic GVHD is the most significant late oral complication seen in allogenic bone marrow transplant recipients. Other late complications of bone marrow transplantation include recurrence of the primary malignancy, occurrence of second primary cancers (especially in long-term survivors), and viral infections, especially VZV. Dental and facial skeletal growth abnormalities have been noted in children younger than 12 years receiving transplants, primarily resulting from damage induced by conditioning regimens, especially total body irradiation.[13-15] Children frequently demonstrate delayed exfoliation of primary teeth, which correlates with the delayed or arrested development of succeeding permanent teeth. Teeth developing after transplantation often exhibit short, conical-shaped roots. Skeletal changes in jaws generally are manifest as decreased jaw length and reduced alveolar ridge height (the latter most likely from decreased root length).

ORAL COMPLICATIONS OF CANCER RADIOTHERAPY

Radiation therapy is a primary treatment modality for head and neck and oral cancer. Oral complications associated with the direct oral toxicity of radiation can be a treatment-limiting complication of radiation therapy, and the most common patient-reported symptom. The oral complications of radiation therapy arise from direct damage to progenitor cells of epithelium, parenchyma, and bone and from vasculitis and endarteritis that additionally adversely affect the oral mucosa, salivary glands, musculature, bone, and connective tissue. These injuries directly or indirectly result in clinical consequences that manifest as mucositis, taste loss, infection, xerostomia, rampant dental decay, soft tissue and bone necrosis, and fibrosis of oral and perioral tissue, including skin and muscles (Box 50-4).

The potential contribution of the oral microflora to established ulcerative mucositis has been suggested, but trials to alter the effect of microflora on oral mucositis with topical or systemic antimicrobials has met with mixed success. Current changes in the management of the primary disease, including accelerated fractionation of radiation therapy, hyperfractionated radiation schedules, and combination of radiation therapy and chemotherapy, have been associated with an increased incidence and severity of many of the oral complications.

Box 50-4

Oral Complications of Radiation Therapy

Acute	Chronic
Oral mucositis	Xerostomia
Infection	Dental caries
Fungal	Infections
Bacterial	Fungal
Salivary gland dysfunction	Bacterial
Sialadenitis	Mucosal fibrosis and atrophy
Xerostomia	Muscular/cutaneous fibrosis
Taste dysfunction	Soft tissue necrosis
	Osteoradionecrosis
	Taste dysfunction
	Dysgeusia
	Ageusia

Ulcerative mucositis occurs in more than 90% of those receiving conventional radiation therapy; however, virtually all patients treated with hyperfractionated radiation or radiation and radiochemotherapy develop ulcerative mucositis. A proposed classification of the late complications of radiation therapy is expected to facilitate reporting and assessment of results of interventions.

The importance of dentistry in the overall management of head and neck cancer patients receiving radiation therapy is well established. The elimination of dental disease and establishment of oral care protocols to maintain maximum oral health must be part of patient assessment and care before radiation therapy. During and after radiation therapy, dental involvement is dictated by the specific care needs of the patient, who may require more frequent assessments and earlier interventions than most general dental patients.

Detailed oral and dental assessment is necessary to identify conditions that should be treated before radiation therapy. Sites of potential mechanical irritation should be eliminated. Dental treatment such as extractions can delay the start of therapy if undertaken late in the preradiation evaluation phase. Early referral and coordination between oncologists and the dental team can reduce this problem. Attempts to reduce the risk of postradiation osteonecrosis, described later in this chapter, generally mandate extraction of nonrestorable or questionable teeth, root tips, and periodontally involved teeth in the planned radiation field with enough time before the start of radiation therapy to allow for adequate initial healing. If time permits, asymptomatic periapical radiolucent lesions can be managed. However, endodontics can be performed or completed after radiation if managed expertly. Detailed review of oral hygiene, oral care during radiation therapy, and oral care after radiotherapy are important components of long-term care. The acquisition of baseline data allows assessment of the trends in oral health after cancer therapy, which may facilitate early intervention.

After a patient has received radiation therapy that includes the jaws, dental treatments that require soft tissue and bone manipulation can result in soft tissue necrosis and osteoradionecrosis. These patients are not candidates for routine dental care but need to be provided care that reduces the risk of postradiation oral complications.

Acute Reactions

Acute reactions arise from direct toxicity to tissues in the radiated treatment volume (see Box 50-4). They generally become apparent shortly after the start of radiation therapy and worsen throughout the course of therapy. After the cessation of therapy, although some complications resolve, several remain and evolve into chronic reactions.

Mucositis

As noted for the high-dose chemotherapy patient, mucositis occurs when the rate of epithelial growth and repair is exceeded by radiation-induced epithelial cell necrosis and inflammation, resulting in epithelial thinning, erythema, erosion, and ulceration. The initial clinical sign of mucosal reaction to radiation can be a white appearance of the mucosa, reflecting early hyperplasia and decreased exfoliation of epithelial cells and hyperkeratinization. This condition may rapidly evolve to an erythematous-appearing surface resulting from hyperemia, epithelial thinning, and ulceration. As in chemotherapy, radiation damage is more marked in rapidly proliferating epithelium, resulting in earlier and more severe mucosal reactions involving the nonkeratinized mucosa. With common fractionation of doses to approximately 200 cGy/day, mucosal erythema is noted 1 to 2 weeks after the start of therapy and increases throughout the course of therapy, often to a maximum in 4 weeks, and persists with healing 2 or more weeks after completion of therapy.[25] The dose, fraction, and duration of radiation are the principal factors affecting the development and severity of radiation mucositis. However, marked individual variability is seen. When the primary radiation beam strikes metallic dental restorations and appliances, a secondary, or backscatter, radiation is produced. Backscatter radiation is of lower energy than the primary beam and only travels a short distance. Thus tissues that contact these metal surfaces are exposed to the primary beam and then the additional backscatter radiation—increasing the total absorbed dose of radiation and thus potentially causing more mucosal breakdown. Consequently, removable dental appliances should be taken out during treatment sessions. Metal restorations need not be removed; efforts to hold tissues away from metal surfaces (use of vinyl mouth guards, cotton rolls, etc.) have been reported anecdotally to reduce mucosal damage.[80] This and other concerns related to the penetration and distribution of radiation to the tumor arise with the increasing use of metal dental implants.

Oral changes elicited by radiation include disruption of the mucosal barrier, reduction of salivary flow rates that result in reduced diluting and clearing effects, and alteration in antimicrobial factors in saliva. Impaired mobility of oral and perioral tissues may lead to decreased clearing of local irritants and food products.

Management of mucositis Management strategies described previously for chemotherapy patients are generally useful for the cancer patient undergoing head or neck radiation. In addition, two radiation-specific issues emerge[48]:

1. Radiation injury is oral site specific and depends on dosage and portals of therapy.
2. Duration of radiation-induced oral mucositis typically extends for 6 to 8 weeks after the cessation of therapy, compared with the approximate 5 to 14 days observed in chemotherapy patients. Extended radiation treatment protocols produce more significant damage to mucosal tissues and submucosal vasculature and connective tissues and thus account for this difference.

An additional, more global issue needs to be addressed for head and neck cancer patients receiving radiation therapy. Because the primary cause of oral cancer is tobacco use, alcohol abuse further escalates risk. Research has shown that patients who do not stop smoking after primary therapy for oral cancer are at increased risk of recurrence or second primary lesions. Patients with head and neck cancer should therefore be encouraged and supported in efforts to permanently cease tobacco use. Additionally, more severe mucositis occurs in patients who smoke and consume alcohol during radiation therapy, and they should be strongly encouraged to discontinue such activities.

Maintenance of oral hygiene and elimination of local irritants may reduce or slow the development of mucositis. Bacterial infection can be a major factor in oral mucositis, as evidenced by studies that used topical antimicrobials to reduce radiation mucositis.[73,75] Although chlorhexidine has a reasonable range of action against many of the normal gram-positive oral bacteria, it has not demonstrated significant efficacy in preventing oral mucositis during radiation therapy.[29,30] Troches or pastilles with a mixture of polymyxin, tobramycin, and amphotericin have shown efficacy in several studies but overall efficacy remains to be demonstrated.[73]

Benzydamine is a nonsteroidal agent that possesses analgesic, antiinflammatory, and mild anesthetic properties. Used topically, benzydamine may stabilize cell membranes, inhibit degranulation of granulocytes, alter synthesis of prostaglandins, and decrease tissue tumor necrosis factor. Signs and symptoms of oral mucositis have been shown to be reduced when benzydamine is used prophylactically throughout the course of radiation therapy.[25] Resolution of mucositis may also be accelerated. Although the phenomenon is not well studied, aspirin and other NSAIDs have been reported to prevent late radiation changes, possibly because of their ability to inhibit prostaglandin synthesis and their effects on platelet adhesion that may reduce vascular complications after radiation therapy.

Palliation of mucositis may be achieved by use of topical anesthetics and coating agents. Normal saline solution (0.9%), sodium bicarbonate solutions, and water have also been suggested for hydration and rinsing. Water-based lubricants or those containing lanolin are preferred for lip moisturizing over petroleum-based products (e.g., petroleum jelly) because long-term use of these latter agents may result in atrophy of epithelium and increase the risk of infection. A number of oral mucosal "coating agents" have been recommended for management of mucositis discomfort; these include kaolin-pectin, aluminum chloride, aluminum hydroxide, milk of magnesia, and sucralfate. Commercial formulations may be diluted 1 : 1 or 1 : 2 with water.

The most frequently used medications for management of mild to moderate mucositis pain are topical anesthetics. These agents provide temporary relief of pain for 15 to 60 minutes, but as the severity of mucositis increases the duration of effective pain relief tends to decrease. Little difference exists among the topical anesthetic agents currently available: dyclonine, lidocaine, benzocaine, and antihistamines (e.g., diphenhydramine). Doxepin suspension has been reported to reduce mucosal pain in cancer patients, does not cause burning on application, and has an extended duration of pain relief up to 4 hours.[26] Caution should be exercised when using topical anesthetic agents. Viscous lidocaine occasionally produces an initial burning sensation with application, taste sensation is abolished, swallowing (and gag reflex) may be adversely affected, and systemic toxicity may be of concern if the substance is swallowed. CNS depression or excitation may follow excessive absorption of topical anesthetic agents (or, additionally, sedation only in the case of antihistamines). Therefore local application to areas of ulceration may be more appropriate than extensive oral rinsing. Concerns about combining agents, such as a coating agent and an analgesic or anesthetic, have been previously described. The combination of kaolin-pectin and diphenhydramine has been reported to reduce radiation mucositis pain. The longest duration of pain relief was reported for dyclonine and lidocaine plus cocaine in radiation mucositis.[8]

Sucralfate is a cytoprotective agent available for the management of gastrointestinal ulceration. The agent protects the surface of ulcerated mucosa in acidic conditions and may provide further protection by stimulating the release of prostaglandins. Controlled studies of sucralfate suspension for the treatment of oral mucositis caused by chemotherapy and radiation therapy have met with mixed success.[43] Sucralfate reduces the growth of streptococcal organisms in culture and thus may have a potential effect on caries risk.

Hydroxypropylcellulose can be applied to isolated ulcers, forming a protective surface barrier that reduces symptoms. The efficacy of benzocaine combined with a film-forming agent was assessed in the management of oral ulcers in patients undergoing cancer therapy and was found to relieve discomfort for at least 3 hours.[40]

A benefit has been reported for topical application of vitamin E, but further studies are needed.[49] Topical application of prostaglandin E_2 to ease mucositis was studied in small groups of patients, with initial results demonstrating that mucositis may be reduced.[44] Additionally, the prostaglandin E_1 analogue misoprostol is currently under study.

A number of investigations have reported successful management of radiation mucositis with corticosteroids used both prophylactically and therapeutically. Corticosteroids can be administered as a spray, as a mouthwash,[1] or as part of combination rinses, and all have shown beneficial effects. These effects may result from inhibition of prostaglandin and leukotriene synthesis, which thereby inhibits inflammation.[1] One concern about the use of topical corticosteroids arises from the reduction of local immunity and the increased risk of secondary infection, but this complication may be overcome by the use of antiseptics or antimicrobial drugs.

When local or topical strategies are not sufficient to control pain, systemic analgesics are necessary (see below). NSAIDs are often useful to manage pain for mild to moderate mucositis; opioids, including such formulations as time-release oral morphine and fentanyl patches, can be used for more severe mucositis pain.

Current research is pursuing the role of biologic response modifiers in preventing or treating oral mucosal damage. In a clinical trial, azelastine, which is thought to suppress neutrophil activity and cytokine release from lymphocytes, was associated with less severe mucositis.[50] Epidermal growth factor and transforming growth factor β_3 have both been studied in animal mucositis models,[71] and clinical trials are planned. Other agents being considered are L-glutamine, interleukin-11,[37] keratinocyte growth factors, and defensins (antimicrobial proteins).

Pain management Head and neck and oral pain may be caused by the tumor, cancer therapy, or its sequelae or may be unrelated to cancer. Pain is commonly reported at the time of diagnosis of head and neck cancer, with up to 85% of those seeking treatment reporting some level of pain, although pain levels are usually described as being low-grade discomfort.[23,25] Oral pain is frequently reported in nearly all patients receiving radiotherapy and surgery. Pain attributable to mucosal sensitivity and musculoskeletal complications of cancer is present in approximately half of patients more than 6 months after cancer therapy.

Pain arising from dental and periodontal disease can initially be controlled with analgesics and antibiotics. However, definitive dental treatment is needed for long-term management. Pain arising from bacterial, fungal, and viral infections is managed with specific antimicrobial agents; analgesics and topical anesthetics are also necessary for more severe infections. Neurologic pain states, including neuropathic pain and neuralgia-like pain, may require the use of antidepressant medications and anticonvulsants. Management of radiation osteonecrosis (see below) may also necessitate pain management. In cases of persistent pain, long-term pain management approaches that include counseling, relaxation therapy, imagery, biofeedback, hypnosis, and transcutaneous nerve stimulation may be considered.

Analgesics should be prescribed according to the degree of pain and the pharmacologic action of the drug and its duration of action. Pain control is improved at a lower total dose if analgesics are provided on a time-contingent basis, not on an as-needed basis. In general, nonopioid analgesics should be initially prescribed and continued even if opioids are later required; again, this may allow a lower dose of opioid medication. The introduction of time-release morphine and fentanyl transdermal patches has made it easier to provide more consistent and convenient pain control for oncology outpatients with severe pain. Adjuvant systemic medications such as tricyclic antidepressants may enhance the analgesic effects of other agents, possess analgesic potential themselves, and promote sleep, which is often disrupted by pain. Use of adjuvant medications directed at the cause of the pain should be used whenever possible. Reassessment of the efficacy of pain control techniques, as well as assessment of their adverse effects, should be conducted regularly. In addition, pain control should not rely on medications alone but should be part of an overall strategy for pain management.

Infection during radiation therapy

Candidiasis is the most common oropharyngeal infection in irradiated patients.[19] Patients receiving head and neck radiation therapy are frequently colonized with *Candida* and demonstrate an increase in quantitative counts and clinical infection. Although the contribution of *Candida* to oral mucositis associated with radiation therapy is not clear, candidiasis may increase the discomfort of mucositis. Treatment of oral candidiasis during radiation therapy has primarily focused on the use of topical antifungals such as nystatin and clotrimazole. Compliance can be a problem with these topical antimicrobial agents for patients with mucositis because of irritation, nausea, pain (nystatin solutions), and difficulty in dissolving the medication forms (nystatin pastilles and clotrimazole troches). More recently, the use of systemic antifungals such as ketoconazole and fluconazole to treat oral candidiasis has proved to be effective and may have advantages over topical agents for patients with mucositis. Systemic antifungals have been shown to be present in the mucosa and in oral secretions.[16] Fluconazole may provide a more rapid effect against C. *albicans* and has been shown to be present in the stratum corneum of the oral epithelium. Fluconazole was also found to reduce fungal adherence to human buccal epithelial cells in addition to its direct antifungal activity.[16]

Bacterial infections should be treated empirically with standard antibiotics and modified if the results of culture and sensitivity tests indicate the need to change antibiotics.

Salivary gland dysfunction

Salivary gland tissue is sensitive to radiation. During the first several weeks of radiation therapy, a nonpainful salivary gland enlargement is noted. Over the following weeks this swelling generally resolves. Shortly after the start of radiation, changes in salivary flow rate and character are noted. The serous acini are more susceptible to radiation damage than mucous acini, which in addition to reducing flow rates also results in saliva having a thicker, more mucous character. Patients report the sensation of dryness and having more difficulty clearing secretions. During the first several weeks of radiation therapy, salivary flow rates modestly recover over days of rest (that is, over weekends) only to decline rapidly during the succeeding 5 days of therapy. After several weeks of therapy, the ability of salivary glands to recover at all after 2 days of rest is lost and flow rates steadily decrease over the course of therapy. After total radiation doses to salivary glands exceed approximately 3000 cGy, the ability for glands to recover is significantly limited. Recently, the radioprotectant drug amifostine has been shown to prevent salivary gland damage when given during radiation therapy.[6,12]

Taste dysfunction

Shortly after the start of external beam radiotherapy to oral fields, including the tongue and posterior oropharyngeal tissues, patients begin to report diminishing senses of taste and smell. A total fractionated dose of more than 3000 cGy reduces the acuity of all tastes: sweet, sour, bitter, and salt.[3,10] Direct damage to the microvilli and outer surface of the taste cells as well as xerostomia and mucosal infection may affect taste. In most instances, taste acuity recovers slowly over 60 to 120 days after treatment, but some patients are left with residual hypogeusia. Zinc supplementation (zinc sulfate, 220 mg twice daily) has been reported to be useful in some patients with taste disturbances. Although animal studies have shown that zinc deficiency can negatively affect the number and size of taste buds and produce fine structure changes in the taste bud cells, the effect of zinc supplementation on recovery of taste receptors in human beings is not known.[9]

Late Reactions

The late oral complications of radiation therapy primarily represent residua from direct damage to the vasculature, salivary glands, mucosa, connective tissue, and bone in the irradiated field. The most common patient symptoms are related to hyposalivation. The types and severity of pathologic changes are directly related to the total dose of radiation, the size of fractions administered, and the time of treatment. Irradiated mucosa demonstrates epithelial atrophy, disrupted vascular supply, and submucosal fibrosis, all of which result in an atrophic, friable mucosa. Fibrosis in skin, muscle, and joint tissue results in limited jaw function and trismus. In salivary glands, loss of acinar cells, alteration in duct epithelium, gland fibrosis, and fatty degeneration occur. In bone, hypervascularity and hypocellularity result in an increased risk of postradiation osteonecrosis.

Xerostomia

Bilateral exposure of the major salivary glands to tumoricidal doses of radiation predictably results in xerostomia. Individuals who receive total radiation doses greater than 3000 cGy are at risk for profound xerostomia if all major glands are in the field; irreversible damage occurs at total doses approaching 5000 cGy over a 5-week period. During radiation, the serous acini are affected earlier than the mucinous acini, resulting in a viscous secretion that can be uncomfortable for patients and can interfere with oral function. As the total dose of radiation increases, saliva production decreases. Some salivary function may recover within 6 months after radiation, but in many cases the loss of function is permanent, and strategies to prevent oral complications related to xerostomia need to be continued indefinitely.

Xerostomia results in a loss of oral mucosal lubrication, reduced pellicle formation (with subsequent reduced resistance to abrasion and chemical damage), and decreased remineralization of hard dental tissue. Changes in total protein and pH also affect the microbial population, resulting in a more cariogenic microflora.

Stimulation of salivary gland function The treatment of radiation-induced salivary gland hyposecretion should begin with an initial assessment of residual function by measurement of whole resting and stimulated saliva volumes.[17] If salivary glands have remaining functional tissue, residual function may be stimulated naturally (i.e., through taste) or with the use of cholinergic or other agents capable of improving gland function. Sugarless chewing gum and candy may help stimulate salivary flow from residual major and minor salivary gland cells that were spared from exposure or able to recover from the irradiation. Citric acid is considered to be the strongest "natural" tastant for stimulation of salivary glands, thus making sugarless lemon candies a reasonable choice for patients with dry mouth. (Many of the "sugarless" candies use sorbitol as a sweetener. Because this sugar can pass through the gastrointestinal tract without being absorbed, patients who consume large quantities of sorbitol may have diarrhea.)

Several drugs are used as sialogogues to provide the protective benefits of saliva. Pilocarpine is the best studied of the sialogogues.[22,40,78] Pilocarpine is a muscarinic receptor agonist (see Chapter 8). Initial divided doses of 15 mg/day (5 mg/dose) are increased to 30 mg/day until effective secretion of saliva occurs or adverse effects intervene. Pilocarpine doses must be individualized carefully for patients to increase drug efficacy and reduce toxicity (e.g., sweating, gastrointestinal disturbance, hypotension). The potential to prevent postradiation xerostomia with prophylactic pilocarpine has been suggested by results from several studies that found less reduction in salivary flow in patients provided with pilocarpine, fewer patient symptoms during radiation, and a potential reduction in mucositis severity.[78] Thus the severity of chronic xerostomia may be reduced with a prophylactic sialogogue during radiation therapy. Cevimeline is a newer cholinergic agent that has a similar mechanism of action and has been recently approved for salivary stimulation.

Bethanechol and bromhexine have received limited study as sialogogues.[17] Bethanechol, a synthetic muscarinic receptor agonist, has been reported to have potential benefits in divided doses of 75 to 200 mg/day without gastrointestinal upset and with a reduced tendency for sweating. Bromhexine has been studied in patients with dry mouth resulting from Sjögren's syndrome; no studies have been conducted in postradiation patients.

Anetholetrithione (not currently available in the United States) has been reported to be beneficial in managing dry mouth. This drug may increase the numbers of muscarinic receptors on salivary acinar cells. Synergistic effects have been suggested with pilocarpine in a study that used both drugs simultaneously.[22,34]

Palliation of xerostomia Saliva substitutes and oral lubricating agents may be used when stimulation of salivary function is not possible. Most commercial products are more viscous than saliva, do not mimic the changing viscosity after secretion of saliva, and do not contain salivary enzymes and antibodies. The majority of products currently available are based on carboxymethylcellulose solutions; animal mucins have been incorporated in some European products. Acceptance of these palliative products can vary and comparative trials have identified patient-preferred products.[4,18,24] A novel line of xerostomia products (Biotène, Laclede, Inc.) is available that provides salivary enzymes that may improve oral health and not merely increase moisturization.[58,81] Unfortunately, the majority of commercial products have not been subjected to controlled clinical study. Because the saliva substitutes have a limited duration of activity, they have to be administered repeatedly, creating problems in patient acceptance and cost. Patients commonly discontinue these products and rely on frequent sipping of water.

Dental caries

Xerostomia increases the risk of dental caries because of such factors as a shift to more cariogenic flora, decreased titers of salivary antimicrobial substances, and loss of mineralizing components.[75] Management of xerostomia decay must address each component of the caries process. Oral hygiene techniques to remove bacterial dental plaque must be scrupulously maintained. Hyposalivation should be managed whenever possible, and thorough trials of sialogogues should be conducted. The tooth structure may be made more caries resistant by the use of topical fluorides, and remineralization may be enhanced by the combined use of fluorides and remineralizing products.[76] Although clinicians have long believed that vinyl fluoride carriers were mandatory for topical fluoride application, brush-on fluoride gels can be effectively used, especially in instances in which compliance with fluoride trays is poor. Comparisons of the various means of fluoride application (brush-on, rinse, or tray) are needed to define the simplest effective protocol. The two forms of topical fluoride that are recommended are stannous fluoride and neutral sodium fluoride. Stannous fluoride can cause staining with persistent use, but this tooth discoloration can generally be removed through standard professional dental cleaning.

The high risk for caries-associated xerostomia is significantly influenced by shifts in resident oral flora, especially increased colonization by *Streptococcus mutans* and *Lactobacillus* species.[20,27] Laboratory assessments to quantify cariogenic organisms should be carried out before proceeding with the use of antimicrobials. Topical fluorides may reduce levels of *S. mutans*, but they may not decrease the numbers of lactobacilli. Chlorhexidine rinses can help control the numbers of *S. mutans;* again, *Lactobacillus* species are more resistant.[20,27] If the underlying risk factors are not controlled, rapid recolonization by cariogenic organisms occurs, necessitating continuing use of topical chlorhexidine and fluoride. A protocol of four initial topical applications of 1% chlorhexidine (given in the first month of therapy), plus daily 1-minute rinses of 0.05% sodium fluoride and 0.2% chlorhexidine, has been reported to prevent radiation caries completely in one group of patients treated for cancer of the head and neck. This approach also produced remineralization of incipient carious lesions. Because of ionic interactions, fluoride (negatively charged ions) bonds with chlorhexidine (positively charged molecules), and thus use of the two agents should be separated by several hours. Additionally, tooth remineralization products high in calcium phosphate and fluoride have been developed and have demonstrated useful in vitro effects that are supported by clinical experience.

Late oral infections

Postradiation therapy oral infections are usually not a major clinical problem for patients recovering from acute radiation toxicities. Oral infections at this time are primarily associated with overgrowth or high carriage rates of bacterial and yeast organisms that are usually attributable to risk factors imposed by reduction or loss of normal salivary function.

Bacterial infections The shift in predominant bacterial species colonizing dental surfaces is noted to involve bacteria associated with dental caries. Other than bacterial infections associated with dental caries and endodontic disease, mucosal bacterial infections are generally not a significant clinical problem. Unless chlorhexidine is used continuously to control gram-positive bacteria in dental plaque, increased colonization of mucosal surfaces by gram-negative organisms is not noted.

Candidiasis With continuing xerostomia, oral candidiasis can persist and may cause discomfort and altered taste. The treatment of choice has been primarily topical antifungal agents. However, systemic antifungals may have some benefits when topical agents are unacceptable or ineffective. Polyene antifungals—nystatin and even amphotericin B—may be used topically. Other topical antifungal drugs currently available include azole derivatives such as clotrimazole. These agents can be applied topically as rinses, troches (or pastilles), or creams—particularly if the patient wears dentures. When prescribing topical antifungal drugs, the clinician should note the presence of sucrose in the product because frequent use of products with sucrose, especially in patients with xerostomia, can promote caries. Limited compliance with the topical agents may be overcome with systemic azoles (e.g., ketoconazole, fluconazole) that can be taken once a day for clinically symptomatic infections and once a week for prophylaxis (see Chapter 40).

Tissue necrosis

Any oral soft tissues included in the field of radiation can potentially be involved with postradiation soft tissue necrosis (PRSTN). The late toxic effects to the oral mucosa (and bone) result from endarteritis and vascular changes that produce a relatively hypervascular, hypocellular, and hypoxic tissue unable to repair or remodel itself effectively if trauma occurs. Additionally, connective tissue changes can produce tissue characteristics that result in soft tissue necrosis. Where PRSTN occurs in tissues over bone, the subsequent exposure of bone can lead to postradiation osteonecrosis (PRON). Risk for tissue necrosis (both PRSTN and PRON) increases as the dose and volume of tissue irradiated increase.

PRON results from the vascular changes that occur in bone as well as from damage to bone cells—osteoblasts, osteocytes, and osteoclasts. Although the mineralized portion of bone is unaffected by radiation, the destruction of the cellular elements of bone and the hypovascularization result in minimally viable bone that is not able to remodel or repair itself. The posterior mandible is the most common site involved with PRON, although necrosis can occur in other areas, including in the maxilla. Symptoms and signs may include discomfort or tenderness at the site, bad taste, paresthesia and anesthesia, fistula formation, and secondary infection. Pathologic fracture can even occur from extensive tissue involvement. As long as a risk for dental or periodontal disease or trauma in irradiated fields exists, so does the risk of PRON. PRON is usually initiated by trauma (e.g., denture trauma) or surgical procedures, but it may also be idiopathic, occurring spontaneously with no identifiable cause. Although PRON lesions may become secondarily infected, PRON is not primarily an infectious process. The risk of necrosis is lifelong and may occur many years after radiation. The overall risk of developing PRON has been estimated to be between 2.6% and 15%.[21]

Prevention of PRON begins with preradiation dental stabilization or elimination of dental disease. Teeth in high-dose fields with questionable prognosis, particularly because of periodontal or endodontic disease or in patients who are unlikely to maintain acceptable oral health, should be extracted before radiotherapy. If at all possible, 7 to 14 days should be allowed for healing; some have even suggested up to 21 days.[21] Surgery should attempt to reduce the degree of trauma to the bone, using primary closure if possible, eliminating infections, and supporting the general health of the patient.

When PRON develops, management includes avoidance of further local irritants, discontinuation of dental appliances if they encroach on the PRON lesion, maintenance of nutritional status, and cessation of smoking and alcohol consumption. Topical antibiotics (e.g., tetracycline) or antiseptics (e.g., chlorhexidine) may reduce the potential local irritation by the microbial flora. For chronic localized PRON, this treatment along with regular follow-up care may be the best approach. Every attempt should be made to promote mucosal coverage of the exposed bone. Appropriate analgesics should be provided. If worsening pain, infection, and PRON progression are noted, hyperbaric oxygen therapy (HBO) is recommended. HBO has been shown to increase oxygenation of irradiated tissue, induce angiogenesis, and promote osteoblast repopulation and fibroblast function. HBO is usually prescribed as 20 to 30 "dives" at 100% oxygen and 2 to 2.5 atm of pressure.[46] If surgery is needed, postsurgical HBO of 10 dives is recommended. Bone sequestra may be managed with local resection, or, in severe cases involving the mandible, mandibulectomy. The mandible can be reconstructed to provide continuity for esthetics and function. In a general cancer clinic, postradiation extractions performed with expert surgery resulted in only 5% of extractions demonstrating delayed healing. This record suggests that when extractions are performed by experienced clinicians, HBO should be reserved for patients in whom osteonecrosis develops.[21,79] However, prophylactic HBO may be considered when extensive surgery is required for a patient who is believed to be at extreme risk from high doses of radiation to bone in the surgical area.

Taste loss

Taste and smell dysfunction can be a chronic disability after exposure to radiation. As noted earlier, taste acuity generally recovers over the 2- to 4-month period after the end of radiation treatment. However, some individuals are left with permanent hypogeusia. Zinc supplementation (220 mg zinc sulfate twice a day) can be used to help recover the sense of taste, but chances of successful recovery appear to be limited. Additionally, if the patient's sense of smell is intact, eating pleasure can be enhanced by trying to make food as "aromatic" as possible to help enhance the taste experience. Nutritional counseling may be necessary to ensure adequate nutritional intake if patients are not able to maintain adequate calorie levels because eating is not enjoyable.

Nutrition

Loss of appetite is common because of radiation-induced complications such as sore mouth, xerostomia, taste loss, dysphagia, nausea, and vomiting. Eating becomes pleasureless and may be painful, resulting in selection of foods that do not aggravate the oral tissues, often at the expense of adequate nutrition. Nutritional complications and deficiencies may be avoided by modifying the texture and consistency of the diet, by adding between-meal snacks to increase protein and caloric intake, and by administering caloric and vitamin and mineral supplements. High-calorie and protein liquid dietary supplements can be used to augment diets to maintain body weight and ensure adequate nutritional intake. Nutritional counseling may be required during and after therapy. Nasogastric feeding tubes or percutaneous esophageal gastrostomy may be required when swallowing is impeded or not possible. After treatment and after mucositis has resolved, nutritional counseling must consider any long-term complications that may be present, including xerostomia, increased caries risk, altered ability to chew, difficulty in forming the food bolus, and dysphagia. Consideration must be given to taste, texture, moisture, and caloric and nutrient content.

Temporomandibular Dysfunction

Musculoskeletal syndromes may arise because of fibrosis of skin and muscles after radiation and surgery, mandibular discontinuity after surgery, and parafunction (clenching/bruxism) associated with the emotional stress caused by the disease and its treatment. Limitation of jaw opening is related to exposure of the lateral pterygoid muscles. Mandibular stretching exercises and prosthetic aids to help reduce the severity of the fibrosis limiting mandibular movement should be instituted before restriction of movement has occurred. Therapy of mandibular dysfunction may include occlusal stabilization appliances, physiotherapy, exercises, trigger-point injections and analgesics, muscle relaxants, tricyclic antidepressants, and other pain management strategies.

SUMMARY

The oral cavity is highly susceptible to the direct and indirect toxic effects of cancer chemotherapy and therapeutic ionizing radiation. Pretreatment oral health stabilization and supportive oral and dental care are crucial components of the patient's overall management, affecting all phases of therapy. Intratherapy and posttherapy oral complications can profoundly add to the suffering of patients, adversely affect the success of therapy, and significantly increase the overall cost of care. Oral care should be both preventive and therapeutic to minimize oral and associated systemic complications.

Oral complications of chemotherapy are generally acute (i.e., during therapy) and resolve shortly after the cessation of therapy. On the other hand, ionizing radiation can cause not only significant intratherapy oral complications, but also general damage and possibly permanent toxic effects. Consequently, the dentist must clearly understand the specifics of the proposed therapy and the potential oral problems based on the patient's current oral health and then develop a plan that covers all phases of therapy.

Future research should be targeted at developing strategies and technologies to address the quality of life and oral function to (1) reduce the incidence and severity of oral mucositis; (2) improve infection prevention, detection, and treatment; (3) prevent salivary gland dysfunction; and (4), specifically for radiation therapy patients, reduce the incidence and severity of chronic oral complications.

CITED REFERENCES

1. Abdelaal AS, Barker DS, Fergusson MM: Treatment for irradiation-induced mucositis, *Lancet* 1:97, 1991.
2. Ballatori E, Roila F, De Angelis V, et al: Clinical and methodological issues in antiemetic therapy: a worldwide survey of experts' opinions. Multinational Association of Supportive Care in Cancer, *Support Care Cancer* 5:269-273, 1997.
3. Bartoshuk LM: Chemosensory alterations and cancer therapies, *NCI Monographs* 9:179-184, 1990.
4. Bellm LA, Epstein JB, Rose-Ped A, et al: Patient reports of complications of bone marrow transplantation, *Support Care Cancer* 8:33-39, 2000.
5. Borowski B, Benhamou E, Pico JL, et al: Prevention of oral mucositis in patients treated with high-dose chemotherapy and bone marrow transplantation: a randomized controlled trial comparing two protocols of dental care, *Oral Oncol Eur J Cancer* 30B:93-97, 1994.
6. Brizel DM, Wasserman TH, Henke M, et al: Phase III randomized trial of amifostine as a radioprotector in head and neck cancer, *J Clin Oncol* 18:3339-3345, 2000.
7. Bustamante CI, Wade JC: Herpes simplex virus infection in the immunocompromised cancer patient, *J Clin Oncol* 9:1903-1915, 1991.
8. Carnel SB, Blakeslee DB, Oswald SG, et al: Treatment of radiation- and chemotherapy-induced stomatitis, *Otolaryngol Head Neck Surg* 102:326-330, 1990.
9. Chou HC, Chien CL, Huang HL, et al: Effects of zinc deficiency on the vallate papillae and taste buds in rats, *J Formos Med Assoc* 100:326-335, 2001.
10. Conger AD: Loss and recovery of taste acuity in patients irradiated to the oral cavity, *Radiat Res* 53:338-347, 1973.
11. Cowen D, Tardieu C, Schubert M, et al: Low energy helium-neon laser in the prevention of oral mucositis in patients undergoing bone marrow transplant: results of a double blind randomized trial, *Int J Radiat Oncol Biol Phys* 38:697-703, 1997.
12. Culy CR, Spencer CM: Amifostine: an update on its clinical status as a cytoprotectant in patients with cancer receiving chemotherapy or radiotherapy and its potential therapeutic application in myelodysplastic syndrome, *Drugs* 61:641-684, 2001.
13. Dahllof G: Craniofacial growth in children treated for malignant diseases, *Acta Odontol Scand* 56:378-382, 1998.

14. Dahllof G, Forsberg CM, Nasman M, et al: Craniofacial growth in bone marrow transplant recipients treated with growth hormone after total body irradiation, *Scand J Dent Res* 99:44-47, 1991.
15. Dahllof G, Forsberg CM, Ringden O, et al: Facial growth and morphology in long-term survivors after bone marrow transplantation, *Eur J Orthod* 11:332-340, 1989.
16. Darwazeh AMG, Lamey PJ, Lewis MA, et al: Systemic fluconazole therapy and in vitro adhesion of *Candida albicans* to human buccal epithelial cells, *J Oral Pathol Med* 20:17-19, 1991.
17. Epstein JB, Burchell JL, Emerton S, et al: A clinical trial of bethanechol in patients with xerostomia after radiation therapy. A pilot study, *Oral Surg Oral Med Oral Pathol* 77:610-614, 1994.
18. Epstein JB, Emerton S, Le ND, et al: A double-blind crossover trial of Oral Balance gel and Biotene toothpaste versus placebo in patients with xerostomia following radiation therapy, *Oral Oncol* 35:132-137, 1999.
19. Epstein JB, Freilich MM, Le ND: Risk factors for oropharyngeal candidiasis in patients who receive radiation therapy for malignant conditions of the head and neck, *Oral Surg Oral Med Oral Pathol* 76:169-174, 1993.
20. Epstein JB, Loh R, Stevenson-Moore P, et al: Chlorhexidine rinse in prevention of dental caries in patients following radiation therapy, *Oral Surg Oral Med Oral Pathol* 68:401-405, 1989.
21. Epstein JB, Rea G, Wong FL, et al: Osteonecrosis: study of the relationship of dental extractions in patients receiving radiotherapy, *Head Neck Surg* 10:48-54, 1987.
22. Epstein JB, Schubert MM: Synergistic effect of sialogogues in management of xerostomia after radiation therapy, *Oral Surg Oral Med Oral Pathol* 64:179-182, 1987.
23. Epstein JB, Schubert MM, Scully C: Evaluation and treatment of pain in patients with orofacial cancer: a review, *Pain Clin* 4:3-20, 1991.
24. Epstein JB, Stevenson-Moore P: A clinical comparative trial of saliva substitutes on radiation-induced salivary gland hypofunction, *Spec Care Dentist* 12:21-23, 1992.
25. Epstein JB, Stevenson-Moore P, Jackson S, et al: Prevention of oral mucositis in radiation therapy: a controlled study with benzydamine hydrochloride rinse, *Int J Radiat Oncol Biol Phys* 16:1571-1575, 1989.
26. Epstein JB, Truelove EL, Oien H, et al: Oral topical doxepin rinse: analgesic effect in patients with oral mucosal pain due to cancer or cancer therapy, *Oral Oncol* 37:632-637, 2001.
27. Epstein JB, Vickars L, Spinelli J, et al: Efficacy of chlorhexidine and nystatin rinses in prevention of oral complications in leukemia and bone marrow transplantation, *Oral Surg Oral Med Oral Pathol* 73:682-689, 1992.
28. Ferretti GA, Ash RC, Brown AT, et al: Control of oral mucositis and candidiasis in marrow transplantation: a prospective, double-blind trial of chlorhexidine digluconate oral rinse, *Bone Marrow Transplant* 3:483-493, 1988.
29. Ferretti GA, Raybould TP, Brown AT, et al: Chlorhexidine prophylaxis for chemotherapy- and radiotherapy-induced stomatitis: a randomized double-blind trial, *Oral Surg Oral Med Oral Pathol* 69:331-338, 1990.
30. Foote RL, Loprinzi CL, Frank AR, et al: Randomized trial of a chlorhexidine mouthwash for alleviation of radiation-induced mucositis, *J Clin Oncol* 12:2630-2633, 1994.
31. Goodman JL, Winston DJ, Greenfield RA, et al: A controlled trial of fluconazole to prevent fungal infections in patients undergoing bone marrow transplantation, *N Engl J Med* 326:845-851, 1992.
32. Graber CJ, de Almeida KN, Atkinson JC, et al: Dental health and viridans streptococcal bacteremia in allogeneic hematopoietic stem cell transplant recipients, *Bone Marrow Transplant* 27:537-542, 2001.
33. Greenberg MS, Cohen SG, McKitrick JC, et al: The oral flora as a source of septicemia in patients with acute leukemia, *Oral Surg Oral Med Oral Pathol* 53:32-36, 1982.
34. Hamada T, Nakane T, Kimura T, et al: Treatment of xerostomia with the bile secretion-stimulating drug anethole trithione: a clinical trial, *Am J Med Sci* 318:146-151, 1999.
35. Holmes S: Food avoidance in patients undergoing cancer chemotherapy, *Support Care Cancer* 1:326-330, 1993.
36. Jankovic L, Jelic S, Filipovic-Ljeskovic I, et al: Salivary immunoglobulins in cancer patients with chemotherapy-related oral mucosa damage, *Eur J Cancer B Oral Oncol* 31B:160-165, 1995.
37. Keith JC, Jr, Albert L, Sonis ST, et al: IL-11, a pleiotropic cytokine: exciting new effects of IL-11 on gastrointestinal mucosal biology, *Stem Cells* 12(suppl 1):79-89, 1994.
38. Kunz M, Wilhelm S, Freund M, et al: Treatment of severe erythrodermic acute graft-versus-host disease with photochemotherapy, *Br J Dermatol* 144:901-902, 2001.
39. LeVeque FG, Montgomery M, Potter D, et al: A multicenter, randomized, double-blind, placebo-controlled, dose-titration study of oral pilocarpine for treatment of radiation-induced xerostomia in head and neck cancer patients, *J Clin Oncol* 11:1124-1131, 1993.
40. LeVeque FG, Parzuchowski JB, Farinacci GC, et al: Clinical evaluation of MGI 209, an anesthetic, film-forming agent for relief from painful oral ulcers associated with chemotherapy, *J Clin Oncol* 10:1963-1968, 1992.
41. Lloid ME, Schubert MM, Myerson D, et al: Cytomegalovirus infection of the tongue following marrow transplantation, *Bone Marrow Transplant* 14:99-104, 1994.
42. Lockhart PB, Sonis ST: Alterations in the oral mucosa caused by chemotherapeutic agents. A histologic study, *J Dermatol Surg Oncol* 7:1019-1025, 1981.
43. Maakonen TA, Bostrom P, Vilja P, et al: Sucralfate mouth washing in the prevention of radiation-induced mucositis: a placebo-controlled double blind randomized study, *Int J Radiat Oncol Biol Phys* 30:177-182, 1994.
44. Matejka M, Nell A, Kment G, et al: Local benefit of prostaglandin E_2 in radiochemotherapy-induced oral mucositis, *Br J Oral Maxillofac Surg* 28:89-91, 1990.
45. McCarthy GM, Skillings JR: A prospective cohort study of the orofacial effects of vincristine neurotoxicity, *J Oral Pathol Med* 20:345-349, 1991.
46. Myers RAM, Marx RE: Hyperbaric oxygen in postradiation head and neck surgery, *NCI Monogr* 9:151-157, 1990.
47. Nagler RM, Nagler A. Major salivary gland involvement in graft-versus-host disease: considerations related to pathogenesis, the role of cytokines and therapy, *Cytokines Cell Mol Ther* 5:227-232, 1999.
48. NCI Supportive Care PDQ: Oral complications of chemotherapy and head/neck radiation, *CancerNet*, http://cancer.gov/cancerinfo/pdq/supportivecare/oralcomplications/healthprofessional/.

49. Oettle H, Riess H: Treatment of chemotherapy-induced nausea and vomiting, *J Cancer Res Clin Oncol* 127:340-345, 2001.
50. Osaki T, Ueta E, Yoneda K, et al: Prophylaxis of oral mucositis associated with chemoradiotherapy for oral carcinoma by azelastine hydrochloride (Azelastine) with other antioxidants, *Head Neck* 16:331-339, 1994.
51. Osoba D, Zee B, Warr D, et al: Effect of postchemotherapy nausea and vomiting on health-related quality of life. The Quality of Life and Symptom Control Committees of the National Cancer Institute of Canada Clinical Trials Group, *Support Care Cancer* 5:307-313, 1997.
52. Peterson DE: Pretreatment strategies for infection prevention in chemotherapy patients, *NCI Monogr* 9:61-71, 1990.
53. Peterson DE: Research advances in oral mucositis, *Curr Opin Oncol* 11:261-266, 1999.
54. Peterson DE, D'Ambrosio JA: Nonsurgical management of head and neck cancer patients, *Dent Clin North Am* 38:425-445, 1994.
55. Pizzo PA: Infections in the cancer patient. In DeVita VT, Hellman S, Rosenberg SA, eds: *Cancer: principles and practice of oncology,* ed 4, Philadelphia, 1993, JB Lippincott.
56. Plevoá P: Prevention and treatment of chemotherapy- and radiotherapy-induced oral mucositis: a review, *Oral Oncol* 35:453-470, 1999.
57. Redding SW, Callander NS, Haveman CW, et al: Treatment of oral chronic graft-versus-host disease with PUVA therapy: case report and literature review, *Oral Surg Oral Med Oral Pathol Oral Radiol Endod* 86:183-187, 1998.
58. Rhodus NL, Bereuter J: Clinical evaluation of a commercially available oral moisturizer in relieving signs and symptoms of xerostomia in postirradiation head and neck cancer patients and patients with Sjögren's syndrome, *J Otolaryngol* 29:28-34, 2000.
59. Rolston KVI, Bodey GP: Infections in patients with cancer. In Holland JF, Frei E, Kufe DW, et al, eds: *Cancer medicine,* ed 3, Philadelphia, 1993, Lea & Febiger.
60. Rossetti F, Dall'Amico R, Crovetti G, et al: Extracorporeal photochemotherapy for the treatment of graft-versus-host disease, *Bone Marrow Transplant* 18(suppl 2):175-181, 1996.
61. Schimpff SC: Infections in patients with cancer: overview and epidemiology. In Moossa AR, Robson MC, Schimpff SC, eds: *Comprehensive textbook of oncology,* ed 2, Baltimore, 1992, Williams & Wilkins.
62. Schubert MM: Oral manifestations of viral infections in immunocompromised patients, *Curr Opin Dent* 1:384-397, 1990.
63. Schubert MM: Oro-pharyngeal mucositis. In Atkinson K, ed: *Clinical bone marrow transplantation: a reference textbook,* Cambridge, 1994, Cambridge University Press.
64. Schubert MM, Epstein JB, Lloid ME, et al: Oral infections due to cytomegalovirus in immunocompromised patients, *J Oral Pathol Med* 22:268-273, 1993.
65. Schubert MM, Peterson DE, Lloid M. Oral complications. In Thomas ED, Blume KG, Forman SJ, eds: *Hematopoietic cell transplantation,* ed 2, Oxford, 1999, Blackwell Science, pp 751-763.
66. Schubert MM, Sullivan KM: Recognition, incidence, and management of oral graft-versus-host disease, *NCI Monogr* 9:135-144, 1990.
67. Silverman S, Jr, Thompson JS: Serum zinc and copper in oral/oropharyngeal carcinoma. A study of seventy-five patients, *Oral Surg Oral Med Oral Pathol* 57:34-36, 1984.
68. Sonis ST. Mucositis as a biological process: a new hypothesis for the development of chemotherapy-induced stomatotoxicity, *Oral Oncol* 34:39-43, 1998.
69. Sonis ST, Costa JW, Evitts SM, et al: Effect of epidermal growth factor on ulcerative mucositis in hamsters that receive cancer chemotherapy, *Oral Surg Oral Med Oral Pathol* 74:749-755, 1992.
70. Sonis ST, Eilers JP, Epstein JB, et al: Validation of a new scoring system for the assessment of clinical trial research of oral mucositis induced by radiation or chemotherapy, *Cancer* 85:2103-2113, 1999.
71. Sonis ST, Lindquist L, Van Vugt A, et al: Prevention of chemotherapy-induced ulcerative mucositis by transforming growth factor β_3, *Cancer Res* 54:1135-1138, 1994.
72. Sonis ST, Oster G, Fuchs H, et al: Oral mucositis and the clinical and economic outcomes of hematopoietic stem-cell transplantation, *J Clin Oncol* 9:2201-2205, 2001.
73. Spijkervet FK, Van Saene HK, Van Saene JJ, et al: Effect of selective elimination of the oral flora on mucositis in irradiated head and neck cancer patients, *J Surg Oncol* 46:167-173, 1991.
74. State FA, Hamed MS, Bondok AA: Effect of vincristine on the histological structure of taste buds, *Acta Anat* 99:445-449, 1977.
75. Stevenson-Moore P, Epstein JB: The management of teeth in irradiated sites, *Oral Oncol Eur J Cancer* 29B:39-43, 1993.
76. Symonds RP: Treatment-induced mucositis: an old problem with new remedies, *Br J Cancer* 7:1689-1695, 1998.
77. Symonds RP, McIlroy P, Khorrami J, et al: The reduction of radiation mucositis by selective decontamination antibiotic pastilles: a placebo-controlled double-blind trial, *Br J Cancer* 74:312-317, 1996.
78. Valdez IH, Wolff A, Atkinson JC, et al: Use of pilocarpine during head and neck radiation therapy to reduce xerostomia and salivary dysfunction, *Cancer* 71:1848-1851, 1993.
79. van Merkesteyn JPR, Bakker DJ, Borgmeijer-Hoelen AMMJ: Hyperbaric oxygen treatment of osteoradionecrosis of the mandible. Experience in 29 patients, *Oral Surg Oral Med Oral Pathol* 80:12-16, 1995.
80. Wang R, Boyle A: A convenient method for guarding against localized mucositis during radiation therapy, *J Prosthodont* 3:198-201, 1994.
81. Warde P, Kroll B, O'Sullivan B, et al: A phase II study of Biotene in the treatment of postradiation xerostomia in patients with head and neck cancer, *Support Care Cancer* 8:203-208, 2000.

General References

National Institutes of Health consensus development conference on oral complications of cancer therapies: diagnosis, prevention, and treatment, Bethesda, Maryland, April 17-19, 1989, *NCI Monogr* 9:1-184, 1990.

NCI Supportive Care PDQ: Oral complications of chemotherapy and head/neck radiation, *CancerNet,* http://cancer.gov/cancerinfo/pdq/supportivecare/oralcomplications/healthprofessional/.

Peterson DE, D'Ambrosio JA: Nonsurgical management of head and neck cancer patients, *Dent Clin North Am* 38:425-445, 1994.

Peterson DE, Schubert MM: Oral toxicity. In Perry MC, ed: *The chemotherapy source book*, Baltimore, 1992, Williams & Wilkins.

Schubert MM: Oro-pharyngeal mucositis. In Atkinson K, ed: *Clinical bone marrow transplantation*, Cambridge, 1994, Cambridge University Press.

Schubert MM, Peterson DE, Lloid M: Oral complications. In Thomas ED, Blume KG, Forman SJ, eds: *Hematopoietic cell transplantation*, ed 2, Oxford, 1999, Blackwell Science, pp 751-763.

CHAPTER • 51

Drugs of Abuse

Charles S. Bockman and Peter W. Abel

Drug abuse can be defined as an inappropriate use of a drug for a nonmedical purpose. Drug abuse is considered to cause harm to the individual abuser and to society as a whole. Many variables not directly related to a drug can influence whether a given individual will become a drug abuser. For example, for those who try nicotine, the risk of developing an addiction is approximately twice that for those who try cocaine.[8] This is not meant to infer that the pharmacologic abuse potential of nicotine is twice that of cocaine. Indeed, many experts argue that cocaine possesses the greatest potential for abuse based on its pharmacologic characteristics alone. Rather, some psychosocial factors are equally important in affecting onset and continuation of drug abuse and addiction. It is beyond the scope of this chapter to cover these factors related to drug users and their environment; this chapter concentrates solely on the pharmacologic aspects of drugs of abuse. A wide variety of different types of drugs and other chemical substances are subject to abuse. For instance, anabolic steroids are abused by bodybuilders and other athletes to add muscle mass and enhance athletic performance. However, the most commonly abused groups of drugs are those that act on the central nervous system (CNS) to alter perception. Therefore this chapter focuses on drugs that are abused because they have effects in the CNS that are perceived by some as desirable.

HISTORIC PERSPECTIVE

Natural products such as hemp flowers, opium, and coca leaves have been used for thousands of years for their ability to cause pleasurable sensations or other alterations in consciousness. Other than alcohol, the first major drugs of abuse in the United States were cocaine and the opioids. Throughout the nineteenth century, unregulated opium use led to a plethora of patent medicines containing opium derivatives. As a result, many middle-class Americans became dependent on opium because of promiscuous use of such preparations. Social attitudes toward drug abuse, nevertheless, remained relaxed until after the Civil War. The widespread use of morphine by injection for dysentery, malaria, and pain resulted in such large numbers of morphine-addicted veterans that morphine dependence became known as "soldier's disease."[11] The chemical isolation of the alkaloid cocaine in 1859 was followed by a rapid increase in the use of that drug. It was enthusiastically promoted for a variety of disorders, and, by the turn of the century, oral abuse of cocaine in the form of patent medicines and tonics was widespread. It was not until 1903, after 17 years in production, that the manufacturers of Coca-Cola stopped using cocaine-containing syrup in their soft drink.

In the early 1900s the mass media developed the myth of cocaine-crazed renegades committing heinous crimes against society. Opioid dependence was still prevalent, and morphine was the major opioid of abuse. During this period, federal laws were enacted to control the widespread drug abuse problem. The introduction of the Pure Food and Drug Act in 1906, the Harrison Narcotic Act in 1914, and the Narcotic Drugs Import and Export Act in 1922, as well as the enforcement of these acts by law enforcement officials, led to the virtual disappearance of cocaine abuse by the 1930s. Unfortunately, the increased cost and reduced street availability of cocaine helped lead to the rise of amphetamine as a stimulant drug of abuse. Intravenous (IV) heroin use was also becoming popular, and by 1935 it was as widely abused as morphine. Between World Wars I and II, addiction began to be widely equated with criminality.[11] In the case of marijuana, sensationalized accounts of murders perpetrated by those under the influence of the "killer weed" led to the passage of the Marihuana Tax Act of 1937, which effectively banned its production, distribution, and sale.

In the 1960s, drug abuse began to make major inroads into middle-class society. The drug-naive, baby-boom generation began "turning on" with lysergic acid diethylamide (LSD) and marijuana. Epidemic amphetamine abuse developed during the 1960s, peaking in 1967 with 32 million legal prescriptions written for amphetamines that suppress appetite and lead to weight loss. To combat the rising tide of drug abuse, the Comprehensive Drug Abuse Prevention and Control Act was enacted in 1970 and replaced previous laws in this area. This act classified drugs into five schedules according to their abuse liability and provided a graded set of penalties for violation of regulations relating to the manufacture, sale, prescription, and record-keeping of drugs of abuse. A summary of the abuse potential and examples of drugs falling under this act are provided in Table 55-5. This act remains as the major regulatory legislation controlling drugs of abuse (see Chapter 55).

In the early 1970s, cocaine was rediscovered as a recreational drug by the young, upwardly mobile, affluent generation. This second cocaine epidemic necessitated a redefinition of the picture of the typical drug abuser as a criminal, unemployed, minority male. For instance, the 1993 *National Household Survey on Drug Abuse* reported that 70% of the current illicit drug abusers are employed, 80% are white, and 75% live in areas outside of the city.[41] In 1983, a glut in the world market for cocaine combined with the development of a smokable, inexpensive, and very addictive form of the drug called "crack" brought the third cocaine epidemic to the inner cities, where availability of powdered forms of the drug was limited because of its cost. In the 1990s, the preparation of a smokable form of methamphetamine led to the widespread abuse of this stimulant, called "ice" and "crank" on the street. More severe abuse patterns than had ever been seen before emerged with the appearance of these smokable, freebase forms of cocaine and methamphetamine. Smoking these drugs results in a more rapid onset of action and a more intense effect, conferring on them more abuse liability than other forms of these drugs that must be sniffed or taken orally. The abuse potential of these drugs increased so dramatically with this mode of administration that drug seeking became more paramount to this population of abusers than it previously had been. As insidious was the emergence of clandestine laboratories that make "designer drugs," synthetic substances that are inexpensive to produce and difficult to detect. These include the amphetamine analogue 3,4-methylenedioxymethamphetamine (MDMA, otherwise known as "ecstasy") and "China white," a synthetic opioid analogue of fentanyl with 1000 to 2000 times its potency.

The economic effect of these new patterns of abuse can be felt both in hospital emergency departments and in board rooms across the United States. For instance, although cocaine and methamphetamine abuse has generally declined since the 1980s, the incidence of cocaine- and methamphetamine-related medical emergencies has increased threefold since 1981.[7] This may reflect the increased toxicity of smokable drug preparations, because smoking leads to a greater concentration of drug in the body than other routes of administration. Some of the potential costs of illicit drug use in the workplace include payment for substance abuse treatment programs, loss of productivity from absenteeism, accidents, disability claims, theft, as well as employee screening for drug use. For instance, half of the largest US companies require some form of drug testing for their employees, and in the employed 18- to 49-year-old age group, 7% reported positive for an illicit drug in the previous month.[5]

In general the incidence of illicit drug use has declined modestly since 1975.[31] For instance, 51% of American high school seniors reported using marijuana annually in 1979; that figure dropped to 38% in 2001. Similar trends were reported for cocaine (6% in 1975 and 5% in 2001), hallucinogens (8% in 1975 and 7% in 2001), amphetamines (16% in 1975 and 9% in 2001), barbiturates and other sedative-hypnotics (10% in 1975 and 6% in 2001), and heroin (1% in 1975 and 1% in 2001). However, there are some important exceptions to the decline in illicit drug use since the 1970s. Annual use of inhalants has nearly doubled among high school seniors, increasing from 3% in 1976 to 5% in 2001. Although overall amphetamine use is down, annual use of the smokable preparation of methamphetamine has increased from 1.5% in 1990 to 3% in 2001. A noteworthy increase in MDMA use from trace levels in 1985 to 3.5% in 1995 to a high of 9% in 2001 reflects the current upward trend in overall use of so-called "club drugs."

DRUG ABUSE CHARACTERISTICS AND TERMINOLOGY

Certain terms used in connection with drug abuse must be defined. The term *psychologic dependence* refers to a compulsion to take a drug on a continuous or periodic basis to experience its psychoactive effects.[4] For psychologic dependence to exist, the abuser must have a mental obsession to continue drug administration to produce pleasure. Additional characteristics of drug dependence, which may or may not be present, are physical dependence and tolerance. When the administration of a drug is discontinued or, in the case of certain drugs, significantly reduced, physical dependence leads to the appearance of a characteristic and specific group of symptoms, termed a *withdrawal* or *abstinence syndrome.*[28] *Tolerance* exists when administration of the same dose of a drug has progressively less effect. This decreased response to the effects of a drug requires that larger and larger doses of a drug be given to produce the same pharmacologic actions. The development of tolerance depends on both the dose of the drug and the frequency of its administration. Tolerance is caused by compensatory responses that act to decrease the body's response to a drug. The cellular basis for drug tolerance may be related to a decrease in receptors for the drug, a reduction in enzyme activity associated with signal transduction pathways, or other effects. *Cross-tolerance* is the phenomenon whereby long-term use of a drug produces tolerance to that drug's effects as well as to other drugs that produce the same effect. Cross-tolerance may be observed among drugs of similar or different chemical types.

On the basis of common pharmacologic actions and of cross-tolerance and cross-dependence, the major drugs of abuse can be divided into relatively distinct categories: opioid analgesics; general depressants of the CNS, including sedative-hypnotics and antianxiety drugs; cocaine, amphetamines, and related psychomotor stimulants; hallucinogens; marijuana; and inhalants. Table 51-1 lists the major abuse characteristics of these six drug groups; that is, the degree of psychologic and physical dependence and tolerance development commonly associated with the abuse of each drug group. In the following discussion, each drug group is described in terms of three major factors: the pharmacologic effects produced by the drug group; the abuse characteristics of the drug group, including tolerance, dependence, withdrawal, and other characteristics; and the toxicity caused by the drug group and how it is treated.

ABUSE OF OPIOID ANALGESICS

The opioid analgesics most commonly abused include heroin, morphine, and, among health care professionals, meperidine and fentanyl. In addition to these agonists, various other synthetic and semisynthetic derivatives are also subject to abuse. These agents differ from each other in their abuse characteristics, their onset and duration of action, the intensity of their effects, and, to some extent, the pattern of their abuse. Many of the mechanisms involved in the analgesic response to opioids also produce euphoria or a perceived state of well-being, and much research has been generated in an attempt

Table 51-1

Abuse Characteristics of Drug Groups

	PSYCHOLOGIC DEPENDENCE	PHYSICAL DEPENDENCE	TOLERANCE
Opioid analgesics	++++	++++	++++
Sedative-hypnotics	+++	++++	+++
Amphetamines	+++	++	++++
Cocaine	++++	++	++
Hallucinogens			
LSD	+	+	++
PCP	+	+	+
Marijuana	++	+	++
Inhalants	+	U	U

++++, Marked; +++, moderate; ++, some; +, slight; *U*, unknown.

to develop efficacious analgesics that are not euphoric and therefore have less abuse potential. Although this research has led to a greater understanding of the physiologic characteristics of pain, at present no opioids or other types of analgesics are superior to morphine. Thus, in the following discussion, morphine is considered the prototype for this group unless another drug is specifically mentioned.

Pharmacologic Effects

In the following discussion, the subjective effects of opioids are those observed in individuals who are opioid abusers. Although opioids produce similar pharmacologic effects in most people (see Chapter 20), not everyone reports the subjective effects of warmth, contentment, orgasm, and euphoria. In nonabusing individuals, the nausea and vomiting caused by opioids are construed as unpleasant and may obfuscate many of the reinforcing characteristics of these drugs. Furthermore, many individuals view the mental clouding produced by opioids as an undesirable inability to concentrate, whereas addicts find this quality appealing. Most important, because opioids are the mainstay in the treatment of moderate to severe pain, it is relevant to know that in the therapeutic setting little substantive evidence suggests that effective pain management with opioids in individuals leads them to develop into opioid abusers.

For people who abuse opioids, the IV administration of heroin causes an immediate overwhelming sense of warmth that permeates the abdominal area and that has been described as orgasmic. Nausea, vomiting, and histamine release occur soon after, causing a sense of itching, reddening of the eyes, and a decrease in blood pressure. Feelings of increased energy with talkativeness ("soapboxing") alternate with periods of relaxation or tranquillity ("coasting"). This intense euphoria may last several minutes. The depressant effects on the CNS then appear and include mental clouding, decreased visual acuity, and sedation accompanied by a feeling of heaviness in the extremities. The abuser has no motivation to participate in physical activity; the individual appears to be asleep, but only the head and facial muscles are relaxed ("nodding"). This period is followed by episodes of light sleeping accompanied by vivid dreaming. Feelings of anxiety and worry are absent, and a pervasive sense of contentment is present. Taken together, the early euphoric period followed by the sedation and sleeping may last from 3 to 5 hours.

Abuse Characteristics

The development of tolerance is a characteristic feature of all opioid agonists. Regardless of whether opioids are administered in a therapeutic setting or are self-administered, repetitive use leads to tolerance or a reduction in response, such that a greater dose of drug is required to achieve the same effect that was produced on initial administration of the drug. Tolerance develops most readily when opioids are given in large doses at short intervals or during constant infusion of the drug; the phenomenon can be observed within days after drug therapy has begun. Tolerance or desensitization to the effects of opioids develops at the cellular level and may be viewed as a homeostatic response by the cell to constant exposure to an agonist. Because the development of tolerance to the effects of opioids is a physiologic phenomenon, it inevitably occurs in patients after repeated drug administration. Therefore the development of tolerance is not a predictor of whether the patient will become an opioid abuser. Because most fatalities resulting from opioid overdose are caused by respiratory depression, the prescribing physician must understand that tolerance develops similarly to the respiratory depressant effect as well as to the analgesic and euphoric effects of opioids. This has important ramifications for the clinician who may be wary about administering, for example, 10 times the normal dose of morphine for adequate pain control in a patient who has developed tolerance to the analgesic effects. Out of concern for the respiratory depressant or addictive properties of morphine, the clinician may not provide adequate pain control even though the patient has developed a similar degree of tolerance to the respiratory depressant and euphoric effects of morphine. Because of this use-induced decrease in the ability of opioids to suppress respiration, considerable tolerance to the lethal effects of opioids may develop. However, tolerance to the respiratory effect of opioids is rapidly lost during abstinence, and death may result if an addict returns to the previously maintained dosage after withdrawal has been completed.

Similar to tolerance, physical dependence on opioids is also a result of repeated administration of an agonist and occurs for all opioids. Physical dependence results from cellular adaptation caused by uninterrupted agonist occupation of opioid receptors. Thus normal function of the individual now requires the presence of an opioid drug at its receptor. When the drug is removed from the receptor during drug withdrawal, an acute withdrawal syndrome ensues. The intensity of the withdrawal syndrome is related to the degree of dependence. As with tolerance, dependence develops most rapidly and to the greatest extent when the opioid receptors are constantly occupied. No outward signs of physical dependence are observed until the drug is withdrawn. Withdrawal symptoms in an opioid-dependent person include rhinorrhea, lacrimation, vomiting, sweating, yawning, diarrhea, irritability, restlessness, chills, piloerection ("cold turkey"), mydriasis, hyperventilation, tachycardia, hypertension, tremors, and involuntary muscle movements. In general, the appearance and severity of withdrawal signs depend on the duration of action of the opioid being taken. For example, signs of withdrawal in a heroin-dependent person appear approximately 6 hours after the last dose, increase in intensity over the next 36 to 72 hours, and subside after about 1 week. In contrast, dependence on a long-acting opioid such as methadone results in a mild but protracted withdrawal syndrome with delayed onset. A withdrawal syndrome can also be precipitated in dependent persons by displacing the opioid from the receptor with either an antagonist (naloxone), an agonist-antagonist (pentazocine), or a partial agonist (buprenorphine). Death from opioid withdrawal is rare; however, when it does occur it is because of cardiovascular collapse from dehydration and acid-base imbalance. The development of physical dependence to opioids is a physiologic response seen in all individuals; it does not predict whether they become abusers. In patients who become dependent, the dose of opioid can be decreased by 50% every other day and eventually stopped without overt signs of withdrawal.

Psychologic dependence on opioids is significant, as exemplified by the high relapse rate among addicts after withdrawal. The euphoria, tranquillity, and abdominal effects, described as orgasmic, promote abuse of opioids. The rapidity with which opioids penetrate the CNS to cause their psychoactive effects correlates with their ability to cause psychologic dependence. Opioid addicts prefer the "rush" sensation produced by the rapid onset of psychoactive effects characteristic of IV administration over the slower onset of effects produced by other routes of administration. Heroin is preferred because its high lipid solubility confers rapid penetration into the brain and thus an intense effect. Conversely, orally administered methadone for control of chronic pain has much less potential for creating psychologic dependence. Psychologic dependence on opioids occurs independently from tolerance and physical dependence and is a result of an addict craving the feelings produced by opioids. This may even happen before, or in the absence of, the development of tolerance and physical dependence. However, the fact that discontinuance of opioids may precipitate a withdrawal syndrome may provide an incentive to continue their use. For example, because of the short duration of action of heroin, the physically dependent addict oscillates between feelings of euphoria and sickness related to withdrawal and exhibits drug-seeking behavior. Drug-seeking behavior is manifested by pleas, complaints, demands, and other activities directed toward obtaining the drug to alleviate the discomfort caused by drug withdrawal. However, an individual may become dependent on the psychologic effects of opioids before developing fear of withdrawal. Patients in need of pain control should not be denied adequate opioid medication because they show evidence of tolerance or exhibit withdrawal symptoms if the medication is stopped because these signs are not indicative of psychologic dependence. In addition, a patient who is in pain and receiving opioids does not respond like a psychologically dependent addict responds to opioids. For example, patients who have the opportunity to self-administer their opioid analgesic take the drug solely to reduce the pain, do not increase the dose greatly over time, and stop administration when the pain goes away.[24]

Toxicity

In acute opioid overdose, the classic triad of coma, respiratory depression, and pinpoint pupils is common to all opioid agonists (except meperidine, in which case the pupils may be dilated in tolerant individuals). Hypoventilation leads to marked hypoxemia and cyanosis, and acute pulmonary edema evidenced by a pink, frothy sputum may occur, especially with heroin overdose. Nausea and vomiting may be prominent. Hypotension, as a result of cerebral ischemia, develops gradually and may eventually lead to circulatory shock. Convulsions do not occur with most opioids, although they have been reported in children with codeine overdose, in addicts in response to meperidine, and in cases of propoxyphene poisoning. The treatment of choice is rapid IV administration of 0.4 mg naloxone, repeated if necessary at 2- to 3-minute intervals. Dramatic improvement occurs within minutes, with enhanced ventilation and dilation of the pinpoint pupils. The patient must be closely monitored because the antagonist's effect lasts only 1 to 4 hours. This is especially important with methadone overdose because respiratory depression may last up to 48 hours. If vital signs return to normal, no attempt should be made to arouse the patient with additional naloxone because, if the patient is an opioid addict, large doses of the antagonist may precipitate an acute withdrawal syndrome.

The toxic effects of long-term abuse of opioids are minimal. Other than constipation, addicts with a stable supply of drug, those enrolled in a methadone maintenance program, or patients taking opioids long term for pain control have few difficulties as long as they continue taking the drug. However, many addicts share unsterile needles and equipment, which increases their risk of contracting acquired immunodeficiency syndrome (AIDS), hepatitis, skin abscesses, deep infections, and endocarditis. When the supply of an addict's preferred drug is compromised, the addict may substitute substances of unknown content and potency or drugs thought to have a similar effect. For example, many addicts like the effects caused by IV injection of the agonist-antagonist pentazocine with the antihistamine tripelennamine. Unfortunately, the talc contained in the crushed tripelennamine tablet has caused deaths as a result of lung emboli. Overdose leading to death may occur when an addict injects a purer sample than that to which he or she is accustomed or a sample containing a much more potent opioid, such as those seen with China white in the 1980s and fentanyl in the 1990s. Unexpected toxic effects also occurred in the late 1970s and early 1980s, when "bathtub chemists" trying to synthesize potent opioids produced a compound contaminated with 1-methyl-4-phenyl-1,2,3,6-tetrahydropyridine, which caused parkinsonlike symptoms in many young abusers. Abuse of prescription opioid analgesics has also resulted in unexpected deaths. In the late 1990s and early 2000s, deaths from overdosage resulted when individuals crushed tablets of the controlled-release formulation of oxycodone to make the entire dose available for intranasal or IV administration.

Opioid withdrawal or detoxification of heroin addicts or other opioid-dependent individuals can be managed with methadone because cross-dependence exists between it and other opioids.[35,42] Because methadone and all other opioid analgesics act at opioid receptors, methadone can be substituted for the opioid being abused without precipitating a withdrawal syndrome. By substituting the longer-acting methadone for a short-acting opioid such as heroin, the addict is spared the undesirable effects of withdrawal because the opioid receptor remains occupied. Methadone can then be withdrawn from the addict over a period of weeks. Methadone, with its long duration of action, produces a protracted but tolerable withdrawal syndrome. The α_2 adrenoceptor agonist clonidine can also be used alone or in combination with methadone to assist in the detoxification of an opioid-dependent individual. Many of the unpleasant effects experienced during opioid withdrawal, such as nausea, vomiting, sweating, tachycardia, cramps, and hypertension, are caused by hyperactivity of the autonomic nervous system. Clonidine, through its action at α_2 adrenoceptors in the brain, suppresses the outflow of sympathetic nervous system activity, thereby reducing the discomfort of opioid withdrawal.

Although management of acute opioid withdrawal is easy, the recidivism rate (i.e., the number of addicts that return to abusing opioids) is very high. Methadone maintenance therapy can also be used in the long-term treatment of opioid abuse. The pharmacologic basis of methadone maintenance depends on its oral effectiveness, long duration of action, and the development of cross-tolerance between it and other opioids, particularly heroin. Recall that tolerance to the effects of opioids is mediated at the cellular level and develops to any opioid acting at the same receptor. The first step in maintenance therapy is to provide an oral dose of methadone that is not sedating yet prevents signs of withdrawal. This is performed at a clinic and is feasible because of the long duration of action of methadone. Patients function normally and do not have the "rush" associated with other routes of administration. If the patient relapses into opioid abuse, the development of cross-tolerance between methadone and heroin or other agents results in a blockade or diminution of the euphoric effect of the abused substance, thereby removing the reinforcing properties of the abused agent. Although the patient is now physically dependent on methadone, withdrawal from a long-acting opioid results in a mild but protracted abstinence syndrome with delayed onset. Thus the dose of methadone is gradually reduced until the patient is opioid free. Of course, methadone maintenance therapy is effective only if the patient wants to quit abusing opioids and, if over the time period of the therapy, the patient breaks the psychologic dependence on opioids.

ABUSE OF SEDATIVE-HYPNOTICS

Drugs in this group are general CNS depressants and include the sedative-hypnotic and antianxiety drugs (discussed in Chapter 13). The older sedative-hypnotic drugs, including the barbiturates, glutethimide, and the widely abused but no longer approved drug methaqualone, have substantial abuse potential. The benzodiazepines and related drugs are now the most commonly used sedative-hypnotic and antianxiety drugs. Although these newer drugs have significant abuse potential, they are less frequently abused than the older sedative-hypnotic agents. Sedative-hypnotic drugs are readily available from illicit sources and by prescription abuse when large amounts of the drugs are accumulated by drug abusers visiting different prescribers.

Pharmacologic Effects

The signs of intoxication with sedative-hypnotic and antianxiety drugs are similar to those produced by alcohol—drowsiness, impairment of motor coordination, ataxia, and slurred speech. Sluggishness, difficulty in reasoning, mood swings, and irritability are also seen. Subjective effects may include sensations of well-being, euphoria, and sometimes stimulation. The next day the abuser may experience nervousness, anxiety, tremor, headache, and insomnia. The exact constellation of effects depends on the dose of the drug, the route of drug administration, the frequency of administration, and the user's expectations.

Abuse Characteristics

The degree of psychologic dependence on sedative-hypnotic drugs depends on the dose of the drug, the frequency of administration, and the duration of drug use. Sedative-hypnotic drugs differ in their onset and duration of action (both short- and long-acting barbiturates and benzodiazepines are available). Psychologic dependence is most commonly associated with abuse of the short-acting drugs such as secobarbital, pentobarbital, oxazepam, and lorazepam. Dependence on longer-acting agents such as phenobarbital and chlordiazepoxide is less common.[3,22] Dependence occurs only rarely with the intravenously administered ultrashort-acting sedative-hypnotics because they cannot be taken frequently enough to maintain adequate plasma concentrations. For the benzodiazepine drugs, those with a higher affinity for the BZ_2 benzodiazepine receptor subtype (e.g., alprazolam) appear to have a greater potential for abuse than drugs with a higher affinity for the BZ_1 benzodiazepine receptor.[30] Initial exposure to sedative-hypnotics may occur when the drug is prescribed to relieve anxiety or insomnia. The dose is slowly increased, and the abuser may become preoccupied with obtaining and using the drug. So called "date rape" drugs such as γ-hydroxybutyrate, a metabolite of γ-aminobutyric acid, and the prescription benzodiazepine flunitrazepam ("roofies") are also subject to misuse. Both drugs have similar effects as sedative-hypnotics; however, their rapid oral absorption, onset of action, and ability to cause anterograde amnesia have resulted in their surreptitious use as sedatives to facilitate rape of unwitting individuals.

Unlike opioids, sedative-hypnotics do not induce physical dependence unless increased doses of drugs are taken over a long period (a month or longer). The onset and severity of the abstinence syndrome also depend, in part, on the dose and the duration of drug use. For instance, minimum withdrawal symptoms are elicited by abrupt withdrawal from long-term daily use of 400 to 500 mg of pentobarbital or secobarbital.[21] With long-term use of larger doses, progressively more severe symptoms of withdrawal can be precipitated, even by abruptly reducing the accustomed dose by half. Although withdrawal from daily doses of 600 to 800 mg of secobarbital after 1 month produces a relatively minor withdrawal syndrome, withdrawal from 800 to 900 mg per day after 2 months or more produces major withdrawal symptoms. Another important determinant of the onset, severity, and duration of the withdrawal syndrome is the half-life of the specific drug. Drugs with relatively short half-lives (8 to 30 hours) tend to produce a severe withdrawal syndrome that develops quite rapidly. Drugs with longer half-lives (40 to 100 hours) produce a slower onset but less severe withdrawal syndrome of long duration.

The withdrawal syndrome after cessation of sedative-hypnotics has some resemblance to that seen after alcohol withdrawal. After a usually symptomless period (8 to 18 hours after the last dose), the person exhibits increasing symptoms of anxiety, insomnia, agitation, and confusion. Anorexia, nausea and vomiting, sweating, and muscle weakness are also seen. Coarse tremors in the face and hands, as well as dilation of the pupils and increases in respiratory rate, heart rate, and blood pressure, may occur. Orthostatic hypotension and syncope may also occur. These symptoms become more severe during the first 24 to 30 hours of drug withdrawal. By the third or fourth day the major manifestations of abstinence may develop, which can include delirium, hallucinations, agitation, hyperthermia, convulsions, and nonspecific symptoms of anxiety. Symptoms associated with benzodiazepine withdrawal also occur; these are persistent tinnitus (up to 8 months), muscle twitching, paresthesias, visual disturbances, and confusion and depersonalization.[36] Of particular dental significance are reports of xerostomia and pain in the jaws and teeth.[9]

Muscle fasciculations and enhanced deep reflexes may progress to frank seizures. One or more grand mal convulsions lasting less than 3 minutes may occur, with consciousness being regained within 5 minutes. In some cases, however, status epilepticus may ensue. The prolonged postictal stupor typical of epileptic seizures is not seen, but confusion may persist for 1 or 2 hours. Delirium develops gradually over 2 to 4 days and is heralded by a period of insomnia. Delirium is characterized by confusion, disorientation of time and place, nightmares, and vivid auditory and visual hallucinations. Paranoid delusions with extreme fear and agitation may develop, especially at night ("night terrors"). The symptoms terminate spontaneously after a prolonged period of sleep. This withdrawal psychosis may be caused by rebound REM sleep, which, having been suppressed during the period of intoxication, intrudes into the waking state. During the phase of delirium, body temperature is elevated. A continuous marked hyperthermia is a life-threatening problem that, if not immediately and vigorously treated, may (along with agitation) lead to fatal exhaustion and cardiovascular collapse. After the acute withdrawal syndrome, recovery is gradual but complete after approximately 8 days, although residual weakness may be noted for 6 to 12 weeks. Abrupt withdrawal from large doses of sedative-hypnotics can precipitate a severe and life-threatening withdrawal syndrome that carries a significant mortality rate. In fact, the withdrawal syndrome from sedative-hypnotics may be more severe than that caused by the opioids.

Tolerance develops to the sedative-hypnotic drugs, and partial cross-tolerance also occurs among the various drugs in this class. Tolerance is usually complete to doses of short-acting barbiturates of up to 500 mg/day, but doses of greater than 800 mg/day are associated with signs of intoxication. The onset of tolerance to benzodiazepines in human beings develops slowly, beginning in 3 to 5 days, with maximal tolerance in 7 to 10 days.[36] The mechanisms of tolerance to these drugs are unclear. Much of the tolerance to large doses of short-acting barbiturates is associated with hepatic enzyme induction that results in enhanced barbiturate elimination. This metabolic tolerance plays less of a role for the benzodiazepine drugs, for which cellular tolerance, a decreased responsiveness of neuronal pathways in the CNS, appears to play a more prominent role.

Toxicity

Ingestion of large doses of sedative-hypnotic drugs may be life-threatening. Coma may develop with progressive deterioration of respiration and blood pressure. The victim exhibits hypoxia, cyanosis, shock, hypothermia, and anuria. Death is usually from cerebral anoxia caused by respiratory failure. Therapy is mainly supportive, consisting of oxygen administered by artificial respiration and fluids or pressor agents (or both) to maintain circulation. For barbiturates, osmotic diuretics with sodium bicarbonate are also used to alkalinize the urine and hasten elimination of the drug. The benzodiazepine receptor antagonist flumazenil has been used to specifically block toxic effects in the treatment of acute benzodiazepine overdose.

Withdrawal from long-term therapeutic abuse of sedative-hypnotics is associated with drug craving, nausea and abdominal cramps, tachycardia, palpitation, and generalized seizures. Panic attacks and disorientation may occur, progressing to paranoid psychosis with aggression, delusions, and visual hallucinations.[9,36] Coma and respiratory depression cause a significant mortality rate. Treatment includes substitution with a long-acting sedative-hypnotic drug, such as phenobarbital, followed by a modest daily reduction in the maintenance dose.[26] Seizures represent a medical emergency and are treated by immediate administration of diazepam, pentobarbital, or carbamazepine. Withdrawal from sedative-hypnotic drugs should be carried out in a hospital setting because life-threatening complications may develop.

Other Sedative-Hypnotic Drugs

Various other sedative-hypnotic drugs may be classified according to chemical structure into aldehyde derivatives (chloral hydrate, paraldehyde), propanediol carbamates (meprobamate), and heterocyclics (glutethimide, methyprylon, methaqualone). All drugs in these groups produce patterns of intoxication, tolerance, and psychologic and physical dependence that are similar to those produced by the barbiturates and benzodiazepine drugs. All these drugs exhibit some degree of cross-tolerance and can suppress the abstinence symptoms of other depressants of the CNS.

ABUSE OF AMPHETAMINES, COCAINE, AND OTHER PSYCHOMOTOR STIMULANTS

Psychomotor stimulants include analogues of phenylethylamine (*d*-amphetamine and methamphetamine), a group of amphetamine derivatives in which the terminal amine nitrogen is part of a heterocyclic group (methylphenidate, phendimetrazine) or a diethylated group (diethylpropion), and cocaine. The chemical structures of some of these drugs are shown in Figure 51-1. Amphetamines and methylphenidate are generally used for treatment of narcolepsy and attention deficit–hyperactivity disorder (ADHD), whereas phendimetrazine and diethylpropion are anorectics. These drugs are available on the street as well as by prescription. Cocaine is the most widely abused member of this class. The chemical structure of cocaine is shown in Figure 51-2. It has been estimated that up to 3 million Americans abuse the various forms of cocaine. In general, the effects of and abuse patterns associated with the individual drugs in this group are quite similar.

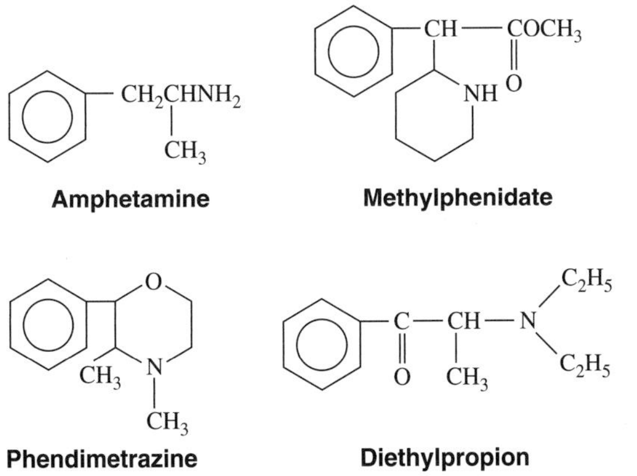

Amphetamine

Methylphenidate

Phendimetrazine

Diethylpropion

Fig. 51-1 Structural formulas of amphetamine and some related stimulant drugs.

Amphetamine and Related Drugs

Pharmacologic effects

Single oral doses of amphetamine and related drugs produce wakefulness, reduced fatigue and reaction times, and improved performance of psychomotor tasks, especially in sleep-deprived individuals. Feelings of enhanced well-being, moderate exhilaration, and euphoria are common. Judgment may be impaired, and irrational behavior may occur. These drugs can cause signs of increased peripheral adrenergic nerve activity such as a rise in blood pressure, tachycardia, mydriasis, sweating, and constipation. These effects probably result from the release of norepinephrine from central and peripheral neurons or the blockade of neuronal uptake of norepinephrine at these sites. High oral doses of CNS stimulants induce feelings of cleverness, enhanced abilities, aggressiveness, and fearlessness and may cause a manic "high," paranoid rage, violent diarrhea, and vomiting.

Abuse characteristics

Patterns of oral use are usually intermittent and involve lower doses causing milder effects. For instance, oral amphetamines have been abused by students who want to study through the night and by truck drivers who want to stay awake for long hauls. Amphetamine abusers also take these drugs intranasally, intravenously, and by smoking. IV administration of methamphetamine results in a markedly pleasurable rush described as an expanding, flashing, vibration feeling, or a total body orgasm. IV administration of amphetamines is more apt to promote repeated use than oral administration. Because the euphoric effect of IV methamphetamine is relatively long, it can be injected every 3 hours to maintain its euphoric effect. The standard hydrochloride salt form of methamphetamine can be converted into its freebase, resulting in a form of the drug called "ice" or "crank" that can be administered by smoking cigarettes laced with the drug. Smoking methamphetamine in its freebase has become the most popular abused form of this drug in recent years. Because smoking the drug is a more acceptable route of administration, the easy availability of this form of the drug has been suggested to be responsible for the recent increase in its abuse. The onset of effects and the intensity of the euphoria produced by smoking "ice" are reported to be at least as great as those seen when methamphetamine is injected intravenously. Both chemical forms of the drug are usually taken continuously for 2 to 5 days, during which time the abuser does not sleep or eat. This is called a "run" or "binge." The next stage is the "crash," during which the abuser sleeps for 24 to 48 hours. This is often followed by hunger, depression, dysphoria, and restlessness.

The degree of psychologic dependence and abuse potential is high for all the drugs in this group. Individuals depend-

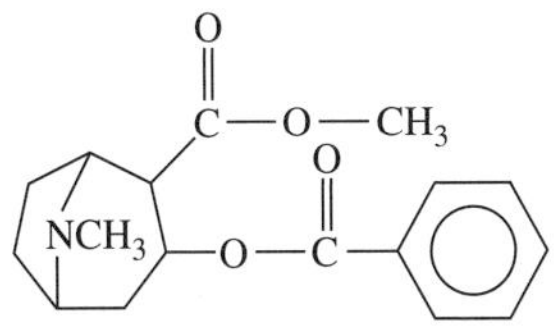

Fig. 51-2 Structural formula of cocaine.

ent on these drugs have a very strong compulsion to engage in drug-seeking behavior. Marked tolerance to the stimulant effects of amphetamine develops readily. Whereas the therapeutic dose of amphetamine is 10 to 15 mg, abusers may inject intravenously up to 2 g/day. The mechanism of tolerance is unknown but has been attributed to the depletion of central catecholamine stores with replacement by *p*-hydroxynorephedrine, a metabolite of amphetamine that may function as a false neurotransmitter in adrenergic nerves. Physical dependence on amphetamine is not easily demonstrable because it may be difficult to differentiate true withdrawal symptoms from the body's response to prolonged sleep and food deprivation and enhanced physical activity. However, withdrawal from the drug after a "run" is followed by a prolonged sleep and then by a ravenous appetite, fatigue, apathy, and depression. This complex of symptoms is interpreted as evidence of physical dependence. In human beings the depression associated with amphetamine withdrawal is correlated with a CNS reduction in 3-methoxy-4-hydroxyphenylglycol, a norepinephrine metabolite, which indicates that CNS catecholamines are depleted. This finding provides a neurochemical mechanism to explain the depression caused by drug withdrawal.

Toxicity

Acute severe overdose, although uncommon, is characterized by CNS and cardiovascular stimulation. Coma and convulsions occur, which may develop into status epilepticus. These convulsions may be controlled with IV diazepam. Cardiac arrhythmias and hypertension, occasionally precipitating subarachnoid hemorrhage or intracerebral hematomas, may lead to cardiovascular collapse. Enhanced autonomic activity, including hyperthermia and dilated pupils, may also be seen.

The long-term amphetamine abuser typically displays anxiety, akathisia, volatile mood, headaches, and cramps. In addition, the abuser frequently shows signs of mental and physical fatigue, poor personal hygiene, and facial twitching. Of particular interest to dentistry are the worn teeth and chewed tongue that result from continuous oral movements. Long-term stimulant abuse leads to stereotypy, psychosis, and overt violence. Stereotypical compulsive behavior is characterized by pleasurable curiosity and fascination with detail. Compulsive, repetitive activity develops, such as cleaning an immaculate home or disassembling and reconstructing mechanical objects. Long-term abuse can cause a drug-induced paranoid psychosis that resembles acute paranoid schizophrenia. Psychosis may develop within 1 to 5 days after beginning drug use and usually lasts 6 to 7 days. The most common symptoms are delusions of persecution; auditory, tactile, and especially visual hallucinations; and hyperactivity. Anxiety, agitation, aggressiveness, and depression are often observed. Paranoia, hallucinations, and terror reactions lead to hostility and difficulty in controlling rage. Amphetamine abusers display a high incidence of unpremeditated, unprovoked, and bizarre acts of violence and assaultive and even homicidal behavior. After amphetamine is discontinued, confusion, delusions, and loss of memory may persist for several weeks or months. Treatment of toxicity is based on enhancing the elimination of the drug from the body. Acidification of the urine with ammonium chloride increases the rate of urinary excretion of amphetamine and causes rapid reduction of psychotic symptoms.[6]

Cocaine

The leaves of the coca plant, which contain up to 1.8% of the pure alkaloid, are the primary source of cocaine. The Andean Indians have chewed coca leaves, mixed with an alkaline substance to promote release of cocaine, for many years. Although peak blood concentrations of 95 ng/ml are achieved, little drug-induced euphoria is reported among Andean Indians who chew coca leaves. The leaves are used to make cocaine paste (30% to 90% cocaine), which is converted to pure cocaine hydrochloride, primarily in South America. Many samples of street cocaine appear to contain adulterants such as amphetamines, mannitol, or lidocaine. The local anesthetic procaine shares some characteristics with cocaine and can produce euphoria. Not surprisingly, procaine powder is frequently used to cut cocaine and, mixed with mannitol or lactose, is sold as cocaine.

Pharmacologic effects

Cocaine is a local anesthetic that produces adrenergic effects by blocking neuronal uptake of norepinephrine. Pharmacologic responses to cocaine are mainly cardiovascular and are similar to those of amphetamine. Cocaine produces a dose-related tachycardia and increase in blood pressure, especially systolic. The onset of action is 2 to 5 minutes by the IV route and approximately 30 minutes by the intranasal route. In both cases the cardiovascular response dissipates over roughly 30 minutes. In IV doses of up to 32 mg, cocaine promotes a moderate mydriasis and hyperglycemia but no effects on the electrocardiogram, respiratory rate, or body temperature.[44]

As a recreational drug, cocaine uniformly causes euphoria and signs of CNS stimulation. The subjective effects of cocaine include elation, arousal, and alertness. Garrulousness and enhanced friendliness facilitate social interaction in group settings. Hunger and fatigue are suppressed. The user has a subjective feeling of increased mental agility. As is true of amphetamine, performance may be enhanced in sleep-deprived, but not in rested, subjects. Cocaine can delay ejaculation, which together with heightened sensory awareness and elevated mood, enhances the sexual experience. The orgasmic rush produced by IV cocaine use may become a substitute for coitus. This essentially pleasant high is produced by doses of about 100, 25, and 10 mg of cocaine by the oral, intranasal, and IV routes, respectively.[44]

Negative subjective effects occur in 3% of intoxications in the early stages of abuse but occur in 82% of compulsive cocaine abusers. The euphoric effects of the drug are followed by restlessness, irritability, and psychomotor agitation. Hyperexcitability and paranoia may occur. Long-term, high-dose cocaine abuse may result in aberrant sexual behavior such as marathons of promiscuity. On the other hand, men may have reduced libido, with an inability to maintain an erection or to ejaculate. Women may be unable to achieve orgasm.[15]

Abuse characteristics

Although ingested cocaine can have stimulant effects, it is rarely taken orally. The intranasal route ("snorting") is more commonly used by cocaine abusers. Cocaine hydrochloride usually is inhaled as a "line" of powder containing 20 to 30 mg of the drug. It produces a maximum effect in 15 to 20 minutes and a duration of effect lasting 1 hour or more. Nasal mucosal vasoconstriction and paralysis of membrane cilia prevent complete absorption by this route, and measurable cocaine remains on the nasal mucosa for 3 hours after use. Snorting of cocaine in solution produces effects in 5 to 15 minutes that last 2 to 4 hours. The euphoric effect of cocaine is less intense when the intranasal route is used compared with IV injection or smoking the drug.

When cocaine is injected, the IV route is preferred over the intramuscular or the subcutaneous route because local vasoconstriction delays the onset of action by the latter routes. IV injection produces an intense orgasmic rush in approximately 1 minute that lasts for 30 to 40 minutes. Abusers average 16 mg of cocaine per injection in a recreational setting. Cocaine is also used intravenously with heroin. The mixture, referred to as a "speedball," is used to attenuate the excessive stimulation caused by large doses of cocaine.

The smoking of cocaine requires conversion of the hydrochloride salt of the drug to the freebase form. The salt form, when heated, decomposes before the vaporization temperature is reached. The freebase volatilizes at temperatures of approximately 90° C and is not destroyed by heating. Smokers may manufacture their own freebase by dissolving the salt in an alkaline solution and extracting the alkaloid with a solvent such as ether. Since the mid 1980s, the freebase form has become commonly available as "crack," a form of freebase melted down into crystalline balls that can be smoked. Crack may be smoked in cigarettes or by heating with an alcohol flame in a pipe. Because the lung-brain circulation time is only 8 seconds, and the inhalation route bypasses the liver, the effects of smoking cocaine base are just as rapid and intense as IV cocaine and last approximately 20 minutes. Smokers average 100 mg of base with each smoke, increasing to 250 mg with rapid tolerance development. Smoking may be repeated every 5 minutes, with intake in compulsive abusers totaling 1.5 g/day. Smoking freebase cocaine has become the most popular method for administration of this drug, and, like methamphetamine freebase, the freebase form of cocaine has contributed significantly to the increase in its abuse.

Used intranasally as a low-dose recreational drug, cocaine produces moderate psychologic dependence. High-dose IV or inhalation use produces compulsive dependence characterized by loss of control over drug use and an inability to stop the drug despite repeated attempts. Cocaine shares with other drugs of dependence a reinforcing property that results in rapid acquisition of self-administration behavior. This reinforcing property may result from activation of a CNS dopaminergic reward system with cell bodies located in the ventral tegmentum projecting to the nucleus accumbens. Cocaine enhances dopaminergic activity at the latter site by blocking dopamine uptake by nerve endings. This endogenous reward system is normally activated by responding to physiologic imperatives such as hunger, thirst, and sex drive. Cocaine directly stimulates this reward circuitry, dominating motivation for essential physiologic needs. Rats given free access to IV cocaine take the drug in preference to food and die of starvation in a few weeks.

Significant tolerance does not develop with occasional cocaine use because of the short half-life of the drug. However, frequent use resulting in constant cocaine concentrations in the body does cause tolerance. Acute tolerance to both subjective and cardiovascular effects is observed within 1 hour after repeated IV dosage. Physical dependence occurs primarily in compulsive, high-dose cocaine abusers. With long-term cocaine use, CNS dopamine depletion may occur, resulting in adverse symptoms during periods of abstinence. Withdrawal results in depression, dysphoria, social withdrawal, craving for the drug, appetite disturbances, tremor, and muscle pain. Such withdrawal phenomena may be severe enough to prevent some abusers from stopping the drug, even though toxic delirium may develop with continued drug use. Oral diazepam has been useful in treating withdrawal anxiety; psychotherapy or cautious use of tricyclic antidepressants is recommended for prolonged depression.

Toxicity

Medical complications of cocaine abuse most often involve the CNS and the cardiovascular system.[15] Among the CNS effects is a toxic psychosis, similar to that caused by amphetamine, which often develops in long-term, heavy abusers of cocaine. The syndrome is characterized by intense anxiety, inability to concentrate, stereotyped compulsive behavior, paranoid delusions, and violent loss of impulse control. Hallucinations may develop that are typically tactile, with sensations of insects burrowing under the skin or snakes crawling over the body. Such psychotic crises are reported in 10% of intoxications in compulsive abusers. Acute depression with suicidal ideation also may develop. Longer-term personality changes include a tendency to paranoia with features of depression, reduced frustration threshold, difficulties in impulse regulation, and social maladjustment.

Cardiovascular complications of cocaine include cardiac arrhythmias, with sinus and ventricular tachycardia, ventricular fibrillation, and fatal cardiac arrest. Acute myocardial infarction is a particular hazard among abusers with preexisting coronary artery disease because of the increased systolic blood pressure, heart rate, and myocardial oxygen consumption engendered by cocaine.[25] Abrupt increases in arterial blood pressure, occurring within minutes of intranasal use of cocaine, have resulted in subarachnoid hemorrhage, particularly in persons with aneurysms of cerebral vessels. One case of fatal rupture of the ascending aorta was reported in a person with preexisting chronic hypertension who had smoked freebase cocaine. Acute cardiac events may occur, even with recreational intranasal use of cocaine, in persons without predisposing cardiac disease.[29] Hepatotoxicity, with clinical findings of elevated titers of serum transaminases and jaundice, has been reported in long-term cocaine abusers. Such liver damage may occur in plasma cholinesterase–deficient persons, in whom cocaine metabolism is shunted through hepatic oxidative pathways, resulting in the production of cytolytic superoxides.[33] A significantly increased rate of spontaneous abortion has been noted in pregnant women. Because cocaine can cross the placental barrier, infants born to cocaine abusers may exhibit tremulousness. Frequent intranasal use leads to chronic rhinitis and rhinorrhea, atrophy of the nasal mucosa, loss of sense of smell, and necrosis and perforation of the nasal septum. These changes, occurring as a result of chronic ischemia, should alert the clinician to possible intranasal cocaine abuse. Bruxism and temporomandibular joint disorders are also more frequent in the cocaine abuser.

Death from cocaine overdose usually is attributable to generalized convulsions, respiratory failure, or cardiac arrhythmias. Deaths have occurred with each route of cocaine administration and may be so rapid that treatment comes too late. Because cocaine is metabolized by plasma esterases, persons with low cholinesterase activity are at high risk of cocaine fatality.[15] Treatment of cocaine overdose is symptomatic. CNS stimulation can be treated with IV diazepam, ventricular arrhythmias with IV lidocaine, and respiratory depression with oxygen and positive-pressure ventilation.

ABUSE OF HALLUCINOGENS

Hallucinogens are defined as drugs that alter perception, mood, and thought without changes in consciousness or orientation. These drugs are also referred to as *psychotomimetics,* because some of their effects mimic naturally occurring psychoses, or as *psychedelics,* because of their use by some people to induce mystical experiences. These drugs are claimed to provide the abuser with enhanced insight and self-knowledge, leading to new ways of looking at life and new insights into personal relationships.

Psychedelic Hallucinogens

The psychedelic hallucinogens can be divided into different chemical classes. The chemical structures of some of the psychedelic hallucinogens are shown in Figure 51-3. The lysergic acid derivative LSD is a semisynthetic chemical that does not occur in nature. LSD is a commonly used hallucinogen and has become the standard to which other hallucinogenic substances are compared. Drugs derived from tryptamine include

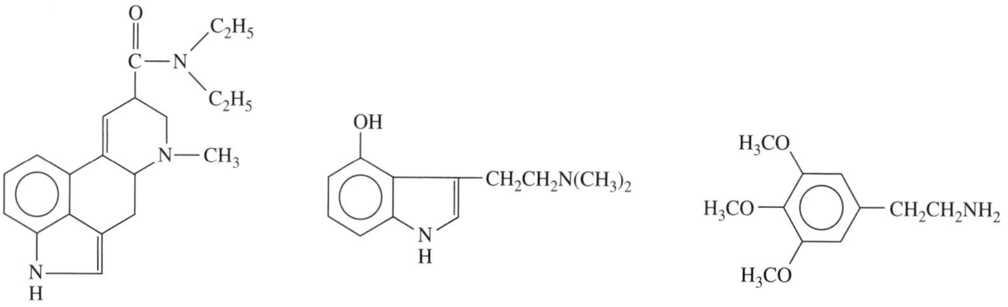

Lysergic acid diethylamide

Psilocin

Mescaline

Fig. 51-3 Structural formulas of representative hallucinogenic drugs.

the synthetic compound dimethyltryptamine and its derivative, psilocin, as well as the naturally occurring phosphorylated form of psilocin, psilocybin. The third class of hallucinogens are amphetamine analogues such as MDMA and mescaline. Mescaline and psilocybin produce effects that are nearly the same as those produced by LSD. MDMA has stimulant effects similar to those of amphetamine as well as some psychedelic effects similar to those of LSD. Because MDMA possesses both mild psychedelic and stimulant properties, it has become popular in club or dance settings, where it can enhance the light and sound experience and enable users to dance vigorously for extended periods. Under these conditions of prolonged physical exertion, MDMA can cause dangerous levels of dehydration and hyperthermia.

Pharmacologic effects

Symptoms associated with the LSD experience occur sequentially, with somatic symptoms developing first, followed by perceptual and mood changes and then by psychic or psychedelic phenomena.[47] Within a half hour of ingestion of LSD, a feeling of inner tension develops, accompanied by somatic symptoms of mild sympathetic stimulation and motor alterations. The individual feels dizzy, weak, vaguely numb, and nauseated. Marked mydriasis is accompanied by a rise in blood pressure and pulse rate, tremor, hyperreflexia, and, at high doses, ataxia. These somatic effects are soon submerged by perceptual and psychic effects, which begin approximately 45 minutes after the drug is taken. Some persons experience euphoria, elation, serenity, or ecstasy, whereas in others the initial tension may progress to anxiety and depression, evoking a panic reaction. A paranoid rage reaction occasionally occurs, although most subjects tend to be passive, quiet, and withdrawn.

Abuse characteristics

The subjective effects of LSD are highly dependent on the psychologic makeup of the person, the environmental influences at the time of the drug experience, the expectations of the person, and the size of the dose. Distortion of sense perception is the most specific symptom of the LSD experience, affecting all modalities but especially vision. Colors seem unusually bright and vivid, and objects appear distorted and seem to undulate and flow. Fixed objects appear to shift from near to far, fine surface details appear in deep relief, and colorful, dreamlike images occur as vivid streaming filmstrips even with the eyes closed. Frank visual hallucinations are rare, but visual illusions are not uncommon, as when a spot on the wall is mistaken for a face. There are distortions of body image, enhanced auditory perception, and, more rarely, alteration of other sensory modalities. Time sense is distorted; it is often described as stopping or going backward. Synesthesias are common, so that music may be experienced visually or colors may be "heard."

The changes in sensory perception are soon followed by the psychedelic "trip." Subjects may experience depersonalization, and the separation between the self and the environment melts away. The user has a sense of profound insight, revelation, and expanded consciousness. This loss of self is interpreted as a "good trip" by psychedelic drug abusers, but, on occasion, loss of control and fear of self-disintegration foster panic and even attempts at self-destruction. The individual remains oriented and alert throughout the experience and often remembers all events during the "trip" even months later.

In general, use of these drugs is not associated with marked physical dependence, and no clear withdrawal syndrome has been reported. If psychologic dependence develops at all, it is mild and infrequent. Tolerance to the effects of LSD is not common but has been reported, and cross-tolerance is seen among members of the psychedelic hallucinogens. With repeated use, tolerance to LSD develops within 1 week but lasts only a few days after discontinuance of the drug.

Toxicity

The adult human lethal dose of LSD has been estimated to be 2 mg/kg, although no deaths caused directly by LSD overdosage have been reported. Adverse psychologic reactions to hallucinogens are common.[48] Panic reactions or "bad trips" are relatively frequent and are related to an overdose of the drug. Often, companionship and reassurance, or "talking down," is sufficient to control this reaction. If this is not sufficient, other treatments include sedation with oral diazepam. Acute depression or psychotic reactions can also occur. Ingestion of up to 50 mg results in hyperactivity, psychosis, amnesia, upper gastrointestinal tract bleeding, and coma.

Approximately one in 20 LSD abusers has "flashbacks," in which episodic visual disturbances resembling previous LSD experiences take place during abstinence from the drug.[2] This alteration is now called *hallucinogen persisting perception disorder.*[4] This disorder may occur months after the previous trip and last from a few minutes to a few hours. It is thought to be caused by a drug-induced permanent change in the visual system. This disorder is treated in the same way as panic reactions. In addition, prolonged psychotic states may be precipitated by LSD use, requiring long-term hospitalization and treatment with antipsychotic drugs.[39]

Deliriant Hallucinogens

The ketamine derivative phencyclidine, also called PCP or "angel dust," is a synthetic drug that produces a unique state characterized by delirium, hallucinations, insomnia, and agitation. PCP produces what is called a "dissociative state" because it is said to dissociate the mind from the body without loss of consciousness. The drug was investigated in 1958 as an anesthetic in human beings but was subsequently abandoned because of severe postanesthetic dysphoria and hallucinations. Derivatives of PCP, such as thienyl and N-ethyl analogues, are also available on the street. The chemical structure of PCP is shown in Figure 51-4.

Pharmacologic effects

To produce its effects, PCP binds to receptors in the CNS that are associated with the N-methyl-d-aspartic acid (NMDA) type of glutamate receptor. NMDA receptors mediate some of the CNS effects of the excitatory amino acid glutamate. The PCP binding site resides within the NMDA-gated calcium channel complex, where PCP acts as a noncompetitive antagonist at the NMDA receptor and thus inhibits some of the CNS effects of glutamate. Receptors that bind PCP have been identified in the CNS in the limbic system and frontal cortex, areas involved in memory, emotion, and behavior. PCP has also been reported to cause dopamine release and inhibit the active reuptake of dopamine into dopaminergic nerves. This enhances and prolongs the effects of dopaminergic nerve stimulation.

In lower doses, PCP abusers usually remain alert and oriented while exhibiting euphoria, agitation, or bizarre behavior. Individuals may be irritable or mute and rigid, stare suspiciously, and exhibit impaired reasoning. They are easily provoked to anger and may exhibit violent behavior. The dissociative state, coupled with effects on limbic-mediated emotional control, may provoke feats of superhuman strength, causing harm to self and others. Inappropriate behavior, such as strolling down a street nude, may occur.[48] Detachment, disorientation, stupor, and coma may also occur but are more common at higher doses.

Abuse characteristics

Currently, the most common route of administration of PCP is by smoking, in which the drug is mixed with tobacco or marijuana. At the burning tip of a cigarette, PCP is converted to 1-phenyl-1-cyclohexene (PC), which is largely inactive. In smoking PCP cigarettes, approximately 40% of the dose is received by the smoker as PCP and approximately 30% as PC. Some abusers snort PCP powder or ingest it mixed with alcoholic beverages or in pill form. A small percentage of abusers inject the drug intravenously. Urine and serum concentrations of PCP do not correlate with the state of intoxication. PCP disappears from urine 2 to 4 hours after a single use (largely because of sequestration in fatty tissues), but it may be detected in the urine of long-term abusers for up to 30 days.[14,46]

The majority of PCP use is intermittent rather than long term. However, some PCP abusers develop psychologic dependence on the drug, although this is less common than with the drugs of abuse previously discussed. No clearly defined physical dependence on PCP has been identified, but withdrawal from long-term use has been reported to result in depression, irritability, confusion, and sleep disturbances along with a strong craving for the drug.

Toxicity

Symptoms of acute intoxication appear 15 to 30 minutes after ingestion. Marked analgesia with shivering, salivation, bronchospasm, urinary retention, hypertension, tachycardia, and hyperpyrexia result. Nystagmus is observed in approximately two thirds of intoxications. Grimacing, localized dystonias, and tremor may progress to grand mal seizures or status epilepticus at doses greater than 70 mg, which also produce deep and prolonged coma with loss of protective reflexes that may last for a week or more. Death has been attributed to intracranial hemorrhage, status epilepticus, and respiratory failure. Life-threatening hyperthermia may also develop, sometimes in association with hepatic necrosis. Those under the influence of PCP act violently with some regularity, and accidents, including drownings, have been documented in a number of cases. Acute treatment centers on acidification of the urine to hasten PCP's renal excretion. IV diazepam is used to control seizures and the agitated or excited state caused by the drug. Prolonged psychotic episodes may require treatment with antipsychotic drugs.

ABUSE OF MARIJUANA

Marijuana is ground up leaves and flowers from the hemp plant, *Cannabis sativa*, and is one of the most frequently abused drugs in the United States. A cannabinoid known as Δ-9-tetrahydrocannabinol (THC; Figure 51-5) appears to be the main psychoactive ingredient. Preparations of marijuana vary widely in their THC content, depending on the variety and part of the plant used and the environment in which the plant is raised. For instance, stalk fibers from any variety of hemp contain no psychoactive agents,[43] and the type of hemp plant from which stalk fibers are used commercially in the production of rope, twine, cord, and clothing is virtually drug free because it is grown under conditions that favor high fiber and low THC content. Conversely, the more potent samples of marijuana are made from the younger, topmost leaves of hemp varieties that can contain approximately 5% THC by weight. Another component of the *C. sativa* plant that is commonly abused is an extract called *hashish*. Unlike marijuana, which is ground-up plant material, hashish is an extract containing only the THC-rich resin that is secreted by the hemp plant. Hashish is more potent than marijuana, and it can contain as much as 12% THC by weight. Marijuana and hashish are usually smoked in the form of cigarettes or from a pipe.

Pharmacologic Effects

Early theories on the mechanism of action of THC in causing effects in the CNS suggested that THC interacted with the lipid component of neuronal membranes affecting their permeability to critical ions. However, with the identification[17] and cloning[38] of a cannabinoid receptor, and the discovery that an arachidonic acid derivative, anandamide, may be the endogenous ligand for the cannabinoid receptor,[18] it is now agreed that THC acts stereospecifically with a G protein–coupled, transmembrane-spanning receptor. Although the physiologic role of the cannabinoid receptor and

N

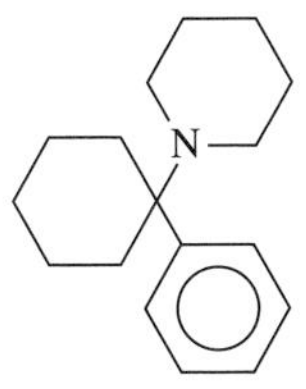

Fig. 51-4 Structural formula of phencyclidine.

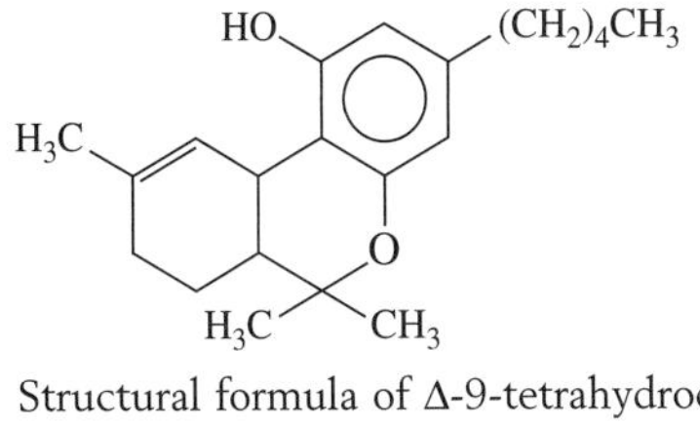

HO $(CH_2)_4CH_3$ H_3C O H_3C CH_3

Fig. 51-5 Structural formula of Δ-9-tetrahydrocannabinol.

its putative ligand remains undefined, these receptors are located in the cerebellum, hippocampus, and basal ganglia.[23]

Intoxication with marijuana is unique, causing changes in mood, motivation, and perception that are similar to some of the effects caused by amphetamines, LSD, alcohol, sedative-hypnotics, and opioids. Within minutes of inhaling marijuana smoke, the typical abuser reports feelings of euphoria, uncontrollable laughter, depersonalization, alterations in judgment of time and space, and sharpened vision. Mild visual hallucinations may occur, particularly when the eyes are closed. Similar to LSD, the abuser knows that these visual disturbances are drug induced. Later, the abuser experiences generalized feelings of well-being, relaxation, and tranquillity that may last from 2 to 3 hours. The abuser experiences a reduction in attention span, difficulty in thinking and concentrating, and impairment of short-term memory. All these effects are considered desirable by the abuser and are described as "mellowing out." Many abusers report that the feelings of intoxication, dreaminess, and sedation can be more easily suppressed voluntarily than the equivalent effects produced by alcohol. The sedative-hypnotic property of marijuana facilitates the onset of sleep and resembles the effects caused by CNS depressants. This property of marijuana is in sharp contrast to the effects of LSD and other hallucinogens. Although it is generally agreed that a dose-related impairment in psychomotor performance occurs, many experienced abusers exhibit no such decrement in their performance. Perhaps this is why no clear correlation has been shown between blood concentrations of THC and an individual's ability to drive a car.[27]

Physiologic effects of smoking marijuana occur within a few minutes, peak in their action in approximately 20 minutes, and wane over 2 to 3 hours.[12] Moderate marijuana use causes reddening of the eyes in association with a euphoric high that is followed by drowsiness.[19,27,40] Autonomic effects of marijuana include xerostomia, tachycardia, reduced peripheral resistance, and, in large doses, orthostatic hypotension.[40] These effects may be deleterious in those with ischemic heart disease or cardiac failure.[27] Marijuana does not affect respiratory rate, blood glucose concentrations, or pupillary diameter[40]; however, marijuana does lower intraocular pressure.

Studies of the potential therapeutic uses of dronabinol, the nonproprietary name of THC, show it to be effective in treating some conditions. Oral administration of dronabinol has been approved as an antiemetic in cancer patients undergoing chemotherapy and as an appetite stimulant in patients with weight loss resulting from AIDS-related anorexia. Smoking marijuana may also have beneficial effects in the treatment of weight loss in patients with AIDS. Whether smoking marijuana has an advantage over orally administered dronabinol in the treatment of AIDS-related anorexia remains to be determined. Although THC is effective in lowering intraocular pressure in patients with glaucoma, its psychoactive properties make THC less desirable than other forms of drug therapy for this indication.

Abuse Characteristics

In human beings the development of tolerance to marijuana is most apparent among heavy long-term abusers and is evidenced by increases in the amount of drug used over time. Although chronic use of marijuana has a long history, whether physical dependence on marijuana develops in human beings remains controversial. Abrupt withdrawal of marijuana from long-term abusers has been reported to cause sleep disturbances, decreased appetite, nausea, and vomiting.[40] Whether these alterations in normal function are alleviated by the readministration of marijuana has not been shown and is necessary to prove that constant exposure to marijuana causes the development of physical dependence. Although the magnitude of psychologic dependence on marijuana is difficult to quantify, marijuana clearly possesses some abuse potential because it is the most commonly used illegal drug in the United States. Perhaps the lack of understanding of the abuse potential of marijuana is related to the fact that few individuals ever seek treatment for marijuana addiction, combined with the knowledge that the extensive and frequent use of this drug has led to few reports of severe toxicity.

Toxicity

Although few reports exist of adverse effects caused by acute administration of marijuana, the most common adverse reaction usually seen in naive abusers is an acute nonpsychotic panic reaction characterized by anxiety and fear of losing one's mind. Many inexperienced elderly abusers interpret the THC-induced tachycardia combined with the psychologic effects of THC as evidence that they are dying. Both of these conditions are best treated with authoritative reassurance or antianxiety agents of the benzodiazepine class. Very high doses of THC may result in self-limiting toxic delirium, acute paranoia, and psychotic episodes.

Long-term use of marijuana appears to cause no functional changes in the CNS; however, heavy smokers may be prone to chronic bronchitis, airway obstruction, poor dentition, and squamous cell metaplasia (as are smokers of tobacco). Contamination of marijuana with *Aspergillus*[32] or the herbicide paraquat can lead to severe pulmonary damage in abusers. Long-term, intensive use of between 5 and 18 marijuana cigarettes weekly is reported to reduce testosterone concentration and cause oligospermia in men.[34] Other studies of shorter exposures to marijuana have not confirmed these findings, although they do show that secondary sexual characteristics in the very young abuser can be suppressed by marijuana.[27] Teratogenic effects of THC are known to occur in animals; no such reports exist for human marijuana smokers. Anecdotal reports suggest marijuana use produces an amotivational syndrome, which is described as an affliction of young abusers of marijuana who drop out of social activities and show little interest in school, work, or other goal-directed activities. Laboratory studies and cross-cultural analyses of marijuana smokers in countries where marijuana use is acceptable do not support the contention that THC use leads to psychosocial deterioration.[37] Others have suggested that the lifestyle and goals of an abuser of any kind of illicit drug may more satisfactorily explain the amotivational syndrome.

ABUSE OF INHALANTS

Modern awareness of the consciousness-altering effects of inhaled compounds began with the discovery of anesthetic agents such as ether, chloroform, and nitrous oxide in the early nineteenth century. Today this list also includes halothane and other halogenated compounds. The use of general anesthetics is discussed in Chapter 18. Although nitrous oxide, halothane, and other volatile anesthetics are usually available only to medical or health care personnel, nitrous oxide can also be found in restaurant supply stores as a propellant for making whipped cream and packaged in small metal canisters called *whippets.* Although ether and chloroform are no longer used as anesthetics, they are available through chemical supply houses. In addition to the volatile anesthetics, three other main classes of inhalants are subject to abuse. The first are volatile solvents, which include glue, paint thinners, cleaning fluids, degreasers, and gasoline. The generalized depressant effects on the CNS caused by these solvents are mediated by ingredients such as trichloroethylene, benzene, toluene, naphthalene, hexane, heptaene, and acetone. This class of inhalants is widely abused because of ready availability. The second class of inhalants includes aerosol propellants such as methanol, ethanol, and isopropanol used, for example, in spray paint and cooking sprays. Trichlorofluoromethane and other fluorocarbons used as refrigerants may also be abused. The alcohols are less rewarding than other volatile solvents, and obviously ethanol is more prone to be abused by the oral route of administration. The third class includes organic nitrites, which include amyl, butyl, and isobutyl nitrite. Amyl nitrite is used as a vasodilator in the treatment of angina pectoris (discussed in Chapter 26) and is packaged in mesh-enclosed glass ampules designed to be crushed between the fingers, allowing for inhalation of the vapors for relief of the pain of angina. Amyl nitrite ampules are commonly referred to as "poppers" because of the popping sound resulting from their being broken. Both amyl nitrite and isobutyl nitrite are perceived to be sexual enhancers, which increases their abuse potential. Although amyl nitrite is available only by prescription, isobutyl nitrite is used as a room deodorizer and can be purchased from shops that sell drug paraphernalia under the names "Locker Room," "Doctor Bananas," and "Rush."

Pharmacologic Effects

With the exception of the organic nitrites, all the abused inhalants have a generalized depressant effect on the CNS similar to that of the volatile general anesthetics. Low doses of these agents first produce signs of stimulation followed by depression, unconsciousness, and, with larger doses, death. The desirable effects of these compounds—euphoria, perceptual distortions, ataxia, giddiness, and slurred speech—occur within seconds of inhalation and last from 5 to 45 minutes. Undesirable effects may be experienced during use, as well as for variable periods afterwards, and include coughing, vomiting, rhinitis, photophobia, irritation of the eyes, tinnitus, nausea, and sneezing. The vasodilatory action of the organic nitrites is immediate and produces a feeling of warmth and lightheadedness that is commonly referred to as a "head rush." The "head rush" is brief and is considered desirable; however, it may result in loss of consciousness as a consequence of postural hypotension if the drug is inhaled while standing. Headaches commonly occur after use of the organic nitrites and are caused by vasodilation of cerebral blood vessels.

Abuse Characteristics

The euphoria, disinhibition, and general feelings of drunkenness are thought to be the reinforcing characteristics of inhaled CNS depressants; abusers take these agents repeatedly, suggesting a psychologic dependence on them. Few controlled studies have been performed on the development of tolerance to solvents, aerosols, and nitrites. However, because solvents, aerosols, ethanol, barbiturates, and benzodiazepines share many of the same pharmacologic effects, considerable interest remains in whether cross-tolerance exists among these agents. There is little evidence that signs of abstinence occur in individuals when inhalants are withdrawn, suggesting that physical dependence is not part of the experience of these abusers.

Toxicity

Ascribing the toxic effects of an abused inhalant to an individual agent is difficult because the toxic effects of inhaled solvents and aerosols may be caused by more than one substance and because solvents typically contain several volatile compounds or may be tainted with heavy metals such as lead and cadmium. However, the major health risks associated with acute use of the anesthetic gases and the volatile liquids are sudden death from asphyxiation, respiratory depression, or arrhythmia-induced cardiopulmonary arrest. The halogenated hydrocarbons, such as trichloroethylene, are particularly likely to cause arrhythmias.

Repeated abuse of inhalation agents may lead to toxic effects caused by long-term exposure. Industrial solvents are known to cause liver and kidney damage, sensory and motor neuropathies, bone marrow suppression, and pulmonary disease. The toxic effects of chloroform on the liver and kidney are so well known that chloroform has not been used as an anesthetic for decades and has been eliminated from commercially available products. Continuous exposure to nitrous oxide can cause megaloblastic anemia, methemoglobinemia, and, in rare instances, peripheral neuropathy. In industrial settings where chronic exposure to organic nitrites occurs, cases of methemoglobinemia have been reported; however, this is rare in abusers of these compounds.

POLYDRUG ABUSE

Drug abuse problems are often compounded by the practice of taking two or more drugs in combination or in sequence. The polydrug abuser may seek additive or potentiated effects (e.g., the simultaneous use of alcohol and another sedative) or the modulation or termination of effects (e.g., the sequential use of amphetamines and barbiturates). Approximately 20% of long-term alcoholics abuse other drugs, especially barbiturates, antianxiety drugs, and marijuana. Primary heavy abusers of marijuana frequently use amphetamines or psychedelic agents, whereas heroin addicts are particularly apt to abuse amphetamines, cocaine, hallucinogens, and barbiturates. The majority of patients in methadone maintenance programs appear to be polydrug abusers. When multiple physical drug dependencies develop, the withdrawal syndrome becomes difficult to treat and is associated with a significantly enhanced mortality rate.

IMPLICATIONS FOR DENTISTRY

It is often claimed that drug abusers have a history of poor employment and academic adjustment and have difficulty with interpersonal relationships. They are characterized as egocentric, immature, impulsive, and self-deprecating and are said to have a psychologic need for approval, respect, and appreciation. Drugs of abuse are used to reverse this state by producing euphoria or to submerge it by eliminating unwanted thoughts.

Certain signs may alert the dentist to the possible parenteral abuse of drugs. Telltale cutaneous lesions may result from the long-term hypodermic administration of drugs of abuse. These lesions include acute septic complications, such as subcutaneous abscesses, cellulitis, and thrombophlebitis, as well as chronic cutaneous complications, including skin tracks and infected lesions, which occur most commonly in the thigh or antecubital or deltoid regions. Skin tracks result from frequent, multiple injections that produce chronic tissue inflammation. These are typically linear or bifurcated erythematous lesions that become indurated and hyperpigmented. Another sign that may alert the clinician to the problem of drug abuse is the presence of an ill-defined febrile illness. This finding often reflects a low-grade bacteremia resulting from the injection of drugs.

In ascertaining whether a patient is abusing drugs, the dentist cannot depend on being able to identify a particular personality type, recognize cutaneous lesions (which may be concealed under clothing), or diagnose a mild febrile illness. Rather, the dentist must rely on careful and thorough questioning of the patient and on the skillful use of a well-designed medical history questionnaire. Drug abuse is a subject of considerable importance to dentists because they are occasionally the unwitting target or victim of the drug abuser's need to secure drugs. Also, drug abuse among health professionals has a long history, a number of medical and dental abnormalities are associated with drug abuse, and interactions may occur between drugs that dentists customarily prescribe and those the patient is abusing.

Dentists as a Target of Drug Abusers

Inevitably drug abusers will, through pretense and subterfuge, attempt to obtain drugs from dentists. Therefore the dentist should be aware of any patient who complains of pain from pulpitis or an abscess and who refuses endodontic or surgical intervention. The opioid abuser may claim to be allergic to codeine or pentazocine in an effort to obtain more positively reinforcing drugs such as meperidine, morphine, or hydrocodone.[1] As a general defense against drug abusers, the dentist should never let patients know where such drugs are kept, never leave prescription pads out where they may be taken, and avoid the use of prewritten prescription forms.

Drug Use Among Dentists

Dentists are not immune to the hazards of drug abuse. Like physicians, they may be in greater danger of developing drug dependencies than the general population because of the ready accessibility of opioid analgesics and sedative-hypnotic drugs. In fact, opioid addiction among medical personnel is much higher than that of the general population. One form of drug abuse common among dentists and other health professionals is the inhalation of nitrous oxide. Evidence suggests that the pleasurable effects of nitrous oxide inhalation can lead to a craving for the drug in some persons.[10] The abuse potential of nitrous oxide coupled with the ease of availability of the drug contributes to its relatively frequent abuse by dentists.

Medical and Dental Complications of Drug Abuse

The most common and serious medical complications in the drug-abusing patient are AIDS, endocarditis, and hepatitis. IV drug abusers represent a population at risk of AIDS. Sharing needles for IV injections spreads the AIDS virus. IV drug abusers are responsible for a significant number of AIDS cases among heterosexuals.

Bacterial endocarditis in the drug abuser is most commonly caused by *Staphylococcus aureus*, which appears to derive from an increase in endogenous pathogens in the addict rather than from contaminated drugs or drug paraphernalia. In drug-abusing patients, the disease often affects the tricuspid valve, which is unusual in nonabusers. *Pseudomonas* endocarditis, although less common, primarily involves the tricuspid valve and has an overall mortality rate of 50%. *Candida albicans* infects the left-sided valves and is almost invariably fatal. Candidiasis may be disseminated to skin, eyes, bones, or joints.

Viral hepatitis is often seen among drug abusers and is probably transmitted by contaminated needles. The disease is usually mild, but persons displaying early signs of elevated prothrombin time, fever, elevated leukocyte count, or encephalopathy have a poor prognosis. In 50% to 80% of cases, the acute infection results in chronic inflammatory hepatic disease.

Opioid drugs have been reported to depress the immune system by interacting with opioid receptors on T lymphocytes and leukocytes. Other drugs of abuse have also been suggested to either suppress or enhance the activity of the immune system. Whether the development of infectious diseases in drug abusers is caused by a direct effect of these drugs on the immune system remains unknown.

Specific dental complications of drug use include rampant caries and rapidly progressing periodontal disorders, probably resulting from nutritional deficiencies and neglect of personal hygiene. Xerostomia with an enhanced rate of dental caries has been reported in those who abuse opioids, amphetamines, sedative-hypnotics, and marijuana. However, in other studies opioid and marijuana use do not appear to reduce the rate of salivary secretion.[20,45] Self-mutilation has occurred among drug abusers; teeth may be deliberately damaged in an effort to obtain drugs. Long-term cocaine and amphetamine abusers may develop facial tics and bruxism, which result in a traumatized tongue and worn teeth.[13] These subjects may also chronically rub the tongue along the inside of the lower lip, producing ulcers on the abraded tissues.[13]

Drug Interactions in Drug Abuse

Drug interactions in abusers are not unique but depend on the drug of abuse.[16] Barbiturates and other sedative-hypnotic agents induce hepatic cytochrome P450 enzyme activity. Therefore abusers of such substances may be resistant to the therapeutic effects of corticosteroids, oral anticoagulants, and many CNS depressants because the metabolism of these drugs is enhanced by enzyme induction. Opioid abusers generally show tolerance to other opioid analgesics. The dentist should beware of giving pentazocine to such patients because this and other agonist-antagonists may precipitate an acute withdrawal syndrome in opioid-dependent patients. Marijuana may intensify the CNS depression produced by barbiturates, general anesthetics, and other CNS depressant drugs. The sympathomimetic effects of cocaine, amphetamine, and marijuana may be enhanced by drugs used in dental practice. Administration of local anesthetics containing epinephrine or gingival retraction cords impregnated with epinephrine may enhance the tachycardia and elevations in blood pressure caused by these drugs.

Pain Control and Drug Abusers

Drug abusers may be more anxious and fearful of dental procedures and may have a lower pain tolerance than patients who do not abuse drugs. To counteract these fears abusers may take their favorite drug of abuse before dental appointments. If the dentist knows that the drug abuser has taken such a drug, the dental procedure should be rescheduled and the patient should be counseled to avoid drug use before the next visit. Complicating this picture is that tolerance to sedative drugs and local anesthetics has also been reported, particularly in parenteral drug abusers. These patients may need somewhat larger amounts of these drugs for pain-free dental treatment. Larger doses of sedatives and local anesthetics carry the risk of enhanced adverse effects caused by these drugs.

Treatment of pain and anxiety in the recovering or reformed substance abuser presents a problem to the dentist.[10] Whether the patient has abused alcohol or other drugs in the past, proper dental care demands a preoperative evaluation of the patient's personal attitude toward drug treatment. Many of these persons refuse mood-altering drugs, and such wishes must be respected. As a rule, it is best never to administer a drug, or another of its class, that has previously been abused by the patient. In cases in which anxiety is predominantly somatic (e.g., tachycardia, breathlessness, and tremulousness), oral propranolol may be of value. Intraoperative pain control can be accomplished with local anesthetics, but systemic exposure to epinephrine should be minimized in patients being treated with neuronal uptake pump inhibitors such as desipramine for postdependence depression. Postoperative pain can usually be adequately controlled with NSAIDs.

Cited References

1. Abbott L: Don't be deceived by a drug addict, *Am Med Assoc News* 19:1-4, 1976.
2. Abraham HD, Aldridge AM: Adverse consequences of lysergic acid diethylamide, *Addiction* 88:1327-1330, 1993.

3. American Psychiatric Association: *Benzodiazepine dependence, toxicity and abuse. A Task Force Report of the American Psychiatric Association*, Washington DC, 1990, American Psychiatric Association.
4. American Psychiatric Association: *Diagnostic and statistical manual of mental disorders* (DSM-IV), ed 4, Washington, DC, 1994, American Psychiatric Association.
5. *An analysis of worker drug use and workplace policies and programs*, NIDA Office of Applied Studies, SAMHSA, US Department of Health and Human Services, Washington, DC, 1997, US Government Printing Office.
6. Anggard E, Sjoquist B, Fryo B, et al: Amphetamine metabolism in amphetamine psychosis, *Clin Pharmacol Ther* 14:870-880, 1973.
7. *Annual emergency room data, Drug Abuse Warning Network (DAWN)*, National Institute on Drug Abuse, Washington, DC, 1991, Department of Health and Human Services, US Government Printing Office.
8. Anthony JC, Warner LA, Kessler KC: Comparative epidemiology of dependence on tobacco, alcohol, controlled substances and the inhalants: basic findings from the national comorbidity survey, *Exp Clin Psychopharmacol* 2:244-268, 1994.
9. Ashton H: Benzodiazepine withdrawal: an unfinished story, *Br Med J* 288:1135-1140, 1984.
10. Aston R: Treating pain and anxiety in the reformed substance abuser, *J Mich Dent Assoc* 69:279-280, 1987.
11. Brill H: The treatment of drug dependence: a brief history. In National Commission on Marihuana and Drug Abuse: *Drug use in America: problem in perspective,* vol 4, Washington, DC, 1973, US Government Printing Office.
12. Cone EJ, Johnson RE: Contact highs and urinary cannabinoid excretion after passive exposure to marijuana smoke, *Clin Pharmacol Ther* 40:247-256, 1986.
13. Connell PH: Clinical manifestations and treatment of amphetamine type of dependence, *JAMA* 196:718-723, 1966.
14. Cook CE, Perez-Reyes M, Jeffcoat AR, et al: Phencyclidine disposition in humans after small doses of radiolabeled drug, *Fed Proc* 42:2566-2569, 1983.
15. Cregler LL, Mark H: Medical complications of cocaine abuse, *N Engl J Med* 315:1495-1500, 1986.
16. Davis JM, Sekerke HJ, Janowsky DS: Drug interactions involving the drugs of abuse. In National Commission on Marihuana and Drug Abuse: *Drug use in America: problem in perspective,* vol 4, Washington DC, 1973, US Government Printing Office.
17. Devane WA, Dysarz FA, Johnson MR, et al: Determination and characterization of a cannabinoid receptor in rat brain, *Mol Pharmacol* 34:605-613, 1988.
18. Devane WA, Hanus L, Breuer A, et al: Isolation and structure of a brain constituent that binds to the cannabinoid receptor, *Science* 258:1946-1949, 1992.
19. Dewey WL: Cannabinoid pharmacology, *Pharmacol Rev* 38:151-178, 1986.
20. DiCugno F, Perec CJ, Tocci AA: Salivary secretion and dental caries experience in drug addicts, *Arch Oral Biol* 26:363-367, 1981.
21. Fraser HF, Wikler A, Essig CF, et al: Degree of physical dependence induced by secobarbital or pentobarbital, *JAMA* 166:126-129, 1958.
22. Griffiths RR, Wolf B: Relative abuse liability of different benzodiazepines in drug abusers, *J Clin Psychopharmacol* 10:237-243, 1990.
23. Herkenham M, Lynn AB, Little MD, et al: Cannabinoid receptor localization in brain, *Proc Natl Acad Sci USA* 87:1932-1936, 1990.
24. Hill HF, Chapman CR, Kornell JA, et al: Self-administration of morphine in bone marrow transplant patients reduces drug requirement, *Pain* 40:121-129, 1990.
25. Hollander JE: The management of cocaine-associated myocardial ischemia, *N Engl J Med* 333:1267-1272, 1995.
26. Hollister LE: Dependence on benzodiazepines. In Szara SI, Ludford JP, eds: *Benzodiazepines: a review of research results, 1980,* NIDA research monograph No. 33, Rockville, MD, 1980, US Department of Health and Human Services.
27. Hollister LE: Health aspects of cannabis, *Pharmacol Rev* 38:1-20, 1986.
28. Isbell H, Chrusciel TL: Dependence liability of "non-narcotic" drugs, *Bull WHO* 43(suppl):1-111, 1970.
29. Isner JM, Estes NA, Thompson PD, et al: Acute cardiac events temporally related to cocaine abuse, *N Engl J Med* 315:1438-1443, 1986.
30. Jaffe JH, Ciraulo DA, Nies A, et al: Abuse potential of halazepam and of diazepam in patients recently treated for acute alcohol withdrawal, *Clin Pharmacol Ther* 34:623-630, 1983.
31. Johnston LD, O'Malley PM, Bachman JG: *Monitoring the future. National results on adolescent drug use: overview of key findings*, NIH Pub No. 02-5105, Washington, DC, 2002, US Government Printing Office.
32. Kagen SI: *Aspergillus*: an inhalable contaminant of marihuana, *N Engl J Med* 304:483-484, 1981.
33. Kloss MW, Rosen GM, Rauckman EJ: Cocaine-mediated hepatotoxicity: a critical review, *Biochem Pharmacol* 33:169-173, 1984.
34. Kolodny RC, Masters WH, Kolodner RM, et al: Depression of plasma testosterone levels after chronic intensive marijuana use, *N Engl J Med* 290:872-874, 1974.
35. Kreek MJ: Rationale for maintenance pharmacotherapy of opiate dependence. In O'Brien CP, Jaffe J, eds: *Addictive states,* New York, 1992, Raven Press.
36. Mackinnon GL, Parker WA: Benzodiazepine withdrawal syndrome: a literature review and evaluation, *Am J Drug Alcohol Abuse* 9:19-33, 1982.
37. *Marihuana: a signal of misunderstanding,* National Commission on Marihuana and Drug Abuse, Washington, DC, 1972, US Government Printing Office.
38. Matsuda LA, Lolait SJ, Brownstein MJ, et al: Structure of a cannabinoid receptor and functional expression of the cloned cDNA, *Nature* 346:561-564, 1990.
39. McLellan AT, Luborsky L, Woody GE, et al: Are the "addiction-related" problems of substance abusers really related?, *J Nerv Ment Dis* 169:232-239, 1981.
40. Meyer RE: Behavioral pharmacology of marihuana. In Lipton MA, DiMascio A, Killam KF, eds: *Psychopharmacology: a generation of progress,* New York, 1978, Raven Press.
41. *National household survey on drug abuse,* National Institute on Drug Abuse, Rockville, MD, 1993, Department of Health and Human Services, US Government Printing Office.
42. O'Brien CP, Childress AR, McLellan AT, et al: Classical conditioning in drug-dependent humans, *Ann NY Acad Sci* 654:400-415, 1992.

43. Paris M, Nahas GG: Botany: the unstabilized species. In Nahas GG, ed: *Marihuana in science and medicine,* New York, 1984, Raven Press.

44. Resnick RB, Kestenbaum RS, Schwartz LK: Acute systemic effects of cocaine in man: a controlled study by intranasal and intravenous routes, *Science* 195:696-698, 1977.

45. Scheutz F: Saliva secretion rate in a group of drug addicts, *Scand J Dent Res* 91:496-498, 1983.

46. Simpson GM, Khajawall AM, Alatorre E, et al: Urinary phencyclidine excretion in chronic abusers, *J Toxicol Clin Toxicol* 19:1051-1059, 1982.

47. Snyder SH: Hallucinogens. In National Commission on Marihuana and Drug Abuse: *Drug use in America: problem in perspective,* vol 1, Washington, DC, 1973, US Government Printing Office.

48. Strassman RJ: Adverse reactions to psychedelic drugs: a review of the literature, *J Nerv Ment Dis* 172:577-595, 1984.

General References

Abbott A, ed: Drugs of abuse, *Trends Pharmacol Sci* 13(special issue):169-219, 1992.

Acute reactions to drugs of abuse, *Med Lett Drug Ther* 44:21-24, 2002.

Aston R: Drug abuse: its relationship to dental practice. In Gage T, ed: Symposium on pharmacology and therapeutics, *Dent Clin North Am* 28:595-610, 1984.

Clouet DH, ed: *Phencyclidine: an update,* NIDA research monograph No. 64, Rockville, MD 1986, US Department of Health and Human Services.

Gawin FH, Ellinwood EH, Jr: Cocaine and other stimulants: actions, abuse, and treatment, *N Engl J Med* 318:1173-1182, 1988.

Grabowski J, ed: *Cocaine: pharmacology, effects, and treatment of abuse,* NIDA research monograph No. 50, Rockville, MD, 1984, US Department of Health and Human Services.

Karch SB: *The pathology of drug abuse,* Boca Raton, FL, 1993, CRC Press.

O'Brien CP: Drug addiction and drug abuse. In Hardman JG, Limbird LE, Gilman AG, eds: *Goodman & Gilman's The pharmacological basis of therapeutics,* ed 10, New York, 2001, McGraw-Hill.

Rees TD: Oral effects of drug abuse, *Crit Rev Oral Biol Med* 3:163-184, 1982.

Winger G, Hofmann FG, Woods JH: *A handbook on drug and alcohol abuse: the biomedical aspects,* ed 3, New York, 1992, Oxford University Press.

CHAPTER • 52

Toxicology

Harrell E. Hurst and Michael D. Martin

Toxicology is a basic science that is concerned with information regarding poisonous substances and their toxic actions. This discipline draws on the fields of biology, chemistry, and medicine to coordinate knowledge regarding toxic materials. Toxicology strives to understand key features of biology relevant to adverse interactions of chemicals with living systems. A principal objective is to promote the safe use of chemicals, particularly among human beings, whether encountered as medicines, food additives or contaminants, industrial materials, household products, or in the environment. Topics of interest to toxicologists include analysis of toxic agents, identification of toxic effects, elucidation of mechanisms of toxicity, management of poisoning, characterization of potential chemical risks, forensic and legal applications, and timely application of knowledge to prevent potentially disastrous consequences of chemical use.

The toxicology of therapeutic agents is integral to their pharmacologic characteristics and is described in appropriate chapters of this text. This chapter reviews general principles of toxicology, summarizes key organ systems that are susceptible to toxic effects, and outlines prevention and management of acute poisoning. It reviews toxic materials not described elsewhere in the text and covers relevant topics related to dental practice.

GENERAL PRINCIPLES

All chemical substances can cause harm or kill if encountered at sufficiently large concentrations over crucial periods of time. This statement embodies insight articulated by Paracelsus in the sixteenth century[27] that *dose* is the major determinant of toxicity. However, a subset of substances have relatively specific toxic effects, are considered very harmful through human experience, and are considered poisons or toxins. Beyond this base of experience exists a vast number of uncharacterized, potential toxicants. As of early 2001 the Chemical Abstracts Service[8] reported counts of more than 17,600,000 organic and inorganic substances, 224,000 inventoried or regulated substances, and some 1,300,000 commercially available chemicals as potentially toxic. This array dictates that toxicologists use some means of triage toward assessment of potential toxicants. At present, selection of chemicals for toxicologic testing is dictated by their potential for use, by funding of basic research on the chemicals, and initial evidence of their specific adverse effects.

The ultimate aim of toxicologic science in our society is to guide safe use of chemicals. The definitions in Box 52-1 can assist in understanding and promoting concise communication in the approach to this objective. Safety is a negative entity, that is, the absence of threat of injury. As such, safety cannot be proved directly. Our society often simplistically considers chemicals "safe" or "toxic." Such naive characterization can preclude the rational judgment that enables safe uses of chemicals. Critical judgment requires understanding of the distinction between the terms *toxicity* and *hazard* to enable assessment of risks (see Box 52-1). Toxicologic assessment promotes safety by defining hazardous situations of use so that the unsafe use of chemicals can be avoided.

A primary concern of toxicology is evaluation of risk. All useful chemicals have some degree of risk associated with their use. Toxicologic science has developed testing paradigms to define toxicity to assess potential risk. Benefits also must be considered relative to the risk of use. A high degree of risk may be acceptable when benefits are great (e.g., use of toxic but potentially life-extending drugs such as chemotherapeutic agents). Otherwise, risk may be unacceptable for less essential uses (e.g., food coloring). In contrast to the science inherent in testing methods, judgment of risk acceptability involves policy. Such judgment invokes economic, social, and ethical values and should consider factors such as needs met by a chemical under consideration, alternative solutions and their risks, anticipated extent of use and public exposure, effects on environmental quality, and conservation of natural resources.

Within such considerations is an issue of major importance to toxicology and to society in general, which is determination of cause-and-effect relationships. This objective of epidemiologic studies is elusive for chronic diseases, such as many types of cancer. Such diseases may involve confounded potential causes, such as chemical or viral exposure as well as genetic susceptibility factors. Uncritical publication of unscientific observations or incomplete studies leads the public to inappropriate conclusions, which should be characterized more correctly as hypotheses. Adequate processes for determination of causation, as opposed to simple unrelated association or correlation, require scientific discipline and judgment based on considerable experience.

The criteria developed by Sir Austin Bradford Hill[33] provide a sound basis for consideration of causal relationships and should be considered a touchstone for expert opinion regarding cause and effect. These are listed in Box 52-2. None of these criteria should be considered as absolutely essential, and they cannot be considered as proof of causal relationships. However, their careful application during evaluation of potential cause-and-effect relationships can assist in organizing knowledge toward a weight-of-evidence judgment and may provide an alternative interpretation for consideration.

Dose-Response Relationships

As mentioned earlier, the relationship between dose and toxic response is the fundamental axiom of the science of

Box 52-1

Basic Definitions Relevant to Principles of Toxicology

Safety	Condition of being secure from threat of danger, harm, or injury
Toxicity	Property of grave harmfulness or deadliness associated with a chemical that is expressed on biologic exposure
Hazard	Threat of danger directly related to circumstances of use of a chemical
Risk	Expected frequency of occurrence of an adverse effect in a given situation

Box 52-2

The Hill Criteria for Consideration of Causal Relationships

Criterion	Explanation
Strength of association	The observed magnitude of the association, compared with other relevant observations, should be considered as a primary indicator in assessment of cause and effect.
Consistency	Can the association of cause and effect be observed repeatedly by others under appropriate circumstances?
Specificity	What particular conditions produce the effect, or what specific group is affected? The bounds of causal relationship should be delimited.
Temporality	Causation generally occurs before effect, whereas correlational effects can vary in temporality.
Biological gradient	Demonstration of a fundamental dose relationship provides convincing evidence of cause and effect.
Plausibility	Some basis in previous knowledge provides a means of common understanding. Remember, however, that all phenomena were novel at some point.
Coherence	Care should be taken that cause and effect interpretation not unduly conflict with scientifically established facts of biology and medicine.
Experiment	What effect does manipulation of accessible variables in the potential cause and effect relationship have?
Analogy	Previously understood examples provide basis for formulation of testable hypotheses.

From Hill A: The environment and disease: association or causation? *Proc Roy Soc Med* 58:295, 1965.

toxicology. Studies are designed to ascertain dose-response functions associated with specific adverse effects. When simple all-or-nothing criteria such as death are used, quantitation of response is relatively simple. More often, however, objectives require more subtle means of assessment that are less readily quantified. Beyond simple indication of the quantity of material required for the toxic effect, dose-response relationships provide evidence of the causal relationship between the observed effect and the chemical under study, as noted previously.

Figure 52-1 indicates three modes of display of idealized dose-response data to illustrate and describe the dose required for median response in subjects tested. These data are typical of quantal or all-or-nothing responses such as lethality. In this example the dose axis is logarithmically spaced, and the data describe a log-normal distribution. Responses that arise from mass action, such as reversible occupancy of receptor by drugs, often are most easily plotted on a logarithmic axis. Alternatively, effects caused by limited biologic capacity, such as irreversible enzyme inhibition, can exhibit abrupt threshold-like effects and may be more easily analyzed on a linear dose axis. The rule is to plot the data to see what type axis is most applicable.

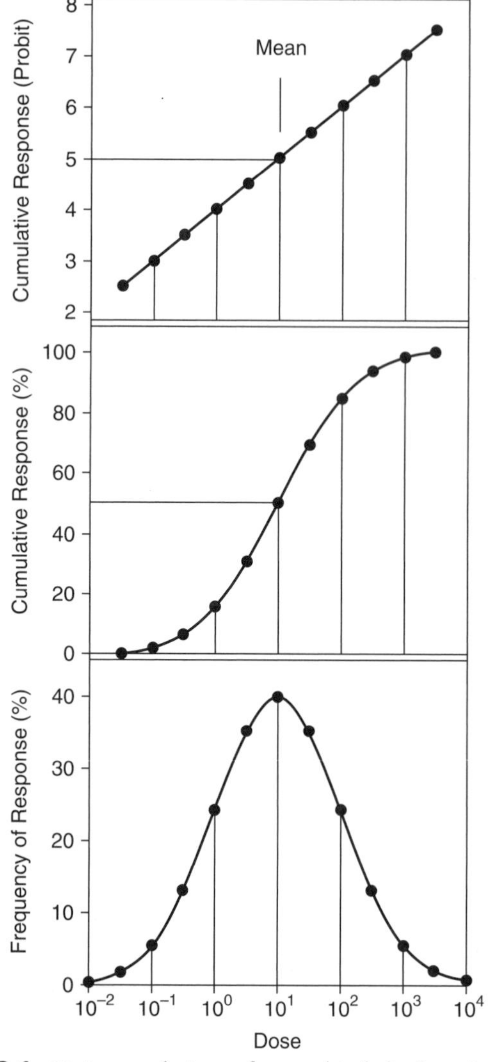

Fig. 52-1 Various techniques for graphical display of quantal response versus dose data, including frequency of response, cumulative response, and cumulative response linearized by probit transformation.

The lower panel indicates distribution of responses across the dose axis, with a mean of 10 and standard deviation (SD) of one $\log_{10}$ unit. Response percentages include approximately 68.3% within ±1 SD of the mean, 95.5% within ±2 SD, and 99.7% within ±3 SD of the mean. The distribution indicates hypersusceptibility for individuals at the lowest doses and resistant responders at the highest doses. Such a plot gives a convenient way to visualize the distribution of responses across dose within the test groups.

The middle panel of Figure 52-1 plots the cumulative response versus dose across all treated groups. Here the response data are practically linear in the range from −1 SD to +1 SD for this ideal data. This plot provides convenient, accurate estimation of dose required for a 50% response, such as the median lethal dose (LD_{50}). However, real data are rarely so well behaved because too few animals may be included for adequate definition of the sigmoid curve. Another disadvantage is that the sigmoid curve presents difficulty in estimating doses that elicit extremes of response, such as 1% or 99%.

An alternative presented in the top panel uses the probit transform[40] for the cumulative response. Probit units are derived by conversion of cumulative response percentages to units of deviation from the mean. The scale uses normal equivalent deviation units (NED), for which the mean is arbitrarily set to a NED value of 5 to give positive values along the axis. As is evident in the example, the probit transform linearizes the extreme values of the response function, which allows accurate estimation of doses affecting 1% or 99% of those exposed. Additionally, the probit transform facilitates determination of the slope, which enables comparison of the dose-response function with other agents or responses.

Such plots are inadequate in dealing with issues of societal risk, however, for which policy often requires estimation of exposure posing a theoretical risk of 1 in 1 million, otherwise described as a 10^{-6} risk factor. Practical problems intervene, including the impracticality of experimental studies involving sufficient animals to define adequately the dose-response function at low response levels. A classic toxicologic experiment conducted at the National Center for Toxicological Research illustrates this point. Officially termed the *ED_{01} Study,*[28] this experiment examined in detail the response function of mice treated with low doses of the experimental carcinogen 2-acetylaminofluorene. The study, sometimes termed the *megamouse study,* involved more than 24,000 mice to determine the dose effective in producing a 1% tumor rate. This work advanced toxicologic understanding of the complexity of genotoxic and proliferative cellular events in chronic cancer bioassays. Additionally, it demonstrated logistic difficulties in conducting such studies and illustrated gaps in the evolving understanding of chemically induced cancer.

Factors That Change Dose-Response Relationships

Dose-response relationships can vary with many factors, including differences within and among individuals. Within an individual, factors responsible for dose-response variations over time may include age and nutritional status, environmental influences, functional status of organs of excretion, concomitant disease, and various combinations of factors. Changes in pharmacokinetics of toxicants are a frequent basis for altered dose-response relationships. Known influences include increased toxicant bioactivation by enzyme induction,[25] such as occurs in certain variants of cytochrome P450[11] with exposure to phenobarbital or polychlorinated biphenyls. Conversely, inhibition of metabolic clearance is possible with interacting chemicals. Such an inhibition of benzodiazepine clearance has been observed with the antifungal drug ketoconazole. Substances are often less toxic by the oral route when administered with food as a consequence of less rapid absorption. The time and frequency of administration can be important in altering dose-response relationships through functional changes. Many compounds induce tolerance on repeated administration, whereas others can become more toxic with closely repeated administration. Receptor densities and sensitivity may vary with time or as a consequence of previous exposure. An example of the latter is the well known tolerance that develops to long-term administration of opioids.

Responses among individuals differ as a consequence of different genetic traits, a subject of intense interest as knowledge emerges from the Human Genome Project and increased use of efficient molecular techniques and transgenic animals becomes widespread in research. Recognition and understanding of relevant aspects of human diversity derived from functional genomic research offer potential for therapeutic gains. The rationale is to use appropriate drugs in those best suited to benefit, and to reduce use in patients with genetic traits that might result in toxicity. These efforts have spawned new terms, including *pharmacogenetics,* representing characterized genetic differences in drug metabolism and disposition, and *pharmacogenomics,* used to describe the broad spectrum of genes that affect drug response. A summary is available[20] that describes progress in determining genetic polymorphisms relevant to drug action and disposition. Known variants linked to altered drug effects in human beings include phase I cytochrome P450 enzymes, phase II enzymes such as *N*-acetyltransferases and glutathione *S*-transferases, small molecule transporters, drug and endogenous substrate receptors, and ion channel variants. Additional information on these topics is available in Chapters 2 and 4.

Similar advances are likely to be applied to understand genetic differences that result in toxic effects aside from those that arise during drug therapy. As an example, some 400 million individuals worldwide exhibit a heritable deficiency in the cytoplasmic enzyme glucose-6-phosphate dehydrogenase. Because this enzyme is essential to the cell's capacity to withstand oxidant stress through production of reducing equivalents, sensitive individuals with this enzymatic deficiency have chemically mediated hemolytic anemia when exposed to oxidants.[4]

Of particular importance to the interpretation of toxicologic studies are interspecies differences, which may confound understanding and interpretation of results from animal models. Well-known differences in physiology, metabolic rates, pharmacokinetics of toxicant metabolism and excretion, and sites of toxicant action mediate these interspecies differences. Advances involving physiologically based pharmacokinetic modeling and use of predictive, mechanistically based biomarkers offer promise of augmenting, or in some cases obviating, conventional toxicity testing.

Acute Versus Chronic Toxicity

Toxicity can be classified by the amount of time required for development of the adverse effect. For this purpose the term *acute* describes toxicity with a sudden onset, whereas *chronic* describes a long latency or duration. In epidemiology this classification typically describes the time between exposure and onset of toxicity. For example, intoxication is an acute effect that results from ingestion of a large quantity of ethanol over a brief time. Alternatively, the progressive diffuse architectural damage to the liver known as *cirrhosis* occurs over years with chronic ethanol exposure. In experimental toxicology, however, these terms are used to refer to experimental paradigms involving the duration of treatment or exposure. Acute testing typically describes a single treatment, whereas chronic toxicity testing usually involves dosing or feeding a chemical over the species' lifetime, as in a rodent carcinogenicity bioassay.

If exposure occurs repeatedly at intervals more frequent than the time required to eliminate a toxicant, the material accumulates in the body throughout the duration of exposure. Although each exposure may be less than toxic, accumulation may produce toxic levels if exposure continues for sufficient time. The primary determinant is the rapidity of elimination versus the frequency and magnitude of exposure. Slowly eliminated toxicants such as lipophilic chemicals or materials readily bound in tissues have the greatest potential for accumulation.

Chronic toxicity may exhibit little or no apparent relation to acute toxicity, as noted in the previous ethanol example. In such cases understanding of cause and effect requires careful study. Of the many chronic toxicities, carcinogenesis currently is of greatest concern in our society. Precancerous cellular changes occur and develop slowly and may remain undetected over long periods. Periodic dental examinations often play a significant role in detection of cancers of the oral cavity. Knowledge of patient habits with adverse potential health effects, such as the link between tobacco use and oral cancer,[32,49] assists the dental practitioner in being vigilant against such chronic toxicity.

Chemically Related Toxicants

Understanding of chemical toxicity can require knowledge of related chemicals that may be present as impurities because of manufacturing or exist as a result of environmental effects. A classic example is 2,3,7,8-tetrachlorodibenzo-*p*-dioxin (dioxin, or TCDD), which was discovered in the herbicide mixture known as Agent Orange used in the Vietnam War. Although dioxin existed at low part-per-million levels in the herbicide mixture, the extreme toxicity of this contaminant in certain species created grave concern for contaminated areas. This led to a ban on the use of the herbicide 2,4,5-trichlorophenoxyacetic acid, because TCDD is formed through a condensation reaction involving two molecules of 2,4,5-trichlorophenol. Dioxin also can be formed from other sources, such as combustion of municipal waste, iron ore sintering, and wood pulp and paper mills. The toxic actions of TCDD are mediated through its binding to the aryl hydrocarbon nuclear receptor,[55] which regulates transcription of genes encoding cytochrome P450 enzymes in the CYP1A subfamily and several other genes that regulate cell growth and differentiation. Despite its extreme toxic potential in some species, epidemiologic studies regarding the effect of TCDD exposure on human beings have been inconclusive to date.

The consequences of metabolism of drugs and chemicals after ingestion are extremely important. An example illustrates the importance of understanding toxic effects relative to drug metabolism. Terfenadine is a nonsedating histamine H_1 receptor antagonist that, until recently, was widely used for relief of symptoms of seasonal allergy. This drug was removed from the market because studies revealed cardiotoxicity when terfenadine was given with erythromycin.[2] The toxic interaction was traced to the antibiotic's inhibition of the high-affinity oxidative enzyme system CYP3A in human liver and intestinal membranes.[42] This interaction inhibited normal clearance of terfenadine, and the abnormally elevated levels produced toxicity in the form of a prolonged QT interval and the cardiac arrhythmia *torsades de pointes*. This antihistamine has been replaced with its active metabolite, fexofenadine, which apparently does not elicit this toxicity (see Chapter 22).

Local Versus Systemic Effects

Toxic effects can occur at a site of exposure, such as dermal contact, or at some site remote from the point of chemical contact or entry. Local effects dependent on applied concentration are usually diminished by dilution with physiologic fluids and diffusion within tissue away from the site of application. The toxic effect depends on the nature of the interaction at the local site. If the effect is caused by reversible interaction with a receptor, such as that of a local anesthetic, toxicity is attenuated by diffusion and the system is returned to a more normal state as the drug dissociates from receptors. For toxicants that act through destruction of normal cellular architecture, such as a caustic agent, return to normality requires repair of membranes and cellular structures.

Systemic effects are facilitated by transport within the body fluids and may be influenced by metabolism. Depending on whether biotransformation activates a protoxicant or detoxifies a toxicant, the effects of systemic processing can increase or attenuate toxicity. Compounds may be more or less toxic by the oral route than by other means of systemic exposure, as the first-pass effect of intestine or liver serves to activate or remove toxicants before distribution in the systemic circulation. Alternative systemic exposures, such as inhalation, are not modulated in this manner because systemic exposure occurs directly.

Target Organ Systems

Most toxic chemicals exhibit specificity in their action on target tissues or organs because these targeted biologic systems reach crucial points in which their physiologic functions are interrupted under the influence of the chemical. The following section presents crucial physiologic systems and their characteristics that are important in understanding organ-specific toxicity.

Nervous system

Given the primary importance in control of integrated function, the central nervous system (CNS) is a most important target for many toxicants. Individual neurons exhibit high metabolic rates and are unable to rely on anaerobic glycolysis. These characteristics make these cells susceptible to toxicants that adversely affect cellular respiration and energy production and lead to neuronal damage when central or peripherally acting toxicants interrupt neuronal metabolism, cerebral circulation, oxygen-carrying capacity of blood, or pulmonary ventilation.

A remarkable cell-selective neurotoxicant is 1-methyl-4-phenyl-1,2,3,6-tetrahydropyridine, an impurity discovered[38] from attempted illicit synthesis and injection of a meperidine analogue. This compound is a protoxicant for 1-methyl-4-phenylpyridinium, which is formed by monoamine oxidase and concentrated by high affinity carrier into dopaminergic neurons. The molecular target of 1-methyl-4-phenylpyridinium is reduced nicotinamide adenine dinucleotide dehydrogenase, and the interaction blocks the cellular respiratory exchange of electrons in mitochondria of cells. Its toxic actions result in destruction of dopaminergic neurons in the substantia nigra (see Chapter 15). Death of these cells produces symptoms strikingly similar to Parkinson's disease, leading to loss of willful motor actions.

Loss of integrity of neuronal cell metabolism can alter neuronal architecture, particularly the myelin sheath of peripheral neurons. Such effects are common to many forms of toxicity expressed in the nervous system. Various compounds, such as tri-*o*-cresyl phosphate, acrylamide, and metabolites of hexane, cause degeneration of long axons that control neuromuscular activities. Termed *central-peripheral distal axonopathy,*[72] this toxicity involves a "dying back" or retrograde degeneration of distal axons and leads to loss of control of motor functions such as gait. Other effects, such as sensory neuropathy and paresthesia, can result from similar effects of toxicants on small sensory fibers.

Blood and hematopoietic system

Given the crucial roles of the elements of blood in delivering oxygen and maintaining immune function, toxic effects on blood or the hematopoietic system can be life threatening. Of these, perhaps no poisoning is more common, preventable, or treatable with timely therapy than the toxic interaction of carbon monoxide (CO) with hemoglobin (Hb). This interaction blocks the vital oxygen-carrying capacity by formation of carboxyhemoglobin (CO-Hb). Characteristics of CO and its toxic effect on various tissues sensitive to anoxia have been concisely reviewed.[86] Details of treatment, which involves displacement of Hb-bound CO with oxygen, are provided in the comprehensive volume of Ellenhorn et al.[19] In mild (CO-Hb <30%) to moderate (CO-Hb 30% to 40%) cases, therapy includes use of 100% oxygen by nonrebreathing mask until CO-Hb is less than 5%. Severe poisoning can mandate hyperbaric use of oxygen to hasten the exchange.

Another toxic effect that alters the oxygen-carrying capacity of erythrocytes is the formation of methemoglobin. In this toxicity, the heme iron is oxidized from the ferrous (Fe^{++}) to ferric (Fe^{+++}) state by exposure to oxidizing chemicals such as nitrites or aromatic amines.[89] As with carboxyhemoglobin, methemoglobin is incapable of carrying molecular oxygen to tissues. Effects of resultant anoxia are similar, but treatment differs. This involves use of methylene blue, as a precursor to its metabolite leukomethylene blue, a cofactor that enables erythrocytes to reduce methemoglobin in the presence of reduced nicotinamide adenine dinucleotide phosphate. This therapy exhibits complications of potential hemolysis for treatment of infants and persons with glucose-6-phosphate dehydrogenase deficiency[89] because this enzyme is essential in the production of reduced nicotinamide adenine dinucleotide phosphate.

Other adverse actions affect the blood-forming cells of the bone marrow. Such effects can cause loss of immune functions mediated through leukocytes, as noted with induction of agranulocytosis during treatment with thioamide antithyroid drugs such as propylthiouracil. Although rare, this adverse effect is devastating because it leaves the patient susceptible to sepsis. Aplastic anemia is a complication of therapy with the antiepileptic drugs felbamate and carbamazepine. This condition is very serious because the marrow loses the ability to produce cells. This potential effect requires vigilance for signs of blood dyscrasias and requires laboratory monitoring of blood cell counts during the first months of treatment. Other adverse effects on the hematopoietic system include overexpression of certain types of cells, such as that noted in the development of acute myelogenous leukemia from benzene. Benzene is a toxicant commonly encountered in petroleum distillates such as gasoline and is considered a causative agent in human leukemia, probably through an active hydroquinone[36] or benzoquinone[48] metabolite. The process of leukemia development appears to involve preferential selection and clonal expansion of stem and progenitor cells through interaction of the toxic benzene metabolites by multiple independent genetic and epigenetic factors.

Respiratory system

The effect of toxicants on the respiratory tract is largely determined by the area of intimate cellular exposure to inhaled chemicals. Such contact is dictated by the structure of the conducting airways and the physical and chemical properties of the toxicant. Larger particles and more water-soluble compounds deposit in the upper regions of the respiratory tract, whereas very fine particles and less soluble gases reach more deeply into the lungs.

Compounds that are rapidly absorbed or highly caustic generally affect the nasal passages. As an example, formaldehyde has a detectable pungent odor at concentrations above 0.5 ppm and is highly irritating to the nasal passages. The nasopharyngeal region serves as a filter for larger particles of size ranging from 5 to 30 μm in diameter. Many of these are cleared upward by mucociliary action. Highly water-soluble gases such as sulfur dioxide dissolve in moisture present in the upper respiratory membranes and form irritating sulfurous acid. Less soluble compounds such as oxides of nitrogen and ozone penetrate more deeply into lung and generally exert effects at membranes in the smallest airways or alveoli. Particles smaller than 5 μm may travel well down into the bronchiolar region, whereas fine particles of 1 μm nominal size reach the alveolar region.[88]

Lung toxicity typically involves damage to the delicate architecture vital for efficient gas exchange. Because lung tissues contain many cytokines and immunologic mechanisms for particle clearance and tissue repair, inflammation is a common result of inspired toxic gases such as ozone. With acute injury, an exudative phase may progress in severe cases to pulmonary edema, which alters ventilation, diffusion of oxygen and carbon dioxide, and perfusion. Severity depends on the extent of damage to bronchiolar and alveolar cells, and the resolution of inflammation through mitogenic or fibrinogenic processes.

Chronic injury to the lung may result from inhalation of fine particles. Phagocytic mechanisms attempting to remove insoluble particles may produce tissue scarring and interstitial fibrosis, in which collagen fibers replace normal membranes and occupy alveolar interstitial space. Such injury is common with inhalation of silicate particles such as asbestos.[62] These actions produce inflexible tissue, diminish surface area, and lead to poor surfaces for gas exchange. Another chronic lung toxicity is emphysema, and its major cause is cigarette smoking. This toxic effect produces distended, enlarged air spaces that are poorly compliant but without fibrosis. The pathogenesis of this condition is not fully understood, but an imbalance between proteolytic activities of lung elastase and antiproteases appears to be involved.[37] Lung cancer became a major concern with the rise in popularity of smoking; this health scourge of today was a rare disease a century ago. Smoking is believed to be the most important single risk factor for this disease, presenting a 10- and 20-fold increase in risk for average and heavy smokers, respectively.[88]

Organs of excretion

Primary organs of toxicant elimination include the liver and kidneys. The liver provides the major site for metabolic transformation, rendering compounds more water soluble and subject to more efficient excretion in urine by the kidney. The unique physiologic features of each organ provide crucial characteristics that are susceptible to toxic actions and subsequent adverse consequences of impaired function.

The liver possesses remarkable capabilities for regeneration. However, hepatotoxicity often results in necrosis and loss of the vital capacities of the liver. Essential functions include protein synthesis, nutrient homeostasis, biotransformation, particle filtration, and formation and excretion of bile.[51] For example, impaired production of proteins such as albumin, clotting factors, and lipoproteins may cause hypoalbuminemia, hemorrhage, and fatty liver. Toxic actions that alter glucose synthesis and storage often lead to hypoglycemia and confusion, whereas effects on cholesterol uptake may produce hypercholesterolemia. Altered biotransformation or biliary excretion of endogenous substrates such as steroid hormones or bilirubin may affect a wide variety of hormonal functions or cause jaundice.

As previously noted, a variety of membrane and cytosolic enzymes in the liver provide the essential metabolic functions of oxidation as well as glucuronide, sulfate, and mercapturate conjugation for removal of toxicants. These reactions usually detoxify compounds, but occasionally metabolic products exhibit enhanced toxicity. Interactions can occur among effects of toxicants within the liver through induction of enzymes or depletion of metabolic resources. As an example, acetaminophen has been widely used without adverse effect as an over-the-counter analgesic. However, in circumstances of glutathione depletion, which occurs with large overdose, malnutrition, or CYP2E1 induction by long-term ethanol use, a reactive, electrophilic intermediate forms in sufficient amounts to produce covalent adducts that severely damage the liver (see Chapter 21).

The kidney plays a vital role in regulating extracellular fluid and excreting soluble wastes through filtration of blood, concentration of wastes, and elimination. To accomplish these vital functions, nephrons are composed of vascular, glomerular, and tubular components. The kidneys possess metabolic and regenerative capabilities, but these resources lead to renal failure when overwhelmed. Nephrotoxicity can be classified as acute or chronic.[29] Acute renal failure can be caused by hypoperfusion from renal vasoconstriction, as elicited by the antifungal amphotericin B, or hypofiltration through glomerular injury resulting from cyclosporine and aminoglycosides. A number of compounds, including nonsteroidal antiinflammatory drugs (NSAIDs), various antibiotics, and heavy metals, cause acute renal failure by nephritis, acute tubular necrosis, or obstruction. Causes of chronic renal failure from many of these toxicants include nephritis from inflammatory and immunologic mechanisms and papillary necrosis through ischemia or cellular injury. Compensatory mechanisms may include hypertrophy and induction of metallothionein synthesis in response to heavy metal exposure.

PREVENTION AND MANAGEMENT OF POISONING

Prevention of chemical toxicity is a responsibility of the entire community. Governmental agencies and private corporations must act in concert to minimize toxic hazards in the workplace and the environment. In the home, parents have a responsibility to protect children from harm as they explore their surroundings. Numerous sources of information are available to aid families in protecting against accidental poisoning. Steps can be taken by practitioners to limit the possibility of accidental poisoning. Patients should be encouraged to keep all medications out of the reach of children, and drugs should always be kept in child-resistant containers. Information on the label of a prescribed drug should be understandable and include the name of the agent and clear directions for use. The prescribing doctor should always indicate the purpose of the medication in the label information on the prescription. This procedure helps reduce confusion about drugs in the medicine cabinet and facilitate rapid identification of the drug involved in cases of accidental ingestion. Patients should be instructed to discard unused medication rather than attempt self-medication with drugs remaining from a previous course of therapy.

Diagnosis and treatment of poisoning are the purview of the physician. Principles of therapy for poisoning are summarized in Box 52-3 and apply to the management of any drug overdose. However, a dentist may well be called on to provide emergency treatment of acute poisoning within the practice environment or because of training as a health care professional.

Box • 52-3

First Aid for Poisoning

1. Summon help.
2. Stabilize the patient.
3. Evaluate the cause.
4. Terminate absorption.
5. Consider specific antidotes.
6. Enhance elimination.
7. Provide for supportive care.

Principles of Therapy for Poisoning

Summon help

When acute poisoning is evident, contact help through the emergency 911 telephone service if available. For less critical situations, the community poison control center provides an invaluable service. These centers are equipped with extensive files describing the signs and symptoms of poisoning and recommended methods of treatment for most toxic substances distributed within the United States. Such poison control centers can be reached by telephone on a 24-hour basis, and phone numbers are usually published inside the cover of telephone directories. If the toxic reaction is serious, expert medical assistance should be sought immediately. Additionally, most major medical centers have drug information centers that provide information to practitioners about drugs and drug interactions.

Stabilize the patient

Give supportive therapy. Because hypoxia and shock are two common manifestations of serious toxicity, respiration and circulation must be monitored and assisted if required. For convulsions, physical protective measures may suffice along with the administration of oxygen to help avoid hypoxia. Intravenous diazepam is a drug of choice for pharmacologic control of continuing seizures.

Evaluate the cause

Proper therapy to eliminate exposure to the toxin or reverse its effects depends on identifying the poison. Questioning the victim or the victim's associates, searching for empty containers, or looking for physical signs on the patient (miosis or needle tracks for opiate or opioid overdose, burn marks in the mouth for ingestion of caustic chemicals) can be important in establishing the cause of poisoning.

Terminate absorption

Remove any obvious means of contact with the poison. For dermal exposure to chemicals, removal of contaminated clothing and repeated washing with soap and water are indicated. With ingested compounds other than petroleum products and corrosive substances, vomiting can be induced, but only in the conscious patient. Poison control centers are able to advise when to use emetics. Vomiting should not be induced for poisoning by petroleum products because of the risk of aspiration. Corrosive damage to the esophagus and gastric perforations may result from emesis induced for corrosive substances. Syrup of ipecac is normally the agent of choice for emesis because, although it requires approximately 20 minutes to act, its effect is self-limiting because the drug is regurgitated with the poison. For home use, a small volume of ipecac can be purchased without a prescription. Depending on body weight, 15 to 30 ml followed closely by a glass of warm water is sufficient. In the unresponsive patient, the induction of vomiting is contraindicated, but gastric lavage can be used by qualified personnel if care is taken to avoid aspiration of stomach contents by the victim. The binding of many drugs within the gastrointestinal tract can be achieved by activated charcoal (10 to 50 g in water), and cathartics may be used to hasten the exit of drugs from the intestine.

Consider specific antidotes
Specific antidotes are available to treat poisoning by certain classes of compounds. Antidotes may be useful in preventing the absorption of ingested agents (e.g., Ca^{++} salts for F^{-}), increasing their rate of elimination (e.g., dimercaprol for inorganic mercury), blocking specific receptors (e.g., naloxone for morphine), or blocking other toxic activity (e.g., *N*-acetylcysteine for acetaminophen overdose). One specific antidote should be remembered by dentists. For ingestion of toxic amounts of fluoride, which might occur with prescribed tablets or with topical liquids or gels, the local antidote to prevent absorption is Ca^{++} (in milk, calcium lactate, calcium gluconate, or lime water). If necessary, 2 to 10 ml of 10% calcium gluconate may be injected intravenously to bind fluoride and overcome hypocalcemia. Dentists who use benzodiazepines and opioid analgesics for conscious sedation must be familiar with the use of flumazenil and naloxone, respectively, to reverse respiratory depression caused by these drugs (see Chapters 13 and 20).

Enhance elimination
Measures to facilitate elimination of toxicants are in the realm of emergency care physicians; they are mentioned here for completeness. The renal excretion of weak electrolytes can often be accelerated by appropriate modification of urinary pH. Administration of an osmotic diuretic in conjunction with large volumes of water is helpful in promoting urinary excretion and reducing the renal concentration of nephrotoxic poisons. In some instances, peritoneal dialysis or hemodialysis may be useful.

Provide for supportive care
Medical assessment of poisoning and continuing treatment, as needed, should be provided by physicians, nurses, and staff in an appropriate health care facility. Professionals with a full range of medical treatment resources may be required to address additional sequelae during the course of recovery.

OCCUPATIONAL SAFETY IN DENTISTRY

Although dentistry is considered to be relatively "occupationally safe," a large number of potentially hazardous substances are used in the dental office or laboratory. Additionally, dental environments may provide exposure to radiation or to blood-borne pathogens. Since 1988 the Occupational Safety and Health Administration (OSHA) has been writing, implementing, and enforcing regulations designed to ensure that employees are informed of hazardous materials in their work environment and given appropriate instruction in the risks and handling of these materials. The primary components of this program include (1) labeling of containers for materials, (2) on-site maintenance of material safety data sheets for materials used in the workplace that contain hazardous chemicals, and (3) employee education and training. For dentistry, the OSHA regulations and guidelines include potential exposures to blood-borne pathogens and biologic agents in addition to chemicals. To assist in fulfilling the requirements of the OSHA regulations, the American Dental Association has published a video seminar program and manual detailing OSHA standards and guidelines.[1]

To meet OSHA regulations, drugs and chemicals must be labeled with the name of the chemical, appropriate risk warnings, and the name and address of the manufacturer or other responsible party. If a hazardous material is transferred to another container at any time other than for immediate use, an appropriate label must be affixed to the new container.

Material safety data sheets are central to the safety program and are the primary source of risk and hazard information. These sheets are required to be provided by the manufacturer on request and must identify the hazardous substances included in the preparation, the physical and chemical characteristics, the fire and explosion danger, and other health-hazard data. They must also provide information on handling, storage, cleanup, disposal, and emergency and first aid procedures. These sheets must be present in the workplace and available to employees at all times. Dentists are required to provide appropriate training for employees in the use and management of hazardous substances when they are hired, whenever new hazardous substances are brought into the workplace, and when new information regarding the use of existing substances becomes available.

SPECIFIC TOXICANTS

The following sections discuss the toxic effects of several classes of substances. Included in each are agents that illustrate general principles presented earlier and that have public health importance or importance in the practice of dentistry.

Metals
Metals as a class are toxic primarily because of their ability to bind with biologic structures such as thiol groups in enzymes and other proteins. The major effect in human beings is the inhibition of enzyme function. Because of this binding affinity, the effect of metals may be widespread in the organism, but usually a primary or most sensitive system in which clinical manifestations may be detected is evident. Metals as a class are important because of their ubiquitous nature in both modern medicine and technology and in nature. Two metals of importance in both public health and dental practice are mercury and lead.

Mercury
Mercury is present virtually everywhere in the environment. An estimated 2700 to 6000 tons are released annually from the oceans and the earth's crust into the atmosphere.[1] An additional 2000 to 3000 tons are released through human activities, including the burning of fossil fuels. Mercury exists in three chemical classes: elemental mercury, which is a liquid at room temperature and is used as a primary component in dental amalgam (Hg^0); inorganic mercury salts; and organic mercury salts. Inorganic mercury salts may exist as mercurous (Hg^{+}) or mercuric (Hg^{++}) forms. Of the many organic forms of mercury, methylmercury is the most important toxicologically because of its ability to permeate membranes and the blood-brain barrier, its potency for biologic damage, and its widespread use in human activities.[56]

Mercury toxicity provides an interesting example of several important toxicologic principles. The first is that a single substance may produce differing effects depending on presentation to the organism. Elemental mercury, for example, is essentially nontoxic when ingested because of a lack of absorption in the gastrointestinal tract. Yet it may be toxic when injected subcutaneously.[74] Additionally, because of its high vapor pressure, it vaporizes readily and is easily inhaled. When inhaled it is absorbed readily into the blood, with absorption rates estimated at between 74% to nearly 100% of inhaled dose.[23,35] Once in the blood it is oxidized and is available for binding to enzymes and other proteins, producing toxic effects. Another important principle demonstrated by Hg is that when a substance can exist in different chemical forms, the forms may present strikingly different health effects. For example, organic mercury typically produces signs of toxicity that are neurologic in nature, whereas inorganic salts often produce gastrointestinal destruction and, secondarily, nephritis. These effects are discussed further below.

Inorganic mercury salts are used widely in industry; mercuric chloride is an example of a mercury compound with a wide variety of industrial uses. These compounds, unlike organic mercury compounds, are not well absorbed through the gastrointestinal tract and do not readily cross biologic membranes once absorbed. Only approximately 10% of an inorganic mercury dose is absorbed through the gastrointestinal tract, compared with more than 90% of a dose of methylmercury ingestion.[30] Nevertheless, inorganic salts such as mercuric chloride are severely corrosive to tissue and once absorbed produce toxic effects through binding of enzymes. Inorganic mercury compounds have been used medicinally and applied dermally in makeup for hundreds of years until recent times. Calomel (a cathartic) and mercurochrome (an antiseptic) are common examples of these. Virtually all such uses have been discontinued.

Organic mercury compounds represent the most important form of mercury from a toxicologic perspective. This is particularly true of methylmercury because of its widespread use and because it is a byproduct of many industrial processes. Organic mercury is known to accumulate in the food chain, and this is particularly evident in seafood, where the pelagic and top-level predators accumulate significant amounts of methylmercury in their flesh.

A number of tragic, inadvertent organic mercury poisonings have occurred in modern times. Two incidents are particularly well documented. From 1932 to 1968, the Chisso Corporation, a company located in Kumamoto, Japan, dumped an estimated 27 tons of mercury compounds into Minamata Bay. Kumamoto is a small town approximately 570 miles southwest of Tokyo. The town consists of mostly farmers and fisherman whose normal diet included fish from the bay. Symptoms of methylmercury poisoning unexpectedly developed in thousands of these people. The illness became known as "Minamata disease." Methylmercury has also been widely used to prevent grain spoilage through its antifungal effect. The second major outbreak occurred in the early 1970s when more than 500 people died and many others were made severely ill in Iraq when grain seed treated with methylmercury was inadvertently ground into flour and consumed. In both of these instances, because organic mercury readily crosses the blood-brain and placental barriers, a significant number of fetal deaths and teratogenic results occurred.

Elemental mercury (Hg^0) is the form of concern in dentistry because it is a primary component of dental amalgam, comprising approximately 50% by volume of the material. The greatest risk of exposure from elemental mercury is by inhalation of the vapor. Elemental mercury vapor is highly lipid soluble and therefore readily crosses membranes. This gives it ready access to the CNS as well as other body components, where it is easily oxidized to the mercuric form. Acute, high-level exposure to Hg^0 vapor produces corrosive inflammation of the upper and lower respiratory tract as well as nephrotoxic and CNS effects. Long-term exposure to low or moderate levels of elemental mercury vapor damages enzymes and structural proteins in the CNS, resulting in blockage of neuromuscular and synaptic transmission. Figure 52-2 shows the currently known range of effects based on urinary mercury concentrations. Urinary mercury concentration is considered a reasonable indicator of recent elemental mercury exposure, but because mercury is sequestered in organ systems, urinary mercury concentration is not a true indicator of total body burden.[45] Although the three forms of mercury (inorganic, organic, and elemental) produce differing toxicologic effects, the two major target organs of any mercury exposure are the CNS and the kidneys.

The earliest indicators of CNS effects of mercury exposure are not always clinically evident yet are measurable with neurobehavioral testing.[5,15] As exposure increases, behavioral changes may be noticed, such as irritability, memory disturbances, personality changes, drowsiness, or depression. Fine muscle tremors are noted, especially of the fingers, eyelids, and lips, and this loss of neuromuscular control increases as exposure levels increase. Renal damage in the form of tubular necrosis increases in a dose-dependent manner. Oral manifestations of mercury intoxication include hypersalivation, gingivitis, and gingival discoloration. Cases of periodontal destruction with tooth loss have been reported at high levels of exposure.[34,47] Also present at high levels of exposure is a yellow-brown discoloration of the lens of the eye.

Mercury in dentistry

Since the introduction of mercury amalgam into dentistry in the early nineteenth century, concerns about its safety have been expressed from time to time. Claims of toxic effects cover virtually the entire spectrum of disease, and a vocal "antiamalgam" contingent currently exists. Much of the confusion regarding the potential health effects of mercury exposure from dental sources is caused by false claims and by flawed studies used to support these claims by antiamalgam proponents. Two areas of potential concern have been the subject of recent and ongoing studies. One is the potential occupational risk to dental personnel working with dental amalgam, and the other is to the consumer or patient who has mercury amalgam placed in the teeth as a treatment.

Both OSHA and the National Institute for Occupational Safety and Health have recognized the need to set occupational thresholds over which exposure must not take place for mercury. These organizations have set a threshold limit value of 50 μg of Hg^0 per cubic meter of air as a time-weighted average based on a 40-hour work week.[13] The World Health Organization (WHO) has set a more restrictive threshold limit value of 25 μg per cubic meter.[16] Elemental mercury, which is readily vaporized, can achieve concentrations as high as 2000 μg/m^3 in a closed room. Studies of ambient air mercury concentrations in dental offices have shown that, under conditions of careless handling of mercury, these levels can be exceeded.[65,68] These high concentrations may occur after contamination through accidental spills of Hg^0. Studies examining occupational exposure among dental personnel show that certain practices in dental offices—now considered outmoded—are the most significant contributors to occupational exposure. These include the use of squeeze cloths to

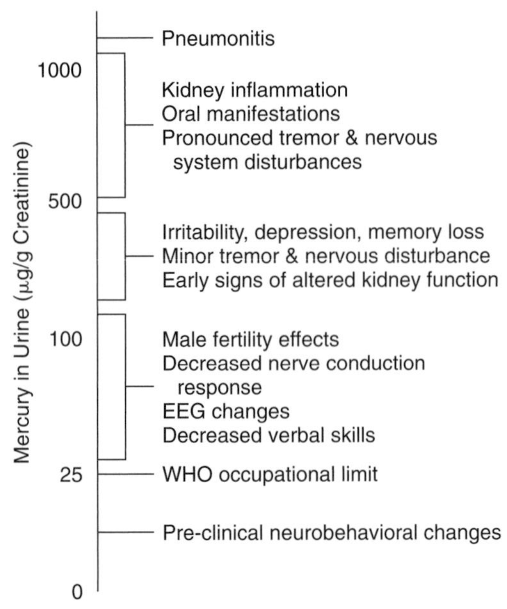

Fig. 52-2 Signs and symptoms of mercury toxicity relative to concentrations in urine. *WHO*, World Health Organization.

express mercury from amalgam; dispensing mercury from a central supply, which leads to accidental spills; and the use of office-prepared capsules.[46] Neurobehavioral changes can result from mercury exposure[15]; however, modern dental offices that have good mercury hygiene practices pose minimal risk to dental personnel. Excellent mercury hygiene remains vital to preventing unnecessary exposure.

With regard to mercury exposure that patients receive from the placement of amalgams in the course of treatment, anecdotal claims of disease states of every sort attributed to such exposure have been reported. Although rare individuals may be sensitive to very low level mercury exposure, little or no valid scientific evidence supports such claims. An important reason for the controversy is the reliance of some individuals on false claims and dubious studies about the dangers of dental amalgams. To date, no scientific studies have supported a health risk from dental amalgams to patients in whom these restorations have been placed.[44] The body of evidence also indicates no detectable negative effect on general health at the levels of mercury exposure produced by the presence of dental amalgam fillings, except in rare cases of allergy to amalgams.[13] Use of the mercury hygiene guidelines listed in Box 52-4 minimizes any exposure to patients beyond that which results from the amalgam itself.

Lead

Lead has been a toxicologic problem for human beings from the earliest times. It was found in early utensils and food storage and preparation vessels. It has been used extensively in plumbing, contaminating drinking water. Occupational exposures to lead occur in miners, smelters, and lead acid battery workers, but the most common chronic exposure is through diet. Perhaps the best recognized sources of lead exposure are from lead-based paint and combustion products of tetraethyl lead antiknock compound added to gasoline before the change to unleaded gasoline. Although Congress produced legislation limiting the lead concentration in paint to 0.06% in the 1970s, many older buildings still contain significant amounts of lead-based paint with very high concentrations of lead. A relatively small chip of this paint may contain up to 100 mg of lead. When consumed by a child, this amount exceeds the daily allowable intake by a factor of at least 30.[30] Because lead compounds that were included in paint formulas have a sweet taste, young children have frequently consumed these paint chips. (The condition of eating unnatural foods is called *pica*.)

Adults absorb approximately 10% of dietary lead, although children may absorb significantly larger amounts. With normal renal function, absorbed lead is primarily excreted by the kidneys. In the body, lead primarily concentrates in the hard tissues such as bone and teeth. Like mercury, lead produces toxic effects primarily by binding with proteins necessary for cellular function. Toxic signs exhibited at various blood levels are illustrated in Figure 52-3. One early effect of lead exposure is inhibition of the heme biosynthetic pathway. Intermediary products of heme biosynthesis called *porphyrins* are excreted in the urine in a characteristic pattern indicative of lead poisoning.[67]

Chronic lead poisoning, known as "plumbism," produces a spectrum of effects depending on the duration and severity of exposure. A microcytic hypochromic anemia may be produced early in exposure and cause lethargy and weakness. Neurologic effects may produce restlessness, irritability, hyperactivity and impaired intellect. Chronic low-level lead exposure can produce deficits in both gross and fine motor development as well as in cognitive and intellectual development. Early detection and management of lead exposure is crucial to prevent

Box • 52-4

Recommended Guidelines for Minimizing Exposure in the Dental Environment

1. Use precapsulated amalgam preparations only. Reclose disposable capsules after use.
2. Do not use squeeze cloths for expressing mercury from amalgam mix.
3. Monitor office levels of Hg^0 yearly or whenever contamination is suspected.
4. Use exposure badges that sample the air for Hg^0 concentration.
5. Provide periodic urinary mercury concentration testing for personnel.
6. If "free" mercury (rather than precapsulated) must be used to mix amalgam, store it away from heat in unbreakable, tightly sealed containers.
7. Store amalgam scrap in a sulfide solution (e.g., used x-ray fixer) or under water.
8. Do not touch amalgam with bare hands.
9. Use a rubber dam for restorative procedures.
10. Use a high-velocity vacuum when manipulating the amalgam and vacuum and water spray when removing old amalgam restorations.
11. In the event of a mercury spill (even a small one) use a mercury spill cleanup kit (commercially available). Do not vacuum the spill because this will hasten the volatilization of the mercury into the air.

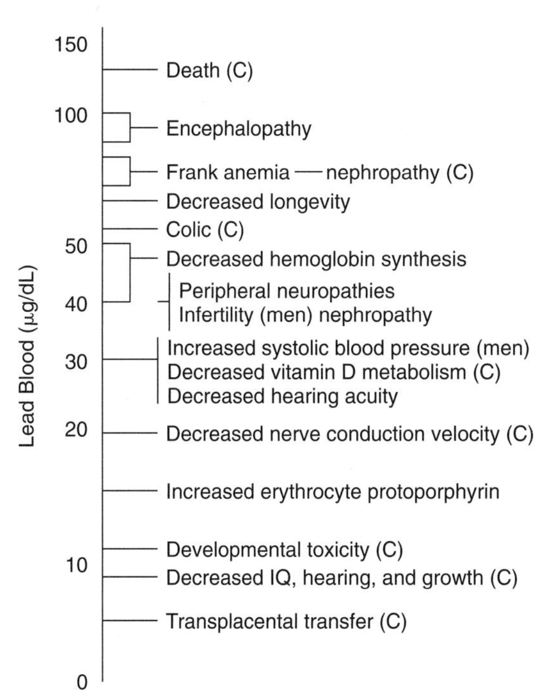

Fig. 52-3 Signs and symptoms of lead toxicity relative to concentrations in blood. Children are represented at the more sensitive end of the designated ranges. *(C)*—Denotes observations in children. (Adapted from Ellenhorn M, Schonwald S, Ordog G, et al: Metals and related compounds: lead. In Cooke D, ed: *Ellenhorn's Medical toxicology: diagnosis and treatment of human poisoning,* ed 2, Baltimore, MD, 1997, Williams & Wilkins.)

these permanent effects in children.[43] Peripheral neuropathies may be seen and are manifested as wrist drop, foot drop, and muscular weakness. Gastrointestinal signs such as intestinal spasms may progress to severe abdominal cramping with increased or continued exposure. The greatest threat from lead poisoning is encephalopathy, which occurs more often in children. Early neurologic signs and symptoms develop as described above and then progress to delirium, convulsions, and coma. As many as one fourth of those with lead encephalopathy do not survive, and up to 40% of survivors are left with severe neurologic dysfunction.[64,69] Lead is toxic to the kidney, and reversible tubular damage as well as irreversible interstitial fibrosis may be seen. Long-term exposure to lead is classically associated with a blue-black line that appears along the gingival margin. This deposit of lead sulfide is known as *Burton's lines* and, although associated with lead exposure, may also be caused by exposures to other metals such as silver, iron, or mercury. For treatment, removal of the subject from the source of lead exposure is paramount. Depending on the blood lead levels, chelation therapy is instituted according to protocols[17] for the treatment of lead poisoning recommended by the Centers for Disease Control and Prevention and the American Academy of Pediatrics. Succimer, edetate calcium disodium, dimercaprol, and penicillamine are all effective but differ in advantages of routes of administration and specificities relative to other essential trace metals.

Iron

The pharmacologic features of iron are discussed in Chapter 30. Iron is a heavy metal that is required to sustain life and is commonly used therapeutically. The daily adult consumption of iron is equivalent to approximately 15 to 40 mg of elemental iron, only a portion of which is actually absorbed. An allowance of 10 mg/day is recommended for children, with small additional increments during puberty to account for rapid growth. However, inappropriate levels of exposure can lead to significant toxicity. Iron toxicity can be either chronic or acute. More than 2000 cases of iron poisoning are reported in the United States each year. Chronic toxicity seems to be more common in people who have a genetic predisposition to absorb excessive amounts of iron taken orally. Pathologic changes include hemosiderin accumulation in the liver and spleen and hemochromatosis. Deferoxamine, a drug that selectively chelates iron (especially the ferric form) and removes iron from hemosiderin, is used to treat chronic toxicity.

Acute toxicity occurs most frequently in children, in whom accidental ingestion is most likely to occur.[21] The lethal dose of ferrous sulfate for a 2-year-old is approximately 3 g. The first signs of acute oral toxicity occur in the gastrointestinal tract. Vomiting and diarrhea are common. The vomitus may appear brown and the stool bloody. Gastric scarring can also occur. Acidosis and shock occur a few hours later. A delayed phase, occurring 24 to 48 hours later, is characterized by convulsions, cardiovascular collapse, and coma. Treatment consists of evacuation of the stomach contents by lavage or induction of vomiting. Support of the cardiovascular system and kidneys by maintaining blood pressure, plasma volume, and correction of acidosis is often necessary. Deferoxamine given intravenously or intramuscularly is effective in chelating iron after it is absorbed. Deferoxamine is not well absorbed by the oral route, and oral administration is not effective in preventing absorption of iron from the gastrointestinal tract.

Treatment of poisoning: heavy metal chelators

Chelators are compounds that form complexes with metal ions. The word *chelator* is derived from the Greek word *chele,* meaning *claw.* A chelator molecule binds a metal ion by two or more polar functions such as sulfhydryl, carbonyl, amino, or hydroxyl groups. These form bonds similar to those of the protein functional units attacked by metal ions. Through this action chelators spare endogenous ligands and promote excretion of metals as the chelator-metal complexes. Dimercaprol, succimer, and penicillamine are drugs currently marketed to promote the excretion of mercury, lead, and other metals. A few additional agents are available to treat poisoning by metals other than mercury, such as edetate calcium disodium for lead and cadmium, and deferoxamine for iron. Structures of these chelators are shown in Figure 52-4. Selectivity for metal ions varies among the chelators. Some such as edetate aggressively remove vital nutrient metals such as calcium and zinc. Such selectivity is important in the choice of the chelator, which should be matched for the heavy metal and circumstances of therapy. Selectivity of chelators for specific heavy metals is presented in Table 52-1.

Dimercaprol (2,3-dimercapto-1-propanol) was developed during World War II as an antidote for the arsenical gas lewisite, and thus it was formerly known as *British antilewisite.* Subsequently, dimercaprol was found to be an active chelator of a variety of heavy metals. Dimercaprol is prepared as a 10% solution in a peanut oil vehicle ***(beware of peanut allergy!)*** and must be injected intramuscularly. It is maximally effective when given shortly after an acute exposure to mercury; however, it is of some value even in chronic mercurialism. Dimercaprol is used with edetate calcium disodium in protocols for treatment of lead poisoning.[17] The drug is usually injected two to three times a day initially, with doses tapering off to once or twice a day over the course of about 10 days. The dimercaprol-mercury complex (actually two dimercaprol molecules to a single mercury atom) is excreted in the

Table • 52-1

Metals and Chelators that Enhance Excretion

METAL	CHELATOR	OTHER NAMES	ADMINISTRATION
Arsenic	Succimer; dimercaprol	Dimercaptosuccinic acid, DMSA; 2,3-dimercapto-1-propanol, BAL	Oral; IM
Cadmium	$CaNa_2$ EDTA	Edetate calcium disodium	IV infusion
Copper	D-Penicillamine	3-mercapto-D-valine	Oral
Iron	Deferoxamine		IM
Lead	Succimer; dimercaprol + $CaNa_2$ EDTA; D-penicillamine		Oral; IM + IV infusion; oral
Mercury	Succimer; dimercaprol; penicillamine		Oral; IM; oral

IM, Intramuscular; *IV,* intravenous.

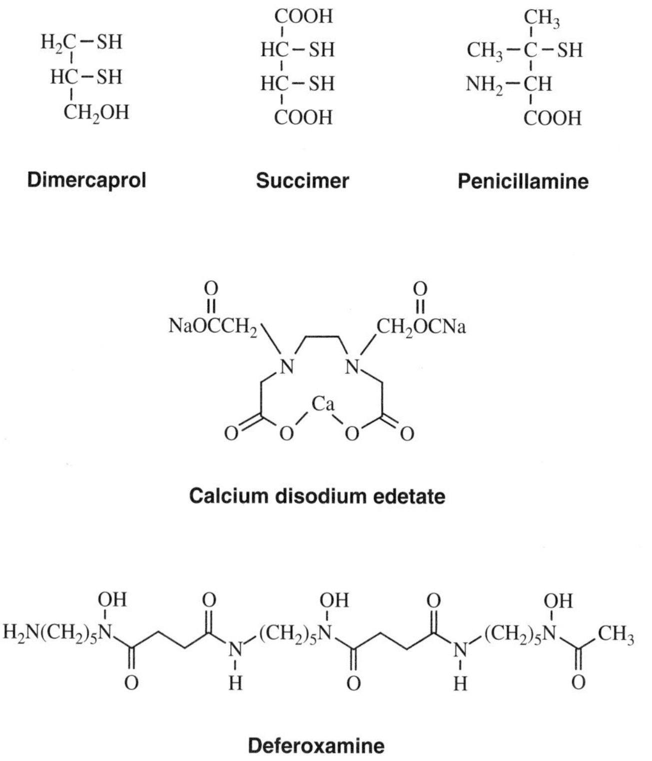

Dimercaprol **Succimer** **Penicillamine**

Calcium disodium edetate

Deferoxamine

Fig. 52-4 Chemical structures of chelating agents.

urine, which must be kept alkaline to avoid dissociation of the conjugate.

Succimer (*meso*-2,3-dimercaptosuccinic acid) is structurally similar to dimercaprol. This drug has the advantage of being effective after oral administration and being somewhat less toxic than dimercaprol. Succimer is more water soluble and is the drug of choice for the treatment of lead poisoning because it is more specific for lead chelation than edetate calcium disodium and removes fewer essential minerals such as calcium, copper, iron, and zinc. The dose for lead chelation is 10 mg/kg every 8 hours for 5 days, then 10 mg/kg every 12 hours for 14 days. In animal studies succimer was more effective than dimercaprol in alleviating acute toxicity and preventing distribution of orally administered mercury from mercuric chloride, particularly to the brain. Additionally, oral administration was more efficient than parenteral administration in reducing retention and organ deposition of oral mercuric chloride, probably because of decreased intestinal uptake.

Penicillamine (3-mercapto-D-valine) is a highly effective chelator of copper and is of primary importance in the management of Wilson's disease (hepatolenticular degeneration). Although less effective against other metals, penicillamine is often a useful drug for asymptomatic patients with a moderate body burden of metal because it is orally effective. Generally, 1 to 2 g/day is administered as needed for therapy of mercury poisoning. The penicillamine-mercury complex (also involving two drug molecules for each mercury atom) is excreted in the urine.

Edetate calcium disodium complex is a chelator for divalent and trivalent metals that can displace calcium from the molecule. Typically these include lead, zinc, cadmium, manganese, iron, and mercury. Edetate calcium disodium is poorly absorbed from the gastrointestinal tract and is therefore given intramuscularly or intravenously. Edetate calcium disodium must be used carefully according to suppliers' protocols because it can produce nephrotoxicity. Edetate calcium disodium can aggravate symptoms of severe lead poisoning, such as cerebral edema and renal tubular necrosis, and in high doses can lead to severe zinc deficiency.

Deferoxamine is a specific chelating agent for iron. It is available only for parenteral administration. The preferred route is intramuscular; acute iron intoxication treatment involves 1 g as an initial dose, followed by 500 mg every 4 hours for two doses and additional doses of 500 mg every 4 to 12 hours as needed based on clinical response.

Treatment of mercury poisoning

Therapy depends on the type of mercury poisoning. Exposure to elemental or inorganic mercury can be treated with dimercaprol (higher mercury levels) or penicillamine (lower mercury levels). Hemodialysis may be needed to protect the kidney. Succimer is also effective. For short-chain organic mercurials such as methylmercury, chelation therapy is not very effective, and dimercaprol is contraindicated because it concentrates mercury in the brain. Hemodialysis is not effective. Methylmercury can possibly be bound in the gut with a polythiol resin.

Gases

Perhaps no other toxic pollution issue stirs such universal concern as does air pollution because gaseous pollutants are dispersed over broad regions and inhalation exposure is insidious. Significant regulatory effort is devoted to decreasing air pollutants by the Clean Air Act, and general information is available from the Internet on topics important in the control of air pollution.[76] The US Environmental Protection Agency uses six "criteria pollutants" as indicators of air quality and has established a maximum concentration for each to preclude adverse effects on human health. The four gaseous criteria pollutants are discussed below; the remaining two are airborne lead and fine particulate material that is 10 μm or smaller in diameter.

Carbon monoxide

The origin of CO, a colorless, odorless gas, is incomplete combustion of carbon. The toxicity of CO results from its combination with Hb and exclusion of oxygen from this vital oxygen transfer mechanism. CO exhibits an affinity for Hb some 210 to 300 times that of oxygen, and the resultant complex with reduced heme iron, CO-Hb, is incapable of combining with oxygen.[85] The relationship between CO air levels and carboxyhemoglobin in blood can be predicted by the Coburn-Foster-Kane equation[71]; typical symptoms associated with varying carboxyhemoglobin levels are presented in the review of Von Burg.[85] The effect of carboxyhemoglobin on oxygen dissociation is shown in Figure 52-5.

Ozone

Ozone (O_3) is an odorless, colorless gas composed of three oxygen atoms. Typically O_3 is not emitted into the air but is created at ground level by photochemical reactions among nitrogen oxides and volatile organic compounds in the presence of heat and sunlight. O_3 occurs naturally in the stratosphere (approximately 10 to 20 miles above the earth) and forms a protective layer that absorbs the sun's harmful ultraviolet rays. In the earth's lower atmosphere and at ground level, however, O_3 is considered unhealthy because of its oxidative effects. Given its relative insolubility, inspired O_3 is carried deep into the lung, where it oxidizes membranes in the alveoli. O_3 irritates lung airways and causes inflammation, reduced lung capacity, and increased susceptibility to respiratory illnesses such as pneumonia and bronchitis. Other symptoms include wheezing, coughing, and pain with deep breathing. Oxidation products arising from O_3 reactions with lung proteins or lipids initiate a number of cellular responses,

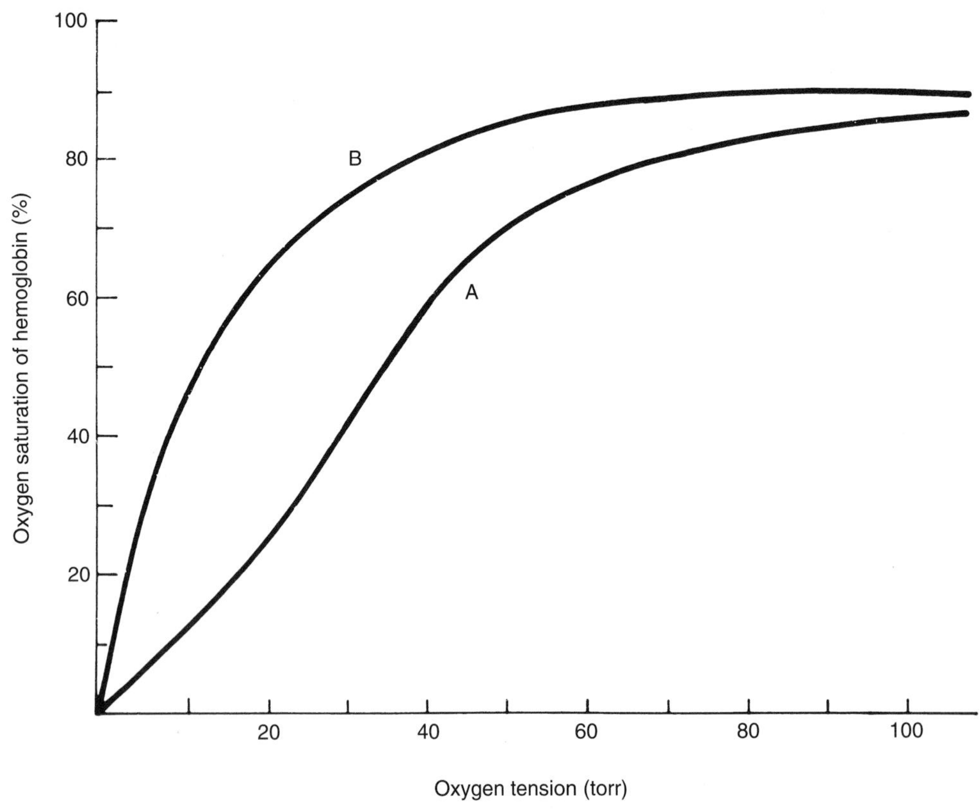

Fig. 52-5 Effect of carbon monoxide on oxygen dissociation. *Curve A* represents the normal desaturation curve for oxyhemoglobin and shows that half of the bound oxygen is made available to tissues as the oxygen tension (Po_2) falls to a little more than 30 torr. In the presence of 50% carboxyhemoglobin *(Curve B)*, the Po_2 must drop to a hypoxic value of 10 torr before a similar percentage of oxygen is released from its hemoglobin binding sites.

including generation of cytokines and expression of adhesion molecules. These responses promote an influx of inflammatory cells to the lung in the absence of a pathogenic challenge, resulting in modification of cellular tight junctions, increased lung permeability, and development of edema.[52] Persons with preexisting respiratory problems such as asthma or chronic obstructive pulmonary disease are most vulnerable. Repeated exposure to O_3 pollution for several months may cause permanent lung damage.

Sulfur dioxide

Sulfur dioxide (SO_2) is a colorless gas with a pungent, irritating odor. SO_2 is used as a preservative of fruits and vegetables, a disinfectant in wineries and breweries, and a bleaching agent in paper and textile industries. It is generated as an air pollutant by industry, such as high-sulfur coal-fired electric power plants, and is largely responsible for the environmental and public health impact of acid rain.[39] In contrast to the properties and site of impact of O_3, SO_2 is highly soluble in aqueous fluids and affects the upper respiratory tract. On dissolution, it forms sulfurous acid, which is extremely irritating to the nasopharyngeal and respiratory tracts. Acute exposure causes dryness of the nose and throat and a decrease in tidal respiratory volume. Coughing, sneezing, choking, and nasal discharge occur. Of note in dentistry, chronic exposure at levels causing these symptoms has been associated with dental caries as well as gingival and periodontal disorders. Patients noted rapid dental destruction, loss of restorations, and increased sensitivity of teeth to temperature change.[86]

Nitrogen oxides

Nitrogen dioxide (NO_2) is a brownish, highly reactive gas that is present in all urban atmospheres. The major mechanism for the formation of NO_2 in the atmosphere is the oxidation of the primary air pollutant nitric oxide (NO). Mixtures of nitrogen oxides (NO_x) play a major role, together with volatile organic hydrocarbons, in complex atmospheric reactions that produce O_3 and are important precursors to acid rain. NO_2 is relatively insoluble in aqueous media and decomposes in water to form nitric acid and nitric oxide, a potent vasodilator. When inspired, it reaches deep into the lungs. NO_2 can cause bronchitis, pneumonia, hemorrhagic pulmonary edema, and diffuse alveolar damage. Exposure also appears to lower resistance to respiratory infections. Acute exposure to nitrogen oxides causes a relatively rare condition known as "silo-filler's disease." Most cases involve young, otherwise healthy farm workers who enter silos freshly filled with corn silage without adequate ventilation. The most common presenting feature is dyspnea, but the disease was fatal in five of 20 cases recently reviewed.[90]

Liquids and Vapors

The organic liquid that presents the greatest risks to humans is ethanol. The toxicologic profile of this compound is unique among organic liquids and is presented in detail with other aliphatic alcohols in Chapter 43. Considered in this section are the organic solvents, including hydrocarbons and chlorinated compounds, and methyl methacrylate (because of its common use in dentistry). Structures of the compounds discussed are illustrated in Figure 52-6.

Solvents

Although transient exposure to solvents may occur in the home, more significant exposure most commonly occurs in the workplace. Exposure most often occurs through inhalation, with absorption through the skin also a common route

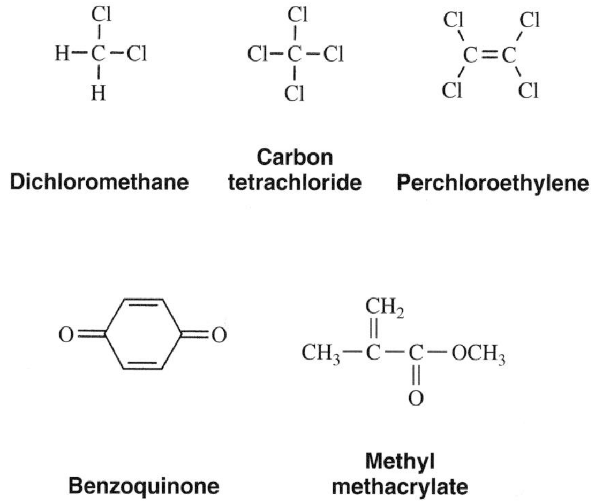

Dichloromethane | Carbon tetrachloride | Perchloroethylene

Benzoquinone | Methyl methacrylate

Fig. 52-6 Chemical structures of chlorinated solvents, the benzene metabolite benzoquinone, and the acrylic plastic monomer methyl methacrylate.

of exposure. Absorption from the gastrointestinal tract is variable. Compounds that are well absorbed, such as benzene or toluene, can produce significant systemic toxicity. Others, such as naphtha or gasoline, are not as well absorbed. A major risk from ingestion of these is the potential for pneumonitis as a result of emesis and aspiration.

Regardless of the site of absorption, the great lipid solubility of this group of compounds allows them to cross the blood-brain barrier very readily. Persons exposed to high concentrations of organic solvents usually demonstrate profound CNS depression. However, chronic exposure to lower concentrations of these chemicals produces toxic effects characteristic of the individual compounds.

Chlorinated solvents

Dichloromethane, otherwise known as *methylene chloride,* is a common solvent in paint remover and is used for liquid-liquid extraction in laboratories. Acute toxicity is caused by CNS depression, and fatalities have resulted from exposure. Symptoms include mental confusion, fatigue, lethargy, headache, and chest pain. Dichloromethane is metabolized to carbon monoxide. Evidence of its carcinogenicity, obtained in mice, appears to be related to metabolites formed by glutathione S-transferase and may be specific to the very high activity and localization of this enzyme in this species.[31]

Carbon tetrachloride is metabolized in the liver to a highly reactive metabolite (a free radical) that, in the presence of oxygen, reacts with proteins and lipids. The resulting hepatotoxicity may take days to develop and be accompanied by severe renal toxicity. Compounds that increase the rate of carbon tetrachloride biotransformation, such as cytochrome P450 enzyme inducers, increase the danger of toxicity. Substances that inhibit its metabolism are protective.

In a similar manner, perchloroethylene (also known as *tetrachloroethylene*) has been found to produce reactive metabolites that are thought to produce renal toxicity. This compound has also been associated with an increased risk of oral, laryngeal, and esophageal cancer in workers occupationally exposed to dry-cleaning processes that use perchloroethylene.[84]

Benzene

Benzene is another widely used industrial solvent commonly encountered in petroleum distillates such as gasoline. Benzene is considered a causative agent in human leukemia, probably through active hydroquinone or benzoquinone metabolites formed at oxidation.[36,48]

Methyl methacrylate

Methyl methacrylate is widely used in dentistry for the production of prosthetic devices and in orthopedic medicine as a luting agent. Although properly cured polymers from methyl methacrylate appear to be biologically inert, a number of adverse effects have been associated with the monomer. Exposure to the monomer can lead to toxicity and allergic reactions.[12] A slight and transient fall in blood pressure has occasionally been reported when methyl methacrylate was used to cement orthopedic devices. The assumption in these cases was that the effects were caused by absorption of the monomer into the patient's vasculature. Adverse effects have also been reported by operating room personnel where, because of improper mixing, concentrations of more than 200 ppm have been measured. Surgeons have developed contact dermatitis and paresthesias[24] and nurses have reported dizziness, nausea, and vomiting.

A survey of dental laboratories suggests that these were exposed to more moderate concentrations (5 ppm or less) of the monomer,[10] although peak concentrations can be double that amount.[54] Although the concentrations to which dental technicians are exposed are moderate, a study of dental technicians suggested that cutaneous absorption of the monomer, a result of dipping the fingers in the liquid to smooth and thus improve the finish of the polymer surface, caused a localized slowing of nerve conduction.[66] Other studies have found more generalized neuropathies attributed to methyl methacrylate exposure in dental technicians.[14,63] Additionally, cutaneous reactions have been reported from both monomer as well as "cured" methacrylate polymer.[41,57]

Pesticides

Pesticides represent a unique segment of the chemical market because these products are designed and produced for their toxic effects. Considerable efforts have been devoted to the concept of selective toxicity, in which products are developed with the objectives of toxic action on pests while affording some advantage to other species. In the United States, pesticides are regulated under the Federal Insecticide, Fungicide, and Rodenticide Act (FIFRA),[77] which delegates regulatory authority to the US Environmental Protection Agency (EPA). Before a pesticide can be legally used, it must be registered with the Office of Pesticide Programs (OPP). Pesticide registration is the process by which the EPA examines the ingredients of a pesticide; the site or crop on which it is to be used; the amount, timing, and frequency of its use; and storage and disposal practices. The EPA OPP evaluates each pesticide to ensure no adverse effects on human beings, nontarget species, or the environment under specified use before initial registration; older, previously registered pesticides undergo re-registration to assess health effects as new information becomes available.

Depending on the toxicity of the marketed product, pesticides are registered for general public use or are classified for restricted use only by a certificated pesticide applicator or under the direct supervision of a certified applicator. Pesticides are restricted from residential or institutional use if the product, as diluted for use, has an oral LD_{50} of 1.5 g/kg or less and restricted for other uses if the product, as diluted for use, has an oral LD_{50} of 50 mg/kg or less.

Certain pesticides have been banned or severely restricted for export or import through the auspices of the United Nations Environment Programme and the Food and Agriculture Organization, which developed internationally accepted guidelines for exchange of information on banned or severely restricted industrial chemicals and pesticides. These guidelines eventually evolved into the United Nations Rotterdam Convention on the Prior Informed Consent Procedure, which lists banned and restricted pesticides.[75]

The Food Quality Protection Act[78] of 1996 amended FIFRA to require evaluation of pesticide safety with consideration of potential aggregate exposures from both nondietary and dietary routes. From this mandate, pesticide registrations are being revised. The current status of pesticides is available electronically.[80] The EPA OPP maintains a web site with extensive information regarding pesticide use, regulation, data sources, consumer alerts, and educational materials[79] and has supported production of a manual, available electronically,[60] that is designed to provide health professionals with current information regarding health hazards of pesticides.

Insecticides

Most insecticides in common use by the public today fall into two classes based on their mode of toxic action. These are the anticholinesterases, characterized by their inhibitory action on acetylcholinesterase, and the pyrethroid insecticides, so named after their origin as pyrethrum extract from flowers of the genus *Chrysanthemum*. Organochlorine insecticides, such as DDT, were widely used from 1945 to 1969 but have been banned for use in the United States because of their adverse effects. These include their biologic and environmental persistence, biomagnification through diet in lipid tissues of higher organisms, demonstrated interaction with estrogen receptors, and enzyme-inducing properties.

The anticholinesterase insecticides are analogues of organophosphate or methylcarbamate esters. Representative structures are shown in Figure 52-7. The mechanism of action of anticholinesterase drugs is described in greater detail in Chapter 8. These compounds inhibit the hydrolytic action of the neurologically essential enzyme system, acetylcholinesterase.[50,59] Anticholinesterases interact with the enzyme in a manner similar to the endogenous substrate but with turnover numbers several orders of magnitude smaller than the substrate, acetylcholine. This leaves the enzyme phosphorylated or carbamylated and inactive regarding physiologic function. Poisoning results in great overabundance of acetylcholine at cholinergic receptors on autonomic nerves, at the neuromuscular junction, in the adrenal medulla, and in the CNS.

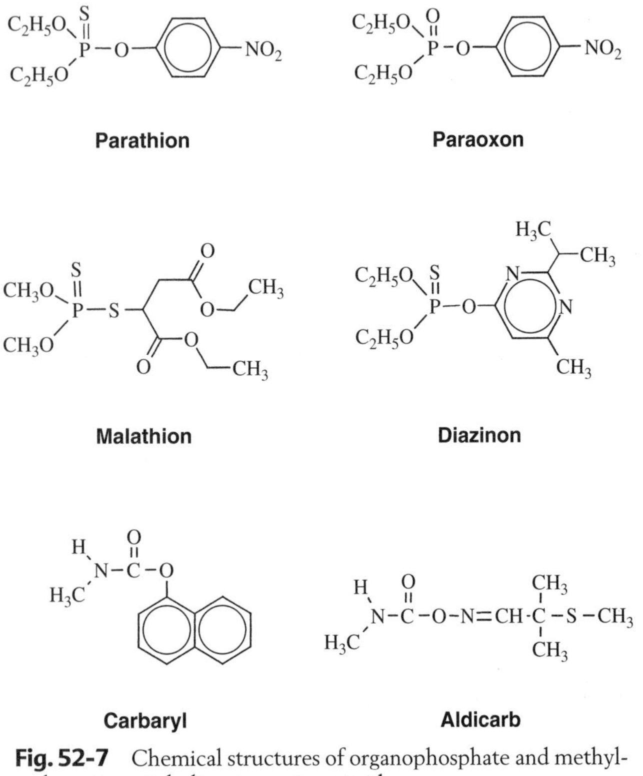

Parathion

Paraoxon

Malathion

Diazinon

Carbaryl

Aldicarb

Fig. 52-7 Chemical structures of organophosphate and methylcarbamate anticholinesterase insecticides.

Approximately 100 organophosphate-class insecticides are currently in use in the United States. Many are analogues of phosphorothioic acid; these are activated preferentially in insects to phosphate homologues by oxidative mechanisms. A classic example of differences in toxicity of thio versus oxo organophosphate homologues is exhibited by parathion (rat oral LD_{50}: 13 mg/kg)[26] versus paraoxon (rat oral LD_{50}: 1.8 mg/kg).[58] The venerable compound malathion has been used widely for nonagricultural applications, whereas chlorpyrifos, diazinon, parathion, and terbufos are now restricted to use only by certified applicators.

Of some 22 methylcarbamates in use, carbaryl (rat oral LD_{50}: 250 mg/kg)[83] has been used most widely in home and garden application. It is relatively nontoxic to mammals but is highly toxic to honeybees. In contrast, aldicarb, a methylcarbamate designed with molecular dimensions based on acetylcholine, is much more toxic to mammals (LD_{50}: approximately 1 mg/kg).[61] Aldicarb is available only to certified applicators; it is applied to the soil and taken up for systemic action in plants. Treatment of acute anticholinesterase poisoning by either organophosphates or methylcarbamates involves liberal use of anticholinergic drugs, particularly atropine, to antagonize muscarinic cholinergic signs. Pralidoxime has been used successfully to reverse cholinesterase inhibition when used early in cases of organophosphate poisoning but may aggravate poisoning with methylcarbamate insecticides.

The pyrethroids consist of a group of natural or synthetic compounds that modify properties of ion channels in nerves. Pyrethroids maintain Na^+ channels open for prolonged periods, leading to hyperexcitation of the nervous system. These compounds elicit repetitive nerve activity, particularly in sensory nerves, along with membrane depolarization, enhanced neurotransmitter release, and eventual block of excitation. These actions occur as a consequence of prolongation of Na^+ ion current in voltage-dependent Na^+ channels. The pyrethroids have remarkably selective toxicity for insects relative to mammals. They are largely contact insecticides with rapid "knock-down" properties. Natural pyrethroids (pyrethrin I, pyrethrin II) are short lived as a consequence of rapid oxidation and photodegradation in the environment and are rapidly hydrolyzed or oxidized when taken orally. These properties have resulted in rapid acceptance with minimal risk of use, but disadvantages are short duration of action and expense of natural product isolation. Synthetic pyrethroids are designed to be more persistent. These include two types, determined by the presence or absence of a cyano function. Two examples are shown in Figure 52-8. Of these, permethrin is stable to light and has low toxicity in adult mammals but is more toxic to neonates with undeveloped hydrolytic and oxidative mechanisms (rat oral LD_{50}: 1500 mg/kg for adults, 340 mg/kg to 8-day-old rats).[7] Other synthetic analogues substituted with a cyano group are more toxic. Cypermethrin, a cyano homologue of permethrin, enables comparison of the effect of the cyano modification (rat oral LD_{50}: 250 mg/kg for adults, 14.9 mg/kg to 8-day-old rats).[7] Occupational exposure to pyrethroid insecticides leads to temporary paresthesia and respiratory irritation. Treatment is generally supportive.

Organochlorine insecticides, once used extensively, are now only of historic importance in the United States, but some are still used in other regions of the world because of their low cost, stability, and efficacy. Structures of some of these organochlorine insecticides are illustrated in Figure 52-9. The prototype, DDT, earned the Nobel Prize for Physiology and Medicine in 1948 for Paul Mueller, who

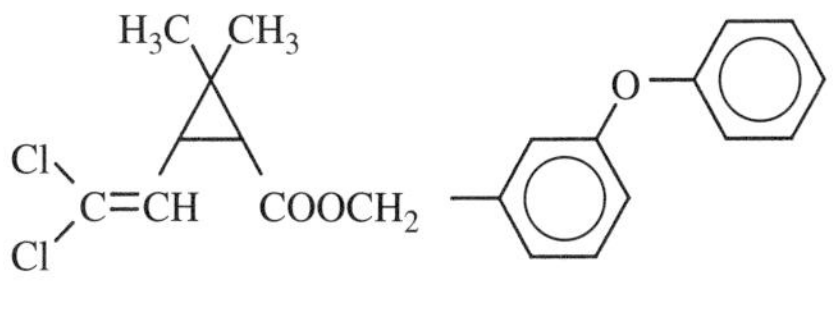

Permethrin

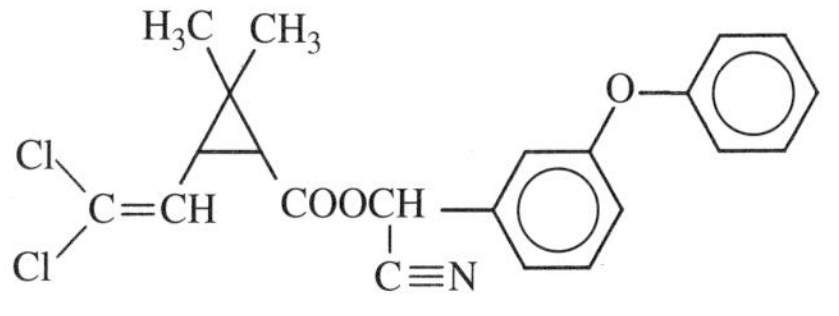

Cypermethrin

Fig. 52-8 Chemical structures of synthetic pyrethroid insecticides.

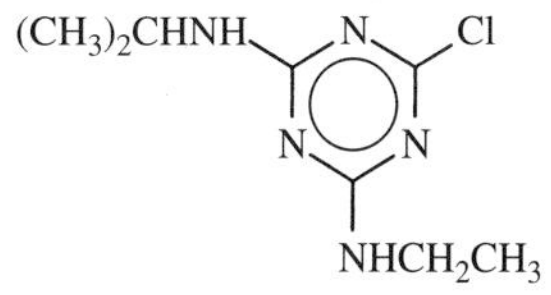

p,p-DDT **Lindane**

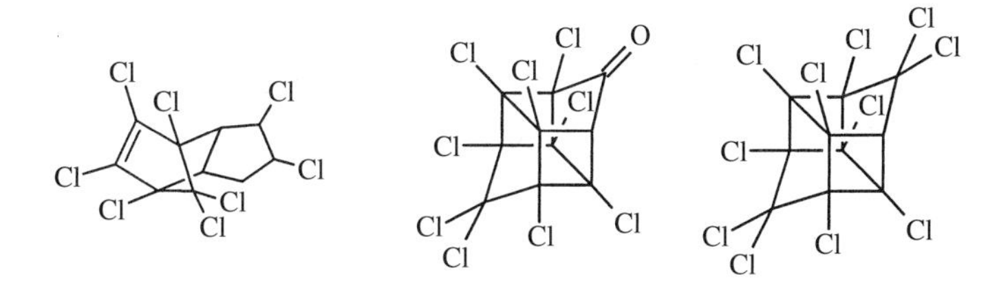

Fig. 52-9 Chemical structures of organochlorine insecticides.

Atrazine 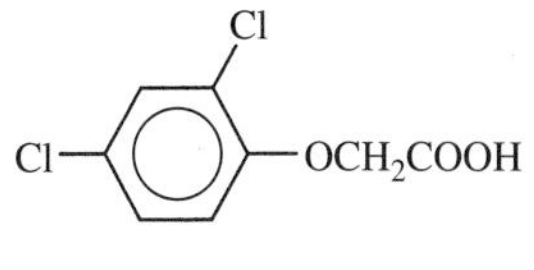 **2,4-dichlorophenoxyacetic acid**

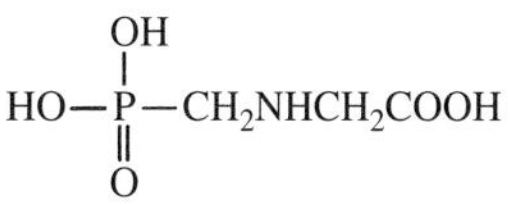

Glyphosate 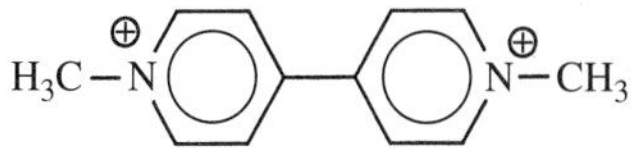 **Paraquat**

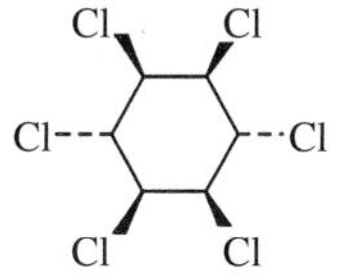

Fig. 52-10 Chemical structures of various herbicides.

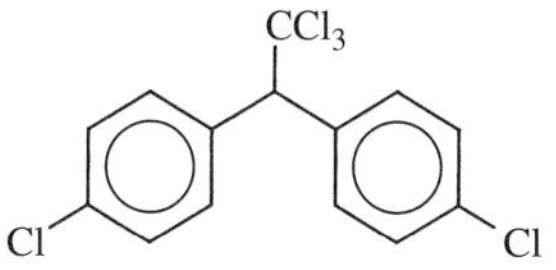

discovered the insecticidal properties. DDT is a member of the dichlorodiphenylethane subclass of organochlorine insecticides but is now restricted under the UN PIC (Prior Informed Consent) procedure.[75] The chlorinated cyclodiene structure subclass includes chlordane, dieldrin, and heptachlor, which also are restricted under the UN PIC procedure. Chlordecone and mirex represent another unique subgroup of cage-like, highly chlorinated C_{10} structures that are restricted from use. The hexachlorocyclohexane-type compounds include lindane, a specific insecticidal isomer that is still used in Kwell shampoo and topical creams as an ectoparasiticide and ovicide for crab and head lice, and in certain home and garden pest control products.

The toxic actions of organochlorines, like pyrethroids, alter conduction in the ion channels of nerves. DDT alters Na^+ and K^+ ion permeability, Na^+- and K^+-dependent adenosine triphosphatase (ATPase) and Ca^{++}-dependent ATPase functions, and inhibition of calmodulin in nerves. These actions reduce the rate of nerve membrane repolarization and increase sensitivity to small stimuli. The chlorinated cyclodienes are somewhat different because their actions appear to be more localized within the CNS. These compounds inhibit Na^+- and K^+-dependent ATPase and Ca^{++}-dependent ATPase and act as GABA antagonists, eliciting uncontrolled neurotoxic excitation.

Fumigants

Fumigants may be gases, volatile liquids, or solids that release toxic gas on treatment with water or acid. Typically fumigants are not selective in toxicity; rather they are used for their asphyxiant, highly reactive, or cytotoxic properties. Examples of gaseous fumigants include carbon dioxide, which is a relatively nontoxic asphyxiant; ethylene oxide, largely used as a sterilizing agent in the health care industry; and methyl bromide, previously in wide use as a soil fumigant but undergoing phaseout as an ozone depletory. Liquids include ethylene dibromide, bromochloropropane, 1,3-dichloropropene, and formaldehyde. Solids that liberate toxic gases for fumigation are zinc phosphide and aluminum phosphide, which produce toxic phosphine. Many of the fumigants form covalent adducts with important protein structures, including enzymes. 1,2-Dibromo-3-chloropropane, perhaps the best known occupational testicular toxin, has been banned for this action. Toxic effects of fumigants have been reviewed with particular attention to mutagenic activities.[22]

Herbicides

Herbicides are the most widely used type of pesticides. Given the broad use of these pesticides with apparently low relative risk in normal use, some herbicides in common use will be presented, with selection based on high usage or significant toxicity where evident. Research efforts by crop scientists in recent decades have produced diverse structures, many of which offer selective toxicity against weeds while sparing economic crops. An example is the use of herbicides in "no-till" production of grains, in which fields are sprayed to kill grasses and seeds are planted without the need for plowing fields. Structures of some herbicides are illustrated in Figure 52-10.

Atrazine is a member of the class of chemically similar compounds known as the triazine herbicides that block photosynthesis in plants. Atrazine is one of the most widely used agricultural pesticides in the United States. Approximately 80 million pounds of the atrazine active ingredient are applied annually to control broadleaf weeds in field corn and sorghum, in lawns and turf, and after production of wheat. Epidemiologic studies of workers exposed in chemical plants and farming populations have not shown a significant incidence of disease related to atrazine use, and little acute toxicity is evident in suicide attempts with atrazine. However, atrazine is currently undergoing review for re-registration by the EPA Health Effects Division.[82] This decision for re-review was based on the high volume of use, persistence of atrazine in surface and ground water, and recent research indicating that atrazine diminished secretion of hypothalamic gonadotropin-releasing hormone in rats. Previous work[9] indicated that atrazine altered luteinizing hormone and prolactin serum levels in two strains of female rats by altering the hypothalamic control of these hormones. Effects of concern are delayed ossification in offspring and prostatitis in adult male offspring through maternal exposure and transmission during gestation or lactation. A scientific panel advisory to the EPA convened to consider potential health consequences of atrazine exposure indicated that "... it is not unreasonable to expect that atrazine might cause adverse effects on hypothalamic-pituitary function in humans."[82] The re-review of atrazine is a work in progress at this writing. It has been included here to indicate the dynamic nature of assessment of potential hazards of chemicals by the agencies charged with this responsibility.

Glyphosate has broad-spectrum herbicidal activity, sometimes called "total kill," against a wide range of weeds. Glyphosate kills plants by inhibiting an essential plant enzyme involved in biosynthesis of aromatic compounds, which is absent in nonplant life forms. As a result, under normal use glyphosate is practically nontoxic to mammals, aquatic organisms, and avian species. Irritation of the oral mucous membrane and gastrointestinal tract was frequently reported with ingestion of the concentrate. Other effects recorded were pulmonary dysfunction, oliguria, metabolic acidosis, hypotension, leukocytosis, and fever. Various reviews, which indicated absence of toxicity in long-term animals studies of glyphosate, have recently been summarized.[87]

Chlorophenoxy compounds, typified by 2,4-dichlorophenoxyacetic acid (2,4-D) and 2-(2-methyl-4-chlorophenoxy) propionic acid, are used to control broadleaf weeds. They act as stimulants of uncontrolled growth in plants by mimicking and disrupting the actions of plant growth regulators such as indole acetic acid. In animals 2,4-D exhibits various mechanisms of toxicity, including uncoupling of oxidative phosphorylation, damage to cell membranes, and disruption of acetylcoenzyme A metabolism. Ingestion of large doses can cause nausea, gastrointestinal hemorrhage, hypotension, muscular twitching and stiffness, metabolic acidosis, and renal failure. Significant dermal exposure and occupational inhalation are associated with progressive sensory and motor peripheral neuropathy.[6] One analogue, 2,4,5-trichlorophenoxyacetic acid (2,4,5-T), was removed from use in the United States in 1979 because of its contamination with the toxic byproduct, 2,3,7,8-tetrachlorodibenzodioxin, as previously noted. The notorious herbicide used in the Vietnam War, Agent Orange, was a 50 : 50 mixture of 2,4-D and 2,4,5-T.

Nitrophenolic compounds formerly used as herbicides, such as dinitrocresol and dinitrophenol, are highly toxic to human beings and animals, with LD_{50} values in the range of 25 to 50 mg/kg.[60] These stimulate energy metabolism in mitochondria by uncoupling oxidative phosphorylation. This leads to hyperthermia, causing profuse sweating, fever, thirst, and tachycardia. Because of this toxicity the registrations for herbicidal uses of dinitrocresol and dinitrophenol, as well as other similar compounds, have been canceled. In contrast, certain dinitroaminobenzene herbicides, including butralin, oryzalin, and pendimethalin, as well as fluorodinitrotoluidine derivatives such as benfluralin, dinitramine, fluchloralin, and triflu-

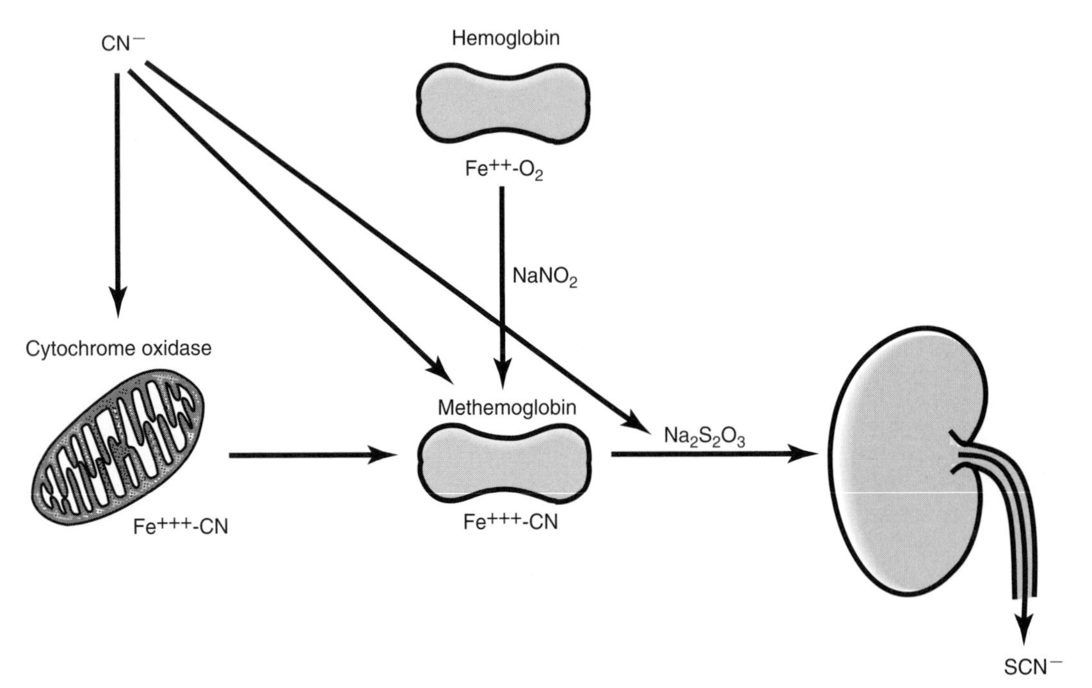

Fig. 52-11 Treatment of cyanide poisoning. Cyanide *(CN^-)*, whether inhaled or ingested, combines with ferric ions *(Fe^{+++})* in cytochrome oxidase to inhibit cellular respiration. Therapy is aimed at eliminating cyanide from the cells by a two-step process: (1) Sodium nitrite *($NaNO_2$)* is administered intravenously to oxidize the iron in hemoglobin from the ferrous *(Fe^{++})* to the ferric state; the methemoglobin thus formed then competes for cyanide, freeing cytochrome oxidase from attack by cyanide. (2) Cyanide is inactivated by the administration of sodium thiosulfate *($Na_2S_2O_3$)* to yield thiocyanate *(SCN^-)*, which is readily excreted in the urine. Experimentally, these steps reduce the lethal potency of cyanide by 80%.

ralin, do not uncouple oxidative phosphorylation or generate methemoglobinemia. These herbicides inhibit cell division in plants. Acute oral LD_{50} values are equal to or greater than that of fluchloralin (1550 mg/kg), and some are greater than 10,000 mg/kg.

Paraquat is the most important dipyridyl herbicide for consideration because it has delayed, severe, and specific pulmonary toxicity. Paraquat exhibits its particular and unique toxicity (LD_{50} in human beings of approximately 3 to 5 mg/kg)[60] in part because of its selective accumulation in lung tissue by a diamine transport system located in the alveolar epithelium. Additionally, paraquat is involved in a single-electron cyclic reduction–oxidation reaction that attacks unsaturated lipids in membranes to form lipid peroxides.[70] The oxidative destruction, and subsequent fibrotic lesions developed during reparative processes, lead to severely diminished lung function, anoxia, and death a period of days after ingestion of paraquat. The comprehensive treatise of Ellenhorn presents pharmacokinetic plots indicating likely survival or death based on blood concentrations versus time after ingestion.[18]

Predicides

Predicides are pesticides used to control predatory animals such as coyote, fox, and wild dog populations that are likely to prey on livestock, poultry, or endangered species or that are vectors of communicable diseases. Sodium cyanide, which liberates hydrogen cyanide, is one such predicide, and this is the only current registered use for sodium cyanide as a pesticide. Because of its extreme toxicity, sodium cyanide is restricted to use only by trained applicators. Cyanide inactivates cellular oxidative phosphorylation by binding to the Fe^{+++} in the cytochrome a-a_3 complex. The inability of cells to use oxygen, particularly in the brain and heart, is rapidly lethal to warm-blooded animals. Therapy for poisoning involves treatment with 100% oxygen and rapid provision of an alternative, less critical source of Fe^{+++} for cyanide binding. This is accomplished by inducing methemoglobinemia by administering amyl nitrite or sodium nitrite. This is followed by treatment with sodium thiosulfate solution to assist conversion of cyanide to thiocyanate by the mitochondrial enzyme rhodanese (Figure 52-11).

Rodenticides

A variety of compounds have been used to attack rodents. Some are quite toxic to rodents, human beings, and wildlife through acute exposure, whereas others require multiple doses to elicit significant toxicity. The majority of these act as anticoagulants, and their structures are shown in Figure 52-12. The oldest, warfarin, is a coumarin derivative that has been used as a rodenticide since 1950. Warfarin derives its action through antagonism of vitamin K action as a cofactor in synthesis of coagulation factors (see Chapter 31). Warfarin exhibits LD_{50} values in the range of 9 to 100 mg/kg in rats, with females being more susceptible.[3] Other multiple-dose anticoagulants are derivatives of 1,3-indandione. These include diphacenone (LD_{50} approximately 2.5 mg/kg) and chlorophacinone (LD_{50} approximately 6.2 mg/kg). Resistant strains of rodents have emerged, which has led to development of new hydroxycoumarin derivatives (so-called "superwarfarins") that are much more potent and do not require repeated doses to kill. Brodifacoum (LD_{50} approximately 0.5 mg/kg) and bromadiolone (LD_{50} approximately 0.7 mg/kg) are characterized as single-dose in use.[77] Necropsies after poisonings support the diagnosis of coagulopathy with findings of hemoperitoneum, hemothorax, and pulmonary hemorrhage. Given the increased potency and increased duration of action in some of these newer rodenticides, poisoning has occurred in pets, wildlife, and exposed human beings.[73] Treatment is based on assessment of prothrombin time, which should be monitored at 24 and 48 hours after ingestion. If prothrombin time is elevated at these times, treatment with phytonadione (phylloquinone, vitamin K_1) should be instituted with continued assessment of prothrombin time over a 4- to 5-day period.[60] Other compounds in use as single-dose rodenticides include strychnine, zinc phosphide, and bromethaline, which is a dinitroaniline derivative that uncouples oxidative phosphorylation.[81]

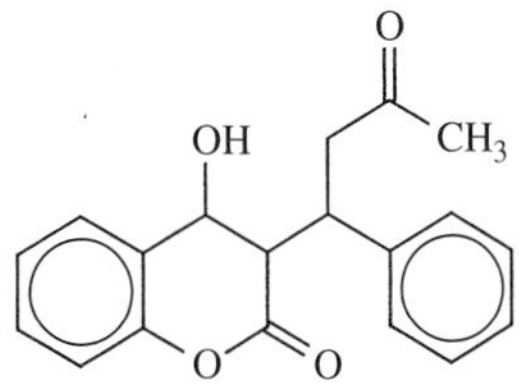

Warfarin

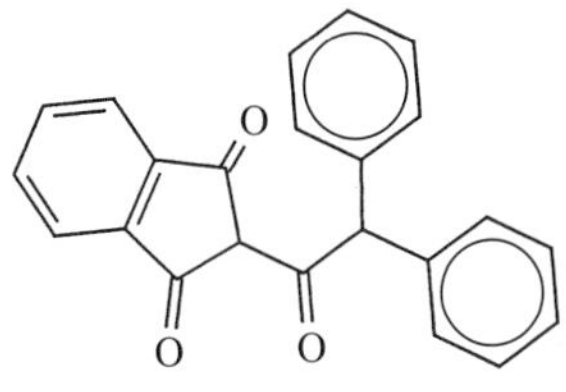

Diphacinone

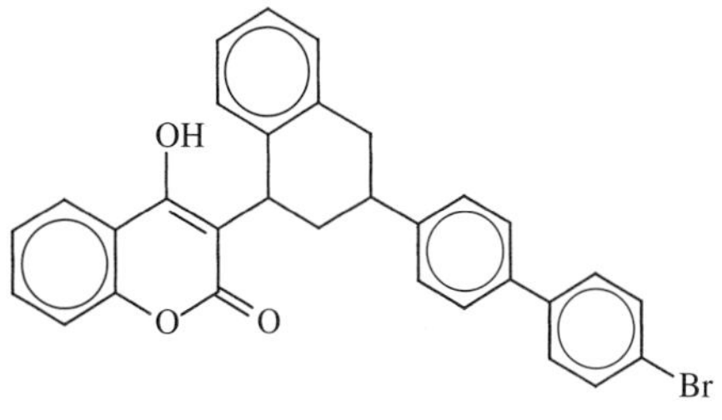

Brodifacoum

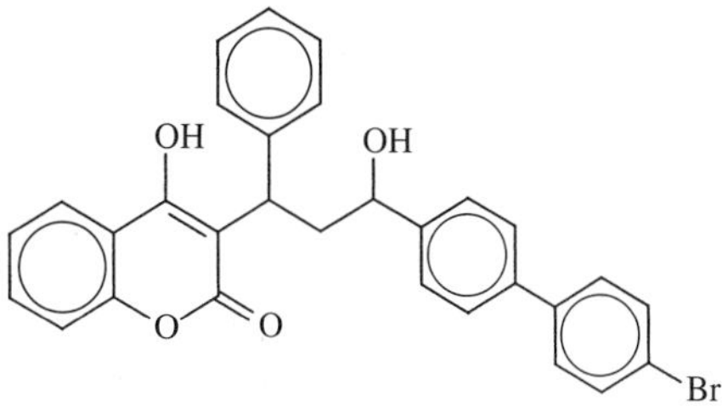

Bromadiolone

Fig. 52-12 Chemical structures of anticoagulant rodenticides.

Cited References

1. American Dental Association: *OSHA: what you must know,* Chicago, 1992, American Dental Association.
2. Ashworth L: Is my antihistamine safe? *Home Care Provid* 2:117-120, 1997.
3. Back N, Steger R, Glassman JM: Comparative acute oral toxicity of sodium warfarin and microcrystalline warfarin in the Sprague-Dawley rat, *Pharmacol Res Commun* 10:445-452, 1978.
4. Beutler E: G6PD deficiency, *Blood* 84:3613, 1994.
5. Bittner AC, Jr, Echeverria D, Woods JS, et al: Behavioral effects of low-level exposure to Hg^0 among dental professionals: a cross-study evaluation of psychomotor effects, *Neurotoxicol Teratol* 20:429-439, 1998.

6. Bradberry SM, Watt BE, Proudfoot AT, et al: Mechanisms of toxicity, clinical features, and management of acute chlorophenoxy herbicide poisoning: a review, *J Toxicol Clin Toxicol* 38:111-122, 2000.
7. Cantalamessa F: Acute toxicity of two pyrethroids, permethrin, and cypermethrin in neonatal and adult rats, *Arch Toxicol* 67:510-513, 1993.
8. Chemical Abstracts Service: Latest CAS registry number and substance count, http://www.cas.org/cgi-bin/regreport.pl, April 17, 2001.
9. Cooper RL, Stoker TE, Tyrey L, et al: Atrazine disrupts the hypothalamic control of pituitary-ovarian function, *Toxicol Sci* 53:297-307, 2000.
10. Cromer J, Kronoveter KA: *Study of methyl methacrylate exposure and employee health*, Washington, DC, 1976, US Government Printing Office.
11. Cupp MJ, Tracy TS: Cytochrome P450: new nomenclature and clinical implications, *Am Fam Physician* 57:107-116, 1998.
12. Danilewicz-Stysiak Z: Experimental investigations on the cytotoxic nature of methyl methacrylate, *J Prosthet Dent* 44:13-16, 1980.
13. Dodes JE: The amalgam controversy. An evidence-based analysis, *J Am Dent Assoc* 132:348-356, 2001.
14. Donaghy M, Rushworth G, Jacobs JM: Generalized peripheral neuropathy in a dental technician exposed to methyl methacrylate monomer, *Neurology* 41:1112-1116, 1991.
15. Echeverria D, Heyer NJ, Martin MD, et al: Behavioral effects of low-level exposure to elemental Hg among dentists, *Neurotoxicol Teratol* 17:161-168, 1995.
16. Eley BM: The future of dental amalgam: a review of the literature. Part 4: mercury exposure hazards and risk assessment, *Br Dent J* 182:373-381, 1997.
17. Ellenhorn M, Schonwald S, Ordog G, et al: Metals and related compounds: lead. In Cooke D, ed: *Ellenhorn's Medical toxicology: diagnosis and treatment of human poisoning*, ed 2, Baltimore, 1997, Williams & Wilkins.
18. Ellenhorn M, Schonwald S, Ordog G, et al: Pesticides: paraquat. In Cooke D, ed: *Ellenhorn's Medical toxicology: diagnosis and treatment of human poisoning*, ed 2, Baltimore, 1997, Williams & Wilkins.
19. Ellenhorn M, Schonwald S, Ordog G, et al: Respiratory toxicology: carbon monoxide. In Cooke D, ed: *Ellenhorn's Medical toxicology: diagnosis and treatment of human poisoning*, ed 2, Baltimore, 1997, Williams & Wilkins.
20. Evans WE, Relling MV: Pharmacogenomics: translating functional genomics into rational therapeutics, http://sciencemag.org/feature/data/1044449.shl, March 13, 2001.
21. Fine JS: Iron poisoning, *Curr Probl Pediatr* 30:71-90, 2000.
22. Fishbein L: Potential hazards of fumigant residues, *Environ Health Perspect* 14:39-45, 1976.
23. Friberg L, Nordberg G: Inorganic mercury: a toxicological and epidemiological appraisal. In Miller W, Clarkson T, eds: *Mercury, mercurials, and mercaptans*, Springfield, IL, 1973, Charles C Thomas.
24. Fries IB, Fisher AA, Salvati EA: Contact dermatitis in surgeons from methylmethacrylate bone cement, *J Bone Joint Surg Am* 57:547-549, 1975.
25. Fuhr U: Induction of drug metabolising enzymes: pharmacokinetic and toxicological consequences in humans, *Clin Pharmacokinet* 38:493-504, 2000.
26. Gaines TB: Acute toxicity of pesticides, *Toxicol Appl Pharmacol* 14:515-534, 1969.
27. Gallo M: History and scope of toxicology. In Klaassen C, ed: *Casarett and Doull's Toxicology: the basic science of poisons*, ed 5, New York, 1996, McGraw-Hill.
28. Gaylor DW: The ED_{01} study: summary and conclusions, *J Environ Pathol Toxicol* 3:179-183, 1980.
29. Goldstein R, Schnellmann R: Toxic responses of the kidney. In Klaassen C, ed: *Casarett & Doull's Toxicology: the basic science of poisons*, ed 5, New York, 1996, McGraw-Hill.
30. Gossel TA, Gricker JD: *Principles of clinical toxicology*, ed 3, New York, 1994, Raven Press.
31. Green T: Methylene chloride induced mouse liver and lung tumours: an overview of the role of mechanistic studies in human safety assessment, *Hum Exp Toxicol* 16:3-13, 1997.
32. Hecht SS, Hoffmann D: N-nitroso compounds and tobacco-induced cancers in man, *IARC Sci Publ* 54-61, 1991.
33. Hill A: The environment and disease: association or causation? *Proc Roy Soc Med* 58:295, 1965.
34. Hunter D: *The diseases of occupations*, ed 6, London, 1978, Hodder and Stoughton.
35. Hursh JB, Cherian MG, Clarkson TW, et al: Clearance of mercury (HG-197, HG-203) vapor inhaled by human subjects, *Arch Environ Health* 31:302-309, 1976.
36. Irons RD, Stillman WS: The effects of benzene and other leukaemogenic agents on haematopoietic stem and progenitor cell differentiation, *Eur J Haematol Suppl* 60:119-124, 1996.
37. Knight KR, Burdon JG, Cook L, et al: The proteinase-antiproteinase theory of emphysema: a speculative analysis of recent advances into the pathogenesis of emphysema, *Respirology* 2:91-95, 1997.
38. Langston JW, Ballard P, Tetrud JW, et al: Chronic parkinsonism in humans due to a product of meperidine-analogue synthesis, *Science* 219:979-980, 1983.
39. Lioy PJ, Waldman JM: Acidic sulfate aerosols: characterization and exposure, *Environ Health Perspect* 79:15-34, 1989.
40. Litchfield JT, Wilcoxon F: A simplified method of evaluating dose-effect experiments, *J Pharmacol Exp Ther* 96:99-113, 1949.
41. Lunder T, Rogl-Butina M: Chronic urticaria from an acrylic dental prosthesis, *Contact Dermatitis* 43:232-233, 2000.
42. Madani S, Howald W, Lawrence R, et al: Analysis of hydroxylated and N-dealkylated metabolites of terfenadine in microsomal incubates by liquid chromatography-mass spectrometry, *J Chromatogr B* 741:145-153, 2000.
43. Markowitz M: Lead poisoning: a disease for the next millennium, *Curr Probl Pediatr* 30:62-70, 2000.
44. Martin MD, DeRouen T, Leroux BG: Is mercury amalgam safe for dental fillings? *Washington Public Health* 15:30-32, 1997.
45. Martin MD, McCann T, Naleway C, et al: The validity of spot urine samples for low-level occupational mercury exposure assessment and relationship to porphyrin and creatinine excretion rates, *J Pharmacol Exp Ther* 277:239-244, 1996.
46. Martin MD, Naleway C, Chou HN: Factors contributing to mercury exposure in dentists, *J Am Dent Assoc* 126:1502-1511, 1995.

47. Martin MD, Williams BJ, Charleston JD, et al: Spontaneous exfoliation of teeth following severe elemental mercury poisoning: case report and histological investigation for mechanism, *Oral Surg Oral Med Oral Pathol Oral Radiol Endod* 84:495-501, 1997.
48. Mason DE, Liebler DC: Characterization of benzoquinone-peptide adducts by electrospray mass spectrometry, *Chem Res Toxicol* 13:976-982, 2000.
49. Massey JD, Moore GF, Yonkers AJ: Smokeless tobacco: a risk factor in oral cancer, *Ear Nose Throat J* 63:453-458, 1984.
50. Moretto A: Experimental and clinical toxicology of anticholinesterase agents, *Toxicol Lett* 102-103:509-513, 1998.
51. Moslen M: Toxic responses of the liver: In Klaassen C, ed: *Casarett & Doul's Toxicology: the basic science of poisons*, ed 5, New York, 1996, McGraw-Hill.
52. Mudway IS, Kelly FJ: Ozone and the lung: a sensitive issue, *Mol Aspects Med* 21:1-48, 2000.
53. Murray KM, Hedgepeth JC: Intravenous self-administration of elemental mercury: efficacy of dimercaprol therapy, *Drug Intell Clin Pharm* 22:972-975, 1988.
54. Nayebzadeh A, Dufresne A: Evaluation of exposure to methyl methacrylate among dental laboratory technicians, *Am Ind Hyg Assoc J* 60:625-628, 1999.
55. Okey AB, Riddick DS, Harper PA: The Ah receptor: mediator of the toxicity of 2,3,7,8-tetrachlorodibenzo-p-dioxin (TCDD) and related compounds, *Toxicol Lett* 70:1-22, 1994.
56. Ozuah PO: Mercury poisoning, *Curr Probl Pediatr* 30:91-99, 2000.
57. Pegum JS, Medhurst FA: Contact dermatitis from penetration of rubber gloves by acrylic monomer, *Br Med J* 2:141-143, 1971.
58. Pickering WR, Malone JC: The acute toxicity of dichloroalkyl aryl phosphates in relation to chemical structure, *Biochem Pharmacol* 16:1183-1194, 1967.
59. Pope CN: Organophosphorus pesticides: do they all have the same mechanism of toxicity? *J Toxicol Environ Health B Crit Rev* 2:161-181, 1999.
60. Reigart JR, Roberts JR: *Recognition and management of pesticide poisonings*, ed 5, http://www.epa.gov/oppfead1/safety/healthcare/handbook/handbook.htm, 1999, US Environmental Protection Agency Office of Pesticide Programs, April 17, 2001.
61. Risher JF, Mink FL, Stara JF: The toxicologic effects of the carbamate insecticide aldicarb in mammals: a review, *Environ Health Perspect* 72:267-281, 1987.
62. Robledo R, Mossman B: Cellular and molecular mechanisms of asbestos-induced fibrosis, *J Cell Physiol* 180:158-166, 1999.
63. Sadoh DR, Sharief MK, Howard RS: Occupational exposure to methyl methacrylate monomer induces generalised neuropathy in a dental technician, *Br Dent J* 186:380-381, 1999.
64. Sanford H: Lead poisoning in young children, *Postgrad Med* 17:162, 1955.
65. Schulein TM, Reinhardt JW, Chan KC: Survey of Des Moines area dental offices for mercury vapor, *Iowa Dent J* 70:35-36, 1984.
66. Seppalainen AM, Rajaniemi R: Local neurotoxicity of methyl methacrylate among dental technicians, *Am J Ind Med* 5:471-477, 1984.
67. Simmonds PL, Luckhurst CL, Woods JS: Quantitative evaluation of heme biosynthetic pathway parameters as biomarkers of low-level lead exposure in rats, *J Toxicol Environ Health* 44:351-367, 1995.
68. Skuba A, Matthew C, Goldhawk M: Survey for mercury vapour in Manitoba dental offices. Summer 1983, *J Can Dent Assoc* 50:517-522, 1984.
69. Smith H, Boehner R, Carney T, et al: The sequelae of pica with and without lead poisoning, *Am J Dis Child* 105:609, 1963.
70. Smith LL: Mechanism of paraquat toxicity in lung and its relevance to treatment, *Hum Toxicol* 6:31-36, 1987.
71. Smith SR, Steinberg S, Gaydos JC: Errors in derivations of the Coburn-Forster-Kane equation for predicting carboxyhemoglobin, *Am Ind Hyg Assoc J* 57:621-625, 1996.
72. Spencer PS, Sabri MI, Schaumburg HH, et al: Does a defect of energy metabolism in the nerve fiber underlie axonal degeneration in polyneuropathies? *Ann Neurol* 5:501-507, 1979.
73. Swigar ME, Clemow LP, Saidi P, et al: "Superwarfarin" ingestion. A new problem in covert anticoagulant overdose, *Gen Hosp Psychiatry* 12:309-312, 1990.
74. Teitelbaum DT, Ott JE: Elemental mercury self-poisoning, *Clin Toxicol* 2:243-248, 1969.
75. United Nations Environment Programme (UNEP) and the Food and Agriculture Organization (FAO): Substances subject to the PIC procedure, http://www.fao.org/waicent/FaoInfo/Agricult/AGP/AGPP/Pesticid/PIC/piclist.htm, April 17, 2001.
76. US Environmental Protection Agency: Air and radiation, http://www.epa.gov/air/, April 7, 2001.
77. US EPA Office of Pesticide Programs: Federal Insecticide, Fungicide, and Rodenticide Act (FIFRA), http://www.epa.gov/pesticides/fifra.htm, April 17, 2001.
78. US EPA Office of Pesticide Programs: Food Quality Protection Act (FQPA) of 1996, http://www.epa.gov/oppfead1/fqpa/, April 17, 2001.
79. US EPA Office of Pesticide Programs: Office of Pesticide Programs, http://www.epa.gov/pesticides/, April 13, 2001.
80. US EPA Office of Pesticide Programs: Pesticide reregistration status, http://www.epa.gov/pesticides/reregistration/status.htm, April 13, 2001.
81. US EPA Office of Pesticide Programs: Reregistration eligibility decision: Rodenticide cluster, EPA738-R98-007, 1998, http://www.epa.gov/oppsrrd1/REDs/2100red.pdf, April 17, 2001.
82. US EPA Office of Pesticide Programs: Atrazine. HED's revised preliminary human health risk assessment for the registration eligibility decision, 2001, http://www.epa.gov/oppsrrd1/reregistration/atrazine/revsd_pra.pdf, April 19, 2001.
83. Vandekar M, Plestina R, Wilhelm K: Toxicity of carbamates for mammals, *Bull World Health Organ* 44:241-249, 1971.
84. Vaughan TL, Stewart PA, Davis S, et al: Work in dry cleaning and the incidence of cancer of the oral cavity, larynx, and oesophagus, *Occup Environ Med* 54:692-695, 1997.
85. Von Burg R: Carbon monoxide, *J Appl Toxicol* 19:379-386, 1999.
86. Von Burg R: Sulfur dioxide, *J Appl Toxicol* 16:365-371, 1996.

87. Williams GM, Kroes R, Munro IC: Safety evaluation and risk assessment of the herbicide Roundup and its active ingredient, glyphosate, for humans, *Regul Toxicol Pharmacol* 31:117-165, 2000.

88. Witschi H, Last J: Toxic responses of the respiratory system. In Klaassen C, ed: *Casarett & Doull's Toxicology: the basic science of poisons*, ed 5, New York, 1996, McGraw-Hill.

89. Wright RO, Lewander WJ, Woolf AD: Methemoglobinemia: etiology, pharmacology, and clinical management, *Ann Emerg Med* 34:646-656, 1999.

90. Zwemer FL, Jr, Pratt DS, May JJ: Silo filler's disease in New York State, *Am Rev Respir Dis* 146:650-653, 1992.

CHAPTER • 53

Geriatric Pharmacology

Marc W. Heft and Angelo J. Mariotti

With the demographic change that has resulted in a "graying" of the population has come a compelling interest in the health and health concerns of older adults. The increasing incidence and prevalence of systemic diseases, especially chronic diseases, among older adults and the concomitant increase in medication use have provided impetus for the subspecialty of geriatric pharmacology. Although it has long been obvious that because children are smaller than adults some reduction of drug dosage is appropriate, it was not understood until recently how elderly patients differ from younger adults. In fact, some misconceptions about aging are widely held, such as the idea that senility or a progressive rise in blood pressure is a normal concomitant of aging. Furthermore, geriatric pharmacology did not emerge out of a specific incident, as occurred with the thalidomide disaster, which highlighted the fetus as an area of special concern for the pharmacologist. Rather, the field of geriatric pharmacology has developed out of changes in demography that have been accompanied by an increasing knowledge of and sensitivity to the special physiologic, pharmacologic, pathologic, psychologic, economic, and emotional problems of older adults.

In 1999 the elderly, considered persons 65 years of age or older, numbered 34.5 million and represented 12.7% of the United States population; by the year 2030, they will represent 20% of the population and number approximately 70 million.[18] Furthermore, not only is the total over-65-year-old group growing faster than the population as a whole, but between the years 2000 and 2030 the group aged 85 years and older will increase from 4.3 million to 7 million.[3,59]

Of special interest to the dentist is the fact that the newer cohorts of older adults are and will be in better oral health.[22] The rate of edentulousness has declined,[40,60,67] and the number of retained teeth among the dentate has increased.[30,38,40,60] With this trend among dentate older adults has emerged an understanding that this population has similar needs for routine restorative and periodontal treatments as do younger adults.[21,30,60] Accordingly, an increasing number of elderly persons will need the kind of dental treatment that was formerly rare in the elderly patient, treatment that will require, among other things, antianxiety drugs, analgesics, local anesthetics, and antiinflammatory drugs. The dentist will be confronted by an increasing number of ambulatory, community-dwelling elderly patients with a significant burden of systemic disease and medication use.

Normative aging studies have shown that the healthy elderly person is substantially and measurably different from his or her younger counterparts. Recently pharmacologists have begun to appreciate how these changes affect the pharmacokinetics and pharmacodynamics of drugs.

As people age, they are more likely to be seen at the dental office with a variety of diseases, especially chronic diseases, for which they take a number of drugs that are strong in effect and potentially toxic. Americans aged 65 years and older take a disproportionately high percentage of all drugs prescribed.[44] Furthermore, studies of ambulatory populations indicate that although 80% to 90% of older adults take at least one medication, most take two or more. The most commonly used drugs are agents affecting the cardiovascular system, analgesic and antiinflammatory drugs, psychotherapeutic medications, and gastrointestinal preparations such as laxatives and antacids. Approximately 40% of the medications are prescribed to patients to be taken "as necessary"—with an average of three drugs per patient.[47]

The number of medications prescribed to individuals of any age increases the risk of adverse drug reactions, drug interactions, and other health-related problems associated with the use and misuse of medications.[28,47] The potential problems in older adults are compounded by age-related physiologic changes that may place these individuals at greater risk. The misuse of medications among the elderly is considered a major health care problem.[20,42] Finally, many segments of our society, not the least important of which is the health care provider, have become sensitized to the nonmedical problems common among the elderly (loneliness, depression, poverty, poor nutritional status) and have come to understand how these can complicate therapeutic management.

This chapter presents a view of geriatric pharmacology that deals mainly with alterations in drug responsiveness that can be attributed directly to aging; it addresses only in passing those psychosocial factors that indirectly influence the way the elderly use and react to drugs.

PHYSIOLOGIC CHANGES ASSOCIATED WITH AGING

Studies of the aging process in community-dwelling, healthy (presumed disease-free) individuals have provided insights into the process of biologic aging. These studies have been either cross-sectional studies, in which different-aged persons are assessed at the same point in time, or longitudinal studies, in which the same individuals are assessed at different times as they "age in place." Although the former studies are easier and quicker to complete, they limit inferences to age differences rather than age-related changes because of the limitations in controlling for and measuring individual differences in biology and behavior. Results of both cross-sectional and longitudinal studies have reported a gradual decline in performance from the third decade through the seventh and eighth decades in a broad range of physiologic functions, including renal function, pulmonary function, cardiac function, and nerve conduction velocity (Figure 53-1).[53] However, findings from these studies have shown that (1) broad indi-

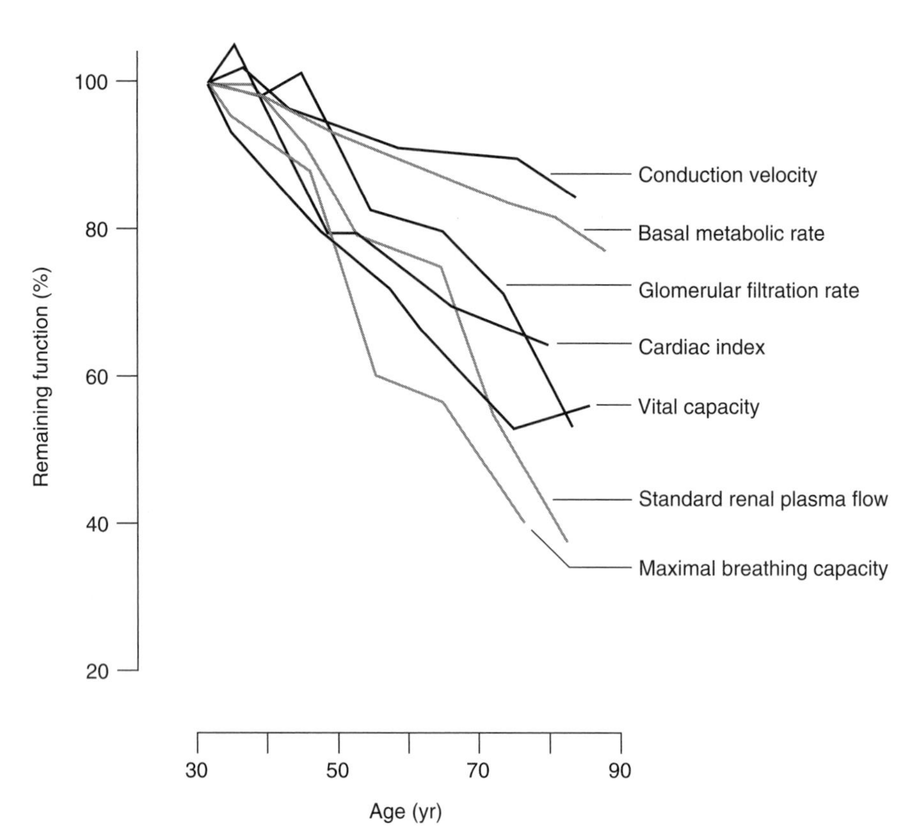

Fig. 53-1 Influence of age on measures of physiologic function beginning at age 30 (100% of remaining function). (From Miller RD: Anesthesia for the elderly. In Miller RD, ed: *Anesthesia*, ed 2, New York, 1986, Churchill Livingstone.)

vidual intersubject differences exist in the rate of aging; (2) not all organ systems age at the same rate; (3) the pattern of age-related declines in organ systems can vary among individuals; (4) with increasing age, greater variability in measures of organ function occurs among individuals within an age cohort; (5) age-associated declines are greater in more complex integrative functions (such as maximum breathing capacity) than in basic functions (such as the velocity of propagation of a nerve impulse along a nerve); and (6) the latency and capacity for achieving adaptive responses are, respectively, greater and smaller for older individuals than younger. Therefore variability is a cardinal feature of the aging process. At least some of the apparent decline in functioning may reflect changes in lifestyle rather than chronologic aging per se (such as declining muscle mass associated with the adaptation of a more quiescent lifestyle).

Age-related changes in drug disposition that have potential importance to drug use are summarized in Table 53-1. These alterations affect the absorption, distribution, biotransformation, and excretion of drugs; the specific features of these changes are considered later. A well-documented decline in homeostatic competence occurs in the elderly, which accounts for the increased incidence of postural hypotension with age,[11] the increasing sluggishness of thermoregulation, and the fact that the elderly are less able to compensate rapidly for the hypotensive effects, for instance, of an antihypertensive drug.[25] Furthermore, the elderly undergo physiologic changes that can be characterized as normal concomitants of the aging process, but they also, to a greater or lesser extent, experience changes related to disease and medication. Because what we consider aging represents an interplay among the physiology of aging, disease, and the cumulative effects of behavioral and lifestyle choices (e.g., sedentary living and tobacco use versus regular exercise and abstention from tobacco), the elderly population are more heterogeneous than, for instance, a population of children between birth and puberty.[62]

NONPHYSIOLOGIC ASPECTS OF AGING

Multiple Disease States

The elderly have more health problems, especially chronic diseases and conditions, than the young. The most prevalent chronic conditions among older adults are listed in Table 53-2. Some of these diseases are degenerative (e.g., cataracts, detached retina), others are caused by cumulative exposure to environmental contaminants (e.g., cases of chronic obstructive pulmonary disease and cancer), and still others are the consequence of metabolic processes commonly seen in aging (e.g., decreased bone density with increasing age). Older adults have an increased incidence of all varieties of heart disease (arrhythmias, myocardial infarction, valvular disease), renal disease, atherosclerosis, arthritis, diabetes, osteoporosis, and a variety of gastrointestinal problems. They also experience declines in both humoral- and cell-mediated immune responses (leading to a decreased resistance to infectious diseases), as well as various sensory and musculoskeletal impairments. More than four out of five persons aged 65 years and older have at least one chronic illness, and multiple coexisting conditions are commonplace among older adults. The leading chronic health conditions for this age group are arthritis, hypertensive disease, and heart disease.[2,13]

Although the elderly represent less than 13% of the population, they account for 30% of hospitalizations[24] and 32% of drug utilizations.[17] Moreover, the symptoms of disease in older adults may often present differently in the elderly than in younger individuals. For example, infections are sometimes manifested not by fever but by tachycardia in older individuals. Furthermore, transient or episodic symptoms may be forgotten, misreported, or misinterpreted.

Numerous studies have shown that older adults, because of the higher prevalence of chronic disease, are the principal consumers of drugs.[44,48] The use of over-the-counter and prescription medications for the treatment of chronic diseases in older adults has dual implications. To begin, these agents can

Table • 53-1

Summary of Age-Related Changes that Affect Drug Disposition in Older Adults

PHARMACOKINETIC PROPERTY	PHYSIOLOGIC CHANGE	POSSIBLE INFLUENCE ON DRUG EFFECT
Absorption	↑Gastric pH	Increased absorption of drugs inactivated by stomach acid
	↓Absorptive surface	Minor effect
	↓Splanchnic blood flow	Minor effect
	↓Gastrointestinal motility	Minor effect
Distribution	↓Cardiac output	Impaired delivery of drugs to organs of elimination; greater acute effects on the central nervous system
	↓Total body water	Increased concentration and effect of drugs distributed in body water
	↓Lean body mass	Increased concentration and effect of drugs distributed in lean body mass
	↓Plasma albumin	Increased effect of, and interaction between, drugs extensively bound to albumin
	↑α_1-Acid glycoprotein	Minor effect
	↑Body fat	Increased sequestration of lipophilic drugs in fat
Metabolism	↓Hepatic mass and enzyme activity	Decreased phase I metabolism of some drugs
	↓Hepatic blood flow	Decreased metabolism of drugs normally rapidly cleared by the liver
Excretion	↓Renal blood flow	Decreased renal elimination of water-soluble drugs and metabolites
	↓Glomerular filtration rate	Decreased renal excretion of water-soluble drugs and metabolites
	↓Tubular secretion	Decreased renal elimination of drugs and metabolites actively secreted into urine

Table • 53-2

Rank Ordering and Prevalence of Selected Reported Chronic Conditions

	PREVALENCE BY AGE (IN YEARS)		
CONDITION	65 TO 74	>75	ALL AGES
Arthritis	444.7	550.4	129.9
Hypertension	372.6	373.6	121.5
Hearing impairment	273.7	380.7	90.8
Heart disease	271.8	333.6	84.1
Chronic sinusitis	176.2	167.8	139.7
Cataract formation	118.1	246.0	25.3
Deformity or orthopedic impairment	151.4	176.6	111.6
Diabetes	95.2	87.8	25.8
Visual impairment	67.4	127.6	34.7
Tinnitus	89.4	75.1	26.4

Prevalence data (number of cases/1000 persons) from Adams PF, Hardy AM: *Current estimates from the National Health Interview Survey, 1988. Vital and health statistics,* Series 10, No 173. Hyattsville, MD, 1989, US Department of Health and Human Services.

provide a cure or palliative treatment of a disease in a relatively nontoxic and economical manner. However, because of the age-related changes in physiologic status and age-dependent and age-related diseases,[10] medications can induce adverse reactions that can be a major source of morbidity or even death.[28,49]

Adverse Drug Reactions

The incidence of adverse drug reactions among older adults is much greater than among younger individuals, and this increase is related for the most part to polypharmacy (multiple drug use). However, other important factors in the occurrence of adverse drug reactions include multiple diseases (especially chronic diseases), hepatic or renal insufficiency, small body size, malnutrition, and previous drug reactions. Important adverse reactions include side effects (e.g., dry mouth with tricyclic antidepressant medication), drug allergy (e.g., pruritus or hives), and toxic reactions[36] (e.g., digitalis toxicity). Toxic reactions are especially important in older adults and may be caused by a broad range of potential pharmacodynamic changes (age-related changes in drug sensitivity) or pharmacokinetic changes (including decreased renal function and changes in lean body mass and water content).

Adverse drug reactions can be categorized into two principal groups: unexpected and unpredictable versus predictable and preventable. An unexpected, unpredictable reaction is an unwanted consequence of drug administration that occurs at appropriate doses for prophylaxis, diagnosis, or therapy. Examples of such reactions include allergic responses, idiosyncratic reactions, and secondary pharmacologic effects. In contrast, predictable, preventable drug reactions involve an unwanted consequence of drug administration that occurs because of failure in decision making by the health care provider. Failure by the physician or dentist to choose the appropriate agent can occur, as in prescribing the wrong drug for a disease or prescribing a drug with known potential adverse effects in a susceptible patient.

Because the majority of adverse drug reactions are preventable, the clinician should be aware of the patient's medical history, drug history, and current list of medications (both over the counter and prescribed), as well as the pharmacologic characteristics of each agent used and any abnormal physiologic factors that can affect drug action. Although the incidence of adverse reactions increases among older patients, in part because of polypharmacy, actions of a single powerful agent can produce severe adverse reactions for the elderly patient. Many of the drugs commonly prescribed by dentists can produce a variety of harmful reactions in their patients.

As illustrated in Table 53-3, a variety of drug classes can be of potential risk to the older patient. For example, cephalosporins commonly prescribed to treat infections can produce deleterious effects. Cefoperazone, cefamandole, and cefotetan can prolong both prothrombin time and partial thromboplastin time, which can impair hemostasis.[16,46] Other antibiotics, such as clindamycin, can markedly increase the incidence of such gastrointestinal problems as diarrhea and colitis in patients older than 60 years.[27,45] In addition to antibiotics, nonsteroidal antiinflammatory drugs (NSAIDs) can also cause morbidity in the elderly. The NSAIDs are commonly used for postoperative pain control in dental practice; however, NSAID use among older adults can be a problem, as documented by an association of NSAID intake with impaired renal function, gastrointestinal toxicity, or hypertension.[1,8,29] Therefore alternatives to NSAIDs can include the use of cyclooxygenaase-2 (COX-2) inhibitors such as celecoxib and rofecoxib. More specifically, because NSAIDs inhibit both the COX-1 and COX-2 pathways, the use of selective COX-2 inhibitors provides antiinflammatory and analgesic properties with less gastrointestinal toxicity.[54]

Another dilemma encountered by older adults that complicates the dental treatment plan are medications that may cause xerostomia. Drug-induced xerostomia is a concern because (1) older adults take prescription and nonprescription medications at a higher rate than the general population; (2) a large number of medications have xerostomic potential (more than 400 medications have been implicated); and (3) the oral health sequelae of xerostomia are consequential. Xerostomia induced by sympathomimetics, diuretics, anticholinergics, tricyclic antidepressants, antihistamines, antiparkinson drugs, psychotropic agents, cardiovascular agents, and muscle relaxants can greatly impair oral health and function.[56] Potential sequelae of xerostomia include rampant dental caries, periodontal problems, difficulty in speech and swallowing, mouth soreness, impaired denture retention, greater likelihood of oral infection, and altered sense of taste.[19,43]

Polypharmacy is a special attribute of drug use among older adults. One fourth of hospitalized patients older than 65 years receive six or more drugs daily[55]; older adults average 13 prescriptions per year[33]; and approximately 90% of patients aged 75 years and older take drugs regularly, with more than one third taking three or more drugs daily.[34] The major consequence of multiple drug use is an increased incidence of adverse drug reactions. These adverse drug reactions result from a number of factors, including incorrect identification of medications, multiple prescriptions from more than one health provider (because of a lack of awareness or communication among providers), and the use of medications prescribed for someone else.

Because the majority of adverse drug reactions are preventable, dentists should take advantage of available resources to minimize the likelihood of these untoward sequelae. Consultation with other health professionals (including physicians and pharmacists) or use of a comprehensive drug reference book assists in determining the appropriate drug and dose schedule. In addition, computer-based data retrieval systems and newsletters can keep the dentist informed regarding appropriate drug selection. Finally, the dentist should always be aware and concerned about the onset of new symptoms that do not normally arise from the anticipated course of the disease process but do follow from dental treatment.

The salient point to remember concerning adverse drug reactions in older adults is that they are largely preventable. A sound approach to avoiding adverse drug reactions involves (1) understanding the physical and psychosocial changes that occur in older adults, (2) knowing the pharmacokinetics and pharmacodynamics of the medications the patient is taking and ones the dentist is planning to use or prescribe, (3) evaluating the existing prescription drug burden of an individual when considering further prescription needs, (4) prudent drug monitoring, and (5) careful record keeping.

Table • 53-3

Age-Related Increased Risk of Toxicity with Some Commonly Prescribed Dental Agents

DRUG	INCREASED RISK FOR ELDERLY PATIENTS
Clindamycin	Diarrhea and colitis
Metronidazole	Toxic plasma concentrations (those older than 70 years)
Cephalosporins	Impaired clotting mechanisms and bleeding problems
NSAIDs	Compromised renal and gastrointestinal function
Opioid analgesics	Increased plasma half-life, respiratory depression
Glucocorticoids	Muscle wasting and osteoporosis with long-term therapy
Benzodiazepines	Impaired memory and decrements in psychomotor performance

Patient Compliance

Patient compliance can be a major source of medication errors. Ample evidence exists that a substantial percentage of the elderly make serious or potentially serious medication errors.[23] Failure to comply with drug regimens consists of omitting medications; using medications not prescribed by the physician or dentist; and making errors of dosage, sequence, and timing. Problems especially identified with the elderly that contribute to compliance errors include poor comprehension and memory, deficits in vision and hearing, financial strictures, inability to cope with the environment, self-neglect, cultural attitudes, and physical obstacles to getting medications out of the bottle (particularly the child-resistant kind) and self-administering them. Therefore, whenever possible, unnecessary medications should be eliminated and drugs with simplified dosing schedules should be selected. Prescription strategies by the dentist, including written instructions, use of drugs that require fewer doses per day (e.g., doxycycline instead of tetracycline), selection of less expensive generic alternatives, and packaging of drugs in easy-open, daily dosing boxes, will increase the likelihood of compliance.

Psychosocial Factors

Any discussion of geriatric pharmacology would be incomplete without mention of the various psychosocial and economic challenges that frequently confront the elderly. Although the elderly no longer inevitably have a serious reduction in income, 10.5% live in poverty, and elderly single women (14% are below the poverty line) are worse off than men or couples. Furthermore, poverty rates are higher for elderly blacks (25%) and Hispanics (24%) than for elderly whites (9%).[58] The elderly may also live in increasing isolation, away from families, children, and spouses, and have depression, loneliness, and sometimes senility. They also receive three times as many prescriptions for psychotropic drugs as do younger people, even though they are more vulnerable to the adverse effects of these drugs and take twice as long to recover from them than do young patients.[32] This constellation of factors places older adults at risk for a number of problems, including inadequate diet, poor nutrition, loss in weight, forgetfulness and inattention to medical and pharmacologic needs, and an inability or lack of desire to fill prescriptions and take them as directed. One widely held belief about the elderly is that their nutritional status is compounded by losses in salivary secretory ability and taste acuity that are presumed to occur with aging and would naturally interfere with the enjoyment of food. Although some studies showed a decrease in parotid gland secretion and salivary amylase activity, as well as morphologic age-related changes in the salivary gland, most studies have not found a diminution of salivary flow in older individuals,[5,6] and the decline in gustatory function is at most modest among the elderly.[66] On the other hand, pathologic aging may have an adverse effect on salivary function and many of the drugs and treatments to which the older person is subject can cause xerostomia of varying degrees of severity.

PHARMACOLOGIC CHANGES ASSOCIATED WITH AGING

Two basic mechanisms have been developed to explain age-related differences in drug effects.[36] The pharmacodynamic mechanism suggests that changes in drug responsiveness account for such differences.[9,26] These changes presumably involve either an alteration in the number or activity of receptors on the target cell or a change in intracellular responses to receptor activation. Documentation in support of this mechanism is modest, involving only a few drug classes. The more widely accepted pharmacokinetic mechanism suggests that age differences in drug response are related to changes in drug disposition as a result of alterations in drug absorption, distribution, metabolism, and excretion or combinations of these processes. A general review of these factors with particular regard to aging is provided in the following sections.

Pharmacokinetics of Drugs

Absorption

Most medications prescribed to patients living independently are taken orally. These medications are absorbed through the gastrointestinal tract. The documented age-related alterations that might predispose older adults to potential declines in absorption are increased gastric pH, decreased absorptive surface, decreased gastric emptying, decreased splanchnic blood flow, and impaired intestinal motility.[7,41] However, little evidence exists to support an age-related decline in absorption.[26] In fact, decreased stomach acidity could improve absorption of drugs normally inactivated by stomach acid. An important consideration for patients of all ages is the possible interaction of medications with food. For example, the absence of food in the gastrointestinal tract improves the efficiency of absorption of some drugs, such as erythromycin. However, the absorption of other medications is relatively unimpaired.[36] Thus although food-drug interactions are not a problem of aging per se, they are important in older adults, who have a heavier medication burden.

Distribution

The distribution of the drug to potential receptor sites occurs after absorption of the drug through the gastrointestinal tract and then into the bloodstream. Distribution is influenced by body composition (lean body mass, body water, and adipose tissue mass), plasma protein binding (particularly albumin), and blood flow to organs. The documented age-related changes that might affect drug distribution in older patients include decreased lean body mass, decreased body water, increased body fat, decreased cardiac output, and decreased albumin level.[41]

The change in lean body mass may reflect other factors, including a potential lifestyle change in physical activity or dietary change, rather than an aging effect per se; nevertheless, this consistent finding in older adults must be considered when evaluating the patient. The net effect is a decrease in both lean body mass and total body water and an increase in total body fat. Thus the respective volumes of distribution for water-soluble medications and fat-soluble medications are decreased and increased, respectively.[41] Water-soluble drugs such as acetaminophen, ethanol, digoxin, and cimetidine are distributed in a smaller volume in older individuals and therefore have higher concentrations at the same dose.[26,41] Similarly, the more lipid-soluble drugs such as diazepam and lidocaine are more widely distributed (yielding a lower concentration at the receptor site) and have a longer terminal half-life in older adults.[26,41]

Although decreased plasma titers of albumin are probably not a concomitant of aging, they may accompany chronic disease seen in an aging population. A decrease in plasma albumin increases the availability of highly bound drug, thereby effectively increasing the drug concentration at the receptor. A higher concentration of free drug in the plasma has been shown for salicylic acid, metronidazole,[37] and phenytoin, but not for warfarin.[61] Theoretically, at least, in situations of reduced plasma albumin, therapeutic and toxic effects should be achieved at lower blood concentrations for drugs that are extensively protein bound.[65] This effect may be especially important with malnutrition. Furthermore, many drugs have no documented age-related difference in protein binding; two examples are diazepam and penicillin G.[14]

Metabolism

The metabolism of most drugs begins with the obligatory passage through the liver after absorption from the gastrointestinal tract. Hepatic metabolism depends on hepatic blood flow, the liver enzymes responsible for biotransformation of the drug, and genetic factors that influence the hepatic enzyme system.[36,41] The reported age-related declines that might be responsible for altered drug disposition include decreased liver mass and decreased hepatic blood flow.[41] Biologic variability, drug utilization, and behavioral factors (such as smoking or alcohol use) or a combination of these factors may exert a greater effect than age on hepatic metabolism.

The documented age-related effects may impair the efficiency of the phase I pathways of metabolism, namely, oxidation, reduction, and hydrolysis. The phase II pathways of glucuronidation, acetylation, and sulfation are relatively unaffected.[41] For drugs that are rapidly cleared by the liver, the rate-limiting step in biotransformation is the hepatic blood flow. Thus the metabolism of high-clearance drugs such as propranolol is reduced when hepatic blood flow is reduced. Caution should be exercised with concurrent administration with drugs (such as some antiarrhythmic medications) that may reduce hepatic blood flow. For low-clearance drugs, metabolism depends on the efficiency of the hepatic enzyme systems. Thus some benzodiazepines (such as desmethyldiazepam) that depend on microsomal oxidation have a prolonged half-life, whereas others (such as lorazepam) that undergo conjugation are relatively unaffected by age. The clinician should also consider the route of administration when assessing the potential for hepatic metabolism. The preceding discussion presumes the oral route of administration, which involves the absorption of the drug from the gastrointestinal tract and then transport through the liver by way of the hepatic portal circulation; however, the parenteral route of administration may eliminate the liver as the organ primarily influencing disposition of the drug.

Excretion

The elimination of drugs by the kidney provides the eventual pathway for removal of most medications. The documented age-related changes that might impair kidney function and excretion include decreased renal blood flow, decreased glomerular filtration rate, and decreased tubular secretion.[41] Renal function is typically evaluated by the creatinine clearance, which has been reported to decline by approximately one third between the ages of 20 and 90 years in the ambulatory, community-dwelling volunteers of the Baltimore Longitudinal Study on Aging.[51] More recent data from the same study, however, have shown that for approximately one third of older subjects, renal function did not decline, and, furthermore, quite variable declines occurred among other older subjects.[35] These latter data underscore the need to establish adequate dosing schedules for medications based on blood concentrations rather than interpretation of age-adjusted "normative" data.

Drugs that are eliminated primarily unchanged in the kidney include digoxin, gentamicin, amantadine, lithium, nadolol, and lisinopril. Dosages for drugs with a high therapeutic index, such as penicillins and cephalosporins, are usually not adjusted for older adults (in the absence of renal disease or polypharmacy). Dosages for medications with active metabolites, such as the benzodiazepines diazepam and flurazepam, should be adjusted.[26]

The response of the elderly to drugs is affected by alterations in renal drug clearance and the fact that altered renal function may make them more sensitive to the nephrotoxicity of drugs such as the NSAIDs and aminoglycosides. Conversely, the decreased activity of the renin-angiotensin system may blunt the effects of drugs that inhibit renin secretion, such as β-adrenergic blocking agents and the angiotensin-converting enzyme inhibitors, diminishing their therapeutic effectiveness in the treatment of hypertension.[39]

The complex and potentially serious alterations in kidney function mandate that consideration be given to renal excretory capacity when prescribing drugs to the elderly. Although a diminution in renal function that is related to age certainly does occur, kidney disease is, of course, not restricted to the elderly.

Pharmacodynamic Changes

Studies investigating age-related changes in pharmacodynamics are quite difficult to pursue, and, consequently, scant data exist in this area. Available evidence suggests no global age-related changes in drug sensitivity. Increased sensitivity to certain benzodiazepine anxiolytic medications and decreased sensitivity to β-adrenergic agonists and antagonists have been reported in older individuals.

There are several possibilities for pharmacodynamic alterations in drug reactivity with aging, including a change in the number of receptors, a change in their affinity for the drug, or a change in tissue responsiveness to drug-receptor binding. Discovering which of these possibilities accounts for a particular reaction is difficult because it requires a knowledge of receptor number, binding affinity, and quantitation of the sequential steps after the drug-receptor interaction to the final observed response. Experimental evidence exists that one or more of these changes does occur with several groups of drugs, but interpretation of the results of some of these experiments is confounded by the fact that the elderly also demonstrate decreases in homeostatic competence, speed of performance, thermoregulation, and immunocompetence.

Changes in sensitivity to β-adrenergic agonists and antagonists have been reported in a number of studies. With the production of cyclic 3′,5′-adenosine monophosphate by lymphocytes as an indicator of responsiveness to isoproterenol in the young and old, a decrease in adenylate cyclase occurs in normal subjects aged 67 to 90 years compared with those 18 to 27 years.[15] Sensitivity of young male subjects to isoproterenol and propranolol was demonstrated to be greater than in elderly men, but the well-documented increase in the blood concentration of norepinephrine in the elderly may possibly create competition for receptor sites.[63] In a series of investigations involving rat myocardial and human lymphocytic β-adrenergic function, a decreased responsiveness of the β receptors to catecholamines was found, along with decreased adenylate cyclase activity but no decline in receptor density.[52]

Increased sensitivity to central nervous system depressants is a recognized fact. In tests involving nitrazepam, age-related decrements in psychomotor performance were described and linked to pharmacodynamic, not pharmacokinetic, changes.[12] Elderly patients who were given diazepam for a surgical procedure required lower doses than younger patients to reach the same level of sedation.[50] This observation has been confirmed in other studies for both diazepam and temazepam.[57] Determination of the minimum alveolar concentration for isoflurane showed an 18% drop in anesthetic requirement in older adults compared with young adults; similar results have been obtained with other anesthetics.[64] In contrast to the generalization that brain function in the elderly appears to be inherently more susceptible to disruption by anesthetic drugs, the greater sensitivity of older patients to etomidate appears to result from a decreased initial distribution of the anesthetic after intravenous injection.[4]

In addition to pharmacodynamic changes, the genetic characteristics of an individual may also influence the behavior of drugs in the elderly. For example, the apparent volume distribution of the acetylator phenotype of isoniazid decreased significantly with age.[31] Hence, pharmacogenetics for the elderly is important because genetically determined enhancement or impairment of drug action in the body can amplify the toxicity of a drug or diminish the efficacy of a drug.

IMPLICATIONS FOR DENTISTRY

The elderly patient differs from the younger adult in ways that have the potential to affect responses to drugs. Changes potentially affecting pharmacokinetics and pharmacodynamics occur during aging, but at this stage in the development of the science of geriatric pharmacology, remarkably few instances have been documented of problems with drugs that arise directly from these changes. On the other hand, responses to drugs in the elderly are confounded by multiple medications, pathologic states, compliance errors, and a variety of psychologic, sociologic, and economic difficulties that beset older people. Some precautions appropriate to dentistry are listed below:

1. The elderly usually take more drugs, both prescription and nonprescription, than the general adult population, and drug interactions as well as adverse drug reactions are more likely to occur in this polypharmaceutical setting. The dentist should take a careful history of the patient's medical and pharmacologic status and update it at regular intervals during treatment.
2. The elderly are more sensitive than are young adults to the depressant effects of drugs. The dosages of analgesics, antianxiety drugs, sedative-hypnotics, and general anesthetics may need to be reduced.
3. Because of the known loss in homeostatic competence, drugs that alter blood pressure, heart rate, and smooth muscle tone should be used with caution in the elderly. Conversely, immunosenescence may dictate a more aggressive antibiotic therapy than normal for the prevention and treatment of infections.
4. The elderly are more susceptible to orthostatic

hypotension than are younger adults. Special attention is called for when they go from a reclining posture in the dental chair to a standing position.

5. A well-known decline in renal function occurs in the healthy elderly patient and an even greater decrease occurs in patients with kidney disease. This fact should be considered when prescribing drugs whose principal route of elimination is the kidney. Conventionally, dosage intervals are increased in such circumstances, but the dose of the drug or drugs may have to be reduced.
6. The dentist should be aware of the psychosocial considerations for the patient and sensitive to such problems as the expense of the medications and the possibility of forgetfulness and poor compliance. Special packaging, clear labeling, and simplified dose regimens may improve compliance because a responsible relative or friend may monitor drug therapy.

CITED REFERENCES

1. Adams DH, Howie AJ, Michael J, et al: Non-steroidal anti-inflammatory drugs and renal failure, *Lancet* 1:57-60, 1986.
2. Adams PF, Hardy AM: *Current estimates from the National Health Interview Survey,* 1988, Vital and Health Statistics, Series 10, Hyattsville, MD, 1989, US Department of Health and Human Services.
3. *Aging America: trends and projections: an information paper to the Special Committee on Aging,* United States Senate, Washington, DC, 1989, US Government Printing Office.
4. Arden JR, Holley FO, Stanski DR: Increased sensitivity to etomidate in the elderly: initial distribution versus altered brain response, *Anesthesiology* 65:19-27, 1986.
5. Atkinson JC, Fox PC: Salivary gland dysfunction, *Clin Geriatr Med* 8:499-511, 1992.
6. Baum BJ: Salivary gland fluid secretion during aging, *J Am Geriatr Soc* 37:453-458, 1989.
7. Bender AD: Pharmacodynamic principles of drug therapy in the aged, *J Am Geriatr Soc* 22:296-303, 1974.
8. Berger RG: Intelligent use of NSAIDs—where do we stand? *Expert Opin Pharmacother* 2:19-30, 2001.
9. Bleich HL, Boro ES, Rowe JW: Clinical research on aging: strategies and directions, *N Engl J Med* 297:1332-1336, 1977.
10. Brody JA, Schneider EL: Diseases and disorders of aging: an hypothesis, *J Chronic Dis* 39:871-876, 1986.
11. Caird FI, Andrews GR, Kennedy RD: Effect of posture on blood pressure in the elderly, *Br Heart J* 35:527-530, 1973.
12. Castleden CM, George CF, Marcer D, et al: Increased sensitivity to nitrazepam in old age, *Br Med J* 1:10-12, 1977.
13. Centers for Disease Control and Prevention. *Unrealized prevention opportunities: reducing the health and economic burden of chronic disease,* Atlanta, 1997, National Center for Chronic Disease Prevention and Health Promotion.
14. Crooks J, O'Malley K, Stevenson IH: Pharmacokinetics in the elderly, *Clin Pharmacokinet* 1:280-296, 1976.
15. Dillon N, Chung S, Kelly J, et al: Age and beta adrenoceptor-mediated function, *Clin Pharmacol Ther* 27:769-772, 1980.
16. Donowitz GR, Mandell GL: Beta-lactam antibiotics. Part 2, *N Engl J Med* 318:490-500, 1988.
17. *Drug utilization in the U.S.—1987: eighth annual review,* Publication no. PB88-146527. Springfield, VA 1987, Food and Drug Administration.
18. Duncker A, Greenberg S. *A profile of older Americans: 2000,* Washington, DC, 2000, Administration on Aging, US Department of Health and Human Services.
19. Fox PC, van der Ven PF, Sonies BC, et al: Xerostomia: evaluation of a symptom with increasing significance, *J Am Dent Assoc* 110:519-525, 1985.
20. German PS, Burton LC: Medication and the elderly. Issues of prescription and use, *J Aging Health* 1:4-34, 1989.
21. Gilbert GH, Duncan RP, Crandall LA, et al: Attitudinal and behavioral characteristics of older Floridians with tooth loss, *Community Dent Oral Epidemiol* 21:384-389, 1993.
22. Gilbert GH, Heft MW: Periodontal status of older Floridians attending senior activity centers, *J Clin Periodontol* 19:249-255, 1992.
23. Gillum RF, Barsky AJ: Diagnosis and management of patient noncompliance, *JAMA* 228:1563-1567, 1974.
24. Graves EJ: *Utilization of short-stay hospitals, United States: annual summary, vital and health statistics,* 1985, Series 13, No. 91. Hyattsville, MD, 1987, US Department of Health and Human Services.
25. Greenblatt DJ, Koch-Weser J: Adverse reactions to propranolol in hospitalized medical patients: a report from the Boston Collaborative Drug Surveillance Program, *Am Heart J* 86:478-484, 1973.
26. Greenblatt DJ, Sellers EM, Shader RI: Drug therapy: drug disposition in old age, *N Engl J Med* 306:1081-1088, 1982.
27. Gurwith MJ, Rabin HR, Love K: Diarrhea associated with clindamycin and ampicillin therapy: preliminary results of a cooperative study, *J Infect Dis* 135:S104-S110, 1977.
28. Gurwitz JH, Avorn J: The ambiguous relation between aging and adverse drug reactions, *Ann Intern Med* 114:956-966, 1991.
29. Gurwitz JH, Avorn J, Bohn RL, et al: Initiation of antihypertensive treatment during nonsteroidal anti-inflammatory drug therapy, *JAMA* 272:781-786, 1994.
30. Heft MW, Gilbert GH: Tooth loss and caries prevalence in older Floridians attending senior activity centers, *Community Dent Oral Epidemiol* 19:228-232, 1991.
31. Kergueris MF, Bourin M, Larousse C: Pharmacokinetics of isoniazid: influence of age, *Eur J Clin Pharmacol* 30:335-340, 1986.
32. Lamy PP: *Prescribing for the elderly,* Littleton, MA, 1980, PSG.
33. Lamy PP, Vestal RE: Drug prescribing for the elderly, *Hosp Pract* 11:111-118, 1976.
34. Law R, Chalmers C: Medicines and elderly people: a general practice survey, *Br Med J* 1:565-568, 1976.
35. Lindeman RD, Tobin J, Shock NW: Longitudinal studies on the rate of decline in renal function with age, *J Am Geriatr Soc* 33:278-285, 1985.
36. Lipton HL, Lee PR: *Drugs and the elderly: clinical, social, and policy perspectives,* Stanford, CA, 1988, Stanford University Press.
37. Ludwig E, Csiba A, Magyar T, et al: Age-associated pharmacokinetic changes of metronidazole, *Int J Clin Pharmacol Ther Toxicol* 21:87-91, 1983.

38. Marcus SE, Drury TF, Brown LF, et al: Tooth retention and tooth loss in the permanent dentition of adults: United States, 1988-94, *J Dent Res* 75 (special issue):684-695, 1996.
39. Meyer BR, Bellucci A: Renal function in the elderly, *Cardiol Clin* 4:227-234, 1986.
40. Miller AJ, Brunelle JA, Carlos JP, et al: *Oral health of U.S. adults: the National Survey of Oral Health in U.S. employed adults and seniors, 1985-1986: national findings*, Publication No. (NIH) 87-2868, Bethesda, MD, 1987, US Department of Health and Human Services.
41. Montamat SC, Cusack BJ, Vestal RE: Management of drug therapy in the elderly, *N Engl J Med* 321:303-309, 1989.
42. Morrow D, Leirer V, Sheikh J: Adherence and medication instructions. Review and recommendations, *J Am Geriatr Soc* 36:1147-1160, 1988.
43. Narhi TO, Meurman JH, Ainamo A: Xerostomia and hyposalivation: causes, consequences and treatment in the elderly, *Drugs Aging* 15:103-116, 1999.
44. Nelson CR, Knapp DE: *Medication therapy in ambulatory medical care: national ambulatory medical care survey and national hospital care survey*, Advance Data from Vital and Health Statistics, No. 290. Hyattsville, MD, 1992, National Center for Health Statistics.
45. Neu HC, Prince A, Neu CO, et al: Incidence of diarrhea and colitis associated with clindamycin therapy, *J Infect Dis* 135:S120-S125, 1977.
46. Nichols RL, Wikler MA, McDevitt JT, et al: Coagulopathy associated with extended-spectrum cephalosporins in patients with serious infections, *Antimicrob Agents Chemother* 31:281-285, 1987.
47. Nolan L, O'Malley K: Prescribing for the elderly: part II. Prescribing patterns: differences due to age, *J Am Geriatr Soc* 36:245-254, 1988.
48. Ouslander JG: Drug therapy in the elderly, *Ann Intern Med* 95:711-722, 1981.
49. Porter J, Jick H: Drug-related deaths among medical inpatients, *JAMA* 237:879-881, 1977.
50. Reidenberg MM, Levy M, Warner H, et al: Relationship between diazepam dose, plasma level, age, and central nervous system depression, *Clin Pharmacol Ther* 23:371-374, 1978.
51. Rowe JW, Andres R, Tobin JD, et al: The effect of age on creatinine clearance in men: a cross-sectional and longitudinal study, *J Gerontol* 31:155-163, 1976.
52. Scarpace PJ: Decreased β-adrenergic responsiveness during senescence, *Fed Proc* 45:51-54, 1986.
53. Shock NW: Aging of regulatory mechanisms. In Cape RDT, Coe RM, Rossman I, eds: *Fundamentals of geriatric medicine*, New York, 1983, Raven Press.
54. Silverstein FE, Faich G, Goldstein JL, et al: Gastrointestinal toxicity with celecoxib vs nonsteroidal anti-inflammatory drugs for osteoarthritis and rheumatoid arthritis: the CLASS study: a randomized controlled trial. Celecoxib Long-term Arthritis Safety Study, *JAMA* 284:1247-1255, 2000.
55. Smith CR: Use of drugs in the aged, *Johns Hopkins Med J* 145:61-64, 1979.
56. Sreebny LM, Schwartz SS: A reference guide to drugs and dry mouth—2nd edition, *Gerodontology* 14:33-47, 1997.
57. Swift CG, Haythorne JM, Clarke P, et al: Chlormethiazole and temazepam, *Br Med J* 280:1322, 1980.
58. Taeuber C: Diversity: the dramatic reality. In Bass S, Kutza EA, Torres-Gil, FM, eds: *Diversity in aging: the issues facing the White House Conference on Aging and Beyond*, Glenview, IL, 1990, Scott, Foresman.
59. US Bureau of the Census: *Population projections of the United States by age, sex, race and Hispanic origin: 1993 to 2050*, Current Population Reports, P25-1104, Washington, DC, 1993, US Government Printing Office.
60. US Department of Health and Human Services, National Center for Health Statistics: *Third National Health and Nutrition Examination Survey, 1988-94*, Public Use Data File No. 7-0627, Hyattsville, MD, 1997, Centers for Disease Control.
61. Verbeeck RK, Cardinal J-A, Wallace SM: Effect of age and sex on the plasma binding of acidic and basic drugs, *Eur J Clin Pharmacol* 27:91-97, 1984.
62. Vestal RE: Drug use in the elderly: a review of problems and special considerations, *Drugs* 16:358-382, 1978.
63. Vestal RE, Wood AJ, Shand DG: Reduced β-adrenoceptor sensitivity in the elderly, *Clin Pharmacol Ther* 26:181-186, 1979.
64. Wade JG, Stevens WC: Isoflurane: an anesthetic for the eighties? *Anesth Analg* 60:666-682, 1981.
65. Wallace S, Whiting B: Factors affecting drug binding in plasma of elderly patients, *Br J Clin Pharmacol* 3:327-330, 1976.
66. Weiffenbach JM, Bartoshuk LM: Taste and smell, *Clin Geriatr Med* 8:543-555, 1992.
67. Weintraub JA, Burt BA: Oral health status in the United States: tooth loss and edentulism, *J Dent Educ* 49:368-378, 1985.

General References

Baum BJ, ed: Oral and dental problems in the elderly, *Clin Geriatr Med* 8:447-699, 1992.

Hazzard WR, Blass JP, Ettinger WH, et al: *Principles of geriatric medicine and gerontology*, ed 4, New York, 1999, McGraw-Hill.

Holm-Pedersen P, Löe H, eds: *Textbook of geriatric dentistry*, ed 2, Copenhagen, 1996, Munksgaard.

Lipton HL, Lee PR: *Drugs and the elderly: clinical, social, and policy perspectives*, Stanford, CA, 1988, Stanford University Press.

Schneider EL, Rowe JW, eds: *Handbook of the biology of aging*, ed 4, San Diego, 1996, Academic Press.

CHAPTER • 54

Drugs for Medical Emergencies

Morton B. Rosenberg

Every dentist can expect to be involved in the diagnosis and treatment of medical emergencies during the course of clinical practice. These emergencies may be directly related to dental therapy, or they may simply occur by chance in the dental environment. In studies surveying the incidence and type of medical emergencies in dental practice, 95.6% of the respondents reported such emergencies. Although the majority of the reported emergencies were minor (e.g., 53% syncopal episodes), life-threatening or major emergencies were also detailed.[10,28] Many medical emergencies occur during the administration of local anesthesia and during potentially painful procedures such as extractions and pulp extirpation.[30] The potential need for acute medical intervention during dental treatment may be increased for those practitioners treating a high percentage of geriatric, special needs, or medically compromised patients, or those using enteral, inhalational, or parenteral sedation or general anesthesia.

It has been postulated that the incidence of medical emergencies in dentistry as a whole is increasing.[29] This increase may be attributed to the following factors.

1. *The increasing age of the general population.* As the number of elderly individuals in the general population increases, the likelihood of encountering a medical emergency as a result of the physiologic and pathologic changes associated with the aging process also increases. In addition to the normal deterioration of major organ systems that occurs with age, the geriatric population is more likely to exhibit chronic clinical manifestations of organ derangement (e.g., angina pectoris, congestive heart failure, chronic obstructive lung disease) that may become acute during the dental visit and require intervention. The elderly take more prescription and over-the-counter drugs than the young, and the effects of these compounds can be significantly different from those seen in the younger population. The pharmacokinetics of many drugs are altered by aging; pharmacodynamic and physiologic changes also may result in greater sensitivity to many drugs, especially central nervous system (CNS) depressants.[6]
2. *Effect of medical advances.* Advances in the diagnosis and treatment of many medical conditions have permitted an increasing population of compromised patients to survive and seek comprehensive dental treatment. Pharmacologic advances in such diverse areas as cancer, cardiovascular disease, and psychiatric illness, and surgical advances such as organ transplants, cardiac valve replacements, coronary artery revascularization, pacemakers, and automatic implantable cardioverter/defibrillators have significant ramifications for dental therapy and can be directly related to acute medical problems in the dental office. In general, the growing number of medically stabilized yet chronically ill patients seeking dental treatment is paralleled by a concomitant increase in the incidence of medical emergencies during dental treatment. Moreover, dental advances such as intraosseous implants and comprehensive periodontal treatment combined with extensive restorative dentistry leading to "life-long dentistry" are attracting an older, less healthy population into the dental environment.
3. *Pharmacologic therapies.* Therapeutic choices for dentists are constantly increasing with the introduction of new generations of antibiotics, analgesics, local anesthetics, and antianxiety drugs. Each new drug has it own inherent indications, contraindications, and possible side effects. These drugs also have the capacity to interact with each other and with other drugs the patient may be taking for medical conditions. Such drug interactions have the potential to elicit acute adverse reactions during the dental appointment.[31] The growing popularity of herbal supplements and other alternative medical therapies have implications that are just being realized and studied. Many of their side effects, such as antihemostatic, hypotensive, and hypoglycemic properties, can directly affect dental treatment.
4. *Drug abuse.* Substance abuse is a fact of life in modern society. Many dental patients "premedicate" themselves with CNS depressants, prescribed or illicit, prior to dental therapy. These drugs may present acute problems by themselves or interact with drugs routinely administered or prescribed by the dentist.

EMERGENCY PREVENTION

Many chronic medical conditions such as asthma, congestive heart failure, coronary artery disease, and cerebrovascular disease may become acute medical emergencies when exacerbated by the stress of the dental appointment. Stress, anxiety, fear, and phobia may be the etiologies for other minor stress-related emergencies such as syncopal episodes and the hyperventilation syndrome. A thorough preoperative evaluation, meticulous detail to achieving profound local anesthesia in a safe manner, consideration of nonpharmacologic stress reduction protocols, or the use of pharmacologic sedative techniques to minimize pain, fear, and anxiety helps reduce this risk.

Preoperative evaluation includes the use of a medical history questionnaire, oral history, review of systems, physical examination, vital signs, and appropriate laboratory tests and consultations. This evaluation should determine the risk/benefit ratio of the contemplated procedure, what drugs should be used or avoided, the potential for a medical emergency, and the type of monitoring best suited for the particular patient.

EMERGENCY PREPAREDNESS

Although just about any medical emergency can occur during the course of dental treatment—which means that dental personnel must be prepared to provide effective basic life support (BLS) and seek emergency medical services in a timely manner—dentists must be able to diagnose and treat common medical problems (e.g., syncope or hyperventilation syndrome) definitively as well as respond effectively to certain less common (or even rare) but potentially life-threatening emergencies, especially those that may arise as a result of dental treatment (e.g., anaphylactic reaction to an administered drug).[5] These emergencies are listed in Box 54-1.

Many factors determine the degree of preparedness for medical emergencies needed in a specific dental practice, but all dental offices must be ready at some minimum level.[25] The use of local anesthesia alone is an indication for the dentist to be prepared to handle medical emergencies, as evidenced by the following language in product literature approved by the Food and Drug Administration: "Dental practitioners who employ local anesthetic agents should be well versed in diagnosis and management of emergencies that may arise from their use. Resuscitative equipment, oxygen and other emergency drugs should be immediately available for immediate use."[3] Clearly an overall emergency preparedness plan, as listed in Box 54-2, is essential for every dental practice. Implicit in Box 54-2 is the necessity to develop a team approach in preparing for and responding to medical emergencies in the dental office, with each staff member (receptionist, dental auxiliary, dental hygienist, and dentist) responsible for a discrete role.

Preparedness must be individually tailored according to the type of patient treated (e.g., young, healthy patients in an orthodontic practice versus medically compromised patients in a periodontal practice), location (an urban setting where emergency help is close at hand versus a rural location where there may be a significant delay until help arrives), and training (whether the dentist and staff are capable of performing advanced emergency procedures and protocols). Although presenting a comprehensive guide to the pathophysiologic characteristics, prevention, diagnosis, and management of specific medical emergencies is beyond the scope of this chapter, several sources for this purpose are listed in the general references. In practices where sedation or general anesthesia is administered, advanced emergency training and equipment is required and often is promulgated by state dental practice acts.

Box • 54-1

Medical Emergencies of Relevance to Dental Practice

Syncope
Hyperventilation
Angina pectoris
Myocardial infarction
Hypertension
Hypotension
Hemorrhage
Cerebrovascular accident
Grand mal seizure
Insulin shock/diabetic coma
Asthma
Anaphylaxis/other allergic reactions

Box • 54-2

Emergency Preparedness Checklist

All staff members have specific assigned duties.
Contingency plans have been made in case of a missing staff member.
All staff members have appropriate training in the management of medical emergencies.
All staff members have a current BLS provider card.
The dental office is equipped with emergency equipment and supplies appropriate for that practice.
Periodic unannounced emergency drills are conducted at least quarterly.
Appropriate emergency phone numbers are placed prominently by each phone.
Oxygen tanks and oxygen delivery systems are checked regularly. Other emergency respiratory support equipment is present, in good working order, and located according to the emergency plan.
All emergency medications are checked monthly to ensure that outdated drugs are replaced.
All emergency supplies are restocked immediately after use.
A specific individual has been assigned to ensure that the above has been completed and to document this checklist review.

Modified from Fast TB, Martin MD, Ellis TM: Emergency preparedness: a survey of dental practitioners, *J Am Dent Assoc* 112:449-501, 1986.

EMERGENCY DRUGS

Even though many medical emergencies may be properly treated without the use of drugs, every dental office must contain an emergency kit with drugs appropriate to the training of the individual dentist, the patient being treated, and the type of procedures being performed.[45] Obviously, no drug can take the place of a properly trained health professional and support staff in diagnosing and treating emergencies. Nevertheless, the design and purchase of an appropriate emergency kit often play an integral role in dictating the course and outcome of emergency treatment.

Besides determining which drugs should be included in an emergency kit, the dentist must understand that he or she must maintain the knowledge base to use them. In the midst of a medical emergency, with the patient by definition in an acutely abnormal or even critical situation, there is no time to begin reading labels, leafing through emergency texts, or administering drugs as suggested by a brochure in the emergency kit. In addition, there is a significant difference between the theoretical knowledge of how to treat an emergency and being able to put such cognitive skills to practical use. Only constant review and training will keep the dental team sharp. Regular continuing education in medical emergencies, review of new advances in pharmacology, certification and recertification in BLS, and emergency drills are the best methods to prepare for emergencies. Many states mandate certification in

BLS for dental licensure, and in offices that use deep sedation/general anesthesia, training in advanced cardiac life support (ACLS) is a standard of care. Without prompt attention to the ABCDs (*a*irway, *b*reathing, *c*irculation, *d*efibrillation) of cardiopulmonary resuscitation, drugs are of little value. The advent of the automatic external defibrillator has placed early defibrillation as an integral part of the BLS "chain of survival" for the treatment of cardiac arrest. Since January 1998, health care provider cardiopulmonary resuscitation courses conducted by the American Heart Association include a mandated module on automatic external defibrillator (AED) application and use.

The role of drugs and the type of intervention that should be attempted by a dentist during a medical emergency are controversial issues. If any consequence of dental treatment is foreseeable and results in harm, liability may be imposed.[42] Emergency drugs are generally powerful, rapidly acting compounds. The correct approach to the use of drugs in any medical emergency should be essentially supportive and conservative. In a review covering the use over a 2-year period of 8500 emergency drug systems purchased by dentists, a 0.75% incidence of use was reported.[41]

Emergency kits can either be organized by the individual practitioner or purchased commercially. Many dentists are not comfortable choosing and purchasing individual drugs for their emergency kits, and the purchase of a high-quality, commercially available emergency drug kit modified for dentistry can provide consistent drug availability (i.e., periodic drug updating) in an organized fashion.

There is a general tendency to overequip basic dental emergency kits with drugs that are beyond the needs and expertise of many general dentists. As a rule, the drugs placed in an office emergency kit should only include drugs familiar to the dentist. Only one agent should be included for each particular need. The fewer drugs in an emergency kit, the easier it is to know their proper use, especially during an emergency.[32] Many authors, state boards of dental registration, commercial vendors, and professional groups have suggested the composition of dental medical emergency kits.[27] The composition of these kits varies greatly and depends on the training and philosophy of emergency care of the creator, whether the kit is dental specific, and whether sedation or anesthesia is employed. The definitive pharmacologic features of these drugs are discussed in other chapters.

Critical Emergency Drugs

All dentists must keep certain drugs readily available in the office in fresh supply for immediate administration (Table 54-1). Dentists must know reflexively when, how, and in what doses to give these specific agents for acutely life-threatening situations.

Oxygen

Oxygen is a primary, if not *the* primary, emergency drug indicated in any medical emergency in which hypoxemia may be present. These emergencies include but are not limited to acute disturbances involving the cardiovascular system, respiratory system, and the CNS. In the hypoxemic patient, breathing enriched oxygen elevates the arterial oxygen tension, which in turn improves oxygenation of peripheral tissues. Because of the steepness of the oxyhemoglobin dissociation curve, a modest increase in oxygen tension can significantly alter hemoglobin saturation in the hypoxemic individual. Hypoxemia leads to anaerobic metabolism and metabolic acidosis, which often adversely affect the efficacy of emergency pharmacologic interventions.

Oxygen can be delivered to the spontaneously breathing patient by full face mask, nasal cannula, or nasal hood. Dental offices must also have the capacity to deliver oxygen by positive-pressure ventilation. Controlled ventilation may be accomplished with the use of a bag-valve-mask device (consisting of a mask, self-inflating bag, and nonrebreathing valve) or with a manually triggered oxygen-powered breathing device (consisting of a mask connected by a valve activated by a lever and high-pressure tubing to the oxygen supply). Each method of providing positive-pressure ventilation requires some practice for effective use. Providing a seal around the nose and mouth while simultaneously ventilating the patient can be difficult with the bag-valve-mask device. The oxygen-powered device is easier to use, but care must be taken not to inflate the stomach. Both techniques, however, are preferred over mouth-to-mouth, mouth-to-nose, or mouth-to-mask techniques.[9] Airway adjuncts such as oropharyngeal and nasopharyngeal airways, endotracheal equipment, laryngeal

Table • 54-1

Critical Emergency Drugs

DRUG	INDICATIONS	PREPARATIONS
Oxygen	For use in all medical emergencies in which hypoxemia may be present	Steel cylinders (green); E tanks, 690 L
Epinephrine	Acute allergic reactions, acute asthma (not responding to adrenergic inhaler)	Ampules, 1 mg; vials, 1 and 30 mg; syringes, 0.3 and 1 mg
Nitroglycerin	Angina pectoris, acute myocardial infarction	Tablets (sublingual), 0.15, 0.3, 0.4, and 0.6 mg; spray, 0.4 mg/actuation
Albuterol	For bronchodilation	Aerosol, 90 μg/actuation
Glucose	Hypoglycemic episode	Various oral/transmucosal preparations (orange juice, cake icing, cola)
Aspirin	For reducing platelet aggregation	Chewable aspirin 81 to 325 mg

Data compiled from Curriculum guidelines for management of medical emergencies in dental education, *J Dent Educ* 54:337-338, 1990; Fast TB, Martin MD, Ellis TM: Emergency preparedness: a survey of dental practitioners, *J Am Dent Assoc* 112:449-501, 1986; Lipp M, Kubota Y, Malamed SF, et al: Management of an emergency: to be prepared for the unwanted event, *Anesth Pain Control Dent* 2:90-102, 1992; Malamed SF: *Medical emergencies in the dental office,* ed 5, St Louis, 2000, Mosby; Malamed SF: Drugs for medical emergencies in the dental office. In Ciancio SG, ed: *ADA Guide to dental therapeutics,* ed 3, Chicago, 2003, ADA Publishing; Moore PA: Review of medical emergencies in dentistry: staff training and prevention. Part 1, *Gen Dent* 36:14-17, 1988; Phero JC: Maintaining preparedness for the life-threatening office medical emergency, *Dent Econ* 81:47-50, 1991; Stewart D: Emergency resuscitation kits, *SAAD Digest* 6:223-231, 1987.

masks, and the means of establishing an emergency airway by cricothyrotomy and transtracheal ventilation can be useful or even life-saving in the hands of a trained and experienced health professional. Without appropriate training, however, their use may prove deleterious in an acute emergency.

Although oxygen toxicity may occur after prolonged therapy with high concentrations of oxygen, it is not an issue during clinical resuscitation. This statement holds true even for the rare patient whose respiratory drive depends on hypoxemia because of chronically elevated carbon dioxide concentrations. If clinically indicated, oxygen should never be withheld during any medical emergency.[4] Inspired oxygen concentrations depend on the delivery system used (Box 54-3).

Epinephrine

Epinephrine is an endogenous catecholamine with both α- and β-adrenergic receptor–stimulating activity. It is the drug of choice for the management of the cardiovascular and respiratory manifestations of acute allergic reactions. The beneficial pharmacologic actions of epinephrine when used in resuscitative dosages include bronchodilation, increased systemic vascular resistance, increased arterial blood pressure, increased heart rate, increased myocardial contractility, and increased myocardial and cerebral blood flow.

For the effective treatment of acute allergic reactions, epinephrine must be administered as soon as the condition is diagnosed. The drug can be injected subcutaneously, 0.3 to 0.5 ml of a 1 : 1000 solution, or intramuscularly (for a more serious emergency), 0.4 to 0.6 ml of the same solution. The intravenous route (slow infusion) is also advocated, but it may induce or exacerbate ventricular ectopy, especially in patients receiving digitalis.

Because of its profound bronchodilating effects, epinephrine is also indicated for the treatment of acute asthmatic attacks unrelieved by sprays or aerosols of β_2-adrenergic receptor agonists. Epinephrine may also be instilled directly into the tracheobronchial tree by an endotracheal tube with good results.[18] Epinephrine is also one of the major vasoactive compounds indicated for use during cardiac arrest because of its ability to elevate coronary perfusion pressure.[36]

Nitroglycerin

Although nitroglycerin is available in many preparations—long-acting oral and transmucosal preparations, transcutaneous patches, and intravenous solutions—the appropriate forms for the dental office are the sublingual tablet and translingual spray. Nitroglycerin is the treatment of choice for acute angina pectoris. It acts primarily by relaxing vascular smooth muscle, dilating systemic venous and arterial vascular beds and leading to a reduction in venous return and systemic vascular resistance. These actions all combine to reduce myocardial oxygen consumption. One tablet or spray (0.4 mg) should be given initially. This dose may be repeated twice at 5-minute intervals to a total dose of three administrations. Relief should occur within 1 to 2 minutes; if the discomfort is not relieved, the diagnosis of evolving myocardial infarction must be considered.[46]

Box 54-3

Inspired Oxygen Concentration with Different Delivery Systems

DELIVERY SYSTEM	INSPIRED OXYGEN CONCENTRATION (%)
Spontaneous Breathing	
Nasal cannula	25 to 45
Face mask	40 to 60
Positive-Pressure Ventilation	
Mouth-to-mouth	17
Mouth-to-mask (oxygen flow to mask of 10 L/min)	80
Bag-valve-mask	75 to 95
Manually triggered, oxygen-powered breathing device	75 to 95

Bronchodilator

Inhalation of a β_2-adrenergic receptor agonist such as metaproterenol, terbutaline, or albuterol is used in the treatment of acute bronchospasm encountered during asthma and anaphylaxis.[34] Their use results in bronchial smooth muscle relaxation and the inhibition of chemical mediators released during hypersensitivity reactions. Albuterol is an excellent choice because it has fewer cardiovascular side effects than other bronchodilators.

Glucose

Glucose preparations are used to treat hypoglycemia that results either from fasting or insulin/carbohydrate imbalance in a patient with diabetes mellitus. If the patient is conscious, oral carbohydrates such orange juice, a chocolate bar, cake icing, or a cola drink act rapidly to restore circulating blood sugar. On the other hand, if the patient is unconscious and acute hypoglycemia is suspected, intravenous administration of 50% dextrose solution, intravenous or intramuscular glucagon (which increases blood glucose by its effects on liver glycogen) are the treatments of choice.

Aspirin

The antiplatelet properties of aspirin have been shown to decrease myocardial ischemia dramatically when administered to patients during myocardial infarction; aspirin is used even in out-of-hospital locations.[17]

Primary Support Drugs

Primary support drugs are helpful for treating medical emergencies that are usually not acutely life threatening (Table 54-2). Although dentists do not have to include these drugs in the emergency kit, they are all useful, particularly for situations in which the dentist is familiar with their use and where emergency medical services may not be immediately available.

Anticonvulsant

Seizures that may require acute medical intervention may be associated with epilepsy, hyperventilation episodes, cerebrovascular accidents, hypoglycemic reactions, or vasodepressor syncope. Local anesthetic overdoses or accidental intravascular injection may also require the administration of an anticonvulsant. Current management of a seizure that interferes with ventilation or persists for longer than 5 minutes includes the use of an intravenous benzodiazepine such as diazepam or the water-soluble benzodiazepine midazolam, which may also be administered intramuscularly.[33,35]

Corticosteroid

Corticosteroids are used in the definitive management of acute allergic reactions and acute adrenal insufficiency. The onset of even an intravenous corticosteroid such as hydrocortisone sodium succinate is delayed, but the drug can be useful in halting the progression of a major allergic or anaphylactoid reaction.[40] The dentist may encounter what initially appears to be a syncopal episode but is in reality the more serious problem of acute adrenal insufficiency in a patient taking sys-

Table • 54-2

Primary Emergency Support Drugs

CATEGORY	REPRESENTATIVE DRUG*	PREPARATIONS
Anticonvulsant	Diazepam (Valium)	Ampules and syringes, 10 mg; vials, 10, 20, and 50 mg
Corticosteroid	Hydrocortisone sodium succinate (Solu-Cortef)	Vials, 100, 250, 500 mg, and 1 g
Antihistamine	Diphenhydramine (Benadryl, Benahist, Nordryl)	Ampules, 50 mg; vials, 50, 100, 300, and 500 mg
Respiratory stimulant	Aromatic ammonia spirit (Aromatic Ammonia Aspirols)	Ampules, 0.4 ml

*Nonproprietary (generic) name (proprietary [trade] names).

temic corticosteroids long term to treat a chronic medical condition or patients suffering from primary adrenal insufficiency such as Addison's disease. For this life-threatening emergency, prompt diagnosis, BLS techniques, and infusion of corticosteroids are needed.[20]

Antihistamine

Antihistamines such as diphenhydramine are useful in the treatment of minor or delayed allergic reactions and as adjuncts in the management of an acute allergic or anaphylactoid reaction. Adverse effects of antihistamines include CNS depression resulting in sedation, thickening of tracheobronchial secretions, and decreased blood pressure.

Respiratory stimulant

Aromatic ammonia is a pungent, noxious irritant to the mucous membranes and stimulates the respiratory and vasomotor centers of the medulla. It is used as a general arousal agent during syncopal episodes.

Drugs for Advanced Cardiac Life Support (ACLS)

ACLS is the standard of care for comprehensive resuscitation by health care providers with advanced skills and training. These guidelines are constantly reviewed and updated and are now subdivided into ACLS[15] and pediatric advanced life support (PALS).[16] Included in this training is the use of many antiarrhythmic and vasoactive drugs (Table 54-3). Training in ACLS is necessary for those dentists administering deep sedation or general anesthesia and is often required by state law for dental anesthesia providers. State regulations should be consulted to determine which of the drugs described here must be available in locations where sedation or anesthesia is administered.

Antiarrhythmics

Lidocaine has long been a major antiarrhythmic drug for the treatment of ventricular ectopy, ventricular tachycardia, and ventricular fibrillation.[14] Amiodarone, a newer agent, has a broader range of indications. Amiodarone exerts its effects on Na^+, K^+, and Ca^{++} channels, as well as exhibiting α- and β-adrenergic blocking properties. In addition to its use as an alternative to lidocaine in the management of ventricular arrhythmias, amiodarone is a drug of choice for several types of supraventricular tachycardia.

Procainamide is recommended for the suppression of premature ventricular contractions and recurrent ventricular tachycardia when lidocaine is contraindicated or has failed to suppress ventricular ectopy.[12] Bretylium is no longer advocated for the treatment of ventricular tachycardia and ventricular fibrillation.[15,24]

Verapamil and diltiazem are Ca^{++}-channel blockers that slow conduction and increase refractoriness in the atrioventricular (AV) node. Verapamil is used to terminate reentrant tachyarrhythmias that require AV nodal conduction for their continuation and to control the ventricular rate in patients with atrial fibrillation or flutter or multifocal atrial tachycardia. Diltiazem is used for the same indications but appears to produce less myocardial depression than verapamil.[43] Because of its narrow safety margin, digitalis has been largely superseded by Ca^{++}-channel blockers and β blockers to manage acute atrial fibrillation.[19]

Adenosine is an endogenous purine nucleoside that acts by depressing AV and sinus node activity. It is an important drug for controlling AV nodal reentrant tachycardia and junctional tachycardias.[8] Bolus administration is indicated for paroxysmal supraventricular tachycardia.

Atropine is used for its anticholinergic effects to increase heart rate during periods of sinus bradycardia resulting from excessive parasympathetic nervous system activity. It is also administered for asystole and slow pulseless electrical activity with the assumption that excessive vagal stimulation was responsible for the cardiovascular collapse. Because atropine can increase myocardial oxygen demand, precipitate tachyarrhythmias, and expand the zone of infarction, it must be used carefully in patients with presumptive myocardial infarction.[44] Isoproterenol, a β-adrenergic agonist with both positive inotropic and chronotropic activity, now has only limited application in ACLS for the treatment of bradycardia.

Mg^{++} replacement is advocated when hypomagnesemia is present. Hypomagnesemia can precipitate polymorphic ventricular tachycardia (torsades de pointes) and fibrillation.[2]

β-Adrenergic blockers such as atenolol, metoprolol, propranolol, and esmolol may enhance the benefits of patients receiving thrombolytic agents and have been shown to reduce the incidence of ventricular fibrillation in postmyocardial infarction patients not receiving thrombolytic agents. These drugs are also used to control the ventricular rate in the presence of atrial tachyarrhythmias. Adverse effects of the β-adrenergic blockers relate to their actions on the cardiac conduction system and to exacerbation of bronchospasm in patients with preexisting lung disease.[47]

Cardiovascular stimulants

These drugs increase peripheral vascular resistance and cardiac output. Indications for their use include ischemic heart disease, acute heart failure, cardiogenic shock, and cardiac arrest. As previously mentioned, epinephrine is the cardiovascular stimulant of choice in the management of cardiac arrest. Its benefits in this application are the drug's ability to cause vasoconstriction, to act as a cardiotonic, and to facilitate cardiac perfusion during cardiopulmonary resuscitation.[39] Vasopressin appears to provide the same benefits of increased cardiac perfusion during cardiopulmonary resuscitation. Unlike epinephrine, only a single dose is required.

Table • 54-3

Advanced Cardiac Life Support Drugs

DRUG	INDICATION
Antiarrhythmics	
Lidocaine	Ventricular tachycardia, pulseless ventricular tachycardia or ventricular fibrillation
Amiodarone	Pulseless ventricular tachycardia or ventricular fibrillation, supraventricular tachycardia (most forms)
Procainamide	Intermittent/recurrent ventricular tachycardia, pulseless ventricular tachycardia or ventricular fibrillation
Verapamil, diltiazem	Atrial flutter or atrial fibrillation, supraventricular tachycardia
Adenosine	Supraventricular tachycardia
Atropine	Bradycardia, asystole, certain types of atrioventricular block
Magnesium sulfate	*Torsades de pointes*, ventricular fibrillation (if hypomagnesemia is present)
β-Blockers (e.g., propranolol)	Atrial flutter or atrial fibrillation, supraventricular tachycardia, refractory ventricular tachycardia
Inotropes	
Epinephrine	Anaphylactic shock, asystole, pulseless electrical activity, pulseless ventricular tachycardia or ventricular fibrillation, bradycardia
Vasopressin	Pulseless ventricular tachycardia or ventricular fibrillation
Norepinephrine	Refractory hypotension
Dopamine	Bradycardia, hypotension
Dobutamine	Congestive heart failure
Isoproterenol	Refractory symptomatic bradycardia, long QT syndrome
Digoxin	Atrial flutter, fibrillation, heart failure
Inamrinone	Refractory congestive heart failure
Milrinone	Refractory congestive heart failure
Vasodilators/Antihypertensives	
Nitroprusside	Hypertension, acute heart failure
Nitroglycerin	Hypertension, acute heart failure, anginal pain
Others	
Sodium bicarbonate	Hyperkalemia, metabolic acidosis with bicarbonate loss, hypoxic lactic acidosis
Morphine	Acute pulmonary edema, pain, and anxiety
Furosemide	Acute pulmonary edema
Thrombolytic agents (e.g., alteplase, streptokinase)	Acute thrombosis

Norepinephrine is indicated in patients with low peripheral resistance and severe hypotension. Under these conditions, the drug is both a potent vasoconstrictor and inotropic agent. Sloughing and necrosis of tissues may occur if extravasation occurs during administration.

Dopamine is a chemical precursor of norepinephrine and has both α_1- and β_1-adrenergic stimulating properties. Specific dopaminergic receptors also contribute to the drug's cardiovascular pharmacologic characteristics. Indications for dopamine include certain types of shock, such as that associated with heart failure.[4,37]

Dobutamine is a synthetic catecholamine and potent inotrope used in the treatment of heart failure when signs and symptoms of shock are absent.[4,37]

Inamrinone and milrinone are nonadrenergic cardiotonic agents that also cause vasodilation with hemodynamic effects similar to dobutamine. They increase cardiac function and induce peripheral vasodilation.[22]

Calcium chloride was initially thought to be of benefit during resuscitation by increasing myocardial contractility, but studies have demonstrated that high concentrations of Ca^{++} may, in fact, be detrimental.[7]

Vasodilators

Intravenous nitroglycerin permits controlled titration in relaxing vascular smooth muscle. This drug may cause severe hypotension when administered to a hypovolemic patient.[21] Sodium nitroprusside is an extremely potent, rapidly acting, direct peripheral vasodilator. It is used for the treatment of acute heart failure and hypertensive emergencies.[38]

Sodium bicarbonate

Sodium bicarbonate is administered to correct metabolic acidosis occurring during protracted resuscitative efforts. The use of this drug should be guided by blood gas analysis if possible.[11]

Diuretics

Diuretics such as furosemide are used for their venodilating and diuretic effects for the treatment of acute pulmonary edema and cerebral edema after cardiac arrest.

Morphine

Morphine is the opioid of choice to manage ischemic chest pain and acute pulmonary edema. The drug is titrated in small intravenous doses to avoid respiratory depression.

Thrombolytic agents

Thrombolytic therapy is often instituted early in the evolving myocardial infarction to promote fibrin digestion and clot dissolution. Many studies are being conducted with streptokinase, urokinase, anistreplase, and alteplase to determine their respective roles in the early treatment of myocardial infarction.[14]

Supplementary Drugs

Supplementary drugs are additional emergency drugs that must be available when certain sedative or anesthetic drugs are administered. They include drugs that are used to reverse untoward effects of anesthetics and others that are used to treat specific medical conditions that may occur during anesthesia.

Naloxone is a specific opioid antagonist that reverses opioid-induced respiratory depression. It is mandatory in practices where parental opioids are administered.[26] Flumazenil is a specific benzodiazepine antagonist that reverses sedation and respiratory depression resulting from benzodiazepine administration.[23] Succinylcholine is used to overcome laryngospasm during general anesthesia by relaxing skeletal muscle controlling the vocal cords. Dantrolene arrests the syndrome of malignant hyperthermia, a genetically transmitted disorder of excessive Ca^{++} release in skeletal muscle occurring during general anesthesia in which succinylcholine or volatile inhalation anesthetics are administered.[1]

The use of parenteral vasopressors to treat hypotension is sometimes indicated during anesthesia. Some vasopressors raise blood pressure by causing peripheral vasoconstriction selectively, such as methoxamine and phenylephrine, and others act by a combination of peripheral vasoconstriction and cardiac stimulation, such as ephedrine and mephentermine.

Cited References

1. Britt BA: Dantrolene, *Can Anaesth Soc J* 31:61-75, 1984.
2. Ceremuzynski L, Jurgiel R, Kulakowski P, et al: Threatening arrhythmias in acute myocardial infarction are prevented by intravenous magnesium sulfate, *Am Heart J* 118:1333-1334, 1989.
3. *Cook-Waite Anesthetics,* Rochester, NY, 1993, Eastman Kodak.
4. Cummins RO, ed: *Textbook of advanced cardiac life support,* Dallas, 1997, American Heart Association.
5. Curriculum guidelines for management of medical emergencies in dental education, *J Dent Educ* 54:337-338, 1990.
6. Davenport HT: *Anaesthesia in the elderly,* New York, 1986, Elsevier Science.
7. Dembo DH: Calcium in advanced life support, *Crit Care Med* 9:358-359, 1981.
8. DiMarco JP, Sellers TD, Berne RM, et al: Adenosine: electrophysiologic effects and therapeutic use for terminating paroxysmal supraventricular tachycardia, *Circulation* 68:1254-1263, 1983.
9. Elam JO: Bag-valve-mask O_2 ventilation. In Safar P, ed: *Advances in cardiopulmonary resuscitation,* New York, 1977, Springer-Verlag.
10. Fast TB, Martin MD, Ellis TM: Emergency preparedness: a survey of dental practitioners, *J Am Dent Assoc* 112:449-501, 1986.
11. Federiuk CS, Sanders AB, Kerb KB, et al: The effect of bicarbonate on resuscitation from cardiac arrest, *Ann Emerg Med* 20:1173-1177, 1991.
12. Giardina E-GV, Heissenbuttel RH, Bigger JT, Jr: Intermittent intravenous procaine amide to treat ventricular arrhythmias. Correlation of plasma concentration with effect on arrhythmia, electrocardiogram, and blood pressure, *Ann Intern Med* 78:183-193, 1973.
13. Gonzalez ER, Kannewurf BS, Ornato JP: Intravenous amiodarone for ventricular arrhythmias: overview and clinical use, *Resuscitation* 39:33-42, 1998.
14. Guidelines for the early management of patients with acute myocardial infarction. A report of the American College of Cardiology/American Heart Association Task Force on Assessment of Diagnostic and Therapeutic Cardiovascular Procedures (Subcommittee to Develop Guidelines for the Early Management of Patients with Acute Myocardial Infarction), *J Am Coll Cardiol* 16:249-292, 1990.
15. International Consensus on Science: Guidelines 2000 for cardiopulmonary resuscitation and emergency cardiovascular care. Part 6: advanced cardiovascular life support, *Circulation* 102(suppl 8):86-166, 2000.
16. International Consensus on Science: Guidelines 2000 for cardiopulmonary resuscitation and emergency cardiovascular care. Part 10: pediatric advanced life support, *Circulation* 102(suppl 8):291-342, 2000.
17. ISIS-2 (Second International Study of Infarct Survival Collaborative Group): Randomized trial of intravenous streptokinase, oral aspirin, both, or neither among 17,187 cases of suspected myocardial infarction: ISIS-2, *Lancet* 2:349-361, 1988.
18. Hasegawa EA: The endotracheal use of emergency drugs, *Heart Lung* 15:60-63, 1986.
19. Heywood JT, Graham B, Marais GE, et al: Effects of intravenous diltiazem on rapid atrial fibrillation accompanied by congestive heart failure, *Am J Cardiol* 67:1150-1152, 1991.
20. Himathongkam T, Newmark SR, Greenfield M, et al: Acute adrenal insufficiency, *JAMA* 230:1317-1318, 1974.
21. Jaffe AS, Roberts R: The use of intravenous nitroglycerin in cardiovascular disease, *Pharmacotherapy* 2:273-280, 1982.
22. Klein NA, Siskind SJ, Frishman WH, et al: Hemodynamic comparison of intravenous amrinone and dobutamine in patients with chronic congestive heart failure, *Am J Cardiol* 48:170-175, 1981.
23. Klotz U, Kanto J: Pharmacokinetics and clinical use of flumazenil (Ro 15-1788), *Clin Pharmacokinet* 14:1-12, 1988.
24. Koch-Weser J: Bretylium, *N Engl J Med* 300:473-477, 1979.
25. Lipp M, Kubota Y, Malamed SF, et al: Management of an emergency: to be prepared for the unwanted event, *Anesth Pain Control Dent* 2:90-102, 1992.
26. Longnecker DE, Grazis PA, Eggers GW, Jr: Naloxone for antagonism of morphine-induced respiratory depression, *Anesth Analg* 52:447-453, 1973.
27. Malamed SF: Drugs for medical emergencies in the dental office. In Ciancio SG, ed: *ADA Guide to dental therapeutics,* ed 3, Chicago, 2003, ADA Publishing.

28. Malamed SF: Managing medical emergencies, *JADA* 124:40-53, 1993.
29. Malamed SF: *Medical emergencies in the dental office,* ed 5, St Louis, 2000, Mosby.
30. Matsuura H: Time and occurrence of systemic complications, *Anesth Prog* 36:219-228, 1989.
31. Miller CS, Kaplan AL, Guest GF, et al: Documenting medication use in adult dental patients: 1987-1991, *J Am Dent Assoc* 123:40-48, 1992.
32. Moore PA: Review of medical emergencies in dentistry: staff training and prevention. Part 1, *Gen Dent* 36:14-17, 1988.
33. Munson ES, Wagman IH: Diazepam treatment of local anesthetic-induced seizures, *Anesthesiology* 37:523-528, 1972.
34. Newhouse MT, Dolovich MB: Control of asthma by aerosols, *N Engl J Med* 315:870-874, 1986.
35. Nordt SP, Clark RF: Midazolam: a review of therapeutic uses and toxicity, *J Emerg Med* 15:357-367, 1997.
36. Otto CW, Yakaitis RW: The role of epinephrine in CPR: a reappraisal, *Ann Emerg Med* 13:840-843, 1984.
37. Otto CW, Yakaitis RW, Redding JS, et al: Comparison of dopamine, dobutamine, and epinephrine in CPR, *Crit Care Med* 9:640-643, 1981.
38. Palmer RF, Lasseter KC: Sodium nitroprusside, *N Engl J Med* 292:294-297, 1975.
39. Paradis NA, Koscove EM: Epinephrine in cardiac arrest: a critical review, *Ann Emerg Med* 19:1288-1301, 1990.
40. Patterson R, Anderson J: Allergic reactions to drugs and biologic agents, *JAMA* 248:2637-2645, 1982.
41. Phero JC: Maintaining preparedness for the life-threatening office medical emergency, *Dent Econ* 81:47-50, 1991.
42. Robbin KS: Medicolegal considerations. In Malamed SF, ed: *Medical emergencies in the dental office,* ed 5, St Louis, 2000, Mosby.
43. Salerno DM, Dias VC, Kleiger RE, et al: Efficacy and safety of intravenous diltiazem for treatment of atrial fibrillation and atrial flutter, *Am J Cardiol* 63:1046-1051, 1989.
44. Scheinman MM, Thorburn D, Abbott JA: Use of atropine in patients with acute myocardial infarction and sinus bradycardia, *Circulation* 52:627-633, 1975.
45. Stewart D: Emergency resuscitation kits, *SAAD Digest* 6:223-231, 1987.
46. Yacobi A, Amann AH, Baaski DM: Pharmaceutical considerations of nitroglycerin, *Drug Intell Clin Pharm* 17:255-263, 1983.
47. Yusuf S, Wittes J, Friedman L: Overview of results of randomized clinical trials in heart disease I. Treatments following myocardial infarction, *JAMA* 260:2088-2093, 1988.

General References

Ciancio SG, ed: *ADA Guide to dental therapeutics,* ed 3, Chicago, 2003, ADA Publishing.

Adler JN, Plantz SH, Stearns DA, et al: *Emergency medicine,* ed 1, Baltimore, MD, 1999, Lippincottt, Williams & Wilkins.

Barsan WG, Jastremski MS, Syverud SA, eds: *Emergency drug therapy,* Philadelphia, 1991, WB Saunders.

Bennett JD, Rosenberg MB, eds: *Medical emergencies in dentistry,* Philadelphia, 2002, WB Saunders.

Cummins RO, Field JM, Hazinski MF, et al, eds: *ACLS provider manual,* Dallas, 2001, American Heart Association.

International Consensus on Science: Guidelines 2000 for cardiopulmonary resuscitation and emergency cardiovascular care, *Circulation* 102(suppl 8):1-384, 2000.

Jenkins JL, Locscatzo J, Braen GR: *Manual of emergency medicine,* ed 3, Boston, 1995, Little, Brown.

Malamed SF: *Medical emergencies in the dental office,* ed 5, St Louis, 2000, Mosby.

McCarthy FM, ed: *Medical emergencies in dentistry,* Philadelphia, 1982, WB Saunders.

Meiller TF, Wynn RL, McMillan AM, et al: *Dental office medical emergencies,* Hudson, OH, 2000, Lexi-Comp.

Terezhalmy GT, Batizy LG, eds: *Urgent care in the dental office: an essential handbook,* 1998, Quintessence Publishing.

CHAPTER • 55

Prescription Writing and Drug Regulations*

Vahn A. Lewis

THE PRESCRIPTION

A prescription is a written or verbal order for medication to be used for the diagnosis, prevention, or treatment of a specific patient's disease by a licensed physician, dentist, podiatrist, or veterinarian. In some states a prescription may also be written by appropriately trained optometrists, physician's assistants, and registered nurses. It is a legal document for which the prescriber and pharmacist are both responsible. A prescription may also be written for a drug to be used in a clinician's practice by designating it "for office use." Prescriptions are subject to state, federal, and local regulations.

The writing of a prescription is but one step in many that must be properly performed to initiate a course of therapy (Figure 55-1). This process starts with establishing a proper prescriber-patient relationship, which includes patient identification, proper diagnostic procedures, presentation and discussion of a treatment plan to the patient, availability of counseling, and follow-up care. These fundamental concepts have recently been reasserted by the medical profession with respect to online prescribing for patients who are unknown to the practitioner. A prescription is prima facie evidence in court that such a relationship exists. Selection of therapy requires a multitude of factors to be considered. These factors include those related to the patient (e.g., has difficulty swallowing tablets) and the therapeutic goal (cure or symptom control); evaluation of drug interactions; recognition of the various relationships among the patient, prescriber, and insurance companies and governmental bodies (that may establish guidelines or limits on payment for medications); and the medication costs and whether the patient can afford to buy it. Prescribing outside the proper prescriber-patient relationship is unprofessional conduct.

Prescribing should be performed in a thoughtful and deliberate way, and the conditions for error-free prescribing must be ensured. In 1999, The Institute of Medicine report "To Err is Human" documented an increasing frequency of medical errors.[6] The report analyzed the nature of errors and categorized them into slips, lapses, and mistakes. Slips and lapses occur when the prescriber knows the correct procedure but fails to perform it properly. Mistakes result from incorrect understanding of the correct course of action. Slips and lapses can be influenced by the conditions under which the prescribing is performed, interruptions during the writing of the prescription, or writing an incorrect drug name from memory, although the intended drug choice was sound. In this regard, several suggestions were made that include standardizing prescribing rules, using automated prescriber drug order entry systems and pharmaceutical software, having necessary patient information available at the point of care, and improving the patient's knowledge about his or her treatment. Some of the areas in which errors often occur include poor handwriting, incorrect calculation of pediatric drug doses, look-alike drug name mix-ups, prescriptions for drugs to which the patient is allergic or intolerant, and inappropriate dosage forms. There is a relationship between increased admissions (practitioner overloading) and increased errors. New errors also occur as new therapeutic entities are introduced. Surveys of prescriptions find errors within single prescriptions but also between multiple prescriptions for the same patient in the form of drug interactions or incompatibilities.

Legal Categories of Drugs

Drugs may be categorized according to legal restrictions governing their use as over-the-counter (OTC), prescription, or controlled drugs. As determined by the Food and Drug Administration (FDA), a prescription drug is one that requires a prescription to be dispensed by a pharmacist, whereas an OTC drug can be purchased without a prescription. The term *legend drug* derives from the requirement that prescription drugs must be identified by the legend, "Caution: Federal law prohibits dispensing without prescription." The 1997 FDA Modernization Act has changed this requirement to having the drugs labeled "RX only" after 2003. Several state laws refer to prescription drugs as "dangerous" drugs, meaning that they are not safe for use except under the supervision of a practitioner licensed to administer them. Drugs such as antibiotics, local anesthetics, and systemic corticosteroids are examples of prescription drugs.

Drugs with an abuse potential, called *controlled substances,* have additional restrictions placed on their use. The Drug Enforcement Administration (DEA) of the Department of Justice is responsible for identifying and regulating such drugs. Controlled substances may be OTC, prescription, or unavailable for medical use. Examples of controlled drugs include cough remedies with codeine, opioids such as morphine that are characterized as having medical use, and opioids such as heroin that are said to have no accepted medical use. Most controlled substances have their principal site of action in the central nervous system. The widely abused anabolic steroids are an important exception to this rule and are controlled substances.

OTC agents are deemed to be safe and effective without professional guidance when used according to their labeled instructions. Examples of OTC, or nonprescription, drugs include some nonopioid analgesics, cold remedies, vitamins, topical antibiotics, and topical corticosteroids. These medications are manufactured under the same quality control

*The authors wish to recognize Dr. Anthony Picozzi for his past contributions to this chapter. See the Acknowledgments.

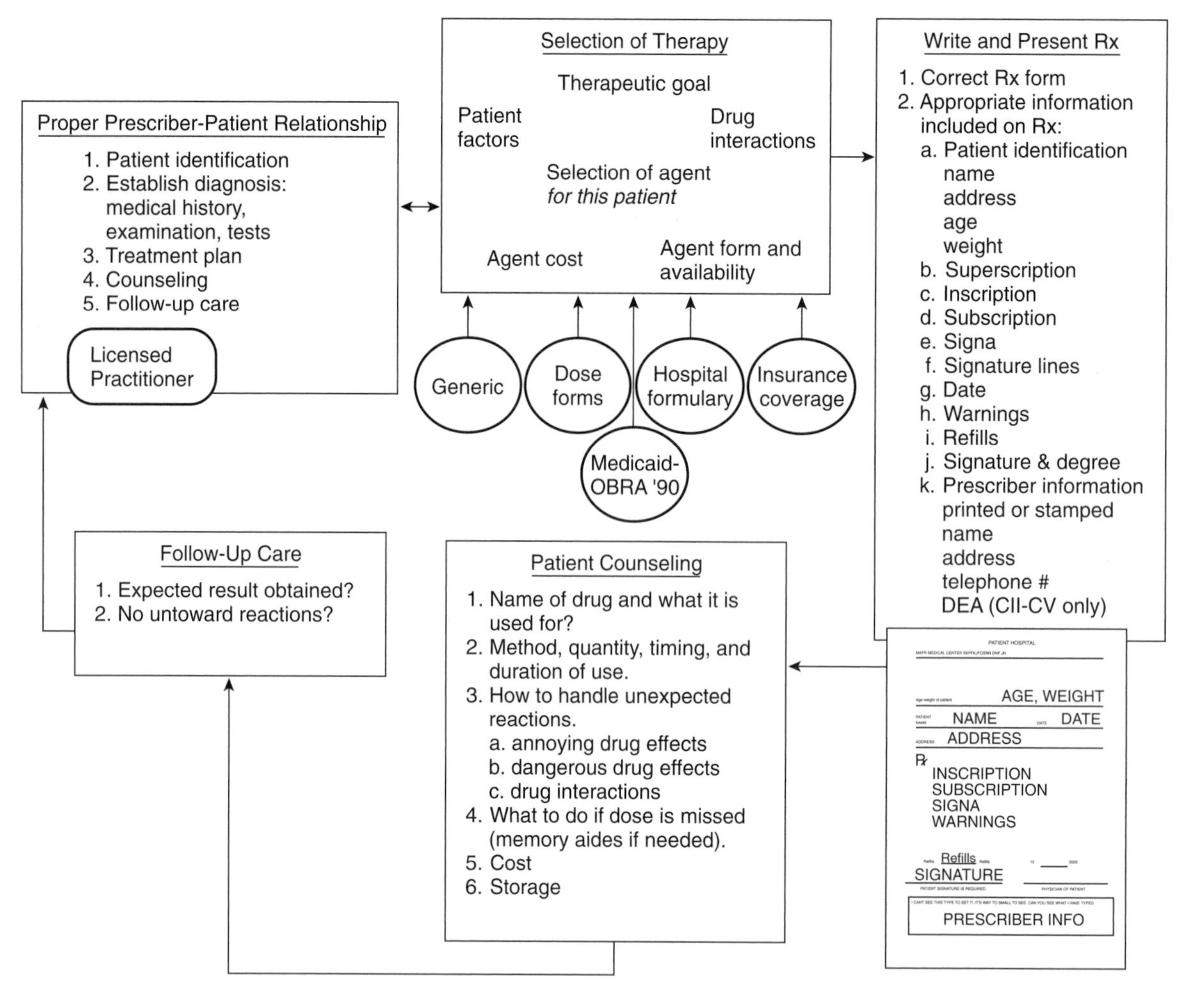

Fig. 55-1 Steps involved in proper prescribing. After selecting the correct therapy, the prescriber must fill out the various components of the prescription to meet both professional and legal requirements established by state, federal, and professional organizations. The next step is to present the prescription to the patient and provide the name of the drug and what it is being prescribed for, how to take it, what kinds of untoward effects the patient might expect, and what they should do about them if they occur. Some discussion of storage and cost of the medication may be included when indicated. After the presentation of the prescription, it is still important to monitor the progress of the patient. If the therapeutic goals are not being achieved, the process may need to be started over. *OBRA*, Omnibus Budget Reconciliation Act.

standards that apply to prescription drugs; their safety and effectiveness are also monitored by the FDA.

As a result of legislative changes during the 1990s (Table 55-1), several additional sources of treatments have become more available. Dietary supplements may contain "dietary ingredients," which can include vitamins, minerals, herbs, amino acids, enzymes, organ tissues, metabolites, extracts, or concentrates. These products must be labeled as *dietary supplements.* The manufacturer is responsible for (1) truthful information, (2) nonmisleading information, and (3) ensuring that the dietary ingredients in the supplements are safe. Manufacturers do not need to register with the FDA or obtain FDA approval. Complementary and alternative medical approaches may use "biologicals," which can include herbal remedies, special diets, or food products used for therapy. *Herbs* are defined as plants or plant products that produce or contain chemicals that act on the body. The National Center for Complementary and Alternative Medicine sponsors many projects to investigate the potential therapeutic value of treatments such as St. John's wort, shark cartilage, and glucosamine. The goal is to determine whether these treatments can aid in the treatment of various disorders. This Center is also concerned with assessing the value of nondrug therapies and nontraditional medical systems such as acupuncture, Eastern medicine, and homeopathic medicine. The FDA can provide guidelines for the therapeutic claims made for these various products through the Center for Food Safety and Applied Nutrition, whose role is primarily educational. The United States Pharmacopeia (USP) has developed a Dietary Supplement Verification (DSV) Program. For a dietary supplement to bear the USP-DSV seal, it must include its ingredients on the label, indicate the strength and amounts of ingredients, prove that the product is demonstrated to be absorbable when taken, and document that it has been screened for heavy metals, microbes, and pesticides and been manufactured in safe, sanitary, and controlled conditions.

Single-Entity versus Combination Prescriptions

A single-entity prescription is one written for a preparation with only one active ingredient, the agent that produces the desired effect (e.g., ibuprofen, 600-mg tablets), compared with a combination prescription, which calls for a preparation

Table • 55-1

Federal Laws Regulating Drugs and Prescribing

LAW	EFFECT
Pure Food and Drug Act 1906 (Wiley Act)	Prohibited mislabeling and adulteration of drugs[15]
Opium Exclusion Act of 1909	Prohibited importation of opium
Amendment (1912) to the Pure Food and Drug Act	Prohibited false or fraudulent advertising claims
Harrison Narcotic Act of 1914	Established regulations for use of opium, opiates, and cocaine (marijuana added in 1937)
Food, Drug and Cosmetic Act of 1938	Required that new drugs be safe as well as pure (but did not require proof of efficacy); enforcement by FDA[16]
Durham-Humphrey Amendment of 1951	Vested in the FDA the power to determine which products could be sold without prescription
Kefauver-Harris Amendments (1962) to the Food, Drug and Cosmetic Act	Required proof of efficacy as well as safety for new drugs and for drugs released since 1938; established guidelines for reporting information about adverse reactions, clinical testing, and advertising of new drugs
Comprehensive Drug Abuse Prevention and Control Act (1970), Controlled Substances Act, as amended	Outlined strict controls in the manufacture, distribution, and prescribing of habit-forming drugs; established programs to prevent and treat drug addiction[17]
Orphan Drug Amendments of 1983	Amended Food, Drug, and Cosmetic Act of 1938, providing incentives for the development of drugs to treat conditions suffered by fewer than 200,000 patients in the United States[18]
Drug Price Competition and Patent Restoration Act of 1984 (Waxman-Hatch Act)	Abbreviated NDA for generic drugs; required bioequivalence data; patent life extended by amount of time delayed by FDA review process; cannot exceed 5 extra years or extend more than 14 years post-NDA approval; authorized abbreviated NDA[19]
Omnibus Budget Reconciliation Act of 1990	Deepened governmental involvement in prescription writing through legislation relating to "best discount prices," rebates, formularies, and pharmacy reimbursements; placed restrictions on payment for prescriptions for barbiturates and benzodiazepines
Generic Drug Debarment Act of 1991 and the Food, Drug, Cosmetic and Device Enforcement Amendment of 1991	Increased penalties for abuses of generic drug regulations
1992 Expedited Drug Approval Act	Allowed accelerated FDA approval for drugs of high medical need; required detailed postmarketing patient surveillance
1992 Prescription Drug User Fee Act	Required manufacturers to pay user fees for certain NDAs; FDA states review time for new chemical entities has dropped from 30 months in 1992 to 20 months in 1994[20]
1994 Dietary Supplements and Health Education Act	Required dietary supplement manufacturers to ensure that a dietary supplement is safe before it is marketed; FDA is responsible for taking action against any unsafe dietary supplement product after it reaches the market; generally, manufacturers do not need to register with FDA or get FDA approval before producing or selling dietary supplements; manufacturers must make sure that product label information is truthful and not misleading[21]
North American Free Trade Act (1994) and General Agreement on Tariffs and Trade (1948), World Trade Organization (1995)	Necessitated harmonization of pharmacopeias and drug regulations between trading partners
1996 Health Insurance Portability and Accountability Act (HIPAA)	Standardized third-party payment for medical treatment and increased confidentiality and privacy for patient information maintained in medical databases[24]
1997 FDA Modernization Act	Replaced "legend" with label "Rx only"; allowed manufacturer to discuss off-label uses of drugs with practitioners; revised accelerated track approval for drugs that treat life-threatening disorders; made provisions for pediatric drug research; revised interaction of agency with individuals doing clinical trials[22]

NDA, New Drug Application.

with more than one active ingredient (e.g., aspirin, 230 mg; acetaminophen, 150 mg; caffeine, 30 mg; and hydrocodone bitartrate, 5 mg).[5] Many combination formulations are available precompounded, in a single fixed-dosage form, and may be prescribed in the same manner as a single drug (e.g., acetaminophen and hydrocodone tablets). When the combination is a rational one (as is the combination of a nonopioid and an opioid analgesic for enhanced pain relief), the ease of prescribing and using the preparation may justify its selection. Too frequently, however, unnecessary drugs (e.g., caffeine) or inappropriate combinations (such as the mixing of two nonopioid analgesics) are used. Fixed-dosage formulations prepared by the manufacturer are not subject to dosage adjustment to suit the needs of the individual patient. Differences in the half-lives of the individual agents may lead to ineffective or excessive action of one or more of the drugs. Nevertheless, at certain times therapeutic advantages can be obtained by using a combination drug to reduce confusion related to taking large numbers of individual medications at irregular times.

Drug Names and Generic Substitution

As discussed in Chapter 3, any drug may be identified by more than one designation in various references, texts, and package inserts. Of special interest here are the nonproprietary and proprietary names. The nonproprietary name is also referred to as the *generic name.* This name is selected by the United States Adopted Names Council. Because of changes in drug laws the number of new drugs available is increasing, and similarities between different drug names is an increasing challenge. The practitioner must be vigilant in prescribing the correct agent and spelling drug names correctly. Because, with few exceptions, individual drugs have only one nonproprietary name, it is this name by which the drug is primarily identified. Nonproprietary names may differ among countries, however. The same agent may also have many proprietary or trade names, which are given to it by the various manufacturers or marketers to identify their brand of the drug. In advertisements and labeling with the trade name, the nonproprietary name of the drug must also be prominently identified.

In recent years, governmental regulatory agencies have had a strong tendency to encourage or even mandate the prescription and dispensation of drugs by nonproprietary name.[10] The principal motivation for these regulations is to control rapidly increasing drug costs. Currently, all states and the District of Columbia have repealed their existing antisubstitution laws and replaced them with drug substitution laws permitting or, in some states, requiring the pharmacist to dispense generic drugs (preparations containing the same active chemicals in identical amounts but sold under the common nonproprietary name) unless specifically prohibited by the prescriber. Also, the federal government has instituted "maximum allowable cost" programs in an effort to contain the cost of prescription drugs to the consumer by limiting prescription by proprietary name. These programs require the prescriber to certify the necessity of prescribing a specific brand of drug rather than its nonproprietary counterpart. On average, the reduction in patient cost is approximately 10%.

Equivalence: Chemical, Pharmaceutical, Biologic, and Therapeutic

If two brands of the same drug are to be considered for substitution, the basis for identifying them as equivalent must be carefully defined.[9] Drug products that contain the same amounts of the same active ingredients in the same dosage forms and meet current official compendium standards are considered chemical equivalents. Pharmaceutical equivalents are drug products that contain the same amounts of the same therapeutic or active ingredients in the same dosage form and meet standards based on the best currently available technology. This description means that pharmaceutical equivalents are formulated identically and must pass certain laboratory tests for equivalent activity, including dissolution tests when appropriate, by standards set for various classes of drugs.

Bioavailability refers to the extent and rate of absorption of a dosage form as reflected by the time-concentration curve of the administered drug in the systemic circulation. Bioequivalent drugs are those that, when administered to the same individual in the same dosage regimen, result in comparable bioavailability. Insofar as the extent of absorption is concerned, pharmaceutical equivalence presumably ensures biologic equivalence.

Therapeutic equivalents are chemical or pharmaceutical equivalents that, when administered to the same individual in the same dosage regimen, provide essentially the same efficacy (and toxicity). Therapeutic equivalency can only be demonstrated by controlled human clinical trials, which are expensive and time consuming. In the absence of contradictory clinical evidence, drugs that are bioequivalent are assumed to be therapeutically equivalent.

Chemically equivalent drugs may not share comparable bioavailability. Problems of bioequivalence can arise from many areas. First, although the amounts of the therapeutic ingredients may be the same in two dosage forms, the preparations may contain different binders, diluents, stabilizers, preservatives, and a variety of other pharmacologically inactive ingredients to give them their physical form. Second, the pressure used to compress the mixture into the tablet or capsule dosage form may vary and alter the dissolution rate. For suspensions or solutions, the method used to dissolve, disperse, or suspend the drug in a liquid formulation may differ. Third, the quality control, age, purity, and physical consistency of any of the chemical constituents contained in different formulations of chemically equivalent products can differ. All these various and sometimes poorly controlled factors can influence the rate at which the product disintegrates or dissolves in the gastrointestinal tract, thereby affecting absorption of the active ingredients.

Variations in bioavailability have been shown to be responsible for some treatment failures with certain categories of drugs. Approximately 5% of drug products pose challenges to generic drug manufacturers. Drugs with poor bioavailability, high lipid solubility, nonlinear pharmacokinetics, or narrow therapeutic ranges cause difficulty[3]; examples include steroids, digitalis glycosides, anticoagulants, thyroid preparations, theophylline, antineoplastic drugs, and anticonvulsants. Advanced or complex dosage forms with coatings or layers are also difficult to match. Drugs with potential bioavailability problems that are likely to be used by dentists include the various dosage forms of erythromycin, diazepam, and ibuprofen.

To facilitate the wider use of generic drugs, the FDA has published a list of all FDA-approved drugs that it regards as therapeutically equivalent, entitled *Approved Drug Products with Therapeutic Equivalence Evaluations* (the "Orange Book").[11] This source can be used as a guide to identifying less expensive generic alternatives that pharmacists can substitute for brand name products designated "reference listed drug," that is, the innovator drug. This list indicates which drugs are considered therapeutically equivalent (termed a *positive formulary*), designated with a rating beginning with the letter *A;* which drugs may not be therapeutically equivalent (a *negative formulary*), designated with a starting letter *B;* and those about which the agency has not yet made a determination (blanks). The FDA's policy is to consider pharmaceutically equivalent drugs as therapeutically equivalent unless scientific evidence to the contrary exists. In the Orange Book (available on the Internet[23]) the reference listed drug, therapeutically equivalent rating, and generic drug rating are provided in tabular form. If a generic oral dosage form preparation is considered therapeutically equivalent, it is given the designation of *AB* (the second letter, *B* in this case, refers to the class of dose form). At the time of this writing, 96% of ibuprofen tablets were judged AB, 100% of diazepam tablets were AB, and all the erythromycin ethyl succinate suspensions were considered AB.

Although FDA recalls of generic drugs greatly outnumber those of brand name drugs, the vast majority of American pharmaceutical firms follow Good Manufacturing Practice regulations and are inspected periodically by the FDA for compliance with quality control standards. Additionally, many generic products are manufactured and distributed by the same company that markets the original proprietary drug. For these reasons, a generic product should not be assumed to be inferior to its brand name counterpart. It is left to the practitioner to know the properties of the drugs used and to decide whether to prescribe by trade or nonproprietary name. If the condition being treated is not serious or life threatening, and if the therapeutic index of the drug category being prescribed is not critical, a generic drug can save the patient a substantial amount of money and should be prescribed by its nonproprietary name.

Component Parts of the Prescription

A complete, ideal prescription is made up of several parts, each of which provides specific information about the prescriber, the patient, and the drug.

The patient's full name and address are required on prescriptions for DEA-controlled substances. Including the patient's age may be required and is especially desirable on prescriptions for children younger than 12 years, permitting the pharmacist to confirm the dosage. The name and full address of the prescriber are necessary. The telephone number may be required and is usually included as a convenience to the pharmacist. The date on which the prescription is written and signed is always desirable and is required on prescriptions for DEA-controlled substances or in states in which prescriptions expire.

The symbol *Rx*, known as the *superscription*, is generally understood to be an abbreviation of the Latin *recipe*, meaning "take thou," but was probably derived from the ancient Roman symbol for Jupiter and used in the physician's prayer for the survival of the patient.

The inscription provides specific information about the drug preparation: (1) the name of the drug, which can be either the nonproprietary or the proprietary name, or possibly both, with the proprietary name following the nonproprietary name in parentheses, as with pentazocine (Talwin); and (2) the unit dosage or amount of the drug in milligrams (as with penicillin VK 500 mg) or other appropriate unit of measure (as with penicillin G 250,000 U) and the dosage form (e.g., tablet, suspension, sprinkles). If the prescription is for a liquid preparation, the individual unit of dosage is usually contained in a teaspoonful or 5 ml (as with amoxicillin 125 mg/5 ml). The inscription should provide an unambiguous identification of the drug and any other ingredients that the pharmacist must assemble to fill the prescription order. Drug products are available in unique strengths and dosage forms. When prescribing, designate a product, strength, and dosage form that is available to the pharmacist. The inscription should be written just below and to the right of the superscription.

Several sources of drug information should be available during selection of drug therapy. Good sources for identifying the drug, dosage form, and dose include *The Physicians' Desk Reference, Facts and Comparisons, Mosby's Drug Consult 2004,* and the *United States Pharmacopeia Dispensing Information* (USP DI). In addition, it is valuable to have a compilation of drug interactions available to screen for possible adverse interactions. A book such as *Drugs in Pregnancy and Lactation* by Briggs et al[2] is helpful when a course of therapy is being planned for a woman of child-bearing potential as well as for pregnant or nursing women. The American Pharmaceutical Association's *Handbook of Nonprescription Drugs* may be useful if the practitioner is uncertain whether an OTC drug might affect therapy. Today, references on herbal drugs and dietary supplements may also be useful (see Chapter 56).

Additional sources of drug information are available as computer software programs, compact disks, and personal digital assistant programs, as well as on the Internet. Electronic resources can have advantages if the text is accompanied by a sophisticated search engine. An innovation in prescribing is the concept of "linked database prescribing" (Figure 55-2).

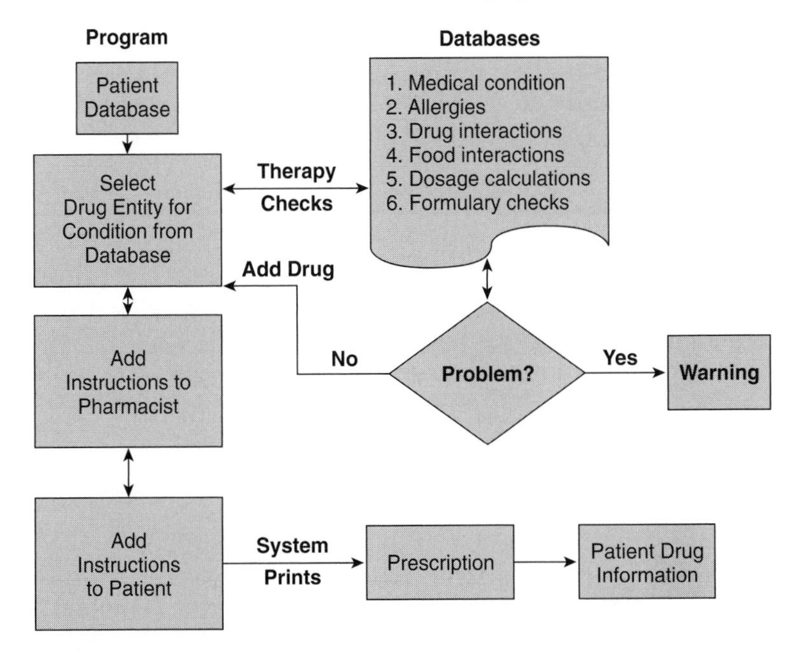

Fig. 55-2 The complex process of prescribing can be facilitated by a linked database prescribing system. These systems can assist the prescriber by putting patient, drug, drug interaction, and formulary information at the prescriber's fingertips. The systems can provide warnings when problems are discovered. Current systems leave the instructions to the pharmacist and patient up to the prescriber. Written drug information for the patient is frequently generated automatically.

This type of system has the potential to reduce several sources of prescribing errors, such as poor handwriting, selection of the wrong drug name (selection is based on therapeutic classification), nonexistent product strengths and dosage forms, orders for drugs to which patients are allergic, and therapeutic incompatibilities. Other errors such as dosing and patient instruction errors could also be reduced by appropriately designed systems.

Although this concept appears to have a bright future, implementation will be challenging for professional, technical, and legal reasons. If patient data are entered into such a system, the system will need to comply with the Health Insurance Portability and Accountability Act of 1996 (HIPAA). Specialties such as dentistry may use drugs in a somewhat different way than are generally used in medicine. This can lead to false rejections or warnings for valid prescriptions. Who will be responsible for programming and maintaining the quality of the databases? Who will pay for the use of such a system? An example of such a system is *Clinical Pharmacology*, an Internet-based program created by Gold Standard Multimedia.

The next part of the prescription is the subscription. The subscription is the prescriber's directions to the pharmacist regarding fulfilling the inscription. Because almost all drugs used by dentists are available in precompounded form, the subscription is usually brief, including only the following:

1. The quantity and dosage form of the drug to be dispensed; that is, the number of tablets or capsules or the volume of a liquid preparation needed for a course of therapy (e.g., "dispense 28 tablets"). This direction is written, preferably in Arabic numerals, for an appropriate amount of the drug as determined by the manner in which it will be used by the patient and the amount of time the patient will need it. The prescriber also considers the toxicity and abuse potential of the drug and the cost to the patient. For DEA-controlled drugs, the quantity must be written in numbers and spelled out (in English, not Latin) to avoid alteration. (Without this precaution, for example, 15 is easily changed to 45, 75, or 150.) In any prescription, no greater quantity of drug than is needed should be ordered. In some cases the amount prescribed should be limited to prevent obscuring symptoms, such as prescribing analgesics for 3 or 4 days rather than the 7 to 10 days common for antibiotics. If multiple appointments are anticipated, it may be more cost effective to write the amount to reflect several appointments. The subscription should be written on the line below the last line of the inscription.
2. The number of authorized refills of the prescription. The number and its time limitation are specified for DEA-controlled drugs but are otherwise left to the discretion of the practitioner. However, some state laws dictate that prescriptions expire at the end of each year. If refill directions are not specified by the prescriber, no refills may be dispensed. With controlled substances, care should be taken to devise a refill authorization system that is not easily altered, such as crossing out all except the desired number in a series (e.g., ~~0,~~ 1, ~~2,~~ ~~3~~). The refill instructions are usually physically located below the transcription (described later) of the prescription.
3. Directions to the pharmacist to list the medication on the container label. The current trend in most states is to require the pharmacist to identify medications on the label unless such identification is not considered to be in the patient's best interest and specifically prohibited by the prescriber. Identifying the drug can prevent allergic reactions or adverse interactions with other medications and misuse of the unused portion of the prescription. It may be especially helpful in directing the management of victims of drug poisoning. When present, this information is often physically located below the transcription on the prescription.

The transcription, or signature (from the Latin *signa*, meaning "label" or "let it be labeled"), indicated on the prescription by "Label:" or "Sig:", is the prescriber's directions to the patient that will appear on the medicine container. At one time, such directions were uniformly written in Latin, but modern practice is to use English. Latin abbreviations are still used by many clinicians in prescriptions and progress notes to save time (Table 55-2); however, such gains are minor in general dental practice and may contribute to prescription errors (e.g., "q4h" instead of "qid" represents a 50% dosage increase). Figure 55-3 depicts the same signature for an analgesic medication, one written entirely in English and the other by Latin abbreviations.

The phrase "use as directed" should not be used. Rather, the transcription should be explicit and include (1) the route

Table • 55-2

Latin Abbreviations Frequently Used in Prescription Writing

ABBREVIATION	LATIN	ENGLISH
ad lib.	*ad libitum*	at pleasure
a.c.	*ante cibum*	before meals
aq.	*aqua*	water
b.i.d.	*bis in die*	twice a day
caps.	*capsula*	capsule
c̄	*cum*	with
d.	*dies*	a day, daily
disp.	*dispensa*	dispense
gtt.	*guttae*	drops
h.	*hora*	hour
h.s.	*hora somni*	at bedtime
non rep.	*non repetatur*	do not repeat (or refill)
no.	*numerus*	number, amount
p.c.	*post cibum*	after meals
p.r.n.	*pro re nata*	as needed
q.h.	*quaque hora*	every hour
q.4h.	*quaque quarta hora*	every 4 hours
q.i.d.	*quater in die*	four times a day
Sig.	*signa*	let it be labeled, label
stat.	*statim*	immediately
tab.	*tabella*	tablet
t.i.d.	*ter in die*	three times a day

Label: Take two tablets immediately. Take one or two tablets every 4 hours as needed for relief of pain.

Sig: Tab 2 stat. Tab 1 or 2 q.4h. p.r.n. for relief of pain.

Fig. 55-3 Sample of the same transcription or signature (instructions to the patient) written in English and with Latin abbreviations.

and method (e.g., take, swallow whole, chew then swallow), (2) the number of dose forms to be taken each time (e.g., swallow one, take two), (3) how frequently to administer the medication (e.g., every 6 hours, at bedtime), (4) for what length of therapy (e.g., for 7 days, until all taken), (5) for what purpose (now required by law in some states; e.g., for an analgesic "to relieve pain" or "for pain"), and (6) any special instructions (e.g., shake well before using, refrigerate). The instructions to the patient should be consistent with the patient characteristics, drug, and dosage form. Prescriptions written for children should use the verb *give* instead of *take* to indicate that the parent or guardian is to administer the drug. Enteric-coated drugs should be swallowed whole to ensure that the coating is still intact when the drug reaches the stomach. Directions for suspensions should include the phrase "shake well then take . . ." to ensure administration of a uniform dose. The transcription should be located on the next line after the subscription. (The arrangement of information on the prescription is by custom, but by observing this order the practitioner is less likely to omit an essential part of the instructions.)

The handwritten signature and professional degree of the prescriber convey the authority of the prescriber to order the medication and of the pharmacist to fill the prescription. Although all prescriptions should be signed, a signature is required by law only for certain controlled substances (schedule II drugs); other prescriptions may be telephoned to a pharmacy, where the pharmacist writes them down. When it appears, the dentist's signature is followed by the prescriber's professional degree rather than preceded by "Dr." as the abbreviation for "Doctor." If several dentists work in a clinic that uses the same prescription form, several states require that the prescriber's name be mechanically printed or stamped on the prescription on an extra line under the signature line. Most state dental practice acts specify that prescriptions may be written only for patients under active care. Many state laws stipulate that only those classes of drugs directly involved with dental treatment may be prescribed by the dentist.

Finally, the prescriber's DEA registration number must appear on any prescription for a controlled or scheduled drug in compliance with the Controlled Substances Act of 1970. This number, however, should not be routinely entered on prescriptions that do not require it in order to prevent its use by potential drug abusers.

Many states have their own acts related to controlled substances. If state, federal, or local regulations governing any drug or procedure differ, the most stringent of the regulations applies. Both the state and federal certificates of registration must be renewed periodically. DEA registration is not required of practitioners in the military or the Public Health Service or of recent graduates in internship or residency programs; in the latter case, the institutional DEA registration number may be used.

After the prescribing of the drug, but before the prescription is filled, another evaluation of the prescription is made by the pharmacist. The pharmacist has responsibility to both the patient and the practitioner to check the prescription for possible errors in drug selection, dosage form and dosage, and patient instructions.

Increasingly, prescriptions are being filled at sites remote from where the patient lives. Prescriptions may be mailed or in some cases submitted by the telephone or Internet to a pharmacy. Remote pharmacies may be used to obtain medications at a better price or required by insurance carriers. In some cases these pharmacies may not be in the United States.

The FDA is charged with regulating the production of prescription drugs from development to distribution. They have set standards that require compliance during drug development (e.g., New Drug Application [NDA]), labeling (package inserts), drug manufacturing (i.e., Good Manufacturing Practices), and drug distribution and post-marketing surveillance (e.g., MedWatch). However, the FDA is challenged by limited funding (Prescription Drug User Fee Act), changes in international agreements (NAFTA and GATT), changes in public attitudes toward regulation of medications (1994 Dietary Supplements and Health Education Act), increased threats to drug and food safety (bioterrorism, "mad cow disease"), and the use of the Internet to market drugs.

Mail order pharmacies

For chronic medications where the cost is covered by an insurance company, patients may be directed to submit the prescription to a central pharmacy if the company is to cover the cost. The medication will be shipped to the patient in the domestic mails, and if the shipment crosses state or national borders the medications must comply with FDA requirements.

Internet prescriptions

The development of Internet drug distribution has added an additional area of challenge for the control of the drug supply. Many of the solicitations for drug sales over the Internet are illegal, and the FDA has moved to close such practices.[25] However, these sites may come and go before the FDA can act. The medications sold may be of unknown quality and may come from distant sources. Cursory Internet health histories may not properly reflect the patient's health status or may not be reviewed by qualified personnel. Drugs can be used more safely when appropriate medical histories are obtained and used by practitioners during the prescribing process. In addition, if a patient has an adverse reaction to a drug obtained from a distant source, recognizing and treating adverse reactions may be difficult. There is also a potential financial risk to the patient when using the Internet because the seller may be unknown to the buyer. Caveat Emptor ("Buyer beware") is very much the operating principle for these transactions. To help reduce some of the risks associated with the use of Internet pharmacies, the National Association of Boards of Pharmacy has developed a voluntary certification program called Verified Internet Pharmacy Practices Site (VIPPS). A VIPPS seal of approval indicates that the pharmacy complies with state licensing and additional requirements, including the patient's right to privacy.

Reimportation of Drugs

Technically no unapproved drugs may be imported into the United States. However, travelers and immigrants may feel more comfortable taking medications they are familiar with from their home countries. The FDA and US Customs Service regulate drug importation for personal use by guidance documents used for interpreting the various laws administered by the FDA.[26] Small quantities of medications not available in the United States, intended to continue a course of treatment begun in a foreign country, may be allowed to enter. The FDA narrows the scope of such drug importations to small amounts (generally less than a 3-month supply) for personal use. If the product's use is properly identified, it is not for a serious condition, and deemed not a health risk, it can be approved. If it is an unapproved product for treatment of a serious illness for which treatment is not available domestically, not for commercial sale, not deemed to pose an unreasonable risk and where the patient can document that a physician is responsible for the patient's care, it may be approvable. These provisions were prompted by the concerns for patients with AIDS who were willing to assume the greater risk of non–FDA approved drugs to treat their often fatal condition.

Commercial importation or re-importation of drugs into the United States is illegal without FDA approval. The Medicine Equity and Drug Safety Act of 2000 does permit re-importation of drugs manufactured in the United States back into this country. However, before the law can go into effect it needs the approval of the U.S. Health and Human Services Secretary. Thus far, approval has not been given. The concern is that once a drug is out of the United States it is no longer subject to US laws and therefore its composition cannot be guaranteed. Although most foreign governments have departments that regulate drugs sold to their own populations, many do not regulate businesses that market drugs to countries beyond their borders. There is a valid concern that for drug entities imported from a variety of sources, assembled into a dosage form in one country, and then sold in another, there would be no way to ensure the purity, safety, efficacy, or proper labeling of the result.

Agents from the FDA may cooperate with the US Customs Service to enforce the Federal Food, Drug and Cosmetics Act with respect to medications that are carried or mailed into the United States. In a pilot survey program, hundreds of packages containing drugs were detained. Some of these packages failed to properly declare medications, which could result in Customs penalties. If the recipient cannot show the FDA that the shipment is in response to valid prescriptions or letters of instruction from a physician, drugs can be destroyed or returned to their source.

There are examples of seized drugs that were previously banned from the United States for safety concerns being illegally imported into the United States. In some cases, labeling for the imported drugs fails to mention offending agents actually contained in the container. Drugs that are outright counterfeits have been discovered. Control over the manufacturing of imported products is unknown and they are sometimes contaminated with bacteria or other "filth." In some cases, drugs that are older than their expiration date are received, resulting in subtherapeutic blood levels, or in worst cases, toxicity from a degraded drug.

However, the cost savings of using drugs from foreign sources can be substantial. A prescription that may cost more than $100 to fill in the United States may be available from Canada for less than half that amount, and may be available from India for pennies per dose. In some cases, these foreign drugs are just as effective as the more expensive versions available in the United States. For patients taking life-saving medications and who have no insurance or have a fixed or low income, their choice may be between no medication or cheaper imported drugs. Programs have been developed for doctors licensed to practice in both the United States and Canada to write prescriptions for busloads of patients who get their prescriptions filled in Canada and then return to the US. In other cases, "storefront" pharmacies have opened that receive prescriptions in various cities in the United States, fax them to Canadian pharmacies for filling, and then deliver the medications to the patients by mail. The FDA has judged the latter operations to be illegal commercial importers and has moved to shut them down.

Noncompliance

A subject of current interest regarding directions on prescriptions is patient compliance or, more accurately, noncompliance. Twenty-five percent to 60% of all patients fail to take medications as intended by their doctors. Noncompliance includes such practices as improper or inappropriate timing of doses or premature discontinuation of the medication. The many possible reasons for patient noncompliance may involve a lack of knowledge or understanding of the drug or the purpose for which it was prescribed, misinformation from nonmedical sources, negative patient attitudes toward illness or "taking drugs," development of an adverse effect, economic factors, or inadequate communication (instruction and emphasis) by the practitioner.

Patient compliance is probably improved when the prescriber explains the condition for which the patient is being treated, what the alternative treatment regimens are, and the anticipated benefits of the selected drug treatment.[1,4,8] After the drug therapy is selected, patients should be informed of the name of the drug and, in layman's terms, its therapeutic purpose. This information helps the patient recognize the importance of each prescription. Specific instructions on drug use should include how and when to take the medication, how much to take, and when to expect the benefits. The patient should also be made aware of possible adverse reactions and side effects. Some side effects such as drowsiness may be disturbing and interfere to an extent with daily living but do not require discontinuation of therapy. Other adverse reactions, such as acute allergic reactions, require immediate discontinuation of therapy. Finally, drug and food interactions should be mentioned. The patient should then be given an opportunity to ask questions or clarify the instructions. A logical presentation of this information, as given above, will improve instruction recall and understanding of the instructions.[13] For patients on a strict budget, a discussion of drug costs may be important. Little is accomplished by prescribing a drug that the patient is unable or unwilling to buy. The patient should also be informed of what to do if a dose is missed and whether the drug should be taken immediately or at the next dosing interval. It is also useful to tell the patient about any special storage requirements, such as the need for keeping the drug refrigerated (emulsions) or at room temperature (syrups). Practitioners need to familiarize themselves with the instructions for use and storage of the medications they prescribe because these instructions can vary between dosage forms and preparations of the same drug entity.

The prescription enhances the doctor-patient relationship and contributes to patient compliance if care is used in presenting it. Writing a prescription in English and in the patient's presence and then explaining it may, in addition to improving compliance, equip the patient to detect any errors that may occur in prescribing or filling the prescription.

Because relatively few patients are able to recall oral instructions accurately, the labeled directions should be specific. Indeed, failure to be specific can provide the basis for malpractice lawsuits. If the patient has many prescriptions or has a special difficulty with oral instructions, a written reminder should accompany the prescription.

Patient compliance may also be improved by selecting drugs that need to be taken only once or twice daily instead of agents that have to be administered more frequently. When multiple drug therapy is necessary, combination products, when appropriate, are helpful in reducing the "confusion over pill profusion," as is prescribing drugs with distinctive physical characteristics (e.g., a red tablet, a white tablet, and a capsule instead of three white tablets).

Prescription Format and Pad Forms

Prescriptions should be written concisely, accurately, and legibly. Ink, indelible pencil, or typing is required for prescriptions for schedule II drugs and is preferable for all prescriptions. With the advent of safe and effective drugs, consumer education, and the concept of informed consent, the need for therapeutic mysticism of an illegible prescription written in a foreign language no longer exists. Furthermore, similarity between the names of some highly active and potentially toxic drugs makes illegibility all the more indefensible.

Blank printed prescription pads should not have the name of a pharmacy or pharmaceutical company imprinted anywhere on the form because such an implicit endorsement may direct the patient to a particular pharmacy or manufacturer's product. Pads should also be kept in a drawer or under similar cover when not in use to avoid loss or theft of prescription blanks by a potential drug abuser. If theft of a prescription pad is suspected, such loss should be reported to the state drug control agency. Additionally, for good dental practice as well as for medicolegal reasons, a duplicate of each prescription or a record thereof should be kept in the patient's chart or record.

Figure 55-4 presents a typical preprinted prescription form used, with minor variations, by most practitioners. Because of state laws permitting or, in some instances, mandating the substitution of a generic preparation for a proprietary drug unless specifically prohibited by the prescriber, the prescription form may have a feature to allow the clinician to indicate whether a substitution is permitted. Because no physical prescription is written in telephone orders, the practitioner must indicate verbally to the pharmacist whether substitution is permitted. Some states also permit the transmission of prescriptions by electronic means (e.g., fax or computer network). In some hospitals, prescriptions are generated by the patient information system and sent directly to the pharmacy. Pharmacists occasionally note prescriptions that make no sense for a particular patient. On review, these prescriptions generally were for agents on the computer medication screen that were adjacent to the desired drugs.

Figure 55-5 presents three sample prescriptions. The first, for antibiotic prophylaxis before dental therapy, is written by nonproprietary name; the second, for postoperative pain relief, is written by proprietary name for the sake of convenience. In the latter case, the dosage is implicit in the particular formulation selected (e.g., Tylenol with Codeine No. 3: acetaminophen [Tylenol] 325 mg and codeine 30 mg, with the notation 3 indicating the 30-mg strength of codeine). The third prescription, for fluoride supplementation in a child (2 years of age) living in a low-fluoride area, is one of the few instances in which long-term drug use is appropriate in clinical dentistry.

Dosage Calculations (Posology)

The dosage of a prescribed drug may vary according to several factors: the degree or severity of the condition for which it is being prescribed; the age, weight, sex, or temperament of the patient; the route, frequency, or timing of administration; concurrent medication; patient suggestibility (placebo effect), habits, sensitivities, or previous medication history (hyperreaction or hyporeaction); and the systemic health of the patient. Important changes in clearance or volume of distribution can produce changes in expected half-lives of drugs. Because drug metabolism and elimination are primarily accomplished by the liver and kidneys, any significant change in the function of these organs may necessitate a change in dosing. For the fluoride prescription in Figure 55-5, the age of the patient and the amount of fluoride in the water supply are the primary determinants of the dosage.

The manufacturer's package insert, pharmacology texts, and the compendial sources mentioned earlier in this chapter list the *official*, *average*, or *usual* adult dose for a drug. A listed dose or dosage range is a guide for prescription purposes, and although it does not carry the weight of a regulation, it does have medicolegal implications if an adverse effect occurs. Practitioners are well advised to stay within the recommended dosage range unless they have a sound reason to go beyond it. Brief resumes of sources of drug information are provided in Chapter 3.

No uniform format is used in references to express dosing information. For most drugs the dose is reported as the amount of drug to be given at a single dose, which is then repeated at a stated interval each day. Alternatively, the manufacturer may indicate the total amount of drug to be administered "in divided doses" per day. The practitioner is expected to know what dosage forms are available and how often to give them on the basis of the pharmacokinetics of the drug and the nature of the patient. For dosage determination, an "adult" is usually interpreted to mean an individual 18 years or older and weighing approximately 70 kg (150 lb).

Children and many underweight, diseased, or elderly patients require a dosage of pharmacologically active agent that is lower than that suggested for the normal adult. Very large or obese patients may require dosage adjustment, but this adjustment can depend on the characteristics of each drug; with some drugs (e.g., gentamicin) the increased dosage can increase the risk of toxicity.[12]

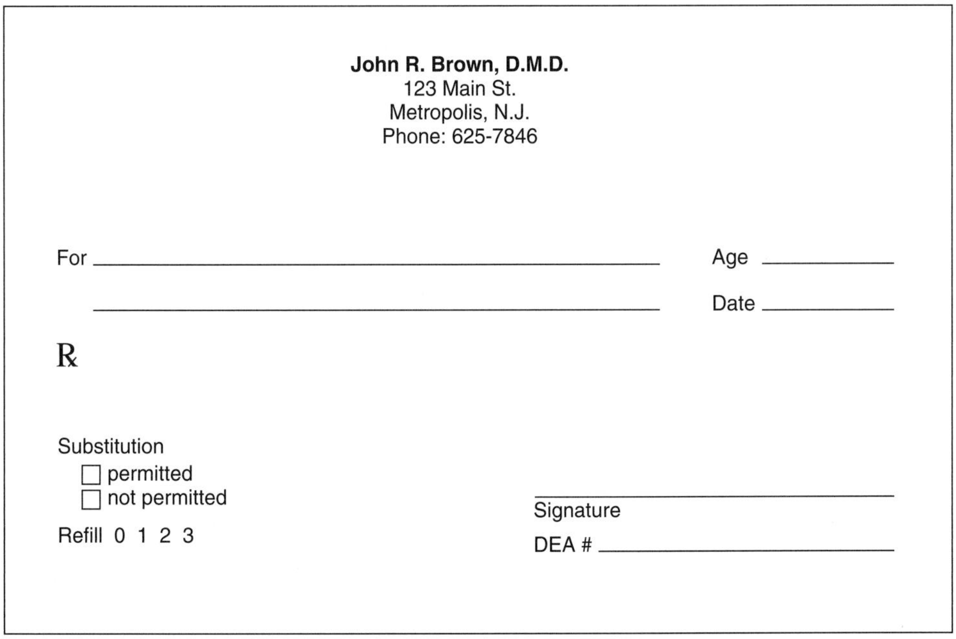

John R. Brown, D.M.D.
123 Main St.
Metropolis, N.J.
Phone: 625-7846

For ______________________ Age ________

______________________ Date ________

℞

Substitution
☐ permitted
☐ not permitted

Refill 0 1 2 3

____
Signature

DEA # ________

Fig. 55-4 Typical prescription form.

℞
Amoxicillin
500 mg
Dispense 4 capsules
Sig: Take 4 capsules with water 1 hour before dental appointment.

Substitution
☐ permitted
☐ not permitted

Signature

Refill 0 1 2 3

DEA#

℞
Tylenol with Codeine #3
Dispense twenty-four (24) tablets
Sig: Take 2 tablets every 4 hours as needed for relief of pain.

Substitution
☒ permitted
☐ not permitted

Signature

Refill 0 1 2 3

DEA# AB1234567

℞
Sodium fluoride oral solution 0.5 mg fluoride/1 ml
Dispense 50 mL
Sig: Give one-half dropperful (0.5 ml) once daily.

Substitution
☐ permitted
☐ not permitted

Signature

Label ☒ Refill 0 1 2 3

DEA#

Fig. 55-5 Sample prescriptions. The top and bottom prescriptions are by nonproprietary name. The middle prescription, for a combination product, is written by trade name for convenience (generic substitution is permitted).

Several rules have been proposed for computing the dosage of a drug for children:

1. Clark's rule,

$$\frac{\text{child's weight (lb [or kg])}}{\text{150 lb (or 70 kg)}} \times \text{adult dose} = \text{child's dose}$$

determines the dose suitable for a child based on the typical adult weight of 150 lb (or 70 kg).

2. Young's rule,

$$\frac{\text{child's age (yr)}}{\text{child's age} + 12\,\text{(yr)}} \times \text{adult dose} = \text{child's dose}$$

calculates the dose for the child based on age, with a 12-year-old receiving half the adult dose.

3. Surface area, extrapolated from the patient's height and weight, is divided by the average adult surface area to determine the fraction of the adult dose. This method is seldom used in dentistry. Dosage tables or graphs such as in Figure 55-6 are available, which obviates time-consuming and error-prone calculations.

Of all these methods, Clark's rule is the most widely used, and Young's rule is the most subject to error. Because physiologic functions dealing with drug disposition are generally proportional to body surface area, the surface area method is probably the most accurate of the three. This distinction is rather dubious, however, because drug responses in children, especially the very young, are modified by factors other than body size (see Chapter 3). When dosage information is unavailable and one of these methods has to be used to estimate the child dose, it is important to monitor the patient carefully to ensure that therapeutic effects are obtained and toxic reactions are held to a minimum.

Weights and Measures

Two systems of designating weights and measures of drugs and preparations are the apothecary and the metric systems. Although the older apothecary measures are still used by some clinicians for some drugs, the metric system is much preferred. Roman numerals are generally used with the apothecary system and Arabic numbers with the metric. The grain is the unit of weight and the minim is the unit of liquid measure

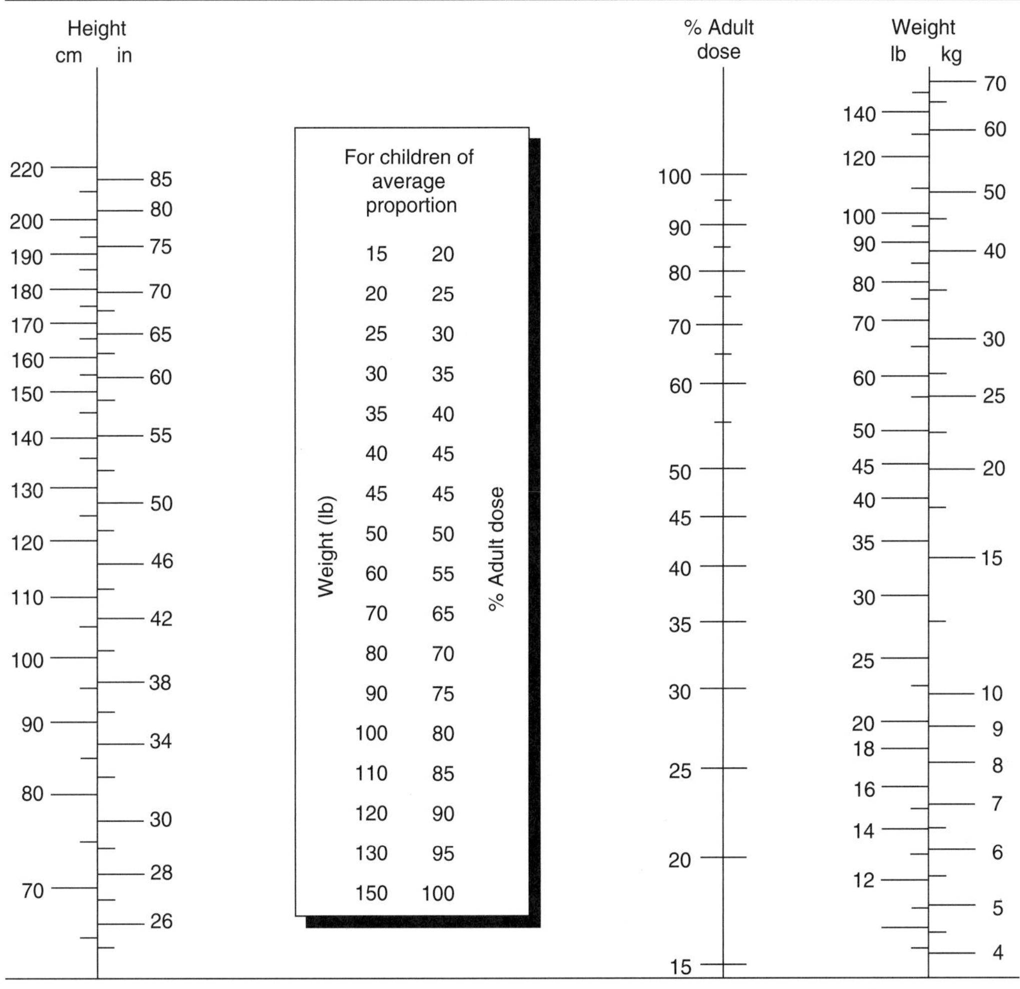

Fig. 55-6 Nomogram for estimating dose based on surface area. A value of 1.73 m^2 is used as the adult surface area standard. The intersection of a *straight line* connecting the patient's height and weight with the dosage column indicates the correct percentage of the adult dose. A simplified table for children of normal height and weight is also provided.

(volume) in the apothecary system. There are 480 grains in 1 ounce and 480 minims in a fluid ounce. In the metric system the gram is the unit of mass and the liter is the unit of volume. Some approximate equivalents between the two systems are given in Table 55-3. Apothecary measures are not equivalent to those used for commercial purposes in the United States, which use the avoirdupois system. Although the grain is the same in avoirdupois, the ounce is 437.5 grains, and there are 16 ounces to the pound in avoirdupois.

Household measures are commonly encountered when liquid preparations are prescribed. If the directions call for the patient to take a certain volume of drug solution, the pharmacist converts the metric value given into its household equivalent, as indicated in Table 55-4. Unfortunately, utensils likely to be used by patients may yield different volumes of medicine than were initially intended. To circumvent this problem, many commercial products are provided with calibrated measuring devices; patients should be encouraged to use these when taking their medications.

Calculating the appropriate patient dose, calculating the amount of drug product needed to achieve this dose, expressing the dose in a household measure, and calculating the total amount of the drug to be dispensed by the pharmacist are common calculations performed in the practice of dentistry. Such calculations are required, for example, when prescribing

Table • 55-3

Approximate Apothecary and Metric Equivalents

APOTHECARY	METRIC
Weight	
1/65 grain	1 mg
1 grain	65 mg
15 grains	1 g
1 dram	4 g
1 ounce	30 g
Volume	
1 minim	0.06 ml
16 minims	1 ml
1 fluid dram	4 ml
1 fluid ounce	30 ml
1 pint	480 ml

Table • 55-4

Metric Equivalents of Some Common Household Measures

HOUSEHOLD MEASURE	METRIC VOLUME
1 USP drop	0.05 ml
1 teaspoon	5 ml
1 tablespoon	15 ml
1 teacup	120 ml
1 glass	240 ml
1 pint	480 ml

an antibiotic suspension for a child. Although the mathematics is simple, teaching experience indicates that 40% of students are unable to perform calculations correctly on examination. The 1999 Institute of Medicine report on medical error noted that dosing errors are frequently made in children's dosing.[13] Students should practice performing such calculations, and any time drug doses are calculated for a patient they should be double-checked for accuracy.

DRUG LAWS

Various federal, state, and local laws have been enacted to control the manufacture, sale, and dispensing of drugs. To comply with these regulations, the clinician should be aware that the most stringent of these laws takes precedence, whether it is federal, state, or local. A summary of federal laws that affect dental prescribing can be found in Table 55-1.

Historic Development of Drug Legislation

One of the major concerns of nations has always been the establishment of criteria for drug identity and purity; to this end, the development of pharmacopeias has proved invaluable. A pharmacopeia is a written description of the source, identification, and preparation of medicinal agents. The first pharmacopeia to gain legal status was one adopted by the city-state of Nuremberg in the early sixteenth century.

The first USP was published in 1820 by a group of physicians, pharmacists, and chemists. This first United States Pharmacopeial Convention established certain policies, notably that only drugs of proven merit would be included in the USP and that regular revisions of the document would be issued. The USP published in 2000 is the twenty-fourth edition. Because most multiple drug entities and various commonly prescribed remedies were excluded from the USP, the need remained for a compendium for standardization of these medicinals. In 1888 the American Pharmaceutical Association began to publish the *National Formulary of Unofficial Preparations*. In 1975 the National Formulary was merged into the USP.

Around the turn of the twentieth century, a growing public clamor over the quality, purity, and safety of food and drug products led to the passage of the Food and Drug Act of 1906. In this legislation the USP and National Formulary were given legal status regarding defining the purity and quality of drugs. Standards were also established for the labeling of medicinal products. In the years that followed, these standards were extended by court decisions and congressional actions to cover promotional materials in addition to the products themselves.

Before 1937 the testing of drugs and ingredients used in the preparation of medications was not necessary before marketing. In 1937 a relatively new solvent, diethylene glycol, was used in an "elixir of sulfonamide." This agent caused the death of many children and was responsible for the swift passage of the Federal Food, Drug, and Cosmetic Act of 1938. This act required manufacturers to provide the FDA with evidence of drug safety in the form of an NDA before distributing the agent. The Act of 1938 also introduced the principle of separating drugs into prescription and nonprescription categories by requiring companies selling OTC drugs to furnish purchasers with the information necessary for their safe and effective use. Questions concerning which drugs could be sold OTC and which had to be reserved for prescription use were not resolved, however, until passage of the Durham-Humphrey Amendment in 1951 (discussed below).

In response to the thalidomide tragedy in Europe, Congress passed the Kefauver-Harris Amendments of 1962. These amendments to the 1938 Act required manufacturers of new drugs to follow set standards of animal and human pharmacologic and toxicologic testing, with the data from each step to be reviewed by the FDA. Requirements for evaluating safety and studying chronic and fetal toxicity and efficacy (omissions of the 1938 Act) were included in this legislation.

Two federal laws controlling prescription drugs are the Durham-Humphrey Amendment (Section 503B) of 1951 to the Food, Drug, and Cosmetic Act of 1938 and the Comprehensive Drug Abuse Prevention and Control Act (Controlled Substances Act) of 1970. The Durham-Humphrey law prohibited the dispensing of certain kinds of drugs (e.g., systemic antibiotics and corticosteroids and other agents whose unsupervised use may not be safe) except on the prescription order of a licensed practitioner. Under this law, a prescription for these drugs may not be refilled unless authorized by the prescriber. The FDA has the responsibility for determining how a drug may be dispensed. The FDA is also responsible for reviewing the labeling and advertising of the use of drugs, both prescription and OTC. This review, based on documented clinical studies, limits the labeled indications and uses of the product, but it does not limit the right of practitioners to use the drug only in these situations, because such action would represent interference with the practice of medicine, which the 1938 Act enjoined the FDA from ever doing. The practitioner, however, can be liable under civil law for mishaps that occur with unlabeled uses of a drug. The USP sponsors a compendium of drug information for prescribers (USP DI), which now includes commonly accepted but not officially approved uses of drugs. A second USP DI for patients is written in a style intended for patient education.

In the 1980s the high cost of drugs became the subject of congressional legislation. Substantive changes in drug substitution laws, simplified approval of generic drugs, and Medicaid drug reimbursement controls were introduced in attempts to curtail explosive drug costs.

One component of the increased cost stems from the development of new drug entities. Because of the complexity of the process, much of the patent protection for a drug can expire before a drug is ever marketed. To recover their investments, manufacturers charge high prices for their new drugs, contributing to the upsurge in medical costs. To blunt this trend, the Drug Price Competition and Patent Term Restoration Act of 1984 (Waxman-Hatch Act) was passed. It extended marketing protection for innovator drugs. An innovator product is an original, newly developed drug that requires an approved NDA for marketing. Under the 1984 Act, innovator drugs may be given extensions of their patent protection. However, the law also simplified the process of obtaining an Abbreviated NDA for approval to market generic drugs to help reduce overall drug costs of known agents. In conjunction with the Orphan Drug Amendment of 1983, this law also made provisions for the development of "orphan drugs"—drugs used for rare diseases. In general, it is economically unfeasible to produce these drugs for the small group of patients (often less than 200,000) who need them. Exclusive rights can be granted under this law for production and marketing of a drug or for specific labeling to permit the use of a drug in a rare disease. No price restrictions are placed on drugs developed under the Orphan Drug Act and these treatments can be expensive. Drug companies have taken an interest in "discovering" new uses of known drugs in small population groups. The drug thalidomide, which was withdrawn from the market when it produced the severe birth defect phocomelia, has been rereleased for use in treating leprosy and aphthous ulcers seen in HIV and Behçet's disease based on data indicating that it increases tumor necrosis factor α. Because of advances in understanding of the human genome and the development of diagnostic gene chips, more populations of disorders will fit within the Orphan Drug Act.

The 1984 Waxman-Hatch Act led to a surge of Abbreviated NDAs by generic manufacturers, and FDA personnel became overloaded with work. In an attempt to speed up the processing of their applications, several generic drug manufactures bribed FDA officials for quick approval, and others submitted samples of the innovator drug as examples of their own product.[7] Other problems that have occurred include the selling of counterfeit drugs and physician drug samples to pharmacists at below-market prices. Their use may lead to therapeutic failure. To discourage these practices, the Generic Drug Debarment Act of 1991 and the Food, Drug, Cosmetic and Device Enforcement Amendment of 1991 were passed to increase substantially the penalties for such activities.

The 1990s represented a revolutionary period for drug regulation. Lawsuits and legal challenges of FDA actions led to substantial changes in the regulation of dietary supplements, natural product drugs, and complementary and alternative medications. In 1994, Congress passed the Dietary Supplements and Health Education Act, which allows a number of agents with pharmaceutical activity to be identified as dietary supplements. In addition, international trade agreements such as the North American Free Trade Agreement and General Agreement on Tariffs and Trade (now the World Trade Organization) necessitated the development of harmonization agreements between member countries by the International Conference on Harmonization. Harmonization seeks to unify pharmacopeias and laws related to the international pharmaceutical trade. Outside these agreements there are additional trade agreements such as those associated with normalization of the United States' relations with China. These changes have led to increased availability of natural products from both domestic and foreign sources. Natural products can have therapeutic potential but also can complicate therapy by inducing unexpected toxic effects and drug interactions. One example is St. John's wort, which has been found to produce an antidepressant effect. However, it can also induce hepatic drug metabolism and decrease blood concentrations of other drugs such as protease inhibitors. In addition, imported natural products are occasionally found to be adulterated with conventional drugs such as phenylbutazone or chlordiazepoxide. This underscores the need for complete patient medical histories, including questions on prescription drugs, OTC drugs, dietary supplements, alternative medicines, and drugs of abuse.

The 1992 Prescription Drug User Fee Act authorized the FDA to charge a drug user fee to be paid by the pharmaceutical companies who are having their NDAs evaluated by the agency. This has doubled the rate of approval of new drug entities. An increased number of postmarketing withdrawals of new drugs has also occurred. The 1997 FDA Modernization Act has further modified the role of the FDA. For dentists, a key provision allows manufacturers to disseminate information about nonlabeled or unapproved uses of drugs and medical devices. This may increase drug company interest in promoting off-label dental uses of medical drugs.

Modern prescribing therapy is complicated by the relationships among the patient, doctor, pharmacist, manufacturer, third-party payer, and government. Today, patients may rely on nontraditional payments for drug purchases. Group purchase plans may require copayments, the use of specific formularies, mail-order pharmacy services, and drug-use reviews. The practitioner who is sensitive to these processes will be better able to elicit patient compliance and accomplish the therapeutic goal.

The Health Insurance Portability and Accountability Act (HIPAA) of 1996 may also affect dental prescribers (see Table 55-1). This legislation is concerned with standardizing the process of third-party payment for medical treatment, but it also substantially tightened the standards for confidentiality and privacy of patient information maintained in medical databases. The fines for violating these new rules can be substantial.

Although the federal government has set no standards concerning which prescription drugs a dentist may use clinically, many state laws regulating the practice of dentistry restrict drugs used to those associated with dental treatment. A typical law of this kind states that dentists can "diagnose, treat, operate, or prescribe for any disease, pain, injury, deficiency, deformity, or physical condition of the human teeth, alveolar process, gums, or jaws."

The dispensing of drugs by physicians and dentists is a recent development in the United States. The Federal Trade Commission has agreed to allow the sale of drugs by practitioners to their patients, and almost all states have recognized physician/dentist dispensing under strict regulatory requirements regarding storage, labeling, and record keeping. The ethical implications of this practice have been questioned on numerous grounds, including conflict of interest, lack of training and facilities for appropriate drug handling, and loss of the traditional practitioner-pharmacist double-checking of prescriptions.

Controlled Substance Laws

In addition to laws regulating drugs in general, special legislation has been enacted pertaining to drugs of abuse. A historic perspective of this legislation is given in Chapter 51. Control of the distribution of commonly abused drugs (e.g., opioids, barbiturates, amphetamines) by the DEA is regulated by the Controlled Substances Act. This act divides drugs of abuse into five Schedules based on the drugs' potential for abuse, their medical usefulness, and the degree to which they may lead to physical or psychologic dependence. The criteria for inclusion within the five Schedules are presented in Table 55-5.

To prescribe controlled substances, the licensed practitioner must register with the DEA. Many of these regulations are administered by the DEA Office of Diversion Control. The registration must be renewed periodically, and the certificate of registration must be retained and displayed by the practitioner.

If controlled drugs are to be administered to patients in the practitioner's office, they can be obtained only on special order forms that are available from the DEA. A record of the dates of acquisition and dispensing of such drugs must be kept, and a biennial inventory of controlled substances on hand must be performed. This inventory must be kept for inspection and copying by officers for at least 2 years.

Schedule I drugs may not be prescribed. Schedule II drug prescriptions may not be refilled. Emergency, partially filled prescriptions must be completely filled within 72 hours. For patients in long-term care facilities or for patients with terminal illnesses, partial filling of Schedule II drugs may be permitted for as long as 60 days after the date on the prescription. In many states, special prescription forms or restrictions are applied to Schedule II drugs. Controlled substances in Schedules III, IV, and V can be refilled up to five times within 6 months, assuming that the prescriber authorizes these refills.

Table • 55-5

Classification of Controlled Substances

SCHEDULE	CRITERIA FOR INCLUSION	EXAMPLES OF DRUGS
I	High abuse potential, no currently accepted medical use, may lead to severe dependence	Research use only: heroin, lysergic acid diethylamide, marijuana, mescaline, methaqualone, peyote, psilocybin
II	High abuse potential, accepted medical use, may lead to severe dependence	Amphetamines, cocaine, codeine, dronabinol, meperidine, methadone, methylphenidate, morphine, oxycodone, pentobarbital, secobarbital
III	Abuse potential less than drugs in Schedules I or II, accepted medical use, moderate to low physical dependence liability, possibly high psychologic dependence	Benzphetamine, butabarbital, methyprylon, mixtures of codeine or hydrocodone with aspirin or acetaminophen, stanozolol
IV	Abuse potential less than drugs in Schedule III, accepted medical use, low dependence liability	Phenobarbital, meprobamate, chlordiazepoxide, ethchlorvynol, diazepam, propoxyphene, chloral hydrate
V	Abuse potential less than drugs in Schedule IV, accepted medical use, limited dependence liability	Cough preparations containing codeine or similar opioid derivatives

After the final permitted refill, a new prescription for the product must be obtained.

Drugs in Schedule V, which consist of preparations containing limited quantities of certain opioid agents, may be sold without a prescription, assuming that the drug is dispensed by a pharmacist to a purchaser who is at least 18 years of age and that a record of the transaction is kept by the pharmacist if permitted by the state.

A pharmacist is permitted to fill oral prescriptions for any prescription drug except Schedule II products, provided they are subsequently committed to writing and filed by the pharmacist. The law does allow for the dispensing of verbal prescriptions for opioid and other Schedule II drugs in emergency situations, but the quantity must be limited to the amount needed for the emergency, the prescription must be put in writing by the pharmacist, and the prescriber must furnish the pharmacist with a signed, written prescription within 72 hours. Labeling of prescriptions for all controlled substances must contain the warning "Caution: Federal law prohibits the transfer of this drug to any person other than the patient for whom it was prescribed."

Small amounts of controlled substances in Schedules II through V may be imported or exported by US citizens for their personal use if the following conditions are met: (1) the controlled substance is in its original container dispensed to the individual, and (2) the prescription is declared to the Customs Service stating that a) the controlled substance is for his/her personal use or for an animal traveling with him/her, and b) the trade name and schedule symbol are on the label or the name and address of the dispensor and the prescription number are on the label. In addition, the total of controlled substance dosage units is not more than 50.

Information and applications for registration may be obtained from the DEA, Office of Diversion Control, Registration Unit, PO Box 28083, Central Station, Washington, DC 20005, online at http://www.deadiversion.usdoj.gov/online_forms.htm, or from the DEA Regional Office in the area in which the applicant practices. The DEA has recently created a website[14] that provides current information on registration and contacts and laws dealing with controlled substances. It is now possible to submit registration documents electronically to this website or to print out forms that can then be mailed to the DEA for registration.

The DEA offers the following suggestions for writing prescriptions for controlled substances:

1. Keep prescription blanks in a safe place where they cannot be stolen easily. Minimize the number of prescription pads in use.
2. Write prescription orders for Schedule II drugs in ink or indelible pencil, or use a typewriter. They must be signed by the clinician. Prescribing controlled substances by telephone is discouraged unless the patient is familiar or the validity of the request can be substantiated.
3. Write out the actual amount prescribed, in addition to giving an arabic number or roman numeral, to discourage the alteration of prescription orders.
4. Avoid writing prescription orders for large quantities of medications, especially controlled drugs, unless such quantities are necessary.
5. Maintain only a minimum stock of controlled drugs in the office.
6. Keep all controlled drugs under lock.
7. Be cautious when a patient says that another clinician has been prescribing a specific controlled drug product or claims that only one product works for him or her. Consult the clinician or the hospital records, or examine the patient thoroughly and decide independently whether the drug product should be prescribed.
8. Prescription blanks should be used only for writing prescription orders, not for notes or memos. A drug abuser could easily erase the message and use the blank to forge a prescription order.
9. Never sign prescription blanks in advance.
10. Maintain an accurate record of controlled drug products that have been dispensed or administered, as required by the Controlled Substances Act of 1970 and its regulations.
11. Assist the pharmacist who telephones in verifying information about a prescription order. A corresponding responsibility rests with the pharmacist who dispenses the prescribed medication.
12. Telephone the nearest office of the DEA to obtain or furnish information. Calls will be held in the strictest confidence.

Cited References

1. Boatwright DE, Clark HW: Safe use of benzodiazepines and other drugs: the pharmacist's duty to counsel, *Am J Hosp Pharm* 48:1291-1296, 1991.
2. Briggs GG, Freeman RK, Yaffe SJ: *Drugs in pregnancy and lactation: a reference guide to fetal and neonatal risk*, ed 6, Baltimore, 2001, Williams & Wilkins.
3. Foster TS: Drug product selection—part 4: selecting therapeutically equivalent products: special cases, *Am Pharm* NS31:49-54, 1991.
4. Hilton S: Does patient education work? *Br J Hosp Med* 47:438-441, 1992.
5. King RE, ed: *Dispensing of medication: a practical manual on the formulation and dispensing of pharmaceutical products*, ed 9, Easton, PA, 1984, Mack.
6. Kohn L, Corrigan J, Donaldson M, eds: *To err is human: building a safer health system*, Washington, DC, 1999, Institute of Medicine, National Academy Press.
7. Major events during the generic drug investigations, *Am Pharm* NS30:38-39, 1990.
8. Morrow DG, Leirer VO, Andrassy JM, et al: Medication instruction design: younger and older adult schemas for taking medications, *Hum Factors* 38:556-573, 1996.
9. Meyer MC: Drug product selection—part 2: scientific basis of bioavailability and bioequivalence testing, *Am Pharm* NS31:47-52, 1991.
10. Parker RE, Martinez DR, Covington TR: Drug product selection—part 1: history and legal overview, *Am Pharm* NS31:72-79, 1991.
11. Parker RE, Martinez DR, Covington TR: Drug product selection—part 3: the Orange Book, *Am Pharm* NS31:47-56, 1991.
12. Salazar DE, Schentag JJ, Corcoran GB: Obesity as a risk factor in drug-induced organ injury. V. Toxicokinetics of gentamicin in the obese overfed rat, *Drug Metab Dispos* 20:402-406, 1992.
13. Talley CR: Counseling patients about drug use, *Am J Hosp Pharm* 48:1196, 1991.
14. www.deadiversion.usdoj.gov/
15. www.fda.gov/opacom/laws/wileyact.htm
16. www.fda.gov/opacom/laws/fdcact/fdctoc.htm
17. www.fda.gov/opacom/laws/cntrlsub/ctlsbtoc.htm
18. www.fda.gov/opacom/laws/orphandg.htm
19. www.fda.gov/oc/oha/patent_term.html
20. www.fda.gov/opacom/7pdufa.html
21. www.fda.gov/opacom/laws/dshea.html
22. www.fda.gov/cder/guidance/105-115.htm
23. www.fda.gov/cder/ob/docs/queryai.htm
24. www.hhs.gov/ocr/hipaa
25. www.fda.gov/cder/drug/consumer/buyonline/guide.htm
26. www.fda.gov/oc/opacom/hottopics/importdrugs/default.htm

CHAPTER • 56

Alternative Medicine in Dentistry

Richard P. Cohan, Peter L. Jacobsen, Mark Blumenthal, and Gretchen J. Bruce

Alternative (integrative, complementary, natural, holistic) medicine is composed of a broad range of treatments that are often preventive in nature and commonly directed at treating the whole person rather than a specific disease. Substances used in alternative therapies are most often derived from natural sources. Many of these modalities have been used for more than 2000 years and are relied on by approximately 80% of the world's population in developing countries. The majority of those who use alternative care modalities do so because they are following traditions handed down from one generation to the next. What we in Western culture call *alternative treatments* are in most cultures often the only available option for health care. Most such treatments lack rigorous scientific evidence of efficacy. In contrast, allopathic, conventional, or Western medicine includes a diverse array of scientific, evidence-based pharmacologic and surgical technologies, which, although described as "mainstream," "conventional," "orthodox," or "traditional," have been practiced for little more than a century. These treatments focus almost exclusively on eliminating disease.

The term *alternative medicine* is used in this chapter to indicate "interventions neither taught widely in medical schools nor generally available in hospitals."[5] This selection is not meant to exclude other terms. Indeed, the term *integrative medicine* may be preferred on occasion because it stresses that these treatment modalities can be effectively integrated with conventional medicine to optimize the health of the patient.

For decades in the United States and in some European countries, alternative medicine—and alternative (or holistic) dentistry, for that matter—has implied care at the "fringe" of accepted medical—or dental—practice. But today there is an increasing trend to incorporate many of these types of care into the mainstream and include them as covered benefits in health insurance plans. Indeed, alternative medical therapies were used by an estimated 42% of the U.S. population in 1997 (Table 56-1),[5] and that number continues to rise.[12] Visits to alternative care practitioners exceed visits to allopathic primary care physicians by more than 200 million annually, and Americans spend an estimated $30 billion a year on these services, the majority of which are not reimbursed.[5] In response to these trends, most medical schools in the United States now provide at least introductory coursework in alternative medicine.

A survey of 46,000 subscribers to *Consumer Reports* magazine found that 60% of those who used alternative therapies told their doctors they were doing so, and most doctors approved of (55%) or were neutral to (40%) their actions.[9] It was also noted that one in four patients tried alternative therapies at the recommendation of a doctor or nurse. Another national survey concluded that individuals who use alternative therapies are better educated but often less healthy than those who do not use them.[3] These individuals are not necessarily dissatisfied with conventional medicine, but they find alternative therapies "more congruent with their own values, beliefs, and philosophical orientations toward health and life."[3]

The health benefits of an increasing number of alternative treatments are being supported by published peer-reviewed research. One such study documented that healthy individuals who regularly consume one or more dietary supplements (such as vitamin C) may have superior health, increased longevity, or both compared with their peers.[14] Chiropractic and acupuncture for both chronic and acute conditions have been accepted by the American Medical Association (AMA), which often is reserved in accepting new or unconventional treatment modalities. Indeed, the majority of alternative therapies are not endorsed by the AMA because of a lack of scientific evidence regarding their efficacy or a lack of knowledge of the existing scientific evidence.

Although some claim that alternative medicine differs from allopathic medicine by virtue of treating the patient as a whole person rather than for their specific disease or collection of diseases, alternative therapies do offer disease-specific methods of care. Alternative treatment modalities also constitute a more self-determined form of health care, especially because they are frequently integrated with nutritional and lifestyle modifications. This chapter focuses on the natural pharmacologic and therapeutic agents—principally botanical (herbal) remedies—that constitute one means of health maintenance and disease treatment.

REGULATIONS AND QUALITY CONTROL

The growth of alternative therapies in the United States has been spurred by the passage of the Dietary Supplement Health and Education Act of 1994 (DSHEA). This act greatly boosted the market for dietary supplements, including vitamins, minerals, and botanical remedies. Under this act (Box 56-1), manufacturers could promote herbal products for the maintenance of health by using "structure/function" claims, such as the product "boosts the immune system" and "improves memory." It also permitted, but does not require, manufacturers to list product safety precautions. Clarification of DSHEA in 1998 allowed herbal product manufacturers/distributors to make some additional claims, primarily to suggest their use for modifying natural life events, including menopause, pregnancy, and aging.

Under DSHEA, dietary supplements, including herbal products, are exempted from the normal review of drugs by the Food and Drug Administration (FDA). New drugs require

Table • 56-1

Alternative Therapies in the United States

THERAPY	USE (%)
Relaxation techniques	16.3
Herbal medicine	12.1
Massage	11.1
Chiropractic	11.0
Spiritual healing by others	7.0
Megavitamins	5.5
Self-help group	4.8
Imagery	4.5
Commercial diet	4.4
Folk remedies	4.2
Lifestyle diet	4.0
Energy healing	3.8
Homeopathy	3.4
Hypnosis	1.2
Biofeedback	1.0
Acupuncture	1.0

Data from Eisenberg DM, Davis RB, Ettner SL, et al: Trends in alternative medicine use in the United States, 1990-1997: results of a follow-up national survey, *JAMA* 280:1569-1575, 1998.

extensive documentation of purity, safety, and efficacy before FDA approval is given. Nonprescription dietary supplements, whole herbs, extracts, and natural compounds are designated as foods under DSHEA, thus they require no prior approval of the manufacturer's claims. Nevertheless, the FDA can rely on third-party research to remove products deemed to be unsafe from the market. The recent ban on the sale of ephedra (ma huang) is the first successful action taken by the FDA since DSHEA to remove a potentially dangerous herbal product from the marketplace. Manufacturers must be able to substantiate, when challenged, all claims made either on the container or in the literature that accompanies the product; however, they are not otherwise required to reveal this evidence unless challenged. The FDA was authorized to establish Good Manufacturing Practices (GMPs) for dietary supplements; however, these rules have not yet been published in final form and will not go into effect fully for several more years. This lack of current regulatory control helps explain why a recent study of 25 commercial ginseng products revealed that the actual total concentration of presumed active ingredients in similar preparations (e.g., liquid extracts) differed by a factor of 200 and that for each individual preparation it equaled 12% to 328% of the labeled value.[7]

Because credibility is an increasingly important factor with consumers, the more reputable manufacturing companies of natural products, eager to gain and retain the public's trust, have voluntarily established more stringent GMPs than generally required for food, and some have voluntarily registered their products with the FDA. The botanical product industry is represented by the American Herbal Products Association (AHPA). AHPA promotes the use of herbal remedies and works with manufacturers to enhance their credibility.

A significant development occurred in 2000 with the launch of ConsumerLab, a for-profit service that procures products at retail outlets in different geographic locations and tests them for adulterants, the presence and quantity of the stated ingredients, and their potential bioavailability.

Box • 56-1

Important Components of DSHEA

Definition of Dietary Supplement

1. A product (other than tobacco) that:
   a. Contains one or more vitamins, minerals, herbs, amino acids
   b. Is formulated in capsules, tablets, liquids, powders, soft gels
   c. Is not a conventional food or sole item of a meal or diet; *and*
   d. Is labeled as a dietary supplement

Safety of Dietary Supplements

1. FDA has burden of proof that the supplement is dangerous.
2. New dietary ingredients introduced into the market after 10/9/1994 must have safety data submitted to the FDA for premarket approval.

Supplement Claims and Labeling

1. Manufacturer must have evidence/research supporting claims but is normally not required to disclose it.
2. FDA has burden of proof that the claim is inadequately substantiated.

Statement of Nutritional Support (on Label and/or in Advertising)

1. Permitted if a classical nutrient-deficiency benefit is claimed.
2. Permitted if role of supplement is to affect structure or function of body.
3. Can include documented mechanism of action.
4. Can describe general well-being from consuming the ingredients.
5. Must prominently display a disclaimer that the statements have not been evaluated by the FDA and that the product is not intended to treat, mitigate, cure, or prevent a disease.

Supplement Ingredient Labeling and Nutrition Information

1. Must include the following (or will be considered misbranded and removed):
   a. Commonly accepted name of each ingredient
   b. Quantity of each ingredient
   c. Total weight of the ingredients
   d. The part(s) of the plant from which ingredients is (are) derived
   e. The term "dietary supplement"

Adapted from Israelsen LD: *Summary of the Dietary Supplement Health and Education Act of 1994. Quarterly review of natural medicine,* Seattle, WA, Spring 1995, Natural Product Research Consultants.

ConsumerLab publishes results of these random tests on its website (www.consumerlab.com). Products approved by ConsumerLab are eligible to receive its "CL" seal of approval if the manufacturer wishes to pay for the privilege. Currently, approximately 7% of these approved products carry this seal, and the number of such products is expected to increase. The United States Pharmacopeia (USP) is also conducting GMP and product quality audits and is offering a seal in its Dietary Supplement Verification Program, and another nonprofit group, NSF International (the world's largest certifier of the purity of drinking water and water filters), also has a program to monitor supplement manufacturers' GMPs adherence and product identity and quality.

In addition to a growing trend within the industry to improve quality control, efforts are being made to document the efficacy of natural products for disease prevention and therapy. American investigators face special challenges regarding herbal and other natural products. Much of the existing scientific evidence is reported in languages other than English. With the FDA prohibited from fully regulating dietary supplements, problems of product purity, standardization, and quality control are potential research confounders in the United States.

Herbal supplement claims are at times based on rather limited scientific data and may contain no detailed information concerning the types and concentrations of known active ingredients in the preparations.[23] Nevertheless, credible information is accumulating for certain herbal remedies. Standardized extracts of *Ginkgo biloba*, for example, have been shown to promote cerebral vasodilation and improve blood flow, thereby reducing short-term memory loss and relieving headache, tinnitus, and depression.[11] Liposterolic extracts of saw palmetto have likewise been documented to decrease the symptoms associated with benign prostatic hyperplasia, although not the enlargement itself.[4]

In industrialized nations the German Commission E (CGE) is generally acknowledged as the leading regulatory model regarding the therapeutic actions of herbs. CGE published 380 monographs between 1983 and 1995 based on extensive research. Its work has promoted product standardization, high manufacturing quality, and prescription herbal medicines in Germany.[4] In the United States, the National Center for Complementary and Alternative Medicine (NCCAM, a division of the National Institutes of Health) is charged with developing unbiased research information on the full range of alternative therapies, including the use of herbal supplements.

TYPES OF ALTERNATIVE PRODUCTS

Natural products of plants are marketed in unmodified forms such as the whole leaf, bark, berry, or root; as powders in capsules and tablets; in herbal teas; and in various extracts and other derivatives. The recorded use of natural preparations for their pharmacologic effects dates from at least 2735 BC, when a Chinese emperor recommended the use of ephedra (which contains ephedrine and at least five other sympathomimetic agents) for a respiratory condition. Approximately 30% of the prescription medications commonly used to treat diseases today are derived from natural sources. Examples include digoxin from the foxglove plant (used to treat congestive heart failure) and quinidine from the cinchona plant (used as an antiarrhythmic drug). Table 56-2 lists some of the more common herbal remedies, their possible uses and indications, and their potential liabilities, including potential adverse drug interactions.

Most therapeutic products used as alternative therapies are the natural herb or extracts of the herb. Water-based extracts include infusions (teas) and decoctions, whereas alcohol extracts are usually marketed as tinctures. A growing number of products are combinations of herbs or a mixture of herbs and nutraceuticals. Nutraceuticals are nutritional compounds used in a therapeutic way to treat or prevent specific problems or diseases. There is also an increasing trend to incorporate herbal derivatives into conventional products ranging from shampoos to toothpastes (which have long relied on herbal essential oils, such as mint, for flavoring). A potential problem is the surreptitious adulteration of imported herbal products by the inclusion of conventional drugs. A few products have been identified, including dong quai combined with estrogen for the management of menopausal symptoms.

Alternative therapies, especially those using pharmacologic or therapeutic agents, may be targeted toward the treatment of specific diseases. There is usually some consensus regarding the specific disease for which a preparation is most appropriate. At the same time, there is a wide range of alternative practitioners, and many natural preparations have multiple uses, so when a patient reveals the use of a particular herbal product, the disease or condition being treated cannot always be predicted.

As previously mentioned, a prominent aspect of alternative therapy is the maintenance of health. The trend toward self-help encourages the use of many alternative preparations, which are considered safer than prescription drugs by the public because they are natural and usually less concentrated than conventional drugs. Quite often this assumption is correct, but some substitute preparations (including the aforementioned adulterated product) may be just as or more powerful than the prescription drug, and injudicious use can lead to untoward effects.

ALTERNATIVE HEALTH CARE AND DENTISTRY

Patient Evaluation

With all dental patients, it is essential to take a thorough health history. A variety of signs and symptoms may be revealed as well as diagnoses of specific diseases that may influence dental care. An important part of the health history is the solicitation of the patient's medication usage. All health history forms should specifically include questions regarding the patient's use of alternative or natural therapeutic agents. Although some patients will provide this information unsolicited under the medication question usually asked in health questionnaires, other patients will not for a variety of reasons. One reason is that they may not believe or understand that their alternative therapy products are considered medications. They also may not feel comfortable telling a conventional health care provider that they are using alternative therapies for fear of disapproval. In either case there is a much greater probability that they will provide the information if it is specifically solicited.

If a dental patient is taking an alternative product, the dentist should inquire about its identity and dose and whether it is being used to treat a specific problem. A variety of natural products may potentially influence dental therapy, but most commonly the dose is low enough, the patient healthy enough, and the dental procedure sufficiently minor that specific interactions between alternative medicines and dental procedures do not occur. Still, it is important to be aware of the potential interactions and, if necessary, to acquire reliable information to advise the patient whether consultation with their health care provider is necessary to determine whether modification of his or her use of the alternative therapy during prescription drug therapy is appropriate. Another aspect of obtaining an accurate alternative medicine health history is that the product and the patient's reason for taking it provide information concerning the patient's overall health. For example, if a patient is taking coenzyme Q_{10} (CoQ_{10}), it provides an opportunity to ask questions regarding the patient's general health and whether sings or

Table • 56-2

Pharmacologic Profiles of Some Common Herbal Products

HERBAL PRODUCT*	USES/EFFECTS	PRECAUTIONS/ADVERSE EFFECTS	DRUG INTERACTIONS
Aloe vera *Aloe vera* (and related species) Aloe, zanzibar	Topical anesthetic (gel). Soothes wounds and burns; accelerates wound healing. Latex form is a laxative.	Topical use to abraded skin may cause a burning sensation. Ingestion of latex derivative causes powerful catharsis by irritating the large intestine; may cause GI cramps and congenital malformation.	Cathartic effect of the latex form hastens passage of oral medications, often inhibiting their absorption, and may potentiate anticoagulant therapy by reducing intestinal absorption of vitamin K.
Asian ginseng *Panax ginseng* Chinese ginseng	Adaptogen and immunomodulator. Fights fatigue; improves concentration and performance; enhances healing; generally increases ability to tolerate stress and recuperate. Principal male adaptogen in Chinese medicine.	Inhibited blood clotting from effects on platelet adhesion and blood coagulation. May reduce blood glucose concentrations. (A "ginseng abuse syndrome," with diarrhea, hypertension, and nervousness, has been described, which may be linked to the concomitant intake of caffeine and large doses of unknown "ginseng" preparations.)	May increase effect of hypoglycemic drugs but promote diuretic resistance when combined with loop diuretics. May potentiate headache, tremors, and mania with MAO inhibitors and increase responses to caffeine. May potentiate bleeding with antiplatelet agents and anticoagulants (but may decrease effect of warfarin).
Astragalus *Astragalus membranaceus* Milk vetch, huang chi	Adaptogen and immunostimulant. Speeds metabolism.	Subject to bacterial degradation when used as a component of denture adhesive. Mutagenic by the Ames test.	May decrease effectiveness of immunosuppressants.
Bilberry fruit *Vaccinium myrtillus* Huckleberry, European blueberry	Mild antiinflammatory of the mucous membranes. Slows cataracts, diabetic retinopathy; leaf used as a tea to treat diarrhea.	Mild antiplatelet effects. May cause diarrhea in some individuals and should be discontinued if it persists for more than 3 days. Bilberry leaf is toxic and can cause hypoglycemia.	Potentiation of antiplatelet and anticoagulant drugs. Effects may be inhibited by phenobarbital. Leaf may increase effect of hypoglycemic drugs.
Cascara sagrada *Rhamnus purshiana* Buckthorn, sacred bark	Laxative/cathartic	K^+ may be lost, causing weakness and coagulation deficits.	Cathartic-induced hypokalemia may potentiate or increase toxicity of muscle relaxants, antiarrhythmics, cardiac glycosides, and K^+-depleting diuretics.
Dong quai *Angelica sinensis* Chinese angelica	Manage pain from injury, arthritis; improve circulation, treat allergic reactions. Principal female remedy in Chinese medicine for overcoming fatigue and treating gynecologic/menopausal symptoms.	Excessive doses may cause hypotension and interfere with platelet activity.	Increased hypotensive effects with antihypertensives and opioids. Potentiation of antiplatelet and anticoagulant drugs.
Echinacea *Echinacea purpurea* (and related species) Purple coneflower	Immunomodulator. Boost immunity and treat symptoms of upper respiratory infection and other viral, bacterial, and fungal diseases.	Possible allergic reactions in individuals with ragweed and related allergies. Potential aggravation of autoimmune illness (e.g., lupus) and progressive diseases (HIV, TB).	Antiinflammatory activity of herb can be inhibited by phenobarbital and other microsomal enzyme inducers. Potential adverse interactions with immunosuppressants (e.g., corticosteroids, cyclosporine).
Ephedra *Ephedra sinica* (and related species) Ma huang	Mixed-acting sympathomimetic. Used to treat asthma and nasal congestion, improve mental and physical performance,	Cardiovascular stimulation may cause potentially fatal arrhythmias, heart attacks, strokes, and hypertensive crises, especially in persons with	Summation of effects with other adrenergic agonists and with methylxanthines, digitalis glycosides, and antiarrhythmic agents. Actions are potentiated

Continued

Table • 56-2

Pharmacologic Profiles of Some Common Herbal Products—cont'd

HERBAL PRODUCT*	USES/EFFECTS	PRECAUTIONS/ADVERSE EFFECTS	DRUG INTERACTIONS
Ephedra—cont'd	and lose weight. *Note: ephedra and related herbal products are banned as a dietary supplement from sale in the United States.*	cardiovascular disease, hyperthyroidism, renal disease, and diabetes.	by MAO inhibitors and possibly propoxyphene.
Feverfew *Tanacetum parthenium*	Antipyretic antiinflammatory. Used for prophylaxis of migraine headache, and to treat arthritis, premenstrual and menstrual discomfort, and fevers.	Chewing fresh leaves or seeds may cause mouth irritation (swelling, ulcers), dysgeusia, nausea, vomiting, and diarrhea. Discontinuation may cause a postfeverfew syndrome of nervousness, tension headaches, insomnia, and joint discomfort. May cause abortion during pregnancy and interfere with platelet aggregation.	Possible increased bleeding with concurrent use of antiplatelet and anticoagulant drugs.
Garlic *Allium sativum* Allium, stinking rose	Used as a digestive aid and to treat hypertension and as a broad-spectrum topical antibiotic. May lower LDL cholesterol and triglycerides and increase HDL cholesterol.	Possible bleeding from inhibition of platelet aggregation and antithrombotic effects. Allergic reactions possible. Ingestion of a large dose may cause burning sensation in mouth and throat. Theoretical risk of increased autoimmune reactions and organ transplant rejection.	Possible increased bleeding with concurrent use of antiplatelet and anticoagulant drugs. Possible increased hypoglycemia in patients taking insulin.
Ginger *Zingiber officinale* Black ginger, zingiberis rhizoma	Antibiotic, antioxidant, antiinflammatory, and antiemetic. Used principally for prophylaxis of motion sickness and to treat digestive disorders, nausea, and vomiting (via local action on stomach receptors).	Possible bleeding from inhibition of platelet aggregation.	Possible increased bleeding with concurrent use of antiplatelet and anticoagulant drugs.
Ginkgo *Ginkgo biloba* Maidenhair tree	The leaf extract is used to improve cerebral and peripheral circulation, for enhanced concentration, memory, and hearing; amelioration of dementia; and relief of peripheral vascular disease.	Possible bleeding from inhibition of platelet aggregation. Mild GI upset and headache, occasional nausea and vomiting.	Possible increased bleeding with concurrent use of antiplatelet and anticoagulant drugs.
Goldenseal *Hydrastis canadensis* Yellowroot, orangeroot, Indian turmeric	Antiinflammatory and broad-spectrum antimicrobial. Treats digestive and respiratory infections; promotes wound healing.	Fresh plant or high doses may cause irritation to the oral mucosa and GI distress.	None documented.
Kava *Piper methysticum* Kava-kava	Anxiolytic, sedative-hypnotic. Used to treat anxiety, insomnia, and muscle tension.	Local anesthetic action causes temporary mouth numbness. May rarely cause hepatotoxicity and liver failure. High doses may cause inebriation, with incoordination, ataxia, and drowsiness. Long-term use may cause a reversible scaly skin rash.	Summation of effects with benzodiazepines and other CNS depressants. High doses may increase dystonic reactions with antipsychotics and levodopa.

Table • 56-2

Pharmacologic Profiles of Some Common Herbal Products—cont'd

HERBAL PRODUCT*	USES/EFFECTS	PRECAUTIONS/ADVERSE EFFECTS	DRUG INTERACTIONS
Red yeast rice *Monascus purpureus* ZhiTai	Antihypercholesterolemic. Blocks cholesterol synthesis and lowers total plasma cholesterol, LDL cholesterol, and triglycerides.	Rarely causes hepatic and skeletal muscle damage. Allergic reactions in persons sensitive to yeast or rice.	Inhibitors of CYP3A4 (e.g., erythromycin, ketoconazole) potentiate hepatic and skeletal muscle toxicity. Risk is also increased with coadministration of other lipid-lowering drugs (statins, fibrates, gemfibrozil, niacin). Oral anticoagulant effects are potentiated.
Saw palmetto *Serenoa repens* Sabal	Treats benign prostatic hypertrophy. May inhibit dihydrotestosterone; may have antiestrogenic effects.	May occasionally cause GI disturbances.	Possible interaction with sex steroids.
St. John's wort *Hypericum perforatum* Klamath weed	Treats mild to moderate depression and anxiety. Antiinflammatory in the GI and respiratory tracts; eases menstrual cramps. Antiviral in large doses against enveloped viruses in vitro. Topical use as an antibacterial and antiinflammatory analgesic for minor wounds and infections.	Photosensitivity in rare cases, such as with high doses, prolonged treatment, and excessive sun exposure. Induces CYP3A4, CYP1A2, and several CYP2 enzymes in the liver and GI tract. May cause drowsiness.	Increased phototoxic/photoallergic reactions with tetracyclines, sulfonamides, and proton pump inhibitors. Summation effects with benzodiazepines, opioids, and other CNS depressants. Serotonergic crisis possible with meperidine, MAO inhibitors, and other antidepressants. Decreases plasma concentrations of protease inhibitors, cyclosporin, digoxin, and warfarin.
Valerian *Valeriana officinalis*	Sedative-hypnotic. Used to reduce anxiety, alleviate motor activity and muscle spasms, and promote sleep.	Drowsiness.	Summation of effects with benzodiazepines, sedative-hypnotics, and other CNS depressants.

Listed in order are the principal **common name,** *scientific name,* and other common names. Some of the uses described in this table have not been validated by well-controlled clinical studies; likewise, many of the adverse effects and drug interactions listed are either speculative or of potential concern but not proved to be clinically significant.
CNS, Central nervous system; *CYP,* cytochrome P450; *GI,* gastrointestinal; *HIV,* human immunodeficiency virus; *LDL,* low-density lipoprotein; *MAO,* monoamine oxidase; *TB,* tuberculosis.

symptoms suggestive of cardiac or other problems have been experienced.

Modifications of Dental Treatment

Sometimes the use of alternative medicines by a dental patient requires modification of the treatment plan. Most commonly, modification involves stopping herbal remedies that inhibit hemostasis prior to surgical procedures. As listed in Tables 56-2 and 56-3, numerous alternative products may potentially exert antiplatelet or anticoagulant activity, but chief among them are garlic and ginger. The practitioner should be aware that the food form of the herb may be just as potent as the supplement. Bleeding can pose a significant problem after major oral and maxillofacial surgery and be a nuisance during the performance of minor surgical procedures.[2] Hospitals are increasingly requiring surgical patients to stop taking specific herbal products for up to 2 weeks before surgery. Although this policy is undoubtedly excessive in most cases, the pervasive lack of knowledge concerning the identity, concentration, and pharmacokinetics of the active principles in most herbal products suggests that a restrictive policy is justified given the risks and benefits involved. A second consideration regarding these herbal medicines is the possibility of postoperative bleeding if the dentist prescribes a nonsteroidal antiinflammatory drug for postoperative pain relief (see Table 56-3). Acetaminophen, opioids, and cyclooxygenase-2–selective analgesics (e.g., rofecoxib) may avoid this potential drug interaction.

Orthostatic hypotension may be more likely to occur in patients taking herbal products capable of lowering arterial blood pressure. Such products include astralagus, dong quai, and sage. Patients taking these remedies—especially the elderly, those with cardiovascular disease, and people fasting for sedation or anesthesia—should be monitored for hypotension. In addition, changes in body position (as in moving from the supine to the standing position) should be made slowly and with careful patient observation.

Several herbal agents, including kava and valerian, can cause sedation.[16] Their combination with standard doses of prescribed anxiolytics, sedative-hypnotics, and so forth may

Table • 56-3

Herbal and Nutraceutical Drug Interactions in Dentistry

DENTAL DRUG	HERBAL/NUTRACEUTICAL PRODUCT	EFFECT	RECOMMENDATION
NSAIDs	Bilberry fruit, bromelain, cat's claw, coleus, cordyceps, devil's claw, evening primrose, feverfew, fish oils, garlic, ginger, ginkgo, ginseng, grapeseed, green tea, guggul, horse chestnut, licorice, prickly ash, red clover, reishi, S-adenosyl methionine, turmeric, vitamin E	Antihemostatic effects (primarily antiplatelet actions) may result in increased bleeding after surgical procedures for which NSAIDs are prescribed	Avoid aspirin; use other NSAIDs cautiously after procedures likely to cause postoperative bleeding
	Deglycyrrhizinated licorice	May reduce or prevent gastrointestinal bleeding	Dissolve deglycyrrhizinated licorice sublingually 20 to 30 minutes before consuming NSAID
Meperidine, tramadol	5-Hydroxytryptophan, L-tryptophan, S-adenosyl methionine, St. John's wort	Theoretical concern of serotonin syndrome	Avoid combined use
Benzodiazepines, barbiturates, opioids, other CNS depressants	Kava, melatonin, St. John's wort, valerian	Increased CNS depression	Avoid combined use
	Astragalus, coleus, hawthorn, dong quai, garlic, parsley, sage	Postural hypotension more likely	Protect patient against postural hypotension: change position slowly; avoid dehydration
Penicillin VK	Guar gum	Penicillin absorption is inhibited	Avoid concurrent administration
Sulfamethoxazole/ trimethoprim	*p*-Aminobenzoic acid	Competitive inhibition of antimicrobial effect	Avoid combination
Sulfamethoxazole/ trimethoprim, tetracyclines	Dong quai (related species), St. John's wort	Phototoxic/photoallergic reactions more likely	Avoid combination
Tetracyclines	Calcium, iron, magnesium, zinc salts	Decreased tetracycline absorption	Avoid concurrent administration
Antibiotics	Probiotic supplements*	Possible decreased gastrointestinal adverse effects	Administer probiotic 20 to 30 minutes before or 2 to 3 hours after antibiotic

*Preparations of normal gut flora used to help restore the normal microbial ecology disrupted by the antibiotic.
NSAIDs, Nonsteroidal antiinflammatory drugs.

yield additive central nervous system depression. Conversely, long-term use of these agents may decrease responsiveness to benzodiazepines and related drugs. Meperidine and tramadol probably should be avoided in patients taking St. John's wort because of the agents' shared potential for increasing 5-hydroxytryptamine activity in the brain, possibly resulting in a serotonergic syndrome of restlessness, motor hyperactivity, and coma.

St. John's wort may interact with a diverse array of medications because of its ability to stimulate microsomal enzyme activity.[8,10] Although increased drug metabolism is less of a problem in dentistry than it is in medicine, the increased first-pass metabolism of triazolam and related benzodiazepines may decrease benzodiazepine effectiveness when given by the oral route. Conversely, fresh garlic may significantly inhibit the first-pass effect, resulting in exaggerated triazolam effects.[6]

Herbal Therapies for Oral Conditions

An important area of interest for dentists, hygienists, and patients is the use of alternative remedies to manage dental and other oral problems. Agents listed in Table 56-2 that have antimicrobial, immunostimulant, and antiinflammatory actions may be used systemically for various oral conditions. In addition, there is a growing range of natural and herbal products formulated for topical oral use, including numerous mouth rinses, toothpastes, and irrigating solutions. Herbal dental products typically include agents that may be classified as astringents, antimicrobials, antiinflammatories, immunostimulants, circulation enhancers, tissue healers and soothers, and breath fresheners. Some of these natural agents are listed in Table 56-4.

Because of the importance of antiplaque/antigingivitis effects on gingival health and because of evidence suggesting antimicrobial effectiveness, a number of natural products for this use are now marketed. Most of these products contain essential oils and other herbal derivatives. Essential oils distilled from plants have been used for centuries as antimicrobials. Specifically, eugenol, thymol, carvacrol, and oil of cloves have a 200-year history of use in dental products. Essential oils are extracted from the glands, veins, sacs, and glandular hairs of aromatic plants. The essential oils are said to penetrate the oral mucosa between cells and through lipids and

Table • 56-4

Herbal Ingredients in Oral Health Care Products

HERBAL INGREDIENT (SCIENTIFIC NAME)	PRODUCTS	POSSIBLE USES AND EFFECTS
Aloe vera (Aloe vera)	Mouth rinse, toothpaste, lubricating gel, antiseptic gel	Antiinflammatory, antiseptic, promotes healing of chancre sores and wounds
Anise (Pimpinella anisum)	Mouth rinse, toothpaste	Breath freshener; may increase bleeding
Bloodroot (Sanguinaria canadensis)	Mouth rinse, toothpaste	Inhibits oral bacteria, used for gingivitis/periodontitis; may cause leukoplakia
Calendula (Calendula officinalis)	Mouth rinse, toothpaste	Antiinflammatory, promotes wound healing
Carrageenan (from red seaweed)	Toothpaste, tooth gel	Stabilizer, thickener
Cinnamon (Cinnamomum verum and related species)	Mouth rinse, toothpaste	Breath freshener
*Clove (Eugenia caryophyllata)**	Toothache balm, mouth rinse, toothpaste, temporary filling material	Antiinflammatory, analgesic, antifungal; may cause increased bleeding
Eucalyptus (Eucalyptus globulus)	Mouth rinse, toothpaste	Antiseptic
Ginkgo (Ginkgo biloba)	Toothpaste	No use reported
Goldenseal (Hydrastis canadensis)	Mouth rinse, toothpaste, antiseptic gel, tooth gel	Immunostimulant, antibiotic, used for cold sores
Green tea (Camellia sinensis)	Toothpaste	Antiviral, cariostatic, antineoplastic, used for gingivitis/periodontitis; if swallowed may decrease absorption of basic drugs
Lemon balm (Melissa officinalis)	Antiseptic gel, lip balm	Antiherpetic; used to treat cold sores, nerve pain; may increase intraocular pressure
Licorice (Glycyrrhiza glabra)	Toothpaste, topical gel	Flavoring, antiherpetic, used to treat cold sores, chancre sores
Myrrh (Commiphora molmol)	Mouth rinse, floss, tincture	Antiinflammatory anticandidal, breath freshener, astringent; used to promote healing and for gingivitis
Neem (Azadirachta indica)	Toothpaste	Antimicrobial, mild abrasive, plaque inhibitor
Peelu (Salvadora persica)	Toothpaste, natural toothbrush	Mild abrasive, antibacterial, hemostatic, breath freshener
Peppermint (Mentha × piperita)†	Mouth rinse, oral gel, dental gum, breath freshener, antiseptic gel, temporary filling material	Antibacterial, breath freshener, used for gingivitis/periodontitis and externally for myalgia and neuralgia; peppermint oil can cause burning sensation; possible tongue spasm; respiratory arrest contraindicates use in young children
Prickly ash (Zanthoxylum americanum)	Mouth rinse	None reported (analgesic and promotes healing?)
Propolis (propolis balsam)	Toothpaste, flossing ribbon, in lysine gel	Analgesic, antibacterial, antifungal, mild antiinflammatory, promotes healing
Spearmint (Mentha spicata)‡	Toothpaste	Breath freshener
Stevia (Stevia rebaudiana)	Dental gel, mouth rinse	Cariostatic sweetener, weak antimicrobial
Tea tree oil (Melaleuca alternifolia)	Mouth rinse, breath freshener, antiseptic (in lozenges, toothpicks, etc)	Antibacterial, antifungal, antiviral; may cause irritation in sensitive individuals
Thyme (Thymus vulgaris)	Mouth rinse	Antiseptic, breath freshener
Vegetable glycerin (glycerol)	Toothpaste, antiseptic gel	Lubricant, soother, sweetener
Witch hazel (Hamamelis virginiana)	Mouth rinse (alcoholic extract)	Antiinflammatory, soothing astringent (from alcoholic content), promotes wound healing; may cause stomach irritation if accidentally ingested
Xylitol (from birch tree bark)	Toothpaste, chewing gum	Cariostatic sweetener§

*Derivatives used in dentistry: eugenol, clove oil.
†Derivatives used in dentistry: menthol, peppermint oil.
‡Distillate used in dentistry: spearmint oil.
§Bacteria cannot metabolize xylitol, which is converted to glucose in the liver.

Table • 56-5

Web-Based Sources of Information on Alternative Medicine

WEBSITE (ORGANIZATION)	COMMENTS
www.consumerlab.com (ConsumerLab)	Free quality ratings of herbal and neutraceutical products. Subscription includes access to *Natural Products Encyclopedia.*
www.factsandcomparisons.com (Facts and Comparisons)	Access for subscription to *Review of Natural Products* and *Drug Interaction Facts: Herbal Supplements and Food* and for purchase of printed versions.
www.herbalgram.org (American Botanical Council)	Membership access to variety of information sources, including *HerbClip*, a biweekly abstract service, *Herbalgram*, a bimonthly journal, *HerbMedPro*, an evidence-based herbal database, and the German Commission E monographs.
www.herbmed.org (Alternative Medicine Foundation)	Subscription access to *HerbMedPro* and free access to *Herbmed* (75 herbal products) and *Resource Guides* on alternative medicine modalities, including herbal medicine.
www.naturaldatabase.com (Therapeutic Research Center)	Subscription access to the *Natural Medicines Comprehensive Database* and purchase access to printed and handheld computer versions.
www.naturalproducts.org (Institute for Natural Products Research)	Purchase access for the *Natural Dietary Supplements Desktop Reference* and the *Natural Dietary Supplements Pocket Reference.*
www.naturalstandard.com (Natural Standard)	Free and expanded subscription access to the *Natural Standard* databases, which provide evidence-based information about alternative therapies, including herbal supplements.
www.nccam.nih.gov (National Center for Complementary and Alternative Medicine)	General information on complementary and alternative medicines, listing of alerts and advisories, and research results.

salivary ducts, thus allowing for enhanced adherence and thereby a longer-lasting effect.[19]

Few of the natural antigingivitis and antiplaque mouth rinses currently available have been scientifically evaluated. As previously mentioned, the quality of herbal extracts can vary greatly from one product to another. In addition, manufacturers may use a wide range of extraction processes,[21] which creates variability among products that are formulated with the same ingredients and for a similar purpose. Nevertheless, there are data indicating the potential for these products to be therapeutically active.

Tinctures of chamomile and myrrh have an inhibitory effect in vitro on certain anaerobic microorganisms comparable to that of chlorhexidine.[15] Derivatives from plants such as goldenseal, rhatany, and sage are also reported to exert antiinflammatory, astringent, and antiseptic actions.[19,22] Echinacea, gotu kola, and calendula are included in oral rinses to provide antiinflammatory and tissue-regenerative properties. The tissue-regenerative action of echinacea is thought to be through the inhibition of hyaluronidase, preventing the breakdown of the connective tissue, and stimulation of fibroblasts that manufacture the ground substance holding the cells together.[18] Goldenseal extracts contain variable quantities of berberine, hydrastine, canadine, and canadaline, one or more of which may be active against herpes labialis, as well as mucositis and gingivitis. These antiinflammatory and antimicrobial benefits have been demonstrated in cell culture and animal studies.[1,17]

Currently, the Council on Scientific Affairs of the American Dental Association (ADA) has four categories of dental therapeutic agents (antiplaque/antigingivitis drugs, anticaries agents, antihypersensitivity agents, and tooth-whitening products), each with specific criteria for evaluating the safety and efficacy of over-the-counter dental products. The potential exists for natural or herbal ingredients to be incorporated in multiple products for use in all these areas. One such example is xylitol (an anticaries agent), found in toothpastes, mints, and gum products, among others. Another is an herbal-related product, Listerine, which has the ADA Seal of Acceptance for antiplaque/antigingivitis activity. Listerine contains the essential oils menthol, thymol, eucalyptol, and methyl salicylate (although these oils are no longer naturally derived).

Kaim et al[13] compared, in vitro, the antimicrobial activities of Listerine, 0.12% chlorhexidine gluconate, and a mouth rinse (Herbal Mouth and Gum Therapy) containing echinacea, goldenseal, and other natural ingredients. All three oral rinses were found to exhibit significant antimicrobial activity against the microorganisms tested. In a separate examiner-blinded, parallel-group clinical trial, the herbal mouth rinse was shown to reduce gingival bleeding compared with a control mouth rinse.[20] For patients who prefer natural remedies, products such as this mouth rinse may offer motivational, psychologic, and self-care benefits along with some specific antiplaque/antigingivitis efficacy.

SOURCES OF INFORMATION

As noted, the field of alternative medicine has grown quickly since 1994. It is expected that this growth will continue. Because the demand for information is coming from both health professionals and laypersons, a number of resources have been developed for each audience. Textbooks such as this can present a brief overview of alternative medicine but cannot provide in-depth information or remain current in such a rapidly developing discipline. Some published sources of pertinent information pertaining to herbal products are listed as general references. Table 56-5 contains a list of websites that provide access, often for a fee, to current, detailed information on alternative therapies. A dental professional wishing to keep abreast of this area may wish to subscribe to one of these sites. One website sponsored by NCCAM can be consulted free of charge for the latest information on research projects that the center is sponsoring.

Cited References

1. Amin AH, Subbaiah TV, Abbasi KM: Berberine sulfate: antimicrobial activity, bioassay, and mode of action, *Can J Microbiol* 15:1067-1076, 1969.
2. Ang-Lee MK, Moss J, Yuan C-S: Herbal medicines and perioperative care, *JAMA* 286:208-216, 2001.
3. Astin JA: Why patients use alternative medicine: results of a national study, *JAMA* 279:1548-1553, 1998.
4. Blumenthal M, Busse WR, Goldberg A, et al, eds: *The complete German Commission E monographs: therapeutic guide to herbal medicines,* Austin, TX, 1998, American Botanical Council.
5. Eisenberg DM, Davis RB, Ettner SL, et al: Trends in alternative medicine use in the United States, 1990-1997: results of a follow-up national survey, *JAMA* 280:1569-1575, 1998.
6. Foster BC, Foster MS, Vandenhoek S, et al: An in vitro evaluation of human cytochrome P4503A4 and P-glycoprotein inhibition by garlic, *J Pharm Pharmaceut Sci* 4:176-184, 2001.
7. Harkey MR, Henderson GL, Gershwin ME, et al: Variability in commercial ginseng products: an analysis of 25 preparations. *Am J Clin Nutr* 73:1101-1106, 2001.
8. Henderson L, Yue QY, Bergquist C, et al: St John's wort *(Hypericum perforatum):* drug interactions and clinical outcomes, *Br J Clin Pharmacol* 54:349-356, 2002.
9. Herbal Rx: the promises and pitfalls, *Consumer Reports* March 19, pp 44-48, 1999.
10. Ioannides C: Pharmacokinetic interactions between herbal remedies and medicinal drugs, *Xenobiotica* 32:451-478, 2002.
11. Jellin JM, Gregory P, Batz F, et al: *Natural medicines comprehensive database,* ed 5, Stockton, CA, 2003, Therapeutic Research Faculty.
12. Johnston BA: Prevention magazine assesses use of dietary supplements, *Herbalgram* 48:65-72, 2000.
13. Kaim JM, Gultz J, Do L, et al: An in vitro investigation of the antimicrobial activity of an herbal mouthrinse, *J Clin Dent* 9:46-48, 1998.
14. Khaw K-T, Bingham S, Welch A, et al: Relation between plasma ascorbic acid and mortality in men and women in EPIC-Norfolk prospective study: a prospective population study, *Lancet* 357:657-663, 2001.
15. Kitagaki K: In vitro herbal inhibition of anaerobes, *Antibact Antifung Agents* 11:451, 1983.
16. Kuhn MA: Herbal remedies: drug-herb interactions, *Crit Care Nurse* 22:22-32, 2002.
17. Kuo CL, Chi CW, Liu TY: The anti-inflammatory potential of berberine in vitro and in vivo, *Cancer Lett* 203:127-137, 2004.
18. Murray MT: *The healing power of herbs,* ed 2, Rocklin, CA, 1995, Prima.
19. Schechter B: Time-tested botanical remedies for modern periodontal therapy, *Dent Today* 17:110-115, 1998.
20. Scherer K, Gultz J, Lee SS, et al: The ability of an herbal mouthrinse to reduce gingival bleeding, *J Clin Dent* 9:97-100, 1998.
21. Van der Weijden GA, Timmer CJ, Timmerman MF, et al: The effect of herbal extracts in an experimental mouthrinse on established plaque and gingivitis, *J Clin Periodontol* 25:399-403, 1998.
22. Willershausen B, Gruber I, Hamm G: The influence of herbal ingredients on the plaque index and bleeding tendency of the gingiva, *J Clin Dent* 2:75-78, 1991.
23. Wyandt CM, Williamson JS: For physicians and pharmacists: a comprehensive overview of popular herbs, their pharmacologic activities and potential uses. In Saltmarsh N, Falcon M, Micozzi MS, et al, eds: *Physician's guide to alternative medicine,* Atlanta, GA, 1999, American Health Consultants.

General References

2004 Mosby's Drug consult, St Louis, 2004, Mosby.

Blumenthal M, ed: *The ABC clinical guide to herbs,* Austin, TX, 2003, American Botanical Council.

Bratman S, Girman AM: *Mosby's Handbook of herbs and supplements and their therapeutic uses,* St Louis, 2003, Mosby.

ESCOP (European Scientific Cooperative on Phytotherapy): *Monographs on the medicinal uses of plant drugs, 1996,* Exeter, UK, 1997, European Scientific Cooperative on Phytotherapy.

Freeman LW, Lawlis GF: *Mosby's Complementary & alternative medicine: a research-based approach,* ed 2, St Louis, 2004, Mosby.

Harkness R, Bratman S: *Mosby's Handbook of drug-herb and drug-supplement interactions,* St Louis, 2003, Mosby.

Jellin JM, Gregory P, Batz F, et al: *Natural medicines comprehensive database,* ed 5, Stockton, CA, 2003, Therapeutic Research Faculty.

Krinsky DL, LaValle JB, Hawkins EB, et al: *Natural therapeutics pocket guide,* ed 2, Hudson, OH, 2003, Lexi-Comp.

Micozzi MS: *Fundamentals of complementary and alternative medicine,* ed 2, New York, 2001, Churchill Livingstone.

Parsa Stay F: *The complete book of dental remedies,* Garden City, NJ, 1996, Avery.

PDR for herbal medicines, ed 2, Montvale, NJ, 2000, Medical Economics.

Pizzorno JE, Jr, Murray MT, Joiner-Bey H: *The clinician's handbook of natural medicine,* London, UK, 2003, Churchill Livingstone.

Yuan C-S, Bieber EJ, eds: *Textbook of complementary and alternative medicine,* New York, 2003, Parthenon.

APPENDIX • 1

Drug Interactions in Clinical Dentistry*

DRUG	INTERACTING DRUG	EFFECT AND RECOMMENDATION
Antibiotics		
Penicillins, cephalosporins	Bacteriostatic antibiotics (e.g., macrolides, tetracyclines, clindamycin)	Bacteriostatic antibiotics (second group) may interfere with the action of bactericidal antibiotics (first group). Consult with other practitioner for optimal therapy.
Penicillins, cephalosporins, tetracyclines, ciprofloxacin	Oral contraceptives	Stimulation of estrogen elimination may decrease effectiveness of the contraceptive agent. Advise patient accordingly.
Penicillins, cephalosporins	Probenecid	Urinary excretion of the antibiotic is retarded. Consult with physician for appropriate dosage schedule.
Penicillins	Enoxaparin, heparin	High-dose penicillins can increase bleeding time. Use cautiously.
	Methotrexate	Urinary secretion of methotrexate may be inhibited. Use cautiously.
Ampicillin	Allopurinol	High incidence of skin rash has been reported. Substitute amoxicillin for ampicillin.
	Atenolol	Atenolol concentrations may be reduced. Use cautiously.
Cephalosporins	Drugs that cause nephrotoxicity or ototoxicity (e.g., aminoglycosides, aspirin, amphotericin B, cisplatin, cephalosporins, colistimethate)	Additive toxicity may occur. Cephalexin and cefoxitin are apparently safe.
Clindamycin, macrolides, tetracyclines	Bactericidal antibiotics (e.g., penicillins, cephalosporins)	The action of bactericidal antibiotics may be inhibited. Avoid concurrent use or consult with other practitioner.
Clindamycin	Erythromycin, clarithromycin, azithromycin	Antagonism can occur between these drugs. Avoid concurrent use. Do not use one agent for prophylaxis of endocarditis after recent use of other agent.

*This appendix lists important interactions that may occur between drugs a patient is taking for nondental conditions and common antimicrobial, analgesic, local anesthetic, and antianxiety-sedative preparations prescribed or used in clinical practice. It is assumed that all prescriptions are for short-term therapy (i.e., 1 week or less) and that all drugs are in conventional dosages. Antimicrobial drugs include oral forms of penicillins (e.g., penicillin V, amoxicillin), cephalosporins (e.g., cephalexin, cefaclor), macrolides (including the various salt forms of erythromycin), tetracyclines (e.g., tetracycline, doxycycline), clindamycin, metronidazole, and parenteral ampicillin. Analgesics covered consist of both peripherally acting and opioid analgesics, agonist-antagonists, and their combinations. Local anesthetics include all formulations currently available for dental use in the United States. Antianxiety-sedative drugs include the short- and ultrashort-acting barbiturates, propofol, benzodiazepines, chloral hydrate, and hydroxyzine. The term *use cautiously* indicates that the interaction is rare and/or not usually dangerous, and that careful administration within recommended dosage limits and increased surveillance of drug effects should suffice to avoid serious toxicity.

DRUG	INTERACTING DRUG	EFFECT AND RECOMMENDATION
Antibiotics—cont'd		
	Kaolin	Absorption of clindamycin is delayed. Avoid concurrent use of clindamycin for endocarditis prophylaxis.
Macrolides	Chloramphenicol, clindamycin, lincomycin	Erythromycin and other macrolides may interfere with the antibacterial effects of the other agents. Avoid concurrent use. Do not give clarithromycin or azithromycin for prophylaxis of endocarditis after recent use of one of these drugs.
Macrolides, tetracyclines	Digoxin	Absorption of digoxin preparations with poor bioavailability is increased. Advise patient accordingly.
Erythromycin, clarithromycin	Cisapride	The antimicrobial drugs impair metabolism of second drug. Serious cardiac toxicity possible. Avoid concurrent use.
	Alfentanil, bromocriptine, caffeine, carbamazepine, corticosteroids, cyclosporine, disopyramide, ergot drugs, felodipine, midazolam, theophylline drugs, triazolam, valproic acid, warfarin	Erythromycin and clarithromycin may interfere with the metabolism of these drugs. Use intravenous agents cautiously. Administration of clarithromycin prophylaxis of endocarditis is probably of little consequence, but a full course of macrolide therapy requires consultation with physician, especially regarding carbamazepine, cyclosporine, and warfarin.
	HMG-CoA reductase inhibitors (statins)	Erythromycin and clarithromycin interfere with the metabolism of these agents, possibly causing rhabdomyolysis. Avoid concurrent use.
Erythromycin	Drugs that cause ototoxicity or especially hepatotoxicity (e.g., furosemide, fluorouracil)	The use of erythromycin for prophylaxis of endocarditis is probably not a problem. Increased risk of ototoxicity or hepatotoxicity may warrant consultation with physician.
Tetracyclines	Antacids, bismuth, calcium, iron, magnesium, or zinc salts, H_2 antihistamines, colestipol	Absorption of the tetracycline is impaired. Space administration schedules to avoid simultaneous ingestion. Occasionally, increased dosage necessary.
	Lithium salts	Plasma Li^+ concentrations may be increased. Advise patient accordingly.
	Anisindione, warfarin	In patients with poor dietary vitamin K, tetracyclines may increase the effect of the oral anticoagulants. Use cautiously.
Doxycycline	Barbiturates, alcohol, carbamazepine, phenytoin	Hepatic clearance of doxycycline is increased. Adjust dosage upward or use alternative tetracycline.
Oxytetracycline	Insulin	Hypoglycemic action of oxytetracycline reduces insulin requirements. Substitute with another antibiotic.
Metronidazole	Alcohol	Alcohol metabolism is altered, leading to the buildup of acetaldehyde. Avoid concurrent use.
	Cimetidine	Hepatic clearance of metronidazole is decreased. Use cautiously.
	Chloroquine, disulfiram	Psychotomimetic reactions possible. Avoid concurrent use.
	Barbiturates, phenytoin	Hepatic clearance of metronidazole is increased. Consider increasing dose if therapy proves to be suboptimal. However, metronidazole may decrease phenytoin, which may warrant consultation with the physician.
	Lithium	Renal toxicity of lithium may occur. Avoid concurrent use.
	Warfarin	Hepatic clearance of warfarin is decreased. A full course of therapy requires consultation with physician.

Continued

DRUG	INTERACTING DRUG	EFFECT AND RECOMMENDATION
Analgesics		
Aspirin and other NSAIDs	NSAIDs	The ulcerogenic and platelet-inhibiting effects of these agents are increased, but not the analgesia. Aspirin may decrease the effectiveness of some NSAIDs. Avoid concurrent use but ensure optimal NSAID therapy.
	Drugs that cause nephrotoxicity and ototoxicity (e.g., aminoglycosides, cyclosporine, furosemide, vancomycin)	Short courses for pain relief are probably of little concern, but avoid or minimize concurrent use.
	Antidiabetic drugs (insulin or oral agents)	Hypoglycemic effects are enhanced. Substitute with acetaminophen.
	Baclofen, methotrexate, lithium, phenytoin, calcium channel blockers	Plasma concentrations of these agents are increased by aspirin-like drugs. Substitute with acetaminophen.
	Probenecid, sulfinpyrazone	Probenecid interferes with the renal and/or biliary excretion of the NSAIDs. Aspirin may block the uricosuric effects of probenecid and sulfinpyrazone. Substitute with acetaminophen.
	Alcohol, corticosteroids	Combination may result in gastrointestinal ulceration and bleeding. Corticosteroid may also increase salicylate clearance. Avoid concurrent use.
	ACE inhibitors, β blockers, diuretics	Hypotensive effect of ACE inhibitors, β blockers, and diuretics may be reduced. Advise patient accordingly.
Aspirin, other NSAIDs, and acetaminophen	Anticoagulants and thrombolytics, broad-spectrum β-lactam antibiotics (e.g., ticarcillin)	Combination may result in increased bleeding, especially with aspirin. Cautious use of acetaminophen acceptable (<2 g/day).
Aspirin	Valproic acid	Increased plasma concentrations of valproic acid and additive antiplatelet effects may increase bleeding tendencies. Use cautiously.
	Carbonic anhydrase inhibitors	Increased CNS toxicity from aspirin or the carbonic anhydrase inhibitor may result. Use cautiously.
	Antacids, griseofulvin	Salicylate concentrations reduced. Use alternative NSAID.
Ibuprofen	Digoxin	Ibuprofen decreases clearance of digoxin. Substitute acetaminophen to avoid possibility of increased toxicity.
Acetaminophen	Alcohol	Acetaminophen hepatotoxicity is more likely in chronic alcoholics. Use cautiously.
	Cholestyramine	Concurrent ingestion inhibits acetaminophen absorption. Administer acetaminophen at least 1 hour before cholestyramine.
	β Blockers, barbiturates, isoniazid, phenytoin, sulfinpyrazone	Alteration of acetaminophen metabolism may increase risk of hepatotoxicity. Use cautiously.
Opioid analgesics and agonist-antagonists	Alcohol, CNS depressants, local anesthetics, antidepressants, antipsychotics, centrally acting antihypertensives, antihistamines, cimetidine, $MgSO_4$ (parenteral)	Increased CNS and respiratory depression may occur. Use cautiously, perhaps in reduced dosage.
	Antimuscarinics, antidiarrheals, antihypertensives	Opioids increase the effects of these drugs. Use cautiously.
	Naltrexone, opioid agonist-antagonists	These drugs block the analgesic effects of opioids. Substitute with ibuprofen or similar NSAID for pain relief.
	Monoamine oxidase inhibitors, furazolidone, procarbazine	Meperidine results in marked toxicity and is absolutely contraindicated. Use other opioids cautiously.

DRUG	INTERACTING DRUG	EFFECT AND RECOMMENDATION
Analgesics—cont'd		
Codeine, hydrocodone, oxycodone	Fluoxetine, paroxetine, quinidine, ritanovir, sertraline	Conversion to analgesic metabolites may be impaired. Avoid use of codeine; may need increased doses of hydrocodone or oxycodone.
Alfentanil	Erythromycin	Erythromycin may interfere with the metabolism of alfentanil. Use cautiously.
Propoxyphene	Alprazolam, carbamazepine, doxepin, warfarin	Propoxyphene inhibits the metabolism of these agents. Substitute with another analgesic.
Opioid agonist/antagonist	Opioid analgesics	Antagonism of the opioid analgesic effect may lead to withdrawal symptoms in dependent patients. Avoid concurrent use.
Local Anesthetic Preparations		
Local anesthetics	Alcohol, CNS depressants, opioids, antidepressants, antipsychotics, centrally acting antihypertensives, antihistamines, $MgSO_4$ (parenteral)	Increased CNS and respiratory depression may occur. Use cautiously.
	Antiarrhythmic drugs	Increased cardiac depression may occur. Use cautiously.
	Anticholinesterases	Local anesthetics may antagonize the effects of anticholinesterases on muscle contractility. Treat myasthenic patients in consultation with physician.
Amides	Amiodarone, β blockers, cimetidine	Metabolism of amides in liver is reduced. Use cautiously.
Esters	Anticholinesterases	Metabolism of esters is reduced. Use cautiously.
	Sulfonamides	Inhibition of sulfonamide action may occur. Avoid concurrent use.
Adrenergic vasoconstrictors	Inhalation anesthetics	Increased possibility of cardiac arrhythmias exists with some agents. Consult with anesthesiologist.
	Methyldopa, tricyclic antidepressants	Sympathomimetic effects may be enhanced. Use epinephrine cautiously. Avoid levonordefrin and norepinephrine.
	β Blockers, adrenergic neuron blockers, entacapone, tolcapone	Hypertensive and/or cardiac reactions are more likely. Use cautiously.
	Antipsychotics	Vasoconstrictor action is inhibited, which may lead to hypotensive responses. Use cautiously.
Antianxiety-Sedative Agents		
Barbiturates, benzodiazepines, chloral hydrate, hydroxyzine, propofol	Alcohol, CNS depressants, opioids, local anesthetics, antidepressants, antipsychotics, centrally acting antihypertensives, antihistamines, $MgSO_4$ (parenteral)	Increased CNS and respiratory depression may occur. Use cautiously, perhaps in reduced dosage.
Barbiturates, benzodiazepines, propofol	Antihypertensives, antipsychotics, IV opioids, lithium	Intravenous administration in patients receiving these medications can lead to hypotension. Use cautiously.
Barbiturates	See below[†]	Barbiturates stimulate metabolism of many drugs. Avoid multidose use. Single administration of short-acting drug (e.g., pentobarbital) is not known to be a problem.
	Antipsychotics	Increased tendency for hypothermia. Evaluate temperature as needed.
	Chloramphenicol, methylphenidate, valproic acid	Metabolism of barbiturate decreased. Avoid multidose use. Advise patient of possibility of postsedation drowsiness.

Continued

DRUG	INTERACTING DRUG	EFFECT AND RECOMMENDATION
Antianxiety-Sedative Agents—cont'd		
	Methsuximide	Metabolism of both drugs decreased. Avoid multidose use. Advise patient of possibility of postsedation drowsiness.
Thiopental, methohexital	Probenecid, sulfonamides	Decreased binding of barbiturate to plasma proteins can potentiate anesthetic effect. Use cautiously.
Benzodiazepines	H_2 antihistamines	Delayed absorption of benzodiazepine. Advise patient accordingly.
	Carbamazepine	Increased metabolism of both agents. Avoid multidose use.
	Cimetidine, disulfiram, fluoxetine, ketoconazole, isoniazid, itraconazole, metoprolol, omeprazole, oral contraceptives, propranolol, probenecid, valproic acid	Metabolism of benzodiazepine may be decreased. Lorazepam and oxazepam least likely to be affected; avoid multidose use of other agents. Advise patient of possibility of postsedation drowsiness.
	Levodopa	Decreased therapeutic effect of levodopa. Advise patient accordingly.
	Amiodarone	Increased cardiovascular toxicity. Avoid concurrent use.
	Digoxin	Digoxin elimination rate may be decreased. Substitute with a short-acting benzodiazepine (e.g., triazolam) and avoid multidose use.
Lorazepam	Alcohol, scopolamine	Increased anxiety with alcohol and irrational behavior with scopolamine. Avoid concurrent use.
Midazolam, triazolam	Diltiazem, erythromycin, fluoxetine, fluvoxamine, ketoconazole, itraconazole, minuprisin/dalfopristin, nefazodone, ritoravir, saquinivir, verapamil	Metabolism of midazolam and triazolan impaired. Avoid concurrent oral use; otherwise use cautiously.
Chloral hydrate	Anisindione, warfarin	Oral anticoagulants are displaced from protein binding sites, which may lead to bleeding. Avoid concurrent use.
	Alcohol	Combination causes increased cardiovascular toxicity. Avoid concurrent use.

†Acetaminophen, anticoagulants (oral), β blockers (except renally excreted congeners), carbamazepine, chloramphenicol, cimetidine, corticosteroids, corticotropin, cyclophosphamide, cyclosporine, dacarbazine, digitalis, digitoxin, disopyramide, doxorubicin, doxycycline, estrogen and estrogen-containing contraceptives, fenoprofen, griseofulvin, guanfacine, haloperidol, hydantoin anticonvulsants, levothyroxine, methadone, metronidazole, mexiletine, phenothiazines, quinidine, theophylline-containing preparations, tricyclic antidepressants, valproic acid, verapamil.

Common examples of drug groups listed in Appendix I.

α Blockers: doxazosin, phenoxybenzamine, prazosin, terazosin

ACE inhibitors (angiotensin-converting enzyme inhibitors): benazepril, captopril, enalapril, fosinopril, lisinopril, perindopril, quinapril, ramipril

Adrenergic neuron blockers: alseroxylon, deserpidine, guanadrel, guanethidine, rauwolfia, rescinnamine, reserpine

Adrenergic vasoconstrictors: epinephrine, levonordefrin, norepinephrine

Aminoglycosides: amikacin, gentamicin, kanamycin, neomycin, netilmicin, streptomycin, tobramycin

Antacids: aluminum hydroxide, aluminum carbonate, magnesium oxide, magaldrate, calcium carbonate, sodium bicarbonate

Antiarrhythmic drugs: amiodarone, β blockers, disopyramide, encainide, flecainide, mexiletine, procainamide, quinidine, verapamil

Anticholinesterases: ambenonium, echothiophate, edrophonium, isoflurophate, neostigmine, physostigmine, pyridostigmine

Anticoagulants and thrombolytics: anticoagulants: anisindione, enoxaparin, heparin, warfarin; thrombolytics: alteplase, anistreplase, streptokinase, urokinase

Antidepressants: bupropion, fluoxetine, MAO inhibitors, paroxetine, sertraline, trazodone, tricyclic antidepressants, venlafaxine

Antidiarrheals: bismuth subsalicylate, difenoxin, diphenoxylate, loperamide

Antihistamines: H_1 antihistamines: brompheniramine, chlorpheniramine, diphenhydramine, promethazine, pyrilamine, tripelennamine, triprolidine; H_2 antihistamines: cimetidine, famotidine, nizatidine, ranitidine

Antihypertensives: ACE inhibitors, adrenergic neuron blockers, α blockers, β blockers, calcium channel blockers, centrally acting antihypertensives, diuretics, hydralazine, mecamylamine, metyrosine, minoxidil

Antimuscarinics: atropine, benztropine, clidinium, dicyclomine, glycopyrrolate, methantheline, propantheline

Antipsychotics: chlorpromazine, chlorprothixene, clozapine, droperidol, haloperidol, perphenazine, prochlorperazine, thioridazine

Barbiturates: amobarbital, butabarbital, mephobarbital, methohexital, pentobarbital, phenobarbital, secobarbital, thiamylal, thiopental

β Blockers: acebutolol, atenolol, betaxolol, bisoprolol, carteolol, labetalol, metoprolol, nadolol, pindolol, propranolol, sotalol, timolol

Benzodiazepines: alprazolam, chlordiazepoxide, clonazepam, clorazepate, diazepam, estazolam, flurazepam, halazepam, lorazepam, midazolam, oxazepam, prazepam, quazepam, temazepam, triazolam

Ca^{++}-channel blockers: amlodipine, diltiazem, felodipine, isradipine, nicardipine, nifedipine, verapamil

Carbonic anhydrase inhibitors: acetazolamide, dichlorphenamide, methazolamide

Centrally acting antihypertensives: clonidine, guanabenz, guanfacine, methyldopa

Centrally acting muscle relaxants: carisoprodol, chlorphenesin, chlorzoxazone, cyclobenzaprine, methocarbamol, orphenadrine, baclofen

Cephalosporins: cefaclor, cefixime, cefotaxime, cefoxitin, ceftazidime, ceftriaxone, cephalexin, cephalothin

CNS depressants: acetylcarbromal, barbiturates, benzodiazepines, centrally acting muscle relaxants, chloral hydrate, ethchlorvynol, ethinamate, etomidate, glutethimide, inhalation anesthetics, ketamine, meprobamate, methyprylon, nitrous oxide, paraldehyde, propofol, propiomazine, zolpidem

Corticosteroids: cortisone, dexamethasone, hydrocortisone, methylprednisolone, prednisolone, prednisone, triamcinolone

Diuretics: amiloride, bumetanide, chlorothiazide, chlorthalidone, ethacrynic acid, furosemide, hydrochlorothiazide, triamterene

Ergot drugs: dihydroergotamine, ergotamine, ergoloid mesylates, methysergide

HMG-CoA reductase inhibitors: atorvastatin, fluvastatin, lovastatin, provastatin, rosuvastatin, simvastatin

Inhalation anesthetics: desflurane, enflurane, halothane, isoflurane, sevoflurane

Local anesthetics: amides: bupivacaine, etidocaine, lidocaine, mepivacaine, prilocaine, ropivacaine; esters: benzocaine, chloroprocaine, cocaine, procaine, propoxycaine, tetracaine

Macrolides: azithromycin, clarithromycin, dirithromycin, erythromycin, troleandomycin

MAO inhibitors: isocarboxazid, phenelzine, tranylcypromine

NSAIDs (nonsteroidal antiinflammatory drugs): aspirin, diclofenac, diflunisal, etodolac, fenoprofen, flurbiprofen, ibuprofen, indomethacin, ketoprofen, ketorolac, meclofenamate, mefenamic acid, nabumetone, naproxen, oxaprozin, piroxicam, sulindac, tolmetin

Opioid agonist-antagonists: buprenorphine, butorphanol, dezocine, nalbuphine, pentazocine

Opioid analgesics: alfentanil, codeine, dihydrocodeine, fentanyl, hydrocodone, hydromorphone, levorphanol, meperidine, methadone, morphine, oxycodone, oxymorphone, remifentanil, sufentanil

Oral antidiabetic agents: acetohexamide, chlorpropamide, glimepiride, glipizide, glyburide, metformin, tolazamide, tolbutamide

Penicillins: amoxicillin, ampicillin, carbenicillin, dicloxacillin, methicillin, mezlocillin, oxacillin, penicillin G, penicillin V, ticarcillin

Sulfonamides: sulfacytine, sulfadiazine, sulfamethizole, sulfamethoxazole, sulfasalazine, sulfisoxazole

Tetracyclines: demeclocycline, doxycycline, minocycline, oxytetracycline, tetracycline

Tricyclic antidepressants: amitriptyline, amoxapine, clomipramine, desipramine, doxepin, imipramine, nortriptyline, trimipramine

APPENDIX • 2

Glossary of Abbreviations

A_1, A_2, A_3	Adenosine receptors
Å	Ångström
ABCD	*A*irway, *b*reathing, *c*irculation, *d*efibrillation
ABO	Antigenic determinants
ABVD	Adriamycin (doxorubicin), bleomycin, vinblastine, dacarbazine (regimen)
AC	Adenylyl cyclase
ACE	Angiotensin-converting enzyme
ACh	Acetylcholine
AChE	Acetylcholinesterase
AChR	Acetylcholine receptor
ACLS	Advanced cardiac life support
ACTH	Adrenocorticotropic hormone
ADA	Adenosine deaminase
ADA	American Dental Association
ADH	Antidiuretic hormone
AD-HD	Attention deficit—hyperactivity disorder
ADP	Adenosine diphosphate
ADT	*Accepted Dental Therapeutics*
AED	Automatic external defibrillator
AHA	American Heart Association
AHPA	American Herbal Products Association
AIDS	Acquired immune deficiency syndrome
AIMs	Abnormal involuntary movements
Al^{+++}	Aluminum ion
ALA	δ-Aminolevulinic acid
ALS	Antilymphocytic serum
ALT	Alanine aminotransferase
AMA	American Medical Association
AMP	Adenosine monophosphate
AMPA	α-Amino-3-hydroxy-5-methyl-4-isoxazole propionate
AMPT	A-Methylparatyrosine
ANUG	Acute necrotizing ulcerative gingivitis
ANS	Autonomic nervous system
AP	Antiplasmin
AP5	2-Amino-5-phosphonovaleric acid
AP7	2-Amino-7-phosphonoheptanoic acid
6-APA	6-β-Aminopenicillanic acid
APC	Aspirin-phenacetin-caffeine
aPC	Activated protein C
APD	Action potential duration
APF	Acidulated phosphate fluoride
APSAC	Anisoylated plasminogen—SK activator complex
aPTT	Activated partial thromboplastin time
AR	Adrenergic receptor
Ara-A	Vidarabine, adenosine arabinoside
ARA-C	Cytosine arabinoside (cytarabine)
ARAS	Ascending reticular activating system

ASA	American Society of Anesthesiologists
AST	Aspartate aminotransferase
ATM	Atmosphere
ATP	Adenosine triphosphate
ATPase	Adenosine triphosphatase
AV	Atrioventricular (node)
AZT	Zidovudine (azidothymidine)
BAC	Blood alcohol concentration
BBB	Blood-brain barrier
BCG	Bacillus Calmette-Guérin
BCL-ABL	Breakpoint cluster region-Abelson
BCNU	Carmustine
BCR	β-Cell antigen receptor
BDP	Beclomethasone dipropionate
BE	Bacterial endocarditis
bFGF	Basic fibroblastic growth factor
BGTI	Basal-ganglia thalamic inhibitor
BHR	Bronchial hyperreactivity
BLS	Basic life support
BMD	Beclamethasone diproprionate
BMP	Beclomethasone monopriopionate
BMT	Bone marrow transplant
BuChE	Butyrocholinesterase
BZ_1, BZ_2	Benzodiazepine receptors
C6	Hexamethonium
Ca^{++}	Calcium ion
cAMP	Cyclic adenosine 3′, 5′-monophosphate
CCB	Calcium-channel blocker
CCNU	Lomustine
CCR5	Cysteine-cysteine chemokine receptor 5
CD	Cluster of differentiation
CD40L	CD40 ligand
CDAC	*Clostridium difficile*–associated colitis
CDAD	*Clostridium difficile*–associated diarrhea
CDC	Centers for Disease Control and Prevention
CDK	Cyolin-dependent kinase
CDR	Complementary-defining region
CG	Chorionic gonadotropin
cGMP	Cyclic guanosine 3′, 5′-monophosphate
CGRP	Calcitonin gene–related peptide
ChAc	Choline acetylase
CL	Clearance
CL	ConsumerLab
Cl^-	Chloride ion
CMI	Cell-mediated immunity
CML	Chronic myeloid leukemia
CMV	Cytomegalovirus
CNS	Central nervous system
CO	Cardiac output
CO_2	Carbon dioxide
CoA	Coenzyme A
CO-Hb	Carboxyhemoglobin
COMT	Catechol-O-methyltransferase
CoNS	Coagulase-negative streptococcus
COX	Cyclooxygenase
CRH	Corticotropin-releasing hormone
CRP	C-reactive protein
CTZ	Chemoreceptor trigger zone
CYP	Cytochrome P450
Cys	Cysteinyl
CXCR4	β-Chemokine receptor 4
D	Dopamine (receptor)
d	Dalton

1,25[OH]D	1,25-Dihydroxycholecalciferol, calcitriol
25[OH]D	Calcifediol
DAG	Diacylglycerol
DATATOP	Deprenyl and Tocopherol Therapy of Parkinsonism
DCC	Day care center
DDAVP	Desmopressin
DDT	Chlorophenothane
DES	Diethylstilbestrol
DFP	Isoflurophate (formerly diisopropylfluorophosphate)
DHFR	Dihydrofolate reductase
DHT	Dihydrotachysterol
DIC	Disseminated intravascular coagulopathy
DIT	Diiodotyrosine
DMARD	Disease-modifying antirheumatic drug
DMFT	Decayed, missing, and filled teeth
DMPP	Dimethylphenylpiperazinium
DMSO	Dimethylsulfoxide
DMT	Dimethyltryptamine
DNA	Deoxyribonucleic acid
Dopa (DOPA)	Dihydroxyphenylalanine
DSHEA	Dietary Supplement Health and Education Act of 1994
DSM-IV-R	*Diagnostic and Statistical Manual of Mental Disorders,* ed 4
DSV	Dietary Supplement Verification Program
DTH	Dihydrotachysterol
DTIC	Dacarbazine
E	Epinephrine
EACA	ε-Aminocaproic acid
EBV	Epstein-Barr virus
ECG	Electrocardiogram
ECL	Enterochromaffinlike cell
ED_{50}	Median effective dose
ED_{99}	Dose effective in 99% of the population
EDRF	Endothelium (endothelially)-derived relaxing factor
EEG	Electroencephalogram
EGFR	Epidermal growth factor
EGFR-TK	Epidermal growth factor tyrosine kinase
eIF-2	Eukaryotic initiation factor
EMLA	Eutectic mixture of local anesthetics
EPA	Environmental Protection Agency
EPO	Erythropoietin
EPP	Endplate potential
EPSP	Excitatory postsynaptic potential
ERP	Effective refractory period
ER/PR	Estrogen receptor/progesterone receptor
erm	Erythromycin-resistant methylase
F	Factor
F^-	Fluoride ion
F_c	Crystallizable fragment (region)
Fe^{++}	Ferrous ion
Fe^{+++}	Ferric ion
FAS	Fetal alcohol syndrome
FDA	Food and Drug Administration
5-FdUTP	5-Fluoro-deoxyuridine triphosphate
FIFRA	Federal Insecticide, Fungicide, and Rodenticide Act
FKBP	Tacrolimus-binding protein
FRAP	FKBP-rapamycin—associated protein
FSH	Follicle-stimulating hormone
5-FU	Fluorouracil
5-FUdR	Floxuridine
FUTP	Fluorouridine-5′-triphosphate
G protein	Guanine nucleotide—binding regulatory protein
GABA	γ-Aminobutyric acid
G-CSF	Granulocyte colony—stimulating factor (filgrastim)

GERD	Gastroesophageal reflux disease
GH	Growth hormone
GHRF	Growth hormone—releasing factor
Gla	Amino-terminal γ-carboxyglutamic acid
GLSA	Glycopeptide *Staphylococcus aureus*
Glut 4	Glucose transporter 4
GM-CSF	Granulocyte macrophage colony—stimulating factor (sargramostim)
GMP	Good Manufacturing Practices
GNB	Gram-negative bacilli
GnRH	Gonadotropin-releasing hormone
GP	Glycoprotein
GPCR	G protein—coupled receptor
GTP	Guanosine triphosphate
GVHD	Graft-versus-host disease
H^+	Hydrogen ion
H_1, H_2, H_3	Histamine receptor
HAART	Highly active antiretroviral therapy
HACEK (group)	*Haemophilus influenzae, Actinomycetum comitans, Cardiobacterium hominis, Eikenella corrodens, Kingsella kingae*
Hb	Hemoglobin
HBO	Hyperbaric oxygen therapy
HBV	Hepatitis B virus
HCG	Human chorionic gonadotropin
HCT	Hematopoietic cell transplantation
HCV	Hepatitis C virus
HDL	High-density lipoprotein
HETE	Hydroxyeicosatetraenoic acid
Hg°	Elemental mercury (dental amalgam)
Hg^+	Mercurous
Hg^{++}	Mercuric
5-HIAA	5-Hydroxyindoleacetic acid
HIO	Hypoiodous acid
HIPPA	Health Insurance Portability and Accountability Act (of 1996)
HIT	Heparin-induced thrombocytopenia
HIV	Human immunodeficiency virus
HLA	Human leukocyte antigen
HMG-CoA	3-Hydroxy-3-methylglutaryl coenzyme A
HMWK	High—molecular-weight kininogen
HPV	Human papillomavirus
HSV	Herpes simplex virus
5-HT	5-Hydroxytryptamine (serotonin)
Hz	Hertz
I^-	Iodide ion
IAP	Inhibitor of apoptosis protein
IBS	Irritable bowel syndrome
IDL	Intermediate-density lipoprotein
IE	Infective endocarditis
IFN	Interferon
Ig	Immunoglobulin
IgG, D, E, M, A	Immunoglobulin isotypes
IGF	Insulinlike growth factor 1
IGF-1	Insulinlike growth factor 1
IL	Interleukin
IL-1	Interleukin-1
IL-2	Interleukin-2
IL-1R	Interleukin-1 receptor
IL-Ira	Interleukin-1 receptor antagonist
IM	Intramuscular
INH	Isonicotinic hydrazide
INR	International Normalized Ratio
IOP	Interocular pressure
IP	*International Pharmacopoeia*
IP	Inositol phosphate

IP_2	Inositol bisphosphate
IP_3	Inositol 1,4,5-trisphosphate
IPG	Inositol phosphoglycan
IPSP	Inhibitory postsynaptic potential
IQ	Intelligence quotient
I_R	Delayed outwardly rectifying current
ISA	Intrinsic sympathomimetic activity
IV	Intravenous
K^+	Potassium ion
KGD	Lysine-glycine-aspartic acid sequence
μl	Microliter
L	Large, long-lasting current
LAK	Lymphokine-activated killer (cell)
LC	Locus ceruleus
LD_{50}	Median lethal dose
LDL	Low-density lipoprotein
Li^+	Lithium ion
LJP	Localized juvenile periodontitis
LH	Luteinizing hormone
LHRH	Luteinizing hormone—releasing hormone
LMWH	Low—molecular-weight heparin
LPH	Lipotropin
LSD	Lysergic acid diethylamide
LT	Leukotriene
LTCF	Long-term care facility
LTOT	Long-term low-flow oxygen therapy
M	Muscarinic receptor (protein)
M	Million
Mab	Monoclonal antibody
MAC	Minimum alveolar concentration
MAO	Monoamine oxidase
MAO-I	Monoamine oxidase inhibitor
MAP	Mean arterial pressure
MCH	Mean corpuscular hemoglobin
MCHC	Mean corpuscular hemoglobin concentration
mChR	Muscarinic cholinergic receptor
MCP	Mean corpuscular volume
MCP-1	Monocyte chemoattractive protein-1
m-CPP	*m*-Chlorophenylpiperazine
M-CSF	Monocyte colony—stimulating factor
MDD	Major depressive disorder
MDMA	3,4-Methylenedioxymethamphetamine
MDP	Maximum diastolic potential
MEOS	Microsomal enzyme oxidation system
MEPP	Miniature endplate potential
MFP	Sodium monofluorophosphate
MG	Myasthenia gravis
Mg^{++}	Magnesium ion
MH	Malignant hyperthermia
MHC	Major histocompatibility gene complex
MHPG	3-Methoxy-4-hydroxyphenylethylene glycol
MI	Myocardial infarction
MIC	Minimum inhibitory concentration
MIT	Moniodotyrosine
MLC	Minimum lethal concentration
MLCK	Myosin light-chain kinase
MLKS (resistance)	*M*acrolide, *l*incosamide, *k*etolide, *s*treptogramin
MMPI	Matrix metalloprotease inhibitor
6-MNA	6-Methoxy-2-naphthylacetic acid
MOPP	*M*echlorethamine, *O*ncovin (vincristine), *p*rocarbazine, *p*rednisone (regimen)
MPHG	3-Methyl-4-phenyl-pyridinium
MPP^+	1-Methyl-4-phenylpyridinium
MPTP	1-Methyl-4-phenyl-1,2,3,6-tetrahydropyridine
MRCoNS	Methicillin-resistant coagulase-negative staphylococci

MRSA	Methicillin-resistant *Staphylococcus aureus*
MSSA	Methicillin-sensitive *Staphylococcus aureus*
MTIC	Monomethyl 5-triazinoimidazole carboxamide
MW	Molecular weight
N	Nicotinic
N_m	Nicotinic receptor on neuromuscular junction
N_n	Nicotinic receptor on postganglionic cells
Na^+	Sodium ion
Na^+,K^+-ATPase	Na^+,K^+-Activated adenosine triphosphatase
NAD(NADH)	Nicotinamide adenine dinucleotide
NADPH	Nicotinamide adenine dinucleotide phosphate
NAM	N-acetylmuramic acid
NAPA	N-acetylprocainamide
NAPQI	N-acetyl-*p*-benzoquinoneimine
NCCLS	National Committee for Clinical Laboratory Standards
NDA	New Drug Application
NE	Norepinephrine
NED	Normal equivalent deviation units
NF	*National Formulary*
NF-ATc	Cytoplasmic component of nuclear factor of activated T cells
NF-ATn	Nuclear component of nuclear factor of activated T cells
NF-κβ	Nuclear factor (κβ)
Ng	Nicotinic receptor, ganglia
NHL	Non-Hodgkin's lymphoma
NI	Nosocomial infection
NK	Natural killer (cell)
NMDA	N-methyl-D-aspartate
NMS	Neuroleptic malignant syndrome
NO	Nitric oxide
N_2O	Nitrous oxide
NOS	Nitric acid synthetase
NPH (insulin)	Neutral protamine Hagedorn
NPY	Neuropeptide Y
NRM	Nucleus raphe magnus
NSAID	Nonsteroidal antiinflammatory drug
NSCLC	Nonsmall-cell lung cancer
NSPH	Nonspecific plaque hypothesis
NTS	Nucleus tractus solitarius
O_3	Ozone
OBRA	Omnibus Budget Reconciliation Act
25[OH]D	Calcifediol
1,25[OH]D	1,25-Dihydroxycholcalciferol
OMPA	Octamethyl pyrophosphamide
OPP	Office of Pesticide Programs
ORL	Opiod-receptorlike
OSHA	Occupational Safety and Health Administration
OTC	Over the counter
P	Peptidergic receptor
P	Purine receptor
PABA	*p*-Aminobenzoic acid
$PaCO_2$	Arterial blood carbon dioxide tension
PAE	Postantibiotic effect
PAF	Platelet-activating factor
PAG	Periaqueductal gray matter
PAI-1	Plasminogen activator inhibitor type 1
PALC	Postantibiotic leukocyte effect
PALS	Pediatric advance life support
PaO_2	Arterial blood oxygen tension
PAR	Protease-activated receptor
PAS	*p*-Aminosalicylic acid
PBP	Penicillin-binding protein
PBSCT	Peripheral blood stem cell transplants
PC	1-Phenyl-1-cyclohexene
PCA	Patient-controlled analgesia

PCMX	Parachlorometaxylenol
PCP	Phencyclidine
PDC	Potential-dependent channel
PDGF	Platelet-derived growth factor
PDR	*Physicians' Desk Reference*
PEG-MGDF	Pegylated megakaryocyte growth and development factor
PET	Positron emission tomography
P-F	Phosphofluoride linkage
PF-3	Platelet factor 3
PFC	Perfluorocarbon
PG	Prostaglandin
PGG_2, PGH_2	Prostaglandin endoperoxides
PGI_2	Prostacyclin
pIgR	Polymeric immunoglobulin receptor
PIP_2	Phosphatidylinositol 4-5-bisphosphate
pK_a	Negative log of the dissociation constant
PLC	Phospholipase C
PLO	Pleuronic lecithin organogel
PMC	Pseudomembranous colitis
PMN	Polymorphonuclear (leukocyte)
PNMT	Phenylethanolamine-N-methyltransferase
PO-IM	Oral/intramuscular potency ratio
PPARα	Peroxisomal proliferators—activated receptor α
PPI	Protein pump inhibitor
ppm	Parts per million
PRH	Prolactin-releasing hormone
prn	Pro re nata (as needed)
PRON	Postradiation osteonecrosis
PRSTN	Postradiation soft tissue necrosis
psi	Pounds per square inch
PT	Prothrombin (time)
PTH	Parathyroid hormone
PTT	Partial thromboplastin time
PUD	Peptic ulcer disease
Ω-3 PUFA	Ω-3 Polyunsaturated fatty acids
PUVA	Psoralen plus ultraviolet-A
R	Resistance factor
RAR	Retinoid acid receptor
REM	Rapid eye movement (sleep)
RGD	Arginine-glycine—aspartic acid sequence
RH	Releasing hormone
RNA	Ribonucleic acid
ROC	Receptor-operated channel
RSV	Respiratory syncytial virus
RTF	Resistance transfer factor
RVM	Rostroventral medulla
RXR	Retinoid X receptor
S	Svedberg unit
SA	Sinoatrial (node)
SAD	Seasonal affective disorder
SAR	Structure-activity relationship
SCF	Stem cell factor
SD	Standard deviation
SERM	Selective estrogen receptor modulator
SHV	Sulfhydryl variable
SIADH	Syndrome of inappropriate antidiuretic hormone secretion
SIF	Small, intensely fluorescent (cell)
SK	Streptokinase
SKF 525A	Proadifen
SLUD	*S*alivation, *l*acrimation, *u*rination, *d*efecation
SNARE (complex)	Synaptobrevin, syntaxin, SNAP-25
SN_C	Substantia nigra pars compacta
SNP	Single nucleotide polymorphism

SNS	Sympathetic nervous system
SO_2	Sulfur dioxide
SP	Substance P
SPA	Stimulation-produced analgesia
SPH	Specific plaque hypothesis
SR	Sarcoplasmic reticulum
SRS	Slow-reacting substance (leukotrienes)
SRS-A	Slow-reacting substance of anaphylaxis (leukotrienes)
SSRI	Selective serotonin reuptake inhibitor
STAT	Signal transducers and activators of transcription
$T_{1/2}$	Half-life, half-time
T_3	Triiodothyronine, liothyronine
T_4	Tetraiodothyronine, thyroxine
TALH	Thick ascending limb of the loop of Henle
TBG	Thyroxine-binding globulin
TBI	Total body irradiation
TCA	Trycyclic antidepressant
TCDD	Dioxin
TCR	T-cell antigen factor
TD_{50}	Median therapeutic dose
TEA	Tetraethylammonium
TF	Tissue factor
TFPI	Tissue factor pathway inhibitor
$TGF\gamma$	Transforming growth factor γ
THC	Tetrahydrocannabinol
THO	Activated T cells that have yet to differentiate
TI	Therapeutic index
TIA	Transient ischemic attack
TIBC	Total iron-binding capacity
TMD	Temporomandibular disorder
TMJ	Temporomandibular joint
TNF	Tumor necrosis factor
TNFR	Tumor necrosis/nerve growth factor receptor
t-PA	Tissue-type plasminogen activator
TPO	Thrombopoietin
TPR	Total peripheral resistance
TRH	Thyrotropin-releasing hormone
TRP	Transient receptor potential (channels)
TRPV1	Transient receptor potential vanilloid receptor 1
TSH	Thyroid-stimulating hormone; thyrotropin
TXA_2	Thromboxane A_2
U	Uptake
UGT	Uridine diphosphate glucuronosyltransferase
UNPIC	Prior Informed Consent (procedure)
u-PA	Urokinase
USAN	United States Adopted Name
USP	*United States Pharmacopeia*
USPDI	*United States Pharmacopeia Dispensing Information*
V_d	Volume of distribution
VEGF	Vascular endothelial growth factor
VGS	Viridans group streptococci
VIP	Vasoactive intestinal peptide
VIPPS	Verified Internet Pharmacy Practices Site
VISA	Vancomycin-intermediate—resistant *Staphylococcus aureus*
VLDL	Very—low-density lipoprotein
VMA	Vanillylmandelic acid
VRE	Vancomycin-resistant enterococci
VRG	Vessel-rich group
vWD	von Willebrand's disease
vWf	von Willebrand factor
VZV	Varicella-zoster virus
WHO	World Health Organization

INDEX*

*Page numbers followed by *f* indicate figures; *t*, tables; *b*, boxes.

O

S